UMPHRED'S NEUROLOGICAL REHABILITATION

UMPHRED'S NEUROLOGICAL REHABILITATION

SIXTH EDITION

Darcy A. Umphred, PT, PhD, FAPTA
Emeritus Professor and Past Chair
Department of Physical Therapy
School of Pharmacy and Health Sciences
University of the Pacific
Stockton, California

Gordon U. Burton, PhD, OTR/L
Professor Emeritus and Past Chair
Department of Occupational Therapy
San Jose State University
San Jose, California

Rolando T. Lazaro, PT, PhD, DPT, GCS
Associate Professor
Department of Physical Therapy
Samuel Merritt University
Oakland, California

Margaret L. Roller, PT, MS, DPT
Professor and Graduate Coordinator
Department of Physical Therapy
California State University, Northridge
Northridge, California
Clinical Instructor
NeuroCom International, a division of Natus
Clackamas, Oregon

ELSEVIER

ELSEVIER
MOSBY

3251 Riverport Lane
St. Louis, Missouri 63043

UMPHRED'S NEUROLOGICAL REHABILITATION

ISBN: 978-0-323-07586-2

Library of Congress Cataloging-in-Publication Data
Umphred's neurological rehabilitation / [edited by] Darcy Umphred ... [et al.].—6th ed.
p. ; cm.
Neurological rehabilitation
Rev. ed. of: Neurological rehabilitation / [edited by] Darcy A. Umphred ; with section editors, Gordon U. Burton, Rolando T. Lazaro, Margaret L. Roller. 5th ed. c2007.
Includes bibliographical references and index.
ISBN 978-0-323-07586-2 (hardcover : alk. paper)
I. Umphred, Darcy Ann. II. Neurological rehabilitation. III. Title: Neurological rehabilitation.
[DNLM: 1. Nervous System Diseases—rehabilitation. WL 140]

616.8'0462—dc23

2012019193

Executive Content Strategist: Kathy Falk
Content Manager: Jolynn Gower
Senior Content Development Specialist: Christie M. Hart
Publishing Services Manager: Catherine Jackson
Senior Project Manager: Carol O'Connell
Design Direction: Kim Denando

Printed in the United States of America

Last digit is the print number: 9 8 7 6 5 4 3 2

Dedicated to: A sequential process of learning from the first to the sixth edition.

To

Gordon, Jeb, Benjamin, my mother, Janet, my daughters-in-law Julianne and Tassie, and our four grandchildren, Jackson, Jelena, Alexander, and Cameron, whose love, patience, and understanding constantly gave and have continued to give me strength and joy.

To

All those special people whose insights, wisdom, guidance, and patience have helped to give the authors of these chapters their unique gifts and talents, as well as their willingness to share their thoughts with all of you.

To

Very dear friends, colleagues, and past chapter authors who gave so much energy, dedication, and service both scholarly as well as practicing clinicians. Over the last 30 years, the book's family has changed, as has the evolution of the text. With great regret we have had to say good-bye to five authors, Mary Jane Bouska, Jane Schneider, Laura Smith, Donna El-Din, and Christine Nelson. The professions will miss all of you, but your gifts continue to make a difference.

To

Life, to each person's journey and to all those who give opportunities for others' growth along that journey. Special thanks to my immediate family and all my friends and colleagues I hold so close to my heart. Because of all of you, my journey has been constantly renewed with love, warmth, and guidance. No one could feel wealthier than I.

To

Each day we are allowed to walk on this earth. Life is very precious, and how long we will be allowed to stay is an unknown. I have learned to appreciate this time and hope none of us become so busy that we forget its finiteness. Enjoy the journey and always find time to stop and appreciate who you are, what you are, and those gifts you have been given to share with the rest of us. We walk alone in physical form but surrounded by all the energies of others as well as our own. Hopefully, as we continue this adventure we share and give positive thoughts and energy to life and leave having given much more than we have taken. Each person we meet, whether as a student, a teacher, a family member, a friend, a colleague or a patient, has something to teach us and, hopefully, we in turn allow those we meet to grow and learn from us. This is a wondrous journey, and I hope all of you enjoy your path as much as I have mine.

To

My fellow editors, Dr. Gordon Burton, Dr. Rolando Lazaro, and Dr. Margaret Roller, for all the time and total commitment they have made to the sixth edition of this text. Few individuals reading and using this book and the complimentary online video site will ever appreciate the hundreds if not thousands of hours these individuals made editing chapters and videos and the totality of their commitment to the future of our professions.

Darcy A. Umphred

Contributors

Paula M. Ackerman, MS, OTR/L
SCI Post Acute Rehab Manager
Shepherd Center
Atlanta, Georgia

Janet Marie Adams, PT, MS, DPT
Professor
Department of Physical Therapy
California State University, Northridge
Northridge, California

Diane D. Allen, PT, PhD
Associate Professor
University of California San Francisco/San Francisco State University
Graduate Program in Physical Therapy
San Francisco, California

Leslie K. Allison, PT, PhD
Assistant Professor
East Carolina University
College of Allied Health Sciences
Department of Physical Therapy
Greenville, North Carolina

Brent D. Anderson, PT, PhD, OCS
President
Polestar Education
Adjunct Professor
University of Miami
Department in Physical Therapy
Miami, Florida

Ellen Zambo Anderson, PT, MA, GCS
Associate Professor
University of Medicine and Dentistry of New Jersey
Newark, New Jersey

Joyce Ann, OTR/L, GCFP
Occupational Therapist, Guild Certified Feldenkrais Practitioner
Highland Park, Illinois

Myrtice B. Atrice, PT, BS
SCI Clinical Manager
Shepherd Center
Atlanta, Georgia

Amy J. Bastian, PT, PhD
Professor
Neuroscience
Johns Hopkins School of Medicine
Director
Motion Analysis Laboratory
Kennedy Krieger Institute
Baltimore, Maryland

Joanna C. Beachy, MD, PhD
Associate Professor
Division of Neonatology
Associate Director NBICU
University of Utah
Salt Lake City, Utah

Sandra G. Bellamy, PT, MS, DPT, PCS
Associate Professor
Department of Physical Therapy
University of the Pacific
Stockton, California

Janet R. Bezner, PT, PhD
Vice President, Education and Governance and Administration
Deputy Executive Director
American Physical Therapy Association
Alexandria, Virginia

William G. Boissonnault, PT, DHSc, FAAOMPT, FAPTA
Professor
Physical Therapy Program
University of Wisconsin-Madison
Madison, Wisconsin

Jennifer M. Bottomley, PT, MS, PhD
Academic ad Clinical Educator in Geriatric Physical Therapy International
Adjunct Professor at the MGH Institute of Health Care Professionals
Coordinates Rehabilitation Services for the Committee to End Elder Homelessness/HEARTH in Boston
Consultant for Amedisys Home Health Care and Hospice
Vice President for International PhysioTherapists Working with Older People (IPTOP)
Independent Educator and Geriatric Rehabilitation Consultant
Boston, Massachusetts

Annie Burke-Doe, PT, MPT, PhD
Associate Professor
University of St. Augustine for Health Science
San Marcos, California

Gordon U. Burton, PhD, OTR/L
Professor Emeritus and Past Chair
Department of Occupational Therapy
San Jose State University
San Jose, California

Katie Byl, PhD
Assistant Professor
University of California, Santa Barbara
Department of Electrical and Computer Engineering
Santa Barbara, California

Marten Byl, PhD
Principal Scientist
Physical Sciences Inc.
Handover, Massachusetts
Visiting Scientist
University of California, Santa Barbara
Santa Barbara, California

Nancy N. Byl, PT, MPH, PhD, FAPTA
Professor and Chair Emeritus
School of Medicine, Department of Physical Therapy and Rehabilitation Science
University of California, San Francisco
San Francisco, California

Beate Carrière, PT, CAPP, CIFK
Physical Therapist, Author, Teacher
Evergreen Physical Therapy Specialist
Pasadena, California

Laurie Ruth Chaikin, MS, OTR/L, OD, FCOVD
Clinical Field Supervisor
VisionCare, Inc.
Saratoga, California

Alain Claudel, PT, DPT, ECS
Board Certified Specialist in Clinical Electrophysiology
Director, Rehabilitation Services
Community Hospital of the Monterey Peninsula
Monterey, California

Carol M. Davis, DPT, EdD, FAPTA
Professor Emerita
Department of Physical Therapy
University of Miami Miller School of Medicine
Myofascial Release Physical Therapist
Polestar Pilates Rehabilitation
Coral Gables, Florida

Judith A. Dewane, PT, DSc, NCS
Assistant Professor (CHS)
Doctor of Physical Therapy Program
Department of Orthopedics and Rehabilitation
University of Wisconsin
Madison,Wisconsin

Peter I. Edgelow, PT, MA, DPT
Assistant Clinical Professor
Graduate Program in Physical Therapy
University of California, San Francisco
San Francisco, California

Barbara Edmison, PT
Center Coordinator of Clinical Education
Therapy Services Department
Santa Barbara Cottage Hospital
Santa Barbara, California

Teresa A. Foy, OT, BS
OT Therapy Manager
SCI Program
Shepherd Center
Atlanta, Georgia

Kenda Fuller, PT, NCS
Owner
South Valley Physical Therapy
Specialist in Neurologic Physical Therapy
Denver, Colorado

Clayton D. Gable, PT, PhD
US Army, Headquarters MEDCOM
Fort Sam Houston, Texas
Private Practice PT
Adult and Pediatric Neuology
San Antonio, Texas
Home Ex Pro
Chief Executive Officer
Odessa, Texas

Mary Lou Galantino, PT, PhD, MSCE
Professor of Physical Therapy
Holistic Health Minor Coordinator
School of Health Sciences
The Richard Stockton College of New Jersey
Galloway, New Jersey
Adjunct Researcher, CCEB
Adjunct Associate Professor of Family Medicine and Community Health
University of Pennsylvania
Philadelphia, Pennsylvania

Teresa Gutierrez, PT, MS, PCS, C/NDT
Pediatric Rehab Northwest, LLC
Gig Harbor, Washington

Ann Hallum, PT, PhD
Dean of Graduate Studies
San Francisco State University
Professor
Graduate Program in Physical Therapy
University of California/San Francisco State University
San Francisco, California

Jeffrey Kauffman, MD
Holistic Health Associate
Sacramento, California

Laura J. Kenny, PT, OCS, FAAOMPT
Clinical Specialist
Occupational Health Department
Oakland, California

David M. Kietrys, PT, PhD, OCS
Associate Professor
Rehabilitation and Movement Sciences
University of Medicine and Dentistry of New Jersey
Newark, New Jersey

Kristin J. Krosschell, PT, DPT, MA, PCS
Assistant Professor
Department of Physical Therapy and Human Movement Sciences
Feinberg School of Medicine
Northwestern University
Chicago, Illinois

Rolando T. Lazaro, PT, PhD, DPT, GCS
Associate Professor
Department of Physical Therapy
Samuel Merritt University
Oakland, California

Preface to the Sixth Edition

Each edition of this book brings new insights, new visions, and new avenues for therapists to advance their respective analytical and clinical skills when assisting individuals with neurological impairments to improve their quality of life. The explosion of new information within neuroscience and its impact on the evidence base of both evaluation and intervention strategies has and will continue to modify and improve services to the many individuals seeking our expertise. With this new knowledge, many individuals within the professions of physical and occupational therapy and other related health care disciplines will assist patients throughout the world to attain a level of life participation that they, as patients, define as quality of life. As the complex interactions of all systems slowly unravel their mysteries in front of the eyes and within the hands of practicing clinician and researchers, the possibilities of new variables that affect outcomes will continue to arise and challenge the mind of the learner. Having a tether to basic neuroscience allows therapists of today and those of the future to stretch to limits and levels of understanding that boggle the rigid linear thinker of yesterday. With the explosion of new research over the last five years, this sixth edition has stretched our professions to the unknowns we might have considered the distant future a few years ago. These doors have led to integration of systems and help us discover what seems like unanswerable questions and continue to ground us to the evidence base of today's practice. This book mirrors a family dedicated to the advancement and quality of life of others. This book does not belong to the publisher, the editor, or even the chapter authors. We are just participants on life's journey and have come together to share what we have learned and to help future colleagues evolve farther than we had at the same age. The book belongs to the learners, those students who are willing to question today's practice and look toward new and innovative ways to provide better and more effective patient care, to prevent loss of life participation, and to enhance the quality of life of all individuals who cross their paths.

Thirty-two years and five previous editions have passed since this book was conceived. In the evolution of a person, the attainment of 32 years usually signifies adulthood approaching middle age. Thirty-two years of evolution of this book has encompassed new visions, greater evidence base to practice within health care delivery, huge advancements in neuroscience and intervention strategies, and without a doubt many more questions. Mastery can never be obtained, because new visions constantly suggest a new beginning while mastery suggests knowledge and wisdom of the whole. The journey has led the reader from a book whose initial problem-solving focus was understanding medical diagnosis and science as it related to neurological problems to a book whose focus is placed on movement diagnosis and the ways to empower individuals in need of our services to the highest quality of life attainable through functional movement. The evolution of the professions encompass in-depth integration of movement science, a comprehension of disease/pathology, a high level of analysis and skill development in objective measurements of functional behavior, and intervention strategies based on best practice and evidence. During the last three and a half decades, the therapeutic management of clients has undergone many stages of evolution. Evidence-based practice that encompasses both effectiveness and efficacy through clinical studies and basic science research should be guiding the choices of intervention procedures today. This shift in paradigm from specific treatment approaches to a problem-solving model that looks at the functional ability, activity limitations, life participation, and quality of life of the client has lead to a transformation of services throughout the world. As these problem-solving approaches become operational, more effective, reliable, and valid therapeutic examinations and management strategies are being presented in the literature. Yet, our understanding of how humans learn, relearn, or adapt is far from reaching closure. Neuroplasticity, once thought impossible, has become widely accepted as fact within the area of neurological rehabilitation. Given the many unknowns and the fact that what is "known" often changes daily, all learners are challenged to keep a mind open to change and to new learning while holding on to a flexible paradigm that allows for effective examination, evaluation, and treatment of clients within a dynamic, ever-changing environment. Client-centered care has shown that willing participation by the consumer of our services leads to the greatest potential outcomes and satisfaction of the client. No longer will therapy be done to the patient but instead will encompass and be enhanced by family's and client's goals and expectations. Master clinicians of the past have always taken these patient goals into consideration whether formally or informally. Thus their outcomes always exceeded others and they never had problems with compliance.

Cost of services, managed care environments, limitations in visits, and practice patterns all create challenges to today's professional. Young therapists are expected to graduate from school and immediately practice as experienced clinical problem solvers. Young colleagues feel they are expected to *know* the answers, not to discover them. Yet, within the clinical arena, problem-solving success is always dependent on one variable, and that variable is the patient. As long as the unique qualities of the patient are considered, a therapist will be able to select examination procedures and appropriate interventions using clinical reasoning. Graduates of today and tomorrow have the knowledge and skill and have practiced clinical problem-solving through their education. The only variables they will always need to add will be those unique characteristics of each patient.

This book is designed to provide the practitioner and advanced therapy student with a variety of problem-solving strategies that can be used to tailor treatment approaches to individual client needs and cognitive style. The treatment of persons with neurological disabilities requires an integrated approach involving therapies and treatment procedures used by physical, occupational, speech and language, music and recreational therapists; nurses; pharmacists; orthotists; physicians; and a variety of other health care providers as well as the family's expectation, values, and social beliefs. Contributors to this book were selected for their expertise and integrated knowledge of various subject areas. The result is, we hope, a blend of state-of-the-art information about the therapeutic management of persons with neurological disabilities.

This book is organized to provide the student with a comprehensive discussion of all aspects of neurological rehabilitation and to facilitate quick reference in a clinical situation. Section I, "Foundations for Clinical Practice in Neurological Rehabilitation," constitutes an overview of foundational theories. This includes the entire diagnostic process used by movement specialists. The basis for this process ranges across many cognitive areas and theories, and thus concepts and integration are presented in a variety of chapters. Additional emphasis has been placed both on health and wellness along with the visual analysis of functional movement development and change across the life span. Theoretical constructs of motor control, motor learning, and neuroplasticity, as well as the limbic components role in movement science and psychosocial variables are again updated and discussed. The complexity of examination tools and treatment categories and techniques have again been edited to help the learner see and analyze the vast opinions available as part of today's practice. To complete this foundational section, discussion ends with the need for reliable and valid documentation, which should lead to reimbursement for services within various clinical environments. Section II, "Rehabilitation Management of Clients with Neurologic System Pathology," offers an in-depth discussion and analysis of the therapeutic management of the most common neurological disabilities encountered by physical and occupational therapists. As professions are becoming autonomous and entry into practice at a doctoral level of study, the importance of the learner comprehending and analyzing each clinical problem confronted when treating individuals with movement dysfunction caused by neurological problems cannot be overemphasized. Hopefully these chapters will clarify how to examine and treat both general and specific movement problems seen in individuals with injury to specific areas of the central and peripheral nervous system. Section III, "Neurological Disorders and Applications Issues," is devoted to recent advances in general approaches to intervention and rehabilitation that might affect any of the diagnostic categories discussed in Section II. The importance of other system problems, such as cardiopulmonary and chronic movement problems, has been emphasized to help the learner integrate the critical nature of an integrated systems model. Two new chapters, one on robotics and one on imaging, have been added in order to enlarge the reader's comprehension of tools and expectations that will become commonplace in years to come.

Special features within all three parts are examinations, evaluations, prognosis, and intervention strategies using sound clinical reasoning. Case studies are presented within each clinical-based chapter to help the reader with the problem-solving process. Online clinical movement examples have been provided to help the learner visually recognize movement problems commonly seen in individuals with specific neurological diagnoses.

The book continues to evolve in order to meet the changing demands placed upon us as clinicians and educators. As we have finally assumed the role of movement specialists both in wellness and in rehabilitation, our clinical observational skill and the ability to compare normal to abnormal movement patterns when formulating a diagnosis, prognosis, and treatment plan has brought both professions to the obvious evolution of clinical doctorates. Our place in health care and the responsibility we assume should positively impact the quality of life of all those individuals for whom we provide service. We hope this book and the online video site will continue to aid all of you as tools to use when confronted with questions regarding movement problems seen in individuals with neurological problems.

During the conceptualization and preparation of all six editions, many individuals gave time, guidance, and emotional support. To all those individuals I extend my sincere appreciation. There are many people to thank in the preparation of this sixth edition: the authors, the researchers, the illustrators, each person assisting during the process of publication, and the patients. No person could have accomplished the end product alone. Yet, during the editing process of this edition, some specific individuals came to deserve special recognition and thanks:

The staff at Elsevier who worked on the publication of this edition: Christie M. Hart and Carol O'Connell. All the teachers and healers who have crossed our paths in the last 40 years and helped us to continually realize that before we can find answers, design research projects, and establish efficacy, we must identify and acknowledge unknowns and formulate questions.

Each family member or significant other who encouraged and supported all of us from the moment we began the editorial process to the day the book reached the learner, we are forever appreciative.

My entire family, all of whom helped me make the time to complete this manuscript.

My two sons, Jeb and Ben, whose support I have had since the beginning of this book. Both are creative and brilliant young professionals in their own right, yet have tirelessly helped me take very complex concepts and ideas and transform them into illustrations that can be comprehended. As small children during the book's conception, their tolerance far exceeded their age. As children, they allowed me to take pictures, many of which have been used to actualize the chapter on movement development across the life span. As young adults, their support and guidance always gives me strength. As successful professionals, they have continued to teach me. Today, they are also husbands and parents. Their wives have given to me two daughters who also help me learn and grow. But, of course the new life found in our grandchildren forever allows me the opportunity to watch development of the mind, body, and spirit of each of them as they have begun their adventure of life.

As a critical aspect of this edition, the three section editors from the fifth edition stepped into the book editor role. Thus, I cannot extend more gratitude, respect, and love to Gordon Burton, Rolando Lazaro, and Margaret Roller. Three leaders, visionaries, and genuinely caring and loving individuals, they have certainly made a significant impact on the direction this book has taken in this edition and will be in the future.

Last, my husband, Gordon, who is the only one who truly knows what demands this book places on me and everyone around me. His support has never dwindled, nor his acceptance of my choices. The demands of this edition as well as life in general has certainly tried both of us as we have entered the later part of our life adventure. But, as always, he is my best friend and present to support me when needed.

This book was conceived 32 years ago. It was presented in print to the world 27 years ago. Both dates signify young adulthood and the evolution from conception to a responsibility as an adult. We are all interconnected in a tapestry that has allowed this book to evolve into what it is today. For that, I give thanks as an author, as the editor, as a consumer but most importantly as a learner. Our lives are finite but the quality of those lives is extremely important to us and those around us. It is hoped that this book will guide colleagues to help consumers in attainment of that quality. It is hoped, with the eyes and minds of so many outstanding colleagues sharing their experiences and their desire to ground what they do into evidence-based practice, that the learner will embrace the adventure with the same vigor and enthusiasm that so many have from the past.

For each of us the journey is today and the adventure tomorrow, no matter how many tomorrows we may have. May all of you have the joy, the challenge, the excitement, and the learning adventure I have had throughout my entire professional career.

Darcy A. Umphred

Rachel M. Lopez, PT, MPT, NCS
Physical Therapist
Barrow Neurological Institute
St. Joseph's Hospital
Phoenix, Arizona

Marilyn MacKay-Lyons, PT, PhD
Associate Professor
School of Physiotherapy
Dalhousie University
Affiliated Clinical Scientist
Physical Medicine and Rehabilitation
QEII Health Sciences Centre
Halifax, Nova Scotia, Canada

Shari L. McDowell, PT, BS
Inpatient Spinal Cord Injury Program Manager
Shepherd Center
Atlanta, Georgia

Rochelle McLaughlin, MS, OTR/L, MBSR
Adjunct Faculty
San Jose State University
San Jose, California
Department of Occupational Therapy
Stanford Hospital Farewell to Falls
Stanford, California
Bay Area Pain and Wellness Center
Los Gatos, California

Marsha E. Melnick, PT, PhD
Professor Emerita
San Francisco State University
Clinical Professor
University of California, San Francisco
UCSF/SFSU Graduate Program in Physical Therapy
San Francisco, California

Sarah A. Morrison, PT, BS
Director Spinal Cord Injury Services
Shepherd Center, Inc.
Atlanta, Georgia

Susanne M. Morton, PT, PhD
Assistant Professor
Department of Physical Therapy and Rehabilitation Science
University of Iowa
Iowa City, Iowa

Mari Jo Pesavento, PT, PCS
Pediatric Physical Therapist
Pediatric Clinical Specialist
Rehabilitation and Development Department
Hope Children's Hospital
Oak Lawn, Illinois

Darbi Breath Philibert, MHS, OTR/L
Pediatric Occupational Therapist
Private Practice
New Orleans, Louisiana

Robert Prue, PhD
Associate Professor
School of Social Work
University of Missouri, Kansas City
Kansas City, Missouri

Myla U. Quiben, PT, PhD, DPT, GCS, NCS, CEEAA
Assistant Professor
Department of Physical Therapy
University of Texas Health Science Center San Antonio
San Antonio, Texas

Walter Racette, CPO
Associate Clinical Professor
University of California San Francisco
Department of Orthopaedics
San Francisco, California

Clinton Robinson, Jr.
Grand Master
9th Dan Taekwondo Black Belt
Department of Physical Education
American River College
Sacramento, California

Margaret L. Roller, PT, MS, DPT
Professor and Graduate Coordinator
Department of Physical Therapy
California State University, Northridge
Northridge, California
Clinical Instructor
NeuroCom International, a division of Natus
Clackamas, Oregon

Susan D. Ryerson, PT, DSc
Owner, Making Progress
Neurological Rehabilitation
Alexandria, Virginia
Research Scientist
Center for Biomechanics and Rehabilitation Research
National Rehabilitation Hospital
Washington, DC

Dale Scalise-Smith, PT, PhD
Dean, School of Health Professions and Education
Professor of Physical Therapy
Utica College
Utica, New York

Osa Jackson Schulte, PT, PhD, GCFP/AT
Executive Director and Continuity Assistant Trainer
Feldenkrais Professional Training Program
Movement and Healing Center
Clarkson, Michigan
Contingent Physical Therapist
Community Care Services
Henry Ford Health System
Detroit, Michigan

Claudia R. Senesac, PT, PhD, PCS
Clinical Assistant Professor
Department of Physical Therapy
University of Florida
Gainesville, Florida

Eunice Yu Chiu Shen, PT, PhD, DPT, PCS
Physical Therapy Education Coordinator
Department of Public Health
County of Los Angeles
California Children's Services
El Monte, California

Timothy J. Smith, RPh, PhD
Professor and Chair
Physiology and Pharmacology
Thomas J. Long School of Pharmacy and Health Sciences
University of the Pacific
Stockton, California

Sebastian Sovero, MS
Doctoral Student
Department of Electrical and Computer Engineering
University of California, Santa Barbara
Santa Barbara, California

Kerri Sowers, PT, DPT
United States Equestrian Federation Paraequestrian National Classifier
Staff Physical Therapist
Atlanticare Regional Medical Center
Atlantic City, New Jersey

Corrie J. Stayner, PT, MS
Adjunct Faculty
Physical Therapy Program
Arizona School of Health Sciences
A.T. Still University
Physical Therapist
Barrow Neurological Institute
Phoenix, Arizona

James Stephens, PT, PhD, CFP
Living Independently for Elders, LIFE
School of Nursing
University of Pennsylvania
Adjunct Assistant Professor
Temple University
Physical Therapy Department
Philadelphia, Pennsylvania
Movement Learning and Rehab
Havertown, Pennsylvania

Bradley W. Stockert, PT, PhD
Professor
Department of Physical Therapy
California State University, Sacramento
Sacramento, California

Jane K. Sweeney, PT, PhD, PCS, C/NDT, FAPTA
Professor and Graduate Program Director
Doctoral Programs in Pediatric Science
Rocky Mountain University of Health Professions
Provo, Utah
Practitioner/Owner
Pediatric Rehab Northwest, LLC
Gig Harbor, Washington

Stacey E. Szklut, MS, OTR/L
Executive Director and Owner
South Shore Therapies
Weymouth and Pembroke, Massachusetts

Candy Tefertiller, DPT, ATP, NCS
Director of Physical Therapy
Craig Hospital
Englewood, Colorado

Marcia Hall Thompson, PT, DPT, DSc
Assistant Professor
Department of Physical Therapy
California State University, Fresno
Fresno, California

Heidi Truman, CPO
Clinical Orthotist/Prosthetist
University of California, San Francisco
Department of Orthopaedic Surgery
San Francisco, California

Karla M. Tuzzolino, PT, NCS
Staff Physical Therapist
Barrow Neurological Institute
St. Joseph's Hospital
Phoenix, Arizona

Darcy A. Umphred, PT, PhD, FAPTA
Emeritus Professor and Past Chair
Department of Physical Therapy
School of Pharmacy and Health Sciences
University of the Pacific
Stockton, California

John Upledger, DO
Developer
Craniosacral Therapy
The Upledger Institute
Palm Beach Gardens, Florida

Richard W. Voss, DPC, MSW, MTS
Professor
West Chester University of Pennsylvania
Department of Undergraduate Social Work
West Chester, Pennsylvania

John G. Wallace, Jr., PT, MS, OCS
Chief Executive Officer
BMS Practice Solutions
Upland, California

Therese Marie West, PhD, MT-BC, FAMI
Board-Certified Music Therapist and Fellow of the Association for Music and Imagery
Retired
Estacade, Oregon

Gail L. Widener, PT, PhD
Associate Professor
Department of Physical Therapy
Samuel Merritt University
Oakland, California

Patricia A. Winkler, PT, DSc, NCS
Assistant Professor (retired)
Regis University
School of Physical Therapy
Denver, Colorado

George Wolfe, PT, PhD
Professor Emeritus
Department of Physical Therapy
California State University
Northridge, California

Contents

Enhance Your Learning and Practice Experience

The images below are QR (Quick Response) codes. The codes will take you to the reference lists for each chapter, videos, and a glossary that can be accessed on your mobile device for quick reference in a lab or clinical setting. References are linked to the Medline abstract where available.

For fast and easy access, right from your mobile device, follow these instructions.

You can also find them at:

http://booksite.elsevier.com/Umphred/neurological6e

What you need:

- A mobile device, such as a smart phone or tablet, equipped with a camera and Internet access
- A QR code reader application (If you do not already have a reader installed on your mobile device, look for free versions in your app store.)

How it works:

- Open the QR code reader application on your mobile device.
- Point the device's camera at the code and scan.
- The codes take you to a main page where you can link to specific chapters for instant viewing of the videos and the references where you can further access the Medline links—no log-on required.

Main Page Code

Reference Code

SECTION I

Foundations for Clinical Practice in Neurological Rehabilitation

CHAPTER 1 Foundations for Clinical Practice*

DARCY A. UMPHRED, PT, PhD, FAPTA, ROLANDO T. LAZARO, PT, PhD, DPT, GCS, and MARGARET L. ROLLER, PT, MS, DPT

KEY TERMS

clinical problem solving
diagnostic model: examination, evaluation, diagnosis, prognosis, intervention
disablement and enablement models
empowerment
holistic model for health care delivery
International Classification of Functioning, Disability and Health (ICF)
learning environment
systems model

OBJECTIVES

After reading this chapter the student or therapist will be able to:

1. Analyze the interlocking concepts of a systems model and discuss how cognitive, affective, sensory, and motor subsystems influence normal and abnormal function of the nervous system.
2. Use an efficacious diagnostic process that considers the whole patient/client and includes evaluation, examination, diagnosis, prognosis, intervention, and related documentation, leading to meaningful, functional outcomes.
3. Apply the International Classification of Functioning, Disability and Health (ICF) to the clinical management of patients/clients with neuromuscular dysfunction.
4. Discuss the evolution of disablement, enablement, and health classification models, neurological therapeutic approaches, and health care environments in the United States and worldwide.
5. Discuss the interactions and importance of the patient, therapist, and environment in the clinical triad.
6. Consider how varying aspects of the clinical therapeutic environment can affect learning, motivation, practice, and ultimate outcomes for patients/clients.
7. Define, discuss, and give examples of a holistic model of health care.

Physical therapists (PTs), occupational therapists (OTs), and other health care individuals involved in improving the function and quality of life of individuals with neuromuscular dysfunction must have a thorough understanding of the client as a total human being. This foundational concept is critical for high-level professional performance. With the use of a clinical problem-solving, diagnosis-prognosis approach, this book orients the student and clinician to the roles that multiple systems within and outside the human body play in the causation, progression, and recovery process of a variety of common neurological problems. A secondary objective is to orient the clinician to a theoretical framework that uses techniques for enhancing functional movement, enlarges the client's repertoire for movement alternatives, and creates an environment that empowers the client to achieve the highest levels of activity, participation, and quality of life.

Methods of examination, evaluation, prognosis, and intervention must incorporate all aspects of the client's nervous system and the influences of the external environment on those individuals. In the clinical management of patients with neurological disabilities, the overlap of basic knowledge and practical application of examination and intervention

*This chapter and the concepts of this book are dedicated to Dr. Donna El-Din, PT, PhD, FAPTA, who has participated in the evolution and vision of where PT practice is today and will be over the next decade. Dr. El-Din had hoped to participate in the writing of this chapter but was taken from us in May 2010. We will forever be grateful for her dedication, teaching, and friendship to thousands of physical therapists across the world.

techniques among all disciplines involved in the care of the client is great. Delineation of individual professional roles in the treatment of these clients is often based on administrative decisions and current billing practices for services provided, rather than distinct boundaries defined by title. This book emphasizes the selection of examination and intervention strategies that have been demonstrated as evidence based. Clinicians must also be open to generating new hypotheses as clinical problems present themselves without clear evidence to guide practice.

A clinical problem-solving approach is used because it is logical and adaptable, and it has been recommended by many professionals during the past 40 years.[1-7] The concept of clinical decision making based in problem-solving theory has been stressed throughout the literature over the past decades and has guided the therapist toward an evidence-based approach to patient management. This approach clearly identifies the therapist's responsibility to examine, evaluate, analyze, draw conclusions, and make decisions regarding prognosis and treatment alternatives.[8-24]

This book is divided into three sections.

Section I lays the foundation of knowledge necessary to understand and implement a problem-solving approach to clinical care across the span of human life. The basic knowledge of the function of the human body in disease and repair is constantly expanding and often changing in content, theory, and clinical focus. This section reflects that change in both philosophy and scientific research.

Roles that therapists are currently playing and will be asked to play in the future are changing.[25-27] Therapists are experts in normal human movement across the life span (see Chapter 3) and how that movement is changed after life events, and with disease or pathological conditions. Therapists realize that health and wellness play a critical role in movement function as a client enters the health care system with a neurological disease or condition (see Chapter 2). In many U.S. states, clients are now able to use direct access for therapy services. In this environment, therapists must medically screen for disease and pathology to determine conditions that are outside of the defined scope of practice, and make appropriate referrals to other medical professionals (see Chapter 7). They must also make a *differential diagnosis* regarding movement dysfunctions within that therapist's respective scope of practice (see Chapter 8). Section I has been designed to weave together the issues of evaluation and intervention with components of central nervous system (CNS) function to consider a holistic approach to each client's needs (see Chapters 4, 5, 6, and 9). This section delineates the conceptual areas that permit the reader to synthesize all aspects of the problem-solving process in the care of a client. Basic to the outcomes of care is accurate documentation of the patient management process, as well as the administration and reimbursement for that process (see Chapter 10).

Section II is composed of chapters that deal with specific clinical problems, beginning with pediatric conditions, progressing through neurological problems common in adults, and ending with aging with dignity and chronic impairments. In Section II each author follows the same problem-solving format to enable the reader either to focus more easily on one specific neurological problem or to address the problem from a broader perspective that includes life impact. The multiple authors of this book use various cognitive strategies and methods of addressing specific neurological deficits. A range of strategies for examining clinical problems is presented to facilitate the reader's ability to identify variations in problem-solving methods. Many of the strategies used by one author may apply to situations presented by other authors. Just as clinicians tend to adapt learning methods to solve specific problems for their clients, readers are encouraged to use flexibility in selecting treatments with which they feel comfortable and to be creative when implementing any therapeutic plan.[16] Although the framework of this text has always focused on evidence-based practice and improvement of quality of life of the patient, the terminology used by professionals has shifted from focusing on impairments and disabilities of an individual after a neurological insult (the International Classification of Impairments, Disability and Health [ICIDH]) to a classification system that considers functioning and health at the forefront: the International Classification of Functioning, Disability and Health (ICF).[28] The ICF considers all health conditions, both pathological and non–disease related; provides a framework for examining the status of body structures and functions for the purpose of identifying impairments; includes activities and limitations in the functional performance of mobility skills; and considers participation in societal and family roles that contribute to quality of life of an individual. The personal characteristics of the individual and the environmental factors to which he or she is exposed and in which he or she must function are included as contextural factors that influence health, pathology, and recovery of function.[29] The ICF provides a common language for worldwide discussion and classification of health-related patterns in human populations. The language of the ICF has been adopted by the American Physical Therapy Association (APTA), and the revised version of the *Guide to Physical Therapist Practice* reflects this change.[30] Each chapter in this book strives to present and use the ICF model, use the language of the ICF, and present a comprehensive, patient-oriented structure for the process of examination, evaluation, diagnosis, prognosis, and intervention for common neurological conditions and resultant functional problems. Consideration of the patient/client as a whole and his or her interactions with the therapist and the learning environment is paramount to this process.

Chapters in Section II also include methods of examination and evaluation for various neurological clinical problems using reliable and valid outcome measures. The psychometric properties of standard outcome measures are continually being established through research methodology. The choice of objective measurement tools that focus on identifying impairments in body structures and functions, activity-based functional limitations, and factors that create restrictions in participation and affect health quality of life and patient empowerment is a critical aspect of each clinical chapter's diagnostic process. Change is inevitable, and the problem-solving philosophy used by each author reflects those changes.

Section III of the text focuses on clinical topics that can be applied to any one of the clinical problems discussed in Section II. Chapters have been added to reflect changes in the focus of therapy as it continues to evolve as an emerging flexible paradigm within a multiple systems approach. A specific body system such as the cardiopulmonary system (see Chapter 30) or complementary approaches used with interactive systems (see Chapter 39) are also presented as part of Section III. These incorporate not only changes in the interactions of professional disciplines within the Western medical allopathic model of health care delivery, but also present additional delivery approaches that emphasize the importance of cultural and ethnic belief systems, family structure, and quality-of-life issues. Two additional chapters have been added to Section III. Chapter 37 on imaging emphasizes the role of doctoring professions' need to analyze how medical imaging matches and mismatches movement function of patients. Chapter 38 reflects changes in the role of PTs and OTs as they integrate more complex technologies into clinical practice.

Examination tools presented throughout the text should help the reader identify many objective measures. The reader is reminded that although a tool may be discussed in one chapter, its use may have application to many other clinical problems. Chapter 8 summarizes the majority of neurological tools available to therapists today, and the authors of each clinical chapter may discuss specific tools used to evaluate specific clinical problems and diagnostic groups. The same concept is true with regard to general treatment suggestions and problem-solving strategies used to analyze motor control impairments as presented in Chapter 9; authors of clinical chapters will focus on evidence-based treatments identified for specific patient populations.

THE CHANGING WORLD OF HEALTH CARE

To understand how and why disablement, enablement, and health classification models have become the accepted models used by PTs and OTs when evaluating, diagnosing, prognosing, and treating clients with body system impairments, activity limitations, and participation restrictions resulting from neurological problems, it is important for the reader to review the evolution of health care within our culture. This review begins with the allopathic medical model because this model has been the dominant model of health care in Western society and forms the conceptual basis for health care in industrialized countries.[31] The allopathic model assumes that illness has an organic base that can be traced to discrete molecular elements. The origin of disease is found at the molecular level of the individual's tissue. The first step toward alleviating the disease is to identify the pathogen that has invaded the tissue and, after proper identification, apply appropriate treatment techniques including surgery, drugs (see Chapter 36), and other proven methods.

It is implicit in the model that specialists who are professionally competent have the sole responsibility for the identification of the cause of the illness and for the judgment as to what constitutes appropriate treatment. The medical knowledge required for these judgments is thought to be the domain of the professional medical specialists and therefore inaccessible to the public. PTs and OTs have never been responsible for the diagnosis or treatment of diseases or pathological conditions of a specific client. Instead, we have always focused on the body system impairments resulting in activity limitations and inability to participate in life that have been caused by the specific disease or pathological condition. Therapists are also responsible for analyzing the interactions of all other systems and how they compensate for or are affected by the original medical problem. As our roles within Western health care delivery have expanded and are becoming clearer, so has the role of the consumer. In today's health care environment, the responsibility of both the therapist and the patient begins with health and wellness and proceeds to regaining optimal health, wellness, and functioning after neurological insult.

Levin[32] points out that there is a lot that consumers can do for themselves. Most people can assume responsibility to care for minor health problems. The use of nonpharmaceutical methods (e.g., hypnosis, biofeedback, meditation, and acupuncture) to control pain is becoming common practice. The recognition and value of a holistic approach to illness are receiving increasing attention in society. Treatment designed to improve both the emotional and physical needs of clients during illness has been recognized and advocated as a way to help individuals regain some control over their lives (see Chapters 5 and 6).

A holistic model (*holos,* from the Greek, meaning "whole") of health care seeks to involve the patient in the process and take the mystery out of health care for the consumer. It acknowledges that multiple factors are operating in disease, trauma, and aging and that there are many interactions among those factors. Social, emotional, environmental, political, economic, psychological, and cultural factors are all acknowledged as influences on the individual's potential to maintain health, to regain health after insult, or to maintain a quality of health in spite of existing disease or illness. Measures of success in health care delivery have shifted from the traditional standard of whether the person lives or dies to the assessment of the extent of the person's quality of life and ability to participate in life after some neurological insult. Moreover, "quality of life" or living implies more than physical health. It implies that the individual is mentally and emotionally healthy as well. It takes all dimensions of a person's being into consideration regarding health. From the beginning, even Hippocrates emphasized treatment of the person as a whole, and the influence of society and of the environment on health.

An approach that takes this holistic perspective centers its philosophy on the patient as an individual.[33] The individual with this orientation is less likely to have the physician look only for the chemical basis of his or her difficulty and ignore the psychological factors that may be present. Similarly, the importance of focusing on an individual's strengths while helping to eliminate body system impairments and functional limitations in spite of existing disease or pathological conditions plays a critical role in this model. This influences the roles PT and OT will play in the future of health care delivery and will continue to inspire expanded practice in these professions.

The health care delivery system in Western society is designed to serve all of its citizens. Given the variety of economic, political, cultural, and religious forces at work in American society, education of the people with regard to their health care is probably the only method that can work in the long run. With limitations placed on delivery of medical care, the client's responsibility for health and healing is constantly increasing. The task of PTs and OTs today is to cultivate people's sense of responsibility toward their own health and the health and well-being of the community. The consumer has to accept and play a critical role in the decision-making process within the entire health care delivery model to more thoroughly guarantee compliance with prescribed treatments and optimal outcomes.[34-40] PTs and many OTs today are entering their professional careers at a doctoral level and beginning to assume the role of primary care providers. A requisite of this new responsibility is the performance of a more diligent examination and evaluation process that includes a comprehensive medical screening of each patient/client.[41,42] Patient education will continue to be an effective and vital approach to client management and has the greatest potential to move health care delivery toward a concept of preventive care. The high cost of health care is a factor that will continue to drive patients and their families to increase their participation in and take responsibility for their own care.[43] Reducing the cost of health care will require providers to empower patients to become active participants in preventing and reducing impairments and practicing methods to regain safe, functional, pain-free control of movement patterns for optimal quality of life.

In-Depth Analysis of the Holistic Model

Carlson[44] thinks that pressure to change to holistic thinking in medicine continues as a result of a societal change in its perspective of the rights of individuals. A concern to keep the individual central in the care process will continue to grow in response to continued technological growth that threatens to dehumanize care even more. The holistic model takes into account each person's unique psychosocial, political, economic, environmental, and spiritual needs as they affect the individual's health.

The nation faces significant social change in the area of health care. The coming years will change access to health care for our citizens, the benefits, the reimbursement process for providers, and the delivery system. Health care providers have a major role in the success of the final product. The Pew Health Professions Commission[45] identified issues that must be addressed as any new system is developed and implemented. Most, if not all, of the issues involve close interactions between the provider and client. These issues include (1) the need of the provider to stay in step with client needs; (2) the need for flexible educational structures to address a system that reassigns certain responsibilities to other personnel; (3) the need to redirect national funding priorities away from narrow, pure research access to include broader concepts of health care; (4) the licensing of health care providers; (5) the need to address the issues of minority groups; (6) the need to emphasize general care and at the same time educate specialists; (7) the issue of promoting teamwork; and (8) the need to emphasize the community as the focus of health care. There are other important issues, but the last to be included here is mentioned in more detail because of its relevance to the consumer. Without the consumer's understanding during development of a new system, the system could omit several opportunities for enrichment of design. Without the understanding of the consumer during implementation of a new system, the consumer might block delivery systems because of lack of knowledge. Thus, the delivery of service must be client centered and client and family driven, and the focus of intervention needs to be in alignment with client objectives and desired outcomes.[33-36,46,47] Today, as stated earlier,[43] this need may be driven more by financial necessity than by ethical and best practice philosophy, but the end result should lead to a higher quality of life for the consumer.

Providers are more willing to include the client by designing individualized plans of care, educating, addressing issues of minority groups, and becoming proactive team caregivers.[37-40] The influence of these methods extends to the community and leads to greater patient/client satisfaction. The research as of 2011 demonstrates the importance of patient participation, and this body of work is expected to grow.

The potential for OTs and PTs to become primary providers of health care in the twenty-first century is becoming a greater reality within the military system as well as in some large health maintenance organizations (HMOs).[48-53] The role a therapist in the future will play as that primary provider will depend on that clinician's ability to screen for disease and pathological conditions, examine and evaluate clinical signs that will lead to diagnoses and prognoses that fall inside and outside of the scope of practice, and select appropriate interventions that will lead to the most efficacious, cost-effective treatment.

The role of therapists in the area of neurological rehabilitation will first be in the area of health and wellness. Medical screening and early detection of neurological problems should facilitate early referral of the consumer to a medical practitioner. This may occur in a wellness center or in physical and occupational therapy clinics where the patient is being seen for some other problem such as back pain. Similarly, patients may reenter physical or occupational therapy after a neurological insult as someone who has a chronic movement dysfunction or degenerative condition that may be getting worse and who needs some instruction to regain motor function.

Neurological rehabilitation is taking place and will continue to take place in a changing health care environment and ever-evolving delivery system. The balance between visionary and pragmatist must be maintained by the practitioner. By the end of the twenty-first century, neurological rehabilitation will have evolved into a new shape and form, will take place within a very different health system, and will involve the client as the center of the dynamic exchange among wellness, disease, function, and empowerment.

THERAPEUTIC MODEL OF NEUROLOGICAL REHABILITATION WITHIN THE HEALTH CARE SYSTEM

Traditional Therapeutic Models

Keen observation of human movement and how impairments in the neuromusculoskeletal system alter motor behavior and functional mobility led several remarkable therapists to develop unique models of therapeutic interventions. These models include those of Ayers (sensory integration), Bobath (NeuroDevelopmental Treatment [NDT]), Brunnstrom (movement therapy approach), Feldenkrais (Functional Integration and Awareness Through Movement), Klein-Vogelbach (Functional Kinetics), Knott and Voss (Proprioceptive Neuromuscular Facilitation [PNF]), and Rood (Rood approach to neuromuscular dysfunction). These were the first behaviorally based models introduced within the health care delivery system, and they have been used by practitioners within the professions of physical and occupational therapy since the middle of the twentieth century. These individuals, as master clinicians, tried to explain what they were doing and why their respective approaches worked using the science of the time. From their teachings, various philosophical models evolved. These models were isolated models of therapeutic intervention that were based on successful treatment procedures as identified through observation and described and demonstrated by the teachers of those approaches. The general model of health care under which these approaches were used was the allopathic model of Western medicine, which begins with disease and pathology. Today, our models must begin with health and wellness, with an understanding of variables that lead a client into the health care delivery system, and an understanding of how the nervous system works and repairs itself.

During the past decades, both short-term and full-semester courses, as well as literature related to treatment of clients with CNS dysfunction, have been divided into units labeled according to these techniques. Often, interrelation and integration among techniques were not explored. Clinicians bound to one specific treatment approach without considering the theoretical understanding of its step-by-step process may have lacked the basis for a change of direction of intervention when a treatment was ineffective. It was difficult, therefore, to adapt alternative treatment techniques to meet the individual needs of clients. As a result, clinical problem solving was impeded, if not stopped, when one approach failed, because little integration of theories and methods of other approaches was never stressed in the learning process. Similarly, because a specific treatment has a potential effect on multiple body systems and interactions with the unique characteristics of each client's clinical problem, establishing efficacy for interventions using a Western research reductionist model became extremely difficult. This does not negate the potential usefulness of any treatment intervention, but it does create a dilemma regarding efficacy of practice. Similarly, the rationale often used to explain these therapeutic models was based on an understanding of the nervous system as described in the 1940s, 1950s, and 1960s. That understanding has dramatically changed. With the basic neurophysiological rationale for explaining these approaches under fire for validity and the inability to demonstrate efficacy of these approaches using traditional research methods, many of these treatment approaches are no longer introduced to the student during academic training. However, if these master clinicians were much more effective than their clinical counterparts, then the hands-on therapeutic nature of their interventions may still be valid in certain clinical situations, but the neurophysiological explanation for the intervention may be very different. To make statements today saying that these masters did not use theories of motor learning or motor control is obvious because those theories and the studies supporting them had not yet been formulated. Yet patients treated by these master clinicians demonstrated improvements for which, it would seem according to our present-day theories, that concepts of motor learning must have been reinforced and repetitive practice encouraged. Although the verbal understanding of behavior sequences used to promote motor learning did not exist, these behavior sequences were often demonstrated by the client, and thus the success of the treatments and the skill of these master clinicians cannot be denied.

Physical and Occupational Therapy Practice Models

Disablement models have been used by clinicians since the 1960s. These models are the foundation for clinical outcomes assessment and create a common language for health care professionals worldwide. The first disablement model was presented in 1965 by Saad Nagi, a sociologist.[54,55] The Nagi model was accepted by APTA and applied in the first *Guide to Physical Therapist Practice,* which was introduced in 2001.[30] In 1980 the ICIDH was published by the World Health Organization (WHO).[56] This model helped expand on the International Classification of Diseases (ICD), which has a narrow focus based on categorizing diseases. The ICIDH was developed to help measure the consequences of health conditions on the individual. The focus of both the Nagi and the ICIDH models was on disablement related to impaired body structures and functions, functional activities, and handicaps in society (Figure 1-1). The WHO ICF model[28] evolved from a linear disablement model (Nagi, ICIDH) to a nonlinear, progressive model (ICF) that encompasses more than disease, impairments, and disablement. It includes personal and environmental factors that contribute to the health condition and well-being of individuals. The ICF model is considered an enablement model as it not only considers dysfunctions, but helps practitioners and researchers understand and use an individual's strengths in the clinical presentation. Each of these models provides an international standard to measure health and disability, with the ICF emphasizing the social aspects of disability. The ICF recognizes disability not only as a medical or biological dysfunction, but as a result of multiple overlapping factors including the impact of the environment on the functioning of individuals and populations. The ICF model is presented in Table 1-1 and discussed in greater depth in Chapters 4, 5, and 8.

It is easy to integrate the ICF model into behavioral models for the examination, evaluation, diagnosis, prognosis, and intervention of individuals with neurological system pathologies (see Figure 1-1). Whether an individual's activity limitations, impairments, and strengths lead to a restriction in the ability to participate in life activities, the perception of poor health, or restriction in the ability to adapt and adjust to the new health condition will determine the eventual quality of life of the person and the amount of empowerment or control he or she will have over daily life. The importance of the unique qualities of each person and the influence of the inherent environment helped to drive changes to world health models. The ICF is widely accepted and used by therapists throughout the world and is now the model for health in professional organizations such as APTA in the United States.[30]

As world health care continues to evolve, so will the WHO models. The sequential evolution of the three models is illustrated in Table 1-1. This evolution has created an alignment with what many therapists and master clinicians have long believed and practiced—focus on the patient, not the disease. The shift from disablement to enablement models of health care is a reflection of this change in perspective.

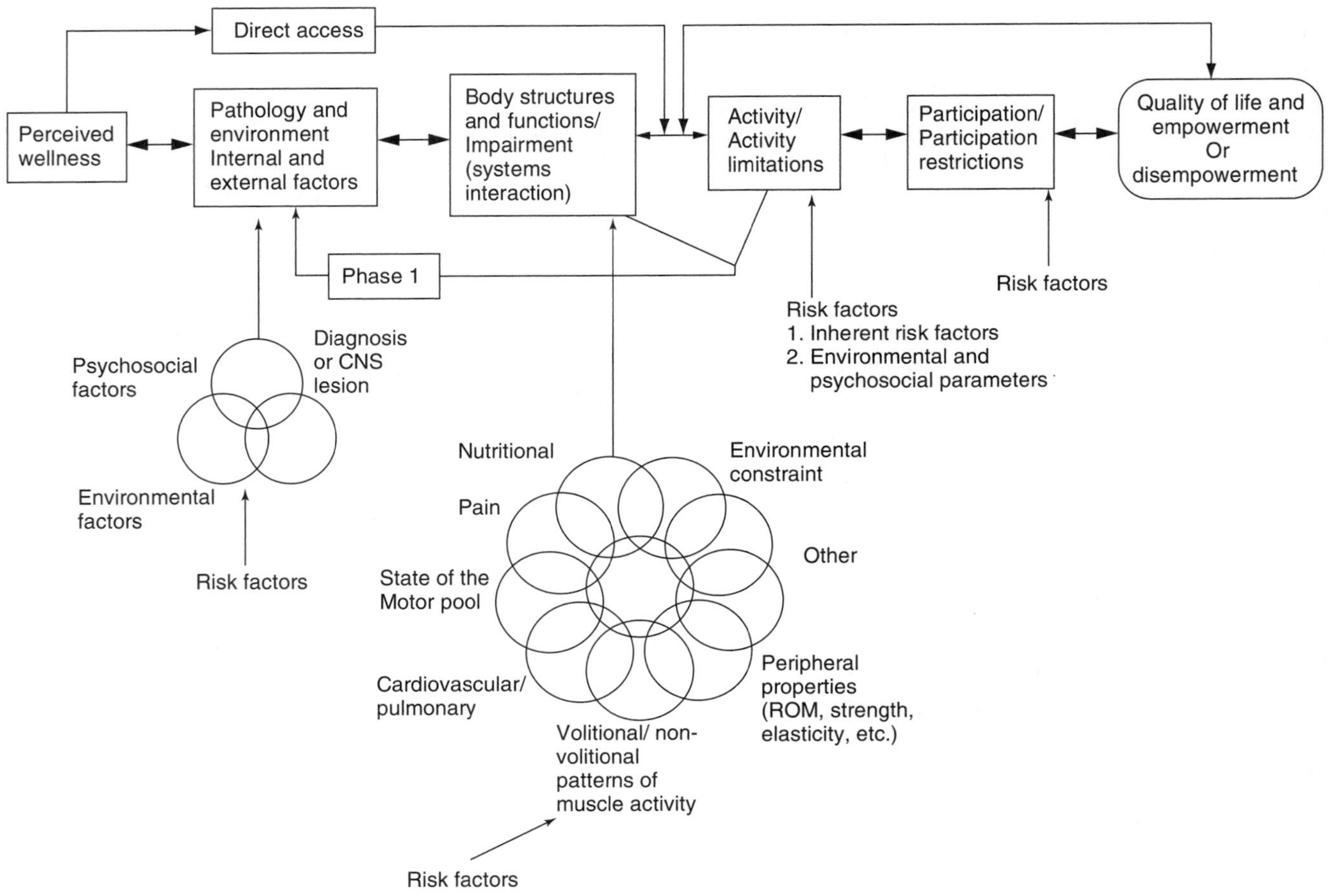

Figure 1-1 ■ Behavioral model for evaluation and treatment based on the International Classification of Functioning, Disability and Health (ICF) enablement schema. *ROM,* Range of motion.

TABLE 1-1 ■ ENABLEMENT AND DISABLEMENT MODELS WIDELY ACCEPTED THROUGHOUT THE WORLD OVER THE LAST 50 YEARS*

ICF model, WHO 2001[30]	Health condition	Body function and structure (impairments)	Activity (limitations)	Participation (restrictions)
ICIDH model, WHO 1980[56]	Disease or pathology	Organ systems (impairments)	Disabilities	Handicaps
Nagi model, 1965[55]	Disease or pathology	Organ systems (impairments)	Functional limitations	Disabilities

ICF, International Classification of Functioning, Disability and Health; *ICIDH,* International Classification of Impairments, Disabilities, and Handicaps; *WHO,* World Health Organization.

*Placed in table form to show similarities in concepts across the models. Please note that the ICF is a nonlinear, progressive model of enablement and includes contextual factors (personal and environmental) that contribute to the well-being of the individual. Also refer to Chapter 8 for a more detailed discussion of the ICF model.

Conceptual Frameworks for Client/Provider Interactions

Three conceptual frameworks for client-provider interactions are commonly used in the current health care delivery system. Each framework serves a different purpose and is used according to the goals of the desired outcome and the group interpreting the results (Figure 1-2). The four primary conceptual frameworks include (1) the statistical model, (2) the medical diagnostic model, (3) the behavioral or enablement model, and (4) the philosophical or belief model.

Statistical Model

The statistical model framework considers some predetermined set of mathematical values as the main driver for patient/client management decisions. For example, in today's health care arena there is often a disconnect between the extent of a patient's clinical problems and the number of approved, predetermined treatment visits needed to remediate these problems. In this situation the clinician must make certain clinical decisions before deciding service and must determine how best to meet the needs of the patient given

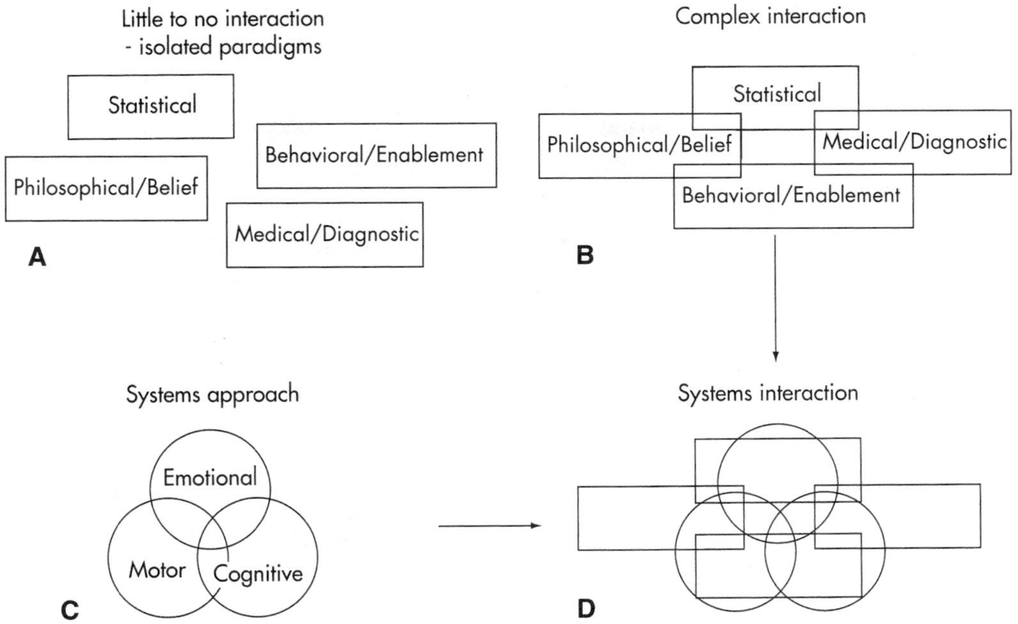

Figure 1-2 ■ Types of clinical models. **A,** Isolated paradigms. **B,** Complex interactive paradigms. **C,** Systems approach or paradigm. **D,** Systems interaction on traditional paradigms.

this limitation. Another illustration of this model involves the use of "numbers" or "grades" obtained from some outcome measure to make a determination on either the extent of functional limitation or the efficacy of a particular intervention. For example, if a patient scores 14 out of 24 points one week and 17 out of 24 points the next, and the payer knows that a score of 19 means the individual's risk of falling is reduced, then the payer often permits additional therapy visits. Those payers generally have little interest in the reasons why the client moved from a score of 14 to 17, only that the person is improving. If clinicians do not provide these types of quantitative measurements, payment for services often is denied. To be able to optimize care under this model, today's therapists need to be flexible critical thinkers who are able to skillfully document and communicate progress to individuals who need numbers, as well to provide this information to patients and their families, who are in emotional crisis because of problems associated with the neurological dysfunction, in a manner that they can understand.

Because efficacy of any intervention may be questioned by anyone, including the client, family, physician, third-party payer, or a lawyer, outcome tools that clearly measure problems in all domains must be carefully selected. Before an evaluation tool is chosen, the specific purpose for the request for examination and the model by which to interpret the meaning of the data must be identified.

Medical Diagnostic Model

Physicians are educated to use a medical disease or pathological condition diagnostic model for setting expectations of improvement or lack thereof. In patients with neurological dysfunction, physicians generally formulate their medical diagnosis on the basis of results from complex, highly technical examinations such as magnetic resonance imaging (MRI), functional magnetic resonance imaging (fMRI), computerized axial tomography (CAT or CT scan), positron emission tomography (PET scan), evoked potentials, and laboratory studies (see Chapter 37). When abnormal test results are correlated with gross clinical signs and patient history such as high blood pressure, diabetes, or head trauma, a medical diagnosis is made along with an anticipated course of recovery or disease progression. This medical diagnostic model is based on an anatomical and physiological belief of how the brain functions and may or may not correlate with the behavioral and enablement models used by therapists.

Behavioral or Enablement Model

The behavioral or enablement model evaluates motor performance on the basis of two types of measurement scales. One type of scale measures functional activities, which range from simple movement patterns such as rolling to complex patterns such as dressing, playing tennis, or using a word processor. These tools identify functional activities or aspects of life performance that the person has been or is able to do and serve as the "strengths" when remediating from activity limitations or participation restrictions. The second scale looks at bodily systems and subsystems and whether they are affecting functional movement. These measurement tools must look at specific components of various systems and measure impairments within those respective areas or bodily systems. For example, if the system to be assessed is biomechanical, a simple tool such as a goniometer that measures joint range of motion might be used, whereas a complex motion analysis tool might be used to look at interactions of all joints during a specific movement. These types of measurements specifically look at movement and can be analyzed from both an impairment and an ability perspective. Chapter 8 has been designed to help the reader clearly differentiate these two types of measurement tools and how they might be used in the diagnosis, prognosis, and selection of intervention strategies when analyzing movement.

Philosophical or Belief Model

A fourth model or framework for client-provider interaction that may still be found in clinical use is a philosophical or belief model such as those described by master clinicians from the past, including Rood, Knott, Bobath, and Ayers, or homeopathic models such as acupuncture or Chinese medicine. These philosophical models, when applied to functional outcomes, would be included with today's behavioral models and encompass a systems approach. The gap between philosophy and practice is narrowing as evidence is slowly showing that many of these approaches positively affect patient outcomes. Research has also identified approaches that have no efficacy. The link is outcome measures and whether a patient changes in participating in and has a quality of life. Thus the change is seen in the patient. Research today has created an alignment with what many therapists and master clinicians have long believed and practiced—focus on the patient, not the disease.

Therapists appreciate a statistical model through research and acceptance of evidence-based practice. A third-party payer also uses numbers to justify payment for services or to set limits on what will be paid and for specific number of visits that will be covered. Therapists also appreciate physicians' knowledge and perspective of disease and pathology because of the effect of disease and pathology on functional behavior and the ability to engage and participate in life. On the other hand, third-party payers and physicians may not be aware of the models used by OTs and PTs. It is therefore critical that therapists make the bridge to physicians and third-party payers because research has shown that interdisciplinary interactions help reduce conflict between professionals and provide better consistency for the patient.[57,58]

It is a medical shift in practice to recognize that patient participation plays a critical role in the delivery of health care. The importance of the patient and what each individual brings to the therapeutic environment has been recognized and incorporated into patient care by rehabilitation professionals.[37-40] This integration and acceptance will guide health care practice well into the next decade.

The need for students to develop problem-solving strategies is accepted by faculty across the country and by the respective accrediting agencies of health professionals. Unfortunately, we may not be educating students to the level of critical thinking that we hope.[59,60] The need for this cognitive skill development in clinicians may be emergent as both physical and occupational therapy professions have moved or plan to move to a doctoring professions.[49] All health-related professions must evolve as patient care demands increase, delineation of professional boundaries become less clear, and collaboration becomes a more integral factor in providing high-quality health care.

All previously presented models (statistical, medical, behavioral, or belief) can stand alone as acceptable models for health care delivery (see Figure 1-2, *A*) or can interact or interconnect (Figure 1-2, *B*). These interconnections should validate the accuracy of the data derived from each model. The concept of an integrated problem-solving model for neurological rehabilitation must also identify the functional components within the CNS (Figure 1-2, *C*).

A model that identifies the three general neurological systems (cognitive, emotional, motor) found within the human nervous system can be incorporated into each of the other models separately or when they are interconnected (Figure 1-2, *D*). A systems or behavioral model that focuses on the neurological systems is much more than just the motor systems and their components, or cognition with its multiple cortical facets, or the affective or emotion limbic system with all its aspects. The complexity of a neurological systems model (Figure 1-3), whether used for statistics, for medical diagnosis, for behavioral or functional diagnosis, or for documentation or billing, cannot be oversimplified. As the knowledge bank regarding central and peripheral system

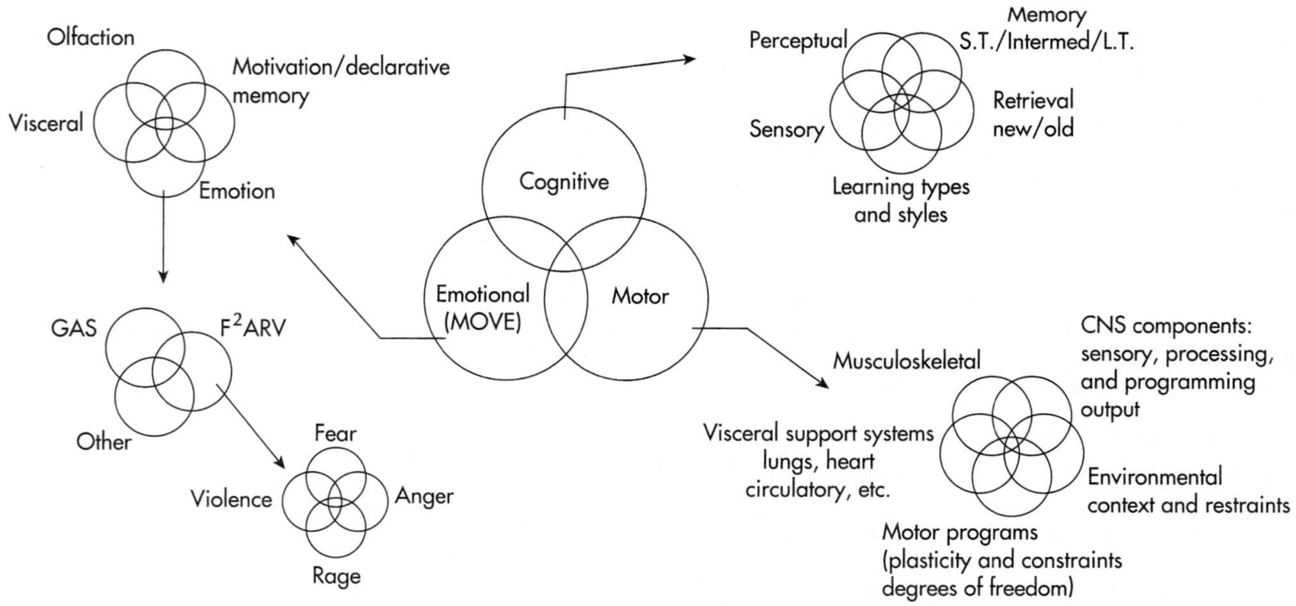

Figure 1-3 ■ Systems model. Dynamic interactive subcomponents: whole to part to whole. *F²ARV*, Fear and frustration, anger, rage, violence; *GAS*, general adaptation syndrome; *L.T.*, long term; *S.T.*, short term.

function increases, as well as knowledge about their interactions with other functions within and outside the body, the complexity of a systems model also enlarges.[61] The reader must remember that each component within the nervous system has many interlocking subcomponents and that each of those components may or may not affect movement. Therapists use these movement problems as guidelines to establish problem lists and intervention sequences. These components, considered impairments or reasons why someone has difficulty moving, are critical to therapists but are of little concern within a general statistics model and may have little bearing on the medical diagnosis made by the physician.

In addition to the Western health care delivery paradigms are the interlocking roles identified within an evolving transdisciplinary model (Figure 1-4). Within this model, the environments experienced by the client both within the Western health care delivery system and those environments external to that system are interlocking and forming additional system components; they influence one another and affect the ultimate outcome demonstrated by the client. Because all these once-separate worlds encroach on or overlay one another and ultimately affect the client, practitioners are now operating in a holistic environment and must become open to alternative ways of practice. Some of those alternatives will fit neatly and comfortably with Western medical philosophy and be seen as complementary. Evidence-based practice, which used linear research to establish its reliability and validity, has provided therapists with many effective tools both for assessment and treatment, but we still are unable to do similar analyses while simultaneously measuring multiple subsystem components. We can measure tools and interventions across multiple sites but are a long way from truly understanding the future of best practice. Other evaluation and treatment tools may sharply contrast with Western research practice, having too many variables or variables that cannot be measured; therefore arriving at evidence-based conclusions seems an insurmountable problem. In time many of these other assessment tools and intervention strategies may be accepted, once research methods have been developed to show evidence of efficacy, or they may be discarded for the same reason. Until these approaches have gone beyond belief in their effects, therapists will always need to expend additional focus measuring quantitative outcomes and analyzing accurately functional responses. Because the research is not available does not mean the approach has no efficacy (see Chapter 39). Thus the clinician needs to learn to be totally honest with outcomes, and quality of care and quality of life remain the primary objective for patient management. Today, models that incorporate health and wellness have been added to these disablement and enablement models to delineate the complexity of the problem-solving process used by therapists[62,63] (see Chapter 2). This delineation should reflect accurate behavioral diagnoses based on functional limitations and strengths, preexisting system strengths and accommodations, and environmental-social-ethnic variables unique to the client. Similarly, it includes the family, caregiver, financial security, or health care delivery support systems. All these variables guide the direction of intervention[64] (Figure 1-5). These variables will affect behavioral outcomes and need to be identified through the examination and evaluation process. Many of these variables may not relate to the CNS disease or pathological condition medical diagnosis to which the patient has been assigned.

The client brings to this environment life experiences. Many of these life events may have just been a life experience; others may have caused slight adjustments to behavior (e.g., running into a tree while skiing out of patrolled downhill ski areas and then never doing it again), some may have caused limitations (e.g., after running into the tree, the left knee needed a brace to support the instability of that knee during any strenuous exercising), or caused adjustments in motor behavior and emotional safety before that individual entered the heath care delivery system after CNS problems occurred. The accommodations or adjustments can dramatically affect both positively and negatively the course of intervention. To quickly accumulate this type of information regarding a client, the therapist must become open to the needs of the client and family. This openness is not just

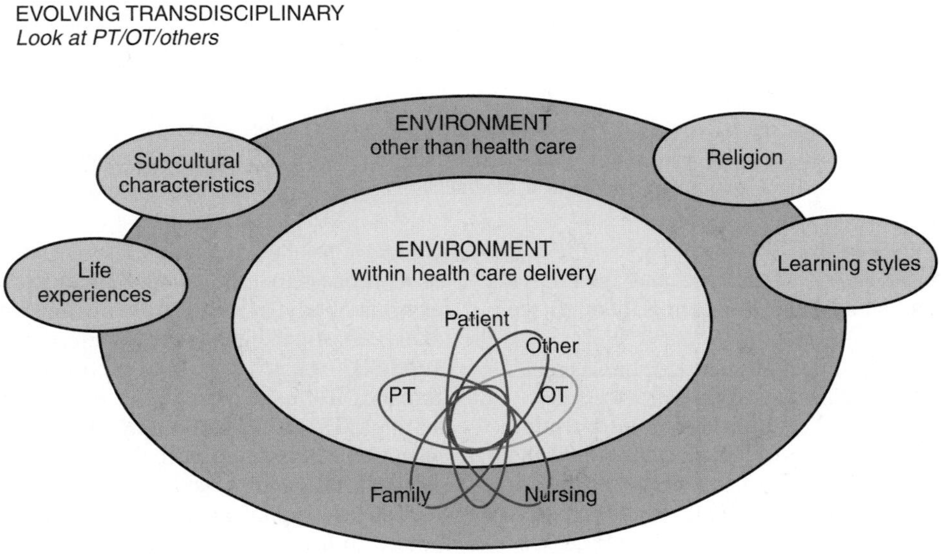

Figure 1-4 ■ Transdisciplinary model for delivery paradigms.

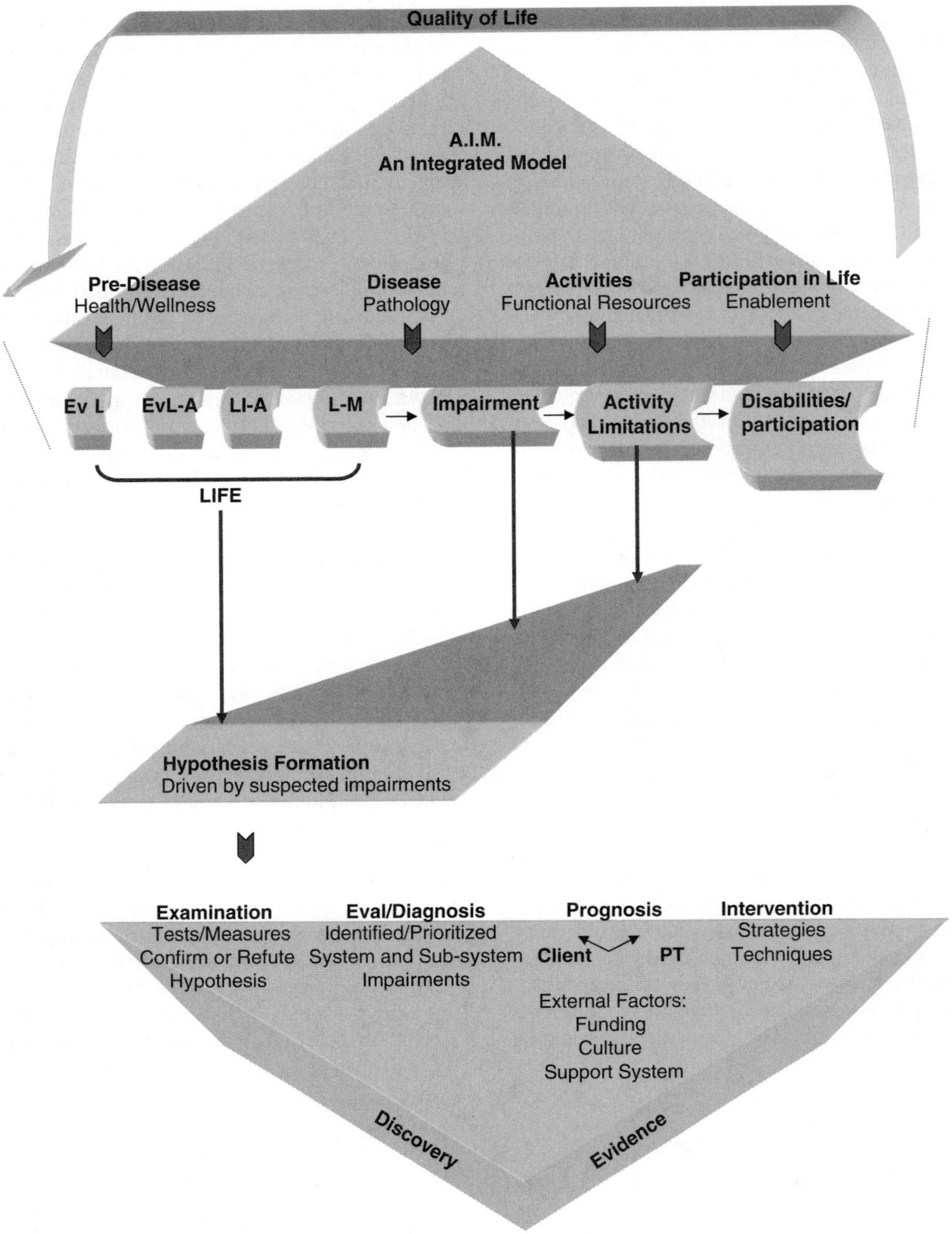

Figure 1-5 ■ Clinical problem-solving process incorporating life events, pathological condition, and postdisease state into a functional diagnosis. *Ev,* Event, disease; *I,* identifiable impairment; *L,* life; *L-A,* life with adaptation; *L-M,* life with modifications.

sensory, using eyes and ears, but holistic and includes a bond that needs to and should develop during therapy (see Chapters 5 and 6).

EFFICACY

Efficacy has been defined as the "ability of an intervention to produce the desired beneficial effect in expert hands and under ideal circumstances."[65] When any model of health care delivery is considered, the question the therapist must ask is "Which model will provide the most efficacious care?" Therapists may not diagnose a pathological disease or its process, but they are in a position of responsibility to examine body systems for existing impairments and to analyze normal movement to determine appropriate interventions for activity-based functional problems. Some differences in this responsibility may exist between practice settings. Therapists in private practice act independently to select both examination tools and intervention approaches that are efficacious and prove beneficial to the patient. Within a hospital-based system, therapists may be expected to use specific tools that are considered a standard of care for that facility, regardless of the therapy diagnosis and treatment rendered. In some hospitals and rehabilitation settings a clinical pathway may be employed that defines the roles and responsibilities of each person on a multidisciplinary team of medical professionals. Regardless of which clinical setting or role the therapist plays, it is always the responsibility of the therapist to be sure that the plan of care is appropriate, is consistent with the medical and therapy diagnoses, meets the needs of the patient, and renders successful outcomes. If the needs of the particular client do not match the progression of the pathway, it is the therapist's responsibility to recommend a change in the client's plan of care. Efficacy does not come because one is *taught* that an examination tool or intervention procedure is efficacious, it comes from the judicious use of tools to establish impairments, activity limitations, and participation restrictions, identify movement diagnoses, create functional improvements, and improve quality of life in those individuals who have come to us for therapy.

Today's health care climate demands that the therapeutic care model be efficient, be cost-effective, and result in measurable outcomes.[66] The message being given today might be considered to reflect the idea that "the end justifies the means." This premise has come to fruition through the linear thought process of established scientific research. Yet when a holistic model is accepted into practice it becomes apparent that outcome tools are not yet available to simultaneously measure the interactions of all body systems that make up the patient, making it difficult to apply models that purport to balance quality and cost of care. Thus we must guard against the reductionist research of today, which has the potential to restrain our evolution and choice of therapeutic interventions. Sometimes the individuals making decisions about what to include and what to eliminate with regard to patient services are not health care providers. They are individuals who are trained to use evidence gained from numbers or statistics to make their decision and do not have knowledge of the patient, his or her situation, or the effect of the neurological condition on function. Therapists should always be able to defend their choice and use of intervention approaches. This becomes even more relevant as the cost of health care rises.

Evidence-based practice is basic to the care process.[30,67,68] Clinicians need to identify which of their therapeutic interventions have demonstrated positive outcomes for particular clinical problems or patient populations and which have not.[69] Those that remain in question may still be judged as useful. The basis for that judgment may be a client satisfaction variable that has become a critical variable for many areas in health care delivery.[70,71] But there is still limited information on patient satisfaction with PT and OT services, although within the last few years more information has become available.[72-76] Although patient satisfaction is a critical variable within the ICF model, there are always problems with satisfaction and outcomes versus identification of specific measurable variables within the CNS that are affecting outcomes. One reason for the problem of integrating patient satisfaction with PT and OT services within a neurorehabilitation environment is the large discrepancy between the variables we can measure and the variables within the environment that are affecting performance. For example, when a neurosurgeon once asked the question to one of the editors, "Do you know how to prove the theories of intervention you are teaching?" The answer was, "Yes, all I need are two dynamic PET units that can be worn on both the client's and the therapist's heads while performing therapeutic interventions. I also need a computer that will simultaneously correlate all synaptic interactions between the therapist and the client to prove the therapeutic effect." The physician said, "We don't have those tools!" The response was, "You did not ask me if the research tools were available, only if I know how to obtain an efficacious result." Thus, the creativity of the therapist will always bring the professions to new visions of reality. That reality, when proven to be efficacious, assists in validating the accepted interventions used by the professional. The therapist today has a responsibility to provide evidence-based practice to the scientific community...but more important, also to the client. Therapeutic discovery usually precedes validation through scientific research. This discovery leads the way to, first, effective interventions, followed by efficacious care. If research and efficacious care always have to come before the application of therapeutic procedures, nothing new will evolve because discovery of care is most often, if not always, found in the clinic during interaction with a client. Thus the range of therapeutic applications will become severely limited and the evolution of neurological care stopped if that discovery is ignored because there is no efficacy as defined by today's research models. However, performing interventions because the approaches "have been typically done in the past" could be wasteful and irresponsible.

DIAGNOSIS: A PROCESS USED BY ALL PROFESSIONALS WHEN DRAWING CONCLUSIONS

Diagnosis is a conclusion drawn regarding specific diseases and pathological processes within the human body; when made by a physician it is considered a medical diagnosis. Diagnosis made by a PT or an OT is a conclusion drawn regarding the status of body systems, activity and participation, and their interactions considering the patient's personal factors and the environment. Specific activity-based functional limitations and the impairments within the body systems that affect the client's ability to control quiet postures or dynamic movement in any activity become a focus in the diagnostic process. The functional loss itself may or may not reflect specific diseases or pathological conditions within the CNS but does reflect specific impairments within that client's body. PTs and OTs, by use of functional behavioral models, are becoming comfortable with the *diagnosis of body system problems (impairments), activity restrictions (functional limitations), and participation* and the conceptual understanding that the diagnosis made by a PT or an OT is very different from that made by a physician.

Once the interpretation has been made, a therapist must draw conclusions regarding those results and their interactions. That interpretation leads to a therapy diagnosis. The interpretation of the evaluation results and their interaction with therapist's and client's desired outcomes, available resources, and client's potential lead to the prognosis. Selection of the best and most efficient resources to achieve the desired outcome will lead to establishment of the treatment intervention plan or "road map."

The diagnostic process used by therapists is complex and is clearly divided into two specific phases of differential diagnosis (Figure 1-6). This is further explained in Chapters 7 and 8.

Phase 1: Differential Diagnosis: System Screening for Possible Disease or Pathology

With the increasing use of direct access and the length of time therapists spend with clients, clinicians have become acutely aware of the need to screen systems for signs of disease and pathological conditions.[51] Accreditation standards for both PTs and OTs require the new learner to develop these skills before graduation. This screening process is used to determine whether the client should be referred to another practitioner, such as a physician, or can progress to diagnosis, prognosis, and intervention within the specific discipline. Thus Phase 1 of this differential diagnosis separates a client's clinical problems into those that fall within a therapist's scope of practice and those that do not. If the Phase 1 differential diagnosis shows signs and symptoms totally outside a therapist's scope of practice, then a referral to an appropriate practitioner must be made. If the signs and symptoms both fall within the clinician's scope of practice and overlap with that of other disciplines, the therapist must refer and decide (1) to treat to prevent problems until the other practitioner's treatment can be performed, (2) to manage the limitations in activity and participation in spite of the pathological process, or (3) to manage functional loss and impairments and therefore correct the pathological cause. In some cases the overlapping with other disciplines may not necessitate an immediate referral, but interactions must be made when needed to ensure the best outcome from intervention. However, when the information obtained by the therapist from this phase of differential diagnosis indicates a possible immediate and life-threatening condition, the therapist must act accordingly by calling 911 and referring the patient to a medical physician. Chapter 7 has been designed to help the reader grasp a better understanding of Phase 1 of differential diagnosis. This form of system screening is part of history taking and may be redone periodically throughout treatment if the therapist has questions regarding changes in body systems. In the *Guide to Physical Therapist Practice*[30] this step is called *systems review* and *review of systems.* There may be times when the therapist has received a referral for a chronic problem and during the medical screen the patient demonstrates signs of a potential medical condition that has nothing to do with the referral. In that situation the therapist may continue with treatment but also should refer the patient back to a physician for a more thorough evaluation of the new problem.

For example, a patient was referred to a PT for treatment of chronic back pain caused by degenerative disc disease. During performance of a system screening the therapist determined that the patient had generalized weakness on the left side. On a return visit 2 days later the patient continued to demonstrate mild weakness on the left side. The therapist referred the patient back to the doctor, and the subsequent MRI showed that the woman had a large tumor in the right lower frontal-temporal lobe area. Over subsequent treatments the therapist was able to eliminate most of the chronic pain in her back. The patient to this day feels the therapist saved her life.[77]

Once a clinician determines that the client's need for service falls within his or her respective scope of practice, then Phase 2 differential diagnosis begins.

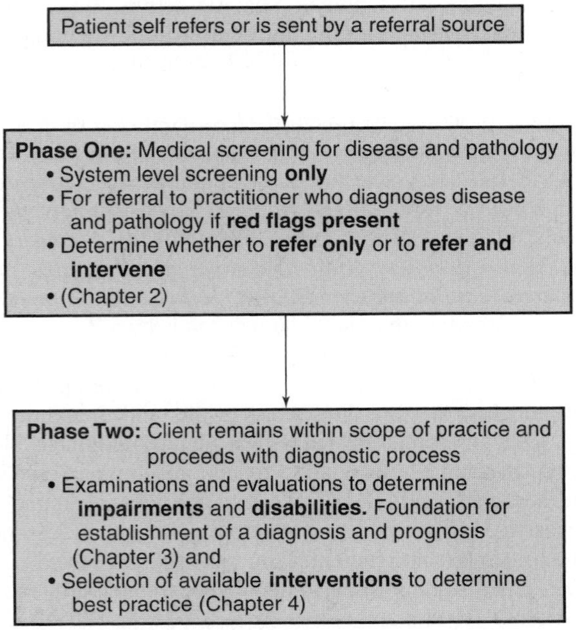

Figure 1-6 ■ The diagnostic process used for best practice by physical and occupational therapists.

Phase 2: Differential Diagnosis within a Therapist's Scope of Practice

Once the client's signs and symptoms have been determined to fall clearly within the scope of PT and OT practice, a definitive therapy diagnosis, prognosis, and plan of care can be established. The use of an enablement model such as the ICF will help the therapist best capture the patient's strengths, impairments, activity limitations, and participation restrictions, which can then be used to determine the patients goals, address the individual's needs, and optimize function and quality of life (see Figure 1-1). The client's functional goals and expectations may include activities of daily living, job skills, recreation and leisure activities, or the skills required for performance of typical societal roles. Each of these goals must have a realistic, objective, measurable outcome that is based on the results of carefully chosen examination tools. An in-depth conceptual framework for selection of appropriate examination procedures needed to evaluate and draw appropriate diagnostic conclusions can be found in Chapter 8.

Two important clinical components affect the accuracy of the diagnostic conclusion. First, the clinician must establish accurate, nonbiased results. This fact seems obvious, but with the pressures of third-party payers, family members, other care providers, and the desire to have the client improve, it is easy to submit to drawing a conclusion based on *desired* outcomes rather than facing what is truly present and realistic. The second factor deals with the honesty of the interaction between the therapist and the client. This "bonding" is critical for obtaining accurate examination results. Safety, trust, and acceptance of the client as a human being play key roles in therapeutic outcomes and thus in efficacy of practice.[78-81] The reader is referred to Chapters 5 and 6 to develop a greater understanding of the impact this bonding has on clinical outcomes.

The specific cognitive process used by therapists before formulation of a therapy diagnosis might be conceptualized as a nine-step process. As the therapist enters into the clinical environment of the client, he or she starts collecting data that might be relevant to the analysis of the clinical problem (step 1). This includes information obtained through observation, history taking, chart review, and interviews. The therapist must take that array of divergent information and determine what data are relevant to the case while disregarding what may be irrelevant information (step 2). This body of knowledge is then differentiated into various body systems that might be affected by the identified problems. If a specific system does not seem to be affected, then it can be eliminated, at least temporarily, from the diagnostic process (step 3). Generally, a clinician performs activity-based testing at this time to obtain a general understanding of the strengths and limitations of the individual in terms of function (step 4). After performing examination procedures and observing patterns of movement and specific normal and abnormal responses, the therapist once again diverges his or her thought processes back to separate large body systems to classify problems in the appropriate system (step 5). The therapist further subdivides these large systems into their components to assess specific subsystem deficits and strengths (step 6). This will allow the therapist to categorize objective measurements of impairments that are recognized as deficits within subsystems. Clusters of specific signs and symptoms will emerge that will help direct the clinicians to a therapy diagnosis. Once the therapist has obtained these clusters of symptoms within specific subsystems, two additional convergent steps need to be completed. First, the presence and lack of impairments and how those impairments interact to cause dysfunction in a major body system are determined (step 7). Second, how those impairments affect the interaction of the major system with other major body systems is determined (step 8). These eight steps tell the therapist exactly why the client has difficulty performing specific functional activities. The problem list that incorporates the severity of impairments that have interacted to cause loss of function gives the clinician the therapy diagnosis. The number and extent of impairments along with an understanding of the cause of loss of function will lead the therapist to establishment of various prognoses and identification of optimal intervention strategies. The last step (step 9) requires the therapist to diverge his or her thought processes back to the client's total environment to determine the accuracy of the diagnosis, prognosis, and selected treatment interventions as they interact with the client as a whole. Although some completion of this diagnostic process may occur within minutes after a client and therapist begin their interactions, the process is continual, and at any time a therapist may need to go back to previous steps to obtain and analyze new and relevant information.

PROGNOSIS: HOW LONG WILL IT TAKE TO GET FROM POINT A TO POINT B?

If a client has a variety of impairments, activity limitations, and participation restrictions, then a variety of appropriate prognoses may be formulated. These prognoses could be used to speculate the amount of time or number of treatments it will take to get from the existing activity limitations and participation restrictions (point A) to the desired outcomes (point B). The outcomes will state whether the intervention will (1) eliminate functional limitations through changes, adaptations, and learning within the client as an organism or (2) improve function through compensation and modification of the external environment. Once the therapy diagnosis has been established, a clinician must consider many factors when making a prognosis. Some factors are related to the internal environment of the client, such as number and extent of impairments, level of physical conditioning or deconditioning of the client, the ability and motivation to learn, participate, and change, and the neurological disease or condition that led to the existing problems. The client's support systems have a dramatic impact on prognosis. Cultural and ethnic pressures, financial support to promote independence, availability of appropriate skilled professional services, prescribed medications, and the interaction of all of these factors need to be considered. Specific environmental factors such as belief in health care and agreement about who has the responsibility for healing can create tremendous conflict among current health care delivery systems; the client; the family; and you, the clinician.[79,82,83] All of these variables affect prognosis. The last aspect of determining prognosis relates to empowerment of the client. Who sets the goals? Who determines function? Who identifies when a therapeutic modality should be used versus a meaningful life activity? If consensus to these questions cannot be found by the therapist and the client, then conflict between anticipated and actual outcome will result and a definitive prognosis will not be achieved.

Once a prognosis has been established, the therapist's next step is to identify the intervention strategies that will guide the client to the desired outcome within the time frame identified. (Refer to Chapter 9 and all chapters in Section II.)

DOCUMENTATION

Documentation of the examination, evaluation, goals, plan, and daily interventions has always been integral to the therapeutic process. However, there is added emphasis in today's health care environment, as well as a renewed respect for the importance of the issue. Documentation must produce a clear framework from which to record and follow client progress. Documentation communicates the process of care and the product or outcome of that process. The outcome is the realistic reflection of the effectiveness of care. The goals should be stated in measurable functional terms and prioritized in order of importance to the client. The number of goals developed by the therapist takes into account the realistic probability of effectiveness of interventions, the environment in which the interventions will likely occur, and support systems available to the client. As the process goes forward, the therapist may add, delete, or change a functional goal, and so states that on the client's record. Refer to Chapter 10 for further information about this process.

INTERVENTION

Clients with neurological diseases or conditions can interact with the medical community for either short or long periods. They possess neurological problems of all types that range from sudden to insidious in onset and presentation. All aspects of human function are represented in the variety of problems. If individual beliefs and values energize and motivate physical behavior, think of the possibilities for stimulating wellness. Return to wellness might be considered return to previous function, maintenance of function, slowing progression of functional loss, habilitation of function never achieved, and striving for excellence in performance. Refer to Chapter 9 for additional discussion.

The established plan of care determines the interventions and the method, or road map, toward the achievement of the agreed-on outcome goals. The therapist, in collaboration with the client, can choose from restrictive and nonrestrictive treatment environments and interventions to best achieve identified goals. The available choices of interventions will depend on the therapist's skill, the level of function and ability of the client to control his or her own neuromuscular system, and treatment tools and strategies that are available in the clinic. Yet freedom within that established environment must exist if learning by the client is to occur. Another way to consider intervention is to refer to it as a clinical road map (Figure 1-7). Within the map, a therapist, through professional education, efficacy of preexisting clinical pathways, and clinical experience can generally identify the most expedient way to guide a client toward the desired outcome. When the specific client enters into this interaction, slight variations off the existing pathway may lead to quicker outcomes. If the client diverges away from the desired end product, it is the therapist's responsibility to guide that individual back into the clinical map. For example, if a therapist and client are working on coming to standing patterns and the client begins to fall, the therapist would need to guide the client back into the desired movement patterns and not allow the fall. In that way the client is working on the identified outcome. Falling as a functional activity should be taught as a different intervention and would be considered part of a different clinical map. The degree to which the therapist needs to control the response of the client will determine the extent to which the intervention would be considered contrived. Contrived interventions can, in time, lead to functional independence of the client, but as long as the therapist needs to control the environment, functional independence has not been achieved. There are many ways to get to a desired outcome. Involving the client in the goal setting and intervention planning process will lead to the best result These interactions require trust of the therapist as a guide and teacher. Refer to Chapter 9 and all chapters in Section II for a more thorough discussion of intervention strategies.

Most treatment interventions used for clients with CNS pathology incorporate principles of neuroplasticity, adaptation, motor control, and motor learning in various environmental contexts. Thus, the consideration of the basic science of central and peripheral nervous system function (see Chapter 4) and a behavioral analysis of movement (see Chapter 3) must be included in any conceptual model used as a foundation for the entire diagnostic process.

Also of considerable significance is the client-therapist interaction, which is labeled the *learning environment.* This may be the critical factor in the success or failure of therapeutic interventions. The concept of human movement as a range of observable behaviors, the complexity of the CNS as a control center, and the interactions between the client and therapist within closed and open learning environments form an abstract conceptual triad. Each part of this triad has unique characteristics that have the ability to influence performance and progress in the clinical setting. Together they allow for the client to be viewed as a total human being, allowing the therapist to consider multiple constructs at once so that a client's responses and movement patterns may all be considered and developed simultaneously. In this way, key signs such as movement in body parts distant to the area being treated, pain, or a response of the autonomic nervous system will not be missed. Attention to these responses

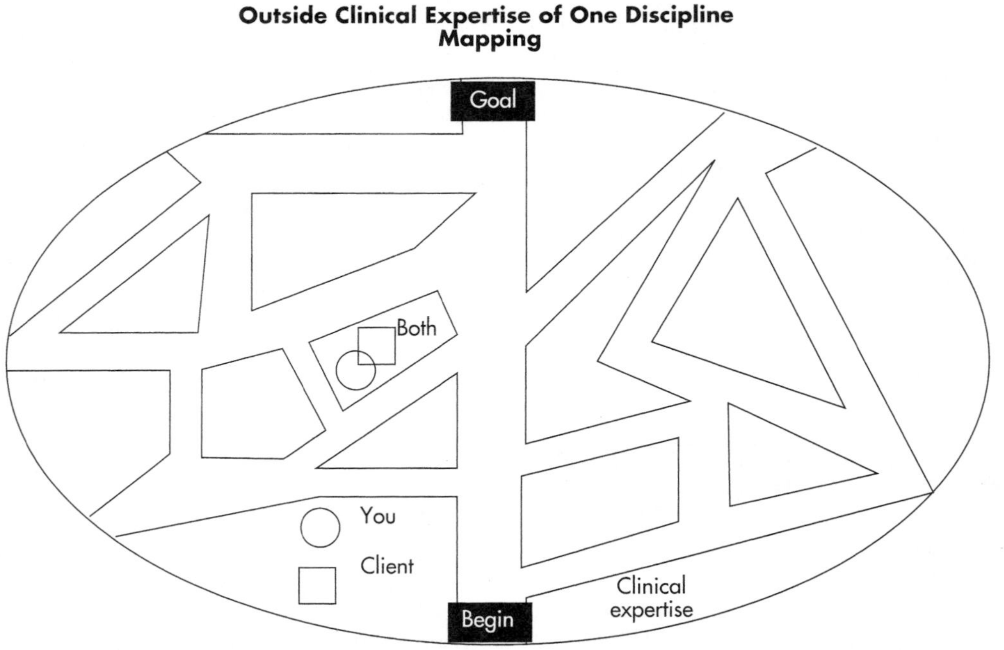

Figure 1-7 ■ Concept of clinical mapping.

may be the answer to attaining goals and successful client-therapist rapport.

Concept of Human Movement as a Range of Observable Behaviors

As researchers continue to unravel the mysteries of brain function and learning, their understanding of how children and adults initially learn or relearn after neurological insult is often explained with new and possibly conflicting theories. Yet behavioral responses observed as functional patterns of movement, whether performed by a child, adolescent, young adult, or older person, are still visually identified by a therapist, family member, or innocent observer as either normal or abnormal.

Human beings exhibit certain movement patterns that may vary in tonal characteristics, amplitude, aspects of the specific movement sequences, and even the sequential nature of development. Yet the range of acceptable behavior does have limitations, and variations beyond those boundaries are recognizable by most people. A 5-year-old child may ask why a little girl walks on her toes with her legs stuck together. If questioned, that same 5-year-old child may have the ability to break down the specific aspects of the movement that seem unacceptable even to that 5-year-old child. From birth a sighted individual observes normal human movement. Because the range of behaviors identified as normal within any functional activity does not vary from individual to individual, human movement patterns are predictable. This concept does provide flexibility in analysis of normal movement and its development. Some children choose creeping as a primary mode of horizontal movement, whereas others may scoot. Both forms of movement are normal for a young child. In both cases each child would have had to develop normal postural function in the head and trunk to carry out the activity in a normal fashion. Thus for the child to develop the specific functional motor behavior, the various components or systems involved in the integrated execution of the act would require modulation in a plan of action. Because the action must be carried out in a variety of environmental contexts, the child would need the opportunity to practice in those contexts, identify errors, self-correct to regulate existing plans, and refine for skill development. Thus each movement has a variety of complex systems interactions, which when summated are expressed by means of the motor neuron pool to striated muscle tissue function. The specifics of that function, whether fine or gross motor control, or full-body or limb-specific movement, still reflect the totality of the interaction of those systems. No matter the age of the individual, the motor response still reflects that interaction, and the behavior can be identified as normal and functional, functional but limited in adaptability, or dysfunctional and abnormal. Because of the simplicity or complexity of various movements and the components necessary to modulate control over various movements, therapists can (1) look at any movement pattern, (2) evaluate its components, (3) identify what is missing, and (4) incorporate treatment strategies that help the client reduce impairments and achieve the desired functional outcome.

One can be confident that no infant will be born, jump out of the womb, walk over to the physician, and shake hands or say "hi" to mom and dad before learning to roll or control posture of the trunk and head. Instead, normal motor development requires new motor plans that lead to the infant's ability to achieve functional movement through motor learning. These new motor programs will be modified and reintegrated along with other programs to develop normal motor control in more complex patterns and environments because of neuroplasticity. Each pattern, and the advancement from one pattern to another, requires time and repetition for mastery.

Two important aspects of the clinical problem-solving process emerge when observing motor behavior. First, the evaluation of motor function is based on the interaction of all components of the motor system and the cognitive and affective influences over this motor system, as stated previously. Second, the therapist needs to recognize which aspects of the movement are deficient, absent, distorted, or inappropriate when cross-referenced with the desired outcome (part of the diagnosis-prognosis process). These behaviors, although dependent on many factors, are consistent regardless of age of the client. Some clients may not have had the opportunity to experience the desired skill, whereas others may have lost the skill as a result of changes within the CNS or disuse. In either case, the normal accepted patterns and range of behaviors remain the same. Refer to Chapter 3 for an additional discussion of movement analysis across the life span.

The Complexity of the Central Nervous System as a Control Center

The concept of the CNS as a control center is based on a therapist's observations and understanding of the sensory-motor performance patterns reflective of that system. This understanding requires an in-depth background in neuroanatomy, neurophysiology, motor control, motor learning, and neuroplasticity and gives the therapist the basis for clinical application and treatment. Understanding the intricacies and complex relationships of these neuromechanisms provides therapists with direction as to when, why, and in what order to use clinical treatment techniques. Motor behaviors emerge based on maturation, potential, and degeneration of the CNS. Each behavior observed, sequenced, and integrated as a treatment protocol should be interpreted according to neurophysiological and neuroanatomical principles as well as the principles of learning and neuroplasticity. As science moves toward a greater understanding of the neuromechanisms by which behaviors occur, therapists will be in a better position to establish efficacy of intervention. Unfortunately, our knowledge of behavior is ahead of our understanding of the intricate mechanisms of the CNS that create it. Thus the future will continue to expand the reliability and validity of therapeutic interventions designed to modify functional movement patterns. First, therapists need to determine what interventions are effective within a clinical environment. Then the efficacy of specific treatment variables can be studied and more clearly identified. The rationale for the use of certain treatment techniques will likely change over time. As our knowledge of the CNS continues to evolve, so will the validation of techniques and approaches used in therapeutic environments. At that point, evidence-based practice will truly be a reality. Chapters 4 and 5 have additional information and references on CNS function. Chapter 9 has an in-depth discussion of intervention options.

Concept of the Learning Environment

The concept of the learning environment is the most abstract and complex of the three concepts in the clinical triad model. For that reason it is by far the most difficult to present in concrete terms. Components of the therapist, the patient, and the clinical environment formulate and maintain this environment.

To comprehend the dynamics of the learning environment and function with optimal success, the clinician must do the following:

- Understand the learning process and provide an environment that promotes learning.
- Investigate the use of sensory input and motor output systems, feed-forward and feedback mechanisms, and cognitive processing as means for higher-order learning.
- Use the principles and theories of motor control, motor learning, and neuroplasticity to facilitate learning and carryover of treatment into real-life environments.
- Obtain knowledge of both the client's and the provider's learning styles. If these learning styles are not compatible, then the clinician is obligated to teach using the client's preferred style.
- Attend to the sensory-motor, cognitive, and affective aspects of each client, regardless of the clinical emphasis at any given time.

At all times there are four distinct components of the learning environment in operation: the internal and external environments of the client, and the internal and external environments of the clinician (Figure 1-8). All four represent interactive components of the learning environment.

The Client

A critical component of the ability to learn is the *client's internal environment.* When a lesion occurs within a body system it affects the entire internal environment of the client both directly and indirectly. If the lesion occurs before initial learning, then habilitation must take place. These clients may possess a genetic predisposition for a specific learning style, even though one has not yet been established. The therapist should test the inexperienced CNS by creating experiences in various contexts that require a variety of types of higher-order processing to discover optimal methods of learning that best suit the CNS of the client. Then the therapist can employ the most effective strategies in treatment. If previous learning has occurred and preferential modes of operating have been established, then the therapist needs to know what those are and whether they have been affected by the neurological insult so that proper rehabilitation can be instituted.[84] The use of preferential sensory input modes such as visual compared with verbal or kinesthetic does not mean that other modes are ineffective, nor do all modes function optimally in any given situation.

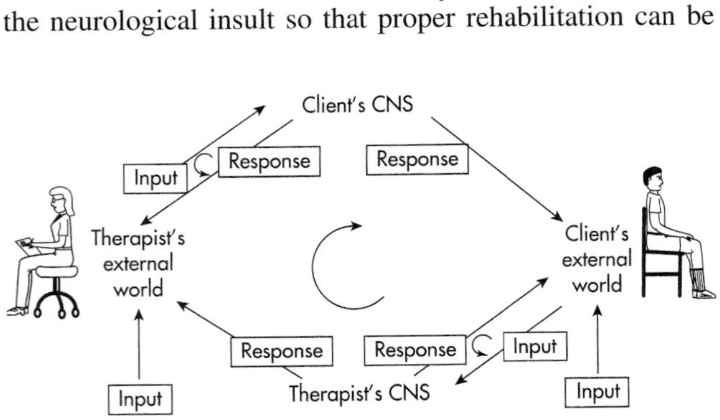

Figure 1-8 ■ Clinical learning environment.

One way to determine preferential learning styles is by taking a thorough history. Leisure activities and job choices often give clues to learning styles. For example, a client who loved to take car engines apart or build model ships demonstrates a preference for the visual-kinesthetic learning style, whereas a client whose preference for pure enjoyment was sitting in a chair with a novel demonstrates a probable preference toward verbal learning. Again, this does not mean that the clients in the examples mentioned could not selectively use all methods, but it does illustrate the issue of preference. Both the position of the lesion and the preferential learning style can play key roles in matching the learner with a particular treatment environment and identifying potential for recovery of function. For example, if a client has had a massive insult to the left temporal lobe and before the trauma showed poor ability in using the right parieto-occipital lobe, then spatial or verbal strategies may be ineffective in the relearning process. However, a client with the same lesion who had high-level right parieto-occipital function before the insult will probably learn at a much faster rate if visual-kinesthetic strategies are used to promote learning.

The *client's external environment* is the second critical component.[85] All external stimuli, including noise, lighting, temperature, touch, humidity, and smell, modulate the client's responses. External inputs can invoke either negative or positive influences on internal mechanisms and alter the client's ability to manipulate the world. A therapist should make every effort to be aware of what externally is influencing the client.[86-89] It is important to know what is happening to the client both within and outside of the hospital or clinic experience. Any behavioral change displayed by the client, such as a change in mood or attitude, or a change in muscle tone could serve as an indicator to the therapist that an environmental effect may have occurred. A follow-up determination of what may have happened can help the therapist understand the situation, help the client deal with the environmental influences, and allow the therapist to obtain additional professional assistance if needed.

The third critical component is the *internal environment of the clinician.*[90] The clinician should be aware of personal internal factors that can influence patient responses. Everyone has preferential styles of teaching and learning; yet many of us may be unaware of what they are and how they affect our outlook on life and interactions with other people. A common example of a mismatch of styles is what happens when two people are arguing opposing sides of a political issue. Although both individuals may process the same data, they may have different learning strategies and come up with very different conclusions.

The interplay of learning styles occurs continually in an academic setting. A student who is asked the question "What do you want out of this course?" would probably say, "A good grade." Getting a good grade requires doing well on course requirements, including tests. High-grade test performance usually depends on not only a knowledgeable demonstration of a subject but also the way in which the teacher formulates the question and the teacher's expectation for a response. In a clinical setting, it is important that the clinician be aware of the client's response to the practitioner's request.

This external-internal environmental interaction concept brings up another important clinical consideration.[91] As students, most of us probably "clashed" with one or two teachers with whose learning styles we could never identify. As learners we cannot or will not adapt to all learning styles. For that reason there may be some clients who do not respond to our teaching. When that seems evident, a shift of therapists is appropriate for the rehabilitation process to succeed.

The fourth component of the learning environment is the *clinician's external environment.* It is generally expected that personal life should never affect professional work. To accept this assumption, however, may be to deny that emotions affect behavioral patterns (see Chapters 5 and 6). Response patterns can vary without cognitive awareness when an individual is emotionally upset or under stress. For example, suppose that Mr. Smith, who has a hypertonic condition because of a stroke, comes down early for therapy each morning, has a cup of coffee, and chats while you write notes. If one day you are under extreme stress and do not feel like interacting as Mr. Smith rolls his wheelchair into your office, you might say, "Mr. Smith, I'll be with you in a few minutes. Go over to the mat, lock your brakes, pick up the pedals, and we'll transfer when I get there." Mr. Smith will quickly sense a change in your behavior. Society has taught him that you are a professional and that your personal life does not affect your job. Thus he may draw a logical conclusion that he must have done something to change your behavior. When you go to transfer him you notice he is more hypertonic than usual and ask, "Is something bothering you? You're tighter than usual," and so goes the interaction. Your external environment altered your internal state and, thus, normal response patterns. In turn, you altered Mr. Smith's external environment, changing his internal balance, and created a change of emotional tone that resulted in increased hypertonicity.[92,93] If instead of interacting with Mr. Smith as if nothing were wrong, you had informed him you were upset over something unrelated to him, you might have avoided creating a negative environment. Mr. Smith's responses may have been different if you had shared with him the fact that there are days that you are upset and have mood changes. As he accepts your changes as normal, you may have created an opportunity for him to also exhibit a range of behavioral moods. You have also given him an opportunity to offer his assistance to comfort or help you if he so desires. Such behavior encourages interdependence and social interaction and facilitates long-term goals for all rehabilitation clients.

Each client is unique. Therefore it is difficult to analyze the specifics related to each individual's learning environment. However, six basic learning principles have been established that are relevant to both the client and the clinician in any learning environment.[94-96] These *six principles of the learning experience* are as follows:

1. Individuals need to be able to solve problems and practice those solutions as motor programs if independence in daily living is desired. This requires the use of intrinsic feedback systems to modulate feed-forward motor plans as well as correct existing plans.
2. The possibility of success must exist in all functional tasks, regardless of the level of challenge to the client.
3. An individual will revert to safer or more familiar motor programs or ways to solve problems and succeed at functional tasks when task demands are new, difficult, or unfamiliar.
4. The learning effect occurs in multiple areas of the CNS simultaneously when teaching and learning are focused within one area of the CNS.
5. Motivation is necessary to drive the individual to try to experience what would be considered unknown. Simultaneously, success at the activity is critical to keep the individual motivated to continue to practice.
6. Clinicians need to be able to analyze an activity as a whole, determine its component parts, and use problem-solving strategies to design effective individualized treatment programs. At the same time, if independence in living skills is an objective, the therapist needs to teach the client those problem-solving strategies rather than teaching the solution to the problem.

Although all six learning principles seem simple, their application within the clinical setting is not always as obvious. *Principles 1 and 2* are intricately linked with the appropriateness and difficulty of tasks presented to clients. If a client is asked to perform a task such as standing, rolling, relaxing, dressing, or maneuvering a wheelchair, a problem has been presented that requires a sequence of acts leading to a solution. To succeed, the client must be able to plan the entire task and modulate all motor control during the sequence of the entire activity. If steps are not mastered, if sequencing is inappropriate or absent, or if motor control systems are not modulated accurately, dependence on the clinician to solve the problem is reinforced. If the clinician can differentiate missing components (impairments) from functioning systems, creating an environment that encourages and allows the CNS to adapt and learn ways to regain that control, it will lead to optimal self-empowerment of the client and will help eliminate disabilities. Error in the ability to intrinsically self-correct during practice is critical for motor learning. Error that always leads to failure does not help the client learn avenues of adaptation. Linked intricately with success is the challenge of the task. The greater the task difficulty or complexity, the greater the challenge and consequently the greater the satisfaction of success.

There is a subtle interplay among degree of difficulty, challenge, and success. Selecting tasks that are age appropriate, clinically relevant, and goal related is a challenge to the therapist. For the patient to be successful, the therapist must be a creative problem solver and knowledgeable about the client's needs, abilities, and goals. If the tasks are too simple or if the client considers them unimportant, boredom will ensue and progress may diminish. If the tasks are too difficult, the client may feel defeated and may turn away from them. In such cases a child tends to withdraw physically, whereas an adult usually avoids the problem. Being late to therapy, having to leave early, needing to go to the bathroom, and scheduling conflicting sessions are all avoidance behaviors that may be linked to inappropriate tasks.

The *third learning principle* describes a behavior inherent in all people: reversal. When confronted by a problem, individuals revert to patterns that produce feelings of comfort and competence when solving the problem. In Figure 1-9, a 2-year-old child is confronted with just such a conflict. The bridge he wants to cross is unstable. The

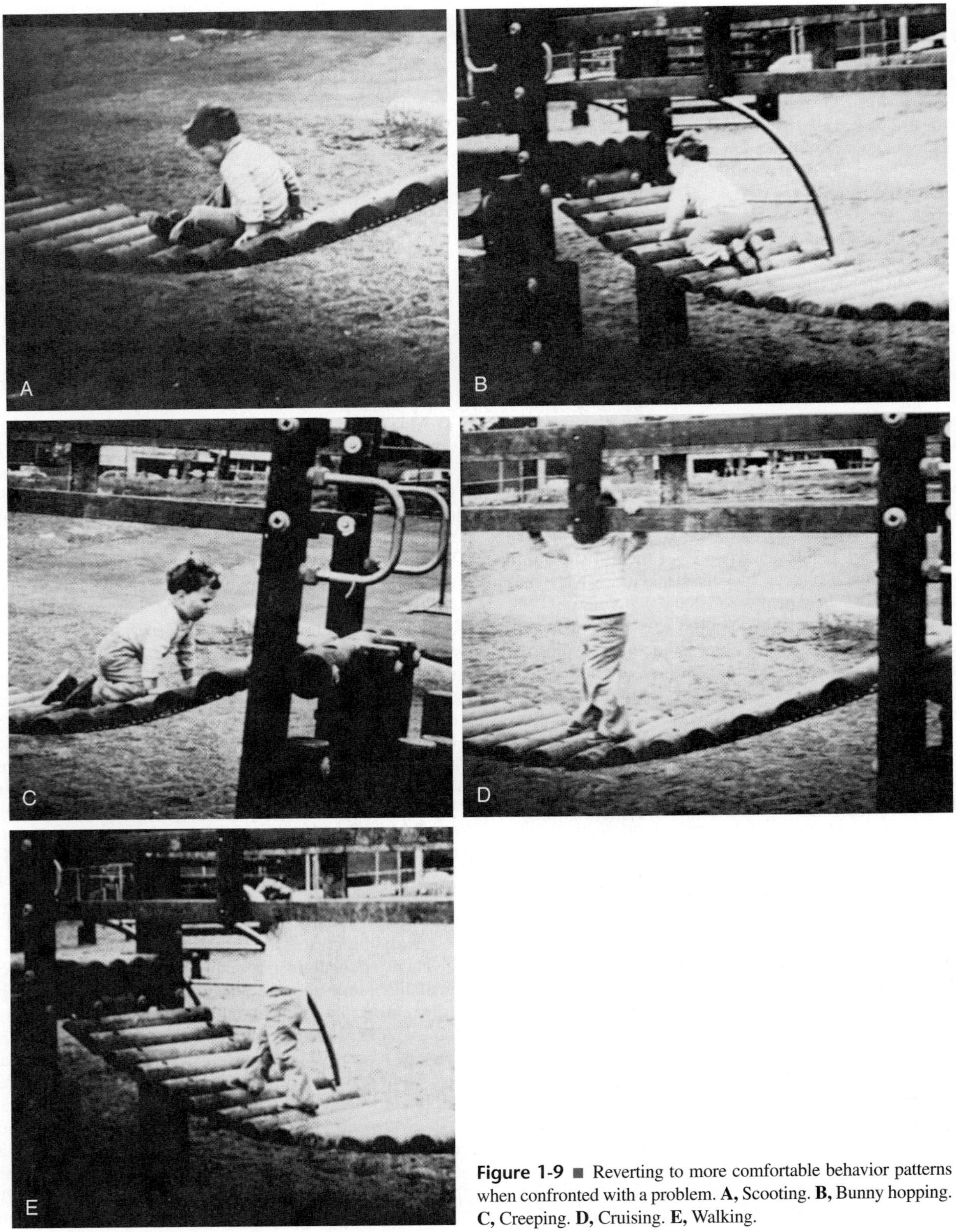

Figure 1-9 ■ Reverting to more comfortable behavior patterns when confronted with a problem. **A,** Scooting. **B,** Bunny hopping. **C,** Creeping. **D,** Cruising. **E,** Walking.

task goal is to cross the bridge; how that is accomplished is not as relevant as the task specificity. Therefore the child chooses a 6-month-old behavior and thus scoots. On gaining confidence, the child sequences from scooting to four-point bunny hopping, then creeping, on to cruising, and finally to reciprocal walking. The child's reversal lasted approximately 2 minutes. Although reverting to more familiar or comfortable ways of solving problems is normal, it creates constant frustration in the clinic if it is prolonged. For example, if a client with residual hemiplegia has spent a week modifying and controlling a hypertonic upper-extremity pattern during a simple task and is now confronted with a more difficult problem, the hypertonia within the limb will most likely return with the added complexity of the task. If another client has successfully worked to obtain the standing position and then is asked to walk, the strong synergistic patterns that had been controlled may return. The pattern or plan for standing is different from that for walking, and the emotional implications of walking are very high. The clinician should anticipate the possibility of the patient returning to a more stereotypical pattern. This possibility must also be explained to the patient. Anticipating that less efficient patterns will usually return as the tasks demanded increase in complexity, the clinician can attempt to modify the unwanted responses and let the patient know that the response is actually normal given the CNS dysfunction, but that movement can be changed and normalized with practice. The key to comprehension of this concept is not the behavior itself; instead, it is the attitude of a therapist toward a new task presented to the client. If the clinician expects the client to be successful, the client will also expect success. If failure occurs, both parties will be disappointed and a potentially negative clinical situation will be created; however, if the client succeeds, both will have expected the result and their attitude will be neither excited nor depressed. On the other hand, a clinician who expects the client to revert to an old behavior can prepare the client. If the client reverts, neither party will be disappointed; but if no reversion occurs, both will be excited, pleased, and encouraged by the higher functional skill. By understanding the concept, the clinician can maintain a very positive clinical environment without the constant negative interference of perceived failure when a client does revert.

The *fourth learning principle* deals with the totality of the client. Whether the area of emphasis is motor performance, emotional balance, or perceptual integration, all areas are affected. Therefore understanding and respect for all areas are important if optimal client function is a primary objective. This does not suggest that therapists should address each aspect of personality; however, integration of the client's physical, mental, and spiritual areas should be a responsibility of the staff. Awareness of possible adverse effects of one learned behavior on other CNS functions can help avoid potential problems. For example, if working on lower extremity patterns creates extreme upper extremity hypertonicity through associated patterns, the clinician is not dealing with the client as a whole.

The unknown creates fear and curiosity for most individuals, and the *fifth learning principle* points out that for most clients the unknown is all encompassing, whatever the degree of prior learning. For a client whose only difficulty is a flaccid upper extremity, functional activities such as toileting, dressing, or eating will be troublesome and unfamiliar. Motivation is a critical factor for success. Maintaining motivation to try while ensuring a high degree of success is an important teaching strategy that tends to encourage present and future learning.

An additional comment regarding clients who lack motivation should be made. If a client chooses to be totally dependent and has no need to become independent, then a therapist will probably fail at whatever task is presented. For example, Mr. Brown, a 63-year-old bank president with a wife, four children, and 10 grandchildren, survives an operable brain tumor with residual right hemiparesis and minimal cognitive-affective deficits. The client's work history indicates that he was highly success oriented. Unknown to most persons is that for 63 years Mr. Brown desired to be a passive-dependent person, but circumstances never allowed him to manifest those behaviors. With the neurological insult, he is in a position to actualize his needs. Until the client desires to improve, therapy will probably be ineffective; thus, motivating the client becomes critical. This might be accomplished in a variety of ways. Knowing that Mr. Brown values privacy, especially with respect to hygiene, that he thoroughly enjoys dancing and birdwatching in the forest, and that he ascribes importance to being accepted in social situations, such as cocktail parties, helps the therapist create a learning environment that motivates this client toward independence. Being independent in hygiene requires certain combinations of motor actions, including sitting, balance, and transfer skills. Being able to birdwatch deep in an unpopulated forest requires ambulation skills, tolerance of the upright position for extended periods of time, and endurance. Being socially accepted depends to a large extent not only on grooming but on normal movement patterns, especially in the upper extremity and trunk. Creating a therapeutic environment that stresses independence in the three goals identified by the client will simultaneously create further independence in other areas. Whether the client decides to return to banking and other activities in conflict with his personality will need to be addressed later. Another way to motivate Mr. Brown is to place him in an environment in which he is not satisfied, such as a nursing home or his own home with an assistant rather than his wife to help him with his needs. Dissatisfaction with the current external environment will generally motivate an individual to change. Obviously, creating a positive environment for change versus a negative one would be the method of choice.

The *sixth learning principle* has been discussed in earlier sections. To be a successful teacher of motor skills and to assist the client in recovery of function, the clinician should be able to break more complex motor plans and functional tasks into smaller component parts. These parts can then be taught successfully and then integrated back into the whole activity for optimal learning to occur. The therapist should always strive to allow each client to solve movement problems and develop strategies for reaching the outcome goals, rather than producing the desired outcome for or with the patient.

Many additional learning principles from the fields of education, development, and psychology can be used to explain the behavioral responses seen in our clients. It is not expected that all therapists will intuitively or automatically know how to create an environment conducive to helping the patient achieve optimal potential. Yet all can become better at creating a beneficial learning environment by understanding how people learn. The critical importance of being honest and accurate with prognosis and how that will ultimately affect function outcomes, participation in life, and quality of life cannot be overemphasized.[97]

The principles presented in this chapter deliver a strong message: individuals need to solve problems and most want to solve the problem given a chance that the solution will be successful. Unless the task fits the individual's current capability, adaptation using whatever is available will become the consensus that drives the motor performance through the CNS. Learning is taking place in all aspects of life, and the client must ultimately take responsibility for the means to solve the problem.[98]

THE CLIENT AND PROVIDER RELATIONSHIP

The Client's Role in the Relationship

Active participation in life and in relationships promotes learning. Rogers[99] defines significant learning as learning that makes a difference and affects all parts of a person. We have spoken of a relationship centered on an individual's health. One of the individuals involved in the relationship (the therapist) has knowledge that is to be imparted to or skills to be practiced by the other. The relationship "works" if the learning environment facilitates exchange between the participants. The concept of equal partners is crucial. The issue and practice of informed consent is not just political or ethical; it is central to client care. Voluntarism has to be practiced by both practitioner and client. Each has a moral obligation to facilitate the process of health care within the moment. Although the Western world of medicine has steadily climbed a path toward excellence in medical technology and clarification of medical diagnosis as seen in WHO's ICD-10,[100] it has not as easily recognized the client's need to assume an equal role in the decision making or for the practitioner to seek the client's help. Consumers are now seeking to play a more active role in their health care. This role has developed out of our scientific understanding of motor learning (see Chapter 4) and the fiscal necessity of decreasing the number of therapeutic visits.

Consumers of health care are becoming aware of the affect of medicine's control over their lives. This awareness has been fueled by the price they are paying for that health care. A recent Surgeon General's report confirms that expenditures for health are increasing. In addition, preventive care assumes major importance in view of the fact that seven out of 10 deaths in the United States today are the result of degenerative diseases, such as heart disease, stroke, and cancer.[101] Like other major causes of death, trauma (cited as the most frequent cause of death in persons younger than age 40 years[102]) is increasingly linked to lifestyles.

During their training, individuals in the health care professions internalize values that reinforce the traditional professional attitude alluded to earlier. Many of these values do not support a partnership relationship with the client. Society is beginning to question the traditional role of the health care professional as the knowledge expert; however, professional educational institutions and organizations resist the pressure to change the image. The professions still hold the image of great authority given to them by the public and fostered through increased political activity. This is true for both those professionals dealing with disease and pathology (physicians, nurses, pharmacists) and those dealing with functional movement problems limiting participation in life (OTs, PTs, Speech Language Pathologists).

The major purpose of the patient's relationship with the health care professional is to exchange information useful to both regarding the health care of the client. McNerney[31] calls health education of the client the missing link in health care delivery. As the gap grows between technology and the users of that technology, client health education becomes more important than ever.[103] McNerney[31] notes that although health care providers are now making efforts to educate their clients, they are doing so with little consistency, enthusiasm, theoretical base, or imagination and often with little coordination with other services. The health care professional continues to receive training and embrace professional organizational membership that places a premium on control of information and control of the decision making. There is and should be a special effort to introduce health education concepts into the basic educational programs of health care professionals. McNerney identified many of the problems three decades ago, and many still exist today.

When patients are given more information about their illnesses and retain the information, they express more satisfaction with their caregivers. A study by Bertakis[104] tested the hypothesis that patients with greater understanding and retention of the information given by the physician would be more satisfied with the physician-patient relationship. The experimental group received feedback and retained 83.5% of the information given to them by the physician. The control group received no feedback and retained 60.5% of the information. Not surprisingly, the experimental group was more satisfied with the physician-patient relationship.

If the client is to be informed and included in the treatment process, client health education will have to go beyond the current styles of information giving. If the client is to assume some of the responsibility for his or her therapy, the therapist will have to facilitate that involvement. The attitude of the therapist toward educating clients about their health could affect his or her ability to facilitate client involvement in the care process.

The more the professional sees himself or herself as the expert, the less likely he or she will be to see the client as capable of responsibility or expertise in the care process. If communication skills and health education were an integral part of medical school and health care professional school curricula, perhaps the health care professionals would temper their assumption of the "expert" professional role. Payton[105] points out that it is the client alone who can ultimately decide whether a goal is worth working for. Careful planning can be influential in helping all providers include the client in the process.

The health care delivery system in the United States has to serve all citizens.[106] That is no easy task. The United States is a society of great pluralism. It is a free society. It is a society that is used to being governed by persuasion, not coercion. Given the variety of economic, political, cultural, and religious forces at work in American society, education of the people with regard to their health care is probably the only method that can work in the long run. The future task of health education will be to "cultivate people's sense of responsibility toward their own health and that of the community." Health education is an effective approach with perhaps the most potential to move us toward a concept of preventive care.

Becker and Maiman[107] discussed Rosenstock's Health Belief model as a framework to account for the individual's decision to use preventive services or engage in preventive health behavior. Action taken by the individual, according to the model, depends on the individual's perceived susceptibility to the illness, his or her perception of the severity of the illness, the benefits to be gained from taking action, and a "cue" of some sort that triggers action. The cue could be advice from a friend, reading an article about the illness, a television commercial, and so on. In some way, the person is motivated to do something.

Mass media has promoted individuals' education, which may correctly guide or misguide consumers' decision making.[108,109] This concept was put forward as early as 1976.[110] Today the consumer thus has a heightened expectation of the quality of care he or she will receive. Similarly, consumers come to receive medical care because of media education, whereas in the past that level of education was not available.[111,112] As of today, the media are just beginning to be used by OT and PT professions, in the hope that this media use will educate the public regarding when, where, and how to decide on whether to seek our services. It will be a few years before research can be done to determine if this use of media will assist in educating the public.

Many aspects of today's lifestyles do not reinforce wellness. The obesity seen throughout the industrialized world proves that point.[113-115] Yet whether the client takes some responsibility for his or her functional problems and recovery depends a great deal on whether the health care provider gives some to him or her. Today's literature certainly reinforces the need for patient responsibility and active participation in one's own functional recovery.[116-124] This change in responsibility may be caused by third-party payers and the lack of funding versus promotion of a new health care model in which the patient is an active participant, but as long as the change occurs, the world will be better served.

Fink[125] in 1980, over three decades ago, recognized the importance of the provider-patient relationship. The state of what is referred to as *health* varies for each client and includes both the simple and complex variables of that client's life, from the last nutritional meal to the totality of the client's life event history (see Figure 1-5). The relationship of the therapist and the client can lead to better use of the health care system by giving responsibility to the consumer.[126,127] The therapist has an advantage over most other health care practitioners, who see the patient at infrequent intervals and who seldom touch the patient as a PT or an OT does.

The illness or trauma of the client that represents a disintegrating force in his or her life may represent an opportunity for the therapist to grow professionally. The client and the therapist may have different psychological backgrounds, and, although the client's presence is usually related to a medical crisis, the therapist's presence may support the purposes of personal growth, financial gain, prestige, and unconscious gratification in influencing the lives of others through professional skill.[128]

As the consumer becomes more involved, so should the family.[129] Patients in therapy have always been happier with the family involved.[130] The therapist must be willing to facilitate the involvement of the family members and help them learn to take responsibility for some of the care and decision making. Most health care professionals are not conditioned to allowing patients and family members to assume responsibility for their own care; however, better outcomes can be achieved if this is permitted and accepted.

Therapists are caught up in the same problems of the health care system as other health care professionals. Inflation has often caused profit to become a more important motive than human care considerations for setting priorities in our clinics. Research is heavily focused on technical procedures, yet the relationship with patients in the care process is vital. Singleton[131] labeled this phenomenon a paradox in therapy. Despite the commitment to humanistic service on which the profession was founded, the service rendered is often mechanistic.

The educational programs should emphasize whole-patient treatment, increased communication skills, interdisciplinary awareness, and patient-centered care.[44-46,132] The change in roles described previously requires a professional who demonstrates a potential for the assumption of many roles, responsibilities, and choices along the care pathway. The therapist working with the client with neurological problems must always be ready to respond to triggers anywhere along the pathway from early intervention, midway during a crisis, or later during long-term care, because these triggers signal a need for change. Of equal importance, the path must be well documented to empower the therapist to reflect on current and prognosticated treatment intervention.

The Provider's Role in the Relationship

Gifted therapists are often thought to have intuition. Yet intuitive behavior is based on experience, a thorough knowledge of the area, sensitivity to the total environment, and ability to ask pertinent questions as the therapist evaluates, conceptualizes about, and treats clients (Chapter 5). How these questions are formulated and the answers documented vary among therapists, but the result is the formulation of a unique profile for each client.

Cognitive-perceptual processing by the client will often determine the learning environment to be used, the sequences for treatment, and the estimated time needed for therapeutic intervention. Thus the client is in a position to play an important role with the therapist within the clinical problem-solving process. In that interactive environment, the therapist can ask questions regarding cognitive, affective, and motor domains that will help clarify, document, and guide future decisions regarding empowerment of the client. (See the client profile questions regarding cognitive, affective, and sensorimotor areas in Boxes 1-1, 1-2, and 1-3.) The motor output area is the main system the client uses to express thoughts and feelings and demonstrate independence to family, therapists, and community. This motor area cannot be evaluated effectively by itself while the cognitive-perceptual and the affective-emotional areas are negated. If that rigidity becomes a standard of care, accurate prognosis and selection of appropriate interventions will continue to be inconsistent and lack effectiveness within the clinical environment. No one will question that therapists today need to use reliable and valid examination tools in order to measure efficacy of our interventions. Finding the link between structured examination and intuitive knowledge is a characteristic of master clinicians. Even therapists who intuitively know a patient's problem need to use objective measures today to verify that intuition. Therefore third-party payers can justify

BOX 1-1 ■ COGNITIVE AREA QUESTIONS FOR CLIENT PROFILE

A. Sensory input: awareness level
   1. What sensory systems are intact, and which have impairments?
   2. Are any sensory systems in conflict with others?
   3. If conflict between systems is present, to which system does the client pay attention?
B. Perceptual awareness and development
   1. What specific perceptual processing deficits does the client have, and how would that affect motor performance?
   2. Do the perceptual problems relate to input distortion, processing deficits, or both? If input distortion is alleviated, is information processed appropriately?
C. Preferential higher-order cognitive system
   1. Was or is the individual's primary preferential system verbal, spatial, or kinesthetic?
   2. Is the client's preferential system different from yours? If so, can you work through the client's system?
   3. Is the client's preferential system affected by the clinical problems?
   4. Can the client adequately use nonpreferred systems?
D. Level of cognition
   1. Is the client functioning on a concrete, abstract, or fragmented level?
   2. Does the client's level of cognition change? If so, when and why?
   3. Is the client realistic? Does the client exercise judgment? If so, when? If not, when and why?
   4. Which inherent systems or outside influences are interfering with or distorting the client's potential? (Systems within the individual and the environment around the client, such as the staff, the family, and the other patients, must be considered.)

BOX 1-2 ■ AFFECTIVE AREA QUESTIONS FOR CLIENT PROFILE

A. Level of adjustment or stage of adjustment to the health condition
   1. At what level or stage of adjustment is the client with respect to the system problem and ability to participate in functional activities?
   2. At what level of adjustment is the family?
   3. Will the level of adjustment of the client or family affect treatment?
   4. If emotions are affecting treatment, what can be done to eliminate this problem?
B. Level of emotional control
   1. Can the client exercise impulse control?
   2. When does the degree of emotional or impulse control vary?
   3. How did and does the client respond to stress?
   4. How did and does the client respond to perceived success and failure?
   5. What types of stresses outside of the specific physical system problems are being placed on the client?
C. Attitude (attitude toward bodily system problems and the functional ability is covered to some degree under level of acceptance, although additional information needs to be gathered)
   1. Before the onset of the bodily system problem, what was the client's attitude toward individuals with cognitive and/or motor system problems, and specifically, those related to his or her primary system problem?
   2. What is the client's attitude toward your professional domain?
   3. What is the family's attitude toward individuals with bodily system limitations and inability to participate in normal life activities, especially those related to its family member?
   4. What is the family's attitude toward your professional domain?
D. Social adjustment
   1. At what social developmental stage is the client's performance?
   2. Is the social interaction in alignment with cognitive and sensorimotor stages of development?
   3. Are the family's social interactions and expectations at the level of the client's performance?
   4. Is the client's level of social adjustment the same as the rehabilitation team's level of expectation?
   5. Is the client aware of his, her, or others' socially appropriate or inappropriate behavior?

BOX 1-3 ■ SENSORIMOTOR AREA QUESTIONS FOR CLIENT PROFILE

A. Level of motor performance with respect to performance
   1. Is the client's level of motor performance or sensory and motor integration congruous with the staff's expected performance level?
   2. Is the client's level of motor control integration congruous with the family's expected performance level?
   3. Is the client's level of motor function congruous with his or her expected level of performance and participation?

B. Functional skills
   1. What functional skills does the client perform in a normal fashion?
   2. What functional skills does the client perform given systems limitations?
   3. What functional skills has the client learned to perform that are reinforcing stereotypical patterns or hindering normal movement and the ability to participate?
   4. What functional skills do the client and family consider of primary importance? Will breaking these down to smaller component skills hinder normal learning?

C. Abnormal patterns
   1. What patterns are present?
   2. When are these normal and abnormal patterns observed? Do they vary according to spatial positions?
   3. Is there ever a shifting or altering in degree of these abnormal patterns? If so, under what circumstances does this variance occur?

D. Degree of cortical override
   1. Does the client need to inhibit abnormal output by intentional thought, or does he or she use procedural adjustment through normal feed-forward mechanisms?
   2. What amount of energy is being used to override abnormal output?
   3. Can the client use cognitive systems to control motor output?
   4. What amount of energy are you demanding the client to use when attending to the task? Are you asking the client to fully attend to the specific motoric task, or are you overloading the system to take away some cortical attention?

payment for services while the patient benefits from the intuitive guidance in the clinical decision making by the therapist.

Once the therapist has a clear understanding of the client's strengths and weaknesses, specific clinical problems can be identified and treatment procedures selected that allow flexibility in treatment sessions. Many treatment suggestions for various problems can be found in Chapter 9 and Chapters 11 to 27.

CONCLUSION

In this sixth edition of the textbook, we hope to bring the reader into the clinical practice of the twenty-first century. As the professions continue to evolve in depth and breadth, the future will encapsulate the knowledge, skill, and lessons of the past and the needs and problems of current and immediate health delivery systems while maintaining unique scopes and parameters of practice in an ever-changing environment. The professions must adapt and grow as they embrace change without losing the integrity and philosophical reasons they came into existence. The only concept that is guaranteed in the future is *change.* Both physical and occupational therapy are dynamic professions with the ability to adapt and evolve to provide the health care service expected and deserved by the consumer. The future is up to every practitioner. The consumer of our services is dependent on our willingness to learn, adapt, and provide a high quality of care at an appropriate cost for the best outcomes. We have done that in the past, are doing it in the present, and will continue doing it in the future.

References

To enhance this text and add value for the reader, all references are included on the companion Evolve site that accompanies this textbook. This online service will, when available, provide a link for the reader to a Medline abstract for the article cited. There are 132 cited references and other general references for this chapter, with the majority of those articles being evidence-based citations.

CHAPTER 2 Health and Wellness: The Beginning of the Paradigm

JANET R. BEZNER, PT, PhD

KEY TERMS

paradigm
perceptions
well-being
wellness
whole person

OBJECTIVES

After reading this chapter the student or therapist will be able to:

1. Define and differentiate the terms *health* and *wellness.*
2. Describe the characteristics of wellness.
3. Compare and contrast illness, prevention, and wellness paradigms.
4. Identify and analyze a variety of wellness measures.
5. Synthesize a wellness approach into neurorehabilitation.

In learning to cope with the often chronic nature of their conditions, individuals with neurological disease, not unlike individuals with health conditions of other systems, learn to rely on their abilities to adapt and compensate for their activity limitations and participation restrictions to regain the ability to participate in life. Although not an uncommon approach to life for any human being, the achievement of health or wellness takes on an increased focus for individuals with chronic health conditions, and it is strongly correlated to the quality of life they achieve. A casual consideration of the terms *health* and *wellness* indicates that they are similar, if not the same, in meaning, a commonly held belief among those without health conditions. This interpretation of the terms becomes problematic, however, in the presence of health conditions. Can an individual with a health condition be well? Can a person without a health condition be ill? The concepts of health and wellness and their associated meanings and measures will be explored in this chapter to provide a perspective for movement specialists that will enhance their ability to promote health and well-being in clients with neurological disease.

DEFINITIONS AND RELATIONSHIPS AMONG TERMS

The classic understanding of the term *health* from a biomedical perspective is "absence of disease." The antonym of *health,* therefore, is disease. The World Health Organization contributed to the confusion between the terms *health* and *wellness* when in 1948 it defined *health* as "a state of complete physical, mental and social well-being, and not merely the absence of disease or infirmity."[1] Indeed, there are numerous illustrations of the influence of the mind and spirit on the body and thus the importance, from a public health perspective, of considering more than the physical state of the body when formulating solutions to health problems. However, there is also value in differentiating health from more global concepts such as wellness and quality of life, if for no other reason than to explain the phenomenon that an individual can be diseased and well or can experience a high quality of life while simultaneously living with a chronic disease. Considering the catastrophic nature of many neurological diseases that compromise physical health, it is even more important to distinguish between health and wellness to recognize and pursue avenues to enhance overall quality of life and well-being.

H. L. Dunn first conceptualized the term *wellness* in 1961 and offered the first definition of the term: "an integrated method of functioning which is oriented toward maximizing the potential of which the individual is capable."[2] Since Dunn's introduction of the term, numerous researchers and educators have attempted to explain wellness by proposing various models and approaches.[3-11] Although the literature is full of references to and information about wellness, including numerous definitions of the term, a universally accepted definition has failed to emerge. Several conclusions can be drawn, however, from the abundance of literature regarding wellness.

For many people, including the public, health and wellness are synonymous with physical health or physical well-being, which commonly consists of physical activity, efforts to eat nutritiously, and adequate sleep. Research has indicated that when the public is asked to rate their general health, they narrowly focus on their physical health status, choosing not to consider their emotional, social, or spiritual health.[12] Referring to the definition of wellness from Dunn, and consistent with numerous other theorists, it is obvious that wellness, as it is defined, includes more than just physical parameters.

The common themes that emerge from the various models and definitions of wellness suggest that wellness is multidimensional,[2,4-13] salutogenic or health causing,* and consistent with a systems view of persons and their environments.[2,15-17] Each of these characteristics will be explored.

First, as a multidimensional construct, wellness is more than simply physical health, as the more common understanding of the term might suggest. Among the dimensions

*References 1, 2, 4, 7, 8, 10, 14.

included in various wellness models are physical, spiritual, intellectual, psychological, social, emotional, occupational, and community or environmental.[18] Adams and colleagues[18] in 1997, toward the aim of devising a wellness measurement tool, proposed six dimensions of wellness on the basis of the strength and quality of the theoretical support in the literature. The six dimensions and their corresponding definitions are shown in Table 2-1.

The second characteristic of wellness is that it has a salutogenic or health-causing focus,[14] in contrast to a pathogenic focus in an illness model. Emphasizing the factors that cause health (e.g., salutogenic) supports Dunn's[2] original definition, which implied that wellness involves "maximizing the potential of which the individual is capable." In other words, wellness is not just preventing illness or injury or maintaining the status quo; rather, it involves choices and behaviors that emphasize optimal health and well-being beyond the status quo. Thus an individual may or may not be well before pathological conditions and health conditions involve the body and similarly may be well during an acute episode or chronic pathology or health condition whether that chronic problem results in static activity limitations or even progressive participation restrictions.

Third, wellness is consistent with a systems perspective. In systems theory each element of a system is independent and contains its own subelements, in addition to being a subelement of a larger system.[12,15,16] Furthermore, the elements in a system are reciprocally interrelated, indicating that a disruption of homeostasis at any level of the system affects the entire system and all its subelements.[15,16] Therefore overall wellness is a reflection of the state of being within each dimension and a result of the interaction among and between the dimensions of wellness. Figure 2-1 illustrates a model of wellness reflecting this concept. Vertical movement in the model occurs between the wellness and illness poles as the magnitude of wellness in each dimension changes. The top of the model represents wellness because it is expanded maximally, whereas the bottom of the model represents illness. Bidirectional horizontal movement occurs within each dimension along the lines extending from the inner circle. As per systems theory, movement in every dimension influences and is influenced by movement in the other dimensions.[18] As an example, an individual who has a knee injury and undergoes surgery to repair the anterior cruciate ligament will probably have at least a short-term decrease in physical wellness. Applying systems theory and according to the model, this individual may also have a decrease in other dimensions such as emotional or social wellness in the postoperative period. The overall effect of these changes in these dimensions will be a decrease in overall wellness, which anecdotally we know occurs when patients have an illness or injury.

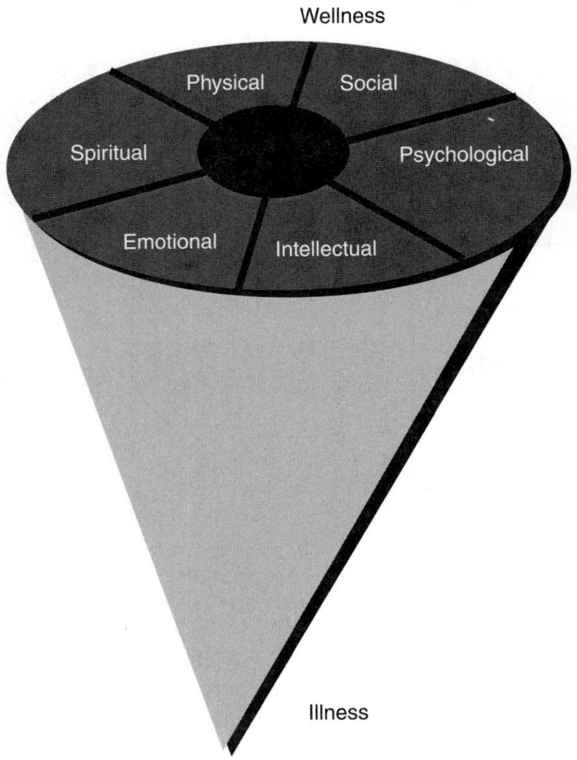

Figure 2-1 ■ The wellness model.

A term related to wellness, *quality of life,* is also used to indicate the subjective experience of an individual in a larger context beyond just physical health. Quality of life has been defined as "an individual's perception of their position in life in the context of the culture and value systems in which they live and in relation to their goals, expectations, standards, and concerns. It is a broad ranging concept affected in a complex way by the person's physical health, psychological state, level of independence, social relationships, and their relationship to salient features of their environment."[19] Parallel to the issues related to the concept of wellness, there is lack of agreement in the literature on the definition of quality of life and its theoretical components,[20-23] as well as variation in the use of subjective or objective quality-of-life indicators.[21] Implied by the World Health Organization definition, and supported by several other authors, quality of life is best conceptualized as a subjective construct that is measured through an examination of a client's perceptions. In other words, quality of life, like wellness, is the subjective experience of health, illness, activity and participation, the environment, social support, and so forth, and it is best measured through an assessment of client perceptions.

TABLE 2-1 ■ DEFINITIONS OF THE DIMENSIONS OF WELLNESS[18]

Emotional	The possession of a secure sense of self-identity and a positive sense of self-regard
Intellectual	The perception that one is internally energized by the appropriate amount of intellectually stimulating activity
Physical	Positive perceptions and expectancies of physical health
Psychological	A general perception that one will experience positive outcomes to the events and circumstances of life
Social	The perception that family or friends are available in times of need, and the perception that one is a valued support provider
Spiritual	A positive sense of meaning and purpose in life

A WELLNESS PARADIGM

The ultimate importance of gaining an understanding of health and wellness is to be able to apply it when interacting with patients/clients. In this sense, the goal would be to improve the health and well-being of the client, in addition to improving movement and participation. A comparison of the traditional "illness" paradigm with both "prevention" and "wellness" paradigms will identify ways in which a physical or occupational therapist can incorporate a wellness paradigm into the treatment of a patient with a neurological condition in the context of rehabilitation. The three approaches or paradigms are contrasted in Table 2-2 on six parameters, including the view of human systems, program orientation, dependent variables, client status, intervention focus, and intervention method.

As stated previously, in a wellness paradigm each dimension or part of the system affects and is affected by every other part, resulting in an integrative view of the human system. In contrast, in a traditional illness or medical model, the systems are independent. There are specialties in medicine by body system (e.g., neurology, orthopedics, gynecology), and in many physical and occupational therapy education programs, courses are arranged by body system (e.g., neurology, orthopedics, cardiopulmonary physical dysfunction, psychosocial), as indicators of the independence of the systems. In a prevention approach, there is recognition that the systems interact, or influence one another, but not in the reciprocal fashion characteristic of wellness.

The program orientation of an illness paradigm is the pathology or disease-causing issue, whereas the orientation of a prevention paradigm is normogenic, meaning efforts are aimed at maintaining a normal state or condition (e.g., normal muscle length, tone). Shifting to a wellness paradigm requires a salutogenic or health-causing approach,[14] with a focus on how to achieve greater well-being, health, or quality of life. This shift emphasizes the capabilities and abilities of the individual rather than the limitations and deficits.

The variables of interest in an illness paradigm are clinical variables, such as blood tests, $\dot{V}O_2max$ (maximum volume of oxygen use), and tests of muscle strength. Changes in these variables result in labeling the patient more or less ill. In a prevention paradigm, the variables measured are behavioral—for example, whether the individual smokes, exercises, or wears a helmet. Positive improvement in a prevention approach typically results in a change in an individual's behavior. In contrast, the variables measured in a wellness paradigm are perceptual, indicating what the patient/client thinks and feels about herself or himself. Although clinical, physiological, and behavioral variables are useful indicators of bodily wellness and are commonly used to plan individual and community interventions, their utility as wellness measures falls short.[24] Clinical and physiological measures assess the status of a single system, most commonly the systems within the physical domain of wellness. It can be argued that behavioral measures are a better reflection of multiple systems because of the importance and influence of motivation and self-efficacy on the adoption of behaviors, but they do not describe the wellness of the mind. On the other hand, perceptual measures, capable of assessing all systems and having been shown to predict effectively a variety of health outcomes,[18,25-29] can complement the information provided by body-centered measures insofar as they are valid, congruent with wellness conceptualizations, and empirically supportable.[24]

TABLE 2-2 ■ THE WELLNESS MATRIX

	ILLNESS	PREVENTION	WELLNESS
View of human systems	Independent	Interactive	Integrative
Program orientation	Pathogenic	Normogenic	Salutogenic
Dependent variables	Clinical	Behavioral	Perceptual
Client status	Patient	Person at risk	Whole person
Intervention focus	Symptoms	Risk factors	Dispositions
Intervention method	Prescription	Lifestyle modification	Values clarification

The influence of perceptions on health and wellness has been demonstrated repeatedly in the literature with a multiplicity of patient/client populations and in a variety of settings. Mossey and Shapiro[25] demonstrated more than 25 years ago that self-rated health was the second strongest predictor of mortality in the elderly, after age. Numerous other researchers have replicated these findings in other populations, lending support to the value of perceptions in understanding health and wellness and indicating that how well you *think* you are may be more important than how well you are as measured by clinical tests and measures or the judgment of a health professional. Wilson and Cleary[24] argued for the use of perceptions in understanding and explaining quality of life, proposing that health perceptions provide an important link between the biomedical model or clinical/illness paradigm, with its focus on "etiological agents, pathological processes, and biological, physiological, and clinical outcomes," and the quality-of-life model or social science paradigm, with its focus on "dimensions of functioning and overall well-being"[24] (Figure 2-2). Citing studies that have used perceptual measures, including the Mossey and Shapiro[25] study, Wilson and Cleary[24] state that health perceptions "are among the best predictors of [outcomes from] general medical and mental health services as well as strong predictors of mortality, even after controlling for clinical factors."[24]

Shifting to client status in each of the three paradigms, the subject receiving treatment in an illness paradigm is called the *patient,* whereas in a prevention paradigm the subject is a *person-at-risk* because of the focus on risk factors and the maintenance of a state of normalcy. In a wellness paradigm, the client is considered a whole person, to emphasize the multiple systems interacting to produce a state of well-being, and, more important, that a high-functioning or intact physical dimension, although important, is not necessary to achieve a state of well-being or a high quality of life.

Consistent with the client status elements, the focus of intervention in an illness paradigm is on symptoms and in a prevention approach on risk factors. Consistent with a whole-person focus in a wellness approach, the intervention focuses on dispositions. Defined as a prevailing tendency,

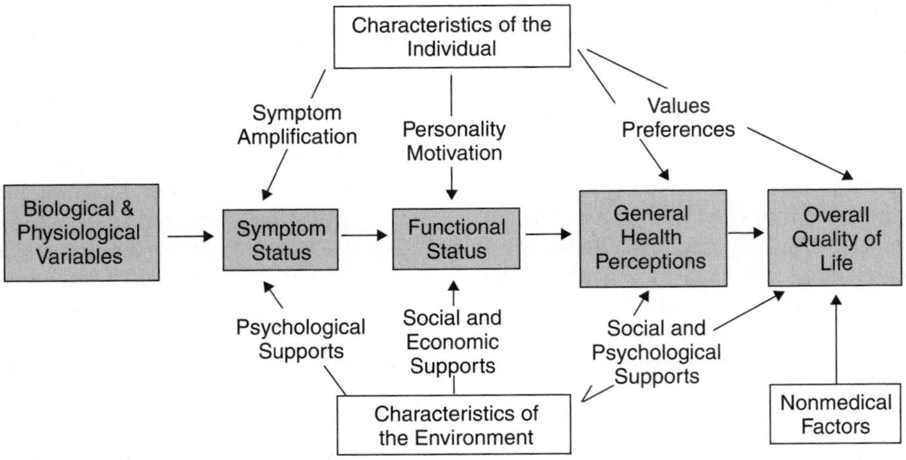

Figure 2-2 ■ Health-related quality-of-life conceptual model. (Modified from Wilson IB, Cleary PD: Linking clinical variables with health-related quality of life. *JAMA* 273:59–65, 1995.)

mood, or inclination or the tendency to act in a certain manner under given circumstances, dispositions produce perceptions, which can be measured to indicate a global or psychosocial assessment of the whole person, given input from all of the systems. Combined with symptom and risk factor assessment, perceptions of the individual provide valuable additional information about a client that can enhance the therapists' ability to intervene and the success of the interventions selected. Table 2-3 lists a few measurement tools that assess client perceptions.

The intervention method used in an illness paradigm is prescriptive. The prescriptive meaning is based on the system affected and symptoms reported. An intervention in an illness paradigm is prescribed to correct or improve the illness. Given that risk factors are the focus in a prevention paradigm and the aim is to maintain or return the person-at-risk to a normal state, the intervention method that is most appropriate is lifestyle modification in an attempt to change the behavior that is producing the identified risk. The intervention method in a wellness approach is called *values clarification,* and it is consistent with the focus on dispositions and measurement of perceptions. The aim of values clarification is to enhance self-understanding by surfacing the person's perceptions of the situation and its impact on his or her life. When values clarification can precede intervention prescription and lifestyle modification, wellness

TABLE 2-3 ■ SAMPLE ITEMS FROM PERCEPTUAL MEASUREMENT TOOLS

INSTRUMENT	PERCEPTUAL CONSTRUCT	SAMPLE ITEMS (RESPONSES)
Short Form 36[32]	General health perceptions	"In general, would you say your health is _______?" (excellent, very good, good, fair, or poor) "Compared with 1 year ago, how would you rate your health in general now?" (much better than 1 year ago, somewhat better, about the same, somewhat worse, much worse)
Satisfaction with Life Scale[45]	Life satisfaction	"In most ways my life is close to my ideal" "I am satisfied with my life" (7-point Likert scale from strongly disagree [1] to strongly agree [7])
Perceived Wellness Survey[28]	Perceived wellness	"I am always optimistic about my future" "I avoid activities that require me to concentrate" (6-point Likert scale from very strongly disagree [1] to very strongly agree [6])
NCHS General Well-Being Schedule[40]	General well-being	"How have you been feeling in general?" (in excellent spirits; in very good spirits; in good spirits mostly; up and down in spirits a lot; in low spirits mostly; in very low spirits) "Has your daily life been full of things that were interesting to you?" (all the time, most of the time, a good bit of the time, some of the time, a little of the time, none of the time)
Philadelphia Geriatric Center Morale Scale[41]	Morale	"Things keep getting worse as I get older" "I am as happy now as when I was younger" (yes, no)
Memorial University of Newfoundland Scale of Happiness[42]	Happiness	"In the past months have you been feeling on top of the world?" "As I look back on my life, I am fairly well satisfied" (yes, no, don't know)

will be enhanced because the intervention will be more targeted and considerate of the person rather than the health condition.

MEASUREMENT OF WELLNESS

As a result of the varied way that wellness has been defined and understood, a variety of wellness measures exist. Consistent with the characteristics of wellness described, a wellness measure should reflect the multidimensionality and systems orientation of the concept and have a salutogenic focus. In the literature, as well as in daily practice, clinical, physiological, behavioral, and perceptual indicators are all touted as wellness measures. Clinical measures include serum cholesterol level and blood pressure, physiological indicators include skinfold measurements and maximum oxygen uptake, behavioral measures include smoking status and physical activity frequency, and perceptual measures include patient/client self-assessment tools such as global indicators of health status ("Compared with other people your age, would you say your health is excellent, good, fair, or poor?")[30] and the Short Form 36 (SF-36) Health Status Questionnaire[31] (see Table 2-3).

Although some perceptual measures assess only single system status (e.g., psychological well-being, mental well-being), numerous multidimensional perceptual measures exist that can serve as wellness measures. Perceptual constructs that have been used as wellness measures include general health status,[31] subjective well-being,[31,32] general well-being,[33,34] morale,[35,36] happiness,[37,38] life satisfaction,[39-41] hardiness,[42,43] and perceived wellness[18,44,45] (see Table 2-3). Refer to Figure 2-3 for the "Perceived Wellness Survey" used by many professionals to help conceptualize

Perceived Wellness Survey

The following statements are designed to provide information about your wellness perceptions. Please carefully and thoughtfully consider each statement, then select the one response option with which you most agree.

	Very Strongly Disagree					Very Strongly Agree
1. I am always optimistic about my future.	1	2	3	4	5	6
2. There have been times when I felt inferior to most of the people I knew.	1	2	3	4	5	6
3. Members of my family come to me for support.	1	2	3	4	5	6
4. My physical health has restricted me in the past.	1	2	3	4	5	6
5. I believe there is a real purpose for my life.	1	2	3	4	5	6
6. I will always seek out activities that challenge me to think and reason.	1	2	3	4	5	6
7. I rarely count on good things happening to me.	1	2	3	4	5	6
8. In general, I feel confident about my abilities.	1	2	3	4	5	6
9. Sometimes I wonder if my family will really be there for me when I am in need.	1	2	3	4	5	6
10. My body seems to resist physical illness very well.	1	2	3	4	5	6
11. Life does not hold much future promise for me.	1	2	3	4	5	6
12. I avoid activities which require me to concentrate.	1	2	3	4	5	6
13. I always look on the bright side of things.	1	2	3	4	5	6
14. I sometimes think I am a worthless individual.	1	2	3	4	5	6
15. My friends know they can always confide in me and ask me for advice.	1	2	3	4	5	6
16. My physical health is excellent.	1	2	3	4	5	6
17. Sometimes I don't understand what life is all about.	1	2	3	4	5	6
18. Generally, I feel pleased with the amount of intellectual stimulation I receive in my daily life.	1	2	3	4	5	6
19. In the past, I have expected the best.	1	2	3	4	5	6
20. I am uncertain about my ability to do things well in the future.	1	2	3	4	5	6
21. My family has been available to support me in the past.	1	2	3	4	5	6
22. Compared to people I know, my past physical health has been excellent.	1	2	3	4	5	6
23. I feel a sense of mission about my future.	1	2	3	4	5	6
24. The amount of information that I process in a typical day is just	1	2	3	4	5	6
about right for me (i.e., not too much and not too little).	1	2	3	4	5	6
25. In the past, I hardly ever expected things to go my way.	1	2	3	4	5	6
26. I will always be secure with who I am.	1	2	3	4	5	6
27. In the past, I have not always had friends with whom I could share my joys and sorrows.	1	2	3	4	5	6
28. I expect to always be physically healthy.	1	2	3	4	5	6
29. I have felt in the past that my life was meaningless.	1	2	3	4	5	6
30. In the past, I have generally found intellectual challenges to be vital to my overall well-being.	1	2	3	4	5	6
31. Things will not work out the way I want them to in the future.	1	2	3	4	5	6
32. In the past, I have felt sure of myself among strangers.	1	2	3	4	5	6
33. My friends will be there for me when I need help.	1	2	3	4	5	6
34. I expect my physical health to get worse.	1	2	3	4	5	6
35. It seems that my life has always had purpose.	1	2	3	4	5	6
36. My life has often seemed void of positive mental stimulation.	1	2	3	4	5	6

Figure 2-3 ■ The Perceived Wellness Survey.[18]

the client's perception of her or his wellness. This survey was first published in the *American Journal of Health Promotion* in 1997.[18]

Physical therapists assess perceptions as a part of the patient/client history, as recommended in the "Guide to Physical Therapist Practice."[46] Occupational therapists assess perceptions as part of their focus on human performance and occupation. Some of the kinds of perceptions that can be assessed include perceptions of general health status, social support systems, role and social functioning, self-efficacy, and functional status in self-care and home management activities and work, community, and leisure activities. Although a few of these categories are included in overall wellness, such as general health status and social and role functioning, measuring wellness perceptions specifically can provide additional and more complete information about the patient that both the physical and occupational therapist can use to formulate a plan that can be insightful to the patient/client. Therefore perceptual tools should be used when measuring wellness.

MERGING WELLNESS INTO REHABILITATION

Incorporating wellness into rehabilitation requires that the therapist or provider modify the traditional approach used to treat patients, which involves changing the focus from illness to wellness, being a role model of wellness, incorporating wellness measures into the examination, considering the client within his or her system, and offering services beyond the traditional patient-provider relationship. Establishing a wellness approach also requires that the provider assume the role of a facilitator or partner rather than that of an authority figure.[47]

When a patient is ill, it is often appropriate for the health care provider to act as the expert because the patient has limited ability to provide self-care and is relying on the provider for information and skills to recover and improve. In a wellness paradigm the best approach is to believe that the client knows best in terms of maximizing her or his potential; therefore assuming a partner or facilitator role is more appropriate and will create a relationship in which the client feels empowered to take control. Rather than "making" the client well, the provider can view the client as a whole person within a biopsychosocial context and partner with the client to discover the most appropriate path to achieve wellness. This approach is consistent with a client-centered perspective, in comparison to a biomedical approach in which the emphasis is on impairment and activity limitations.[48-50] Recent discussions in the literature by a variety of health care providers suggest there is an important role for a client-centered approach within traditional medical settings.[48-52] Client-centered care requires the following:

- Assessment of and consideration for client thoughts, feelings, and expectations
- Education about the client's condition to enhance the client's ability to take responsibility for her or his own well-being
- A shift in professional identity from expert advisor to partner and facilitator
- Excellent communication skills, including the use of language the client can understand and effective listening skills
- Providers who have a high level of confidence in their knowledge and skill to guide clients to optimize their potential (e.g., achieve greater wellness)[49,50]
- Providers who are role models and who assume the role of facilitator, which will establish a relationship and an environment in which clients can attain greater wellness

It may be most instructive to consider first how a wellness approach could be adopted with clients who are seemingly healthy or without pathology. As experts in movement problems associated with the causes and consequences of pathological conditions, physical and occupational therapists should play a significant role in primary and secondary prevention. Indeed, intervention programs designed by therapists for patients/clients with pathology generally include instruction in preventive behaviors and activities (secondary prevention). Although appropriate and worthwhile, these efforts do not produce the significant outcomes that primary prevention programs might because they are applied after the onset of risk, illness, or injury. Contemporary practice includes a role for the physical and occupational therapist in primary prevention—that is, interacting with clients to promote health and improve wellness *before* they become patients.

Because individuals without overt disease are typically unmotivated to seek professional assistance, consideration must be given to how a provider recruits those without disease. A focus on wellness and health-causing activities is a powerful solution to this dilemma. In a sports or athletic context, this approach would be considered "performance enhancing" and would be marketed to individuals who have goals and ambitions related to improving athletic performance in a specific context (e.g., improving 10K time, increasing cycling distance or speed). In a general wellness context, an appropriate marketing message might be to improve quality of life or productivity, or any subjective measure that a client deems important. The same knowledge and skills therapists use when intervening to prevent injury, delay or prevent the progression of disease, or enhance quality of movement are useful in a primary prevention context in which the goal is to improve quality of life, well-being, and productivity. The difference is the context in which the knowledge and skills are applied. Adopting a wellness paradigm and a client-centered perspective or focus creates an environment surrounding the client-provider relationship that both empowers the client to make meaningful changes and establishes a partnership that is most conducive to change and improvement. The improvement of quality of life or wellness requires a consideration of the client as a whole person, by definition, as discussed previously in this chapter. Using a client-centered, whole-person approach to the design of an intervention program requires a considerably different approach than the traditional, biomedical approach of measuring clinical and behavioral variables to identify impairments and functional loss and creating an intervention aimed at ameliorating the impairment.[49,50] Suddenly clients are more than their diseases, which sends a much different message and creates a much different relationship between the provider and the client.

Applying this same approach to individuals with chronic health conditions implies that the therapist must attend to more than just impairments and activity limitations and their causes when designing intervention programs and determining the best approach to adopt with an individual client. It requires consideration of issues such as social support given and received, intellectual curiosity, physical self-esteem, general self-esteem, optimism, and so forth. Recognition of these dimensions of the individual provides a unique opportunity to keep the client at the focus of the intervention and design interventions in partnership with the client that will stand a greater chance of producing positive, meaningful outcomes.[49] The following examples attempt to illustrate the adoption and application of a wellness paradigm within neurorehabilitation.

CASE STUDY 2-1 ■ WELLNESS INTERVENTION CONCEPTS IN NEUROREHABILITATION

The client is a 56-year-old poststroke (cerebrovascular accident [CVA]) man who expresses a desire to return to a pre-CVA hobby, fly fishing. In addition to the physical requirements necessary to fly fish, which the therapist would typically assess and then incorporate into the intervention plan for the goal of independence in fly fishing, a wellness approach requires additional considerations. Recognizing the client's desire to fly fish requires the therapist to explore the client's goals and expectations and incorporate them into the intervention plan, as well as to appreciate the role of fly fishing in the achievement of well-being for this client. After the therapist provides education about living after a CVA, the client is aware that fly fishing is a realistic expectation. To understand the biomechanics and physical requirements of fly fishing, the therapist partners with the client to learn the process of fly fishing, thus gaining from the "expertise" of the client for the purpose of helping the client achieve his goal. The partnership relationship established in this case requires the therapist to be confident that she or he can identify the motor control, motor programming, and perceptual and cognitive aspects of the movement program such as the strength, motion, postural requirements, axial-distal motor relationships for fly fishing, and the client's self-efficacy post-CVA, even though the therapist had never participated in or observed the activity. Throughout the process, excellent communication is required between the therapist and client to ensure that expectations are clear and that understanding is achieved to establish and meet goals. The task of learning how to fly fish may have also required the therapist to go beyond the typical boundaries of traditional care, including challenging reimbursement limitations, to assist the client in his quest for enhanced well-being.

CASE STUDY 2-2

The client is a 25-year-old man with a posttraumatic brain injury who would like to be able to spend more time with his friends. During the discussion about his desires, the therapist, learning that the group plays basketball one or two times per week, inquires about the client's interest in joining the group. The client indicates that he used to play basketball but is concerned about his ability to run and produce the movements necessary to play now. The therapist, in the role of facilitator and partner, assures the client that playing basketball is a realistic goal and expresses a willingness to assist the client in achieving his goal. To provide the interventions necessary, the therapist must understand the physical requirements of basketball, obtain access to a basket and ball, interact with the client's friends, be open to learning about basketball from the "expertise" of the client, and support and motivate the client. The therapist recognizes that playing basketball with his friends will contribute greatly to the client's overall well-being and is thus a worthwhile goal.

In both cases the therapist functions as the movement specialist, also recognizing, however, the role of movement in the enhancement of emotional and social well-being within a paradigm of overall wellness. The potential contributions this approach can make to the overall quality of life of individuals living with neurological disease are immense and within the scope of practice and abilities of the physical and occupational therapist. Viewing the client within a larger context than the narrowly focused physical dimension provides increased opportunity to have an impact on well-being and quality of life.

References

To enhance this text and add value for the reader, all references are included on the companion Evolve site that accompanies this textbook. This online service will, when available, provide a link for the reader to a Medline abstract for the article cited. There are 52 cited references and other general references for this chapter, with the majority of those articles being evidence-based citations.

CHAPTER 3 Movement Analysis across the Life Span

DALE SCALISE-SMITH, PT, PhD, and DARCY A. UMPHRED, PT, PhD, FAPTA

KEY TERMS

abnormal movement strategies
developmental theory
neuroconstructivism
nonlinear dynamics
normal movement strategies
stages of motor development
systems theory

OBJECTIVES

After reading this chapter, the student or therapist will be able to:

1. Comprehend the complexity and interlocking nature of human development over a lifetime.
2. Differentiate traditional theories of development from contemporary theories.
3. Analyze the differences among various subsystems within the human organism.
4. Identify elements of physiological changes over a lifetime.
5. Analyze normal movement strategies and identify subsystems responsibility for success of a motor task.
6. Identify normal changes in motor strategies over a lifetime and synthesize differences between normal movement patterns and pathological movement problems across the life cycle.

As physical and occupational therapists assume greater roles in primary care of patients/clients, they recognize the importance of a multifactorial approach. To competently evaluate functional movement across the life span, clinicians must possess knowledge and skills in the development of skilled, refined movement across domains. Only then will therapists be prepared to perform the necessary evaluative and diagnostic testing and effectively develop and implement plans of care aimed at minimizing impairments, maintaining or regaining functional skills, and improving quality of life.

Throughout much of the twentieth century, developmental researchers were heavily focused on skill acquisition from infancy through early childhood.[1-3] In the 1970s, as research paradigms directed at motor development and motor learning evolved, it became evident that changes in motor skills were not limited to childhood but occurred throughout the life span. Consequently, the concept of life span development came to incorporate the prenatal period through older adulthood.

During infancy (birth to 1 year) and childhood (1 year to 10 years) acquisition of motor skills coupled with cognitive and perceptual development are the primary foci of developmental researchers and clinicians. As the young child transitions to adolescence (11 to 19 years) and has the opportunity to experience motor behaviors across different environmental contexts, more complex behaviors emerge. Adulthood (20 to 59 years) signals a period when skills are refined and motor behaviors mature. Only through practice and repetition are skills attained and retained. Individuals who continue to use motor learning strategies into late adulthood (60 years through death) often report more successful aging than those who do not engage in such motor skills.[4]

Identifying mechanisms that enable individuals to be successful in acquisition and retention of functional motor behaviors is critical to examining variables that alter or impair these same behaviors in other individuals. Kandel and colleagues[5] suggested that "the task of neural science is to understand the mental processes by which we perceive, act, learn, and remember" (p. 3). This view supports the interactive and collaborative nature of intrinsic and extrinsic systems to accomplish motor learning tasks.

Given the interactive nature of different subsystems, it would seem most effective for clinicians to recognize the need for implementing a multidimensional approach when devising intervention programs. To discuss the interactive nature of these issues, this chapter will (1) briefly provide a historical perspective of theories of motor development, (2) discuss domains (cognition, memory, perception, and so on) associated with life span motor development from prenatal development through older adulthood, (3) discuss the impact of various body systems on motor skill acquisition, and (4) describe behavioral changes that may positively or negatively influence motor performance across the life span.

With the focus of this book on neurological rehabilitation, it is imperative to incorporate the complex and interactive nature of the physiological, cognitive, and perceptual systems. Although readers can read about movement development across the life span, it will not integrate into clinical practice until the therapist understands movements of the client and how those movements reflect the summation of systems interacting to allow that individual to express movement, whether that be as a functional task, a written script, or the use of verbal language. Without that link between identified movement and motor control expressing that movement, often the therapist misses critical clues to the analysis of the central nervous system (CNS) of the client and how best to provide an environment that provides the opportunity for that individual to improve functional skills and quality of life. For that reason, figures have been inserted to help the reader understand the differences among movement patterns across the life span.

THEORIES OF DEVELOPMENT

Development is often portrayed as a series of stages through which an infant progresses, with a fixed order to the sequence.[6] A developmental theory may be characterized as a systematic statement of principles and generalizations that provides a coherent framework for studying development. Historically, development was thought to be linear, occurring in an invariant sequence and resulting in behavioral changes that are direct reflections of the maturation of anatomical and physiological systems.[7,8] Development is generally examined in terms of quantitative and qualitative change. Although it is universally accepted that acquisition of developmental skills is not reversible, the underlying principles surrounding the emergence of these behaviors has evolved over the past 50 to 75 years.

Early developmental theorists used neuromaturational models of CNS organization as the framework for conceptualizing development.[1,2] These researchers provided elaborate descriptions of posture acquisition and a blueprint delineating skill development. Research focused on the emergence of cognitive and affective behaviors and ignored the processes and mechanisms involved in acquiring motor skills.[9] Several investigators attributed developmental changes to intrinsic variables such as maturation of the CNS, whereas others associated changes with extrinsic variables involving the environment.[1,2,10,11]

During the 1930s and 1940s, Arnold Gesell and Myrtle McGraw led a cadre of avant-garde researchers exploring the field of infant motor development. Gesell[1,12] described the normative time frame for when behaviors emerge, and McGraw[2] examined the underlying mechanisms responsible for the emergence of these behaviors. The underlying premise, the foundation for their elaborate descriptions of motor development, was based on maturational processes in the CNS.

Gesell, a pioneer in developmental research, was a proponent of the theory that nature drives development.[13] He proposed that growth is a process so complicated and so sensitive that intrinsic factors are solely responsible for influencing development. He used the evolutional thinking of Darwin and Coghill to explain changes in motor behaviors. Coghill,[14] in his work with salamander embryos, reported that motor behaviors, like swimming, emerge in an orderly sequence as connections of specific neural structures appear. Coghill concluded from his observations of emergence of behaviors in the salamanders that human infant motor behaviors appear in a predictable sequence and at predictable chronological ages.

With Coghill's research as the foundation for his thinking, Gesell embraced the concept of a hierarchical organization of the CNS. He believed that the emergence of motor behaviors was contingent on maturation in the CNS and concluded that only after the emergence of higher-level neural structures would complex motor behaviors appear. Within this constrained theoretical perspective, extrinsic or environmental stimuli, human or otherwise, were thought to have little impact on the appearance of motor behaviors. Gesell concluded that infant development is preprogrammed and linear, emerging at predetermined stages or periods in time.[13] Perhaps his greatest contribution to motor development was the conceptualization of milestones as markers to evaluate infant behavior.

Although McGraw was a proponent of ontogenic development as one variable influencing motor development, she did not believe, as Gesell did, that it was the sole determinant.[15] Rather, McGraw attempted to explain the emergence of motor behaviors through environmental influences as well as CNS maturation.[2] She examined the temporal and qualitative aspects of motor skill acquisition through her study of Jimmy and Johnny,[16] a study of twin brothers in which one twin was provided an exercise program, whereas no intervention was afforded the other twin. She found temporal and qualitative differences in the boys' acquisition of motor skills and attributed differences in acquisition of these behaviors to disparities in practice opportunities.

McGraw believed that the acquisition of the movement (process) is as important as when (chronological time frame) the behavior is acquired (the outcome). She further elaborated that, within the constraints imposed by the developing CNS, a rich and challenging environment can and does facilitate temporal efficiency in acquisition of motor behaviors. And finally, she proposed that practicing motor skills influences emergence of the same behavior.

Sufficient evidence exists to support the premise that although some predetermined processes occur at relatively similar points in development, not all motor behaviors emerge at the same biological, chronological, or psychological age in every individual. Although motor milestones provide information regarding outcome, no information can be derived about the process of attaining motor skills from those specific milestones. Perhaps a more realistic explanation may be that emergence of new skills occurs out of a need to solve specific problems within the environment. Working within this context, it is evident that traditional theories of development and maturation fail to adequately encapsulate the innate variability in human development.[9,10]

Within the last few decades, researchers have used more current theories of development when designing studies involving infants and young children.[17-19] These investigators examined the process of skill acquisition rather than using traditional methods that assess outcome as a measure of motor development.[20]

Although early pioneers in developmental research described development as linear, uniform, and sequential, Thelan and Smith[21] depict development as "messy," "fluid," context-sensitive, and nonlinear. Linear and nonlinear dynamics are derived from mathematics. Linear dynamics is described by the proportional relationship of the initial condition to the outcome, whereas no such proportional relationship exists in nonlinear dynamics. Nonlinearity is used to describe complex systems, in this case biological or more specifically human systems.[22] Within these complex systems exists a level of unpredictability, given the interactive and interdependent nature of biological systems.

Thelan and Smith[21] suggested that, although traditional theories of development support the premise that behaviors emerge in accordance with a relatively fixed temporal sequence, an organism may exhibit "precocial" abilities when the context is altered and the behavior emerges earlier than expected. These authors stated that immature systems exhibit behaviors that are variable and easily disrupted.

Although development of some organisms in a controlled laboratory environment may reflect more traditional perceptions of development, outside, in a more naturalistic environment, development is more likely to be flexible, fluid, and tentative. Thelan and Smith also found that factors most likely to have an impact on performance are the "immediacy of the situation" and the "task at hand" rather than "rules" of the performance. Given this perspective, Thelan and Smith[21] identified six goals as essential to developmental theory. These goals are as follows:

1. To understand the origins of novelty.
2. To reconcile global regularities with local variability, complexity, and context-specificity.
3. To integrate developmental data at many levels of explanation.
4. To improve a biologically plausible yet non-reductionist account of the development of behavior.
5. To understand how local processes lead to global outcomes.
6. To establish a theoretical basis for generating and interpreting empirical research.[21] (p. xviii)

Thelan and Smith urged developmental researchers to devise paradigms that attempt to explain development in terms of diversity, flexibility, asynchrony, and "the ability of even young organisms to reorganize their behavior around context and task" (p. 18).[21]

Contemporary theorists inferred that developmental changes are nonlinear and emergent and may be the result of the interactive effects of intrinsic and extrinsic variables. This divergence from traditional thinking compelled avant-garde scholars to propose new theories.[21,23,24] Investigators described behaviors as complex, interactive, cooperative, and reflects an ability to organize and regroup around task and context, rather than conforming to a rigid structure and rule-driven hierarchy, as many earlier cognitive researchers believed.[21,24] Contemporary theorists exploit technology to derive a model to explain variability and flexibility in developing, mature, and aging populations.[24]

GENERAL SYSTEMS THEORY

Systems theory, first described by von Bertalanffy in 1936, was not discussed in great detail until 1948. In 1954 von Bertalanffy and colleagues from three other professions met to discuss systems movement.[25] Theorists then applied systems theory to a variety of human and nonhuman systems. As theorists became acquainted with systems theory, they became more receptive to alternate theoretical proposals of growth and development in living organisms.

Systems theory may be applied as a transdisciplinary model examining relationships of structures as a whole.[26] "The notion of a system may be seen as simply a more self-conscious and generic term for the dynamic interrelatedness of components"[26]; von Bertalanffy proposed this theory to more adequately describe biological systems, investigate principles common to all complex organisms, and develop models that can be used to describe them.[26]

Principles that embody general systems theory include nonsummative wholeness, self-regulation, equifinality, and self-organization.[26] Contrary to systems theory in disciplines such as traditional physics, in which systems are said to be *closed,* von Bertalanffy suggested that biological systems are open and modifiable and that changes in the system are the result of the dynamic interplay among elements of the system.[26]

Embedded in the general systems theory is nonlinear dynamics, a concept in which behaviors are not described as the sum of their parts. Thus within a nonlinear model, a mathematical model is derived.[24,27] Characterized within this model is the notion that systems may change in a sudden, discontinuous fashion. During development a small increase or decrease in one parameter leads to changes in the behavior. This abrupt change, identified as a bifurcation, causes the system to move out of its previous state and toward a new state of being.

Throughout development, periods of rapid differentiation or change occur when an organism is most easily altered or modified. These periods were identified by Scott[28] as "critical periods." Physiological systems are most vulnerable during these periods and may be seriously affected by both intrinsic and extrinsic factors acting on the system. These periods occur at different times for different body systems. Understanding systems theory and the concept of critical periods is crucial to all aspects of motor development.

As scientists began to revisit theories of motor development, they discarded some of the traditional theories and embraced contemporary concepts of nonlinear dynamics.[24,25,27] Proponents of nonlinear dynamics contend that modifications in motor behaviors are the result of dynamic interactions among the musculoskeletal, peripheral and central neuromuscular, cardiovascular and pulmonary, and cognitive and emotional systems.[26] These interactive, multidimensional elements are vulnerable to changes in organizational and behavioral abilities (system) over time.[28,29] Some theorists propose that as skills are acquired and organizational or behavioral changes occur, the system is driven to identify the most efficient and effective strategy to produce motor behavior(s).[28,29] Yet others purport that variability implies that typical healthy individuals may use a variety of strategies to produce the same behavioral outcome and that variability is an indication of the individuals' flexibility in responding to unpredictable perturbations.[24,30] Implicit in nonlinear dynamics is the concept of critical periods in development.[28,29,31] Investigators suggested that interventions imposed during a critical period may more easily positively or negatively modify the behavior. Recognizing the crucial role systems theory and critical periods play in development is vital to comprehending how developmental skills emerge. The multifactorial nature of nonlinear dynamics illustrates the complexity of development and the difficulty in identifying the appropriate variables that influence motor skill development.

With use of concepts previously described, it is reasonable to expect that a small change in any subsystem may result in a large change in a motor behavior. This is evident in work by Thelan and colleagues examining stepping in infants 8 weeks of age.[29,31-34] They reported that introducing a small change in one element of the system, identified as a small weight applied to an infant's leg, resulted in the infant being unable to step. The authors deduced that small changes in one subsystem, in this case the musculoskeletal system, may result in a change in the outcome. This lends support to the hypothesis that modifying one aspect of a multicomponent system, especially during a critical period, may cause the system to evolve into an entirely new behavior.

Periods of rapid differentiation, although often observed during early life, have also been observed across the life span. Changes in anthropometric measures, such as weight gain during pregnancy, influence coordination between limbs and cause emergence of a different gait pattern. Changes in one system, in this case the endocrine system, result in increased ligamentous laxity at the pelvis and also contribute to gait alterations.

Menopause may be another critical period. During menopause, decreases in hormone production are thought to lead to osteoporosis and cardiac disease.[35] Examples described previously provide evidence across the life span that the dynamic interplay within a system and among systems may significantly influence emergence and disappearance of behaviors.

Although research in the beginning of the twentieth century was heavily focused on development of the very young, studies during the latter part of the century were directed toward research on aging. Technological advances in medicine have dramatically increased life expectancies. During the twentieth century, the number of individuals in the United States older than 65 years old grew from 3 million to 35 million.[36] Perhaps the most significant statistic is that the oldest old grew from 100,000 in 1900 to 4.2 million in 2000.[36] By 2011 the Baby Boomer generation will begin turning 65 years old, and the number of older individuals will increase sharply between 2010 and 2030.[36] By 2030, Americans over the age of 65 years will represent nearly 20% of the population, and by 2050 the number of individuals over the age of 85 years could grow to 21 million.[36] Given this incredible demographic transformation and that current policymakers are, in large part, the generation directly affected by these statistics, a significant paradigm shift in funded research has evolved over the past quarter century. "As such, aging and death are inseparable partners to growth and development"[37] (p. 32). Recognizing that a critical mass of Americans are entering older adulthood, terminology that operationally defines and is then applied consistently when referring to the aging population or an individual is imperative.

Biological and Chronological Age

Age can be described in terms of chronological age and biological age.[38] Chronological age is the period of time that a person has been alive, beginning at birth. In infants it is measured in days, weeks, or months, whereas in adults it is expressed in terms of years and at times decades.

Although chronological age is measured in terms of temporal sequencing, biological age is related more to functioning and physiological aging of organ systems.[39] For example, a triathlete may have biologically younger cardiovascular and pulmonary systems than same-age peers who do not perform high-level aerobic activities. Another example might be a child who underwent precocious puberty. Precocious puberty, identified as puberty earlier than 8 years of age in girls and 9.5 years in boys, results in acceleration in a biological system before same-chronological-age peers.[40] Physiological changes include elevated hormonal levels, which would then stimulate development of breast tissue and early menstruation in girls. Changes in the musculoskeletal system include early closure of the epiphyseal plates, resulting in significantly smaller stature. Conversely, these young women's reproductive cycles are significantly skewed. Women would also have menopause and aging issues associated with hormonal changes earlier than other women of the same chronological age. Although no consistent method has been established for measuring biological age, there is general agreement that a wide variability of biological aging exists and that a number of factors contribute to accelerated or decelerated biological aging.

Aging

"Aging refers to the time-sequential deterioration that occurs in most animals including weakness, increased susceptibility to disease and adverse environmental conditions, loss of mobility and agility, and age-related physiological changes" (p. 9).[41] Although Goldsmith's description of aging is typically viewed as an inevitable fact of life, there is scientific evidence and theoretical support for the idea that age-related changes will eventually be more medically treatable than previously thought.[38,41,42]

Scientists are hesitant to attribute a decline in functional movement in older adults to a decline in physiological systems or to diminished opportunities for practice or conditioning.[4] Rowe and Kahn reported that "with advancing age the relative contribution of genetic factors decreases and [of] the nongenetic factors increases" (p. 446).[4] Age-related factors that are modifiable may be used to identify individuals who may or may not age successfully. For instance, lifestyle choices, including diet, physical activity, and other health habits, and behavioral and social factors have a potent effect and accelerate or decelerate aging. Evidence to support this was initially derived from a 10-year study conducted by Rowe and Kahn.[43] The authors identified three critical factors that contribute to aging successfully: avoidance and absence of disease, maintaining cognitive and physical functioning, and "sustained engagement in life."[43] Recently researchers suggested that Rowe and Kahn's classification of successful aging is too restrictive and may lead to classifying individuals with relatively minor health problems as unhealthy. McLaughlin and colleagues[44] suggested that a critical variable in defining successful aging is first identifying what the goal is for measuring successful aging. Only then can researchers determine how best to define and measure successful aging. Although controversy exists regarding defining successful aging, factors that contribute to successful aging hinge on higher levels of physical activity, increased social interactions, and positive perception of health, as well as no smoking, chronic diseases (arthritis, diabetes), or impaired cognition.[45,46] Consequently, developing healthy behaviors early in life may be critical to maintaining good health and may play a significant role in successful aging. Factors associated with aging are generally identified as either age related or age dependent. Age-dependent changes within organ systems are observed in individuals at a similar age, whereas age-related changes may be accelerated or decelerated in same-age individuals on the basis of intrinsic or extrinsic factors related to lifestyle. Just as variables associated with lifestyle (extrinsic factors) influence aging, genetics (intrinsic factors) also play a significant role. From a genetic perspective, structural and functional changes are generally thought to be a consequence of aging and are therefore predictable and consistent across physiological systems. Variables thought to influence the genetic potential for longevity include environmental factors such as toxins, radiation, and oxygen free radicals. Free radicals are highly reactive molecules produced as cells turn food and oxygen into energy.[47] In summary, the use of biological age rather than chronological age may be a more accurate reflection of an individual's true age.

Theories of Aging

Throughout the twentieth century, the average life expectancy of individuals living in the United States increased. The second half of the twentieth century signaled a shift in the focus of human development research, from infant and child development to older adult development.

Scientists view aging as a progressive accumulation of changes over time that increases the probability of disease and death.[48] Given that portrayal of aging, researchers have proposed myriad hypotheses regarding aging. Aging theories evolved because there is no single factor or mechanism responsible for physiological aging.[38] Biological aging theories, similar to developmental theories, are attributed to complex, underlying mechanisms.[38,41,42,49] Although theorists attempt to classify aging theories, these theories are rarely mutually exclusive. Some theories were formulated around control of physiological functioning, others around cellular changes, and still others around genetic causes.

Neuroendocrine theory is based on the premise that hormones play a significant role in aging.[42,49] Hormones are vital to repairing and regulating bodily functions. Hormone production decreases significantly during aging and limits the body's ability to repair and regulate itself as effectively. Although hormonal decline is one plausible explanation for age-related changes, it does not account for all changes. Harman[50] proposed the free radical theory on the basis of his investigations that examined the effects of radioactive materials on human tissue.[50]

Harman reported that when human tissue is exposed to radiation, a byproduct is formed. He identified the byproduct, an unstable compound, as a free radical. Over time, human tissue with free radicals showed evidence of biological defects consistent with accelerated aging. Harman postulated that accumulation of free radicals in human tissue may also occur as a part of the normal aging process. This became known as the free radical theory of aging.[50-52]

Free radicals are highly reactive molecules that damage proteins, lipids, and deoxyribonucleic acid (DNA). In some instances the free radicals combine with enzymes and turn into water and a harmless form of oxygen that moves harmlessly through the cells.[51] In other instances the oxygen binds with intrinsic or extrinsic sources that influence the aging process.

Scientists have suggested several different ways that free radicals influence aging through intrinsic and extrinsic mechanisms.[51,52] An example of an intrinsic mechanism would be chronic infections that extend phagocytic activity and expose tissues to oxidants, creating cumulative oxidative changes in collagen and elastin. Extrinsic sources of free radicals include environmental toxins—for example, industrial waste and cigarette smoke.

Human exposure to intrinsic and extrinsic free radicals causes large numbers of reactive oxygen molecules to interact with DNA, leading to mutations thought to be the cause of a variety of diseases, including cancer, atherosclerosis, amyloidosis, age-related immune deficiency, senile dementia, and hypertension. Although some scientists suggest that aging has many factors that can accelerate or decelerate the process, other scientists suggest a much simpler, preprogrammed theory, known as the Hayflick limit.[38,51-53]

Hayflick and Moorhead[53,54] proposed that there is a finite number of times that a normal cell is capable of dividing. Current thinking is that cells are capable of dividing up to 50 times. Cell division is recognized as one way in which cells age and, after attaining the maximum number of divisions, finally die.

The factor thought to limit a cell's ability to divide infinitely is the presence of telomeres. Telomeres are minute units at the end of the DNA chain.[53] Each time a cell divides a small amount of the telomere is used in the process. Eventually, when cells have exhausted the supply of telomeres available, the cell is unable to divide and cell death ensues.

Telomerase, a substance that can lengthen telomeres, is available in human cells. Typically, telomerase is switched off in all cells except the reproductive cells. The availability of telomerase in reproductive cells allows for many more divisions than previously observed in the Hayflick limit. In addition to the presence of telomerase in reproductive cells, scientists have also discovered that telomerase remains active in cancer cells. Both reproductive and cancer cells divide well beyond the 50-division limit. Consequently, scientists are now working toward activating telomerase in all cells to slow or stop aging. If scientists are successful in activating telomerase in other cells, it may stimulate skin cell regrowth for burn patients and cure diseases that result from failure of aging cells to divide, as in macular degeneration or Hutchinson-Guilford progeria syndrome.[55,56] The downside of this is that scientists may have a difficult time controlling the telomerase and in fact may see more uncontrolled cell growth—cancer—one of the greatest threats to prolonged existence.

Although many aging theories are directed at mechanisms that negatively influence aging, other theories are focused on factors that have a positive impact on aging processes. One such process is the caloric restriction theory.[50,52,53,57] Liang and colleagues,[57] with use of several genetic mouse models, investigated the impact of dietary control on the life span. The authors reported that the mice did, in fact, have their life spans extended when their dietary intake was controlled. Although these findings are potentially significant, given the small sample size and model examined, these data were not generalizable to all species. The researchers suggested that these preliminary data provide a foundation for scientists to examine whether dietary control will extend the life span in humans as it did in the mouse models.

Although a large body of literature exists examining the underlying mechanisms associated with aging, it seems inconceivable that any one mechanism is responsible for age-related changes. More likely is that aging may be attributed to multiple factors, including lifestyle choices, in combination with the physiological and environmental factors.[58]

Garilov and Gavrilova[58] conducted an exhaustive review of aging theories and concluded that additional research is necessary to further elaborate and validate existing aging theories and dispel unlikely theories.

In summary, scientists are unsure how much of the decline in motor behaviors in older adults is attributable to true decline in physiological systems, how much is attributable to expected decline, how much to a decreased ability to perform skilled behaviors under variable conditions, and how much to decreased practice or conditioning.[59-62] This suggests that physical or occupational therapy intervention may provide older adults with strategies to positively influence successful aging rather than being applied only after a negative outcome of aging is realized or a neurological insult has occurred.

The exogenous and endogenous variables of aging are thought to be interrelated and provide an expansive description of the deleterious changes at the cellular, organ, and system level that accompany both aging and many age-associated diseases. The accumulation of damage is in DNA, proteins, membranes, and organelles, as well as the formation of insoluble protein aggregates. Many organ systems, such as the cardiovascular system, the brain, and the eye, are not programmed for indefinite survival. Consequently, the inability to maintain the integrity of tissues and organs is the end result of the multidimensional aspect of aging.

PHYSIOLOGICAL CHANGES IN BODY SYSTEMS ACROSS THE LIFE SPAN

Organ systems undergo critical physiological changes across the life span. These alterations are observed most often during periods of rapid differentiation. Applying concepts of dynamic systems theory to life span development may help to explain how small changes in biologic systems have a significant impact on the individual as a whole.

Examining interactions among variables within different body systems may provide insight into when one system may play a greater or lesser role in acquisition, retention, or deterioration of functional motor behaviors. The next section will examine how different systems develop and their contribution to functional movement.

Musculoskeletal System

Structural and functional adaptations in the musculoskeletal system are evident across the life span. The musculoskeletal system provides a structural framework for the body to move and serves as protection for the internal organs.

Skeletal muscle tissue first appears during the fifth week of embryonic development and continues to develop into adulthood.[53,63] During this early period of embryonic development, the differentiation of musculoskeletal system is rapid: during the fifth week of embryonic life the limb buds appear, by the seventh week muscle tissue is present in the limbs, and limb movements emerge as early as the eighth week of prenatal life.[40,64,65]

Whereas many of the structural aspects of the musculoskeletal system are formed prenatally, muscle and bone continue to grow into adulthood. Motor skill acquisition involves considerable variability among young children from age 5 months through 3 years. During this time, the rate of growth of muscle tissue is reportedly two times faster than that of bone.[66]

Structural and functional differences in the musculoskeletal system of a child versus an adult are attributed to the presence and predominance of muscle fiber types. For example, infant muscles are composed predominantly of type I (slow-twitch) fibers, whereas adult muscles contain types I and II (fast-twitch) fibers. Behaviorally, infant movements are characterized predominantly by postural movements. The capacity to produce a greater repertoire of movements, including rapid or ballistic movements, emerges later in development.

Distinct differences also exist in temporal differentiation of the muscular systems of males and females of the same chronological age. Through adolescence, boys show evidence of a significantly greater increase in fiber size compared with girls.[67] In addition, differences exist in the age at which the number of muscle fibers dramatically increases. Girls reportedly have a steady increase in the muscle fibers from 3.5 to 10 years of age. In contrast, boys have two periods of rapid differentiation in the number of muscle fibers. The first period occurs from birth until 2 years of age and the second from ages 10 to 16 years.[67] Although the pace slows considerably, muscle fiber development continues in men and women well into middle adulthood.

Age-related changes evident in the musculoskeletal system include decreased fiber size, loss of muscle mass, denervation of muscle fibers, decline of total muscle fiber number, and decreased quantity of fast-twitch fibers.[68-70] Muscle mass decreases beginning at around age 50 years, and by age 80 years up to 40% of muscle mass has been lost.[71] Muscle force production likewise decreases at a rate of about 30% between 60 and 90 years of age. Additional musculoskeletal changes documented in older adults include decreased tensile strength in bone, reduced joint flexibility, and limited speed of movement. Decreased muscle mass in a person older than 60 years may be attributed to decreased size, fewer type II muscle fibers, and an increase in fat infiltration into the muscle tissue.[72,73] Clinically these factors manifest as reduced muscle force production during high-velocity movements.

Currently, scientists are examining the premise that, as an individual ages, muscular changes are more likely attributable to decreased motor activity levels and are age related rather than being solely age dependent.[69,72] Acknowledging that investigators had previously found that muscle power deteriorates more quickly with age, scientists set out to measure training effects in older adults.[61,74] These investigators concluded that with training older adults were capable of improving strength, power, and endurance.

The skeletal system, similar to the muscular system, experiences periods of growth, stability, and degeneration. The immature skeletal system is composed primarily of preosseous cartilage and physes (growth plates).[75] More simply, bone in infants and young children is flexible, porous (lower mineral count), and strong with a thick periosteum.[75,76] Given these properties of immature bone, a child is less likely to have a fracture because the periosteum is strong and consequently the bones absorb more energy before the break point is reached. In addition, if a fracture does occur, healing is usually quicker because callus is formed faster and in greater amounts in children than in adults.

A primary difference between the child's and the adult's skeletal system is the presence of the growth plate complex in children. Whereas primary ossification occurs prenatally, secondary ossification is not complete until the child reaches skeletal maturity, generally at age 14 years in girls and 16 years in boys.[76,77]

Even after bones have attained their full length, they continue to grow on the surface. This is termed *appositional growth* and continues throughout most of life. During childhood and adolescence, new bone growth exceeds bone resorption and bone density increases. Until age 30 years, bone density increases in most individuals, and bone growth and reabsorption remain stable through middle adulthood. Later in adulthood, resorption exceeds new bone growth and bone density declines.[78]

Women exhibit more loss of bone mass than men do.[79] Decreased bone density in women is generally attributed to differences in the types and levels of hormones present. Although the difference is most significant during menopause, premenopausal women still lose bone density at a higher rate than their male peers do.

Osteopenia is the presence of a less-than-normal amount of bone and, if not treated, may result in osteoporosis. Progressive loss of bone density, observed into older adulthood, is commonly identified as osteoporosis. Osteoporosis is more common in women than in men and is a major cause of fractures and postural changes in both sexes.[80]

Overall, much of the growth in the musculoskeletal system is related to demands placed on the system. Intrinsic and extrinsic forces imposed on the musculoskeletal systems of typically and atypically developing children may lead to structural and functional differences in their respective skeletal structures. Consequently, temporal sequencing, acquisition, and characteristics of motor behaviors emerge differently in typically and atypically developing children. Similarly, age-related changes in older adulthood may be accelerated in direct proportion to decreased levels of activity.[81] Older adults who maintain more active lifestyles and place greater physical demands on their musculoskeletal systems are more likely to have an improved bone density and muscle mass than their peers who are not as active.[82]

Sarcopenia, the age-related loss of muscle mass, affects strength, power, and functional independence in older adults.[72,82] Although these changes are observed in many older adults, the degree of the muscular changes varies.[70] Researchers examining sarcopenia in older adults reported that men are affected more by sarcopenia than women are.[72,83] In fact, men with sarcopenia manifest four times the rate of activity limitations than do men with a normal muscle mass. Changes in the cross-sectional area of muscles directly affect the force production of a given muscle; consequently, as the cross-section of a muscle diminishes, its ability to produce force decreases. As an individual ages the number and size of the muscle fibers decrease, resulting in a reduction in strength.[80] Although this is true in all muscles, the impact is greater on muscles of the lower extremities than in those of the upper extremities.[72]

Although strength is critical to musculoskeletal function, flexibility is equally as important. Flexibility incorporates joint motion and the extensibility of the tissues that cross the joint. The degree of flexibility changes across the life span as a direct result of aging and activity level.[10] Changes in flexibility are evident throughout life: limited at birth, increasing until the individual approaches adolescence, and then gradually decreasing. Exceptions may be seen in athletes, dancers, and other individuals involved in activities that incorporate flexibility training. Loss of flexibility as a consequence of age may have a negative impact on functional independence in older adults. Flexibility is thought to be directly proportional to the amount, frequency, and variability of motor activities performed. As activity increases, so does flexibility. Conversely, as individuals exhibit decreased levels of motor activity, often associated with age, flexibility decreases.[78]

By age 70 years, flexibility is thought to have decreased by 25% to 30%.[70] Although this was purported to be age dependent, it may be more likely that it is age related.[69] Regularly performing exercise directed toward improving strength and flexibility can reverse the effects of inactivity for most individuals, even those older than 90 years of age.[69,81]

Although it may take longer for older individuals to regain strength or flexibility than a young adult or child, musculoskeletal tissue is modifiable throughout life. Modifying the strength and flexibility of an older adult requires that other bodily systems be capable of modifying performance levels to meet the increased needs of the musculoskeletal system.

As scientists continue to examine functional changes across different systems as a consequence of age, physical and occupational therapists must educate individuals regarding the importance of embracing a physically active lifestyle and methods to enhance quality of life at each stage in an individual's life (see Chapter 2). Although all systems contribute to an individual's health and wellness across the life span, the cardiovascular and pulmonary systems play a key role (see Chapter 30).

Cardiovascular and Pulmonary Systems

The cardiovascular system is composed of the heart, lungs, and associated vascular complex. It is responsible for pumping blood through the coronary, pulmonary, cerebral, and systemic circulations, with the goal of perfusing all bodily tissues for the delivery of oxygen and vital nutrients and picking up waste products for elimination. The pulmonary system is responsible for oxygen transport, gas exchange, and removal of airborne pollutants that may enter during respiration (see Chapter 30).

The interdependent nature of the cardiovascular and pulmonary systems is evident in the fact that, each minute, all of the body's blood travels through the lungs before being returned to the left side of the heart for ejection into the systemic circulation.[84] Because of this relationship, changes in heart function can dramatically affect lung function, and vice versa. In addition, these two systems are connected as part of a larger closed pressure-volume loop through the peripheral circulatory structures. Likewise, any alteration in the function of the peripheral vessels will affect both the heart and lungs, and vice versa.

The function and homeostasis of the cardiovascular, pulmonary, and peripheral vascular systems are influenced by both internal and external forces.[84] Internal mechanisms of control are based on the autonomic nervous system, the relative health of the anatomic structures involved, the growth and development of the structures, and the behavioral and emotional adaptations of a particular individual.

All those internal mechanisms are subject to changes with growth and development, aging, and the unique life experiences of an individual. Growth and development primarily affect the physics of the system by altering volumes, lengths, smooth and myocardial muscular tension, and physiological capacitance within the system to support the growing body. Numerous effects of aging have an impact on the adaptability of the system. Behavioral and emotional responses influence both autonomic and volitional cardiovascular and pulmonary reactions to stress. External forces include movement environment and activity level, which alter the gravitational forces on the closed pressure-volume system. An increased activity level causes exercise stress, which requires an altered demand for oxygen and nutrients to the structures providing the work. Finally, emotional stress needs to be considered as an external factor. Behavioral responses to stress can affect functional movement and cause maladaptive coping mechanisms on any or all systems. As with anything, the age, cognitive status, and relative health of an individual will dictate the potential success of these endeavors.

Because oxygen transport and exchange are the primary requirements for sustaining life, efforts toward maximizing the efficiency of the cardiovascular and pulmonary systems represent a fundamental component of therapeutic practice. It is critical that no matter where a patient falls in the life span, strategies for screening, prevention, and rehabilitation of the cardiovascular and pulmonary systems be incorporated into a comprehensive plan to promote optimal mobility and independence.[85] It is essential for therapists to keep in mind that all interventions have a direct or indirect impact on these systems and that it is their responsibility to monitor and manage those responses to maintain safety.

A detailed understanding of the anatomy of the heart, lungs, and vessels, as well as the physiology and interrelationship of the organs involved, is essential to the practice of both physical and occupational therapy. Refer to Chapter 30 for additional information. For pediatric therapists, the added knowledge of normal growth and development of these structures is critical.

From weeks 3 to 8 of fetal life, the cardiac structures are formed.[63,64,86] All other structures of the cardiovascular system are fully developed and functional shortly after birth. Although the left and right ventricles are of similar size at birth, by 2 months of age the muscle wall of the left ventricle is thicker than that of the right ventricle.[87] This is attributable to the fact that the left ventricle is responsible for pumping blood to the whole body, requiring a higher internal pressure and contractile force, whereas the right ventricle is responsible for pumping blood only to the lungs, a relatively low-pressure function in a healthy individual.

It bears mentioning that the heart's function begets structure. Therefore if function becomes impaired, the structure is likely to adaptively change. For example, if the resistance in the vascular system from the right ventricle to the lungs becomes increased, the right ventricle must pump harder, with a greater volume of blood, to overcome the resistance.[88] Over time, this will increase the size of the ventricular walls because the myocardium is muscular tissue that is as equally capable of hypertrophy as skeletal muscle tissue.

Structurally, the heart doubles in size by year 1, and its size increases fourfold by year 5. Many of the changes associated with size are complete by the time the child has reached maturity. Recall that cardiac output (CO) is equal to stroke volume times heart rate. As the size of the heart increases (increasing the volume capacity for each stroke), the heartbeat decreases and the blood pressure increases.[89] Heart rate in a newborn infant is generally 120 to 200 beats per minute (bpm), 80 bpm by 6 years of age, and 70 bpm by 10 years of age.[87,90] Systolic blood pressure (defined as maximal pressure on the artery during left ventricular contraction or systole) is 40 to 75 mm Hg at birth and increases to 95 mm Hg by 5 years of age.[87] Blood pressure continues to rise into adolescence. The capacity to maintain exercise for longer periods and greater intensities increases through early childhood. Although cardiovascular disease is generally associated with adults, children as young as 5 years of age may show signs of or be at risk for cardiovascular disease if they do not engage in regular aerobic activity.[87,91]

Development of the pulmonary system occurs late in prenatal and early postnatal life.[90] As the lungs increase in size, tripling in weight during year 1, the capacity and efficiency increase while the respiratory rate decreases.[90] Although the vital capacity of a 5-year-old child is 20% of an adult's, this is not usually a limiting factor during exercise.[89] Overall, aerobic capacity increases during childhood and is slightly higher in boys than in girls. The overall work capacity of children increases most dramatically from 6 through 12 years of age.[89] Peak oxygen consumption is achieved early in adulthood and changes in direct relation to activity levels. Lungs of an average adult at rest take in about 250 mL of oxygen every minute and excrete about 200 mL of carbon dioxide.[92]

As activity decreases in older adulthood, so do the structural and functional capacities of the cardiovascular and pulmonary systems. Many of these changes are a result of decreased elasticity of the tissues, decreased efficiency of the structures, and decreased ability to increase workload. CO decreases approximately 0.7% per year after age 20 years so that by age 75 years the CO is 3.5 L/min, down from 5 L/min at age 20 years.[92] Functional changes include a decrease in the overall maximum heart rate from 200+ bpm through young adulthood to 170 bpm by age 65 years.[87] Older adults have less elastic vessels, and resistance to the blood volume increases. Consequently, older adults reach peak CO at lower levels than do younger individuals. These cardiovascular changes may be compounded by inactivity, resulting in decreased capacity to perform activities that raise metabolic demands and increase the requirement for oxygen transport.[93] The impact of these normal aging responses, however, can be reduced through structured aerobic and anaerobic activities. Conversely, physiological performance of the cardiovascular and pulmonary systems improves in response to growth and development.

Throughout life, performance of motor activities and activities of daily living (ADLs) is highly dependent on the integrity of an individual's cardiopulmonary and cardiovascular systems. Introduction of aerobic activities during early childhood has implications for improved health and wellness across the life span. Although aging has a negative impact on performance and efficiency of the cardiovascular and pulmonary systems, aerobic exercise has a positive impact on these systems. Changes in the cardiovascular and pulmonary systems have a significant impact on other systems and consequently on overall body function. Information from these systems, including blood pressure and oxygen saturation rates, is communicated through the nervous system. The nervous system, in turn, regulates responses of the cardiovascular and pulmonary systems through the autonomic nervous system.

Neurological System

The nervous system encompasses the CNS and the peripheral nervous system (PNS). The CNS includes the brain and spinal cord, and it is responsible for all bodily functions. The PNS includes both the autonomic and the somatic nerves and is responsible for transporting impulses to and from the CNS.[5] The capacity for humans to produce behaviors far beyond those of other animals is directly related to the complex abilities of the CNS and interneuronal communications.

Over the past two decades, technological advances have enabled neuroscientists to dramatically improve their understanding of the molecular changes in the nervous system over time.[94] Development of the CNS is coordinated through intrinsic influences involving the temporal and spatial coordination of synaptic connections with genetic processes, along with extrinsic or environmental factors. Initially, development of the CNS is dependent on precise connections formed between specific types of nerve cells and begins with the recruitment of cells that form the neural plate, which gives rise to the neural tube, and then differentiation of regions of the brain begins.[5,95] Changes in the nervous system are predicated on critical periods, or times when different regions of the brain are sensitive to change, and occur across the life span.[5,28]

Each region of the brain is thought to undergo critical or sensitive periods at different ages. One of the most critical periods in development of the CNS occurs from birth through 1 year of age. During this period, when the system is most vulnerable to change, intrinsic and extrinsic variables may influence the nervous system structurally and functionally.

Differentiation of cells in the nervous system begins during the embryonic period and continues throughout adulthood.[5,94] Development of the nervous system during embryonic life involves the overproduction of glial cells and neurons that, after they are no longer useful, die. Additional developmental changes noted in the nervous system include increased myelination within the brain and an increase in neuronal size.[63] Much of the growth may be attributed to these changes in the nervous system and may account for the development of the infant's brain, which increases to one half the size of the adult brain during the first year of life. Neural development, particularly in the cerebral cortex, documented early in development may emerge out of environmental demands and the need to solve problems (tasks). Consequently, experiences can alter neural networks, and more complex experiences lead to increasing complexity of the neural structures.[96] Whereas researchers long supported the premise that decline of the nervous system begins generally after age 30 years, more recent studies indicate that adults, even older adults, can form new neural connections and grow new neurons as an outgrowth of learning and training.[94,97] Before the work of Eriksson and colleagues, researchers and clinicians believed that structural changes in older adults, such as decreased numbers of corticospinal fibers, intracortical inhibition, and neuronal degradation in centers in the CNS, particularly the cerebellum and basal ganglia, were inevitable.[98] In contrast, findings from a study conducted by Draganski and colleagues[99] challenged traditional constructs that the only possible changes in the adult human brain were the result of negative changes caused by aging or pathology. Instead these researchers suggested that a direct relationship existed between learning a novel task, juggling, and structural changes in the gray matter. The authors caution that these structural changes were task specific and limited to the training period. Reexamination of magnetic resonance imaging (MRI) scans, after 3 months of no training, demonstrated that subjects no longer displayed the same structural changes as during juggler training.

Loss of neurons in the centers controlling sensory information, long-term memory, abstract reasoning, and coordination of sensorimotor information negatively affects function. For some individuals this may not have significant implications. For others, CNS changes create serious functional losses. Alterations in the CNS, including altered neural control and decreased efficiency in temporal sequencing of muscle synergies, may play a role in postural instability and impaired sensation. Together these changes can result in falls.[68]

Although the CNS, similar to other bodily systems, may have the capacity to compensate for some age-related changes, the degree of compensation may be modulated by the complexity of the task and continuation of "practice" over time. Although some investigators have reported that neuromuscular systems in older adults may not be as flexible as systems in younger adults, new studies examining changes in mature and aging systems are still in the early stages. Neuromuscular systems in older adults may not be as capable of rapidly reorganizing muscle synergies to produce variable functional responses.[98] The researchers did say that this may be related not solely to the aging neurological system but to other factors including experience, cardiovascular and musculoskeletal fitness, and current level of functional independence. Other scientists suggested an alternative view that repetition of motor activities may stimulate new growth in dendrites located proximal to neurons previously lost.[68] The authors were quick to add that, although the pathways or connections may be activated, this may or may not result in improved functional ability. Implicit in performance of many functional activities is cognition. If changes in cognition coexist with changes in other systems, it may be difficult to accurately interpret the underlying causes.

Cognitive System

Cognition may be defined as awareness, perception, reasoning, and judgment.[100] Cognitive development involves processes of perception, action, attention, problem solving, memory, and mental imagery. Action, from the perspective of physical or occupational therapy, may be referred to as *functional movement(s)* and incorporates all the processes described previously to successfully perform a specific task.

Jean Piaget, one of the most recognized scientists in developmental psychology of the twentieth century, was particularly intrigued with how biological systems affect what individuals "know."[100,101] He observed interactions among children of different ages and hypothesized that younger children's thought processes were different from those of older children as evidenced through the differences in responses between them to the same questions.

Piaget proposed that cognitive development moved in a linear, stagelike progression, each stage of which involves radically different schemes.[101] He suggested four stages of cognitive development, identified as sensorimotor state (infancy), preoperational (toddler and early childhood), concrete operational (childhood and early adolescence), and formal operational (adolescence and adulthood).[100] He proposed that (1) sensorimotor behaviors stimulate cognitive development and (2) problem solving as a measure of cognition enables infants and young children to identify and modify motor behaviors.

Piaget's theory of cognitive development focused around how humans adapt within the environment and how these adaptations or behaviors are controlled.[101] He postulated that behavioral control is mediated through schemas or plans, generated centrally. These schemas provide a representation of the world in an effort to formulate an action plan. At birth, infants' earliest schemas are organized around reflexive behaviors that are modified as the infant adapts to the affordances and constraints of the environment.

Piaget suggested that adaptations occur through two processes: assimilation and accommodation.[101] He defines *assimilation* as a process of altering the environment around cognitive structures. An example of assimilation is when an infant, initially breast-fed, is transitioned to bottle feeding. *Accommodation* refers to changes of the cognitive structures to meet changing demands of the environment. Accommodation may be involved when an infant transitions from nutritive sucking (breast or bottle) to nonnutritive sucking (pacifier).

Much of Piaget's work was based on descriptive case studies. Although some aspects of his theory were supported by subsequent studies, other aspects of his work have not been shown to have empirical evidence. The inconsistencies of research findings examining Piaget's stages of development may be indicative of the dynamic and nonlinear nature of development and, more specifically, cognition.

Rather than postulating that infants are reflexive beings with little or no volitional movements early on, it may be more appropriate to view infants as competent beings with volitional and complex behaviors present at birth.[102] Brazelton reported that a newborn infant turns toward the mother's voice rather than toward an unfamiliar voice. In addition, research conducted by Meltzoff and Moore[103] provides evidence supporting the complex nature of infant behavior. They found that infants as young as 2 to 3 weeks of age can imitate facial gestures performed by adults. Their work was supported by subsequent studies performed by independent investigators using different procedures and in different environments.[104] These findings, contrary to Piaget's proposal that infants were not capable of imitative behaviors until 1 year of age, provided scientists with a new perspective on infant behavior.

Contemporary researchers approach developmental theory from a dynamic and nonlinear model.[21,95,96,105] Over the past 10 years, advances in technology (e.g., diagnostic imaging, functional magnetic resonance imaging [fMRI], magnetoencephalography [MEG], event-related potentials [ERPs]) have dramatically improved the ability to document change within the developing brain.[95] These technological advances coupled with developmental paradigm shifts and computer modeling have led developmentalists to propose new theoretical frameworks to explain cognitive development. One model, called *neuroconstructivism,* incorporates intrinsic constraints and abilities of the CNS at the most basic cellular level with extrinsic influences involving environmental experiences and interactions.[95,96] Fundamental to the neuroconstructivist theory is the principle of context dependence, in which representations emerge in direct response to the structural changes in the cognitive system. Embedded within neuroconstructivism is the concept of the infant as interactive, in contrast to more traditional developmentalists' perception of the infant as passive. Experiences that individual infants engage in vary through processes involving competition and cooperation. The processes employed during development may result in differing pathways or trajectories of development through which the outcome or behavior is realized. Despite the variability in the individual developmental trajectories, the behavioral outcome is often similar.

This model is purportedly applicable to typical and atypical development as well as mature and aging systems. In contrast, whereas the processes and interactions among multiple interactive constraints (biological and environmental) may be similar in typical and atypically developing systems, the constraints may differ. Hence, the outcome or emergent behavior may be different.

Current theories lend support to the concept that the cognitive system integrates multimodal input to process, interpret, store, and retrieve information as a mechanism for information processing and problem solving.[100] Changes in cognition, defined as relatively permanent changes in behavior, cannot be measured directly but rather must be inferred from changes observed across multiple systems.

As the ability of infants to act on the environment develops, their ability to accurately detect and process relevant information becomes more efficient, lending support to the interdependence of the motor, cognitive, and perceptual systems.

Information processing, defined as the ability to understand human thinking, is a critical factor that must be examined within the cognitive system. Initially, infants and young children cannot recognize relevant cues or chunk information for storage. As children's developing systems become more adept at integrating information from multiple systems and more efficient at processing information, they begin to process relevant information more effectively. Consequently, infants and young children may not use or interpret information as efficiently as older children.

The integrative nature of movement, cognition, and perception is evident in developmental psychology literature.[106] Given that these domains are interrelated, one area cannot be examined in isolation of other interrelated systems. Acquisition of motor skills is the primary mechanism for evaluating cognition and perception in prelinguistic children. In addition, as individuals grow older, changes in any system may influence functional movement. Finally, when examining functional movements, therapists must always consider the individual's cognitive and perceptual abilities.

As higher-level cognitive processing skills become apparent, the child can accurately identify relevant cues, filter irrelevant cues, and process information more efficiently. One such higher-level cognitive processing skill is executive functioning. Adolescence signals a period during which executive functioning begins to mature.[107] This period may be characterized as critical in CNS development. During this critical period, production of mature, adult-like decisions requires selective attention and increased integration of information via the prefrontal cortex. During the maturation process, adolescents may exhibit inconsistent decision making, resulting in less-than-optimal outcomes. By young adulthood, as the individual approaches maturity, optimal executive decision making becomes more consistent.

Human systems are continuously pelted with sensory information through some or all of the sensory modalities. At any one time much more sensory information is available than can possibly be processed. Consequently, the individual must learn to select information relevant to the task and chunk the information for processing.

Another example of the multidimensional processes involved in higher-order tasks such as functional movement is found in a study conducted by Hazlett and Woldorff.[108] They proposed that implicit in motor tasks are concepts of cognition including attention, perception, and information processes. This multimethodological approach examined (1) the influence of attention on sensory and perceptual processing, (2) the executive control of attention by higher centers of the brain, and (3) the processes underlying multisensory integration and the mechanisms by which attention interacts with such integration processes.[108]

Throughout the life span, physical growth and development of many systems have an impact on the acquisition and performance of motor skills. Changes in one system and the interactive effects on all other systems can lead to deleterious changes in motor performance as a whole.

A new paradigm that embraces the concept that memory and cognition do not deteriorate as part of normal aging is a topic of discussion in scientific literature.[109] This perspective was proposed after Gould and colleagues[109] conducted a study that found that adult primates continue to develop new brain cells throughout life. The addition of new neocortical neurons throughout adulthood provides a continuum of neurons of different ages that may form a basis for marking the temporal dimension of memory. These late-generated neurons play an important role in learning and memory of older adults.

Changes in cognitive function are often revealed during tasks that require processing and retrieval of cognitive or motor memory. Consequences of aging include slowed information processing and increased time necessary to perform motor skills. Even though learning may take more time in older adults, once a behavior is learned, retention is similar to that of younger individuals. Of significance for older adults is delayed performance of long-standing tasks such as driving a car, which may have serious consequences for the driver, passengers, or others in the immediate vicinity of the vehicle. Delays in processing and task execution pose risks to the older adult or individuals with CNS deficits and may affect the individual's level of independence and quality of life.[110]

Although older adults experience deterioration in the processing and retrieval of information, the extent of the decline is unpredictable. Cognitive deficits most frequently observed in older adults include word retrieval, recall, dual-task execution, and activities involving rapid processing or working memory.

Memory

Memory can be broken down to three types: working, declarative, and procedural. Working memory, short-term memory, is the equivalent of the RAM of a computer.[100] This is the mechanism that enables a child who does not appear to be attending to what the parent is saying to repeat what the parent has just said. Given the temporary nature of this memory, no space in the hippocampus or amygdala is required. Working memory may in fact be more of a cortical phenomenon. Declarative memory is what is typically envisioned when we think of intermediate or long-term memory. Declarative memory is the area where long-term information about everything an individual has ever learned or information acquired is stored, including facts, figures, and names.[100] An example of declarative memory is a second-grade teacher recalling the name of a student she had in her class 15 years previously. Declarative memory is analogous to the hard drive in the computer. The third type of memory is procedural memory. Procedural memory involves all motor activities, actions, habits, or skills that are learned through repetition in motor practice.[100] Examples of procedural memory include walking, playing an instrument, and driving a car.

Rovee-Collier and colleagues[111-113] have conducted numerous studies related to memory retention in prelinguistic children. Evidence exists to support the premise that infants as young as 2 to 3 months of age are capable of identifying relevant cues and chunking this information for later retrieval. One caveat is that retrieval of such information is possible only when the specifics of the behavior are retained. Infant memories are tightly linked to the specific information related to the task, environment, and stimulus. Consequently, a slight change in any of these three components may result in an inability to retrieve information from infant memory. Retention of information is directly proportional to the infant's age. As an infant grows older, the period for which information is retained increases.

As children grow older, they develop more effective and efficient strategies to retain information. During adolescence the brain enters a plastic period, particularly in the frontal lobes. Neuronal connections that control sleeping and eating habits, regulate motor behavior, and modulate impulses, decision making, memory, and other high-level cognitive functions change significantly during adolescence. Given the plasticity of the adolescent's brain, it is highly probable that environmental stimuli influence intrinsic changes in the adolescent's CNS.

Across the life span, some aspects of cognition seem to be impaired or changed before others. One area most susceptible to age-associated changes is the prefrontal cortex.

This particular area of the brain is where information critical to executive function, attention, and working memory is stored.[114] Although memory is one component of cognition that is generally acknowledged to deteriorate as an individual moves toward older adulthood, not all aspects of memory are affected at the same time or in the same way.

Episodic memory is reportedly the first to be impaired, then working memory (short-term memory).[114] Implicit memory and semantic memory remain intact for a much longer period of time. Little information is available about procedural memory, memory of how to perform tasks. Researchers have suggested that an older adult's declarative memory is also affected by normal and neuropathological aging.[42,114] These investigators suggested that although older adults with deterioration in declarative memory are able to perform tasks, the individual is unable to retain information and consequently unable to learn tasks.[42] Many factors negatively or positively influence memory, including the nature of encoding or processing that information, such as the source of the material or time of day material is presented.[114]

Although evidence exists that many aspects of memory decline with age, recent evidence supports the premise that variables other than encoding and retrieving information may have a significant impact on memory and remembering in older adults.[115,116] Researchers at the University of Kuopio examined memory in older persons and focused on neuropsychological processes as a method for evaluating memory and other functions of the frontal lobe.[116] The investigators reported that elderly subjects with subsequent degradation of the frontal lobe had memory loss. These researchers suggested that some aspects of memory loss could be staved off through memory-sharpening activities and games, limitation of alcohol consumption, and participation in activities designed to retain details of skills and tasks. Similar to these findings are the conclusions of May and colleagues,[115] who examined the role of emotion in memory tasks for older adults. They reported that older adults seem to be motivated to remember information that is emotionally relevant and meaningful. These findings lend support to yet another system, the emotive system, which could add vital information to an older adult's memory and task performance.

Emotional System

Although current literature does examine the emotional development of children,[117-125] the normal emotional development of adults over a life span remains a mystery. Zinck and Newen[126] proposed a classification of emotion that might provide a clearer understanding of responses within and between individuals and factors that affect emotion. The authors characterized emotion into four categories based on when the emotions appear developmentally. Emotion is characterized as a means of communicating state, expectations, and reactions of an individual.[126] Emotions are "interpersonal/interactive" behaviors that enable the individual to communicate to the world. The four categories are pre-emotions, basic emotions, primary cognitive emotions, and secondary cognitive emotions. Pre-emotions and basic emotions function as basic mental representations, whereas primary cognitive and secondary cognitive emotions are categorized as cognitive attitudes.

Pre-emotions are characterized as innate behaviors, present at birth, nonspecific, nonintentional, and used for communication to others about the state of the infant.[126] Pre-emotions are identified as comfort and distress. These responses may be positive or negative responses depending on the situations. Pre-emotions are the most fundamental sensations followed by basic emotions.

Basic emotions and developmental timing of basic emotions include joy at 2 to 3 months, anger at 3 to 4 months, sadness at 3 to 7 months, and fear at 7 to 9 months. These emotions are said to emerge in the absence of conscious processing of stimuli. These responses are shared by other mammals, and do not involve complex cognitive processing. These behaviors lead to faster and more stereotypic responses.[126]

Primary cognitive emotions are characterized as basic emotions with more specificity, in addition to a cognitive component. Primary cognitive emotions are highly dependent on the individual's cognitive development as well as cultural variations and socialization.

Secondary cognitive emotions are depicted as complex constructs that involve social relations, with consideration for expectations of the future. Consequently, secondary cognitive emotions are highly dependent on personal experiences and culture. The authors provide an example of how one situation—high performance in academics—would be perceived by different cultures. Whereas a child from one culture might receive praise for and exhibit pride in high academic performance, a child from another culture could have such performance deemphasized and display shame. In addition to cognition, secondary cognitive emotions incorporate social constructs of family, culture, previous experiences, and environment in formulating complex responses. These responses are cumulative, using previous experiences to render new responses.

Typically, emotional "development" emerges in childhood. Examination of emotion in adults often involves a retrospective analysis of the behavior over a specified period of time. Although the focus of the research may be directed toward emotion, memory cannot be disentangled from the emotion. With regard to aging in older adults, researchers generally have reported that emotions—in particular, negative emotions—diminish later in life. Some researchers have suggested that diminished negative emotions may be attributed to decreased functioning in the amygdala.[127] Still other investigators have suggested that, rather, a decline in the functioning of the amygdala and decreased ability to recall negative experiences may be attributed to the socioemotional selectivity theory (SST).[128] The SST involves prioritization of memories and which temporal boundaries play a role in prioritization. Specifically, older adults do not perceive negative emotions as a priority; hence older adults are more likely to process positive emotions than negative.

A literature search of "normal emotional development across the life span" was limited in scope and volume.[129] Problems in normal emotional development can be identified throughout medical literature, but again the emphasis is on children and adulthood emotional problems stemming from either pathological conditions or environmental conditions during childhood.[130-135] Within the literature, the reader can find discussions of emotional intelligence in adults and how emotional skills such as empathy or cultural sensitivity might be taught.[136-142] Specific aspects of an emotion or mood change and how that might assist or hinder an individual within a psychosocial environment can be located,[143-146] but the integration of the entire emotional system and its normal changes throughout life still eludes researchers. Future research directed toward aging and emotion has potential to broaden the theoretical perspective by examining emotional experiences in an ecological context.[147] In addition, identifying, measuring, and analyzing variables that appear to make a difference in social and professional success will be future scholars' dissertation studies.[148] (See Chapter 5 on the limbic system and its influence on motor control and Chapter 9 on psychosocial adaptation and adjustment for additional information.)

Language

Consistent with all areas of development, acquisition of language, receptive and expressive, is measured quantitatively and qualitatively. Critical to the acquisition of receptive and expressive language is sensory, cognitive, perceptual, and motor development in the infant and child. Researchers have found evidence that language development emerges through nonverbal gestures or "signs"[149-153] and is evident as early as 6 months of age.[152,153] As the number of nonverbal gestures increases, verbal communication reportedly emerges earlier than in infants who do not use nonverbal gestures.[150,152,153] "Gesture thus serves as a signal that a child will soon be ready to begin producing multi-word sentences."[154] Having a large number of gestures at 18 months of age positively affects later language development and is the foundation for later linguistic abilities.[151]

Imitation, such as "mama" or "dada," is often the first form of verbal communication, progressing to spontaneous single-word utterances. Infants produce their first spoken single-word utterances as early as 12 to 15 months of age.[155] During this time the child's brain is undergoing rapid differentiation in Broca's area; at the same time, motoric ability to communicate verbally is emerging. Consequently it is evident that intrinsic (neurodevelopmental) constraints and extrinsic (environmental) factors affect the emergence of receptive and expressive language. Investigators examining utterances in children and adults reported that utterances produced by children do not approximate those of adults until 14 years of age.[156,157] Recently researchers reported that, consistent with findings of earlier investigators, articulatory movement speed increases from birth to adulthood.[157] Throughout childhood, as language acquisition emerges, children become more sophisticated in communicating and more fully integrate information from intrinsic and extrinsic sources to produce more complex utterances.[155]

Maner and colleagues[156] reported that children exhibited increased variability when a five-word sentence was embedded in longer sentences than when the child spoke only the five-word sentence. These findings led the investigators to infer that a relationship existed between language processing and movement in young children.[158] In addition, adults reportedly modified the five-word sentence when it was embedded in the longer sentence, but 5-year-olds did not modify the utterance. Sadagopan and Smith[159] replicated the work of Maner and colleagues[156] and found that children aged 5 to 16 years exhibited more variability when the five-word sentence was embedded in a more complex sentence compared with when the five-word sentence was spoken in isolation. Young adults (21 to 22 years old) reportedly did not exhibit this same variability. In addition, investigators reported that the duration of the simple and complex utterances differed between children and adults. Unlike the youngest children (5 and 7 years), duration of the utterances decreased in adults. This finding provided evidence for the investigators' theory that adults altered or shortened the complex utterances, given the shorter duration taken to utter the complex sentence. Whereas earlier researchers reported that both adults and children decrease their rate of speech during complex sentences,[160] more recently investigators suggested that adults may increase their rate of speech production. Sadagopan and Smith[159] reported that although both children and adults slow the rate of speech production, children exhibited a much slower rate than adults in producing complex sentences. Hence investigators concluded that whereas adults' rate of speech production did explain some of the difference in utterance duration for the simple and complex sentences, it did not fully explain the differences. This led investigators to suggest that differences in utterance duration may be attributed to both faster rate of speech and altered or shortened complex sentences containing the simple five-word phrase.

The dynamic nature of language is grounded in the constructs of dynamical systems theory involving intrinsic and extrinsic mechanisms. These mechanisms evolve over time and are highly sensitive to changes within and between systems.

Perceptual System

As researchers continue to examine the interactive and interdependent roles of body systems, the perceptual system must not be omitted. Perception, yet another process important to performance of functional movements, involves acquisition, interpretation, selection, and organization of sensory information. Perception is the very essence of the interaction between organism and environment. Every movement gives rise to perceptual information and in turn guides the organism to adapt movements accordingly.[10,161]

Initially perception revolves around the infant's visual exploration of people, objects, and environmental activities. Infants are capable, at birth, of visually exploring their environment, people, and objects.[101] Investigators have suggested that infants use information acquired through visual exploration to develop new methods of exploring and discovering cues about the environment such as depth, distance, surface definition, and dimensionality of objects.[162]

A second phase of perceptual exploration emerges as an infant's exploratory behaviors transition to functional movements such as reaching and kicking. Through these exploratory behaviors emerge additional mechanisms for acquiring information about the environment.[6,161] Throughout development, active exploration enhances perceptual information through each new encounter and enables the infant to recognize distinctive features and similar characteristics that allow the infant to differentiate between objects. The information generated from exploration provides new input to many subsystems, in particular the sensory, motor, and cognitive systems that enable the individual to gain new knowledge about the environment and the action.

Development of the infant's perceptual system is dependent on acquiring new information about the affordances of the task that may influence performance of the action. As the infant develops the capacity for independent mobility, the expanse of the environment increases, as do the opportunities to integrate prior knowledge with newly acquired information to discover unchartered surroundings. This again supports the interactive and interdependent nature of systems throughout development. As maturation progresses, infants develop the ability to evaluate information acquired from various systems and to make decisions about the optimal strategy for successfully navigating over or around a surface. With maturation, successful navigation of new environments depends on opportunities for exploration that may involve other processes in addition to motor processes. An example of this may be seen in a person trying to locate a building in an unfamiliar city. Adults typically use maps as a visual representation of the surroundings that allow them to find the location. Infants and young children are most accurate in locating desired targets through active exploration. This allows the child to acquire spatial information critical to locating the destination at a future time.

If perception is the process of integrating and organizing intrinsic and extrinsic input, then changes in sensory systems as a consequence of aging are certain to affect perception.[163] The visual perceptual processing system is most often identified as altered in older adults. Specifically, researchers have reported that although older adults are capable of discriminating between variation in depth perception in a manner similar to that of younger adults, they are less able to discriminate between three-dimensional shapes of objects.[164] Clearly the perceptual system is closely associated with many other body systems, and therefore age-related or age-associated structural and functional changes in associated systems will affect the perceptual system.

In addition, May and colleagues[115] found that older adults placed less emphasis on perceptual aspects of an event than they did on the emotional components when encoding information. They suggested that older adults may find emotional information to be more meaningful than perceptual information and may retain more elaborate, detailed processing of emotional data than perceptual information.

Although there is no conclusive evidence regarding age-related changes in perception, evidence may be emerging that supports age-associated or individual differences.[165] Nonetheless, the role of perception in aging should continue to be investigated and should not be underestimated or minimized until such time as adequate evidence exists.

MOTOR DEVELOPMENT

Movement is the primary mechanism by which prelinguistic children communicate with their environment. That said, it is no wonder that development of motor skills is greatest during the first 2 years of life. Motor development may be defined as the acquisition, refinement, and integration of biomechanical principles of movement in an effort to achieve a motor behavior that is proficient.[11]

Early developmental researchers referred to infants as *reactive,* inferring that, early on, infants are responsive to stimuli rather than capable of initiating functional movements. Young infants were characterized as "reflexive" beings producing stereotypic primitive and postural responses to stimuli. Emergence of these reflexive motor behaviors was based on traditional models of CNS organization and motor development theories. Traditional theories of human development emerged from animal models and studies involving spontaneously aborted fetuses.[14,166] Traditionally, sucking and stepping behaviors were examples of developmental reflexes. By definition, a reflex is a consistent response to a consistent stimulus. By use of traditional models of CNS organization, developmental reflexes, present at birth, become integrated as higher centers assume control over lower centers and then volitional movements begin to emerge.

Over the past two to three decades, advances in technology have enabled scientists to gain more insight into fetal and infant motor abilities. More recently, research has generated evidence that behaviors emerge out of a need to solve a problem in the environment rather than solely as a result of maturation in the CNS.[167] Given this evidence supporting the premise that newborn infants are capable of producing complex volitional movements, previous views of the infant as passive and "reflexive" are no longer accurate. In addition, continuing to refer to early infant motor behaviors as "reflexes" may also not accurately reflect the behavior. A reflex is defined as a consistent response given in response to a consistent stimulus. Perhaps use of the term *innate motor behaviors* to reflect behaviors that are present at birth may be more appropriate. See Figure 3-1, *A* to *C,* for a visual explanation of how the complexity of the stepping reaction of a newborn infant and the learned programming for upright posture and balance, including biomechanical range and force production, will lead to the integration of stepping in standing. Similarly, as an individual ages, loss of some of the postural power, effectiveness of balance reactions, and fear can create a potentially dangerous environment for an elderly person (Figure 3-1, *D* to *E*). Likewise, an individual with an abnormal or inefficient stepping pattern (Figure 3-1, *F*) should automatically stand out to a therapist analyzing movement dysfunction. If a clinician does not have a clear picture in his or her mind of the movement pattern desired, then easily or quickly identifying the system or subsystem motor impairments seen in a client's movement dysfunction may be outside a therapist's analytical repertoire.

Contemporary research refutes the assertion that infants are reactive organisms.[95,96] In contrast, contemporary studies purport that infants are competent and capable of producing complex interactive behaviors at birth.[101,168] Additional support for the complex nature of a newborn infant is evident in the infant's ability to discriminate and turn toward his or her mother's voice rather than toward the voice of an adult with whom the infant is unfamiliar.

Evidence from studies examining motor development indicate that motor behaviors do not always emerge in a linear and predictable sequence, nor do all individuals achieve the same skills at the same chronological age.[8,168] Rather, emergence of motor behaviors in an alternate sequence may be attributed to the intrinsic and extrinsic constraints that contribute to motor development in a nonlinear fashion and is not necessarily indicative of atypical development. Figure 3-2, *A* is an example of a child who had a very large head at birth. His head circumference was in the

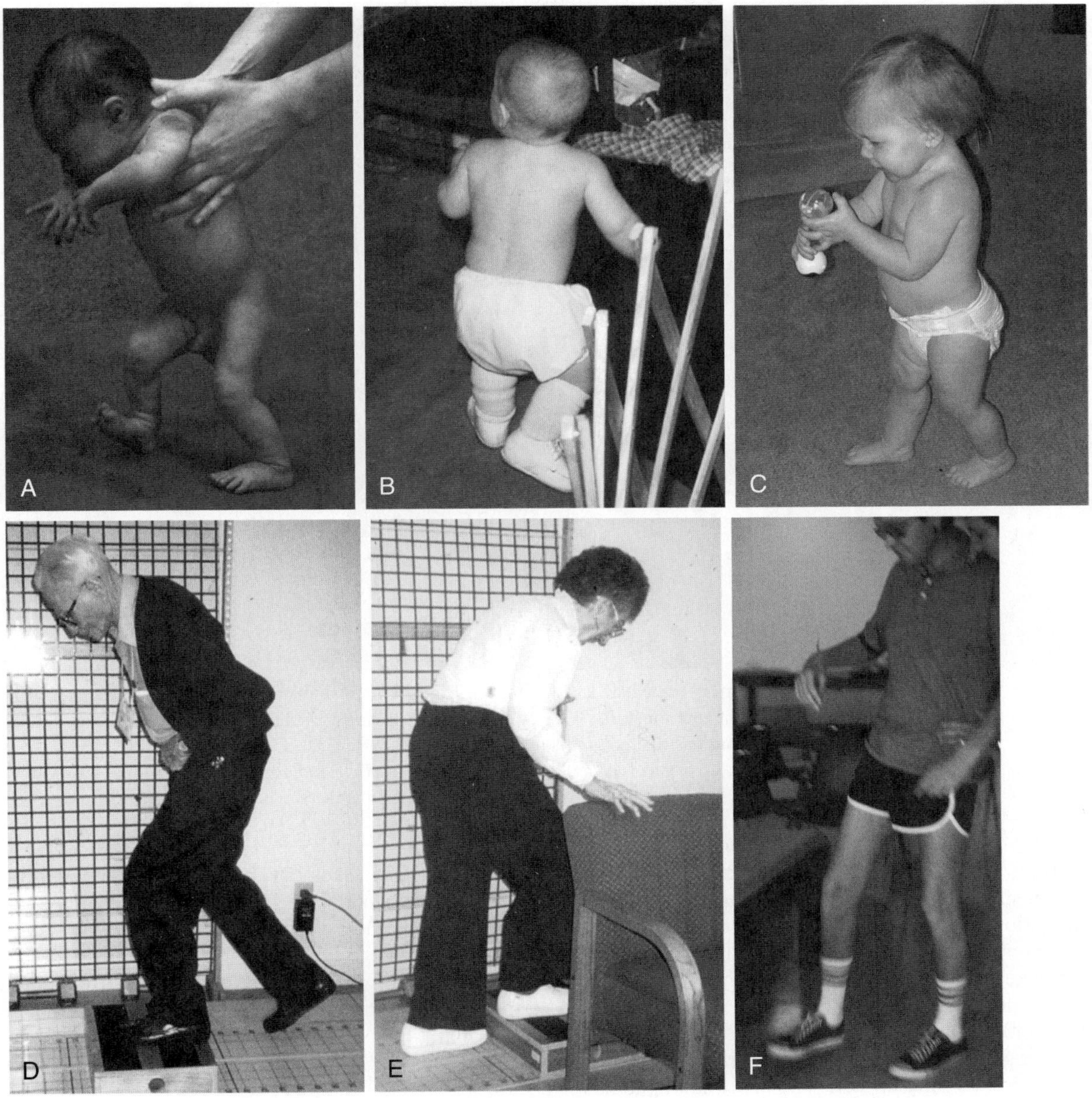

Figure 3-1 ■ Development and integration of stepping, upright vertical posture, and vertical balance reaction: **A,** automatic stepping in a newborn infant; **B,** early cruising or side-stepping using multiple points of support; **C,** early bipedal independent stepping; **D,** 90-year-old client stepping; **E,** 78-year-old client with falling problems; **F,** abnormal stepping after traumatic brain injury.

99.9th percentile and remained so for the first 3 years of his life. His Apgar score at birth was 10, or normal. He was slow in rolling over and coming to sit and spent much of his time playing with his hands and feet and visually exploring the environment. Figure 3-2, *B* and *C* illustrate that his focus was on fine motor development throughout his first year, especially when he was placed in a vertical position. He loved to play catch when placed in a sitting position and accurately trajected the ball toward a partner when playing by age 1 year. His early gross motor development was within the normal range but below the mean. He started independently walking at age 14 months and began running on the same day. Figure 3-2, *D* through *F* illustrate that once he gained control over the heavy weight of his head, he quickly caught up in gross motor skill. And, like any child, he has taken full advantage of his environment to play and learn.

Motor performance, measured both qualitatively and quantitatively, is highly dependent on the task, the environment, and the individual. Changes in motor performance emerge in accordance with age-dependent changes, within different systems, and with respect to environmental affordances and constraints. As skills emerge in speech, language, and cognition, other previously achieved skills may "regress." In reality, acquisition of a new skill requires more attention than the previously attained skills; consequently, the infant or child's attention is divided between the tasks. Lindenberger and colleagues[169-171] conducted studies investigating life span changes in resource allocation during multitask activities. The researchers found that for young

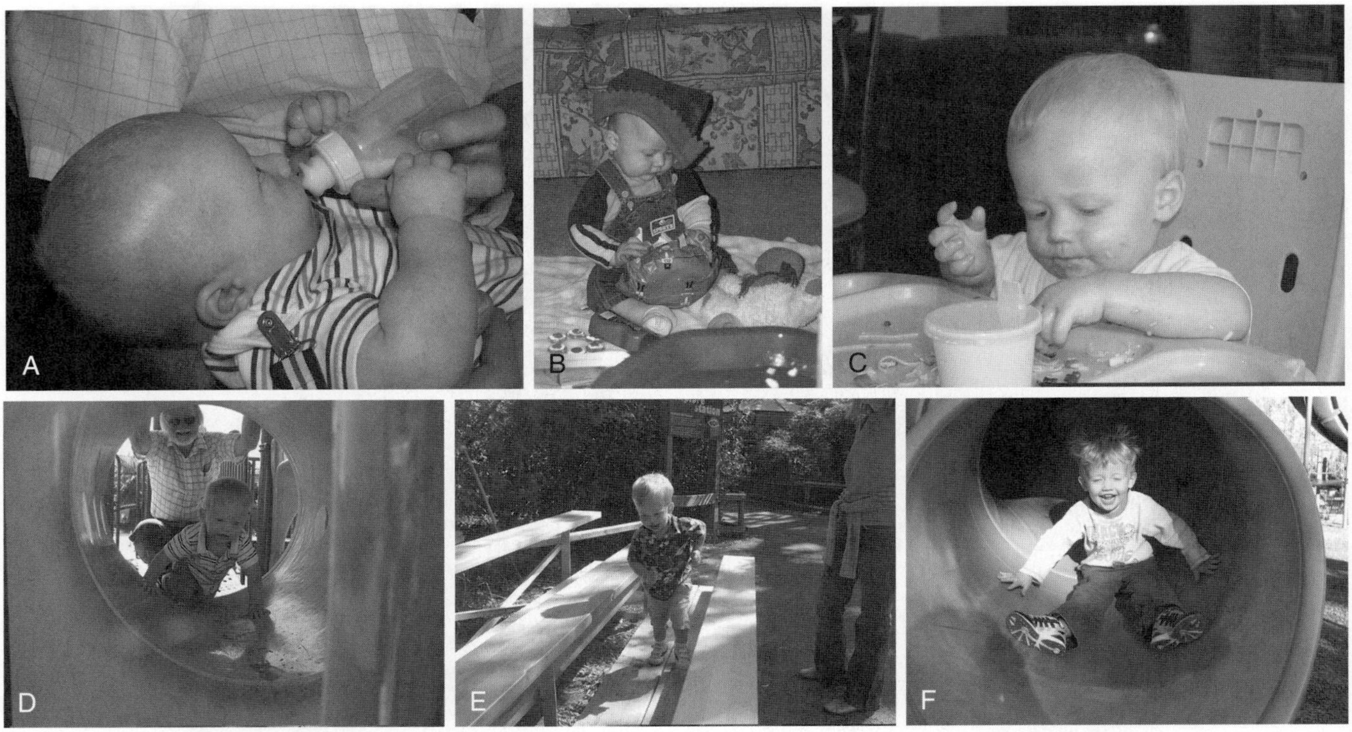

Figure 3-2 ■ Head size can affect when a child initiates independent movement activities and whether he develops gross or fine motor skills. **A,** A 2-month-old being fed (note large head). **B,** Child at 5 months old placed in sitting has overcome delayed head control in vertical. **C,** By 9 months old, the child has gained normal head control as well as fine motor skills. **D**, Head control in horizontal crawling. **E,** Child running at 2 years of age. **F,** Normal head control on slide. By 1 year of age, head size is no longer a variable.

children certain tasks require more attention, and attempting to perform such a task in conjunction with a task requiring less attention causes deterioration in performance of both tasks. Hence, deterioration of a previously attained skill is more likely a result of attentional demands of young children performing high-attention tasks rather than a true "regression" of the skill (see Chapter 1, Figure 1-9, p. 18). This progression is illustrated by a child confronted with a new environment, who will seem as if he or she has regressed in motor performance while confronting and solving a task-specific challenge—for example, crossing over a suspension bridge that moves from side to side, is compliant to body weight, and creates a perceptual challenge from the visual surround. Once the child understands the task, his attention is directed toward developing effective strategies to solve a problem and successfully perform the motor behavior of crossing the bridge. Stability or consistency in performing a skilled movement is achieved by self-organization through practice and repetition.[21] Performance of skilled movements, such as those observed in athletes, is measured not only on the consistency in performing the task but also on the skilled performance of the task under variable conditions.[21] Conversely, decreased frequency in performing a motor skill as an effect of age may result in a less rich repertoire of normal variability and may be a contributing factor to a decline in motor skills.[30] Just as motor skills emerge from a multifactorial interweaving of maturation and experience, deterioration in motor performance may be attributable to alterations in various systems that occur as part of the aging process. Emergence of motor behaviors is never the same for any two individuals, nor does decline in functional motor behaviors follow the same time line. Figure 3-3 illustrates how standing patterns will change with practice, be maintained as long as practice continues, become extremely efficient within a specific environmental context, or become deficient after CNS injury.

Prenatal (0 to 40 Weeks' Gestation) Development

Motor behaviors emerge early in embryonic life. By the tenth week of fetal life the variety of observed movements increases, as does the frequency of the movements. Complex movements are present by gestational age (GA) 12 weeks, and goal-directed movements may be seen as early as GA 13 weeks. Facial movements, including sucking, swallowing, and yawning, are evident in the second and third trimesters. The fetal activity level increases so that by week 14 GA, periods of quiet (no activity) are only 5 to 6 minutes in duration. Investigators have documented 15 fetal movements visible by 15 weeks of age.[172] After initial observation of a motor behavior, it remains part of the fetal repertoire. Pooh and Ogura's[172] research lends support to the premise that before delivery fetuses are in fact capable of producing complex motor behaviors.

The dynamic nature of birth and the associated change from the intrauterine to the extrauterine environment alter the production of movements previously observed in fetal life.[65] As the newborn infant adapts to the forces in the extrauterine environment, motor behaviors emerge. These

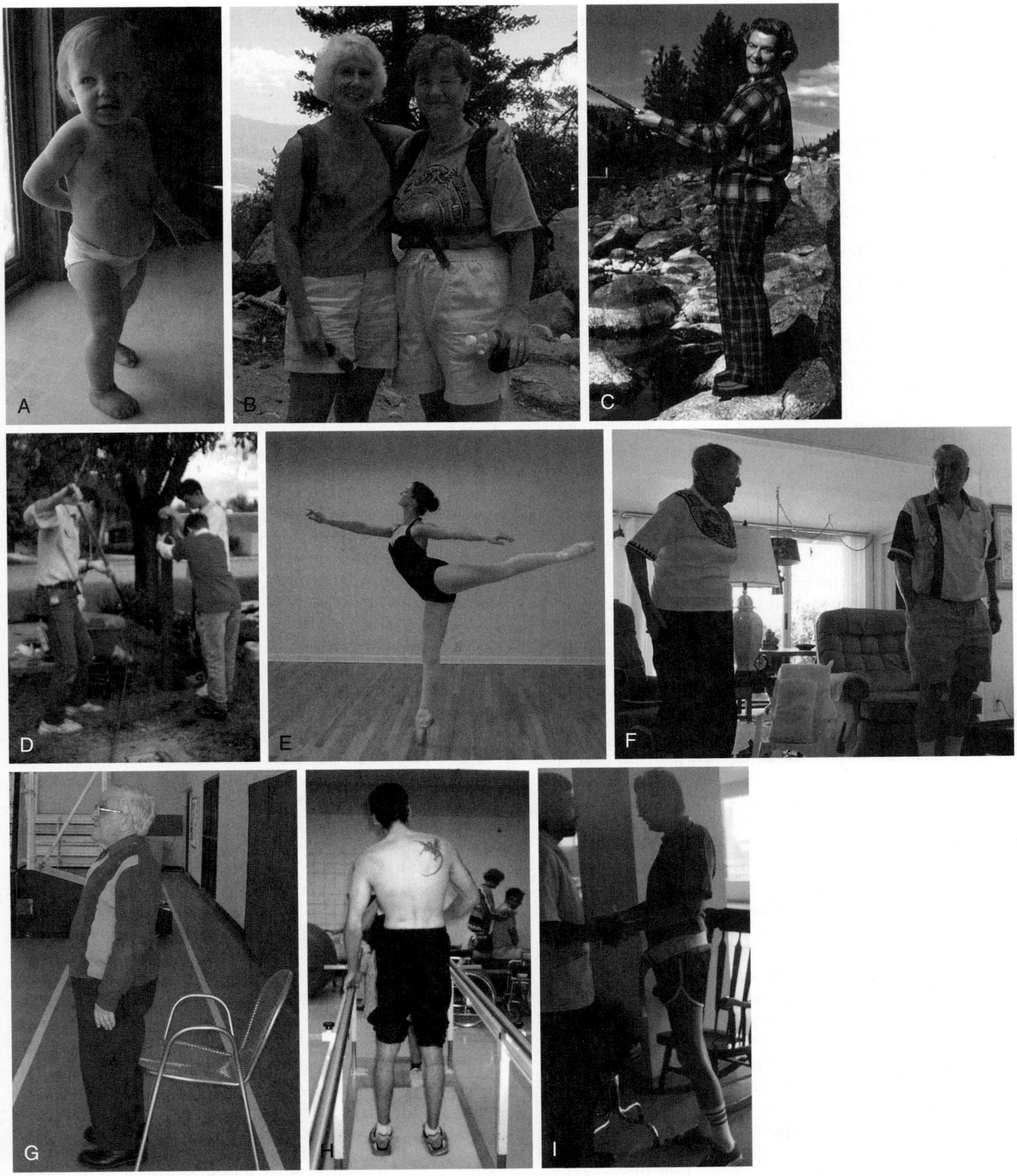

Figure 3-3 ■ Standing as a functional activity will become procedural with practice and be maintained over a lifetime as long as impairments do not preclude practice or injury to the central nervous system (CNS): **A,** early standing; **B,** relaxed standing as adults; **C,** standing on uneven surfaces; **D,** procedural standing during a functional activity; **E,** advanced skill in standing as ballet dancer; **F,** maintained functional standing in healthy 83-year-old elderly couple; **G,** elderly man developing verticality impairment; **H,** subtle abnormal standing after head injury; and **I,** multiple subsystem problems in standing after CNS injury.

complex behaviors lend additional evidence to the premise that at birth infants are competent beings.

The extrauterine environment poses many challenges for the newborn infant. Consequently, fetal behaviors observed by ultrasonography may not be evident postnatally until the infant learns to adapt to the new environment by modifying movements to accommodate to the new forces imposed by gravity. Newborn infants must learn to use new strategies to generate functional motor behaviors, given the different environmental constraints.

Infancy (Birth to 12 Months)

As alluded to earlier, newborn infants possess a rich array of motor behaviors. During the first year of life, motor behaviors are the primary mechanism for learning. Every movement is a new and unique opportunity to gain knowledge about the environment. During each movement, new information is gathered in an effort to solve environmental problems, and as a result this motor planning fosters cognitive development. Similarly, each movement provides feedback that intrinsically enables the infant to modify movements in accordance with changes in the environment, the skill, or growth parameters.[173] This interdependence between perception and motor behaviors allows one domain to facilitate acquisition of skills in the other domain in a reciprocal fashion.

Given the capabilities of a newborn infant, many behaviors previously identified as reflexes are in fact functional motor behaviors that the infant is capable of modifying. Evidence that one such behavior, sucking, is not a reflex was supported by studies examining sucking rates when stimuli were varied.[174,175] Researchers reported that the sucking response varied depending on the level of hunger or environmental stimuli. In addition, when the stimulus is introduced after feeding, after the infant is satiated, the stimulus may produce no response or a diminished response, thus refuting the idea that sucking is reflexive.

Consequently, rather than refer to these behaviors as *developmental reflexes,* it seems more accurate to refer to such motor behaviors, evident at birth, as *innate motor behaviors.* Innate motor behaviors are, in essence, functional behaviors present at birth that are modifiable given alterations in feedback from intrinsic or extrinsic mechanisms.

Additional evidence exists to refute the concept that other motor behaviors are reflexes. Stepping is one such behavior. Thelan and Fisher[18,32,33] conducted a series of experiments examining the stepping reflex in young infants. Early developmentalists hypothesized that stepping reflexes, present at birth, became integrated and then later emerged as a volitionally controlled movement. Thelan and Fisher[18,33] found that when one variable, weight, was altered, infants mimicked "integration" or emergence of the behavior. Young infants who were stepping had weights added to their lower extremities, to simulate weight gain over the first few months. These infants stopped stepping. Similarly, infants who did not step were submersed in chest deep water, simulating less weight in the lower extremities, and stepping appeared. Obviously, the presence and absence of this behavior was mediated by weight gain in the lower extremities and not by CNS control as early developmental researchers had postulated. Consequently, upright mobility emerges when the infant is able to garner the force production in the lower extremities to modulate stepping. This is just one example of the significance of one system on another and the interdependent nature of body systems. Recognizing the interdependence of systems may provide one explanation for the presence or absence of motor behaviors at any given time. These concepts have been transferred into the therapeutic practice environment when working with individuals who cannot generate enough force to produce the movement given the body size or cannot produce the postural stability to reinforce the stepping pattern or one of a variety of other motor components that support normal upright stepping or walking. (See Chapter 4 for theories of motor control and learning, Chapter 8 for therapeutic approaches to assist a client with learning or relearning motor control, and Chapter 37, which introduces emerging practices to bridge the gap between normal human movement development and technologies.)

At birth, an infant is capable of turning toward the sound of her or his mother's voice and visually focusing on objects 8 to 12 inches from the face.[101] These behaviors are apparent when the infant's head is supported, given that at birth the newborn infant does not have the neck strength to maintain head control against gravity. Similarly, auditory and visual stimuli continue to bombard the infant and challenge the motor system, fostering the need to attain head control.

Infant motor behaviors during the first 3 months of life are focused on acquisition of head control in all planes of movement. Once the infant has achieved head control in the supine and prone positions, the complexity of the tasks increases exponentially on the basis of the new challenges and stimuli presented to the infant. For example, while in the prone position an infant may reach for an object out of reach and then roll to attain the desired object. Improvements in visual acuity enable an infant to visually track people and objects at greater distances while challenging the infant to seek out the stimuli.

By age 3 to 4 months, as the infant is able to maintain head control in the upright position for longer periods, coordinated eye-hand activities begin to emerge. Acquisition of manipulative skills involves perception and lends support for the coupling of developing cognitive, sensory, and motor systems.[23,161] Bushnell and Boudreau[6] added that if the infant is unable to achieve a motor skill and this skill is coupled with a sensory or cognitive task, that task may not be attained. Bushnell and Boudreau's[6] research focused on the role of motor development in achieving skills in other domains.

Reaching is one such task that the researchers suggest may serve to promote skills in cognitive and sensory domains. Initial reaching activities enable the infant to gain information relevant to depth perception, and coupling this information then allows the infant to modulate parameters associated with reaching. For example, the infant must learn to vary the distance moved and force necessary to attain an object given a series of opportunities. Infant grasping and reaching may initially seem inefficient, but with practice under varying situations efficiency and accuracy improve across multiple domains with varying rates. Figure 3-4 illustrates both the error that provides feedback and the success during complex movement patterns after practice.

As infants develop an upright sitting posture, they use their upper extremities for support. Sitting, a functional motor

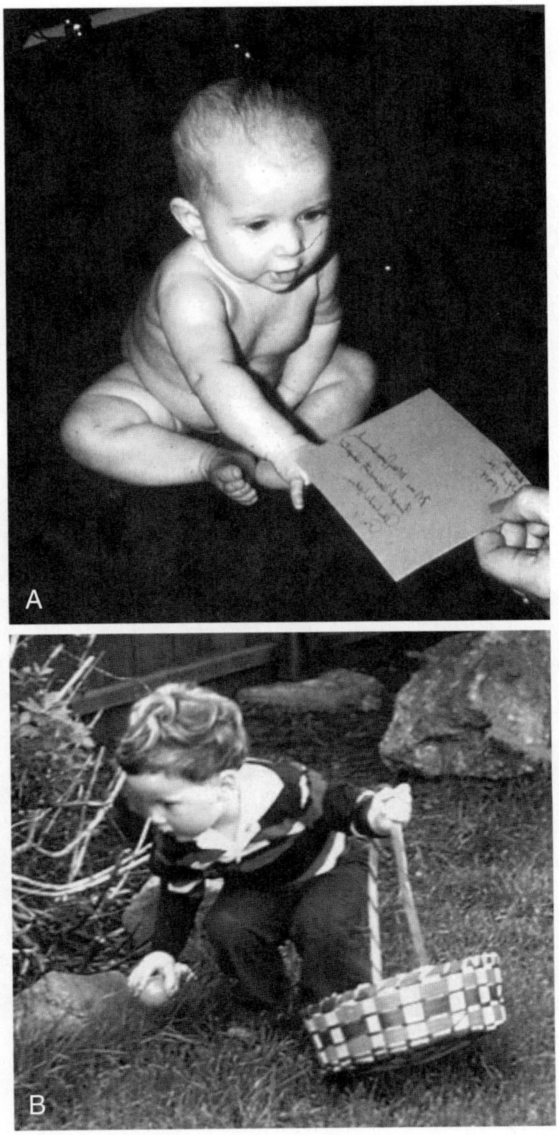

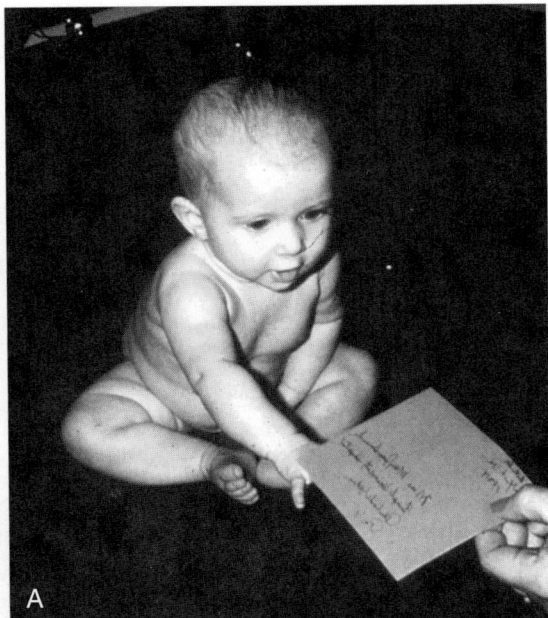

Figure 3-4 ■ Reaching activity. **A,** Error in reaching leads to learning, and **B,** reaching becomes accurate during a complex motor task.

behavior, is tightly linked to the performance of most ADLs and occupational and leisure-time activities. Figure 3-5 depicts development of functional sitting over a lifetime. A delay in attaining independent sitting may directly affect upper extremity control, alter attainment of skills in other domains, and ultimately affect an individual's level of functional independence.

As upright trunk posture is attained and independent sitting emerges, usually by 6 months of age, and infants then begin to explore using their manipulative skills. Manipulative skills are composed of reaching and grasping behaviors. Upper-extremity interlimb coordination bimanual and unimanual tasks include retrieving objects (placed within reach); holding two objects, one in each hand; using two hands to hold an object (bottle); and holding a toy in one hand while retrieving another object with the free hand.[176]

During the second half of year 1, the infant is focused on mobility, initially prone (rolling, crawling), then creeping on all fours, and then upright (cruising and ambulation). Adolph and Berger[23] reported that as coordination of upper- and lower-extremity movements with trunk control emerges and infants begin upright mobility, they spend up to 50% of their day performing balance- and mobility-based activities, varying the surface, distance, and other parameters each time the task is performed (Figure 3-6). On the basis of research conducted with infants acquiring independent mobility, Adolph and Berger[23] estimate that an infant walks up to 29 football fields each day.

Acquisition of independent mobility is complicated by new manipulative skills, as discussed by Corbetta and Thelan.[176] They found that while infants are achieving independent mobility, their manipulative skills are highly variable and vacillate between bimanual and unimanual tasks depending on the nature of other tasks with which the infant is involved. Infants may revert to performing bimanual activities, with upper extremities coupled and movements synchronized, during early acquisition of independent mobility, signaling the presence of multiple tasks requiring attention. Unimanual control signals uncoupling of the upper extremities and asynchronous manipulation in young children.

Analyzing the early development of a child is often done at specific times over the first year, such as at birth, 2 months, 6 months, and 9 months. As important as understanding and analyzing a complex phase of development such as 3 months is analyzing the changes in motor control and learning of a specific motor function over a period of time. The development of head control is a good example of how the nervous system adapts and learns given different environmental restraints over a period of time. The complexity and integration of movement patterns involved in a child gaining functional control over the head in all spatial environments can be delineated into many components. Each component can then become a variable in determining how and if a child has or will develop a specific movement pattern such as head control (see Figure 3-2).

Early Childhood (1 Year to 5 Years)

Whereas the first year of life is characterized by periods of rapid physical growth and acquisition of motor skills, the second year signals a slower rate of growth, refinement of current skills, and acquisition of new motor skills.[177] Concurrently the toddler experiences rapid differentiation in other domains including cognition, speech, and social-emotional domains.

At the onset of the second year of life, independent ambulation becomes refined as other forms of mobility wane. Dynamic balance in an upright bipedal posture evolves as the infant develops more mature gait characteristics. Modification of parameters indicative of a more mature gait include narrowing of the base of support, decreased co-contraction in the lower extremities, and improved intralimb coordination, as well as learning to modulate displacement and velocity.[23] As gait matures and toddlers have more opportunity to explore their environment, more challenges appear. Attempts to solve these problems and challenges result in the appearance of more complex motor behaviors that include running, climbing, and jumping. Toddlers find particular pleasure in throwing, kicking, and catching balls. In addition, toddlers assert their independence through such activities as propelling themselves with riding toys.

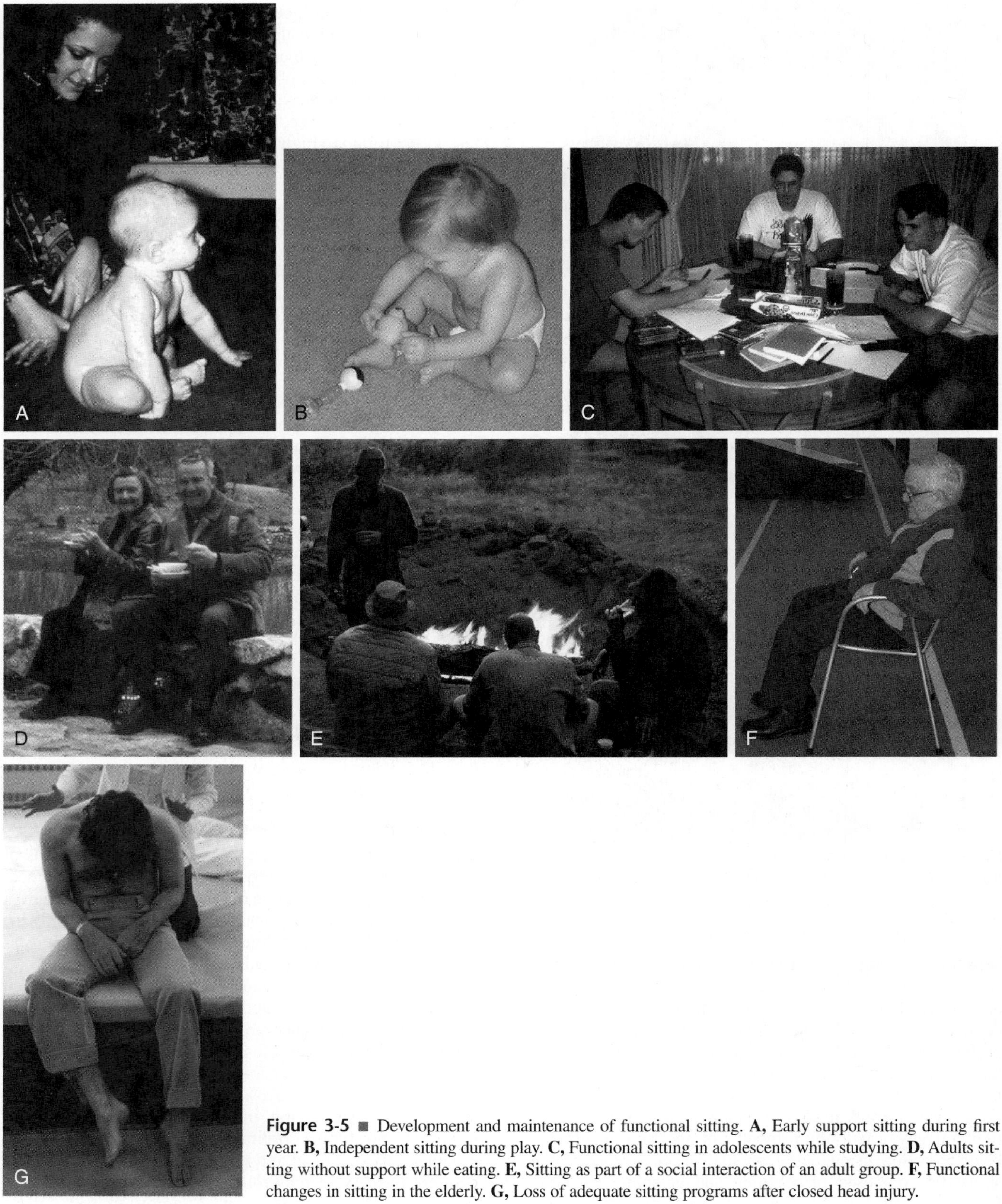

Figure 3-5 ■ Development and maintenance of functional sitting. **A,** Early support sitting during first year. **B,** Independent sitting during play. **C,** Functional sitting in adolescents while studying. **D,** Adults sitting without support while eating. **E,** Sitting as part of a social interaction of an adult group. **F,** Functional changes in sitting in the elderly. **G,** Loss of adequate sitting programs after closed head injury.

Toddlers continue to explore and assert independence through activities involving bimanual and unimanual tasks. Challenges to fine motor skills of toddlers involve manipulating functional objects (large buttons, eating utensils, crayons, door knobs, and blocks; opening and closing jars to retrieve small objects [cereal, raisins]). Achieving these tasks enables the toddler to perform rudimentary aspects of ADLs such as eating and dressing and adds another degree of independence. Figure 3-7 illustrates development of ambulatory skill over a lifetime.

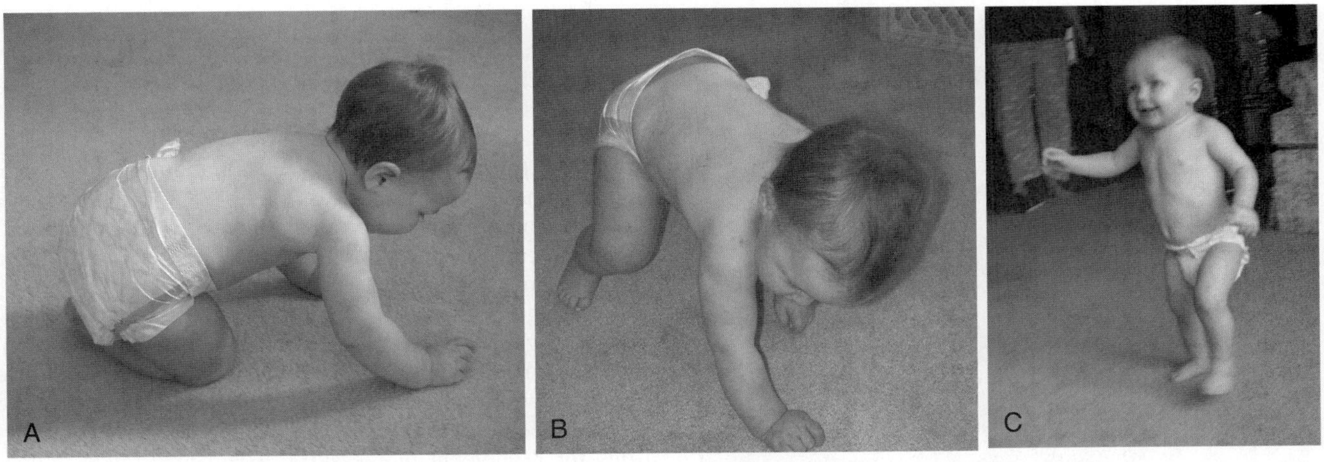

Figure 3-6 ■ Emergence of upright mobility: **A,** quadruped in preparation for quadrupedal creeping, **B,** moving from quadruped into standing, and **C,** moving in vertical.

Preschool-age children pedal a tricycle and use a narrow base of support to walk along a balance beam. By age 3 years most children ascend stairs using alternating feet and by 4 years most descend stairs alternately. Figure 3-8 shows a preschooler descending stairs. The gait pattern matures with reciprocal arm swing and a heel-to-toe gait pattern. Early in the preschool period, children mimic a "true" run and have difficulty efficiently controlling all aspects of the behavior. Finally, receipt and propulsion of balls of all shapes and sizes improve qualitatively.

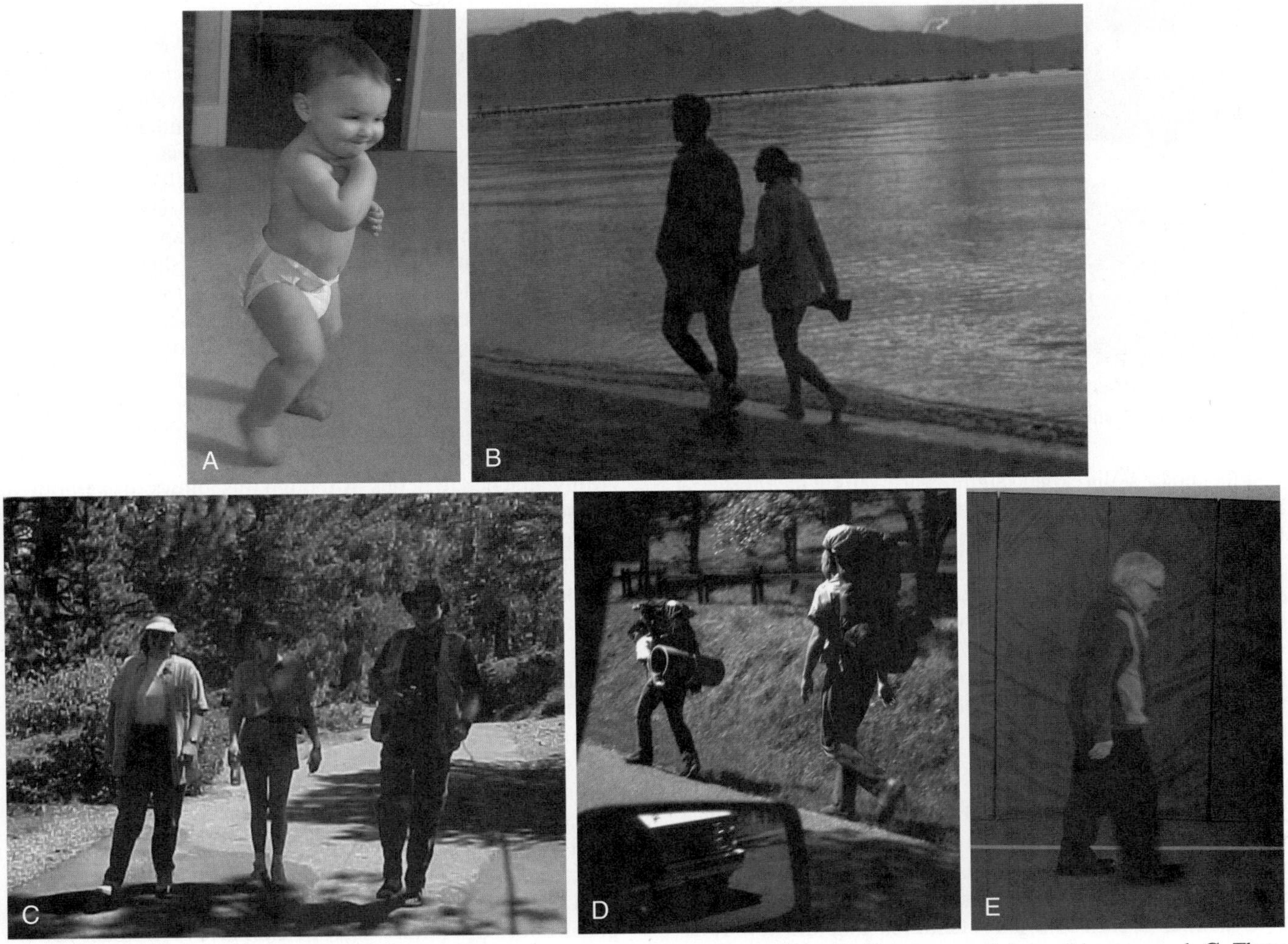

Figure 3-7 ■ Functional ambulation over the life span. **A,** Early independent walking. **B,** Two young adults walking on sand. **C,** Three adults of different body sizes, each walking independently. **D,** Hiking with backpacks requires motor adaptations. **E,** Elderly man walking with visual guidance instead of visual anticipation, creating potential functional impairments.

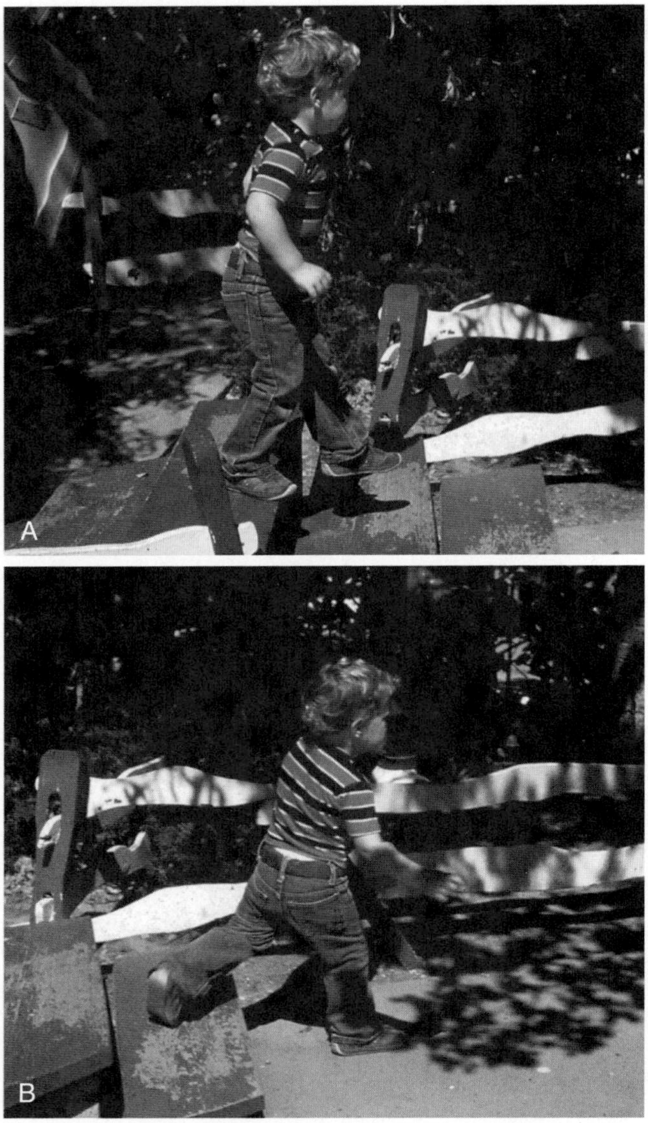

Figure 3-8 ■ Child descending stairs successfully: **A,** attention on stepping down and **B,** success at the task.

Fine motor skills expand significantly during the preschool period. The environmental demands of preschool and day care preparation for entering primary grades are the driving force behind acquisition of many manipulative behaviors. Most children begin to cut with scissors, copy circles or crosses, use a crayon to trace a circle, match colors, and often demonstrate hand preference. Although maturity certainly plays a role in skill performance, the efficiency with which skills are performed is also influenced by genetics, affordances and constraints of the environment, practice, and intrinsic motivation.

Childhood (5 to 10 Years)

Childhood is characterized as a period when children begin their formalized education, usually in a structured environment separate from their families. Consequently, a new set of dynamics comes into play. Children take on new roles with peers and adults outside of the family. During this period of social-emotional change, other systems also undergo changes.

Motor skills that children display during this period include galloping, hopping on one foot for up to 10 hops (hopscotch), jumping rope, kicking a ball with improved control (soccer), and bouncing a large ball (basketball). Often these skills emerge while playing with peers during directed (physical education or community-based team sports) and nondirected (recess) periods. Mobility, balance, and fine motor skills improve dramatically. Girls and boys exhibit similar abilities in speed up to age 7 years but by age 8 years boys begin to outperform girls.[177]

During childhood, manipulative skills increase exponentially. Figure 3-9, *A* through *E,* shows the amazing skill developed between birth and age 4 years. Manipulative skills assume a predominant role as part of the academic experience, requiring high levels of practice and opportunities for refinement of the skills. Hand preference is confirmed by this age. As components of independence, many of the manipulative skills achieved are directly related to self-care activities. Skills that improve dramatically include dressing, including fastening and unfastening clothing; tying shoes; using an implement for writing (coloring and handwriting); and successfully manipulating utensils not only to eat, but to socially interact while eating. As children approach preadolescence (9 to 12 years of age), manipulative skills improve dramatically. Children produce cursive handwriting and complex drawings.

Perceptual development often improves significantly, often in direct relationship to the demands of the tasks along with practice, feedback, and motivation.[177] Visual-perceptual systems are nearing maturity and allow children to participate in sophisticated activities such as archery, baseball, dance, and swimming. Figure 3-10 helps bring to light complex skill development during a lifetime. That skill development may begin with a fun team sport activity and lead to a lifetime of professional accomplishment.

The musculoskeletal system enters a period when muscle growth is rapidly increased, accounting for a large percentage of the weight gained during this period.[177] Constraints and affordances of the musculoskeletal system along with demands of the tasks and environment are highly interactive and influential in skilled activities. Children are generally flexible because muscle and ligamentous structures are not firmly attached to bones. Although this allows for flexibility, it also poses risks for musculoskeletal injury. Care should be taken when participation in high-level athletic activities is a consideration.

Qualitative changes in coordination, balance, speed, and strength improve while existing motor skills become more refined and controlled, more efficient, and more complex.[177] Qualitative improvements of motor skills may be attributed to an asynchronous growth in children's limbs in relation to the trunk. Consequently, better leverage is attained. Motor skills strongly influence social domains as boys and girls begin to perform in organized sports teams in school and the community. Competition within sports becomes a powerful force in motivating children to practice motor skills or directing children away from organized sports. Children with poorly developed motor skills, as a result of either genetics or opportunity, may be excluded from team activities and experience social isolation.[177] Similarly, a child may have the genetic potential to become a master in an area that uses a specific motor task, but if he or she is never introduced

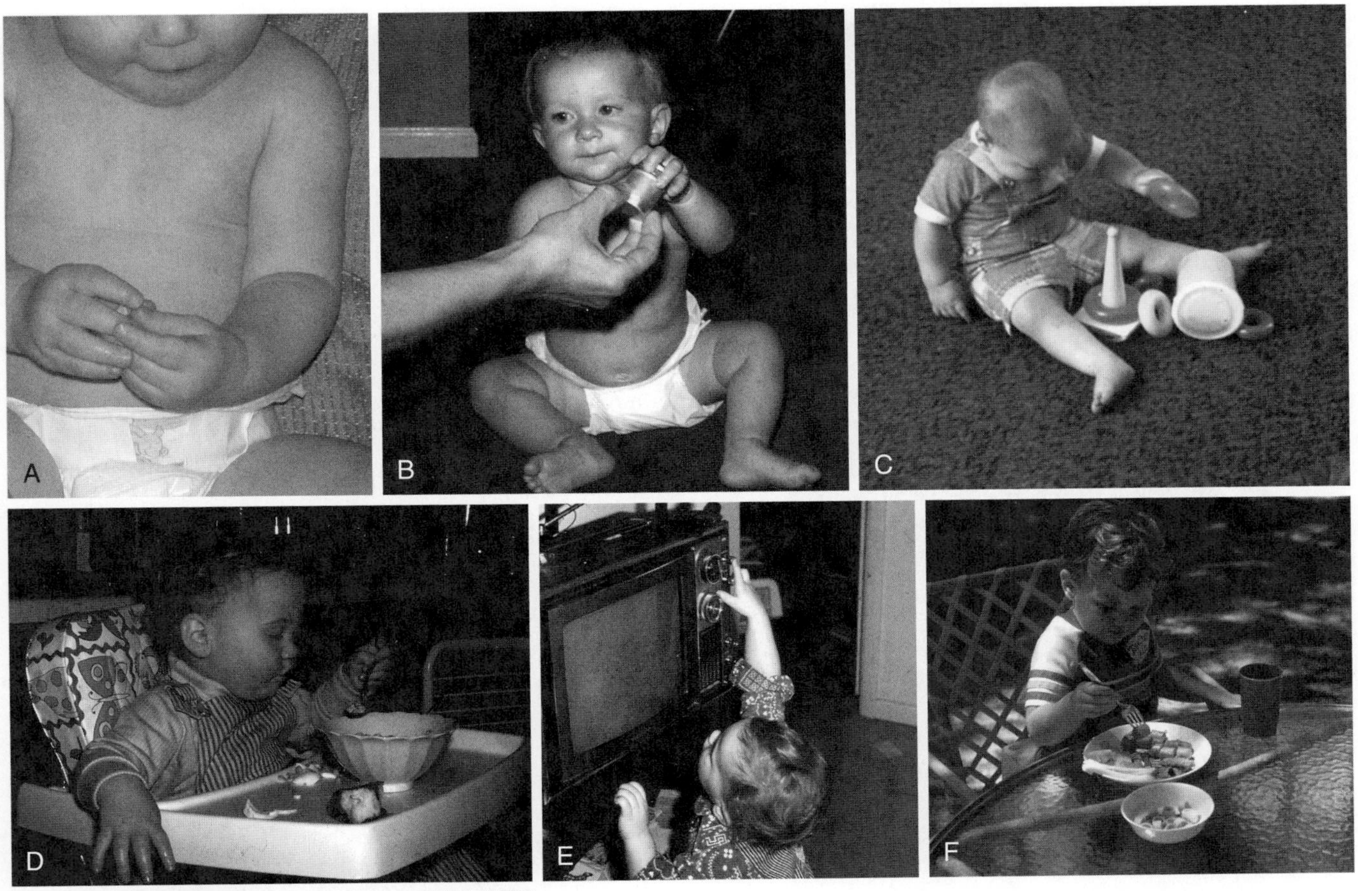

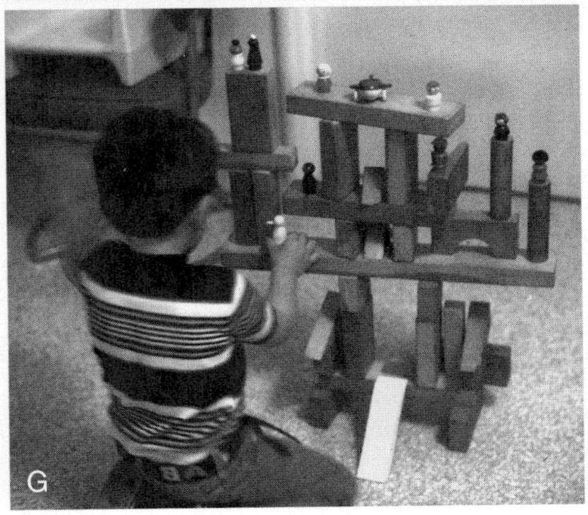

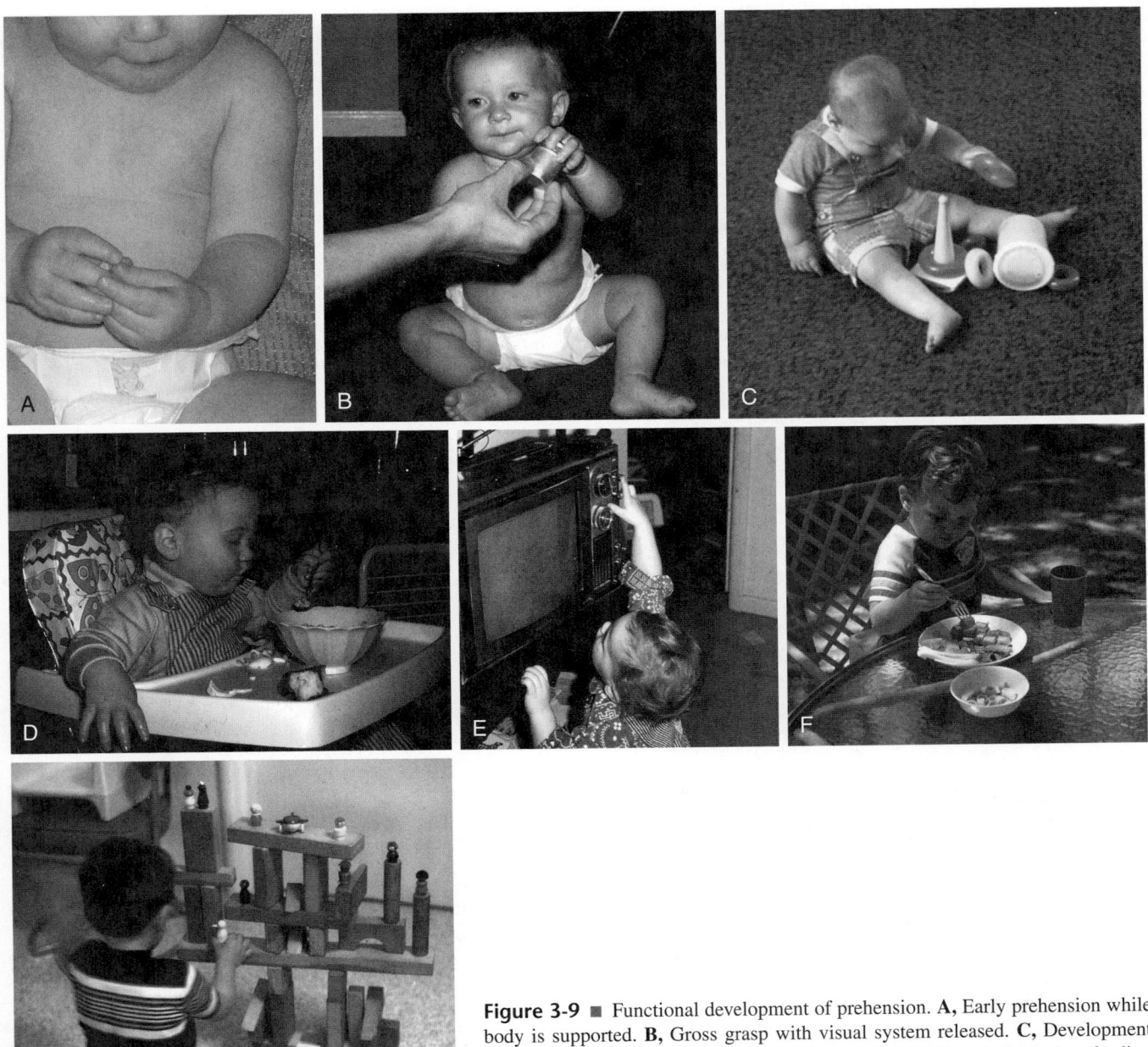

Figure 3-9 ■ Functional development of prehension. **A,** Early prehension while body is supported. **B,** Gross grasp with visual system released. **C,** Development and practice of eye-hand coordination during play. **D,** Early independent feeding with error. **E,** Functional use of individual digit. **F,** Eating with few errors while using utensils. **G,** Fine motor prehension while simultaneously using force and direction of the upper extremity with little error during play.

to the specific environment, such as playing a piano, and the motor skill is never actualized.

Adolescence (11 to 19 Years)

Early adolescence signifies a period characterized by improved quantitative performance and qualitative changes in skills along with physical growth (size and strength).[11] By age 12 years, reaction times closely resemble those of the mature adult. Although skills involving balance, coordination, and eye-hand coordination also continue to improve with respect to perceptual development and information processing, the rate is not as dramatic. Elite athletes, in contrast, often continue to show steady improvement in qualitative and quantitative skill performance well into adulthood.

During later adolescence, when periods of physical growth have stabilized, motor skills acquired previously continue to develop in speed, distance, accuracy, and power. Many adolescents are involved in competitive sports. However, few exhibit performance levels identified with elite athletes. Those athletes that do reach this high level of skill often have a genetic predisposition, environmental affordances, adequate opportunities for high-level practice and performance, and strong motivation. More often, adolescents performing in competitive sports will find this is their avocation rather than their vocation (see Figure 3-10).

Manipulative skills of adolescents resemble those of adults. Greater dexterity of the fingers for more complex tasks including art, sewing, crafts, knitting, wood carving,

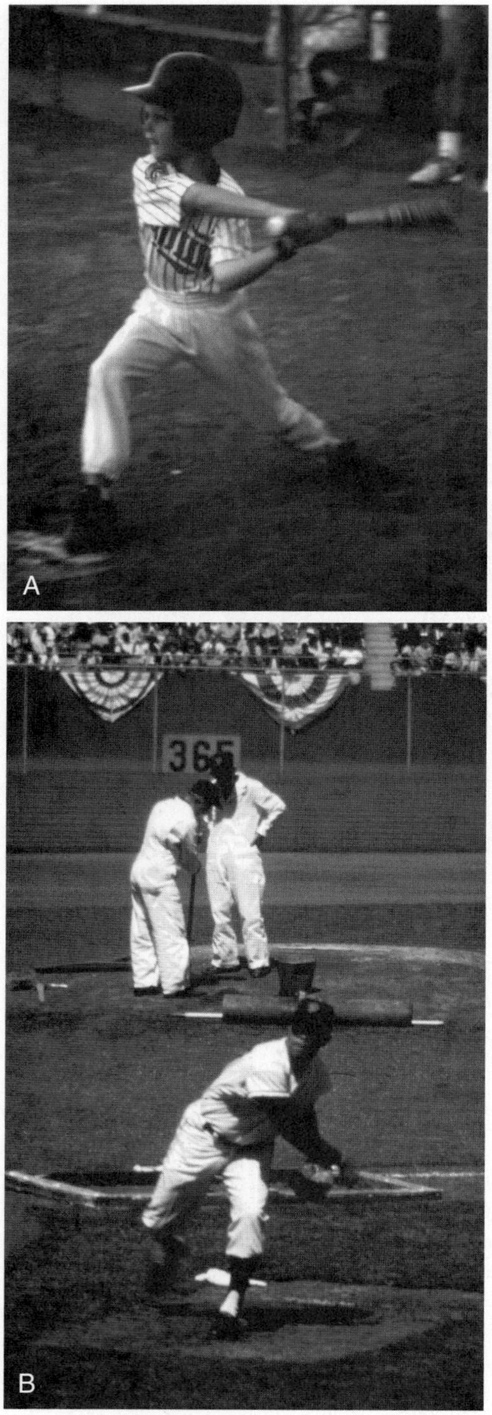

Figure 3-10 ■ Complex skill development. **A,** Child participating in a team sport. **B,** Adult demonstrating advanced skill development as a professional baseball player.

and musical performance enables adolescents to perform these motor tasks with greater precision and proficiency.

Adulthood (20 to 39 Years)

Motor performance is relatively consistent in adulthood. Skillful performance of movements may be characterized not only through consistency, but also through the infinite ways in which the skill is performed. Hence, change is generally focused on leisure activities or elite athletic competition. Leisure activities of many adults involve exercise of some form. Maintaining a healthy lifestyle through exercise and fitness is one method for staving off effects of aging and degenerative diseases. Although many adults participate in exercise for health and wellness (refer to Chapter 2 for additional information), others who do not routinely exercise are at risk for obesity and associated health problems. Often some of the physical activity expressed through the motor system is an example of parent-child bonds and creates a fun environment for play. When a task-specific activity is selected and challenged by family members, the motivation to perform becomes high. In Figure 3-11, *A,* the observer might think that all three individuals are performing similarly with similar strategies. In reality, single-leg stance increases in difficulty as the base of support decreases and the body size changes. Note that the smallest individual has the smallest foot and the largest base of support in proportion to his body size. The adolescent is not as tall as his father, but his foot size is significantly larger, which (1) increases his base of support, (2) gives him less input proportional to his foot size or representation on the somatosensory cortex, and (3) gives him higher degrees of freedom when shifting his weight, which can either increase or decrease the task difficulty depending on practice. Figure 3-11, *B* shows the way both taller individuals use strategies to initially assume the upright stance position while the smaller child attained the single leg stance by stepping from a table. Body height, weight, and amount of practice all are variables that will help determine outcome. All three individuals achieve success, although the specific motor patterns and strategies used to succeed may be different. In Figure 3-11, *C,* a child with severe sensory organization problems would not be able to solve the challenge presented in Figure 3-11, *A,* because he cannot even begin to stand independently on a large, stable surface. Again, therapists need to be able to match the motor program impairments causing the child with learning disabilities to fail at the task and identify what programs are needed or expressed in the success of all three individuals in Figure 3-11, *A.*

The peak of muscular strength occurs at 25 to 30 years of age in both men and women. After that period, muscle strength decreases as result of a reduction in the number and size of the muscle fibers.[178] Loss is related to genetic factors, nutritional intake, exercise regimen, and daily activities.

Middle Adulthood (40 to 59 Years)

Changes associated with aging have been identified in the neuromuscular, musculoskeletal, and cardiovascular and pulmonary systems. These age-associated changes can greatly affect motor performance, although the degree is highly variable. Between 30 and 70 years of age, strength loss is moderate, with about 10% to 20% of total strength lost, for most activities—insignificant and undetectable by the individual.[68,179] Participating in regularly scheduled exercise regimens that emphasize aerobic and strengthening activities may reduce effects associated with aging. Furthermore, developing muscle mass and competence in motor skills early in life may have long-term positive effects on adult skills and reduce the risk of disability and frailty later in life.[180]

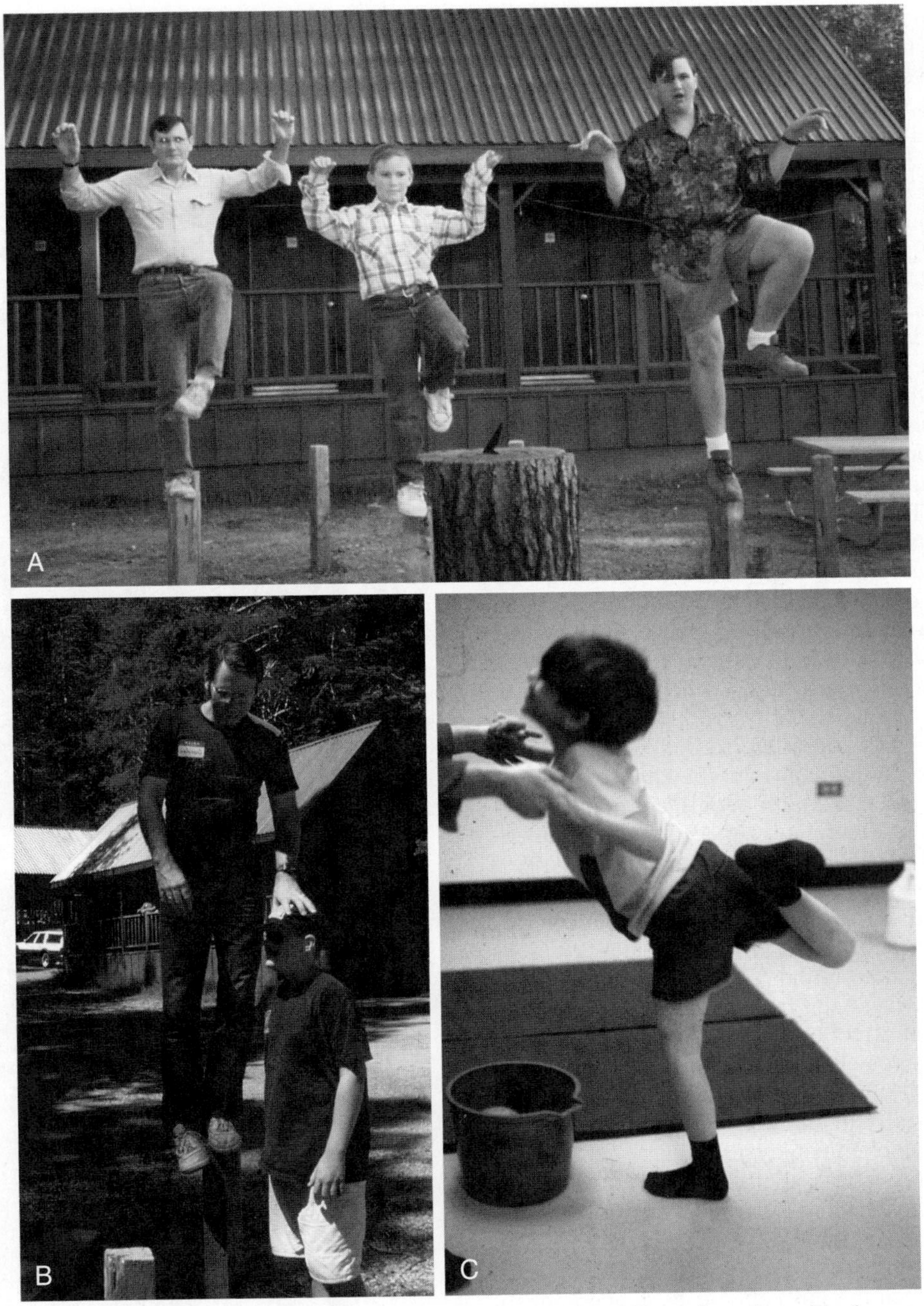

Figure 3-11 ■ A complex task performed by individuals with different foot size and body composition. **A,** Three individuals of differing age, body composition, and experience successfully performing the same task. **B,** The strategy used by the adolescent and adult to find verticality. **C,** A child with learning difficulties failing at independent one-legged stance.

Older Adulthood (60+ Years)

Age-related changes may be attributed to alteration in perception, compensations in the neural mechanisms, and changes between and within the different systems involved in motor skill performance.[181] Integrated effects may include slowing in movement production and increased activation of agonist-antagonist muscle groups. An example of agonist-antagonist activation is during dynamic balance activities.[182] After age 70 years, most individuals incur losses in muscle strength of up to 30% over the next 10 years. Overall, the loss of muscle strength through adulthood may be as much as 40% to 50% by the time an individual reaches 80 years of age.[65] The percentage decline is inversely related to the demand by the individual for repetition of the movements. For example, repetitive movements, such as playing tennis daily, running, playing golf, or downhill skiing, may significantly decrease the percentage of loss of strength compared with individuals who do not participate in such activities.

Although some effects are age associated and may be reduced with regular exercise and increased motor activity, not all are modifiable. Willardson[82] reported that older adults who maintain more active lifestyles are more likely to have a more favorable outcome than are peers who were not as active. Findings by Voelcker-Rehage and Willimczik[97] supported the findings of Willardson[82] in regard to older adults and lifestyle. In addition, Voelcker-Rehage and Willimczik[97] found that older adults aged 60 to 69 years were able to acquire and refine a novel task (juggling) at a level comparable to children 10 to 14 years old and adults 30 to 59 years old. Only young adults aged 15 to 29 years performed at a higher skill level. Furthermore, adults older than age 70 years were found to have limitations in their ability to learn the novel motor skill. Moreover, as individuals age, they generally have a decreased ability to produce force, and they tend to coactivate agonist-antagonist muscles.[183] The researchers suggested that older adults may coactivate agonist-antagonist muscles as a strategy to (1) modulate movement variability and (2) maintain accuracy in movement. The investigators also reported that older adults' coactivation strategy compromised the subjects' ability to rapidly accelerate their limbs in exchange for improved accuracy of control.

In addition, information processing appears to be slowed in older adults.[181] Motor times have also been found to be delayed in older adults, particularly when a higher-level force is required.

Temporal coupling also appears to be altered in older adults.[181] Perhaps as individuals age, they are less able to modulate timing of muscles during contraction and relaxation phases and are more likely to coactivate agonist-antagonist muscles. The outcome behaviors are typified by poorly coordinated motor activities and increased time to produce adequate muscle force to elicit the behavior.

In addition to reduced efficiency in movement production, variability in performance of motor skills also increases with age. Although small changes in individual systems may not have a significant effect on functional movements, the compounding effects of changes in several systems may have serious implications for older adults and place them at increased risk for falls and injuries.[58] Figure 3-12, *A* and *B* are examples of movement dysfunctions seen within an elderly population. These alterations are limiting the individual's ability to respond to a given motor task. As individuals age, there can be a large number of potential alterations in the body systems that limit CNS and musculoskeletal options when the individual tries to accomplish a motor activity. These limitations can place individuals at high risk of failure of any one motor task. The greatest fear within this group is not death; it is falling, and as a result losing independence. Prevention, as discussed in Chapter 2, will be more and more important as the world's population of elderly individuals enlarges on a yearly basis.

Thirty percent of all community-dwelling elderly persons fall at least once each year.[179,184] Factors contributing to falls include intrinsic and extrinsic variables.[185-187] Intrinsic alterations in the older adult have implications for performance of motor skills and potential for falls. Risks associated with falls increase with age and when functions of the neuromuscular, musculoskeletal, cardiovascular and pulmonary, and sensory systems deteriorate. This deterioration of covariant factors and not age itself is more closely related

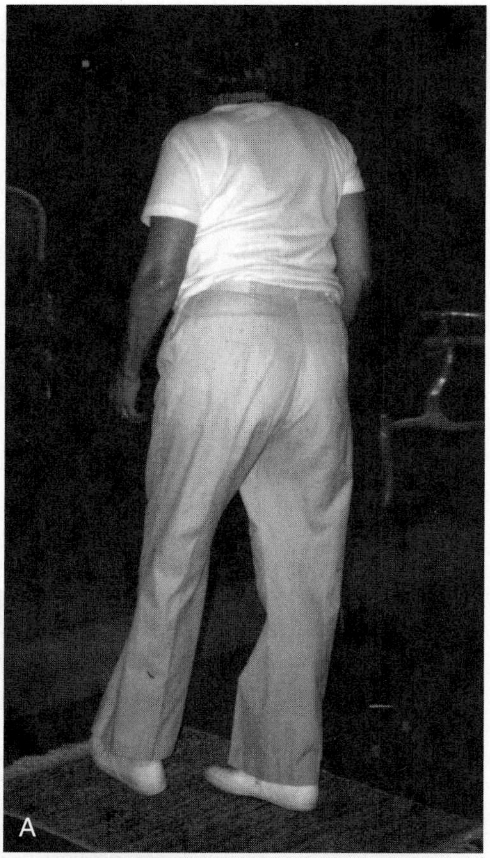

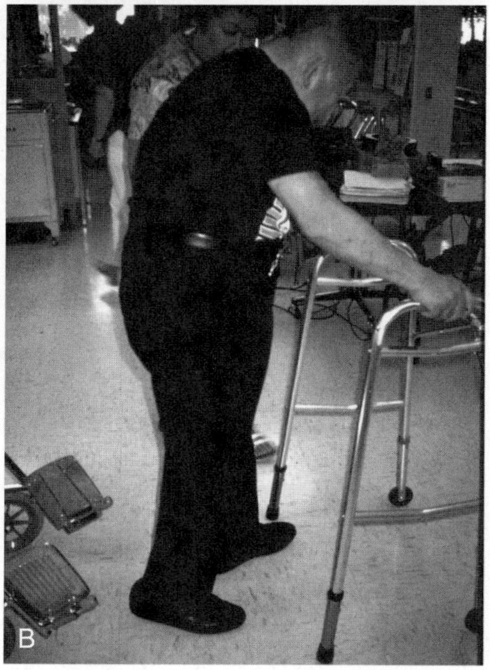

Figure 3-12 ■ As individuals age, more sedentary lifestyles, preexisting long-term health issues such as chronic obstructive pulmonary disease or chronic back pain, and a decrease in environmental challenges can lead to a higher risk of falls. **A,** Woman with chronic back problems leading to a fixed trunk. **B,** Man with chronic obstructive pulmonary disease and a fixed flexed posture resulting from inactivity.

to health and wellness and end-of-life age.[188] Another critical variable that is closely associated with motor decline in the aging is the individual's social interactions and participation in life.[189] Research has yet to determine whether a decrease in motor performance results from a decrease in participation in life.

Researchers have examined manipulative skills in older adults and reported changes in muscle performance and flexibility.[56,190,191] These changes resulted in decreased hand function associated with impaired performance of ADLs.

STRATEGIES FOR FOSTERING ACQUISITION AND RETENTION OF MOTOR BEHAVIORS ACROSS THE LIFE SPAN

Movements occur out of a need to solve problems in the environment. Solving these problems is not dependent on any one system but rather is a collaborative effort of multiple systems. The clinician is responsible for examining the patient's performance by evaluating the underlying conditions and the strategies that the individual may use to modify a behavior. Figure 3-13, *A* to *F*, presents an example of individuals standing up from a chair. The first panels (Figure 3-13, *A* and *B*) show a child whose feet are not on the surface because the child's legs are not long enough. No matter the variance of the task, the child was motivated to succeed. The second individual (Figure 3-13, *C* and *D*), an elderly man, has lost the ability to shift his weight forward over his feet and thus is rising posterior on his heels, which will require anterior flexor power to prevent him from falling backward. The third individual (Figure 3-13, *E* and *F*) has residual motor problems after a stroke. She has been taught to come to stand over her less-involved leg versus centering her base of support between her two feet. The specific way an individual learns, maintains, and relearns a specific motor task as a functional activity will vary, but the important principle will be to empower the individual to succeed with fluid, dynamic motor pattern options. Therapists need to visualize movement and place the movement pattern of the individual on top of that image. The specific motor impairments will then become obvious and treatment options will be generated. Examination is vital to this process, although it often occurs in an environment far removed from the client's natural surroundings.

Through acquisition of motor skills, individuals of all ages are afforded the opportunity to meet the environmental demands imposed by work, play, family, or personal activities. Refer to Figure 3-13 as an example of common motor activities used at work, play, and home. Motor skill acquisition, retention, and decline are influenced by constraints or affordances that affect opportunities for practice in an environment that challenges and drives the individual to perform optimally. The client's investment in achieving a successful outcome can help foster persistence in reaching the desired outcome.

Practice, the primary method for acquisition and retention of motor tasks, is exciting for very young children because each attempt is a new opportunity to achieve the outcome and reach a new level of independence. In contrast, practice in adolescent and adult populations may not be seen in the same light but rather as tedious and boring. Instead, physical and occupational therapists have the responsibility to challenge the cognitive, affective, motor, perceptual, sensory, and physiological systems through client-selected activities. Activities directed toward the age and needs of the individual, such as interactive dance mats for adolescent clients or ballroom dancing for the older adult, may provide the motivation necessary to practice the task a sufficient number of times to achieve the desired outcome. Figure 3-14, *A* to *H* show age-appropriate challenges to individuals. The activity used with a child may be inappropriate for use with an adult, although a similar motor behavior may be the desired outcome. If the individual identifies the activity, he will be more motivated and more likely to practice a desired skill. Carryover from a clinical setting to a home or environmental setting is critical when looking at movement function over a life span.

Strategies used to achieve desired motor outcomes may include a variety of feedback mechanisms to correct errors and identify more efficient strategies to attain the motor skill. Embracing the concept of enablement rather than disablement may also serve to motivate the client because individual abilities are acknowledged and promoted while strategies are used for acquisition or relearning of motor skills. The needs of adolescent and adult clients are unique and differ significantly from those of the young infant or child.

Opportunities for exploration that engage the infant or young child are the primary motivation for movement. Although motor activities serve as the primary focus, engaging the infant or child provides stimulation that promotes development across multiple domains (e.g., cognition, social, communication). Environmentally challenging activities place demands on the child that maintain a level of curiosity or motivation and encourage persistence in attaining a motor skill that is successful and efficient. As the child matures, play-based activities shift the focus, depending on the expected outcomes. Overall, play is the primary mechanism that children use to mimic adult-like behaviors. Finally, children and adults use play or leisure activities as a means of promoting skill acquisition and proficiency across all developmental domains.

Development of Head Control as an Example of Movement Development across the Life Span and Its Impact on Quality of Life

When analyzing the development of head control by viewing movement of a young child over the first few years, it becomes clear that the motor control of the head in all spatial positions is very complex, requiring the integration of a variety of movement patterns. The infant needs to develop both the flexors that bend the head forward as well as the flexors that tuck the chin. These flexor patterns will be integrated into diagonal movements in order to roll over from supine to prone. A neck-righting program orients the body to the head when the head is initially moving. Although the neck-righting program is present at birth, it will take the child a couple of months to gain the power necessary to independently flex and rotate the head against gravity with the body following the head in order to roll over. As the flexor power improves, it will be integrated into patterns of coactivation with postural extensors. The extensor movements of the head include (1) extension from a flexion position through hyperextension and/or rotation of the head in

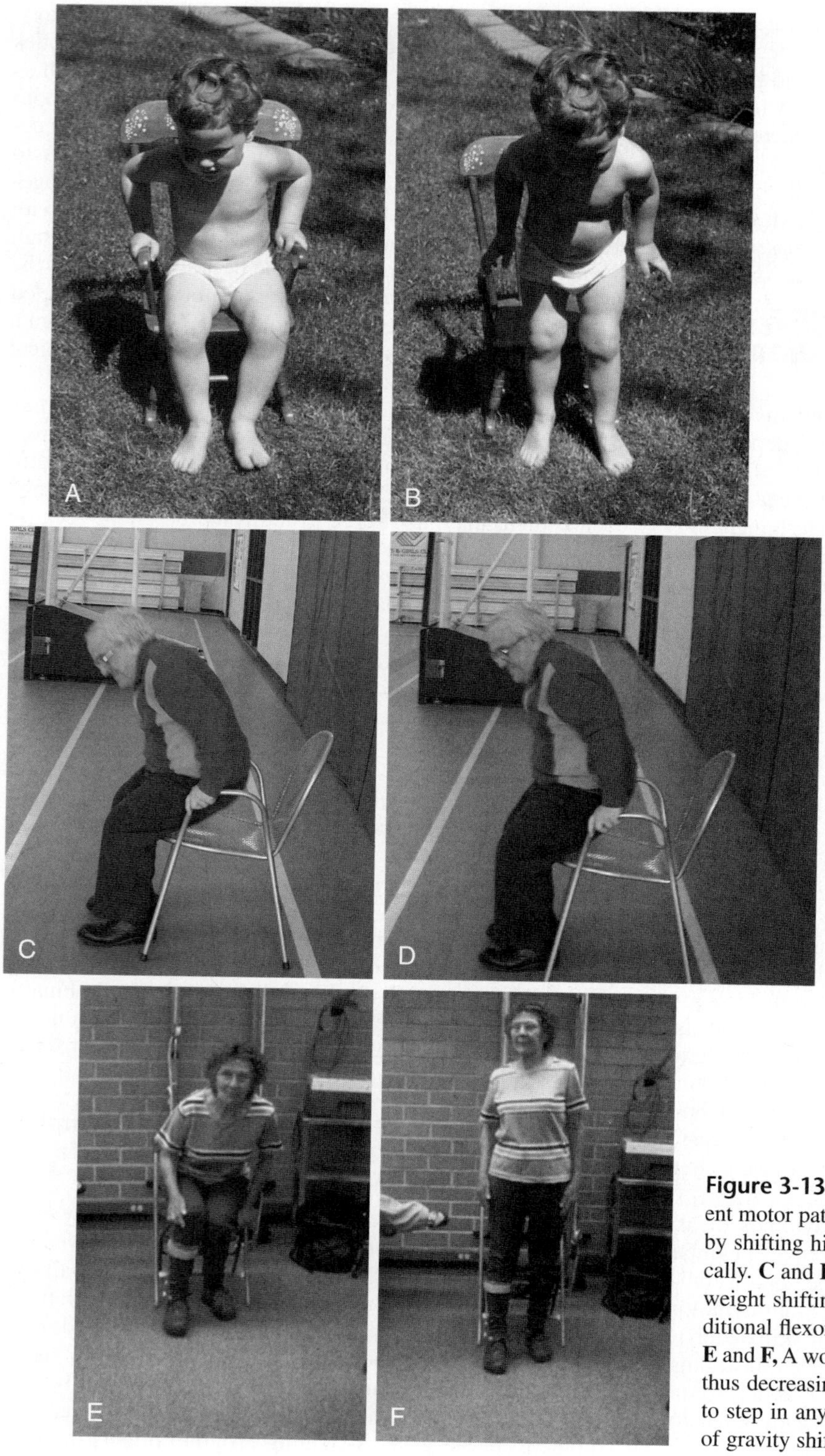

Figure 3-13 ■ Three individuals coming to stand using different motor patterns. **A** and **B,** A child rising to stand from a chair by shifting his weight over his base of support and rising vertically. **C** and **D,** An elderly man rising to stand without adequate weight shifting forward over his base of support, requiring additional flexor power to prevent falling backward into the chair. **E** and **F,** A woman after a stroke rising over her less involved leg, thus decreasing her symmetrical weight distribution and ability to step in any direction with either foot as a response to center of gravity shifting outside her base of support.

all spatial planes, and (2) postural extension, holding and/or stabilizing each vertebra within the spinal column. These postural programs help coactivate the flexors and postural extensors simultaneously to stabilize the head in space. There are a variety of motor programs that assist in gaining this control of the head. Head-righting reactions, using the semicircular canals, are programmed to right the head, or bring it to face vertical, no matter where the head is in space.

The righting programs need the underlying power to produce the force necessary to right the head. The heavier the head, whether in weight of the cranium or its positioning against gravity, the harder it is to right the head to vertical. Thus it could be hypothesized that if the head were in a vertical position or vertical in reference to gravity, it would be easier to control the head in space. The force production would be nominal compared with the force production

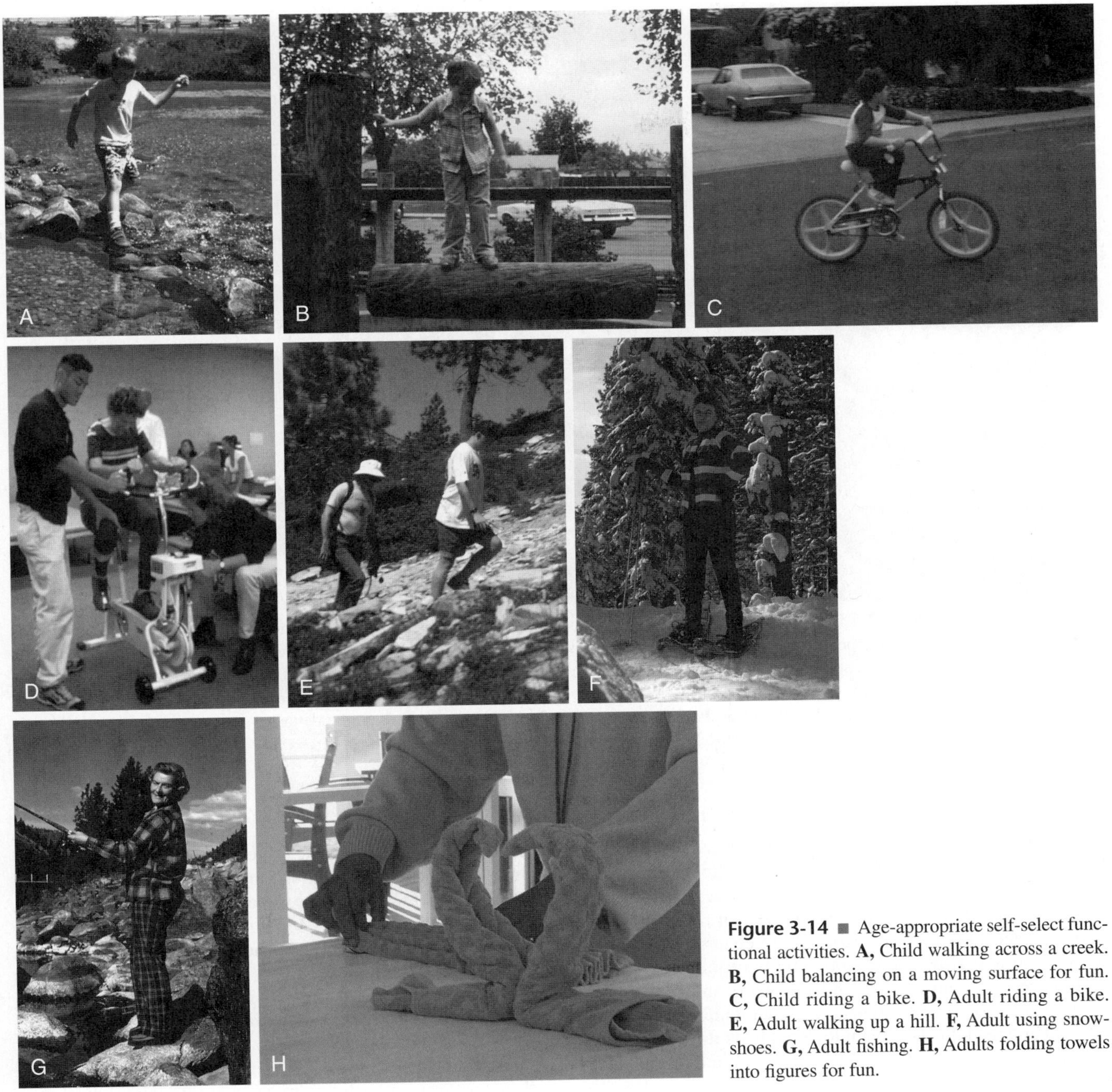

Figure 3-14 ■ Age-appropriate self-select functional activities. **A,** Child walking across a creek. **B,** Child balancing on a moving surface for fun. **C,** Child riding a bike. **D,** Adult riding a bike. **E,** Adult walking up a hill. **F,** Adult using snowshoes. **G,** Adult fishing. **H,** Adults folding towels into figures for fun.

needed when bringing the head up from horizontal or just holding it against gravity when horizontal. There are motor programs triggering extensor tone due to the position of the otoliths in the inner ear. The degree of tone will depend upon whether the head is horizontal in supine, vertical, or in between. This response has been labeled the *tonic labyrinthine reaction* (TLR). The TLR is strongest in the supine position because of the optimal pull of the otoliths by gravity. When an individual is supine, the tactile input from pressure to the surface of the skin increases extensor tone. Thus, in the supine position the tactile input and the information from the hair cells of the otoliths are activating the motor pool of the extensors and simultaneously decrease the motor pool of the flexors. These systems decrease the ability of the motor control system to generate flexor tone in supine. When the child is placed prone, the skin sensitivity decreases extensor tone.

Flexor Control

Figure 3-15, *A* through *F,* illustrates the patterns of a healthy 4-week-old when being pulled to sit and returned to the floor. Initially the child has difficulty flexing his head when trying to pull the head into flexion from the supine position because of both the extensor tactile system and the labyrinthine mechanism, which inhibit the flexors while facilitating the extensor muscles. This can be seen in Figure 3-15, *A* through *C*. This lack of adequate flexor control would be considered normal for the child's age but also defined as a head lag

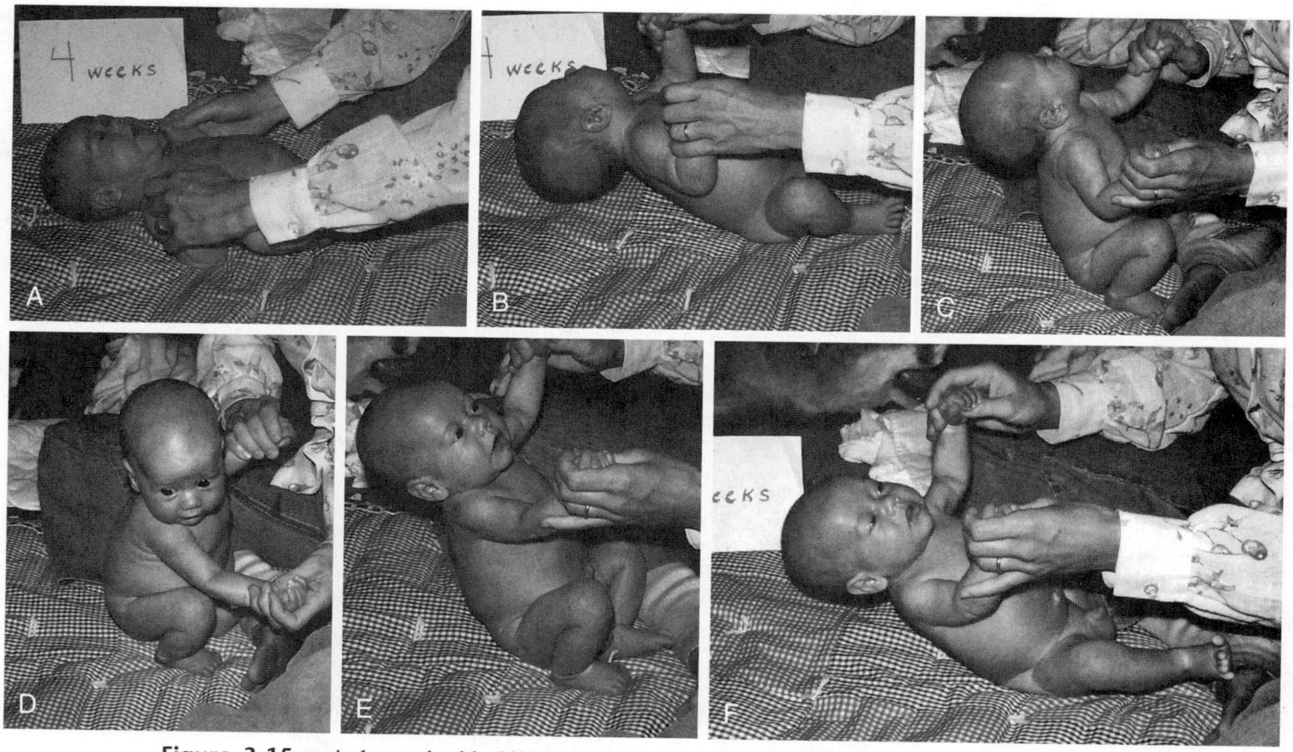

Figure 3-15 ■ A 1-month-old child being pulled to sit from supine and lowered back down. **A,** Starting position in supine. **B,** Pulled toward vertical, maximal resistance from gravity, inadequate response to stretch by neck flexors. **C,** Position of ears and otoliths inhibits flexors; thus inadequate head righting is still seen. **D,** Child in vertical, weight through hips, quick stretch to head in all directions facilitates head control. **E,** Child lowered back toward horizontal continues to have adequate head control. **F,** Maximal stretch from gravity; child still retains adequate neck flexion.

(Figure 3-15, *A* through *C*). As the child approaches vertical, his weight is shifted down through his buttocks and over his base of support. At that point the head control kicks in (Figure 3-15, *D* and *E*). This motor control of the head in vertical incorporates both postural extensors and flexors while optimizing the use of optic and labyrinthine righting and stretch to both flexors and extensors muscle groups (Figure 3-15, *D*). The child is able to maintain better control of head and neck flexors when lowered back down to supine (Figure 3-15, *E* and *F*). This ability to control the head while transitioning from sitting to supine illustrates the fan swing principle: once the flexor program is elicited in the vertical position, it can maintain head control for a longer period of time and through more degrees of motion as the head movement progresses from vertical to horizontal.

Over the next month the child will develop flexor control in space by using head righting, muscle strength, and facilitation of the nervous system to keep the head and eyes oriented toward an object as the head travels through space. Motor control over flexor patterns becomes more flexible, and the power needed to perform tasks increases. Figure 3-16, *A* through *C*, demonstrates the pull to sit pattern in a healthy 3-month-old infant. She not only has learned to dampen the influence of the TLR in the supine position and the skin's influence on the extensor motor pool, but also has learned that by flexing most of her body parts (flexion facilitates flexion) she will gain additional flexor control of the head when pulled from supine (Figure 3-16, *A*). This flexion continues as the child goes through midrange (Figure 3-16, *B*) and continues as the child approaches vertical (Figure 3-16, *C*). Unfortunately, the child does not have the integrated motor control over flexion and extension or the balance reactions in sitting to extend the legs as she approaches vertical. This movement is a prerequisite for gaining control of long sitting in vertical. These new motor movements will become the foundation for balance reactions in vertical sitting.

A month later the child's nervous system integrates the flexor patterns into smooth movement through 90 degrees of motion from supine to sitting (Figure 3-17, *A* through *C*). The child also demonstrates a more integrated response to being lowered backward from vertical (Figure 3-17, *D*). Yet the child's motor system has not developed the rotatory aspects or control of the diagonal flexor patterns as shown in Figure 3-17, *E*. These rotatory patterns will develop as the child practices rotation in rolling and then incorporates that rotation when coming to sit in a partial rotation pattern.

The child will not be able to independently initiate motor control over the adult pattern of coming to a sitting position for at least 3 to 5 years but certainly should gain that control by age 6 (Figure 3-18). As the child's age increases, the movement patterns become more complex, and additional motor programs are learned and integrated. This aspect of head control will be maintained and integrated in movement patterns as the individual explores the environment.

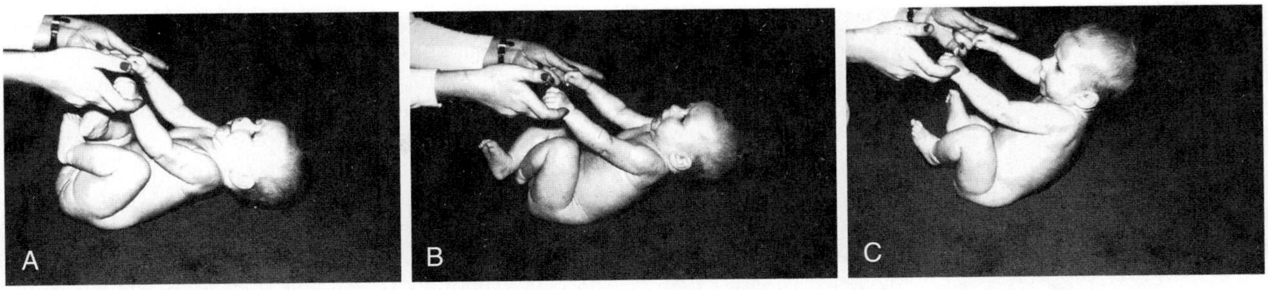

Figure 3-16 ■ A 3-month-old healthy child pulled to sit. **A,** Initial stretch in horizontal pulls in neck flexion along with flexion of the hips and knee. **B,** Adequate neck flexion persists as child looks at therapist while being pulled to sit: midrange. **C,** Transitioning to vertical; less stress on neck flexors, yet flexion persists in lower extremities.

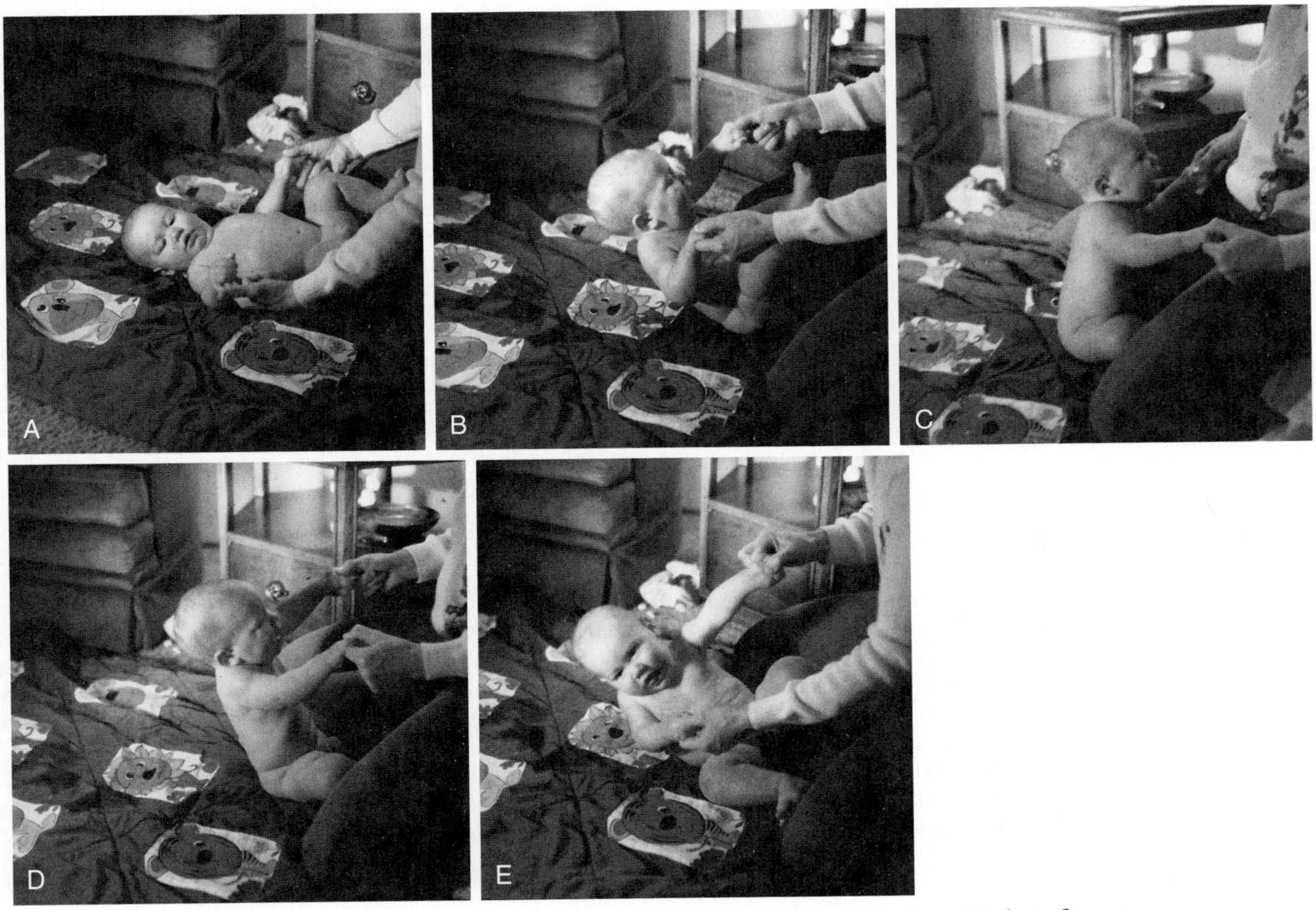

Figure 3-17 ■ Pull to sit in 4 month-old-healthy child. **A,** Child looks as therapist places finger to the child's head—recognized tactile stimulus, relaxed supine. **B,** Child pulled to sit, neck tucked and hips flexed. **C,** In vertical, child relaxes hip flexors in order to have sitting balance. **D,** Child lowered toward supine maintains neck and trunk control. **E,** Rotation added into lowering to supine pattern; neck response is inadequate.

Extensor Control

As the child develops flexion, the child also needs to develop the extensor control of the head. There are two extensor component patterns used by the CNS to control extension. The first pattern is controlling extension of the head from a totally flexed position (as if an individual were looking down at his shoes) to a hyperextension position (as if an individual in a standing position were looking up at the stars). This pattern has a large range of motion, and the power needed will change depending on the head's position in space, in relation to gravity, as well as the weight of the head itself. The second pattern is considered "postural" and requires the small muscles of the neck and the shoulder and trunk to hold each vertebra in relation to the vertebra above

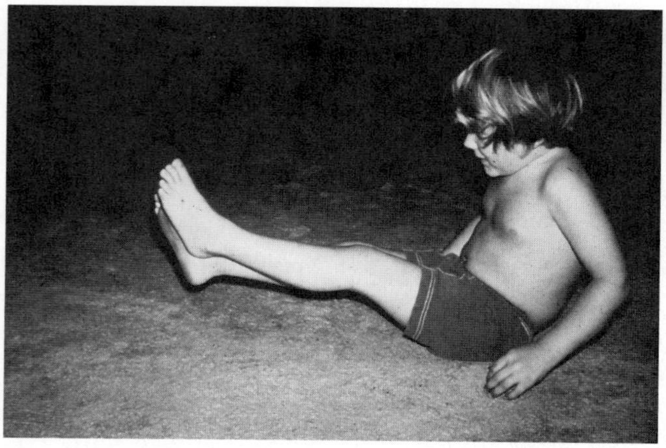

Figure 3-18 ■ Normal 6-year-old using adult independent coming-to-sit pattern.

and the vertebrae below. This is the boney support encompassing the spinal cord. Similarly, in the upper cervical region as the flexor and extensor patterns work together in a coactivation pattern, chin tucking occurs. This pattern allows the head to remain stable in space, keeping the eyes and the ears horizontal to the surroundings, a key component for perceptual learning. This movement pattern is often called *optic and labyrinthine righting of the head* because both the eyes and the ears provide stimuli to trigger this motor response.

Assessment of Head Control

Most individuals analyze the development of postural control by evaluating the extensor aspect of head control in the prone position. But the prone position is not the first position in which a child begins to achieve independent head control. Figure 3-19, *A* through *C,* illustrates a newborn (2 days old) extending both the long extensors (Figure 3-19, *A* and *B*) as well as moving into the postural extensor pattern component when tucking the chin (Figure 3-19, *C*). While prone the newborn child has very little independent control over extension and can just clear the airways (Figure 3-20). This same limitation is not present when the child is in a supported vertical position. After a week the extensor patterns in the vertical position have already become more functional and demonstrate better motor control and greater power. Figure 3-21, *A* through *C*, shows the same child at 1 week of age while supported in a vertical position. Figure 3-21, *C* is a beautiful example of the postural pattern one expects to see consistently later in the child's development. Obviously, he is practicing these movements every time he is vertical and given these limited degrees of freedom. Looking at the same child at 1 month of age (Figure 3-22), the integration of these postural movements is continuing down his entire spine. This does not mean he can hold this pattern for an extended period of time but does illustrate his ability to move with control into a total postural extension pattern and hold it at least briefly. On the same day and about 15 minutes later, the child (Figure 3-23) was placed prone on the floor, clearly demonstrating that he has not developed the necessary power to control his head or upper trunk for postural extension in the prone position. Although he is more relaxed prone at 1 month than at birth (see Figure 3-20) and can lift and turn his head in both directions, it will still be 1 or 2 additional months before he can extend his head and trunk enough to prop on his elbows. It will take more time to roll from prone to supine.

While the cervical and upper thoracic muscles are developing postural power, they need to learn to hold the head in space against gravity for longer periods of time. Postural function requires coordination and coactivation of the short extensors of the neck and the neck flexors—especially the sternocleidomastoid, hyoid, and scalene muscles—in order to tuck the chin and balance the head in space. These movement patterns play a key role in stabilization of the head in order to move the head in and out of vertical space. The motor control system uses both righting and balance reactions in order to gain full head and neck control of vertical space. The movements become more and more complex, modifying and integrating various additional motor programs in order to have greater flexibility to control and move the head. These patterns give the eyes and ears the visual and auditory orientation needed to process consistent external environmental information. Figure 3-24 illustrates an individual after head injury who has lost his automatic righting of the head in vertical. He has the ability to bring his head to vertical by hyperextension of the neck but does not do so automatically. This hyperextension pattern dramatically changes the motor patterns of head, neck, and trunk control which will affect his upright behaviors including balance, gait, feeding, and social interactions.

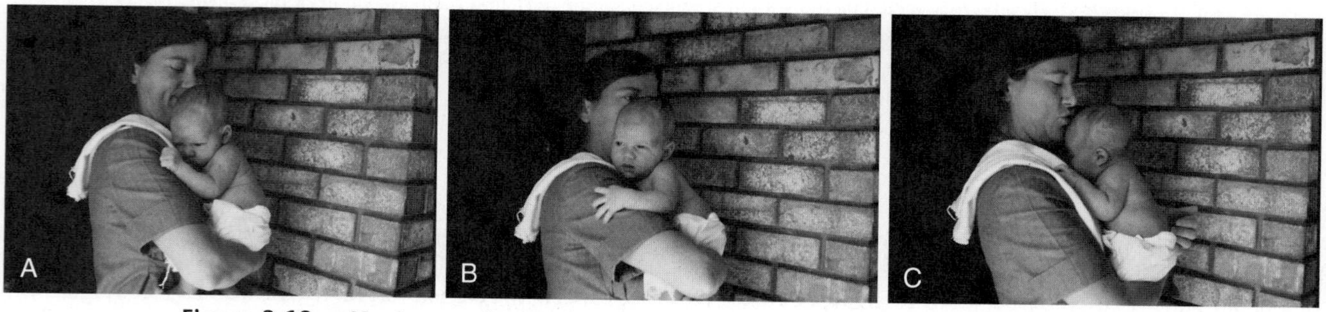

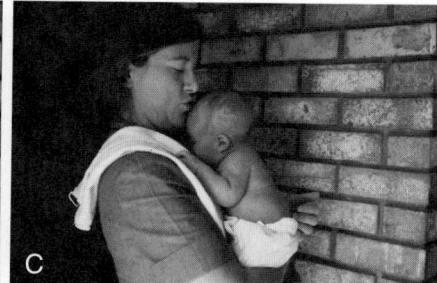

Figure 3-19 ■ Newborn neck extension in supported vertical position. **A,** Newborn lacks postural extension of trunk and head. **B,** Newborn initiates neck extension, showing that patterns exist. **C,** Newborn moves into postural extension of upper cervical region.

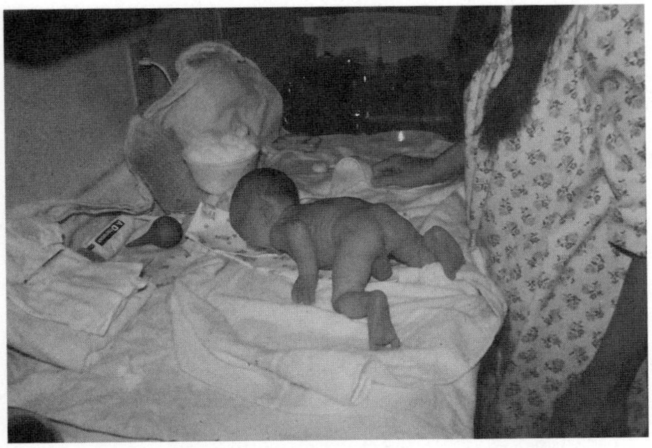

Figure 3-20 ■ When placed prone, the newborn has excessive flexion.

Application of the Development of Head Control to Rehabilitation

The reason the patterns of head extension in vertical have been presented is to illustrate that motor control progresses from vertical to horizontal and then from horizontal to vertical. Therapists think of the prone position as the first position in which the child develops extensor control because it is the first position in which an observer sees independent selection of extensor movement. However, extensor control begins when an individual passively brings a young baby to sitting or standing. The baby learns to control the head with small movements that displace the center of gravity. Understanding this stage of head control may be a critical component of working with a neurologically impaired youngster or an adult.

Analysis between Normal and Impaired Motor Function

Differentiating normal age-related reactions of any movement impairment is the responsibility of a movement specialist. For example, differentiating the movement of a normal child who has a lag in head control (see Figure 3-15, *B* and *C*) from the movement of a child who does not demonstrate any head control (Figure 3-25, *A* through *E*) should guide the therapist in a decision about where to begin treatment. It is an unrealistic expectation for the child in Figure 3-25 to gain flexor head control by starting at supine. After the child has been pulled to sit, flexor power production is beyond the control of the child's motor system. Once the child is vertical, the influence of gravity on the weight of the head has decreased. The vertical position also inhibits any influence of the otoliths when supine. The upright position helps to facilitate the labyrinthine and optic righting of the head. Figure 3-25, *D* and *E* demonstrates how the tone within the neck and shoulder girdle changes once the head attains a vertical position. A therapist should not only see a change to more normal tonal patterns but also observe relaxation of the facial muscles—closure of the mouth and a more functional position of the eyes in space for visual processing.

Movement demonstrates the ease or difficulty the motor system is experiencing while trying to complete an activity. The activity analyzed may be a basic pattern such as head control or a complex one as seen in Figure 3-3, *E*. Differentiating between the movements in Figure 3-15, *A* and Figure 3-25, *A* should guide the clinician in establishing realistic prognoses. The first child, with practice and CNS maturity, should automatically develop head control, whereas the second child has gone beyond his age-appropriate movement delays and has abnormal responses to the stretch stimuli.

Similar analysis can be made when looking at the extensor component of head control. The vertical position that optimizes extension is kneeling or standing because compression down through the joints and spine facilitates extension. Using kneeling or standing may pull in too much extension, especially if it results in hyperextension. In that case sitting may be appropriate even though it may facilitate flexion. When kneeling or standing, if inadequate extension still exists, then adding additional compression (see Chapter 9, p. 207) down though the head or shoulder girdle may help. Using an apparatus that takes away some of the weight of the head or trunk reduces the demand on the nervous system and may help the individual regain postural neck, shoulder girdle, and upper trunk control (see Chapter 9, p. 232). As the individual begins to demonstrate that control, the therapist can slowly take away the assistance with the expectations that the individual will gain independence in that activity.

As the individual ages, changes in the control of the head can lead to new problems. Figure 3-12, *B*, is an example of a man who has a fixed flexed posture. If the flexed posture is permanent, treatment alternatives must take into consideration

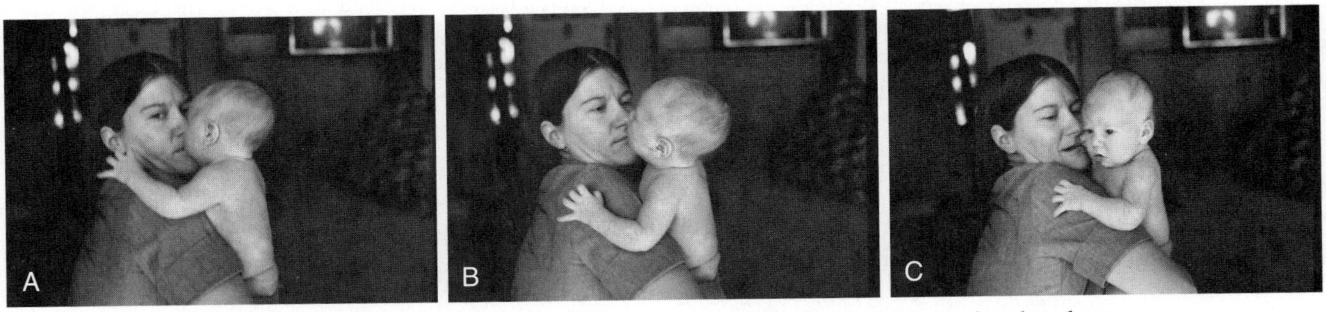

Figure 3-21 ■ Child 7 days old in vertical extension. **A,** Child eliciting active neck and truck extension in vertical at 7 days. **B,** Child does not have adequate righting of the head in vertical at 7 days but is responding. **C,** Child pulls into postural extension of the neck and trunk, allowing for binocular vision at 7 days.

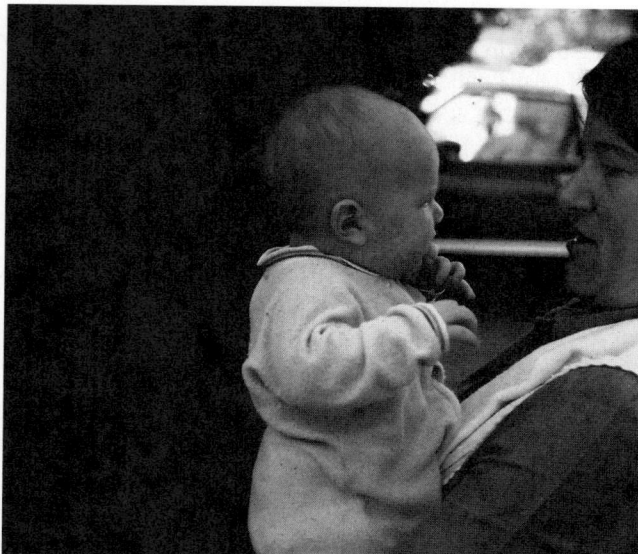

Figure 3-22 ■ A 1-month-old child, when supported in a vertical position, shows postural extension of the neck and trunk while looking at his mother.

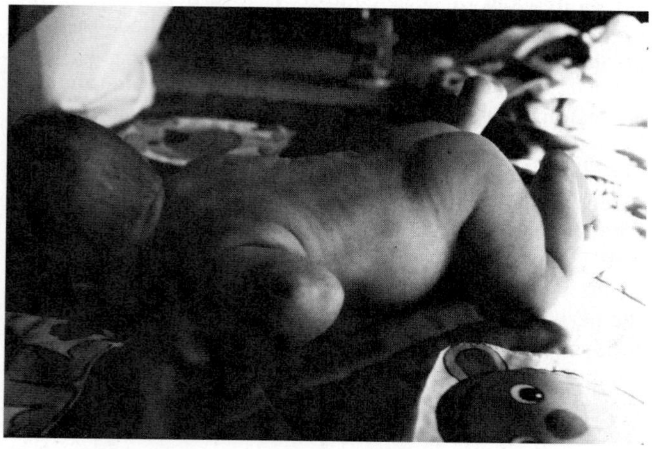

Figure 3-23 ■ Same child when placed prone, 15 minutes after Figure 3-22 was taken. This child demonstrates that when prone he still has a flexor bias and has little adequate postural extension in this position.

the impact this posturing will have on all ADLs. As stated earlier, any patient can exhibit a range of problems in head control. How those movement impairments present themselves and which treatment alternatives a therapist might select will depend on the clinician's ability to analyze normal movement and create an optimal environment for patients to engage and practice those patterns.

Clinical Example

Cervical torticollis in a child is an imbalance in rotation of the neck and muscle groups secondary to position of the fetus in utero. Cervical torticollis in adults is a focal dystonia or an imbalance of excitation and inhibition of the neck muscles. These patients have impaired integrative balance responses. Standard medical intervention is botulinum toxin injections followed by physical therapy focusing on range of motion and strengthening exercise. The emphasis needs

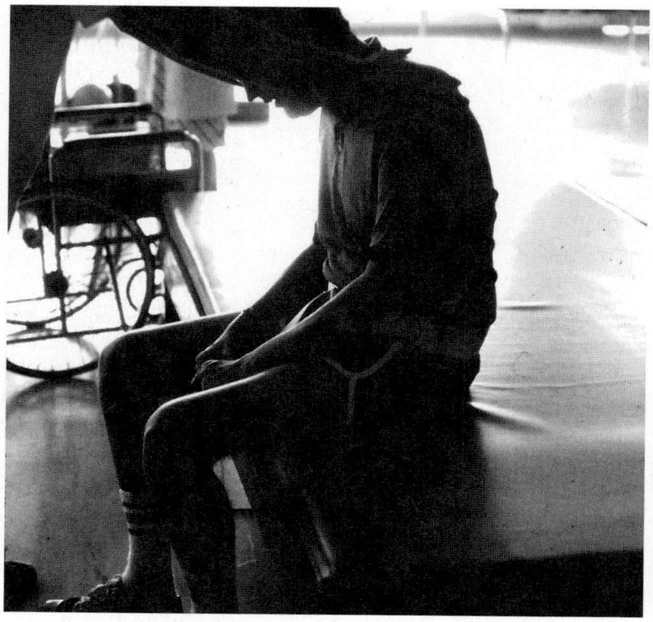

Figure 3-24 ■ An individual who sustained a closed head injury with residual lack of postural neck extension has poor head control in vertical.

to be on restoring and progressing head control from vertical to supine—that is, trying to help the neck muscles to retrain a stable condition in the vertical position by using a collar for support. Compression down through the cervical and thoracic spine can facilitate flexors, extensors, and rotator muscles. Then, as in the infant, with arms fixed on a stable support surface, slowly let the patient move out of vertical toward horizontal, moving only as far as head control is maintained, which may be as limited as 10 to 20 degrees. Repeat this activity many times in order for this activity to become procedural. Patients can hold onto some stable support object at home in order to practice. The challenge for both the therapist and the patient is to retrain head control in order for the individual to be able to participate in life.

Summary

Normal development of head control has been highlighted because so many clinicians become frustrated with clients who do not have adequate head control. The examples of the development of head control serve as a foundation for every movement pattern that people use, whether stationary or in motion. The process used to analyze the development of head control can be used to analyze all movement patterns, whether the movement problem is caused by a bodily system (biomechanical, cardiopulmonary, CNS or another system problem) or by some environmental factor.

SUMMARY

Clinicians must focus best practice toward successful client management geared toward promotion of function and prevention of chronic illness or disability for the youngest of the young to the oldest of the old. As practitioners, we must embrace tenets central to the *Healthy People 2020* project. Physical and occupational therapists serve as role models for individuals of all ages and educate diverse groups of individuals about the multifaceted, interactive systems involved in the acquisition, retention, and deterioration of motor

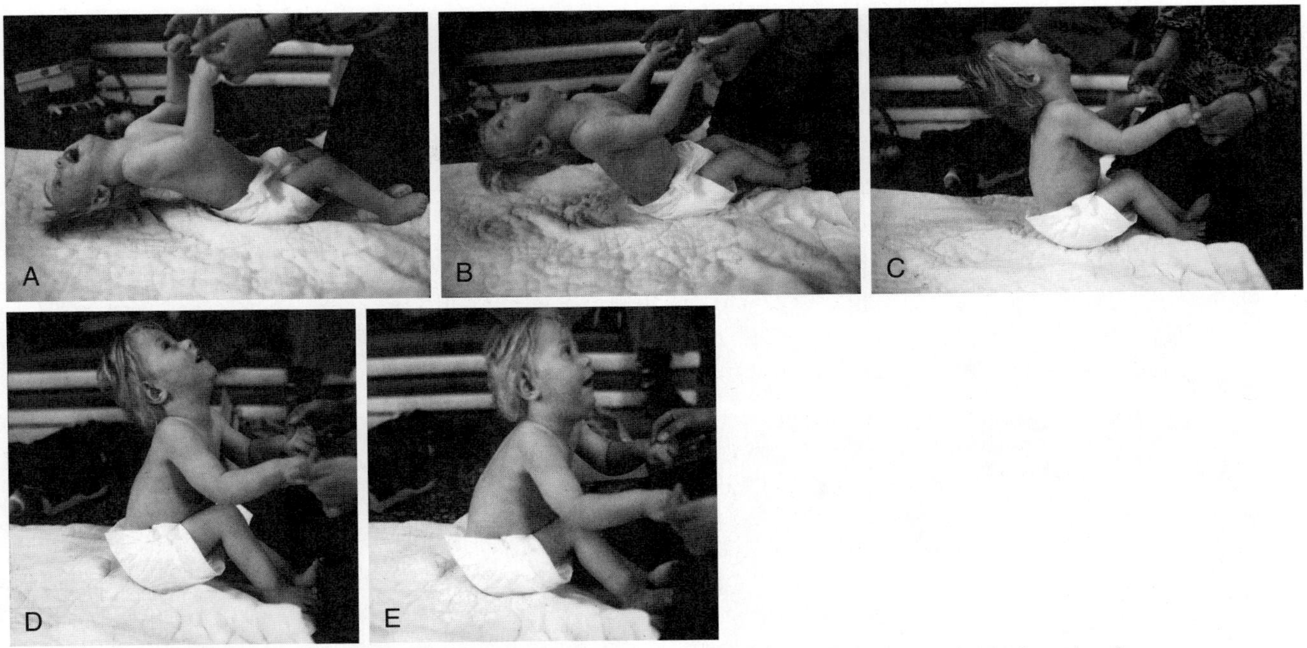

Figure 3-25 ■ Child 2½ years old with cerebral palsy being pulled to sit, and muscle action facilitated once vertical. **A,** Initial pull toward sit; no response to stretch of neck flexors. **B,** Continued pull toward vertical, head at end range of neck extension. **C,** Trunk in vertical but neck remains in horizontal; no flexor response. **D,** Child pulled beyond vertical as trunk extensors begin to activate from stretch and mouth closure is beginning. **E,** Therapist facilitates head into vertical as mouth continues to relax and close and eyes are looking at a target.

behaviors. Recognizing internal and external constraints or affordances that influence motor behaviors enables the clinician to devise a plan of care and the scientist to design a study targeting the needs of the whole person. Analyzing, understanding, and visually recognizing movement patterns that are efficient, fluid, and goal oriented and that vary across the life span are the first steps or prerequisites to evaluating abnormal movement patterns that do not fall within a normal parameter. Figure 3-26, *A* to *G,* shows an example of rolling, a basic movement strategy controlled by the child midway through the first year of life that can become an extremely challenging activity after a CNS insult. Differentiating between components of a normal movement and deviations that prohibit normal movement falls into the clinical expertise of occupational and physical therapists (see Chapter 9, Figure 9-1, p. 199) Without the knowledge of normal movement, analysis of the causation of abnormal movement would be difficult if not impossible. This chapter has been written to help the reader understand normal movement across the life span. It is the first step, and in sighted individuals the analysis begins as soon as visual images are recorded in the visual cortex.

Scientists acknowledge that development is characterized as nonlinear, emergent, and dynamic, rather than sequential, predictable, and stagelike. Dynamic systems theory, although it does have certain limitations, provides a better explanation for development than do neuromaturational theories. The emphasis or responsibility does not lie with any one system but varies across different systems as a consequence of age, genetics, or experience.[104] That said, future studies directed at examining human movement and optimal variability through nonlinear dynamics may provide new perspectives in motor development and control.

Human behavior is by nature complex. As such, no one system or skill develops in isolation but rather emerges from a complex interaction among multiple systems. Complex behaviors are evident beginning in utero and continuing throughout life. No one theory explains the development of complex motor behaviors, and none encompass the essence of interindividual and intraindividual variability in aging. Aspects of various theories provide evidence that an integrative perspective is a more accurate reflection of aging. As theorized earlier, lifestyle choices and other modifiable behaviors have potent effects on aging. Interventions designed to provide older adults with strategies to positively influence successful aging, rather than being sought after a negative outcome of aging is realized, may improve the quality of life. Optimal quality of life is what all individuals hope to obtain, whether learning to reach a cracker, climbing the highest mountain, or playing a game of bridge. Maintaining that quality before the end of life, no matter the age, is often based on movement function. The client, whenever possible, should determine identification of the specific function. Identification of the necessary steps to get from existing skill to desired skill is the role of a movement specialist, whether that therapist is dealing with preventive care or postinsult care.

References

To enhance this text and add value for the reader, all references are included on the companion Evolve site that accompanies this textbook. This online service will, when available, provide a link for the reader to a Medline abstract for the article cited. There are 191 cited references and other general references for this chapter, with the majority of those articles being evidence-based citations.

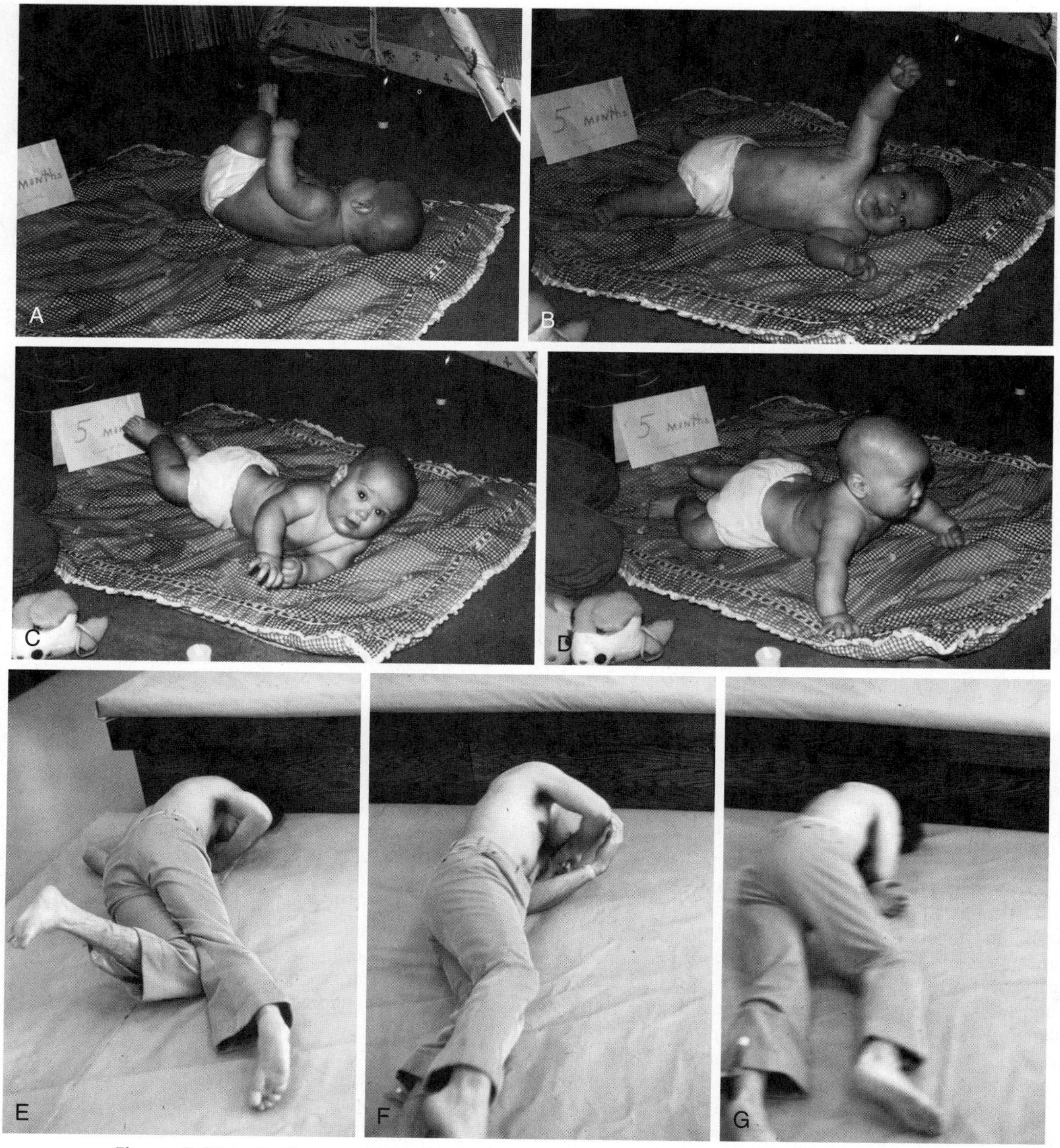

Figure 3-26 ■ Rolling—an activity achieved within the first year. **A,** Child beginning rolling in supine position. **B,** Child semiprone with trunk rotation. **C,** Child brings arm through to become symmetrical while proceeding toward prone position. **D,** Child prone with postural extension. **E,** Adult with traumatic brain injury; first try at rolling toward prone position from supine. **F,** Adult's second try at rolling, changing programming. **G,** Once prone, he is stuck, unable to extend.

CHAPTER 4

Contemporary Issues and Theories of Motor Control, Motor Learning, and Neuroplasticity

MARGARET L. ROLLER, PT, MS, DPT, ROLANDO T. LAZARO, PT, PhD, DPT, GCS, NANCY N. BYL, PT, MPH, PhD, FAPTA, and DARCY A. UMPHRED, PT, PhD, FAPTA

KEY TERMS

motor control theory
motor learning
neuroplasticity

OBJECTIVES

After reading this chapter the student or therapist will be able to:

1. Identify the evolution of motor control theories and discuss the utility of current theory in clinical practice.
2. Identify body structures and functions that contribute to the control of human posture and movement.
3. Relate the cognitive, associative, and autonomous stages of motor learning to behavior and skill performance.
4. Describe the variety of practice conditions that may be used to enhance motor learning within a practice session.
5. Apply motor learning variables related to person, task, and environment within the therapeutic setting.
6. Discuss neuroplasticity theories that explain how the nervous system adapts to demands placed on learning and performance.
7. Discuss the relationship among motor control, motor learning, and neuroplasticity in the production of functional movement behaviors.

The production and control of human movement is a process that varies from a simple reflex loop to a complex network of neural patterns that communicate throughout the central nervous system (CNS) and peripheral nervous system (PNS). Neural networks and motor pattern generators develop as the fetus develops in utero and are active before birth. These simple patterns become building blocks for more skillful, complex, goal-directed motor patterns as a person develops throughout life. New motor patterns are learned through movement, interactions with rich sensory environments, and challenging experiences that drive a person to solve problems. Personal desires and goals of the individual shape the process of learning new motor skills at all stages of life. If a condition exists or develops, or if an event occurs that damages the nervous system and prevents normal transmission, processing, and perception of information in the PNS and CNS, movement control becomes abnormal, slow, labored, uncoordinated, or weak, or movement may not be produced at all. The damaged nervous system is able to repair itself, change, and adapt to some extent by means of nerve regeneration and neuroplasticity. However, when nerve cells die and neural connections are not viable, alternative pathways within the nervous system exist to take the place of the normal process and provide some means of meeting the movement goal—whether it is to walk, use an arm to eat, or make a facial expression. This process of change, healing, or motor learning depends on many factors including inherent elements of the individual such as age, the extent of tissue damage, and other physiological and cognitive processes, as well as external factors such as interactions with sensory and motor system challenges, and goal-directed practice of meaningful, functional motor skills.

This chapter introduces the reader to basic concepts of motor control, motor learning, and neuroplasticity. Figures and tables are provided within each section to emphasize and summarize concepts. A patient case example is used to illustrate concepts in this chapter as they apply to the evaluation and management of people with neurological conditions. This chapter provides a foundation for chapters in Section II: Rehabilitation Management of Clients with Neurological System Pathology, and acts as a foundation for interacting with and treating patients in any clinical setting.

MOTOR CONTROL

Motor control is defined as "the systematic transmission of nerve impulses from the motor cortex to motor units, resulting in coordinated contractions of muscles."[1]

This definition describes motor control in the simplest terms—as a top-down direction of action through the nervous system. In reality, the process of controlling movement begins before the plan is executed, and ends after the muscles have contracted. The essential details of a movement plan must be determined by the individual before the actual execution of the plan. The nervous system actively adjusts muscle force, timing, and tone before the muscles begin to contract, continues to make adjustments throughout the motor action, and compares movement performance with the goal and neural code (directions) of the initial motor plan. This extension of the definition takes into account that the body *accesses sensory information* from the environment, *perceives* the situation and *chooses a movement plan* that it believes to be the appropriate plan to meet the outcome goal of the task that the person is attempting to complete, *coordinates this plan* within the CNS, and finally *executes* the plan through motor neurons in the brain stem and spinal cord to communicate with muscles in postural and limb synergies, plus muscles in the head and neck that are timed to fire in a specific manner. The movement that is produced supplies *sensory feedback* to the CNS to allow the person to (1) modify the plan during performance, (2) know whether the goal of the task has been achieved, and (3) store the information for future performance of the same task-goal combination. Repeated performance of the same movement plan tends to create a preferred pattern that becomes more automatic in nature and less variable in performance. If this movement pattern is designed and executed well, then it is determined that the person has developed a skill. If this pattern is incorrect and does not efficiently accomplish the movement goal, then it is considered abnormal.

Theories and Models of Motor Control

We begin this section with a summary and historical perspective of motor control theories (Table 4-1). The control of human movement has been described in many different ways. The production of reflexive, automatic, adaptive, and voluntary movements and the performance of efficient, coordinated, goal-directed movement patterns involve multiple body systems (input, output, and central processing) and multiple levels within the nervous system. Each model of motor control that is discussed in this section has both merit and disadvantage in its ability to supply a comprehensive picture of motor behavior. These theories serve as a basis for predicting motor responses during patient examination and treatment. They help explain motor skill performance, potential, constraints, limitations, and deficits. They allow the clinician to (1) identify problems in motor performance, (2) develop treatment strategies to help clients remediate performance problems, and (3) evaluate the effectiveness of intervention strategies employed in the clinic. Selecting and using an appropriate model of motor control is important for the analysis and treatment of clients with dysfunctions of posture and movement. As long as the environment and task demands affect changes in the CNS and the individual has the desire to learn, the adaptable nervous system will continue to learn, modify, and adapt motor plans throughout life.

Motor Programs and Central Pattern Generators

A motor program (MP) is a learned behavioral pattern defined as a neural network that can produce rhythmic output patterns with or without sensory input or central control.[2] MPs are sets of movement commands, or "rules," that define the details of skilled motor actions. An MP defines the specific muscles that are needed, the order of muscle activation, and the force, timing, sequence, and duration of muscle contractions. MPs help control the degrees of freedom of interacting body structures, and the number of ways each individual component acts. A generalized motor program (GMP) defines a pattern of movement, rather than every individual aspect of a movement. GMPs allow for the adjustment, flexibility, and adaptation of movement features according to environmental demands. The existence of MPs and GMPs is a generally accepted concept; however, hard evidence that an MP or a GMP exists has yet to

TABLE 4-1 ■ THEORIES OF MOTOR CONTROL

MOTOR CONTROL THEORY	AUTHOR AND DATE	PREMISE
Reflex Theory	Sherrington 1906[244]	Movement is controlled by stimulus-response. Reflexes are combined into actions that create behavior.
Hierarchical Theories	Adams 1971[245]	Cortical centers control movement in a top-down manner throughout the nervous system. Closed-loop mode: sensory feedback is needed and used to control the movement. Open-loop mode: movements are preprogrammed and no feedback is used.
Dynamical Systems Theory	Bernstein 1967[10] Turvey 1977[246] Kelso and Tuller 1984[247] Thelen 1987[248]	Movement emerges to control degrees of freedom. Patterns of movements self-organize within the characteristics of environmental conditions and the existing body systems of the individual. Functional synergies are developed naturally through practice and experience and help solve the problem of coordinating multiple muscles and joint movements at once.
Motor Program Theory	Schmidt 1976[249]	Adaptive, flexible motor programs (MPs) and generalized motor programs (GMPs) exist to control actions that have common characteristics.
Ecological Theories	Gibson and Pick 2000[250]	The person, the task, and the environment interact to influence motor behavior and learning. The interaction of the person with any given environment provides perceptual information used to control movement. The motivation to solve problems to accomplish a desired movement task goal facilitates learning.
Systems Model	Shumway-Cook 2007[35]	Multiple body systems overlap to activate synergies for the production of movements that are organized around functional goals. Considers interaction of the person with the environment.

be found. Advancements in brain imaging techniques may substantiate this theory in the future.[2,3]

In contrast to MPs, a central pattern generator (CPG) is a genetically predetermined movement pattern.[4] CPGs exist as neural networks within the CNS and have the capability of producing rhythmic, patterned outputs resembling normal movement. These movements have the capability of occurring without sensory feedback inputs or descending motor inputs. Two characteristic signs of CPGs are that they result in the repetition of movements in a rhythmic manner and that the system returns to its starting condition when the process ceases.[5] Both MPs and CPGs contribute to the development, refinement, production, and recovery of motor control throughout life.

The Person, the Task, and the Environment: An Ecological Model for Motor Control

Motor control evolves so that people can cope with the environment around them. A person must focus on detecting information in the immediate environment (perception) that is determined to be necessary for performance of the task and achievement of the desired outcome goal. The individual is an active observer and explorer of the environment, which allows the development of multiple ways in which to accomplish (choose and execute) any given task. The individual analyzes a particular sensory environment and chooses the most suitable and efficient way to complete the task. The *person* consists of all functional and dysfunctional body structures and functions that exist and interact with one another. The *task* is the goal-directed behavior, challenge, or problem to be solved. The *environment* consists of everything outside of the body that exists, or is perceived to exist, in the external world. All three of these motor control constructs (person, task, environment) are dynamic and variable, and they interact with one another during learning and production of a goal-directed, effective motor plan.

Body Structures and Functions that Contribute to the Control of Human Posture and Movement

Keen observation of motor output quality during the performance of functional movement patterns helps the therapist determine activity limitations and begin to hypothesize impairments within sensory, motor, musculoskeletal, cardiopulmonary, and other body systems. The following section presents and defines some of these key factors, including sensory input systems, motor output systems, and structures and functions involved in the integration of information in the CNS.

Role of Sensory Information in Motor Control

Sensory receptors from somatosensory (exteroceptors and proprioceptors), visual, and vestibular systems and taste, smell, and hearing fire in response to interaction with the external environment and to movement created by the body. Information about these various modalities is transmitted along afferent peripheral nerves to cells in the spinal cord and brain stem of the CNS. All sensory tracts, with the exception of smell, then synapse in respective sensory nuclei of the thalamus, which acts as a filter and relays this information to the appropriate lobe of the cerebral cortex (e.g., somatosensory to parietal lobe, visual to occipital lobe, vestibular, hearing, and taste to temporal lobe). Sensory information is first received and perceived, then associated with other sensory modalities and memory in the association cortex. Once multiple sensory inputs are associated with one another, the person is then able to *perceive* the body, its posture and movement, the environment and its challenges, and the interaction and position of the body with objects within the environment. The person uses this perceptual information to create an internal representation of the body (internal model) and to choose a movement program, driven by motivation and desire, to meet a final outcome goal. Although the sensory input and motor output systems operate differently, they are inseparable in function within the healthy nervous system. Agility, dexterity, and the ability to produce movement plans that are adaptable to environmental demands reflect the accuracy, flexibility, and plasticity of the sensory-motor system.

The CNS uses sensory information in a variety of ways to regulate posture and movement. Before movement is initiated, information about the position of the body in space, body parts in relation to one another, and environmental conditions is obtained from multiple sensory systems. Special senses of vision, vestibular inputs that respond to gravity and movement, and visual-vestibular interactions supply additional information necessary for static and dynamic balance and postural control as well as visual tracking. Auditory information is integrated with other sensory inputs and plays an important role in the timing of motor responses with environmental signals, reaction time, response latency, and comprehension of spoken word. This information is integrated and used in the selection and execution of the movement strategy. During movement performance, the cerebellum and other neural centers use feedback to compare the actual motor behavior with the intended motor plan. If the actual and intended motor behaviors do not match, an error signal is produced and alterations in the motor behavior are triggered. In some instances, the control system anticipates and makes corrective changes before the detection of the error signal. This anticipatory correction is termed *feed-forward control.* Changing one's gait path while walking in a busy shopping mall to avoid a collision is an example of how visual information about the location of people and objects can be used in a feed-forward manner.

Another role of sensory information is to revise the reference of correctness (central representation) of the MP before it is executed again. For example, a young child standing on a balance beam with the feet close together falls off of the beam. An error signal occurs because of the mismatch between the intended motor behavior and the actual motor result. If the child knows that the feet were too close together when the fall occurred, then the child will space the feet farther apart on the next trial. The information about what happened, falling or not falling, is used in planning movement strategies for balancing on any narrow object such as a balance beam, log, or wall in the future.

Sensory information is necessary during the acquisition phase of learning a new motor skill and is useful for controlling movements during the execution of the motor plan.[6-8] However, sensory information is not always necessary when performing well-learned motor behaviors in a stable and familiar context.[6,7] Rothwell and colleagues[7] studied a man with severe sensory neuropathy in the upper extremity. He could write sentences with his eyes closed and drive a car with a manual transmission without watching the gear shift. He did, however, have difficulty with fine motor tasks such as buttoning his shirt and using a knife and fork to eat when denied visual information. The importance of sensory information must be weighed by the individual, unconsciously filtering and choosing appropriate and accurate sensory inputs to use to meet the movement goal.

Sensory experiences and learning alter sensory representations, or cortical "maps," in the primary somatosensory, visual, and auditory areas of the brain. Training, as well as use and disuse of sensory information, has the potential to drive long-term structural changes in the CNS, including the formation, removal, and remodeling of synapses and dendritic connections in the cortex. This process of cortical plasticity is complex and involves multiple cellular and synaptic mechanisms.[9] Plasticity in the nervous system is discussed further in the third section of this chapter.

Choice of Motor Pattern and the Control of Voluntary Movement

A choice of body movement is made based on the person's perception of the environment, his or her relationship to objects within it, and a goal to be met. The person chooses from a collection of plans that have been developed and refined over his or her lifetime. If a movement plan does not exist, a similar plan is chosen and modified to meet the needs of the task. Once the plan has been chosen it is customized by the CNS with what are determined to be the correct actions to execute given the perceived situation and goal of the individual.

Coordination

The movement plan is customized by communications among the frontal lobes, basal ganglia, and cerebellum, with functional connections through the brain stem and thalamus. During this process specific details of the plan are determined. Postural tone, coactivation, and timing of trunk muscle firing are set for proximal stability, balance, and postural control. Force, timing, and tone of limb synergies are set to allow for smooth, coordinated movements that are accurate in direction of trajectory, order, and sequence. The balance between agonist and antagonist muscle activity is determined so that fine distal movements are precise and skilled. This process is complicated by the number of possible combinations of musculoskeletal elements. The CNS must solve this "degrees of freedom" problem so that rapid execution of the goal-directed movement can proceed and reliably meet the desired outcome.[10] Once these movement details are complete the motor plan is executed by the primary motor area in the precentral gyrus of the frontal lobe.

Execution

Pyramidal cells in the corticospinal and corticobulbar tracts *execute* the voluntary motor plan. Neural impulses travel down these central efferent systems and communicate with motor neurons in the brain stem and spinal cord. The corticobulbar tract communicates with brain stem motor nuclei to control muscles of facial expression, mouth and tongue for speaking and eating, larynx and pharynx for voice and swallow, voluntary eye movements for visual tracking and saccades, and muscles of the upper trapezius for shoulder girdle elevation. The corticospinal tract communicates with motor neurons in the spinal cord. The ventral corticospinal tract system communicates primarily with proximal muscle groups to provide the appropriate amount of activation to stabilize the trunk and limb girdles, thus allowing for dexterous distal limb movements. The lateral corticospinal tract system communicates primarily with muscles of the arms and legs—firing alpha motor neurons in coordinated synergy patterns with appropriate activity in agonist and antagonist muscles so that movements are smooth and precise. Other motor nuclei in the brain stem are programmed to fire just before corticospinal tract activity in order to supply postural tone. These include lateral and medial vestibular spinal tracts, reticulospinal tract, and rubrospinal tract systems. Adequate and balanced muscle tone of flexors and extensors in the trunk and limbs occurs automatically, without the need for conscious control. These brain stem nuclei have tonic firing rates that are modulated up or down to effectively provide more or less muscle tone in body areas depending on stimulation from gravity, limbic system activity, external perturbations, or other neuronal activity.

Adaptation

Adaptation is the process of using sensory inputs from multiple systems to adapt motor plans, decrease performance errors, and predict or estimate consequences of movement choices. The goal of adaptation is the production of consistently effective and efficient skilled motor actions. When all possible body systems and environmental conditions are considered in the motor control process, it is easy to understand why there is often a mismatch between the movement plan that is chosen and how it is actually executed. Errors in movements occur and cause problems that the nervous system must solve in order to deliver effective, efficient, accurate plans that meet the task goal. To solve this problem the CNS creates an internal representation of the body and the surrounding world. This acts as a model that can be adapted and changed in the presence of varying environmental demands. It allows for the ability to predict and estimate the differences between similar situations. This ability is learned by practicing various task configurations in real-life environments. Without experience, accurate movement patterns that consistently meet desired task goals are difficult to achieve.[11]

Anticipatory Control

Anticipatory control of posture and postural adjustments stabilizes the body by minimizing displacement of the center of gravity. Anticipatory control involves motor plans that are programmed to act in advance of movement. A comparison between incoming sensory information and knowledge of prior movement successes and failures enables the system to choose the appropriate course of action.[3]

Flexibility

A person should have enough flexibility in performance to vary the details of a simple or complex motor plan to meet the challenge presented by any given environmental context. This is a beneficial characteristic of motor control. When considering postural control, for example, a person will typically display a random sway pattern during standing that may ensure continuous, dynamic sensory inputs to multiple sensory systems.[12] The person is constantly adjusting posture and position to meet the demand of standing upright (earth vertical), as well as to seek information from the environment. Rhythmic, oscillating, or stereotypical sway patterns that are unidirectional in nature are not considered flexible and are not as readily adaptable to changes in the environment. Lack of flexibility or randomness in postural sway may actually render the person at greater risk for loss of balance and falls.

Control of Voluntary Movement

Table 4-2 shows the body system processes involved in motor control, their actions, and the body structures included. The following section explains these processes in more detail.

Role of the Cerebellum

The primary roles of the cerebellum are to maintain posture and balance during static and dynamic tasks and to coordinate movements before execution and during performance. The cerebellum processes multiple neural signals from (1) motor areas of the cerebral cortex for motor planning, (2) sensory tract systems (dorsal spinal cerebellar tract, ventral spinal cerebellar tract) from muscle and joint receptors for proprioceptive and kinesthetic sense information resulting from movement performance, and (3) vestibular system information for the regulation of upright control and balance at rest and during movements. It compares motor plan signals driven by the cortex with what is received from muscles and joints in the periphery and makes necessary adjustments and adaptations to achieve the intended coordinated movement sequence. Movements that are frequently repeated "instructions" are stored in the cerebellum as procedural memory traces. This increases the efficiency of its role in coordinating movement. The cerebellum also plays a role in function of the reticular activating system (RAS). The RAS network exists in the brain stem tegmentum and consists of a network of nerve cells that maintain consciousness in humans and help people focus attention and block out distractions that may affect motor performance. Damage to the cerebellum, its tract systems, or its structure creates problems of movement coordination, not execution or choice of which program to run. The cerebellum also plays a role in language, attention, and mental imagery functions that are not considered to take place in motor areas of the cerebral cortex (see Table 4-2).

The cerebellum plays four important roles in motor control[13]:

1. *Feed-forward processing*: The cerebellum receives neural signals, processes them in a sequential order, and sends information out, providing a rapid response to any incoming information. It is not designed to act like the cerebral cortex and does not have the capability of generating self-sustaining neural patterns.
2. *Divergence and convergence*: The cerebellum receives a great number of inputs from multiple body structures, processes this information extensively through a structured internal network, and sends the results out through a limited number of output cells.
3. *Modularity*: The cerebellum is functionally divided into independent modules—hundreds to thousands—all with different inputs and outputs. Each module appears to function independently, although they each share neurons with the inferior olives, Purkinje cells, mossy and parallel fibers, and deep cerebellar nuclei.
4. *Plasticity*: Synapses within the cerebellar system (between parallel fibers and Purkinje cells, and synapses between mossy fibers and deep nuclear cells) are susceptible to modification of their output strength. The influence of input on nuclear cells is adjustable, which gives great flexibility to adjust and fine-tune the relationship between cerebellar inputs and outputs.

Role of the Basal Ganglia

The basal ganglia are a collection of nuclei located in the forebrain and midbrain and consisting of the globus pallidus, putamen, caudate nucleus, substantia nigra, and subthalamic nuclei. It has primary functions in motor control and motor learning. It plays a role in deciding which motor plan

TABLE 4-2 ■ COMPONENTS OF MOTOR CONTROL: BODY SYSTEM PROCESSES INVOLVED IN MOTOR CONTROL, THEIR ACTIONS, AND THE BODY STRUCTURES INCLUDED

PROCESS	ACTION	BODY STRUCTURES INVOLVED
Sensation	Sensory information, feedback from exteroceptors and proprioceptors	Peripheral afferent neurons, brain stem, cerebellum, thalamus, sensory receiving areas in the parietal, occipital, and temporal lobes
Perception	Combining, comparing, and filtering sensory inputs	Brain stem, thalamus, sensory association areas in the parietal, occipital, visual, and temporal lobes
Choice of movement plan	Use of the perceptual map to access the appropriate motor plan	Association areas, frontal lobe, basal ganglia
Coordination	Determining the details of the plan including force, timing, tone, direction, and extent of the movement of postural and limb synergies and actions	Frontal lobe, basal ganglia, cerebellum, thalamus
Execution	Execution of the motor plan	Corticospinal and corticobulbar tract systems, brain stem motor nuclei, and alpha and gamma motor neurons
Adaptation	Compare movement with the motor plan and adjust the plan during performance	Spinal neural networks, cerebellum

or behavior to execute at any given time. It has connections to the limbic system and is therefore believed to be involved in "reward learning." It plays a key role in eye movements through midbrain connections with the superior colliculus and helps to regulate postural tone as a basis for the control of body positions, preparedness, and central set. Refer to Chapter 20 for additional information on the basal ganglia.

Information Processing

The processing of information through the sensory input, motor output, and central integrative structures occurs by various methods to produce movement behaviors. These methods allow us to deal with the temporal and spatial components necessary for coordinated motor output and allow us to anticipate so that a response pattern may be prepared in advance. *Serial processing* is a specific, sequential order of processing of information (Figure 4-1) through various centers. Information proceeds lockstep through each center. *Parallel processing* is processing of information that can be used for more than one activity by more than one center simultaneously or nearly simultaneously. A third and more flexible type of processing of information is *parallel-distributed processing.*[14] This type of processing combines the best attributes of serial and parallel processing. When the situation demands serial processing, this type of activity occurs. At other times parallel processing is the mode of choice. For optimal processing of intrinsic and extrinsic sensory information by various regions of the brain, a combination of both serial and parallel processing is the most efficient mode. The type of processing depends on the constraints of the situation. For example, maintaining balance after an unexpected external perturbation requires rapid processing, whereas learning to voluntarily shift the center of gravity to the limits of stability requires a different combination of processing modes.

In summary, information processing reinforces and refines motor patterns. It allows the organism to initiate compensatory strategies if an ineffective motor pattern is selected or if an unexpected perturbation occurs. And, most important, information processing facilitates motor learning.

Movement Patterns Arising from Self-Organizing Subsystems

Coordinated movement patterns are developed and refined via dynamic interaction among body systems and subsystems in response to internal and external constraints. Movement patterns used to accomplish a goal are contextually appropriate and arise as an emergent property of subsystem interaction. Several principles relate to self-organizing systems: reciprocity, distributed function, consensus, and emergent properties.[15]

Reciprocity implies information flow between two or more neural networks. These networks can represent specific brain centers, for example, the cerebellum and basal ganglia (Figure 4-2). Alternatively, the neural networks can be interacting neuronal clusters located within a single center, for example, the basal ganglia. One model to demonstrate reciprocity is the basal ganglia regulation of motor behavior through direct and indirect pathways to cortical areas. The more direct pathway from the putamen to the globus pallidus internal segment provides net inhibitory effects. The more indirect pathway from the putamen through the globus pallidus external segment and subthalamic nucleus provides a net excitatory effect on the globus pallidus internal segment. Alteration of the balance between these pathways is postulated to produce motor dysfunction.[16,17] An abnormally decreased outflow from the basal ganglia is postulated to produce involuntary motor patterns, which produce excessive motion such as chorea, hemiballism, or nonintentional tremor. Alternatively, an abnormally increased outflow from the basal ganglia is postulated to produce a paucity of motions, as seen in the rigidity observed in individuals with Parkinson disease (see Chapter 20).

Distributed function presupposes that a single center or neural network has more than one function. The concept also implies that several centers share the same function. For example, a center may serve as the coordinating unit of an activity in one task and may serve as a pattern generator or oscillator to maintain the activity in another task. An advantage of distributing function among groups of neurons or centers is to provide centers with overlapping or redundant functions. Neuroscientists believe such redundancy is a safety feature. If a neuronal lesion occurs, other centers can

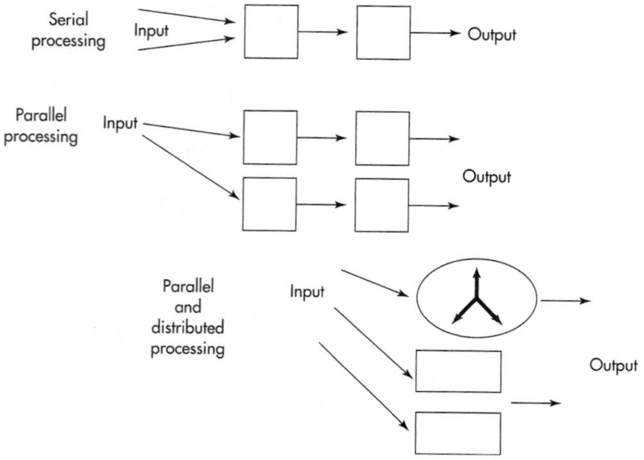

Figure 4-1 ■ Methods of information processing.

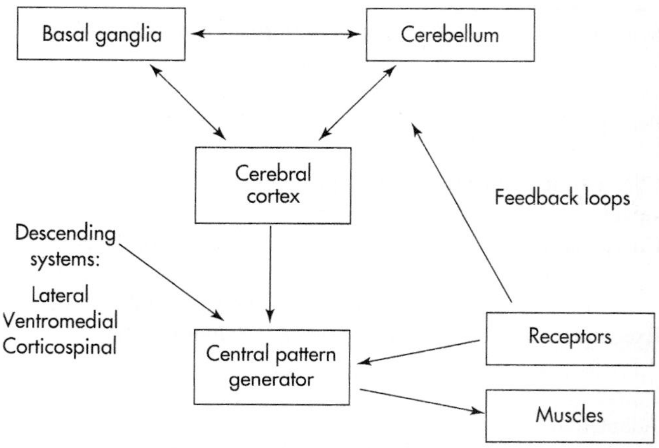

Figure 4-2 ■ Systems model of motor control.

assume critical functional roles, thereby producing recovery from CNS dysfunction.[18-22]

Consensus implies that motor behavior occurs when a majority of brain centers or regions reach a critical threshold to produce activation. Also, through consensus extraneous information or information that does require immediate attention is filtered. If, however, a novel stimulus enters the system, it carries more weight and receives immediate attention. A novel stimulus may be new to the system, may reflect a potentially harmful situation, or may result from the conflict of multiple inputs.

Emergent properties may be understood by the adage "the whole is greater than the sum of its parts." This concept implies that brain *centers,* not a single brain center, work together to produce movement. An example of the emergent properties concept is continuous repetitive activity (oscillation). In Figure 4-3, *A,* a hierarchy is represented by three neurons arranged in tandem. The last neuron ends on a responder. If a single stimulus activates this network, a single response occurs. What is the response if the neurons are arranged so that the third neuron sends a collateral branch to the first neuron in addition to the ending on the responder? In this case (Figure 4-3, *B*), a single stimulus activates neuron No. 1, which in turn activates neurons No. 2 and No. 3, causing a response as well as reactivating neuron No. 1. This neuronal arrangement produces a series of responses rather than a single response. This process is also termed *endogenous activity.*

Another example of an emergent property is the production of motor behavior. Rather than having every MP stored in the brain, an abstract representation of the intended goal is stored. At the time of motor performance, various brain centers use the present sensory information, combined with past memory of the task, to develop the appropriate motor strategy. This concept negates a hardwired MP concept. If MPs were hardwired and if an MP existed for every movement ever performed, the brain would need a huge storage capacity and would lack the adaptability necessary for complex function.

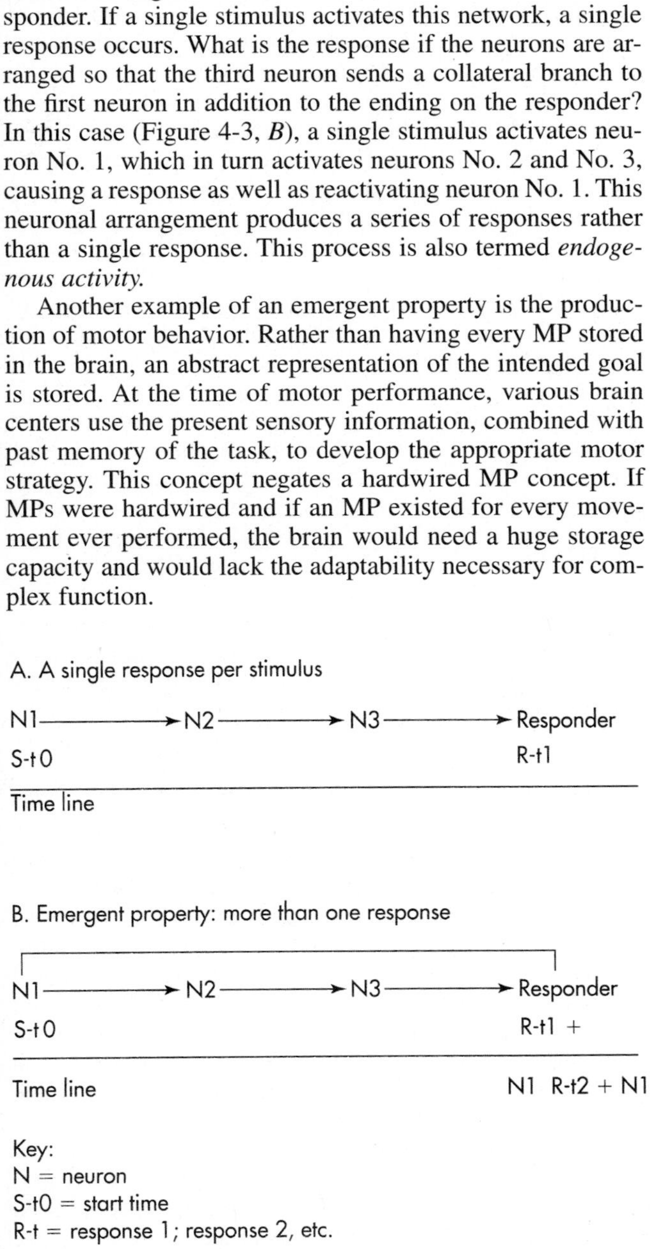

Figure 4-3 ■ Emergent property.

Controlling the Degrees of Freedom

Combinations of muscle and joint action permit a large number of degrees of freedom that contribute to movement. A system with a large number of degrees of freedom is called a *high-dimensional system.* For a contextually appropriate movement to occur, the number of degrees of freedom needs to be constrained. Bernstein[10] suggested that the number of degrees of freedom could be reduced by muscles working in synergies, that is, coupling muscles and joints of a limb to produce functional patterns of movement. The functional unit of motor behavior is then a *synergy.* Synergies help to reduce the degrees of freedom, transforming a high-dimensional system into a low-dimensional system. For example, a step is considered to be a functional synergy pattern for the lower extremity. Linking together stepping synergies with the functional synergies of other limbs creates locomotion (interlimb coordination).

Functional synergy implies that muscles are activated in an appropriate sequence and with appropriate force, timing, and directional components. These components can be represented as fixed or "relative" ratios, and the control comes from input given to the cerebellum from higher centers in the brain and the peripheral or spinal system and from prior learning (see Chapter 21).[20,22,23] The relative parameters are also termed *control parameters.* Scaling control parameters leads to a change in motor behavior to accomplish the task. For example, writing your name on the blackboard exemplifies scaling force, timing, and amplitude. Scaling is the proportional increase or decrease of the parameter to produce the intended motor activity.

Coordinated movement is defined as an orderly sequence of muscle activity in a single functional synergy or the orderly sequence of functional synergies with appropriate scaling of activation parameters necessary to produce the intended motor behavior. Uncoordinated movement can occur at the level of the scaling of control parameters in one functional synergy or inappropriate coupling of functional synergies. The control parameter of duration will be used to illustrate scaling. If muscle A is active for 10% of the duration of the motor activity and muscle B is active 50% of the time, the fixed ratio of A/B is 1:5. If the movement is performed slowly, the relative time for the entire movement increases. Fixed ratios also increase proportionally. Writing your name on a blackboard very small or very large yields the same results—your name.

Timing of muscle on/off activation for antagonistic muscles such as biceps and triceps, or hamstrings and quadriceps, needs to be accurate for coordination and control of movement patterns. If one muscle group demonstrates a delayed onset or maintains a longer duration of activity, overlapping with triceps "on" time, the movement will appear uncoordinated. Patients with neurological dysfunction often demonstrate alterations in the timing of muscle activity within functional synergies and in coupling functional synergies to produce movement.[24,25] These functional movement synergies are not hardwired but represent emergent properties. They are flexible and adaptable to meet the challenges of the task and the environmental constraints.

Finite Number of Movement Strategies

The concept of *emergent properties* could conceivably imply an unlimited number of movement strategies available to perform a particular task. However, limiting the degrees of freedom decreases the number of strategies available for selection. In addition, constraints imposed by the internal environment (e.g., musculoskeletal system, cardiovascular system, metabolic activity, cognition) and external environment (e.g., support surface, obstacles, lighting) limit the number of movement strategies. Horak and Nashner[26] observed that a finite number of balance strategies were used by individuals in response to externally applied linear perturbations on a force plate system. With use of a life span approach, VanSant[27] identified a limited number of movement patterns for the upper limb, head-trunk, and lower limb for the task of rising from supine to standing.

The combination of these strategies produces the necessary variability in motor behavior. Although an individual has a preferred or modal profile, the healthy person with an intact neuromuscular system can combine strategies in various body regions to produce different movement patterns that also accomplish the task. Persons with neurological deficits may be unable to produce a successful, efficient movement pattern because of their inability to combine strategies or adapt a strategy for a given environmental change (e.g., differing chair height for sit-to-stand transitions).

Variability of Movements Implies Normalcy

A key to the assessment and treatment of individuals with neurological dysfunction lies in variability of movement and in the notion that variability is a sign of normalcy, and stereotypical behavior is a sign of dysfunction.

Age, activity level, the environment, constraints of a goal, and neuropathological conditions affect the selection of patterns available for use during movement tasks. When change occurs in one or more of the neural subsystems, a new movement pattern emerges. The element that causes change is called a *control parameter.* For example, an increase in the speed of walking occurs until a critical speed and degree of hip extension are reached, thereby switching the movement pattern to a run. When the speed of the run is decreased, there is a shift back to the preferred movement pattern of walking. A control parameter shifts the individual into a different pattern of motor behavior.

This concept underlies theories of development and learning. Development and learning can be viewed as moving the system from a stable state to a more unstable state. When the control variable is removed, the system moves back to the early, more stable state. As the control variable continues to push the system, the individual spends more time in the new state and less time in the earlier state until the individual spends most of the time in the new state. When this occurs, the new state becomes the preferred state. Moving or shifting to the new, preferred state does not obviate the ability of the individual to use the earlier state of motor behavior. Therefore new movement patterns take place when critical changes occur in the system because of a control parameter but do not eliminate older, less-preferred patterns of movement.

Motivation to accomplish a task in spite of functional limitations and neuropathological conditions can also shift the individual's CNS to select different patterns of motor behavior. The musculoskeletal system, by nature of the architecture of the joints and muscle attachments, can be a constraint on the movement pattern. An individual with a functional contracture may be limited in the ability to bend a joint only into a desired range, thereby decreasing the movement repertoire available to the individual. Such a constraint produces adaptive motor behavior. Dorsiflexion of the foot needs to meet a critical degree of toe clearance during gait. If there is a range of motion limitation in dorsiflexion, then biomechanical constraints imposed on the nervous system will produce adaptive motor behaviors (e.g., toe clearance during gait). Changes in motor patterns during the task of rising from supine to standing are observed when healthy individuals wear an orthosis to limit dorsiflexion.[28] The inability to easily open and close the hand with rotation may lead to adaptations that require the shoulder musculature to place the hand in a more functional position. This adaptation uses axial and trunk muscles and will limit the use of that limb in both fine and gross motor performance. Refer to Chapter 23.

Preferred, nonobligatory movement patterns that are stable yet flexible enough to meet ever-changing environmental conditions are considered *attractor states.* Individuals can choose from a variety of movement patterns to accomplish a given task. For example, older adults may choose from a variety of fall-prevention movement patterns when faced with the risk of falling. The choice of motor plan may be negatively influenced by age-related declines in the sensory input systems or a fear of falling. For example, when performing the Multi-Directional Reach Test,[29] an older adult may choose to reach forward, backward (lean), or laterally without shifting the center of gravity toward the limits of stability. This person has the capability of performing a different reaching pattern if asked, but prefers a more stable pattern.

Obligatory and stereotypical movement patterns suggest that the individual does not have the capability of adapting to new situations or cannot use different movement patterns to accomplish a given task. This inability may be a result of internal constraints that are functional or pathophysiological. The patient who has had a stroke has CNS constraints that limit the number of different movement patterns that can emerge from the self-organizing system. With recovery, the patient may be able to select and use additional movement strategies. Cognition and the capability to learn may also limit the number of movement patterns available to the individual and the ability of the person to select and use new or different movement patterns.

Obligatory and stereotypical movement patterns also arise from external constraints imposed on the organism. Consider the external constraints placed on a concert violin player. These external constraints include, for example, the length of the bow and the position of the violin. Repetitive movement patterns leading to cumulative trauma disorder in healthy individuals can lead to muscular and neurological changes.[30-33] Over time, changes in dystonic posturing and changes in the somatosensory cortex have been observed. Although one hypothesis considers that the focal dystonia results from sensory integrative problems, the observable result is a stereotypical motor problem.

To review, the nervous system responds to a variety of internal and external constraints to develop and execute motor behavior that is efficient to accomplish a specific task. Efficiency can be examined in terms of metabolic cost to the individual, type of movement pattern used, preferred or habitual movement (habit) used by the individual, and time to complete the task. The term *attractor state* is used in dynamical systems theory to describe the preferred pattern or habitual movement.

Individuals with neurological deficits may have limited repertoires of movement strategies available. Patients experiment with various motor patterns in order to learn the most efficient, energy-conscious motor strategy to accomplish the task. Therapists can plan interventions that help to facilitate refinement of the task to match the patient's capability, allowing the task to be completed using a variety of movement strategies rather than limited stereotypical strategies, leading to an increase in function.

Errors in Motor Control

When the actual motor behavior does not match the intended motor plan, an error in motor control is detected by the CNS. Common examples of errors in motor control are loss of balance; inappropriate scaling of force, timing, or directional control; and inability to ignore unreliable sensory information, resulting in sensory conflict. Any one or combination of these errors may be the cause of a fall or error in performance accuracy.

Errors also occur when unexpected factors disrupt the execution of the program. For example, when the surface is unreliable (sand, unstable, moving), this will force the individual to adapt motor responses to meet the demand of the environment. Switching between closed environments (more stable) and open environments (more unpredictable) will challenge the individual to adapt motor responses. When an individual steps off of a moving sidewalk, a disruption in walking occurs. The first few steps are not smooth because the person needs to switch movement strategies from one incorporating a moving support surface to one incorporating a stationary support surface.

Errors occur in the perception of sensory information, in selection of the appropriate MP, in selection of the appropriate variable parameters, or in the response execution. Patients with neurological deficits may demonstrate a combination of these errors. Therefore an assessment of motor deficits in clients includes analysis of these types of errors. If a therapist observes a motor control problem, there is no guarantee that the central problem arises from within the motor system. Somatosensory problems can drive motor dysfunction; cognitive and emotional problems express themselves through motor output. Thus it is up to the movement specialist to differentiate the cause of the problem through valid and reliable examination tools (see Chapter 8). Once the cause of the motor problem has been identified, selection of interventions should lead to more outcomes.

All individuals, both healthy and those with CNS dysfunction, make errors in motor programming. These errors are assessed by the CNS and are stored in past memory of the experience. Errors in motor programming are extremely useful in learning. Learning can be viewed as decreasing the mismatch between the intended and actual motor behavior. This mismatch is a measure of the error; therefore a decrease in the degree of the error is indicative of learning. Errors, then, are an important part of the rehabilitation process. However, this does not mean that the therapist allows the client to practice errors over and over. The ability of the patient to detect an error and correct it to produce appropriate and efficient motor behavior is one key to recovery and an important consideration when intervention strategies are developed. This will be discussed further in the next section of this chapter.

Motor Control Section Summary

Motor control theories have been developed and have evolved over many years as our understanding of nervous system structure and function has become more advanced. The control of posture and movement is a complex process that involves many structures and levels within the human body. It requires accurate sensory inputs, coordinated motor outputs, and central integrative processes to produce skillful, goal-directed patterns of movement that achieve desired movement goals. We must integrate and filter multiple sensory inputs from both the internal environment of the body and the external world around us to determine position in space and choose the appropriate motor plan to accomplish a given task. We combine individual biomechanical and muscle segments of the body into complex movement synergies to deal with the infinite "degrees of freedom" available during the production of voluntary movement. Well learned motor plans are stored and retrieved and modified to allow for flexibility and variety of movement patterns and postures. When the PNS or CNS is damaged and the control of movement is impaired, new, modified, or substitute motor plans can be generated to accomplish goal-directed behaviors, remain adaptable to changing environments, and produce variable movement patterns. The process of learning new motor plans and refining existing behaviors by driving neuroplastic changes in the nervous system is discussed in the next sections of this chapter. The control of posture and balance is also discussed in Chapter 22.

MOTOR LEARNING

Therapeutic interventions that are focused on restoring functional skills to individuals with various forms of neurological problems have been part of the scope of practice of physical therapists (PTs) and occupational therapists (OTs) since the beginning of both professions. These two professions have emerged with a complementary background to examine, evaluate, determine a prognosis, and implement interventions that empower clients to regain functional control of activities of daily living (ADLs) (e.g., getting out of bed, bathing, walking, and eating, as well as working, playing, and socially interacting) and resume active participation in life after neurological insult. These two professions specialize in the analysis of movement and possess knowledge of the scientific background to understand why the movement is occurring, what strengths and limitations exist within body systems to produce that movement, and how different therapeutic interventions can facilitate or enhance functional movement strategies that remediate dysfunction and ultimately carry over into improved performance of daily activities and participation in life of an individual. PTs and OTs are also knowledgeable about diseases of body systems (neurological, musculoskeletal, integumentary, cardiopulmonary, and integumentary systems) and how the existence or progression of these pathological states affects motor performance and quality of life. Consideration and training of individuals who give assistance and support needed to help clients maintain functional skills during transitional disease states is also a component of practice and of treating the client in a holistic manner.

It is therefore important for clinicians to understand how individuals learn or relearn motor tasks and how learning of motor skills can best be achieved to optimize outcomes.

Motor learning results in a permanent change in the performance of a skill because of experience or practice.[34] The end result of motor learning is the acquisition of a new movement, or the reacquisition and/or modification of movement.[35] The patient must be able to prepare and carry out a particular learned movement[36] in a manner that is efficient (optimal movement with the least amount of time, energy, and effort),[37] consistent (same movement over repeated trials),[38] and transferrable (ability to perform movement under different environments and conditions) to be considered to have learned a skill.

Long-term learning of a particular motor task allows the patient to use this particular skill to optimize function. This type of learning is expressed in declarative and procedural memory. Declarative or explicit memory is expressed by conscious recall of facts or knowledge. An example of this could be the patient verbally stating the steps needed when going up the stairs with the use of crutches. This is opposed to procedural (or nondeclarative) learning, in which movement is performed without conscious thought (e.g., riding a bike or rollerblading). The interplay of conscious (cognitive and emotional) and unconscious memory affects ultimate learning and may decrease the time needed to learn or relearn a functional movement and its use in everyday activity.

The ability of an individual to have learned a motor skill is measured indirectly by testing the ability of a patient to perform a particular task or activity both over time and in different environmental contexts (performance). The testing must be done over a period of time to determine long-term learning and minimize the temporary effects of practice. In *retention tests,* the patient performs the task under the same conditions in which the task was practiced. This type of test evaluates the patient's ability to learn the task. This is in contrast to *transfer tests,* in which the patient performs the activity under different conditions from those in which the skill was practiced. This evaluates the ability of the patient to use a previously learned motor skill to solve a different motor problem.

Motor skills can be categorized as discrete, continuous, or serial. Discrete motor skills pertain to tasks that have a specific start and finish. Tasks that are repetitive are classified as *continuous* motor skills. Serial skills involve several discrete tasks connected in a particular sequence that rapidly progress from one part to the next.[37] The category of a particular motor skill is a major factor in making clinical decisions regarding the person-, task-, and environment-related variables that affect motor learning. This is discussed later in the chapter.

An Illustration of Motor Learning Principles

Motor learning is the product of an intricate balance between the feed-forward and feedback sensorimotor systems and the complex central processor—the brain—for the end result of acquiring and refining motor skills. People go through distinct phases when they learn new motor skills.

Observe the sequential activities of the child walking off the park bench in Figure 4-4, *A* through *C.* A clear understanding of this relationship of walking and falling is established. In frame *A,* the child is running a feed-forward program for walking. The cerebellum is procedurally responsible for modulating appropriate motor control over the activity and will correct or modify the program of walking when necessary to attain the directed goal. Unfortunately, a simple correction of walking is not adequate for the environment presented in frame *B.* The cerebellum has no prior knowledge of the feedback presented in this second frame and thus is still running a feed-forward program for stance on the

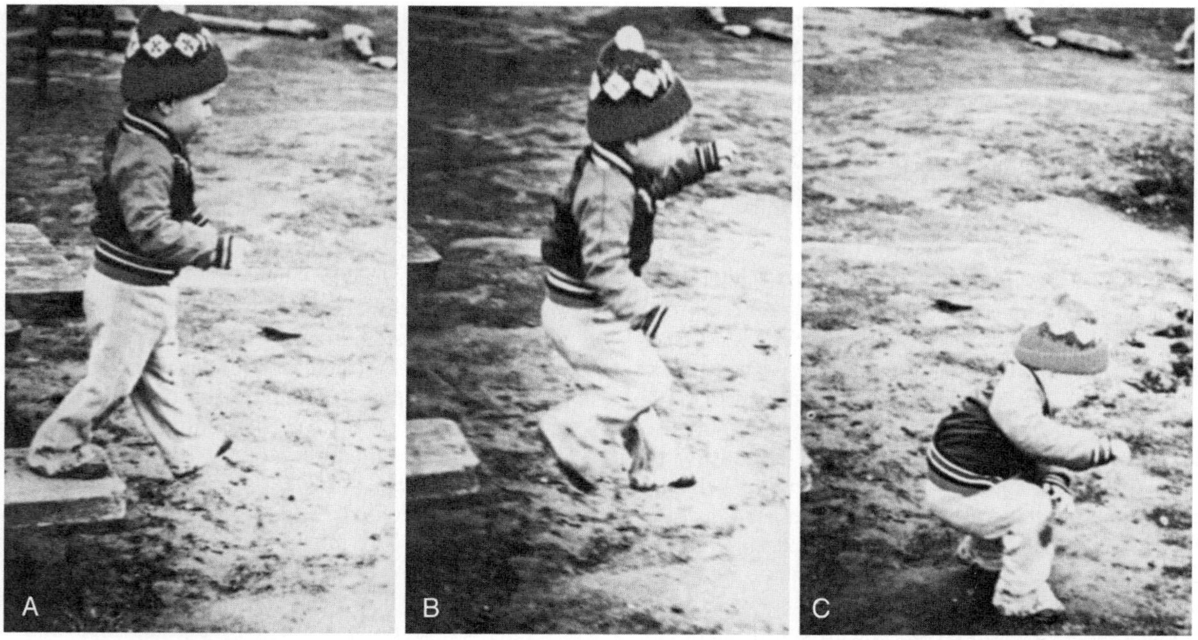

Figure 4-4 ■ **A,** Experiencing the unknown. **B,** Identifying the problem. **C,** Solving the problem.

left leg and swing on the right leg. The cerebellum and somatosensory cortices are processing a massive amount of mismatched information from the proprioceptive, vestibular, and visual receptors. In addition, the dopamine receptors are activated during the goal-driven behaviors, creating a balance of inhibition and excitation. Once the executive or higher cognitive system recognizes that the body is falling (which has been experienced from falling off a chair or bed), a shift in motor control focus from walking to falling must take place. To prepare for falling, the somatosensory system must generate a sensory plan and then relay that plan to the motor system through the sensorimotor feedback loops. The frontal lobe will tell the basal ganglia and the cerebellum to brace and prepare for impact. The basal ganglia are responsible for initiating the new program, and the cerebellum carries out the procedure, as observed in Figure 4-4, *C*. The child succeeds at the task and receives positive peripheral and central feedback in the process. It is possible that this experience has created a new procedural program that in time will be verbally labeled "jumping." The entire process of the initial motor learning takes 1 to 2 seconds. Because of the child's motivation and interest (see Chapter 5), the program is practiced for the next 30 to 45 minutes. This is the initial acquisition phase and helps the nervous system store the MP to be used for the rest of the child's life. If this program is to become a procedural skill, practice must continue within similar environments and conditions. Ultimately the errors will be reduced and the skill will be refined. Finally, with practice, the program will enter the retention phase as a high-level skill. The skill can be modified in terms of force, timing, sequencing, and speed and is transferrable to different settings. This ongoing modification and improvement are the hallmarks of true procedural learning. Modifications within the program will be a function of the plasticity that occurs within the CNS throughout life as the child ages and changes body size and distribution. Similar plasticity and the ability to change, modify, and reprogram motor plans will be demanded by individuals who age with chronic sensorimotor limitations. Unfortunately, in many of these individuals, the CNS is not capable of producing and accommodating change, which creates new challenges as they age with long-term movement dysfunctions (see Chapters 27, 32, and 35).

Stages of Motor Learning

Several authors have developed models to describe the stages of motor learning. These models are presented in Table 4-3. Regardless of the model, it is widely accepted that the process of learning a motor task occurs in stages. During the initial stages of learning a motor skill, the intent of the learner is to understand the task. To be able to develop this understanding requires a high level of concentration and cognitive processing. In the middle and later stages, the individual learns to refine the movement, improve efficiency and coordination, and perform the skill within different environmental contexts. The later stages are characterized by automaticity and a decreased level of attention needed for successful completion of the task. It is important to emphasize early that because the activities performed by a learner during each stage of learning will be different, the role of the clinician, the types of learning activities, and the clinical environment must also be different.

TABLE 4-3 ■ STAGES OF MOTOR LEARNING—THREE MODELS

MOTOR LEARNING MODEL	STAGE ONE	STAGE TWO	STAGE THREE
Fitts and Posner (1967)[39]	Cognitive	Associative	Autonomous
Bernstein (1967)[10]	Novice	Advanced	Expert
Gentile (1998)[46]	Acquire the plan	Develop consistency and adaptability	

The learning model described by Fitts and Posner[39] consists of a continuous progression through three stages: cognitive, associative, and autonomous.

A learner functions in the *cognitive stage* at the beginning of the learning process. The person is highly focused on the task, is attentive to all that it demands, and develops an understanding of what is expected and involved in performance of the skill. Many errors are made in performance; questions are asked; cues, instructions, and guidance are given by the clinician; and demonstrations are found to be helpful in this phase of learning. Performance outcomes are variable and inconsistent, but the improvements achieved can be profound.

During the *associative stage* the learner refines movement strategies, detects errors and problem solves independent of therapist feedback, and is becoming more efficient and reliable at achieving the task goal. The length of time spent in this phase tends to be dependent on the complexity of the task. The ability to associate existing environmental inputs with motor plans for improved timing, accuracy, and coordination of activities to accomplish a task goal is improved. Although variability in performance decreases, the client continues to explore solutions to best solve a movement problem.

Focused practice with repetition over time leads to the automatic performance of motor skills in the *autonomous stage* of learning. The individual is in control of the learned movement plan and is able to use it with little cognitive attention while involved in other activities. Skills are performed with preferred, appropriate, and flexible speed, amplitude, direction, timing, and force. Consistency of performance is a hallmark of this phase, as is the ability to detect and self-correct performance errors. Individuals who do not have the cognitive skill to remember the learning can go through a much longer repetitive practice schedule to learn the motor skill, but there will be very little carryover into other functional movements or activities.[40-42]

In summary, the overall process of the stages of motor learning as introduced by Fitts and Posner[39] suggests that first a basic understanding of a task be established, along with a motor pattern. Practice of the task then leads to problem solving and a decrease in the degrees of freedom during performance, resulting in improved coordination and accuracy. As the learner continues to practice and solves the motor task problem in different ways and with different physical and environmental constraints, the movement plan becomes more flexible and adaptable to a wide range of task demands.

Bernstein[10] presented a more biomechanical perspective as he addressed the problem of degrees of freedom during motor learning. He also broke the motor learning process down into three stages: novice, advanced, and expert. He proposed that these three stages are necessary to allow a learner to reduce the large number of degrees of freedom that are inherent in the musculoskeletal system, including structure and function of muscles, tendons, joints. He proposed that as a person learns a new motor skill, he or she gains coordination and control over the multiple interacting variables that exist in the human body to master the target skill.

The *novice stage* is defined by the coupling of movement parameters—degrees of freedom—into synergies. During this stage some joints and movements may be "frozen" or restrained to allow successful completion of the task. An example of this is posturally holding the head, neck, and trunk rigid while learning to walk on a narrow surface.

The *advanced stage* is achieved by combining body parts to act as a functional unit, further reducing the degrees of freedom while allowing better interaction and consideration for environmental factors. He considers that motor plans must be adapted to the dynamic environmental conditions in which the task must be performed. In this stage the learner explores many movement solutions, reduces some degrees of freedom, develops more variable movement patterns, and learns to select appropriate strategies to accomplish a given task. This stage of motor learning is accomplished through practice and experience in performing a task in various environments. To achieve this stage the learner progressively releases some couplings, allowing more degrees of freedom, greater speed and amplitude of movement, and less constraints on the action. Performance of the task becomes more efficient, is less taxing on the individual, and is executed with decreased cognitive effort. Variability of performance becomes an indicator that a level of independence in the activation of component body parts during a given task has indeed been achieved.

In Bernstein's *expert stage,* degrees of freedom are now released and reorganized to allow the body to react to all of the internal and external mechanisms that may act on it at any given time. At the same time, enhanced coactivation of proximal structures is learned and used to allow for greater force, speed, and dexterity of limb movements.[43]

Gentile presented a two-stage model of motor learning.[44,45] She considered motor learning from the goal of the learner and strongly considered how environmental conditions influence performance and learning.

Stage one requires the client to problem solve strategies to get the idea of a movement and establish a motor pattern that will successfully meet the demands of the task. As with the models presented previously, this process demands conscious attention to the components of the task and environmental variables to formulate a "map" or framework of the movement pattern. Once this framework is established, the client has a mechanism for performing the task; however, errors and inconsistency in performance accuracy are often present.[46]

During *stage two* the client attains improved consistency of performance and the ability to adapt the movement pattern to demands of specific physical and environmental situations. Greater economy of movement is achieved, and less cognitive and physical effort is expended to reach the task goal. Practice in appropriately challenging conditions leads to consistent, efficient, correct execution while maintaining adaptive flexibility within the motor plan, allowing the client to react quickly to changing conditions of the task.

The three motor learning theories just presented simplify a complex process into simple stages to give a broad picture of the development of skilled movement performance. Each theory can be used to assist the therapist in the process of teaching and facilitating long-term learning or relearning of motor skills before and after insult to the nervous system. The ultimate goal of motor learning is the permanent acquisition of adaptable movement plans that are efficient, require little cognitive effort, and produce consistent and accurate movement outcomes.

Variables that Affect Motor Learning

The ecological model (constraints theory) of motor control and learning states that motor learning involves the person, the task, and the environment.[47] For a purposeful and functional movement to occur, the *individual* must generate movement to successfully meet the *task* at hand, as well as the demands of the *environment* where the task must be performed. For motor learning to be successful, several variables related to each of these three constructs must be taken into account.

Variables Related to the Individual

The clinician must first differentiate general motor performance factors that are under the control of the individual's cognitive and emotional systems and those that are controlled by the motor system itself. These concepts are presented in Figure 4-5. There are many cognitive factors such as arousal, attention, and memory, as well as cortical pathways related to declarative or executive learning, that have specific influences over behaviors that are observed after neurological insult.[48,49] Other factors such as limbic connections to cortical pathways affected by motivation, fear and belief, and emotional stability and instability also dramatically affect motor performance and declarative learning. Some of these factors may also limit activity and participation. Therapists need to learn how to discriminate among motor output, somatosensory input, cortical processing, and limbic emotional state problems and identify how the latter two systems affect motor output. With that differentiation,

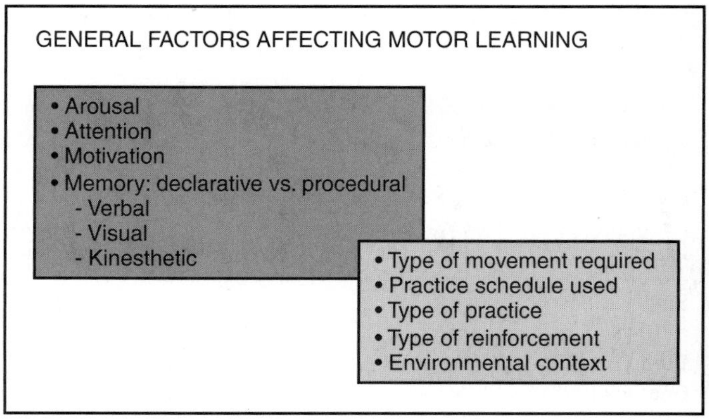

GENERAL FACTORS AFFECTING MOTOR LEARNING
• Arousal
• Attention
• Motivation
• Memory: declarative vs. procedural
- Verbal
- Visual
- Kinesthetic
• Type of movement required
• Practice schedule used
• Type of practice
• Type of reinforcement
• Environmental context

Figure 4-5 ■ Concepts affecting motor learning.

clinicians should also be able to separate specific motor system deficits from motor control problems arising from dysfunction within other areas of the CNS. Last, the patient's fitness level; current limitations in strength, endurance, power, and range of motion; or pain level may also influence learning.[35,50-55]

Variables Related to the Task

The two major variables related to the task itself that must be considered when facilitating motor learning include practice of the task and feedback related to task performance.

Practice. Practice is defined as "repeated performance in order to acquire a "skill."[56] As the definition implies, several repetitions of the task are usually required to be able to achieve skillful performance of a task. With other variables being constant, more practice results in more learning.[35] To be effective, these repetitions must involve a process of problem solving rather than just repetition of the activity.[57] The therapist can manipulate several variables related to practice to optimize motor learning of an individual with a movement dysfunction secondary to a neurological insult.

Practice Conditions. The term *practice conditions* refers to the manner in which the task or exercise is repeated with respect to rest periods, the amount of exercise, and the sequence in which these tasks or exercises are performed.

According to apportionment of practice in relation to rest periods, massed tasks or exercises can be classified as *massed practice* or *distributed practice.* Massed practice is when the rest period is much shorter in relation to the amount of time the task or exercise is practiced.[58] This is contrasted against distributed practice, in which the time between practice sets is equal to or greater than the amount of time devoted to practicing a particular task or activity, such that the rest period is spread out throughout the practice.[59] In terms of neurological physical therapy practice, it is important to consider the effect of physical and mental fatigue when training. For example, physical fatigue sets in during massed practice of a particular balance exercise activity in standing and may cause a patient to fall. Moreover, individuals who are cognitively impaired may not respond positively to sustained activity that requires considerable concentration and therefore might fail in the performance of the skill. On the other hand, to be functional and useful in daily life, certain activities have to be performed without significant amounts of rest periods. For example, taking significant rest breaks when ambulating for even a short distance limits an individual's ability to use walking in a functional manner. Sometimes a patient needs more rest periods in the initial stages of learning a skill to compensate for impairments in muscular endurance or cardiopulmonary function, with the intent of decreasing these rest periods to achieve skill performance that reflect how that activity is used in real-life situations. Therefore therapists should consider the skill demands and the desired results when choosing one practice type versus another.[59]

Complete tasks or activities can usually be divided into smaller subcomponents. The way those subcomponents are practiced relative to the entire task or activity can also be manipulated to optimize motor learning. To practice the entire task or parts of the task, whole learning, pure-part learning, progressive-part learning, or whole-part learning may be used. Figure 4-6 summarizes these concepts.

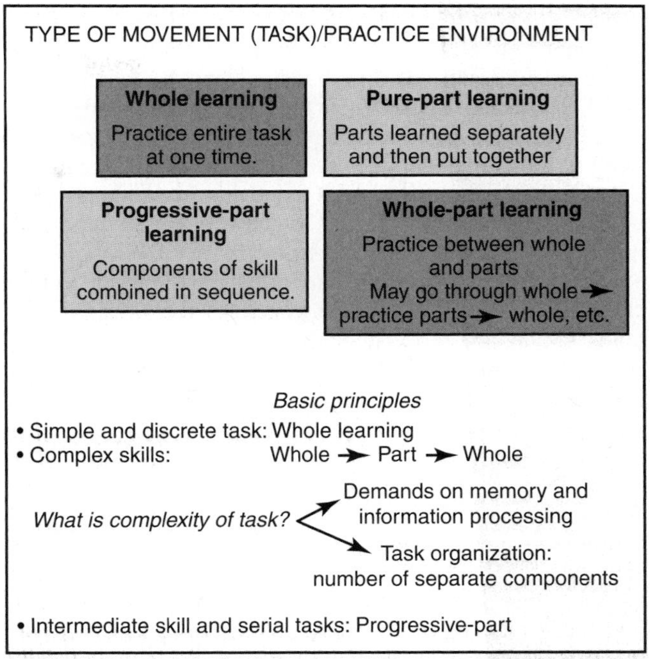

Figure 4-6 ■ Type of movement (task) and practice environment.

Whole learning suggests that the learner practice the entire movement as one activity. Asking a person to stand up incorporates the entire activity of coming to stand from sitting. Simple movements such as rolling, coming to sit, coming to stand, and walking might best be taught as a whole activity as long as the individual has all the component parts to practice the whole.

In pure-part learning the therapist introduces one part first, then this part is practiced by the learner before another new part is introduced and practiced. Each part is critical to the whole movement, but which one is learned first does not matter. Learning a tennis serve is an excellent example of an activity that can be taught as a pure-part. Learning to toss the ball vertically to a specific spot in space is a very different and a separate part from swinging the tennis racket as part of the serve. Learning to squeeze the toothpaste onto the brush is a very different movement strategy from brushing the teeth.

Progressive-part learning is used when the sequence of the learning and the component parts need to be programmed in a specific order. Line dancing is an activity taught using progressive parts. Individuals with sequencing deficits often need to be taught using progressive parts or the individual will mix up the ordering of parts during an activity. Therapists see this in the clinical arena when an individual stands up from a wheelchair and then tries to pick up the foot pedals and lock the brakes. Given that problem, that patient needs to practice progressive part learning by first locking the brake, then picking up the foot pedals and finally standing. If the activity is not practiced using progressive-part learning, the patient will have little consistency in how the parts are put together, thereby placing that individual at high risk of failing at the functional task.

Whole-part learning can be used when the skill or activity can be practiced between the whole and the parts. In the clinical environment, a common application of this concept is *whole to part to whole learning.*[60] First the therapist has the client try the whole activity, such as coming to stand or reaching out to turn the door handle. Next, the therapist has the client practice a component part. Finally the whole activity is practiced as a functional pattern. In this way therapists work on the functional activity, then work on correcting the impairment or limitation, such as power production, range, or balance, and then go back to the functional activity in order to incorporate the part learning into the whole. An example might be asking a patient to first stand up from a chair. As he tries to stand he generates too much power, holds his breath, and cannot repeat the activity more than once. The therapist decides to practice a component part by first assisting the patient to a relaxed standing posture, then having him eccentrically begin to sit into a partial squat, and then having him return to standing. As the patient practices, he will increase the range of lengthening and eventually will sit and return to stand. Once that is accomplished, he will continue to practice sit to stand to sit to stand as a whole activity.

According to the sequence in which component tasks are practiced, blocked or random practice may be used. In *blocked practice* the patient first practices a single task over and over before moving to the next task. On the other hand, in *random practice,* the component tasks are practiced without any particular sequence. The contextual interference effect explains the difference in motor performance found when comparing these two types of practice. Studies have shown performance may be enhanced by using blocked practice; however, learning is not enhanced by using this type of practice. Random practice has been shown to enhance learning because this type of practice forces the learners to come up with a motor solution each time a task is performed.[61,62]

Feedback. The use of feedback is another important variable related to motor learning. Feedback is defined as the use of sensory information—visual, auditory, or somatosensory—to improve performance, retention, or transfer of a task. Internal feedback pertains to sensory information that the patient receives that can be used to improve performance of that particular task or activity in the future. The therapist provides extrinsic or augmented feedback with the intent of improving learning of the task. In people with neurological dysfunctions, extrinsic feedback is important because the patient's intrinsic feedback system may be impaired or absent.

Extrinsic feedback can further be classified as knowledge of performance (KP) or knowledge of results (KR). KP is given concurrently while the task is being performed and can therefore also be called *concurrent feedback.* Feedback given concurrently, especially during the critical portions of the task, allows the patient to successfully perform the activity.

KR pertains to feedback given at the conclusion of the task (therefore also called *terminal feedback*) and provides the patient information about the success of his or her actions with respect to the activity. KR can be classified as faded, delayed, or summary. In faded feedback the therapist provides more information in the beginning stages of learning of the skill and slowly withdraws that information as the patient demonstrates improvement in the performance of the task. With delayed feedback, information is given to the patient when a period of time has elapsed after the task has been completed. The intent of this pause between the termination of task and feedback is to give the patient some time to process the activity and generate possible solutions to the difficulties encountered in the previous performance of the task. In contrast, summary feedback is provided after the patient has performed several trials of a particular task without receiving feedback. Previous studies showed that subjects who were given more frequent feedback performed better during the task acquisition stage of learning but worse on retention tests compared with those who received summary feedback.[63,64]

Additional concepts related to long-term learning are presented in Figure 4-7.

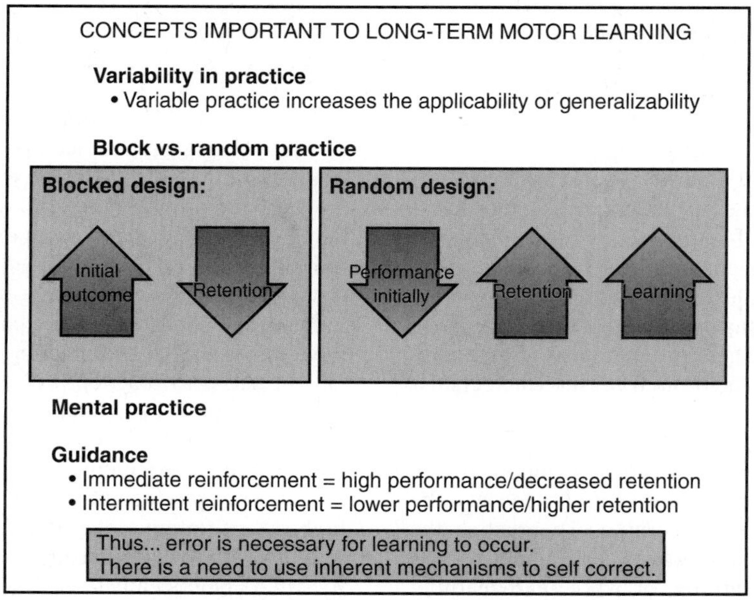

Figure 4-7 ■ Concepts important to long-term learning.

Variables Related to the Environment

Therapists can alter the environmental conditions to optimize motor learning. Gentile[44,45] described the manipulation of the environment in which a task is performed to make an activity more appropriate for what the patient is able to do. A *closed environment* is stationary; it allows the patient to practice the skill in a predictable manner, with minimal distractions from the environment. On the other hand, an *open environment* is one that is in motion or unpredictable. In patients with neurological dysfunctions, clinicians may decide to have a patient practice a skill in a closed environment to allow the patient to plan the movement in advance and to perform the movement with minimal distractions or challenges. An example of this would be performing gait training in a quiet and empty therapy gym. As the patient improves, it may be important to practice this activity in an open environment to provide a real-world application of a task. Going back to the previous example, the therapist may have the patient ambulate in an open environment such as a busy gym with crowds and noise, a crowded cafeteria, or a moving walkway.

If prior procedural learning has occurred, then creating an environment that allows the program to run in the least restrictive environment should lead to the most efficient outcome in the shortest time.[51,52] If a patient needs to learn a new program, such as walking with a stereotypical extension pattern, then goal-directed, attended practice with guided feedback is necessary. It may be easier to bring back an old ambulatory pattern by creating an environment to elicit that program than to teach a client to use a new inefficient movement program.[53-55]

A therapist must identify what MPs are available and under what conditions. This allows the therapist to (1) determine whether deficits are present, (2) anticipate problems in performance, and (3) match existing programs with functional activities during training. Similarly, knowing available MPs and the component body systems necessary to run those programs aids the therapist in the selection of intervention procedures.

If the client has permanent damage to either the basal ganglia or the cerebellum, then retaining the memory of new MPs may be difficult and substitution approaches may become necessary. Through evaluation the clinician needs to determine whether anatomical disease or a pathological condition is actually causing procedural learning problems and whether identifying and teaching a substitution pattern or teaching the patient to compensate with an old pattern will allow the individual to succeed at the task. However, therapists should never forget that the plasticity of the CNS can promote significant recovery and adaptation through the performance of attended, goal-directed, repetitive behavior.[65,66]

Providing an appropriate level of challenge to the learner optimizes motor learning. The clinician must learn to expertly manipulate the environment to best facilitate learning. A task that is too difficult for the client will result in persistent failure of performance, frustration, and lack of learning, and the only option will be to compensate through available patterns of movement that limit function. An activity that is too easy and routinely results in 100% success also does not result in learning because the learner becomes bored and no longer attends to the learning. The most beneficial level of challenge for training will create some errors in performance, require the client to solve problems to meet the demands presented, and allow a level of success that inspires continued motivation to practice and achieve a higher standard of skill.

Systems Interactions: Motor Responses Represent Consensus of Central Nervous System Components

Motor behavior reflects not only motor programming but also the interaction of cognitive, affective, and somatosensory variables. Without a motor system, neither the cognitive nor the emotional systems have a way to express and communicate inner thoughts to the world. The cognitive and emotional systems can positively or negatively affect motor responses. The significance of the somatosensory or perceptual-cognitive cortical system must be emphasized. The somatosensory association areas play a critical role in the ideational and constructional aspects of the MP itself. When there are deficits within this system, clients will often demonstrate significant distortions in motor control even without a specific motor impairment. An example of this problem might be an individual who had a stroke and developed a "pusher syndrome." The motor behavior shown by this client would be pushing off vertical generally in a lateral or posterolateral direction.[67] Physically correcting the client's posture to vertical or asking the patient to self-correct will not eliminate the original behavior. Pusher syndrome does not stem from a motor problem but rather from a perceptual problem of verticality from thalamic nuclei radiating false information to the somatosensory cortices. Although a therapist might want to augment intervention by trying to push the patient to vertical, the patient will resist that movement pattern. Functional training becomes frustrating to both the patient and the therapist because the impairment does not fall within the motor system itself. Reliance on the use of vision and environmental cues might be the best intervention strategy for this type of problem because the impairment is within the sensory processing centers.[68] Asking the patient to find midline and reach across midline, then acknowledging success, along with a lack of falling help the somatosensory system to relearn and thus begin to inherently correct to vertical. Verbalizing to the patient that you (the therapist) acknowledge that she or he feels as if she or he is falling when placed in the vertical position demonstrates to the client that you have accepted the patient and his or her perceptions. Simultaneously maintaining tactile contact to prevent the patient from falling effectively lets the limbic system relax and reduces its need to trigger motor reactions. This example creates conflict between the cognitive system's information from the thalamus and motor system feedback. The thalamus is saying vertical is "X," and the motor system is saying "if X then I am falling." When the goal is not to fall, then the cognitive system will generally override the thalamic information and learn to accept a new concept of vertical. Taking all these variables into the treatment environment optimizes the potential that the patient will self-correct during a functional activity such as reaching with weight shift.

If a patient's insult falls within the limbic or emotional system, then motor behavior could also be affected. The motor dysfunction will be different from the dysfunction reflecting damage either in the sensory cortices or associated with information sent to them. For years it has been common knowledge that individuals who are depressed will demonstrate motor signs of withdrawal (e.g., flexion). If the posture of flexion was created by a chemical response related to depression, then somatosensory retraining would have a limited effect on behavior. Similarly, functional training may initially modify the impairments, but without changes within the limbic system itself no permanent change will be achieved. Instead, augmenting the input to alter the emotional system and then reinforcing self-control could create the best potential outcome.

For many clinical problems, functional retraining of the motor system through attended, sequenced, repetitive practice could lead to greater functional gains, although the body system impairment(s) may never be eliminated. That is, muscle strengthening and programming coactivation to enable joint stability could restore client independence. Given the complexity of impairments and function in a patient with a neurological insult, a therapist may need to use all three types of intervention procedures to affect all areas of the CNS simultaneously. The decision of which intervention is most appropriate or which should be emphasized falls within the professional judgment of the clinician. There is no easy recipe to decide which intervention is best for all people. It is the problem-solving skills of the therapist and one's keen analysis of movement function and dysfunction that lead to the best solution. Obviously, patient involvement and desired outcomes are also critical components leading to this decision.

PRINCIPLES OF NEUROPLASTICITY: IMPLICATIONS FOR NEUROREHABILITATION

Rehabilitation, Research, and Practice

Rehabilitation is the process of maximizing functional learning. The integration of basic neuroscience into clinical practice is critical for guiding the questioning of researchers and maximizing the recovery of patients. The 1990s were referred to as the "Decade of the Brain." For the last 20 years, researchers have made enormous advances in understanding the adaptability of the CNS. Because of this revolution, clinicians must focus on recovery rather than compensation. There is sufficient evidence that the CNS not only develops and matures during adolescence, but also recovers from serious disease and injury and maintains sensory, motor, and cognitive competency through spontaneous healing, appropriate medical management, physical exercise, balanced nutrition, and learning. Across the life span, individuals can maximize independence and quality of life by taking advantage of learning from enriched environments, task-specific training, and attended, progressive, goal-oriented, repetitive behaviors. In addition, the nervous system can adapt negatively to repetitive and abnormal patterns of movement based on structural anomalies, pain, abnormal biomechanics, or bad habits (see the section on motor learning in this chapter).

The paradigm shift in rehabilitative intervention strategies based on neuroplasticity has just begun. Basic science researchers cannot ignore the impact of their findings on the health and function of the consumer. Clinical researchers must collaborate in clinical studies to determine the impact of basic science findings with patients.[69-71] Clinicians cannot simply provide the same, familiar treatment of yesterday because it is comfortable and easy and requires minimal effort. Physical therapy professionals must be dynamic, enthusiastic, evidence-based and committed to lifelong learning, ready to accept the challenge and unique opportunity to work with other members of the health care team to translate neuroscience to practice. Failure to translate basic science findings into clinical practice will significantly impair the potential for patient recovery.

During the last 45 years, three large conferences[72-74] focused on these issues in neuroscience. In 1966 the Northwestern University Special Therapeutic Exercise Project (NUSTEP) conference in Chicago, Illinois, brought researchers, basic scientists, educators, and master clinicians together for 6 weeks to identify commonalities in approaches to interventions and to integrate basic science into those commonalities. A huge shift from specific philosophies to a bodily systems model occurred in 1990 at Norman, Oklahoma, the site of the Second Special Therapeutic Exercise Project conference (II STEP). During the next 15 years, concepts of motor learning and motor control were beginning to affect the methodology and intervention philosophies of both occupational and physical therapy. Simultaneously, newer approaches such as locomotion training with partial weight bearing on a treadmill,[75,76] task-specific training,[77,78] constraint-induced movement training,[79,80] neuroprotective effect of exercise,[81] mental and physical practice,[82,83] patient-centered therapy,[84-86] and sensorimotor training[87] were frequently seen in peer-reviewed literature. The third STEP conference, Summer Institute on Translating Evidence into Practice (III STEP), occurred in July 2005 in Salt Lake City, Utah. At this conference, unique clinical models for intervention were embraced that will direct professional education for decades. Changes in practice over the next 15 years will lead to embracing many older intervention techniques with current evidence-based practice.

Four primary conclusions were summarized from the III STEP conference: (1) client-centered, empowerment models needed to be the platform for all neurorehabilitation and postdisease models of care; (2) evidence-based practice needs to start with the documentation of clinical effectiveness based on reliable and valid measurement tools followed by efficacy studies; (3) a strong link is needed among basic science, clinical science, and disease-specific motor dysfunction research to develop the best patient management environments; and (4) movement science belongs to a broad community that requires integration of the goals, cultural beliefs, ethnic values, emotional understanding, and scientific knowledge of many individuals, including but not limited to health care providers (physicians, PTs and OTs, psychologists), clinical research practitioners, basic science researchers, educators, clients, families, and employers.

There are a variety of challenges to implementing effective, neuroscience-based interventions. The first is the patient. Patient-centered therapy is critical for effective therapeutic outcomes. The patient can be both the obstacle to successful recovery[88,89] and the critical link to success.[90,91] To achieve optimum neural adaptation, the patient must be engaged in attended, goal-directed, novel, progressive behaviors. There is no measurable neural adaptation with passive movements or passive stimuli. For a change in neural response to be achieved, the stimulus needs to be novel or a surprise and the individual has to attend to the stimulus, make a decision about what to do, and receive some feedback regarding the appropriateness or accuracy of the outcome.[92] This progressive decision making has to be done repetitively and progressed in difficulty over time. These behaviors may be difficult to achieve when a person is depressed, feels hopeless, lacks motivation or cognition, or has emotional instability or there is neglect of one or more parts of the body.

Another obstacle to bringing scientific evidence into practice is the barrier created by living in a society in which the economics of health care rather than the science or the patient benefits drive the delivery of services (see Chapter 10). When a physician or a therapist recommends a new approach to intervention, the third-party payer may deny payment for service because it is "experimental." Furthermore, third-party payers may deny the opportunity to apply findings from animal studies to human subjects. Another example of constraint from the third-party payer is the timing of intervention. Despite the evidence that the CNS can be modified under conditions of goal-oriented, repetitive, task-relevant behaviors even years poststroke, insurance companies deny coverage of service late in the recovery process. The insurance company may interpret "medically necessary services" as the services provided during the first 30 days postinjury, the time after a cerebrovascular accident when the greatest spontaneous recovery occurs. Furthermore, even though neural adaptation research confirms that enriched environmental conditions and sensory inputs can facilitate both greater and continued recovery, the insurance company may claim that the services[93-95] are simply for maintenance. Thus, as the science of neuroplasticity continues to develop, it is critical to improve the interface among the scientist, the practitioner, the patient, and the third-party payer. Clinicians and researchers must regularly inform third-party payers about current research evidence.

Integration of Sensory Information in Motor Control

Understanding neural adaptation must include attention to sensory as well as motor systems. In virtually all higher-order perceptual processes, the brain must correlate sensory input with motor output to assess the body's interaction with the environment accurately. A problem in the somatic motor system affects the motor output system. Both systems are independently adaptive, but functional neural adaptation involves the interaction of both sensory and motor processing.

The sensory system provides an internal representation of both the inside and outside worlds to guide the movements that make up our behavioral repertoire. These movements are controlled by the motor systems of the brain and the spinal cord. Our perceptual skills are a reflection of the capabilities of the sensory systems to detect, analyze, and estimate the significance of physical stimuli. (See the section on augmented therapeutic intervention in Chapter 9 for a detailed discussion of each sensory system.) Our agility and dexterity represent a reflection of the capabilities of the motor systems to plan, coordinate, and execute movements. The task of the motor systems in controlling movement is the reverse of the task of sensory systems in generating an internal representation. Perception is the end product of sensory processing, whereas an internal representation (an image of the desired movement) is the beginning of motor processing.

Sensory psychophysics looks at the attributes of a stimulus: its quality, intensity, location, and duration. Motor psychophysics considers the organization of action, the intensity of the contraction, the recruitment of distinct populations of motor neurons, the accuracy of the movements, the coordination of the movements, and the speed of movement. In both the sensory and motor systems, the complexity of behaviors depends on the multiplicity of modalities available. In sensation, there are the distinct modalities of pain, temperature, light touch, deep touch, vibration, and stretch, whereas in the motor system can be found the modalities of reflex responses, rhythmic motor patterns within and between limbs, automatic and adaptive motor responses, and voluntary fine and gross movements.[96-116] Although all motor movements require integration of sensory information for motor learning, once motor control is attained the system can run on very little feedback. The relationship of incoming sensory information is particularly complex in voluntary motor movements that constantly adapt to environmental variance. For voluntary motor movements, the motor system requires contraction and relaxation of muscles, recruitment of appropriate muscles and their synergies, appropriate timing and sequencing of muscle contraction and relaxation, the distribution of the body mass, and appropriate postural adjustments. As stated, once an MP is learned, it does not take the same amount of sensory information to run the program in a feed-forward manner within the motor system as long as the information to the cerebellum is able to run and adjust all aspects of the program. (See Chapter 21 and the section on motor control in this chapter.) To learn new programs, the CNS must go through the process of receipt of sensory input, perceptual processing, communication with the frontal lobes, and relays to basal ganglia and cerebellum, followed by intentional, goal-directed execution of the motor plan.

Within each movement, there must be adjustments to compensate for the inertia of the limbs and the mechanical arrangement of the muscles, bones, and joints both before and during movement to ensure and maintain accuracy. The control systems for voluntary movement include (1) the continuous flow of sensory information about the environment, position, and orientation of the body and limbs and the degree of contraction of the muscles; (2) the spinal cord; (3) the descending systems of the brain stem; and (4) the pathways of the motor areas of the cerebral cortex, cerebellum, and basal ganglia. Each level of control is based on the sensory information that is relevant for the functions it controls. This information is provided by feedback, feed-forward, and adaptive mechanisms. These control systems are organized both hierarchically and in parallel. These systems also control activation of sensations and motor movements as well as inhibition (e.g., globus pallidus). Furthermore, some parts of the brain are needed for new learning (e.g., cerebellum) and others for maintained learning (e.g., globus pallidus, hippocampus). The hierarchical but interactive organization permits lower levels to generate reflexes without involving higher centers, whereas the parallel system allows the brain to process the flow of discrete types of sensory information to produce discrete types of movements.[117,118]

Ultimately, the control of graded fine motor movements involves the sensory organ of the muscle, the muscle spindle, which contains the specialized elements that sense muscle length and the velocity or changes in spindle length. In conjunction with the tendon organ, which senses muscle tension, the muscle spindle provides the CNS with continuous information on the mechanical state of the muscle. Ultimately the firing of the muscle spindles depends on both muscle length and the level of gamma motor activation of the intrafusal fibers. Similarly, joint proprioceptors relay both closed and open chain input and mobility (range) information from within the joint structures to the CNS. This illustrates the close relationship between sensory and motor processing and the integral relationship between the two.[119]

Foundation for the Study of Neuroplasticity

The principal models for studying cortical plasticity have been based on the representations of hand skin and hand movements in the New World owl monkey *(Aotus)* and the squirrel monkey *(Saimiri)*. These primate models have been chosen because their central sulci usually do not extend into the hand representational zone in the anterior parietal (S1) or posterior frontal (M1) cortical fields. In other primates the sulci are deep and interfere with accurate mapping. Albeit there are differences in hand use among primates, in all of the primates the hand has the largest topographical representation for the actual size of the extremity, the detail of this representation is distinct, and the hand has the greatest potential for skilled movements and sensory discrimination. However, the findings from studies of this cortical area are applicable across the different cortices as well as the other cornerstones of the brain such as the thalamus, basal ganglia, brain stem, and cerebellum.[120,121] See Figure 4-8 to identify specific anatomical locations and their respective classifications.

To understand neural adaptation and to be able to apply the principles to practice, it is necessary to objectively measure the changes. Positive changes in neural structure can be measured by using a variety of imaging techniques (e.g., magnetic resonance imaging [MRI], functional MRI [fMRI], magnetoencephalography, magnetic source imaging [MSI]). The types of outcomes that can be expected electrophysiologically and functionally are summarized in Table 4-4. At this time, imaging techniques are applied primarily for research purposes or to rule out other pathology. The specific type of intervention to address the principles of neuroplasticity may vary, but the outcomes must be clearly documented.

Principles of Neural Adaptation

To achieve maximum neural adaptation, there are some basic principles to follow (Box 4-1). Learning is the key to neural adaptation. Plasticity is the mechanism for encoding, the changing of behaviors, and both implicit and explicit learning. During neural adaptation, the fundamental questions are as follows: As we learn, how does the brain change its representations of inputs and actions? What is the nature of the processes that control the progressive elaboration of performance abilities? In different individuals, what are the sources of variance for emergence of improved performance? What changes in cortical plasticity facilitate the development of "automatic" motor behaviors? Why are some behaviors hard

TABLE 4-4 ■ NEUROPROTECTIVE MOTOR ENRICHMENT FACTORS AFFECTING OUTCOMES

	NEGATIVE PLASTICITY	POSITIVE PLASTICITY
Stimulation	Disuse, unskilled	Intensive, skilled
Quality of sensory input	Noisy, nonspecific	Appropriate, specific
Modulation	Not challenging	High stakes, novel, challenging
Outcome	Negative behaviors	Positive behaviors

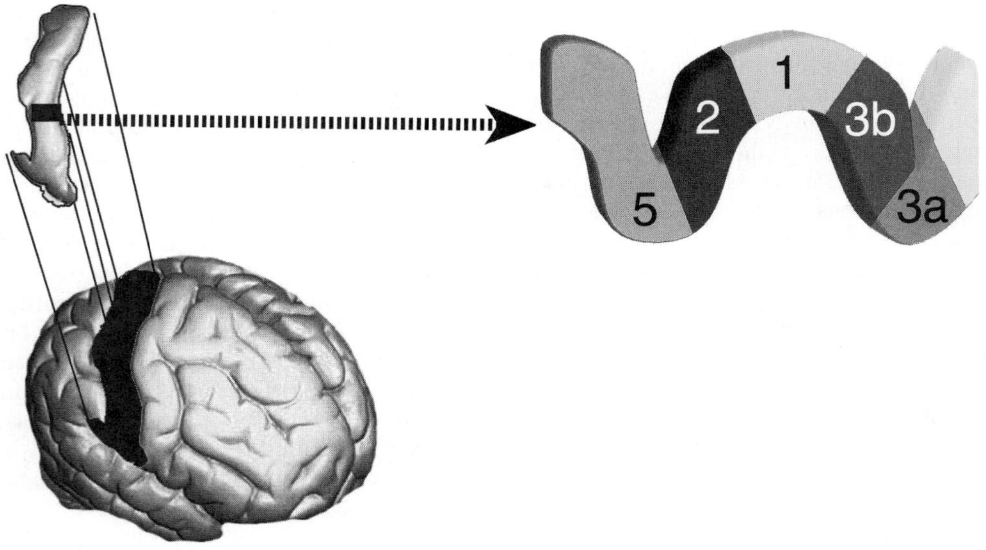

Figure 4-8 ■ Classification and anatomical locations of cortical map.

to change? What limits plasticity processes? What are the critical elements of brain circuitry, genes, synapses, neural chemistry, neuronal networks, and neural connections for restoration of lost function? What guidelines need to be followed to drive the greatest change in brain structure and function? How do spontaneous compensatory behavioral strategies contribute to or interfere with restoring lost neuronal function? How does the unaffected side contribute to or interfere with neuroplastic changes and restoration of function? Does damage to the brain alter the neuronal response to learning (e.g., cascade of cellular activity for healing altered circuitry, new neural connections)?

BOX 4-1 ■ NEUROPLASTICITY PRINCIPLES TRANSLATED TO GUIDE CLINICAL PRACTICE

BASIC PRINCIPLES

Translating basic science to clinical practice is a challenge over time. There is no exact protocol. Learning activities need to be adapted and matched to the abilities, goals, and objectives of each individual. Based on research evidence, the following principles can help guide training:

1. *Use it or lose it*—Stay active and keep challenging learning. Failure to regularly engage specific and general brain functions can lead to functional degradation.
2. *Use it and improve it*—Engaging in training behaviors that drive specific brain functions can lead to an enhancement of the function.
3. *Be specific*—The training experience must match the desired outcome; the nature of neural plasticity is dictated by the nature of the training.
4. *Repetition is essential*—Learning requires repetition progressed in difficulty and spaced over time.
5. *Intensity matters*—Plasticity changes require a sufficient training intensity to ensure durability of pathways.
6. *Salience is important*—The training must be salient and match the outcome behavior desired and the goals of the individual.
7. *Age must be addressed*—Training-induced plasticity occurs most readily in a young brain, but neural adaptation continues across the life span with learning-based training. With aging, greater efforts at variety, integration, and discovery may be needed.
8. *Transference*—Plasticity in response to one training experience can also enhance acquisition of similar behaviors and adaptation in other experiences and other parts of the body.
9. *Interference*—Plastic changes after one training experience may interfere with the acquisition of changes in similar systems.
10. *Patient expectation*—Patient expectation can facilitate the outcomes of training; patients who expect to get better can enhance their learning.
11. *Reward or feedback*—Feedback allows modification of training behaviors, correcting errors and improving accuracy of learning.
12. *Environment*—Enrich the environment by simply noticing everything in the environment, expanding the environment to include new opportunities and interacting with others.
13. *Fun*—Learning is greatest when it is associated with discovery and fun.
14. *Helping others*—Maintaining the fitness of the brain is best when individuals look beyond themselves to help and involve others.

INTEGRATE THE PRINCIPLES OF NEURAL ADAPTATION INTO NEUROREHABILITATION

When embarking on a rehabilitation program with someone, match the principles of neuroplasticity to interactions with the patient, the family, the health care team, and the job, emphasizing the importance of the following:

1. Thinking positively about health and recovery; expect to get better
2. Setting clear goals and objectives for retraining
3. Encouraging the family to be involved in the retraining activities.
4. Creating learning activities that are attended-goal directed, repetitive, progressed in difficulty, increased in variety and depth, spaced over time, rewarded, and complemented with feedback on accuracy
5. Linking activities temporally (in time) and spatially but progressively sequenced; making the stimulus strength adequate for detection and appropriate to avoid abnormal behaviors
6. Integrating training behaviors into meaningful functional activities
7. Making training activities age appropriate
8. Integrating training activities across multiple sensory modalities appropriate for desired outputs
9. Performing training activities in different postural orientations and different environments, which facilitate the best performance
10. Matching training behaviors with progression of healing and recovery as well as development
11. Strengthening positive responses with meaningful rewards
12. Making it difficult to use the unaffected side (e.g., wearing a glove)
13. Avoiding activities that stimulate repetition of abnormal movements
14. Maintaining high levels of attention and cognitive function within the context of all daily activities; avoiding habitual unattended behaviors
15. Maintaining self-esteem
16. Avoiding an egocentric focus; thinking about how to help and be involved with others
17. Being fit, thinking "tall," and challenging balance by interacting in new unstable environments

RESEARCH VALIDATED OUTCOMES FOLLOWING CENTRAL NERVOUS SYSTEM TRAINING

With thoughtful, attentive regular physical exercise, integrated learning-based activities, daily learning, and specific

Continued

BOX 4-1 ■ NEUROPLASTICITY PRINCIPLES TRANSLATED TO GUIDE CLINICAL PRACTICE—cont'd

practice to improve skills, there is scientific evidence confirming the following positive outcomes:

1. Strengthened and elaborated neuronal interconnections
2. Improved health and vigor of nerve cell populations (including neurotransmitters, nerve brain growth factors, dopamine)
3. Increased physical size of brain centers and a slowing down of shrinkage and atrophy of the brain with aging and disuse
4. Increased accuracy of neuronal processing
5. Improved strength of associative memory processes and the capacity for the brain to remember what is seen, heard, felt, or learned
6. Faster brain processing and more reliable connections to improve sharpness and completeness of how our brain represents and records information
7. Improved coordination of neuronal activities across brain subsystems
8. Improved abilities to broaden and control our attention, shift attention, and take in more information with better acuity
9. Improved integration in vision, listening, feeling, and awareness of joint and trunk position in space
10. Improved ability to suppress noise and distractions to stay on track
11. Improved security of mobility and more reliable postural reactions to protect from falling in familiar and stable as well as unfamiliar and unstable environments
12. Reactivation of long underpracticed skills that support independent mental and physical actions (e.g., riding a bike, skipping, throwing and catching balls, playing an instrument)
13. Restoration of fluency, self-confidence, liveliness, and happiness
14. Increased longevity
15. Increased blood flow and oxygen to the heart and nervous system
16. Physical exercise combined with attended learning-based exercise for decreased risk of heart disease, cancer, metabolic failure, and Alzheimer disease

METHODS OF MEASURING NEURAL ADAPTATION

Neurophysiological and Neuroanatomical Outcomes

Neurophysiological and neuroanatomical changes can be measured in the central nervous system (CNS) with learning. Measurements have been made with a variety of techniques (e.g., neurophysiological mapping after craniotomies, electroencephalography, magnetic source imaging [MSI], functional magnetic resonance imaging [fMRI], electromyography, cortical response mapping with positron emission tomography, and spectroscopy with the potential for neurochemical analysis of neurotransmitters, growth hormones, inhibitors, corticosteroids). With learning it is possible to measure the following:

1. Achievement of specialized cortical representations of behaviorally important inputs
2. Growth in the number of neuron populations excited with progressively greater specificity in the neuronal representations, and stronger temporal coordination
3. Strengthening of neural connections (synapses) following important behavioral inputs
4. Increased oxygenation
5. Decreased atrophy of the brain
6. Shortening of the time between the stimulus and neuronal activation (latency)
7. Modification of the amplitude of neuronal firing
8. Improvement in the ability to turn off neurons once fired
9. Increased ability to inhibit unwanted neuronal firing in response to an input
10. Shortened integration time between processing inputs and production of outputs
11. Specialization of representational firing in response to familiar inputs
12. Improved temporal sequencing of firing following familiar inputs
13. Increased myelination
14. Increased complexity of dendrites and change in number and complexity of synapses
15. Increased consistency of response (e.g., density of neuronal responses)
16. Improved selective excitation
17. Increased specificity of neuronal response
18. Increased salience of the response
19. Change in cortical (and noncortical) topography
20. Increased area of representation
21. Smaller receptive fields
22. Increased density of receptive fields
23. Improved precision and order of receptive fields

Clinical Documentation of Outcomes after Learning-Based Training

Basic science and clinical research studies report positive correlations between functional outcomes and neural adaptation. With timely prevention, appropriate management of acute insults to the CNS, spontaneous recovery, and thoughtful attention to activities of daily living (ADLs) and task practice, disabling CNS problems can be minimized. Furthermore, early treatment after CNS injury or onset of disease may prevent more extensive damage to the brain. Learning activities may not only be neuroprotective but also drive more complete recovery of function. Changes in neural adaptation can be measured clinically in terms of improvement in function including the following:

1. Fine and gross motor coordination
2. Sensory discrimination
3. Balance and postural control
4. Reaction time
5. Accuracy of movements
6. Rhythm and timing of movements
7. Memory storage, organization, and retrieval
8. Alertness and attention

BOX 4-1 ■ NEUROPLASTICITY PRINCIPLES TRANSLATED TO GUIDE CLINICAL PRACTICE—cont'd

9. Sequencing
10. Logic, complexity, and sophistication of problem solving
11. Language skills (verbal and nonverbal)
12. Interpersonal communication
13. Positive sense of well-being
14. Insight
15. Self-confidence
16. Self-image
17. Signal/noise detection; able to make finer distinctions
18. Ability to "chunk" information for memory and use
19. Learning skills including faster learning
20. Achievement of developmental milestones
21. Appropriate sensitivity of the nervous system (e.g., reduction in hyperactivity and sensory defensiveness)
22. Ability to perform a skill from memory
23. Flexible behaviors; variability in task performance
24. Flexibility for experience-based learning

PRACTICAL SUGGESTIONS FOR MAINTAINING PHYSICAL AND BRAIN HEALTH ACROSS THE LIFE SPAN[35,128]

Make living a learning experience by creating goal-directed activities that require attention and can be progressed in difficulty or variety over time. Where possible, provide conditions where feedback about performance is received. Try to maintain variability in activities and vary the environments for performing the same and different tasks. Take some risks by changing activities that are familiar and comfortable. Walk around on unstable surfaces as well as familiar surfaces with the eyes closed to challenge balance and postural reactions. Assume different positions to perform common tasks. More specifically:

1. Integrate low intensity to moderate physical exercise into the day, balanced with healthy eating, good hydration, and stress management.
2. Stop all negative learning behaviors; minimize or eliminate bad habits.
3. Be actively engaged at the cutting edge of all activities; minimize habitual behaviors.
4. Improve skills; progressively practice to perform each task better and use mistakes to guide practice.
5. Improve language listening skills and expand the words and the language used.
6. Be a lifelong learner; take classes, go to lectures, listen to audio books, and discuss what was learned with others.
7. Engage in conversational listening (review what is remembered about a conversation right after the conversation ends).
8. Keep hobbies alive; mix life with work and play.
9. Consider learning to play a musical instrument (e.g., take lessons, practice and carefully listen while playing).
10. Sing along with music; sing out loud in the car (loud, clearly, and slowly), and consider joining a choir to share the joy of singing with others.
11. Take time and opportunities to dance; consider taking some lessons.
12. Volunteer in the community to interact with others.
13. Wear a hearing aid if one has been prescribed; wear glasses if they are needed.
14. Improve everyday activities by learning something new or by challenging observation and recall skills: have a puzzle out and add pieces, or have challenging crossword puzzles to work on.
15. Play games that require fine motor skills (e.g., shuffling cards, Ping-Pong, bowling, tennis).
16. After walking to the store, reconstruct all of the things that were seen on the way and at the store and what was accomplished.
17. When waiting for scheduled appointments, review the details of the environment; examine what has changed since the last visit.
18. Before going to social gatherings, try to remember the names of the people who are expected to be there; afterward, review who was there by name.
19. When idle or waiting, instead of sitting, walk around and mentally review items in the environment, organize these items, review tasks that need to be done (including steps required), play a game.
20. Find different ways to get to common places; evaluate which way is fastest, easiest, most interesting, most fun.
21. Constantly read and listen to the news, attend lectures, listen to or watch educational programs.
22. When with others, especially with children or grandchildren, play progressive or problem-solving games (e.g., Boggle, chess, card games, checkers).
23. Look beyond the self; think what you can to do make others happy.
24. Avoid stress; instead enjoy life and share joy with others.
25. Take a walk or ride a bike every day.
26. Find something fun to do every day.

Data from Byl N, Merzenich MM, Cheung S, et al: A primate model for studying focal dystonia and repetitive strain injury: effects on the primary somatosensory cortex, *Phys Ther* 77:269-284, 1997; Kleim J, Jones TA: Principles of experience-dependent neural plasticity: implications for rehabilitation after brain damage. *J Speech Lang Hear Res* 51(1):S225-S239, 2008; and Merzenich M: *The brain revolution* (in press), 2010.

The most informative studies on neuroplasticity are those specifically directed toward defining the changes induced by learning. One approach has been to document the patterns of distributed neural response representation of specific inputs before and after learning. In particular, neuronal responses have been measured in the primary auditory, somatosensory, and motor cortices in animals. These animal studies have been paired with behavioral studies in humans. Both the animal and the human studies provide strong evidence documenting the ability of the brain to functionally self-organize. This capacity for change occurs not only during development but also in adulthood, specifically after learning-based activities. The basic processes for neural adaptation are discussed in the following paragraphs.

1. *Neural circuits must be actively engaged in learning-based activities if degradation and atrophy are to be prevented.*

We know that if infants are deprived of sensory and motor experiences during development, the brain does not develop normally. For example, without exposure to light, there is a reduction in the number of neurons in the visual cortex.[122] Similarly, if infants are not exposed to sound, there is a reduction in the neurons in the auditory cortex.[123] Even in adults, when neural circuits are not used over an extended period of time, they begin to degrade, and the unused area of the brain is allocated to serve another part of the body.[124] Similarly, if task performance is practiced, then the topography expands and becomes more detailed, as might occur in someone who is blind and reads Braille.[125] It is also interesting to note that although a person is blind, the visual cortical areas may become active when the individual is reading Braille.[126] Similarly a person who is deaf may demonstrate activation of the auditory cortex when visual stimuli are presented.

2. *With learning, the distributed cortical representations of inputs and brain actions "specialize" in their representations of behaviorally important inputs and actions in skill learning.*

There seems to be a minimal level of repetitive practice needed to acquire a new skill that will be maintained over time. In fact, this may lead to specialization or change in the underlying neurophysiological processing.[127-129] This specialization develops in response to selective cortical neuron responses specialized to demands of sensory, perceptual, cognitive, and motor skill learning.[130-133] This adaptation has been clearly documented in animal studies. For example, if an animal is trained to make progressively finer distinctions about specific sensory stimuli, then cortical neurons come to represent those stimuli in a progressively more specific and progressively "amplified" manner.

3. *There are important behavioral conditions that must be met in the learning phase of plasticity.*
   a. If behaviorally important stimuli repeatedly excite cortical neuron populations, the neurons will progressively grow in number.
   b. Repetitive, behaviorally important stimuli processed in skill learning lead to progressively greater specificity in the spectral (spatial) and temporal dimensions.
4. *The growing numbers of selectively responding neurons discharge with progressively stronger temporal coordination (distributed synchronicity).*

Through the course of progressive skill learning, a more refined basis for processing stimuli and generating actions critical to skilled tasks is enabled by the multidimensional changes in cortical responses. Consequently, specific aspects of these changes in distributed neuronal response are highly correlated with learning-based improvements in perception, motor control, and cognition.[134-137] In these processes the brain is not simply changing to record and store content, but the cerebral cortex is also selectively refining its processing capacities to fit each task at hand by adjusting its spectral or spatial and temporal filters. Ultimately it establishes its own general processing capabilities. This "learning to learn" determines the facility with which specific classes of information can be stored, associated, and manipulated. These powerful self-shaping processes of the forebrain machinery are operating not only on a large scale during development but also during experience-based management of externally and internally generated information in adults. This self-shaping with experience allows the development of hierarchical organization of perception, cognition, motor, and executive management skills.

5. *In learning, selection of behaviorally important inputs is a product of strengthening input coincidence-based connections (synapses).*

The process of coincidence-based input co-selection leads to changes in cortical representation. Coincident, temporally and spatially related events that fire together are strengthened together. In skill learning, this principle of concurrent input co-selection results from repetitive practice that includes the following:

   a. A progressive amplification of cell numbers engaged by repetitive inputs.[136-138]
   b. An increase in the temporal coordination of distributed neuronal discharges evoked by successive events to mark features of behaviorally important inputs is a consequence of a progressive increase in positive coupling between nearly simultaneously engaged neurons within cortical networks.[136,139]
   c. A progressively more specific "selection" of all input features that collectively represent behaviorally important inputs, expressed moment by moment in time.[138,139] Thus skill learning results in mapping temporal neighbors in representational networks at adjacent spatial locations when they regularly occur successively in time.[65,140,141] Changes in activation patterns, dendritic growth, synapses, and neuronal activities may also be observed.

The basis of the functional creation of the detailed, representational cortical maps converting temporal to spatial representations is related to the Hebbian change principle.[142] The Hebbian plasticity principle applies to the development of interconnections between excitatory and inhibitory inputs within the cortical pyramidal neurons and their connections to extrinsic inputs and outputs. On the basis of the Hebbian principle, the operation of coincidence-based synaptic plasticity in cortical networks results in the formation, strengthening, and continuous recruitment of neurons within neuronal "assemblies" that "cooperatively" represent behaviorally important stimuli.

6. *Plasticity is constrained by anatomical sources and convergent-divergent spreads of inputs.* Every cortical field has the following:
   a. Specific extrinsic and intrinsic input sources
   b. Dimensions of anatomical divergence and convergence of its inputs, limiting dynamic combination Hebbian input co-selection capacities[143,144]

Anatomical input sources and limited projection overlap both to enable change by establishing input-selection repertoires and to determine the limits for change. There are relatively strict anatomical constraints at the "lower" system levels, where only spatially (spectrally) limited input coincidence-based combined outcomes are possible. In the "higher" system hierarchies, anatomical projection topographies are more powerful, with neurons and neuronal assemblies developing that respond to complex combinations of features of real-world objects, events, and actions.

7. *Plasticity is constrained by the time constants governing coincident input co-selection and by the time structures and potentially achievable coherence of extrinsic and intrinsic cortical input sources.*

To effectively drive representational changes with coincident input-dependent Hebbian mechanisms, temporally coordinated inputs are prerequisite, given the short durations (milliseconds to tens of milliseconds) of the time constants that govern synaptic plasticity in the adaptive cortical machinery (see reference 145 for review). Consistently uncorrelated or low–discharge-rate inputs induce negative changes in synaptic effectiveness. In addition, stimuli occurring repetitively simultaneously can also degrade the representation. These negative effects also contribute importantly to the learning-driven "election" of behaviorally important inputs.

8. *Cortical field–specific differences in input sources, distributions, and time-structured inputs create different representational structures.*
   a. There are significant differences in the activity from afferent inputs from the retina, skin, or cochlea generated in a relatively strictly topographically wired V1 (area 17), S1 proper (area 3b), or A1 (area 43) compared with the inferotemporal visual, insular somatosensory, dorsotemporal auditory, or prefrontal cortical areas that receive highly diffuse inputs (see Figure 4-8). In the former cases, heavy schedules of repetitive, temporally coherent inputs are delivered from powerful, redundant projections from relatively strictly topographically organized thalamic nuclei and lower-level, associated cortical areas. Whereas neighboring neurons can share some response properties, neurons or clusters of neurons respond selectively to learned inputs. These neurons are distributed widely across cortical areas and share less information with neighboring neurons. In the "lower" levels, afferent input projections from any given source are greatly dispersed. Highly repetitive inputs are uncommon, inputs from multiple diffuse cortical sources are more common as well as more varied, and complex input combinations are in play. These differences in input schedules, spreads, and combinations presumably largely account for the dramatic differences in the patterns of representation of behaviorally important stimuli at "lower" and "higher" levels.[146]
   b. Despite these differences in representational organization across the cortex, the cortex does progressively differentiate cortical cells to accomplish specific operational tasks. There is a serial progression of differentiation to allow the development of functional organization that allows an individual to progressively master more and more elaborated and differentiated perceptual, cognitive, monitoring, and executive skills.
   c. The sources of inputs and their field-specific spreads and boundary limits, the distributions of modulatory inputs differentiated by cortical layers in different cortical regions, the basic elements and their basic interconnections in the cortical processing machine, and crucial aspects of input combination and processing at subcortical levels are inherited (see reference 147 for review). Although these inherited aspects of sensory, motor, and cortical processing circuit development constrain the potential learning-based modification of processing within each cortical area, representation changes can occur as a result of environmental interaction and purposeful behavioral practice.

9. *Temporal dimensions of behaviorally important inputs also influence representational "specialization."* In at least four ways, the cortex refines its representations of the temporal aspects of behaviorally important inputs during learning.
   a. First,
      1) The cortex generates more synchronous representations of sequenced and coincident associative input perturbations or events, not only recording their identities but also marking their occurrences (for examples, see references 132, 136, 139, and 148 to 151). These changes in representation appear to be primarily achieved through increases in positive coupling strengths between interconnected neurons participating in stimulus- or action-specific neuronal cell assemblies.[132,150,152-171] The strength of the interconnectedness increases representational salience as a result of downstream neurons being excited as a direct function of the degree of temporal synchronization of their inputs.
      2) Increasing the power of the outputs of a cortical area drives downstream plasticity. Hebbian plasticity mechanisms operating within downstream cortical (or other) targets also have relatively short time constants. The greater the synchronicity of inputs, the more powerfully those change mechanisms are engaged. The strength of the interconnections also helps protect against noise. For example, by simple information abstraction and coding, the distributed neuronal representation of the "signal" (a temporally coordinated, distributed neuronal response pattern representing the input or action) is converted at the entry levels in the cortex into a form that is not as easily degraded or altered by "noise." The strength of the interconnectedness also confers robustness of complex signal representation for spatially or spectrally incomplete or degraded inputs.
   b. Second,
      1) The cortex can select specific inputs through learning to exaggerate the representation of specific input time structures. Conditioning a monkey or a rat with stimuli that have a consistent, specific temporal modulation rate or interstimulus time, for example, results in a selective exaggeration of the responses of neurons at that rate or time separation. In effect, the cortex "specializes" for expected

relatively higher-speed or relatively lower-speed signal event reception.

2) Both electrophysiological recording studies and theoretical studies suggest that cortical networks richly encode the temporal interval as a simple consequence of cortical network dynamics.[172,173] It is hypothesized that the cortex accomplishes time interval and duration selectivity in learning by positively changing synaptic connection strengths for input circuits that can respond with recovery times and circuit delays that match behaviorally important modulation frequency periods, intervals, or durations. However, studies on including excessive, rapid, repetitive fine motor movements can sometimes lead to serious degradation in representation if the adjacent digits are driven nearly simultaneous in time. This may be associated with negative learning and a loss of motor control.[174]

c. Third,

1) The cortex links representations of immediately successive inputs that are presented in a learning context.

2) As a result of Hebbian plasticity, it establishes overlapping and neighboring relationships between immediately successive parts of rapidly changing inputs yet retains its individualized, distinct cortical representation.[65,175]

d. Fourth,

1) The cortex generates stimulus sequence-specific ("combination-sensitive") responses, with neuronal responses selectively modulated by the prior application of stimuli in the learned sequence of temporally separated events.

2) These "associative" or "combination-sensitive" responses have been correlated with evidence of strengthened interconnections between cortical cell assemblies representing successive event elements separated by hundreds of milliseconds to seconds in time.[176,177] The mechanisms of origin of these effects have not yet been established.

10. *The integration time ("processing time") in the cortex is itself subject to powerful learning-based plasticity.*

a. Cortical networks engage both excitatory and inhibitory neurons by strong input perturbations. Within a given processing "channel," cortical pyramidal cells cannot be effectively reexcited by a following perturbation for tens to hundreds of milliseconds. These integration "times" are primarily dictated by the time for recovery from inhibition, which ordinarily dominates poststimulus excitability. This "integration time," "processing time," or "recovery time" is commonly measured by deriving a "modulation transfer function," which defines the ability of cortical neurons to respond to identical successive stimuli within cortical "processing channels." For example, these "integration" times normally range from about 15 to about 200 ms in the primary auditory receiving areas.[178-180] Progressively longer processing times are recorded at higher system levels (e.g., in the auditory cortex, they are approximately a syllable in length, 200 to 500 ms in duration) in the "belt cortex" surrounding the primary auditory cortex.[181]

b. These time constants govern—and limit—the cortex's ability to "chunk" (i.e., to separately represent by distributed, coordinated discharge) successive events within its processing channels. Both neurophysiological studies in animals and behavioral training studies in human adults and children have shown that the time constants governing event-by-event complex signal representation are highly plastic. With intensive training in the right form, cortical "processing times" reflected by the ability to accurately and separately process events occurring at different input rates can be dramatically shortened or lengthened.[182-185]

11. *Plasticity processes are competitive.*

a. If two spatially or spectrally different inputs are consistently delivered nonsimultaneously to the cortex, cortical networks generate input-selective cell assemblies for each input and actively segregate them from one another.[139,184,186-188] Boundaries between such inputs grow to be sharp and are substantially intensity independent. Computational models of Hebbian network behaviors indicate that this sharp segregation of nonidentical, temporally separated inputs is accomplished as a result of a wider distribution of inhibitory instead of excitatory responses in the emerging, competing cortical cell assemblies that represent them.

b. This Hebbian network cell assembly formation and competition appear to account for how the cortex creates sharply sorted representations of the fingers in the primary somatosensory cortex.[140,189] The Hebbian network probably accounts for how the cortex creates sharply sorted representations of native aural language-specific phonemes in lower-level auditory cortical areas in the auditory and speech processing system of humans. If inputs are delivered in a constant and stereotyped way from a limited region of the skin or cochlea in a learning context, that skin surface or cochlear sector is an evident competitive "winner."[136,190] By Hebbian plasticity, the cortical networks will co-select that specific combination of inputs and represent it within a competitively growing Hebbian cell assembly. The competitive strength of that cooperative cell assembly will grow progressively because more and more neurons are excited by behaviorally important stimuli with increasingly coordinated discharges. That means that neurons outside of this cooperative group have greater numbers of more coordinated outputs contributing to their later competitive recruitment. Through progressive functional remodeling, the cortex clusters and competitively sorts information across sharp boundaries dictated by the spectrotemporal statistics of its inputs. If it receives information on a heavy schedule that sets up competition for a limited input set, it will sort competitive inputs into a correspondingly small number of largely discontinuous response regions.[191,192]

c. Competitive outcomes are, again, cortical level dependent. The cortex links events that occur in different competitive groups if they are consistently excited synchronously in time. At the same time, competitively formed groups of neurons come to be synchronously linked in their representations of different parts of the complex stimulus and collectively represent successive complex features of the vocalization through the coordinated activities of many groups.

d. Neurons within the two levels of the cortex surrounding A1 (see Figure 4-8) have greater spectral input convergence and longer integration times that enable their facile combination of information representing different spectrotemporal details. Their information extraction is greatly facilitated by the learning-based linkages of cooperative groups that deliver behaviorally important inputs in a highly salient, temporally coordinated form to these fields. With their progressively greater space and time constants, still higher-level areas organize competitive cell assemblies that represent still more complex spectral and serial-event combinations. Note that these organizational changes apply over a large cortical scale. In skill learning over a limited period of training, participating neuronal members of such assemblies can easily be increased by many hundredfold, even within a primary sensory area such as S1, area 3b, or A1.[136,139,174,184,193]

e. In extensive training in complex signal recognition, more than 10% of neurons within temporal cortical areas can come to respond highly selectively to a specific, normally rare, complex training stimulus. The distributed cell assemblies representing those specific complex inputs involve tens or hundreds of millions of neurons and are achieved by enduring effectiveness changes in many billions of synapses.

12. *Learning is modulated as a function of behavioral state.*
   a. At "lower" levels of the cortex, changes are generated only in attended behaviors.[137,138,146,193-195] Trial-by-trial change magnitudes are a function of the importance of the input to the animal as signaled by the level of attention, the cognitive values of behavioral rewards or punishments, and internal judgments of practice trial precision or error based on the relative success or failure of achieving a target goal or expectation. Little or no enduring change is induced when a well-learned "automatic" behavior is performed from memory without attention. It is also interesting to note that at some levels within the cortex, activity changes can be induced even in nonattending subjects under conditions in which "priming" effects of nonattended reception of information can be demonstrated.
   b. The modulation of progressive learning is also achieved by the activation of powerful reward systems releasing the neurotransmitters norepinephrine and dopamine (among others) through widespread projections to the cerebral cortex. Norepinephrine plays a particularly important role in modulating learning-induced changes in the cortex.[148,184,195]
   c. The cortex is a "learning machine." During the learning of a new skill, neurotransmitters are released trial by trial with application of a behaviorally important stimulus or behavioral rewards. If the skill can be mastered and thereafter replayed from memory, its performance can be generated without attention (habituation). Habituation results in a profound attenuation of the modulation signals from these neurotransmitter sources; plasticity is no longer positively enabled in cortical networks.

13. *Top-down influences constrain cortical representational plasticity.*

Attentional control flexibly defines an enabling "window" for change in learning.[182] Progressive learning generates progressively more strongly represented goals, expectations, and feedback[196,197] across all representational systems that are undergoing change and to modulatory control systems weighing performance success and error. Strong intermodal behavioral and representational effects have also been recorded in experiments that might be interpreted as shaping expectations.[198,199] These shaping expectations would be similar to those observed in a human subject using multisensory inputs such as auditory, visual, and somesthetic information to create integrated phonological representations, to create fine motor movement trajectory patterns that underlie precise hand control, or to make a vocal production.

14. *The scale of plasticity in progressive skill learning is massive.*
   a. Cortical representational plasticity must be viewed as arising from multiple-level systems that are broadly engaged in learning, perceiving, remembering, thinking, and acting. Any behaviorally important input (or consistent internally generated activity) engages many cortical areas. Repetitive training drives all cortical areas to change.[131,144,200] Different aspects of any acquired skill are contributed from field-specific changes in the multiple cortical areas that are remodeled in its learning.
   b. In this kind of continuously evolving representational machine, perceptual constancy cannot be accounted for by locationally constant brain representations; relational representational principles must be invoked to account for it.[131,201] Moreover, representational changes must obviously be coordinated level to level. It should also be understood that plastic changes are also induced extracortically. Although it is believed that learning at the cortical level is usually predominant, plasticity induced by learning within many extracortical structures significantly contributes to learning-induced changes that are expressed within the cortex.

15. *Enduring cortical plasticity changes appear to be accounted for by local changes in neural anatomy.*

Changes in synapse turnover, synapse number, synaptic active zones, dendritic spines, and the elaboration of terminal dendrites have been demonstrated to occur in a behaviorally engaged cortical zone.[144,202-207] Through many changes in local structural detail, the learning brain is continuously physically remodeling its processing machinery, not only across the course of child development but also after behavioral training in an adult who has had a neural insult.

16. *Cortical plasticity processes in child development represent progressive, multiple-staged skill learning.*
   a. There are two remarkable achievements of brain plasticity in child development. The first is the progressive shaping of the processing to handle the accurate, high-speed reception of the rapidly changing streams of information that flow into the brain. In the cerebral cortex, shaping appears to begin most powerfully within the primary receiving areas of the cortex. With early myelination, the main gateways for information into the cortex are receiving strongly coherent inputs from subcortical nuclei, and they can quickly organize their local networks on the basis of coincident input co-selection (Hebbian) plasticity

mechanisms. The self-organization of the cortical processing machinery spreads outward from these primary receiving areas over time to ultimately refine the basic processing machinery of all the cortex. The second great achievement, which is strongly dependent on the first, is the efficient storage of massive content compendia in richly associated forms.

b. During development, the brain accomplishes its functional self-organization through a long parallel series of small steps. At each step, the brain masters a series of elementary processing skills and establishes reliable information repertoires that enable the accomplishment of subsequent skills. Second- and higher-order skills can be viewed as both elaborations of more basic mastered skills and the creation of new skills dependent on combined second- and higher-order processing. That hierarchical processing is enabled by greater cortical anatomical spreads, by more complexly convergent anatomical sources of inputs, and by longer integration (processing, recovery) times at progressively higher cortical system levels. This hierarchical but integrating processing allows for progressively more complex combinations of information integrated over progressively longer time epochs as one ascends across cortical processing hierarchies.
c. As the cortical machinery functionally evolves and consequently physically "matures" through childhood developmental stages, information repertories are represented in progressively more salient forms (i.e., with more powerful distributed response coordination). Growing agreement directly controls the power of emerging information repertoires for driving the next level of elaborative and combinatorial changes. It is hypothesized that saliency enables the maturation of the myelination of projection tracts delivering outputs from functionally refined cortical areas. More mature myelination of output projections also contributes to the power of this newly organized activity to drive strong, downstream plastic change through the operation of Hebbian plasticity processes.
d. As each elaboration of skill is practiced, in a learning phase, neuromodulatory transmitters enable change in the cortical machinery. The cortex functionally and physically adapts to generate the neurological representations of the skill in progressively more selective, predictable, and statistically reliable forms. Ultimately, the performance of the skill concurs with the brain's own accumulated, learning-derived "expectations." The skill can then be performed from memory, without attention. With this consolidation of the remembered skill and information repertoire, the modulatory nuclei enable no further change in the cortical machinery. The learning machine, the cerebral cortex, moves on to the next elaboration. In this way the cortex constructs highly specialized processing machinery that can progressively produce great towers of automatically performable behaviors and great progressively maturing hierarchies of information-processing machinery that can achieve progressively more powerful complex signal representations, retrievals, and associations. With this machinery in a mature and thereby efficiently operating form, there is a remarkable capacity for reception, storage, and analysis of diverse and complexly associated information.
e. The flexible, self-adjusting capacity for refinement of the processing capabilities of the nervous system confers the ability of our species to represent complex language structures. This self-adjusting capacity also allows humans to develop high-speed reading abilities; remarkably varied complex modern-era motor abilities; and abstract logic structures characteristic of a mathematician, software engineer, or philosopher. This nervous system refinement also creates elaborate, idiosyncratic, experience-based behavioral abilities in all of us.

Neuroplasticity and Learning

How Are Learning Sequences Controlled? What Constrains Learning Progressions? Perhaps the most important basis of control of learning progressions is representational consolidation. Through specialization, the trained cortex creates progressively more specific and more salient distributed representations of behaviorally important inputs. Growing representational salience increases the power of a cortical area to effectively drive change wherever outputs from this evolving cortical processing machinery are distributed (e.g., in "higher system levels distributed and coordinated [synchronized] responses" more powerfully drive downstream Hebbian-based plasticity changes).

A second powerful basis for sequenced learning is progressive myelination. At the time of birth, only the core "primary" extrinsic information entry zones (A1, S1, V1) in the cortex are heavily myelinated.[208,209] Across childhood, connections to and interconnections between cortical areas are progressively myelinated, proceeding from these core areas out to progressively "higher" system levels. Myelination in the posterior parietal, anterior, and inferior temporal and prefrontal cortical areas is not "mature" in the human forebrain until 8 to 20 years of age. Even in the mature state, it is far less developed at the "highest" processing levels.

Myelination controls the conduction times and therefore the temporal dispersions of input sources to and within cortical areas. Poor myelination at "higher" levels in the young brain is associated with temporally diffuse inputs. They cannot generate reliable representational constructs of an adult quality because they do not as effectively engage input-coincidence–based Hebbian plasticity mechanisms. That ensures, in effect, that plasticity is not enabled for complex combinatorial processing until "lower" level input repertoires are consolidated (i.e., become stable, statistically reliable forms).

Although myelination is thought to be genetically programmed, some scientists hypothesize that myelination in the CNS is also controlled by emerging temporal response coherence and is achieved through temporally coordinated signaling from the multiple branches of oligodendrocytes that terminate on different projection axons in central tracts and networks. It has been argued that central myelination is positively and negatively activity dependent and that distributed synchronization may contribute to positive change.[210] If the hypothesis that coherent activity controls myelination proves to be true, then the emerging temporal correlation of distributed representations of behaviorally important stimuli is generated level by level. This is done by changes in coupling in local cortical networks in the developing cortex. It would also directly drive changes in myelination for the outputs of that cortical area. These two events in turn would enable the generation of reliable and salient representational constructs at that higher level. By this kind of progression, skill learning is hypothesized to directly control progressive functional and physical brain development through the course of child development. This is accomplished both by refining ("maturing") local interconnections through response dynamics of information processing machinery at successive cortical levels and by coordinated refinement ("maturing") of the critical information transmission pathways that interconnect different processing levels.

Another constraint in the development of neural adaptation may be the development of mature sleeping patterns, especially within the first year of life.[211] Sleep both enables the strengthening of learning-based plastic changes and resets the learning machinery by "erasing" temporary unreinforced and unrewarded input-generated changes produced over the preceding waking period.[212-214] The dramatic shift in the percentage of time spent in rapid-eye-movement sleep is consistent with a strong early bias toward noise removal in an immature and poorly functionally unorganized brain. Sleep patterns change dramatically in the older child, in parallel with a strong increase in the daily schedule of closely attended, rewarded, and goal-oriented behaviors. This research will need to be explored in greater detail when these data are related to patients with CNS damage. This population often has poor breathing habits and capabilities that lead to decreased oxygenation and often broken sleep cycles. How much either impairment, breakdown, or the interaction of the two diminishes neuroplasticity has yet to be determined.

Top-down modulation controlling attentional windows and learned predictions (expectations and behavioral goals) must all be constructed by learning. Delays in goal development could also create an important constraint for the progression of early learning. In the very young brain, prediction and error-estimation processes would be weakened because stored higher-level information repertoires are ill formed and statistically unreliable. As the brain matures, stored information progressively more strongly and reliably enables top-down attentional and predictive controls, progressively providing a stronger basis for success and error signaling for modulatory control nuclei and progressively enabling top-down syntactic feedback to increase representational reliability.

Attention, reward and punishment, accuracy of achievement of goals, and error feedback gate learning through a modulatory control system are critical for learning. The modulatory control systems that enable learning are also plastic, with their process of maturation providing constraint or facilitation for progressive learning. These subcortical nuclei are signaled by complex information feedback from the cortex itself. The salience and specificity of that feedback information grow over time. The ability to provide accurate error judging or goal-achievement signaling must grow progressively. The nucleus basalis, nucleus accumbens, ventral tegmentum, and locus coeruleus must undergo their own functional self-organization on the basis of Hebbian plasticity principles to achieve "mature" modulatory selectivity and power. The progressive maturation of the modulatory control system occurs naturally with development or training. This system can provide another important constraint on skill development progression and regulation of axial or trunk postural and balance control and fine motor coordination.

What Facilitates the Development of Permanent "Automatic" Motor Behaviors? The creation and maintenance of cortical representations are functions of the animal's or human's level of attention at a task. Cortical representational plasticity in skill acquisition is self-limiting. Because the behavior comes to be more "automatic," it is less closely attended, and representational changes induced in the cortex fade and ultimately disappear or reverse (unlearning effects).[215,216] The element of behavioral performance that enables maintenance of the behavior with minimum involvement of the cortical learning machinery is probably stereotypical movement sequence repetition. As a movement behavior is practiced, an effective, highly statistically predictable movement sequence is adopted that enables the storage of the learned behavior in a permanent form that requires only minimal or no behavioral attention. If behavioral performance declines or behavioral or brain conditions change to render a task more difficult, attention to the behavior will again need to increase, producing an invigorated cortical response to the new learning challenge.

By this view, the cerebral cortex is clearly a learning machine. William James[217] was the first to point out that the great practical advantage for a self-organizing cortex was the development of what he called "habits." When a skill is overlearned, it will engage pathways that are so reliable that they can be followed without attention.

Why are some habits retained and others lost? Can sensorimotor learning be sustained when the adaptive representations of the learned behavior "fade" in the cerebral cortex? These areas have not been well researched. However, there are several possibilities. Habits could come to be represented in an enduring form extracortically. The cortex could modify processing in the spinal cord, the basal ganglia, the red nucleus, or the cerebellum. For example, the learning of manual skills requires a motor cortex, but overlearned motor skills may not be significantly reduced by the induction of a wide area 4 lesion.

Another possibility is that behaviorally induced cortical changes endure in a highly efficient representational form that can sustain the representation of its key features on the cortex itself, engaging only limited distributed populations of cortical neurons to represent the behavior with high fidelity. Thus, recall of past learning may take less time to restructure than to reformat entirely new learning, whether it be a cognitive or motor task. The fact that a monkey improves discriminative abilities or movement performance after modifying the cortical neuron response with heavily practiced behaviors supports this alternative. However, many behaviors, such as musical performance, require constant, attended practice at a highly cognitive level to maintain both the representational changes and the performance. It also appears that continued learning with heavily practiced behaviors may be neuroprotective with aging, maintaining function despite loss of cortical neurons as a natural part of aging.

SUMMARY

Over the years, learning has been tied to critical periods of development, with the assumption that if a particular skill or behavior was not learned during the critical period, the opportunity to acquire that skill was lost. In addition, after this critical period of development, aging was associated with inevitable deterioration of brain and neurophysiological function. However, today there is substantial evidence that the brain is an incredibly specialized representational machine that can adapt to meet the specific inputs that engage it. The beauty of the brain is that it not only self-organizes but stores the contents of its learning to create a foundation that increases in depth and breadth and makes predictions on even novel inputs to facilitate acute and efficient operations. The earlier the exposure to multisensory stimuli, the easier it is for the competitive neuronal processes to adapt and to make extensive connections. With growing neuronal specificity and salience, more powerful predictions are continued until there is greater learning and mastery.

Among the important findings of the twentieth century was the validation that the brain is a learning machine that operates throughout life. The aging process can take a toll on the ability to store information and may reduce both the complexity of the information that is processed and the individual's ability to remember. But if an individual is conscious of good hydration, balanced nutrition, physical exercise, and regularly goal-directed progressive learning, CNS pathways of representation and prediction can not only be preserved but also continue to adapt. These activities can also slow the aging process. Thus it is possible to drive improvement in function in individuals with abnormalities related to development, disease, injury, or aging. Learning is not necessarily specifically staged, but rather represents complex abilities developed mostly from systems interaction and integration. Therapists must develop the ability to determine what inputs are reliable and salient to effectively create functional and physical brain maturation, adaptation, and learning. In the face of different types of challenges (structural, emotional, pathological), clinicians must develop more effective strategies that can be used to facilitate neural adaptation, learning, substitution, and representational changes that will allow meaningful maintenance and improvement in function despite anatomical or physiological variances in structure. Although strong behavioral events can be associated with measurable neural adaptability, new, more permanent neural connections and synapses must be strengthened with repetition and increased complexity. Clients with CNS disorders may have damaged certain areas of the brain, which may not recover; however, with learning-based activities it is possible to reorganize the brain, stimulate neurons from adjacent areas, establish new synapses and dendritic pathways,[218] and activate neurons in the contralateral, uninjured parts of the brain.[219-225] Creating the best environment to learn a skill may initially need to be contrived, with limitations controlled externally by the therapist's hands or clinical arena. In time, those limitations must be eliminated and variability within the natural environment reintroduced to achieve true learning and ultimate neuroplasticity.

The elements of neuroscience research on neural adaptation have been summarized into 14 principles to guide rehabilitation programs designed to facilitate experience-dependent plasticity.[96,226,227] These principles, outlined in Box 4-1, are similar to those suggested by Nudo[129] as well as Kleim and Jones[128] and Byl and colleagues.[228] Although these principles are particularly relevant to patients with a head injury or stroke, they are also relevant for aging adults,[229-233] and those with neurodegenerative disease. These principles are not meant to be exhaustive or mutually exclusive but to highlight the principles of experience-dependent plasticity. However, they can serve as a reference for therapists who are designing creative intervention programs based on the translation of basic science to clinical practice and to help organize the extensive research on neuroplasticity.

These principles can be applied across a broad range of exercises—not just "brain exercises" to improve cognition and intellect, but also physical exercise. For example, we know that brain derivative neural factor (BDNF) is necessary for learning. BDNF decreases with aging and is severely reduced in animals with dementia. However, BDNF can be increased with moderate and aerobic exercise.[234,235] Furthermore, it is clear that timing of enrichment (e.g., mental stimulation, physical exercise, sensory and motor training) is important, not only during development but across the life span. Initiating an exercise program too early (e.g., in less than 24 hours acute post neural injury) may be associated with an exaggeration of cellular injury.[236] However, waiting too long to intervene can limit the efficacy of the learning-based training experience.[237] It also appears that the efficacy of learning-based training may be enhanced with cortical stimulation,[238] repetitive transcranial magnetic stimulation (TMS),[239] and imagery. It is critical to create a positive foundation to maximize learning (e.g., good hydration to maximize blood flow and oxygenation of tissues, adequate nutrition to energize the body, and aerobic activity to increase endorphins and BDNF, as well as positive expectations of getting better [limbic system]). Rehabilitation specialists must not only translate basic neuroscience into practice but participate in clinical research, serve as advocates for patients, ensure access to appropriate rehabilitative services, and be politically active in health care reform.

To ensure maximum neural adaptation, rehabilitation programs must include strong, carefully outlined home programs. Therapists must educate patients and their families about the principles of neuroplasticity to empower them to create progressive learning activities at home and in the community. Patients should revisit health care team members to facilitate ongoing learning. Patients must become their own best therapist, consistently motivating themselves to learn something new, perform attended behavioral activities, observe and integrate new information from their environment, have fun, stay engaged with family, friends, and community and avoid habitual stereotypical behaviors. Learning should be an excuse to travel to new places and learn new skills. Every day should include a new learning experience. Learning and aerobic exercise may not only be neuroprotective but could be critical for slowing down the natural neurodegenerative aspects of aging. Computer gaming, new technology, and robotics can be integrated to expand daily learning-based activities at home (see Chapter 38).

The maximum attainment of skilled performance cannot necessarily be determined. The original injury can be used only as an estimate of the damage with some indicators for prognosis and recovery. The rest of the success of rehabilitation and restoration of function will reside with the motivation and commitment of the individual. How that motivation and commitment are initially established and continually reinforced is based on the patient, the therapist's interactive skills and emotional bond (see Chapter 5),

CASE STUDY 4-1 ■ PERSON WITH PARKINSON DISEASE

People with Parkinson disease develop an array of deficits in motor control that interfere with multiple ADLs and can eventually degrade quality of life. When motor control deficits are evaluated in this population, the severity of the disease, the activity level of the person, and the medication schedule are important considerations. Following are several motor control deficits that are evident in this disease.

Motor control impairments of rigid tone and bradykinesia create alterations in stride length, speed, and step frequency in the gait pattern of persons with Parkinson disease. The person may demonstrate a gait pattern characterized by decreased amplitude of leg movement, duration of the gait cycle, trunk rotation, and arm swing. Difficulty initiating gait, or "freezing," is an observable motor control problem, and small shuffling steps and a festinating gait pattern are also common.[240] Impaired righting and balance reactions can contribute to gait instability. When the demands on gait velocity and frequency are altered, metabolic cost increases and the ability of the individual to safely complete the functional movement with appropriate coordination of postural and motor control is challenged.

A practical outcome measure that can be used to capture the effect of these motor deficits on functional mobility is the Timed Up-and-Go Test (TUG). This quick test can be used to capture the time it takes for a person to initiate sit to stand, transition from sit to stand, walk 3 meters, turn around, walk back, turn, and sit down. During the performance of these sequential movement patterns the clinician can observe gait deviations, postural abnormalities, movement amplitude, and safety awareness. Episodes and duration of "freezing," or failed initiation, can be accounted for, and the number of steps to turn 180 degrees can be documented.[241] The overall time to complete the test can supply the clinician with objective data related to fall risk.

Overshooting or undershooting the 3-meter line before turning may be demonstrated. Although clients with Parkinson disease are able to prepare the motor strategy and use advance information, the primary problem is slow onset of execution of movement; therefore changing motor patterns (e.g., switching from walking to turning) can be quite difficult.

To illustrate the multiple motor control deficits, imagine a patient performing the TUG.[242] The person may have difficulty accelerating to walk and decelerating to turn around and may have difficulty decelerating when approaching the chair and sitting down. Postural instability may be observed during transfers and turning, and a loss of balance in the backward direction without the activation of an automatic stepping response may occur. The motor control deficits exhibited in the patient with Parkinson disease are numerous and intertwined and their severity is influenced by the progression of the disease. As mentioned earlier, the client cannot appropriately control the increase and decrease in the rate of force production, which is evident in the acceleration and deceleration phases of the movement. If the rate of force production is altered; amplitude of force production may also be affected.

The person may have a decreased ability to predict and prepare the motor pattern for turning before the actual turn. There appears to be a slow initiation of the turning task. This phenomenon could be caused by an inability to sequence the motor behavior as a whole. Several researchers have observed that the person completes one movement before starting the next movement in the sequence rather than executing a smooth, continuing movement pattern.[25] Another reason for the decrease in the ability to perform this task smoothly is the patient's dependence on visual feedback. Relying more heavily on visual feedback to accomplish a task slows the movement.

The movement deficits observed may also be a result of the inability to effectively coordinate movements such as those observed between postural and motile components of the task. Postural strategies may be classified on a continuum that includes postural preparations, postural adaptations, and postural reactions.[243] The person with Parkinson disease may not predict and make appropriate postural adjustments before the movement and may have deficits in adaptive and reactive postural responses (e.g., righting and equilibrium reactions, and adapting to environmental demands). In the case of the TUG, movement and balance strategies are assessed when the client stands up and sits down. If the client does not use a controlled descent into the chair but rather falls backward, what are the possible causes for the sudden descent? The client's goal may be to land in the chair, but the preferred pattern may be to fall into the chair. The individual may not be able to predict the time and force needed to activate the muscles for a smooth descent, the individual may be deconditioned and not have the strength or endurance to perform a smooth descent, or the individual may not have the balance strategies required to perform this maneuver.

The client with Parkinson disease is one example of a client with a neurological condition that affects motor output and control. Regardless of the diagnosis, all aspects of motor control need to be examined and activity-based tests must be conducted to determine how the impairments interact to affect the execution of functional tasks. A few key deficits in gross and fine motor control and postural control were examined in this example. It is not within the scope of this section to present all the motor and postural control deficits but to highlight the complexity of patients with neurological pathology. Accurate identification of motor control problems in clients assists the therapist and the client in the development of realistic functional goals and effective intervention programs (see Section II for recommendations regarding specific diseases or pathological conditions and their related body system impairments and activity-based functional limitations).

and the family and other support systems surrounding the client (see Chapter 6).

Acknowledgment

All the present authors and the editors would like to thank both Roberta Newton, PT, PhD, and Sharon Gorman, PT, DPTSc, GCS for their commitment to this text's evolution, as well as to the delivery of best practices to the elderly population.

References

To enhance this text and add value for the reader, all references are included on the companion Evolve site that accompanies this textbook. This online service will, when available, provide a link for the reader to a Medline abstract for the article cited. There are 250 cited references and other general references for this chapter, with the majority of those articles being evidence-based citations.

CHAPTER 5 The Limbic System: Influence over Motor Control and Learning

DARCY A. UMPHRED, PT, PhD, FAPTA, MARCIA HALL THOMPSON, PT, DPT, DSc, and THERESE MARIE WEST, PhD, MT-BC, FAMI

KEY TERMS

amygdala
declarative memory
emotional behavior
F²ARV (*f*ear and *f*rustration, *a*nger, *r*age, *v*iolence/withdrawal) continuum
general adaptation syndrome (GAS)
hippocampus
hypothalamus
limbic network
motor learning
MOVE (*m*otivation or *m*emory, *o*lfaction, *v*isceral, autonomic nervous system, *e*motional)

OBJECTIVES

After reading this chapter the student or therapist will be able to:

1. Understand the complexity of the limbic network and the influence of the limbic network on behavioral and functional responses.
2. Describe the behavioral responses directly influenced by the limbic network.
3. Describe the structures of the limbic network.
4. Describe the interaction between the limbic network and body systems responsible for behavioral responses.
5. Differentiate between limbic-driven motor control responses and frontal, cerebellar, and basal ganglia motor regulation.
6. Differentiate between declarative and procedural learning.
7. Identify signs of both positive and negative limbic network influence on a client's observable behavior and functional responses.
8. Describe appropriate treatment interventions or program modifications for both the limbic high and limbic low client.
9. Understand the influence of the therapist over the limbic network and behavioral and functional responses, and effectively integrate limbic network treatment techniques into current treatment models.

Since the publication of the fifth edition of this book, the limbic network has emerged as a key component of central nervous system (CNS) function, becoming one of the most researched areas of the CNS when analyzing behavior, learning, emotions, and their influence on activities and participation. In the past, review of the literature on the limbic network was limited to investigating potential interactions of other systems with nuclei within the limbic network. This is no longer the case, as neuroscience research has helped to identify the critical nature of behaviors controlled or influenced by the limbic network. Based on research at a cellular level,[1-3] a consciousness level,[4-7] a bodily systems level,[8-10] and a quantum level[11-13] it is now clear that the motor system is just one of the many systems affected by the complex limbic network.[14-21]

Although far from yielding a complete understanding, this research and knowledge are increasing daily and force today's therapist not only to recognize limbic behavior but also to develop an understanding of how involvement of the limbic network will positively and negatively affect each patient. Therapists can no longer think of motor control and motor learning as controlled exclusively by an anatomically unique motor system, nor can we understand movement using motor control or motor learning principles alone. Therapists must consider how emotions may influence selection of health care services and how the limbic network strongly influences treatment participation and outcomes, such as motivation and cooperation, responsibility for and compliance with home programs, levels of functional activity, and empowerment over treatment planning and life activities.

Obviously, the human organism is a complex totality made up of many interlocking parts. The medical system has traditionally divided the body into systems and has forgotten that each specific system is co-dependent on many other systems for function. Today the medical profession is rediscovering the importance of how the systems interact with and influence one another.[22,23] It is very important that movement specialists do not fall into the same trap as medicine in the past and look at movement from only a biomechanical, muscular, neurological, cardiopulmonary, or integumentary system perspective. They must consider the interaction among systems and their subsystems within an individual. For example, the motor system is a system in and of itself. But cognitive impairment and limbic network involvement can lead to tremendous errors in motor responses even when the motor system is intact. In our clients with CNS dysfunction, impairments exist in the motor and limbic network and in cognition, thus creating the potential for a complex set of behavioral responses to internal or external environmental influences.

Again, the totality of these problems is like interlocking pieces of a complicated puzzle. The therapist learner must always maintain clear visualization of the entire puzzle (the client and all his or her systems) while analyzing any one piece or component system. The process of unraveling the multisystem "puzzle" and adding new pieces of learning is the journey a therapist learner begins in school and can continue throughout his or her career. This is one example of the limbic network's influence in our own work as therapists. The decision to continue on a learning journey is driven by desire to learn and answer questions regarding the unknown. The emotions felt by the therapist learner in pursuit of mastery and the ability to have the intellectual memory of the learning are also limbic functions. These behavioral responses play an important role in all our lives and in the lives and recovery of our patients/clients, as we will continue to investigate in this chapter.

A patient example of these interactions can be found in a case description of a middle-aged woman admitted to the intensive care unit (ICU) with multiple pelvic fractures and diagnosed with severe internal bleeding, kidney failure, pneumonia, pulmonary emboli, and severe clotting in the lower extremities. The physician took her husband aside to let him know that she was going to die, to which her husband replied, "I understand. Juggling one system problem is easy, juggling two systems takes a little practice, and three-system involvement may challenge the best medical skill. She is presenting four or five body system failures and you are sure no one can juggle that many problems." The doctor said yes and the patient's husband then said, "Please keep juggling and don't worry about me, because if you do, I would then be one more ball to juggle." And it did seem that every time the doctors got a handle on a body system problem, another system would fail. She required services from an endocrinologist, infection control specialists, interventional radiologists, a pulmonologist, a hematologist, a vascular surgeon, an internal medicine specialist, a urologist, and a nephrologist. Each specialist shared his or her limited experience with a complex clinical problem like this and that there was nothing in the literature to help his or her respective understanding. After 2½ months in the ICU, the woman survived. The physician who had foretold her death met again with the patient and her family. He stated, "How are you still alive? I know what we did medically, but that was not enough to keep you alive." And he was right. No model within each respective field could account for her recovery. However, the piece not considered within her medical management was the beliefs and spiritual strength of the patient and her family, a positive limbic network influence on the function of each failing body systems. This concept of limbic influence will be further discussed in the third section of this chapter.

So why has this chapter been positioned so prominently within a textbook on basic neurological rehabilitation? In many curricula the limbic network is discussed only in a basic science course of neuroanatomy and neurophysiology. In others, the limbic role in declarative memory and emotional responses is presented as part of a discussion on memory or cognitive function within a psychology course. Yet today's curricula do stress and accept "motivation and attention" by the patient as key factors in neuroplasticity and motor learning. Similarly, discussions about the negative effects of "fear of falling" on balance and function in the elderly population are stressed. Both components are controlled by the limbic network, yet the science behind how the system works is often not presented as a critical element in a student's education or background for identifying the rationale for behavioral responses. This chapter has been written to provide the reader with the realization that without an understanding of limbic interactions and modulations over motor expression, patient outcomes will always be variable even with consistent and accepted interventions. Similarly, the reliability and validity of measurements of motor performance will always be in question and often inconsistent. And, given the limitations in today's health care delivery models, stresses, and the growing dependence on home programs, without a keen awareness of the limbic responses of both the patient and the provider, a therapist will have little guarantee of the best possible functional outcome for patients.

For the student learner, the first section of the chapter is a discussion of limbic behavior and how to begin to differentiate true motor responses from those entangled in limbic interactions. For the therapist learner desiring ongoing clinical mastery, the second section delves into the anatomy and physiology of the limbic network, the biology of learning and memory, neurochemistry, and neuroplasticity. The third section discusses the immediate relevance to both the student and practicing clinician—how can we apply our understanding of the limbic network to our patient assessments, treatment, and interactions? In other words, how might it change what we do "come Monday morning"? And finally, in the last section, current advances and future research possibilities in the role of the limbic network are explored.

The concept of patient/client-centered therapy has evolved to become an important aspect of health care delivery.[24-34] The desire to improve or regain function can be self-motivated, but very often it is instilled through the clinician to the patient that his or her best interests and unique goals are the focus of the health care team. This belief is based on trust, hope, and attainable steps toward desired and realistic goals. Patients know that their desires, interests, and needs as unique and valued members of society are considered. They first believe and then recognize that they are persons with specific problems and desired outcomes. Although they may have specific medical diagnoses, be placed on clinical pathways, administered drugs, and sent off to the next facility in a couple of days, patients need to feel that they, as individuals, have not lost all individuality and that someone cares. That need is a feeling of security and safety that bonds a patient to a therapist along the journey of learning.[35-37]

Before understanding and becoming compassionate regarding the needs of other people, such as patients with signs and symptoms of neurological problems, therapists need to understand their own limbic network and how it affects others who might interact with them.[38-43] Because both occupational and physical therapy professions have evolved to using enablement models and systems interactions to explain movement responses of their respective client populations, separating limbic from true motor or cognitive impairments will help guide the clinician toward intervention strategies that will lead to the quickest and most effective outcomes.

The complexity of the limbic anatomy, physiology, and neurochemistry baffles the minds of basic science doctoral students. The changes in understanding of cellular metabolism, membrane potentials, and the new mysteries of cell communication and memory perplex the world of science and neuroscience.[44-47] How this microcosm relates to the macroworld and how the external environments influence not only consciousness but all levels of CNS function are slowly unraveling but still remain mysteries. Yet a therapist deals with the limbic network of clients on a moment-to-moment functional level throughout the day. Figure 5-1 illustrates the interlocking co-dependency of all major CNS components with the environment. At no time does any system stand in isolation. Thus from a clinical perspective the therapist should always maintain focus on the whole environment and all major interactive components within it, while directing attention to any specific component. How the feedback (internal and external) to the patient's CNS changes the neurochemistry and membrane potential, triggers memory, creates new pathways, or elicits other potential responses is not the responsibility of the clinician or therapist. The responsibility of the clinician is accurate documentation of changes and consistency of those changes toward desired patient outcomes. The professions that focus on movement science are interacting more closely with the neurosciences and other biological sciences and many related professions to unravel many of these mysteries and create better assessment and intervention procedures for future patients.

The primary purpose of this chapter is to discuss the influence of the limbic network on motor learning, motor performance, neuroplasticity, and functional independence in life activities. If a person is fearful or apprehensive, motor performance and the ability to learn either a motor skill or intellectual information will be very different[48-55] from that of an individual who feels safe, is given respect, and becomes part of the decision-making process and thus functions inherently with control.[52,56-61]

An individual will naturally have feelings of loss and reservations or fears about the unknown future after injury to any part of the body, but especially the CNS (see Chapter 6).

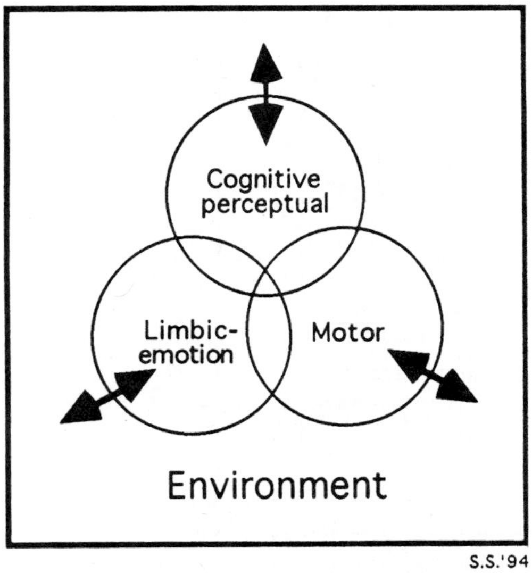

Figure 5-1 ■ Interlocking co-dependence of all major central nervous system components.

Yet that individual needs to be willing to experience the unknown to learn and adapt. The willingness, drive, and adaptability of that individual will affect the optimal plasticity of the CNS.[62] The limbic network is a key player that drives and motivates that individual. The lack of awareness of that variable or its effect on patient performance will ultimately lead to questions and doubts about the effectiveness and efficacy of both assessment and intervention results. Similarly, if this system is overwhelmed either internally or externally, it will dramatically affect neuroplasticity and motor learning as well as cognitive, syntactical learning (see Chapter 4). At the conclusion of this chapter it is hoped that therapists will comprehend why there is a need to learn to modulate or neutralize the limbic network so that patients can functionally control movement and experience cognitive learning. Then therapists need to reintroduce emotions into the activity and allow the patient to once again experience movement and cognitive success during various levels of emotional demands and environments. This change in the emotional environment will create novelty of the task. This novelty is a critical motivator for learning and will drive neuroplasticity.[63-65]

THE FUNCTIONAL RELATIONSHIP OF THE LIMBIC NETWORK TO CLINICAL PERFORMANCE

The Limbic Network's Role in Motor Control, Memory, and Learning

It is not easy to find a generally accepted definition of the "limbic network or complex," its boundaries, and the components that should be included. Mesulam[66] likens this to a fifth-century BCE philosopher's quotation, "the nature of God is like a circle of which the center is everywhere and the circumference is nowhere." Brodal[67] suggests that functional separation of brain regions becomes less clear as we discover the interrelatedness through continuing research. He sees the limbic network reaching out and encompassing the entire brain and all its functional components and sees no purpose in defining such subdivision. Although the anatomical descriptions of the limbic network may vary from author to author, the functional significance of this system is widely acknowledged in defining human behavior and behavioral neurology.[68]

Brooks[69] divides the brain into the limbic brain and the nonlimbic sensorimotor brain. He also defines the two limbic and nonlimbic systems functionally, not anatomically, because their anatomical separation according to function is almost impossible and task specific (Figure 5-2). The sensorimotor portion is involved in perception of nonlimbic somatosensory sensations and motor performance. Brooks defines the limbic brain component as primitive and essential for survival, sensing the "need" to act. The limbic brain is also responsible for memory and the ability to select what to learn from each experience, either positive or negative. Thus the overall purpose of the limbic network is to initiate need-directed motor activity for survival, based on experience. The limbic network therefore initiates and can send neurons up to the frontal lobe or down to the brainstem and thus regulates motor output.

Kandel and colleagues[56] state that functional behavior requires three major systems: the sensory, the motor, and the motivational or limbic systems. When a seemingly simple

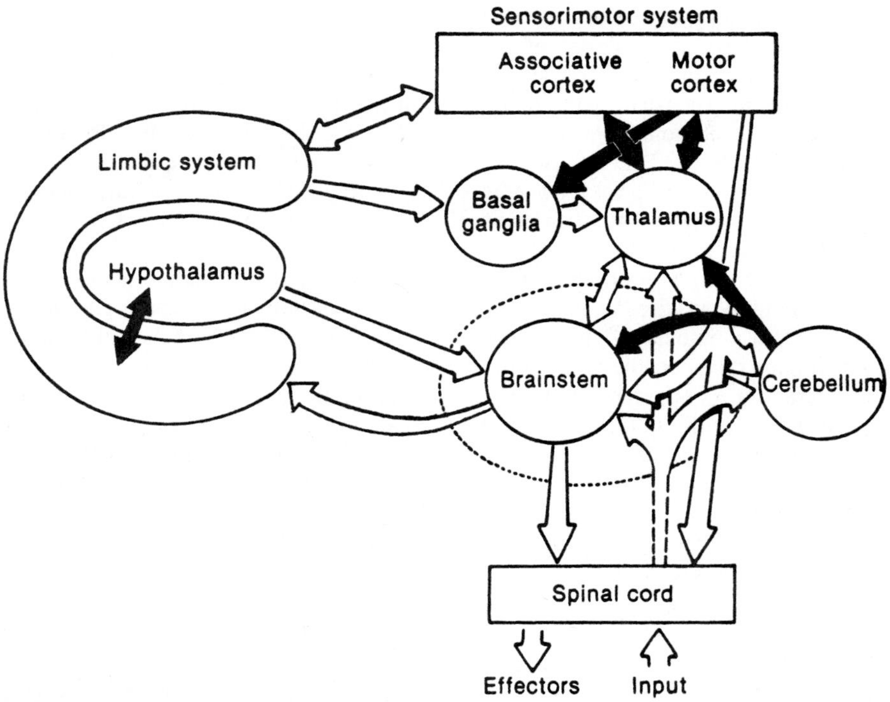

Figure 5-2 ■ Divisions and interconnections between the limbic and nonlimbic cortices (sensory and motor areas).

action, such as swinging a golf club, is analyzed, the sensory system is recruited for visual, tactile, and proprioceptive input to guide the motor systems for precise, coordinated muscle recruitment and postural control. The motivational (limbic) system does the following: (1) provides intentional drive for the movement initiation, (2) integrates the total motor input, and (3) modifies motor expression accordingly, influencing both the autonomic and the somatic sensorimotor systems. It thereby plays a role in controlling the skeletal muscles through input to the frontal lobe and brain stem and the smooth muscles and glands through the hypothalamus, which lies at the "heart" of the limbic network (Figure 5-3).

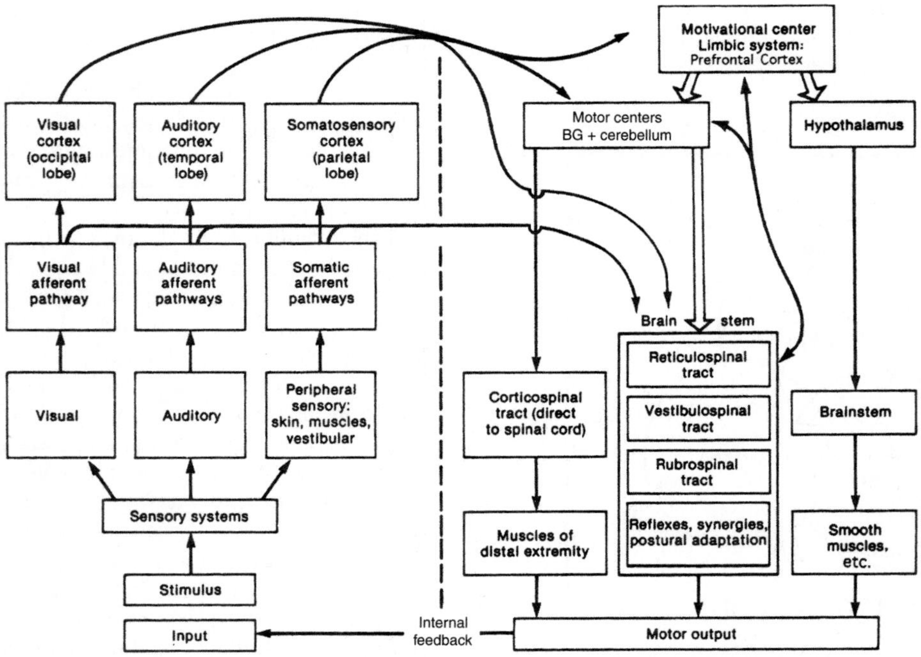

Figure 5-3 ■ Motivational system's influence over the sensorimotor and autonomic nervous systems. (Adapted from Kandel ER, Schwartz JH, Jessell TM: *Principles of neural science,* ed 4, New York, 2000, McGraw-Hill.)

Noback and co-workers[70] state that the limbic network is involved with many of the expressions that make us human; namely, emotions, behaviors, and feeling states. That humanness also has individuality. Our unique memory storage, our variable responses to different environmental contexts, and our control or lack thereof over our emotional sensitivity to environmental stimuli all play roles in molding each one of us. Because of this uniqueness, each therapist and each client need to be accepted for their own individuality.

Broca[71] first conceptualized the anatomical regions of the limbic lobe as forming a ring around the brain stem. Today, neuroanatomists do not differentiate an anatomical lobe as limbic, but rather refer to a complex system that encompasses cortical, diencephalon, and brain stem structures.[56] This description is less precise and encompasses but is not limited to the orbitofrontal and prefrontal cortex, hippocampus, parahippocampal gyrus, cingulate gyrus, dentate gyrus, amygdaloid body, septal area, hypothalamus, and some nuclei of the thalamus.[56,72-76] Anatomists stress the importance of looking at the interrelated structures and segments or loops within the complex limbic region.[77,78]

These multiple nuclei and interlinking circuits play crucial roles in behavioral and emotional changes[77,79,80] and declarative memory.[79-96] The loss of any link can affect the outcome activity of the whole circuit. Thus damage to any area of the brain can potentially cause malfunctions in any or all other areas, and the entire circuit may need reorganization to restore function.

Researchers do not ascribe a specific single function to CNS formations but see each as part of a system participating to various degrees in the multitude of behavioral responses (see Chapters 3 and 4 for additional information). Therefore the loss of any part of higher centers or the limbic network may not be clearly definable functionally, and the return of function is not always easy to predict.

Recovery of function after injury may involve mechanisms that allow reorganizing of the structure and function of cortical, subcortical, and spinal circuits. In very young infants, areas within opposite hemispheres may "take over" function, whereas in more mature brains reorganization of existing systems seems to be the current accepted hypothesis within the expanding knowledge of neuroplasticity.[97-100] For complex behavior, such as in motor functioning requiring many steps, the limbic network, cortex, hypothalamus, basal ganglia, and brain stem work as an integrated unit, with any damaged area causing the whole system to initially malfunction. Without change or encouragement of appropriate external and internal environmental changes that will create neuroplasticity, the initial malfunction can become permanent.[101] The timing for optimal neuroplasticity has not yet been established. The medical use of drugs to alter cellular activity and plasticity after CNS damage has become a huge pharmaceutical research area (see Chapter 36). Early as well as later drug therapy may encourage neuroplasticity.[102-108] The same questions must be asked about early instead of later rehabilitation intervention, as well as the limbic influence over the motor system. A loss of function or a change in behavior cannot necessarily be localized as to the underlying cause. A lesion in one area may cause secondary dysfunction of a different area that is not actually damaged.

The complexity of the limbic network and its associative influence over both the motor control system and cortical structures are enormous. A therapist dealing with a client with motor control or cognitive learning problems needs to understand how the limbic network affects behavioral responses. The knowledge base focuses not only on the client's deficits but also on the integrative function of the therapist. This understanding should lead to a greater awareness of the clinical environment and the factors within the environment that cause change. Without this knowledge of how to differentiate systems, objective measurements of motor performance or cognitive abilities may be inconsistent without any explanation. Similarly, with excessive limbic activity, clients' ability to store and retrieve either declarative or procedural learning may be negatively affected, thus limiting the patients' ability to benefit from traditional interventions and from potentially regaining their respective highest quality of life.

The Limbic Network's Influence on Behavior: Its Relevance to the Therapeutic Environment

Levels of Behavioral Hierarchies: Where Does the Limbic Network Belong?

Strub and Black[109] view behavior as occurring on distinct interrelated levels that represent behavioral hierarchies. Starting at level 1, a state of alertness to the internal and external environment must be maintained for motor or mental activity to occur. The brain stem reticular activating system brings about this state of general arousal by relaying in an ascending pathway to the thalamus, the limbic network, and the cerebral cortex. To proceed from a state of general arousal to one of "selective attention" requires the communication of information to and from the cortex, the thalamus, and the limbic network and its modulation over the brain stem and spinal pattern generators.[56,110]

Level 2 of this hierarchy lies in the domain of the hypothalamus and its closely associated limbic structures. This level deals with subconscious drives and innate instincts. The survival-oriented drives of hunger, thirst, temperature regulation, and survival of the species (reproduction) and the steps necessary for drive reduction are processed here, as well as learning and memory. Most of these activities relate to limbic functioning. If an individual or patient is in a perceived survival mode, little long-term learning regarding either cognition or motor programming will occur. Thus, making the patient feel safe is initially a critical role for the therapist. This approach may require placing the therapist's hands on the patient initially to take away any possibility of falling. The therapist would first deal with the emotional aspect of the patient's environment and then shift to the motor learning and control component, in which the patient is empowered to practice and self-correct within the program she or he can control.

On level 3 only cerebral cortical areas are activated. This level deals with abstract conceptualization of verbal or quantitative entities. It is at this level that the somatosensory and frontal motor cortices work together to perceptually and procedurally develop motor programs. The prefrontal areas of the frontal lobe can influence the development of these motor programs, thus again illustrating the limbic influence over the motor system.[111,112]

Level 4 behavior is concerned with the expression of social aspects of behavior, personality, and lifestyle. Again, the limbic network and its relationship to the frontal lobe are vital. The shift to the World Health Organization International Classification of Functioning, Disability and Health (WHO-ICF) model, which reflects patient-centered therapy, has actualized the critical importance of this level of human behavior.[24,28,31,113,114]

The interaction of all four levels leads to the integrative and adaptable behavior seen in the human. Our ability to become alert and protectively react is balanced by our previous learning, whether it is cognitive-perceptive, social, or affective. Adaptability to rapid changes in the physical environment, in lifestyles, and in personal relationships results from the interrelationships or complex neurocircuitry of the human brain. When insult occurs at any one level within these behavioral hierarchies, all levels may be affected.

As Western medicine is unraveling the mysteries behind the neurochemistry of the limbic network[58,115-117] and alternative medicine is establishing effectiveness and efficacy for various interventions and philosophies (see Chapter 39), a fifth level of limbic function may become the link between the hard science of today and the unexplained mysteries. Those medical mysteries would be defined as unexplained yet identified events that have either been forgotten or been hidden from the world by those scientists—mysteries such as why some people heal from terminal illnesses spontaneously, various others heal in ways not accepted by traditional medicine,[60,118] and still others just die without any known disease or pathological condition.[119-122] One critical component everyone identifies as part of that unexplained healing is a belief by the client that he or she will heal. That belief has a strong emotional component,[120] and that may be the fifth level of limbic function. How conscious intent drives hypothalamic autoimmune function is being unraveled scientifically, and clinicians often observe these changes in their patients. Through observation it becomes apparent that clients who believe they will get better often do, and those who believe they will not generally do not. Whether belief comes from a religious, spiritual, or hard science paradigm, that belief drives behavior, and that drive has a large limbic component.

The Limbic Network MOVEs Us

Moore[123] eloquently describes the limbic network as the area of the brain that moves us. The word *MOVE* can be used as a mnemonic for the functions of the limbic network.

Limbic Network Function.

Memory and motivation: drive
- Memory: attention and retrieval, declarative learning
- Motivation: desire to learn, try, or benefit from the external environment

Olfaction (especially in infants)
- Only sensory system that does not have to go through the thalamus as a second-order synapse in the sensory pathway before it gets to the cerebral cortex

Visceral (drives: thirst, hunger, and temperature regulation; endocrine functions)
- Sympathetic and parasympathetic reactions
- Hypothalamic regulation over autoimmune system
- Peripheral autonomic nervous system (ANS) responses that reflect limbic function

Emotion: feelings and attitude
- Self-concept and worth
- Emotional body image
- Tonal responses of motor system affected by limbic descending pathways
- Attitude, social skills, opinions

As seen in this outline, the *M* (memory, motivation) depicts the drive component of the limbic network. Before learning, an individual must be motivated to learn, to try to succeed at the task, to solve the problem, or to benefit from the environment. Without motivation the brain will not orient itself to the problem and learn. Motivation drives both our cortical structures to develop higher cognitive associations and the motor system to develop procedures or motor programs that will enable us to perform movement with the least energy expenditure and the most efficient patterns available. Once motivated, the individual must be able to pay attention and process the sequential and simultaneous nature of the component parts to be learned, as well as the whole. Thus there is an interlocking dependence among somatosensory mapping of the functional skills[124] (cognitive), attention (limbic) necessary for any type of learning, and the sequential, multiple, and simultaneous programming of functional movement (motor). The limbic amygdala and hippocampal structures and their intricate circuitries play a key role in the declarative aspect of memory.[125-128] Once this syntactical, intellectual memory is learned and taken out of short-term memory by passing through limbic nuclei, the information is stored in cortical areas and can be retrieved at a later time without limbic involvement.[129]

The *O* refers to olfaction, or the incoming sense of smell, which exerts a strong influence on alertness and drive. This is clearly illustrated by the billions of dollars spent annually on perfumes, deodorants, mouthwashes, and soap as well as scents used in stores to increase customers' desires to purchase. This input tract can be used effectively by therapists who have clients with CNS lesions such as internal capsule and thalamic involvement. The olfactory system synapses within the olfactory bulb and then with the limbic structures and then may go directly to the cerebral cortex without synapsing in the thalamus. Although collaterals do project to the thalamus, unlike all other sensory information, olfaction does not need to use the thalamus as a necessary relay center to access the cortical structures, although many collaterals also project there.[56,130] Other senses may not be reaching the cortical levels, and the client may have a sensory-deprived environment. Olfactory sensations, which enter the limbic network, may be used to calm or arouse the client. The specific olfactory input may determine whether the person remains calm or emotionally aroused.[131,132] Pleasant odors would be preferable to most people. With the limbic network's influence on tone production through brain stem modulation, this is one reason aromatherapy causes relaxation and is used by many massage therapists.

A comatose, seemingly nonresponsive client may respond to or be highly sensitive to odor.[133] The therapist needs to be acutely aware of the responses of these patients because these responses may be autonomic instead of somatomotor and may be reflected in a higher heart rate or an increase in blood pressure. Using noxious stimuli to try to "wake up" a patient in a vegetative state has the possibility of causing negative arousal, fear, withdrawal, or anxiety and an increase in base tone within the motor generators.[132] Using this type of input places the patient at level 2 in a "protective state of survival." Using a pleasant and personal desirable smell will more likely place a client at level 2 "safety." The former can lead to strong emotions such as anger, whereas the latter often leads to bonding and motivation to learn. Research has shown that retrieval processing and retrieval of memory have a distinctive emotionality when they are linked to odor-evoked memories.[134-136]

The *V* represents visceral or autonomic drives. As noted earlier, the hypothalamus is nestled within the limbic network. Thus, regulation of sympathetic and parasympathetic reactions, both of the internal organ systems and the periphery, reflects continuing limbic activity. Obviously, drives such as thirst, hunger, temperature regulation, and sexuality are controlled by this system. Clients demonstrating total lack of inhibitory control over eating or drinking or manifesting very unstable body temperature regulation may be exhibiting signs of hypothalamic-pituitary involvement or direct pathways from hypothalamus to midbrain structures.[56] Today, this interaction of the hypothalamus with motor neurons that change or support movement has clearly been established.[137]

Less obvious autonomic responses that may reflect limbic imbalances often go unnoticed by therapists. When the stress of an activity is becoming overwhelming to a client, she or he may react with severe sweating of the palms or an increase in dysreflexic activity in the mouth rather than with heightened motor activity. A therapist must continually monitor this aspect of the client's response behaviors to ascertain that the behaviors observed reflect motor control and not limbic influences over that motor system.

If the sensory input to the client is excessive whether through internal or external feedback, the limbic network may go into an alert, protective mode and will not function at the optimal level, and learning will diminish. The client may withdraw physically or mentally, lose focus or attention, decrease motivation, and become frustrated or even angry. The overload on the reticular system may be the reason for the shutdown of the limbic network and not the limbic network itself. Both are part of the same neuroloop circuitry. All these behaviors may be expressed within the hypothalamic-autonomic system as motor output, no matter where in the loop the dysfunction occurs. Having a functional understanding of the neuroanatomy and their relationships with each other helps therapists unravel some of the mysteries patients present after CNS insult.[138,139] The evaluation of this system seems even more critical when a client's motor control system is locked, with no volitional movement present. Therapists often try to increase motor activity through sensory input; however, they must cautiously avoid indiscriminately bombarding the sensory systems. The limbic network may demonstrate overload while at the same time the spinal motor generators reflect inadequate activation. How a therapist might assess this overload would be to closely monitor the ANS's responses such as blood pressure, heart rate, internal temperature, and sweating versus observing or measuring muscle tone. Although the somatosensory system and the ANS are different, they are intricately connected. The concept of massively bombarding one system while ignoring the other does not make sense in any learning paradigm, especially from a systems model in which consensus creates the observed behavior. To illustrate this concept, think of an orchestra leader conducting a symphony. It would make no sense for the conductor to ask the string section to play louder if half the brass section got sick. Instead, the conductor would need to quiet the string section and all other sections to allow the brass component to be heard.

E relates to emotions, the feelings, attitudes, and beliefs that are unique to that individual. These beliefs include psychosocial attitudes and prejudices, ethnic upbringing, cultural experiences, religious convictions, and concepts of spirituality.[120] All these aspects of emotions link especially to the amygdaloid complex of the limbic network and orbitofrontal activity within the frontal lobe.[140-142] This is a primary emotional center, and it regulates not only our self-concept but our attitudes and opinions toward our external environment and the people within it.

To appreciate the sensory system's influential interaction with the limbic network directly, the reader need only look at the literature on music and how it interacts with emotions.[143,144] Most people can give examples of instances where music has elicited immediate and compelling emotional responses of various types. Pleasant and unpleasant musical stimuli have been found to increase or decrease limbic activity and influence both cognitive and motor responses. Although the neurological mechanisms are not yet well understood, the limbic network seems to be implicated in both "positive" and "negative" emotions in response to musical stimuli.[145-148] The clinical implications are huge. Excessive noise, loudspeaker announcements, piped in music, and all the therapists' voices can affect the CNS of a client. These responses can be highly emotional, cause changes in visceral behavior, and affect striated motor expression. Level of musical consonance or dissonance is just one element of the auditory stimulus that is subjectively experienced by the listener as pleasant or unpleasant. The implications not only that listening to music affects limbic emotional states but that the influence may direct the hypothalamus in regulation of blood flow within the CNS have also been shown.[148] With music or sound being just one input system, the therapist must realize that sensory influence from smell, taste, touch, proprioception, and vestibular and organ system dysfunction can lead to potential limbic involvement in all aspects of CNS function and directly affect the emotional stability of the patient.

Another very important concept linked to the emotional system is the emotional aspect of body image or the concept of SELF. For example, assume that one morning I look in the mirror and say, "The poor world, I will not subject it to me today." I then go back to bed and eat nothing for the rest of the day. The next day I get up and look in the same mirror and say, "What a change, I look trim and beautiful. Look out world, here I come!" In reality, my physical body has not been altered drastically, if at all, but my attitude toward that body has changed. That is, the emotional component of my body image has perceptually changed.

A second self-concept deals with my attitude about my worth or value to society and the world and my role within it.[149] Again, this attitude can change with mood, but more often it seems to change with experience. This aspect of client-therapist interaction can be critical to the success of a therapeutic environment. The two following examples illustrate this point, with the focus of bringing perceived roles into the therapeutic setting:

Your client is Mrs. S., a 72-year-old woman with a left cerebrovascular accident (CVA). She comes from a low socioeconomic background and was a housekeeper for 40 years for a wealthy family of high social standing. When addressing you (the therapist), she always says "yes, ma'am" or "no, ma'am" and does just what is asked, no more and no less. It may be very hard to empower this client to assume responsibility for self-direction in the therapeutic setting. Her perceived role in life may not be to take responsibility or authority within a setting that may, from her perception, have high social status, such as a medical facility. She also may feel that she does not have the right or the power to assume such responsibilities. Success in the therapeutic setting may be based more on changing her attitudes than on her potential to relearn motor control. That is, the concept of empowerment may play a crucial role in regaining independent functional skill and control over her environment.[24,28,31,150-153]

Your client is a 24-year-old lumberjack who sustained a closed-head injury during a fall at work. It is now 1 month since his accident, and he is alert, verbal, and angry and has moderate to severe motor control problems. During your initial treatment you note that he responds very well to handling. He seems to flow with your movement, and with your assistance is able to practice a much higher level of motor control within a narrow biomechanical window; although at times he needs your assistance, you release that control whenever possible to empower him to control his body. At the end of therapy he sits back in his chair with much better residual motor function. Then he turns to you (the female therapist) and instead of saying, "That was great," he says, "You witch, I hate you." The inconsistency between how his body responded to your handling and his attitude toward you as a person may seem baffling until you realize that he has always perceived himself as a dominant male. Similarly, he perceives women as weak, to be protected, and in need of control. If his attitude toward you cannot be changed to see you in a generic professional role, he will most likely not benefit as much from your clinical skills and guidance as a teacher. Before the accident the patient may have suppressed that verbal response but not tone and body language. After a traumatic brain injury affecting the orbitofrontal system, the inhibition of the behavioral response itself may be lost, further embarrassing the patient emotionally.

Preconceived attitudes, social behaviors, and opinions have been learned by filtering the input through the limbic network. If new attitudes and behaviors need to be learned after a neurological insult, the status of the amygdaloid pathways seems crucial. Damage to these limbic structures may prevent learning[154]; thus, socially maladaptive behavior may persist, making the individual less likely to adapt to the social environment. It is often harder to change learned social behaviors than any other type of learning.[155-158] Because our feelings, attitudes, values, and beliefs drive our behaviors through both attention and motor responses, the emotional aspect of the limbic network has great impact on our learning and motor control. If a patient is not motivated and places little value on a motor output, then complacency results and little learning will occur.[159-161] On the other hand, if a therapist places an extremely high value on a motor output as a pure expression of motor control without interlocking that control with the patient's limbic influence, the behavioral response may lead to inconsistency, lack of compliance, and thus lack of motor learning and carryover.[159] Similarly, it can cause extreme stress, which even the general public knows causes disease.[162]

Motivation and Reward. Moore[123] considers motivation and memory as part of the MOVE system. Esch and Stefano[163] link motivation with reward and help, illustrating how the limbic network learns through repetition and reward. They state that the concept of motivation includes drive and satiation, goal-directed behavior, and incentive. They recognize that these behaviors maintain homeostasis and ensure the survival of the individual and the species. Although the frontal lobe region appears to play an important role in self-control and execution activities, these functions seem to require a close interlocking neuronetwork between cognitive representation within the frontal regions and motivational control provided by limbic and subcortical structures.[140,164] An important aspect of motivated behavior is linked to patient- and family-centered therapy.* "The most powerful force in rehabilitation is motivation."[167] These words are strong and reflect the importance of the limbic network in rehabilitation.

Motivated behavior is geared toward reinforcement and reward, which are based on both internal and external feedback systems. Repeated experience of reinforcement and reward leads to learning, changed expectancy, changed behavior, and maintained performance.[168] Emotional learning, which certainly involves the limbic network, is very hard to unlearn once the behavior has been reinforced over and over.[169,170] For that reason, motor behavior that is strongly linked to a negative emotional response might be a very difficult behavior to unlearn. For example, a patient who is willing to stand up and practice transfers just to get the therapist off his back is eliciting a movement sequence that is based on frustration or anger. When that same patient gets home and his spouse asks him to perform the same motor behavior, he may not be able to be successful. The spouse may say, "The therapist said you could." The patient may respond, "I never did like him!" Thus repetition of motor performance with either the feeling of emotional neutrality or the feeling of success (positive reinforcement) is a critical element in the therapeutic setting. Consistently making the motor task more difficult just when the client feels ready to succeed will tend to decrease positive reinforcement or reward, lessen the client's motivation to try, and decrease the probability of true independence once the patient leaves the clinical setting. When pressure is placed on therapists to produce changes quickly, repetition and thus long-term learning are often jeopardized, which may have a dramatic effect on the quality of the client's life and the long-term treatment effects once he or she leaves the medical facility. Motor control theory (see Chapter 4) coincides with limbic

*References 24, 27, 28, 31, 34, 135, 150, 165, 166.

research regarding reinforcement. Inherent feedback within a variety of environmental contexts allowing for error with correction leads to greater retention.[171] Repetition or the opportunity to practice a task (motor or cognitive) in which the individual desires to succeed will lead to long-term learning.[172] Without practice or motivation the chance of successful motor learning is minimal to nonexistent.

Positive emotional states may create a limbic environment in which the therapist can link reward and pleasure associations to new motor sequences. Although it is well known that appropriate selections of music can stimulate states of highly pleasant positive affects and physical relaxation, the neurological mechanisms for these effects are not well understood. In an early study by Goldstein[173a] subjects reported pleasant physical sensations of tingling or "thrills" in response to music listening. After subjects were injected with naloxone, which blocks opiate receptors, thrill scores and tingling sensations were attenuated in some subjects. Although responses to music are highly individualized and this study has not been replicated, it suggests that endorphins may be released under certain music listening conditions that elicit pleasant physical sensations. In a positron emission tomography (PET) study of cerebral blood flow (CBF) changes measured during highly pleasurable "shivers or chills" in response to subject-selected music, Blood and colleagues[147] found that as the intensity of the chills increased, CBF increases occurred in the left ventral striatum, dorsomedial midbrain, bilateral insula, right orbitofrontal cortex, thalamus, anterior cingulate cortex, supplementary motor area, and bilateral cerebellum. As the intensity of chills increased, significant CBF decreases were also observed in the right amygdala, left hippocampus and amygdala, and ventral medial prefrontal cortex. The increases found in brain structures associated with reward or pleasant emotions and decreases in areas associated with negative emotional states suggest that music (1) must be carefully selected according to individual preferences and responses, in order to reliably elicit such highly pleasurable experiences as "shivers down the spine" and (2) might be used therapeutically to positively affect limbic activity.

Other studies provide additional support for the notion that music may activate limbic and paralimbic areas associated with reward or pleasurable emotions. Brown and colleagues[145] conducted a PET study of 10 nonmusicians who listened passively to unfamiliar music, which they later reported had elicited strongly pleasant feelings. Unlike previous studies of music, emotion, and limbic activity, this research design called for subjects to listen passively without engaging in any task such as evaluating affective components during the music. The authors noted that the music stimuli used was musically complex and strongly liked by the subjects. When the CBF during the music was compared with silent rest conditions in the same subjects, activations were seen, as expected, in areas presumed to represent perceptual and cognitive responses to music (primary auditory cortex, auditory association cortex, superior temporal sulcus bilaterally, temporal gyrus of the right hemisphere, in the right superior temporal pole, and adjacent insula). In addition, responses were found in limbic and paralimbic areas, which included the left subcallosal cingulate, the anterior cingulate, left retrosplenial cortex and right hippocampus, and the left nucleus accumbens and cerebellum. The researchers compared these results with those from the earlier studies by members of the same team[147,148] and suggest that areas such as the subcallosal cingulate are related to the direct experience of occurrent emotions rather than discriminate processing for emotion and that different areas are specifically activated during the pleasant physical responses known as "chills." They go on to propose that the superior temporal pole and adjacent insula may serve as a point of bifurcation in neural circuitry for processing music. They also suggest that neurons from that region project to limbic and paralimbic areas involved in emotional processing and to premotor areas possibly involved in discrimination and structural processing of music. Although research has increased our appreciation of the complexity of brain activation by music, much more study is needed to validate a model of limbic network activity in human emotional responses to musical stimuli. Clinically, music can be used to improve mood and increase patient motivation to participate in rehabilitation treatment. Case studies[174,175] suggest that music can be used to decrease crying by infants and toddlers during physical therapy treatment. West has participated in both developmental and rehabilitation settings as a music therapist in co-treatment with physical and occupational therapists. The music therapist first does a thorough assessment of the individual's preferences and responses to music, then provides music selected or composed specifically to provide motivating energy, pleasant associations, and positive affective states to accompany the motor activity. This individualized, live-music approach allows the music therapist to modify the musical elements as needed in the moment, working in a real-time limbic partnership with both the client and the physical or occupational therapist. Music or pleasure sounds can be used to help neutralize or balance the limbic influence on motor expression. Obtaining a limbic-neutral impact is critical before evaluating functional movement in order to accurately determine true motor system involvement.

Many types of emotions create motivation, such as pleasure, reward processes, emotions associated with addiction, appreciation of financial benefits, amusement, sadness, humor, happiness, and depression.[163,173b,176-179] Some emotions tend to drive learning, whereas others may discourage learning, whether that learning be cognitive or motor.

Integration of the Limbic Network as Part of a Whole Functioning Brain

Motivation, alertness, and concentration are critical in motor learning because they determine how well we pay attention to the learning and execution of any motor task. These processes of learning and doing are inevitably intertwined: "We learn as we do, and we do only as well as we have learned."[180]

Both motivation ("feeling the need to act") and concentration ("ability to focus on the task") are interlinked with the limbic network. The amygdaloid complex with its multitude of afferent and efferent interlinkages is specially adapted for recognizing the significance of a stimulus, and it assigns the emotional aspect of feeling the need to act. These neuroanatomical loops have tremendous connections with the reticular system. Hence, some authors call it the reticulolimbic network.[56,157] The interaction of the limbic network and the motor generators of the brain stem and ultimate direct and indirect modulation over the spinal system lead to need-directed and therefore goal-directed motor activity. It also filters out significant from insignificant information by selective processing and storing the significant for memory, learning, and recall. These interconnected neuroloop circuitries reinforce the concept that areas have both specialization and generalization and thus work closely together with other areas of the brain.[169,181]

Goal-directed or need-directed motor actions are the result of the nervous system structures acting as an interactive system. Within this system (Figure 5-4), all components share responsibilities. The limbic network and its cortical and subcortical components represent the most important level. In response to stimuli from the internal or external environment, the limbic network initiates motor activity out of the emotional aspect of feeling the need to act. This message is relayed to the sensory areas of the cerebral cortex, which could entail any one or all association areas for visual, auditory, olfactory, gustatory, tactile, or proprioceptive input. These areas are located in the prefrontal, occipital, parietal, and temporal lobes, where they analyze and integrate sensory input into an overall strategy of action or a general plan that meets the requirements of the task. Therefore these cortices recognize, select, and prepare to act as a response to relevant sensory cues when a state of arousal is provided by reticular input. The limbic cortex (uncus, parahippocampal gyrus /isthmus, cingulate gyrus, and septal nucleus) has even greater influence over the sensorimotor cortices through the cingulate gyrus, both directly and indirectly through association areas.[182-184] The thalamus, cerebellum, and basal ganglia contribute to the production of the specific motor plans. These messages of the general plan are relayed to the projection system. The limbic structures through the cingulate gyrus also have direct connections with the primary motor cortex. These circuits certainly have the potential to assist in driving fine motor activities through corticobulbar and corticospinal tract interactions. The thalamus, cerebellum, basal ganglia, and motor cortices (premotor, supplementary motor, and primary motor) contribute to the production of the specific motor plans.[56] Messages regarding the sensory component of the general plan are relayed to the projection system, where they are transformed into refined motor programs. These plans are then projected throughout the motor system to modulate motor generators throughout the brain stem and spinal system.[56] Limbic connections with (1) the cerebellum, basal ganglia, and frontal lobe[56,185-189] and (2) the motor generator within the brain stem enable further control of limbic instructions over motor control or expression. If the limbic and the cognitive systems decide not to act, goal-driven motor behavior will cease. An individual's belief (emotional and spiritual) can inhibit even the most basic survival skills, as has been clearly shown in history when individuals with particular

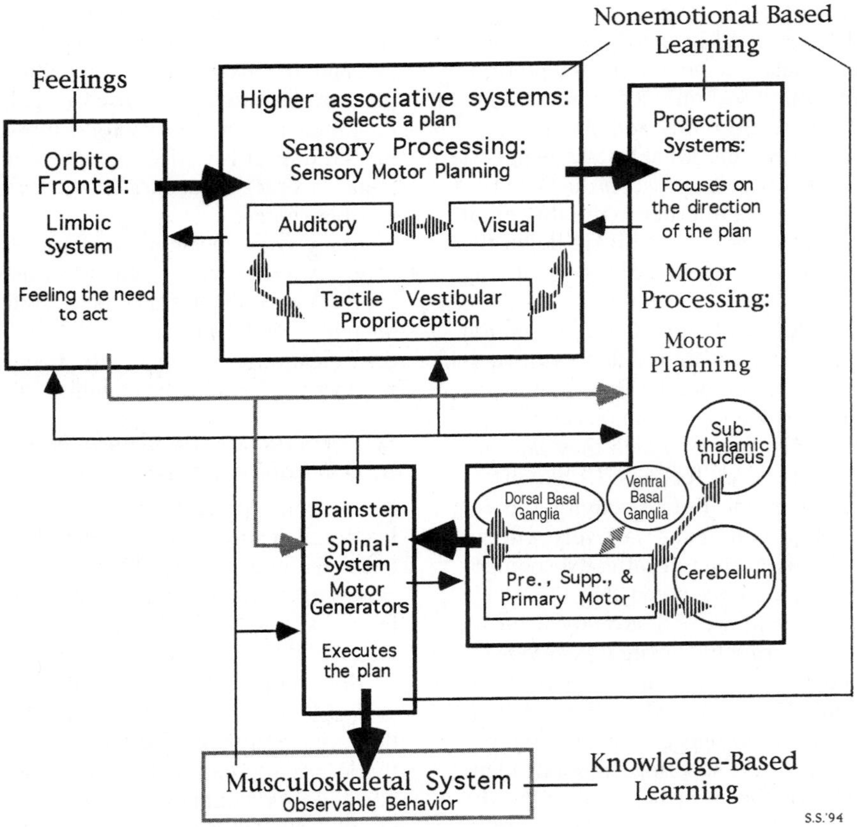

Figure 5-4 ■ Functional and dynamic hierarchy of systems based on both limbic and motor control interactions. (Adapted from Brooks VB: *The neural basis of motor control,* New York, 1986, Oxford University Press.)

religious beliefs were pitted against vicious predators and those people chose not to defend themselves.

Within the projection system and motor planning complexes, the specifics are programmed and the tactics are given a strategy. In general, "what" is turned into "how" and "when." The necessary parameters for coordinated movement are programmed within the motor complex as to intensity, sequencing, and timing to carry out the motor task. These programs, which incorporate upper motor neurons and interneurons, are then sent to the brain stem and spinal motor generators, which in turn, through lower motor neurons, send orders regarding the specific motor tasks to the musculoskeletal system. (See Chapters 3, 4, and 8 for more specific in-depth discussion.) The actions performed by each subsystem within the entire limbic–motor control complex constantly loop back and communicate to all subsystems to allow for adjustments of intensity and duration and to determine whether the plan remains the best choice of responses to an ever-changing three-dimensional world.[138,186,187]

The limbic network has one more opportunity to modify and control the central pattern generators and control the body and limbs through direct connections to the spinal neuronetwork.[110,190-193] That is, the limbic network can alter existing motor plans by modulating those generators up and down or altering specific nuclear clusters and varying the patterns themselves. Therapists as well as the general public see this in sports activities when emotions are high, no matter the emotion itself. Individuals who have excellent motor control over a specific sport may find high-level performance difficult as the stress of competition increases. Having control over emotional variance as well as motor variance with a functional activity is an accurate example of empowerment. Thus, for a therapist to get a true picture of a patient's motor system's function, the limbic network should be flowing in a neutral or balanced state without strong emotions of any kind. Generally, that balance seems to reflect itself in a state of safety, trust, and compliance. Once the motor control has been achieved then the therapist must reintroduce various emotional environments during the motor activity to be able to state that the patient is independent.

In summary, the limbic complex generates need-directed motor activity and communicates that intent throughout the motor system.[110,191,194,195] This step is vital to normal motor function and thus client care. Clients need the opportunity to analyze correctly both their internal environment (their present and feed-forward motor plans and their emotional state) and the external world around them requiring action on a task. The integration of all this information should produce the most appropriate strategy available to the patient for the current activity. These instructions must be correct, and the system capable of carrying out the motor activity, for effortless, coordinated movement expression to be observed. If the motor system is deficient, lack of adaptability will be observed in the client. If the limbic complex is faulty, the same motor deficits might present themselves. The therapist must differentiate what is truly a motor system problem versus a limbic influence over the motor system problem.

Schmidt[196] stresses the significance of "knowledge of results feedback" as being the information from the environment that provides the individual with insights into task requirements. This insight helps the motor system correctly select strategies that will successfully initiate and support the appropriate movement for accomplishing the task. This knowledge of results feedback is required for effective motor learning and for forming the correct motor programs for storage.[197,198]

The reader may better understand the role of the limbic network in motor programming through a nonmedical example. Imagine that you are sitting in your new car. The dealer has filled the tank with necessary fuel. The engine, with all its wires and interlocking components, is totally functional. However, the engine will not perform without a mechanism to initiate its strategies or turn on the system. The basal ganglia or frontal lobe motor mechanism plays this role in the brain. The car has a starter motor. Yet the starter motor will not activate the motor system without the driver's intent and motivation to turn the key and turn on the engine. The limbic complex serves this function in the brain. Once the key has been turned, the car is running and ready for guidance. Whether the driver chooses reverse or drive usually depends on prior learning unless this is a totally new experience. Once the gear has been selected, the motor system will program the car to run according to the driver's desires. It can run fast or slow, but for the plan to change, both a purpose and a recognition that change is necessary are required. The car has the ability to adapt and self-regulate to many environmental variables, such as ruts or slick pavement, to continue running the feed-forward program, just as many motor systems within the CNS, especially the cerebellum, perform that function. The limbic network may emotionally choose to drive fast, whereas one's cognitive judgment may choose otherwise. The interactive result will drive the pedal and brake pressure and ultimately regulate the car. The components discussed play a critical role in the total function of the car, just as all the systems within the CNS play a vital role in regulating behavioral responses to the environment.

Brooks[69] distinguishes insightful learning, which is programmed and leads to skills when the performer has gained insight into the requirements, from discontinuous movements, which need to be replaced by continuous ones. This process is hastened when clients understand and can demonstrate their understanding of what "they were expected to do." Improvement of motor skills is possible by using programmed movement in goal-directed behavior. The reader must be cautioned to make sure that the client's attention is on the goal of the task and not on the components of the movement itself. The motor plan needs programming and practice without constant cognitive overriding. The limbic/frontal system helps drive the motor toward the identified task or abstract representation of a match between the motor planning sequence and the desired outcome. The importance of the goal being self-driven by the patient cannot be overemphasized.*

Without knowledge of results, feedback, and insight into the requirements for goal-directed activity, the learning is performing by "rote," which merely uses repetition without analysis, and meaningful learning or building of effective motor memory in the form of motor holograms

*References 24, 28, 31, 111, 199, 200.

will be minimal. Children with cognitive and limbic deficits can learn basic motor skills through repetition of practice, but the insights and ability to transfer that motor learning into other contexts will not be high (see Chapters 12, 13, and 14).

Schmidt[196] suggests that to elicit the highest level of function within the motor system and to enable insightful learning, therapy programs should be developed around goal-directed activities, which means a strong emotional context. These activities direct the client to analyze the environmental requirements (both internal and external) by placing the client in a situation that forces development of "appropriate strategies." Goal-directed activities should be functional and thus involve motivation, meaningfulness, and selective attention. Functional and somatosensory retraining uses these concepts as part of the intervention (see Chapters 4 and 9). Specific techniques such as proprioceptive neuromuscular facilitation, neurodevelopmental therapy, the Rood method, and the Feldenkrais method can be incorporated into goal-directed activities in the therapy programs, as can any treatment approach, as long as it identifies those aspects of motor control and learning that lead to retention and future performance and allows the patient to self-correct.[196] With insights into the learned skills, clients will be better able to adjust these to meet the specific requirements of different environments and needs, using knowledge of response feedback to guide them. The message then is to design exercise activities or programs that are meaningful and need directed, to motivate clients into insightful goal-directed learning. Thus, understanding the specific goals of the client, patient-centered learning, is critical and will be obtained only by interaction with that client as a person with needs, desires, and anticipated outcomes.[201,202] A therapist cannot assume that "someone wants to do something." The goal of running a bank may seem very different from that of birdwatching in the mountains, yet both may require ambulatory skills. If a client does not wish to return to work, then a friendly smile and the statement, "Hi, I'm your therapist and I'm going to get you up and walking so you can get back to work," may lead to resistance and decreased motivation. In contrast, a therapist who knows the goal of the client may help him or her become highly motivated to ambulate; that client may be present in the clinic every day to meet the goal of birdwatching in the mountains although never wishing to walk back into the office again.

Clinical Perspectives

The Client's Internal System Influences Observable Behavior. At least once a year almost any local newspaper will carry a story that generally reads as follows: "Seventy-nine-year-old, 109-pound arthritic grandmother picks up car by bumper to free trapped 3-year-old grandson."

We read these articles and at first doubt their validity, questioning the sensationalism used by the reporter. But we know that these events are real. That elderly lady picked up the car out of fear of severe injury to her grandchild. Emotions can create tremendously high tonal responses, either in a postural pattern such as in a temper tantrum or during a movement strategy such as picking up a car. Conversely, fear can immobilize a person and make it impossible to create enough tone to run a motor program or actually move. Evaluating muscle power or tone production in relation to emotional state (versus a pure reflection of motor control) is an aspect of evaluation often overlooked.

Limbic Influence on Emotional Output: The F^2ARV and GAS Continua

Some of the earliest understanding of the limbic network was of its role in "fight or flight." It is important that clinicians not only understand but also recognize two powerful limbic motor response programs: the fear and frustration, anger, rage, and violence continuum (F^2ARV) and the general adaptation syndrome (GAS).

F^2ARV (Fear and Frustration, Anger, Rage, and Violence or Withdrawal) Continuum. One sequence of behaviors used to describe the emotional circuitry of the limbic network through the amygdala is the F^2ARV continuum[157,203,204] (Figure 5-5). This continuum begins with fear or frustration. This fear can lead to avoidance behavior.[205] If the event inducing the fear or frustration continues to heighten, avoidance behaviors can continue to develop.[205] In a simple example, we recall or have seen these behaviors in our teens and as young adults, when the challenges faced in high school can lead to *avoidance* of activities. Alternately, extreme fear and frustration can also lead to *anger*. Anger is a neurochemical response that is perceived and defined cognitively (at the cortical level) as anger. If the neurochemical response continues to build or is prolonged, the anger displayed by the person may advance to *rage* (internal chaos) and finally into *violence* (strong motor response). A common societal example is in the case of domestic discord and violence. Women who attain the level of rage may become withdrawn and thus become victimized by a partner who is also in rage or inflicting physical or emotional violence.[206] Another current example is posttraumatic stress disorder (PTSD), in which the prolonged stress of deployment and unique challenges of warfare lead to limited adaptive reserves in warriors and returning veterans. Suicide and domestic violence have become a more common occurrence between deployments, necessitating a dramatic shift in mental health policy in the last 5 years.[207-210]

How quickly and completely any individual will progress from fear to violence is dependent on several factors. First, the genetic neurochemical predisposition (initial wiring) will influence behavioral responses.[204] Second, "soft-wired" or conditioned responses resulting from experiences and reinforced patterns will influence output. For example, it is commonly known that abusive parents were usually abused children[203,211]; they learned that anger quickly leads

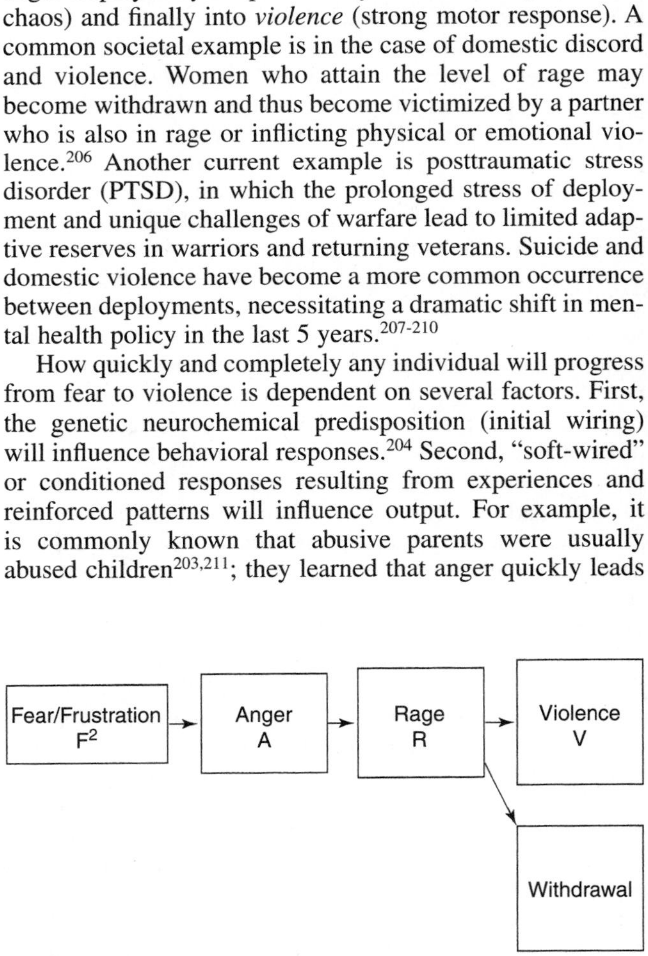

Figure 5-5 ■ Fear and frustration, anger, rage, and violence or withdrawal: F^2ARV continuum.

to violence and that the behavior of violence was somehow acceptable. Last, the quality and intensity of the stimulus initiating the continuum will influence the level of response.

The neurochemistry within an individual's CNS, whether inherently active or altered through drugs or injury, will have great influence on the plasticity of the existing wiring.[40,212] Repetitive or prolonged exposure to negative environmental stimuli may also lead to a chronically imbalanced neurochemical state that results in a lowered threshold or tolerance to a given stimulus. Chemistry or wiring can become imbalanced from damage, environmental stress, learning, or other potentially altering situations, changing an individual's control over this continuum.[56,106-108,213,214] When neurochemical imbalance exists, these behaviors will persist, and balance may be restored only through natural neurochemical activity (e.g., sleep, exercise, diet, spirituality) or medication support (chemical replacement).

Therapists need to be acutely aware of this continuum in clients who have diffuse axonal shearing within the limbic complex. Diffuse axonal shearing is most commonly seen and reported in research on individuals with head trauma[215,216] (see Chapter 24). Resulting lesions within the limbic structures may cause an individual to progress down this continuum at a rapid speed. This point cannot be overemphasized. Patients with an accelerated F^2ARV continuum may physically strike out at a clinician or caregiver out of simple frustration during care. Knowing the social history of the client and the causation of the injury often can help the therapist gain insight into how an individual patient might progress down this continuum. Not all head-injured patients had prior difficulty with the F^2ARV continuum; however, it is important to note that many individuals received their head injuries in violent confrontational situations or in wartime conflict. Some individuals, primarily females, when confronted with stress, anger, and potential violence from another, will withdraw and become depressed. This behavior, similar to violence, will change the structure of the limbic network.[55]

GAS (General Adaptation Syndrome). The autonomic responses to stress also follow a specific sequence of behavioral changes and are referred to as the *general adaptation syndrome.*[217-223] The sequential stages of GAS are a direct result of limbic imbalance and can play a dramatic role in determining client progress.

Stress can be caused by many internal or external factors, often unique to the individual. Examples include pain, acute or chronic illness or the ramification of illness, confusion, sensory overload, and a large variety of other potential sources. The initial reaction to a stressor is a neurochemical change or "alarm" that triggers a strong sympathetic nervous system reaction. Heart rate, blood pressure, respiration, metabolism, and muscle tonus will increase. It is at this stage that the grandmother lifts the car off the child as in our previous example. If the overstimulation or stress does not diminish, the body will protect itself from self-destruction and trigger a subsequent parasympathetic response. At this time, all the symptoms reverse and the client exhibits a decrease in heart rate, blood pressure, and muscle tonus. The bronchi become constricted, and the patient may hyperventilate and become dizzy, confused, and less alert. As the blood flow returns to the periphery, the face may flush and the skin may become hot. The patient will have no energy to move, will withdraw, and again will exhibit decreased postural tone and increased flexion.

This stress or overstimulation syndrome is characterized by common symptoms as described earlier.[140,224-231] If the acute symptoms are not eliminated, they will become chronic and the behavior patterns much more resistant to change.

GAS is often seen in the elderly, with various precipitating health crises,[221] and also in neonatal high-risk infants (see Chapter 11), victims of head trauma, and other clients with neurological conditions. The initial alarm can be precipitated by moderate to maximal internal instability with less intensive external stress, or by minimal internal instability with severe external sensory bombardment. For instance, in the elderly, stresses such as change of environment, loss of loved ones, failing health, and fears of financial problems can each cause the client's system to react as if overloaded.[223] As another example, individuals with head trauma (Chapter 24), vestibular dysfunction (Chapter 22B), inflammatory CNS problems (Chapter 26), and brain tumors (Chapter 25) often possess hypersensitivity to external input such as visual environments, noise, touch, or light. In these individuals, typical clinical environments and therapeutic activities may create a sensory overload and trigger a GAS response.

Stress, no matter what the specific precipitating incident (confusion, fear, anxiety, grief, or pain), has the potential to trigger the first steps in the sequence of this syndrome.[224-229,232] The clinician's sensitivity to the client's emotional system will be the therapeutic technique that best controls and reverses the acute condition.

Similarly, patients with dizziness and instability, particularly within visually stimulating environments, can develop feelings of panic, which can evolve into full attacks and agoraphobic responses.[233] These individuals avoid participating in activities that put them within visually overstimulating environments in an effort to control the dizziness and prevent the associated autonomic reactions. Similar types of reactions have been documented, such as space-motion discomfort (SMD),[234] postural phobic vertigo,[233] visual vertigo,[235] and dizziness of "psychogenic" origin. Often these individuals are referred first to psychology or psychiatry. However, there is an underlying physiologic explanation for these symptoms. In a majority of individuals with SMD, there is a documented increase in vestibular sensitivity (increased vestibulo-ocular reflex [VOR] gain) and an impairment in velocity storage (shorter VOR time constant).[236] In addition, the dorsal raphe nucleus (DRN of the midbrain and rostral pons) is the largest serotonin-containing nucleus in the brain and directly modulates the firing activity of the superior and medial vestibular nuclei. It is this interaction between serotonin and vestibular function that helps to explain the link between vestibular and anxiety disorders. It can also help explain how patients with sleep disorders or other serotonin-depleting disorders develop vestibular-like symptoms and anxiety.[237,238]

Although there are physiological reasons underlying the vestibular system disorder in a majority of these cases, the symptoms triggered are part of a spectrum of limbic responses to aberrant vestibular, cerebellar, and brain stem interactions. Normal clinic activity or typically appropriate therapeutic activity may trigger an autonomic cascade versus the desired somatomotor response. The rehabilitation of the resultant visual and postural movement dysfunction is typically more complicated in the absence of limbic network management. The clinician's strategic prescription (or "dosing") of therapeutic activities with careful monitoring of the client's emotional system and physiological response will be one of the therapeutic techniques that best controls the aberrant responses and allows vestibular adaptation and compensation to occur. This must be done to manage limbic network activity for successful motor learning to occur.

The F^2ARV and GAS continua are often interrelated in individuals who have direct or indirect limbic network involvement. The therapist needs to be aware that a patient may overrespond to stress, frustration, or fear of failure in both cognitive and motor activities. The initial response may be an escalation of the F^2ARV continuum with what then seems like a rapid withdrawal or a heightened state of anger (GAS). There are many ways to help the patient balance these autonomic reactions and continue to learn within the therapeutic setting. The Bonny Method of Guided Imagery and Music is a music-centered psychotherapy method that has been used extensively with individuals recovering from various types of trauma.[239-242] In reviewing specific Bonny Method treatment approaches used with trauma patients, Körlin[242] describes a cyclical process whereby an important initial treatment period emphasizes the mobilization of inner resources, alleviating vulnerability and increasing the patient's self-confidence. This phase uses carefully selected music that elicits positive limbic states and "bodily manifestations with qualities of warmth, energy, strength, movement, nourishing, and healing, all belonging to the implicit realm of positive vitality affects and mental models" (p. 398). The individual is then better equipped to face a period of confrontation with painful or traumatic material or the challenges faced within a therapeutic rehabilitation environment. Successful confrontation of difficult realities is then followed by a new phase of resource mobilization and consolidation of healthier behaviors that begin to replace dysfunctional defenses such as avoidance, behavioral extremes, or substance abuse.

This process continues in repeated cycles of rest-resourcing and working-confronting. The clinical success of this approach suggests that for some patients it may be advantageous to purposefully facilitate positive or pleasant physical and affective experiences before engaging in more challenging work. Although it may be impractical to provide appropriate music selections on the basis of individual assessment in the therapeutic environment (e.g., physical, occupational, music), other modalities such as heat, massage, or ultrasound treatment may also elicit relaxed, receptive physical states. The treating professional can also become aware during assessments or treatments of environmental auditory input that may trigger stress responses in patients who have limbic network involvement or who may have experienced traumatic physical or emotional injuries. These triggers can be something as simple as the therapist's tone of the voice in a sentence to the patient or as complex as the multiple-noise environment of a busy rehabilitation setting. Some patients may need to be scheduled for early morning, during lunchtime, or in the late afternoon to provide a decrease in the auditory environment.

Decreasing stimulation versus increasing facilitation may lead to attention, calmness, and receptiveness to therapy. When the client feels that control over her or his life has been returned, or at least the individual is consulted regarding decisions (informed consent, forced choices), resistance to therapy or movement is often released and stress is reduced. Even clients in a semicomatose state can participate to some extent. As a clinician begins to move a minimally responsive client, resistance may be encountered. If slight changes are made in rotation or trajectory of the movement pattern, the resistance is often lessened. If the clinician initially feels the resistance and overpowers it, total control has been taken from the client. Instead, if the clinician moves the patient in ways her or his body is willing to be moved, respect has been shown and overstimulation potentially avoided.

No single input causes these limbic responses, nor does one treatment counteract their progression. Being aware of clinical signs is critical. In a time when therapists are often rushed by the realities of a full schedule or stressed by third-party or short discharge demands, a clinician may inadvertently miss key signs and opportunities to treat. In addition, he or she may actually create a less optimal environment by physically moving faster than the pace best tolerated by the patient, who may need more time to process stimuli or to practice a target skill. The challenge for both the therapist and the patient is to find harmony within the given environment to allow for optimal outcomes.

Developing limbic network assessment tools (or repurposing existing tools) for their ability to screen or identify the presence of direct or indirect limbic involvement is of critical value. In addition, the ability to discriminate the type of limbic involvement (decreased responsiveness and withdrawal from increased responsiveness or overresponsiveness) is important to treatment planning. Treatment techniques will be discussed later in the chapter. However, the specific techniques appropriate for treating these syndromes are tools all therapists possess. These tools range from simple variations in approach (e.g., lighting, sound, smell) to more formal therapeutic techniques, such as the Feldenkrais approach, or The Bonny Method of Guided Imagery and Music.[239] How each clinician uses those tools is a critical link to success or failure in clinical interaction.

Specific Limbic influences on Motor System Output. Throughout the existence of humankind, emotions have been identified in all cultures. A child knows when a parent is angry without a word being spoken. A stranger can recognize a person who is sad or depressed. People walk to the other side of the road to avoid being close to someone who seems enraged. Emotions are easily recognizable as they are expressed through motor output of the face and body. Emotions similarly have an impact on functional motor control. The effect and intensity of emotions and limbic influence on motor control are an important part of the therapy evaluation. Table 5-1 helps differentiate the level of limbic activity with observed behavioral states cross-referenced with various medical conditions.

Fear. Fear is often associated with pain, be it somatic or emotional. To the individual in pain, pain is just pain. Figure 5-6, *A* illustrates two people who are on a roller-coaster which could create automatic responses of fear. The boy looks scared and obviously exhibits fear. The woman

TABLE 5-1 ■ INTERACTIONS AMONG LIMBIC STATE, MEDICAL CONDITIONS, AND BEHAVIORS*

LIMBIC STATE	OFTEN ASSOCIATED WITH	OBSERVED BEHAVIORS
Neutral	Health and wellness	Relaxed state
Low	Depression, stroke	Decreased eye contact, crying Lack of motivation
High	Anxiety and panic disorders Vestibular disorders Mild or traumatic head injury Blast injury, PTSD	Anxiety, anger, fear, increased respiratory rate, higher blood pressure, high muscle tension or tone, hyperactivity
Overload (F^2ARV, GAS)	Traumatic head injury Blast injury, PTSD, frail individual (either young or old), physiologically unstable individual	Violence, extreme withdrawal, loss of inhibition, reversal of expected behavior

GAS, General adaptation syndrome; *F^2ARV,* fear and frustration, anger, rage, violence; *PTSD,* posttraumatic stress disorder.
*Many individuals with neurological dysfunction fall into these categories.

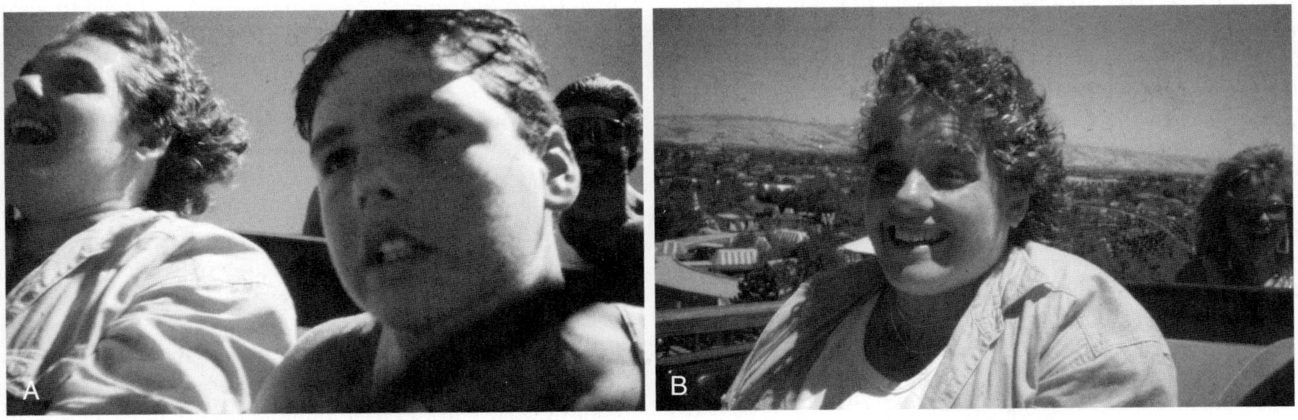

Figure 5-6 ■ **A,** Two individuals riding a rollercoaster. Individual on right looks scared; this facial expression represents fear. The facial expression of the individual on the left could represent enjoyment, with eyes open and a smile, or extreme fear, with hyperextension of her head causing her mouth to open. **B,** Individual's facial expression after the rollercoaster stopped. She was unable to relax her facial muscles for over 2 minutes because she had been so scared or demonstrated extreme fear.

could be expressing joy or fear given her motor responses. Her eyes seem fixed, which might lead to the assumption that she is truly in fear. She may not have control over her facial responses and could be exhibiting an extreme reaction to fear. If that were the case, this would be a limbic motor reaction, which could be semiautomatic. This extension pattern, if limbic, could trigger hyperextension of the neck, causing opening of the mouth. In Figure 5-6, *B,* the rollercoaster has stopped, and she still has the same expression. In fact, it took over a minute before she was able to relax her face and regain the feeling that she had some control over her emotional reaction. Her next reaction to occur was crying and observable frustration in her inability to control her initial response. The amygdala nuclei plays a critical role in regulation of facial responses to fear, pain, and other incoming stimuli.[243] This is often observed in healthy normal individuals such as seen in Figure 5-6 and similarly can be seen in patients who are extremely fearful, no matter the cause.

Fear of falling is a common problem with the elderly, especially the elderly who have various neurological diagnoses.[244,245] Therapists working with individuals who have a fear of falling need to first acknowledge that the fear is normal and then make sure that when the individual moves, he or she does not fall. Trust will be discussed later in the chapter, but fear often precedes the development of trust. Fear is an emotional response and thus is initiated and controlled by the limbic network.

Fear of pain is another emotional response housed within the limbic network that drives many individuals' motor responses. Whether individuals have fear of movement after a musculoskeletal injury,[243] fear of going to the dentist after a dental procedure,[246] fear of pain intensity after a chronic pain problem,[247] or fear of falling,[248] fear will drive motor responses, and that fear will often lead to a lower quality of life.[244] For that reason alone, therapists need to differentiate the limbic system's and the motor system's summated responses when observing the movement patterns of the individual in therapy.

Anger. Anger itself creates muscle tone through the amygdala's influence over the basal ganglia and the sensory and motor cortices and their influence over the motor control system. This is clearly exhibited in a child throwing a temper tantrum (Figure 5-7) or an adult putting his fist through a wall. How far a client or a friend will progress through the F²ARV continuum (discussed in the previous section) depends on a large number of variables. When a client loses control, the therapist must first determine whether the intervention forced the client beyond her or his ability to control. If so, changes within the therapeutic environment need to be made to allow the client opportunities to develop control and modulation over that continuum.

Creating opportunities to confront frustration and fear or even anger in real situations while the client practices modulation will lead to independence or self-empowerment. The client simultaneously needs to practice self-directed motor programming without these emotional overlays. Thus, true motor learning can result. In time, practicing the same motor control over functional programs when confronted with a large variety of emotional situations should lead to independence in life activities and thus meet a therapeutic goal.

Similarly, being unaware of a client's anger may lead the therapist to the false assumption that that individual has adequate inherent postural tone to perform activities such as independent transfers. If the client is angry with the therapist and performs the transfer only to get the therapist "off my case," when the client is sent home she or he may be unable to create enough postural extension to perform the transfer. Thus this transfer skill was never functionally independent because the test measurements were based on limbic or frontal influence over the extensor component of the motor system. The client needs to learn how to do the activity without the emotional overlay. When a therapist is unwilling, unaware, or unable to attend to these variables, the reliability or accuracy of functional test results becomes questionable.

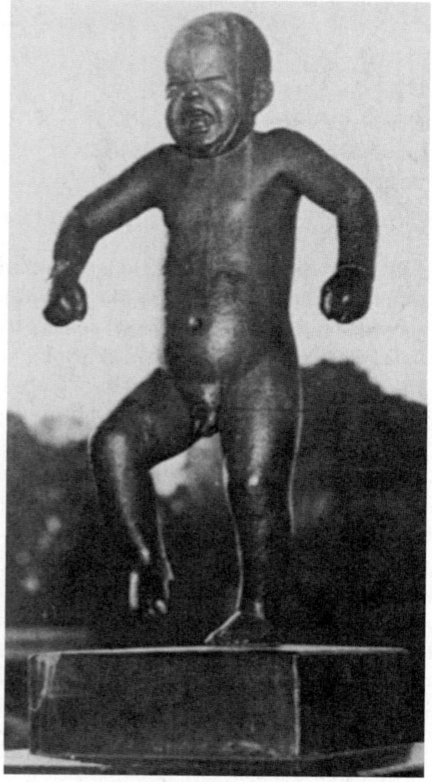

Figure 5-7 ■ Extensor behavior responses caused by anger. ("Angry Boy," Vigelund Sculpture Grounds in the Frogner Park, Oslo, Norway. Adapted from photo by Normann.)

For example, West was asked to consult with a rehabilitation team to devise a treatment program to address violent rage episodes in a 40-year-old man with moderate physical and severe cognitive functioning deficits resulting from a brain aneurysm. He would escalate very rapidly along the F²ARV continuum when presented with environmental challenges such as passing another patient with his wheelchair in the hallway. Although his physical rehabilitation had progressed well and he had regained much independence in mobility, because his assaultive outbursts posed risks to other patients as well as to caregivers, this patient appeared to be heading for placement in a locked facility, a more restrictive environment than he would need considering his level of physical limitation. Although this unfortunate man had no short-term memory function and no insight about his behaviors, West found during her assessment that he was highly responsive to calming music and was able to access some intact long-term memories that could be used to elicit a relaxation response. A highly positive limbic state of deep relaxation was thus elicited, and simple verbal cues were then presented to develop a conditioned response that any staff member could then call forth with the verbal cue alone. The entire rehabilitation team was briefed on the use of this intervention and reported success using this approach in the milieu as well as during physical therapy and occupational therapy treatments when the patient would become resistant and angry in response to therapist instructions. The patient was trained to self-regulate by giving himself the same verbal cue when confronted with challenging situations. This treatment supported the patient's ability to regain emotional controls and allowed him the opportunity to be placed in a less-restrictive community environment. West observed this individual maintaining his progress in positive behavioral adaptation in a group home environment more than a year after the intensive inpatient rehabilitation treatment protocol had been completed. The patient never recalled a previous music therapy treatment session and asked each time to have the purpose of the treatment explained to him. But his body remembered the set of behavioral experiences, and he quickly complied with the relaxation procedure. The success of this approach demonstrates that even in the absence of short-term memory and other cognitive functions usually considered essential for new learning, the skillful engagement of positive limbic states and intact areas of patient functioning (strengths) can support development of new adaptive skills, which can be generalized to new environments.

Grief, Depression, or Pain. Emotions such as grief or depression can be expressed by the motor system.[56,249] The behavioral responses are usually withdrawal, decreased postural extension, and often a feeling of tiredness and exhaustion (Figure 5-8). Sensory overload, especially in the elderly, can create low muscle tone and excessive flexion. Again, because of the strong emotional factor, these motor responses are considered to be the result of the limbic network's influence over motor control.[110] Learned helplessness is another problem that therapists need to avoid.[250] When patients are encouraged to become dependent, their chances of benefiting from services and regaining motor function are drastically reduced.[251,252]

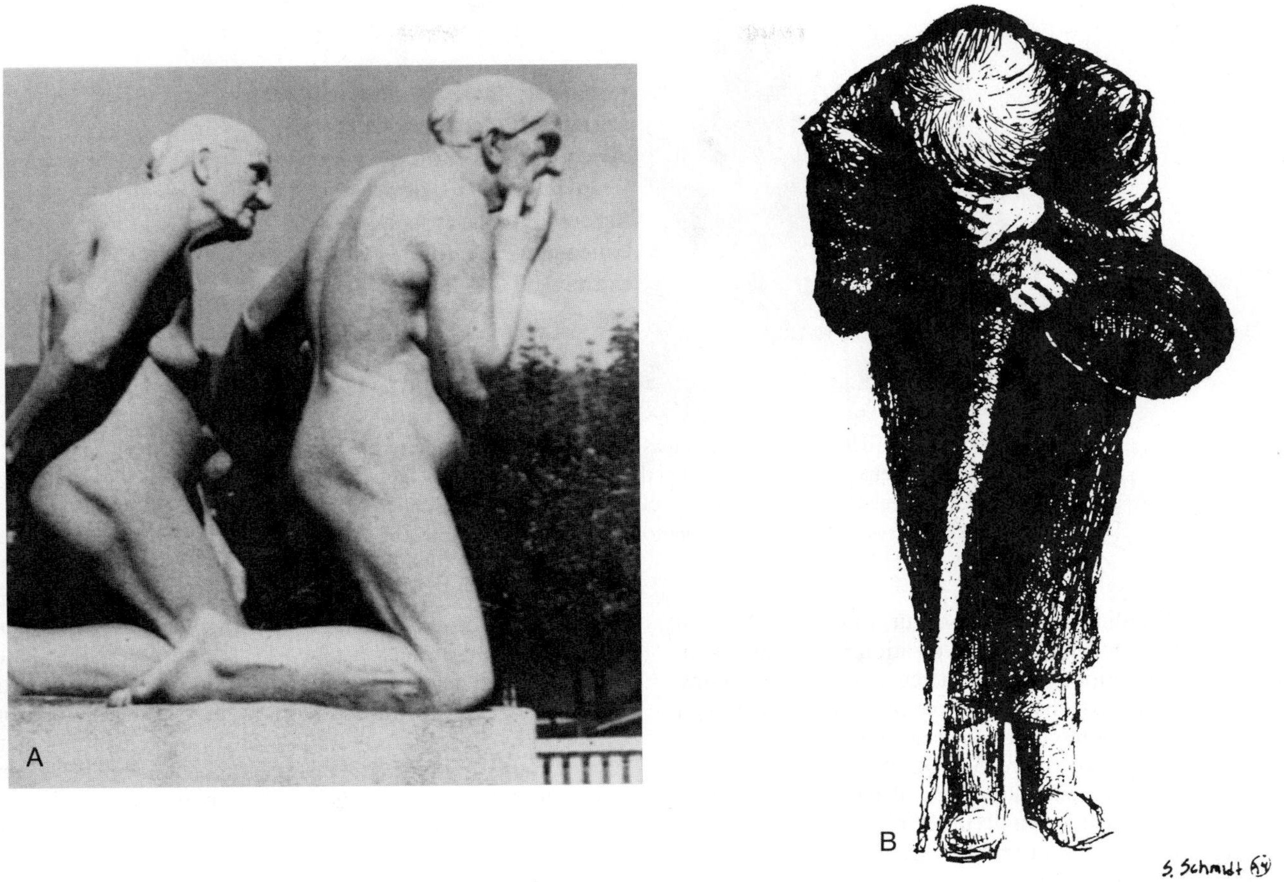

Figure 5-8 ■ **A,** Behavior responses elicited by concern, pain, and grief. **B,** Pain or grief elicits flexion and can modify postural extension. (**A** from Vigelund Sculpture Grounds in the Frogner Park, Oslo, Norway. Adapted from photo by Normann.)

Pain is a complex phenomenon, and the more it is understood, the more complex it becomes[253-257] (see Chapter 32). The concept of pain and pain management is discussed in detail in both Chapters 18 and 32. Hippocampal volume has been identified as a variable in pain ratings in the elderly.[258] Whether the pain is peripherally induced or centrally induced because of trauma or emotional overload, often the same motor responses will exist. A withdrawn flexor pattern from pain makes postural activities exhausting because of the work it takes to override the existing central pattern generators. Thus, daily living activities, which constantly require postural extension against gravity, may be perceived as overwhelming and just not worth the effort. The therapist needs to learn to differentiate between peripheral physical pain and central or emotional pain and between mixed peripheral and central induced pain. To the patient, "pain is pain!"[259-266]

Client-Therapist Bonding. Bonding projects relaxation, whereas lack of bonding reflects isolation. Because of the potency of the limbic network's connections into the motor system, a therapist's sensitivity to the client's emotional state would obviously be a key factor in understanding the motor responses observed during therapy. This requires that a therapist first understand her or his own feelings, emotional responses, and communication styles that are being used within any given clinical or social environment.[267-274]

In Figure 5-9 an entire spectrum of motor responses can be observed in four statues. A client who feels safe can relax and participate in learning without strong emotional reactions. The woman being held in Figure 5-9, *A* is safe and relaxed. The man and woman are interacting through touch with the warmth and compassion that are often observed in the client-therapist interaction of an experienced or master clinician. In Figure 5-9, *B,* the client and clinician seem to flow together during the treatment as if they shared one motor system. When looking at the therapist and client or looking at the man and woman in the statue, it becomes obvious that the two figures seem to flow together. In the statue, those two figures make one piece of art.

With clinical emphasis on clients generating and self-correcting motor programming, it would perhaps seem reasonable for a therapist to conclude that he or she need not, or should not, touch the patient. This conclusion may be accurate when considering the motor system in isolation and assuming that patients can self-correct errors in motor programs. When correction by the therapist is through words rather than touch, external feedback through the auditory system has replaced internal feedback from the somatosensory system. The voice, as well as touch, can be soothing and instill confidence.[275] Yet language in and of itself will not replace the trust and safety felt both physically and emotionally through the deep pressure of touch as illustrated in

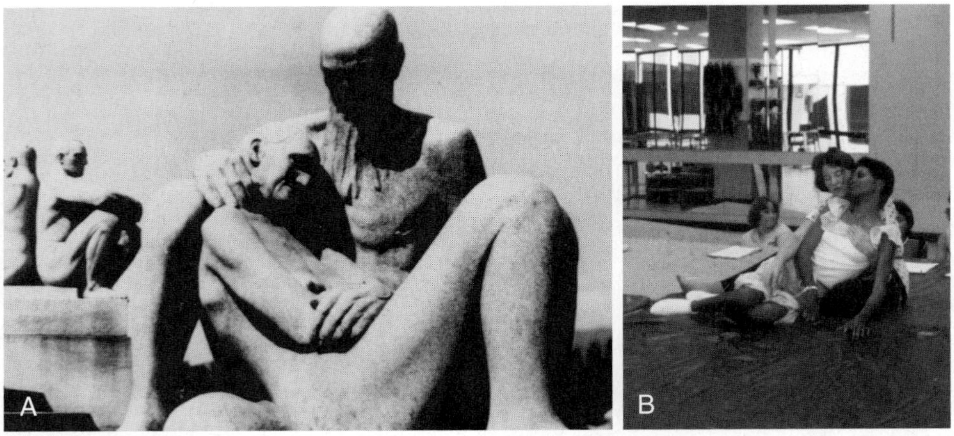

Figure 5-9 ■ **A,** Grief, depression, and compassion responses are seen in the center figures, and rigid, stoic, distancing behaviors are observed in the two left statues. **B,** Compassion is easily recognized in the clinic between a therapist and the client. (**A** from Vigelund Sculpture Grounds in the Frogner Park, Oslo, Norway. Adapted from photo by Normann.)

Figure 5-9. Bonding and trust occur much more often through touch than through conversation.[276] Recall, also, that verbal instructions require intact auditory processing and translation from declarative to procedural information, a cognitive ability that the client may not possess.

Referring again to Figure 5-9, *A,* the two men in the statue on the left demonstrate a lack of bonding. In fact, if the artist could have brought them closer together, they might just have rejected or repelled each other with greater intensity. If one of the men were the therapist and one the patient, little interaction would be occurring, and thus an assumption that learning is occurring is probably false. The therapist could do nothing to the other person (and vice versa) without that person perceiving the act as invasive, negative, or even disrespectful, with little consideration of the person's individual values. The therapist's responsibility is to open the patient's receptiveness to learning, not to close it.[277,278]

These pictures clearly illustrate two types of therapist-client interactions. If an artist can clearly depict the tonal characteristics of emotion, certainly the therapist should be able to recognize those behaviors in the client.[279] If a client is frustrated or angry and simultaneously has rigidity, spasticity, or general high tone, then a therapist might spend the entire session trying to decrease the motor response. If the client could be helped to deal with the anger or frustration during the therapy session and neutralize the emotion and achieve a *limbic neutral* state, then the specific problems could be treated effectively. Differentiating the limbic network component from the motor control system when establishing treatment protocols has not typically been within the spectrum of a therapist's skills. It is a skill that must be developed and practiced, as it is clear that the influence of an overactive or overloaded *(limbic high)* or underactive *(limbic low)* limbic network state may drastically alter the consistent responses of the motor systems and thus dampen the procedural learning and limit the success of the therapeutic setting. Carryover of procedural learning (Chapter 4) into adaptive motor responses needs to be practiced with consistency.[56]

Many factors in an interactive setting, such as therapy, cannot be identified, but certain limbic or emotional factors may play a role in that gifted clinician's skill. Although therapists are trained to be skilled observers of patient behavior, the development of "master clinician" capabilities also requires self-awareness on the part of the helping professional. "Behavioral activity can often tell us about the inner state of another or ourselves" (p. 19).[280] The willingness to be aware of one's own internal state increases the therapist's ability to perceive subtleties in the patient's responses.

Achieving a limbic neutral state in the client by carefully modifying the therapeutic environment will facilitate effective motor learning. There are many core tenets and techniques necessary to effectively achieve this neutral state, internal and external therapeutic environment, and optimal learning in the client.

Trust. Trust is a critical component of a successful therapy session.[281] The therapist gains the client's trust by his or her actions. The therapist may also build trust through sincere acknowledgment that the patient has life-limiting functional problems and that those problems are limiting normal participation. Trust is further developed when the therapist's words can be supported by data. When the therapist can illustrate the presence of functional limitations and generate a treatment plan with the patient using objective data, a bond and trust between the patient and the therapist are created.[282] In today's environment the use of reliable, valid, objective tests and measures allows for this form of communication, which has not existed to the same extent in the past. Honesty and truth lead to trust.[119,283-287]

A trusting relationship is strengthened when an agreement or "contract" can be established that sets the boundaries for discomfort (fatigue, dizziness, nausea, imbalance) or pain that the patient will experience within a therapeutic session. As one example, telling a person that you will not hurt them is a therapist-patient contract. If the therapist continually ranges a joint beyond a pain-free range, that behavior is dishonest and untruthful and will not lead to trust. Trust can be earned by stopping as soon as the client verbalizes symptoms or shows pain with a body response such as a grimace. Being sensitive to a patient's pain, no matter the cause, and working with the patient to eliminate that pain often lead to very strong bonding and trust that will lead to compliance and learning. Ignoring the pain may be perceived as insensitivity and lack of caring, which can lead to distrust and often resistance to learning or performance.

As another example, a patient with vestibular dysfunction associated with significant dizziness and nausea will experience symptoms within the course of recovery (adaptation and compensation), but those symptoms must be carefully controlled in intensity and duration. Symptoms poorly controlled can trigger an ANS or GAS cascade and elevate the limbic state, preventing learning and recovery and destroying trust.

Because these symptoms can be overt or covert, the therapist needs to be aware of both the physical and emotional responses of the patient. The use of analog or perceived exertion scales can be a valuable way to make the covert more overt to the therapist. Symptoms are valuable to the therapist as well as the patient to create environments for change, but the intensity of those stimuli need close monitoring because they can dramatically affect motor responses and ultimately overwhelm the CNS and prevent learning. Compliance to participate is limbic, and the limbic system has tremendous control over intentional movement, no matter the context of the environment.[119]

Once a client gives his or her trust, a clinician can freely move with the client and little resistance caused by fear, reservations, or need to protect the self will be felt or observed. When the patient is *limbic neutral* (the limbic network is emotionally neutralized), the tightness or limitations in movement that are present on examination can be considered true impairments within those systems or subsystems. Examination and interventions at this time will more consistently reflect true motor performance. Once limbic neutral has been achieved and examination is complete, it is recommended, for example, that if the pain is a result of peripheral tightness or joint immobility, the therapist does not elicit pain during that session. Deal with those issues in the next session after gaining the trust of the client. Trust by the therapist or the client does not mean lack of awareness of potential danger. Trust means acceptance that although the danger is present, the potential for harm, pain, or disaster is very slight and the expected gain is worth the risk (in this case, delay in intervention). In Figure 5-10, the student's trust that the instructor will not hurt her can be seen by her lack of protective responses and by her calm, relaxed body posture. The student is aware of the potential of the kick but trusts her life to the skills, control, and personal integrity of the teacher. Those same qualities are easily observed in patient-therapist interactions when watching a gifted clinician treat clients. The motor activities in a therapeutic setting may be less complex than in Figure 5-10, but in no way are they less stressful, less potentially harmful, or less frightening from the client's point of view.

In addition, therapists must first trust themselves enough to know that they can effect changes in their clients.[7,288] Understanding one's own motor system, how it responds, and how to use one's hands, arms, or entire body to move someone else is based partly on procedural skills, partly on declarative learning, and partly on self-confidence or self-trust. Trusting that one, as a therapist, has the skill to influence the motor response within the patient has a limbic component. If a therapist has self-doubts about therapeutic skills, that doubt will change performance, which will alter input to the client. This altered input can potentially alter the client's output and vary the desired responses if the client's motor system cannot run independently.

Responsibility. Very close to the concept of trust is the idea of responsibility. Accepting responsibility for our own behavior seems obvious and is accepted as part of a professional role.[289] Accepting and allowing the client the right to accept responsibility for her or his own motor environment are also key elements in creating a successful clinical environment and an independent person.*

Figure 5-11 illustrates the concept through the following example: The instructor asked the student to perform a

*References 24, 28, 31, 150, 290, 291.

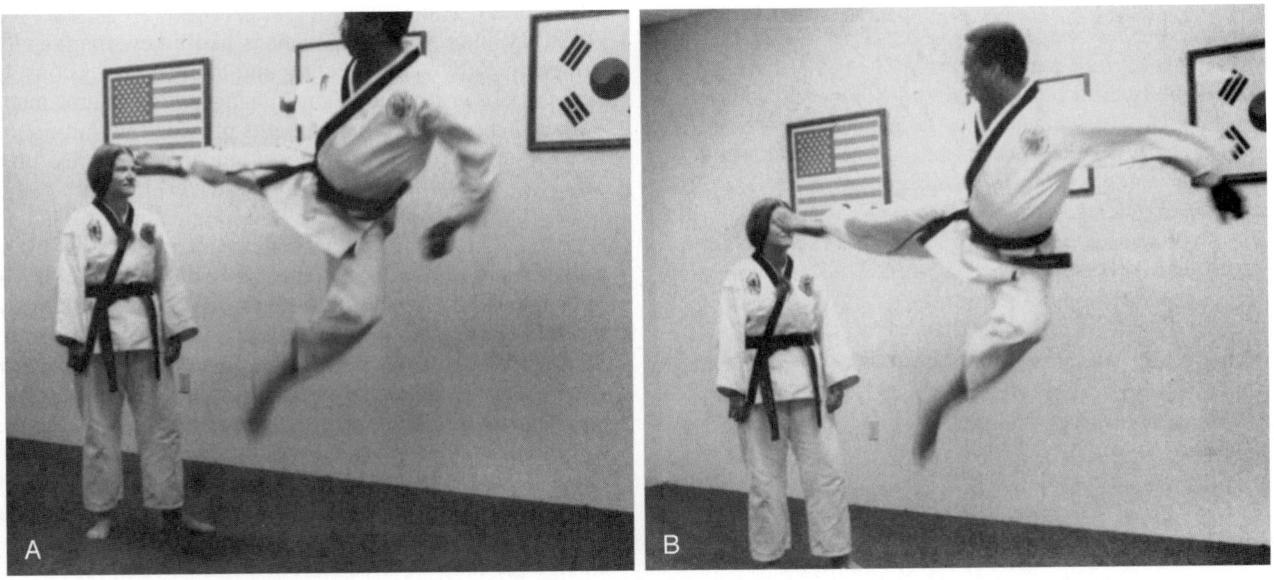

Figure 5-10 ■ Trust relaxes the limbic network's need to protect. **A,** The skill of the teacher is obvious. **B,** The student trusts that she is in no danger.

motor act, in this case, to perform a kick to the teacher's head. The kick was to be very strong or forceful and completed. The student was instructed not to hold back or stop the kick in any way, even though the kick was to come within a few inches of the teacher's head. This placed tremendous responsibility on the student. One inch too far might dangerously hurt the instructor, yet one inch too short was not acceptable. The teacher knew the student had the skill, power, and control to perform the task and then passed the responsibility to the student. The student was hesitant to assume the responsibility, for the consequence of failure could have been very traumatic. However, the student trusted that the teacher would not ask for the behavior unless success was fairly guaranteed. That trust reduced anxiety and thus neutralized the neurochemical limbic effect on the motor system of the student, giving her optimal motor control over the act.[292] Once the task was completed successfully, the student gained confidence and could repeat the task with less fear or emotional influence while gaining refinement over the motor skill.

Although the motor activities described in this example are complex and different from functional activities practiced within the clinic by therapists and clients, the dynamics of the environment relate consistently with client-therapist roles and expectations. A gifted clinician knows that the client has the potential to succeed. When asked to perform, the client trusts the therapist and assumes responsibility for the act. The therapist can facilitate the movement or postural pattern, thereby ensuring that the client succeeds. This feeling of success stimulates motivation for task repetition, which ultimately leads to learning. The incentive to repeat and learn becomes self-motivating and then becomes the responsibility of the client. As the therapist relinquishes control and empowers the client to more and more of the function, novelty to the learning is occurring.

Current literature has shown that people are more motivated by novelty and change than by success at mastery or

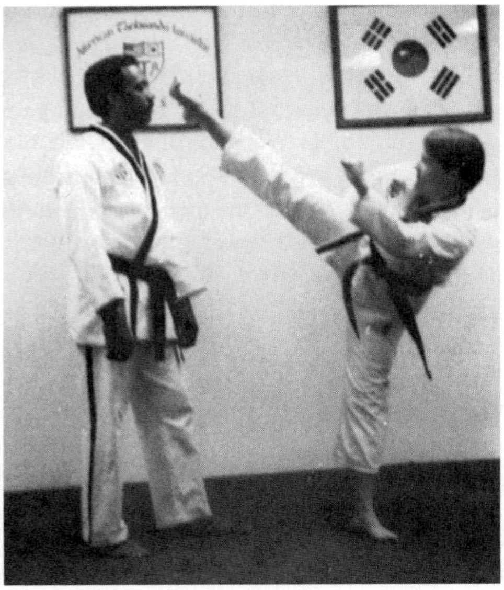

Figure 5-11 ■ The teacher relinquishes the task to the student, and the student trusts the teacher is right even if self-doubt exists.

accomplishment of a goal.[90,292,293] The limbic complex and its interwoven network throughout the nervous system play a key role in this behavioral drive.[294] The task itself can be simple, such as a weight shift, or as complex as getting dressed or climbing onto and off of a bus. No matter what the activity, the client needs to accept responsibility for her or his own behavior before independence in motor functioning can be achieved. Although the motor function itself is not limbic, many variables that lead to success, self-motivation, and feelings of independence are directly related to limbic and prefrontal lobe circuitry. The variance and self-correction within the movement expression also create novelty and motivation to continue to practice.[90,292-295]

As another clinical example of responsibility, in a patient with vestibular dysfunction and dizziness compounded by anxiety, symptoms of dizziness are necessary during treatment to drive CNS change. The therapist has a responsibility to prescribe the appropriate activities, dosage (intensity, timing, and so on), and environment to retrain sensory organization and balance (motor output). The patient can be given the responsibility of monitoring and managing her or his own symptoms within these activities, for instance, by agreeing on the maximal level of dizziness the patient and therapist are willing to accept within the therapeutic activity. A tool as simple as a verbal or visual analog scale can empower the patient to manage symptoms, dampen the limbic network response, and improve motor output for balance control.

Flexibility and Openness. Another component of a successful clinical environment deals with learning and flexibility on the part of the therapist. A master clinician sees and feels what is happening within the motor control output system of the client. Letting go of preestablished belief of what will happen is difficult.[296,297] It is important for a clinician to be open to what is present as the motor expression. This openness is critical to actually identifying what is being expressed by the nervous system of the patient. Master clinicians do not get stuck on what they have been taught but use that as a foundation or springboard for additional learning. Learning is constantly correlated to memories and new experiences.

To the therapist, each client is like a new map, sparsely drawn or sketchy at the beginning, but one that is constantly revised as the terrain (client) changes. The initial medical diagnosis may link to many paths provided within the map, but the comorbidities can result in great variance among patients.[298] That initial map might be a critical care pathway for the client, given her or his neurological insult. That pathway is a map, but only a sketchy one, and may not even be a map that a particular patient falls within in spite of his or her medical diagnosis. It is the therapist's responsibility to evaluate the patient and determine whether that pathway or map will work or is working and when changes in that map need to be altered. That is, the therapist must let go of an outdated map or treatment technique and create a new one as the environment and motor control system of the client change. This transference or letting go of old maps or ideas is true for both the client and therapist. If a position, pattern, or technique is not working, then the clinician needs to change the map or directions of treatment and let the client teach the therapist what will work. The ability to change and select new or alternative treatment techniques is based on the attitude of the therapist toward selecting alternative approaches. Willingness to be flexible and open to learning is based on confidence in oneself, a truly emotional strategy or limbic behavior. Master clinicians have learned that the answers to the patient's puzzle are within the patient, not the textbooks.

Figure 5-12 depicts two maps with a beginning point and a terminal outcome or goal in each. The parameters of the first map illustrate the boundaries of that therapist's experience and education. The clinician, through training, can identify what would seem to be the most direct and efficient way or path toward the mutually identified goal of the therapist and client. When the client becomes a participant within the environment or map, what would seem like a direct path toward a goal might not be the easiest or most direct path for the client. If empowerment of the client leads to independence, then allowing and encouraging the client to direct therapy may provide greater variability, force the client to problem solve, and lead to greater learning. The therapist needs to recognize when the client is not going in the direction of the goal. For example, the client is trying to perform a stand-pivot transfer and instead is falling. If it is important to practice transfers, then practicing falling is inappropriate and the environment (either internal or external) needs modification. Falling can be learned and practiced at another time. Once both strategies are learned, the therapist must empower the patient to take ownership of the map. In the examples of transferring, if the therapist asks the client to practice transfers and if the client starts to fall, a change in required motor behavior must be made and the opportunity given to the client to self-correct. In that way the client is gaining independent control over a variety of environmental contexts and outcomes. Within the same figure (Figure 5-12) is a second map. That second map might represent another professional's interaction and goal with the same client. It is during these overlapping interactions that both professionals can empower the patient to practice, and that practice will help lead to those functional goals established by both practitioners. In some situations a clinician from one profession may guide a client toward obtaining the functional skill necessary for a member of the second profession to begin guiding the client toward the expected outcomes of the second profession. These interlocking dependencies of the client and the professions are illustrated in Figure 5-12. If the client begins therapy striving for the first goal and ends at the functional outcome of the second goal, then additional functional outcomes have been achieved and both professions interacted for the ultimate prognosis for the patient. That interaction requires respect and openness of both professionals toward each other as well as toward the client. Those attitudes and ultimate behaviors are limbic driven.

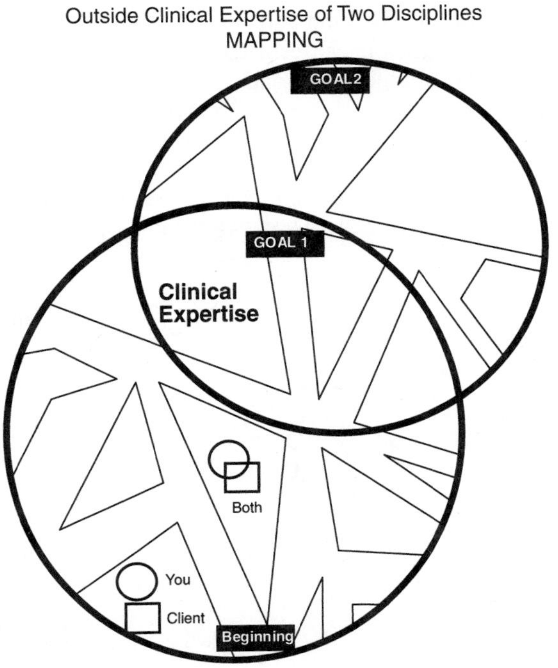

Figure 5-12 ■ Concept of clinical mapping including client and therapist and the interactions and importance of overlapping professional goals and staying within the professional expertise.

Matching maps should be a collaborative effort instead of coincidence. These collaborative efforts include interactions with all professions within the rehabilitation setting. Occupational and physical therapists are very familiar with collaboration, and both often approach interventions as a team effort. There are many additional therapists and individuals within that same setting who could also collaborate. Recreational therapists, psychologists, nurses, family members, and music therapists are but a few. Within a profession such as music therapy, the existence of two maps may overlap within a multidimensional environment. When a physical or occupational therapist needs to challenge a patient, the music therapist may be able to calm the system at the same time (overlapping maps). Research on affective responses to consonance and dissonance in music supports the creation of a map within a rehabilitation environment that could overlap with either physical, occupational, or speech therapy. Words such as *relaxed* or *calm* correlated positively with higher levels of consonance in the music, whereas adjectives associated with negative emotions *(unpleasant, tense, irritable, annoying, dissonant, angry)* were found to correlate positively with higher levels of dissonance.[133] Creating a whole environment where potential frustrations within motor learning could be balanced with higher levels of consonance in the music would potentially balance the limbic network emotional response within the overlapping maps and bring balance or stability to the limbic network's influence on motor learning and control. A later study by Peretz and colleagues[148] related the same variables to a happy-sad rating task. Given the research evidence for activity within the limbic network as it relates to music,[144,299] motor learning,[300] and cognitive enhancement,[301] a natural multiple map system would be easy to incorporate within a therapeutic setting. The clinician needs to appreciate the uniqueness of each map while holding onto the concept of the interaction of the two maps.

Vulnerability. To receive input from a client that is multivariable and simultaneous, a therapist has to be open to that information. If a clinician believes that he or she knows what each client needs and how to get those behaviors before meeting the client, then the client falls into a category of a recipe for treating the problem. Using the recipe does not mean the client cannot learn or gain better perceptual and cognitive, affective, or motor control, but it does mean that the individuality of the person may be lost. A more individualized approach would allow the clinician to identify through behavioral responses the best way for the client to learn how to sequence the learning, when to make demands of the client, when to nurture, when to stop, when to continue, when to assist, when to have fun, when to laugh, or when to cry. An analogy might be going to a fast food restaurant versus a restaurant where each aspect of the meal is tailored to one's taste. It does not mean that both restaurants are not selling digestible foods. It does mean that at one eating place the food is mass produced with some choices, but individuality, with respect to the consumer, is not an aspect of the service. Unfortunately, managed care, limited visits, reduced time for treatment, and therapists' level of frustration all are pushing therapeutic interventions toward a "one size fits all" philosophy that may increase the time needed for learning, not reduce it.

To be open totally to processing the individual differences of the client, the clinician must be relaxed and nonthreatened, and feel no need to protect himself or herself from the external environment. This environment needs to project beyond the therapist-client relations and envelope all disciplines interacting with the client.[302] In order for these interactions to occur, the clinician's emotional state requires some vulnerability, allowing him or her to be open to new and as-yet-unanalyzed or unprocessed input. This vulnerability implies the role not of an expert who knows the answers beforehand but of an expert investigator. Being open must incorporate being sensitive not only to the variability of motor responses but also to the variability of emotional responses on the part of the client.[303,304] This vulnerability leads to compassion, understanding, and acceptance of the client as a unique human being. It can also be exhausting. Therapists need to learn ways to allow openness without taking on the emotional responsibility of each patient.

Limbic Lesions and Their Influence on the Therapeutic Environment

Many lesions or neurochemical imbalances within the limbic network drastically affect the success or failure of physical, occupational, and other therapy programs. This chapter does not discuss in detail specific problems and their treatment, but instead it is hoped that identification of limbic involvement may help the reader develop a better understanding of specific neurological conditions and carry that knowledge into Section II, where the specific clinical problems are discussed.

Substance Abuse (See Chapter 24). The anterior temporal lobe (especially the hippocampus and amygdala) has a lower threshold for epileptic seizures than do other cortical structures.[56] This type of epilepsy is produced by use of systemic drugs such as cocaine and alcohol. The seizure is often accompanied by sensory auras and alterations in behavior, with specific focus on mood shifts and cognitive dysfunction.[305] Obviously, the precise association between behavior and emotions or temporolimbic and frontolimbic activity is not understood, yet the associations and thus their impact on a therapeutic setting cannot be ignored.[217,306]

Whether street bought, medically administered, or ingested for private or social reasons (such as in alcohol consumption), drugs and alcohol can have dramatic effects on the CNS and often are associated with limbic behavior.[307] Korsakoff syndrome, caused by chronic alcoholism and its related nutritional deficiency, is identified by the structural involvement of the diencephalon with specific focus on the mammillary bodies, and the dorsal medial and anterior nucleus of the thalamus[56] usually shows involvement (see the anatomy section and Figure 5-13). This syndrome is not a dementia but rather a discrete, localized pathological state with specific clinical signs. The most dramatic sign observed in a client with Korsakoff syndrome is severe memory deficits.[252,308-310] These deficits involve declarative memory and learning losses, but the most predominant problem is short-term memory loss.[311] As the disease progresses, clients generally become totally unaware of their memory loss and are unconcerned. Initially, confabulation may be observed,[312] but in time most clients with a chronic condition become apathetic and somewhat withdrawn and are in a profound amnesic state. They are trapped in time, unable to learn from new experiences because they cannot retain memories for more than a few minutes and are unable to maintain their independence[252,308-310,313]; many may become social isolates and homeless.

The use of alcohol affects not only adults but also children and adolescents. Still another population of children affected by alcohol abuse has surfaced as a specific clinical problem. These children are infants who have the effects of fetal alcohol syndrome. A variety of researchers have investigated the effects of alcohol and other toxic drugs on neuromotor and cognitive development.[314-319]

Alzheimer Disease (See Chapter 27). In Alzheimer disease, the hippocampus and nucleus basalis are the most severely involved structures, followed by neurofibrillar degeneration of the anterotemporal, parietal, and frontal lobes.[252,320-323]

Initially the symptoms fall into several categories: emotional, social, and cognitive. Usually the symptoms have a gradual onset. Depression and anxiety often are seen during the early phases because of the neuronal degeneration within the prefrontal lobes and limbic network.[322,324-326] During the second stage, the emotional, social, and intellectual changes become more marked. Clients have difficulty with demands, business affairs, and personal management. Their memory and cognitive processing continue to deteriorate, whereas their awareness of the problem is often

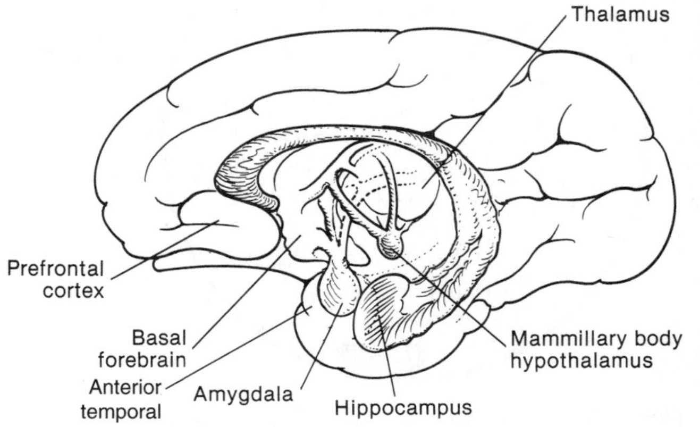

Figure 5-13 ■ Anatomy of the limbic network: schematic illustration.

still insightful, causing additional anxiety and depression. During this phase clients may be unable to recognize familiar objects and become scared because they are losing control of the environment both internally and externally. Thus the client may become combative out of a defensive (fight-or-flight) autonomic response. For that reason, therapists need to make sure the client feels safe during therapy to optimize the learning and compliance. The third phase manifests itself with moderate to severe aphasic, apraxic, and agnosic problems. Object agnosia, the failure to recognize objects, is a typical sign of advancing Alzheimer disease. Distractibility and inattentiveness are also common signs of this third stage. The final stage of Alzheimer disease is marked by an individual who is uncommunicative, with little meaningful social interaction, who often takes on the features of the Klüver-Bucy syndrome (see Chapter 13). Thus they exhibit emotional outbursts, inappropriate sexual behaviors, severe memory loss, constant mouth movements, and often a flexor-type postural pattern. In this latter phase, the client is virtually decorticate and clinically indistinguishable from persons with other dementias. The prognosis of Alzheimer disease was only a few years ago totally bleak, but today there are hopes that in the future, pharmacological interventions may slow and even reverse the damage inflicted by this disease.[327-330]

In spite of future treatments, the continual degeneration of the limbic network is a key distinguishing factor in Alzheimer disease.[109,331-333] Many clients in the past have been misdiagnosed as having other problems such as intracranial tumors, normal pressure hydrocephalus, multiinfarct dementia, or alcoholic or chronic drug intoxication.[334-337] Similarly, many clients with tumors, multifaceted dementias, alcoholism, or heart attacks resulting in hippocampal damage may be diagnosed with Alzheimer disease. When the disease is correctly evaluated and diagnosed, however, it becomes obvious that the limbic-cortical area involved from phase 1 through the last phase is interacting with other areas of the brain and constantly affecting the behavioral patterns of the patient.[338-341] Owing to the neurochemical sensitivity and production within the limbic network, drugs are often used to prevent or slow the progression of Alzheimer disease (see Chapter 36).[342-346] Similarly, a genetic predisposition has been found in some patients with Alzheimer disease[56,347-349]; thus, gene therapy may prove to have great therapeutic value.[350] Because music is able to activate many different brain areas, it is particularly valuable in the treatment of persons at all stages of Alzheimer disease[351] and can effectively be used during physical or occupational therapy. Long after declarative memory is lost, individuals can sing entire songs (procedural memory), dance with a loved one they no longer recognize (procedural memory), or be soothed and calmed by hearing someone who cares about them singing familiar favorite songs or lullabies (limbic response). This is why the power of music is so great, especially as observed in individuals with Alzheimer disease who have lost declarative memory. In earlier phases of the disease, individuals who have lost words can recall words such as song lyrics through the linking with melody. When melody is lost, individuals still retain rhythmic responses. At the palliative stage of Alzheimer disease care, agitated patients are observed to calm to simple music such as familiar lullabies. Thus Alzheimer disease patients are able to continue to respond to music through the progression of the disease, and the response to rhythm may represent overlearned motor responses that are tied to positive limbic states. For example, nonambulatory individuals, when presented with familiar and preferred music, may stand and move with the rhythm of the sound. Their bodies may remember how to dance with the spouse whose name they no longer know.[352] A physical or occupational therapist can instruct a caregiver to use music as part of everyday activities. The therapeutic effects of music to engage and maintain attention, activate long-term memory, and modulate emotion states are well suited to the needs of both the person with Alzheimer disease and his or her caregivers.[352]

Head Injury (See Chapter 24).

Traumatic Injury. One potentially severe limbic problem that can be present after traumatic closed head injury is diffuse axonal injury.[215,216,353-356] The long associative bundles or fibers that transverse the cortex on a curved route can be sheared by an impact or a blow to the head. One of these long associative bundles is the cingulate fasciculus, which coordinates the amygdala and hippocampal projections to and from the prefrontal cortex. Many basic perceptual strategies, such as body schema, hearing, vision, and smell, are linked into the emotional and learning centers of the limbic network through the cingulate fasciculus.[357] Thus, declarative learning through sensory and cognitive processing can become impossible. If the pathways to and from the hippocampus and amygdala are sheared bilaterally, total and permanent global anterograde amnesia will be present.[109,358,359] If destruction of both tracts on one side occurs, but the contralateral side is left intact, the individual can compensate, but learning will be slower or the rate of processing delayed.[157] If only one tract on one side is damaged, such as the tract to and from the hippocampus, the amygdaloid system on the same side will compensate but be slower than without the lesion.[157] Thus the specific degree of involvement will vary and depend on the extent of shearing. Those with total shearing on both sides will usually be in a deep coma and will not survive the injury.[360] Those with less severe insult will show signs ranging from total amnesia to minor delays in declarative learning.[361] The emotional problems of traumatic head injury can often be associated with other limbic problems such as posttraumatic stress syndrome. This problem is especially apparent when treating soldiers injured on the battlefield who have returned home.[362]

Integrating various professions becomes a critical aspect of an injured soldier's rehabilitation. When the interaction of the limbic network and higher control is considered, additional variables can be taken into consideration within the therapeutic environment. In treating more than 200 patients who had trauma, Körlin[242] found that certain kinds of musical elements often triggered intrusive and traumatic reexperiences of the event. (For a theoretical discussion of this phenomenon, see Goldberg.[363]) The phenomenon of auditory triggering has implications for the rehabilitation setting, where patients may be recovering from traumas related to accident, injury, or difficult medical procedures. Both environmental noise and "background" music may present auditory triggers that elicit limbic network and ANS activity. Thus the potential for eliciting the F^2ARV continuum during a physical or occupational therapy treatment session is always present, and the therapists need to be acutely aware of background noise.

Cerebral contusions (bruises) have long been a primary sign of traumatic head injury.[364] Regardless of area of impact, the contusions are generally found in the frontal and temporal regions. There are long-term neuropsychological ramifications after mild traumatic brain injury even when there is no loss of consciousness.[365] The regions most frequently involved are orbitofrontal, frontopolar, anterotemporal, and lateral temporal surfaces.

The limbic network's connection to these areas would suggest the potential for direct and indirect limbic involvement. The greater the contusion, the greater the likelihood that the limbic structures might simultaneously be involved. Impulsiveness, lack of inhibition, and hyperactivity are a few of the clinical signs associated with orbitofrontal or limbic involvement.[366] The dorsomedial frontal region, involved in the hippocampal-fornix circuit (once referred to as the *Papez circuit*),[367] when damaged seems to induce a pseudodepressed state, including slowness, lack of initiation, and perseveration.

Nontraumatic Head Injuries: Anoxic or Hypoxic Brain Injury. Lack of oxygen to the brain, regardless of the cause, seems not only to have a dramatic effect throughout the cortex but also selectively damages the hippocampal regions.[368] The loss of hippocampal declarative memory systems bilaterally would certainly provide one reason for the slowness in processing so commonly observed in head injury.[369] A hypothesis could also be made regarding the limbic network's interrelation with other cortical and brain stem structures. In cases of hypoxia, many structures interconnecting in the limbic network are potentially affected, so information sent to the limbic network may be distorted. These distortions could cause tremendous imbalances within the limbic processing system, with not only attention and learning problems but also the hypothalamic irregularity often seen in head trauma. Individuals who demonstrate obstructive sleep apnea, another cause of hypoxia, have been shown to have an imbalance in the hippocampal area.[370] This imbalance may lead to severe cognitive dysfunction.[371] This preexisting hypoxic environment certainly can have a long-term effect on any patient who has CNS damage at any age.

A therapist always needs to understand the environment within which the injury occurred as well as being aware of preexisting complications. If the injury was sustained in a violent confrontation, such as a fight or a frightful experience such as a near-drowning, the emotional system had to be at a high level of metabolic activity at the time of the insult. If the event was anoxic, then those areas with the highest oxygen need or at the highest metabolic state might be the most affected or damaged after the event. Knowing that information, a therapist's analytical problem-solving strategies should guide her or him toward limbic assessment.

Summary of Limbic Problems with Head-Injured Clients. The behavioral sequelae after any head injury reflect many signs of limbic involvement. In studies of both the pediatric and adult populations,[353-355,357,365,372,373] behaviors of impulsiveness, restlessness, overactivity, destructiveness, aggression, increased tantrums, and socially uninhibited behaviors (lack of social skills) are frequently reported. These behaviors all reflect a strong emotional or limbic component. Given Moore's concept of a limbic network that MOVEs us and the F^2ARV continuum regarding emotional control over noxious or negative input, it is no wonder so many clients have difficulty with personal and emotional control over their reactions to the therapeutic world. If the imbalance were within the client, then the external environment would be one possible way to help center the client emotionally.[374,375] This centering requires that the therapist be sensitive to the emotional level of the client. As the client begins to regain control, an increase in external environmental demands would challenge the limbic network. If the demand is excessive, the client's emotional reaction as expressed by motor behavior should alert the therapist to downgrade the activity level.

Head injuries affect many areas of the CNS. A client with spasticity, rigidity, or ataxia may exhibit an increase in those motor responses when the limbic network becomes stressed. Learning to differentiate a motor control problem from a limbic problem that influences the motor control systems requires that the therapist be willing to address the cause of the problems and their respective treatments.[376] Each client is different, no matter the commonalities of the site or extent of the lesions, because of prior learning, conditioning of the limbic network, and their respective perception of quality of life.[377] The response of two clients to the same clinical learning environment may have great variance and should not surprise the clinician. Thus the therapist needs to give undivided attention to the client at all times and be willing to make moment-to-moment adjustments within the external environment to help the client maintain focus on the desired learning.

Vestibular Disorders. The vestibular system has extensive neuronal connections and commissural influences on the limbic network and structures; conversely, the limbic network has significant influence on the vestibular nuclei. Details of the neuroanatomical connections are described later in this chapter.

It is generally accepted that vestibular dysfunction results in erroneous input to the CNS. This erroneous sensory information creates a mismatch between the external (afferent) cues and the internal conceptual model for movement contained by the cerebellum. This mismatch creates an imbalance in vestibular and cerebellar signals to the CNS, flooding the central limbic structures and resulting in symptoms such as vertigo, motion sickness, nausea, or decreased postural control. Detection of this mismatch results in an attempt by the cerebellum to compensate for the imbalance, which becomes a core tenet of recovery.[378] Alternately, this neural stimulation may create an internal stressor, and trigger an adverse limbic response, such as a GAS response.

Newer evidence from animal research has demonstrated that vestibular lesions result in dramatic changes in the morphology and function of the hippocampus. Of note is that bilateral vestibular lesions have been associated with hippocampal atrophy. The hippocampus makes unique contributions to memory, both spatial and nonspatial. Thus vestibular lesions impair learning and memory, particularly those tasks that require spatial processing. In addition to the more well known deficits in spatial and gravitational orientation for balance control, vestibular lesions can also result in impaired cognition, learning, and memory through damage to this connection. Decreased concentration, thought processes, and memory are among the most common complaints in patients with vestibular disorders. In the past these complaints were often attributed to competitive resources, suggesting that cognitive resources were being devoted to the basic tasks of staying balanced during function. It is now clear that there is a true physiologic explanation for these secondary symptoms, which are quite limiting to activity and participation in normal daily activities, particularly working. It has also been suggested that treatment activities that stimulate the function of the vestibular system also stimulate activity within the hippocampus and can improve memory, which has important implications for treatment.[379-387]

Thus vestibular dysfunction can influence the therapeutic environment both in the assessment and the treatment of this system. However, the vestibular system is not a primary consideration of most physicians and therapists during evaluation. On the basis of benchmarking data from within specialized balance centers, the average patient with a vestibular disorder (dizziness or imbalance) travels within the medical system an average of 52 months before finding a solution. During this time, he or she has seen on average four physicians. There is also at least one visit to the emergency department in crisis and one visit to a psychiatrist. Typically there has been no rehabilitation referral or intervention during this time.[388]

The patient with a chronic vestibular disorder can have myriad symptoms, including vegetative, autonomic, motoric, cognitive, psychological, and behavioral symptoms that are often misdiagnosed during this search for an outcome as other, more serious medical diagnoses. As an example, of those patients diagnosed with dizziness or imbalance of a psychologic origin, evidence has determined that more than 70% of these patients have underlying vestibular dysfunction on key vestibular function tests (electronystagmography and calorics, rotary chair, computerized dynamic posturography, auditory brain stem response, and acoustic reflexes).[233,235,389-391] Conversely, of those patients with chronic dizziness and imbalance, only 16% were found to have dizziness of a true psychogenic origin.[392] Acknowledgment of a patient's symptoms, use of data, and explanation (in understandable detail) that there is a physiologic explanation for his or her complaints builds the client-therapist relationship and begins to neutralize the client's abnormal limbic state (anxiety versus depression). It can lower the GAS or autonomic cascade, maximizing the treatment time before the onset of limiting symptoms (i.e., raise the symptom threshold).

Even patients with motion sickness have documentable physiologic and functional changes. Some of the best current evidence is in our military personnel with symptoms of motion sickness. On examination, these soldiers have physiological changes identifiable by results of rotary chair (60% with abnormally long time constants) and computerized dynamic posturography (70% with abnormal sensory organization test [SOT] condition 5 and 6).[393]

Patients who have sustained a mild head injury, postconcussive syndrome, blast exposure or injury (positive or negative pressure event), or whiplash often have concomitant involvement of the vestibular apparatus or nuclei. This often goes undetected within the initial medical workup and management plan excepting in specialty vestibular practices.[393-397] When the disorder is undetected and left unchecked, the patients do not respond to standard treatment interventions. They also complain of atypical symptoms or responses to these typical treatments. When the patient does not respond in predictable ways to standard treatment, the label "aphysiological" is applied, particularly in situations where disability or secondary gain is a factor. Fortunately there are well established performance criteria that can effectively differentiate true balance or vestibular impairment from embellishment for secondary gain.[398] (Refer to Chapters 22A and 22B.)

In treatment, recovery is based on long-term compensation mediated by the cerebellum, and symptoms must be reproduced for recovery to occur. However, stimulation of the vestibular system must be controlled, with every effort made to maintain a limbic (emotional) neutral state. Some patients have true vestibular dysfunction that affects only motor responses, whereas other patients have true limbic psychiatric problems that do not manifest themselves with vestibular symptoms. These two behaviors are located at the polar ends of the curve between limbic motor and vestibular motor dysfunction. Before prescribing appropriate intervention strategies, the clinician must be clear regarding the degree of limbic overlay on the vestibular dysfunction, and the question "What are the best vestibular and limbic interactive environments that will challenge and drive neuroplastic change?" must be answered. Although researchers[233,390] have identified tools that differentiate the two extremes, today researchers are trying to clarify the midrange of patients who clearly have symptoms on the basis of the interaction of both systems.[398,399] Development of tools that can further discriminate whether the behaviors are first driven by vestibular and followed by limbic responses, or vice versa, is a key to treatment planning.

Parkinson Disease. The motor impairments seen in individuals with Parkinson disease are widely accepted, understood, and treated by physical and occupational therapists (see Chapter 20). What is not commonly synthesized by physical and occupational therapists, no matter the working environment (hospital, outpatient, rehabilitation, home health), is that individuals diagnosed with Parkinson disease often have limbic involvement.

Masked expression is accepted as a motor sign of this disease and is linked directly to the rigidity expressed within the motor system. Yet, a masked expression is also associated with fear as an emotion (see Figure 5-6). Similarly, the ability to extinguish this fear response or masked expression is also based on the infralimbic prefrontal lobe and the number of dopamine receptors.[400] These areas may not be directly damaged by Parkinson disease, but the amount of available dopamine is dramatically reduced. Given this interaction, patients with Parkinson disease may have difficulty facially expressing what they are feeling. Thus, when a therapist sees a patient with a fixed facial expression, that therapist cannot draw a conclusion from that facial expression.

Similarly, depression is commonly associated with any individual with a degenerative disease.[401,402] Obviously, depression from a neuroanatomical perspective is housed with the limbic system. Depression from a motor response perspective causes lower postural tone with increased flexion in the neck (see Figure 5-8, *B*). This pattern within the trunk is also often described as the postural patterns of an individual with Parkinson disease. The question arises, "Is the tone generated from the motor system alone, from the limbic influence on the motor system alone, or from a combination of the two?"

Individuals working in a psychological setting (inpatient and outpatient) may focus on the psychoemotional problems without addressing the functional motor involvement. It is not infrequent that an individual with this disease may simultaneously exhibit signs of psychosis and other potential psychiatric problems.[403-407] It is critical for therapists, despite the physical setting, to develop and understand the entire spectrum of the problems associated with this disease.

Cerebrovascular Accidents (See Chapter 23). The most common insult in CVA results in occlusions within tributaries of the middle cerebral artery.[56] When this occlusion is in the right hemisphere, studies have shown that clients are often confused and exhibit metabolic imbalance.[408] The primary problem of this confused state is inattention. After brain scans, it has been shown that focal lesions existed within both the reticulocortical and limbic cortical tracts, suggesting direct limbic involvement in many middle cerebral artery problems.[66]

With the use of magnetic resonance imaging (MRI), specific lesion deficits after CVA can help physicians and therapists identify specific motor and limbic behavioral problems that would limit quality of life of the patients.[409-411] Many clients who have had a CVA do not have direct limbic involvement, yet the stresses placed on the client,[412,413] whether external or internal, are often reflected in the limbic network's influence over cognition and the motor control systems.[414] Everyday existence as well as performance of motor tasks required during therapy are usually valued highly in the client's life. This value or stress placed on the limbic network overflows into the motor system and never allows it to relax, as observed by noting the increase of tonus in the unaffected leg. The client is usually unaware of this buildup of tonus but can release it once attention is drawn to it. If attention is never directed toward these tension buildups, a therapist trying to decrease tonus in the affected arm or leg will always be interacting with the associated patterns from the less-involved extremities.

Tumor (See Chapter 25). Any brain tumor, regardless of whether it directly affects the limbic structures, will certainly arouse the limbic network because of the stress, anxiety, and emotional overlays of the diagnosis. The degree of emotional involvement will obviously affect the declarative learning of the client as well as the limbic network's influence over motor response.

Tumors specifically arising within limbic structures[415,416] can cause dramatic changes in the client's emotional behavior and level of alertness, especially with hypothalamic tumors.[417] The behaviors reported include aggressiveness, hyperphagia, paranoia, sloppiness, manic symptoms, and eventual confusion.[56] Tumors within the hypothalamus cause not only behavioral abnormalities but also autonomic endocrine imbalances, including body temperature changes, menstrual abnormalities, and diabetes insipidus.[109]

When the tumor is located within the frontal and temporal lobes, associated with limbic structures, psychiatric problems may manifest, ranging from depression to anorexia to psychosis.[109,418] Obsessive-compulsive disorder resulting from limbic tumor has been used as a tumor marker for relapse.[419] Amnesia has been reported in patients with dorsomedial thalamus, fornix, midbrain, and reticulolimbic pathway lesions. This again reinforces the importance of the limbic network's role in storage.[109,420,421]

The neurochemistry within the limbic network is very complex and will be discussed within the next large section, but even without a keen understanding of the specific chemistry, therapists need to recognize behavior and mood changes within the client. These changes often signal neurochemical problems affecting the individual's motor system. If medical intervention includes medicine, pharmacists should be able to explain how those behaviors are being regulated by pharmacological intervention. Literature is now reporting that what were once thought idiopathic seizures are now believed to be neurochemical imbalances with the limbic structure and may someday be controlled with medications that directly affect the immune system.[422]

Ventricular Swelling after Spinal Defects in Utero, Central Nervous System Trauma, and Inflammation (See Chapters 15, 24, and 26). Although the effects of ventricular swelling after trauma, inflammation, and in utero cerebrospinal malformations are not discussed in great detail in the literature with respect to limbic involvement, the proximity of the lateral and third ventricle to limbic structures cannot be ignored. It is common knowledge that most people exposed to hot, humid weather begin to swell; become more irritable, less tolerant, and moody; and may complain of headaches. Some people become aggressive, others lethargic. All these behaviors are linked to some extent with limbic function. Thus, ventricular swelling causing hydrocephalus, whether caused by trauma, inflammation, or obstruction, would potentially affect the limbic structures. Reported behavioral changes such as seizures, memory and learning problems, personality alterations, alertness, dementia, and amnesia can be tied to direct or indirect limbic activity.[56]

Summary of Clinical Problems Affected by Limbic Involvement. It is easy to identify limbic problems when the behaviors deviate drastically from normal responses. It is much more difficult to determine subtle behavior shifts in clients. The therapist should be sensitive to these minor mood shifts because they may represent early signs of future problems. Similarly, noting that a particular client is always irritable and has difficulty learning on hot days should help direct the therapist toward establishing a treatment session that regulates humidity and temperature to optimize the learning environment. The limbic network is not just a neurochemical bundle of nuclei and axons found within the brain. It is a pulsating center that links perception of the world and the way an individual responds to that perception. Quality of life is a value, and that value has a strong limbic component. If functional outcomes leading to maintaining or improving the quality of life of our clients is the goal of both physical and occupational therapy,[291,423,424] then the limbic network is no less important during examination, evaluation, prognosis, and intervention than the motor system itself.

THE NEUROSCIENCE OF THE LIMBIC NETWORK

Basic Anatomy and Physiology

A brief overview of the anatomy and physiology of the limbic network is presented in the following sections. The reader is referred to a variety of textbooks and websites for a more in-depth understanding of this system[56,119] and how higher thought might be much more complex than previously identified.[44,68,425-427]

Basic Structure and Function

The limbic network can best be visualized as consisting of cortical and subcortical structures with the hypothalamus located at the central position (Figures 5-13 and 5-14). The hypothalamus is surrounded by the circular alignment of the subcortical limbic structures vitally linked with one another and the hypothalamus. These structures are the amygdaloid complex, the hippocampal formation, the nucleus accumbens, the anterior nuclei of the thalamus, and the septal nuclei (see Figure 5-13). These structures are again surrounded by a ring of cortical structures collectively called the "limbic lobe," which includes the orbitofrontal cortex, the cingulate gyrus, the parahippocampal gyrus, and the uncus. Other neuroanatomists also include the olfactory system and the basal forebrain area (see Figure 5-14). Vitally linked and often included in the limbic network as the "mesolimbic" part is the excitatory component of the reticular activating system and other brain stem nuclei of the midbrain. Some consider components of the midbrain a very important region for emotional expression.[86] Derryberry and Tucker[86] found that attack behavior aroused by hypothalamic stimulation is blocked when the midbrain is damaged and that midbrain stimulation can be made to elicit "attack behavior" even when the hypothalamus has been surgically disconnected from other brain regions. Recent research has clearly identified the neurochemical precursors to this aggressive behavior.[53,56,428-430] This "septo-hypothalamic-mesencephalic" continuum, connected by the medial forebrain bundle, seems to be vital to the integration and expression of emotional behavior.[431] The linking of other brain structures to emotions came initially from the work of Papez,[367] who first identified the hippocampal-fornix circuit. He saw this as a way of combining the "subjective" cortical experiences with the emotional hypothalamic contribution. Earlier, Broca[71] labeled the cingulate gyrus and hippocampus "circle" as "the great limbic lobe." Today, the concept of the limbic network and its interaction with sensory inputs and motor expression has become extremely complex.[432] Mood can change motor output, and motor activity can change mood.[421,433]

Klüver and Bucy[434] linked the anterior half of the temporal lobes and the amygdaloid complex to the limbic network. They showed changes in behavior, with specific loss of the amygdaloid complex and anterior hippocampus input, resulting in (1) restless overresponsiveness, (2) hyperorality of examining objects by placing them in the mouth, (3) psychic blindness of seeing and not recognizing objects and the possible harm they may entail, (4) sexual hyperactivity, and (5) emotional changes characterized by loss of aggressiveness. These changes have been named the *Klüver-Bucy syndrome* (see Chapter 13).[435] Myriad connections link the amygdala to the olfactory pathways, the frontal lobe and cingulate gyrus, the thalamus, the hypothalamus, the septum, and the midbrain structures of the substantia nigra, locus coeruleus, periaqueductal gray matter and the reticular formation. The amygdala receives feedback from many of these structures it projects to by reciprocal pathways.

At the heart of the limbic network is the hypothalamus. The hypothalamus, in close reciprocal interaction with most

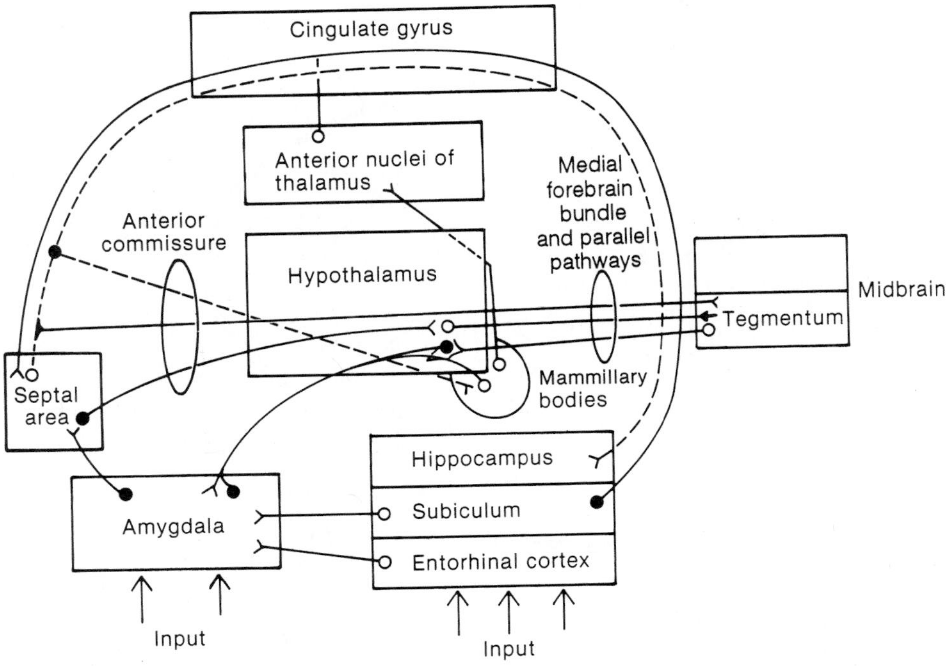

Figure 5-14 ■ Limbic network circuitry with parallel and reverberating connections and with medial forebrain bundle.

centers of the cerebral cortex and the amygdala, hippocampus, pituitary gland, brain stem, and spinal cord, is a primary regulator of autonomic and endocrine functions and controls and balances homeostatic mechanisms. Autonomic and somatomotor responses controlled by the hypothalamus are closely aligned with the expression of emotions.[429,436-438]

In the temporal lobe, anteromedially is the amygdaloid complex of nuclei, with the hippocampal formation situated posterior to it. Located medial to the amygdala is the basal forebrain nuclei, which receive afferent neurons from the reticular formation, the hypothalamus, and the limbic cortex. From this basal forebrain, efferents project to all areas of the cerebral cortex, the hippocampus, and the amygdaloid body, providing an important connection between the neocortex and the limbic network. These nuclei represent the center of the cholinergic system, which supplies acetylcholine to limbic and cortical structures involved in memory formation. Depletion of acetylcholine in clients with Alzheimer disease relates to their memory loss.[192,320,321,439]

Interlinking the Components of the System

The limbic network has many reciprocating interlinking circuits among its component structures, which provide for much functional interaction and also allow for continuing adjustments with continuous feedback (Figure 5-15).[56,429] The largest pathway is the fornix.[440]

Another limbic pathway is the stria terminalis, which originates in the amygdaloid complex and follows a course close to the fornix to end in the hypothalamus and septal regions. The amygdala and the septal region are also connected by a short direct pathway called the *diagonal band of Broca.* A third pathway, the uncinate fasciculus, runs between the amygdala and the orbitofrontal cortex.[56,441,442]

The medial forebrain bundle and other parallel circuits (see Figure 5-14) are vital connections of the limbic network.[443] These pathways course through the lateral hypothalamus to terminate in the cingulate gyrus in its ascending limb and in the reticular formation of the midbrain in its descending part; these pathways have strong interconnections and control over the periaqueductal gray area.[192] These links enable the limbic network itself and the non–limbic-associated structures to act as one neural task system. No portion of the brain, whether limbic or nonlimbic, has only one function.[56] Each area acts as an input-output station. At no time is it totally the center of a particular effect, and each site depends on the cooperation and interaction with other regions. For therapists the concept of neuroplasticity within the motor system is incorporated into our theories of motor learning, but we still have difficulty integrating sensory, emotional, and motor components as interactive elements in motor performance. Yet research is identifying that these neurocircuitries are present and interactive.[444]

The parvicellular reticular formation (PCRF, or lateral medullary reticular formation), together with the nucleus tractus solitarius, receives both vestibular and nonvestibular input from the cortex, cerebellum, and limbic network and is considered functionally as the vomiting center. It also receives input from the area postrema (floor of the fourth ventricle), which contains the chemoreceptor region for the production of vomiting in response to noxious chemicals. Commissural fibers from the vestibular nuclei complexes run through the PCRF and connect the vestibular nucleus to the reticular formation through axon collaterals. The PCRF also projects fibers to the parabrachial nuclei that contain the respiratory centers and to the hypoglossal nucleus.[378] Visceral autonomic input from multiple sources, including the vestibular nuclei, converges in the parabrachial nucleus. The locus ceruleus and autonomic brain stem nuclei also receive vestibular nuclear input.[234,445-448] Thus, cardiovascular activity and respiration (brain stem–mediated autonomic

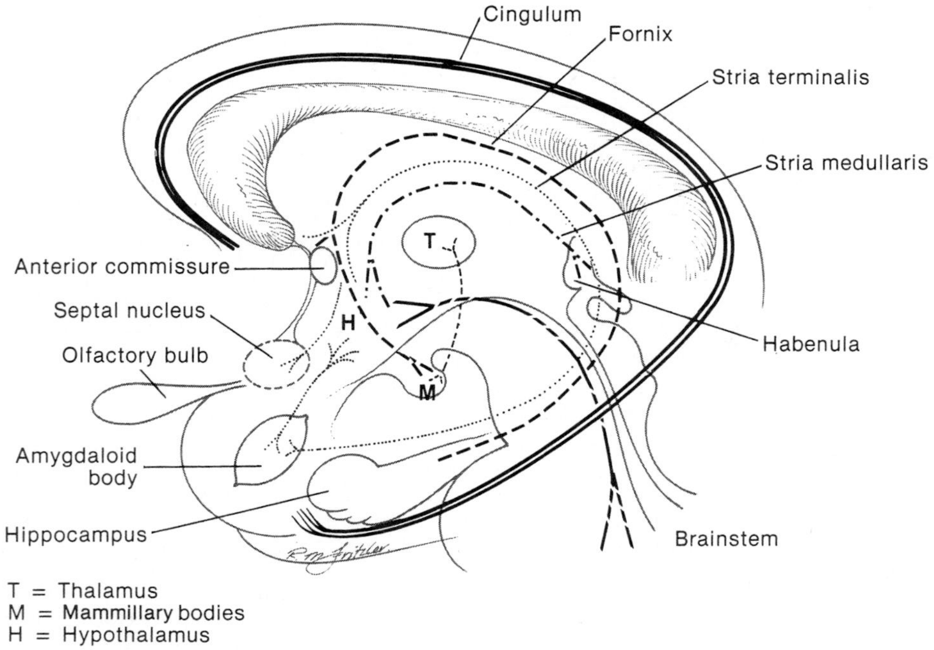

Figure 5-15 ■ Interlinking neuron network within the limbic network. (Adapted from Kandel ER, Schwartz JH, Jessell TM: *Principles of neural science,* ed 4, New York, 2000, McGraw-Hill.)

activity), as well as vomiting, are highly influenced by the status of the vestibular system. If we could understand how cold to the neck or forehead, pressure to the wrist, or taste or olfactory input of ginger interacts with known autonomic reactions and nausea in response to chronic vestibular or interneuronal connections problems, the synthesis of many aspects of health care delivery would no longer be a mystery. Obviously, these older treatment techniques are effective and have been for thousands of years, but to today's researchers the "why" drives the desire to better understand the neuromechanisms underlying the observable responses. There are three different types of drugs that neuroanatomically suppress or modulate vestibular input and thus have a dramatic effect on dizziness and nausea.[449]

Research involving functional MRI (fMRI) supports the concept that there is increased activity within the inferior frontal cortex when nausea is induced by either vestibular stimulation or ingestion of an emetic.[450] This research verifies that there is a strong interconnection among vestibular input, limbic nuclei, and autonomic responses.[451]

There are also connections between the parabrachial nucleus and higher brain centers, including the amygdala, which is known to be critical in the development of conditioned avoidance, such as found in agoraphobia, as an example. Thus, vestibular input results in a sensory stimulus that may induce a state of general autonomic discomfort as a trigger of avoidance that precedes the onset of a panic attack.[378,445,451,452]

Vestibular firing rates are modulated and regulated from the DRN of the midbrain and rostral pons. The DRN is the largest producer of serotonin in the brain and explains the significant linkage between vestibular dysfunction and anxiety, and sleep deprivation and anxiety.[237]

Vestibular lesions in animals result in dramatic changes in the morphology and function of the hippocampus. Of note is that bilateral vestibular lesions have been associated with hippocampal atrophy. The hippocampus is responsible for spatial and gravitational orientation, cognition, learning, and memory (spatial and nonspatial).[379-387]

During the past decade anatomical pathways have been identified that are descending motor tracts that terminate in the caudal brain stem and spinal cord.[453-455] These pathways help modulate the activity level of somatic and autonomic motor neurons. Some of these tracts receive direct and indirect afferent information from the periphery and are part of the interneuronal projection system to motor neurons. They are found in the caudal brain stem, in the spinal cord, and between the two and play a role in the generation of fixed action patterns such as biting and swallowing, which have a strong emotion context linked to the motor program.[456,457] Some of the pathways are linked with the ventromedial and lateral systems, identified for many years as part of the proximal and axial and distal motor control system, modulated by a variety of structures.[192,457] They connect the limbic network to the brain stem and spinal neuronal pools. These tracts do not seem to synapse on what would be considered true motor nuclei of the brain stem (e.g., red nucleus, vestibular nuclei, lateral reticular nuclei, interstitial nuclei of Cajal, or inferior olive). However, these pathways do connect with raphe nuclei, periaqueductal gray matter, and locus coeruleus. The medial components of these tracts originate within the medial portion of the hypothalamus, and the lateral portion originates in the limbic network (lateral hypothalamus, amygdala, and bed nucleus of the stria terminalis). The prefrontal area may be the master controller over this regulatory system.[458-461] The functional motor implication of these tracts is determined by whether the fibers project as part of a medial or lateral descending system. The medial system, through the locus coeruleus, periaqueductal gray matter, and raphe spinal pathways, plays a role in the general level of activity of both somatosensory and motor neurons. Thus the emotional brain or limbic network has an effect on both somatosensory input and motor output. These fibers can alter the level of excitation to the first synapse of somatosensory information, thus altering the processing or importance of that information as it enters the nervous system. Similarly, it can alter the level of motor generators involved in motor expression, which may account for the extension with anger and flexion with depression. The lateral system seems to be involved in more specific motor output related to emotional behavior and may explain some of the loss of fine motor skill when one is placed in an emotional situation such as competition. To differentiate whether the tonal conditions of a client are a result of limbic imbalance or problems within the traditionally accepted motor system, the clinician would need to observe the emotional state and how it changes within the client. If the abnormal state consistently alters with mood shifts, then limbic involvement causing motor control disturbances would be identified. Human social behavior requires motor expression, yet that behavior is driven through the limbic circuitry.[444,462-464] Neuroimaging has helped to reduce uncertainty concerning the anatomical pathways, and neurochemistry has widened the possibilities of variations across synaptic connections.[465-467]

Neurobiology of Learning and Memory

Functional Applications for an Intact System

"Ultimately, to be sure, memory is a series of molecular events. What we chart is the territory within which those events take place."[123] Although expressed more than four decades ago, these words are still accurate. They were expressed by a master clinician and researcher, a clinician who watched behavior, emphasized neuroscience, stressed accurate documentation, and always was respectful and aware of patient interaction and how that affected motor behavior.

The brain stores sensory and motor experiences as memory. In processing incoming information, most sensory pathways from receptors to cortical areas send vital information to the components of the limbic network. For example, extensions can be found from the visual pathways into the inferior temporal lobe (limbic network).[56,468,469] Visual information is "processed sequentially" at each synapse along its entire pathway, in response to size, shape, color, and texture of objects. In the inferior temporal cortex, the total image of the item viewed is projected. In this way the sensory inputs are converted to become "perceptual experiences." This also applies to other sensory stimuli, such as tactile, proprioceptive, and vestibular. The process of translating the integrated perceptions into memory occurs bilaterally in the limbic network structures of the amygdala and the hippocampus.[56,470-481]

Before the limbic network's impact on learning and memory can be delved into, a clear understanding of what is meant by these functions is needed. Current theories support a "dual memory system" that uses different pathways in the nervous system. Terms such as *verbal* and *nonverbal, habit* versus *recognition, intrinsic* and *extrinsic,* and *procedural* and *declarative* have been given to these two memory systems. These systems do not operate autonomously, and many therapeutic activities seem to combine these memory systems to achieve functional behavior.[56] In reality, the complexity of memory is not a two-category system. Verbal and nonverbal memory both interact with declarative function.[482] Even within spatial memory, additional areas of integration and parallel circuitry have been identified.[483,484]

For this discussion, two specific categories of learning—procedural and declarative—will be used, although in today's neuroscience environment, the terms *implicit* and *explicit memory* are used as frequently. Both categories of learning have been correlated to limbic function.[485-487] Declarative (explicit) memory entails the capability to recall and verbally report experiences. This recall requires deliberate conscious effect, whereas the procedural counterpart is the recall of "rules, skills, and procedures (implicit),"[56] which can be recalled unconsciously.

Procedural learning is vital to the development of motor control. A child first receives sensory input from the various modalities through the thalamus, terminating at the appropriate sensory cortex. That information is processed, a functional somatosensory map is formulated,[124,488] and the information is programmed and relayed to the motor cortex. From there, it is sent to both the basal ganglia and the cerebellum to establish plans for postural adaptations, refinement of motor programs, and coordination of direction, extent, timing, force, and tone necessary throughout the entire sequence of the motor act. Storage and thus retrieval of memory of these semiautomatic motor plans are thought to occur throughout the motor control system.[56] The complexity of this process has had an impact on the study of motor control and variables that might affect that control.[489]

The frontal lobe, basal ganglia, and cerebellum are critical nuclei for changing and modulating existing programs.[56] Many interlocking neuronetworks establish pathways allowing for the conceptualization of research on motor theory concepts of reciprocity, distributed function, consensus, and so on (see Chapter 4). Procedural learning and memory do not *necessitate* limbic network involvement as long as an emotional value is not placed on the task. This memory deals with skills, habits, and stereotyped behaviors. This motor system is involved in developing procedural plans used in moving us from place to place or holding us in a position when we need to stop.[56]

Unlike procedural learning and memory, declarative (explicit) learning and memory require the wiring of the limbic network. Recent literature has clearly identified that the basal ganglia and cerebellum both play roles in cognitive function, especially as it relates to category learning tasks.[490] This type of learning is closely associated with limbic function, further identifying the complexity of what was considered two entirely separate systems. Declarative thought deals with factual, material, semantic, and categorical aspects of higher cognitive and affective processing. A strong emotional and judgmental component is linked with declarative thought. Thus as soon as a motor behavior has value placed on the act, it becomes declarative as well as procedural, and the limbic network may become a key element in the success or failure of that movement.[491,492] Most functional tasks or activities practiced in a clinical setting have value attached to them. That value can be clearly seen by observing the emotional intent placed on the activity by the client.[493]

The two reverberating or reciprocal pathways, or circuits, within the limbic network most intimately involved in declarative learning are (1) the amygdaloid, dorsomedial thalamic nucleus, and cortical pathways and (2) the hippocampal, fornix, anterior thalamic nucleus, and cortical pathways.

The hippocampus may be more concerned with sensory and motor signals relating to the external environment, whereas the amygdala is concerned more with those of the internal environment. They both contribute in relation to the significance of external or internal environmental influences.[475,494-499] The hippocampus is rich in stem cells and may be a primary nuclear mass that directs the bodily systems to heal after injury. This is especially true when the external environment is enriched and nurtures the emotional environment for that healing.[500,595]

The amygdaloid circuits seem to deal with strongly emotional and judgmental thoughts, whereas the hippocampal circuits are less emotional and more factual. The amygdala may be more involved in emotional arousal and attention, as well as motor regulation, whereas the hippocampus may deal with less emotionally charged learning. These limbic circuits seem crucial in the initial processing of material that leads to learning and memory. Once the thought has been laid down within the cortical structures, retrieval of that specific intermediate and long-term memory does not seem to require the limbic network, although new associations will need to be run through the system.[56,471,473,475]

A third component in the memory pathway involves the medial diencephalon, a structure that contains the thalamic nucleus. When this region is destroyed by neurotrauma such as strokes, neoplasms, infections, or chronic alcoholism, global amnesias result, owing to the destruction of the amygdala and hippocampus. The amygdala and hippocampus send fibers to specific target nuclei in the thalamus, and the destruction of these tracts also causes the same amnesic effect. It appears that the limbic network and the diencephalon cooperate in the memory circuits. The medial diencephalon seems to be another relay station along the pathway that leads from the specific sensory cortical region to the limbic structures in the temporal lobe to the medial diencephalic structures and ends in the ventromedial part of the prefrontal cortex (Figure 5-16).[56,501,502]

As shown in Figure 5-16, memories may be stored in the sensory cortex area, where the original sensory input was interpreted into "sensory impressions." Today, concepts regarding memory storage suggest that declarative memory is stored in categories similar to a filing system. Those categories or files seem to be stored in several cortical areas bilaterally depending on the context.[503,504] This system allows for easy retrieval from multiple areas. Memory has stages and is continually changing. It was once thought that the hippocampus only dealt with long-term memory, but it is now accepted that it also supports multi-item working memory.[505] To go from short-term to long-term memory, the brain must physically change its chemical structure (a plastic phenomenon). Memory first begins with a representation

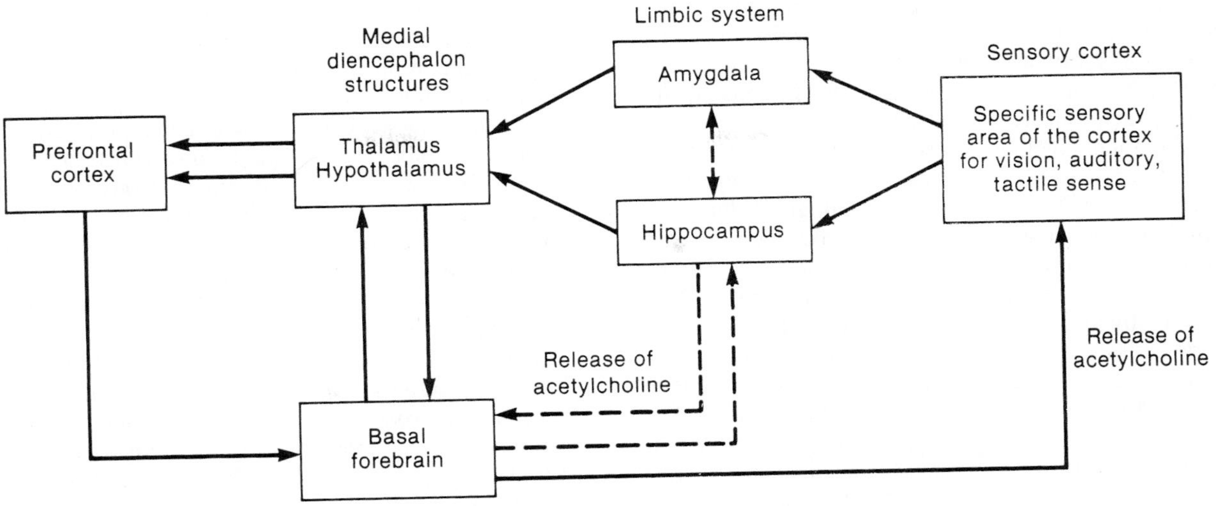

Figure 5-16 ■ The basal forebrain closes the circuit and causes changes in sensory area neurons, which could lead to correct perception and stored memory. This is neurochemical dependent.

of information that has been transformed through processing of perceptual systems. The transferring of this new memory into a long-lasting chemical bond requires the neuronetwork of the limbic complex. Owing to the multiple tracts or parallel circuits in and out of the limbic network and throughout neocortical systems, clients, even with extensive lesions, can often learn and store new information.[56,506] This may also explain why damage to the limbic network structures does not destroy existing memory nor make it unavailable because it is actually stored in many places throughout the neocortex. The circular memory circuit illustrated in Figure 5-16 shows only one system. The reader must remember that many parallel circuits function simultaneously. The circular memory circuit shown reverts to the original sensory area after activation of the limbic structures to cause the necessary neuronal changes that would inscribe the event into retrievable stored memory.[507] This information can be recognized and retrieved by activation of storage sites anywhere along the pathway.[56,508]

The last station or system to be added to the circuit is the "basal forebrain cholinergic system," which delivers the neurochemical acetylcholine to the cortical centers and to the limbic network, with which it is richly linked. The loss of this neurotransmitter is linked to memory malfunctioning in Alzheimer disease. Currently, many chemicals are being studied for their influence on brain structures and specially limbic structures.[509,510] Similarly, loss of this cholinergic system plays a key role in dementia problems in Parkinsonism.[511] Performance of visual recognition memory can be augmented or impaired by administration of drugs that enhance or block the action of acetylcholine.[512-514]

It has also been shown that the amygdala and hippocampus are interchangeably involved in recognition memory.[515] The hippocampus is vital for memory of location of objects in space, whereas the amygdala is necessary for the association of memories derived through the various senses with a specific recognition recall. For example, a whiff of ether might bring to mind a painful surgical experience or the sight of some food may cause a recall of its pleasant smell. Removal of the amygdala brings out the behavior shown in Klüver-Bucy syndrome. For clients with this neurological problem, familiar objects do not bring forth the correct associations of memories experienced by sight, smell, taste, and touch and relate them to objects presented.[516] Association of previously presented stimuli and their responses appear to be lost. Animals without amygdaloid input had different response patterns that ignored previous fears and aversions. Thus the amygdala adds the "emotional weight" to sensory experience. Loss of the amygdala takes away many positive associations and potential rewards, thereby altering the shaping of perceptions that lead to memory storage.

When stimuli are endowed with emotional value or significance, attention is drawn to those possessing emotional significance, selecting these for attention and learning. This would give the amygdala a "gatekeeping" function of selective filtering. The amygdala may enable emotions to influence what is perceived and learned by reciprocal connection with the cortex. Emotionally charged events will leave a more significant impression and subsequent recall. The amygdala alters perception of afferent sensory input and thereby affects subsequent actions.[126,517,518]

In the human, memory functioning has been associated with the phenomenon of long-term potentiation observed in hippocampal pathways.[56] This potentiation of synaptic transmission, lasting for hours, days, and weeks, occurs after brief trains of high-frequency stimulation of hippocampal excitatory pathways. Whether this phenomenon is caused by alteration at the presynaptic or postsynaptic terminals has not been established, and the complexity continues to evolve.[250] The question remains whether there is an increased amount of neurotransmitter released presynaptically (glutamate) or whether the expected amount is producing a heightened postsynaptic response. Or, are both sites involved[56]? Even a third hypothesis regarding nonsynaptic neurotransmission or exocytoses with receptor sites on the surface of neurons beyond postsynaptic sites may help guide our understanding of memory and memory storage in the future.[56,192] Recent literature has linked a neurotropic factor usually considered for long-term potentiation within the hippocampus as a factor in amygdala-dependent learning, thus reiterating the interaction between these two nuclei and their role in memory and learning.[126]

Learning and memory evoke alterations in behavior that reflect neuroanatomical and neurophysiological changes.[56,115] These alterations include the phenomenon of long-term potentiation as an example of such changes. The hippocampus demonstrates the importance of input of long-term potentiation in associative learning. In this type of learning, two or more stimuli are combined. Tetanizing of more than one pathway needs to occur simultaneously. When only one pathway is tetanized, the effect is decreased synaptic transmission. Long-term potentiation, requiring the cooperative action of numbers of coactive fibers, is engendered and formed by the "associative" interaction of afferent inputs. Thus, long-term potentiation serves as one model for understanding the neural mechanism for associative learning. Interacting with this neural mechanism are hormones,which, combined with stress, can change the specific circuitry active during the experience.[519] As our understanding of the complexity of the limbic network evolves, limbic responses to input stimuli need to be differentiated from limbic memory and initiation of a response without the stimuli. Recent research has shown that the amygdala is not only involved in learning related to emotional experiences but is also responsible for changing motor expression or conditioned response generated as part of an autonomic fear expression.[444,520]

Learning and Memory Problems after Limbic Involvement

For initial declarative learning and memory, the combination of hippocampus and amygdala of the limbic network is required.[56] For memory formation to occur, there must be a storing of the "neural representation" of the stimuli in the association and the processing areas of the cortex. This storage occurs when sensory stimuli activate a "cortico-limbo-thalamo-cortical" circuit.[56] Although there is not one single all-purpose memory storage system, this circuit serves as the "imprinting mechanism," reinforcing the pathway that activated it. On subsequent stimulation, a stimulus recognition or recall would be elicited. In associative recall, stored representations of any interconnected imprints could be evoked simultaneously.[56]

A vital processing area for all sensory modalities is located in the region of the anterior temporal lobe. This area is directly linked with the amygdala and indirectly with the hippocampus. The hippocampus and amygdala are also linked both structurally and functionally to each other and to specific thalamic nuclei. Clients with temporal epileptic seizures and whose temporal lobes have been surgically removed develop global anterograde amnesia—that is, amnesia develops for all senses, and no new memories can be formed. Experimental removal of only the hippocampus does not bring about these changes, although processing is slowed down. When both the hippocampus and the amygdala are removed bilaterally, the amnesia is both retrograde and global. It is postulated that the amygdala is the area of the brain that adds a "positive association," the reward part to stimuli received and passed through processing. In this way, stimulus and reward are associated by the amygdala, and an emotional value is placed on them.[521,522]

It appears that limbic involvement in the declarative memory creates a chemical bond that allows cortical storage of "stimulus representation" necessary for subsequent recognition and recall of the information.[56,471,473,474,494]

When declarative and procedural learning from a clinical reference is analyzed, a separation of functional mediation can be observed. Clients with brain lesions localized in the limbic network components of the amygdala and hippocampus have the ability to acquire and function with "rule-based" games and skills but have lost the capacity to recall how, when, or where they gained this knowledge or to give a description of the games and skills learned. Relating this to clinical performance, clients may develop the skill in a functional activity but not the problem-solving strategies necessary to associate danger or other potentially harmful aspects of a situation that may develop once out of the purely clinical setting.[212,428,523-525] Similarly, if a client needs to learn a procedural task such as walking, transfers, eating, and so on, it may be extremely important to direct the attention off the task while the task is being practiced procedurally. As knowledge about the complexity of memory evolves, the clear dichotomy between explicit and implicit learning or declarative and procedural learning is being questioned by current research.[526] This study clearly demonstrates that anterograde amnesia affects learning that is dependent on combining a novel association with the development of memory compared with its accessibility to consciousness. As the specificity and generalizability of memory come under scrutiny, a question arises regarding the differentiation of semantic memory from music perception, music production, and music memory.[527] If emotional and associational aspects of music memory are different from declarative memory and if both are different from procedural memory, then perhaps music may be used to activate existing robust and rich neural networks linking different kinds of memory and learning, and/or elicit neuroplasticity potentials, to address therapeutic goals.[528]

Neurochemistry

Discussion of the limbic network's intricate regulation of many neurochemical substances is not within the scope of this chapter. Yet therapists need to appreciate how potent this system can be with respect to neurochemical reactions. The amount of research reflecting new understanding of the role of neurochemistry in brain function is inundating the pharmacological research literature on a monthly basis.[479,529-536]

The hypothalamus, the physiological center of the limbic network (see Figures 5-2 and 5-14), is involved in neurochemical production and is geared for passage of information along specific neurochemical pathways.

Squire and colleagues[537] consider it the major motor output pathway of the limbic network, which also communicates with every part of this system. Certain nuclei of the hypothalamus produce and release neuroactive peptides that have a long-acting effectiveness as neuromodulators. As such, they control the levels of neuronal excitation and effective functioning at the synapses. By their long-lasting effects, they regulate motivational levels, mood states, and learning. These peptide-producing neurons extend from the hypothalamic nuclei to the ANS components and to the nuclei of the limbic network, where they modulate neuroendocrine and autonomic activities. The importance of these neuropeptides is being recognized as research begins to unravel the mysteries of the limbic network's role in the regulation of affective and motivated behaviors.[56,140,192,538-540] Lesions in the medial hypothalamus affect hormone production and thus alter regulation of many hormonal control systems.[56] For example, clients with medial hypothalamic lesions may have huge weight gain because of the increase of insulin in the blood, which increases feeding and converts nutrients into fat. Similarly, this weight gain may be caused by hyperphagic responses resulting from the loss of satiety. General hyperactivity and signs of hostility after minimal provocation can also be observed. These problems are often encountered in patients with head trauma.

Lesions in the lateral hypothalamus lead to damage of dopamine-carrying fibers that begin in the substantia nigra and filter through the hypothalamus to the striatum. Lesions, either along this tract or within the lateral hypothalamus, lead to aphagia and hypoarousal. Decreased sensory awareness contributing to sensory neglect is also present in lateral hypothalamic lesions. The decreased awareness may be caused by a decrease of orientation to the stimuli versus awareness of the stimuli once they are brought to conscious attention. These lesions cause the client to exhibit marked passivity with decreased functioning. Bilateral infarcts within the mammillothalamic tract create an acute Korsakoff syndrome.[541]

As noted earlier, depression is clearly identified as a limbic function. A functional deficiency in monoamines, especially serotonin, is hypothesized to be a primary cause of depression.[542,543] The serotonin systems originate in the rostral and caudal raphe nuclei in the midbrain. Ascending serotonergic tracts start in the midbrain and ascend to the limbic forebrain and hypothalamus; they are concerned with mood and behavior regulation. Damage with direct or indirect limbic involvement results in the client exhibiting depression. Descending pathways to the substantia gelatinosa are involved in pain mechanisms and have also been linked through a complex sequence of biochemical steps to the increased sensitization of the presynaptic terminals of the cutaneous sensory neurons, leading to a hyperactive withdrawal reflex or hypersensitivity to cutaneous input.[56] This would account for the behavior patterns seen in clients with head trauma, when the therapist sees a flexed posture with a withdrawn or depressed affect yet with an extremely sensitive tactile system.

It is hypothesized that the underlying pathophysiological mechanism of one form of schizophrenia involves an excessive transmission of dopamine within the mesolimbic tract system.[56] The dopaminergic cell bodies are located in the ventral tegmental area and the substantia nigra. Some of these neurons project to the limbic network. These projections go to the nucleus accumbens, the stria terminalis nuclei, parts of the amygdala, and the frontal entorhinal and anterior cingulate cortex. It is the projection to the nucleus accumbens that seems critical because of its influence over the hippocampus, frontal lobe, and hypothalamus. This nucleus may act as a filtering system with respect to affect and certain types of memory, and the dopaminergic projections may modulate the flow of neural activity.[56] The masked facies caused by the impaired motor activity seen in clients with Parkinson disease and the paranoid-schizophrenic behaviors observed in some clients with CNS damage may directly reflect these mesolimbic dopaminergic systems.

The specific roles of the noradrenergic pathway are numerous and affect almost all parts of the CNS. The center for the noradrenergic pathways is located within the caudal midbrain and upper pons. Its nucleus is referred to as the *locus coeruleus*. This nucleus sends at least five tracts rostrally to the diencephalon and telencephalon.[56] Of specific interest for this discussion are the projections to the hippocampus and amygdala. The axons of these neurons modulate an excitatory effect on the regions where they terminate.[56] Thus the activation of this system will heighten the excitation of the two nuclei within the limbic network intricately involved in declarative learning and memory. Hyperactivation may cause overload or the lack of focus of attention.[544] Decreased activity may prevent the desired responses. Attention to task may depend on continuing noradrenergic stimulation. These tracts from the midbrain rostrally play a key role in alertness. The correlation of alertness and attention to performance of motor tasks as well as to learning can be demonstrated.[56] Again, these research findings reiterate previous statements regarding a therapist's role in balancing the neurochemistry within the client's limbic network. From a clinical perspective, a therapist will observe a relaxed, motivated, alert participant in the learning environment and will observe better carryover because the chemical interactions will only enhance the learning.

More than 200 neurotransmitters have been identified within the nervous system.[56] How each transmitter and the interaction of multiple transmitters on one synapse affect any portion of the CNS is still unclear. Certainly, some relationships have been identified. Novelty-seeking behavior of the limbic network seems to be dopamine dependent,[545] whereas melatonin receptors seem to coordinate circadian body rhythm.[546] Adrenal corticosteroids modulate hippocampal long-term potentiation.[547] The complexity of this system still challenges many researchers.

In conclusion, the neurochemistry of the limbic network is intricately linked to the neurochemistry of the brain and the body organs regulated by the hypothalamus. All systems within the limbic circuitry seem to be interdependent, with the summation of all the neurochemistry being the determinants of the specific processing of information. Similarly, the interdependence of the limbic network with almost all other areas of the brain and the activities of those areas at any time reflect the complexity of this system.

THE LIMBIC CONNECTIONS TO THE "MIND, BODY, SPIRIT" PARADIGM

As neuroscientists, safe and deep within a Western allopathic model of linear research, establishing efficacy and evidence-based practice for what is taught to new learners is critically important.[290,291,548] Yet there are too many unexplainable behavioral unknowns occurring daily in the clinical environment that cannot be researched using standard Western research tools common to physical or occupational therapists. Identifying with treatment approaches that base their philosophy on energy fields, flow patterns of those fields through the body, rhythms that do not seem to be proven as existing, or planes of consciousness and belief seems to contradict that comfortable groundedness of basic science. Thus for many health care practitioners, denial of all those potential parameters that might affect evaluation and intervention outcomes is an easy way to feel safe and linked to what is believed to be efficacy- or evidence-based practice within respective professions. Most allopathic medical physicians within the clinical environment are the first to reject what seem like irrational claims or ideas regarding philosophical approaches. Therapists are not far behind those physicians with their attitudes and verbal expressions toward both patients and colleagues who bring in ideas regarding potential approaches that seem to be outside of our reductionistic, linear research models used to establish efficacy. In the clinical arena, clinicians are realizing that effectiveness of practice with objective outcome measures is another way to establish evidence. Similarly, effectiveness can be subdivided into variables that pose questions. Researchers might be able to select variables that can be researched to establish efficacy of treatment approaches used within a clinical environment. Western medicine has taught both medical practitioners and therapists to strongly question anything that reflects concepts of energy, healing, or spiritual beliefs with regard to outcomes of therapy. Yet electromagnetic tools have been embraced by physicians and neuroscience researchers in the form of computed tomography, MRI, PET, and fMRI to diagnose and study neurological damage and neuroplasticity. These evaluation and research tools create their own electromagnetic field while the human body is placed within that field.[549,550] Practitioners can still deny that there is a natural energy field and that this field has anything to do with health, but it is getting harder and harder to deny the presence of such a force. All of us have received an electric shock between our body and a metal surface. That shock is called an *electromagnetic charge*, and the voltage depends on the inherent voltage of that individual. Where did this voltage come from? What is meant by *inherent voltage of an individual?* We all have learned that there is a static electromagnetic field around us, but it is very hard to identify how that charge might affect our body systems. As long as practitioners do not inquire about the physics of these energy fields and the bioelectric or biochemical reactions of our human cells to these fields, the idea that the electromagnetic and electrochemical fields have nothing to do with neuroplasticity and changes with patients after neurological insults unfortunately can remain a myth. Over a decade ago, some allopathic physicians stepped out of their established model and developed a subspecialty in psychoneuroimmunology. Checking PubMed for articles from 2012, a reader can find over 1120 published articles under the term *psychoneuroimmunology.* This subspecialty incorporates the relationships among emotion, the endocrine and immune systems, and the CNS and peripheral nervous system.[22,113,114,551] As the limbic neuronetwork intricately links various nuclei that deal with emotion, endocrine production, and autoimmunity, there is little doubt that this system is involved with belief in healing, emotions, and spirituality. "Despite such conceptual progress, the biological, psychological, social and spiritual components of illness are seldom managed as an integrated whole in conventional medical practice."[23]

Fortunately or unfortunately, there are scientists and therapists who are "myth busters" and challenging the rigid paradigm of linear research, stating that there are many more variables and multiple systems involved in neurorecovery or neuroplasticity than have yet been identified. Physicians and neuroscientists studying the effects of disease and neuroplasticity after trauma[549] or application of drugs[552-554] are trying to unravel a complex maze of chemical and electrical reactions at a level of the cell membrane.[44] Quantum physicists are studying the universe and the electromagnetic pull of suns on planets and solar systems on one another.[555-557]

Science is a long way from unraveling the mysteries explored by cellular biologists and quantum physicists and how they might relate to each other. But many scientists trust that there is a relationship. As humans, we are made up of billions of these cells; each cell has a membrane potential and the ability to adapt and change; and they play an important role in the existence of our species. Similarly, the universe is made up of billions of masses; each has some relationship to energy pull, whether that be one solar system in relation to another, one planet in relationship to a sun, one moon in relationship to a planet's oceans, one person in relationship to the gravity on a planet, or one person in relationship to another person. If those cells are what makes a person human, and if what holds the person together is electromagnetic energy, then it is hard to ignore the possibility that one person might affect another person just by being present.[553]

Therapists want to study the interaction of brain responses between a practitioner and the client during a therapeutic treatment session.[558] It is obvious that this interaction cannot be explained by one variable within linear space, nor that it is one variable alone that is causing all change over a linear set in time. Establishing efficacy on what seems to be a multidimensional construct using a basic science research model is not realistic. Thus efficacy research on the totality of the mind, the physical body, and the human spirit eludes basic scientist researchers in a manner similar to the way that researching the effectiveness of intuition eludes psychiatric researchers.

As research practitioners we use various tools to manipulate both the internal and external environments within which our clients function to measure effectiveness of specific or generalized outcomes. Each person is so complex and unique that finding the best combination of tools and environments has a very person-specific answer.[554,559] Thus what we as researchers are trying to do is find evidence that shows that one treatment paradigm has a better chance of creating change than another, without placing rigid restrictions that say all persons will optimally benefit from any one particular approach.[560-567] MRI, PET, and fMRI tools are certainly capable of identifying changes in the CNS after interventions. Even when researchers or clinicians try to control as many variables as possible, many additional external and internal input possibilities exist.

This brings us full circle to the question regarding additional variables that might affect health, well-being, and recovery outcomes from therapeutic interventions.[568-575]

After 30 years of clinical practice and hearing Western physicians say, "Physical therapy and occupational therapy just make the patients *feel* better," it is obvious, first, that many physicians do not understand the depth and breadth of our professions or what is provided to the clients. Second, those physicians do not understand the limbic interconnections to "feel better" and how that might drive the neuroplasticity of the CNS and the autoimmune system's response to disease or pathology.[575-582] Similarly, after many patients have been observed over the last 40 years regaining consciousness, whether the vegetative state lasted 6 months, 9 months, a year, or 4 years, the fact remains that each individual shifted from what might be considered a level 2, 3, or 4 on the Rancho Levels of Cognitive Functioning to a 6, 7, or 8 on the same scale after 5 to 20 minutes. This reality made me ask the question from the beginning of my professional career, "What are the variables that cause changes in these clients?" The answers are not yet fully understood, although the behavioral outcomes keep presenting themselves. Every time a patient comes out of this vegetative state, I [DAU] feel wondrous, emotional, and humbled. Something happens that is far beyond our scientific understanding, something simple but extremely complex, cellular and universal, all at the same time. Similarly, the bond between that therapist and that client is very strong and deeply spiritual. The memory of those patients stays forever embedded in the mind of the therapist even if the clinical environment existed for only 30 minutes. All the words used to explain such clinical experiences link closely to the limbic network and its role in creating change, both within the therapist and the patient; certainly at this time, these experiences fall outside the paradigm of Western medical science. According to a report on the BBC, the use of appropriate fMRIs shows that many individuals in a vegetative state are awake but still have little to no awareness because of the severe brain injury.[583] This explains the fact that a therapist "feels" that a patient is aware but does not explain how the therapist-patient interaction brings that client to a conscious state of attention.

Medical schools and health science programs are becoming increasingly aware of the need to train the practitioners of the future to enter into a healing relationship with the whole patient,[584] a relationship that empowers the patient to engage endogenous healing capacities, even while we work to better understand these mechanisms through both basic and applied research. Master clinicians have long appreciated this dynamic healing relationship, which affects both the therapist and patient. Thus even when our patients can verbally communicate with the therapist, it is still important to listen directly to the body, and on a deeper level, to more subtle input that we do not yet have the ability to describe and quantify with scientific method. It has been demonstrated that even for persons in very low awareness and response states, appropriately selected music can provide time-organized and emotionally meaningful stimuli to gently activate intact neural networks, and to communicate with the person still alive inside the disabled body.[585] The sounds we make and the way we touch communicate to the deeper levels of being and do not require words to convey caring, instill hope, and motivate the will to keep trying to get better.

The success or failure of many forms of alternative medical practice, and for that matter Western allopathic medicine and therapeutic practices, may depend on the limbic network.[557,573,586] At times research can prove unequivocally that certain variables do not show a healing effect, after double blind studies.[587] If a patient "believes" an intervention will work, even if it is a placebo, the chances of success far exceed those when the patient does not think it will work.[588-591] If it is a placebo and the body heals, then logic dictates that the body and the mind did the healing. Similarly, when the drug itself aided in neuroplasticity and change, is it the drug itself or the individual's belief that the drug will work that creates the change or both? How these changes occur is yet to be totally understood, but research substantiates that both neurochemical and neuroelectrical changes occur within an individual's physical body when the individual believes that change is possible.[119,120,570,576,587,590]

When I was a novice therapist, a nurse once said, "I am very glad you are not a nurse because you are so idealistic. You believe these patients in comas are going to wake up and walk out of here. And what is even worse is that most of them do!" That moment should have told me that I would be clashing with allopathic doctrine throughout my professional career, but instead I was confused about the nurse's use of the term *idealistic*. If the patients awoke and walked back into life with function and quality, then should that not be considered a *realistic* expectation? In that same job situation, my boss asked me to treat all the patients who were considered vegetative; once they were awake, my colleagues would treat them from there. My response was, "Emotionally for both the patient and myself, I could not do that. Once I bonded with a person, gained his or her trust, and found the patient was willing and capable of regaining consciousness, I could not just abandon the patient and go on to another person." The significance of that statement took many years to understand, and it was not until I began my study of the limbic network that I truly comprehended the accuracy of that perception, once considered naïve.[570,578,586,592,593] It was not until the writing of this edition that I could shrug off comments such as "This has nothing to do with physical therapy."[3,22,23,60,594]

After 45 years of practice and often treating individuals in front of colleagues in workshop situations, I cannot deny that something more than just "feeling good" occurs during physical or occupational therapy interventions although that feeling good is certainly a limbic response. When working with clients, I find myself feeling very open and bonding in some way that is neither "physical" nor "mental"—and thus the only option left is a definition of "spiritual." If, when treating a patient in a vegetative state, that bond tells me that the patient is lost within another plane of consciousness and wants to regain consciousness as defined by healthy people, and the physical body of the patient seems capable, then the treatment is goal directed, the direction of the intervention is identified, and thus the outcome is selected by the patient. The map has been established, and together the patient and the therapist proceed. As with all therapists, the intervention will be guided by the motor responses and control of the patient and the window within which the patient can run those programs independently. At times, when treating clients in a vegetative state, I feel unable to locate the "spirit"; at other times it feels as if that person has not decided whether to venture to an awake state, but more often I sense a frightened, confused individual who just wants to find her or his way back to what we call "life or reality." Those patients often gain consciousness during therapy. It is not a miracle, nor can I ever say, "I healed something."[595] The term *healing* refers to a concept of "whole." The only person who can regain the structure of the whole is the patient.[596]

As a therapist, I am a teacher or a guide, helping others relearn and regain control over their respective lives. If after a 30-minute treatment session a person regains feeling and control of an extremity 18 years after a CVA or regains functional use of a hand 6 years after incomplete spinal cord injury, there is more to the intervention than merely following a clinical pathway or a treatment regimen geared to all individuals at a specific stage of a disease process or a specific motor impairment.

One variable that always seems to be present when clients achieve dramatic recovery is strong motivation by the patient to retain the control and an appreciation for the instruction on how to do that. A strong bond or compassionate appreciation for each other always seems to be present as another interlocking variable. Thus the clinical question "What is spirituality?" presented itself to me more than 30 years ago. It is a variable that is very difficult to define. That variable, when researched, has been shown to affect health and healing in individuals with health problems. *Spirituality* and *healing* are both words that each individual defines according to her or his own beliefs, cultural experiences, and use of verbal language.[425,426,597-601] The literature is available for those who wish to pursue this topic.[360,516,602-609]

Over the last 5 years since the fifth edition was published, thousands of articles dealing with health, healing, spirituality, energy fields, quality of life, energy medicine, and emotional balance have been published in a large variety of types of journals.[610,611] Within this chapter a system that affects all areas of the CNS and peripheral function has been discussed. How this system is affected by or affects one's spirituality is open for many lifetimes of future study.[612,613] Yet if spirituality affects healing and an individual believes that this potential is available, then this variable may play a critical role in patient compliance, neuroplasticity, and the limbic interface with other treatment procedures.[614,615] Ignoring this variable is no different from ignoring cognitive perceptual deficits when dealing with abnormal motor behavior. Owing to the strong emotional foundation for an individual's spirituality, one could easily assume that the limbic network plays a strong role in establishing and storing memories that reflect these beliefs.

Until we can measure simultaneous synaptic activity of all interactions within the therapist's and the client's CNS, we will not, from a grounded neuroscience efficacy base, be able to demonstrate exactly what occupational, speech, music, cognitive, or physical therapists do, even though we know they play a role.[616] Until then, outcomes need to be measured objectively. Even if interactions seem unmeasurable and subjective, clinicians still need to record the event change in the patient record and not bury that outcome deep somewhere in the subconscious level of the therapist's mind. The mind, the body, and the spirit are connected as a whole. If therapists treat only one part, it may help the whole, but if the whole is treated simultaneously, the outcome is more likely to change the whole.[617,618] The concept is no different from focusing on strengthening an isolated muscle and hoping it will lead to functional use versus strengthening that muscle in functional patterns and in relation to other muscles that also work together within that movement sequence.

After years of clinical experience and thousands of patients responding positively to various interventions, the question arises regarding clinical decision making and choice of interventions. There is not a "variable" that has been identified that guides that decision. It has been shown that humans bring to consciousness about 10% of all incoming information. Yet the human brain is making decisions using 100% of the input information. Given that relationship, quite a bit of human decision making may be based on nonconscious information regarding the external and internal world.[119] Thus the word all neuroscientists shudder over—*intuition*—may to a large extent be the unraveling of that nonconsciously received data.[619] I have effectively taught colleagues how to feel blood pressure and heartbeats of clinical partners by just barely touching the top of the hand, which might be explained by the high level of sensitivity of Meissner corpuscles within our skin.[618] If a clinician can sense an autonomic response such as heart rate when touching a patient's skin, then knowing how the limbic network is interacting within a motor response can also be deduced. This would allow the clinician to modulate the rate used to move the patient during an activity such as bed mobility, while maintaining a consistent state of the motor generators. That steady state should decrease any need for limbic fear by the patient. Fear has been shown to be very detrimental to motor performance.[620-622] Therapists may interpret these tactile responses as intuitive, but they are not. When one clinician seems to know how fast to move the patient and another clinician has no idea how to determine that decision or control that variable, we say it is the *art* of therapy and not the *science*. Yet it is the science of therapy. Similarly, helping someone shift consciousness levels seems similar to hypnosis. The exact identification of these variables is very hard, let alone finding reliable and valid research tools. This may just be a case of one clinician being open to receiving information and processing it. The other therapist, for some reason, is either not receiving or not processing the available information. This is not an example of "intuition."

Intuition has been a source of fascination over centuries. Recently, with consumer dissatisfaction with health care and the assurgency of alternative medical practices, intuition has again sparked the interest of scholars and the public. To many it reflects mystery, magic, and even voodoo. Individuals with a strong ethnic, cultural, and even religious bias may find it hard to scientifically analyze this human strategy. For more than 35 years my husband has answered questions I have posed in my mind. It took at least the first decade for my left brain to actually accept that I was not subvocalizing the thought or that he could not have extrapolated the thought from an environmental stimulus. Yet he consistently has told me he hears me ask the question or state a fact. Obviously, my thoughts have traveled to the primary and associative receiving areas of his left temporal lobe and he "hears" the thought in my voice. The dilemma that confronted me as a scientist is, if the information was not input through his eighth cranial nerve, how did it enter into his system? The answer would seem to be intuition. A definition might be knowing something without entering the data through traditional input systems. The next question is "What is intuition?"

Unfortunately, after 35 years of study, I cannot answer that question. I do acknowledge that it is something, it can be learned, and master clinicians use it as a part of their clinical decision making, even if they choose not to verbalize it to their colleagues or even acknowledge it within their conscious mind. Much research and literature are available regarding intuition.[119,623-646] Yet the answer to that simple question "What is intuition?" is unavailable and does not seem so simple. No answer exists that has shown to be definitively efficacious and reliable, although research over the last 10 years has begun to identify components of intuition.[623-642] It may be that intuition is more than one variable and can be accessed in more than one way. In fact, after studying various alternative medical practices, all using very different interventions based on different philosophies and belief systems, it seems as if all approaches may be tapping into the same human system, just opening to that system through different paradigms.

In the late 1960s, I [DAU] was beginning to present an integrated approach to neurological disabilities and integrating various treatment philosophies using the behavioral responses of patients and known science to guide intervention. I was told at that time that integrating approaches could not be done and that I would potentially injure patients by using approaches from different philosophical techniques. Today, of course, with our understanding of motor control, motor learning, and neuroplasticity, an integrated approach from the 1960s based on a systems model is what we do. I now present the same model when looking at complementary approaches to intervention and the concept of intuition. There are a number of variables that seem to open one's intuition: bonding, being dedicated to the patient, having openness in listening to the patient, letting preconceived knowledge be a springboard from which to expand that knowledge, having not only a willingness to learn but an insatiable appetite to continue learning, and possessing the ability to let go of one's importance and just be another person within the environment. These variables may be the best place for a learner to begin learning how to develop this skill. It would seem as if intuition is like an aptitude. Some individuals come into this life already with a high level of potential, others are nurtured to develop that potential, and still others never have an opportunity or an environment in which to develop those strategies. Some individuals have had strong intuitive senses from childhood but share those experiences with few, if any, other people. Experiencing intuition is an all-knowing experience. One knows something first, then one becomes emotional regarding that knowledge. It is a knowledge that has a "wholeness" component and then has a strong emotional base. For example, I *knew* I was going to lose a parent. Which parent, I did not know, but I moved home for a year to make sure there wasn't anything I should have said to either parent before I went on with my life. A year later I was married and home for a holiday. When I left I cried all the way back to my and my husband's dwelling across the country because I knew I would never see my father again. I was right; he passed 2 weeks before I was to return home. My father had been a very healthy man with no health issue that would indicate any life-threatening health problems. I had known what was going to happen as a whole (intuition) and then had had a very strong emotional response to that intuition. Also, when my brother called to say that our father was critically ill, I had already adjusted to the probability of his loss and was the one individual within the family who could make cognitive decisions or answer press questions by phone. If I were to hazard a guess, the intuitive center is probably in the right anterior temporal lobe owing to the "whole" understanding and its strong emotional connection. If that proves true, it will solidify the limbic network's connection to intuition. Experiences often create the first questions that lead to hypotheses and later to research that establishes efficacy.

Until 40 years ago, I [DAU] hid from most people that aspect of my person because I was becoming a neuroscientist and wanted to be grounded in scientific efficacy like all my colleagues. Unfortunately, my clinical experiences did not allow me to hide that intuitive aspect of my clinical decision making from my family or close colleagues or those colleagues who recognized that something had happened during a treatment that made no sense whatsoever. Those individuals recognized changes within the patient that, although very positive, should not have happened or were very far from our basic scientific understanding. I treated a woman who had a severe head injury and who after 6 months was at a Rancho level III. After 30 minutes of intervention the woman volitionally moved all of her limbs and trunk without cognitive confusion. That motor function and cognition might be partially explained by recent research using fMRI.[583] But something that goes far beyond today's fMRI followed the intervention. I innocently stepped out of the safety of scientific understanding. I shared with my colleagues this woman's medical and social history. That information was critical to their understanding the course of progression of this woman through the rehabilitation process. I discussed the patient's social background, her education, her family, her children, and her husband, who had shot her in the head. This all made perfect sense, until the head of the department asked me how I knew that information. I said, "I read it in the chart." The director informed me that I had not seen the chart. I said, "You told me?" The director responded with, "We did not discuss the case!" I asked if I had been wrong, and the director said "no." In fact, she was amazed at how accurate I had been and just wondered how I had known that about the patient.

At that moment, my life was changed. I could no longer hide whatever this "intuition" was, nor could I truthfully tell colleagues what I had done during interventions without bringing up this topic. Also, I could only tell them ways to develop intuition but had no understanding of the basic neuroscience behind its function. I could not tell anyone exactly what it was because I did not know. That unknown is still present. although some of the variables may have been identified. The future will unravel those answers. What I have found since that day is that "masters," whether they are physicians, therapists, or teachers, often use this additional source of information gathering to help them in their clinical reasoning. I do not make this statement lightly nor without tremendous professional risk. I will leave you with an interaction that solidified my belief that this direction of scientific study needs to be pursued. Two decades ago, I was a keynote speaker at an international neurosurgical conference on brain tumors. I was the token "other," and the only speaker who was not a neurosurgeon. I presented the topic "The Limbic System's Influence on Motor Output." With this audience of 500 neurosurgeons and 50 token others, I, of course, used charts and pictures and based every sentence on efficacy-based scientific research. At dinner that night when all the speakers were together, the master neurosurgeon whom everyone acknowledged asked if he could sit next to me. I was aghast—a little nervous but honored nonetheless. He opened by saying, "I think many physical and occupational therapists are intuitive." With that, I knew him, his life, his experiences, and so on. I let my left brain validate my intuition and said, "Yes, it is like walking into a room, looking at a patient, knowing where and what type of tumor he has, and using instruments such as PET studies to validate what you already know!" He responded with a smile and said, "Yes, it is exactly like that!" I do not need to continue to discuss the fascinating interactions of that night but leave the reader with the thought that even the master of the masters in neurosurgery uses intuition as a variable in clinical decision making, and it gave this man one additional bit of information that his colleagues could not use in clinical reasoning. No physician or therapist uses intuition as the only variable; intuition just gives additional information that helps in the process of clinical reasoning. It would seem as though intuition is highly integrated into the limbic network.

As said previously, intuition is knowing something and as a result experiencing great emotion, such as "I know, thus I fear." If the sequence of events begins with an emotion or fear and leads to what is perceived as knowledge or truth, one might question whether intuition was the driving force behind the belief. When emotions become elevated an individual may progress with "I fear, thus I think I know." Research that looks at intuition assumes that when the limbic network is involved, the experience is highly emotional, and one might argue that an individual can be highly emotionally charged and still be neutral as far as a balance in emotions. Fear is not what drives intuition; instead it is emotional balance. Emotional balance or centering is not a state of being without emotion but rather a heightened state of emotional awareness without emotion, all at the same time. To become truly intuitive, one needs to become emotionally centered. In our everyday world where each of us is overstimulated as a day-to-day experience, this emotional balance is extremely difficult to achieve. It is even harder to find that balance in a clinical arena where patients are arriving with more acute diseases along with chronic secondary problems, often patients' schedules overlap with other patients' time, and therapists not only are limited with time for intervention but also find that the number of allowed visits falls well short for optimal opportunity for learning by the patient. That reality does not mean that the therapists' responsibility has changed. It is always up to the therapist to find those avenues by which better care may be provided within the existing environment. This reality just says that the challenges and questions are enormous. Finding emotional balance within that environment is very hard. Yet intuition seems to be a variable that gives some colleagues additional information that is then used as part of the clinical reasoning process.

Intuition as a variable needs to be identified, studied, researched, and taught once it is clearly understood. It is up to all of us to find the answers to these questions and the solutions to today's clinical problems and develop evidence-based practice to progress into the twenty-first century.[647,648]

The concept of integration of mind, body, and spirit as a critical element in maintaining or regaining quality of life between birth and death is not new.[649-652] Western society has tried to separate this concept into three distinct categories. The mind is made up of perception, cognition, and emotion. The body is made up of all systems external to the nervous system such as peripheral organs, muscles, bones, and skin. Both the peripheral and central motor systems, which control the body, are also included in the concept of body. The last component, the spirit, is a transcendental concept and is thought to depend on individuals' beliefs. Some individuals believe that spirit means belonging to a religious order. Others define spirit or spirituality as beyond religion—the essence that links the person to a greater energy force. For decades this last category has been considered outside the domain of responsibilities of Western allopathic health care delivery and was comfortably relegated to religious leaders or spiritual guides.

Today, everything is changing. Some scientists refer to energy fields around cells; others talk about energy fields around solar systems. Complementary practitioners talk about energy fields around the living organisms. Physicians are being taught cultural sensitivity training while in medical school to be more empathetic to the populations of people they will service. Physical therapy curricula are responsible for creating culturally sensitive professionals.[653] Occupational therapy programs are responsible for including spirituality as one of the competencies a graduate is to have met.[654] None of these professions has identified how these competencies relate to evaluation and intervention outcomes after treatment, but even the accrediting bodies believe they are important. Thus even at the entry level, for student therapists, emphasis is placed on making sure not only that the therapists' limbic systems have become sensitive to spirituality, but also that they be able to identify its significance in their clients' lives. Where does the interaction of the mind, body, and spirit play a critical role in quality-of-life issues and empowerment of the patient? The answers to that question cannot be found within this text or any other text in print today. Individuals with strong beliefs in a specific paradigm that includes spirituality can project the answer to this question, but establishing efficacy is an entirely different issue. Our professions are tethered to research, science, behavioral observations, and current knowledge. We as clinicians can stretch that tether. Much of our early treatments developed from behavioral observations that included individuals' beliefs that clearly required the limbic network for processing, storage, and direct effect on bodily system reactions. If a patient lacks motivation, a therapist knows part of the job is to motivate the person. If the person believes his "God" will heal him, the therapist should never undermine that belief because everyone knows it cannot hurt and often creates a positive change.[655] How that interaction occurs is unknown today, but clinical observation would reinforce that it does help. Because spirituality uses belief and hope, memory of those feelings must be processed and later stored with the help of the limbic network.

These dilemmas exist with every professional dealing with health and wellness and quality-of-life issues. I [DAU] will leave you with one additional example. I spent over 2 months in the ICU a few years ago after a severe fall that caused two fractures to the pelvis, followed by severe internal hemorrhages. To summate the medical problems, I had 18 initial arterial ruptures treated with radiological interventional surgery, followed by four more ruptures 1 week later leading to more surgery. I also had bilateral kidney failure, a large pulmonary embolism on the right side, pulmonary collapse in the left inferior lobe, massive internal infections, infusion of 12 units of blood, thrombophebitis, fevers of over 105° F, very low blood pressure, and low oxygen absorption, along with external bleeds through most external orifices. In addition, the two bleeds destroyed my adrenal glands bilaterally, throwing me into another life-threatening imbalance of chemistry within my body. The doctor kept telling my husband with confidence that I would die. As my husband had been told this many times before, he kept telling the doctor he would wait for 3 days after I had been declared dead before he would accept that conclusion. Two weeks after the initial hospitalization, the doctor came into the room. He shut the door, sat down in a chair, addressed both of us and asked, "I know what medical problems you have had, I know that we did everything medically that we could, but it was not enough, so *how come you are still alive*?" I responded with, "There is a lot more to healing than what we understand, and that is what is fun about being a health professional." Life has taught me the lesson, whether as an intuitive, as a neuroscientist, or as a therapist, that there will be unknowns or mysteries along one's life journey. Sometimes one can solve the problems or answer the questions, but more often than not one just has to file them in memory with the hope that one will sometime find an answer. The unknowns are always present even as answers are discovered. Having those unknowns creates an exciting challenge and adventure for every clinician who has or will have the opportunity to interact with individuals who have been brought into the health care delivery system because of a CNS problem. Those individuals want to be considered as a whole human being even if part of their physical body is dysfunctional. A circle has been drawn, and this chapter needs to end with a question. What is that whole? Refer to Case Study 5-1 as a clinical example.

SUMMARY

The complexity and interwoven neurological arrangement of the limbic network may seem overwhelming. A reader who tries to grasp all parts on first study will feel lost and defeated, which is a true limbic emotion. Thus this chapter has been presented in three parts. The first part introduces the system and its potential clinical application. This section, in and of itself, has many interwoven components, for nothing in the limbic network functions in isolation. Yet the mysteries of this complex neurological network, when identified, may hold the answers to many clinical questions regarding the art and gift of a master clinician. The second part introduces in more detail the basic anatomy and physiology of the limbic network. It is hoped that once the student or clinician has been drawn to the conclusion that this system may be a key to clinical success, she or he might be willing to delve into the science of the system. This path of exploration is challenging, difficult, and frustrating at times but certainly worth the effort once understanding has been achieved. The last section opens up the minds of the readers when and if they so choose to address these unknown variables. The limbic network is very complex, is very interactive with all parts of the human body, and may hold many answers about patients' responses and recovery. The reader's journey has just begun, and the future will open up many more avenues of research and clinical study as well as many more questions.

References

To enhance this text and add value for the reader, all references are included on the companion Evolve site that accompanies this textbook. This online service will, when available, provide a link for the reader to a Medline abstract for the article cited. There are 659 cited references and other general references for this chapter, with the majority of those articles being evidence-based citations.

CASE STUDY 5-1

A 25-year-old first-grade teacher with a history of whiplash has been referred by the neurology department 5 months after a motor vehicle accident with complaints of severe dizziness and imbalance. She is unable to recall the accident; however, there was evidence to suggest that she struck her head on the steering wheel and briefly lost consciousness. Results of diagnostic testing (MRI, electroencephalography) are inconclusive. Medical management to date has been limited to central depressant medications (alprazolam [Xanax], diazepam [Valium]; see Chapter 36). She has received physical therapy since the accident for neck and back pain, which exacerbated her symptoms. She denies specific assessment or treatment of her dizziness or imbalance until this time. Her medical history includes a hospitalization 3 months after the motor vehicle accident with "intractable migraine, postconcussive syndrome." Of note is a previous head injury 2 years before with moderate to severe postconcussive syndrome, including vertigo and migraines. She has been referred for psychological assessment and management and was recently diagnosed with obsessive-compulsive disorder. She is now referred to physical therapy for a full postural control and vestibular assessment. The differential medical diagnosis is postconcussive syndrome, rule out aphysiological performance (psychogenic, secondary gain). The physician believes that a large part of her problem is based within the medical psychiatric domain, but he is willing to widen his paradigm to include other possibilities and obtain additional data to assist in his patient's management. The patient's goal is to eliminate the dizziness and imbalance and return to normal activity and work.

PHASE I: EVALUATION

Unaware of being observed, the patient walks into physical therapy extremely slowly, holding the wall, watching the ground, and stopping periodically to close her eyes. Her color is pale, her build small and thin, and her clothing loose. She is, however, well groomed. Her steps are shortened in length, widened in width, and limited in swing time. She demonstrates no segmental movement of the head or trunk, walking en bloc (rigidly) without arm swing. As she sits down to begin the evaluation session, she smiles. She periodically closes her eyes as people move around her. There is visible extraneous eye movement, although no immediate visualization of nystagmus (eyes opened or closed). She is pleasant and cooperative with no overt signs of anxiety in quiet sitting.

System Impairment

- Dizziness with severe nausea and vomiting (at least once weekly)
- Dizziness Visual Analog Scale 7.5/10 and Dysequilibrium Visual Analog Scale 7.0/10 (with 10 representing the most severe symptoms imaginable)
- Decreased concentration and memory; forgetfulness
- Visual diplopia and blurriness with visual headaches
- Depression of central vestibular function (treated with medication)

Continued

CASE STUDY 5-1—cont'd

- Decreasing body mass as observed by loose clothing and supported by reports of severe nausea
- Emotional stability: fight or flight; in both active F^2ARV and active GAS (autonomic) states:
  - She reported that she was capable of rapid change from a state of calm to fits of rage with her family and other support systems.
  - Anger and rage alternated with reports of depression and avoidance.
  - She reported photophobia with hypersensitivity to light and sound.

Activity: Client Report

- Impaired balance for function, with near falls in dark and eyes-closed environments. Patient reports one true fall in the shower with her eyes closed.
- Impaired balance within visually challenging environments.
- Sleep deprivation and extreme fatigue.
- Long-term stress and sensory intolerance and overstimulation

It is important for a clinician to remember that the long-term *stress* associated with a chronic disability of this nature can result in a decrease in serotonin, which influences the hypothalamus and modulation of the vestibular nuclei through the DRN. Loss of sleep can alter levels of serotonin and other neurotransmitters. A decrease in serotonin results in further depression and *loss of sleep,* resulting in a physiological *fatigue.* It also can result in an increase in sensitization of presynaptic terminals of the cutaneous sensory nerves, contributing to the *sensory bombardment* and overstimulation.[656]

Participation in Life (Client Report)

- She attempted to return to work as a first-grade teacher but had a severe exacerbation of all symptoms in the classroom.
- She is unable to drive and requires assistance for shopping.
- She lives alone in an apartment and is independent in function, modified by her symptoms.
- Disability Rating is 4/5 (recent severe disability, medical leave).[657]
- Dizziness Handicap Inventory (DHI) score is significant for physical and emotional impact of her dizziness, including depression. (Total disability score is 78/100, functional subscore 28/32, emotional subscore 30/40, and physical subscore 20/28.[390])

Based on the signs and symptoms obtained in the intake phase and subjective reporting, the preliminary physical therapy hypothesis would be the presence of a probable vestibular dysfunction of a mixed central and peripheral cause, a sensory integration dysfunction, and anxiety overlay. The patient clearly has limbic network overload. It will be the therapist's responsibility to differentiate that from physical motor system problems with the assessment and treatment. The examination phase is designed to confirm or refute and redirect this hypothesis. (See Chapter 22b for clarification of these specific vestibular tests and measures.)

Oculomotor

Oculomotor examination was performed, with results supportive of the hypothesis of vestibular involvement, although inconclusive for peripheral versus central versus combination.

Gaze instability—Clinical dynamic visual acuity test revealed a significant five- to six-line deterioration in dynamic visual acuity when head was moving, with loss of postural control in posterior-left direction and symptom exacerbation during testing.

Balance Stability

- SOT of sensory balance function[658] showed an across-the-board dysfunction pattern,[14] although results were incomplete because the patient was not able to complete all 18 trials of the test protocol as a result of extreme symptoms (nausea, respiratory, and anxiety symptoms, particularly on conditions 2, 3, 5, and 6).
- Total dependence (overreliance) on visual information for balance stability.
- Center of gravity position shift significantly leftward and anterior of midline.
- Excessive use of a hip strategy for basic equilibrium (versus ankle), even with stable surfaces or the smallest perturbation.
- Inability to effectively:
  - Use somatosensory or vestibular sensory cues on functional demand (reweight)
  - Organize the sensory inputs to the CNS to facilitate appropriate motor output
  - Dampen ANS/vegetative response, particularly in visual-vestibular mismatch conditions (SOT 3 and 6)
- Aphysiological criteria—Aphysiological responses on SOT raw data traces (exaggerated sway frequency and lateral sway responses). Motor Control Test (of automatic motor responses) results would have strengthened conclusions made regarding an aphysiological component but were unavailable to this clinician at the time of the examination.[658]

Function and Gait

Self-selected velocity of 1.82 ft/sec (normal preferred gait speeds in a 20- to 30-year-old woman should be closer to 3.47 ft/sec).[14] The patient watched the floor for the entire distance with no head or trunk or arm movement. Thus vision was clearly directing each step and was adjusted to decrease extraneous visual flow or input. When she was encouraged to focus on a distant object, velocity declined to 1.34 ft/sec and the patient veered consistently leftward 100% of the distance. She could be encouraged to walk at 2.86 ft/sec (normal encouraged gait speeds should approach 6.43 ft/sec), with an increase in instability and a leftward loss of balance, not requiring assistance to regain necessitating assistance.

The interactions of the patient and therapist (limbic bonding, as referred to previously within this chapter) became a critical element in the examination. The patient had to trust the therapist that if she followed the therapist's direction in examination, she would not fall or incur additional symptoms outside her control. The therapist, during the evaluation, empowered the patient to take responsibility for her functional movement while making sure the patient was successful if willing to take the risk. This aspect of the therapeutic interaction is a limbic-neutral technique, and its success or failure will be reflected in the motor responses of the patient.

Confirmatory Tests and Measures

- Intact sensation but extreme hypersensitivity to vibratory input (with strong ANS response)
- Normal strength and range of motion

Multiple rests were required throughout the examination to decrease symptomatology (nausea, increased respiration, sweating) to patient tolerance. Testing reproduced all subjective dizziness, and there was a resultant gross instability with loss of balance in the posterior direction, necessitating assistance. Imbalance, nausea, and anxiety were residual for 10 minutes after testing.

CASE STUDY 5-1—cont'd

In the evaluative phase, the working hypothesis after the examination phase was as follows:

- **Diagnoses** as identified by therapist:
- *Medical*—mixed central and peripheral vestibular presentation without confirmatory medical diagnostics or diagnosis. Further medical workup required.
- *PT Rehabilitation*[291]—Primary Problem: Practice Pattern 5D: Acquired impairment of the central nervous system; Secondary Problem: Practice Pattern 5A: Primary prevention of falls
- **Characterized** by (1) SMD with VOR impairment, probable high gain, with gaze instability, (2) central processing impairment, (3) postural control impairment with somatosensory dependence, and (4) limbic high state with autonomic response to testing procedures and frequent rests required.
- **Prognosis:** Fair for modified community level independence, physiologically complicated by history and chronicity. Improvement intratrial is a positive physiological sign. However, anxiety overlay and history may have psychogenic versus physiological impact on recovery.
- **Red Flags:** Watch for (1) additional central signs, (2) signs of secondary gain, (3) F^2ARV and GAS limbic cascade, or (3) social service issues.

PHASE II: INTERVENTION

1. There are three objectives of the treatment phase driven by findings in the clinical assessment:
   a. Monitor and manage limbic symptoms through environment change of input systems (vision, auditory, kinesthetic) with the goal of the limbic network going neutral if possible.
   b. Maximize sensory integration, central processing, compensatory impairments of the vestibulospinal reflex (balance control) and VOR (gaze control).
   c. Integrate gains in balance and gaze control into functional activity with and without emotional overlays.
2. Treatment approach:
   a. Patient-oriented (limbic) approach.
   Goal: Maximize internal locus of control and trust; quiet the limbic influence (facilitate limbic neutral) to set an environment appropriate for motor learning and functional change.
   Techniques:
      - Awareness and validation of the problem. Provide the patient with objective findings of organic and functional involvement (sensory organization, dynamic visual acuity, and other testing). Many of these patients have been told for years that it is "in their head." The statement is accurate but the intent is condescending and implies some psychological dysfunction.
      - Awareness of and participation in the plan and approach. The treatment plan should have strong emotional meaning to the patient to turn the "limbic key" to maximize involvement and motivation. It should be goal directed intrasession and intersession. Achieving proper motivation and reward maximizes neuroplastic change.[659]
      - The correct patient-therapist pairing for effective execution of the plan. Safe clinician contact may actually be part of the rehabilitation plan, with gradual reduction based on limbic and functional improvements.
      - The correct environment to effect change. Use appropriate voice (timber, pitch, volume), appropriate pacing (onset of sound or other stimuli), sound, light, consistency, and predictability.
   b. Balance retraining using sensory reorganization (reweighting).
   Gaze stability (VOR) retraining
   Goal: Appropriate timing and predictability of sensory treatment: "dose" to achieve desired limbic and functional outcomes.
      - Expose the patient to the problem sensory conditions identified during the examination, presenting first the easier conditions and progressing the difficulty and complexity on the basis of patient response. Force the development of sensory integration, compensation, or substitution, as well as the development of new and appropriate movement strategies.
      - Provide for selective attention through predictable, short segments of sensory integrative challenge.
      - Avoid sensory overload through proper exercise prescription (intensity, duration, repetitions, frequency) during sensory integrative treatment.
      - Provide for maximal motor learning environment by keeping the limbic network quiet while achieving the correct balance between error detection and correction versus demotivation through making mistakes.
      - Provide knowledge of performance and knowledge of results frequently. As one example, computerized visual biofeedback provides direct one-on-one feedback of body position in space and motor performance.
   c. Functional activity requires complex integration of balance and gaze control.
      - Gait training at controlled pacing in stable environments, progressing to changing pace within predictable visual environments, to unstable visual environments and variable surface environment.
      - Hippotherapy (an activity meaningful to the patient), at a controlled cadence provided by the animal, provides predictable sensory input (somatosensory, vestibular, auditory, and olfactory), controlled rhythmic visual flow, and neutral warmth in a meaningful, goal-directed activity (as identified by the patient). This can be a very limbic-neutralizing activity when fear is controlled as a factor.
   d. If the patient does not progress in a physiologically normal manner or limbic signs remain unchanged (or increase) then psychological management may take precedent over (or be required before) recovery in

Continued

CASE STUDY 5-1—cont'd

rehabilitation (motor learning and neuroplasticity within the CNS) can be achieved.

- Successful life outcome is affected by early management. The extent to which a mild dizziness problem becomes chronic is dependent mainly on the psychological reaction to the symptoms.[233]
- There are specific management strategies associated with anxiety-type disorders within psychology, including use of medications. One theory of recovery from psychology problems is referred to as exposure. Although exposure is meant to cause habituation of the patient to the triggering events, in our case exposure actually will lead to forced use of the appropriate sensory system(s) as required in activities of daily living.

CONCLUSION

What makes this a clinical problem within the domain of the limbic network is that this woman's limbic network was overriding all other systems. At first glance this person was referred to therapy with typical vestibular and balance dysfunction. She was anything but typical and could not be approached with a "standard protocol," or failure for both the therapist and the patient was inevitable. The role of the patient within this setting was to gain an appreciation and integration of how her vestibular, motor, and limbic networks were interacting and when she went into system overload and why. The therapist's role was to (1) help the patient gain this body awareness, (2) empower the patient with regard to her potential for recovery, (3) design interventions that would nurture patient success, (4) collaborate with the patient on needed interventions regarding practice and novelty within the environment along with consistency of practice, and (5) allow the patient to improve at a pace her CNS could manage.

After 4 months of intervention the therapist moved and thus did not follow up on the long-term outcome of this case. Although the therapist does not know whether the patient reached her ultimate goals, it was obvious after 4 months that the client was changing in the direction of functional control and participation in life.

The long-term permanent changes that may or may not have occurred with this patient's vestibular, motor, or limbic networks are not known. The essential role of complete history taking and dedication to reality by the therapist is obvious. The therapist's success within this case was dependent on her ability to listen and watch (visually, auditorily, and emotionally [limbic]) as the patient unfolded the mystery of her CNS problems. The patient was the key to successfully unlocking her complex subsystem problems. In the health care world of stress, limited visits, and expected outcomes after intervention, it is far too easy to blame the patient for our failure as clinicians. It is also easy to quickly identify that the patient has problems in other system areas outside our scope of practice and thus infer that it is those areas that are limiting improvement. The difficulty is that all professions are doing the same thing, and the patient is drowning in the repercussions of the waves. Partnering interventions both with other professionals and with the client should optimize an environment that nurtures long-term learning and plastic changes within the CNS. The limbic network drives our attention, our motivation, and our willingness to take risks into unknown environments. How you as a clinician accompany those patients throughout the learning experience will depend on your limbic network as much as theirs.

CHAPTER 6 Psychosocial Aspects of Adaptation and Adjustment during Various Phases of Neurological Disability

ROCHELLE McLAUGHLIN, MS, OTR/L, MBSR, and GORDON U. BURTON, PhD, OTR/L

KEY TERMS

adaptation
adjustment
bonding
coping
family network
loss and grief
mindfulness
problem solving
sexuality
support systems

OBJECTIVES

After reading this chapter the student or therapist will be able to:

1. Describe adaptation and adjustment as parts of a flexible and flowing process, not as static stages.
2. Describe elements of the grief process that deal with age, cognition, and developmental level.
3. Integrate the elements of mindfulness, problem solving, loss, cognitive functioning, and coping, as well as significant others' coping and learning styles, into the treatment process to encourage adaptation.
4. Integrate the family of the client and the client's styles of coping into therapeutic treatment strategies to be used in the clinic.
5. Respect aspects of sexuality in treatment and consider them when treating the client.
6. Accept the role of patient advocate and the responsibility to report any abuse. Each clinician is responsible for knowing state law as part of her or his state licensure requirements.

It is a part of the human condition to have intense life experiences. There are a variety of ways in which we can respond and adjust to these kinds of life experiences. Adjusting to a disability is an ongoing process, just as adjusting to all other aspects of life is for everyone. This process of moving forward is a lifelong one. In moving forward with a disability it is important to turn toward and confront the situation, thereby opening up to the potential hidden within the situation. If we turn away and deny the situation, we are at risk of never fully coming to terms with and adjusting to the life experience. Adjusting to a disability is not unilateral. The family and support system must be involved in this process. Therapists may be tempted to treat the impairment in isolation and not be involved in the adjustment process for the individual or their support system. This would be a major mistake. Technicians address the mechanical (technical) aspects of treatment, but clinical professionals must treat the whole person and must be involved in the process of adjustment at all times. It is a fatal flaw to reduce the individual to just the impairment and not see or try to understand the bigger picture with regard to what is really needed during treatment intervention. A technician may obtain good physical results, but if the individual has not adapted to the life-altering event, the physical results may never be maximized. If the individual's support system has not adjusted to the impairment, those individuals may hold the client back from optimal functioning or put unnecessary pressure on the individual simply out of a lack of knowledge. Proper training and practice can allow for the empowerment of the client and the support system. In this chapter we will pursue topics that cover important aspects of the adjustment process for the individual with a disability and his or her support system.

PSYCHOLOGICAL ADJUSTMENT

In clinical practice, theoretical foundations for adjustment to disability appear to be elusive because they represent a fluid process: all people are constantly changing. This is especially true for people who have recently become physically disabled. They do not reach a certain state of adjustment and stay there but progress through a series of adaptations. Therapists see clients in a crisis state[1-6] and therefore identify their adjustment patterns from this frame of reference. How well the individual adjusts to the crisis, however, does not necessarily indicate how well he or she will adjust to all aspects of the disability, or the rate of progress from one point of adaptation to another.[6-15] Disabilities are an unimaginable insult to an individual's self-perception.[16-19] A month or even a year after the injury may not be long enough to put the disability into perspective.[10,16,17,19-22]

For most people, progressing from the shock of injury to the acceptance of and later adaptation to disability is a process filled with psychological ups and downs. Several authors have discussed the possible stages of adjustment and grieving.[10,14] The research of Kübler-Ross[23] into death and dying has application to this topic of adjustment to disability. She discussed the concept of loss and grief in relation to life; loss of function may result in just as profound a reaction. The practice of mindfulness may be important in disengaging individuals from automatic thoughts, habits, and unhealthy behavior patterns and thus could play a key role in fostering informed and self-endorsed behavioral regulation, and adjustment to catastrophic life events.[24] Peretz[25] and others[26-28] discuss the grieving process in relation to the loss of role function as well as loss of body function. These losses must be grieved for before the client can fully benefit from therapy or adjust to a changed body and lifestyle. Therapists must be aware that the client can and must deal with the death of certain functional abilities.

Some authors have questioned the concept of stages of adjustment,[1,29] and call for more empirical research into adaptation and adjustment; this has been started.[30] One alternative concept that has been developed is cognitive adaptation theory.[31] This concept examines self-esteem, optimism, and control. In this theory, if the individual feels good about himself or herself and has an optimistic view of life and a sense of control over life, the individual will adapt to the functional limitations and will participate in life. Cognitive adaptation theory does not consider the organic changes that may take place when brain damage has occurred, but the basic goals are very much worth taking into consideration. These should be examined in relation to the limbic system (see Chapter 5) because limbic involvement is crucial to reaching all goals and plays a key role in establishment of motivation.

The components of successful psychological adjustment to a physical disability (activity limitations) are varied. To bring a client to a level of function that is of the highest quality possible for that individual, therapists must look holistically at the psychosocial aspects and at the adjustment processes involved, evaluate each component, and integrate the processes into the therapeutic milieu to promote growth in all areas. There is much more to evaluation and treatment than just the physical component; the mind and body have incredibly interrelated influences, and both must be understood, evaluated, and treated individually and as a whole.

WE UNDERSTAND MORE ABOUT SUFFERING THAN WE THINK

Clinical professionals have a wellspring of knowledge to draw from beyond their extensive traditional education. We are all human beings, and being human comes with a great deal of innate suffering. If we bring awareness to the fact that we have all suffered in our lives, we may not feel so separate from our clients. We may realize that we have more to offer our clients than just the knowledge we have gained about their disability and how we might help them gain function. The more we allow ourselves to slow down and be present with suffering—our own or that of another—the more we will be able to be open to the mystery and joy of our lives just as they are without requiring them to be any different.[32] It may be our lifetime's journey to be servants of the healing arts; this is our job, and it also takes enormous skill and bravery to bear witness to the full catastrophe of the human condition.[32] One of the benefits of our profession is the stimulus to examine our lives through the experiences of others. This can improve our function and help us grow as professionals and individuals, but if we are not open to the clients' experiences we may not find a reason to examine and grow from our own experiences.

If we haven't endured great suffering personally, we have borne witness to it—"9/11" is a perfect example of this. If we acknowledge this fact, then maybe we can acknowledge that we are more connected to our clients than we once thought and that we have more to offer our clients in terms of their ability to adjust to their disability than we once imagined.

AWARENESS OF PSYCHOLOGICAL ADJUSTMENT IN THE CLINIC, SOCIETY, AND CULTURE

Working with individuals with functional limitations requires that we cultivate a holistic and all-encompassing perspective: to visualize how they might best participate within their own homes and communities, and in the context of their society and a given time. This is a dynamic and constantly changing process. The clinician must develop an intervention that will appropriately stimulate the individual and all their potential caregivers to maximize the potential for the highest-quality life possible. The skilled clinician initially evaluates the individual's physical and cognitive capabilities depending on the type of functional limitations. The more subtle psychological aspects of the client's ability to function need to be assessed at some level. These include the individual's support system and/or family network and its ability to adjust to the imminent changes in lifestyle. It would be a tragic situation for a clinician to ignore the individual's psychological adjustment or consider it to be less important in any way.[19,33-36]

Livneh and Antonak[37] have introduced a consolidated way to look at adaptation as a primer for counselors, which should be examined by therapists. They use some of the same basic concepts, such as stress, crisis, loss and grief, body image, self-concept, stigma, uncertainty or unpredictability, and quality of life, to frame their approach. They also consider the concepts of shock, anxiety, denial, depression, anger and hostility, and adjustment in a format that is usable by the therapist.

Livneh and Antonak[37] mention that one of the aspects that the therapist must watch out for is a form of coping called *disengagement.* This style of coping may be demonstrated through denial or avoidance behavior that can take many forms. It can result in substance abuse, blame, or just refusal to interact. Research regarding people with head injuries has demonstrated that if a premorbid coping style for a person was to use alcohol or other drugs, the client may revert to these same styles of coping, which can result in poor physical and emotional rehabilitation.[38] It is important to help the individual out of this quagmire. The skills of a therapist are likely not enough to do this in the short time that the client is in treatment, so a referral to social work, psychology, or psychiatry is required to help support the long-term process. It is still the therapist's job to understand the process of adjustment, the indications regarding how an individual is adjusting, key concepts for how to engage with an individual who is adjusting, and how to set personal boundaries so that the clinician is less likely to be overwhelmed by the process of adjustment and disability. In light of all this, it is still the primary job of the therapist to help promote and maximize the engagement in functional activities. These activities are behaviors that must be goal oriented (patient, family, and therapist driven), demonstrating problem solving and information seeking and involving completion of steps to positively move forward into life with the disability and to maximize independence (promoting function).

The rest of this section introduces the reader to some of the psychological change components that may be assessed and acknowledged. The last section will attempt to demonstrate possible ways that these components can be taken into account as an aspect of therapy.

Growth and Adaptation

The clinician must keep in mind the context from which the client is coming. Just days or even hours ago the individual may have been going about daily life without difficulty. The trauma may be multifaceted: (1) physical trauma, (2) emotional trauma occurring to the individual's support system, and (3) trauma of each of these systems interacting (the support system trying to protect the individual, and the client trying to protect the support system). The interaction of these multifaceted components of the trauma may lead to posttraumatic distress syndrome. This syndrome usually happens within the first 6 months after the injury. This syndrome may be observed more often in women[39] but because of cultural barriers it can be hidden in men. It happens more often when there has been a near-death situation.[40,41] The client may blame others, try to protect others, or be so self-absorbed that little else in the world may be seen or heard. It may be helpful to get psychological help for the individual early in therapy if this is preventing optimal outcomes or creating obstacles in therapy.[4,15,42-45]

It is the therapist's job to develop a trusting relationship with the client. Through this relationship the individual can be guided to focus on the goals of therapy and work on a positive perspective about the future. One of the errors of the medical system is that of focusing on the disease outcomes and pathology and not on the person and the positive capabilities still within the individual's grasp.[19] This focus on the negative or loss may cause the individual to see only the injury, disease, or pathological condition and nothing else. In a Veterans Administration hospital, spouses of people with spinal cord injuries formed a group in which the group's focus was on why the partners got married in the first place; the group never looked at the physical limitations as disabling. After a little while people came to the conclusion that they did not marry their spouses for their legs and the fact that the legs no longer worked was not a major issue after all. This started the decentering from the medical disability model and the focus started to be placed on the people and the families' future. If we can help clients focus on their functions and not their dysfunctions, the effect of therapy after treatment will be much better. More work needs to be done to help clients see the potential they will have in the future to live their lives with the highest quality possible.[34,46-50] The World Health Organization developed a model that differentiates the disease pathology model of medicine and focuses on individuals' activities in life and the ability to participate in those interactions. This model, the International Classification of Functioning, Disability and Health (ICF), has been enthusiastically accepted by the therapy world, and the professions of both occupational and physical therapy use it as a reference model for practice.

Focusing on how to participate, move, and function in the world is one of the keys to helping the client and the family work toward its future.[33,49,51-54]

The therapist needs to help the client focus on the direction of treatment objectives and to demonstrate how therapy translates into meeting the client's goals.[19,55] To discover the client's true goals, the therapist must gain the trust of the client and establish sound lines of communication. Distrust from health professionals may obstruct the adjustment process and lead to negative consequences.[56] Whenever possible, the client's support system should be enlisted to help establish realistic support for the client and the goals of both the client and the family. It has been found that if the client trusts the health professional, the client will be more adherent and will seek assistance when it is needed (see Chapter 5 for additional information).[57,58]

A New Normal

When we experience a decline in our ability to carry out our everyday routine tasks, regardless of the cause of our "disability," we may experience incredible degrees of despair. Many societies emphasize a very specific idea of what it means to be normal. There doesn't appear to be a great deal of flexibility in what this standard of normal is, regardless of one's cultural background. When an individual fails to live up to or no longer fits this norm, there can exist a tremendous amount of mental and emotional suffering. Because our bodies and minds are so intricately connected, our physical being is adversely affected by the mental and emotional anguish. On top of what the individual may already be experiencing physically, suddenly there is another layer of mental-physical anguish that is far too easily ignored and unattended to by clinical professionals. However, once we are aware of the multifaceted potential for human suffering with regard to adjusting to a disability, we may be empowered to assist the individual with a nonlinear, multifaceted approach. Researchers and theorists from various psychotherapy traditions have begun to explore the potential value of the therapeutic relationship by making direct references to different levels of validation as a means of demonstrating warmth, genuineness, empathy, and acceptance and reiterate how important it is for therapists to reflect back to the patient that their feelings, thoughts, and actions make sense in the context of their current experience. The therapist articulates an expectation that the treatment collaboration will be effective in an attempt to convey hope and confidence in their ability to work together.[59]

We can guide our clients in identifying a new normal for themselves, all the while allowing them and their support system to grieve the loss of the old normal. As the Harvard psychologist Ellen Langer described in her book *Mindfulness,* "if we are offered a new use for a door or a new view of old age [or disability], we can erase the old mindsets without difficulty."[60] We can offer our clients a new view of themselves by showing them what they are capable of as they rebuild their lives. We can also help them acknowledge what is present in this moment and what the reality of the situation is. This does not have to be a problem to be suffered over but is a situation to be dealt with carefully and fully in the present moment. A woman who has lived with multiple sclerosis for over 30 years described how the relief of suffering does not require restoring physical function to some perceived level of normality. "Suffering is relieved to the extent that patients can learn to integrate bodily disorder and physical incapacity into their lives, to accommodate to a different way of being" (p. 591).[61] According to research by De Souza and Frank,[61] their subjects with chronic back pain expressed regret at the loss of capabilities and distress at the functional consequences of those losses. They found that facilitating "adjustment" to "loss" was more helpful than implying the potential for a life free of pain as a result of therapeutic interventions.

Guiding the individual through practice and repetition of basic functional activities will allow the client to identify for himself or herself how to live successfully in this world again and cultivate this "different way of being." At the same time we can encourage these clients to mindfully plan for and visualize their future (see practice later) during specific times of their day so that their minds are not in constant worry mode or rehearsing, which can cause a great deal of anxiety about the future. We can assist our clients in planning for that future, especially in a medical environment where shorter rehabilitation stays are the norm.

Without any need to apologize for their loss, just simply being with them in the moment in a nonjudgmental way and allowing them to grieve can be a powerful tool for healing. Acknowledging the loss and the suffering may help clients move forward with their lives in a new way. "Acceptance [of what is] doesn't, by any stretch of the imagination, mean passive resignation. Quite the opposite. It takes a huge amount of fortitude and motivation to accept what is—especially when we don't like it—and then work wisely and effectively as best we possibly can with the circumstances we find ourselves in and with the resources at our disposal, both inner and outer, to mitigate, heal, redirect, and change what can be changed."[62]

Practice: Mindful Planning and Visualization of Future

- Find a time when you are alone; you need only a few minutes every day for this practice.
- Allow this time to be specifically for future planning and visualization, not worrying.
- If you find yourself worrying about the future at other times during the day, acknowledge that there will be a specific time devoted to planning and visualizing. Worrying throughout the day will bring a great deal of mental anguish during times when you need to focus attention on an important task or rehabilitation intervention.
- Use a journal to record thoughts and ideas on paper so that the thoughts do not have to stay in the mind and be rehearsed. Write down concerns as well as plans.
- Try to let go of planning during daily activities and tasks until the next scheduled Mindful Planning Session, or, if necessary, allow this moment to be the next planning session but be sure to stop whatever else you are doing and be fully present in the planning process.

Societal and Cultural Influences

Culture, subcultures, and the culture and beliefs of the given family are all aspects of the client that the therapist must be aware of.[22,52,63-69] This concept gets into the beliefs about the world and maybe a belief about the cause of the disability or at least how the client is viewing the disability. Asking "why do you think this happened to you?" can lead to an enlightening experience. "Causes" may range from "God is punishing me" to "I deserved it" to "life is against me."

From an early age, people in our society are exposed to misconceptions regarding the disabled person.[70-73] If in the therapeutic environment, however, the client and family have their misconceptions challenged constantly, they may start reformulating their concept of the role of the disabled person. As this process progresses, therapists and other staff can help make the expectations of the disabled person more realistic. Therapists can schedule their clients at times when they will be exposed to people making realistic adjustments to disabilities. Use of individuals who have been successfully rehabilitated as staff members (role models) can help to dispel the misconception that people with disabilities are not employable.[74-76]

This process of adaptation to a new disability can be considered as a cultural change from a majority status (able bodied) to a minority status (disabled). Part of the adaptation process can be considered as an acculturation process, and the therapist can help facilitate this process.[16,72,77,78]

The cultural background of the individual also contributes to the perception of disability and to the acceptance of the disabled person. Trombly[79] states that perception and expression of pain, physical attractiveness, valuing of body parts, and acceptability of types of disabilities can be culturally influenced. One's ethnic background can also affect intensity of feelings toward specific handicaps, trust of staff,[79] and acceptance of therapeutic modalities.[80-84]

The successful therapist will be sensitive to the cultural values of the client and will attempt to present therapy to the client in the most acceptable way. For example, in the Mexican culture it is not polite to just start to work with a client; rapport must first be established. Sharing of food may provide the vehicle to accomplish rapport. Thus, the therapist might schedule the first visit with a Mexican client during a coffee break. The therapist must remember that the dysfunctional client may be the one who can least be expected to adjust to the therapist and that the therapist may need to adjust to the client, especially in the early stages of therapy.

Gaining trust is one of the crucial links in any meaningful therapeutic situation.[58,85,86] Trust will create an environment that facilitates communication, productive learning, and exchange of information.[75,86] Trust is important in all cultures and will be fostered by the therapist who is sensitive to the needs of the client. This sensitivity is necessary with every client but will be manifested in many different ways, depending on the background and needs of the individual in therapy. A client of one culture may feel that looking another person in the eyes is offensive, whereas in another culture refusal to look into someone's eyes is a sign of weakness or lack of honesty (shifty eyed).[87] Thus although it is impossible to know every culture or subculture with which the therapist may come into contact, the therapist must attempt to be sensitive to the background of the client. Even if the therapist knows the cultural norms, not every person follows the cultural patterns, and thus every client needs to be treated as an individual in the therapeutic relationship. It should be the therapist's job to be sensitive to the subtle nonverbal and verbal cues that indicate the level of trust in the relationship. The therapist will obtain this information by being open to the client, not open to a textbook. The client is the owner of this information and will share it with everyone he or she trusts.

Trust is often established in the therapeutic relationship through physical activities. The act of asking a client to transfer from the chair to the bed can either build trust or destroy the potential relationship. If the client trusts the therapist just enough to follow instructions to transfer but then falls in the process, it may take quite some time to reestablish the same level of trust, assuming that it can ever be reestablished. This trusting relationship is so complex and involves such a variety of levels that the therapist should be as aware of attending to the client's security in the relationship as to the physical safety of the client in the clinic.[58,85] If the client believes that the therapist is not trustworthy in the relationship, then it may follow that the therapist is not to be trusted when it comes to physical manipulation of a disabled body. If the client does not know how to use the damaged physical body and thus cannot trust the body, then lacking trust in the therapist will only compound the stress of the situation.[58,85,88] Chapter 8 provides more information on the neurological components of this interaction during the intervention process.

The client's culture may be alien to the therapist, even though both the clinician and client may be from the same geographical region. A client's problems of poverty, unemployment, and a lack of educational opportunities[76,86,89,90] can all result in the therapist and client feeling that therapy will be unsuccessful, even before the first session has begun. Such preconceived concepts held by both parties may not be warranted and must be examined. These preconceived concepts can be more reflective of failure of rehabilitation than any physical limitation of the client.

Cultural and religious values may also result in the client feeling that he or she must pay for past sins by being disabled and that the disability will be overcome after atonement for these sins. Such a client may not be inclined to participate in or enjoy therapy. The successful therapist does not assault the client's basic cultural or religious values but may recognize them in the therapy sessions. If the therapist feels that the culturally defined problems are impeding the therapeutic process, the therapist may offer the client opportunities to reexamine these cultural "truths" in a nonjudgmental way and may help the client redefine the way the physical limitations and therapy are seen.[91] Religious counseling could be recommended by the therapist, and follow-up support in the clinic may be given to the client to view therapy not as undoing what "God has done" but as a way of proving religious strength. Reworking a person's cultural and religious (cognitive) structure is a sensitive area, and it should be handled with care and respect and with the use of other professionals (social workers and religious and psychological counselors) as appropriate.

The hospital staff can be encouraged to establish groups in which commonly held values of clients can be examined and possibly challenged.[16,91-97] Such groups can lead the client to a better understanding of priorities and may help the person see the relevance of therapy and the need to continue the adjustment process. This can also prepare the client to better accept the need for support groups after discharge. The therapist may be able to use information from such group sessions to adjust the way therapy sessions are presented and structured to make therapy more relevant to the client's values and needs. Value groups or exercises[98] can be another means used by the therapist for evaluation and understanding of the client.

Beliefs and values of cultures and families can play a profound role in the course of treatment. Such things as physical difficulties, which can be seen, are usually better accepted than problems that cannot be seen, such as brain damage that changed an individual's cognitive abilities or personality.[99] A person with a back injury may be seen as lazy, whereas a person with a double amputation will be perceived as needing help. At the same time, in some cultures a person who has lost a body part may be seen as "not all there" and should be avoided socially. Therefore being attuned to the culture and beliefs of the client is imperative in therapy. The reader is encouraged to refer to texts on cultural issues in health care such as *Culture in Clinical Care* by Bonder, Martin, and Miracle[100]; *Cultural Competence in Health Care: A Practical Guide* by Rundle, Carvalho, and Robinson[101]; and *Caring for Patients from Different Cultures* by Galanti[102] for more detailed discussions on how culture and beliefs affect health care.

Establishment of Self-Worth and Accurate Body Image

> *"The true value of a human being is determined primarily by the measure and the sense in which he has attained liberation from the self."*
>
> **—Albert Einstein**

Self-worth is composed of many aspects, such as body image, sexuality, and the ability to help others and to affect the environment. The body image of a client is a composite of past and present experiences and of the individual's perception of those experiences. Because body image is based on experience, it is a constantly changing concept. An adult's body image is substantially different from the body image of a child and will no doubt change again as the aging process continues. A newly disabled person is suddenly exposed to a radically new body, and it is that individual's job to assess the body's capabilities and develop a new body image. Because the therapist is at least partially responsible for creating the environmental experiences from which the client learns about this new body, the therapist must be aware of the concept. In the case of an acute injury, the client has a new body from which to learn. The therapist can promote positive feelings as the therapist instructs the client how to use this new body and to accept its changes.[1,16,20,27,103,104]

Because in "normal" life we slowly observe changes in our bodies, such as finding one gray hair today and watching it take years for our hair to turn totally white, we have the luxury of slowly adapting to the "new me." Change usually does not happen quite so slowly and "naturally" when trauma or a disease affects the nervous system. This sudden loss of function creates a void that only new experiences and new role models can fill.

The loss of use of body parts can cause a person to perceive the body as an "enemy" that needs to be forced to work or to compensate for its disability. In all cases the body is the reason for the disability and the cause of all problems. The need for appliances and adaptive equipment can create a sense of alienation and lack of perceived "lovability" resulting from the "hardness of the hardware." People tend to avoid hugging someone who is in a wheelchair or who has braces around the body because of the physical barrier and because of the person's perceived fragility; a person with physical limitations is certainly not perceived as soft and cuddly.[20,27,52,102,103] Both the perception that these individuals are not lovable and their labored movements can sap the energy of the disabled and discourage social interaction or life participation. To accept the appliances and the dysfunctional body in a way that also allows the disabled person to feel loved is surely a major challenge.

In the case of a person who will be disabled for the long term, such as the person with cerebral palsy or Parkinson disease, the therapist is attempting to teach the client how to change the previously accepted body image to one that would allow and encourage more normal function. In short, the therapist has two roles. One role is to help lessen the disabled body image. The second is to teach a functional disabled body image to a newly disabled person. The techniques may be the same, but in both cases the client will have to undergo a great amount of change. The person with a neurological disorder or neurologically based disability may assume that he or she will not be capable of accomplishing many things with his or her life. The therapist is in a unique position to encourage development of and maximize the client's level of functional ability. The individual may then expect more of himself or herself. The newly disabled person must change the expectations; however, he or she has little concept of what is realistic to expect of this new body. At this point, role models can be used to help shape the client's expectations. If the client is unable to adjust to the new body and change the body image and self-expectations, life may be impoverished for that individual. Pedretti[105] states that the client with low self-esteem often devalues his or her whole life in all respects, not just in the area of physical dysfunction.[1,16,20,27,103,104]

One way the client can start exploring this new body is by exploring its sensations and performance. Dr. Jon Kabat-Zinn developed a guided "body scan" meditation that can help individuals learn how to become more connected and in tune with the sensations of the body.[62] This kind of practice is about learning to pay attention to the body in a new way and can be very helpful in developing an accurate body image and improve self-awareness. The client with a spinal cord injury may also use the sensation of touch to "map out" the body to see how it reacts.[106] They may ask themselves the following questions: Is there a way to get the legs to move using reflexes? Can positioning the legs in a certain way aid in rolling the wheelchair or make spasms decrease? What, if anything, stimulates an erection or lubrication? Such exploration will start the client on the road to an informed evaluation of his or her abilities.

The therapist's role is to maximize the client's perceptions of realistic body functioning. Exercises can be developed that encourage exploration of the body by the individual and, if appropriate, the significant partner. Functioning and building an appropriate body image will be more difficult if intimate knowledge of the new body is not as complete as before injury.[9] The successes the client experiences in the clinical setting coupled with the client's familiarity with his or her new body will result in a more accurate body image and will contribute to the client's feelings of self-worth.

The last aspect of self-worth is often overlooked in the health fields. This aspect is the need that people have to help others.[107] People often discover that they are valuable through the act of giving. Seeing others enjoy and benefit from the individual's presence or offering increases self-worth. Situations in which others can appreciate the client's worth may be needed. Unless the client can contribute to others, the client is in a relatively dependent role, with everyone else giving to him or her without the opportunity of giving back. Achieving independence and then reaching out to others, with therapeutic assistance if necessary, facilitates the individual's more rapid reintegration into society. The therapist should take every opportunity to allow the client to express self-worth to others through helping.

The ability to expand one's definition of oneself is a key factor in adjusting to a disability. Expanding the definition of oneself in terms of all the roles and responsibilities one has can help the individual comprehend the enormity of who he or she is. The individual may begin to understand how he or she is so much greater than just the job he or she once performed and so much greater than the role he or she once played. This practice can cultivate understanding of how complex our species is and how much we have to offer the world, differently abled or not (see journal activity, Box 6-1).

Sense of Control

"Oh, I've had my moments, and if I had to do it over again, I'd have more of them. In fact, I'd try to have nothing else. Just moments, one after another, instead of living so many years ahead of each day."
—Nadine Stair, 85 years old, Louisville, Kentucky

As Drs. Roizen, and Oz stated in their book *You: The Owner's Manual,* we can control our health destiny.[108] Although we can't always control what happens to us (no matter how fit we are), there are some things we can control: our attitude, our determination, and our willingness to take our own health into our own hands.[108]

Adjusting to a disability can make clients feel as though they have very little control over their lives; they may feel

BOX 6-1 ■ JOURNAL ACTIVITY

Write down three words that someone who loves you would choose to describe you. Choose qualities that you think others appreciate about you, such as *intelligent, funny, kind, organized.*

Write down the ways that you express those qualities in your life. Maybe it is when you garden, write, draw, or listen.

Write down your ideal vision of the world. Maybe it is, "I envision a world that is free of violence" or "where everyone has access to knowledge about how to keep our oceans clean" or "where children are well cared for."

Put it all together in one statement: "I will use my intelligence, humor, organization, and kindness, through writing, drawing, gardening, and listening to help create a world that is peaceful, where children are well cared for, and where the oceans are clean." Then do it!

helpless, as though their health is in everyone else's hands but their own. This feeling can cause incredible suffering and emotional anguish on top of their physical or cognitive disability. If we focus solely on treating the disability and ignore what may be going on for our clients mentally and emotionally, we may be creating even more suffering for them. Clinical professionals have the opportunity to guide their clients toward a new way of relating to their disability by focusing on what they do have control over as well as identifying ways in which they may relate differently to those situations over which they do not have control.

Dr. Jill Bolte-Taylor says this eloquently in a passage from her book:

> *"I've often wondered, if it's a choice, then why would anyone choose anything other than happiness? I can only speculate, but my guess is that many of us don't exercise our ability to choose. Before my stroke, I thought I was a product of my brain and had no idea that I had some say about how I responded to the emotions surging through me. On an intellectual level, I realized that I could monitor and shift my cognitive thoughts, but it never dawned on me that I had some say in how I perceived my emotions. . . . What an enormous difference this awareness has made in how I live my life."*[109]

As Dr. Bolte-Taylor describes, all of us have the choice to be in relation to the present moment fully, or we can allow our thoughts and emotions to "take us for a ride" as though we were on automatic pilot.[109] If we allow our minds and emotions to take over our experience of the present moment, we can easily be dragged along into rehashing our past events that led up to the disability, which can create more suffering and emotional anguish. We also may be rehearsing what our lives will be like without allowing the dust to settle, without waiting until we have a clearer picture of what implications the disability may have for us. An unacknowledged rehashing and rehearsing can create an incredible sense of lack of control over one's life, thereby increasing anxiety and depression. Approximately 70% of our thoughts in any particular waking state can be considered to be daydreams, and they can often be unconstructive.[110] In an experience sampling method, Klinger and his colleagues found that "active, focused problem-solving thought"[111] made up only 6% of the waking state. According to Baruss, "it would make more sense to say that our subjective life consists of irrational thinking with occasional patches of reason"[110] while we are participating in our daily activities. Especially when one is participating in menial, basic self-care activities, our mind is often in another place. If an individual is frequently disconnected from the present moment, tending to ruminate over the past or future events, he or she may experience significant negative effects from this distraction. Rumination, absorption in the past, rehashing, or fantasies and anxieties about the future can pull one away from what is taking place in the present moment. Awareness or attention can be divided, such as when people occupy themselves with multiple tasks at one time or preoccupy themselves with concerns that detract from the quality of engagement with what is focally present, and this can increase anxiety and depression.[112]

According to Drs. Oz and Roizen,[108] these emotions can cause high blood pressure, as well as disrupting the body's normal repair mechanism, and also constrict our blood vessels, making it even harder for enough blood to work its way through the body. They go on to say that learning relaxation techniques such as yoga and meditation can help us handle these damaging feelings in a healthier way. We know now that these mind states affect our bodies profoundly—for example, a feeling of helplessness appears to weaken the immune system.[108] If we can teach our clients to be mindful of and pay attention to their "mind states"—also known as "thoughts"—at any given moment during therapeutic intervention, we may be able to encourage a greater sense of control and facilitate greater mental and emotional adjustment to the individual's disability. According to a 2008 article by Ludwig and Kabat-Zinn in *JAMA,* "the goal of mindfulness is to maintain awareness moment by moment, disengaging oneself from strong attachment to beliefs, thoughts, or emotions, thereby developing a greater sense of emotional balance and well-being."[113] Anat Baniel, in her book *Move into Life,* describes how research shows that the moment we bring attention and awareness to our movements moment by moment, the brain resumes growing new connections and creating new pathways and possibilities for us.[114]

According to a research study by Dr. Jon Kabat-Zinn[115] of the Stress Reduction Program at the Center for Mindfulness in Medicine, Health Care, and Society, the practice of mindfulness meditation used by chronic pain patients over a 10-week period showed a 65% reduction on a pain rating index. Large and significant reductions in mood disturbance and psychiatric symptoms accompanied these changes and were stable on follow-up. Another study looked at brain imaging and immune function after an 8-week training program in mindfulness meditation.[116] The study demonstrated that this short program in mindfulness meditation produced demonstrable effects on brain and immune function. The results of a clinical intervention study by Brown and Ryan[112] showed that higher levels of mindfulness were related to lower levels of both mood disturbance and stress before and after the Mindfulness-Based Stress Reduction (MBSR) intervention. Increases in mindfulness over the course of the intervention predicted decreases in these two indicators of psychological disturbance. Evidence has indicated that those faced with a life-threatening illness often reconsider the ways in which they have been living their lives, and many choose to refocus their priorities on existential issues such as personal growth and mindful living.[117]

These findings suggest that meditation may change brain function and immune function in positive ways. "Meditation" as it is taught in this 8-week program is simply an awareness and attention training: a way of learning how to pay attention in the present moment to our thoughts and emotions and coming to understand how our thoughts and emotions affect our bodies. It may sound simple but actually can be incredibly challenging. However, an instant stress reliever can be bringing awareness to the breath. Deep breathing can act as a mini-meditation and from a longevity standpoint is an important stress reliever.[108] Shifting to slower breathing in times of tension can help calm us and allow us to perform, whether mentally or physically, at higher levels.[108]

Another study, focused on Coping Effectiveness Training (CET), consisted of weekly 60-minute psychoeducational group intervention sessions focused into six topic areas and was adapted from the protocol Coping Effectively with Spinal Cord Injury.[118] The treatment protocol was structured to provide education and skill building in areas of awareness of reactions to stress; situation appraisal; coping strategy choice; interaction among thoughts, emotions, and behaviors; relaxation; problem solving; communication; and social support.[119] There was a significantly positive correlation between the learned coping strategies and the disabled individual's ability to adjust in a healthy way.

Hope and Spiritual Aspects to Adjustment

Through great suffering there is incredible potential for us to transcend the mental and emotional limits of the physical body. As clinical professionals we need to be aware of this capability. As described by Dr. E. Cassel in the *New England Journal of Medicine,* "Transcendence is probably the most powerful way in which one is restored to wholeness after an injury of personhood. When experienced, transcendence locates a person in a far larger landscape. The sufferer is not isolated by pain but is brought closer to a transpersonal source of meaning and to the human community that shares those meanings. Such an experience need not involve religion in any formal sense; however, in its transpersonal dimension, it is deeply spiritual."[120] Parker Palmer, a writer and teacher, describes it this way: "Treacherous terrain, bad weather, taking a fall, getting lost—challenges of that sort, largely beyond our control, can strip the ego of the illusion that it is in charge and make space for true self to emerge."[121] Eckhart Tolle describes the ego as complete identification with form—physical form, thought form, emotional form.[122] The more we are identified with the physical realm, the more we will suffer when our attachment to stuff or "form" becomes torn.

"For all of us, our willingness to explore our fears, to live inside helplessness, confusion, and uncertainty, is a powerful ally. Acknowledging our repeated exposure to human suffering—our own and others'—and the seductive draw of numbness and melancholy that provides temporary escape is necessary if we are to be renewed."[32] Dr. Santorelli goes on to say that "there is no way out of one's inner life, so one had better get into it."[32] "On the inward and downward spiritual journey, the only way out is in and through."[121]

Practice: The Willingness to Embrace What Is

1. Become aware of the moments when "resistance to what is" is noticed. This may manifest itself as anxiety, sadness, fear, depression, anger.
2. As soon as anger arises (for example), notice how it manifests itself physically in the body. It may be tension in the muscles, a quickened or palpitating heartbeat, or sweating.
3. Note what the sensation feels like in the body without trying to make the moment different than it is. Acknowledge whatever is present in the moment.
4. Note that we are not the anger, we are the awareness of it.
5. Note what the awareness does. Journal any thoughts or feelings about the practice.

Dr. Jon Kabat-Zinn, in his book *Coming to Our Senses,* states, "It seems as if awareness itself, holding the sensations without judging them or reacting to them, is healing our view of the body and allowing it to come to terms, at least to some degree, with conditions as they are in the present moment in ways that no longer overwhelmingly erode our quality of life, even in the face of pain or disease."[62]

"Mystery surrounds every deep experience of the human heart: the deeper we go into the heart's darkness or its light, the closer we get to the ultimate mystery of God [the Universe]."[121]

Religious and spiritual beliefs can be assistive in the process of adjusting to a disability. Johnstone, Glass, and Oliver highlight that religion and spirituality are important coping strategies for persons with disabilities.[67] According to Dr. Jill Bolte-Taylor in her book *My Stroke of Insight: A Brain Scientist's Personal Journey,* "Enlightenment is not a process of learning but a process of unlearning."[109] Western society rewards the skills of the "doing" left brain much more than the "being" right brain, which can significantly hinder our process of spiritual growth. The focus of our lives becomes more about obtaining positions, roles, and "stuff." We begin to identify ourselves with all of this when in reality the positions, roles, and stuff can be taken from us at any moment. "When we are obsessed with . . . productivity, with efficiency of time and motion, with projecting reasonable goals and making a beeline toward them, it seems unlikely that our work will ever bear fruit, unlikely that we will ever know the fullness of spring in our lives."[121]

There is a much deeper definition of ourselves that goes beyond all of the material possessions and the roles that we may ever play. According to Eckhart Tolle,[122] when forms that we identify with, that give us a sense of self—such as our physical bodies—collapse or are taken away, it can lead to a collapse of the ego, because ego is identification with "form." When there is nothing to identify with anymore, who are we? When forms around us die, or death approaches, Spirit is released from its imprisonment in matter. We can finally understand that our essential identity is formless, spiritual.[122] Cultivating greater understanding of these concepts and delving more into the spirit can provide a great deal of relief for all of us who are suffering.

There is a wonderful quote by former Secretary-General of the United Nations U Thant, as he describes how he envisions the spiritual:

> *"Spirituality is a state of connectedness to life.*
> *It is an experience of being, belonging and caring.*
> *It is sensitivity and compassion, joy and hope.*
> *It is harmony between the innermost life and the outer life or the life of the world and the life of the universe.*
> *It is the supreme comprehension of life in time and space, tuning of the inner person with the great mysteries and secrets that are around us.*
> *It is the belief in the goodness of life and the possibility for each human person to contribute goodness to it.*
> *It is the belief in life as part of the eternal stream of time, that each of us came from somewhere and is destined to somewhere, that without such belief there could be no prayer, no meditation, no peace, and no happiness."*[123]

Spirituality is something that provides hope, connection with others, and reason or meaning of existence for many (if not most) people. It is amazing that the medical community has been slow to accept the power of spirituality because this is an area that gives meaning to so many peoples' lives. Spirituality has been linked to health perception, a sense of connection with others, and well-being.[66,67,124-130]

Anything that helps the client put the disability into perspective and helps the client move on with life in a healthy way is good. The Western medical system was based on diagnosis of pathology and how best to cure disease, but there has been a slow but fruitful shift toward a more holistic view of the healing process and prevention. The National Institutes of Health now has a National Center for Complementary and Alternative Medicine (http://nccam.nih.gov). Almost every major hospital and university in the country now has an integrative health center (e.g., http://stanfordhospital.org/clinicsmedServices/clinics/complementaryMedicine and www.osher.hms.harvard.edu). Although this small but steady shift in the focus of medicine has gained momentum, one of the dangers of the medical system is still the entrapment in pathology to the point where the client may not see anything but his or her pathology. Spirituality can help the client and the family to see that there is more to life than pathology, stimulate interaction with others, put the functional limitations in perspective, give meaning to life (and the disability), and give the person hope and a sense of well-being.* This is what we all want for the client and the family. Refer to Chapters 1, 5, and 39 for additional content.

Adjustment Using the Stage Concept

Each person has his or her own coping style, and each should be allowed to be unique. Kerr[133] describes five possible stages of adjustment:

Shock: "This really isn't happening to me."
Expectancy for recovery: "I will be well soon."
Mourning: "There is no hope."
Defense: "I will live with this obstacle and beat it." (healthy attitude) "I am adjusted, but you fail to see it." (neurotic attitude)
Adjustment: "It is part of me now, but it is not necessarily a bad thing."

In light of current research, it is important for the therapist to realize that these are not lockstep stages and are to be thought of as concepts to help with the understanding of common reactions of all individuals.[134,135] Some individuals may settle in one stage for quite some time or may even skip stages altogether, whereas others may move through the stages quickly. This is an incredibly individual process.

Shock

The individual in shock does not recognize that anything is actually wrong. The client may totally refuse to accept the diagnosis. The client may even laugh at the concern expressed by others. This stage is altered when the person has an opportunity to test reality and finds that the physical or cognitive condition is actually limiting the ability to participate in functional activities. If this stage continues, it may signify either a lack of mental health or an inability to cognitively realize the situation.

Expectancy for Recovery

The client in the stage of expectancy for recovery is aware that he or she is disabled but also believes that recovery will be quick and complete. The person may look for a "miracle cure" and may make future plans that require total return of function. Total recovery is the only goal, even if it takes a great deal of time and effort to achieve. Key signs of this stage are resentment of loss of function and the feeling that the whole body or mind is necessary to do anything worthwhile. The staff can stimulate a change from this stage by giving clear statements to the client that the damage is permanent (if in fact that is true), by transferring the person home or to the rehabilitation unit, or by discontinuing therapy. Any one of these occurrences can help make the client realize the permanence of the disability. It is also important to not take away an individual's hope. In the case of an individual who has experienced a stroke or a brain injury, we know now that the brain is capable of repairing itself throughout a lifetime—though we need to be clear that we do not know how much recovery will occur, if any. This all depends on the severity of the damage and the lifestyle of the client—for example, smoking, stress, and/or lack of participation in meaningful activity, all of which impede progress.

Mourning

During the stage of mourning the individual feels that all is lost, that he or she will never achieve anything in life. Suicide is often considered. The individual may feel that characteristics of the personality (such as courage or will) have also been lost and must be mourned as well. Thus, motivation to continue therapy or the will to improve may be impeded. The prospect of total recovery may no longer be held, but at the same time there appears to be no other acceptable alternative. This feeling of despair may be expressed as hostility, and as a result therapists may view the individual as a "problem patient." It is possible for a client to remain at this stage with feelings of inadequacy, dependence, and hostility. However, it is also possible for therapeutic intervention to facilitate movement to the next stage by creating situations in which the client may feel that "normal" aspirations and goals can be achieved. In this circumstance, normal would not include such "low-level" activities as dressing or walking; these are all activities that were taken for granted before the injury. Normal, though, would include performing the job the client was trained to do. Such activities would also include playing with or caring for a child or family. This would be seen as self-actualization by Maslow.[136]

Defense

The defense stage has two components. The first represents a healthy attitude in which the client actually starts coping with the disability. The individual takes pride in his or her accomplishments and works to improve independence and become as "normal" as possible. The person is still very much aware that barriers to normal functioning exist and is bothered by this fact but also realizes that some of the barriers can be circumvented. This healthy stage can be undermined and possibly destroyed by well-meaning family,

*References 66, 67, 124, 126, 127, 131, 132.

friends, and therapists who encourage the individual to see only the positive aspects and who do not allow the client to examine feelings about the restrictions and barriers of the condition. Conditions that lead to the final stage of adjustment are the realization that the whole body or mind is not needed to actualize his or her life goals and that needs can be actualized in other ways. A therapist should watch for opportunities to facilitate this transition. There is a fine line between hopelessness and hope of regaining function. Taking away any hope of regaining quality of life leads to helplessness and may take away the motivation for neuroplasticity within the patient's central nervous system. Thus, helping the patient be realistic and reality oriented while not taking away hope is a skill all therapists need to cultivate.

The negative alternative during the defensive stage is the neurotic defensive reaction. The client refusing to recognize that even a partial barrier exists to meeting normal goals typifies this. The client may try to convince everyone that he or she has adjusted.

Adjustment

In the final stage, adjustment, the person sees the disability as neither an asset nor a liability but as an aspect of the person, much like a large nose or big feet. He or she is accepting what is, not resisting what is. Functional limitation or inability to participate in any life activity is not something to be overcome, apologized for, or defended. Kerr[133] refers to two aspects or goals of this stage. The first goal is for the person to feel at peace with his or her god or greater power: the client does not feel that he or she is being punished or tested. The second goal is for the client to feel that he or she is an adequate person, not a second-class citizen. Kerr[137] believes that "It is essential that the paths to those more 'abstract goals' be structured if the person is to make a genuine adjustment." She also believes that it is the health care professional's job to offer that structure.

Acceptance or adjustment is at least as hard to achieve and maintain in life for the disabled person as happiness and harmony are for all people.[138] Adjustment connotes putting the disability into perspective, seeing it as one of the many characteristics of that person. It does not mean negating the existence of or focusing on the condition. Successful adjustment may be defined as a continuing process in which the person adapts to the environment in a satisfying and efficient manner. This is true for all human beings, able-bodied or disabled. There are always obstacles to overcome in attempting the goal of a happy and successful life.[16,92,138,139]

People and circumstances change. Maintaining a balanced state of adjustment is not easy, especially for the person with limitations. I recall a woman who had achieved a stable state of acceptance of her quadriplegic condition. One day she called in a panic because, as she saw it, she "wasn't adjusted anymore." She had moved into a college dormitory and wanted to go out for a friendly game of football with her new friends but suddenly saw how physically limited she was. She had grown up in a hospital and had never had to face this situation. After discussing this, she was able to put things into perspective and was able to talk over her feelings of isolation with her friends, who, without hesitation, altered the game to include her. Keeping a balanced perspective is hard in a world that changes constantly.

White[140] stated that without some participation, there can be no affecting the environment and thus no sense of self-satisfaction. Fine[141] and King[142] point out that without satisfaction from affecting the environment, reinforcement is insufficient to carry on the behavior, and the behavior will be extinguished. Thus satisfaction and performance must be linked. If the patient has not adjusted to his or her new body, however, little satisfaction can be gained from such everyday activities as walking, eating, or rolling over in bed.[143] To define adjustment on a purely performance basis is to run the risk of creating a "mechanical person" who might be physically rehabilitated but, once discharged, may find that he or she lacks satisfaction, incentive, and purpose. The psychological state of adjustment is what makes self-satisfaction possible.

Body Image

"Self-care is never a selfish act—it is simply good stewardship of the only gift I have, the gift I was put on this earth to offer to others. Anytime we can listen to true self and give it the care it requires, we do so not only for ourselves but for the many others whose lives we touch."[121]

Body image is an all-encompassing concept that looks at how the person and to some extent the support systems view the person and roles that are expected to be assumed. Taleporos and McCabe[20] found that clients had negative feelings about their bodies and general negative psychological experiences after injury. Even when clients do not have disfigurements that are readily observable, they often still report changes in body image and negative feelings of self-worth.

One of the issues that may arise relating to body image is sexuality. This concept may take many behavioral forms: flirting, harassment, questions about fertility, or questions regarding whether the client is capable of performing the sex act at all. Flirting may be a sign that clients have had assaults on their femininity or masculinity. By flirting, clients are often trying to determine whether they still are seen as a sensual being. In this case the therapist may need to set boundaries by saying that he or she is not allowed to date or flirt with clients. This is to make sure that the client does not think that it is something about the disability that is the "turnoff." Sensitivity must be used because the client could think that "if a medical person finds me repulsive then no one will ever see me as attractive." It is important for the therapist to try to ascertain the intent behind the behavior. Usually this can be accomplished by evaluating how he or she feels about the interaction. If the therapist feels unthreatened and does not feel demeaned when the client is flirting, he or she still needs to report this to the therapist of record. If the therapist feels defensive, demeaned, or very uncomfortable, then he or she may be experiencing harassment. It is never warranted or "part of the job" to be harassed, and the client's behavior must be stopped immediately by alerting the client that the behavior is making the therapist feel uncomfortable and that it must stop now. Again, the therapist needs to go to the supervisor or team to mention this behavior. It can often be the case that other team members are experiencing the same behavior and it can be dealt with as a team. If the behavior is considered a chronic problem by the team, a treatment plan needs to be designed to stop the behavior. It is important to remember that sexual health should not be a neglected area of client treatment. It may take time for the appropriate questions to be asked by the client.[28,144-148]

Questions about any physical performance are within the domain of therapy. If the client is asking for information regarding sex (e.g., positioning options) it is a subject that needs to be addressed in a respectful manner. If the questions are regarding fertility, capability, and the like, then these should be referred to an appropriate medical person. None of these questions should be discouraged or neglected, because this area is important for your clients' motivation and sexual health.[149,150] It is important for the therapist to know that in spinal cord injury, fertility will generally not be impaired for a woman, but issues of lubrication before sex should be addressed by the appropriate person. Men may have erection problems and ejaculation issues, but these too can be addressed by the appropriate person. It is now known that fertility in spinal cord–injured men may be possible and should not be ruled out.[146,151-154]

Awareness of Sexual Issues

Sexuality is usually one of the last areas to be assessed by clinical staff, but it is one area mentioned as having great importance to family members and the client.[83,104,155,156] Sexuality involves more than just the sex act; it incorporates characteristics such as sexual attraction, sexual identification, sexual confidence, and sexual validation.[104,155,156] It is a predictor of adjustment to disability, of success in vocational training, and of marital satisfaction when the woman is disabled.[28,73,147,148,156-162]

Sexuality (sensuality) is representative of how the person is dealing with his or her world. If the person feels inadequate as a sexual, sensual, and lovable human being, there is little chance that the person will also feel motivated to pursue other avenues of life.[83,156,163] This area of function must be assessed with great sensitivity to the individual's feelings.[143,148,163-165]

The framework for assessing sexuality differs with the therapist. Some therapists see sexuality as an activity of daily living and incorporate it into the evaluation. Others feel the client needs information about body mechanics to perform the sex act; thus positioning and reflex inhibiting patterns are assessed. Still others have found it a motivating force when range of motion and muscle control are worked on. A further discussion of these concerns follows in the section on adult sexuality.

Development of Sensuality (Sexuality)

Even before birth, the sense of touch[166] and the ability to distinguish pleasurable and unpleasurable tactile sensations begin to develop. Pleasurable feelings are comforting, and attempts are made to prolong them; for example, a baby cries when nursing is stopped. If satisfaction is not derived from this interaction on a regular basis, a feeling of anxiety may develop, the child may withdraw from interaction with others, and distrust may develop.[166] If pleasure in interaction with others is obtained in the first 3 years, the ability to maintain the warmth of being close and being nourished is translated into trust (that all needs will be satisfied by the caretaker) and lovability (bonding). It is here that a sense of intimacy is initiated.[106,167] By the age of 5 years, the ability to explore the world by using the hands and mouth, as well as other parts of the body, allows the individual to develop communication, self-gratification, and a feeling of compete nce.[106,140,167]

This feeling of competence is derived from the effective use of the body to meet its needs and to accomplish tasks. By the age of 8 years, body parts and body processes are usually named and the child perceives the body as good. At this time intimacy between the self and another person is further refined, as are roles. During puberty, body changes and sexual tension are heightened. Self-acceptance is based on the person's perception of how effectively he or she has accomplished the previous tasks.[106,167-169]

The preceding is an oversimplification of the first 20 years of life, but the role of sensuality and sensation cannot be overemphasized. This is especially true for those professionals who constantly interact with clients in a physical manner such as handling. The intervention the therapist provides when the client is, or feels he or she is, in a dependent state can have a direct impact on how the client may perceive himself or herself in the future.

Pediatric Sensuality

The child needs to learn to enjoy the body. The therapist should help the client to distinguish between therapeutic touch and "fun" sensual touch, such as tickling or cuddling. It is important for clients to distinguish between the two so that they do not "turn their bodies off" to touch. For example, a woman with cerebral palsy stated during an interview that therapy was either painful or so clinical that she disassociated herself from sensations in her body during therapy. Later in life this became a problem when she was married. She stated that it took 7 years of marriage before she could enjoy the sensations of being touched by her husband.

The therapy session should also help the client develop a sense of personal ownership of the body.[81,155,170] This aspect is often neglected when working with children.[81,167] The therapist often does not ask permission to touch a client, thus suggesting that the client lacks the right to control being touched by others. The last thing the therapist would desire to communicate, especially to a child, is that any person has the right to handle and touch the client's body. Child molestation with a disabled population is just beginning to be recognized as a problem in this country, with possibly one third of the female and male population being victimized.[81] It is hard to think of a more likely victim than a person who has (unintentionally) been taught that he or she does not have the right to say "No" to being touched and who cannot physically resist unwanted advances and in some cases cannot even communicate that abuse has taken place. The effects of this can be seen in adults. When one client was asked why tone increased in her lower extremities when she was touched, her response was, "I was sexually abused by my father in the name of therapy, and therapy and sexual abuse are synonymous at this point." No wonder she had not wanted to reenter therapy!

One way of helping clients "own" their respective bodies (besides asking permission to touch) is by naming body parts and body processes using correct terminology (as opposed to baby talk), thus making it possible for the client to communicate and relate appropriately.[81,167,170,171] This can be accomplished as the need arises, or it can be encouraged through the use of anatomically correct puzzles or dolls during therapy sessions.

One goal of therapy may be to develop the concept that the body (in the case of persons with the congenital disabilities) or the "new body" (in the case of those with acquired disabilities) is acceptable and good,[167-171] thus giving the client a more positive attitude toward his or her body and toward therapy. Pointing out a particularly positive aspect of the client's body and mentioning this regularly can encourage this attitude. This feature could be the hair, the eyes, or a smile, but it should be an aspect of the client that can be seen and commented on by others as well. Commenting on how well the body feels when it is relaxed or how good the sun feels on the body helps the client recognize that the body can be a positive source of pleasure.

Another message that can negatively affect the client in later life is the concept that individuals with movement dysfunction are asexual and will never have sexual needs or partners.[73,148,169-173] Although it may not be appropriate to deal directly with the concept in therapy with a child, the therapist might mention that he or she knows of a person with a functional problem such as the client's movement limitations who is married or who has children. In this way the therapist communicates that there is a possibility that the "normal" sex roles of the child may be fulfilled in the future. Without this possibility being presented, the child may think that there is no chance that all the movies, books, and television programs that deal with normal adult interactions apply to individuals with functional limitations, a belief that leads to poor socialization and further alienation from participating in life.*

Adult Sexuality

Discussing positioning to reduce pain and spasticity or to enable the client to more comfortably engage in sexual relations will help the client deal with problems before they reveal themselves. Because sexual hygiene may be considered as an activity of daily living, it may fall within the domain of therapy.

The client may feel that his or her sexual identity is threatened by a newly acquired disability and may try to assert sexuality through jokes, flirting, or even passes toward the therapist. In these cases it is important for the therapist to realize that what is often being looked for is the confirmation that the client is still a sexual and sensual human being; thus the therapist's response is very important.[106,170,171,173,174] If the therapist rejects or even ridicules the client, it may be a very long time before the client can even think of attempting such a confirmation of personal attractiveness. The client may feel that because the therapist rejects the client and the therapist is familiar with the disabled, there is little chance anyone who is not familiar with the disabled could accept the client as lovable.[175] The therapist should not be surprised by such advances and should deal with the situation in a professional manner. The therapist should also realize that approximately 10% of the population is homosexual and be prepared for advances from clients of the same sex. The therapist needs to be as professional as possible in acknowledging this client as with any other. All of the therapist's interactions should be directed toward creating an environment that will promote a stronger and more well-adjusted client.[106,170,171,173]

The therapist's response to sexual advances must be tempered with an understanding of the possible cause for the behavior. The client may be cognitively impaired and may not even be aware of the inappropriateness of some forms of sexual behavior, or the client may be trying to control others through acting-out behaviors. The client may have been sexually aggressive even before the injury. At no time should the therapist allow himself or herself to be sexually harassed. If the therapist feels harassed, the therapist must take control of the situation and find a way to stop the client's behavior. This is usually achieved by confronting the issue. Not dealing with inappropriate behavior will allow it to continue and may be detrimental to the medical team and to the client's normal participation in life.[145,156,170,171]

The therapist can assist the client in moving through the stages of self-awareness to appreciate that the client is still sensual, sexual, and huggable. This process can be done through everyday interaction; it may entail encouraging the family to embrace the client and may even call for the therapist to role model these behaviors at times.[174] The therapist may provide reading materials to the client and family directly by reviewing and answering questions or indirectly by having such books as *Reproductive Issues for Persons with Physical Disabilities,*[175] *Sexuality and the Person with Traumatic Brain Injury: A Guide for Families,*[176] and *Sexual Function in People with Disability and Chronic Illness*[177] available for their reading. In this way, the individual and significant others are made aware of possible options for the expression of intimacy and of the fact that this part of life is not over.

Because the therapist is in a situation of one-to-one treatment involving touching, moving, and handling the client's body, he or she may frequently be the natural person from whom the individual may seek information. If this natural curiosity does not appear to be forthcoming, however, the therapist can give the client an opening. For example, during an evaluation of motor skills, the person may be asked if there are any problems in such areas as sexual positioning. The topic need not be pursued any further by the therapist, but when the client is ready to deal with the subject area, he or she will probably remember that the therapist brought it up and may be a person to approach when dealing with these issues.[163,170,178]

Other ways of presenting sexual information are to have literature available on the client's ward so that those who are interested may pursue the topic in private, to have a group discussion (interested clients, clients and significant others, or whatever group the client and therapist might choose to assemble), or to have literature in the department waiting room.

It is important for the therapist to be aware of some of the aspects of sexuality that may or may not affect the client as a result of trauma or disease. Fertility is seldom affected in women.[179-183] Men, on the other hand, may experience dysfunction of the penis and testicles and/or fertility.[55,69,184-186]

Devices may be used and adapted to allow for sexual gratification of the client (masturbation) or significant others. Stimulant drugs such as sildenafil citrate (Viagra) or other aids may be used to enhance a person's sex life. Sensation

*References 73, 106, 148, 171, 173, 174.

should be checked and sexual activities modified (or the client should be alerted to the problem) to avoid breakdowns or medical complications. Positioning modifications may be needed to allow for better energy conservation, joint protection, motor control, maintenance of muscle and skin integrity, and pleasure. Clients may have questions regarding modifications that may be needed for the use of birth control devices or contraindications regarding the use of such devices. Clients may also need equipment (e.g., vibrators) modified if hand function is involved. Complications that may affect function and mobility of the client may arise as a result of pregnancy. Delivery may present some unique situations that may also need to be addressed. After delivery the disabled parent may require modifications to the wheelchair, or consultations may be needed to achieve an optimal level of function in the parenting role. All of these possibilities point to the fact that sexual issues must be dealt with throughout the treatment of all individuals with disabilities, whether the functional limitations are progressive, stable, or correctable.[175,179,187] The therapist may approach these needs or aspects of function while taking a client's sexual history. Clients have repeatedly called for more attention to be paid to sexual concerns. This is not sex counseling or therapy, and the therapist should not try to deal with deep psychosexual issues. The therapist must be informed and needs to provide information that relates to the therapist's areas of expertise, especially because other medical personnel may not have the knowledge to correctly analyze the components of some of these activities.[45,55,69,175,182,183,188-190]

Any of these issues may present themselves during the medical screening phase of evaluation, whereas others become issues as the patient is adjusting to and questioning functional limitations caused by the disease or condition. Once the patient has identified the need for this information, the therapist, whether through referral, group work, or individual discussions, needs to address the questions and must not deny the patient answers because the therapist is uncomfortable.

All the clinical problem areas that need assessment and evaluation and that have been mentioned previously are examined in relation to treatment planning in the clinical setting in the following sections.

Support System

Earlier literature hinted that partner relationships may be negatively affected by a member being disabled. Within the last few years this concept has been questioned in regard to some disabilities such as adult-onset spinal cord injuries,[189] whereas pediatric spinal cord injury and other disabilities may result in relationship problems.[191,192] It has been shown that adjustment and quality of life can be adversely affected by the physical environment being inadequate, thus making the person more dependent. The result of the dependence appears to be poor relationships.[193-195] This can also be seen with the families in which a member has had a brain injury.[196,197] In studies on muscular dystrophy it was found that physical dependence is not the only variable needing to be considered. Psychological issues need to be identified and considered as part of intervention.[198,199] Recent literature has identified a number of elements that the client and the family may need help to work on, such as "to assist them to develop new views of vulnerability and strength, make changes in relationships, and facilitate philosophical, physical and spiritual growth."[198] Turner and Cox[198] also felt that the medical staff could facilitate "recognizing the worth of each individual, helping them to envision a future that is full of promise and potential, actively involving each person in their own care trajectory, and celebrating changes to each person's sense of self."[198] Man[199] observed that each family copes differently in relation to a brain-injured family member and that the family's structure should be explored to develop intervention guidelines. It has also been noted that health care professionals should view the situation from the family's perspective to approach and support the family's adaptation.[200] This should be done to help the client and the family accept the disability but at the same time to help them keep the negative views of society in perspective.[70] In general, it has also been found that family support is a significant factor in the client's subjective functioning[201,202] and that social engagement is productive.[89,203] According to Franzén-Dahlin, Larson, and colleagues,[204] enhancing psychological health and preventing medical problems in the caregiver are essential considerations to enable individuals with disabilities to continue to live at home. Their research found that evaluating the situation for spouses of stroke patients was an important component when planning for the future care of the patient.

When working with children it is important to realize that they often feel responsible for almost anything that happens in life, such as divorce, siblings getting hurt, or general arguments between parents. It is important that the therapist help the client and the siblings realize that they are not responsible for the client's condition. Part of this magical thinking that often appears is the concept that "bad things happen to bad people." Thus, the child is bad because a bad thing has happened or the adult is bad just because the disease or trauma has occurred. It is important to be sensitive to this ideation and help dispel this maladaptive thought pattern because it is not true or productive for the client, the siblings, parents, or spouses within a family and may cause further adjustment problems later in treatment. Siblings of the client should be helped to see their roles as good siblings and should not be placed in the role of caretakers of a sibling with special needs. In this way all children can grow naturally without any one of the children being overly focused on. At the same time, it is a fact of life that the disabled child will probably need physical assistance, therapy, increased medical care, and thus more time devoted to him or her, and this is just a fact of life.

It should always be noted by the medical establishment that having a disability is expensive in ways that we are often not aware of. There are the obvious medical costs of therapy, surgery, drugs, wheelchairs, or orthoses, but there are other costs such as the possibility of extra cost of transportation, catheters for urination, wheelchair maintenance, adaptive clothing, and the like that are continuing costs not covered by most insurance plans. These costs add up and contribute to the emotional costs and demands on the family. The significant others may feel the need to work more to have the money to cover such expenses, but then that person is not around to help out. This is but one of the many dilemmas that must be acknowledged for the support system of the disabled person. The family may be encouraged to contact such groups as the Family Caregiver Support Network (www.caregiversupportnetwork.org) to get information and assistance with such diverse topics as being a caregiver, legal and financial aid, and communications (this group tends to focus on the adult but still may be a wonderful aid). Such groups will give information to all who need it and help to empower the family. This takes the focus off of the medical condition and may help the family to gain a better, more balanced perspective on the condition.

Loss and the Family

In this chapter the client's support system is referred to as the *family*. The family may be composed of spouses, parents, children, lovers (especially in gay and lesbian relationships), friends, employers, or interested others such as church groups, civic organizations, or individuals. The people in the support system may go through the same stages of reaction and adjustment to loss that the client does.[1,9,141,205-207]

Family Needs

The family will, at least temporarily, experience the loss of a loved family member from the normal routine. During the acute stage the family may not have concrete answers to basic questions regarding the extent of injury, the length of time before the injured person will be back in the family unit, or possibly whether the person will live.

During this phase, the family network will be in a state of crisis.[9] New roles will have to be assumed by the family members, and the "experts" will not even tell them for how long these roles must be endured. If children are involved, they will probably demand more attention to reassure themselves that they will remain loved. Depending on the child's age, the child will have differing capabilities in understanding the loss (see the section on examination of loss). Each member of the family may react differently to bereavement, and each may be at a different stage of adjustment to the disability (see the section on adjustment). One member may be in shock and deny the disability, whereas another member may be in mourning and may verbalize a lack of hope. The family crisis that is caused by a severe injury cannot be overstated.[98,206-209]

Role changes in the family may be dramatic.[64,74,92,210-212] Members who have never driven may need to learn that motor skill; one who has never balanced a checkbook may now be responsible for managing the family budget; and those who have never been assertive may have to deal forcefully with insurance companies and the medical establishment.[9,57,173,213,214]

The family may feel resentment toward the injured member. This attitude may seem justified to them because they see the person lying in bed all day while the family members must take over new responsibilities in addition to their old ones. In a study by Lobato, Kao, and Plante,[215] Latino siblings of children with chronic disabilities were at risk for internalizing psychological problems. The medical staff may not always understand the stress that family members are under and may react to the resentment expressed either verbally or nonverbally with a protective stance toward the client. Siding with the "hurt" client may alienate the family from the medical staff and may also drive a permanent wedge between family members. This long-term situation may undermine the compliance of family members' involvement in home programs and ultimately the successful outcome of long-term intervention.

Parental Bonding and the Disabled Child

The parental bonding process is complicated and is still being studied.[48] The process may start well before the child is even conceived. The parents often think about having a child and plan and fantasize about future interactions with the child; after conception the planning and fantasizing increase. During the pregnancy the mother and father accept the fetus as an individual, and after the birth of the child the attachment process is greatly intensified. The "sensitive period" is the first few minutes to hours after the birth. During this time the parents should have close physical contact with the child to strongly establish the attachment that will later grow deeper.[216,217] There is an almost symbiotic relationship between mother and child at this time: infant and mother behaviors complement each other (e.g., nursing stimulates uterine contraction). It is important at this point for the child to respond to the parents in some way so that there is an interaction. In the early stages of bonding, seeing, touching, caring for, and interacting with the child allow for the bonding process. When this process is disturbed for any reason, such as congenital malformations or hospital procedures for high-risk infants, problems may occur later.

When the parents are told that their child is going to be malformed or disabled, it is a massive shock. The parents must start a process of grieving. The dream of a "normal" child must be given up, and the parents must go through the loss or "death" of the child they expected before they can accept the new child. Parents often feel guilty. Shellabarger and Thompson[218] state that parents feel the deformed child was their failure.[1] The disabled child will always have a strong impact on the family, sometimes a catastrophic one.[1,8,9,218,219] A study by Ha, Hong, Seltzer, and Greenberg[220] found that compared with parents of nondisabled children, parents of disabled children experienced significantly higher levels of negative affect, poorer psychological well-being, and significantly more somatic symptoms. Older parents were significantly less likely to experience the negative effect of having a disabled child than younger parents.

In a study by Arnaud, White-Koning, and colleagues[221] greater severity of impairment was found to not always be associated with poorer quality of life; in the moods and emotions, self-perception, social acceptance, and school environment domains, less severely impaired children appeared to be more likely to have poor quality of life. Pain was associated with poor quality of life in the physical and psychological well-being and self-perception domains. Parents with higher levels of stress were more likely to report poor quality of life in all domains, which suggests that factors other than the severity of the child's impairment may influence the way in which parents report quality of life.

Parents must be encouraged to express their emotions, and they must be taught how to deal with the issues at hand. Techniques for accomplishing these goals are discussed in later sections.[48,217,219]

The Child Dealing with Loss

If a parent is injured, the young child may experience an overwhelming sense of loss. Child care may be a problem, especially if the primary caregiver is injured. The child will probably feel deserted by the injured parent and may demand the attention of the remaining parent. This will increase the strain on all family members.[64]

If the child is the client, his or her life will have undergone a radical change: every aspect of the child's world will have altered. Loved objects and people will help to restore the child's feeling of security. It is of major importance to explain to the child in very simple terms what is going on and to allow the child the opportunity to express feelings both verbally and nonverbally. It is important to use play and art as the medium of communication for children.

The hospital setting is threatening to all people, but children are especially susceptible to loss of autonomy, feelings of isolation, and loss of independence. Senesac (see Chapter 12) has stated that the severity of the disability is not as important a variable in the emotional development of the child as are the attitudes of parents and family.[2,8] Parents must attempt to be aware of the child's inability to understand the permanence (or transience) of the loss of function.[8] They will also need to help the child feel secure by bringing in familiar and cherished objects. A schedule should be established and kept to promote consistency. Play and art should be encouraged, especially types that allow the child to vent feelings and deal with the new environment. Any procedures or therapies should be presented in a relaxed and playful way so that the child has time to think and to feel as comfortable as possible about the change. The parents may often need to be reminded to pay attention to the children in the family without disabilities during this acute stage.

The Adolescent Dealing with Loss

The adolescent is subject to all of the feelings and fears that other clients express. Adolescents are in a struggle to achieve autonomy and independence, and they often are ambivalent about these feelings. When an adolescent is suddenly injured and has to cope with being disabled, it can be a massive assault on the individual's development.[139,222] According to research conducted by Kinavey,[50] findings imply that youth born with spina bifida face biological, psychological, and social challenges that interfere with developmental tasks of adolescence, including identity formation. Therapists are urged to direct intervention toward humanizing and emancipating the physical and social environment for youth with physical disabilities to maximize developmental opportunities and potential while fostering positive identity.

Kingsnorth, Healy, and Macarthur[49] stated that with advances in health care, an increasing number of youth with physical disabilities are surviving into adulthood. For youth to reach their full potential, a number of critical life skills must be learned. Specific learning opportunities are important, as youth with physical disabilities may be limited in the life experiences necessary to acquire these skills. Therapists are in the unique position of fostering these kinds of environments to encourage adolescents to engage in critical life skills such as problem solving, decision making, goal setting, critical thinking, communication skills, assertiveness, self-awareness, and skills for coping with stress. Life skills differ from instrumental daily living skills. Daily living skills are the activities required to function independently in the community and include skills such as financial management, meal preparation, or navigation in the community. An approach emphasizing life skill development can, however, be used to acquire daily living skills.

The adolescent appears to react differently from other age groups to the knowledge of his or her own terminal illness. The adolescent often feels that he or she has gone through a very painful process (initiation) that will soon lead to the "joys and rights" of adulthood. Unlike persons in older age groups, who might feel that they can look back and gain solace from the past, the adolescent feels that he or she will have what Britto and colleagues[222] term "death before fulfillment" and thus may react by feeling cheated by life. This same pattern may occur with the disabled adolescent.[223] The therapist must be acutely aware of these feelings so that therapy may be presented in the most effective manner for the client to find challenge and fulfillment in life.[224]

Family Maturation

The family also has a maturational aspect. If the injured person is a child and if the family is young with dependent children at home, the adjustment may not be the problem that it would be for a family whose children are older. In the latter case, parents have begun to experience freedom and independence, and they may find adjusting to a return to a restricted lifestyle difficult or even intolerable. They may have the feeling that they have already "put in their time" and should now be free. If the disability interrupts the child's developmental process, future conflict may arise because the parents will eventually want retirement, relaxation, and freedom. Parents may feel guilty and try to repress this normal response.

The reverse may also be true. The parents may be feeling that the children have left them ("empty nest syndrome"), and they may be too willing to welcome a "dependent" family member back into the home. This may lead to excessive dependence or anger toward the parents on the part of the client. All these factors must be taken into consideration by the therapist when therapy is presented to the client and family.

The therapist can develop a greater understanding of the client and family by being aware of the normal human developmental patterns. These patterns identify some of the major hurdles that must be overcome in the client's life.

Coping with Transition

In the acute stage of a family member's injury, the family must be helped to deal with the crisis at hand. During this phase, the family must first be allowed to cope with the emotional impact of what is happening with a loved one. Second, the family should be helped to see the situation as a challenge that if overcome will facilitate growth. Third, adaptation within the family unit must occur for the situation to be overcome.

Brammer and Abrego[224] have developed a list of basic coping skills that they have broken into five levels. In the first level the person becomes aware of and mobilizes skills in perceiving and responding to transition and attempts to handle the situation. In the second level the person mobilizes the skills for assessing, developing, and using external support systems. In level three the person can possess, develop, and use internal support systems (develop positive self-regard and use the situation to grow). The person in level four must find ways to reduce emotional and physiological distress (relaxation, control stimulation, and verbal expression of feelings). In level five the person must plan and implement change (analyze discrepancies, plan new options, and successfully implement the plan). Using this model, the therapist and family can evaluate the coping skill level of the family. The therapist and staff can then help promote movement toward the next level of coping with the transition. These levels are also broken into specific skills and subskills so that the therapist can grade them further.

One of the more damaging aspects of hospitalization to all involved is that the hospital staff focuses on the disability rather than on the individual's strengths.[76,206,225] Centering on the disability can lead to a situation in which client, family, and staff see only the functional limitations and not the potential ability of the client.

Decentering from the loss of function will be examined further in this chapter. If the family relationship was positive before the insult and if the client is cognitively intact, then the focus must be directed toward the relationship's strengths as well as toward the client's and family's individual cognitive and emotional strengths.[91] In the initial acute stage of adjustment, crisis intervention may help the family use its strengths and at the same time deal with the situation at hand.

To adequately deal with the crisis, the family should do the following:

1. Be helped to focus on the crisis caused by the disability; identify the situation to stimulate problem solving; identify and deal with doubts of adequacy, guilt, and self-blame; identify and address grief; identify and deal with anticipatory worry; be offered basic information and education regarding the crisis situation; and be helped to create a bridge to resources in the hospital and in the community for support and to see their own family resources.[48,226-229]
2. Be helped to remember how they have dealt successfully with crises in the past and to implement some of the same strategies in the present situation.
3. Work with the family as a unit during crisis to help strengthen the family and facilitate more positive attitudes toward the client. These attitudes by the family will improve the client's attitudes or feelings toward the injury and hospitalization.[92,212,230-233] Encouraging family-unit functioning in this situation will decrease the amount of regression displayed by the client. If the family is encouraged to function without the client, however, more damage than good may be done.[1,139]

TREATMENT VARIABLES IN RELATION TO THERAPY

Skilled therapy intervention focuses on maximizing participation in functional activities, participation in life, and behavioral change. Livneh and Antonak[134] promote the following activities for the health professional:

1. Assisting clients to explore the personal meaning of the disability. "Training clients to attain a sense of mastery over their emotional experiences." A way of doing this would be to help the client not to demonstrate emotional outbursts or to help the client look at his or her emotions and to put them into perspective.
2. Providing clients with relevant medical information. "These strategies emphasize imparting accurate information to clients on their medical condition, including its present status, prognosis, anticipated future functional limitations, and when applicable, vocational implications." This may be done by helping the client and family access resources such as PubMed (www.ncbi.nlm.nih.gov/pubmed) online or find medical references in the library.
3. Providing clients with supportive family and group experiences. "These strategies permit clients (usually with similar disabilities or common life experiences) and, if applicable, their family members or significant others, to share common fears, concerns, needs, and wishes." This can be done in rather unobtrusive ways such as scheduling clients with the same disability at the same time so that they meet in the waiting room or while doing group mat activities. Another option is hiring individuals with limitations who are health care professionals and can discuss and role model positive behaviors and answer relevant questions from the client's perspective. Remember that clients are all potential teachers for you as well as other clients.
4. Teaching clients adaptive coping skills for successful community functioning. "These skills include assertiveness, interpersonal relations, decision making, problem solving, stigma management, and time management skills." This would entail role-playing situations that may occur in the community, such as an able-bodied person asking why the client is in a wheelchair; preaching to the wheelchair user because he or she must have offended God in some way—otherwise the person would not be in a wheelchair; or telling a woman that it is such a shame that she is disabled because she is so good looking and could have found a man if it were not for the disability. Role playing can also be used to help a person deal with the possibly awkward experience of going to bed with a new partner and having to explain how to be undressed, or what those tubes coming out of the body are for, or what positions are best for someone with this condition.

ROLE OF THE THERAPEUTIC ENVIRONMENT

Whenever possible in therapy the functional activity should be presented and structured to promote empowerment, problem solving, and adjustment. Adjustment and adaptation to life form a dynamic process that allows for the person to interact with life in a meaningful and productive way that encourages the person to enjoy life (Figure 6-1).[17,80,234-237] We see the client at a very stressful time, and we need to make this time as productive for the client and the family as possible.

This section examines issues the therapist and staff should know to create a therapeutic environment that will facilitate psychological adjustment and independence of the client with activity limitations. The physical and the attitudinal environment of the treatment facility plays a major role in the way the client views the services that are rendered.

Recall a time before you became a member of the medical community. Think about how awe inspiring the people in white coats were, how strange the smells of the hospitals were, how busy it all seemed, and how puzzling the secret

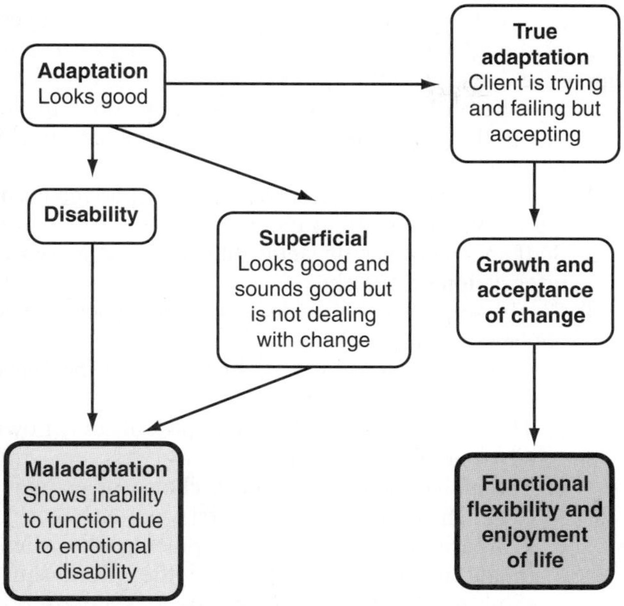

Figure 6-1 ■ Possible directions of the adaptive process.

medical language was. It all seemed overwhelming then, and it still is to newcomers, especially newly admitted patients and their families. The hospital usually appears impersonal,[238] sterile, monotonous, and confusing, and all status accumulated outside the hospital means little inside.

The therapist needs to take the setting into account when dealing with the client. The environment can be altered in a variety of ways. Therapy staff could wear street clothes, decorate the department or hospital with posters and lively colors, and allow clients to bring some personal items into the hospital.

The nature of the therapy process can often lead the therapist to see only the disability and not the person—as occurs, for example, when a client is referred to by his or her disability rather than by name. This stereotyping of those with disabilities can lead the therapist to concentrate on the lack of abilities rather than on the strengths of the clients. The real danger is that the client and family will also start to focus on the functional limitations of the client and feel that their family relationship is now permanently altered. The accuracy of this perception may have to be evaluated as part of the adjustment process. The wife of a man with paraplegia said with a sudden burst of insight, "I didn't marry him for his legs—this doesn't change the relationship." Often so much attention is directed toward the disability that tunnel vision develops. One way to try to get a better perspective is to look at the bigger picture. A variety of questions can be asked that may help the therapist gain a greater insight into the client as a person (Box 6-2).

After the therapist is aware of the strengths of the client, these strengths may be capitalized on in therapy to help the client realize them and build confidence. Clients often reported that they were not complimented in therapy and especially that they never received feedback that their bodies were desirable[239] or that they were doing things correctly.[11,76,175,176,240] A logical thought by the client is, "If the therapist cannot see anything desirable about me, and the therapist deals with the individuals with similar problems all the time, then there must not be anything good about me." Positive, sincere comments to client and family can add a motivational factor to treatment that may have been missing.[76,232]

Providing opportunities to be outdoors can help clients cultivate a sense of connection with something that is larger than themselves. At the most basic level there is more oxygen outside, and in general the air is fresher than indoors. "And looking at a faraway horizon or sky can help us gain needed perspective on our small world, bounded by our bodies and our lives."[241]

The last and possibly the most important aspect in creating an environment that will foster growth and adjustment in the client is a staff whose members are well adjusted and aware of their own personal needs. Just as coping skills are necessary for the client, the staff, too, must be capable of coping with the stresses of the emotional and physical pain of the client and the client's family. The therapist must also deal with his or her own personal reactions to the sometimes devastating situations others are in.[76,232,242] Exposure to such

BOX 6-2 ■ QUESTIONS TO HELP GAIN INSIGHT INTO THE CLIENT AS A PERSON

The following questions can be asked:

- What would this person be doing if he or she did not have this condition?
- What is stopping the person from reaching these goals now?
- Who will marry this person and why?
- What are his or her positive traits?
- What will this person do for a living?
- What will this person do for enjoyment?
- How will this person bring others enjoyment?
- What would this person be doing if there was no disability?
- How is the disability stopping the person from actualizing their goals? (These are the goals that need to be worked on.)

Similar questions can be asked of the client to explore ways of helping the client have a meaningful life:

- What do you look like and function like now?
- What will you look like after therapy?
- What important things would you be doing now if you were not in need of treatment?
- What activities or forms of productivity were you involved in before, and which were important to you?
- Which of these things do you still do?
- What if anything is preventing you from doing these things now?
- How does this condition affect your being a lover of life, family, significant other, and so on?
- How will this condition affect your important life goals, your activities, and your ability to do meaningful activities?
- How much different would your life look if it were not for this condition?
- Will any of the above be stopped by your condition, and if so how?

situations often elicits introspection on the part of the staff that can result in emotional turmoil for staff members and affect their own personal relationships. This emotional energy needs to be directed in a productive way so that the energy does not turn into chaos within the staff interaction or become a destructive force for the client.

To decrease the possibly distractive nature of this emotional energy, the staff should be made aware of their own coping styles, and they should be allowed to vent their reactions to particularly distressing client case loads in a positive, supportive group. Group meetings can be used to handle some of the inevitable tension, especially if there is a respected member who is skilled in group work. This is not a psychotherapy session (although psychotherapy may be warranted in some situations) but rather an opportunity to test reality and remove tension before it is incorrectly directed toward fellow staff members. These sessions can make use of the four elements of crisis intervention mentioned in the previous section, as well as information from others.[177,232] Other times that this stress reduction can be achieved are in supervision or during coffee breaks, as long as the sessions are productive.

The staff can use these sessions to better understand their various reactions to stress and to explore their coping styles.[211,232,243,244] Ideally, this knowledge of coping styles and stress reduction will decrease staff burnout and aid the staff to help clients and their families deal with stress more successfully.[139,240-244] There are also MBSR courses held in most hospitals, universities, and communities and can be found online at www.umassmed.edu/cfm/mbsr.

The need to have a staff that is supportive is of paramount importance because the attitude of rehabilitation personnel has emerged as one of the chief motivating factors in rehabilitation.[1,92,137] In fact, the use of humor has been found to be assistive in the process of adjustment. In a study by Solomon,[245] aging well was related to aspects of humor. It seemed to affect aging well through its relationship with perceived control. Physical health, satisfaction with housing, and relationships with family and friends were also positively influenced by humor. One suggestion by McCreaddie and Wiggins[246] is that stress can be coped with through distraction, which lessens the negative physical effects of stress. Humor is also known to have a number of potential benefits in relation to interpersonal skills or social support.[247] Specific aspects such as empathy, intimacy, and interpersonal trust have all been positively correlated with a sense of humor and subsequently with interpersonal relationships. According to McCreaddie and Wiggins,[246] a degree of rapport with the patient is necessary before humor can be used, and humor should be used only after a level of empathy, caring, and competence has been clearly demonstrated. This interaction of therapy and societal interactions explains why the World Health Organization model went from a disability or handicap model to a model of functional ability and participation in life. Although the International Classification of Diseases (ICD-9 or ICD-10) deals with physicians and disease categories, therapy clearly separates itself into a clear model that stresses the strength of an individual and his or her potential to participate in and have quality of life (www.who.int/classifications/icf).

Rogers and Figone[143] developed the following suggestions that could benefit the therapist when trying to create a supportive environment:

1. It is helpful to use the same staff member to develop the relationship and to provide continuity of care.
2. Concerned silence is most appreciated, although pushing is sometimes necessary.
3. Staff members should anticipate the need to repeat information graciously.
4. Cumbersome, hard-to-repair adaptive equipment should not be used after discharge.
5. Give clients responsibility so that they feel they have some control over therapy.
   a. The client should be allowed to pick his or her own advocate from the team.
   b. The client should be given a choice of activities (e.g., which exercise comes first).
   c. Professionals should avoid placing the client in an inferior status. In time the client starts thinking this way (feeling like a "second-class citizen").
6. Psychological support is attributed to noncounseling personnel. Personal matters are better discussed with staff members with whom the client has developed a relationship.[2,173,227]
7. Willingness to allow the client to try and fail is more helpful than controlling the client.

Bolte-Taylor[109] developed "forty things I needed the most" during her rehabilitation for her stroke. Here are a few:

1. I am not stupid, I am wounded. Please respect me.
2. Come close, speak clearly, repeat yourself if necessary, and enunciate.
3. Approach me with an open heart, slow your energy down, take your time.
4. Be aware of what your body language and facial expressions are communicating to me.
5. Make eye contact with me, encourage me.
6. Honor the healing power of sleep.
7. Protect my energy. No talk radio, TV, or nervous visitors! Keep my visitations brief.
8. Speak to me directly, not about me to others.
9. Clarify for me what the next step or level is so I know what I am working toward.
10. Celebrate all of my little successes. They inspire me.

CONCEPTUALIZATION OF ASSESSMENT AND TREATMENT

Assessment

The one component that weaves through all of Rogers and Figone's[143] seven points is the need for the therapist to be involved with the client in a therapeutic relationship—that is, to know where the client is "coming from." To know where the client is coming from is to be aware of and sensitive to the person's total psychosocial frame of reference.[2,227]

The therapist who knows his or her own beliefs, reference points, and prejudices can evaluate whether an assessment result or treatment sequence reflects the client's needs and values or those of the therapist. In the first half of this chapter, several assessments were discussed that could be summarized into the following three major components:

1. Preinjury
   a. Values and prejudices (value systems, culture, and prejudgments) of the client and family members before the injury
   b. Developmental stage of the client and family members
   c. Cognitive level of the client and family members
   d. Ability of the client and family members to handle crisis
2. Components to be evaluated leading to adjustment
   a. Loss and grief process for the client and family members
   b. Adjustment process for the client and family members
   c. Transitional stages for the client and family members
   d. Role changes for the client and family members
   e. Age or cognitive level of client and family members[9,139,227,248]
   f. Sexual adjustment for the client and spouse
3. Techniques used to elicit adjustment and independence
   a. Crisis intervention strategies
   b. Letting the client and family take control
   c. Expression of emotion, both verbally and nonverbally
   d. Problem solving
   e. Role playing
   f. Praise
   g. Education
   h. Support groups

Once an assessment has been made of the client and family members' stages of psychological adjustment, the client's occupational history and roles, and their preinjury attitudes and beliefs, a treatment protocol can be established. This protocol will need to incorporate steps toward stage change and possibly attitudinal change. Because these changes require learning on the part of the client and family, an environment that optimally facilitates these changes must be established.*

Therapy can be seen as a form of education in which the client and the client's family are taught how the client should use his or her body. The education process is not limited to the physical aspects of therapy, however. The client is also taught how to look at and think about the body and the disability. If the staff is nonverbally telling the client and the family that the client is not capable of making decisions and of being independent, it follows that the client may indeed feel dependent and incapable of making decisions. Giles[211] and others[207,211,249,252,253] stated that there was an inverse relationship between independence and distress. Distress causes further anxiety and decreases the learning potential of the client. There are ways, however, for the therapist to encourage independence on the part of the client and his family.

Specific Therapeutic Interventions

"Engagement in leisure-like activities may not only help people 'feel better' in the immediate context of coping with rehabilitation treatments, but may help sustain coping efforts as individuals learn to live with ongoing functional limitations."[254]

*References 9, 75, 92, 98, 195, 210, 249-251.

Problem-Solving Process

The family unit, including the client, should be encouraged to take active control over as much of the client's care and decision making as possible.* This can be done in every phase of the rehabilitation process. A family conference with the rehabilitation staff should actively involve the client and family in all stages of planning and treatment, up to and including discharge. The family (including the client) should be briefed ahead of time to prepare questions that they want answered or problems that need to be addressed. Rogers and Figone[143] report that conferences with family members that excluded the client engendered suspicion[2,211]; therefore if the client is capable, the client may educate the family in regard to what is happening in the hospital and in rehabilitation. Conversely, family involvement facilitates and shortens the rehabilitation process and encourages reintegration into the community.[8,207,249,253] The family can also be educated regarding the side effects and interactions of medication with publications such as the *Physicians' Desk Reference.*[258] Later in the rehabilitation process the client and family can be encouraged to arrange transportation services, find and evaluate housing, and supervise attendant care. All these activities allow the client and the family to be more in control of the environment and thus to feel independent.

In the context of one-on-one therapy, giving choices can foster client responsibility and independence. Making a decision about the order of treatment activities (such as on which side of the bed to transfer out of or which direction to roll one's wheelchair first) can give the individual a sense of self-worth that can continue to grow. This will cultivate a belief by the client and family that they are strong, with rights that need to be met. Moving out of the role of the victim, the client begins to exercise responsibility and to take action, such as applying for extended health benefits or getting a second consultation when an important medical decision needs to be made. If the client and family start to realize that they do not have to be a casualty of the medical establishment and if they find ways to control the medical establishment,[92,234,259] they are better able to discard the role of victim.

In some centers, such as the occupational therapy clinic at San Jose State University, clients have been taught the art of self-defense to make sure that they never have to fall into the victim (dependent) role. It should be noted, however, that this knowledge on the part of the client and family can be used in ways that the therapist may not always agree with. At such times it may help to adopt a philosophical attitude toward the situation and to view it as a positive direction for the client in terms of moving from victim to advocate in the rehabilitation process.

The steps of crisis intervention, which were mentioned in the previous section, can be used to help the family understand and analyze their needs in the crisis situation. Once the family has discovered that they are in crisis, they will then be able to create strategies that they can use to overcome present and future problems.

Problem solving is another element the therapist may use to help the client and family gain independence and control.†

*References 19, 22, 52, 208, 211, 248-250, 252, 253, 255-257.
†References 19, 52, 207, 211, 249, 250, 252, 253, 255, 256.

Persson and Rydén[22] acknowledged the importance of this when they found that there were a few significant categories to adjustment: self-trust, problem-reducing actions (problem solving), change of values, and social trust. Acknowledgement of reality and trust in oneself was found to be significant, and they identified the importance of understanding coping processes from the disabled person's point of view. In a phenomenological study by Bontje, Kinébanian, Josephsson, and Tamura,[260] participants stated they used already familiar problem-solving strategies and personal resources as well as resources in their social and physical environments to identify prospects of potential solutions and to create solutions to overcome constraints on occupational functioning.

Rather than having the client routinely learn how to accomplish a specific task, the client or family must be encouraged to think through the process from the problem to the solution and to accomplishment of the task. To achieve this activity analysis, the client would have to know the basic principles behind the activity[143] and may then be responsible for educating the family. An example of this would be a transfer from the wheelchair to the toilet. If the therapist simply has the client memorize the steps in the task, the client or family members will not necessarily be able to generalize this procedure to a transfer to the car. If the client learns the principles of proper body mechanics, work simplification, and movement, the client or family member may be more able to generalize this information to almost any situation and to solve problems later when the therapist is unavailable.[252] Rogers and Figone[143] have noted that although the client and family may fail at times during these trials, the therapist should let them be as independent and responsible as possible: let them try it their way, even if they are not successful the first time.

Pictures or slides of a restaurant, movie theater, or public building can be used to facilitate discussion and problem solving by the family unit when analyzing potential architectural barriers in the environment. Thus in the future when the family is presented with a problem or a barrier, they will have the resources to overcome it rather than be devastated by it.

Role playing in combination with support groups can also be used to defuse potentially painful situations and operate independently. While the client is still in the safe environment of the rehabilitation setting, simulations of incidents can be created for them to practice problem solving with supervision to help anticipate potential situations. They can be asked what they would do when a stranger (possibly a child) approaches the client and asks why he or she is in a wheelchair or is disabled or what they would do when a waiter asks the family member to order for the disabled client. All of these situations are potentially devastating for all involved; however, if role playing and support groups are used in advance to help all members of the family (client included) to satisfactorily handle and feel in control of the situation, the family will not be as likely to be traumatized by a similar occurrence. The result is that the family will not be as inclined to be overwhelmed by social situations and will be able to socialize in a much freer, more gratifying way.[77,79,261]

Cognitive-behavioral therapy has been used for clients and spouses with success.[93-95] Psychosocial support groups have been called for throughout the literature.* Throughout the therapeutic process, the client and the family need to be praised frequently, and credit needs to be given for the gains made by the client and family members. Granted, the therapist may have engineered the gains, but the family and client are the ones who need the reinforcement. As Bolte-Taylor[109] suggested, celebrate all of the little successes—they can help inspire the client and their family. Through gratifying experiences the family will unite to overcome the disability. They need to know that they can survive in the world without having the medical staff constantly there to solve the family's problems. In short, they need the strategies and resources that will allow them to be independent outside the medical model.

Yet another way to encourage independence can be applied to working with parents of disabled children.[13] The parents should be educated about normal and abnormal growth and development, including physical, cognitive, and emotional growth, so that the family can maintain some perspective and objectivity about their child's various levels.[8,92,167,236] The parents can then better understand the needs of those children with disabilities and those without in the family. Armed with this knowledge, the parents and children will not be frustrated with unreal expectations or unreal demands. Education of the parents could take place at local colleges, at the hospital, or even in a parent's group.

Support Systems

Groups are often used to increase motivation, provide support, increase social skills, instill hope, and help the client and family realize that they are not the only ones who have a disabled family member. This will help the client and family establish a more accurate set of perceptions about the disabled individual and allow for greater independence of the client and family.[1,9,92,135,261,265] Problem solving can be encouraged and value systems can be clarified. Client or family support groups can be used to relieve pressure that might otherwise be vented in therapy. Lawrie Williams, a mother of two daughters who experienced serious medical challenges, is the author of a series of articles about parental roles in family-centered care. One article in particular highlights the role parents can play in helping other families through parent-to-parent support programs. Williams first experienced the support of another parent when one of her daughters was young, and later realized she could use her own experiences professionally. For the past 6 years, Williams has been the coordinator of the Parent Support Program at the Center for Children with Special Needs, Children's Hospital and Regional Medical Center in Seattle, Washington.[266]

Livneh and Antonak[134] found that in a chronic-care ward family involvement helped the client and the family improve their status. Schwartzberg[249] and Schulz[128] and others[1,98,107,248,267-269] have reported great success in the use of support groups with individuals who had brain damage. Support groups can also be used to educate the client about the client's disability to increase independence.†

*References 91, 226, 229, 236, 249, 262-264.

†References 1, 207, 248, 253, 270, 271.

Kreuter and colleagues[271] and Taanila and colleagues[13,270] found that independent physical functioning and knowledge about one's condition were exceedingly important in moving through the phases of the rehabilitation process.[75,234,265,272] A guide to facilitating support groups has been published by Boreing and Adler,[274] and it has been found to be useful, especially by laypeople establishing such groups.*

The Adult Client with Brain Damage

The adult client with brain damage and the needs of the family will be specifically, yet briefly, examined here. Brain damage can affect the cognitive, perceptual, emotional, social, and neurological systems of the individual and can be incredibly disruptive and catastrophic to the client's and family's lives. When a person sustains a brain injury and is hospitalized, emotional support for the family (client included) is the primary need to be met initially. The therapist should attempt to convey warmth and a caring attitude, especially during the family's initial contacts.[275] Typical complaints about the acute period involve impersonal hospital routines and lack of definite information about the patient's status.[13,92,175,229,276] Unfortunately, definite information is usually not available at the earliest stages.

Later the family must deal with the physical changes in the client's body; what may be even more injurious to the family are the psychological, cognitive, and social changes in the client.† People with cerebrovascular accidents have been found to be more clinically depressed than orthopedic patients are. The libido[263] and the emotional systems are also affected.[75,176-178,226] It has further been shown that persons who survive a cerebrovascular accident or other impairment and who have a full return of function do not return to normal life because of a lack of social and emotional skills.‡ Families of cerebrovascular accident victims have also reported that social reintegration is the most difficult phase of rehabilitation.[277] Lack of socially appropriate behaviors has been one of the most troublesome complaints of people who deal with the person with a traumatic brain injury.[176] Therapists may be able to help alter this syndrome by encouraging appropriate behavior and by structuring therapy situations to reteach the client appropriate behavioral and social interaction skills. A technique called *dialectical behavioral therapy* has been used with people with mental health disorders, and it appears to be a promising approach. One study by Miller and colleagues[278] found significant reductions in suicidal symptoms; the most highly rated skills included distress tolerance and mindfulness skills. The goals of a dialectical behavioral therapy program designed for individuals with mild traumatic brain injury include decreasing the individual's self-defeating behaviors and cognitions, cultivating understanding of the individual's abilities and impairments, and increasing behavioral and cognitive skills that will lead to a greater sense of self and feelings of self-esteem. The program is designed to improve each patient's ability to accept his or her life as it is and to function independently.[279]

Better follow-up care needs to be implemented when dealing with the adult with brain damage.[1,98,107,248,267-269] In some areas there are outpatient, privately funded programs that can help support the brain-injured individual and his or her family on discharge from hospital settings. These resources must be recommended for follow-up care as needed.

It may not be possible for the client and family to constantly come to the clinic for support and follow-up, but telephone conversations can be scheduled on a periodic basis, or the exchange of letters or audiotapes can also be used. With the increased availability of video recorders, the day may come when a follow-up may be performed on videotapes and sent via the Internet by clients living in rural areas. Support groups are being used increasingly to facilitate client and family adjustment and accommodation to disability, as well as reentry into the community.*

References

To enhance this text and add value for the reader, all references are included on the companion Evolve site that accompanies this textbook. This online service will, when available, provide a link for the reader to a Medline abstract for the article cited. There are 281 cited references and other general references for this chapter, with the majority of those articles being evidence-based citations.

*References 75, 92, 98, 207, 249, 270-274.
†References 1, 8, 9, 16, 18, 19, 262.
‡References 1, 9, 92, 135, 261, 265.

*References 1, 16, 92, 232, 248, 239, 270, 280.

CASE STUDY 6-1 ■ PUTTING EVALUATIONS AND TECHNIQUES INTO PRACTICE

Joan, a married 30-year-old woman, has had a T2 spinal cord injury. She has worked as a computer programmer for the past 8 years, except for a short maternity leave when she gave birth to her daughter, who is now 6 years old. Joan was always very active physically and often stated that she felt sorry for her physically disabled neighbor because the neighbor could not hike, be active, or enjoy the outdoors. Joan's husband, age 33 years, is attempting to visit Joan regularly and care for their daughter, a role that is new for him.

The therapist has assessed several things regarding Joan's developmental stage, adjustment stage, social and cultural influences, and family adjustment reactions. The two adult family members are probably in Sheehy's[281] "catch-30" stage, in which the person reevaluates his or her life and relationships. Joan already "knows" that the physically disabled cannot enjoy a physically active life and is also feeling that everything she has worked for in her career is lost. She appears to be in the mourning stage of adjustment. Her daughter and husband have to adjust to radical role changes. Cognitively, Joan's young daughter is not going to understand the permanence of the disability and may be inclined to act out as the result of the turmoil. The husband will have to be assessed to determine his stage of adjustment to her disability.

Continued

CASE STUDY 6-1 ■ PUTTING EVALUATIONS AND TECHNIQUES INTO PRACTICE—cont'd

The therapist has determined that Joan's transfers need further work but would like to use the adaptive process to stimulate adjustment. The therapist has devised a treatment session to meet the goals of promoting the defense stage of adjustment, decreasing Joan's prejudice against the disabled, encouraging problem solving, increasing her feelings of self-worth, proving to her that she can take care of her daughter through interacting with children, and having her decenter her focus from her disability to her ability. The therapist has contacted the recreational therapist (who has paraplegia) to plan a collaborative session at the park across the street from the hospital. Because the recreational therapist works in the pediatrics ward, it is determined that the children with spina bifida should come and play tag, transferring from log to log in the playground.

The stage is now set. Joan will be asked to help supervise the children. The adaptive process will be used to teach Joan how to transfer using the environment. The transfer will be organized subcortically because she will be attending cortically to the children's needs and to the game itself. Joan will be actively affecting her personal environment, and if everything goes well, the act of helping the children will increase her self-worth and will also be self-reinforcing. Within this treatment session, the therapist has used the recreational therapist as a role model to change Joan's prejudice against the disabled being active in the outdoors and to show Joan that she can still be a parent although she is disabled. The therapist may also increase Joan's knowledge of how to interact with children from a wheelchair by giving a few hints and then having Joan transfer up a set of stairs to reach one of the children.

If we want to carry this scenario further, the therapist could introduce Joan to a child who is interested in computers and who needs help with a programming problem (Joan's computer background will be used, which will increase Joan's feelings of self-worth and help her focus on her abilities rather than her disabilities). On the way back to the ward, the therapist and Joan may discuss how the family is dealing with the crisis they are in and help her realize how the family has made it through other crises in the past and how those previously successful strategies could be used in this situation. Support groups and psychological counseling are mentioned as resources. The session may end with Joan planning the next therapy session and thus starting to take control of her life.

CHAPTER 7 Differential Diagnosis Phase 1: Medical Screening by the Therapist

WILLIAM G. BOISSONNAULT, PT, DHSc, FAAOMPT, FAPTA, and DARCY A. UMPHRED, PT, PhD, FAPTA

KEY TERMS

Differential Diagnosis Phase 1
Differential Diagnosis Phase 2
Medical screening
Patient referral
Review of systems screening
Causational systems interaction

OBJECTIVES

After reading this chapter the student or therapist will be able to:

1. Identify the difference between Differential Diagnosis Phase 1, medical screening, and Phase 2, diagnosis of impairments and functional limitations.
2. Analyze the concept of body system and subsystem screening.
3. Develop a mechanism for body system screening to be used with clients with preexisting neurological dysfunction.
4. Analyze the significance and importance of performing a medical screening for all clients who interact in a therapeutic environment with occupational or physical therapists.
5. Differentiate between direct causation of a clinical symptom as opposed to system causation of a clinical problem.

Traditionally, the term *differential diagnosis* has referred to a process used by physicians to diagnose disease. This process typically involves three distinct steps. Step 1 is taking a thorough history, including an investigation of the patient's medical history, presenting complaints, and a review of systems. Step 2 is the performance of the physical examination. This history and the findings of the physical examination will lead to a diagnosis or to step 3, the identification of necessary tests, including laboratory tests, diagnostic imaging modalities, and so on. The goal of the three steps is the formulation of a specific diagnosis that will lead to the implementation of the appropriate medical treatment and an accurate prognosis.

For the professions of physical and occupational therapy the concepts associated with and use of the term *differential diagnosis* are still evolving and under debate. A recent editorial describes diagnosis in physical therapy as complex and controversial, with diverse views existing.[1] For physical therapists (PTs), the guiding premise is that the differential diagnostic process fits within the Patient/Client Management Model described in the *Guide to Physical Therapist Practice*[2] (Figure 7-1) and within *The Guide to Occupational Therapy Practice*.[3] The therapist attempts to organize the history and physical examination (including tests and measures) findings into clusters, syndromes, or categories. There are certain clusters of findings that suggest the presence of disease or an adverse drug event and warrant communication with a physician. There are other symptoms and signs that are consistent with conditions that still fit into the older disablement framework. In the world today, the model of choice of all therapists is the World Health Organization (WHO) International Classification of Functioning, Disability and Health (ICF), which moves away from the consequences of disease classification to a health focus classification. Thus a shift in how one looks at disease and its impact on health and wellness not only has changed the words used by therapists but also incorporates external societal limitations that our clients face.[4] These changes do not affect the way a therapist should medically screen before formulating a clinical diagnoses based on movement dysfunction. These conditions are inherent in the interrelationships among impairments, functional or activity limitations, and participation in life and are appropriate for physical or occupational therapy interventions.[2,3,5,6]

The process of differentiating the cluster of findings that warrant communication with a physician regarding concerns about a patient's health status compared with those that do not will be called *Differential Diagnosis Phase 1*.[7] In this scenario a physician will ultimately diagnose the patient's illness, but the PT's and occupational therapist's (OT's) examination findings and subsequent patient referral contribute to the diagnosis being generated. For many of these illnesses, the use of advanced imaging, laboratory testing, and/or tissue biopsy is necessary for the diagnosis to be made.[8] Numerous examples exist in *Physical Therapy Journal* and *Journal of Orthopaedic and Sports Physical Therapy* of published case reports and case series describing such action taken by PTs.

If the decision is reached that the symptoms and signs do fall within the scope of practice of PTs and OTs, a second level of differential diagnosis occurs. Now the therapist attempts to categorize the examination findings into the specific diagnostic categories that will specifically guide the choice of treatment interventions and the development of a prognosis. This second level of diagnosis is called *Differential Diagnosis Phase 2*[7] and is the focus of Chapters 8 and 9. Figure 7-2 illustrates where Differential Diagnosis Phase 1 and Phase 2 fit into the Patient/Client Management Model.

The purpose of this chapter is to discuss the medical screening components associated with Differential Diagnosis

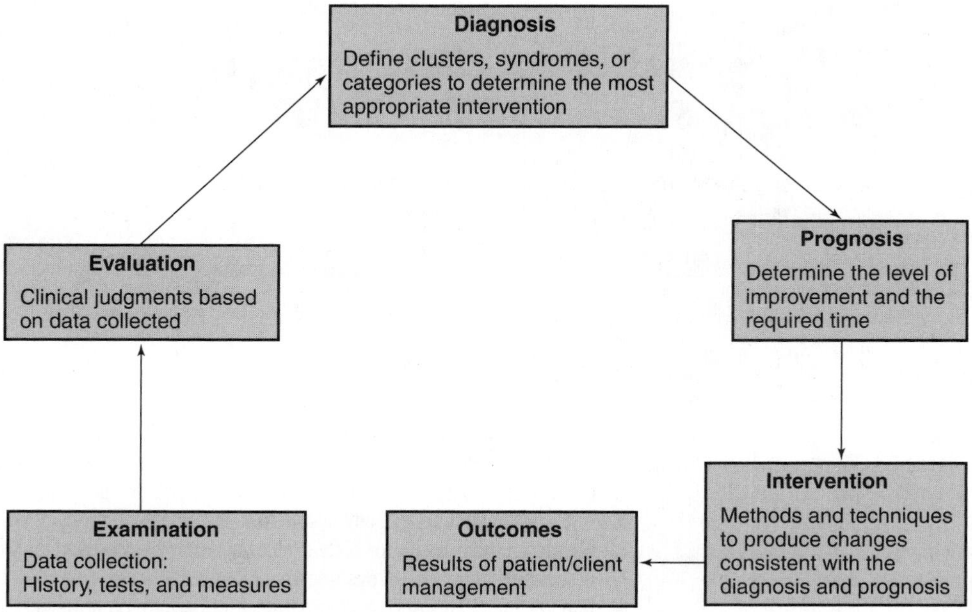

Figure 7-1 ■ Patient/client management model. (Adapted from American Physical Therapy Association: Guide to physical therapist practice. *Phys Ther* 81:43, 2001, with permission of the American Physical Therapy Association.)

Phase 1, including identification of patient health risk factors, recognition of atypical symptoms and signs, review of systems, and within-systems review. Methods to collect this information during a patient examination are also presented. The critical importance of therapists developing these visual and analytical skills is that they can lead to identification of the differences between direct causation of movement dysfunction pain syndromes arising from disease versus a system causation that may or may not be directly connected to a specific disease. The therapist referral often plays a critical role in providing the doctor the patient behaviors observed as system causation with or without a disease

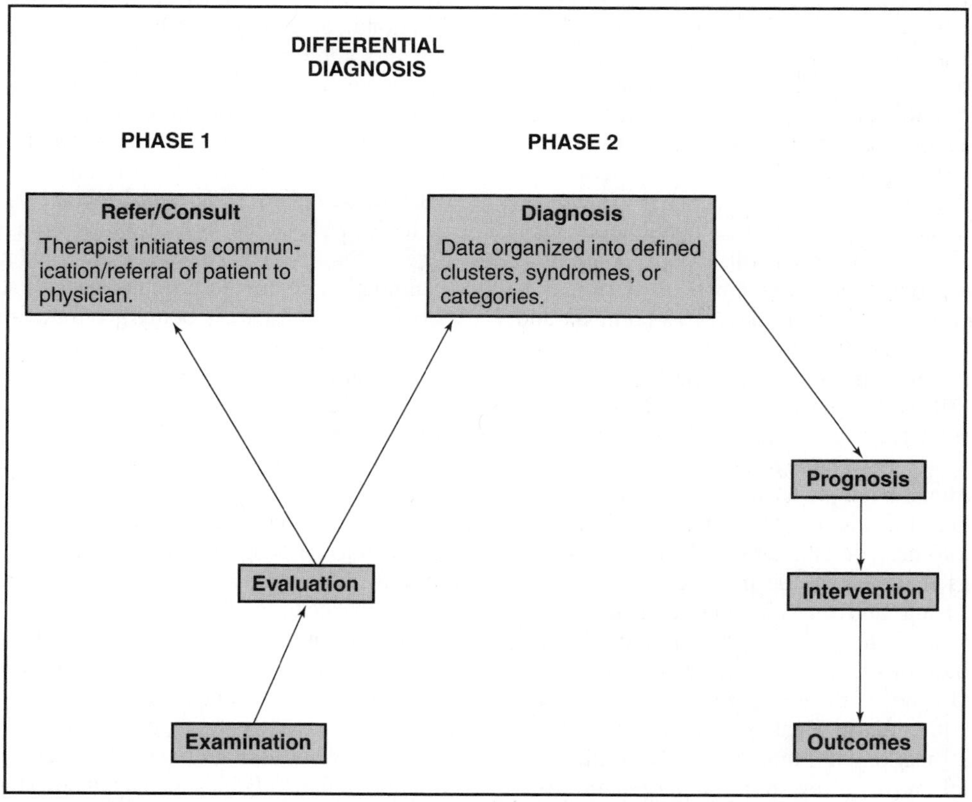

Figure 7-2 ■ Patient/client management model showing Differential Diagnosis Phase 1 and Phase 2. (Modified from Umphred DA [Chair]: Diagnostic Task Force, State of California, 1996–2000, California Chapter of American Physical Therapy Association.)

classification. Patient case scenarios are used to illustrate the important medical screening principles.

DIFFERENTIAL DIAGNOSIS PHASE 1: MEDICAL SCREENING

The *Guide to Physical Therapy Practice*[2,9] and *The Guide to Occupational Therapy Practice*[3] clearly describe the therapists' responsibility to refer patients/clients with health concerns to other practitioners. The emphasis of the following discussion is detecting clinical manifestations that suggest the specific need for physician intervention. Typically the initial warning signs associated with these scenarios include a recent onset or exacerbation of symptoms such as pain, weakness, numbness, dizziness, falls, confusion, and so on—common complaints of patients with neurological disorders. Therapists may also detect symptoms or signs unrelated to the primary medical neurological condition but that could be related to an existing comorbidity or a medication side effect. In addition, a general health and wellness screen may reveal a need for a psychological, dermatological, or other nonneurological medical consultation.

As opposed to Phase 2, the goal of Differential Diagnosis Phase 1 is *not* to formulate a specific diagnosis on the basis of these clinical manifestations. A therapist's Phase 2 diagnosis is primarily a group of motor behaviors representing movement dysfunction and how it limits independence in life activities and an individual's ability to participate in life. The Phase 1 process identifies signs and symptoms that are health or disease and pathology driven and, when they have been identified, directs a referral to a medical specialist. In fact, providing a specific diagnosis or labeling a cluster of examination findings when referring a patient to a physician because of health status concerns (e.g., peptic ulcer disease, endometriosis, new or progressive neurological problems) could place the therapist outside the scope of his or her practice. Having the ability to formulate such a specific systemic, neurological, or visceral disease or pathology diagnosis is not necessary to meet the responsibilities described in the Guides to Practice. Once the therapist's concerns have been communicated, it is then up to the physician to diagnose the presence of such disease entities.

The purpose of the therapist's medical screening is to (1) identify existing medical conditions, (2) identify symptoms and signs suggesting that an existing medical condition may be worsening, (3) identify neurological manifestations that suggest an acute or life-threatening crisis, and (4) identify symptoms and signs suggestive of the presence of an occult disorder or medication side effect. This medical screening has always taken place within the clinical framework of PTs' and OTs' practices, but as practitioners become more autonomous, this screening must become more comprehensive, requiring tools and documented evaluation results. Figure 7-3 is an example of an examination scheme leading to the decision to treat the patient, to treat *and* refer the patient, or to refer the patient. Phase 2 may also include the decision to refer the patient to another practitioner (e.g., dietician, social worker, clinical psychologist) for services augmenting the therapy or to social programs such as wellness clinics that will encourage the patient to participate in movement activities even though he may need individualized therapeutic intervention. The following material focuses on the components of this scheme most directly related to the medical screening process leading to a patient referral.

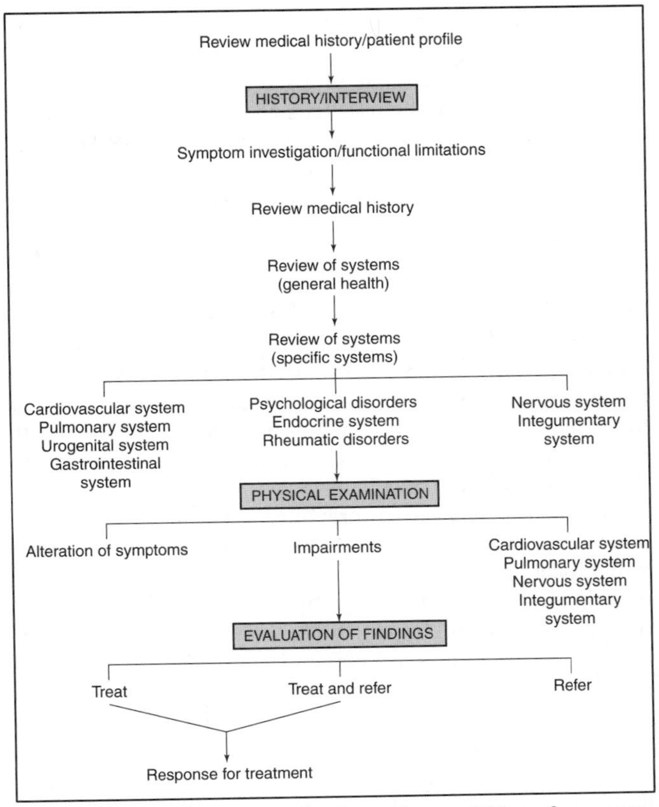

Figure 7-3 ■ Patient examination scheme. (Taken from notes from course by W. G. Boissonnault, 1998.)

Identifying Patients' Health Risk Factors and Previous Conditions

Owing to the considerable overlap in symptomatic presentation of impairment-related conditions and those requiring physician examination, identifying existing health risk factors for occult diseases is important. Numerous factors have an effect on the patient's risk for compromised health status, including age, sex, race, occupation, leisure activities, preexisting medical conditions, medication usage (over-the-counter and prescription drugs), tobacco use, and substance abuse or the interaction of some of these conditions, and family medical history.

Of these, a personal history of a current or recent medical condition, current medication use, and a positive family history (e.g., mother and aunt with a history of breast cancer, father diagnosed with prostate cancer at the age of 58 years) are the most relevant risk factors for the potential presence of an occult condition. For example, the history of a previous episode of depression significantly increases the risk of a second episode compared with the risk that someone who has never had an episode of depression will have his or her first such episode.[10] The greater the number of existing risk factors, the more vigilant the therapist should be for the presence of warning signs suggestive of disease and the more extensive the other medical screening components will need to be. Those increased risk factors, whether within one system or multiple systems, can lead to clinical behaviors that are the summation of the systems problems and their interactions that affect movement. Physicians should be able to depend on the therapist to recognize these interactive symptoms and refer the patient back to either the referring physician or to another specialist.

There are different methods to collect this medical history and patient profile information, including a review of the medical record and use of a self-administered questionnaire, depending on the practice setting and patient population. Figure 7-4 is an example of a self-administered questionnaire that could be completed by the adult patient, a family member, or a caregiver. As noted in Figure 7-3, a quick scanning review of this information should occur, if possible, before the patient interview is begun. The therapist will have a head start in organizing the history and physical examination, knowing what to prioritize and at least initially what parts of the examination can be deemphasized. The utility and accuracy of a self-administered questionnaire in patient populations germane to therapists' practice, similar to the one illustrated in Figure 7-4, have been described, with the conclusion that such a tool can be a valuable adjunct to the oral patient interview.[11]

Affirmative answers to previous or current illness questions should direct the therapist to consider what the potential impact may be on the patient's symptoms, choice of examination and treatment techniques, rehabilitation potential, and risk for additional illness. For example, the presence of existing chronic kidney disease (e.g., renal failure) should alert the therapist to numerous potential complications including patient fatigue, weakness, and impaired concentration, all of which could interfere with rehabilitation efforts. Chronic renal failure is also marked by paresthesia and muscle weakness, which could mistakenly be associated with other neurological conditions. Renal osteodystrophy is yet another complication associated with chronic renal failure. The concern of compromised bone density should direct the therapist to use techniques that carry a reduced risk of skeletal injury. A series of follow-up questions for the affirmative answers will assist the therapist in determining the relevance (if any) of each item (see Figure 7-5 for examples of follow-up questions for selected information categories).

Having the self-administered questionnaire completed before the scheduled time of the initial visit will improve the therapist's efficiency. Mailing the questionnaire to the patient before the visit or having the patient arrive 10 to 15 minutes before the appointment would allow for the form's completion without taking time away from the actual examination itself. Once the questionnaire has been completed, taking 1 to 2 minutes to scan it before the interview should be all that is necessary for the therapist to begin formulating questions and organizing the physical examination. The inability of the patient to recall information or complete the questionnaire may be another sign that medical clearance is necessary before progression to Phase 2.

Symptomatic Investigation of Functional Restriction

The chief presenting symptoms or functional restriction typically provides the reason for therapy services being sought and can provide the initial warning sign(s) of potential medical issues needing to be addressed. Despite pain not typically being the chief complaint of many patients with primary neurological conditions, a relatively mild pain is often the initial complaint associated with a serious pathological condition; a dull diffuse ache is often the initial presenting complaint associated with tumors of the musculoskeletal (MSK) system.[12] This relatively minor complaint can easily be overlooked by therapists working with patients who have neurological involvement and signs and symptoms (e.g., weakness, numbness) that are much more debilitating and cause more functional limitations than the pain complaints do. Although investigating pain complaints may not be the initial priority for these therapists, at a later visit such questioning is very important, especially if it continues, increases in intensity, shifts, or enlarges its region with no causation. Effective medical screening involves the interpretation of a patient's description of symptoms, functional limitations, and the corresponding physical examination findings. Descriptions of symptoms associated with neuromusculoskeletal impairments (loss or abnormality of physiological, psychological, or anatomical structure or function) generally reveal a fairly consistent and predictable pattern of onset and change over a defined period of time. In addition, the neurological and MSK impairments noted during the physical examination should match with the functional limitations described by the patient or the caregiver. If these expectations are not met, it does not necessarily mean the patient has cancer or an infection, but doubt should be raised on the therapist's part whether therapy is indicated.

Patients many times are not aware that presenting symptoms or signs suggest a condition better addressed by a physician as opposed to a PT or an OT. For example, Mr. S. had a cerebrovascular accident 6 months ago with resultant mild residual left hemiplegia. At the time of discharge from rehabilitation services he was independent in all activities of daily living, but residual left upper extremity weakness remained. When visiting his internist for a routine checkup, he complained that over the prior 3 weeks he had lost some functional skills and was having difficulty with self-care. The physician then referred Mr. S. to the therapy clinic for evaluation and treatment. Mr. S. states he has been less active and just needs some help regaining his motor function. During the history taking he states that he is experiencing a deep, dull, aching sensation in the lower lumbar spine and right buttock. He assumes it has developed as a result of his inactivity and thus saw no reason to bother the physician with this problem. As Mr. S. continues to describe his difficulties, he also notes a constant deep ache in the right shoulder that he relates to increased use of his right arm to compensate for the left arm weakness. The physical examination of the low back, pelvis, and right shoulder reveals that the existing symptoms do not vary with active or passive range of motion, resisted testing, or postural holding. In addition, quantity of motion is normal for these regions and motor programming appears intact. At this point the therapist cannot explain the symptoms from an impairment standpoint; therefore, depending on other examination findings, including the patient profile and medical history, communication with the internist may be warranted. The following information describes some of the subcategories associated with symptom investigation.

Location of Symptoms

A body diagram can be a valuable tool to document the location of symptoms expressed verbally or nonverbally by patients with identified neurological deficits. Besides pain and altered sensation, patterns of abnormal tone, asymmetrical posturing, and areas of weakness can also be noted on the body diagram (Figure 7-6). Numerous body structures are potential pain generators, including visceral structures.

Medical History Questionnaire

Name:______________________ Age ____________
SS#: ____________ Occupation: ______________________
Leisure activities: ______________________

I. Are you currently being seen by any of the following professionals:

A. General medical doctor (MD)	Yes	No
B. Medical specialist (MD)	Yes	No
If yes: please specify ____________		
C. Osteopathic doctor	Yes	No
D. Physical/occupational therapist	Yes	No
E. Chiropractor	Yes	No
F. Psychiatrist/psychologist	Yes	No
G. Alternative medical practitioner	Yes	No
If yes: please specify ____________		

If you have been seen by any of the above practitioners within the last year, please discuss the reasons:
____
____
____

II. Have you EVER been diagnosed as having the following condition(s)?

A. Stroke	Yes	No
B. Seizure disorders	Yes	No
C. Migraines	Yes	No
D. Other neurologic problems:	Yes	No
Specify ____________		
E. Depression	Yes	No
F. Cancer: Specify ____________	Yes	No
G. High blood pressure	Yes	No
H. Heart condition	Yes	No
I. Emphysema	Yes	No
J. Asthma	Yes	No
K. Tuberculosis	Yes	No
L. Diabetes	Yes	No
M. Rheumatoid arthritis	Yes	No
N. Other arthritic disease	Yes	No
O. Kidney disease	Yes	No
P. Anemia	Yes	No
Q. Hepatitis	Yes	No
R. Circulatory problems	Yes	No
S. Thyroid problems	Yes	No
T. Skin problems	Yes	No
U. Digestive problems	Yes	No
V. Bowel or bladder problems	Yes	No
W. Chemical dependency (e.g., alcoholism)	Yes	No
X. Unexplained falls	Yes	No
Y. Cognitive dysfunction	Yes	No
Z. Genetic disorders	Yes	No
AA. Other ____________	Yes	No

Please list all surgeries/hospitalizations including dates and reasons.
Date Surgery/hospitalization/reason
_____ ______________________
_____ ______________________

Are you being or have you been treated for musculoskeletal injuries (fracture, dislocations, repetitive strains, joint instability)? If so, please state:
Date Injury
_____ ______________________
_____ ______________________

Are you being or have you been treated for neuromuscular problems (weakness, pain, spasticity, incoordination, dizziness, tremor)? If so, please state:
Date Injury
_____ ______________________
_____ ______________________

Has anyone in your immediate family (parents, sisters, brothers) ever been treated for any of the following:

A. Stroke	Yes	No
B. Seizure disorders	Yes	No
C. Parkinson's disease	Yes	No
D. Multiple sclerosis	Yes	No
E. Other neurologic problems ____________	Yes	No
F. Mental illness	Yes	No
G. Cancer	Yes	No
H. High blood pressure	Yes	No
I. Heart condition	Yes	No
J. Breathing problems	Yes	No
K. Diabetes	Yes	No
L. Arthritic disease	Yes	No
M. Kidney disease	Yes	No
N. Anemia	Yes	No
O. Vascular problems	Yes	No
P. Thyroid problems	Yes	No
Q. Skin problems	Yes	No
R. Chemical dependency (e.g., alcoholism)	Yes	No
S. Learning disabilities	Yes	No
T. Cognitive dysfunction	Yes	No
U. Genetic disorders	Yes	No

Please list any PRESCRIPTION medications you are currently taking (include pills, injections, patches, etc.)
____
____
____
____

Please list any OVER-THE-COUNTER MEDICATIONS you are taking:
____
____
____
____

Please list any *prescriptions* or *over-the-counter* medications you were taking prior to your current problems
____
____

How much caffeinated coffee or other caffeinated beverages do you drink per day? (number of cups/cans/bottles) ______

Do you smoke? Yes No
If yes: How many packs per day? ______

Do you drink alcohol?
If yes: How many days per week do you drink? ______ days/week
If yes: How many drinks per sitting? ______ drinks/sitting
(Note: one beer or one glass of wine equals 1 drink)

If you use marijuana or other substances, how often? ______ days/week

Figure 7-4 ■ Self-administered questionnaire to collect medical history information. (Modified from Boissonnault WG, Koopmeiners MB: Medical history profile: orthopaedic physical therapy outpatients. *J Orthop Sports Phys Ther* 20:2–10, 1994, with permission of the Orthopaedic and Sports Sections of the American Physical Therapy Association.)

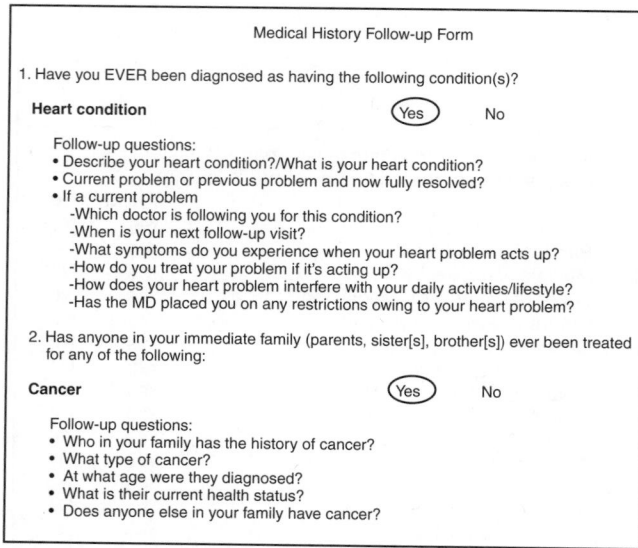

Medical History Follow-up Form

1. Have you EVER been diagnosed as having the following condition(s)?

Heart condition Yes No

Follow-up questions:
- Describe your heart condition?/What is your heart condition?
- Current problem or previous problem and now fully resolved?
- If a current problem
  - -Which doctor is following you for this condition?
  - -When is your next follow-up visit?
  - -What symptoms do you experience when your heart problem acts up?
  - -How do you treat your problem if it's acting up?
  - -How does your heart problem interfere with your daily activities/lifestyle?
  - -Has the MD placed you on any restrictions owing to your heart problem?

2. Has anyone in your immediate family (parents, sister[s], brother[s]) ever been treated for any of the following:

Cancer Yes No

Follow-up questions:
- Who in your family has the history of cancer?
- What type of cancer?
- At what age were they diagnosed?
- What is their current health status?
- Does anyone else in your family have cancer?

Figure 7-5 ■ Potential follow-up questions for affirmative answers on the self-administered questionnaire. (From W. G. Boissonnault, course notes, 1998.)

Figure 7-7 and Table 7-1 illustrate local and referred pain patterns from various visceral organs. Although the presented pain patterns illustrate those most commonly noted, clinicians should be aware of other potential patterns. For example, ischemic heart disease—the complaint of left chest wall and left upper extremity pain, pressure, or tightness—is not the classic presentation for women and many of the elderly. Besides what is noted in Figure 7-7 and Table 7-1, pain from the heart can also be experienced in the right shoulder or biceps, jaw and tooth, epigastric, and interscapular regions.[13,13a]

Because there is so much overlap between pain locations associated with visceral disease and neuromusculoskeletal conditions, the results obtained in and of themselves have minimal use in differentiating MSK from non-MSK conditions. Being familiar with the visceral pain patterns will be extremely important, however, when deciding which body systems to screen during the review of systems. Besides noting where symptoms are located, it is equally important to document areas of no complaints (see Figure 7-6). Once the patient has reported symptoms (e.g., low back and right buttock aching, see Figure 7-6), therapists should clarify. Screening to eliminate the possibility of symptoms being present down the back and up the front of the legs; in the pelvis, stomach, chest, neck and face areas; or between the shoulder blades and in the arms is critical. If there is one

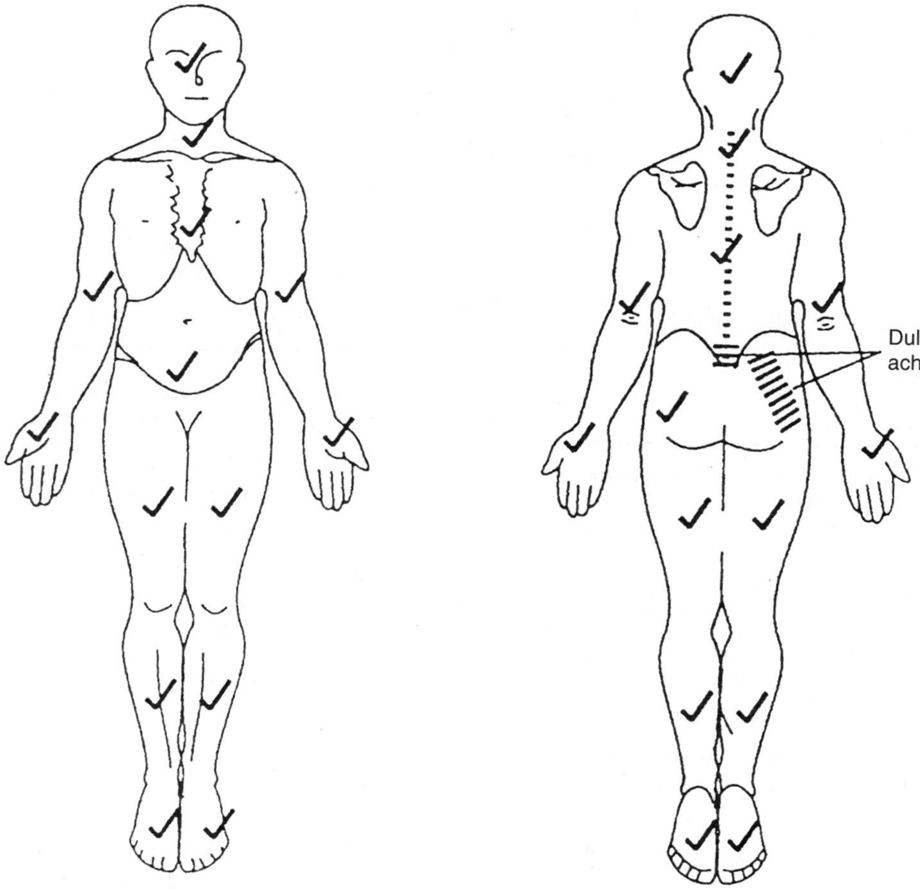

Figure 7-6 ■ Body diagram illustrating symptom location. Body areas with no known symptoms or abnormalities are marked with a checkmark. (From Boissonnault WG, editor: *Examination in physical therapy practice—screening for medical disease,* ed 2, New York, 1995, Churchill Livingstone.)

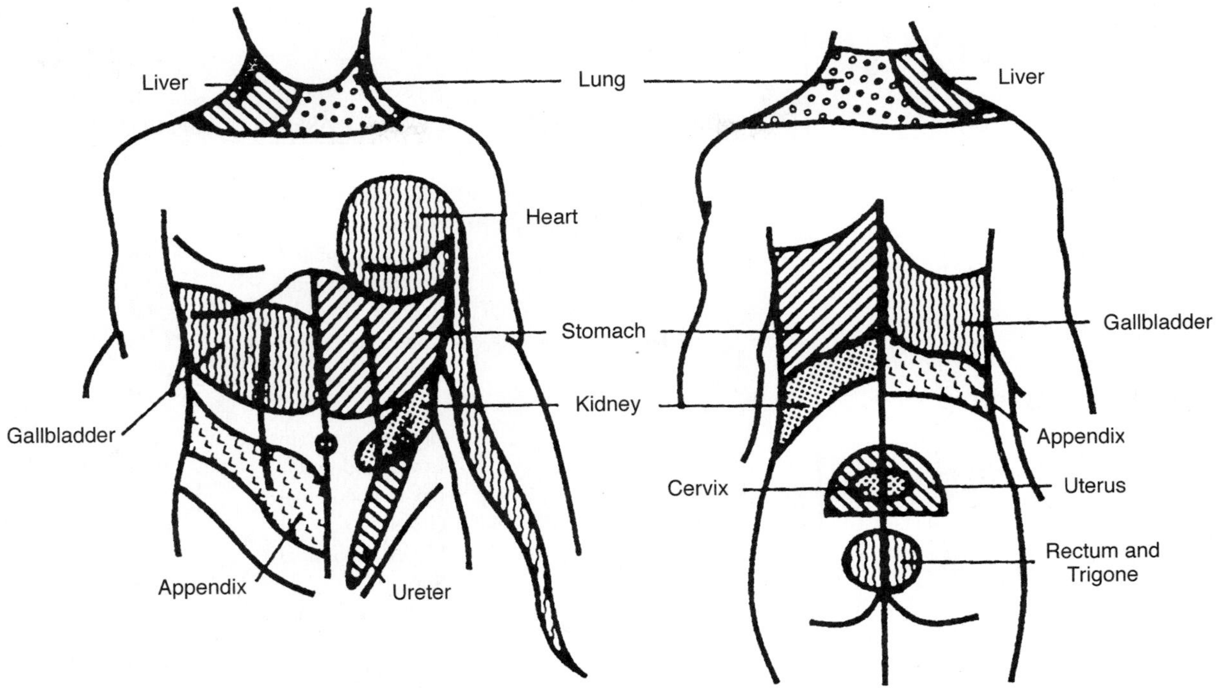

Figure 7-7 ■ Possible local and referred pain patterns of visceral structures. (From Boissonnault WG, editor: *Examination in physical therapy practice—screening for medical disease,* ed 2, New York, 1995, Churchill Livingstone.)

body area so involved that all the patient's and practitioner's attention is focused on it, a relatively mild but potentially serious symptom may be overlooked elsewhere. Placing a checkmark over each body region devoid of symptoms or other abnormal findings is one way to document such information and record change over time.

Symptom Pattern

Aspects of the patient's chief complaint other than symptom location are very relevant to the process of differential diagnosis, in particular a description of how and when the symptoms changed over a defined period of time. Complaints of pain, paresthesia, and numbness associated with primary MSK conditions typically change in a consistent manner over a 24-hour period. The patient will report that the symptom intensity increases with the assumption of specific postures such as left side lying or sitting or with specific activities such as walking, driving, or 2 hours of computer work. Conversely, patients typically can relate paresthesia or pain relief with avoiding certain postures or activities, the assumption of certain postures, wearing an arm sling, and so on. Night pain investigation also falls under this subcategory of patient data. Pain that wakes an individual from sleep and for which changing positions in bed does not provide relief is more concerning than if the pain is positionally related. If the pattern of symptom aggravation and alleviation is that there is no consistent pattern, such as pain that comes and goes independently of the patient's posture, activities, or time of day; night pain is the patient's most intense pain; or paresthesia or pain moves from one body region to another inconsistently with common pain referral patterns or identified medical conditions, then the therapist should start thinking whether physical or occupational therapy is what the patient truly needs.[14]

In general, when symptoms such as weakness or numbness associated with primary neurological conditions are investigated, the 24-hour reference point to assess symptom change is not realistic. Except for an acute onset or exacerbation, these symptoms tend not to fluctuate that quickly with change in posture or position. Understanding the pathogenesis of primary neurological disorders will allow for detection of symptom change unusual for the patient. This will lead to follow-up questions to determine whether this change may represent a medically serious situation. Similarly, a change in the biomechanical alignment of a joint (e.g., the shoulder), may immediately alter the patient's pain response, indicating a direct relationship between MSK imbalance in joint stabilization and gravitational pull, for which therapy would be appropriate.

History of Symptoms

The therapist must also scrutinize the patient's report of the onset of the symptoms. Pain and paresthesia or numbness associated with neuromusculoskeletal impairments typically can be related to trauma, either on a macro or a micro level, or to a medical event such as a cerebrovascular accident. More often than not it is repetitive overuse or cumulative trauma that leads to tissue breakdown and inflammation (see Chapter 18). Patients with neurological impairments resulting in postural abnormalities and abnormal movement patterns are at risk for such conditions. If a patient's symptoms are truly insidious, meaning not related to macro or micro trauma, or there has not been a significant change in activity level that reasonably accounts for

TABLE 7-1 ■ VISCERAL PAIN PATTERNS

STRUCTURE	SEGMENTAL INNERVATION	POSSIBLE AREAS OF PAIN REFERRAL
PELVIC ORGANS		
Uterus including uterine ligaments	T10-L1, S2-4	Lumbosacral junction Sacral Thoracolumbar
Ovaries	T10-11	Lower abdominal Sacral
Testes	T10-11	Lower abdominal Sacral
RETROPERITONEAL REGION		
Kidney	T10-L1	Lumbar spine (ipsilateral) Lower abdominal Upper abdominal
Ureter	T11-L2, S2-4	Groin Upper abdominal Suprapubic Medial, proximal thigh Thoracolumbar
Urinary bladder	T11-L2, S2-4	Sacral apex Suprapubic Thoracolumbar
Prostate gland	T11-L1, S2-4	Sacral Testes Thoracolumbar
DIGESTIVE SYSTEM ORGANS		
Esophagus	T6-10	Substernal and upper abdominal
Stomach	T6-10	Upper abdominal Middle and lower thoracic spine
Small intestine	T7-10	Middle thoracic spine
Pancreas	T6-10	Upper abdominal Lower thoracic spine Upper lumbar spine
Gallbladder	T7-9	Right upper abdominal Right middle and lower thoracic spine, including caudal aspect scapula
Liver	T7-9	Right middle and lower thoracic spine
Common bile duct	T6-10	Upper abdominal Middle thoracic spine
Large intestine	T11-12	Lower abdominal Middle lumbar spine
Sigmoid colon	T11-12	Upper sacral Suprapubic Left lower quadrant of abdomen
CARDIOPULMONARY SYSTEM		
Heart	T1-5	Cervical anterior Upper thorax Left upper extremity
Lungs and bronchi	T5-6	Ipsilateral thoracic spine Cervical (diaphragm involved)
Diaphragm (central portion)	C3-5	Cervical spine

Modified from Boissonnault WG, Bass C: Pathological origins of trunk and neck pain, I. Pelvic and abdominal visceral disorders. *J Orthop Sports Phys Ther* 12:192–207, 1990, with permission of the Orthopaedic and Sports Sections of the American Physical Therapy Association.

the complaints, the therapist should again be concerned about the source of the symptoms. A worsening of symptoms (e.g., numbness, weakness, spasticity, swelling) associated with an existing medical condition should be investigated by the therapist with the same scrutiny. The therapist always needs to ask, "Is there a reasonable explanation for the worsening?" An increase in the intensity of the complaints or the involvement of additional body regions could signal a progression of the disease.

Review of Body Systems

By design, *review of systems* screening allows the therapist to detect symptoms secondary (and maybe unrelated) to the reason therapy has been initiated.[15] The review of systems allows for a general screening of body systems for symptoms suggesting the presence of an adverse drug reaction, occult disease, or worsening of an existing medical condition. Suspicions of any of these scenarios would warrant communication with a physician. Checklists of symptoms and signs for each body system can be used by the PT or OT during the patient interview (Box 7-1). To keep the checklists manageable in length, the therapist should investigate presenting complaints and symptoms and the patient's medical history before the review of systems, as noted in Figure 7-3. For example, on review of the cardiovascular and peripheral vascular system checklist items associated with heart conditions in Box 7-1, important items appear to be omitted, such as chest pain, claudication, a history of heart problems, hypertension, high cholesterol levels, and circulatory problems. If symptoms have already been investigated by use of a body diagram, the therapist would already know whether the patient has chest pain. If symptom change (aggravation or alleviation) over a 24-hour period has already been investigated, the therapist would know whether claudication is an issue. Finally, if the patient's medical history has already been discussed, the therapist would know whether heart problems, hypertension, or circulatory problems existed.[13a]

All of the checklists in Box 7-1 need not be used for every patient. The location of symptoms will direct the therapist in deciding which checklists should be included in the initial examination. Figure 7-7 and Table 7-1 can be used to link pain location with visceral systems that could be the source of the complaints. Table 7-2 provides a summary of potential pain locations and diseases of the pulmonary, cardiovascular, gastrointestinal, and urogenital systems. Other symptom characteristics can also alert the therapist to the possible involvement of the endocrine, nervous, and psychological systems. Symptoms, including pain and paresthesias that come and go irrespective of posture, activity, or time of day and that appear to move among the various body regions, can be associated with these systems as well as the visceral systems. In addition to the identification of the location and characteristics of symptoms, a patient's medical history will also help the therapist decide which systems to screen. A positive medical history, such as a heart problem, would direct the therapist to investigate the patient's condition, including possible use of the cardiovascular and peripheral vascular checklist as well as the questions listed in Figure 7-5. The therapist also needs to be aware of the medications taken by the patient to medically manage these pathological conditions. Similarly, therapists need to be able to analyze how the drugs potentially affect functional movements and functional loss. Often, that means a therapist must have a working professional relationship with a clinical pharmacist (see Chapter 36). Use of a general health checklist (Box 7-2) can assist the therapist in prioritizing the inclusion of the checklists in the systems review checklists box during the initial visit. The symptoms noted in this checklist can be associated with disease of most of the body's systems, as well as with systemic disease and adverse drug events.

If the patient or caregiver (on the patient's behalf) replies yes to any *review of systems* question, the therapist must determine whether there is a reasonable explanation for the complaint, whether the physician is aware of the complaint, and, if so, whether the complaint has worsened since the patient last saw the physician. When the given explanation is not satisfactory, the physician is unaware of the complaint, or the symptom is worsening, communication with the physician is warranted. Similarly, most physicians look at direct causation: complaint to disease. Therapists need to look at system causation because we see the end result of the combinations of the problems: disease, maturation, environmental factors, and other nondisease causations. All the checklists do not need to be covered during the initial visit. If the patient says "no" for each of the general health items, the patient's health history is uneventful, and the therapist is comfortable with the description of the chief complaints (including pattern and onset), then the therapist can proceed with the evaluation of specific impairments and functional limitations with some confidence that Differential Diagnosis Phase 2 and therapy intervention are very likely appropriate. The review of systems then takes a lower priority. The result is that the therapist could decide to delay the use of the appropriate systems review checklists until the patient's second or third visit. If the patient answers "yes" to general health items and has an inconsistent pain pattern, the appropriate review of systems then takes a higher priority and should be covered during the initial visit.

Musculoskeletal System

Box 7-3 provides the checklist for the MSK system. In addition, as with all other body systems, the general health checklist also provides a level of screening for conditions of the MSK system such as infections, metastatic cancers, and rheumatic disorders (e.g., rheumatoid arthritis). Identifying patient risk factors for these conditions is a key for recognizing when to be suspicious. For example, those at highest risk for MSK cancers are those (1) over the age of 50 years and under 20 years, (2) having a previous history of cancer (e.g., breast, lung, prostate, thyroid, and kidney—the most common cancers to metastasize to the axial skeleton), (3) having a positive family history of cancer, and (4) having had exposure to environmental toxins. Those individuals at highest risk for MSK infections report or demonstrate (1) current or recent infection (e.g., urinary tract, tooth abscess, skin infection), (2) history of diabetes with use of large doses of steroids or immunosuppressive drugs, (3) elderly age, and (4) spinal cord injury with complete motor and sensory loss.[16] Last, the primary risk factors for rheumatoid arthritis include (1) female sex, (2) age (peak) 30 to 40 years, and (3) positive family history.[17]

The other category of MSK conditions for which therapists need to be vigilant is fractures. The pain and deformity

BOX 7-1 ■ REVIEW OF SYSTEMS CHECKLISTS

CARDIOVASCULAR AND PERIPHERAL VASCULAR
dyspnea
orthopnea
palpitations
pain with sweating
syncope
peripheral edema
cold feet or hands
peripheral sensory loss
skin discoloration
open wounds or gangrene
cough

GASTROINTESTINAL
difficulty with swallowing
heartburn, indigestion
specific food intolerance
bowel dysfunction
- color (black and tarry, light slate colored)
- frequency
- shape, caliber (flat ribbon-like, thin-caliber pencil-like)
- constipation or diarrhea
- incontinence

UROGENITAL
urinary
- frequency
- urgency
- incontinence

reduced force of stream
difficulty initiating or attention needed to urinate
dysuria
color (hematuria, dark, brownish tea color)

REPRODUCTIVE: MALE
urethral discharge
impotence
dyspareunia

REPRODUCTIVE: FEMALE
vaginal discharge
dyspareunia
change in menstruation
frequency and length of cycle
dysmenorrhea
blood flow
date of last period
number of pregnancies
number of deliveries
menopause

PSYCHOLOGICAL (DEPRESSION)
depressed or irritable mood
psychomotor agitation or retardation
apathy
sleep disturbance
weight gain or loss
fatigue
feelings of worthlessness
impaired concentration
suicide ideation (recurrent)
recent loss of family member

PULMONARY
dyspnea
onset of cough
change in cough
sputum
hemoptysis
clubbing of the nails
stridor
wheezing

SENSORY AND MOTOR (NERVOUS)
sudden or slow onset of sensory loss
impaired balance
unexplainable frequent falls
impaired gross movement patterns
decrease in or difficulty with fine motor skill
impaired mentation
tremors: intentional or unintentional
muscle atrophy: symmetrical vs asymmetrical
asymmetrical facial features
asymmetrical tongue patterns
facial contour
ptosis
pupil abnormalities
strabismus

ENDOCRINE
arthralgias
myalgias
neuropathies
cold or heat intolerance
skin or hair changes
fatigue
weight gain or loss
polyuria
polydipsia

associated with most sudden-impact, traumatic fractures make for an obvious presentation. However, trauma sufficient to cause a fracture may not be so obvious in a patient with decreased bone density. Lifting a gallon of milk, experiencing a mild slip or bump, or trying to open a window that is stuck may be sufficient to cause a fracture in a patient with a history of chronic renal failure, multiple sclerosis, rheumatoid arthritis, hyperparathyroidism, gastrointestinal malabsorption syndrome, and long-term corticosteroid, heparin, anticonvulsant, and cytotoxic medication use. The most common locations for such fractures include vertebral bodies, the neck of the femur, and the radius. Observation of posture and body position may provide a clue that something may have changed structurally. For example, with vertebral compression fractures the thoracic kyphotic curve may be accentuated, accompanied by a very pronounced

TABLE 7-2 ■ LINKING PAIN PATTERNS AND VISCERAL SYSTEMS

PAIN LOCATION	VISCERAL SYSTEMS
Right shoulder (including shoulder girdle)	Pulmonary Cardiovascular Gastrointestinal
Left shoulder (including shoulder girdle)	Cardiovascular Pulmonary
Upper thoracic or midthoracic spine	Cardiovascular Pulmonary Gastrointestinal
Lower thoracic and upper lumbar or midlumbar spine	Peripheral vascular Pulmonary Gastrointestinal Urogenital
Lumbopelvic region	Gastrointestinal Urogenital Peripheral vascular

BOX 7-2 ■ GENERAL HEALTH CHECKLIST

Fatigue
Malaise
Fever, chills, sweats
Nausea
Unexplained weight change
Dizziness, lightheadedness
Unexplained paresthesia, numbness
Unexplained weakness
Unexplained cognitive and emotional changes

BOX 7-3 ■ MUSCULOSKELETAL SYSTEM SCREENING

Insidious onset of symptoms
Atypical pain pattern (aggravating or alleviating factors)
Night pain (progressive and/or nonpositional)
Early morning stiffness lasting longer than 30 to 60 minutes
Inadequate relief of symptoms with rest or rehabilitation
Inability to alter symptoms during the physical examination
Lack of impairments that match patient's functional limitations
Atypical physical examination findings (e.g., masses, unexplained atrophy, or weakness)

apex of the curve that was not present before. With femoral neck fracture the lower extremity is often positioned in external rotation and appears shortened compared with its counterpart.[18]

Causing potential confusion for the clinician are diseases (especially in the early stages) of the MSK system, which may mimic mechanical MSK conditions. The patient may report a specific event or time of onset of symptoms, and a pain pattern of increasing pain with weight bearing on the involved extremity over time and lessoning relief of pain with assumption of non–weight-bearing positions—all typical findings with impairment-driven symptoms. The therapist may also be able to provoke symptoms during the physical examination as the involved bony area is mechanically loaded. When the history and physical examination findings are evaluated, an unusual finding or pattern will emerge, or the patient will not respond to treatment as expected, making the therapist step back and consider alternative hypotheses regarding the origin of patient symptoms, especially if the risk factors listed earlier are present.

Integumentary System

Screening of the integumentary system is not typically based on the presence or absence of pain, paresthesia, or numbness. As with the nervous system, some degree of screening of the integumentary system occurs with every patient regardless of the presenting diagnosis. Skin cancer has the highest incidence of all the cancers,[19] and therapists generally see a number of exposed body areas during the postural assessment and regional examination that make up the physical examination. In fact, as noted in Figure 7-3, screening the skin begins during the patient interview. During the interview the therapist can be looking at areas of exposed skin such as the face, neck, arms, and feet. As with screening of the other body systems, the therapist's goal is not to identify a melanoma or differentiate squamous cell and basal cell carcinoma but simply to identify skin lesions with atypical presentations. Once the patient has been referred to the physician, disease will be ruled out or diagnosed. Box 7-4 can be used to assess any mole or other skin marking. The items noted are atypical for a benign lesion, more suggestive of a pathological condition.[20] Selected items from Box 7-4 have been highlighted, resulting in an acronym—*A* (asymmetry), *B* (borders), *C* (color), *D* (diameter), and *E* (evolving)—that has been used to educate the public for self-screening.[21] If the therapist notes any of these findings and the patient reports a recent change in the size, color, or shape of the lesion and that a physician has not looked at the lesion, a referral would be warranted.

Besides skin lesions, abnormal general skin color can be a manifestation of a number of conditions. Table 7-3 summarizes abnormal skin color changes. Occasionally, some of

BOX 7-4 ■ SKIN LESION SCREENING—PATHOLOGICAL CHARACTERISTICS

Multivariant color
Black or blue-black color
Irregular borders
Nondistinct ("fuzzy") borders
Size: 6 mm or larger in diameter
Asymmetrical shape
Friable tissue
Ulcerations
Evolving (changing size, shape, color)

TABLE 7-3 ■ ABNORMAL COLOR CHANGES OF THE SKIN

COLOR CHANGE	PHYSIOLOGICAL CHANGE	COMMON CAUSES
White, pale (pallor)	Absence of pigment or pigment changes	Albinism, lack of sunlight
	Blood abnormality	Anemia, lead poisoning
	Temporary interruption or diversion of blood flow	Vasospasm, syncope, stress, internal bleeding
	Internal disease	Chronic gastrointestinal disease, cancer, parasitic disease, tuberculosis
Blue (cyanosis)	Decreased oxygen in blood (deoxyhemoglobin)	Methemoglobinemia (oxidation of hemoglobin), high blood iron level, cold exposure, vasomotor instability, cerebrospinal disease
Yellow	Jaundice, excess bilirubin in blood, excess bile	Liver disease, gallstone blockage of bile duct, hepatitis pigment (conjunctivae are also yellow)
	High levels of carotene in blood (carotenemia)	Ingestion of food high in carotene and vitamin A
Gray	High level of metals in body	Increased iron, bronze-gray; increased silver, blue-gray
Brown (hyperpigmentation)	Disturbances of adrenocortical hormones	Adrenal pituitary Addison disease

From Shapiro C, Skopit S: Screening for skin disorders. In Boissonnault WG, editor: *Examination in physical therapy practice—screening for medical disease,* ed 2, New York, 1995, Churchill Livingstone.

the most obvious abnormalities are the most difficult to note when one is so focused on items more directly related to therapeutic intervention.

Nervous System

As with the integumentary system, the nervous system is screened to a degree for all patients. The systems review checklists in Box 7-1 include items that provide a very gross, general screening of the nervous system. The therapist should be vigilant for the presence of any of these items in all patients during the initial and subsequent visits. For patients with preexisting findings from this checklist, the therapist must be vigilant for a worsening of the observed abnormalities. Covering the items in the nervous system checklist should add little time to the therapist's initial examination. Assessing for facial asymmetries and tremors can take place during the interview. Observing balance, movement patterns, and muscle atrophy can occur while watching the patient ambulate into the examination area, during the interview, and as the patient changes positions during the physical examination. Last, impaired mentation may become apparent during the interview or the physical examination as the patient struggles to appropriately answer questions or follow directions. Case Studies 7-1 and 7-2 illustrate the importance of this general screening.

CASE STUDY 7-1

A 55-year-old elementary school teacher was referred with a diagnosis of cervical degenerative disk disease at C5-6 and C6-7. Her chief complaint was posterior cervical aching and a sense of neck weakness. Functionally, the patient's primary concern was her increasingly difficult time making it through her workday. She taught first-grade students, so much of her workday was spent with her neck and trunk in a forward flexed position. The patient stated that this persistent flexion posturing was a significant factor for the worsening of her symptoms as her workday progressed. As the interview continued, a tremor of the patient's right hand and forearm was observed as the arm rested on her thigh. When questioned about the observed tremor she stated it started 4 or 5 months ago. She admitted the tremor appeared to be getting worse and that she did not mention it to her physician. No other positive neurological findings were noted. After the initial examination was completed, the concern about the tremor was discussed and the patient consented to allow her primary care physician (the referring physician) to be called to discuss the finding. The physician facilitated a referral of the patient to a neurologist. Approximately 1 month later, after the neurology consultation and tests, the patient was diagnosed with Parkinson disease. During that month the patient continued to receive physical therapy care for her cervical complaints. In this example, performance of Differential Diagnosis Phase 1 showed the presence of a new symptom (tremor of the right hand) that was not consistent with the medical diagnosis of degenerative disk disease. This symptom triggered the decision by the therapist to refer the patient back to the physician for that specific clinical sign, which led to the additional diagnosis of Parkinson disease. With the patient having been referred to the physician, therapy was also initiated. Differential Diagnosis Phase 2 was performed, which resulted in the decision to treat the cervical complaints of the patient.

CASE STUDY 7-2

A 75-year-old woman was sent to physical therapy with the diagnosis of moderate to severe osteomalacia of the spine. The physician referred her to a PT. The therapist evaluated her spine and noted weakness, pain, and tightness. The plan of care included strengthening and stretching, with the assumption that the pain would subside once the muscles could better support the spine. The therapist did not do a medical screen, and for much of the therapy program the patient exercised without supervision. Both the patient and the husband felt physical therapy was not helping at all. The patient and her husband discussed this problem with a neighbor who was also a PT. The neighbor referred them to another PT who had extensive manual therapy background and used the *Guide to Physical Therapy Practice* as a cornerstone to practice. The new therapist performed a medical screen as part of the examination and noticed that the woman had some general weakness in her left side that did not coincide with the original diagnosis. The symptoms were very subtle and the therapist asked her if she was having any difficulty with daily living activities. She said "no," so the therapist treated her for her back impairments but monitored her neurological signs. The treatment went far beyond strengthening and stretching muscles, and the patient was very excited about therapy and how much improvement she was making. At the next treatment session her neurological signs were still subtle but enhanced, so the patient was told that she needed to see her primary care physician for examination and consideration of diagnostic imaging. She continued with PT for three more sessions with her pain almost resolved.
Per the therapist's recommendation she saw her physician after the second treatment. The physician ordered magnetic resonance imaging, and it revealed a grapefruit-sized nonmalignant tumor in her right lower frontal-temporal area. The tumor was removed and the patient recovered after 2 weeks of rehabilitation. The woman and her family believe that it was the PT that saved not only her quality of life, but also her life itself. The first PT, by not doing a medical screening examination, did not identify the occult neurological problem. If the second therapist's medical screening and referral to the doctor had not been performed, the first therapist could have been deemed negligent and cited in a liability suit; importantly, the patient's tumor may have caused more permanent damage as it grew undiagnosed within her cranium.

Depression. Depression is a commonly encountered psychological disorder that is associated with significant morbidity and mortality.[10,22-24] The systems review checklists in Box 7-1 contain items the therapist can use to help make the decision to refer a patient for consultation. If the patient has suicide ideation, the physician should be contacted before the patient leaves the clinic. For the first eight items on the depression checklist, concern should be raised when the therapist detects four or five of the items present daily for a minimum of 2 weeks and resulting in the patient having difficulty functioning at home, work, or school, socially, or in rehabilitation. Of the four or five items, one of them should be depressed or irritable affect or apathy. An exception to the 2-week time frame is during periods of bereavement. When people are faced with a significant loss, it is not uncommon for them to experience a number of the checklist items as they work through the grieving process (refer to Chapter 6).[10] It is reasonable for these people to experience these symptoms for up to 2 months. A neurological event such as a cerebrovascular accident could easily trigger a major clinical depressive disorder, and the depression could significantly impede rehabilitation progress. The therapist may be in a position to facilitate a psychological consultation.

Considering that approximately 15% of people with true major clinical depression commit suicide,[10] therapists need to be vigilant for warning signs that the patient may be considering this action. See the suicide screening shown in Box 7-5 for a list of warning signs. Once the patient acknowledges suicidal ideation, follow-up questions would be appropriate to investigate the patient's plan and how readily available the resources are regarding the reported method of attempt. This is all-important information to be reported when the therapist contacts the physician. Therapists should be very familiar with their facility's "suicide protocol or procedure" in terms of what information should be collected from the patient and who should be contacted.

BOX 7-5 ■ SUICIDE WARNING SIGNS

- History of major clinical depression, chemical dependency, schizophrenia, or previous suicide attempt
- Expressions of hopelessness
- The sense that the patient is "giving up"
- An abrupt improvement in patient mood

PHYSICAL EXAMINATION

In addition to this discussion of observation screening for the integumentary and nervous systems, other screening principles are associated with the physical examination. The therapist should have expectations of physical examination findings based on the existing medical diagnosis and data from the history. There should be a correlation between the described functional limitations and the noted impairments. Using the clinical example previously described, the right shoulder pain Mr. S. was experiencing would be expected to increase or decrease in intensity with palpation, movement assessment, or special tests. Not only was the therapist unable to alter the ache, but the shoulder motion and motor control also appeared intact. Essentially there is nothing for the therapist to treat. The inability to alter a patient's complaints and the lack of neuromusculoskeletal impairments one would expect with the medical diagnosis and the reported functional limitations should again raise concern about the source of the symptoms. The physical examination also includes elements of the systems review.

The *Guide to Physical Therapy Practice* describes the systems review, in part, as a brief or limited examination of the anatomical and physiological status of the cardiovascular and pulmonary, integumentary, MSK, and neuromuscular systems.[1] For the purposes of this chapter the discussion will focus on assessment of height and weight and assessing heart rate and blood pressure. Being overweight or obese can significantly increase the risk of development of a number of serious conditions (Table 7-4). Using patient height and weight to calculate body mass index (BMI) can be a valuable measure to identify patients who may need a dietary consultation to prevent disease states or minimize morbidity associated with current illnesses. BMI is calculated by dividing body weight (in kilograms) by height (in meters). Table 7-4 provides a summary of disease risk associated with BMI and waist circumference.

Resting blood pressure and pulse rate and rhythm are also important values to be routinely measured. See Table 7-5 for a summary of blood pressure values for adults. Table 7-6 presents normal resting pulse rate parameters for therapists to consider when examining a patient. A 30-second monitoring period after a 2- to 5-minute rest period is recommended to obtain baseline rate values.[25] Resting blood pressure values can also provide important screening information. As with assessing pulse rate, resting blood pressure should be assessed after a 5-minute rest period. Variations from the normative values may lead therapists to additional assessment of the vascular system and the central autonomic nervous system and then to a patient referral.

Examination Summary

For many patients a single red flag finding does not warrant a referral, but a cluster of history and physical examination findings does increase disease probability to the point where a referral is indicated. Two examples that are germane to a number of individuals with neurological conditions are deep venous thrombosis (DVT) and pulmonary embolus (PE). DVT affects approximately 2 million individuals in the United States annually, making it the third most common

TABLE 7-4 ■ DISEASE RISK RELATIVE TO NORMAL WEIGHT AND WAIST CIRCUMFERENCE

	BMI (KG/M²)	OBESITY CLASS	MEN ≤102 CM (≤40 INCHES) WOMEN ≤88 CM (≤35 INCHES)	>102 CM(>40 INCHES) >88 CM (>35 INCHES)
Underweight	<18.5		—	—
Normal	18.5-24.9		—	—
Overweight	25.0-29.9		Increased	High
Obesity	30.0-34.9	I	High	Very high
	35.0-39.9	II	Very high	Very high
Extreme obesity	≥40	III	Extremely high	Extremely high

From the National Heart, Lung, and Blood Institute: Clinical guidelines on the identification, evaluation, and treatment of overweight and obesity in adults. Available at: www.nhlbi.nih.gov/health/public/heart/obesity/lose_wt/risk.htm/. Accessed July 20, 2011.

BMI, Body mass index. Classification by Body Mass Index (BMI), waist circumference, and associated disease risks.

TABLE 7-5 ■ CLASSIFICATION OF BLOOD PRESSURE FOR ADULTS 18 YEARS OLD OR OLDER*†

CATEGORY	SYSTOLIC BLOOD PRESSURE (mm Hg)		DIASTOLIC BLOOD PRESSURE (mm Hg)
Optimal‡	<120	and	>80
Normal	120-129	and	80-84
High normal	130-139	or	85-89
Hypertension			
Stage 1	140-159	or	90-99
Stage 2	160-179	or	100-109
Stage 3	≥180	or	≥110

From The Sixth Report of the Joint National Committee on Prevention, Detection, Evaluation, and Treatment of High Blood Pressure. *Hypertension* 23:275–285, 1994, and The Sixth Report of the U.S. Department of Health and Human Services, Public Health Service, National Institutes of Health, National Heart, Lung and Blood Institute, Bethesda, MD, 1997.

*Not taking antihypertensive drugs and not acutely ill. When systolic and diastolic blood pressures fall into different categories, the high category should be selected to classify the individual's blood pressure status. In addition to classifying stages of hypertension on the basis of average blood pressure levels, clinicians should specify presence or absence of target organ disease and additional risk factors. This specificity is important for risk classification and treatment.

†Based on the average of two or more readings taken at each of two or more visits after an initial screening.

‡Optimal blood pressure regarding cardiovascular risk is less than 120/80 mm Hg. However, unusually low readings should be evaluated for clinical significance.

TABLE 7-6 ■ RESTING PULSE RATE IN BEATS PER MINUTE

	AVERAGE	LIMITS
Norms	120-160	—
Fetal	120	70-190
Newborn	120	80-160
1 year old	110	80-130
2 years old	100	80-120
4 years old	100	75-115
6 years old	90	70-110
8-10 years old		
12 years old		
Female	90	70-110
Male	85	65-105
14 years old		
Female	85	65-105
Male	80	60-100
16 years old		
Female	80	60-100
Male	75	55-95
18 years old		
Female	75	55-95
Male	70	50-90
Well-conditioned athlete	50-60	50-100
Adult	—	60-100
Aging	—	60-100

Modified from Jarvis C: *Physical examination and health assessment,* ed 4, Philadelphia, 1992, WB Saunders.

cardiovascular disease.[26] A sobering estimation is that approximately 50% of those with a DVT are asymptomatic in early stages.[27] Clinicians are challenged to identify patients at greater risk for this condition who do not have the obvious signs and symptoms of calf pain, swelling, and redness. The following clinical decision rule has been validated in ambulatory patient populations (Table 7-7). Of note for the neurological population, a history of spinal cord injury does not appear in this rule even though it is considered a strong risk factor for DVT. The authors assume there were very few patients with spinal cord injury in the validation research.

Similarly for PE, a clinical decision rule exists for screening (Table 7-8). PE is associated with high morbidity and mortality, highlighting the critical nature of timely detection. Hull describes PE as one of the "great masqueraders" of medicine because of the often nonspecific presenting symptoms and signs.[28] Wells and colleagues estimate that 50% of PEs go undiagnosed.[29]

Clinician concern regarding the possibility of a DVT and/or a PE being present would warrant urgent communication with the patient's physician.

RESPONSE TO TREATMENT

Frequently during Differential Diagnosis Phase 1 the therapist will decide referral of the patient to a physician is not warranted and will proceed to Differential Diagnosis Phase 2 and determine whether physical therapy is warranted or no intervention recommended. As treatment is initiated and progresses, the therapist must remain vigilant for the appearance of symptoms and signs discussed throughout this chapter. In addition, correlating subjective and objective changes as treatment progresses will help the therapist decide whether further intervention is warranted or whether referral back to the physician or other health care practitioner is appropriate. For example, if a patient reports a significant improvement or worsening, one would expect the therapist to note a corresponding change in posture, movement ability, palpatory findings, or neurological status. If the expected correlation between patient report and physical examination findings is not found, the therapist should begin considering that therapy may not be warranted. A careful review of systems and symptom investigation would again be necessary as part of the return to Differential Diagnosis Phase 1.

TABLE 7-7 ■ CLINICAL DECISION RULE FOR DEEP VENOUS THROMBOSIS (DVT)

CLINICAL CHARACTERISTIC	SCORE
Active cancer (treatment ongoing, or within previous 6 months or palliative)	1
Paralysis, paresis, or recent plaster immobilization of lower extremities	1
Recently bedridden >3 days, or major surgery in past 12 weeks requiring general or regional anesthesia	1
Localized tenderness along distribution of deep venous system	1
Swelling of entire leg	1
Calf swelling >3 cm greater than asymptomatic side (measured at 10 cm below tibial tuberosity	1
Pitting edema confined to symptomatic leg	1
Collateral superficial veins (nonvaricosed)	1
Alternative diagnosis is as likely as or more likely than DVT	−2

KEY

SCORE	SIGNIFICANCE
−2 to zero	Low probability of DVT: 5% (95% confidence interval [CI], 4.0%-8.0%)
1-2	Moderate probability of DVT: 17% (95% CI, 13%-23%)
3 or greater	High probability: 53% (95% CI, 44%-61%)

From Wells PS, Anderson DR, Bormanis J, et al: Value of assessment of pretest probability of deep-vein thrombosis in clinical management, *Lancet* 350(9094; Dec 20-27):1795-1798, 1997.

TABLE 7-8 ■ "WELLS" CRITERIA FOR DETERMINING PROBABILITY OF PULMONARY EMBOLISM (PE)

CRITERION	POINT VALUE FOR CRITERION
Clinical signs of deep venous thrombosis (DVT)	3.0
Heart rate >100 beats per minute	1.5
Immobilization for 3 days or longer, or surgery in previous 4 weeks	1.5
Previous diagnosis of PE or DVT	1.5
Hemoptysis	1.0
Patients with cancer receiving treatment, treatment stopped in past 6 months, or receiving palliative care	1.0
Alternative diagnosis less likely than PE	3.0
Pretest probability of PE is low with a score <2 points; moderate with a score 2 to 6 points; and high with a score >6 points.	

Data from Wells PS, Anderson DR, Rodger M, et al: Excluding pulmonary embolism at the bedside without diagnostic imaging: management of patients with suspected pulmonary embolism presenting to the emergency department by using a simple clinical model and a d-dimer. *Ann Intern Med* 135:98–107, 2001.

CONCLUSION

If all diseases manifested with a high fever, coughing up blood, and blood in the urine, the medical screening process would be a simple one. Unfortunately, many diseases initially manifest with subtle complaints, intermittent symptoms or mild pain, stiffness, subtle weakness or paresthesias, or acute dementia. If these complaints are brought to a physician's attention by the patient, they often are not severe enough to warrant extensive diagnostic testing. Many patients or family members simply ignore symptoms or physiological changes, rationalizing that everything is okay, the family member is just old, or he or she simply does not like to see physicians or is too busy. All of the scenarios can account for patients with occult disease seeing therapists. The fact that PTs and OTs tend to spend a moderate amount of time with patients over a period of weeks or months can facilitate the detection of subtle manifestations. In addition, as therapists develop rapport with patients and family members, information may be shared that they were uncomfortable disclosing initially. Always remember that acute dementia is never normal and is reflective of an acute problem rather than simply of aging.

The responsibilities of the PT and OT related to screening for symptoms and signs that indicate the involvement of another health care practitioner are clearly stated in the *Guide to Physical Therapy Practice*[2] and *The Guide to Occupational Therapy Practice.*[3] The process associated with Differential Diagnosis Phase 1 allows for the appropriate medical screening yet keeps therapists within their scope of practice. The therapist simply communicates to the physician the list of clinical findings. The physician will determine whether new or additional medical tests are needed to rule out or diagnose specific diseases. Facilitating the timely referral of patients to physicians is an important role for therapists working within a collaborative medical model. It is this model that best serves the needs of our patients. For additional information related to the medical screening process, the readers are directed to four other textbooks.[25,30-32]

With changes in health care delivery and physicians also being asked to see more patients in less time, it is critical that all health care practitioners include an adequate medical screening component to their examinations. If quality-of-life issues are truly an important component of health care delivery, then Differential Diagnosis Phase 1, medical screening, has and will continue to be a professional expectation and responsibility placed on each PT and OT. Because consumers are accessing therapeutic services through more direct means, that responsibility will remain and grow in importance as part of both professions' education and practice. Over the next few years PTs' and OTs' roles will continue to evolve in the arena of primary care. Medical screening performed by the therapist will guide patients to a physician and could become a key component of maintaining the health and quality of life of that consumer.

In the future another choice will have to be considered as part of the role of a movement specialist. The results of Phase 1 and 2 assessments may determine that neither a medical referral nor therapeutic intervention itself is appropriate. In this situation, the patient might benefit from community activities but would not need a movement specialist, especially if the physician also has determined that medical intervention is not necessary.

References

To enhance this text and add value for the reader, all references are included on the companion Evolve site that accompanies this textbook. This online service will, when available, provide a link for the reader to a Medline abstract for the article cited. There are 32 cited references and other general references for this chapter, with the majority of those articles being evidence-based citations.

CHAPTER 8

Differential Diagnosis Phase 2: Examination and Evaluation of Functional Movement Activities, Body Functions and Structures, and Participation

ROLANDO T. LAZARO, PT, PhD, DPT, GCS, MARGARET L. ROLLER, PT, MS, DPT, and DARCY A. UMPHRED, PT, PhD, FAPTA

KEY TERMS

activity limitations
body system problems and impairments
evaluation
examination
participation restrictions

OBJECTIVES

After reading this chapter the student or therapist will be able to:

1. Differentiate the medical diagnosis made by the physician from the diagnosis made by a movement specialist.
2. Identify the differences among activity limitations, participation restrictions, and impairments in specific body structure and function.
3. Choose appropriate examination tool(s) from each category of the ICF model—body system problems and impairments, activity limitations, and participation restrictions.
4. Identify resources used to analyze the usefulness and psychometric properties of outcome measures that address body system impairments, activity limitations, and participation restrictions.
5. Discuss the role of support personnel and assistants in the examination process.
6. Evaluate the results of the clinical examination to establish a therapy diagnosis that drives intervention planning.

Since the beginning of the evolution of practice for movement specialists within the health care arena, clinicians have been expected to examine a client's functional performance and draw conclusions from the examination. The synthesis of information gathered has led to the establishment of short- and long-term goals, a prognosis concerning the likelihood of the goals being achieved, and the time it will take to achieve those goals. Similarly, the selection of the most effective and appropriate intervention strategies will guide the therapist and patient toward the desired outcomes. Today, clients are referred for physical and occupational therapy with "evaluate and treat" orders as the common referral pattern used by physicians or other health care providers. With direct access to physical and occupational therapy becoming a reality in many states across the United States and other countries, many patients are walking into clinics because they have decided that therapy is the best alternative to assist with their functional problems. Whether through self-referral or referral from another medical or health care practitioner, once a client enters into a therapeutic environment, clinicians must first determine whether the individual is medically stable at a body system level (see Chapter 7) and an appropriate candidate for therapeutic intervention. Once medical screening has been completed and the therapist determines that there are no red flags to suggest that the client needs to be referred for additional disease or pathology examination or does not need therapeutic intervention, then the client enters into Phase 2 of the evaluation process (Figure 8-1). In this phase it is important to examine and identify the client's strengths that will facilitate recovery of functional movement, as well as what the client is unable to do functionally.

Numerous tools are used to examine clients with physical complaints and problems with functional movement. Many of these tools directly measure specific strengths and weaknesses of *body system structures and functions,* helping the clinician to identify specific impairments of a client that are causes of functional loss. Each body system or impairment tool is intended for a specific purpose and is designed to supply the user with a given outcome measure in a predetermined set of values.

Other tools measure a client's ability or limitation for performing functional *activities.* These tools are designed to examine the performance of a client during various functional skills and activities of daily living. Functional tools also provide the user with a predetermined set of values. These tools, however, do not directly supply information about the cause of the client's functional movement problems. The user must extrapolate information from the results of each functional test and then choose the appropriate body system or impairment measurement tools to determine the combination of impairments that may be contributing to the limitations in the client's ability to perform daily living activities or participate in normal life interactions.

A third category of assessment is the administration of *participation* outcome measures. These are designed to

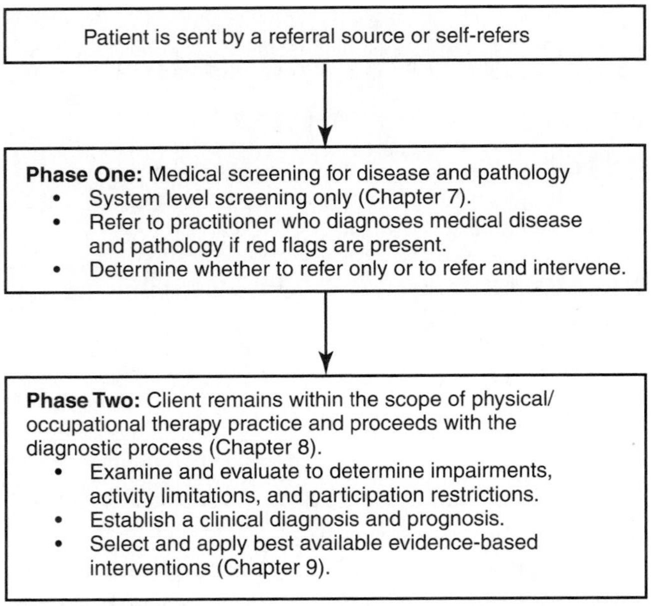
Patient is sent by a referral source or self-refers
Phase One: Medical screening for disease and pathology
• System level screening only (Chapter 7).
• Refer to practitioner who diagnoses medical disease and pathology if red flags are present.
• Determine whether to refer only or to refer and intervene.
Phase Two: Client remains within the scope of physical/ occupational therapy practice and proceeds with the diagnostic process (Chapter 8).
• Examine and evaluate to determine impairments, activity limitations, and participation restrictions.
• Establish a clinical diagnosis and prognosis.
• Select and apply best available evidence-based interventions (Chapter 9).

Figure 8-1 ■ The diagnostic process used for best practice by physical and occupational therapists.

assess a client's involvement or restriction in domestic, community, social, and civic life situations. These tools examine the client's perspective on the effects of his or her health condition on the ability to function in major life areas, interpersonal interactions and relationships, and quality of life.

The process of examination and evaluation occurs throughout the entire episode of care. The therapist must be constantly assessing the patient's health status during each encounter. Initially the therapist may miss something important that does not become identified until more complex activities are introduced. Once the subtle body system problems become obvious, the therapist may need to go back to identify more in-depth causes and fine-tune intervention strategies. The intervention strategy may proceed in various directions depending on whether the patient and therapist mutually agree that the goal should stress adaptation and compensation versus regaining function through motor learning.

To be able to provide information that is meaningful in determining the best possible intervention for a particular patient, the examination tools selected by the clinician must be objective, reliable, valid, and appropriately matched with patient expectations. These tools should also communicate necessary information in a language that is understandable to all health care professionals and the payer responsible for funding the services (see Chapter 10). With the limitations on visits within the clinical setting and the critically important variable of motivation and adherence of the patient, the setting of goals and the selection of intervention strategies need to be established through patient-centered participation.[1-10]

This chapter has been developed to help the reader work through the problem-solving and decision-making process for selecting appropriate tests. It is not within the scope of this chapter or text to explain each examination tool in detail. However, the reader is presented with an extensive list of tests for body function and structure, activity, and participation in Appendix 8-A.

SELECTION OF APPROPRIATE TESTS AND MEASURES

After the patient history and interview and the review of systems, the next step in the patient/client management process is the selection of appropriate tests and measures that will identify the most important patient problems that require therapeutic intervention. In the clinical environment, the therapist often approaches this process by first identifying the functional activities that the patient is able and not able to do (activity limitation or functional limitation), hypothesizing the possible impairments causing this activity or functional limitation, and then testing the body systems and subsystems to identify the nature and extent of the impairments. Consistent with the International Classification of Functioning, Disability and Health (ICF) model, the client's strengths are often emphasized as the foundation for this process. The approach is proactive and collaborative, truly capitalizing on the client's potential and goals, and highlights the therapist-client partnership.

TESTS OF ACTIVITY AND FUNCTIONAL PERFORMANCE

As mentioned previously, the therapist typically starts with the examination of functional activities. This step will allow the therapist to understand the specific functional tasks that the patient can do, as well as those activities or functions that the patient is unable to perform. It is important to observe the client during the performance of these tasks and to note the motor patterns used. Many functional assessment tools have been developed to provide a more objective assessment of everyday skills and tasks. Each tool is designed to measure and score a specific type of functional ability. Several tools test a range of skills from balance skills to walking ability during the performance of functional tasks. Some tests are quick and easy to set up and perform, such as the Functional Reach Test and Timed Up and Go (TUG) Test, whereas other tools may take longer to administer, such as the Berg Balance Scale or Fugl-Meyer Assessment. There are advantages and disadvantages to both of these types of tests. Those that are the quickest to administer tend to measure fewer functional skills and do not supply information on the total functioning of a client. However, if the clinician properly identifies the client's problems and is able to focus on the most efficient way of measuring them, a quick functional test can be the most beneficial one to use. Tests that take a bit longer to administer typically assess multiple skills and supply the user with a more comprehensive picture of the client's functional abilities including those in various domains such as gross mobility, self-care, cognitive ability, and communication ability, among others. Often the decision on the complexity of the assessment tool used is based on the client and family's objectives and long-term goals.

Outcome scales for functional tests may be found in ordinal format (e.g., Functional Independence Measure [FIM], Barthel Index, Katz Index of Independence in Activities of Daily Living). Each has its own unique point value and range, varying from a two- to three-point scale (e.g., Tinetti Performance-Oriented Mobility Assessment [POMA]) to a seven-point scale (e.g., FIM). A few tools supply ratio scale data (e.g., the TUG, Functional Reach Test, and measures of gait velocity). Test data presented in ratio scale format will more clearly show incremental changes, thereby facilitating the comparison of pretherapy to posttherapy performance.

TESTS OF BODY FUNCTIONS AND STRUCTURES

After identifying problems with functional performance of activities, the clinician then focuses on the performance of appropriate tests for body functions and structures. Consistent with the ICF model, the intent is to identify which body systems or subsystems are intact and functioning normally and could be optimized as the patient works on regaining the ability to perform functional tasks or participate in life. In this step, it is also important to identify which body systems and subsystems are not normal. These body system impairments may be the cause of the functional loss.

Impairment (ICF; International Classification of Impairments, Disabilities, and Handicaps [ICIDH]; Nagi)[11] is defined as the loss or abnormality of physiological, psychological, or anatomical structure or function at the organ system level.[12] The clinician needs to make the distinction between primary impairments, which are a direct consequence of the client's specific disease or pathological condition, and secondary impairments, which occur as sequelae to the disease or rehabilitation process or as the result of aging, disuse, repetitive strain, lifestyle, and so on. Moreover, the clinician must remember that, although functional limitations are usually caused by a combination of specific impairments, it is possible that impairments may not contribute to specific functional problems for a particular client. If this is the case, the clinician should make a determination regarding whether these impairments, if left uncorrected, will result in the development of activity limitations at a later time. Simultaneously, the patient needs to be a part of this discussion because the therapist may not have the time to address all impairments. The correction of particular impairments may have more meaning or value to the patient. To the consumer some impairments may lead to limitation of functions that are important to them, whereas other impairments may restrict an activity in which the patient would never want to participate.

The ultimate goal of any therapeutic intervention program is to attain the highest level of health and wellness possible. Measurement tools that the clinician chooses to use also need to reflect this end result. For example, "traditional" impairment measurements may indicate that a client demonstrates shoulder range of motion (ROM) that is decreased by 25 degrees. The more important question should be how this decrease in ROM affects the client's ability to perform a functional task such as dressing or any other activity that the client perceives as important. The clinician is therefore encouraged to consider the functional implications of these measurements to obtain results that are more meaningful for the client.

The clinician is always faced with the challenge of identifying and administering examination tools that will not only reflect the client's level of health and wellness but also reflect the client's functional improvement as a result of the intervention provided. Functional measurement tools can be used as a baseline measure for those functional skills. However, these tools typically require a large improvement in a client's functional performance for a clinically significant change to be seen. Results obtained from impairment tests can fill in the large gaps between numerical scores on functional scales, demonstrating objective measurements and trends in the direction toward improvement before any change is demonstrated on the functional examination.

Box 8-1 illustrates impairments that may be seen in patients/clients with movement disorders caused by neurological dysfunctions. These impairments are further classified as those that are within the central nervous system and those that are outside the central nervous system and result from interaction with the environment. These impairments are further discussed in detail in various sections of this book.

Range of motion testing is one example of a common neuromusculoskeletal system examination procedure. Clinicians depend heavily on ROM measurements as an essential component of their examination and consequent evaluation process. It is imperative that the data obtained from this procedure be reliable. It has been suggested that the main source of variation in the performance of this procedure is method and that reliability can be improved by standardizing the procedure.[13]

An impairment in ROM can be the result of other body system impairments. ROM measurements may be used to

BOX 8-1 ■ IDENTIFICATION AND CLASSIFICATION OF IMPAIRMENTS

IMPAIRMENTS WITHIN THE CENTRAL NERVOUS SYSTEM

1. Tone, reflexes, and abnormal state of the motor neuron pool
2. Synergies (volitional or reflexive)
3. Sensory integration and organization
4. Balance and postural control
5. Speed of movement
6. Timing
7. Reciprocal movement
8. Directional control, trajectory or pattern of movement
9. Accuracy
10. Emotional influences
11. Perception
12. Cognition, memory, and ability to learn
13. Levels of consciousness

IMPAIRMENTS OUTSIDE OF THE CENTRAL NERVOUS SYSTEM AND INTERACTION WITH THE ENVIRONMENT

1. Range of motion
2. Muscle strength or power production
3. Endurance
4. Cardiac function
5. Circulatory function
6. Respiratory function
7. Other organ system interactions
8. Hormonal and nutritional factors
9. Psychosocial factors
10. Task content
11. Environmental construct

determine the effect of tone, balance, movement synergies, pain, and so forth on the neuromuscular system and ultimately on behavior. Most important, the clinician needs to remember that the ROM needed to perform a functional activity is more critical than "normal," anatomical, biomechanical ROM values and must be considered when labeling and measuring impairments. For example, full ROM in the shoulder is seldom needed unless activities of daily living, work, or leisure activities require it, such as performing a tennis serve or reaching overhead to paint a ceiling. When needed for specific tasks, goniometric measurements of ROM are appropriate, but at other times a functional range measurement may be sufficient.

Muscle strength testing is another commonly used examination procedure. Clinicians use various methods of quantifying strength including "traditional" manual muscle testing (MMT) and the use of a dynamometer. As with ROM, strength should be correlated with the patient's functional performance. Again, the clinician may find a client to have 3/5 strength in the shoulder flexor muscle groups or find grip strength to be 35 kg, but the more important question should be "What does this mean in terms of the client's ability to perform activities of daily living, and/or can he use that power in a functional activity?" The clinician is also advised to make the distinction between muscle strength and muscular endurance as it relates to function. A client may have sufficient lower-extremity strength and power to get up from the seated position; however, this does not necessarily mean that the client has muscular endurance to perform the task repeatedly during the day as part of normal everyday activities.

The status of the cardiac, respiratory, and circulatory systems significantly affects a client's functional performance (see Chapter 30). Blood pressure, heart rate, and respiration give the clinician signs of the patient's medical stability and the ability to tolerate exercise. The clinician may also obtain the results of pulmonary function tests for ventilation, pulmonary mechanics, lung diffusion capacity, or blood gas analysis after determining that the client's pulmonary system is a major factor affecting medical stability and functional progress. Various exercise tolerance tests also attempt to quantify functional work capacity and serve as a guide for the clinician performing cardiac and pulmonary rehabilitation.

A client who has difficulty performing activities of daily living and who has neurological impairments in the central motor, sensory, perceptual, or integrative systems needs to undergo examination procedures to establish the level of impairment of each involved system and to determine if and how that system is contributing to the deficit motor behaviors. Functional evaluation tools used may include the FIM, the Barthel Index, the Tinetti POMA, or the TUG test. The results of these tests will help to steer the clinician toward the most useful impairment tools to use to evaluate limitations in the various body systems. Impairment tools may include the Modified Ashworth Scale for spasticity, the Upright Motor Control Test for lower-extremity motor control, the Clinical Test of Sensory Interaction on Balance (CTSIB), or the Sensory Organization Test (SOT) for balance and sensory integrative problems, or computerized tests of limits of stability on the NeuroCom Balance Master, among others (see Appendices 8-A, 8-B, and 8-C).

The clinician is also advised to investigate the interaction of other organs and systems as they relate to the patient's functional limitations. For example, electrolyte imbalance, hormonal disorders, or adverse drug reactions (see Chapter 36) may explain impairments and activity limitations noted in other interacting systems.

TESTS FOR PARTICIPATION AND SELF-EFFICACY

In ICF terminology, *participation* is defined as an individual's involvement in a life situation. Domestic life, interpersonal interactions and relationships, and community, social, and civic life are some examples of aspects of participation that can be examined for each individual. *Participation restriction* is the term used to denote problems that individuals may experience in involvement in life situations. When considering participation it is important to obtain the individual's perception of how the medical condition, impairments, and activity limitations affect his or her involvement in life and community. Therefore many of the tests for participation and self-efficacy are in self-report format. The Activities-specific Balance Confidence Scale (ABC), Short Form 36 (SF-36), and Dizziness Handicap Inventory (DHI) are examples of tests that can be used to gather information under this domain. These tests allow an individual to assess his or her health quality of life after an incident that affected activity and participation. Appendices 8-A, 8-B, and 8-D include tools that measure participation and quality of life.

CHOOSING THE APPROPRIATE EXAMINATION TOOL

The ability to choose the appropriate examination tool(s) for a particular client will depend on several factors:

1. The client's current functional status (ambulatory vs nonambulatory)
2. The client's current cognitive status (intact vs confused or disoriented)
3. The clinical setting in which the person is being evaluated for treatment (acute hospital, rehabilitation, outpatient, skilled care, or home care)
4. The client's primary complaints (pain vs weakness vs impaired balance)
5. The client's goals and realistic expectation of recovery, maintenance, or prevention of functional loss (acute injury, chronic problem, or progressive disease process)
6. The type of information desired from the test (discriminative or predictive)

The evaluator should select examination tools that will measure the client's primary problems (activity limitations, impairments, and participation restrictions) and supply outcome values that are needed to set realistic treatment goals in accordance with those of the client and family and to plan efficient and effective intervention strategies. The clinician is advised to select functional tools that contain component skills that the particular client is having difficulty performing. Skills the client performs poorly will disclose the activity limitations. Skills the client performs well determine the client's strengths and abilities. The evaluator must then focus on the client's functional activity limitations as determined by the test(s) to determine the impairment tests that will be performed next. For example, if the client demonstrates difficulty in rising from a chair during a functional test and scores low on this skill on the outcome measure (the Tinetti POMA or Berg Balance Scale), the clinician must then closely examine the skill of coming to stand to determine the cause of the mobility limitation. The problem may be that the client cannot generate adequate muscle power to push up from the chair, does not have adequate ROM in the hip or the ankle joints to rise from the chair, or no longer sees a reason to get out of the chair, or that it hurts too much to even try. It may be a problem with dynamic balance during or after the transitional movement. Any impairment that is hypothesized by observing performance of the functional skill needs to be measured more specifically. It is up to the examiner to determine the next best steps to take to target the client's problems as efficiently as possible, to measure and record the needed outcomes as objectively as possible, and then to set treatment goals in consultation with the client to design the best intervention to remediate or manage the problems.

Many of the examination tools that measure a client's ability to perform functional activities have been accepted as valid, reliable, and useful for the justification of payment for services rendered. The number of activity limitations and the extent of the client's participation limitation are often reasons why an individual either has accessed therapy services directly or was referred by a medical practitioner. For this reason, the third-party payer expects to receive reports concerning positive changes in the client's functional status for therapeutic services to be justifiable (see Chapter 10). The initial list of functional or activity limitations or participation restrictions helps the therapist determine the extent of, expectations for, and direction of intervention, but it does not determine why those limitations exist. This is the question that is critical to answer as part of the evaluation process. Examination tests and procedures that identify specific system and subsystem impairments help the therapist determine causes for existing participation and activity limitations. These tools need to be objective, reliable, and sensitive enough to provide needed communication to third-party payers to explain the subsystem's baseline progress during and after the intervention. These tools should also supply explanations for residual difficulties in the event that the functional problems themselves do not demonstrate significant objective change or show progress within the time frame estimated.

USING THE EVALUATION PROCESS TO LINK BODY SYSTEM PROBLEMS, ACTIVITY LIMITATIONS, AND PARTICIPATION RESTRICTIONS TO INTERVENTION

After objective measures have been obtained for activity limitations, body system and subsystem impairments, and participation restrictions, clinicians must determine whether the impairments or the functional problems are changeable to a more independent, safe, and functional level. In certain situations a mobility limitation may be remediated and become more functional, although the contributing component impairments may remain unchanged. In other situations, impairment measures may significantly improve but the functional problem may remain unaltered. This is especially true when one impairment is significantly improved but functional progress is masked by the contribution of other impairments. The examiner must be able to come to a conclusion regarding the relationship between the client's activity limitations and the existing body systems impairments. Without an understanding of this relationship, it is difficult to assess the effect of the treatment intervention(s) on an individual.

The interactions and interrelationships of the identified functional problems and impairments provide the clinician with an initial status or problem list specific to that individual. That list helps the clinician formulate a diagnosis for the movement dysfunction. Through consideration of the objective values obtained during the examination process, a target status to be reached at the conclusion of therapeutic intervention can be estimated. That target status is both impairment and function driven and traditionally would be considered a list of outcome goals. The interactions between impairments and their related activity and participation limitations make up the unique problem map of that individual and direct the clinician toward selecting optimal interventions.

The prognosis made by the clinician is based on the assessment of the likelihood that the patient will achieve the target outcome in a given time frame and estimated number of visits needed to reach the treatment goal. Once the clinician has measured and identified specific activity limitations and their respective impairments, he or she then has an excellent opportunity to conceptually understand how various impairments affect multiple functional problems and which impairments are activity specific.

The following case scenario synthesizes the clinical examination and evaluation process used by physical and occupational therapists.

Assume that a clinician has been called in to examine a client who has sustained an anoxic brain injury during heart surgery. The client's cognitive ability is within normal limits, and he is highly motivated to get back to his normal activities. He is retired; he loves to walk in the park with his wife and to go on birdwatching experiences in the mountains with their group of friends. The clinician must select which functional tests to use to obtain an objective initial status and target the client's problems. Currently the client requires assistance with all gross mobility skills and is demonstrating difficulty balancing in various postures and performing activities of daily living. Results of functional testing reveal that the client demonstrates significant limitations, requiring moderate assistance in the activities of coming to sit, sitting, coming to stand, standing, walking, dressing, and grooming. Assume that the client also displays impairment limitations in flexion ROM at the hip joints caused by both muscle and fascia tightness and hypertonicity within the extensor muscle groups. He has compensated to some degree and is able to perform bed mobility independently. Upper-extremity motor control is within normal limits, and thus the client is capable of performing many activities of daily living as long as his lower trunk and hips are placed in a supportive position and hip flexion beyond 90 degrees is not required. The client has general weakness from inactivity, and power production problems in his abdominals and hip flexor muscles owing to the dominance of extensor muscle tonicity. Once he is helped to stand, the extensor patterns of hip and knee extension, internal rotation, slight adduction, and plantarflexion are present. He can actively extend both legs after being placed in flexion, but he is limited in the production of specific fine and gross motor patterns. Thus a resulting balance impairment is present owing to the inability to adequately access appropriate balance strategies caused by the presence of tone, limb synergy production, and weakness in the antagonists to the trunk and hip extensors. Through the use of augmented intervention (see Chapter 9) the client is noted to possess intact postural and procedural balance programming; however, both functions are being masked by existing impairments. The decision is made to perform impairment measures, including assessments of ROM at the hip, knee, and ankle joints; the ability to produce strength in both the abdominal and hip flexor muscle groups; and volitional and nonvolitional synergic programming, balance, and posture, and volitional control over muscle tone. The demand on ROM, power production, and specific synergic programming will vary according to the requirements of the functional activities performed.

Using a clinical decision-making process, the clinician will conclude that the impairments that are being targeted to measure will vary from one functional activity to the next. For instance, if this client is demonstrating difficulty rising from a chair, the target impairment may be a ROM measurement. This same ROM impairment may also contribute to problems with moving about the base of support in functional sitting. The clinician makes the determination as to the extent to which the impairment interferes with each functional problem for that particular client.

These objective measurements help the clinician explain which outcomes would be expected to be achieved first and why. These measurements are recorded as part of intervention charting and help to objectively demonstrate that the client is improving toward functional independence. They also give an indication of what the client still needs to reach the desired outcome, the rate of learning that is taking place, and an estimation of recovery time that is still required. These objective measurements give to the clinician and the client a better avenue to discuss expectations with family members, other medical practitioners, and third-party payers. In this example, assume that, after intervention, functional ROM in the hip was achieved. However, this improvement did not result in an improvement in the activity problems because synergic programming prevented adequate hip flexion during one or more functional activities. Understanding and measuring the difference between lack of ROM as a result of muscle or fascia tightness versus lack of range from abnormal synergic patterning helps the clinician communicate why a client is successful in one activity and may still need assistance in another.

Scores obtained from tests of activity, participation, and impairments supply statistically important measurements that can then be used to discuss the limitations placed on the therapeutic environment by fiscal intermediaries. Therapists must be clear when documenting the initial status and the target status for clients so that the recommended intervention and length of stay may be justified (see Chapter 10).

When making a determination of the potential impact of an intervention on improving a client's problems, clinicians must remember that a key factor in this process of examination and evaluation is the acceptance of the movement dysfunction or impairment by the client. A mobility problem or impairment may be clearly identified by a functional test or impairment test; however, the client may deny that the problem even exists. Acceptance of the problems by the client and a willingness to change are critical to the client's adherence to the intervention strategy.

As mentioned earlier, the identification of potential impairments was done after functional testing to streamline the examination process. After performing the functional examination, the therapist postulated that the client might have impaired motor control, muscle weakness, sensory deficits, pain, and decreased endurance that may have been causing the functional limitations. MMT revealed lower-extremity strength of 1/5 in both ankle motions, 2/5 in both knees, and 3−/5 in both hips. Upper extremities tested as 1/5 finger flexors (incomplete grip), 2/5 wrist motions, and 3+/5 in both elbow motions. Shoulder and trunk strength were within functional limits for all motions. Sensory testing indicated absent touch and proprioceptive sensations from the foot to the knee of both lower extremities, with impaired sensation from the thighs to the hips. Both hands and wrists tested absent to touch and proprioception, with the elbows and shoulders testing intact. The client's endurance was limited to short bouts of activity (3 to 5 minutes), with rapid muscular and cardiovascular fatigue. The presence of these impairments helped to explain the resultant functional limitations tested earlier.

In terms of standardized functional tests, the multidisciplinary FIM could give insight into this patient's ability to function in multiple domains and categories. Baseline scores on the Tinetti POMA and the Berg Balance Scale could be collected because this client is expected to regain further function in balance and postural control as recovery from the condition occurs. As the client regains strength and peripheral sensory ability, he may be able to perform the TUG and the 10-Meter Walk Test. These functional assessments paint a better picture of what the client can and cannot do, as well as providing a way to measure functional progress in various activities throughout rehabilitation.

When determining an appropriate tool to examine a client's functional status, the clinician must also consider the "ceiling and floor effect" of the functional tools. In this particular case, the patient is probably unable to perform the Functional Gait Assessment (FGA) but may be appropriate for beginning the balance portion of the Tinetti POMA. As the patient progresses, the predictive and discriminative properties of some of these tests could provide information regarding the patient's likelihood of falling, or ability to safely perform selected functional tasks.

References

To enhance this text and add value for the reader, all references are included on the companion Evolve site that accompanies this textbook. This online service will, when available, provide a link for the reader to a Medline abstract for the article cited. There are 209 cited references and other general references for this chapter, with the majority of those articles being evidence-based citations.

CASE STUDY 8-1*

The patient is a 30-year-old man who was referred to outpatient physical therapy after a 1-week stay in an acute care facility following an exacerbation of relapsing-remitting multiple sclerosis (MS). His height was 2.05 m (6 feet 9 inches) and his weight was 133.81 kg (295 pounds). The patient was first diagnosed with MS 4 years ago. He developed optic neuritis during the exacerbation and was treated with corticosteroid pulse therapy. The patient's past medical history included depression, gastroesophageal reflux disease (GERD), migraine headaches, and hyperlipidemia. After being diagnosed with MS, the patient had to stop working. Before the most recent hospitalization, the patient lived with his sister in a single-story home with five stairs to enter with a railing. At that time he was able to ambulate independently without an assistive device and to complete all activities of daily living without any assistance.

An outpatient physical therapy initial examination was conducted 1 week after the patient was discharged from the hospital. He reported that he was using a wheelchair to get to and from appointments, and inside his home. He was alert and oriented to person, place, and time, although responses were delayed and speech was slightly slurred. There were no complaints of pain, and the patient stated that fatigue and temperature had not affected him.

Several tests of functional movement activities were performed first. The patient was able to roll to the right and left with minimal assistance, with rolling to the right being less difficult for the patient. He needed supervision to move from supine to sitting.

The patient required moderate assistance to perform a sit-to-stand transfer. He was able to ambulate five steps with a front-wheeled walker (FWW) and moderate assistance of one person.

After examination of the patient's functional movement activities, several tests of body function and structures were then administered. Passive ROM for all joints in both upper and lower extremities was within normal limits. The patient presented with 3/5 (fair) strength of the right upper and lower extremities and good (4/5) strength of the left upper and lower extremities during MMT. Light touch and superficial pain sensations tested intact from C4-S2 dermatomes bilaterally.

Sitting balance was scored as 3/4 (good), as the patient was able to accept moderate challenges. Standing static balance was 1+/4 (poor plus); the patient was able to maintain balance with handheld support and occasional minimal assistance.

Observational gait analysis was performed, and impairments in gait included the following: decreased step length bilaterally, wide base of support, decreased weight bearing through the right lower extremity, and lack of toe-off. It was also noted that ataxic type movements were present with ambulation.

The Gait Abnormality Rating Scale (GARS) was performed, and the patient scored a 32/48, indicating increased fall risk. The Tinetti POMA was also administered. The patient scored 8/28, indicating a high risk for falls. Several tests were performed using the NeuroCom Balance Master. The sit-to-stand test showed that the patient had difficulty maintaining balance immediately after rising and had more weight on his left lower extremity. The results were abnormal, based on the norms for the patient's gender and age. Next, the weight-bearing squat test was done. During this test the patient was not able to maintain equal weight through bilateral lower extremities, with the patient bearing weight more on the left side. The patient then performed the limits of stability test, which revealed an inability to lean his center of gravity (COG) over his right lower extremity, or forward onto his toes. The patient then performed the rhythmic weight-shift test; he was not able to complete the forward-backward component of the rhythmic weight-shift test without falling, and he also had difficulty with directional control and velocity during lateral weight shifting.

Last, tests for participation and self-efficacy were administered. The Activities-specific Balance Confidence (ABC) Scale questionnaire was given to the patient to assess the patient's balance self-efficacy. The patient had a score of 20%, indicating a low level of physical functioning. He scored 10% on being able to bend down, pick a slipper up off the floor, and reach for a can on a shelf at eye level with the use of a FWW.

The data collected at initial examination revealed limitations in functional performance resulting from impairments in balance, gait, strength, and motor control, giving the therapist the various movement diagnoses that reflected problems. The *Guide to Physical Therapist Practice* was used to classify the patient in the neuromuscular practice pattern E (impaired motor function and sensory integrity associated with progressive disorders of the central nervous system). The *Guide* indicates a range of 6 to 50 visits needed to reach anticipated outcomes for patients who are classified in this practice pattern. Intervention frequency and duration was set at three times per week for 8 weeks. The prognosis that the patient would be able to ambulate independently in the community with an assistive device in 8 weeks was good, given the patient's willingness to participate in physical therapy, positive outlook, family support, and positive response to medical interventions. The plan of care that was developed focused on improving activity limitations such as transfers and gait and impairments such as weakness and imbalance. The long-term goals were set to be achieved in 8 weeks, and short-term goals were set to be achieved in 4 weeks.

*Case study modified from Larsen-Merrill J, Lazaro R: Use of the NeuroCom balance master training protocols to improve functional performance in a person with multiple sclerosis. *J Stud Phys Ther Res* 21:1–16, 2009.

APPENDIX 8-A ■ Outcome Measures from the Neurology Section of the American Physical Therapy Association (APTA) Special Interest Groups (SIGs) from *Neurologic Practice Essentials: A Measurement Toolbox,** Organized by Categories of the World Health Organization (WHO) International Classification of Functioning, Disability and Health (ICF)[14-17]

ICF Category	Outcome Measures
Balance and Falls SIG	
Body Structure/Function	None submitted
Activity	Berg Balance Scale Fregly-Graybiel Ataxia Test Battery Functional Reach Test Gait Abnormality Rating Scale, Modified (mGARS) Gait Speed—10 Meter Walk Test Limits of Stability Test (LOS) Physical Performance Battery Sensory Organization Test (SOT) Tinetti Performance-Oriented Mobility Assessment (POMA) Walky-Talky Test
Participation	Activities-specific Balance Confidence Scale (ABC) Tinetti Falls Efficacy Scale (FES)
Brain Injury SIG	
Body Structure/Function	Agitated Behavior Scale Awareness Questionnaire Coma/Near Coma Scale Disorders of Consciousness Scale Glasgow Coma Scale (GCS) JFK Coma Recovery Scale, Revised Modified Ashworth Scale Patient Competency Rating Scale Rancho Levels of Cognitive Functioning
Activity	Berg Balance Test Brunel Balance Test Functional Independence Measure (FIM) Functional Independence Measure/Functional Assessment Measure (FIM/FAM) High-level Mobility Assessment Test (HiMAT)
Participation	Community Integration Questionnaire Craig Handicap Assessment and Reporting Technique (CHART) Disability Rating Scale Mayo Portland Adaptability Inventory Participation Objective, Participation Subjective
Degenerative Diseases SIG	
Body Structure/Function	ALS Functional Rating Scale Hoehn and Yahr Stage Kurtzke Extended Disability Status Scale Modified Ashworth Scale Modified Mini-Mental State Examination (MMSE) Unified Huntington's Disease Rating Scale (UHDRS) Unified Parkinson's Disease Rating Scale (UPDRS)
Activity	2- or 6-Minute Walk Test 360-Degree Turn Test Berg Balance Scale Dynamic Gait Index (DGI) Functional Independence Measure (FIM) Functional Reach Test Gait Speed—Self-Paced and Fast Modified Gait Abnormality Rating Scale Schwab and England Scale Timed Up and Go Test (TUG) Tinetti Performance-Oriented Mobility Assessment (POMA)
Participation	Fatigue Severity Scale Modified Falls Efficacy Scale Modified Fatigue Impact Scale Parkinson's Disease Questionnaire–39 (PDQ-39) Short Form 36 (SF-36) or Short Form 12 (SF-12)
Spinal Cord Injury SIG	
Body Structure/Function	American Spinal Injury Association (ASIA) Impairment Classification Scale Manual Muscle Testing (MMT) Modified Ashworth Scale Myometry Penn Spasm Frequency Scale
Activity	Functional Evaluation in Wheelchair (FEW) Functional Independence Measure (FIM) Quadriplegia Index of Function (QIF) Spinal Cord Injury Functional Ambulation Inventory (SCI-FAI) Spinal Cord Injury Measure (SCIM) Walking Index for Spinal Cord Injury–II (WISCI-II) Wheelchair Assessment Tool (WAT)
Participation	Craig Handicap Assessment and Reporting Technique (CHART) Impact on Participation and Autonomy (IPA) Life Habits and Handicap (LIFE-H)
Stroke SIG	
Body Structure/Function	Fugl-Meyer Assessment of Sensorimotor Recovery After Stroke (FMA) Hand-Held Dynamometry Mini-Mental State Examination (MMSE) Modified Ashworth Scale National Institutes of Health Stroke Scale (NIHSS) Neurobehavioral Cognitive Status Examination Postural Assessment Scale for Stroke (PASS) Stroke Rehabilitation Assessment of Movement (STREAM) Trunk Control Test Trunk Impairment Scale

APPENDIX 8-A ■ Outcome Measures from the Neurology Section of the American Physical Therapy Association (APTA) Special Interest Groups (SIGs) from *Neurologic Practice Essentials: A Measurement Toolbox,** Organized by Categories of the World Health Organization (WHO) International Classification of Functioning, Disability and Health (ICF)[14-17]—cont'd

ICF Category	Outcome Measures
Activity	10-Meter Walk Test (10MWT) 6-Minute Walk Test (6MWT) Barthel Index Berg Balance Scale Chedoke-McMaster Stroke Assessment Scale Frenchay Activities Index (FAI) Functional Independence Measure (FIM) Modified Rankin Handicap Scale Motor Assessment Scale (MAS) Rivermead Motor Assessment (RMA) Timed Up and Go Test (TUG)
Participation	Euro Quality of Life–5D (EuroQol-5D) Short Form 36 (SF-36) Stroke Impact Scale (SIS) Stroke Specific Quality of Life (SS-QOL) Stroke-Adapted Sickness Impact Profile (SA-SIP30)

Vestibular SIG

ICF Category	Outcome Measures

Body Structure/Function	Clinical Test of Sensory Interaction on Balance (CTSIB)
	Romberg Test and Sharpened Romberg Test
	Sensory Organization Test (SOT)
	Single-Leg Stance Test
	Nystagmus Tests
	Gaze-Evoked Nystagmus
	Post–Head Shaking Nystagmus Test
	Spontaneous Nystagmus
	Vibration-Induced Nystagmus
	Positional Testing
	Dix-Hallpike Test
	Motion Sensitivity Quotient (MSQ)
	Tests of Voluntary Eye Movement
	  Saccades
	  Smooth Pursuit
	  Vergence
	  VOR Cancellation Test
	Vestibular Ocular Reflex Tests (VOR)
	Dynamic Visual Acuity Test (DVA)
	Gaze Stabilization Test (GST)
	Head Thrust Test (HTT)

Activity	Dynamic Gait Index (DGI) Functional Gait Assessment (FGA) Timed Up and Go Test (TUG)
Participation	Dizziness Handicap Inventory (DHI) Physical Activities Scale for the Elderly Short Form 36 (SF-36) Vestibular Disorders Activities of Daily Living Scale (VADL)

Generic Measures

ICF Category	Outcome Measures
Body Structure/Function	Mini-Mental State Examination (MMSE)
Activity	5- or 10-Meter Walk Test 6-Minute Walk Test Clinical Test of Sensory Interaction on Balance (CTSIB) Four Square Step Test (FSST) Functional Ambulation Categories Functional Gait Assessment (FGA) Trunk Impairment Scale
Participation	Activities-specific Balance Confidence Scale (ABC) Short Form 36 (SF-36)

**Neurologic Practice Essentials: A Measurement Toolbox* Development Team: Jane Sullivan (lead), Bill Andrews, Richard Bohannon, George Fulk, Desiree Lanzino, Aimee Perron, Peggy Roller, Kirsten Potter, Yasser Salem, Teresa Steffen. Neurology Section Support and Coordinators: Nancy Fell, Karen McCulloch, Dorian Rose.

APPENDIX 8-B ■ Sample Outcome Measures According to the Examination Areas in the Guide to Physical Therapist Practice, from: Neurologic Practice Essentials: A Measurement Toolbox*

Body Structures and Functions—List of Measures

Cognition

- Ability to follow multistep commands
- Alert, oriented × 4
- Kokman Short Test of Mental Status
- Mini-Mental State Examination (MMSE)
- Montreal Cognitive Assessment
- Scales to detect behavioral and cognitive impairments often seen in patients with brain injury:
  - Agitated Behavior Scale
  - Apathy Evaluation Scale
  - Awareness Questionnaire
  - Cognitive Log
  - Coma Recovery Scale–Revised
  - Coma/Near Coma Scale
  - Confusion Assessment Protocol
  - Disorders of Consciousness Scale
  - Glasgow Coma Scale (GCS)
  - Glasgow Outcome Scale (GOS)
  - JFK Coma Recovery Scale–Revised
  - Neurobehavioral Cognitive Exam
  - Neurobehavioral Functioning Inventory
  - Patient Competency Rating Scale
  - Rancho Los Amigos Levels of Cognitive Functioning
- Tests for depression
  - Beck Depression Inventory
  - Geriatric Depression Scale (GDS)
- Tests for inattention and neglect
  - Behavioral Inattention Test
  - Clock Drawing Test
  - Line Bisection Test
  - Motor-Free Visual Perceptual Test
  - Star Cancellation Test

Fatigue

- Fatigue Severity Scale
- Modified Fatigue Impact Score

Joint Integrity and Mobility

- Glenohumeral joint positioning
- Palpation of subluxation

Muscle Performance and Motor Control

- Reflexive motor and involuntary responses
  - Babinski
  - Clonus (ankle, wrist)
  - Deep tendon reflexes (DTRs)
  - Modified Ashworth Scale (tone, spasticity)
  - Motor Control Test (MCT) on force platform
  - Penn Spasm Frequency Scale
- Automatic motor
  - Adaptation Test (ADT) on force platform
  - Nudge-push test (postural reactions to perturbations)
  - Shoulder tug test (STT) (Parkinson disease)
- Voluntary motor
  - American Spinal Injury Association (ASIA) Scale (spinal cord injury)
  - Coordination tests
    - Detection of tremor
    - Finger-to-nose and rapid alternating movement tests (and other nonequilibrium coordination tests)
    - Fregly-Graybiel Ataxia Test Battery
    - Tandem walking (and other equilibrium coordination tests)
  - Five-Times Sit-to-Stand Test (FTSST)
  - Hand-held dynamometry
  - Manual muscle testing (MMT)
  - Motor Assessment Scale (MAS)
  - Motricity Index
  - Rivermead Motor Assessment
  - Stroke Rehabilitation Assessment of Movement (STREAM)
  - Tests of endurance
    - 2-Minute Walk Test
    - 3-Minute Walk Test
    - 6-Minute Walk Test
    - Borg Scale of Perceived Exertion
    - Maximum distance ambulated or propelled in wheelchair
  - Trunk Control Test
  - Trunk Impairment Scale

Posture

- Observational description of posture

Range of Motion

- End feel assessment
- Goniometry
- Neural tension tests

Sensory Integrity

- Sensory organization
  - Modified Clinical Test of Sensory Interaction on Balance (mCTSIB)
  - Sensory Organization Test (SOT)
- Somatosensory
  - Exteroception
    - Monofilament testing
    - Superficial pain (sharp or dull)
    - Superficial touch (light touch)
    - Temperature (can be left out if pain is normal per Goodman and Snyder)
    - Two-point discrimination
    - Vibration
  - Proprioception
    - Joint position sense testing
    - Kinesthesia Test (Mirroring Test)
    - Thumb-finding test
  - Rivermead Assessment of Somatosensory Performance
  - Cortical Sensory Tests
    - Graphesthesia
    - Stereognosis

APPENDIX 8-B ■ Sample Outcome Measures According to the Examination Areas in the Guide to Physical Therapist Practice, from: Neurologic Practice Essentials: A Measurement Toolbox*—cont'd

- Vestibular system testing
  - Dix-Hallpike Test (for benign paroxysmal positional vertigo [BPPV])
  - Fukuda Step Test—50-step protocol
  - Head-Shaking Nystagmus Test
  - Head Thrust Test
  - Motion Sensitivity Quotient (MSQ) (positional testing)
  - Vibration-Induced Nystagmus
- Visual system testing and vestibuloocular reflex (VOR) tests
  - Dynamic visual acuity (DVA) (clinical or computerized)
  - Gaze stabilization test (GST) (clinical or computerized)
  - Oculomotor tests (saccades, smooth pursuit, vergence)
  - Perception time test (computerized)
  - Static visual acuity
  - Visual field test (i.e., confrontation testing)

Pain

- FACES Pain Scale
- Visual Analog Pain Scale (0 to 10 numerical scale versus line bisection)
- Wheelchair User's Shoulder Pain Index (WUSPI)

Multi-Categorical Measures of Body Structure and Function

- ALS Functional Rating Scale
- Canadian Neurological Scale (stroke)
- Chedoke-McMaster Stroke Assessment Scale
- Fugl-Meyer Assessment of Motor Recovery After Stroke
- Hoehn and Yahr Staging of Parkinson's Disease
- Kurtzke Expanded Disability Status Scale (multiple sclerosis)
- NIH Stroke Scale
- Stroke Impact Scale (also addresses activity and participation on ICF)
- Unified Huntington's Disease Rating Scale (UHDRS)
- Unified Parkinson's Disease Rating Scale (UPDRS)

Activity—List of Measures

Balance and Mobility

- Berg Balance Scale
- Dynamic Gait Index (DGI)
- Functional Gait Index (FGA)
- Tinetti Performance-Oriented Mobility Assessment (POMA) (balance and gait)
- Gait speed—10-meter walk test

Participation—List of Measures

- Activities-specific Balance Confidence Scale (ABC)
- Craig Handicap Assessment and Reporting Technique (CHART)
- CHART-19—SF
- Dizziness Handicap Inventory (DHI)
- Geriatric Depression Scale
- Modified Fatigue Impact Scale (mFIS)
- Multiple Sclerosis Quality of Life–54 (MSQOL-54)
- Parkinson's Disease Quality of Life Questionaire-39 (PDQ-39)
- Satisfaction With Life Scale (SWLS)
- Short Form 36 (SF-36)
- Stroke Impact Scale (SIS)
- Stroke Impact Scale–16 (SIS-16) Physical Performance Short Form
- Tinetti Falls Efficacy Scale (FES)
- Vestibular Activities of Daily Living Scale (VADL)

**Neurologic Practice Essentials: A Measurement Toolbox* Development Team: Jane Sullivan (lead), Bill Andrews, Richard Bohannon, George Fulk, Desiree Lanzino, Aimee Perron, Peggy Roller, Kirsten Potter, Yasser Salem, Teresa Steffen. Neurology Section Support and Coordinators: Nancy Fell, Karen McCulloch, Dorian Rose.

APPENDIX 8-C ■ Pediatric Tools

Ages and Stages Questionnaire[18,19]
Alberta Infant Motor Scale[20-25]
Assessment, Evaluation, and Programming System for Infants and Children[26]
Battelle Developmental Inventory[27-31]
Bayley Infant Neurodevelopmental Screener[32-36]
Bayley Scales of Infant Development[37-59]
Bruininks-Oseretsky Test of Motor Proficiency[60-69]
Canadian Occupational Performance Measure[2,70-84]
The Carolina Curriculum for Infants and Toddlers with Special Needs[85]
The Carolina Curriculum for Preschoolers with Special Needs[86]
Child Health Questionnaire[87-99]
Childhood Health Assessment Questionnaire[100]
Children's Orientation and Amnesia Test[101]
Clinical Observation of Motor and Postural Skills Test[102]
DENVER II[103-112]
Energy Expenditure Index (EEI)[113]
Early Intervention Developmental Profile[114]
Erhardt Developmental Prehension Assessment[115]
Functional Independence Measure for Children (WeeFIM)[116-124]
Gillette Functional Assessment Questionnaire[125]
Goal Attainment Scaling[126]
Gross Motor Function Measure[127-139]
Harris Infant Neuromotor Test (HINT)[140]
Health Utilities Index Mark 3[141]
Infant Motor Screen[142,143]
Infant Neurological International Battery[144-146]
Milani-Comparetti Motor Development Screening Test[147]
Movement Assessment of Infants[148-153]
Neurological Assessment of the Preterm and Full-Term Newborn Infant[154]
Neurobehavioral Assessment of the Preterm Infant[155]
Neonatal Behavioral Assessment Scale[156-168]
Neonatal Neurobehavioral Examination[169]
Neonatal Oral Motor Assessment Scale[170]
Peabody Developmental Motor Scales[54,171-175]
Pediatric Clinical Test of Sensory Interaction for Balance[176]
Pediatric Evaluation of Disability Inventory[136,177-185]
Pediatric Outcomes Data Collection Instrument (PODCI)[186]
Pediatric Quality of Life Inventory[187]
Infant/Toddler Sensory Profile[188-191]
School Function Assessment[192]
Sensory Integration and Praxis Test[193,194]
Sensory Profile[195]
Test of Infant Motor Performance[21,22,196-198]
Test of Sensory Functions in Infants[199]
Toddler and Infant Motor Evaluation[200,201]

APPENDIX 8-D ■ Quality-of-Life Tools from the World Health Organization

World Health Organization Quality of Life instrument (short form) (WHOQOL-BREF)[202-206]
World Health Organization Quality of Life instrument (long form) (WHOQOL-100)[205]
World Health Organization Disability Assessment Schedule 2.0—36 items[202,207-209]

Special note: Condition-specific examination tools can be found in the respective chapters:
Spinal Cord Injury: Chapter 15, Chapter 16
Neuromuscular Diseases: Chapter 17
Multiple Sclerosis: Chapter 19
Basal Ganglia Disorders: Chapter 20
Cerebellar Disorders: Chapter 21
Balance and Vestibular Disorders: Chapter 22
Hemiplegia: Chapter 23
Head Injury: Chapter 24
Aging, Dementia, and Disorders of Conditions: Chapter 27

CHAPTER 9

Interventions for Clients with Movement Limitations

DARCY A. UMPHRED, PT, PhD, FAPTA, NANCY N. BYL, PT, MPH, PhD, FAPTA, ROLANDO T. LAZARO, PT, PhD, DPT, GCS, and MARGARET L. ROLLER, PT, MS, DPT

KEY TERMS

augmented intervention
evidence-based practice
functional training
impairment training
neuromuscular retraining

OBJECTIVES

After reading this chapter the student or therapist will be able to:

1. Appreciate the complexity of motor responses, and discuss methods used to influence body systems and their effects on functional behaviors.
2. Outline the differences in recovery related to healing, compensation, substitution, habituation, and adaptation.
3. Analyze the similarities and differences among impairment training of specific body systems, functional training, augmented feedback training, and learning-based sensorimotor retraining.
4. Select appropriate intervention strategies to optimize desired outcomes.
5. Analyze variables that may both positively and negatively affect complex motor responses and a patient's ability to participate in functional activities.
6. Identify procedures and sequences required to attain the most successful therapeutic outcome that best meets the needs and goals of the client and the family.
7. Consider the contribution of the client, the client's support systems, research evidence, neurophysiology, and the best practice standards available to optimize outcomes.

Before discussing therapeutic intervention procedures, the therapist must identify the learning environment within which the client will perform. As discussed in Chapter 1, that environment is made up of the therapist and the client, all internal body control mechanisms of the client, and the external restraints and demands of the world. Although this text focuses on relearning functional movement, the reader must always consider all aspects of the client including how other organs or body systems will be affected by or will affect the therapeutic outcome both during rehabilitation and in relation to long-term quality of life. An examination and evaluation (see Chapter 8) are performed before intervention to establish movement diagnoses. These examinations lead to movement diagnoses that must link to functional limitations or restrictions in activities and their causations (body system problems). Movement diagnoses and the degree and extent of the system or subsystem dysfunction or impairments determine prognosis of the outcomes on the basis of the client's potential for functional improvement. Factors such as motivation, family support, financial support, and cultural biases must be considered as part of the prognosis.[1] This process guides the selection of intervention strategies. Although it could be assumed that some of these impairments would be directly correlated to the central nervous system (CNS) trauma experienced by the client, it must also be determined whether some or most of these impairments have developed over a lifetime as a result of small traumas and adjustments to life. This insidious cause of impairments needs to be differentiated from acute causation of activity limitations because goal setting and expectations related to prognosis and recovery can be different.

Both the American Occupational Therapy Association (AOTA) and the American Physical Therapy Association (APTA) have developed guides to practice that help to direct therapists entering the professions and should help to guide practice throughout their working lives.[2,3] APTA, through the initiation of the California Physical Therapy Association, has been collecting and classifying evidence-based articles through the Hooked on Evidence project.[4] Through the use of current evidence-based practice; sensorimotor processing, motor control, motor learning, and neuroplasticity theories (see Chapter 4); and body systems models, the therapist must determine the flexibility or inherent motor control the client demonstrates while executing functional activities and participating in life. This chapter or other chapters in the book cannot establish for the reader the exact treatment sequence that should be used for every patient, but an example of a decision-making pathway has been given in Box 9-1. Functional goals must be established that lead to the client's ability to participate in life within his or her environment and whenever possible lead to or maintain the quality of life desired by the client. Similarly, the therapist must differentiate whether the observed motor problems are based on acute or longstanding impairments before establishing timelines for prognosis.

Before beginning any intervention, the therapist must determine the treatment strategies that will be used to help the client attain the desired functional outcomes. The specific environment used by the therapist to optimize patient performance will depend on the functional level and amount of motor control exhibited by the patient. The following

BOX 9-1 ■ TREATMENT STRATEGY CATEGORIES

COMPENSATION TRAINING

Use of an assistive device or orthotic to compensate for a permanent impairment or lost body system function.

SUBSTITUTION TRAINING

Teaching the client to use a different sensory system or muscle(s) group to substitute for lost function of another system. An example of sensory substitution might be teaching the client to use vision to substitute for an impaired vestibular system or somatosensory system for balance function. Substitution within the motor system might be teaching hip hiking to substitute for lack of dorsiflexion of the ankle during swing phase of gait.

HABITUATION TRAINING

Activity-based provocation of symptoms with the goal of symptom reduction with repetitive practice. An example would be teaching head movement to a patient who has a chronic labyrinthitis and severe nausea with any head movement.

NEURAL ADAPTATION

Driving changes in structure and function of the central or peripheral nervous system with repetitive, attended practice. This category would be considered neural plasticity. This category of treatment strategy takes the greatest repetition of practice and requires a strong desire by the individual to gain the functional ability and realize the potential of the central nervous system to change.

classifications can be used to document the specific role of the therapist within the training session (refer to Chapter 4 for additional detail):

Functional training: Practice of a functional skill that is meaningful, goal directed, and task oriented. Patient will experience errors and self-correct as the program becomes more automatic and integrated. An example would be gait training on a tile surface, rugs, inclined surfaces, compliant surfaces such as grass, and so on to practice ambulation.

Body system or impairment training: Treatment focus is on correcting a body system problem during an activity (e.g., pure muscle strengthening, stretching, sensory training, endurance training).

Augmented feedback training: Patient needs external feedback (auditory, visual, kinesthetic) and control over the motor program running the target task. This will limit the response patterns (e.g., reducing degrees of freedom, reduction or enhancement of tone) for successful performance of the desired movement (e.g., handling techniques, body-supported treadmill training, constraint-induced training).

Learning-based sensorimotor retraining: Treatment focus is placed on improving sensory discrimination dysfunction as a consequence of somatosensory, premotor, and motor cortical disorganization resulting from trauma, degeneration, or overuse.

Clients with CNS damage often benefit from combining interventions from the above categories. An example of this might be the early phase of partial body-weight supported treadmill training. In the early phases, a therapist or assistant is guiding the client's leg during swing and stance phases while the body harness supports a proportion of the client's total weight (augmented feedback) to assist the postural system in running appropriate programs to maintain balance and decrease the power needed to generate a more normal gait pattern. This augmented intervention is being done in a functional pattern within an environment that perturbs the client's base of support under the normal center of gravity. Thus, this perturbation moves each foot reciprocally backwards and the body forward, triggering a stepping reaction. In the case of an individual after a cerebrovascular accident (CVA), one leg will still respond normally, thus helping to trigger a between-limb reciprocal stepping action of the involved leg. In the case of bilateral involvement, both legs may need placement, requiring two people to assist. The activity may be classified as impairment training, with the focus on appropriate power production or cardiovascular fitness, leading to functional training to trigger normal motor programs necessary for gait. Simultaneously, augmented training done by a therapist includes manual assistance in the direction, rate, and placement of the involved leg throughout the gait cycle. In this previous example, therapists need to make sure they are aware of the patient's center of gravity and do not move the foot before it should be at "push off" during the gait cycle. This activity would not be considered functional training until the client could reciprocally move both legs during the gait pattern without the need of the harnass for postural support and the therapist to guide the movement.

When selecting from a variety of treatment interventions (neuromuscular retraining, functional training, impairment training, and augmented feedback training), it is important for the therapist to consider that each one is based on different strategies and rationales that contribute to the expected outcome. All interventions should address the needs of the patient and must consider any emotional and cognitive restraints. Although these intervention methods can be used simultaneously or in various combinations, the clinician needs to consider which aspect of the intervention falls into which treatment classification. Although various treatment outcomes can be measured, if classification of each treatment variable is not identified, the determination of how and why the outcomes were influenced by the intervention becomes confusing and difficult to distinguish. Without understanding the interactions of intervention methods and the outcome, treatment effectiveness and future clinical decision making remain unpredictable, and unique practice patterns and pathways are hard to identify with consistency. A master clinician who is effective with all patients but does not know how and why the decisions are made along the intervention pathway cannot leave a legacy of effectiveness that will ever lead to efficacy. Although not all graduates or inexperienced clinicians may have the innate aptitude or potential to become master clinicians, if professionals understand the verbal, spatial, cognitive, fine and gross motor, and emotional sensitivity variables that play a role in the evolution toward mastery, educational experiences might be able to nurture future colleagues along this pathway and help those with mastership potential reach that level of function earlier in their professional careers.

The reader must also remember that intervention encompasses multiple interactive environments where intervention decisions are often made moment by moment during any treatment period. The challenge to the educated clinical professional is to determine what is being done, why it is working, how to continue its effectiveness, and how to determine the progress of the successful intervention. The clinician must also determine how to empower the client (emotionally, cognitively, and motorically) to take over the intervention with inherent, automatic mechanisms that lead to fluid, flexible, functional outcomes independent of both the therapist and the environment within which the activity is occurring. It is not until clinicians can determine effective treatment outcomes from various interventions that efficacy within a research laboratory can be studied without speculation and hypothesis formation based on speculation.[1] Effectiveness is the first way to determine evidence-based practice. Once effectiveness has been established through case studies and larger controlled studies within the clinical environment, researchers can begin to tease out separate variables and establish efficacy as part of evidence to justify clinical decision making.

HISTORY OF DEVELOPMENT OF INTERVENTIONS FOR NEUROLOGICAL DISABILITIES

In the mid 1900s the interventions by physical therapists (PTs) and occupational therapists (OTs) were separate. Generally, PTs worked on gross motor activities with specific emphasis on the lower extremities and the trunk, whereas OTs worked on the upper extremities and fine motor activities. Both professions focused on daily living skills, with those involving the arms falling within the domain of the OT and those involving the legs falling within the domain of the PT. Activities that required gross motor skills such as sitting, coming to stand, walking, walking with assistive devices, and running fell within the purview of the PT, whereas grooming, hygiene, and eating were the responsibility of the OT. Today, this approach is considered ridiculous owing to our understanding of motor learning, neuroplasticity, and motor programming and control. In the past it was also accepted that the PT worked on specific system problems such as weakness, inflexibility, lack of coordination, and voluntary control, whereas the OT worked on functional activities integrated within the environment (such as dressing) and the patient's emotional needs and desires (occupational expectations). According to the terminology of the mid to late twentieth century, PTs were trained to identify and correct impairments that caused functional limitations, whereas OTs were trained in activity analysis and treatment that identified and optimized the functional activities that resulted from the impairments. Few clinicians seemed to focus on the sequential or interactive aspect of lack of function with specific impairments. Thus after the onset of a stroke the PT would strengthen and evaluate range of motion (ROM) of the leg and trunk, whereas the OT would encourage the patient to try to functionally use the arm. The PT would be preparing the patient to transfer out of bed and get into and out of a chair and then helping the patient walk, whereas the OT would be preparing the patient to use the arm in functional activities such as grooming or eating. Both therapists hoped the patient would accept responsibility for continued improvement through practice. What both professions discovered was that the patient generally did not regain normal motor control. He or she might be able to walk and might be able to move the shoulder, but the movement strategies were generally stereotypical, were abnormal in patterns, and took tremendous effort by and energy from the patient to perform. Over time, clients lost the motivation to even try, and thus what had been gained through therapy may have been lost from lack of practice once they got home. There was also minimal recovery of functional hand use, often because of the tremendous effort a patient had to use to move the shoulder to place the hand somewhere. Once that effort had been used the tightness and increased tone in the hand prevented functional use. Although functionally independent skills as measured on the Functional Independence Measure were achieved, normal movement patterns and normal motor control were rarely restored, and quality of life was clearly affected for the patient and family.

During the decade or two before the 1960s, some talented and intelligent clinicians began to question the traditional intervention strategies used by the OT and PT. These pioneers[5-29] in neurological rehabilitation set the stage for the development of new concepts that allowed basic science to infiltrate the clinical arena. The intervention strategies of Jean Ayers, Berta Bobath, Signe Brunnstrom, Margaret Johnstone, Susanne Klein-Vogelbach, Margaret Knott, Dorothy Voss, Margaret Rood, and others became popular. Colleagues observed these master clinicians and could easily see that the "new" interventions were much more effective and provided better outcomes than previous interventions. Each approach focused on multisensory inputs introduced to the client in controlled and identified sequences. These sequences were based on the inherent nature of synergistic patterns[5,21,30,31] and motor patterns observed in humans[5,7,32] and lower-order animals[33] or a combination of the two.[19,21] Each method focused on the individual client, the specific clinical problems, and the availability of alternative treatment approaches within an established framework. Some of these approaches focused on specific neurological medical diagnoses. The treatment emphasis was then on specific patients and their related movement disorders. Children with cerebral palsy and head injuries[7,23,28] and adults with hemiplegia[8,9,21,32] were the three most frequently identified medical diagnostic categories. In 1968 at Northwestern University a large conference was held and laid the foundation for the first STEP conference (Northwest University Special Therapeutic Exercise Project [NUSTEP]). Most of these master clinicians, along with research scientists of the day, came together to try to (1) identify the commonalities and differences between these approaches, and (2) integrate and use the neuroscience of the day to explain why these approaches worked.[34] Since the 1970s, substantial clinical attention has also been paid to children with learning and language difficulties.[5,13,35] Now these concepts and treatment procedures have been applied across the age spectrum for all types of medically diagnosed neurological problems seen in the clinical setting (refer to Section II of this text). This expansion of the use of any of the methods for any pathological condition manifested by insults from disease, injury, or degeneration of the brain seems to be a natural evolution given the structure and function of the CNS and commonalities in system problems and activity limitations that take the individual away from participating in life.

Fortunately, most dogmatism no longer persists with respect to territorial boundaries identified by clinicians using some specific intervention methods. A conference in 1990[36] played a significant role in challenging the relevance of these territorial boundaries and stressed the adoption of a systems model when looking at impairments, activity limitations, and participation in life interactions.[37] As the boundaries for interventions began blurring, intervention approaches such as proprioceptive neuromuscular facilitation (PNF) were then integrated into the care of clients with orthopedic problems and patients with neurological impairments. Today, few universities within the United States teach separate sections or units on specific approaches, but rather teach students to identify problems, when they are occurring in functional programs, and what bodily systems might be the cause of those activity limitations.

For example, assume that a client with hemiplegia exhibited signs of a hypertonic upper-extremity pattern of shoulder adduction, internal rotation, elbow flexion, and forearm pronation with wrist and finger flexion. Brunnstrom[8] would have identified that pattern as the stronger of her two upper-extremity synergies. Michels,[21] although using an explanation similar to Brunnstrom's to describe the pattern, would have elaborated and described additional upper-extremity synergy patterns. Bobath would have asserted that the client was stuck in a mass-movement pattern resulting from abnormal postural reflex activity.[30] Although the conceptualization of the problem certainly determined treatment protocols, the pattern all three clinicians would have worked toward was shoulder abduction, external rotation, elbow extension, forearm supination, and wrist and finger extension. The rationale for the use of this pattern within an intervention period would vary according to the philosophical approach. One clinician might describe the pattern as a reflex-inhibiting position (Bobath).[31] Another would describe the pattern as the weakest component of the various synergies (Brunnstrom),[8] whereas still another might identify the pattern as producing an extreme stretch and rotational element that inhibited the spastic pattern (Rood).[25] How those master clinicians sequenced treatment from the original hypertonic pattern to the opposite pattern and then to the goal-directed functional pattern would vary. Some would facilitate push-pull patterns in the supine and side-lying positions and rolling. Others would look at propping patterns in sitting clients or at weight-bearing patterns of clients in the prone position, over a ball or bolster, or in partial kneeling. All have the potential of improving the functional pattern of the upper extremity and modifying the hypertonic pattern. One method may have been better than the others given a particular patient, but in truth improved patient performance may have stemmed not from the method itself, but rather from the preferential CNS biases of the client and the variability of application skills among the clinicians themselves. That is, when a therapist intentionally uses specific augmented feedback to modulate the motor system's response to an environment but does not identify the other external feedback present within that environment (e.g., lighting, sound, touch, environmental constraints), therapeutic results will vary. Because of variance, efficacy of intervention is often questionable, although the effectiveness of that therapist may be easily recognized.

Because of the overlap of treatment methods and the infiltration of therapeutic management into all avenues of neurological dysfunction, various multisensory models were developed during the early 1980s.[13,38-41] These have continued to evolve into acceptable methods in today's clinical arena. Although these models attempted to integrate existing techniques, in reality they have created a new set of holistic treatment approaches. In July 2005 the III STEP conference[42] was held in Utah to again bring current theories and evidence-based practice into today's clinical environment. The history of the three STEP conferences demonstrates the evolution of evidence-based practice from the first conference, where basic science was the only evidence to justify treatment, to the second conference, where evidence in motor learning and motor control began to bring efficacy to intervention. By the time the third conference was held, the research in neuro/movement science regarding true efficacy within practice and the reliability and validity of our examination tools set the stage for standards in practice.[43] Where the next conference will take the professions and how soon that will occur is up to colleagues in the future. No proceedings from that third conference were published, but over the preceding years articles covering most of the presentations had been published in the *Journal of Physical Therapy.* The ultimate goal would be to develop one all-encompassing methodology that allows the clinician the freedom to use any method that is appropriate for the needs and individual learning styles of the client as well as to tap the unique individual differences of the clinician. Although intervention today is based on an integrated model, the influence of third-party payers, the need for efficacy of practice, and time constraints often factor into the therapist's choice of intervention. Visionary and entrepreneurial practice ideas that have the potential to be effective will always be a challenge to future therapists. Those ideas generally originate within the clinical environment and not the research laboratory. For that reason, clinicians need to communicate ideas to the researcher, and then those researchers can develop research studies that test the established efficacy or refute that effectiveness. Few researchers are master clinicians, and few clinicians are master researchers; thus collaboration is needed as the professions move forward in establishing evidence-based practice.

Today's therapists have replaced many of the existing philosophical approaches with patient-centered therapeutic intervention. Patient performance, available evidence, and the expertise of the clinician often play a key role in the specific decision regarding an intervention. When confronted with an abnormal upper-extremity pattern, today's therapist may choose to work on improving the movement pattern using a functional activity. Control of the combination of movement responses and modulation over specific central pattern generators or learned behavior programs will allow the patient opportunities to experience functional movement that is task oriented and environmentally specific. With goal-directed practice of the functional activity, neuroplastic changes, motor learning, and carryover can be achieved.[44] With a better scientific basis for understanding the function of the human nervous system, how the motor system learns and is controlled, and how other body systems, both internal and external to the CNS, modulate response patterns, today's clinicians have many additional options for selection of intervention strategies.[45-54] Whether a patient would initially benefit best from neuromuscular retraining, functional retraining, or a more traditional augmented or contrived treatment environment is up to the clinician and is based on the specific needs identified during the examination and evaluation process.

No matter what treatment method is selected by a clinician, all intervention should focus on the active learning process of the client. The client should never be a passive participant, even if the level of consciousness is considered vegetative, nor should the client be asked to perform an activity when the system problems only create distortion or demonstrate total lack of control of the desired movement. With all interventions requiring an active motor response, whether to change a body system impairment such as by increasing or reducing the rate of a motor response, modulate the tonal state of the central pattern generators and learned motor behaviors, or influence a functional response during an activity, the client's CNS is being asked to process and respond to the external world. That response needs to become procedural and controlled by the patient without any augmentation to be measured as functionally independent. In time, the ultimate goal is for the client to self-regulate and orchestrate modulation over this adaptable and dynamic integrated sensorimotor system in all functional activities and in all external environments.

A problem-oriented approach to the treatment of any impairment or activity limitation implies that flexibility and neural adaptation are key elements in recovery. However, adaptation should not be random, disjointed, or non–goal oriented. It should be based on methods that provide the best combination of available treatment alternatives to meet the specific needs of the individual. Development of a clinical knowledge bank enables the therapist to match treatment alternatives with the patient's impairments, activity limitations, objectives for improved function, and desired quality of life. A professionally educated therapist no longer bases treatment on identified approaches, although specific aspects of those approaches may be treatment tools that will meet the client's needs and assist him or her in regaining functional control of movement. Treatment is based on an interaction among basic science, applied science, the therapist's skills, and the client's desired outcomes.[49-52,55,56] In most cases, multiple intervention strategies must be included, but the therapist needs to be able to identify why those selected treatments will lead to system improvement as well as documenting those findings using reliable standardized and acceptable clinical methods and terminology. These intervention strategies must be dynamic yet also understandable and repeatable. As new scientific theories are discovered, new information must be integrated to continue to modify treatment approaches.

INTERVENTION STRATEGIES

Functional Training

Functional training is a method of retraining the motor system using repetitive practice of functional tasks in an attempt to reestablish the client's ability to perform activities of daily living (ADLs) and participate in specific life activities such as golfing, fly-fishing, basketball, or bridge. This method of training is a common and popular intervention strategy used by clinicians owing to the fact that it is a relatively simple and straightforward approach to improving deficits in function. A system problem such as weakness in the quadriceps muscle of the leg can be treated by muscle strengthening in a functional pattern that can be easily measured. Because of its inherent simplicity, functional training is sometimes misused or abused by clinicians. Most patients with neurological deficits have multiple subsystem problems within multiple areas, which forces the CNS to use alternative movement patterns in order to try to accomplish the functional task presented. If the therapist accesses a motor plan such as transfers but allows the patient to use programs that are inefficient, inappropriate, or stereotypical, then the activity itself is often beyond the patient's ability. The patient may learn something, but it will not be the normal program for transfers. This activity often leads to additional problems for the client.

In Chapter 8 the steps involved in the examination process are explained in detail. The intricate relationship of body system problems, impairments, and functional limitations that decrease participation in the rehabilitation process are discussed. Functional training can be implemented once the clinician has identified the client's activity limitations. The clinician must first answer the questions "What can the client do?" "What limitations does the client have when engaging in functional activities?" "Are there motor programs that are being used to substitute for normal motor function?" and "Can the therapist use functional training to improve body system problems within the context of the functional skill?" Once the therapist has an understanding of the reasons for any activity limitation and can alleviate substitution and compensation for the deficit, functional tasks should be identified and practiced.

The Effect of Functional Training on Task Performance and Participation

The main focus of functional training is the correction of activity limitations that prevent an individual from participating in life. However, through repetitive practice of functional tasks and gross motor patterns, many of the client's impairments can also be affected. For example, if a therapist practices sit-to-stand transfers with a client in a variety of environments and performs multiple repetitions of each type of transfer, not only can learning be reinforced, but the client can also gain strength in the synergistic patterns of the lower extremities that work against gravity to concentrically lift the client off of the support surface and eccentrically lower him or her down. Weight bearing through the feet in a variety of degrees of ankle dorsiflexion during transfer training will effectively place the ankles in functional positions. The act of standing also helps the trunk and neck extensors to engage in postural control. Varying the speed of the activity during the treatment can stimulate cerebellar adaptation to the movement task. Moving from one position to another with the head in a variety of positions stimulates the vestibular apparatus and may assist in habituating a hypersensitive vestibular system, allowing the client to change body positions without symptoms of dizziness, resulting in a higher quality of life. Repetitive practice also affects the vasomotor system and may assist in habituating postural hypotensive responses.

A good example of the misuse of functional training is the "nag-and-drag" method of gait training in the parallel bars. This method finds the therapist literally dragging the client through the length of the parallel bars in an attempt to elicit some sort of movement response from the client. The therapist then labels this procedure "gait training." Clearly, this approach will result in the client eventually learning dysfunctional, inefficient motor programs. Before long, as the client learns to run these dysfunctional programs procedurally, the clinician will realize that he or she has created a bigger problem, and a considerable amount of time and resources may be required to undo the damage that was created by limiting the available movement strategies, limiting the variability within practice, and ultimately restricting the plasticity of the nervous system. Similarly, forcing the axial trunk musculature to compensate for lack of motor control within the elbow and wrist will result in dysfunctional upper-extremity movement patterns.

Functional training is the best method of intervention when the client can run normal programs that have some limitation such as poor ROM or inadequate muscle power from disuse. In that way, functional training will run normal programming until fatigue sets in, which may be after only one or two repetitions. Increasing the repetitions and/or the power necessary to run the programs will lead to functional improvement. In using functional training, accurate standardized measurement tools that clearly illustrate change will quickly tell the therapist whether the change is in the direction of more functional control or additional limitation.

An intervention approach in the early 1990s that evolved as an offshoot of functional training was labeled *clinical pathways.* These pathways were established by health care institutions to improve consistency of management of patients who met specific medical diagnostic criteria. It has been proven that the implementation of these pathways reduces variability in clinical practice and improves patient outcomes.[67] Health care practitioners also became aware that some individuals do not fall into these pathways and need to be treated according to the specific clinical problems that the patients were presenting.

Selection of Functional Training Strategies

What is the "ideal" procedure for effectively and efficiently using functional training as a treatment intervention? First, it is suggested that the clinician identify and select procedures that will use the client's strengths to regain lost function and correct system limitations—"What can the client do?" The clinician is also advised to avoid activities that may be too difficult and elicit compensatory strategies that may result in the development of abnormal, stereotypical movement and potentially create additional impairments. An example of this is using transfer training when the patient is unable to keep the program within the limits that define it as a transfer. What instead happens is that the patient would begin to fall. Once in that situation, the patient is then working on approaches to prevent from falling, not activities that allow the patient to safely transfer. The therapist's decision regarding what functional patterns or activities to practice, and in what order, will depend on several factors. The therapist must choose functional activities that are necessary for the client to perform independently or manage with less help before being discharged home. For PTs, safe transfers and ambulation are generally the focus of functional training. For OTs, independent bathing, dressing, and feeding are major foci. Yet both PTs and OTs also need to be sensitive to the activities that the patient or the patient's family want to improve to enhance the quality of life for everyone involved in the person's case. The ability to get in and out of a car might be the most important activity for the client to learn because he or she needs to make frequent trips to the physician's office and the primary caregiver has cardiac problems and is unable to assist the patient in transferring without placing his or her own cardiac system at extreme risk.

It is suggested that the clinician modify or "shrink" the environment to allow normal motor programs to run. An example of this might be to limit the ROM an individual is allowed while performing a rolling pattern. The therapist may opt to start this movement with the patient in a sidelying position. The amount of patient movement may be even further limited by the therapist stabilizing the patient's hips by using the therapist's one leg in kneeling position against the patient's posterior pelvis and the therapist's other leg in half-kneeling position with the top leg of the patient over the therapist's half-kneeling leg. In this way the individual's body can be totally controlled by the therapist; the patient can be encouraged to roll the upper part of his trunk both backward with the arm reaching back and then forward with the arm coming across the body toward a weight-bearing pattern on the hand. The therapist can change the rate of movement and also use his or her knees to control the range that the patient is allowed. The environment can be progressively "enlarged" to allow the client to perform the activity in a functional context. Although this narrowing of the functional environment would be considered a contrived environment and must not be recorded as functional as defined in a functional or activities-based examination, it may allow the nervous system the opportunity to control and modify the motor programs within the limitations of its plasticity at the moment. Therefore this therapeutic technique could be used within a functional training environment or may fall into an augmented treatment approach category, given an individual who has neurological problems that prevent normal movement.

The goal of therapy is to move toward functional training as quickly as the client's motor system can control the movement. As learning and repetition assist the CNS in widening the response pattern during a functional activity, the client's ability to respond to variance within the environment will enlarge and assist in gaining greater independence.

An example of this application of functional training might be asking a client to perform a stand-to-sit transfer. The client is first guided down to sitting onto a large gym ball, a high-low table, or a stool that allows the client to sit only one fourth to one half of the way down before returning to stand. As the client develops increased strength and balance and improved control over abnormal limb synergies and tone in this pattern, then a smaller gym ball or a lower point on a high-low table can be used. Finally, the client is asked to sit down onto a ball/mat or chair that results in the patient sitting with the hips and knees at 90 degrees. Once the client can sit down and return to a vertical position, the next task will be to sit down, relax, and then stand up. Once that activity is done easily, the client will be functionally able to stand to sit and to reverse the movement pattern to sit to stand.

Although many clinicians understand the importance of running motor tasks within an appropriate biomechanical, musculoskeletal, and sensorimotor window in which the client has the ability to perform procedures functionally, it may be argued that in many cases this particular type of treatment strategy is simply not possible in a real-world situation. For example, given the current health care environment, if the client is given a limited number of visits to achieve the desired outcome, the clinician may conclude that there is no choice but to "allow as many degrees of freedom as possible" or, in other words, to "force the window open" no matter the abnormal movement patterns used or the limitations in independent functional control that they may produce.

In summary, the clinician should first identify and emphasize the client's strengths ("What can the client do?") and use those strengths to efficiently and effectively achieve functional change. Next, the clinician must prioritize what systems or activities the client truly needs to change. The choice of what activities to emphasize during therapeutic training always poses a dilemma to therapists. Although it may be ideal for the client to eventually be able to ambulate independently on all surfaces without any assistance or reach for any object in and from any spatial position, it may be more important initially for the client to be able to safely transfer from the bed to the wheelchair, sit independently while someone assists with dressing, or walk and transfer onto and off of the commode independently at home. One should keep in mind that although several skills may be learned by training them simultaneously, it may make more sense to concentrate on the safe performance of one or two necessary functional tasks rather than having the client end up being able to perform multiple tasks that require considerable outside assistance for safety. The need to work functionally on additional activities may also be an opportunity for the clinician to request additional therapy visits for the client, arguing that there is a reasonable expectation that more intervention would result in a greater increase in function and a greater decrease in the risk for potential injury than if the intervention were not continued. The use of valid and reliable functional outcome measures becomes critically important in case management. These tools objectively measure the effect of the intervention, help predict the potential risks if the therapy is not continued, and ultimately aid in the justification to continue therapeutic intervention.

CASE STUDY 9-1 ■ FUNCTIONAL TRAINING: AMBULATION

Teaching a client to ambulate can be approached in many ways. Assume that the objective for a particular session is ambulation. First, the client may be asked to ambulate in the parallel bars using the upper extremities to assist in forward progression of the movement to decrease fear and to assist in maintaining balance. Once the patient can perform this ambulatory activity, the therapist might decide to progress the patient's ambulation by introducing a walker, which has four points of support. Ambulating with the walker will again increase power production in the legs and create an environment of safety for the client. Once walking with the walker can be performed at various speeds and distances, the therapist may advance the activity to using two canes, then one cane depending on the client's balance, coordination, and need. While the patient is practicing ambulating with cane(s), he may also be walking on a treadmill to increase endurance, velocity of gait, and power. Once the patient can ambulate safely with a cane, the therapist may decide to transition to walking without any assistive devices. Again the patient may first be asked to walk on a treadmill while holding on with his arms until he feels safe walking and no longer needs an assistive device. The therapist could transition to ramps, obstacles, uneven ground, and so on. All these activities would require the individual to begin with functional control over the program for ambulation. All the activities are focused on regaining independence in the functional activity of walking, using repetitive practice. These therapeutic devices assist the patient in successfully practicing the entire gait cycle on both legs. In time, the patient is asked to continue walking without the need of the assistive devices and will continue to practice that activity as functional movement or is considered functionally independent with the use of an assistive device. The therapist must also remember that when introducing an assistive device, that device itself will usually limit the environments within which a patient can ambulate independently.

Conclusion

One important variable that has clearly been identified with respect to functional training is "task specificity."[47,68-76] Although it is important that a patient be independent in as many ADLs as possible, often the therapist, the patient, and the family need to prioritize which activities are most important to the quality of life of the patient. If walking into the mountains to do "birdwatching" is one important goal to the patient, then creating an environment that would closely resemble the environment of that activity is crucial. Similarly, practice within that environment is a key to successful carryover (see Chapter 4). If the patient wants to walk into the mountains and the family expects the patient to walk into his or her old job, a therapist must accept that motivation will drive behavior and task specificity will drive learning. Carryover into any other functional activity such as walking into the office building in order to go back to work may not be the motivating factor that will guide that individual's desire to perform that motor task. Whether the patient ever goes back to work is not the variable that should be used as part of the motivational environment for task-specific gait training geared to walking in the mountains and is not a decision for which the therapist is responsible. Therapists need to allow the patient to tell them what will be the most important task and the specificity of that task to optimize motor learning and functional recovery.

Body System and Impairment Training

As mentioned in Chapter 8, the therapeutic examination results in the identification of activity limitations and possible body system and subsystem impairments that are causing the functional movement disorders. Impairment training is another intervention strategy that involves the correction of impairments with the expectation that improving these impairments will result in a corresponding improvement in function. For example, when a client has the inability to stand up without assistance (activity limitation) and the clinician determines the cause to be lower-extremity weakness, an appropriate approach may be to strengthen the lower extremities (impairment training). Numerous studies have shown the effectiveness of impairment training in improving the functional performance of individuals with neurological conditions such as cerebral palsy,[77,78] stroke,[79-87] multiple sclerosis,[88-93] Parkinson disease,[94-98] and other neuromuscular diagnoses.[99-110] The strengthening intervention selected should reflect the task and the environment within which the impairment was identified. The clinician should attempt to create a training situation so that the client may be able to run the necessary motor programs with all the required subsystems in place. For example, training sit to stand with weakness in the hip and knee extensors is much less likely to automatically result in the improvement of sit-to-stand function if the therapist begins the activity in sitting where generation of extension is most difficult, than if the strengthening training was performed with repetition of practice starting in standing and going to sit and back again to stand. By decreasing the degrees of freedom of the eccentric control of the hips and knees when going from stand to sit, the functional training activity has turned into specific impairment training. The therapist can ask the patient to eccentrically lengthen the extensors only in a limited range and then concentrically contract back to standing. As the power increases, the degrees of freedom can also be enlarged until the patient is able to complete the task of stand to sit while simultaneously regaining the sit to stand pattern. In pure impairment training a patient might also be asked to straighten the knee when sitting or to extend the hip when prone. These three exercises have the potential of training impaired strength, but only the first example forces the training within a functional pattern. Similarly, the therapist could train the sit-to-stand pattern using various seat heights that encompass many of the components that force the use of normal movement synergies and postural control, using the environment in which that activity is typically performed, versus performance of strengthening exercises against resistance in an open chain exercise program.

The decision to treat the impairments causing the activity limitations or to correct the functional problems themselves is influenced by myriad factors. It would appear that for certain tasks to be completed the client must possess the "threshold amount" of basic movement components required for the task. Task specificity within this limited environment will result in more meaningful changes in function. Impairment training can be a very effective treatment approach. It can lead to functional gains after an improvement in a specific body system problem. This can lead to improved participation in not only normal functional activities but also activities that should lead to a better quality of life.

Often, clients with neurological trauma or disease cannot begin therapy with functional or impairment training because of the degree and extent of impairments within the entire CNS. Therapists must then choose augmented therapeutic interventions that externally guide the client's learning through hands-on and environmentally controlled techniques such as a body-weight–supported treadmill training (BWSTT). It is cautioned that the therapist should not consider these interventions as functionally independent until the individual's success is based on internal self-regulation of movement. The clinician must continually strive to transfer control to the client by widening the window of independence and limiting the manual or verbal guidance used during therapy.

Augmented Therapeutic Intervention

As discussed in the previous section, some treatment alternatives require little if any hands-on therapeutic manipulation of the client during the activity. For example, the patient practices transfers on and off many support surfaces with standby guarding only. Thus the client self-corrects or uses inherent feedback mechanisms to self-correct error to refine the motor skill. This ultimate empowerment of the client allows each individual to adapt and succeed at self-identified and self-motivated objectives first with augmented intervention and finally without any assistance. Often, allowing the client to try to succeed without assistance enables the therapist to evaluate what components of the task the client can control and what components are not within the client's current capabilities, especially if normal, fluid, efficient, and effortless movement is the desired outcome. In some cases the therapist may use hands-on skills or augmented aids such as BWSTT, which would substitute for many aspects of the environment and allow the client to succeed at the task—*but* the control and feedback during the activity would be considered augmented feedback and fall into that classification.

These augmented techniques make up a large component of the therapist's specific interventions tool box. The difference between augmented and functional training might be the need for the therapist or piece of equipment to be part of the client's external environment for the client to succeed at the task. For example, in BWSTT a harness is used to take away the demand of gravity on the limbs during gait and the demand of the postural trunk and hip muscles for stability. Before the therapist or the patient can consider the movement as independent, those aspects must be removed from the environment. In the previous example, the individual needs to transition from maximal body weight support during ambulation to not needing any external support during ambulation. The client must assume *total ownership* of the functional responses. Then and only then has independence been achieved. At that time, functional retraining can be used with the intent of enlarging the environmental parameters to allow for maximal independence. Figure 9-1 illustrates this concept of functional versus contrived

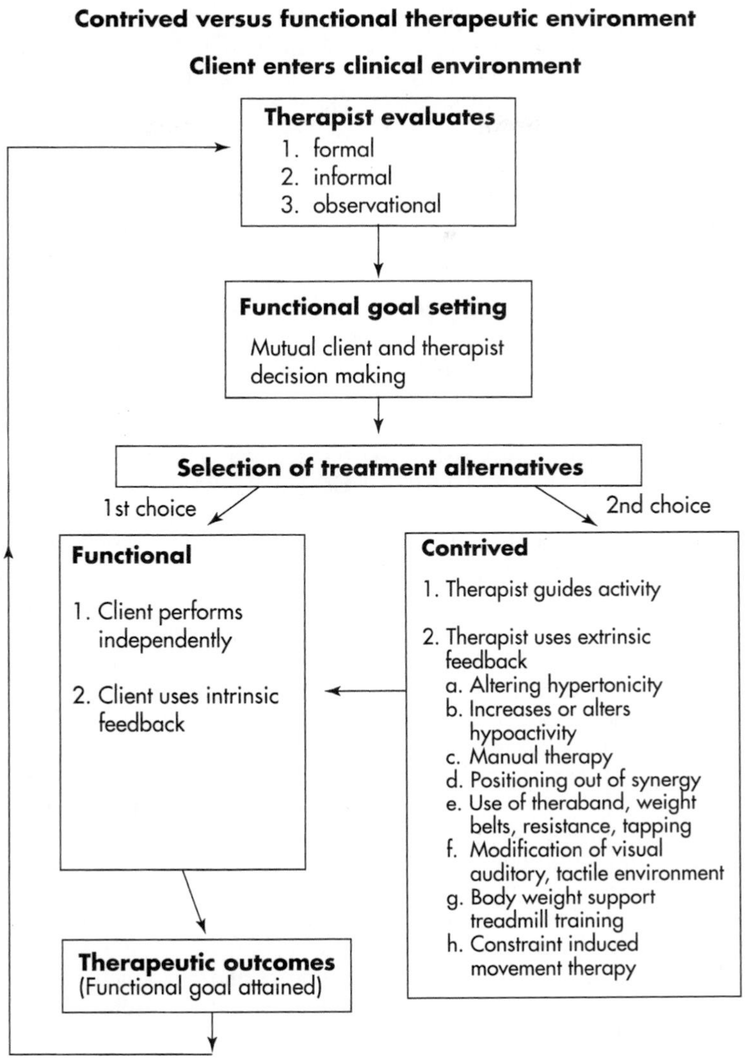

Figure 9-1 ■ Contrived versus functional therapeutics. (Modified from the original work of Jan Davis, OTR, San Jose State University.)

intervention, which must be constantly considered throughout any treatment session. Augmented techniques are often the early choices for treatment of patients who have neurological insults. It cannot be emphasized enough that once the client has the ability to perform without augmented methods and does so in functional, efficient ways, those augmented techniques need to be selectively eliminated.

Once a clinician has chosen to augment the clinical environment, the client needs to learn efficient motor behaviors within the limitations of that environment. The client influences the therapist's decision-making strategies by selecting inefficient or ineffective motor responses to a given task demand. If the response is effortless, efficient, and noninjurious to any part of the body and meets the client's expectations and goals, then the therapist knows the strategies selected were effective even if the therapist augmented the intervention. If the movement itself is available to the client, then there is a high probability that the client will be able to regain that movement control, regardless of the need for early augmentation to achieve the skill. If the response does not meet the desired goal for any reason, then the therapist must determine why. Often, it is because the therapist did not identify the correct body system problems. Many correct solutions may answer the question. Which solution is best may be more client than approach dependent. Yet if flexibility means that the therapist selects any component of any method that helps the client reach an objective, then the therapist is confronted with hundreds—if not thousands—of various treatment choices. If the treatment procedures used introduce information to the client through sensory systems, then from a neurological perspective a limited number of input systems or modalities are available. The myriad treatment procedures are transformed into neurochemical and electrophysiological responses that must travel along a limited number of pathways in the nervous system. Thus, many different treatment procedures may produce similar types of neurotransmission. The temporal and spatial sequencing or timing of the input will vary according to the technique and the specific application. The clinician has little basis for decision making without a comprehensive understanding of the neurophysiological mechanisms of (1) the various techniques introduced to modify input, (2) where that information will be processed and how that might affect motor output, (3) prior learning and the ability for new learning, and (4) the client's willingness and motivation to adapt. The reader is referred to Chapter 1 (Figure 1-1); Chapter 4 on motor control, motor learning, and neuroplasticity; and Chapter 5 for a discussion on motivation.

The number of available contrived or augmented feedback techniques is almost infinite. This section presents an overview of a classification system that can be used to help the reader develop a greater understanding of why certain responses occur and why the selection of certain techniques is appropriate and should positively affect the desired motor responses. This section focuses on intervention strategies that have been accepted, have been used within the traditional Western health care model, and are efficacious. Some alternative approaches to intervention that are not necessarily classified as traditional within this chapter are introduced in Chapter 39. There are other classification systems a clinician might use when analyzing movement problems seen in patients with neurological dysfunction. For example, a therapist may see in a patient a problem primarily with tone, such as hypertonicity, hypotonicity, rigidity, dystonia, flaccidity, intentional and nonintentional tremors, ataxia, and combinations of or fluctuations in the total movement strategies. Given this specific classification schema, one still uses the available treatment strategies or uses an input modality that may modify the specific tone problem that was causing the movement dysfunction.

The primary goal of this section is to help the reader develop a classification system based on the primary input modality used when introducing an augmented treatment technique to facilitate a sensory system and provide feedback to the CNS in order to help a client learn or relearn motor control. The reader has been provided with an in-depth reference to the specific neurophysiological approaches in the past also discussed in Chapter 1, and only a brief overview has been included within this chapter. In-depth discussion of some basic treatment strategies, explanations of less familiar techniques, and current approaches gaining popularity within the clinical area of movement analysis are found within the body of this section.

When the primary input system for a technique is identified, at no time do we suggest that it is the only input system affected. For example, when a proprioceptive technique is introduced, tactile cutaneous receptors are also simultaneously firing. If there is a "noise" component (such as with vibration or tapping with the fingers), then auditory input has been triggered as well. There is evidence that a given sensory modality may "cross over" or fuse with a completely different modality, helping in the synthesis of motor responses. In addition, there is evidence that the principles of neuroplasticity are applicable across modalities (e.g., auditory, visual, vestibular, somatosensory). Sometimes responses occur in a modality that does not appear to be related. For example, olfaction may improve tactile sensitivity of the hand. This concept is called *cross-modal training* or *stimulation.*[111,112] Yet a classification schema based on a primary modality promotes logical problem solving because the therapist can select from available treatment procedures that theoretically provide similar information to the CNS and help in the organization of appropriate motor responses. The motor system and its various motor programmers adapt to the environment to achieve functional motor output toward a goal. Both external and internal feedback are critical for adaptation and change. External feedback in this chapter is considered a mechanism to help the client's CNS optimally learn and adapt. Obviously, as the patient learns, internal feedback will allow the person to run feed-forward motor programs without the need for external feedback for control. External feedback will, it is hoped, be used only when the outside surrounding needs the feed-forward program to change to adapt to a new environment (refer to the Chapter 4 section on motor learning). Therapists must realize that even if the primary goal may be to facilitate or dampen a motor system response, diverging pathways may also connect with endocrine, immune, and autonomic systems. According to motor control theory, the clinical picture is a consensus of all interacting body systems (see Chapter 4). Research tools are not yet available to measure those systems interacting simultaneously, although functional magnetic resonance imaging (fMRI) studies are beginning to help researchers and clinicians identify what happens to the nervous system with input from the environment and how that information is processed. Efficacy using reliable and valid measurement tools must then be based on outcomes, with an understanding of the best available scientific knowledge as a rationale for why the outcome is present.

This classification system is based on identified input, observed responses, current research on the function of the CNS, and the various systems involved in the control and modification of responses. An understanding of normal processing of input and its effect on the motor systems helps the clinician evaluate and use the intact systems as part of treatment. Research with fMRI is now allowing greater insight into specific brain regions that are being used during various cognitive and motor activities.[113-128] Yet the specific interactive nature of multisensory input, memory, motivation, and motor function is still unknown. When the response to certain stimuli does not help the client select or adapt a desired motor response, then the classification schema for augmented input provides the clinician with flexibility to select additional options. This can be done by spatially summating input, such as using stretch, vibration, and resistance simultaneously, or temporally summating input, such as increasing the rate of the quick stretch or increasing the time between inputs to give the system ample time to respond.

Many factors can influence motor behavior, such as the methods of instruction, the resting condition of the nervous system, synaptic connections, cerebellar or basal ganglia or cortical processing, retrieval from past learning, motor output systems, or internal influences and neuroendocrine balance. Figure 9-2 illustrates and simplifies this total system. Its clinical implications become clearer if the therapist retains a visual image of the client's total nervous system, including afferent input, intersystem processing, efferent response, and the multiple interactions on one another. At any moment in time, multiple stimuli are admitted into a client's input system. Before that information reaches a level of primary processing, it will cross at least one if not many synaptic junctions. At that time the information may be inhibited, excited, changed or distorted, or allowed to continue without modification. If the information is at the first synapse, the patient will have no sensation. If it is inhibited at the thalamus, again the patient will not perceive sensation,

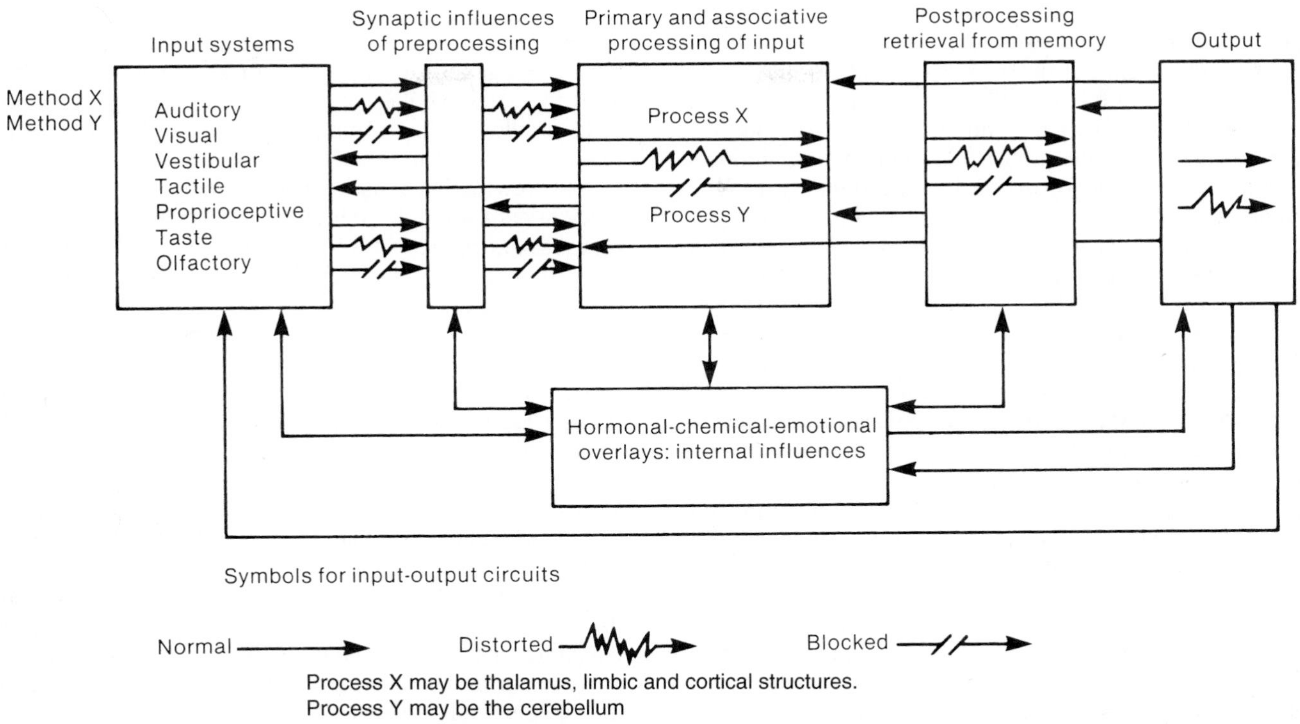

Figure 9-2 ■ Model of possible interactive effects among methods of treatment, input systems, processing and output systems, internal influences, and feedback systems.

but that does not mean other areas of the brain will not be sent that information, because sensory information is also sent to a variety of areas after that initial synapse. Research studies have found that sensory input information may even affect gait and other movement patterns even if the patient has no perception of the input.[129,130] If the input is changed, then the processing of the input will vary from the one normally anticipated. The end product after multiple system interactions will be close to, will be farther away from, or will seem to have no effect on the desired motor pattern. Furthermore, sensory processing can take place at many segments of the nervous system. Although the CNS is not hierarchical, with one level in total control over another, certain systems are biased to affect various motor responses. At the spinal level the response may be phasic and synergistic. Brain stem mechanisms may evoke flexor or extensor biases, depending on various motor systems and their modulation. Cerebellar, basal ganglia, thalamic, and cortical responses may be more adaptive and purposeful.[130-133] Thus the therapist must try to discern where the input or the feedback is being affective or short circuited.

Remembering input as a possible option for intervention will always allow the therapist to differentiate the same five alternatives—no response, facilitating (heightening), inhibiting (dampening), distorting, or normal processing. These alternatives can occur anywhere in the system at synaptic junctions. Finally, motor output is programmed and a response is observed. If the response is considered normal, the clinician assumes that the system is intact with regard to the use and processing of the inputs. If the response is distorted or absent, little is known other than there is a lack of the normal processing somewhere in the CNS or an insufficient amount of input was used. One way to differentiate motor problems from problems with other systems is to use other functional activities that have programs similar to the body system program identified as impaired. If a program, such as posture, demonstrates deficiencies in one functional pattern, then the therapist must determine if it is also deficient in other patterns. If the postural motor problem affects all motor performance, then the therapist had determined that a motor program deficit exists and will have to determine how to correct that problem. If, on the other hand, the program runs smoothly and effortlessly when certain demands are taken away, such as resistance from gravity, position in space, need for quick responses, and so forth, then it may be that the problem is within another subsystem such as cognition, perception, the biomechanical system, or the cardiopulmonary system or is a power-production problem that can be corrected by slowly increasing the demand on the postural system through repetitive practice using various additional input interventions. Differentially screening motor impairments as pure CNS motor problems (muscle recruitment, firing rate, balance) versus problems with another system (perception of vertical) becomes critical in a managed-care system that funds only a certain number of treatment sessions. Internal influences also need to be considered because they affect each aspect of the system. Once normal processing has been identified, understanding of deficit systems and potential problems can be analyzed more easily. To reiterate, this requires awareness of the totality of the individual—that is, the client's personal preference of stimuli and the uniqueness of processing and internal influences.

A systems model requires simultaneous processing of multiple areas, with interactions being relayed in all directions. A client's CNS and peripheral nervous system (PNS) are doing just that, and the therapist must develop a sensitivity toward the client as a whole while interacting with specific components (see Chapters 1, 4, 5, 6, and 39 for additional information). With input from the client and family, it is the therapist's responsibility to select methods most efficacious and effective for each client's needs in relation to that person's specific neurological problems. (See all clinical chapters in Section II.) This viewpoint, based on a variety of questions, leads to a problem-oriented approach to intervention. Because the output or response pattern is based on alpha motor neuron discharge and thus extrafusal muscle contraction, the *first question* is posed: what can be done to alter the state of the alpha motor neuronal pool or motor generators? *Second*, what input systems are available, either directly or indirectly, that will alter the state of the motor pool? *Third*, which techniques use these various input systems as their primary modes of entry into the CNS? *Fourth*, what internal mechanisms need modification or adaptation to produce a desired behavior response from the client? *Fifth*, which input systems are available to alter the internal mechanism and what outcomes are expected? *Sixth*, what combination of input stimuli will provide the best internal homeostatic environment for the client to learn and rehearse a more optimal response pattern? For example, assume that a client with a residual hemiplegia resulting from an anterior cerebral artery problem has a hypertonic lower extremity that produces the pattern of extension, adduction, internal rotation of the hip, extension of the knee, and plantarflexion inversion of the foot. The answers to the first two questions are based on the knowledge that the proprioceptive and exteroceptive systems can drastically affect spinal central pattern generators and that these input systems are intact at spinal, brain stem, cerebellum, and thalamic levels and may even project to the cortex.

Appropriate selection of specific techniques—such as prolonged stretch using the tendon organ to modulate the hypertonic pattern, quick stretch or light touch to the antagonistic muscle, or any other treatment modality within the classification schema—will provide viable treatment alternatives. Awareness that a client's response pattern is an inherent synergistic pattern and that it is further elicited by pressure to the ball of the foot leads to a better understanding of the clinical problem. Knowing that the client is unable to combine the alternative patterns, such as hip flexion with knee extension needed for the late stage of swing phase through the early aspects of stance phase during gait, the therapist can use the other inherent processes to elicit these and other patterns. BWSTT is an example of an augmented treatment intervention in which the clinician assists the patient to place the leg and foot with each step while the apparatus controls balance and posture to provide an experience of normal gait while requiring the patient to have only the strength to manage partial body weight.[134-139] Finally, techniques such as combining standing and walking with the application of quick stretch, vibration, or rotation, or having the client reach for a target or follow a visual stimulus while walking, provide a variety of combinations of therapeutic procedures to help the client learn or relearn normal response patterns. Furthermore, combining techniques gives the clinician a choice of various procedures and promotes a learning environment that is flexible, changing, and interesting. The therapist must, again, make the transition from applying contrived therapeutic procedures during functional tasks to allowing the client to practice the task without the therapist interceding and without external feedback.[140] In that way the client uses inherent feedback to self-correct feed-forward motor programming and then to continue running the appropriate movement strategies. This self-correction leads to independence, adaptability, and long-term learning (see Figure 9-2).

To avoid confusion about which peripheral sensory nerve fiber coming from the surface of the body or extremities is being discussed, the two primary methods of classifications (Gasser-Erlanger and Lloyd), along with a description of the functional component, have been included in Table 9-1 for easy referral. The other sensory systems will be presented separately to help the reader establish an appropriate classification scheme. The primary sensory input systems presented include proprioception, exteroception, vestibular, vision, auditory, taste, and smell. These sensory inputs have the potential to influence CNS structures including the thalamus, sensory and motor cortices, the cerebellum, the reticular formation, and the basal ganglia and thus to affect the descending fibers under their control.

Proprioceptive System Integration of Stretch, Joint, and Tendon Receptors

Proprioception as an input system has a direct effect on program generators at the spinal level.[141] Because of its importance in motor learning and motor adaptation to new or changing environments, however, proprioception also has significant connections to the cortical and cerebellar neural networks. Its divergent pathways have synapses within the brain stem, diencephalon, and spinal system. Proprioceptive input can potentially influence multiple levels of CNS function, and all those levels can potentially modulate the intensity or importance of that information through many different mechanisms.[141,142] Proprioceptors are found in three peripheral anatomical locations: the stretch receptors, the tendon, and the joint. The afferent receptors responsible for relaying sensory information through those sites are discussed in the following subsections.

Muscle Stretch Receptors

Stretch. Stretch, quick stretch, and maintained stretch are all sensory input systems that use the stretch receptors in the muscles and heighten the motor pool.[143-145] Stretch simultaneously heightens both the muscle response to that stretch and potentially heightens the sensitivity of the agonistic synergy. It will also lower the excitation of the antagonistic muscle and those muscles that are part of the antagonistic synergy. Stretch information will be sent to higher centers for sensory integration and perception. The cerebellum uses this incoming feedback to maintain and/or regulate motor nuclei in the brain stem that will influence the state of the alpha and gamma motor neurons. This allows for cerebellar feed-forward regulation (refer to Chapter 21). There are many ways to apply stretch to the muscles. The therapist can use (1) the hands and their respective muscle power to apply a stretch, (2) a manual weight system of some sort that maintains the stretch through the range, (3) a suspension system such as used in Pilates exercises (see

TABLE 9-1 ■ CLASSIFICATIONS OF PERIPHERAL NERVES ACCORDING TO SIZE

GASSER-ERLANGER	LLOYD	MOTOR (FUNCTIONAL COMPONENT)	SENSORY (FUNCTIONAL COMPONENT)
A fibers: large myelinated fibers with a high conduction rate			
A alpha	Ia	Large, fast fibers of alpha motor system (large cells of anterior horn to extrafusal motor fibers)	Muscle spindle; primary afferent endings (primary stretch or low threshold stretch; Ia tonic fibers respond to length, Ia phasic fibers respond to rate)
	Ib		Tendon organ for contraction; respond to tendon stretch or tension
A beta	II		Muscle spindle; secondary afferent endings; tonic receptors responding to length Exteroceptive afferent endings from skin and joints; respond to light or low threshold stretch
A gamma 1 and 2	II	Gamma motor system (small cells of anterior horn to intrafusal motor fibers)	Bare nerve endings; joint receptors, mechanoreception of soft tissues; exteroceptors for pain, touch, and cold (low threshold)
A delta	III		
B fibers: medium-sized myelinated fibers with a fairly rapid conduction rate			
B beta		Preganglionic fibers of autonomic system (effective on glands and smooth muscle; motor branch of alpha): unknown function	
C fibers: small, poorly myelinated or unmyelinated fibers having slowest conduction rate; augmentation and recruiting occur within the nervous system after stimulation of these fibers has ceased			
	IV	Postganglionic fibers of sympathetic system	Exteroceptors; pain, temperature, touch

Chapter 39), (4) the patient's own body weight against gravity, (5) a complex robotic system that computerizes the amount of stretch depending on the individual's specific data (see Chapter 38), or many other creative ways to apply stretch to muscle fibers within the belly of the muscle tissue. As stated previously, stretch can also be applied to the antagonist muscle or muscle synergy in order to dampen agonist function. Thus stretch can be used to enhance tone in the agonist or to decrease tone of the agonist through the antagonist. The therapist should always remember that even though a response may not look obvious, as long as the peripheral nerves and motor neurons within the spinal system are intact, these approaches will change the state of the motor pool.

Table 9-2 lists a variety of treatment procedures believed to use proprioceptive input from the muscles as a primary mode of sensory stimulation. The varying intensity, amount of tension, or rate of the stimuli, in addition to the original length of the muscle before application of the stimulus, will determine its firing. Remember, afferent information is projecting to many areas above the spinal system, and the result will be regulation or modulation, ultimately affecting activity.[141]

Resistance and Strengthening. Resistance is often used to facilitate intrafusal and extrafusal muscle contraction. Resistance can be applied manually, mechanically, and by the use of gravity. Resistance recruits more motor units in the target muscles. Although muscles can contract both in an isometric and an isotonic fashion, most contractions consist of a mixture of the two. Certain muscle groups, such as the flexors, benefit from isometric exercise, as well as isotonic exercise in both eccentric and concentric modes. Under normal circumstances, the flexors are used for repetitive or rhythmical activities. The extensors, on the other hand, usually remain contracted in an effort to act against the forces of gravity. Therefore the extensor groups benefit best from isometric and eccentric resistance.[146]

When resistance is applied to a voluntary muscle, spindle afferent fibers and tendon organs fire in proportion to the magnitude of the resistance. Resistance is more facilitative to an isometrically contracted muscle than in an isotonic contraction.[35] As isometric resistance is increased or continued, more motor units are recruited, thereby increasing the strength of extrafusal contraction.[26] Eccentric isotonic contraction refers to the lengthening of muscle fibers with resistance added to the distal segment, as in lowering the arms while holding a heavy weight. Eccentric contraction uses less metabolic output and promotes strength gains in less time.[26] However, all types of muscle contraction will promote increased strength. Resistance is an important clinical treatment and has been used and will continue to be used by clinicians within multiple treatment philosophies over the next millennium.[8,19,25,29,77,147-153] The complexity of neural adaptation after resistive exercises may lead to a different training environment depending on age, athletic status, and specific body system deficits.[154] Combining resistive training with guided imagery or other types of adjunct interactions has conflicting results.[154-156] Yet there are still questions regarding optimal resistive training and

TABLE 9-2 ■ PROPRIOCEPTIVE STRETCH RECEPTORS

RECEPTOR	STIMULUS	NATURE OF RESPONSE
Ia tonic	Length	Monosynaptic and polysynaptic facilitation of agonist
Ia phasic	Rate of change in length	Polysynaptic inhibition of antagonist and antagonistic synergy
		Polysynaptic facilitation of agonistic synergy
		Input to cerebellum
		Input to opposite parietal lobe
		Specific parietal lobe responses open for question
II	Length	Monosynaptic facilitation of agonist
		Polysynaptic facilitation of specific muscle groups, depending on muscle function of tissue where II fibers originate
		Transmittal of information to higher centers

POSSIBLE TREATMENT ALTERNATIVES

1. Resistance
2. Quick stretch to agonist
3. Tapping: tendon and/or muscle belly
4. Reverse tapping: gravity stretches; tapping agonist into shortened range
5. Positioning (range)
6. Electrical stimulation
7. Pressure or sustained stretch
8. Stretch pressure
9. Stretch release
10. Vibration: facilitatory frequency for small vibrator, relaxation for total body vibration
11. Gravity as a prolonged stretch
12. Active motion

whether one resistive technique is better than another.[157,158] Research certainly has shown that resistance training does enhance functional abilities across age groups,[150,159,160] but again the specifics regarding resistive training techniques are often not identified. The terms *resistive training, weight training,* and *strength training* are often used synonymously, and thus specifics are yet to be identified in the research. How all these uses of resistive exercises will play out in the future is up to future researchers in the field of movement science. Very costly high-technology tools have been added to aid in resistive training (see the discussion of Pilates in Chapter 39 and robotics in Chapter 38).[161,162] Given the needs of individuals after neurological insults, cost becomes a major factor, and finding creative and cost-efficient ways to apply resistance may become a common research question in the future.

Tapping. Three types of tapping techniques are commonly used by therapists. Tapping of the tendon is a fairly nondiscriminatory stimulus. Physicians use this technique to determine the degree of stretch sensitivity of a muscle. A normal response would be a brisk muscle contraction. Because of the magnitude of the stimulus and the direct effect on the alpha motor neuron, this technique is not highly effective in teaching a client to control or grade muscle contraction.[163] Instead, tapping of the muscle belly, a lower-intensity stimulus, is more satisfactory. Reverse tapping is a less frequently described technique, but it can be used. The extremity is positioned so gravity promotes the stretch, instead of the therapist manually tapping or actively inducing muscle stretch. Once the muscle responds, the therapist taps or passively moves the extremity to help the muscle obtain a shortened range. An example of reverse tapping would be tapping the triceps muscle when the client is bearing weight on the extended elbow and actively trying to achieve full elbow extension. Gravity quickly stretches the triceps. Timing of this technique is important. If the therapist taps the elbow toward extension when the flexors' motor neurons are sensitive, then those flexor muscles may respond to the stretch and contract, taking the arm farther into flexion. If the timing follows the quick stretch to the extensor, then the flexors will be dampened and active extension more likely a motor response.

Positioning (Range). The concept of submaximal and maximal range of muscles is highly significant to clinical application. Bessou and colleagues[164] monitored the neuronal firing of muscle spindles at different ranges of motion. Upper motor neuron lesions can alter the sensitivity of the spindle afferent reflex arc fibers by not using presynaptic inhibition to normally dampen incoming afferent activity.[165] Therefore ROM should be carefully assessed on an individual basis, particularly in a patient with an upper motor neuron lesion, to determine the maximal or submaximal range for an individual. Therapists always need to determine whether the difference between optimal range and functional ROM is different. If a patient will never need to use full ROM, then spending long periods of time trying to stretch a shoulder or hip may not be the best decision with regard to intervention. As well as the ROM itself, therapists need to carefully evaluate excessive range resulting from hypermobility and hypotonicity. In those situations, external support of the affected joint or limb needs to be considered in all functional positions in order to prevent complications such as pain.[166-168]

Electrical Stimulation. For an in-depth discussion of the use of electrical stimulation both as an evaluation and a treatment modality, see Chapter 16 and Chapter 33. Electrical stimulation has the potential to be an excellent muscle spindle facilitatory technique, especially if additional therapeutic tools, such as resistance, are included. Electrical stimulation delivered to create muscle contraction is beneficial, but electrical stimulation as a sensory stimulus is less effective as a learning tool because there are no sensory receptors for electrical currents and thus they are not represented as a unique stimulus on the somatosensory cortex. Functional electrical stimulation (FES) is a technique that applies electrical stimulation during functional movement. Chapter 16 discusses this technique with traumatic spinal cord injury, but the application has gone beyond those individuals diagnosed with spinal injury. Individuals poststroke have also been studied using FES. The results were inconsistent. Some studies showed there was no difference in the stroke groups during or directly after intervention but that the long-term effect remained with those individuals who received FES, whereas those who did not regressed in function.[169,170] Studies have shown that FES training increased walking ability and speed during and after the training.[171,172] Studies that have looked at other neurological problems have also used FES and certainly are showing that this type of intervention may become a standard of practice in the future.[173-175] Combined modulation of voluntary movement, proprioceptive sensory feedback, and electrical stimulation might play an important role in improving impaired sensorimotor integration by power-assisted FES therapy.[176] The use of FES over acupressure points has been shown to significantly reduce pain.[177]

Stretch Pressure. The muscle belly is the stimulus focus of stretch pressure. The therapist slowly applies pressure to the muscle belly. It is used to decrease or release tone in the target muscle, allowing for the (temporary) recovery of voluntary movement.[111,178] Generally this type of stimulus is applied and maintained for a period of time (e.g., 5 to 10 seconds). It is not a quick stimulus and may be using the tendon organ to dampen tone. This type of pressure technique is also used in a variety of complementary approaches (see Chapter 39).

Stretch Release. This technique is performed by placing the fingertips over the belly of larger muscles and spreading the fingers in an effort to stretch the skin and the underlying muscle. The stretch is done firmly enough to temporarily deform the soft tissue so the cutaneous receptors and Ia afferent fibers may produce facilitation of the target muscle. It is easy to determine quickly whether the response is efficacious by just feeling and looking at the response of the patient.

Manual Pressure. Manual pressure can be facilitatory when it is applied as a brisk stretch or friction-like massage over muscle bellies. The speed and duration at which the manual pressure is applied determine the extent of recruitment from receptors. Paired with volitional efforts, manual pressure can lead to motor function, and with repetition, motor learning.

Vibration. There are two types of vibratory methods used therapeutically. The first deals with the use of a handheld vibrator to facilitate Ia receptors to enhance agonistic muscle contraction in hypotonic muscles or to facilitate Ia receptors of antagonistic muscle fibers to inhibit hypertonic agonists. Currently the use of vibration to facilitate Ia responses within specific muscle function has been used to show how proprioception can be used to alter upright standing.[179,180] The second type of vibratory method is a total-body vibration to facilitate postural tone and balance and is applied through the feet in a standing position.[181-184]

Bishop[185,186] wrote an excellent series of articles on the neurophysiology and therapeutic application of vibration in the 1970s. High-frequency vibration (100 to 300 Hz or cycles per second) applied to the muscle or tendon elicits a reflex response referred to as the *tonic vibratory response.* Tension within the muscle will increase slowly and progressively for 30 to 60 seconds and then plateau for the duration of the stimulus.[187] Some researchers found that at cessation of the input the contractibility of the muscle was enhanced for approximately 3 minutes.[187,188] The discrepancy in the research may reflect the way the individual is using the input, both from a direct effect on the motor generator and from supraspinal modulation over the importance of the input, which may affect the overall learning and plasticity of the CNS. To facilitate hypotonic muscle, the muscle belly is first put on stretch, and then vibratory stimuli are applied.[189] To inhibit a hypertonic muscle, the antagonistic muscle could be vibrated.[185,189] The use of vibration can be enhanced by combining it with additional modalities such as resistance, position, and visually directed movement. Vibration also stimulates cutaneous receptors, specifically the Pacinian corpuscles, and thus can also be classified as an exteroceptive modality.[190] Because of its ability to decrease hypersensitive tactile receptors through supraspinal regulation, local vibration is considered an inhibitory technique (it is also discussed later in the section on exteroceptor-maintained stimulus). Therapists have reported that vibration over acupressure points can modulate localized pain syndromes. It seems to trigger A delta exteroceptive fibers, which in turn dampen the effect of C fibers. (See Chapter 32 for more information on the treatment of pain.)

Farber[111] summarized the use of vibration and clearly identified precautions that must be taken. Frequencies greater than 200 Hz can be damaging to the skin. We have found frequencies greater than 150 Hz to cause discomfort and even pain. Therefore it is recommended that vibrators registering 100 to 125 Hz be used. Most battery-operated hand vibrators function at 50 to 90 Hz.[11] Frequencies less than 75 Hz are thought to have an inhibitory effect on normal muscle,[187] although a study showed that some muscle groups, especially the lateral gastrocnemius, do respond positively to frequencies of 40 to 60 Hz.[191] Another researcher[192] studying vibration found similar results that frequencies of 50 Hz generated more neuromuscular facilitation than lower frequencies (30 Hz) when studying improvements in upper body resistance exercise performance. Cutaneous pressure is also known to cause inhibition, so if it is combined with a vibration technique that is being used to augment a muscle contraction, it can only serve to cancel the desired effects.

Amplitude or amount of displacement must also be considered when vibration is analyzed as a modality. It has been reported that high amplitude causes adverse effects, especially in clients with cerebellar dysfunction.[186] Vibration is not recommended for infants because the nervous system is not yet fully myelinated and the vibration might cause too much stimulation. The reader is also cautioned about using vibration over areas that have been immobilized because of the underlying vascular tissue potential for clotting. Vibration on or near these blood vessels could dislodge a clot, causing an embolism. Vibration also needs to be used cautiously over skin that has lost its elasticity and is thin (e.g., that in older persons) because the friction itself from the vibration can cause tearing. The therapist must always keep in mind the environment and the functionality of an intervention procedure. The use of vibration may assist the client in contractions and somatosensory awareness, but it is an unnatural way to facilitate either system and thus needs to be removed as part of an intervention as soon as the patient demonstrates some sensory awareness and/or volitional control over a movement component.

Within the last decade the use of vibration of specific muscle groups of the neck has been studied in order to determine its effect on upright standing and the interaction with and without eyes open.[179,180] These studies showed that by vibrating specific muscle groups, those muscles would actively contract and change the position of the head in space but that with eyes open the effect was minimized in relation to global postural control. A similar study examined the effect of vibration on various muscles within the lower extremities and how that affected various postural responses.[191,193] These researchers found that different frequencies affected different muscle groups. The one consistent thing all studies have shown is that vibration does facilitate Ia muscle fibers, which in turn affect muscle contraction of the agonist receiving the vibration. Other sensory systems can assist or override the effect of vibration, but that is because of superspinal influence over motor generators.

Total-body vibration is currently being used to determine if it affects motor performance. Studies have shown that whole-body vibration can enhance motor performance in high-level athletes performing sprints and jumps,[181,182] as well as improve trunk stability, muscle tone, and postural control in individuals after stroke while in geriatric rehabilitation.[184] Its application for individuals with neurological dysfunction is inconclusive.[194,195] Studies specifically directed toward the elderly again show promise, but further research is needed for specificity.[196,197] Future research will need to determine the effect of total-body vibration when introduced to all populations of individuals with neurological dysfunction. At that time both amplitude and magnitude will need to be identified in order to replicate studies. Total-body vibration certainly falls under primarily proprioception but also could be classified under combined proprioceptive techniques or multisensory classification techniques because the input affects the muscle spindles, the joints, the vestibular system, and possibly the auditory system with the low frequency noise. And every time vibration is applied, the skin receptors will initially fire although most will adapt quickly to prolonged use of any stimuli.

The Tendon. The tendon receptors are specialized receptors located in both the proximal and the distal musculotendinous insertions. In conjunction with the stretch receptors, the tendon plays an important role in the mediation of proprioception.[141,142,198-203]

The principal role of the tendon is to monitor muscle tension exerted by the contraction of the muscles or by tension applied to the muscle itself. Research has demonstrated that the tendon is highly sensitive to tension and acts conjointly with the stretch receptors to inform higher centers of continuing environmental demands to modulate or change existing plans; these higher centers in turn regulate tonicity and the state of the motor pool.[43,141] The tendon (Ib) signals not only tension but also the rate of change of tension and provides the sensation of force as the muscle is working.[198] A fundamental difference between the tendon organ and the stretch receptors is that the stretch receptors detect length, whereas the tendon monitors tension and force. Sensory input from the stretch receptors and the tendon are mostly opposites.[43,202] The stretch receptors regulate reciprocal inhibition, whereas the tendon modulates autogenic inhibition. Table 9-3 lists a variety of known treatment approaches that use the tendon to inform higher centers regarding needed change and regulation over spinal generators.

Maintained Stretch to the Tendon Organ. Maintained stretch to a muscle has the potential for triggering the tendon organ if tension is great enough. Once the maintained stretch fires the tendon organ, autogenic inhibition of the same muscle occurs. A therapist will feel a release of the agonist muscle, allowing for elongation of the contractile components. Simultaneously, the tendon organ's sensory neurons will facilitate motor neurons to the antagonist muscle, thus heightening its sensitivity and potential for activity. This is the technique used when a joint has developed range restriction. The clinician always needs to differentiate whether the tightness found within the joint is caused by compensatory muscles considered *movers* protecting injured postural muscles beneath or by tightness just from positioning, disuse, or fear.

Inhibitory Pressure. Pressure has been used therapeutically to alter motor responses. Mechanical pressure (force), such as from cones, pads, or the orthokinetic cuff developed by Blashy and Fuchs,[204] provided continuously is inhibitory. That pressure seems most effective on tendinous insertions. It is hypothesized that this deep, maintained pressure activates Pacinian corpuscles, which are rapidly adapting receptors. A variety of researchers have studied these receptors and their relationship to regulating vasomotor reflexes,[205] modulating pain,[206-210] and dampening other sensory system influence on the CNS.[188,209]

This inhibitory pressure technique also works when pressure is applied across the longitudinal axis of a tendon. The pressure is applied across the tendon with increasing pressure until the muscle relaxes. Constant pressure applied over the tendons of the wrist flexors may dampen flexor hypertonicity and elongate the tight fascia over the tendinous insertion (see Chapter 39 for additional information).

Pressure over bony prominences has modulatory effects. A common example is pressure on the medial aspect of the calcaneus, which dampens plantarflexors and allows contraction of the lateral dorsiflexor muscles. Pressure over the lateral aspect of the calcaneus also dampens calf muscles to allow for contraction of the medial dorsiflexor muscles.[25] Localized finger pressure applied bilaterally to acupuncture points has been shown to relieve pain and reduce muscle tone.[210-214] This technique has also been found to be particularly effective when used in a low-stimulus environment and when combined with deep breathing.

This combination of pressure (manually applied), environmental demands (low), and parasympathetic activity (slow, relaxed breathing) illustrates various systems interacting

TABLE 9-3 ■ PROPRIOCEPTIVE RECEPTORS OF TENDONS AND JOINTS

RECEPTOR	STIMULUS	RESPONSE
TENDON		
Tendon organ Ib	Tension on extrafusal muscle	Polysynaptic inhibition of agonist, facilitation of antagonist spinal level circuitry; supraspinal regulation
Possible Treatment Suggestions 1. Extreme stretch 2. Deep pressure to tendon 3. Passive positioning in extreme lengthened range 4. Extreme resistance: more effective in lengthened and shortened range 5. Deep pressure to muscle belly to put stretch on tendon 6. Small repeated contractions with gravity eliminated		
TYPE OF JOINT		
I (6-9 μ)	Static and dynamic joint tension: muscle pull	Thought to facilitate postural holding and joint awareness
II (9-12 μ)	Dynamic: sudden change in joint tension	Thought to facilitate agonist and awareness of joint range of motion
III (13-17 μ)	Dynamic: linked to Golgi tendon organ traction; activates in extreme range	Thought to inhibit agonist
IV (5 μ >2 μ)	Pain	Thought to inhibit agonist
Possible Treatment Suggestions 1. Manual traction (distraction) to joint surfaces to facilitate joint motion 2. Manual approximation (compression) to joint surfaces to facilitate co-contraction or postural holding 3. Positioning: gravity used to approximate or apply traction 4. Weight belts, shoulder harnesses, and helmets to increase approximation 5. Wrist and ankle cuffs to increase traction 6. Wall pulleys, weights, manual resistance 7. Manual therapy[20] 8. Elastic tubing to provide compression during movement		

together to create the best motor response. The real world requires the client to respond to many environmental conditions while relaxed or under stress. Thus, once a client begins to demonstrate normal adaptable motor responses, the therapist needs to change the conditions and the stress level to allow the client to practice variability. That practice should incorporate motor error, especially error or distortions in the plan, yet still achieve the desired goal. As the client self-corrects, greater demand and variability should be introduced.[215]

Joint Receptor Approximation. Approximation of the joint mimics weight bearing and facilitates the postural extensor system. Gravity creates approximation and its greatest force is produced down through the body in vertical postures. Approximation should help to stabilize any joint that is in a load-bearing situation by eliciting coactivation of the muscles around the joint in question. In standing, gravity creates approximation down through the entire spine, hips, knees, and ankles. When in a prone position on elbows, the load goes down again through the upper spine while simultaneous going down through the shoulder girdles of both arms. If a therapist increases that load by adding pressure down through the joints in question, then an augmented intervention has been added to the therapeutic environment. Using weight belts around the waist or a weighted vest on the trunk can facilitate the postural coactivation needed during standing or walking.[216-218] At times, approximation can be used to heighten normal postural tone while simultaneously dampening excessive tone in the other leg. For example, clients who have CNS insult often have an imbalance in function within the two lower extremities. This can be very frustrating for the therapist because bringing the patient to standing to assist in regaining normal postural extension of one leg triggers the other into a strong extensor pattern, causing plantarflexion and inversion of that foot. One way to use approximation in treating both legs simultaneously might be to first bring the patient from sitting onto a high-low mat. Then the therapist can raise the mat high enough that the patient can be lowered into standing on the normal-functioning leg. At the same time the patient's other leg can be bent at the knee, and that knee placed on a stool or chair. This allows approximation down through the entire leg that is in standing position while approximating the trunk, hip, and knee of the other leg in the kneeling position. The therapist can work on standing and weight shifting in one leg while dampening abnormal tone in the kneeling leg. As the kneeling leg starts to regain postural coactivation in its hip, postural function will often be felt in the knee and ankle.

One very effective way to apply approximation and resistance simultaneously is to use the product similar to a cut large elastic rubber band: Thera-Bands. The rubber material is attached under the heel on the right and left side; both ends of the band are brought up across the ankle and then crossed over the lower leg, once more over the back of the thigh, and then anchored onto a belt around the patient's waist. A similar pattern can be used for the arm; the band is first placed across the palm and then crossed in the forearm and then the arm. Finally one end is brought across the upper chest and the other comes around from the back of the arm. Then the two ends of the band are tied together across the neck.These techniques can be graded by the elasticity of the material.[219-221]

Traction and Distraction. One or more joints are distracted by a force that causes it or them to separate or pull apart, similar to the swing phase of the leg during ambulation or the arms in a reciprocal pattern to each leg. This distraction of the joint receptors also puts stretch on the muscles, which combines to facilitate the pattern into which the limb is moving. Simultaneously, distraction dampens the antagonistic movement pattern, which allows the agonist movement to continue. A therapist will often use manual traction to get relaxation of hyperactive extensor muscles or for limited mobility.[222] Often therapists do not think of the traction when applying resistance to a limb. For example, a mistake made is placing ankle weights to facilitate limbs that are ataxic. Ataxia is an imbalance in coactivation and smooth movement of both agonist and antagonist muscle groups.[223] The weight itself slows down the excessive movement by the resistance. However, weight on the ankle creates traction that will facilitate only the flexor group and often creates an additional imbalance in the ataxic leg.[224] When the weights are removed, the patient often is more ataxic.

Combined Proprioceptive Input Techniques. Many techniques succeed because of the combined effects of multiple inputs. Some of these combined techniques include jamming; ballistic movements; total-body positioning; PNF patterns; postexcitatory inhibition (PEI) with stretch, range, rotation, and shaking; heavy work patterns; Feldenkrais (see Chapter 39)[225-227]; and manual therapy.[20,208,228]

Jamming. Jamming is usually applied to the ankle and knee with the intent of dampening plantarflexion while facilitating postural co-contraction around the ankle. The client can be placed in a side-lying position, can sit on a chair or mat, or can be positioned over a bolster with the hip and knee in some degree of flexion. This flexion dampens the total extension pattern, including the plantarflexor muscles. With release of plantarflexion these muscles are placed on extreme stretch to maintain the modulation. In this position, intermittent joint approximation and compression of considerable force is applied between the *heel* and *knee.* If the client is sitting, this approximation can easily be applied by pounding the heel on the floor and controlling a counterforce at the knee. Once coactivation is minimally palpated, the clinician should initiate a movement pattern such as partial weight bearing to further encourage the CNS to readapt with postural control. This technique can also be used to dampen flexion of the wrist and fingers by applying force to the appropriate upper-extremity patterns, modulating flexor reflex afferent activity, and applying a large amount of joint approximation between the heel of the hand and the elbow. To augment functional outcomes, the technique should be incorporated into functional training to achieve better sensorimotor responses, improved cortical representation of the involved body part, and greater functional carryover.

Ballistic Movement. Ballistic movements are effective because of their combined proprioceptive interaction. The client is asked to initiate a movement, such as shoulder flexion while prone over a table with the arm hanging over the side. This component is volitional, but the client then maintains a passive role. As the patient relaxes, the movement patterns become automatic. The physiology behind the automatic movement is easy to understand. As the muscle approaches the shortened range, the amount of ongoing gamma afferent activity decreases. Thus both the agonist alpha motor neuron bias and the inhibition of Ia and II receptors of the antagonistic alpha motor neurons decrease. Simultaneously, the antagonistic muscle is being placed on more and more stretch. This stretch, as well as the lack of inhibition on the antagonistic alpha motor neurons, will encourage the antagonistic muscle to begin contraction and reverse the movement pattern. The tendon organs also play a key role in ongoing inhibition. As the muscle approaches the shortened range and tension on the tendon becomes intense, the tendon organ increases its firing, thus inhibiting the agonistic muscle in the shortened range while facilitating the antagonistic muscle. This technique is highly movement oriented, and the traction applied by gravity to the shoulder joint while swinging the arm further facilitates the movement. These ballistic movements are part of the program generators within the spinal system that facilitate reciprocal movements of the limb. As the client performs the movement, there is little need for conscious attention to drive the movement; it will run automatically. The role of the Ib fibers during this open chain or movement pattern is definitely different from its role in a closed chain or weight-bearing environment.[199] Supraspinal influence over programmed activity also plays a role in the effectiveness of this treatment.[229] The specific rationale for why ballistic movements have functional carryover may be explained by recent research into cerebellar function and the importance of mechanical afferent input in regulation of movement (see Chapter 21).

The clinician using this technique must exercise caution. ROM can easily be obtained through ballistic movement. Consequently, the clinician must always determine before therapy the reasons for specific clinical signs and whether the total problem will be corrected through an activity such as a ballistic movement. This is the diagnostic responsibility of the professional. If one component of the problem is alleviated, such as limitation of range, while other components are ignored, this can be a dangerous technique. If the lack of range is a result of muscle splinting because there is lack of postural tone or joint stability, then ballistic movement has the possibly increasing the problem. For example, assume that the rotator cuff muscles are slightly torn and the movers of the shoulder are superficially splinting to prevent further tearing. Instructing the client to perform ballistic movement that causes relaxation of more superficial muscles will then place more responsibility for shoulder stabilization on the rotator cuff muscles. If those stabilizers are torn, traction along with relaxation of muscles that are splinting may increase the tear on the rotator cuff muscles and thus increase the problem. The patient may never return to therapy, but if he does, he will complain of more pain than before.

Total-Body Positioning. Total-body positioning implies the use of positioning and gravity to dampen afferent activity on the alpha motor neurons and thus cause a decrease in tone, or relaxation.[230] Today, the rationale for why relaxation of striated muscle occurs after this treatment implies that the effect of the flexor reflex afferents is being dampened by a combination of input and interneuronal activity. These changes in the state of the muscle tone will not be permanent and will revert to the original posturing unless motor learning and adaptation within the central programmer occur simultaneously. Thus for this treatment to effect permanent change, a large number of systems need modification. This modification can be augmented by techniques that facilitate autogenic inhibition, reciprocal innervation, labyrinthine and somatosensory influences, and cerebellar regulation over tone.[231] Changing the degree of flexion of the head also alters vestibular input and the state of the motor pool. But again, the CNS of the client needs to be an active participant and will ultimately determine whether permanent learning and change are programmed.

Proprioceptive Neuromuscular Facilitation. To analyze and learn the principles, techniques, and patterns that constitute PNF, a total approach to treatment, refer to the texts by Adler,[232] Voss,[233] and Sullivan and colleagues.[29] This approach is being used extensively for patients with musculoskeletal and neuromuscular problems, with research on this method encompassing more populations with lower motor neuron and musculoskeletal problems than upper motor neuron lesions.[154,228,234-242] When proprioceptive techniques are packaged in specific movement patterns, it may be referred to as PNF. When individual proprioceptive techniques are discussed alone, the specific sensory function is being acknowledged, and these techniques can be integrated into many rehabilitation intervention strategies.

Postexcitatory Inhibition with Stretch, Range, Rotation, and Shaking. The concept of PEI is based on the action potential or electrical response pattern of a neuron at the time of stimulation and on the entire phase response until the neuron returns to normal. At the time of stimulation, the action potential will build and go through an excitatory phase. The neuron then enters an inhibitory phase or refractory period during which further stimulation is not possible. This is referred to as the *PEI phase* or *postsynaptic afferent depolarization.*[111] These phase changes are extremely short and, in normal muscle, asynchronous with respect to multiple neuronal firing. In a hypertonic muscle more simultaneous firing occurs. When the muscle is lengthened, and thus tension is created, more fibers will be discharged. It is hypothesized that if the hypertonic muscle is placed at the end of its spastic range and a quick stretch is applied and held, then total facilitation followed by total inhibition will occur because of PEI. As the inhibition phase is felt, the therapist can passively lengthen the spastic muscle until the facilitatory phase sets in repolarization. At that time the clinician holds the lengthened position. Increased tone will ensue, followed by inhibition and continued lengthening. Holding the range (not allowing concentric contraction during the excitatory phase) is critical. If the muscle is held as the tone increases, the resistance and stretch are then maximal and probably further facilitate the inhibitory phase.

At a certain point in the range, if the muscle is not limited by fascial tightness, the hypertonic muscle will become dampened and tone will disappear. It is thought that at this time either the tendon organ activity takes over and maintains inhibition or flexor reflex afferents are modified, thus creating an inhibitory range in which antagonistic muscles can be more easily initiated and controlled by the client. If this technique is performed in a pure plane of motion, the clinician will find it a time-consuming procedure. Range can be achieved quickly by integrating a few additional techniques, that is, incorporating rotational patterns of movement. For example, if the spastic upper extremity is positioned in the pattern of shoulder adduction, internal rotation, elbow flexion, forearm pronation, and wrist and finger flexion, then a pattern in the opposite direction can be incorporated to include external rotation of the shoulder and supination of the forearm. Every time the clinician begins to lengthen the spastic extremity, those rotational patterns should be used. This should be done both on initial stretch and when resisting movement during excitation and then lengthening (allowing movement) during the inhibitory phase. Rotation seems to lengthen the inhibitory phase and allows additional range. If the clinician adds a quick stretch to the antagonistic muscle during the inhibitory phase of the agonistic muscle, then further facilitation of the antagonistic muscle will occur. Because the agonistic muscle is in an inhibitory phase, movement in and out of its spastic range should not affect it. Yet the quick stretch facilitation of the antagonistic muscle inhibits the spastic agonistic muscle and again lengthens the inhibitory phase. This entire procedure occurs very quickly. An observer might say that the clinician "shakes the hypertonicity out of the arm." The shaking action is thought to be the quick stretch as well as joint oscillations. The degree of success depends on the therapist's sensitivity to the tonal shifts or phase changes occurring in the client. These tonal shifts are automatic at the hundredth-of-a-millisecond level and not under the client's conscious control. But the sensitivity of the Meissner corpuscles are at approximately 2 hundredths of a millisecond and provide adequate input to the therapist. If a master clinician responds to each inhibitory phase, it will look like the tone melts away. Most clinicians do not have that keen sensitivity, and the interventions will look more jerky because not every inhibitory phase is sensed and thus there will be a lot of stop-and-go movement in very small ranges of movement out of synergy until the hypertonic muscles finally relax.

Rood's Heavy Work Patterns. Rood's concepts of co-contraction in weight-bearing positions such as on elbows, on extended elbows, kneeling, and standing blend with today's concepts of motor learning. Concepts explain why postural holding in shortened range for periods of time are valid treatment procedures. Rood stressed the need for patients to work in and out of those shortened ranges in order to gain postural control as well as to practice directing the limbs during both closed and open chain activities.

Feldenkrais. The Feldenkrais concepts[225,226] of sensory awareness through movement place emphasis on relaxation of muscles on stretch, and distracting and compressing joints for sensory awareness. Both techniques reflect combined proprioceptive techniques. Taking muscles off stretch slows general afferent firing and thus overload to the CNS. Compression and distraction of joints enhance specific input from a body part while simultaneously facilitating input of a lesser intensity from other body segments. This combined proprioceptive approach enhances body schema awareness in a relaxed environment. It also integrates empowerment of the client by use of visualization and asking for volitional control. (See Chapters 27 and 39 for additional information.)

Manual Therapy, Specifically Maitland's. "The peripheral and central nervous systems need to be considered as one because they form a continuous tissue tract."[208,225,243-246] Manual therapy or mobilization of joint or soft tissue structures is not specific to orthopedic conditions, nor are neurological treatment principles ineffective on orthopedic patients. Regardless of the diagnosis or pathological body system leading to joint immobility, the functional consequences can be synonymous. Joint immobility can cause the peripheral nerves to lose their adaptability to change in the length of the nerve bed. This change in neural elasticity then creates additional problems in connective tissue function, which in turn may affect the function of the motor system's control over the musculoskeletal component.[228,247] For this reason alone, discussion of musculoskeletal mobilization needs to be included in this section as a component of classification.

"Pathological processes may interfere with both of these mechanisms: extraneural pathology will affect the nerve/interface relationship and intraneural pathology will affect the intrinsic elasticity of the nervous system."[247] Patient complaints of pain that limits functional movements constitute the primary reason clients are referred to a therapist for a musculoskeletal evaluation. During the physical examination, tension tests can be used to determine the degree of pain and joint limitation, to differentiate between somatic and radicular symptoms, and to identify adverse neurophysiological changes in the PNS.[247] "The increased muscle tone (in a peripheral injury) is considered to be a protective mechanism for the inflamed tissue."[248] This increase in tone may be caused by a dampening of presynaptic activity of the flexor reflex afferent by supraspinal mechanisms. This same mechanism may be triggered by a CNS injury. The difference between the orthopedic patient and the neurological patient may be the trigger to the CNS. In a central lesion the motor generators are often not adequately maintained after injury, which results in hypotonicity. The hypotonicity causes peripheral instability, stretches peripheral tissue, and potentially causes peripheral damage. In both orthopedic and neurological cases, there is peripheral instability, the first the result of peripheral damage and the second the result of hypotonicity. The CNS response to the instability may be the same: an increase in muscle tone by dampening of presynaptic inhibition. A decrease in presynaptic inhibition on incoming afferents would cause an increase in spinal generator activity. With an isolated musculoskeletal problem and an intact CNS, the motor system would have the adaptability and control to modulate the spinal generators and isolate only those components in which an increase in tone might directly affect the problems. The client with CNS involvement may lose some of the flexibility of the motor system's control over the pattern generators, and thus high-tone synergistic patterns may develop.

In either case, the peripheral system needs to be evaluated and intervention provided when necessary. Tension tests look for adverse responses to physical examination of neural tissues. These adverse responses are muscle tone increases as a result of painful provocation of sensitized neural tissue nociceptors attempting to prevent further pain by limiting the movement of the neural tissue.[248] Pain increases tone and leads to limited range of passive movement.[248,249] Pain-free range suggests CNS sensitivity to the large, highly myelinated alpha fibers and functions in a discriminatory manner. Pain range encompasses the degree of joint motion where neural length, as well as nociceptors in the skin, fascia, muscles, and joints, plays a primary role in CNS attention and protection. Inflammation of neural tissue can also cause the nociceptors to become hypersensitized or more reactive to mechanical or chemical changes. This is particularly true in the joint when the nociceptors react significantly to movement at the end ranges.[248]

Treatment will be based on the degree of immobility, the pain range, the site of the irritability, and the degree of pain. Butler[228] not only looks at joint problems but also considers many joint problems as having adverse neural dynamics (tension on the PNS). Treatment still incorporates Maitland's grades of passive movement, but with consideration across the length of the neural tissue across multiple joints.

Butler[247,250] divides treatment of the joint into three categories: limitations, pain, and adverse mechanical tension. When analyzing selective nervous system mobilization as identified by Butler, the therapist needs to mobilize the nervous system and its surrounding fascia rather than stretching it. These techniques may be either gentle (grade I) or strong (grade IV), through the range (grades II and III), or at end range only (grade IV). Different disorders (irritable compared with nonirritable) will require different treatment approaches (Figure 9-3).

Treatment must interface with related tissues. When joint immobility is interfaced with muscle and fascia tightness, all components must be treated simultaneously. If the focus of treatment is the correction of joint and muscle signs, then constant reassessment of the effect on the nervous system is crucial. This aspect would seem even more crucial in clients with CNS and PNS injuries. The treatment may be direct or indirect. Direct intervention involves procedures aimed at rebalancing the neuromusculoskeletal system through strengthening and increasing ROM to improve motor control. Indirect treatment includes the use of movement patterns, especially posture-based patterns. When individuals have nervous system changes, static and dynamic postural patterns often emerge as compensatory reactions to the problem state. Pain posturing, tension, or stiffness from prolonged positioning, and forced postures that are the result of synergy patterns, to name a few, all seem to respond well to indirect treatment with or without passive CNS mobilization. The use of posture-based movement patterns during functional activities also provides for variability and repetition and thus should lead to greater carryover in motor learning.

Many manual therapy approaches affect and use the proprioceptive system as a means to change motor responses. The reader is again reminded that the proprioceptive system affects all systems within the CNS and vice versa. The end effect of all system interactions will be intrinsic reinforcement of existing behavior or changes in and adaptations of behavior to meet intrinsic and extrinsic demands. The

Grades of Movement

Grade I A small amplitude movement performed near the beginning of range.

Grade II A large amplitude movement carried well into range. It's a movement that occupies any part of the range that is free of pain or resistance.

Grade III A large amplitude movement that moves up to the limit of range or into resistance.

Grade IV A small amplitude movement performed near the end of range or slightly into resistance.

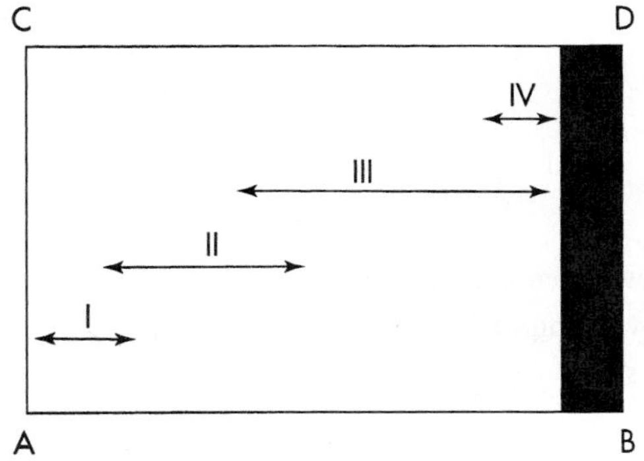

Maitland has also been using the pluses (1) and minuses (2) in his grades of movement for many years now. It enables the therapist to communicate better with other therapists as well as treat the patient with accuracy and skill.

Grade IV−−: just nicking resistance

Grade IV−: touching resistance

Grade IV: into resistance about 25%

Grade IV+: into resistance about 50%

Grade IV++: into resistance about 75%

Figure 9-3 ■ Grades of movement. (Modified from Maitland's theory of joint and tissue mobilization by John Sievert, PT, GDMT. From Course notes, Graduate Diploma in Manipulative Therapy, Curtin University of Technology, Perth, Western Australia, 1990; and from Maitland GD: *Peripheral manipulation,* ed 3, Boston, 1991, Butterworth Heinemann.)

behavior observed by the therapist as the client initiates motor strategies in response to functional goals will be a consensus of all these interactions.

Exteroceptive or Cutaneous Sensory System

Differentiation of Receptor Site as Augmented Intervention. Humans have many different types of tactile receptors. Some are superficial, and others are deep within the layers of the skin. These receptors have been identified within the chapter on motor learning. Their use as augmented intervention strategies is discussed in the following section.

A list of treatment techniques using the exteroceptive (tactile) input system as their primary mode of entry can be found in Table 9-4.

Treatment Alternatives Using the Exteroceptive System. The function of the exteroceptive system is to inform the nervous system about the surrounding world. The CNS will adapt behavior to coexist and survive within this environment. Although many protective responses are patterned within the motor system, these patterned responses can be changed or modulated according to momentary inherent chemistry, attitude, motivation, alertness, and so on. Different from some of the other treatment approaches, the function of the exteroceptive input system is not reflexive but rather informative and adaptable.

Quick Phasic Withdrawal. The human organism reacts to painful or noxious stimuli at both conscious and unconscious levels. If the stimulus is brief and of noxious quality, it will elicit a protective reaction of short duration with use of the long-chain spinal reflex loops. Simultaneously, afferent impulses ascend to higher centers to evoke prolonged emotional-behavioral responses. Stimuli such as pain, extremes in temperature, rapid movement, light touch, and hair displacement are the most likely to cause this reaction by activating free nerve endings. These stimuli are perceived as potentially dangerous and communicate directly with the reticular-activating system and nonspecific thalamic nuclei. These structures have diffuse interconnections with all regions of the cerebral cortex, ANS, limbic system, cerebellum, and motor centers in the brain stem. Research has shown that children who exhibit hyperactive withdrawal reactions also develop negative emotional reactivity and show significantly more avoidance behavior and in time show right frontal asymmetry.[251] These alerting stimuli have been linked to motor seizures in critically ill patients.[252] As indicated by these research studies, therapists need to be aware of these potential responses, especially in patients with severe neurological insult that has resulted in a lower level of consciousness. These low-functioning clients cannot express their feelings nor how their nervous system is reacting to the input. Thus therapists need to be very aware of any motor response a patient may express and try to avoid using stimuli that might trigger these avoidance behaviors. From observance of the behavior of clients with chronic pain, these responses seem to become habitual and may lead to somatosensory remapping, making it hard to differentiate protective from discriminatory information. Thus, any movement or touch triggers pain. Patients need to be taught to discriminate between tightness and true pain, and therapists need to feel when the muscle response has shifted from muscle gliding to muscle restriction. Therapists need to gain trust, and one way is to not elicit a lot of pain. For example, if a therapist tells a patient to say something when it hurts, and the patient says, "Now," the therapist should never respond with "Well, just a little more." In that instant the patient has learned that the therapist lied (because the patient was told to tell the therapist when it hurt, suggesting that the therapist would stop then) or that the therapist is a masochist. If the therapist had stopped when the patient said that it hurt, the patient would then know that he does not need to tell the therapist to stop 10 degrees before it hurts because the therapist is not going to range him that 10 extra degrees. Often the therapist will find that without any effort the patient now has that extra range and has no need to splint the limb because it is not going to hurt to have therapy.

TABLE 9-4 ■ EXTEROCEPTIVE INPUT TECHNIQUES

RECEPTORS	STIMULI	RESPONSE*
Free nerve endings: C + A fibers	Pain, temperature, touch	Seem to protect and alert, perception of temperatures, protective withdrawal
Hair follicles	Mechanical displacement of hair receptors	Increased tone of muscle below stimulus site
Merkel disk	Touch: pressure receptors	Touch identification
Meissner corpuscles	Discriminative touch	Postural tone; two-point discrimination
Pacinian corpuscles	Deep pressure and quick stretch to tissue, vibration	Position sense, postural tone and movement
Ruffini corpuscles	Touch mechanoreceptor	Touch and spatial discrimination

SUGGESTED TREATMENT PROCEDURES USING CUTANEOUS STIMULI

Quick Phasic Withdrawal

1. Stimulus
   a. Pain
   b. Cold: one-sweep with ice cubes, Rood's quick ice
   c. Light touch: brush (quick stroking), finger, feather
2. Response
   a. Stimulus applied to an extensor surface: elicits a flexor withdrawal
   b. Stimulus applied to flexor surface: may elicit flexor withdrawal or withdrawal from stimulus into extension

Prolonged Icing (Repetitive Icing Should Be Used with Caution Because of Rebound Effect)

1. Stimulus
   a. Ice cube
   b. Ice chips and wet towel
   c. Bucket of ice water
   d. Ice pack
   e. Immersion of body part or total body
2. Response: inhibition of muscles below skin areas iced

Neutral Warmth

1. Stimulus
   a. Air bag splints
   b. Wrapping entire body or individual body part with towel
   c. Tight clothing such as tights, fitted turtleneck jerseys, Lycra clothing
   d. Tepid water or shower
2. Response: inhibition of area under which neutral warmth was applied

Light Touch, Rapid Stroking

1. Stimulus
   a. Light intermittent tactile stimulus to an identified dermatome-myotome interaction area
2. Response: facilitation of muscle(s) related to the stimulus area

Maintained Pressure or Slow, Continuous Stroking with Pressure

1. Stimulus
   a. Slowly rubbing the target area with a towel
   b. Wearing Lycra or spandex clothing
2. Response: sensory receptor adaptation and decrease in afferent firing

*Response: adaptation of many cutaneous receptors to stimulus, thus decreasing exteroceptive input, decreasing reticular activity, and decreasing facilitation of muscles underlying stimulated skin.

There are some real therapeutic limitations to using stimuli that "load" the spinothalamic system. A painful stimulus will be excitatory to the nervous system and produce a prolonged reaction after discharge. According to Wall's gate-control theory,[253-257] all sensory afferent neurons converge and synapse in the dorsal horn in an area called the *substantia gelatinosa.* Curiously, the large, more discriminatory fibers do outnumber the small fibers.[258] Therefore, physical activity, frequent positioning, deep pressure, and proprioceptive and cutaneous stimulation should cause enough impulses to converge on cells within the substantia gelatinosa to close the gate and thus block transmission of pain messages to the brain. Studies have demonstrated that physical activity (types of physical stress) stimulates the production of endorphins, which in turn release opiate receptors and act as the body's own morphine for pain control[20,212,259-262] (see Chapters 18 and 32).

Because light touch has both a protective and a discriminatory function, techniques such as brushing or stroking the skin with a soft brush have the potential of informing the CNS about (1) texture, object specificity, and error in fine motor responses or (2) danger (eliciting a protective response). If a protective response is triggered, the specific withdrawal pattern will depend on a variety of circumstances. If the stimulus is applied to an extensor surface, then a flexor withdrawal will be facilitated. If the stimulus is placed on a flexor surface, one of two responses occurs. First, the client might withdraw from the stimulus, thus going into an extensor pattern. Second, the stimulus may elicit a flexor withdrawal and cause the client to go into a flexor pattern. Which pattern occurs depends on preexisting motor programming bias as a result of positioning and the predisposition of the client's CNS. Both responses would be considered normal. The condition or emotional state of the nervous system and whether the stimulus is considered threatening also determine the sensitivity of the response, again reinforcing the systems' interdependence. These responses are protective and do not lead to repetition of movement or motor learning. For that reason, along with the emotional and autonomic reactions, a phasic withdrawal to facilitate flexion or extension is not recommended as a treatment approach unless all other possibilities have been eliminated.

Short Duration, High-Intensity Icing. Cold is another stimulus that the nervous system perceives as potentially dangerous. The use of ice as a stimulus to elicit desired motor patterns is an early technique developed by Rood. Her technique was referred to as *repetitive icing.* An ice cube is rubbed with pressure for 3 to 5 seconds or used in a quick-sweep motion over the muscle bellies to be facilitated. This method activates both exteroceptors and proprioceptors and causes a brief arousal of the cortex. This method can produce unpredictable results. Although initially a phasic withdrawal pattern generator response will be activated immediately after the reflex has taken place, the "rebound" phenomenon deactivates the muscle that has been stimulated and lowers the resting potential of the antagonistic muscle.[263] Therefore a second stimulus to the same dermatome-myotome neural network may not elicit a second response. But, because of reciprocal innervation, the antagonistic muscle may effect a rebound movement in the opposite direction. Icing may also cause prolonged reaction after discharge because of the connections to the reticular system, limbic system, and ANS. Thus the ANS would be shifted toward the sympathetic end. Too much sympathetic tone causes a desynchronization of the cortex.[264] Although the resting state of the spinal generator may be altered briefly, if the heightened state persists the cause is most likely fear or sympathetic overflow (see Chapter 5). This state is destabilizing to the system and most likely will not lead to any motor learning. Because of unpredictable response patterns to Rood's repetitive icing, this technique is seldom used.

The therapist is cautioned not to use short-duration, high-intensity icing to the facial region above the level of the lips, to the forehead, or to the midline of the trunk. These areas have a high concentration of pain fibers and a strong connection to the reticular system.[10,265]

Ice should not be used behind the ear because it may produce a sudden lowering of blood pressure.[266] The therapist should also avoid using ice in the left shoulder region in patients with a history of heart disease because referred pain from angina pectoris manifests itself in the left shoulder area, indicating that the cold stimulus might cause a reflexive constriction of the coronary arteries.[267] In addition, the primary rami located along the midline of the dorsum of the trunk have sympathetic connections to internal organs. The cold stimulus may alter organ activity and perhaps produce vasoconstriction, causing increased blood pressure and reduced blood supply to the viscera.[268,269]

Brief administration of ice can have beneficial effects if the nervous system's inhibitory mechanisms are in place. For instance, in children with learning disabilities or adults with sensorimotor delays, the application of ice to the palmar surface of the hands will cause arousal at the cortical level because of the increased activity of the reticular activating system. This arousal response presumably produces increased adrenal medullary secretions, resulting in various metabolic changes. Therefore icing should be used selectively. If the patient has an unstable ANS, icing should be eliminated as a potential sensory modality.[270]

Prolonged Use of Ice. Physicians have used therapeutic cold for the treatment of individuals with high fever and/or intracranial pressure with the intent of reducing the body temperature or brain swelling to prevent brain damage.[271] This procedure is done with cooling pans or blankets. Whole-body cryotherapy has been used to reduce inflammation and pain and overcome symptoms that prevent normal movement. This type of therapy consists of the use of very cold air maintained for 2 minutes in cryochambers. A recent study looked at this type of therapy for injured athletes. It was found that the procedure did not cause harm to the individual.[272] This approach does not seem realistic for use in occupational or physical therapy clinics.

A variety of approaches that incorporate prolonged icing techniques have been used in therapy clinics for decades. The PNF approach may be the most common.[19] Inhibition of hypertonicity or pain is the goal for the use of any of these methods. With prolonged cold the neurotransmission of impulses, both afferent and efferent, is reduced. Simultaneously the metabolic rate within the cooled tissue is reduced (see Chapter 32). Caution must be exercised with regard to the use of this modality. However, for effective treatment results, the client (1) should be receptive to the modality, (2) should be able to monitor the cold stimulus (sensory deficits should not be present), and (3) should have a stable autonomic system to prevent unnecessary adverse effects of hypothermia. Research of the last decade has consistently shown that cryotherapy is an effective tool for reducing pain and has helped individuals regain integration of axial musculature after neurological insults.[273-276] Individuals of all ages seem to respond similarly, which allows therapists to use this therapeutic tool across generations.[277]

Ice immersion of the contralateral limb was used decades ago in order to get a reflexive decrease in temperature in the affected limb. It was believed that this intralimb reflex was an effective way of treating pain without directly treating the limb. Recent research has validated that belief.[278]

Ice massage is another form of prolonged icing and is often used to treat somatic pain problems.[279] It is also used over high-toned muscles to dampen striated muscle contractions. Caution must be used when eliminating pain without correcting the problem causing pain. For example, if instability causes muscle tone and pain, then icing might decrease pain while causing additional joint instability and potential damage. The end result would be an increase, not a decrease, in pain and motor dysfunction.

Neutral Warmth. Like icing, neutral warmth alters the state of the motor generators, either directly or indirectly through afferent input. According to Farber,[12] the length of application depends on the client. A 3- to 4-minute tepid bath may create the same results as a 15-minute total-body-wrapping procedure. As with any input procedure, the effects should be incorporated into the therapeutic session to maximize the results and promote client learning. The Johnstone approach uses air splints effectively as a neutral warm treatment intervention while clients work on functional activities.[17] If neutral warmth is applied as an isolated intervention, the client may feel relaxation or a decrease in discomfort, but neuroplastic CNS changes are unlikely, owing to the lack of repetition, attention, and error correction by the client during activities. A recent study looked at blood pressure, heart rate, and other autonomic mechanisms in subjects using compression hose. The researchers did not look at neutral warmth as a mechanism to maintain a homeostatic state of the nervous system. Yet the use of compression hose does create a state of neutral warmth, and the link to homeostasis can easily be made.[280]

Maintained Stimulus or Pressure. Because of the rapid adaptation of many cutaneous receptors, a maintained stimulus will effectively cause inhibition by preventing further stimuli from entering the system. This technique is applied to hypersensitive areas to normalize skin responses. Vibration used alternately with maintained pressure can be highly effective. It should be remembered that these combined inputs use different neurophysiological mechanisms. It is often observed that low-frequency maintained vibration is especially effective with learning-disabled children who have hypersensitive tactile systems that prevent them from comfortable exploration of their environment. When children themselves use vibration on the extremities, their hypersensitive systems seem to normalize and they become receptive to exploring objects. If that exploration is accompanied by additional prolonged pressure, such as digging in a sandbox, the technique seems to be more effective because of the adaptive responses of the nervous system.

Maintained pressure approaches using elastic stockings, tight form-fitting clothing (e.g., wet suits, expanded polytetrafluoroethylene [Gore-Tex] biking clothing), air splints, and other techniques can be incorporated into a client's daily activity without altering lifestyle. The use of TheraTogs in children with various hyperactivity conditions has become an accepted therapeutic tool. They add some resistance, some support, and maintained pressure.[281] TheraTogs have also been shown to be effective in assisting individuals with hemiplegia to regain abductor control.[282]

In this way clients can self-regulate their systems, allowing greater variability in adapting to the environment. Owing to the multisensory and multineuronal pathways used when peripheral input is augmented, traditional linear, allopathic research on human subjects is extremely difficult to design or measure with control. But outcome studies demonstrating efficacy are possible. Initially, efficacy confirmed by observation was acceptable. Now it is time to repeat studies and use objective measures to demonstrate the same outcome.

Light Discriminatory Touch. Once an individual can discriminate light touch both for protection and for discriminatory learning, a lot of therapeutic tools become available to the therapist. Using boxes with an opening so the individual can insert a hand and arm but cannot see what is inside, a patient can work on discriminating textures, objects, letter, numbers, and so on while working on higher-order processing. Once this touch has been integrated, the patient can also use light touch to determine balance, position in space, and various other types of perceptual tasks.[283]

Vestibular System (Refer to Chapter 22B)

Vestibular Treatment Techniques. The vestibular system is a unique sensory system, critical for multisensory functioning, making it a viable and powerful input modality for therapeutic intervention (see Chapter 22B). Any static position and any movement pattern will facilitate the labyrinthine system; therefore vestibular function and dysfunction play a role in all therapeutic activities. To conceptualize vestibular stimulation as spinning or angular acceleration minimizes its therapeutic potential and also negates an entire progression of vestibular treatment techniques.[12,41,284-286] Linear movements in horizontal and vertical postures and forward-backward directions occur early in development and should be considered one viable treatment modality. These movements seem to precede side-to-side and diagonal movements, which are followed by linear acceleration and end with rotational movements. All these movements can be done with assistance or independently by the client in all functional activities. It is important to remember that the rate of vestibular stimulation determines the effects. A constant, slow, repetitive rocking pattern, irrespective of plan or direction, generally causes inhibition of total-body responses via the alpha motor neuron but not the spindles,[287] whereas a fast spin or fast linear movement tends to heighten both alertness and the motor responses. Again, the vestibular mechanism is only one of many that influence the motor system. Thus, the system interaction must be constantly reassessed.

As already indicated, constant, slow, repetitive rocking patterns, irrespective of plane or direction, generally cause inhibition of the total-body responses. Yet any stimulus has the potential of causing undesired responses, such as increased or decreased tone. When this occurs, the procedure should be stopped and reanalyzed to determine the reason for the observed or palpated response. For example, assume that a client, whether a child with cerebral palsy, an adolescent with head trauma, or an adult with anoxia, exhibits signs of severe generalized extensor hypertonicity in the supine position. To dampen the general motor response, the therapist decides to use a slow, gentle rocking procedure in supine position and discovers that the hypertonicity has increased. Obviously, the procedure did not elicit the desired response and alternative treatment is selected, but the reason for the increased hypertonicity needs to be addressed.

It is possible that the static positioning of the vestibular system is causing the release of the original tone and that through increasing of the vestibular input the tone also increases. It may also be that the facilitatory input did indeed cause inhibition, but the movement itself caused fear and anxiety, thus increasing preexisting tone and overriding the inhibitory technique. Instead of selecting an entirely new treatment approach, a therapist could use the same procedure in a different spatial plane, such as a side-lying, prone, or sitting position. Each position affects the static position of the vestibular system differently and may differentially affect the excessive extensor tone observed in the client. The vertical sitting position adds flexion to the system, which has the potential of further dampening extensor tone. This additional inhibition may be necessary to determine whether the slow rocking pattern will be effective with this client. It would seem obvious that if a vestibular procedure was ineffective in modifying the preexisting extensor tone, then use of a powerful procedure, such as spinning, would be inappropriate. Selection of treatment techniques should be determined according to client needs and disability. Clients either with an acoustic tumor that perforates into the brain stem or with generalized inflammatory disorders may be hypersensitive to vestibular stimulation, whereas other clients, such as a child with a learning disability, may be in need of massive input through this system. Heiniger and Randolph[41] and Farber[12,111] present in-depth analyses of various specific vestibular treatment procedures commonly used in the clinic. A general summary of the treatment suggestions is summarized in Table 9-5.

The literature clearly establishes the causation of one vestibular imbalance, dizziness, for all age groups.[288-291] Certainly individuals can have vestibular problems and will present themselves as being dizzy or hyperactive to movement of the head. There is a lot of literature discussing treatment of dizziness, and only a few publications are listed here.[292-294] There is certainly evidence to show how the vestibular system links to the autonomic nervous system and especially the sympathetic pathways.[295] In Chapter 22B the reader will be able to find in-depth discussion of vestibular rehabilitation and the role movement scientists play in that rehabilitation.

General Body Responses Leading to Relaxation. Any technique performed in a slow, continuous, even pattern will cause a generalized dampening of the motor output.[296] During handling techniques, these procedures can be performed with the client in bed, on a mat while horizontal, sitting at bedside or in a chair, or standing. The movement can be done passively by the therapist or actively by the client. Carryover into motor learning will best be accomplished when the client performs the movement actively, without therapeutic assistance. In a clinical or school setting, a client who is extremely anxious, hyperactive, and hypertonic may initiate slow rocking to decrease tone or feel less anxious or hyperactive. The reduction of clinical signs allows the client to sit with less effort and to be more attentive to the environment, thus promoting the ability to learn and adapt.

It is the type of movement, not the technique, that is critical. The concept of slow, continuous patterns is used in Brunnstrom's rocking patterns[8] in early sitting, in PNF mat programs, and in therapeutic ball exercise programs; the use of these patterns can be observed in every clinic. Although the therapist may be unaware of why Mr. Smith gets so relaxed when slowly rocked from side to side in sitting, this procedure elicits an appropriate response. The nurse taking Mr. Smith for a slow wheelchair ride around the hospital grounds may do the same thing. Once the relaxation or inhibition has occurred, the groundwork for a therapeutic environment has been created to promote further learning, such as learning of ADL skills. The technique in and of itself will relax the individual but not create change or learning.

Pelvic mobilization techniques in sitting use relaxation from slow rocking to release the fixed pelvis. This release allows for joint mobility and thus creates the potential for pelvic movement performed passively by the therapist, with the assistance of the therapist, or actively by the client. This technique often combines vestibular with proprioceptive techniques, such as rotation and elongation of muscle groups, which physiologically modify existing fixed tonal response through motor mechanisms or systems interactions. Simultaneously, slow, rhythmic rocking, especially on diagonals, is used to incorporate all planes of motion and thus all vestibular receptor sites to get maximal dampening effect, whether directly through the vestibulospinal system or indirectly through the cerebellum and reticular spinal motor system. The same pelvic mobility can be achieved by placing the patient (child or adult) over a large ball. The ball must be large enough for the patient to be semiprone while arms are abducted and externally rotated and legs relaxed (either draped over the ball or in the therapist's arms). Again, this position allows for maintained or prolonged stretch to tight muscles both in the extremities and in the trunk while doing slow, rhythmical rocking over the ball. The pelvis often releases, and the patient can be rolled off the large ball to stand on a relaxed pelvis preliminary to gait activities. A word of caution must be given regarding use of a large ball for relaxation. It is much easier to control the ball when someone is assisting that control from the opposite direction (in front of the patient). If slow rocking is done and the therapist is keeping his or her voice monotonous for further relaxation, the individual assisting will also relax. One author has had family members fall asleep and slowly or quickly fall to the floor.

Techniques to Heighten Postural Extensors. Any technique that uses rapid anteroposterior or angular acceleration of the head and body while the client is prone will facilitate a postural extensor response. Scooter boards down inclines, rapid acceleration forward over a ball or bolster, going down slides prone, and using a platform or mesh net to propel someone will all facilitate a similar vestibular response of righting of the head with postural overflow down into the shoulder girdle, trunk, hips, and lower extremities. Rapid movements while on elbows, on extended elbows, and in a crawling position can also facilitate a similar response. Depending on the intensity of the stimulus, the response will vary. In addition, the client's emotional level during introduction to various types of stimuli may cause differences in tonal patterns. Clinical experience has shown that facilitatory vestibular stimulation promotes verbal responses and affects oral-motor mechanisms. Children with speech delays will speak out spontaneously and respond verbally.

Because facilitatory vestibular stimulation biases the sympathetic branch of the ANS, drooling diminishes and a generalized arousal response occurs at the cortical level. Therefore the appropriate time to teach adaptive rehabilitative techniques is after vestibular stimulation.[297]

Facilitatory Techniques Influencing Whole-Body Responses. Tactile, vestibular, and proprioceptive inputs also assist in the regulation of the body's responses to movement.[35,111] As stated previously, the vestibular system, when facilitated with fast, irregular, or angular movement, such as spinning, not only induces tonal responses but also causes massive reticular activity and overflow into higher centers.

TABLE 9-5 ■ COMBINED INPUT SENSORY SYSTEMS: TREATMENT MODALITIES

									INHERENT RESPONSE	
TECHNIQUE	PROPRIOCEPTIVE: JOINT, TENDON SPINDLE	EXTEROCEPTIVE	VESTIBULAR	GUSTATORY	OLFACTORY	AUDITORY	VISUAL	ANS	LABELED	NOT LABELED
Sweep tapping[620]	X	X								
Brunnstrom rolling (hand)[40]	X	X							Automatic extension of hand	
Raimiste sign[40]	X	X								?
Stretch pressure[620]	X	X								
Digging in sand, and so on	X	X					?			
Gentle shaking[620]	X		X							
Prone activities over ball[51,620,621]	X	X	X				X		Automatic righting of head (tectospinal or vestibulospinal)	
Sitting activities on ball[51]	X	?	X				X	X	OLR and balance (all systems)	
Mat activities	X	X	X			?	?			
Resistive exercises	X	X								
1. Resistive rolling	X	X	X			If verbal command	If visual leads			Rotatory integration
2. Resistive patterns: PNF[622-624]	X	X	Depends on pattern			X	X			
3. Resistive gait[625]	X	?	Depends on pattern			If verbal command	X			
4. Isokinetics[626,627]	X	Some					X			
5. Wall pulleys	X		X (if done in body rotation)				X (if guided toward target)			
6. Rowing[40]	X	?	X			If verbal command	X			Body rotation
Feeding[51,99,620]										
1. Maintained pressure: walking to back of tongue	X	X		?	?					
2. Resistive sucking										
a. Straw	X	X		?	?					
b. Popsicle	X	X		X	X				X	

a. Peanut butter								
b. Applesauce								
4. Maintained pressure to top lip	X	X				X		Automatic closing of mouth
Inverted TLR[620,628]	X		X	?	X	X		
Touch bombardment[620]	X	X	X			X	Decreased hypersensitive tactile system and thus withdrawal pattern: stereognosis	
1. Tactile discrimination in sand, and so on								
2. Pool therapy								
Joint compression more than body weight[629,630]	X	X				X		
Throwing and catching								
1. Balloon	?	X			X	?	? (withdrawal to light touch)	
2. Heavy ball	X	?			X	Result of light touch		
Variance in movement								
1. Quick action directed by vision	X		X		X			
2. Postural activities in front of mirror	X		?		X			
3. Therapist using voice command to assist client with movement	X		X	X				
High-level movement								
1. Walking balance beam	X		X	?	? If visually corrected	X	Labyrithine righting and equilibrium; possible OLR	
2. Trampoline activities	X		X		If visually corrected	X	OLR and equilibrium	
3. Running, jumping, skipping	X		X					

OLR, Optic and labyrinthine righting reactions; *PNF*, proprioceptive neuromuscular facilitation; *TLR*, tonic labyrinthine reflex.

Thus increased attention and alertness are often the outcome. The tracts going from the spinal cord, brain stem, and higher subcortical structures must be sufficiently intact to permit the desired responses from this type of input. If a lesion in the brain stem blocks higher-center communication with the vestibular apparatus, then massive input may cause a large increase in abnormal tone. The therapist needs to closely monitor any distress or ANS anomalies.[295]

Total-Body Relaxation Followed by Selective Postural Facilitation. The use of the inverted position in therapy has become very popular as a way to relax postural muscles and decrease compression between vertebrae.[298] Not only does this decrease pain, but it also causes relaxation. Earlier research on the labyrinth's influence on posture and the influence of the inverted position showed that total inversion (angle of 0 degrees) produced maximal postural extensor tone, and the normal upright position elicited maximal flexor tonicity.[230] There seems to be confusion in the literature about the clinical effects of inversion. The initial research was performed on anesthetized animals and cannot be representative of how the human CNS responds to inversion as a system. Kottke[299] reports that the static labyrinthine reflex is maximal when the head is tilted back in the semireclining position at an angle of 60 degrees above the horizontal. Conversely, minimal stimulation occurs when the head is prone and down 60 degrees below the horizontal position. Stejskal[297] studied the effects of the tonic labyrinthine position in hypertonic patients. This study failed to show labyrinthine reflexes in subjects with hypertonia. The problem with use of the inverted position is its lack of permanency. It is a contrived technique used to relieve pain or to achieve total relaxation. The effectiveness of this approach comes with the next set of therapeutic activities that allow the CNS to maintain that relaxation for a period of time and hopefully indefinitely over a series of multiple treatments.

The explanation for the incongruity in the literature over decades seems to be one of interpretation. Any time a subject is put on a tilt table or even a scooter board, the weight bearing of the body on the surface must cause firing of the underlying exteroceptors while gravity pulls on the proprioceptors. This position also has the potential to create fear.[300] As the body shifts and presses onto the underlying surface, stretch reflexes associated with posture and movement must contribute some bias to muscle tone.[301] In addition, if the subject is in supine and the neck flexors are activated eccentrically (being lowered to supine) or concentrically (being pulled toward sitting or actively lifting the head), or if the subject is in prone and the neck extensors are activated eccentrically (lowering the head toward the ground) or concentrically (holding the head up in prone), the proprioceptors of the neck could alter the muscle tone of the limbs.[302]

Another factor that contributes to tonal changes in the extremities is the cervicoocular reflex.[303,304] Reflex eye movements to center the eyes as the body or neck rotates also exert influences on the muscles of the limbs. Because all the influences brought about by gravity and postural mechanisms in a clinical situation cannot be controlled, the inverted position appears to be an interplay of cutaneous receptors, proprioceptors, and tonal changes in the labyrinthine system.[305]

Several highly recognized therapists have reported using the inverted position as a therapeutic modality.[12,28,41] Generally the inverted position produces three major changes. First, because of the gravitational forces on circulation, the carotid sinus sends messages to the medulla and cardiac centers that ultimately lower heart rate, respiration, and resting blood pressure through peripheral dilation, creating a parasympathetic response pattern. This position may be contraindicated for certain patients with a history of cardiovascular disease, glaucoma, or completed stroke. Clients with unstable intracranial pressure—for example, those with traumatic head injuries, coma, tumor, or postinflammatory disorders—and many children with congenital spinal cord lesions would also be at high risk for further injury if the inverted position were used. However, this position has been used with some success for adult patients with hypertension. In any case, scrupulous recording of blood pressure and other ANS effects should be taken before, during, and after positioning.

Another benefit of the inverted position is generalized relaxation. Farber[12] recommends its use as an inhibitory technique. Because the carotid sinus stimulates the parasympathetic system, the trophotropic system is influenced and muscle tonicity is reduced. This has been found to be beneficial to patients with upper motor neuron lesions and also to children who exhibit hyperkinetic behavior. Heiniger and Randolph[41] report that severe hypertonicity in the upper extremities is noticeably reduced.

The third benefit of the inverted position is an increased tonicity of certain extensor muscles. This phenomenon is not purely a function of the labyrinth; it is also a result of activation of the exteroceptors being stimulated by the body's contact with the positioning apparatus.[305] Therapists have capitalized on this reaction to activate specific extensor muscles of the neck, trunk, and limb girdles.[27,297,299]

Because the inverted position decreases hypertonicity and hyperactivity and facilitates normal postural extensor patterns, the responses to the technique should be incorporated into meaningful functional activities. For example, if the position of total inversion over a ball is used, then postural extension of the head, trunk, and shoulder girdles and hips should be facilitated next. Additional facilitation techniques, such as vibration or tapping, could help summate the response. Resistance to the pattern in a functional or play activity would be the ultimate goal. If the inverted position is used in a squat pattern, then squatting to standing against resistance would probably be a primary goal. This can be accomplished by the therapist positioning his or her body behind and over the child, not only to direct the child initially into the inverted position but also to resist the child coming to stand. If the inverted position is used in sitting, activities of the neck, trunk, and upper extremities would be the major focus after the initial responses.

Because the inverted position elicits both labyrinthine and ANS responses, this technique needs to be cross-referenced within the classification schema. Because of its ANS influence, close monitoring is important for all clients placed in an inverted position. As with all labyrinthine treatment techniques, this approach, considered a normal, inherent human response, is used outside the therapeutic setting. For example, standing on one's head in a yoga exercise causes the same physiological state as that observed in the clinic. In many respects the yoga stance is done for the same reasons: decreasing hypertonicity (generally caused by tension), achieving relaxation, and increasing postural tone and altered states of consciousness. Clients can certainly be taught to control their own ANS activity and hypertonicity by placing their hands between their legs when they need a generalized dampening effect on motor generators. Thus, when accessing and incorporating other approaches, the therapist analyzes each specific technique with use of a critical neuroscientific frame of reference.

This section has described procedures that use the vestibular system as a primary input modality to alter the client's CNS. If the client's vestibular system itself is dysfunctional, this dysfunction has the potential to alter the functional state of the motor system. See Chapter 22A for additional information on balance and Chapter 22B for information on the vestibular system.

The therapist must always remember that in combining vestibular and proprioceptive input or asking the CNS to process this information, a variety of results can develop. When the two input systems are congruent, the response will be summated and the CNS will not need to make a lot of adjustment. However, if the inputs are in conflict, then the CNS needs to update the differences and weigh which stimulus is more relevant. Then the updating and response will be in direct proportion to how both inputs were weighted.[306]

Autonomic Nervous System

The ability to differentiate tone created by emotional responses versus tone resulting from CNS damage is a critical aspect of the evaluation process. Emotional tone can be reduced when stress, anxiety, and fear of the unknown have been reduced. This is true for all individuals. The client with brain damage is no exception. Six treatment modalities[307] that normally produce a parasympathetic or decreased sympathetic (flight or fight) response are as follows:

1. Slow, continuous stroking for 3 to 5 minutes over the paravertebral area of the spine
2. Inversion, eliciting carotid sinus reflex along with other somatosensory receptors (refer to the discussion of vestibular system earlier in the chapter).
3. Slow, smooth, passive and active assistive movement within a pain-free range (refer to Maitland's grade II movements (see Figure 9-3)[20]
4. Deep breathing exercises (see Chapter 18)
5. Progressive muscle relaxation
6. Cranial sacral manipulation (see Chapter 39)

When pressure is applied to both the anterior and posterior surfaces of the body, measurable reductions may be recorded in pulse rate, metabolic activity, oxygen consumption, and muscle tone.[266,308] These pressure techniques are identified as an intricate part of the many intervention approaches such as therapeutic touch,[24,267] Feldenkrais,[225-227,309] Maitland,[20] massage,[310,311] and myofascial release.[6,212,312-314] Although not verbally identified, other techniques (e.g., neurodevelopmental treatment (NDT),[31,32] Rood,[29,41,111] Brunnstrom,[8] and PNF[29]) also place an important emphasis on the response of the patient to the therapist's touch.

Treatment Alternatives Using the Autonomic Nervous System

Slow Stroking. Slow stroking over the paravertebral areas along the spine from the cervical through lumbar components will cause inhibition or a dampening of the sympathetic nervous system. The technique is performed while the client is in the prone position. The therapist begins by stroking the cervical paravertebral region in the direction of the thoracic area, using a slow, continuous motion with one hand. Usually a lubricant is applied to the skin, and the index and middle fingers are used to stroke both sides of the spinal column simultaneously. Once the first hand is approaching the end of the lumbar section, the second hand should begin a downward stroking at the cervical region. This maintains at least one point of contact with the client's skin at all times during the procedure. The technique is applied for 3 to 5 minutes—and no longer—because of the potential for massive inhibition or rebound of the autonomic responses.[35,296] It is also recommended that at the end of the range of the last stroking pattern, the therapist maintain pressure for a few seconds to alert both the somatic and visceral systems that the procedure has concluded. Eastern medicine recognizes the importance of the ANS in total-body regulation to a greater extent than Western medicine does. The concepts of meridians and acupressure and acupuncture points are all intricately intertwined with the ANS (see Chapter 39). For that reason, a technique such as slow stroking would potentially interact with meridians and does extend over the row of acupuncture points referred to as *shu points* and relates to visceral reflexes connecting smooth muscle and specific organ systems. It is believed that this continuous, slow, downward pressure modulates the sympathetic outflow, causing a shift to a parasympathetic reaction or relaxation. Whether a result of the pressure on the sympathetic chain, some energy pressure over meridian points, a pleasant sensation, or something unknown, slow stroking does elicit relaxation and calming.[41,111] Clients with large amounts of body hair or hair whorls are poor candidates for this procedure because of the irritating effect of stroking against the growth patterns and the sensitivity of hair follicles.

Slow, Smooth, Passive Movement within Pain-Free Range. Increasing ROM in painful joints is a dilemma frequently encountered by therapists caring for clients with neurological damage. Having the client communicate the first perception of pain and then moving the limb in a slow, smooth motion toward the pain range elicits a variety of behaviors. First, the client generally gestures or verbalizes that pain is present 10 to 15 degrees before it may, in reality, exist. This behavior may occur because the patient during previous treatment interventions learned that therapists often responded to the client's statement of pain by saying, "Let's just go a little farther." That additional range is usually 10 to 15 degrees. If the therapist stops at the stated point of pain, retreats back into a pain-free area, and approaches again, possibly with a slight variation in rotation or direction, the client will often relinquish the safety range and a true picture of the pain range will be obtained. The second finding is that if the motion toward the pain range is slow, smooth, and continuous, then frequently much of the range that was initially painful becomes pain free. The hypothesis is that slow, continuous motion is critical feedback for the ANS to handle imminent discomfort. The slow pattern provides the ANS time to release endorphins, thus modifying the perception of pain and allowing for increased motion. If the therapist stabilizes the painful joint and prevents the possibility of that joint going into the pain range, rapid, oscillating movements can often be obtained within the pain-free range. This maintains joint mobility and often, as an end result, increases the pain-free range. This technique is not unique to the treatment of clients with neurological problems; it is often used as a manual therapy procedure.[212,253,315] Furthermore, one can move slowly into a range that actually shortens muscles. If held for 30 seconds, the muscle that is too short can relax, promoting greater motion in the opposite direction. This can be called *strain-counterstrain*—inhibiting firing by maintaining a position of active insufficiency, making the muscle too short.

Manual therapy[20,148,316-319] can be used to describe the pain and joint changes occurring at the joint level. As the fields of orthopedics and neurology merge into one system,[228] with the brain acting as an organ controlling the entire system and its components, the question of whether the pain reduction is centrally or peripherally triggered may be an important one. The answer is probably both. For example, thumb pain can increase the sensation of the nervous system to the point that even cutaneous and proprioceptive receptors act as nociceptors.

Maintained Pressure. Farber[12] discusses a variety of techniques that facilitate a reduction of tone or hyperactivity. Pressure to the palm of the hand or sole of the foot, to the tip of the upper lip, and to the abdomen all seem to produce this effect. The pressure need not be forceful, but it should be firm and maintained.[320] This same technique is defined as inhibitory casting when applied through the use of an orthosis (see Chapter 34).

Progressive Muscle Relaxation. Progressive muscle relaxation is practiced during both meditation and treatment approaches such as Feldenkrais.[309,320,321] These methods of relaxation tend to trigger parasympathetic reactions, which in turn slow down heart rate and blood pressure and trigger slow, deep breathing (see Chapters 18 and 39). The Alexander technique has also been shown to cause relaxation while simultaneously increasing postural tone.[322]

Cranial Sacral Manipulation. Summarizing the complexity of cranial sacral theory is not within the scope of this book. The reader is referred to references to gain a global understanding of the treatment interactions and the ANS response to cranial therapy as well as a brief discussion in Chapter 39.[307,312] This treatment approach needs to be more intensively researched in terms of physiological effects and clinical effectiveness.

Olfactory System: Smell

The complexity of the olfactory system and how it interacts with nuclei that direct emotion in humans is still not totally understood. Yet quality of life in patients without smell (dysosmic) is often impaired. How the neuroanatomy and neurophysiology of human smell lead to a decreased quality of life is still under investigation.[323-326]

Smell evokes different responses by means of the limbic system's control over behavior. Pleasant odors, such as vanilla or perfume, can evoke strong moods. Unpleasant odors can facilitate primitive protective reflexes, such as sneezing and choking. Sharp-smelling substances such as ammonia can elicit a reflex interruption of breathing.[327,328]

As a result of arousal, protective reflexes, and mood changes caused by odors, the use of smell as a treatment modality has been implemented, especially during feeding procedures. Odors such as vanilla and banana have been used to facilitate sucking and licking motions.[329,330] Ammonia and vinegar have been used clinically to elicit withdrawal patterns and increase arousal in semicomatose patients.[331] When odors are used as a stimulant, the therapist must be aware of all behavior changes occurring within the client. Arousal, level of consciousness, tonal patterns, reflex behavior, and emotional levels all can be affected by odor. Because of limited research in this area, caution must be exercised to avoid indiscriminate use of the olfactory system. Odors such as body odor, perfumes, hairspray, and urine can affect the client's behavior although the smell was not intended as a therapeutic procedure. Some clients, especially those with head traumas and inflammatory disorders of the CNS, often seem to be hypersensitive to smell. In these cases the therapist needs to be aware of the external olfactory environment surrounding the client and to make sure those odors that are present facilitate or at least do not hinder desired response patterns.[332]

Many clinical questions arise regarding smell as a therapeutic modality. If the choice of odors is between pleasant and noxious, a pleasant odor will theoretically be perceived in a way that should be enjoyable, relaxing, and thus potentially tone reducing. On the other hand, noxious odors should cause a sympathetic reaction and, although producing alertness, may also create a fight-or-flight internal reaction that if repeated frequently could cause an adverse response to the client's perception of the world. This has the potential for having a profound effect on her or his feelings toward the therapist and the therapeutic environment. The effect may not be observable until the client reaches a level of consciousness or motor skill in which there is some ability to react.

Individuals' perception of smell is not correlated to their actual olfactory ability.[333] Because of the complex neuronetwork of the olfactory system, the specifics between emotional responses and olfactory environment cannot be established, and determining which olfactory input will drive a pleasant, unpleasant, or neutral response is variable. There may be a cultural sensitivity to various smells that would suggest a cultural learning linked with emotional responses to smell.[334-336] Therefore if a therapist is going to use smell as part of therapy, identification of the individual's prior likes and dislikes is very important. Family members and close friends will be the best people to consult in order to get this information.

Without a sense of smell an individual may not be able to respond appropriately to various olfactory environments, which may increase a client's feeling of isolation and lack of social interactive skills.[337-339] Smell is intricately linked to the sense of taste. Without these sensory systems, individuals tend to stop eating, thus creating an entirely different health care issue.[340,341]

Gustatory Sense: Taste

Gustatory input is generally used as part of feeding and prefeeding activities. As already mentioned, the oral region is sensitive not only to taste but also to pressure, texture, and temperature. For that reason feeding would be classified as a multisensory technique that uses gustatory input as one of its entry modalities. Specific input modalities are based on the combined taste, texture, temperature, and affective response pattern—that is, both a banana and an apple may be sweet, yet the textures vary greatly. When mashed, both fruits may have a pudding-like texture, yet the client's emotional response may differ. Disliking the taste of banana but enjoying apple may cause startling differences in the client's response during a feeding session. Thus the importance of the clinician's sensitivity to the client's response patterns within each sensory modality cannot be overemphasized.[111] Similarly, a therapist needs to take into consideration normal changes with taste and smell that occur as a result of aging and adjust the input threshold appropriately.[342,343] The interrelationship of taste and smell leads to the perception of flavor. Current research has shown that the role of taste may be guided more by taste than by smell, but with each a client will not be able to differentiate flavors of food.[344] Understanding this sensory system will lead to a greater understanding of some patient problems that follow CNS damage.[345]

Auditory System

Treatment Alternatives with Use of the Auditory System. Because of the complexity of the auditory system, a potentially large number of types of input modalities exists. Although some of them might not be considered traditional therapeutic tools, they are nonetheless techniques that affect the CNS. Some treatment alternatives focus on the following:

- Quality of voice (pitch and tone)[346]
- Quantity of voice (level and intensity)[347]
- Affect of voice (emotional overtones)[348,349]
- Spatial and temporal sound (how fast a stimulus occurs, and how frequently)[350-354]
- Extraneous noise (sound)[355]
- Auditory biofeedback[356-362]
- Language[363]
- Volume, level, and affect of voice[364-366]
- Auditory perception[367-369]

The therapist's voice can be considered one of the most powerful therapeutic tools. Even constant sound has the ability to cause adaptation of the auditory system and thus inhibition of auditory sensitivity.[141,355] Similarly, intermittent, changing, or random auditory input can cause an increase in auditory sensitivity.[346,370] Because of auditory system connections, an increase or decrease in initial input or auditory sensitivity has the potential for drastically affecting many other areas of the CNS.[371] The connections to the cerebellum could affect the regulation of muscle tone. The collaterals projecting into the reticular formation could affect arousal, alertness, and attention, in addition to muscular tone. The importance of voice level has been acknowledged by colleagues for decades with respect to encouraging clients to achieve optimal output or maximal effort. The use of voice levels is a critical aspect of the entire PNF approach.[29] Yet the volume or intensity of a therapist's voice is only one aspect of this important clinical tool. Through clinical observation, it has been observed that clients respond differently to various pitches.[346] The response patterns and specific range of comfortable pitch seem to be client dependent. The concept that each individual may have a range within the musical scale or even a specific note that is optimal for biorhythm function has been proposed by one composer-musician.[372] This concept needs research verification but may prove to relate to one of those innate talents some therapists have that distinguish them as gifted therapists.

The emotional inflections used by the clinician certainly have the potential to alter client response.[348,349] For example, assume the therapist asks Tim, a child with cerebral palsy, to walk. The specific response from the child may vary if the clinician's voice expresses anger, frustration, encouragement, disgust, understanding, or empathy. Knowing which emotional tone best coincides with a client's need at a particular moment may come with experience or sensitivity to others' unique needs.

Extraneous Noise. The varying level of sound or extraneous noise in a clinical setting can at times be overwhelming. Dropping of foot pedals, messages over loudspeakers, conversations, computers, printers, telephones, moans, a jackhammer outside the clinic, water filling in a tank, a drip in a faucet, whirlpool agitators, a burn patient screaming, and a child crying all are encountered in the clinical environment, and all could be occurring simultaneously. A therapist whose CNS is intact usually can inhibit or screen out most of the irrelevant sound, although his or her voice may rise according to the surrounding noise and the therapist may not even be aware of the vocal change.[347] Clients with CNS damage may not have the ability to filter sensitivity to all these intermittent noise sensations.[361] The protective arousal responses these sounds might produce in a client could certainly elevate tone, block attention to the task, heighten irritability, and generally destroy client progress during a therapy session. Awareness of the noisy environment and the client's response to it not only is important for treatment modalities but also is critical to the problem-solving process.

Decreasing auditory distracters or sudden noises can drastically improve the client's ability to attend to a task or to succeed at a desired movement.[343,373] The therapist is reminded that if the environment has been externally adapted for a client to procedurally and successfully practice the goal, then independence in that functional skill has not been achieved. Reintroduction of the noises of the external world must be incorporated into the client's repertoire of responses so that the individual can feel competent in dealing with any auditory environment the world might present.

Music. Music as an adjunct to therapy has been suggested as a viable way to help clients develop timing and rhythm in a movement sequence (see Chapter 20 for a discussion of basal ganglia disorders and Chapters 5 and 39 for a discussion of music therapy). Consistent sound waves and tempos, such as soft music, allow the patient to develop a neuronal model or an engram for the stimulus. The use of background music during therapy sessions enables the patient to make an association to the sounds, producing an autonomically induced relaxation response to a particular musical composition.[374-376] Therapists must remember that music has a very strong emotional link to all other areas of the nervous system.[377] For that reason, the use of music needs to be discriminative and not randomly introduced because the therapist likes the sound. Similarly, the music selected should be a piece that assists the patient and does not become a deterrent to succeeding at the current motor task. The clinician will easily tell the difference by the tone the music creates (increase or decrease) and the success made toward achieving the desired task.

Music is used for encouraging not only motor function but also memory[378,379] and socialization.[380-382] Rhythmic sound perceived as an enjoyable sensation certainly has the effect of creating motor patterns in response to that rhythm. Individuals, young and old, will tap their fingers or feet to a beat. If the beat has words, people will often sing along, recalling from memory the appropriate words. The movement, memory, and willingness to interact are all critical aspects of the therapeutic environment. Having clients dance with a significant other twice a day to music they have enjoyed in the past encourages both the physical function and the social bonding so important for quality of life.[383] Music affects heart rate, blood pressure, and respiration.[384,385] It has even been suggested that easy listening music may bolster the immune system.[386-390]

Auditory Biofeedback. Biofeedback as a total therapeutic modality is discussed under the treatment sections in Chapters 33 and 39. Auditory biofeedback is generally thought of as a procedure in which sound is used to inform the client of specific muscle activity.[360,362] The level or pitch may change in relation to strength of muscle contraction or specific muscle group activity. Yet auditory biofeedback also encompasses feedback as simple as a foot slap that communicates that a client's foot is on the floor or verbal praise after a successful therapeutic session.[359] The importance of the auditory feedback system as a regulatory mechanism between internal and external homeostasis cannot be overlooked. However, the clinician should not assume that this system is intact and can automatically be used as a normal feedback mechanism for clients with CNS damage.[112,361,391]

Language. Although most therapists thoroughly appreciate the complexity of the language system as a whole, they have little if any in-depth background to help them understand the components or the sequences leading to the development of language.[364,392,393] Thus many therapists are extremely frustrated when confronted with clients who show perceptual or cognitive deficits involving the auditory processing system.

Therapists easily identify language comprehension difficulties with adults who have first language differences and with young children because of their age and lack of language experience. Nevertheless, many clients have a language processing dysfunction that leads to communication difficulties, both in reception and appropriate expression.[351] The elderly often can understand a conversation in a quiet room but have difficulty in rooms that are noisy.[371,394,395] The environment within which communication occurs can drastically affect both reception and the ability to express to the world inner feelings and thoughts.[387] Creating an environment conducive to that exchange will dramatically affect the motivation and drive of a patient within the therapeutic setting.[388] The complexity of auditory reception, processing, and responses is extremely extensive and could be overwhelming to a PT or OT, but developing an understanding of how auditory information affects motor performance will certainly enhance the therapist's analysis of movement problems.[396,397]

Visual System

Treatment Alternatives with Use of the Visual System. Because light is an adequate stimulus for vision, any light, no matter the degree of complexity, has the potential to affect a client's CNS. That input not only reaches the optic cortex for sight recognition and processing but also projects to the brain stem and to the cerebellum through the tectocerebellar tract. Simultaneously, these afferents activate the reticular-activating and limbic spinal generators through the tectospinal tract.[296,398] Thus, as long as light is entering a client's CNS, it has the potential to alter response patterns either directly—through the tectospinal system or the corticospinal system through occipitofrontal radiations—or indirectly through the influence of the ANS and limbic system on muscle tone resulting from emotional responses to light.[399]

The five categories of visual-system treatment alternatives should not be considered fixed, all-inclusive, or without overlap. The first three categories (color, lighting, and visual complexity) are common everyday visual stimuli. Combined, they make up the visual world.

Colors. When colors, hues, tones, the type of lighting, and the degree of complexity of the combined visual stimuli are varied, the treatment modality and the way the CNS processes it change.[400-407] Because the visual system tends to adapt to sustained, repetitive, even patterns, any input falling under those parameters should elicit visual adaptation.[141,408,409] This adaptation response will lead to decreased firing of sensory afferent fibers and have an overall effect of decreasing CNS excitation. A clinician would expect to see or palpate a decrease in muscle tone, a calming of the client's affective mood, and a generalized inhibitory response. Cool colors, a darkened room, and monotone color schemes all seem to have an inhibitory effect. What a therapist might look for is a change in a patient's behavior. For example, four days ago Patient A was placed on the green mat for therapy and he seemed interactive, calm, and involved in producing motor function. On the next day, he came to therapy and the red mat was available. When Patient A got on the mat he became agitated and inattentive. The next day again Patient A was placed on the red mat and again was agitated and distracted. On day four, Patient A was placed on the green mat and had a great therapy session. On this fourth day he was calm, interactive, and involved in regaining motor function. It would be easy for a therapist to miss behavioral changes occurring when a patient is placed on a green or a red mat. These problems should be anticipated when treating patients with emotional instability (see Chapters 5, 14, 23, 24, and 26).

In contrast, intermittent visual stimuli, bright colors, bright lights, and a random color scheme seem to alert the CNS and have a generalized facilitatory effect.[410-412] Research in the 1980s in the area of criminology has produced evidence to suggest that specific shades of colors can produce either a sedating response (such as certain pinks) or general arousal (certain blues).[413] Although a tremendous amount of research is required to substantiate these results if the clinician is to apply them with confidence, research is beginning to show that specific shades of colors and hues may drastically affect a client's general response to the world and specific response to a therapy session.[403,404,407,414] Within the next few years, many facts regarding the reaction of the CNS to specific visual stimuli may be uncovered, and the clinician will be responsible for integrating this new information into the present categorization scheme.[415] Although a person without body system problems may react in specific ways to color, intensity, and visual distracters, individuals with CNS may not respond with the same behavior.[416] In the Netherlands at the Institut de Hartenbuer, playrooms have been designed in different colors.[14] Except for color, all rooms are exactly the same and originate from a central hub or core.[14] Children are allowed to select which room they wish to play or be treated in. Children seem to pick the color room that most suits their moods and alertness and creates an environment in which they can learn.[14]

Lighting. Two types of lighting are found in a clinical environment. Fluorescent or luminescent lighting comes by definition from a nonthermal cold source. This type of lighting is generally emitted by a high-frequency pulse. Umphred (clinical observations, 1967 to 2005) has found that many individuals within a normal population complain that this high-frequency flutter is irritating and causes distraction. For this reason, it is recommended that each clinician observe clients' responses to various types of lighting to determine whether fluorescent visual stimuli cause undesirable output.[417] This is especially true with clients who already have an irritated CNS, such as those with inflammatory disorders (see Chapter 26), head trauma (see Chapter 24), or seizure disorders.[418,419] The clinician should also remember that clients frequently lie supine and look directly at overhead lighting, whereas the therapist looking at the client is unaware of that particular visual stimulus. The types of visual stimuli that may cause seizures and are seen by clients within rehabilitation settings include computers, videogames, television, and venetian blinds.[417] For that reason, any change in lighting should alert the clinicians to watch for changes in their clients' behavior.

Incandescent lights by definition come from hot sources and emit a constant light without a frequency. The brightness of this type of lighting has the potential to alter CNS response. The visual system quickly responds to bright lights with pupil constriction. After prolonged exposure to a bright environment, the visual system adapts and becomes progressively less sensitive to it.[141,408] Similarly, when exposed to darkness the retina becomes more sensitive to small amounts of light. Because of the response of the visual system to incandescent lighting, it is recommended that a therapist monitor the brightness of the lighting, especially before any type of visual-perceptual training or visually directed movement.

Although the sun is a natural source of light, it is not generally the primary source in a clinical setting. The sun can effectively be used as indirect lighting, thus eliminating the problems produced by artificial lighting. Sunlight is also more acceptable psychologically. Some clinics have designed the buildings to allow for maximum use of natural light.[13]

Visual Complexity. The visual system is the primary spatial sense for monitoring moving and stationary objects in space.[420,421] An infant continually refines the ability to discriminate objects in external space until capable of identifying specific objects amid a complex visual array.[409] When brain damage occurs, the ability to identify objects, localize them in space, pick them out from other things, and adapt to their presence may be drastically diminished.[268] Because of the distractibility of many clients, reducing the visual stimuli within their external space can help them cope with the stimuli to which they are trying to pay attention. Using rooms that have been stripped of such stimuli as furniture and pictures can reduce not only distractibility but also hyperactivity and emotional tone. If this method of reduction of stimuli is used, the clinician must remember that this procedure has a sequential component. The client must once again adapt to extraneous visual stimuli. Thus as the client's coping mechanisms improve, the therapist needs to monitor and change the visual environment. The therapist can monitor the amount of input according to the response patterns of the client but in time needs to have the client function in everyday environments and practice adaptation.

Cognitive-Perceptual Sequencing with the Visual System. In sighted individuals the visual system is important for integrating many areas of perceptual development, such as body schemes, body image, position in space, and spatial relationships.[268,422,423] Vision as a processing system is so highly developed and interrelated with other sensory systems that when intact it can be used to help integrate other systems.[395,424] Conversely, if the visual system is neurologically damaged, it can cause problems in the processing of other systems.

For example, assume that a child is asked to walk a balance beam while fixating on a target. The child is observed falling off the beam. On initial assessment vestibular-proprioceptive involvement would be primarily suspected. On further testing the therapist might discover that the child, while looking at the target, switches the lead eye in conjunction with the ipsilateral leg. As the child switches from right to left eye, the target will seem to move. Knowing the wall is stationary, the child will assume the movement is caused by body sway, will counter the force, and will fall off the beam. The problem is a lack of bilateral integration of the visual system in contrast to other sensory modalities. The visual system deficit is overriding normal proprioceptive-vestibular input to avoid CNS confusion. Unfortunately, the client is attending to a deficit system and negating intact ones. This visual conflict would be overriding the normal processing of intact systems.[425]

An intact visual system can be overridden by deficits in other systems. This can be seen in clients who are trying to relearn the concept of verticality. Clients with hemiplegia who demonstrate a "pusher" syndrome illustrate this conflict. This clinical problem originates from a posterior thalamic stroke and less frequently with extrathalamic lesions.[426,427] An intact visual system can often be used to help reintegrate other sensory systems. First teaching clients to attend to vestibular-proprioceptive cues while vision is occluded or visual stimuli tremendously reduced will help present a kinesthetic conflict. Individuals feel straight at 20 degrees or more to the ipsilesional side yet when not supported they fall. This conflict does not need to be verbally discussed. The patients' nervous systems will interpret the conflict. The intent of the CNS is not to fall. If the patient does not automatically self-correct, the therapist can add reaching patterns across midline to assist. Then vision can be reintroduced to assist orientation to vertical or upright posture. The pusher syndrome is not just a posterior thalamic problem and can be combined with neglect. When additional perceptual problems are added, the testing results and direction of the backward push can change.[428] Once the orientation has been reestablished, visual input will often be perceived in a more normal fashion. This syndrome has been linked to the posterior thalamus as well as other integrative cortical areas within the brain.[427,429-432]

Familiarity with the visual-perceptual system and its interrelationships with all aspects of the therapeutic environment is crucial if the clinician is to have a thorough concept of the client's problem. (See Chapter 28 for specific information regarding visual deficits and treatment alternatives.)

Mental Imagery. As is mentioned in the discussion of neuroplasticity in Chapter 4, and as is discussed further in the section on somatosensory retraining within this chapter, having patients visualize the sensory awareness of input from the environment has a positive effect on treatment outcomes. Similar positive effects have been shown to be effective when having patients practice motor imagery as part of the treatment protocol.[137,433-436] It is known today that using mental imagery to retrieve past information or experiences does use a variety of pathways within the CNS, depending on the specific task.[437] Having some cognitive understanding of the correlation between cortical deficits in specific patients and their visual-spatial problems helps the clinician avoid task-specific activities that will lead to failure while introducing task-specific mental imagery that will lead to success.[438] Having the patient practice mental imagery of the functional activity practiced during a therapeutic session can be an excellent way to empower patients to practice when they cannot perform the activity itself independently, without extreme effort and abnormal movement strategies.[155,439] A therapist will know whether the patient has mentally practiced the movement strategies by the carryover within the next session. The neurophysiological reason for this perceived contradiction may lie in neuroanatomy, site of the lesion, specificity of the individual client.[156,439,440] Although imagery usually insinuates visualization, there are also other forms of imagery that can be used as part of intervention.[155,437,439,441-443] Refer to the music therapy section in Chapter 39 for information on mental imagery.

One extension of mental imagery that came into common usage in the 1990s as a result of videogame popularity was "virtual reality." Over the last two decades the interface between virtual reality and medical education has included the use of a virtual environment to teach surgeons fine motor skill without having them practice on a live subject.[444] An inevitable link has currently been identified between virtual reality and motor rehabilitation.[445-448] Today the literature certainly reflects the potential advantage virtual reality may have with regard to not only motor learning but also the use of these environments as an adjunct to therapy in individuals with CNS damage.[449-455] The future realization of the potential of this type of augmented intervention will be up to visionary thinkers who "push the envelope" of traditional therapeutic interventions.

Compensatory Treatment Alternatives with Use of the Visual System. The visual system can be used effectively as a compensatory input system if the sensory component of the tactile, proprioceptive, or vestibular system has been lost or severely damaged. The procedure for using vision in a compensatory manner should not be attempted until the clinician is convinced the primary systems will not regain needed input for normal processing. Although vision can direct and control many aspects of a movement, it is not extremely efficient and seems to take a tremendous amount of cortical concentration and effort.[418,456,457] Vision was meant to lead and direct movement sequences.[297,420,458] If it is used to modify each aspect of a movement, it cannot warn or inform the CNS about what to expect when advancing to the next movement sequence. Thus, using vision to compensate eliminates one problem but also takes the visual system away from its normal function. For example, if a hemiplegic man is taught to use vision to tell him the placement of his cane and feet, his need to attend to proprioceptive cues will decrease. When advancing to ambulatory skills such as crossing the street, the client may be caught in a dilemma. As he is crossing the street, if he attends to the truck coming rapidly down the road, he will not know where his cane or foot is and thus will become anxious and possibly fall. If, on the other hand, he attends to his foot and cane, he will not know if the truck is going to hit him. That may increase emotional tone and make it difficult to move. If normal sensory mechanisms could be reintegrated, this client would have freedom to respond flexibly to the situation. Thus caution should be exercised to avoid automatic use of this high-level system to compensate for what seem to be depressed or deficit systems.[225,226,309,459,460]

Visual input should be used to check or correct errors if other systems are not available. Movement should be programmed in a feed-forward mode unless change is indicated. Vision often recognizes the need for that change. If a client is taught a motor strategy in which vision is used as feedback to direct each component of the pattern, the pattern itself will generally be inefficient and disorganized and will lack the automatic nature of feed-forward procedural motor plans. If the client is too anxious to practice the procedure physically without overusing vision, then visual mental practice can be introduced.

Internal Visual Processing: "Visualization Techniques." A previous section discussed mental imagery as a substitute in the presence of a sensory deficit or as a practice method for when a patient cannot perform a motor task. The use of visualization of some aspect of bodily function goes far beyond just mental practice. Visualization has been and continues to be used in many forms of therapy.[459] In a randomized controlled study that looked at normal bone healing versus the use of a specific type of yoga that involves breath control, chanting, and visualization as an adjunct treatment, the individuals who practiced this yoga-based approach had accelerated fracture healing.[461] It has been shown that individuals can modulate their immune responses and that others can change that response through visualization.[460,462] Smith and colleagues[460] showed that individuals could exercise through their thoughts and visualization various degrees of control over what had been thought to be mindless internal processes. These concepts have been used therapeutically but usually when the client is resting or totally relaxed.[225,226,309]

More recently, technology in neuroscience has allowed for the measure of tissue metabolism (positron emission transaxial tomography [PET])[463] and changes in blood flow (fMRI) while the brain is engaged in functional mental tasks.[464,465] All areas of the brain except the cerebellum appear to be activated during intense goal-directed mental imagery. Given that the task is not motorically executed, errors in rhythm and accuracy are not made, and thus the cerebellum is not recruited for correction. This suggests that mental imagery can be used to restore a function that might have been lost as the result of a stroke or other type of injury because the individual may be able to use kinesthetic memory to facilitate learning even if current kinesthetic recognition is impaired.[466] Visual imagination has the benefit of allowing correct task performance when physical limitations may prevent normal task completion. This could prevent abnormal learning (e.g., like that developing from abnormal posturing in gait in a stroke patient who lacks the voluntary control to ambulate and integrate a primitive synergy). For additional information, see the section on somatosensory discrimination.

Today these concepts can be integrated during active treatment in a variety of ways. Before a client begins to initiate a plan of movement, the therapist could ask the client to close the eyes and imagine the movement and what it felt like in that functional activity before the CNS injury. In this way, the patient is using prior memory and visualization to access the motor systems and hopefully initiate better motor plans. Similarly, if during a movement plan the state of the motor generators builds to such a level that the client is becoming dysfunctional, the therapist can stop the movement; ask the client to visualize a calm, quiet place; and then continue with the movement pattern when the tone is reduced or extraneous patterns cease.[467] The client can be asked to practice mental imagery of the task until she or he can accomplish it normally and then finally carry it over to the real environment.[468,469] For example, a client may have practiced transferring during an intervention session in which the therapist, using augmented treatment, kept the patient within a biomechanical window or limits of stability. During the interval between sessions, the patient is asked to visualize performing transfers initially from the same surface practiced and later to other surfaces at least a couple of times an hour. At the follow-up session, the therapist will often be able to tell if the patient has done the visualization. If the patient did practice, there is often carryover into the skill performance. If the patient forgot to practice, often the skill has reverted back to the initial level of learning, with little carryover from the last intervention.

Another way to use the visual system to access the processing strategies of the client is to observe eye gaze. Neurolinguistic theory postulates that the eyes gaze in the direction of brain processing.[264,468] Figure 9-4 illustrates the eye gaze direction along with the suggested processing activity. For example, a client who needs to access and process motor plans through the frontal lobe will look down. A client who needs to visually construct an idea of something new will look up and to the right. Various cortical lobes and hemispheres serve specific global processing functions. There are many ways to apply and interpret this theory. By observing the patient's eye gaze, the therapist can determine whether processing is conducted in what would be believed to be the appropriate areas. Even more clinically relevant is observing where the eyes are gazing before and during successful functional activities. It may be that the area once used in processing is no longer available to do the function. If gazing to the right and down always leads to motor success, then the therapist can empower the patient to look down and right before dressing or transferring. Similarly, if a patient always looks down at the feet during ambulation, the reason may not be "to look at the feet" but instead may be to access the motor cortex to gain better motor function. If the client is asked to visualize the movement before and during the activity, the head often comes to a posturally correct position as the eyes gaze upward toward the occipital lobe and the body automatically orients to vertical. If the client is asked to walk while visualizing the movement, again the result may be a more upright, posturally efficient pattern. Once the program is set and practice scheduling begun, the patient may no longer need to look down and into the frontal lobe. Thus in this case the client not only learned the procedure but also avoided practicing and learning a posturally incorrect ambulation strategy.

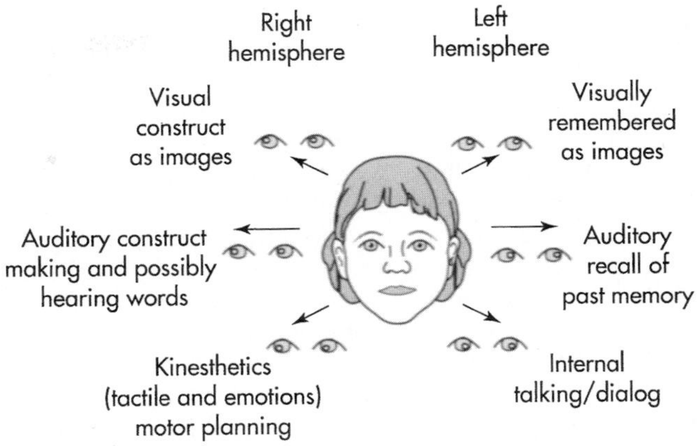

Figure 9-4 ■ Eye gaze: correlation with lobe and hemispheric processing based on right-handed individuals. (Modified from a handout from New Learning Pathways, Denver, 1988. Illustrations by Ben Burton.)

Combined Multisensory Approaches. Although all techniques have the potential to be multisensory, the specific mode of entry may focus on one sensory system, as already described, or it may target two or more input modalities along with automatic motor programming. As stated before, Table 9-5 categorizes a variety of treatment techniques that are clearly multisensory. The therapist, analyzing how the summated effect of the combined input and automatic responses influences client performance, gains direction in anticipating treatment outcomes in terms of the problem-solving process. Because the potential combinations of multisensory input classification are enormous, only a few examples of combinations are included in the text to illustrate the process a clinician might use when classifying a new technique or a new approach to intervention. When clinicians select augmented treatment interventions to help a client as part of somatosensory retraining or functional retraining or to establish a procedural program, the basic science understanding behind the clinical decision helps develop questions for future research, determine a prognosis regarding outcomes, and rationally explain why or why not an intervention was effective. Clinical decisions must ultimately be made regarding which techniques or component of an approach should be eliminated first as the patient progresses. These decisions must be based on understanding and integration of neurophysiological mechanisms, learning environments, concepts of motor learning and control, and what motor impairment or body system problems are affecting functional performance and on the client's and family's needs, motivations, and goals. A simple rule a therapist might follow would be to take away the least natural technique first. That technique would be the most artificial or contrived. An example using only one sensory system might help to clarify this point. For example, a therapist might assist a client with elbow flexion during a feeding pattern by (1) vibrating the biceps, (2) quickly tapping the biceps, or (3) quickly stretching the biceps a little beyond midrange by using gravity. The first option would be the least natural and obviously the least socially acceptable at a dinner party. The third option is the most natural and closest to what might occur in the real environment in which the client will need to function. Remember, these contrived techniques are used to assist clients who cannot control or perform the motor programs or functional activities without assistance or who need assistance in learning to modulate motor control for greater functional adaptability. If the therapist added verbal feedback or music as well as asking the patient to visually look at the target, the example would become multisensory.

Within the following section are examples of combined multisensory approaches that might be used to augment sensory feedback to obtain a better environment for regaining functional control.

Sweep Tapping. Sweep tapping is usually used to open a hypertonic flexor-biased hand. Many isolated techniques, such as sweep tapping[111] or rolling,[8] would be considered primarily proprioceptive-tactile in sensory origin. During sweep tapping the clinician first uses a light-touch sweep pattern over the back of the fingers of one of the hands. This stimulus is applied quickly over the dermatome area that relates to muscles the client is being asked to contract. Second, the therapist applies some quick tapping over the muscle belly of the hypotonic muscle. The first technique is tactile and believed to stimulate the reflex mechanism within the cord to heighten motor generators and increase the potential for muscle contraction of the hypotonic muscle or to dampen the hypertonic flexors. The second aspect, tapping, is a proprioceptive stimulus used to facilitate afferent activity within the muscle spindle of the extensors, thus further enhancing the client's potential for muscle contraction. At the same time the client will be asked to voluntarily activate the extensor motor system, which then automatically augments tactile, proprioceptive, and auditory input with functional control.

Rolling of the Hand. Before Brunnstrom's rolling pattern is implemented, the client's upper extremity is placed above 90 degrees to elicit a Souque's sign. This decreases abnormal, excessive tone in the arm, wrist, and hand.[8] This phenomenon may well be a proprioceptive reaction of joints and muscle. The rolling technique consists of two alternating stimulus patterns. The wrist and fingers are placed on extensor stretch. The ulnar side of the volar component of the hand is the stimulus target. A light-touch sweeping pattern is applied to the hypothenar aspect, which has the potential to elicit an automatic opening of the hand beginning with the fifth digit.[8] Immediately after the light touch, a quick stretch is applied to the wrist and finger extensors. These two techniques are applied quickly and repeatedly, thus giving the visual impression that the therapist is rolling his or her hand over the ulnar aspect of the dorsum of the client's hand. In reality, tactile and proprioceptive stimuli are being effectively combined to facilitate the central pattern generators responsible for the extensor motor neurons controlling the wrist and finger musculature. Because the tone is felt in the client's extensors and thus induces relaxation of the hypertonic flexors, the therapist can more easily open the client's hand. As the client obtains volitional control, some resistance can be added by the therapist to further facilitate wrist and finger extension. A hemiplegic client can also be taught to use this combined approach to open the affected hand and give it increased range. This technique is a noninvasive, relaxing approach to opening the hand stuck in wrist and finger flexion hypertonicity. The technique itself also seems to trigger spinal generator patterns that dampen the existing neuron network. It does not teach the patient anything unless that individual begins to assist or take over control of the extensor pattern. This usually occurs first when the therapist feels the flexors relax while the patient is trying to extend the wrist and fingers even if no active extension is palpated. Encouraging the patient at this time, confirming that he or she is thinking correctly, and urging him or her to continue doing it provide important motivation for continued practice.

Withdrawal with Resistance. A therapist could combine the technique of eliciting a withdrawal with resistance to the withdrawal pattern. This can be an effective way to release hypertonicity, especially in the lower extremities. The withdrawal can be elicited by a thumbnail, a sharp instrument, a piece of ice, or any adequate light-touch stimulus to the sole of the foot. As soon as the flexor withdrawal is initiated, the therapist must resist the entire pattern. Once the resistance is applied, the input neuron network changes and the flexor pattern is maintained through the proprioceptive input caused by resistance to the movement pattern. The one difficulty with this technique is the application of resistance. The withdrawal pattern directly affects alpha motor neurons innervating those muscles responding in the flexor pattern and simultaneously suppresses alpha motor neurons going to the antagonistic muscles. If the antagonistic muscles are hypertonic, then initially the hypertonicity is dampened within the alpha motor neurons' neuronal pool. Because of the pattern itself, as soon as the flexor response begins, a high-intensity quick stretch is applied to the extensor muscles. If resistance is not applied to the flexors to maintain inhibition over the antagonistic muscles, the extensors will respond to the stretch. The client will quickly return to the predisposed hypertonic pattern and may even exhibit an increase in abnormal tone. This extensor response is a complex reaction within the spinal generators. The therapist should instruct the patient if appropriate to assist with the flexor pattern to recruit other components of the motor system to enhance the system's modulation over the spinal generators. This can be a way to generate the early component of rolling when leading from the lower extremity and can get the patient out of an extreme extensor pattern in the supine position.

Touch Bombardment. Another example of a proprioceptive-tactile treatment technique is modification of a hypersensitive touch system through a touch-bombardment approach. The goal of this approach is to bombard the tactile system with continuous input to elicit light-touch sensory adaptation or desensitization. Deep pressure is applied simultaneously to facilitate proprioceptive input and conscious awareness. Proprioceptive discrimination and tactile-pressure sensitivity are thought to be critical for high-level tactile discrimination and stereognosis. A hypersensitive light-touch system elicits a protective, altering, withdrawal pattern that prevents development of this discriminatory system and the integrated use of these systems in higher thought. This method of treatment can be implemented by having an individual dig in sand or rice. The continuous pressure forces adaptation of the touch system, and the resistance and deep pressure enhance the proprioceptive-discriminatory touch system by a complex adaptation process that most likely affects all areas involved in light and discriminatory touch, as well as the complex interaction of all motor system components. Whereas sand is often used in the clinic or outside, rice can be used inside and vacuumed easily whether in the clinic or in a patient's home.

Pool therapy can be used effectively for the same purpose, with the added advantage of neutral warmth, as long as the temperature is in the neutral warmth parameters. Heat increases the sensitivity of light touch, whereas cold initially heightens the nervous system. In time cold can suppress the state of the motor pool (refer to the section on cold). Any client perceiving touch as noxious, dangerous, and even life-threatening will not greatly benefit from any therapeutic session in which touch is a component. Touch includes contacts such as touching the floor with a foot, reaching out and touching the parallel bar railings, and touching the mat. The client may not respond with verbal clues such as "Don't touch me" or "When I touch the floor it hurts" but will often respond with increased tone, emotional or attitude changes, and avoidance responses. Nevertheless, this treatment approach has application in many areas of intervention with clients having neurological deficits. As an adjunct to this method, a clinician should cautiously apply light touch when in contact with the client. Deep pressure or a firm hold should elicit a more desirable response for the client even if the light-touch system is functional.[212,320] The use of Gore-Tex material for clothing can greatly enhance the client's ability to tolerate the external world, where light-touch encounters cannot be avoided. Similarly, socks can decrease the hyperactive tactile system in the foot and may allow the patient to stand or transfer without the feeling that he is standing on pins or that it is a noxious stimulus.

The therapist may also consider systematic desensitization as a strategy to integrate the touch system. By allowing patients to apply the stimuli to themselves, they can grade the amount that they can tolerate. In this respect they are empowered to control their own environment. They can practice adaptation in many situations. When the environment seems overwhelming, they have learned techniques to dampen the input both from within their own systems and by controlling the external world. For example, the therapist may place a box containing objects of different textures before the patient and encourage exploration and active participation to learn which textures are acceptable or offensive. A gradual exposure to the offensive stimuli will raise the threshold of the mechanoreceptors in the skin. There are also the benefits to the patient of being in control of the stimulus and having awareness of the treatment objectives. In addition, vibratory stimuli through a folded towel provide proprioceptive input to desensitize the touch system.[188,268,320] Desensitizing the touch system from a need to protectively withdraw is an important process within the CNS if normal stereognosis is to develop.

Taping. Taping procedures normally used in peripheral orthopedic muscle imbalances and pain have the same potential for patients with neurological problems. This adaptation would be a modification of both splinting and slings. Research has been done to demonstrate efficacy of taping to offset peripheral instability in individuals with neurological system impairments.[282,470-474] The concepts and ideas remain that taping has implications when treating individuals with neurological problems. Taping hypotonic muscle groups into a shortened range should effectively reduce the mechanical pull of gravity on both the muscle groups and joints and prevent the CNS from developing the need for compensatory stabilization or hypertonicity. If hypertonicity is the result of peripheral instability, then taping a hypertonic muscle into its shortened range should stabilize the peripheral system and eliminate the need for the CNS to create the hypertonic pattern. On the other hand, taping can also be used to heighten information about proprioception and joint position, providing feedback to avoid hyperextension or hypermobility of a joint. This is especially true when there is an imbalance of intrinsics and extrinsics in the hand.

Oral-Motor Interventions. There are more research articles available on specific oral-motor dysfunctions in patients with neurological problems[475-480] than on intervention. These are studies using fMRI of the CNS during oral-motor activity, but the transition to intervention again is limited.[481,482] Systematic reviews of potential oral-motor interventions are even fewer.[483]

When dealing with oral-motor intervention, the complexity of combined proprioceptive-tactile input becomes enhanced by adding another sensory input, such as taste. Implementation of one of a variety of feeding techniques clearly identifies the complexity of the total input system. When taste is used, smell cannot be eliminated as a potential input, nor can vision if the client visually addresses the food. The following explanation of feeding techniques is included to encourage the reader to analyze the sensory input, processing, and motor response patterns necessary to accomplish this ADL task. The complexity of the interaction of all the various systems within the CNS is mind-boggling, but if the motor response is functional, effortless, and acceptable to the client and the environment, then the adaptation should be facilitated after attended repetitive behaviors.

Several feeding techniques have been developed in the past by master clinicians such as Mueller,[301] Farber,[111] Rood,[25] and Huss.[296] These techniques were not easily mastered or understood through reading alone. Competence in feeding techniques is best achieved through empirical experience under the guidance of a skilled instructor. Today, some evidence base for implementation of feeding techniques or related motor activities can be found in the literature.[52,484,485]

The facial and oral region plays an important role in survival. Facial stimulation can elicit the rooting reaction. Oral stimulation facilitates reflexive behaviors, such as sucking and swallowing. Deeper stimulation to the midline of the tongue elicits a gag reflex. These reactions and reflexes are normal patterns for the neonate. When these reactions and reflexes are depressed or hyperactive, therapeutic intervention is a necessity. Oral facilitation is an important treatment modality for infants and children with CNS dysfunction. Therapeutic intervention during the early stages of myelination can be crucial to the development of more normalized feeding and speech patterns.

Similarly, adults with neurological impairment often have difficulty with oral-motor integration. Problems with swallowing, tongue control, and hypersensitive and desensitive areas within the oral cavity and also with mouth closure and chewing are frequently observed in adults with CNS damage.[475,476]

Before basic feeding techniques are implemented, clinicians need to understand how the CNS and PNS work collaboratively with the musculoskeletal system to control and perform these complex oral-motor functional movements.[141,486,487] Feeding therapy is preceded by observation and examination. With a pediatric client the therapist should observe breathing patterns while the client is feeding to determine whether the child can breathe through the nose while sucking on a nipple. In addition, the child's lips should form a tight seal around the nipple. Formal assessments should include functional assessments, developmental milestones, and behavioral manifestations. Medical charts and results from neurological examinations should be consulted for baseline data.

Postural mechanisms can influence feeding and speech patterns in clients with neurological dysfunction.[28,485,488] A client with a strong extensor pattern may have to be placed in the side-lying, flexed position to inhibit the forces of the extensor pattern. The ideal pattern for feeding is the flexed position, which promotes sucking and oral activity. Basic reflexes such as rooting, sucking, swallowing, and bite and gag reactions should be elicited and graded in children and evaluated in adults. The head needs to be in slight ventroflexion to pull in the postural stabilization of the neck and tongue. This is necessary to effectively facilitate programs that provide functional swallowing and control of foods by the tongue.

The facial region and the mouth have an extraordinary arrangement of sensory innervation. Therefore oral techniques must be used with utmost care. Anyone who has visited the dentist can attest to the feeling of invasiveness when foreign objects are placed in the mouth. With this in mind, the therapist should begin each treatment session by moving the autonomic continuum toward the parasympathetic end. Activation of the parasympathetic system should lower blood pressure, decrease heart rate, and, more important, increase the activity of the gastrointestinal system. Neutral warmth, the inverted position, and slow vestibular stimulation should help to promote parasympathetic "loading." Another approach that is applicable to feeding techniques is the application of sustained and firm pressure to the upper lip. An effective inhibitory device is a pacifier with a plastic shield that applies firm pressure on the lips. Perhaps this is why a pacifier is a "pacifier." Adults can acquire resistive sucking patterns with a straw and plastic shield and achieve the same results.

Sometimes children or adults are not cooperative and will not open their mouths.[489,490] Rather than the mouth being pried open, the jaw is pushed closed and held firmly for a few seconds. On release of the pressure, the jaw reflexively relaxes. The receptors in the temporomandibular joint and tooth sockets may be involved in the production of this response.

A common problem seen in neurologically impaired infants and adults with head trauma is the "hyperactive tongue," which is often accompanied by a hyperactive gag reflex. To alleviate this problem, the receptors have to be systematically desensitized. The technique called *tongue walking* has met with clinical success.[12,41] It entails using an instrument such as a swizzle stick or tongue depressor to apply firm pressure to the midline of the tongue. The pressure is first applied near the tip of the tongue and progressively "walked back" in small steps. As the instrument reaches the back of the tongue, the stimulus sets off an automatic swallow response. The instrument is withdrawn the instant the swallow is triggered. This technique is repeated anywhere from five to 30 times a session, depending on individual responses.

Another technique, which might be called *deep stroking,* is used to either elicit or desensitize the gag reflex. Again, an instrument such as a swizzle stick is used to apply a light stroking stimulus to the posterior arc of the mouth. The instrument should lightly stretch the lateral walls of the palatoglossal arch of the uvula. Normally, the palatoglossal muscle elevates the tongue and narrows the fauces (the opening between the mouth and the oropharynx). Just behind the palatoglossal arch lies another arch, called the *palatopharyngeal arch.* Normally, this structure elevates the pharynx, closes off the nasopharynx, and aids in swallowing. Touch pressure to either arc incites the gag reflex. This touch pressure should be carefully calibrated. A hyperactive gag reflex may be best diminished by prolonged pressure to the arcs, whereas light, continuous stroking may be more facilitatory in activating a hypoactive gag reflex. A child or adult who has been fed by tube for extended periods of time will often have both hypersensitive reactions in various parts of the oral cavity and hyposensitive areas in other locations. This problem needs to be assessed to formulate a complete picture of the client's difficulties.

The use of vibration over the muscles of mastication appears to be physiologically valid. Muscle spindles have been identified in the temporal and masseter muscles.[39] Selected use of vibration on the muscles of mastication enhances jaw stability and retraction. For protraction to be facilitated, the mandible is manually pushed in.[111]

To promote swallowing, some therapists use manual finger oscillations in downward strokes along the laryngopharyngeal muscles and follow up with stretch pressure. Ice is beneficial as a quick stimulus to the ventral portion of the neck or the sternal notch. In addition, chewing ice chips provides a thermal stimulus to the oral cavity and a proprioceptive stimulus to the jaw and teeth; it also increases salivation for swallowing.

It is recommended that a therapist work closely with a colleague who has experience working with functional feeding before independently beginning to work with clients. The possible complications that might develop with individuals aspirating food cannot be overemphasized.[491]

The therapist can quickly realize that feeding as a proprioceptive, tactile, and gustatory input modality is extremely complex and often incorporates other sensory systems. Breaking down the specific approaches into finite techniques helps the clinician categorize each component and then reassemble them into a whole. The job of dividing and reassembling the parts becomes more and more difficult as the number of input systems enlarges.[267]

Head and Body Movements in Space. Proprioceptive and vestibular input is one of the most frequent combination techniques used by therapists. In fact, client success in almost all therapeutic tasks depends on the coordinated input of these two sensory modalities.

If the head is moving in space and gravity has not been eliminated from the environment, vestibular and proprioceptive receptors will be firing to inform the CNS whether it should continue its feed-forward pattern or adapt the plan because the environment no longer matches the programmed movement. Depending on the direction of the head motion and the way gravity is affecting joints, tendons, and muscles, the specific body response will vary according to the degree of flexibility within the motor system. Bed mobility, transfers, mat activities, and gait all incorporate these two modalities. Although all these functional movements can be performed without these feedback mechanisms, the CNS cannot adapt effectively to changing environments without input from these systems. For that reason alone, a thorough examination of the integrity of both systems and the effect of their combined input seems critical if any ADL is to be used as a treatment goal.

The use of a large ball or a gymnastic exercise ball can be classified under the category of proprioceptive-vestibular input. Many activities can be initiated over a ball. When a child or adult is prone on a ball, righting of the head can often be elicited by quickly projecting the child forward while the therapist exerts control through the feet, knees, or hips. If the weight of the head is greater than the available power, then a more vertical and less gravitationally demanding position can be used. As the head begins to come up, approximation of the neck can be added. Vibration of the paravertebral muscles might also assist. Rocking forward or bouncing the client who is weight bearing on elbows or extended elbows will facilitate postural weight-bearing patterns through the two identified sensory input systems. Having a client sitting on a therapy ball doing almost any exercise will require vestibular and proprioceptive feedback for appropriate adaptive responses to be made. The combination seems to play a delicate role in the maintenance of normal righting and the equilibrium response so important in functional independence.

A trampoline, balance board, or similar apparatus has the potential to channel a large amount of vestibular-proprioceptive input into the client's CNS. In fact, a trampoline is so powerful it can often overstimulate the client and cause excitation or arousal in the CNS.

The trampoline and balance board are generally used to increase balance reactions, orient the client to position in space and to verticality, and increase postural tone. A client with poor balance, poor postural tone, or inadequate position in space and verticality perception may be justifiably fearful of these two apparatus because of the rate, intensity, and skill necessary to accomplish the task. Because fear creates tone and that tone may be in conflict with the motor response from the client, caution must be exercised with either modality. (See Chapter 22A for further discussion of the interactions of sensory systems and balance.)

Gentle Shaking. A specific technique of gentle shaking can be listed under a combined vestibular, muscle spindle, and tendon category. This technique is performed while the client is in a supine position and the head ventroflexed in midline. The head is flexed 35 to 40 degrees to reduce the influence of the otoliths and unnecessary extensor tone through the lateral vestibulospinal tract. This flexed position should be maintained throughout the procedure. The therapist places one hand under the client's occiput and the other on the forehead. Light compression is applied to the cervical vertebrae. This technique activates the deep-joint receptors (C1 to C3) and muscle spindles in the neck along with the vestibular mechanism, which in turn connects with the cerebellum and motor nuclei with the brain stem. If the technique is performed slowly and continuously in a rhythmical motion, total-body inhibition will occur. If the pattern is irregular and fast, facilitation of the spinal motor generators will be observed.

Any one of these techniques can be implemented as a viable treatment approach in considering vestibular-proprioceptive stimuli. The selection of an approach or a method will depend on client preference, client response, the clinician's application skills, and the need for therapeutic assistance.

Summary of Techniques Incorporating Auditory, Visual, Vestibular, Tactile, and Proprioceptive Senses

Most therapeutic activities activate five sensory modalities: auditory, visual, vestibular, tactile, and proprioceptive. Auditory and visual inputs are used as the therapist talks to the client, asks the patient to look, and/or demonstrates the various movement or response patterns to be accomplished during an activity. As the client moves, vestibular, tactile, and proprioceptive receptors are firing as inherent feedback systems. Thus the complexity of any activity with respect to analysis of primary input systems is enormous. Even a sedentary activity such as card playing requires a certain amount of proprioception for postural background adaptations, tactile input from supporting body parts and limbs, and visual input for perception and cognition. When treating an individual with CNS damage, one or a number of sensory systems may not be processing at all or may be processing incorrectly, which confounds the clinical problem even farther.

Thus when the categorization of techniques—such as a PNF slow reversal,[19] a Brunnstrom marking time,[8] marking time with music,[492] Feldenkrais's sensory awareness through movement,[225,226] NDT,[31,493] Rood's mobility on stability,[25,28] or any mat or ADL activity—is considered, the therapist must observe the sensory systems being bombarded during the activity. At the same time, if the therapist has determined which sensory systems are intact, which are suppressed or dysfunctional, and which seem to be registering faulty data, then altering duration and intensity of the input environment through any one system and the combined input through multiple systems creates tremendous flexibility in the clinical learning environment. Understanding this diagnostic process leads to more accurate prognosis and selection of appropriate interventions. Highly gifted therapists seem to instinctively go through this diagnostic process. One skill that seems consistent among master clinicians is a highly developed sensitivity to the client's responses, which represents a summation of expression of all systems within the CNS. Simultaneously, they adjust the quantity and duration of combined input to best meet the needs of the client. These masters release external control and encourage the client to use normal, inherent monitoring systems to adapt to changing environments as soon as the client is able to function independently, no matter if that is only 5 degrees of motion or an entire functional pattern made up of many motor programs. Control may begin within a part of the range of a functional skill and not necessarily the entire functional activity itself. Therapists must remember that when the control comes from the clinician and not the patient, it is then augmented. The key to carryover will be the client's empowerment over the motor control system and the degree of practice, self-monitoring, and adaptation available to the client. By analyzing and categorizing input and patient responses, many therapists may develop skills that were initially considered out of reach. Today, clinicians have the examination tools to validate changes in their patients' motor behavior (refer to Chapter 8).

Innate Central Nervous System Programming

The responses of the PNS and CNS to various external stimuli determine the individuality of an organism and its survival potential within the environment. As organisms become more and more complex, the types of external stimuli and the internal mechanisms designed to deal with that input also increase in complexity. As the CNS develops structurally and functionally, inherent control over responses to certain common environmental stimuli seems to be manifested. Different areas of the motor system play different roles in the regulation of motor output. No area is dominant over another. Each area is interdependent on both the input from the environment and the intrinsic mechanisms and function of the nervous system.

As mentioned earlier, the PNS is intricately linked to the CNS and vice versa. Damage to one could potentially alter the neuropathways, their function, and ultimately behavior anywhere along the dynamic loops. Nevertheless, although researchers today emphasize the dynamic interactions of all components,[494-501] clinicians have observed for decades different motor problems when different areas of the brain are damaged. Thus, when clients with neurological damage are discussed, it seems paramount to identify inherent synergy patterns available to humans, especially if those patterns become stereotypical and limit the client's ability to adapt to a changing environment.

The authors do not recommend or discredit the use of any stereotypical or patterned response as a treatment procedure. Acknowledging the presence and stressing the importance of knowing how these motor programs affect clients' functional skills are important. Without this knowledge, therapists working with either children or adults with CNS dysfunction limit their understanding of the normal CNS, the normal motor control mechanism and its components, and the interactive effect of all systems on the end product: a motor response to a behavioral goal.

To conceptualize a systems model, the reader must replace the hypothesis of a stimulus response–based concept of reflexes[308] with a theory of neuronetworks that may be more or less receptive to environmental influences (see Chapter 4).[502] That sensitivity is modulated by a large number of interconnecting systems throughout the CNS and by the internal molecular sensitivity of the neurons themselves. Specific motor patterns seem to be organized or programmed at various levels or areas within the CNS. These synergies or patterned responses are thought to limit the degrees of freedom available to programming centers such as the basal ganglia and cerebellum[11,231] and to enable more control over the entire body. Having soft-wired, preprogrammed, patterned responses allows organizing systems to activate entire sequences of plans and modify any components within the total plan. Modification and adaptation then become the goal or function of the motor system in response to both internal and external goal-directed activities. The specific location of soft-wired programs is open to controversy, as is the complexity of programming at any level within the CNS. Recognizing that these neuronetworks exist with or without external environmental influences would suggest that patterns can and will present themselves without an identified stimulus. In the past, when an external influence was not correlated with an identifiable stereotypical motor pattern, it was referred to as a *synergy.* When a stimulus was identifiable, the entire loop was called a *reflex.* Reflexes and preprogrammed, soft-wired neuronetworks such as walking are interactive or superimposed on one another to form the background combinations for more complex program interactions. This superimposed network may encompass spinal and supraspinal coactivity, which makes it difficult to specify a level of processing. The exact control mechanisms that regulate the specific pattern may again be a shared responsibility throughout the nervous system, thus providing the plasticity observed when disease, trauma, or environmental circumstances force adaptation of existing plans, as discussed in the neuroplasticity section (see Chapter 4).

One way to conceptualize this complex neuronetwork is to picture a telephone system linking your home to any other home in any city in any country on the planet. If the relay between a friend in New York and you in California develops static, the system may self-correct, relay through another area, or even route through a nonwired mechanism such as a satellite. The options are infinite, but priorities for efficiency and adaptability exist within both the telephone network and the brain. If the wires to your home are cut, the phone will not ring. If your peripheral nerve is cut or the alpha motor neuron damaged, the muscle will not contract. If the relay centers at one end of your block are short-circuited and not working properly, then your phone and those of your neighbors may still function, but not in a fluid or specific manner. That is, someone may be calling your neighbor but both your phone and your neighbor's phone might ring. Spinal involvement can create a similar problem. The muscles are innervated and the input from the environment is accurate, but the neuronetwork is faulty. Regulation or modulation may be less efficient or controlled, but the system will use all available resources to try to respond to internal and external environmental requirements. This rule seems consistent throughout the nervous system, and the degree of plasticity is tremendous.[503]

When specific patterned responses are observed, the reader must always hold simultaneously the interaction of all other motor programming options. In this way the therapist can easily conceptualize the variations within one response and the reason why, under different environmental and internal constraints, the motor response pattern may show great variations within the same general plan. Similarly, the expected motor response may not be observable, although it would seem appropriate and anticipated. The clinician must remember that the more complex the action (e.g., rolling compared with dressing compared with playing hockey), the greater the need for integration and coordination over pattern generators. Similarly, the more complex the desired action (especially in new learning), the greater the potential for needed perceptual-cognitive and affective interactions and the greater the potential for gratification and also for failure.

Certain patterned responses or neuronetworks might be considered more simplistic or protective in function. These patterns were once thought to be hard-wired spinal reflexes. It is now known that these reflexes, as well as complex pattern generators, exist at the spinal level and that their responses affect brain stem, cerebellar, and cortical actions. These centers simultaneously affect the specifics of the spinal neuronetwork responses.[129,130,504] With clients who have low functional control over the spinal or brain stem motor networks, identifying existing patterns, optional patterns as a response to environmental demands, and obligatory patterns not within the control of the client's intentional repertoire of patterns becomes a critical evaluative component before prognosing or identifying the most appropriate interventions.

Recognizing specific patterns and how those patterns and others might affect functional movement or positional patterns has clinical significance. A child with spastic cerebral palsy, for instance, shows extension and "scissoring" when the pads of the feet are stimulated. Sometimes the extension pattern is so strong that the child will arch backward. Sustained positions that oppose pathological patterns are believed to elicit autogenic inhibition. Contraction-relaxation techniques also work on the autogenic inhibition principle.[19]

Just as afferent input can be used to alter tone and elicit movement, it can also become an obstacle when the therapist tries to coordinate complex movement patterns. The human palmar and plantar grasp patterns are often thought of as reflexive patterns, as seen in a newborn.[505-507] A persistent grasp pattern is a common occurrence in children and adults with a CNS insult. This dominant grasp is often reinforced by the client's own fingers and frequently prevents functional use of the hand. If a withdrawal pattern is elicited every time a client is touched, the client not only will be unable to explore the environment through the tactile-proprioceptive systems but also will experience arousal by the influence of the cutaneous system over the reticular activating system. Severe agitation could likely be a behavioral outcome from such a persistent reflex.

As with any treatment procedure, a clinician should determine whether the technique will help the client obtain a higher level of function. The clinician must learn to recognize not only specific patterns but also what combinations of responses of pattern generators would look like. If the reader overlaid the map of the pattern generators for any combination of programs, a complex neuronetwork would result. To some it would verify chaos theory, and to others it would verify the end result of multiple systems interacting. The neuronetwork complexity of multiple input can be overwhelming. Thus a therapist must always be observant of the specific behavioral response and the moment-to-moment changes in behavior during a treatment session, even if the specific neuronetwork is not understood.

The clinician needs to observe whether the specific patterned response is (1) triggered by afferent input, (2) triggered by volitional intent, or (3) activated without environmental input including position in space or cortical intent. In the third case, the entire motor system needs to be evaluated to determine which portion might be modulating the observable behavior. Differentiating these motor components will help in selecting appropriate examination tools, making the movement diagnosis, prognosing, and selecting interventions.

Holistic Treatment Techniques Based on Multisensory Input

As already mentioned, a variety of accepted treatment methods exist. Each approach focuses on multisensory input introduced to the client in controlled and identified sequences. These sequences are based on the inherent nature of synergistic patterns,[5,30] the patterns observed in humans[5,7,249] and lower-order animals,[33] or a combination of the two.[19,28] Each method focuses on the total client, the specific clinical problems, and alternative treatment approaches available within each established framework. Certain methods have traditionally emphasized specific neurological disabilities. Cerebral palsy in children[7,23,28,508-510] and hemiplegia in adults[8,9,21,31,511,512] are the two most frequently identified. In the past two decades, substantial clinical attention has been paid to children with learning difficulties.[12,35,513-515] Yet the concepts and treatment procedures specific to all the techniques have been applied to almost every neurological disability seen in the clinical setting. This expansion of the use of each method seems to be a natural evolution because of the structure and function of the CNS and commonalities in clinical signs manifested by brain insult. Literature in occupational and physical therapy management of individuals with various other neurological problems has also enriched therapists' identification of efficacious interventions as well as those that should be removed from the toolbox.[519,516-521]

Additional Augmented Interventions: Today's Focus

Four augmented therapeutic intervention approaches that have become accepted over the last decade are (1) BWSTT, (2) constraint-induced movement therapy (CIMT), (3) imagery (discussed in the section on the visual system) and virtual reality, and (4) robotic training. Each is discussed as a separate intervention philosophy, but the reader must remember that these are *augmented intervention* programs. Before an individual would be considered functionally independent, the patient must be able to perform the functional activity in a natural environment, such as ambulation within a home setting or eating using the more involved extremity without having the unaffected extremity restrained. A fourth augmented intervention approach, robotics, will also be presented briefly within this chapter in order to illustrate how therapists and patients have the capabilities to interface with new and sophisticated technology. The reader is also referred to Chapter 38 for more in-depth detail. One additional augmented approach, the Accelerated Skill Acquisition Program (ASAP), has been described here. This approach is currently undergoing, and research is still needed to establish efficacy. This approach is impairment oriented, emphasizes bimanual activities, and focuses on active, patient-centered collaboration reinforced with self-management and self-efficacy.[522-525] This approach emphasizes attended, repetitive task practice progressing in difficult situations and meets the principles for neuroplasticity.

Body-Weight–Supported Treadmill Training. Over the last decade BWSTT has been accepted within the therapeutic community as an alternative approach to teaching gait training for individuals with CNS damage and residual motor dysfunction. Students are introduced to the treatment procedures and potential sequences from total dependence to independence of the patient. Colleagues take continuing education courses to learn to position and drive the various motor components of the gait program while using BWSTT. Both a vertical support (harness) or air-distributed positive pressure to unweight the body and a treadmill are combined for BWSTT. The treadmill perturbs the feet backward or shifts the center of gravity forward, and the ground reaction forces are reduced by the support. The clinical environment unloads the CNS's need to (1) provide protection from falling; (2) trigger and control an effective and efficient postural system reaction; (3) reflexively drive the power stepping reaction necessary to perform upright ambulation; (4) control the balance strategy of stepping to prevent falling; (5) facilitate rhythmic, symmetrical, bilateral stepping; and (6) have a cognitive interface with the various motor programs necessary to run this functional activity. The treadmill perturbation of the lower limb into extension facilitates the transfer of weight to the forefoot. This forward translation forces the feet backward and optimizes the stepping reaction forward. If the moving treadmill is not a sufficient stimulus to trigger a step, this component can be controlled by one or two therapists depending on whether it is a unilateral or bilateral problem. If the patient does not step, has a delayed stepping response, or steps effectively with only one foot, the therapist(s) can help to initiate the desired response at the patient's feet. The rate of movement or speed of the treadmill can also be controlled, as well as the length of time spent on the affected leg. This treadmill strategy may encourage more symmetrical and faster gait speed in patients after stroke[526] and with Parkinson disease[527-529] compared with standard physical therapy. This control by the therapist helps to facilitate a patient's response even if it is slow or inadequate for normal over-ground ambulation. The question remains whether this type of augmented therapeutic intervention does create the best environment to empower the patient to learn or relearn normal locomotion after a neurological insult.

The literature is mixed with regard to this question. The literature supports BWSTT for individuals with incomplete spinal injury,[520] the elderly with Parkinson disease,[521] and some individuals after stroke,[138,522] but other literature suggests that BWSTT is equivalent to or maybe less effective than over-ground gait training with a PT,[533,534] and still other researchers report that there is no difference among different forms of ambulation training.[534] With the literature so inconsistent, the clinician could be confused as to the effectiveness of BWSTT and whether this type of augmented intervention should even be considered. One primary problem with the research literature is the great variance in training and the identified variables selected by researchers within their respective studies.[136,532,535-537] The following are examples of potential variables:

- Walking speeds
- Frequency of training
- Length of training
- Aerobic levels of training
- Type of unweighting
- Endurance
- Type and severity of the patient's neurological dysfunction
- Presence of hypertonicity
- Age of patient
- Time since injury
- Level of independence
- Assistance needed during ambulation

There have been some excellent systematic reviews of BWSTT in the literature that help identify many of the reasons the literature seems so inconsistent.[136,538] The research indicates that the two populations of individuals who most often benefit from use of BWSTT are people with incomplete spinal cord injuries and individuals poststroke. Another problem in BWSTT research is that the harness systems can be uncomfortable at 20% to 30% unweighting.[539] Thus, as stated, the huge number of possible variables and functional ways to measure outcomes using BWSTT or other types of training along with BWSTT has led to confusion in the literature.[532,534,537,540,541] Even with all the confusion regarding these variables, this form of augmented intervention seems to show promise as a protocol for gait training. Future research studies will still need to determine which patients, their degree of motor involvement, the optimal dosage, the time after insult, the best combination of other interactive interventions (e.g., pharmacological, robotic), the specific type of gait impairments, and where within the gait cycle the clients would most likely benefit from this type of augmented intervention. It is important to continue to obtain evidence to more precisely define the practice guidelines for BWSTT. As has been shown in the past, new treatment ideas gain popularity and become standards of practice without the rigor of establishing an evidence-based practice.[35,36,42,542] Physical therapy and occupational therapy need to establish that evidence as proof of the evolving effectiveness of clinical practice.

Constraint-Induced Movement Therapy. CIMT (or CI therapy) is a type of treatment of clients with motor system limitations that combines constraint or immobilization of the unaffected arm with forced use of the affected limb. A hand mitt or sling is used to constrain the use of the unaffected upper limb while the affected limb is engaged in a forced-use, mass practice meaningful motor task. The treatment focus of CIMT is on shaping behavior to improve functional use of the impaired upper limb.[543,544] CIMT is based on the theory that impairment in hand and arm function in clients after a stroke is compounded by learned nonuse of that affected upper extremity, which leads to a physical change in the cortical representation of the upper limb in the primary sensory cortex.[545] Learned nonuse develops in the early stages after a stroke in humans as the patient compensates for difficulty using the impaired limb by increasing reliance on the intact limb. This compensation has been shown to hinder recovery of function in the impaired limb.[546]

CIMT and the learned nonuse theory are based on deafferentation experiments in monkeys done by Dr. Edward Taub.[547,548] Early primate studies demonstrated that if the upper limb was surgically impaired by dorsal rhizotomy to disrupt afferent input to the sensory cortex, the animal stopped using the limb for function. Active mobility was restored by immobilizing the intact upper limb for several days while training the animal to use the affected limb.[546] The first report of CIMT for hemiparesis in humans was by Ostendorf and Wolf in 1981.[549] Since then, investigations have demonstrated the effectiveness of CIMT with individuals who have residual upper-extremity weakness as the result of an upper motor neuron lesion.[549-559] CIMT has been shown to be an effective therapy in persons with chronic stroke who have sufficient residual motor control to benefit from the exercises,[550-552,557,560-565] in brain-injured patients,[566,567] in children with hemiplegic cerebral palsy,[543,568-573] and in patients with Parkinson disease.[574] The CI therapy approach has also been used successfully for the lower-limb rehabilitation of patients with stroke hemiparesis, incomplete spinal cord injury, and fractured hip.[553] Other diverse chronic disabling conditions, including nonmotor disorders such as phantom limb pain and aphasia, may also benefit from CIMT.[553]

The criteria for the inclusion of subjects in most CIMT research studies have focused on voluntary movement ability in the involved upper extremity.[549,543-560,565] These criteria included the ability to start from a resting position of forearm pronation and wrist flexion and actively extend each metacarpal-phalangeal and interphalangeal joint at least 10 degrees and extend the wrist at least 20 degrees through a ROM.[561] It is estimated that approximately 20% to 25% of the population of patients with chronic stroke with residual motor deficit meet this motor criterion.[575]

Not all patients with hemiparesis have been found to benefit from CIMT. It has not been shown to be beneficial for clients with severe chronic upper-extremity hemiplegia after a stroke.[576] Attempts to include individuals who did not meet the minimal motor criteria (at least 10 degrees of finger extension and 20 degrees of wrist extension) have failed to demonstrate significant or lasting functional improvements in the involved upper extremity after CIMT.[553,576]

The criteria associated with successful therapeutic components of CIMT therapy are (1) restraint of the unaffected arm with a mitt, sling, or glove for 90% of waking hours for a 2- to 3-week period; and (2) therapeutic sessions with physical and occupational therapy in which patients concentrate on intense, repetitive task training of the more affected upper extremity for 8 hours a day.*

Clients typically participate in 6 to 7 hours of therapy a day; in addition, clients must reinforce this training in home activities and ADLs.[546,564,572,575] The therapist-client ratio is typically 1:1, with the therapist present to give tactile and verbal feedback and instruction, along with assistance for the desired skill training. Clients also typically keep a daily treatment diary to document the amount and intensity of therapeutic intervention and the amount of time spent wearing the mitt or sling each day for the duration of the intervention.[572]

*References 550, 551, 554, 555, 557, 558, 560, 565, 573, 574.

Subjects with chronic stroke hemiparesis who have participated in CIMT rehabilitation programs have demonstrated significant gains in functional use of the stroke-affected upper extremity as measured by the Motor Activity Log,[575] significant reductions in motor impairment on the upper-extremity motor component of the Fugl-Meyer Test,[576] and more efficient task performance as measured by the Wolf Motor Function Test.[577-581] Fine motor improvements have also been measured with use of the Grooved Pegboard Test and other dexterity tests.[545,546] These improvements in impairment and function have been shown to persist at follow-up evaluations up to 2 years after training.[545,559,573,580] Individuals participating in CIMT studies have demonstrated improvements in the amount of use and quality of movement in the more involved upper extremity and carryover of skills from the clinic to real-world activities.[549-551,572] This functional improvement may be significant even if the patient has previously participated in a conventional rehabilitation program.[582]

The question of when to begin CIMT after a stroke has not yet been definitively answered. CIMT has been applied to clients with subacute strokes. This early use of CIMT is based on the hypothesis that earlier intervention may prevent learned nonuse and may have a greater impact on overall function. Investigators have found no adverse effects of CIMT in the subacute phase and only slightly greater improvement in motor function of the affected upper extremity.[583] There is some evidence from animal studies to suggest that if CIMT is introduced too early (e.g., 24 hours poststroke), it may be detrimental and potentially harmful to humans. It may cause an increase in the size of the cortical lesion. This is based on studies of "forced overuse" in animals.[584-587] Kozlowski and colleagues[587] found that early forced overuse of the affected limb within the first 7 days after a sensorimotor cortex lesion impeded motor recovery of the affected limb and enlarged lesion volume. Bland and co-workers[584] also forced overuse of the affected forelimb immediately after a focal cortical middle cerebral artery stroke, which increased the lesion size and impaired motor recovery. The relative risks and benefits of "acute" CIMT, and its optimal timing, remain to be determined.[546]

The neurophysiological mechanisms that are believed to underlie the treatment benefit of CIMT include overcoming learned nonuse and plastic brain reorganization.[582,588] Studies have confirmed that CIMT produces use-dependent cortical reorganization in humans with stroke-related paresis of an upper limb.[551,559,588,589] There is some question, however, as to whether the improvements in upper-extremity motor function after CIMT are a result of the reduction of learned nonuse or of overcoming a sense of increased effort during movement.[545] Thus, task-specific, goal-oriented training with the affected limb might be similarly beneficial, even without the constraint of the less affected side.

Neuroimaging studies such as transcranial magnetic stimulation (TMS), fMRI, and electroencephalography[411,545] have been used to provide cortical evidence of neuroplasticity and cortical changes after CIMT.[554,559,572,590] These studies have validated that massed practice of CIMT produces a massive use-dependent cortical reorganization. This change increases the area in which the cortex is involved during voluntary movements of an affected limb, even in patients with chronic stroke.[546,591]

The application of CIMT to real-life clinical environments presents some challenges, including the time and physical demands on therapists, the cost to the patient, and the resources required during rehabilitation. This limits its cost-effectiveness and overall effect.[546] Many patients in the acute rehabilitation setting do not qualify for CIMT on the basis of limited motor function.[546] CIMT, by its nature, can prove to be difficult, frustrating, and intense, and progress can be slow. It will create beneficial effects only if all participants put in the time and effort to make it successful.[572] Many subjects who have been presented with the opportunity to participate in CIMT programs and studies have refused because of the intense practice schedule and the necessity of the restrictive device.[592] Therapists have also voiced concerns about patient adherence and safety.[592] Although it has been shown to be effective in laboratory research, CIMT may have limited practicality in some clinical environments.[592]

The future success of CIMT will depend on its ability to be modified according to disease factors, economic considerations, limitations of the practice setting, and the cognitive and physical status of the patient. Less intense practice schedule models[590,593,594] and combining CIMT with pharmacological interventions or robotic assistance may help increase its effectiveness and decrease costs without sacrificing the benefits.[546,595] Studies are now underway to determine if massed task-specific practice without constraint can be equally beneficial.[596,597] Patient satisfaction, overall cost, and the impact on quality of life are other areas that require further evaluation.[598]

Robotics, Gaming, and Virtual Reality (See Chapter 38). The most recent augmented intervention procedures involve the use of technology to regain control over functional movement and are the third and fourth approaches mentioned in the first sentence in this section. The use of robotics,[599-602] virtual reality,[603-606] and gaming[607-610] in the clinical environment continues to gain popularity as such technology continues to be more affordable, and their applications are becoming more widespread. A thorough discussion of these technologies can be found in Chapter 38.

Summary of Augmented Intervention Strategies. As with many interventions, the therapist may need to start with augmented approaches to reduce impairments and/or gain functional movement in a controlled environment. As the patient demonstrates improvement in this narrow window of movement or function, the clinician could then increase the challenge with the goal of optimizing functional performance and improving quality of life. A summary of the augmented intervention strategies that facilitate neuroplasticity can be found in Box 9-2.

Case Examples: Using Augmented Intervention Strategies to Optimize Functional Performance

Case Study 1: *Client with Lack of Head Control.* There is a potential for lack of head control in young, developmentally delayed children or in individuals who have sustained a severe injury to the CNS. For that reason it is a common clinical problem. Furthermore, because of the importance of head and neck control, virtually all functional activities are affected by its absence.

The client is Timothy, a 16-year-old adolescent male with a closed-head injury. He had a lesion in his CNS 3 months ago and currently demonstrates the following attributes regarding head control:

- Mild extensor hypertonicity is present in the supine position, and Timothy is unable to flex and rotate his head off the mat.
- In prone position, extensor hypertonicity is absent and hypotonicity prevails. The client is able to briefly bob his head off the mat in a hyperextension pattern. Mild tonal shifts occur to either side when the head is turned and when it is symmetrically flexed or extended.
- Timothy is unable to roll or perform any functional activity in the horizontal plane.
- When placed in a long sitting position, he is unable to hold the position or sit with flexed hips and extended knees. His head remains in total flexion with his chin on his chest.
- When placed in a short sitting position on a mat table, he is unable to hold the position. General hypotonicity prevails, although slightly more flexion is palpable. His head remains flexed. When asked to pick up his head, he extends into a hyperextension pattern followed by extensor relaxation into flexion.
- He is unable to hold the head in a neutral postural coactivation pattern in a vertical position.
- Timothy does not mind being touched and responds well to handling techniques.

From the analysis of these clinical signs, the following clinical interpretations are presented:

1. In the horizontal position, Timothy has persistence of a motor program that is enhanced by the spatial position and its influence on the vestibular system. The result might be considered persistence of a tonic labyrinthine reflex (TLR). In this client the dominant synergic pattern is extension. While he is supine, extension prevails. While he is prone, extension is inhibited, although flexion tone is not dominant. Because of the persistence of hyperactivity among the extensor motor generators, the ability to initiate rolling using a neck-righting pattern is prevented. The presence of a mild, asymmetrical tonic neck reflex to both sides and a symmetrical tonic neck reflex has been noted. Because of his instability and low tone, Timothy seems to be using these stereotypical patterns volitionally to assist in gaining some control over his motor patterns. In prone position, Timothy has the ability to move into a neck extension or optic and labyrinthine righting (OLR) pattern but is unable to hold it. Thus movement and range are present but postural holding is missing.
2. As a result of ventroflexion of the head in sitting, the vestibular apparatus is placed in a position similar to that when prone. In a like manner, the total patterns remain fairly consistent. The increase in flexor tone may result from the positioning of hip and knee flexion and kyphosis of the back. The inability to flex the hips with knee extension suggests that total tonal patterns or synergies are dominant. The client is unable to break out of those dominant patterns. Dominant OLR is not present.
3. When asked, Timothy carries out the command to the best of his motor ability. This suggests the presence of

BOX 9-2 ■ SUMMARY OF INTERVENTION STRATEGIES TO FACILITATE NEUROPLASTICITY

There are many different intervention strategies to use when working with patients with neurological problems. These interventions need to be matched to the needs of the individual patient and be consistent with the patient's goals and objectives. All the intervention strategies should be goal directed and repeated with attention to both the input mechanisms (motivation, sensory) and the output mechanisms (movement). The input and output mechanisms are multifactorial, and they also involve all components of the sensory, emotional, sensorimotor, and motor systems. Although evidence is increasing about the benefit of learning-based activities, research is still needed to help define more precisely when intervention should occur, how intense the intervention should be, how much repetition is needed, how long the learning-based activities need to be continued and spaced, how specific the training needs to be, how quickly behaviors can be progressed and the magnitude of gradation needed, how to keep patients interested, motivated, and compliant in learning, and the magnitude of interference in learning relative to depression, stress, and loss of self-esteem. The intervention strategies can be broadly classified as follows:

1. General body responses leading to quieting of the nervous system[8,296]
   a. Slow rocking in a rocking chair or hammock.
   b. Slow anterior-posterior, horizontal, or vertical movements (chair, hassock, mesh net, swing, ball bolster, riding in a carriage, glider chair).
   c. Rotating equipment such as a bed, chair, stool, hammock, or therapeutic or gymnastic ball (e.g., rhythmical bouncing).
   d. Slow linear, undulating movements, such as in a carriage, stroller, wheelchair, or wagon.
   e. Wrapping up tightly before rocking (e.g., roll self in sheet; put both arms inside tight tee shirt).
   f. Listening to quiet music or natural environmental sounds (e.g., waves).
   g. Repeating activities listed above first with eyes open and then closed.
2. Techniques to heighten postural righting reactions[141]
   a. Rapid or unexpected anterior-posterior or angular acceleration.
      i. Scooter board: pulled or projected down inclines.
      ii. Prone over ball: rapid acceleration forward.
      iii. Platform or mesh net: prone.
      iv. Slides.
      v. Any proprioceptive input that heightens postural extensors (e.g., quick stretch, tapping, resistance, vibration, joint compression). Remember to use the most natural first, such as quick stretch versus vibration.
   b. Rapid anterior-posterior motion in prone position, weight-bearing patterns such as on elbows or extended elbows while rocking and crawling.
   c. Weight-shifting in kneeling, half-kneel, or standing positions (first in vertical and then off vertical within limits of stability by an activity itself [reaching]).
   d. Do activities with eyes closed.
   e. Create dual-task activities such as walking and talking, stepping over obstacles while on unstable surfaces, reading while maintaining balance in a confusing environment.
   f. Challenge balance in distracting environments (e.g., moving surround, multisensory stimuli in visual surround).
3. Facilitatory techniques to influence whole-body responses[30,111,295]
   a. Movement patterns in specific sequences.
      i. Rolling patterns.
      ii. Prop on elbows (prone and side-lying positions) and extend and flex elbows as well as crawling (e.g., side by side, or linear and angular motion).
      iii. Coming to sit (side-lying to sit [using upper trunk and head rotation], prone to four-point position to sit [four-point position to lower trunk rotation to side sit to sit], adult sit [full flexion leading with head]).
      iv. Coming to stand (squat to stand, half-kneel to stand, standing from a chair or stool).
   b. Spinning.
      i. Mesh net.
      ii. Sit and spin toy.
      iii. Office chair on universal joint.
   c. Any activity that uses acceleration and deceleration of head.
      i. Sitting and reaching.
      ii. Walking.
      iii. Running.
      iv. Moving from sit to stand.
      v. Doing activities with eyes closed, head still, and then eyes closed, head turning.
   d. Performing activities that require attention, memory, and cognitive processing at the same time.
4. Combined facilitatory and inhibitory technique: inverted tonic labyrinthine activities
   a. Inverted tonic labyrinthine activities.
      i. Semiinverted in-sitting (head between the legs).
      ii. Squatting to stand (head below heart).
      iii. Thirty degrees to total inverted vertical position beginning in supine.

Continued

BOX 9-2 ■ SUMMARY OF INTERVENTION STRATEGIES TO FACILITATE NEUROPLASTICITY—cont'd

b. Somatosensory and sensorimotor stimulation (refer to earlier in this chapter).
    i. See detailed progressive learning-based sensorimotor training (Appendices 9-B and 9-C).
    ii. Proprioceptive stimulation.
        (a) Vibration over joints.
        (b) Vibration in opposite direction of movement.
        (c) Wear weights around ankles or on belt.
        (d) Position the limbs and the trunk to match a position visually presented.
        (e) Move slowly to the count of a metronome and then change speeds.
        (f) Look at pictures and position the body to match the pictures.
c. Auditory discrimination (localization).

5. Techniques to facilitate specific task performance
    a. Forced use.
        i. Create training activities in which patients must use the affected extremity.
        ii. Minimize the need to use the unaffected side.
        iii. Use bilateral activities in which both hands and upper extremities are required.
    b. Constraint-induced movement therapy (CIMT) (forced use)[550-552,591,631,632] emphasizes the repetitive use of an impaired limb in regular functional activities by restricting the movement of the less affected or unaffected side.
        i. The patient is constrained from using the unimpaired limb on a concentrated task basis.
        ii. The impaired limb is used on a concentrated basis.
        iii. The theory is to reduce motor deficits early in the recovery period (learned disuse).
        iv. The assumption is that the nervous system is adaptable and training for recovery should begin as soon as possible.
        v. If the good arm is constrained, the patient must use the affected limb.
        vi. Set time limits to use the constraint; in one large randomized clinical trial the patients were asked to wear a protective safety mitt on the less affected upper limb for a goal of 90% of the waking hours for 14 consecutive days.
        vii. During constraint, the individual works under supervision on designated functional tasks for 6 hours a day.
        viii. The patient is encouraged to try to use the affected limb during waking hours.
        ix. The constraint is paired with motor or behavioral objectives.
        x. Tasks are practiced and progressed in difficulty or speed.
    c. Mass task practice (see Chapter 4).
    d. Mental imagery.
    e. Mental practice.
    f. Body-weight–supported treadmill training (BWSTT)[524-527,633]
    g. Integration of robotics and technology (see Chapter 38)
    h. Use of gaming (Wii Fit, Brain Fit)[604,607-610]

some intact verbal processing, which is translated into appropriate motor acts. Similarly, when asked to pick up his head, he does just that, suggesting some perceptual integrity of body image, body schema, and position in space. Knowing where his head is in space and where to reposition it also suggests that some proprioceptive-vestibular input and processing are occurring.

4. Timothy's enjoyment of being moved in space as related to handling techniques suggests proprioceptive-vestibular integrity. Similarly, his tactile systems seem to be functioning in a discriminatory manner and modifying negative responses of withdrawal and arousal. However, specific tactile perception would need a great deal of further testing. Thus he demonstrates functional strengths in cognition and perception, in limbic motivation, in some areas of sensory integrity, and in control over available but limited motor programming. Yet performance on any functional test would result in identification of an individual whose functional limitations prevent him from independence in any activity. Prognosis must be guarded until the therapist has had an opportunity to augment the environment to determine how quickly he will regain control and retain the learning. The initial plan of care is assumed to focus on development of head control as a preliminary and necessary motor program for all functional daily living activity. The estimated time it will take to regain this function will not be identified until after the first intervention session.

Movement Diagnosis. The client is unable to functionally control his head in any position in space, which limits independence in all functional activities. Lack of postural coactivation and adequate control over the motor generators has led to imbalances in the tonal characteristics of flexor and extensor patterns with the compensatory development of stereotypical patterns of movement.

Goal of Intervention Program. The goal is development of independent head control, initially in a vertical midline posture with the intent of enlarging that biomechanical window to include all positions in space.

Now that the clinical problem has been analyzed and the goal of development of head control set, an intervention sequence or protocol must be established. Timothy lacks head control in all planes and in all patterns of movement. Thus, flexors and extensors must be facilitated to develop a dynamic coactivation or postural holding pattern of the neck. The categorization scheme can now be of some assistance. The therapist can ask, "Are there any inherent mechanisms that enhance flexors or extensors in a holding pattern?" The optic and labyrinthine righting (OLR) reaction should elicit the desired response. Similarly, the clinician can ask, "Are there any inherent motor programs that would prevent righting of the head to face vertical OLR?" The TLR would block or modify the facilitation of OLR. Knowing that the TLR is most dominant in horizontal and least dominant (if at all affected) in vertical is of clinical significance. It is also important to know that the OLR is most frequently tested in a vertical position and seems most active in that position. Awareness that the client is sensitive to total patterns (e.g., flexion facilitates flexion or extension facilitates extension) gives additional treatment clues.

After all this information has been assimilated, the following treatment could be established.

For enhancement of neck flexors, the client will be placed in a totally flexed position in vertical, with the head positioned in neutral. The client will be rocked backward toward supine, allowing gravity to quick stretch the flexors (Figure 9-5, *A*). As soon as the neck flexors are stretched, the head should be tapped forward and then back to vertical but not beyond. This avoids hyperextension, extreme stretch to the proprioceptors, and the horizontal supine position of the labyrinths, all of which dampen the flexors and facilitate the extensors. The quick stretch and position should optimally facilitate OLR, which should activate the neck flexors. The total flexion of the body similarly facilitates the neck flexors. Once the neck flexors respond, Timothy can be rocked farther and farther backward while maintaining the head in vertical or ventroflexion (Figure 9-5, *B*). Once Timothy can be rocked from vertical to horizontal and back to vertical while maintaining good flexor neck control, his CNS has demonstrated inherent control and modification over the stereotypical patterns, such as the TLR in supine with respect to its influence over the neck musculature. This rocking maneuver can be done on diagonals to practice flexion and rotation (Figure 9-5, *C*), the key to eliciting a neck-righting, rolling pattern from supine to prone. The total flexed pattern can also be altered by adding more and more extension of the extremities. This decreases the external facilitation to the flexors and demands that Timothy's CNS take more and more control (internal regulation). Additional treatment procedures can be extracted from a variety of sensory categories. To add additional proprioceptive input, any one of those listed techniques might be used. The rotation and speed of the rocking pattern affect the vestibular mechanism. Auditory and visual stimuli can be used effectively. If the therapist takes a position slightly below the client's horizontal eye level, the client (to look at the therapist) will need to look down and flex his head, thus encouraging the desired pattern. Any type of visual or auditory stimulus that directs the client into the desired pattern would be appropriate. The therapist must remember that neck flexion is one of the identified goals. Rotation was added to incorporate and set the stage for inherent programming that will lead to rolling, coming to sit, and reaching while sitting. Because the postural extensor component still needs integration, total head control has not been attained. To facilitate neck extension, a procedure similar to the one for flexion can be established. A vertical position, thus eliminating the influence of the TLR, would again be the starting position of choice. For additional visual feedback on the development of flexor head control, refer to Chapter 3, Figures 3-15 through 3-18.

With extension facilitating extension, the client should be placed in as much extension as possible without eliciting excessive extensor tone. An inverted labyrinthine position, a kneeling position, or a standing position would be viable spatial patterns to facilitate OLR of the head and coactivation of postural extensors. The vestibular system sensory category can be checked to identify the treatment procedure for use with an inverted labyrinthine position. The kneeling or standing position places the client in a vertical position with hip and trunk extension. Kneeling rather than standing is used first because of the influence of the positive supporting reaction in standing and the massive facilitation of total extension. Kneeling avoids total extension while maintaining a predominant extensor pattern. As a result of the gravitational pull of body weight through the joints,

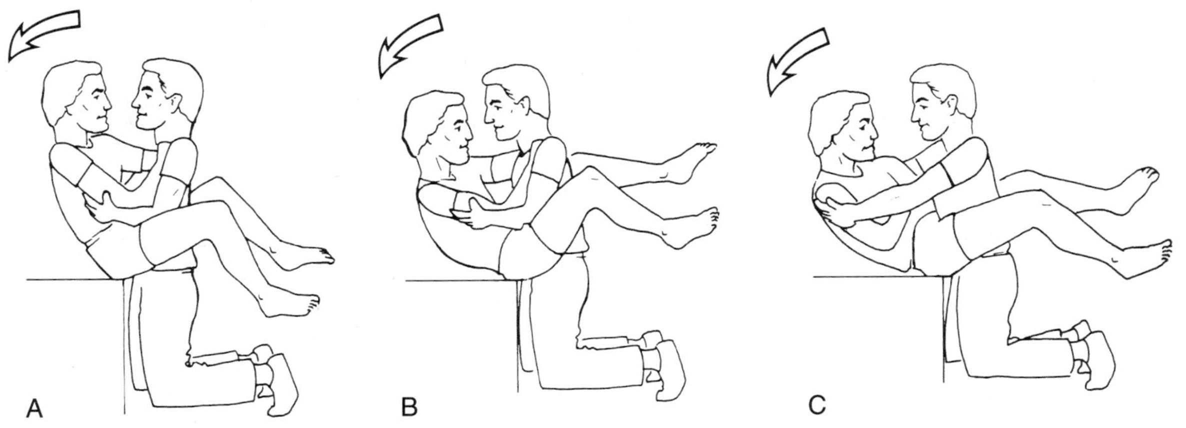

Figure 9-5 ■ Development of flexor aspect of head control. **A,** Vertical position: head at midline and midrange (total-body flexion) to optimally facilitate neck flexors. **B,** Facilitating symmetrical neck flexion, using position, gravity, and flexor positions. **C,** Facilitating flexion and rotation to develop pattern necessary for neck-righting pattern.

approximation to facilitate postural extension is constantly maintained. The upper extremities can be placed in shoulder abduction and external rotation, which tends to inhibit abnormal upper-extremity flexor tone and facilitate postural tone into the shoulder. This extensor tone has the potential through associated spinal reactions to facilitate neck and trunk extension. The arms can be placed in this position over a bolster or ball or by the therapist handling the client from the rear (Figure 9-6, *A*). The head should begin again in a neutral position. The client is rocked forward (Figure 9-6, *B*) to facilitate OLR of the head and to elicit a quick stretch to the postural extensors. If the head begins to fall forward, the therapist can tap the client's forehead immediately after the quick stretch. This tapping action is the reverse tap procedure described under the proprioceptive stretch receptors category. The tapping is done to passively move the head back to vertical.

A variety of additional procedures can easily be combined to summate facilitation to the postural extensors. Tapping, vibration, and approximation through the head to the shoulders are only a few of the proprioceptive modalities. All would be facilitatory. A variety of auditory and visual stimuli could be used to orient the client to a position in space and thus righting of the head. Techniques listed under the exteroceptive and vestibular systems could also be part of the treatment protocol. The therapist would want to sequence the client toward prone while the head remained in a vertical postural holding pattern. As the therapist rocks the client toward prone again, a rotational component should be added (Figure 9-6, *C*). The client will extend and rotate to counterbalance the movement, thus incorporating the neck-righting pattern of extension and rotation necessary when rolling from prone to supine. Resistance to neck extension with or without rotation is an important element in regaining normal functional control. The client is alert and has some functional use of the arms and legs. This rocking pattern in kneeling can be done as a functional activity. The therapist asks the client to assist in reaching toward an object with one upper extremity. The therapist can guide the client in the reaching pattern in a forward, sideward, or cross-midline direction. While reaching, the client can be rocked forward to elicit right and equilibrium reactions. In incorporating an activity into the treatment of head control, the client not only is entertained but also attends to the task rather than cognitively trying to keep his head up. In this way automatic head control is facilitated, and often postural patterns follow. In a partial kneeling pattern the client can be sequenced to on-elbow over a bolster or ball or on a chair. These activities should be sequenced from vertical to prone to ensure both total postural programming in prone and optimal integration of OLR, as well as to let the client experience control of various motor strategies in many different environmental contexts. For more analysis of the development of extensor head control, refer to Chapter 3, Figures 3-19, 3-21, and 3-22.

Once the client can maintain good flexor, extensor, and rotational components of head control, the activity should, if possible, be practiced with the client's eyes closed. If the client can still maintain head control, labyrinthine righting would be adequate for any functional activity. If the client loses head control, then additional labyrinthine facilitation would be indicated. If a client uses only vision to right the head, then any time vision is needed to lead or direct another activity, head control might be lost. Because symmetrical vestibular stimulation plays a key role in activating the neck muscles to hold the head in vertical, it also is a key element leading to the perception of vertical and all the directional activities sequencing out of the concept of verticality. The postural extensor programming for head control needs to be practiced in a standing position and a sitting position. The client needs to be able to stand quietly without excessive extension to run both postural and balance programs. Similarly, he needs to be able to sit with hip flexion while coactivating postural extension in the trunk and neck.

Head control is a complex motor response. A therapist can facilitate inherent mechanisms to assist a client in regaining function. Simultaneously, multitudinous external input techniques classified under the various sensory modalities and combined modalities can be used to give the client additional information. Awareness of one technique and the ability to categorize it appropriately allow easy identification and implementation of many additional approaches. The therapist always needs to remember that the client must practice the behavior (head control) in a variety of spatial positions during various functional activities. This practice must be functional and no longer contrived.

The reader is referred to Chapter 3 in order to understand the normal development of head control and how the nervous system demonstrates motor learning and control.

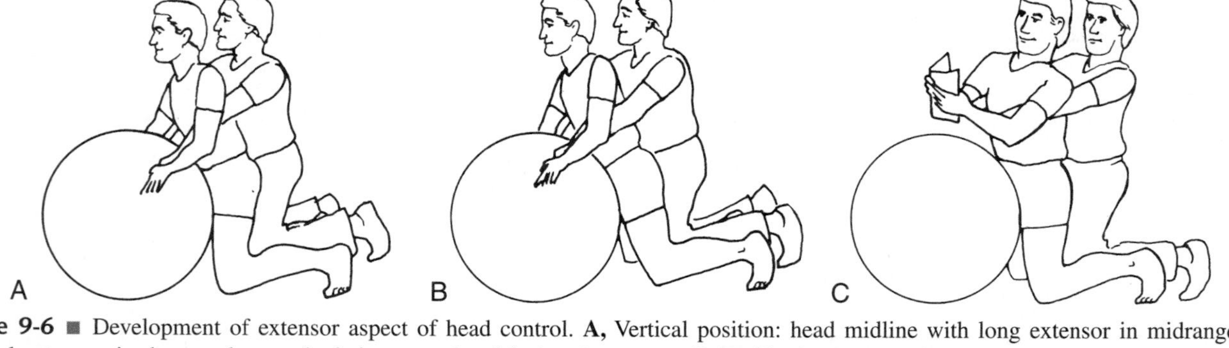

Figure 9-6 ■ Development of extensor aspect of head control. **A,** Vertical position: head midline with long extensor in midrange and postural extensors in shortened range; body in postural weight-bearing pattern. **B,** Facilitating symmetrical extension of head, trunk, and hips while inhibiting abnormal upper-extremity tone. **C,** Facilitating head and trunk extension and rotation to encourage neck righting pattern; client reaches for an object, which is then placed on the opposite side.

Case Study ***2: Initial Augmented Intervention Transitioning to Independence in Bed Mobility.*** Teaching the client to roll in bed can be approached in a variety of ways to accomplish the goal. The entire rolling pattern may be practiced with enough assistance for the client to be able to accomplish the goal, but also limiting help so that the client must use the maximum amount of power and ROM available within the key movement pattern.

Rolling. The patient is a 73-year-old man, status post–ischemic infarct in the frontoparietal cortex with resultant left hemiplegia, hemisensory deficit, and left homonymous hemianopia. The patient demonstrates visual-spatial inattention to the left environment. The client must learn to roll independently in bed for comfort and function. An example of a treatment session aimed at reaching the goal of independent rolling to the right and left may include the following sequence of activities: (1) begin in side-lying on one side; (2) ask patient to tip back a few degrees and then return to the side-lying position (impairment training within limited ROM); and (3) progressively increase the degree the patient must roll backward, assisting (augmenting) him as needed. By the end of several repetitions the patient may be rolling from supine to side lying and the movement is functional because he is performing independently. The client will need to practice many times to relearn the activity before that activity would be considered functional training within the environment practiced. Rolling on a therapeutic mat table is not the same as rolling on a soft mattress at home. There may or may not be carryover. That needs to be identified by the therapist and appropriate steps taken to ensure that independence in all environments is obtained.

Refer to the video for a demonstration of handling while working on rolling for bed mobility.

Case Study ***3: An Individual post Stroke.*** A 66-year-old man after a stroke has mild extensor synergic hypertonicity within the right lower extremity and hypotonicity within the right upper extremity except within the shoulder girdle, which has weak but functional movement patterns. His stroke was medically considered mild and his prognosis good in relation to the potential of the CNS regarding function. It has been agreed that the therapeutic goals after physical rehabilitation are to ambulate independently and use the right upper extremity to fly-fish, an activity that he loves and has done daily since he retired.

In terms of occupational and physical therapy intervention, the patient would be taught to regain independent functional skills in dressing, feeding, hygiene, transfers, and other ADLs. To facilitate the patient's goal of fly-fishing, his family is asked to bring in the rod and reel to augment a real situation with the functional skill he possessed within his right shoulder girdle.

Specific Physical Therapy Task Training: Fly-fishing. In addition to ADL training, it is decided to use BWSTT as a training tool for his right lower extremity. Manual assistance is used to guide the placement of the right foot into dorsiflexion at heel strike. The training begins with a 30% weight reduction, and the patient is relaxed into the gait pattern. His right arm is suspended with the use of a shoulder harness and a robotic aid that swings through the arm in a reciprocal pattern to the left leg. This intervention is performed twice daily for 3 weeks. During weeks 2 and 3, the patient's body weight support is reduced to 15%. By the end of the second week the patient is actively assisting the therapist with the entire gait cycle of both legs. By the end of week 3, the patient is able to walk on the treadmill independently. During the second week, over-ground ambulation is begun to transfer the treadmill learning into a functional activity. By the end of the fourth week, the patient is independent on noncompliant surfaces. Over the next month the patient is in an outpatient environment with the primary goal of independent ambulation on compliant surfaces such as sand, dirt hills, and gravel environments.

Specific Occupational Therapy Intervention with Regard to Fly-Fishing. It is determined that the OT will work on postural endurance of the trunk and lower extremities while facilitating the right upper extremity to practice fly-fishing. Initially the training is done in sitting to create a stable environment for the right upper extremity. The arm is placed over a ball that the patient can roll back and forth as he visualizes fly-fishing. His right hand is placed in a glove that has a wrist support and is fastened to the rod with Velcro. The rod is placed in a bucket with a hinge joint that allows for anterior and posterior movement of the rod attached to its base of support. Using this adaptation of the ball, rod brace, and wrist support and glove, the patient is able to mimic one half of the range needed to fly-fish. He so enjoys the activity that his family takes it up to the room to allow him to practice between therapy visits. After a week, the patient is brought to stand, and the apparatus is adjusted for height. The ball is still used but placed on an adjustable bedside table. As normal motor programs begin to be generated within the right upper extremity, modifications in size of the ball, angle of the wrist and hand, and range allowed within the hinge joint are made to allow for error and self-correction. Within the 3-week period of inpatient rehabilitation, the patient becomes able to perform the activity normally with only the use of the ball for postural support within the shoulder girdle. The apparatus is taken home and the patient adjusts all components depending on his fatigue level. Within a 2-month period of the patient working at home, he goes from a totally augmented intervention program to functionally being able to stand by a river or lake and fly-fish independently. His endurance for this activity improves as he continues to practice.

SOMATOSENSORY RETRAINING

Somatosensory retraining is a multisensory approach to retraining target-specific skills for patients with movement dysfunction that manifests with measurable levels of sensory impairments. This type of therapy is based on the principles of learning and plasticity and progresses from a strong sensory emphasis to sensorimotor practice to motor learning. This approach has been used with patients with various types of hypertonicity resulting from congenital deficits (see Chapter 15) to degeneration (see Chapters 13, 17, 19, and 20) and disease (see Chapters 21, 23, 25, and 26). It has been most commonly used in patients with dystonia and chronic pain. This approach combines a variety of the strategies summarized in the augmented intervention section as well as Box 9-3. The principles for retraining can be found in Appendix 9-A. The progression of specific learning-based sensorimotor training is summarized in Appendix 9-B. Additional ways to enhance sensorimotor training can be found in Appendix 9-C.

BOX 9-3 ■ CONCEPTUAL GUIDELINES FOR CLINICAL DECISION MAKING: HOW TO SELECT TREATMENT OPTIONS FOR PATIENTS WITH NEUROLOGICAL IMPAIRMENTS

After performing examination procedures in which you identify problems with activities and participation, you will then be able to classify these into clusters or syndromes (i.e., the physical therapy diagnosis). You then need to formulate a prognosis and determine the intervention options.

In order to determine the *best* treatment options for a patient with a neurological condition with movement problems, you must simultaneously consider non–physical therapy–based as well as non–neurological system–based limitations along with the specific neurological impairments.

Assume the *best case scenario* (which never exists) in which there are no limitations in health benefits, from cultural beliefs or family, caused by conflict with other care providers, or in systems other than motor such as cognitive, emotional, vascular, integumentary, pulmonary, cardiac, and so on.

First, what does the patient want to do compared with what his or her motor system can do? Can you work on improvement of impairments and function within activities the patient is motivated to do? *If so, do it!*

Second, without altering the patient's normal feedback (intrinsic) mechanisms, can he or she perform the functional activity without causing program adaptations that are so stereotypical that those programs may limit future movement functions and carryover?

For example: can you create an activity that will do the following without contriving the environment and while still running flexible, malleable motor programs?

1. Improve range of motion (ROM) or
2. Improve power or
3. Improve coordination or
4. Improve balance or
5. Improve endurance or
6. Any or all of the above
7. Have any similar effect

If so, do it!

If not, you will need to contrive the environment in order to create functional change through treatment intervention.

ASK YOURSELF

1. Where in the activity can you optimize biomechanics, and where are biomechanics deoptimized? If the body was placed at a better biomechanical advantage:
   a. Would the client be able to run and power the program?
   b. Would the motor program run more fluidly and procedurally?
   c. Would there be greater endurance?

   If your answer is *yes,* then try running the program that way initially and then increase the range and challenge all components of the program.
2. Throughout the activity, where would the least and greatest power be needed? Does the program run differently at different points throughout the activity depending on power production? Optimize what power you have, while maintaining fluid, relaxed program generators. Hypertonicity will often be observed if you ask for more power than the generators can create in a normal fashion.
3. Look at the program itself.
   a. What central nervous system (CNS) components are missing (impairments or functional problems)? These are usually your neurological diagnoses (physical therapy diagnoses).
   b. Can you elicit through treatment intervention corrections of the impairments in any aspect of the program? *If so, how?*
      - ❑ Caused by biomechanical advantage
      - ❑ Caused by musculoskeletal advantage
      - ❑ Caused by the program advantage itself

   Optimize:
      - ❑ Synergistic advantage
      - ❑ Balance synergies
      - ❑ Sensory processing
      - ❑ And so on

   These treatment answers will lay the foundations for your specific intervention strategies.
   c. Can you elicit those components in any other movement programs? If so, these are treatment alternatives, although they will not be task specific and have less immediate carryover.
4. Select movement activities that use existing components procedurally and facilitate or elicit function from impairment component of subsystems.
5. Prioritize functional activities by identifying daily living needs of the patient, goals of the patient, and functional skill of the patient. Determine which impairments affect the greatest number of functional activities. Similarly determine which impairments can be quickly changed in order to gain functional skill. Decide within the limits of the environment which activities to focus on first.

BOX 9-3 ■ CONCEPTUAL GUIDELINES FOR CLINICAL DECISION MAKING: HOW TO SELECT TREATMENT OPTIONS FOR PATIENTS WITH NEUROLOGICAL IMPAIRMENTS—cont'd

For example: Assume the patient has poor balance in sitting and standing. He plans to sit in the lounge chair most of the day but walk to the toilet when necessary. Although range, power, and postural control would need to be considered, you might decide to work on standing balance and balance during walking before sitting balance owing to task specificity and functional need. This is not stating that sitting balance is not important; it is prioritizing the activities according to need. Power, range, posture, and so on may determine the specific intervention strategies used to work on standing and walking balance.

6. If normal programming cannot be elicited, look at adaptations and determine alternative interventions such as the following:
   a. Adaptive equipment: biofeedback, orthotics, canes, and so on
   b. Adaptive environments: ramps, rails, lights, changing walkways, changing surfaces (e.g., removing shag carpets)
   c. Encouraging stereotypical and inflexible programs
   d. Combination of a, b, or c

Make sure that when selection of alternative approaches or adaptations is made, consideration is given to what will be given up by adapting the environment and CNS. Consider whether that decision is truly cost efficient and the best alternative to meet the needs and goals of the patient, his or her family, and the physical and cultural environment within which he or she will function.

Neural Mobilization

Neural mobilization is often needed as an intervention strategy before somatosensory retraining is begun. Often there is increased sensitivity in a limb from pain,[611] neurovascular restrictions, or soft tissue adhesions limiting the ability of the peripheral nerve to move through the tissue (see Chapter 18). This sensitivity can increase hypertonicity and further interfere with retraining motor control. In order to address this, it is important to quiet the nervous system and then gently mobilize the neural tissue. One way to quiet the nervous system is by "swaddling." This is often used in newborns to quiet their nervous system. For an older child or an adult, the patient is wrapped similar to the way a baby would be; then gentle rocking in a rocking chair or a swing is added. Patients can do this themselves by putting on a t-shirt with the arms tight to the trunk and then wrapping even further with a blanket. This technique can be used periodically on days that the nervous system appears to be responding primarily to adrenaline rather than purposeful heightened activity. There are a variety of ways to mobilize the PNS. Detailed examples of this can be found in textbooks on the hand.[612]

NATURAL ENVIRONMENTS AND QUALITY OF LIFE

Research has already been identified in the discussions of the various sensory input systems that recognizes that changes in external sensory input such as decreasing sound, light, tactile contact, or color of mats can change the processing of CNS of the clients. The present and future research will recommend that therapists apply changes that affect not only the patient's inherent sensory systems, but also the environments within which the therapy is done. Therapists are going to have to adapt to change. At this time it is unrealistic to think that acute management of patients after a neurological insult will occur anywhere but in a large medical institution, but treatment needs after that acute stage may better be served in a more natural environment of the individual needing service.[613-618] Not only has this conclusion been accepted conceptually in postacute pediatric settings, but federal law has ordered that individuals up to 21 years of age must receive educational experiences in the least restrictive environment. This amendment was made to the Individuals with Disabilities Educational Act (IDEA) in 1997.[619] These changes have been mandated within the school systems and have affected therapy environments for clinicians who work in those situations. It is realistic to assume those changes will in time affect all therapy environments.

As the World Health Organization has moved toward an individual-friendly focus and thus a focus on body system strengths as well as impairments, participation in life, and its quality, the term *patient* may also need to be changed to *participant.* As can be seen in Chapter 8, examination tools have been included that deal with quality of life and not just functional outcomes from therapy. Therapists, if they have not done so already, are going to have to learn to deal with individuals coming to them for assistance as a partner in the process and not a patient who receives services. Change will come. That is one of the exciting aspects of being an OT or PT in the coming decades.

CONCLUSION

There are treatment techniques that are universally applied to the very young and the very old. As discussed in Chapter 4, the CNS is in a constant state of change throughout life. The brain is unique to each individual. Each brain has idiosyncrasies but also has an enormous number of predictable responses. These factors affect the success or failure of a client-therapist interaction. In Box 9-3 the reader will find guidelines that may assist in determining the type of interventions (functional, impairment, augmented, or somatosensory training) that will best match the patient's functional movement capability. In answering the questions presented, the therapist will gain a better idea of which examination tools will best help objectively measure the progress of the patient toward that patient's specific goals. From that thorough evaluation process (see Chapter 8), the therapist must decide which treatment is appropriate and the most efficient course of intervention on the basis of the goals of the patient and family, the movement diagnosis, the prognosis, the resources available, and the skills of the therapist. Once a decision is made regarding whether the interventions should be based on compensation, substitution, habituation, neural adaptation, or a combination of the four, the team must select the best options available given all the resources. The options include functional retraining, impairment training, augmented and contrived interventions, and somatosensory reintegration. No matter the specifics of the intervention selection, the therapist must cognitively organize intervention options in a sequential process, be willing to change direction or options as the patient changes, and develop a greater clinical repertoire of intervention strategies.

When specific augmented interventions are needed, the therapist must select specific treatments according to the needs of the client, the time available for therapy, the level and extent of the functional involvement, the motivation of the client and family, the creativity of the therapist, and, of course, the existing pathology, whether it be stable or an active disease process. A therapist must choose whether somatosensory retraining, functional training, impairment training, augmented treatment interventions, or any combination of these four will provide the client with the most environmentally effective, cost-efficient, and quickest map to functional independence or maximal quality of life. How each therapist combines the interventions with the client's specific needs will vary according to education, belief, skill, and openness to learning from the total environment itself. Learning should lead to further learning. Answers to unknowns will be found, with new unknowns coming to consciousness. The brain is still more mystery than not, so for most OTs and PTs beginning or ending their practice, the adventure has just begun. *Enjoy the experience.*

References

To enhance this text and add value for the reader, all references are included on the companion Evolve site that accompanies this textbook. This online service will, when available, provide a link for the reader to a Medline abstract for the article cited. There are 636 cited references and other general references for this chapter, with the majority of those articles being evidence-based citations.

APPENDIX 9-A ■ Principles Used by Therapists for Retraining Clients with Pain and Motor Control Problems of the Hand

Nancy N. Byl, PT, PhD, FAPTA, Professor Emeritus, Department of Physical Therapy and Rehabilitation Science, School of Medicine, University of California, San Francisco

A. Positive Foundation for Retraining

1. Carry out a regular exercise program, be well hydrated, eat balanced meals, get adequate sleep, make time to have fun, minimize habitual repetitions, and effectively manage stress.
2. Engage in challenging balance to improve posture and integrating diaphragmatic breathing, neural mobilization, and core trunk strengthening to maintain a healthy posture.
3. Create learning strategies that emphasize sensory input and feedback. You can do this by placing sticky, coarse, or rough surfaces on tools that are used in functional activities (e.g., pen, keyboard, glass, hammer, utensils).
4. Set goals and objectives to guide your training.
5. Think positively about learning to be as good as you can be or to recover after injury; expect to regain function.
6. Analyze and break down the tasks you want to learn or to improve into manageable components.
7. Perform each component of functional tasks without abnormal movements (e.g., pathological synergies, extraneous movements, excessive muscle firing, involuntary movements, strain, pain).
8. Be sure each activity is designed to require attention, repetition, progression of difficulty, feedback regarding accuracy of performance, and positive reinforcement (reward).

B. Stress-Free Hand Use Strategies

1. Strengthen the small muscles inside the hand (intrinsic muscles) to facilitate stability of functional hand use.
   i. Give resistance to spreading fingers apart (try not to use muscles that straighten the fingers).
   ii. Try to hold the fingers together while you use your other hand to try and spread them apart.
   iii. Bend the fingers at the large knuckle (metacarpophalangeal joint) to 90 degrees by placing the back of the hand against the edge of a table. Now, one finger at a time, try to keep the fingers straight as you use the other hand to try and bend the finger, giving resistance at the distal segment of the finger.
2. Concentrate on using the small muscles of the hands in all functional activities.
   i. Initiate bending the fingers from the base joint (the large metacarpophalangeal joint that joins the finger to the palm); try to do this without bending the fingers at the other joints, especially without using the muscles that bend the distal finger joints.
   ii. Avoid heavy gripping; squeeze the fingers in a power grip only when necessary. For example, do not (1) squeeze the steering wheel, (2) exercise while holding on to free weights, or (3) squeeze a ball or strengthen the grip in other ways.
   iii. Practice reaching for common objects with the eyes closed and the hand relaxed. When you contact the object, let the sensation of the surface of the object open the hand. For example, when you reach for your cup, let the cup open the hand (e.g., do not actively spread the fingers first). Do not use the handle of the cup.
3. When practicing tool use, let the sensation of the object teach your hand how hard to squeeze.
   i. Modify the sensation of the object (e.g., very rough, slightly rough, coarse, smooth, silky).
   ii. Take practice lifts of the object to determine how heavy it is.
   iii. Manipulate the object in your hands without visual monitoring before beginning functional use of the tool.
4. Avoid aggressive, precise, rapid, alternating, forceful finger flexion and extension movements of the hand.
   i. Transfer some of the work of the hand from the fingers to the forearm. For example,
      - Lift the fingers by rotating the forearm into supination (e.g., turn palm up). If forearm rotation is limited, let the shoulder externally rotate if necessary.
      - When the hand needs to be palm down (pronated), let the elbow swing away from the trunk if necessary to keep the hand relaxed (e.g., internal rotation of the shoulder can take the stress off the forearm).
   ii. Use the hand in a *natural functional position* (e.g., rounded palm from the base of the thumb to the base of the fifth finger and rounded from the tips of the fingers to the wrist). Thus all the finger joints are slightly bent, the palm is round, and the wrist is extended about 15 degrees. When your arms are at your side, this will usually be the position of the hand.
   iii. Do not let the joints of the fingers collapse or hyperextend when they are down on a surface. This can be difficult if the joints are hypermobile or the intrinsic muscles (muscles inside the hand) are weak.
      - Practice dropping the hand onto a surface and maintaining the roundness of the hand (a small soft ball under the palm may be used for assistance).
      - Lean lightly onto the hand while it is on a flat surface, pronated and keep the round shape of the hand (e.g., may need to initially keep small round ball under palm).
      - Thread the fingers of one hand through the fingers of the other hand to help stabilize the hand when placing weight onto the hand as noted previously.
      - Put a soft, rubber ball about 2 inches in diameter on the table; roll the palm of the hand over the ball while letting the finger pads (not the tips) drop onto the surface.

C. Using the Computer Keyboard Safely

1. Position yourself comfortably to use the computer.
   i. Sit with feet flat on the floor. Sit tall with hips about 90 degrees (vary this posture throughout the day).
   ii. Place the computer screen at or slightly below eye level.
   iii. Keyboard height should be adjusted to maintain elbow flexion at about 80 degrees (positioned in approximately 100 degrees of extension).
   iv. Forearms should be angled toward the floor and not resting on the table. If it is difficult to let your hands rest lightly on the keyboard with the wrist floating, it may be helpful to have a pillow on your lap (or a lumbar roll around the waist), where the forearms receive positive sensory information to help them relax.

Continued

APPENDIX 9-A ■ Principles Used by Therapists for Retraining Clients with Pain and Motor Control Problems of the Hand—cont'd

v. Place the screen about 2 feet away from the eyes for most work; pull the screen closer as necessary for close work.
vi. Consider getting special antiglare glasses for computer terminal display work or use a screen glare protector.

2. Use your hands in a functional (e.g., round, not flat or angular) position on the keyboard.
   i. Look at the contour of the hand when it is at your side; maintain that position as the finger pads (not the tips) are dropped on the keyboard.
   ii. Place a rough surface on the keys (e.g., Velcro) to make it easier to feel the pads on the keys.
   iii. Avoid placing the tips of the fingers on the keys. This creates an obligatory co-coactivation of the finger flexors and extensors.
3. Keep the wrist in a neutral position (0 to 10 degrees of extension) while working on the keyboard (e.g., a floating wrist).
   i. Do not rest the wrist on a "wrist rest." Resting the wrist and forearm on the work surface will increase the pressure in the carpal tunnel and force all the work to be done with the fingers.
   ii. If there is a wrist pad on the computer keyboard tray, think of the pad as a "sensory tickle" to let you know that your wrists should be floating above the rest.
4. Have all the fingers resting on the keyboard.
   i. Do not let any of the fingers fly up.
   ii. Continue to keep the fingers resting down even when one finger is engaged in depressing a key.
   iii. Avoid allowing the adjacent fingers to extend to get them away from the finger actively pressing down.
5. It is not necessary to actively lift the fingers after pressing down. Usually it is sufficient to release the pressure without actively lifting up the digits.
6. Avoid resting the fingers on the keyboard with the finger tips. This leads to a contraction of the fingers and the wrist.
   i. Do not keep your fingers excessively curled. In that position it is impossible to keep the fingers on their pads.
   ii. Initiate the movement down from the base joint of the fingers.
   iii. Imagine that you are using the muscles inside your hand and not the long muscles that bend the fingers.
   iv. Avoid reaching one finger out in isolation from the others.
7. In general, change the primary fulcrum of movement from the fingers of the hand to the elbow and shoulder.
   i. Allow the elbow to move freely in flexion, extension, and rotation.
   ii. Use the trunk with a little shoulder movement when reaching for an object or a paper or to move closer to or away from the computer keyboard or screen.
8. Use the mouse by using forearm rotation rather than individual finger movements.
   i. Do not squeeze the mouse; drape your hand on the mouse.
   ii. Keep your wrist in neutral position.
   iii. Avoid clicking the button by lifting and bending the index finger.
   iv. Use rotation of the forearm to activate the button on the mouse.
   v. Make sure the mouse is close to you and that the arm is not extended to the side. Place a cover for the mouse over the number keys, if necessary, to keep the arm closer to your trunk.
   vi. Consider interfaces other than a mouse (e.g., roller ball, a movement-sensitive pad, pen).
   vii. If it is not possible to use the hand in a stress-free way when on the computer, then consider voice-activated software to use your computer.
      - Use your voice carefully and without excessive force or strain (e.g., loudness).
      - Be careful to prevent co-contractions and stressful use of the vocal cords.
9. Take regular breaks (e.g., every 15 minutes).
   i. Consider obtaining the software that forces a computer breakthrough screen reminder.
   ii. Do diaphragmatic breathing continually while working on your computer to minimize tension and facilitate good oxygen exchange.
   iii. When taking a break and staying at the desk, get your hands off the computer and change your sitting posture while doing gentle range-of-motion exercises. Occasionally place the arms on the desk and bend the trunk over the arms.
10. At least every 20 minutes, stand up for a few minutes and stretch.

D. Writing

1. The fulcrum for the movement of writing should be the shoulder and elbow, not the fingers.
2. The hand should be round and relaxed.
3. Try putting a sticky or a rough surface on the pen or pencil before you begin to practice.
   a. A sticky surface (e.g., tape with the sticky side facing out) can be strong enough to hold the pen in place without any squeezing.
   b. A fatter pen is not as helpful as a sticky or a rough surface. It is possible to excessively grip a large pen.
4. Practice writing when you are not at work or at a store when you have to write your name.
5. Practice writing non–work-related words and sentences and then progress to meaningful writing.
6. Try holding the pen by different fingers or using different movements.
   i. Try to hold the pen between the second (index) and third (middle) finger rather than the thumb (D1), index finger (D2), and middle finger (D3). The hand should be open, thumb resting down.
   ii. If you must hold the pen in the traditional way, try to hold the pen lightly among D1, D2, and D3, with D1 and D2 moving toward the thumb from the base joint with all joints of the digits extended.
   iii. With a sticky surface on the pen, it is possible to control the pen with minimal squeezing.
7. Practice picking up the pen and putting it down without feeling any tension in your hand.
8. Control the movement of the pen primarily from the elbow and shoulder; keep wrist and fingers quietly positioned on the pen.
   i. Let the arm rest lightly on the table and comfortably on the ulnar (fifth finger) side of your hand. Avoid resting the elbow on the surface. If there is inadequate pronation (e.g., it is uncomfortable to have the hand be palm side down), allow the shoulder to move out away from the trunk (e.g., shoulder abduction or rotation).

APPENDIX 9-A ■ Principles Used by Therapists for Retraining Clients with Pain and Motor Control Problems of the Hand—cont'd

   ii. Let all fingers rest down on the pen or the support surface. Do not hold any fingers up off the pen or the support surface.
   iii. Mentally review relaxed writing before beginning to write with a new technique.
   iv. Practice making circles, loops, large numbers, and letters. Consider practicing by writing in shaving cream, finger paints, or water.
   v. If you see your fingers moving and your knuckles turning white, you are squeezing too hard and you are using only your fingers.
9. Use a mirror to get some feedback to retrain your style of writing.
   i. Place a mirror in front of your affected hand as you write and notice whether it appears relaxed.
   ii. Place the unaffected hand in front of the mirror and the affected hand behind the mirror. Look at the image of the unaffected hand (e.g., looks like the affected side), and then have the affected hand behind the mirror copy the mirror image.
10. Put the pen down if any signs of stress develop.

E. Daily Activities in the Kitchen

1. Use two hands to hold a pot or a frying pan.
2. Use an electronic can opener and jar opener.
3. Use an electronic blender rather than hand stirring.
4. Use a chopper to avoid heavy cutting.
5. Stand close to the sink and the work surface so you do not have to have your arms out too far in front of you.
6. Get close to the table for setting the table; avoid having to lean over; bend at the knees.
7. If you are short, stand on a stool to work at the sink.
8. If you are tall, consider raising the refrigerator up higher so you do not have to lean over.
9. Concentrate on eating and using utensils without stress in your hands.
   i. Consider putting a sticky or a rough surface on the utensils (e.g., Velcro or flooring with a sticky back).
   ii. When eating, hold the utensils lightly, even when trying to cut.
   iii. When cutting, move the whole arm from the shoulder; use the weight of the trunk to assist putting force down on the knife.

F. Driving

1. Use a lumbar roll in the back of your seat to support your lower back. Also consider placing a wedge in your seat (varying the placement of the wedge with the high side in front and then toward the back).
2. Pull the seat close to the steering wheel so that you do not have to reach out so far for the gas pedal.
3. Sit tall to ensure good visibility, and try to drive without stress.
4. Consider putting a rough surface on the wheel so you do not tend to squeeze it (you can buy ergonomic steering wheel covers).
5. When you need to look behind you, shift your weight in the opposite direction that you want to look. This will allow you to turn your whole trunk in the desired direction and avoid the isolated neck strain that occurs when you only turn your head.
6. Mentally rehearse and review calm, alert driving.
7. Do not squeeze the wheel in a death grip. Hold the steering wheel by gently pushing your arms together. You only need to hold the wheel with a palmar squeeze when turning.
8. Keep your arms comfortably at your sides.
9. Do not grip the shift knob; press the palm of your hand down on the shift bar to change gears. You may even want to allow your trunk to move with your arm while shifting.
10. If you continue to experience stress with driving, practice braking and turning the wheel in your garage and imagine different scenarios.
11. Also, if you need a diversion to avoid emotional confrontation with rude drivers, bring a plastic bag of buttons that you can manipulate and match to decrease your stress.

G. Other Household Activities

1. As before, do not grip objects too firmly; keep hands open and work with your arms close to the trunk.
2. Always bend your knees to pick up objects from the floor.
3. Be careful to avoid leaning over and straightening the bedding (e.g., when making the bed, ask someone to do it with you; otherwise, make one side of the bed at a time).
4. Put items at eye level; avoid putting things over your head for which you have to reach out and up.
5. Walk close to the vacuum cleaner; try to hold it where you do not have to reach your arms out (e.g., step forward and backward with the movement of the vacuum cleaner).
6. Do not lean over from the waist for dusting; if necessary, dust while kneeling or wipe the floor while you are on your knees; hold the dust cloth lightly.

APPENDIX 9-B ■ Specific Learning-Based Sensorimotor Training

A. Instructions

Patients

We use our hands for many skilled fine motor and functional tasks. It is important for these movements to be smooth, efficient, and accurate. When there is dysfunction in the central or peripheral nervous system from congenital anomalies, injury, disease, overuse, degeneration, or chronic pain, skilled and functional movements can be impaired. Although it is still important to strengthen the muscles, increase flexibility, and restore normal motor control, it is critical to improve sensory processing. The purpose of learning-based sensorimotor activities is to place demands on the sensory receptors of the skin, the muscle, and the joints to restore normal sensitivity and accuracy of sensory input and feedback. Your brain can change with training. By improving the accuracy of sensory discrimination under conditions of high levels of attention, repetitive activities progressed in difficulty and reinforced with feedback and reward should improve how the hand is mapped on your brain (e.g., primary sensory cortex). When specific tasks involve motor practice, topographical changes will also occur in other parts of the brain (e.g., thalamus, motor cortex, limbic system, basal ganglia, prefrontal cortex, supplementary motor cortex, brain stem). Although most think about the motor requirements for performing a task, it is essential to have accurate sensory information and feedback, which comes from accurate sensory differentiation of the hand. Dynamic sensory topography and function are requisite for the restoration of fine motor control.

Research also suggests that positive expectations can facilitate recovery and maximize performance.[634] Physical impairments can lead to significant handicaps and disability. In these cases it is challenging to maintain a positive attitude and be motivated for recovery and rehabilitation. Depression, anxiety, loss of self-worth, and compromised self-esteem can significantly impair the recovery process, especially when training activities are demanding, intensive, and possibly associated with discomfort or frustration. It is essential to progress activities without causing unnecessary anxiety, apprehension, or pain. With these issues in mind, the initial steps in sensorimotor training may seem unusually simple and involve imagery in lieu of motor practice. Also, although the suggestions here focus on the hand, the principles apply to sensorimotor retraining for other parts of the body as well.

Specific randomized clinical trials have not been carried out on this series of training activities. However, Moseley[611] carried out several studies establishing the procedures to perform recognition training of hand laterality, imagined hand movements, and mirror movements. He also carried out a randomized clinical trial for patients with complex regional pain syndrome using these training techniques. He randomly assigned 20 subjects to one of three different groups: hand laterality recognition, imagined movements, mirror training, or imagined movements; hand laterality recognition, imagined movements, or hand lateral recognition; mirror movements or hand recognition laterality. At 6 and 18 weeks after training for 2 weeks on these behaviors, subjects in all groups had a significant reduction in pain and disability ($P < .05$), with the group doing hand laterality recognition, imagined movements, and mirror training making significantly greater gains than the other two groups. Byl and co-workers[635,636] also reported significant gains in patients with focal hand dystonia after 6 weeks of learning-based training. Candia and colleagues[634] also reported significant gains in performance for musicians with focal hand dystonia after 1 year of training focusing on task practice while controlling the fingers with a splint to improve isolated control of the dystonic fingers. For patients who are stable after a stroke, Byl and colleagues[44] also reported significant gains in fine motor performance after a sensory retraining program similar to the activities described here.

Therapists and Family Members

When giving these instructions to patients, it is important to supplement the written instructions with pictures or even videos. For patients with significant cognitive impairments, these instructions are almost more important for the family members who are helping reinforce the supervised therapy program.

B. Principles of Learning-Based Sensorimotor Training

1. Learning strategies focus on improving the discrimination of the somatosensory system in a range of tasks that focus primarily on sensory processing during sensory discrimination tasks and fine motor tasks.
2. Successful recovery is contingent on being able to imagine using the hands normally again without abnormal movements, apprehension, or pain.
3. The injured hand (affected limb) needs to recover laterality (right and left).
4. The patient needs to be able to look at a hand and imagine integrating the image of the hand into the movement or positioning of his or her own hand.
5. The hand must be able to interface with the target surface without creating tension, pain, or abnormal movement.
6. It is essential to be able to mentally imagine performing related and target tasks without abnormal movements or pain.
7. Sensory processing must achieve a minimum level of accuracy before functional fine motor movements are integrated.
8. Functional fine motor tasks need to be mentally practiced before they are physically practiced.
9. Tasks must be divided into the smallest components that can be normally executed (e.g., partial task performance), which will serve as the foundation for building skill-based learning on the whole task.
10. Learning requires attention and repetition of behaviors progressed over time.
11. Feedback and reward must be integrated into all learning activities, either by mental imagery, mirror imagery, visual reinforcement, auditory feedback, or objective, accurate task performance.
12. Feedback from error correction may be critical for enhancing learning.
13. Each component of a functional task must be performed as normally as possible before progressing to a more difficult task (e.g., without pathological synergies, extraneous movements, excessive muscle firing, involuntary movements, strain, pain).
14. Repetitive activities must avoid stereotypical movements that occur nearly simultaneously in time.
15. Sensory discriminative retraining should eliminate visual cues to facilitate somatosensory learning (e.g., eyes closed, blindfolded, distorting lenses).

APPENDIX 9-B ■ Specific Learning-Based Sensorimotor Training—cont'd

16. Begin sensory training on nontarget surfaces or with easy tasks that do not trigger abnormal responses (e.g., nontarget tasks).
    i. Practice on nontarget tasks until sensory processing is improved and the task can be performed without any abnormal movement.
    ii. Integrate sensory retraining in tasks that historically have been associated with abnormal movement (e.g., writer's cramp, keyboarder's cramp, hand functions associated with abnormal synergies related to hypertonicity, tremors, dystonia).

C. Preliminary Activities to Improve Readiness for Learning-Based Sensorimotor Discrimination Training

1. Restore hand laterality recognition.
    i. Follow the guidelines developed by Moseley[611] to be able to quickly see the hand in different positions and identify whether the hand is right or left.
    ii. See pictures of the hand in different orientations and different positions of the wrist and fingers and identify whether right or left.
    iii. See the pictures in random order, faster and faster, and be able to accurately determine the side.[611]
2. Restore ability to mentally imagine putting the affected hand into different positions.[611]
    i. See pictures of the appropriate hand (affected) in different positions.
    ii. When picture is shown, mentally put your hand into the same position as the one in the picture.
    iii. Practice doing this while changing the order of the positions and the time the position is visualized.
3. Restore the ability to imagine performing normal movements while observing a video of the hands of someone else performing target and nontarget tasks.
    i. Record video of different people performing target and nontarget tasks.
    ii. Watch the videos and imagine that the hands being observed are your hands performing the tasks without pain or abnormal movements.
4. Learn how to copy a mirror image of the affected side.[635]
    i. Place the unaffected hand in front of a vertical mirror and the affected hand behind the mirror (out of sight).
    ii. Look in the mirror and note that the mirror image of the unaffected hand looks like the affected hand.
    iii. Do simple tasks using the mirror image to guide the movement of the affected side.
        - ❑ Take the pictures from the visualization training and assume the position of the hand and wrist.[635]
        - ❑ Put different sensory objects within the reach of both hands; pick up an object and make the object feel the same on both sides.[635]
        - ❑ Do simple functional tasks with both hands simultaneously (e.g., turn hand up and down, tap a finger, bring thumb to each finger, pick up a pen, circle the pen, pick up objects of different size or same size but different surfaces).[635]

D. Initiate Specific Learning-Based Sensorimotor Training

1. Retrain cutaneous, muscle, and joint receptors at nontarget tasks.
    i. Develop a variety of active sensory discrimination activities that you can do by yourself (e.g., actively exploring to interpret different object surfaces—stereognosis).
        - ❑ Take the opportunity to feel objects in your environment and identify the objects without looking at the object.
        - ❑ Put small objects in bowls of rice or beans and reach in and try to find and match the objects.
        - ❑ Hang different objects from a string on a door jamb; start the objects swinging and allow them to stimulate your hand. See whether you can differentiate the different objects as they move across your hand.
    ii. Modify the difficulty of the sensory task.
        - ❑ Change the intensity of the sensory stimuli (e.g., make the surfaces less distinct).
        - ❑ Increase the challenge or the complexity of the stimuli you are trying to identify.
        - ❑ Change the environment in which you are exploring the sensory stimuli (e.g., hand in water, still or agitated; in shaving soap; in whipped cream as you discriminate an object or manipulate a pen).
        - ❑ Change the position you assume when discriminating the stimulus (e.g., lie down on your back or your stomach, stand instead of sitting).
    iii. Palpate objects in water or other media for identification; have the water be still and then agitate the water.
    iv. Put pairs of coins and objects in your pocket (or a plastic bag) and try to match them or discriminate between them.
    v. Purchase clay that can be molded and shaped and then heated until firm.
        - ❑ Place or draw different shapes on the clay.
        - ❑ Always include a pair of designs that can be matched.
    vi. Paste matched pairs of items on a card and try to find the matched pairs.
        - ❑ Paste stickers with shapes on cards and try to find matched pairs.
        - ❑ Paste matched pairs of buttons on a card.
        - ❑ Paste alphabet soup letters on a card and match letters or spell words.
        - ❑ Put magnetic letters and other shapes on a card or a refrigerator and move them to spell words.
    vii. Take construction paper and create pairs of letters, shapes, or other designs by pressing heavily with the pen; this will create a raised surface on the other side.
        - ❑ With eyes closed, palpate and try to find matching pairs.
        - ❑ Turn the paper in different directions to make the exploration different.
    viii. Make a grab bag of items and reach into the bag and identify the objects by gentle touch.
    ix. Obtain Braille workbooks and learn to read Braille.
        - ❑ If you have trouble learning Braille with the affected side, try with the unaffected side.
        - ❑ Do not tense your hand as you feel the letters, and do not extend the adjacent digits away.

Continued

APPENDIX 9-B ■ Specific Learning-Based Sensorimotor Training—cont'd

- Work your hands smoothly over the dots. You can improve your skill, getting other workbooks for the blind and ultimately purchasing books in Braille.
- Obtain "Braille object cards" where the object is described in Braille. Palpate the letters and sentences.

x. Place raised numbers and designs on the computer keyboard and try to determine what the number or shape is before striking the key; make some labeled letters match or mismatch the key itself.

2. Practice activities requiring the interpretation of sensory information delivered to the skin (interpretation of sensory inputs without active exploration of the stimulus, graphesthesia).

i. Ask a friend to stimulate your skin with different stimuli (e.g., hot, cold, sharp, dull, rough) and try to identify the stimuli.

ii. Ask this friend to draw numbers, letters, words (upper and lower case or cursive), and designs on your forearm, hands, and fingers when you are not looking.

- Identify the letters, numbers, words, and shapes verbally (e.g., start with capital letters).
- When it is easy to be correct on capital letters, have your friend draw lowercase letters, including words.
- Progress to having designs drawn on your skin; replicate the design by drawing it on a piece of paper or on your own skin.
  - Ask your friend to give you feedback about the drawing to make sure the drawing matches the stimulus.
  - Check the angles where the lines meet.
  - Note accuracy of detection of curves.
  - Note whether all parts of the design are placed in the right relationship and orientation (spatial accuracy).
  - Note whether the design is the correct size.
  - Check whether the drawing has some elaborate components that were not actually drawn on the surface of the skin.
  - Your friend should make the drawings smaller and smaller to increase the challenge of detection (e.g., 2 to 3 mm).
  - The drawing or the stimuli should be delivered two or three times. If the design is still missed, look at the design. After viewing the design, repeat the design at the next trial (or the alternate trial), and before progressing determine whether you can recognize the drawing). Use a friend to check on your accuracy.

3. Use other stimuli to reinforce somatosensory learning.

i. Develop tasks to improve sound discrimination (either location or determination of whether you hear one or two sounds delivered).

ii. Have a visual stimulus provided at the same time an object is touched to the skin (on the affected and unaffected side); the goal is for you to accurately describe the cutaneous stimulus (e.g., sharp, dull, smooth, rough, silky, hard, soft).

4. Develop activities to emphasize proprioceptive and kinesthetic learning.

i. Where necessary, use tape on the skin, use electrical or auditory biofeedback, or put weights around the wrist and ankle to increase feedback from joint, tendon, and muscle receptors.

ii. Create games in which a part of an object has to be accurately placed on a topographical picture.

iii. Create games in which objects have to be moved accurately across specific distances on a variable surface.

iv. Create objects of the same weight and place different types of surfaces on the object (e.g., Velcro, sandpaper, flooring). Then practice picking up, moving, and putting down the object with minimal effort.

v. Assemble puzzles by feeling the matching pieces rather than looking with the eyes.

vi. Work with a friend and practice copying movements together (first by looking and then by feeling).

- Tap one finger while the other fingers are resting down.
- Bring arms up over head and tap one finger at a time.
- Bend wrist with one arm and bend elbow with other arm.
- Circle wrist to the right (right hand) and circle to the left with left hand.

vii. Have a friend give you some resistance as you move one finger, the wrist, or the forearm up and down.

viii. On a piece of paper, draw hand diagrams with different angles of each finger and different angles of the wrist. Then put up a vertical screen where you cannot see your hand. Look at each picture and try to copy the pictures with your own hand. Look behind the screen to check to see how accurate you are.

ix. See if you can rent a continuous passive motion machine.

- Set the machine at different speeds.
- Try to follow the movements of the machine.
- Apply vibration to the skin over the joint in the direction opposite to the movement.
- Carefully time the movements to enable success.

x. Practice grasping objects with a light grip on the object. Use a spherical group (thumb pad to the pads of other fingers). Practice this with objects of different size with minimum graded force.

xi. Practice bending and straightening the elbow, wrist, or fingers while applying vibration to the appropriate joint.

- When bending (flexing) the joint, apply vibration on the extensor surface.
- When straightening the joint, apply vibration on the flexor surface.

E. Sensory and Fine Motor Activities at Nontarget Tasks

1. Move in normal patterns in desired directions without excessive firing of the muscles.

i. Consider a number of strategies to allow you to move the most difficult finger more easily (e.g., stabilize adjacent digits).

- Use a soft splint to stabilize the fingers adjacent to the finger you want to move.
- Mold a piece of clay; keep an area clear under the finger you want to move, and place a hole in the clay for the other fingers to rest in.
- Put a buddy strap on fingers adjacent to most dystonic or painful finger.
- Put tape on the fingers on the surface that would be most likely to improve movement (e.g., on the flexor surface if the finger extends; on the extensor surface if the finger flexes; on the side of the finger if having difficulty with isolation).
- Use a finger interphalangeal splint on fingers adjacent to dystonic fingers.

ii. Increase sensory feedback on the finger you are trying to move (e.g., use tape on the finger).

APPENDIX 9-B ■ Specific Learning-Based Sensorimotor Training—cont'd

2. With the eyes closed, play games that require discrimination of sensory information through the skin of the fingers.
   i. Play dominoes.
   ii. Play pick-up sticks.
   iii. Play shape games (e.g., match a shape to an opening, such as in Perfection).
   iv. Put together puzzles that have a raised surface.
   v. Play Scrabble with raised or indented letters.
   vi. Play games that require orientation in place without the benefit of vision.
      - Play pin the tail on the donkey.
      - Walk through the house with your eyes closed and hands out to feel objects in your way and to catch yourself if needed.
   vii. Get a Braille deck of cards and play cards (e.g., Solitaire can be played alone; play hearts, bridge, pinochle, or poker with others).
   viii. Create other sensory games that require planning and control and that can be played without vision.

F. Learning-Based Sensorimotor Retraining (Praxis)

1. Feel objects and then define and demonstrate what to do with the objects.
2. Have a friend provide a sensory stimulus and ask you to do something that indicates you felt the stimulus (e.g., "when I tap with this sharp object, I want you to tap once, but when I touch you with this dull object, I want you to tap twice").
3. Feel a number of items in a bag that are related to performing a task, and put the items together to do the task.
4. Feel a number of objects put together in a specific design; have someone give you a second set of the objects to replicate or match the design.
5. Practice throwing objects of different size; practice throwing them to a particular spot.
6. Get accustomed to grading movements without uncontrollable contractions.
   i. Place the hand on a moving target and do not stop the movement.
   ii. Manipulate objects without excessive force.
   iii. Put your hand on a record player and do not stop the record movement (e.g., do not change the sound).
   iv. Put your hand on the moving belt of a treadmill and feel the moving belt.
      - Feel the belt moving under the hand.
      - Hold objects under the fingers.
      - Pass objects back and forth between the fingers, and make the objects feel the same.
7. When it is possible to perform the sensory activities in nontarget tasks, begin placing the hand on the target instrument without abnormal movements.
   i. With the hand on the target instrument, mentally rehearse the movements and the tasks you should perform.
   ii. Add rough surfaces to the target instrument if necessary to change the interface with the hand.

G. Sensorimotor and Fine Motor Training at Target Tasks

1. Emphasize the sensory aspects of the task even when beginning to perform the target task.
2. Perform a selected component of the task (e.g., drop one finger down on the keyboard).
3. Progress the ability to complete more and more of a target task, emphasizing sensory exploration as long as the tasks can be done normally.
4. Be sure to get reinforcement for performing all tasks normally (e.g., use a mirror, use biofeedback, get verbal feedback).
5. Have someone make a video performing the target task with which you are having trouble. Then try to copy the movements. Watch the movements carefully and imagine that the movements are your hands moving.
6. Perform the target task in different, nontraditional positions (e.g., practice in nontraditional positions such as lying on the back, lying on the stomach, reaching hand behind you or over your head).
7. Do the target task in different media (e.g., if having a problem with writing, draw shapes and letters in shaving soap; draw big letters and then small letters and then words).
8. Provide external support of the affected hand to appropriately position the digits (e.g., a splint if necessary to prevent movement of adjacent digits) while doing sensory and sensorimotor tasks on the target instrument.
   i. Begin with a single digit adjacent to the most involved digit, but not the most involved digit.
   ii. When you can do complex sensory exploration with a single finger without abnormal movement, combine sensory exploration with more complete target movements.
   iii. Add multiple digits to the sensorimotor tasks.
9. Without externally supporting the position of the digits (e.g., all digits free) perform one simple movement on the target task.
   i. Integrate sensory exploration with the simple movements and do the movements slowly, in time with a metronome.
   ii. Increase the complexity of the sensory-driven motor tasks (e.g., tapping single note to playing scales and chords to playing new music or performing new keyboard tasks).
   iii. Increase the speed of the movements on the target task, keeping up with the metronome.
   iv. Perform the target task normally for brief periods, and progress the practice time slowly with frequent breaks.

H. Reinforcing Sensorimotor Learning with Feedback

1. Biofeedback can include visual, cutaneous, muscle, vibration, auditory, or stretch stimuli.
2. Biofeedback can be supervised by another person, facilitated with robotic movements, controlled by electronic contraction (activation of muscles), or controlled by a physical constraint of a limb; guided repetitive passive movements can be supplemented with active movements to control motor output.
   i. Put tape on the top of the skin over the extensor surface of the digits to limit motion or emphasize somatosensory input and feedback.
   ii. Use multichannel biofeedback to learn how to avoid abnormal movement strategies.
      - Practice isolated movements and stop practice of unnecessary co-contractions of agonists and antagonists.
      - Use the small muscles inside the hand (intrinsic muscles) to move the digits instead of the extrinsic muscles.
      - Use imagery with mental rehearsal and practice to help restore the image of performing the task normally (see Appendix 9-C).

I. Return to Work

1. Try to return to work part time.
2. Discuss other work options if you cannot resume the original job tasks.
3. Make ergonomic modifications at the workplace.
4. Integrate stress-free techniques.
5. Take frequent brief breaks.
6. Walk or do other exercises at lunch time.

APPENDIX 9-C ■ Enhancing Learning-Based Sensorimotor Training: Use of Imagery, Mental Rehearsal, and Mental Practice

A. General Comments about Imagery

It is critical to restore confidence, a sense of wellness, and normal control of the movements of the extremities and trunk. Initially this may be difficult because of pain, lack of accurate sensory information, and difficulty with the control of movement or imagining that the hand or arm could be normal again. One way to begin to restore the accuracy of the information processing system so you can use your hand normally is to begin by changing how the hand and the functional task you are trying to perform are represented on your brain (the internal representation of that injured part).

It is important to be able to restore the normal image of the involved limb, that is, how it used to be and how it will be normal again. In the process of restoring normal control, it is also important to begin to use the hand normally and not increase the pain or repeat the abnormal movements. Thus, visually imagine your hand and how it looks. Making your hand look like the other hand is a good beginning. Then begin to create an image of the hand and the task you want to perform. Imagine using the hand normally to perform all the usual and target tasks. You can start by imaging small parts of a larger task and then finally the whole task and then related skills and activities that would be associated with performing the task.

With advances in magnetic resonance imaging, we can more readily confirm the recruitment of brain processes with imagery. It is possible to activate functional, motor, and sensory representations of the hand with mental imagery. The area of the brain recruited is dependent on the activities imagined by the individual. For example, you have many different maps of your body. Some of the topographical maps may be redundant across different parts of the central nervous system (e.g., motor cortex, sensory cortex, prefrontal cortex, thalamus, basal ganglia). Well-learned functions are also mapped separately from sensory and motor topography. When you visualize a body part, you will activate the somatosensory cortex. When you imagine doing the task (motor imagery), you will also activate the motor cortex. When you can visually and motorically imagine completing the task in your mind, you will activate the cortical areas representing the part of your body that is moving and the part of the brain that is devoted to completing that task (e.g., walking, writing, playing an instrument). The intensity with which the neurons fire when you are imaging is less than the intensity of firing when you are actually performing the task. Try to imagine performing your tasks without mistakes. This will reinforce the positive aspects of the sensorimotor feedback. You must imagine without interruption (e.g., attention), and you must repeat the imaging process with a high level of concentration to help the nervous system learn. If you are imaging and you run into difficulty completing a task normally, try to focus on the source of the difficulty, including asking your inner self what barriers are getting in the way. Once you can get insight into these barriers, you should be able to break them down.

During imaging or mental practice, approximately 30% of the neurons are recruited as would be recruited when the task is physically executed. Furthermore, when learning a new task, more neurons are recruited than when the task is learned. An impairment of structure (e.g., neurological or musculoskeletal) could modify the ability to image performing a task normally. On the other hand, imaging normal function and task performance could be easier than actually executing normal performance. In addition, repetitive imaging could begin to drive neural adaptation and recovery.

When there are conditions of chronic pain, there are changes in the organization and representation of the painful part in the central nervous system (e.g., cortex, thalamus, prefrontal cortex, supplemental motor cortex). Similarly, repetitive, abnormal patterns of movement also can dedifferentiate the representation of the body part. Thus, intervention must focus on restoring the normal representation of the brain. Sometimes it is easier to imagine normal movement or pain reduction than it is to actually change the pattern of movement or turn off the "on cells" for pain.

B. Suggestions for Goal-Directed Imaging

1. Set goals for yourself to specifically improve the function of your hand.
2. Follow a sequence for learning.
   a. Imagine that you are healthy and fit and have full normal control of all of your extremities.
   b. Focus on healing the involved tissues, particularly if you have signs of inflammation and pain.
      i. Focus on diaphragmatic breathing and bringing blood to the tissues.
      ii. Imagine the blood carrying important elements to the area of injury (e.g., the growth factors and oxygen that are requisites for healing tissues).
      iii. Imagine that an injury causes inflammation that triggers the healing response (e.g., laying down collagen [scar]). Also imagine that the body modifies the scar tissue and tries to keep it mobile.
   c. Visualize the anatomy, physiology, and kinesiology of the hand.
      i. Imagine the bones gliding smoothly on one another.
      ii. Imagine the muscles being strong, with a balance between the intrinsic and extrinsic muscles that serve the hand.
      iii. Imagine normal movement patterns.
      iv. Imagine normal sensation in the hand.
   d. Imagine pain-free movement.
   e. Imagine the hand being quiet and relaxed.
   f. Imagine smooth control of the hand without involuntary extraneous movements.
   g. Imagine that the affected hand is working just like the unaffected hand.
   h. Imagine using the hand as you used to use it. Go back in time to when your hand felt good and you did not have any problems.
   i. When mentally practicing and imaging, there should be no distractions. Spend at least 30 to 60 minutes a day normalizing the hand and imagining how good it feels.
   j. Mentally practice and perform the target task without any signs of strain or pain.
   k. Concentrate and mentally review each of the components of the hand working normally.
   l. Concentrate on the free flow of rhythmic movements of the hand and arm as you walk.
   m. Recapture the excitement of using your hand while playing your instrument or working at your job without pain or strain.
   n. Reinforce the image of a normal hand by continuing to progress learning, including more complex tasks and public performances.

CHAPTER 10 Payment Systems for Services: Documentation through the Care Continuum

BARBARA EDMISON, PT, and JOHN G. WALLACE, JR., PT, MS, OCS

KEY TERMS

capitation
CMS
CPT
HIPAA
ICD-9-CM
ICD-10-CM
Medicaid
Medicare
prospective payment system
reasonable and necessary
skilled services
third-party payer

OBJECTIVES

After reading this chapter the student or therapist will be able to:

1. Value the importance of documentation and its relationship to payment for services.
2. Synthesize different inpatient and outpatient payment systems.
3. Differentiate the continuum of care and documentation needed in different treatment settings.
4. Appropriately assign an ICD-9-CM code to medical and functional diagnoses.
5. Identify and select the CPT codes that best describe therapeutic interventions used in treating patients.
6. Analyze how payment policy can affect patient outcomes.

IMPORTANCE OF DOCUMENTATION

Physical therapists (PTs) and occupational therapists (OTs) are in the business of providing a health care service to improve quality of life. Because of the myriad insurance options available from both private and government-run programs, people rarely pay cash (self-pay) for physical and occupational therapy. Therapists want to be paid a "fair" amount for their skills and knowledge, but they generally rely on a third party to provide this payment. Clinicians must convince the third-party payer, an entity that was not present and did not receive the therapeutic interventions, that the patient received valuable, unique, and worthwhile services. Documentation is one method used to persuade the third-party payers to pay for the professional services provided.

Documentation is a skill a therapist must acquire. Its importance is equivalent to other forms of therapy skills. Documentation creates a lasting impression of the practitioners who represent the profession. Occupational therapy and physical therapy are an imperative and integral part of patient care; the documentation must reflect that. In addition, PTs and OTs are legally responsible for interventions provided by personnel under their supervision. Therapists then depend on other people to interpret their documentation and, on the basis of contracted rates, determine how much should be paid for each service. Third-party payers often submit documentation to peer reviewers to ascertain excessive, useless, or fraudulent treatments.

Securing payment for services rendered is, and will continue to be, a crucial element for the therapist as a professional as well as for the therapist's livelihood. Documentation, which is a legal and professional responsibility, is the basis for billing and is the proof that treatment was provided. Documentation is critical for success in the payment appeals process. For these reasons, documentation and payment for services are tightly linked together. This chapter will look at the payer sources at the national level and their required documentation components for payment.

It is important to remember that all the federal programs mentioned in this chapter are constantly changing. The process of legislating health care is dynamic and will be significantly modified in the next several years because there are not enough dollars available to cover the projected total costs. The supply of funds is in direct conflict with both the increased numbers of patients and their need for services. Major changes must occur in the future to enable health care, as expected by the public, to survive. One of the keys to these changes lies in documentation. A new national health policy plan for United States citizens was voted on and accepted in the spring of 2010, and new payment schedules or structure may be the outcome; but the need for documentation will remain constant, and documentation will always be a tool used for evaluating and justifying payment for services.

Why document? Documentation provides baseline status, records pertinent information, measures progress and success, fulfills predictions, and declares the final outcomes. It creates a record of the appointments the patient or client had. It provides data for concurrent or retrospective audits as well as evidence for research. It serves as an itemized bill for services rendered. The medical record may also become evidence in legal proceedings, which can either defend or incriminate the clinician. Documentation provides a snapshot of a period of time that gives the reviewer a full and practical description of the status of patients and the impact care has made on their quality of life.

Who reads the medical record? Although many therapists seem to believe that documenting is a necessary evil with no particular purpose, the information that therapists provide is vitally important. Physical and occupational therapy documentation is read by colleagues in the same or related disciplines to affect or continue the plan of care (POC). It is also read by physicians and discharge planners to assist in determining additional treatment or surgical options or placement opportunities. Insurance case managers rely on documentation for the assessment of proper use of services. OT and PT documentation is read by employees of third-party payers who may be screening for proper dates and codes or for predicted outcomes in a reasonable time frame. Therapists do not want to have payment denied for any reason; therefore it is extr emely important that the documentation clearly present all the pertinent information in a manner that is easily understood by all parties.

DEFINITION OF TERMS

There is an entire language of terms regarding payment issues. Please refer to the Quick Reference Guide to Acronyms (Appendix 10-A) for assistance. When therapy services are received, either the person pays the therapist directly or someone else pays the bill. Generally a patient will pay directly for therapy in three circumstances: (1) having a need for skilled services and not having insurance; (2) having had therapy interventions, understanding their value, and wishing to continue beyond what insurance is willing to cover; or (3) having a preference for a specific therapist who accepts only cash payment or who is not a preferred provider of the insurance company. When someone else pays the bill, it is the third-party payer that is billed for the services. Third-party payers are usually insurance carriers who, by contract or written agreement, may determine the maximum amount of money paid and under what circumstances.

Private health insurance is either purchased by a consumer or provided to people as a benefit of employment. People may have additional coverage by paying for it or as a result of being a dependent on someone else's insurance plan. This secondary insurance may pay for the portion of the bill that is unpaid by the patient's primary insurance. In the case of Medicare coverage, Medicare beneficiaries can purchase supplemental insurance that will pay some or all of the charges that are not part of their Medicare benefit. As the federal government is taking on a larger role in making sure individuals are insured by setting up a National Health Insurance System, the payer for the therapeutic services may change, but the fact remains that someone or a group of insurance carriers will pay for services rendered.

Health care services, for purposes of payment, are generally divided into three groups: inpatient, outpatient, and home health services. Inpatient services are delivered to patients staying in a hospital or health care facility. Outpatient services are delivered to patients who receive service by going to a health care provider. Home health agencies (HHAs) deliver services to patients in their own homes. Medicare services are processed and paid for by Medicare Administrative Contractors (MACs). MACs are responsible for administrating Medicare programs in 15 jurisdictions comprised of two or more states. MACs are private companies that have been awarded contracts by the Centers for Medicare and Medicaid Services (CMS) for processing all Part A and Part B claims within their geographical jurisdictions. MACs have the ability to accept or deny claims made to them for payment on the basis of their interpretations of the CMS guidelines. Medicare Parts A and B are discussed in more detail later in this chapter.

COBRA (from the Consolidated Omnibus Budget Reconciliation Act of 1985) refers to short-term interim insurance coverage. It allows people whose employment benefits have been terminated to have continuing employer-sponsored group health coverage temporarily. The American Recovery and Reinvestment Act of 2009 (ARRA) has expanded premium assistance to some people who qualify.

Workers' compensation is coverage for people who have been injured on the job. These regulations are determined at both national and state levels. Workers' compensation is discussed in greater detail later in this chapter.

Correct billing and claims processing are also dependent on accurately communicating treatment diagnoses and interventions to third-party payers. Three primary coding systems are used to communicate diagnoses and interventions in health care. The International Classification of Diseases, Ninth Revision, Clinical Modification (ICD-9-CM) is a tabular list of medical diagnoses approved for use by CMS based on the World Health Organization's ICD-9, originally published in 1977. Current Procedural Terminology (CPT) (a registered trademark of the American Medical Association [AMA]) is a coding system that describes health care interventions. CMS has developed its own coding system to meet the specific requirements of the Medicare and Medicaid programs. The Healthcare Common Procedure Coding System uses CPT and alphanumerical codes developed by CMS in conjunction with the AMA to describe interventions, procedures, and supplies for the Medicare and Medicaid programs.[1] Use of these coding systems is discussed in greater detail later in this chapter.

FEDERAL PROGRAMS

Medicare and Medicaid

"Medicare is a health insurance program for people age 65 or older, people under age 65 with certain disabilities, and people of all ages with end-stage renal disease . . . (permanent kidney failure requiring dialysis or a kidney transplant)."[2] The Medicaid program provides medical benefits to groups of low-income people, some of whom may have no medical insurance or inadequate medical insurance.[3] Although the federal government establishes general guidelines for the program, the Medicaid program requirements are actually established by each state. Whether or not a person is eligible for Medicaid will depend on the state where he or she lives.

"President Truman was the first President to propose a national health insurance plan."[4] Congressional debate about federal health care coverage continued for 20 years. In 1965, HR 6675, the "Mills Bill," was introduced. "Congressman Wilbur Mills, Chairman of the House Ways and Means Committee, created what was called the 'three-layer cake' by starting with President Johnson's Medicare proposal (Part A), adding to it physician and other outpatient services (Part B), and creating Medicaid which significantly expanded federal support for health care services for poor elderly, disabled, and families with dependent children. Medicare became Title 18 of the Social Security Act and

Medicaid became Title 19."[4] Although HR 6675 passed the House without a single amendment, the Senate version required much more discussion and many amendments. Finally, Medicare Part A, which involves basic hospital benefits and other institutional services for the elderly; Medicare Part B, a voluntary program; and Medicaid were approved by both the House and Senate.

Medicare and Medicaid implementation did not begin until 1966. Initially, "Medicare was the responsibility of the Social Security Administration (SSA), the agency that controlled the retirement social insurance program through which most people became eligible for Medicare. Federal assistance to the State Medicaid programs was administered by the Social and Rehabilitation Service (SRS). SRS oversaw welfare programs including Aid to Families with Dependent Children (AFDC), through which many people became eligible for Medicaid. SSA and SRS were agencies in the Department of Health, Education, and Welfare (HEW). In 1977, HEW Secretary Joseph Califano reorganized the department to create the Health Care Financing Administration (HCFA). HCFA was designed to improve administration of both Medicare and Medicaid by moving both health programs together, to improve the staffing of the Medicaid program, and to create a new administrative structure to implement national health insurance. In 1980, HEW was divided into the Department of Education and the Department of Health and Human Services (HHS). In 2001, Secretary Tommy G. Thompson renamed HCFA to become the Centers for Medicare and Medicaid Services (CMS) as part of his initiative to create a new culture of responsiveness in the agency."[4]

"Coverage for Medicare Part A is automatic for people age 65 or older (and for certain disabled persons) who have insured status under Social Security or Railroad Retirement. Most people don't pay a monthly premium for Part A. Coverage for Part A may be purchased by individuals who do not have insured status through the payment of monthly Part A premiums. Coverage for Part B also requires payment of monthly premiums. People with Medicare who have limited income and resources may get help paying for their out-of-pocket medical expenses from their state Medicaid program. There are various benefits available to 'dual eligibles' who are entitled to Medicare and are eligible for some type of Medicaid benefit. These benefits are sometimes also called Medicare Savings Programs (MSPs). For people who are eligible for full Medicaid coverage, the Medicaid program supplements Medicare coverage by providing services and supplies that are available under their state's Medicaid program. Services that are covered by both programs will be paid first by Medicare and the difference by Medicaid, up to the state's payment limit. Medicaid also covers additional services (e.g., nursing facility care beyond the 100-day limit covered by Medicare, prescription drugs, eyeglasses, and hearing aids). Limited Medicaid benefits are also available to pay out-of-pocket Medicare cost-sharing expenses for certain other Medicare beneficiaries. The Medicaid program will assume their Medicare payment liability if they qualify."[5]

The Balanced Budget Act of 1997 (BBA) made the most significant changes to the Medicare and Medicaid programs since their implementation. One goal was to shift some of the financial stress to the private sector, which was accomplished by allowing Medicare beneficiaries options for additional types of health plans. The BBA also reduced hospital payments, which had considerable consequences in the health care industry. This was one reason that the Balanced Budget Refinement Act of 1999 (BBRA) was introduced. The BBA was also designed to address fraud, abuse, and waste in the federal health care programs.

The BBA also created the Children's Health Insurance Program (CHIP), also known as Title XXI of the Social Security Act. "CMS administers this program, which helped states expand health care coverage to over 5 million of the nation's uninsured children. The program was reauthorized on February 4, 2009, when President Obama signed into law the Children's Health Insurance Program Reauthorization Act of 2009 (CHIPRA or Public Law 111-3). CHIPRA finances CHIP through fiscal year 2013. It will preserve coverage for the millions of children who rely on CHIP today and provides the resources for states to reach millions of additional uninsured children. CHIP is jointly financed by the federal and state governments and is administered by the states. Within broad federal guidelines, each state determines the design of its program, eligibility groups, benefit packages, payment levels for coverage, and administrative and operating procedures. CHIP provides a capped amount of funds to states on a matching basis. Federal payments under CHIP to states are based on state expenditures under approved plans effective on or after October 1, 1997."[6]

At least two other federal laws affect children who may not have sufficient health care coverage. The Elementary and Secondary Education Act of 1965 (ESEA), reauthorized as the No Child Left Behind Act of 2001 (NCLB), is standards-based education reform that is directed at disadvantaged students. IDEA, the Individuals with Disabilities Education Act, provides for early intervention, special education, and related services to children with disabilities.[7]

Health Insurance Portability and Accountability Act of 1996

The Health Insurance Portability and Accountability Act of 1996 (HIPAA) is a legislative effort to improve insurance coverage of the work force and also to improve the continuum of care by switching health care records away from paper and into the computer age.

Title I of HIPAA refers to health insurance reform. This reform increases the opportunities for workers to maintain or acquire insurance coverage when they lose or change jobs.

Title II of HIPAA relates to administrative simplification. These provisions are more closely associated with documentation and payment for services. The purpose of administrative simplification is to create a national database for medical records to ease communication among health care agencies. However, this led to concerns about privacy and security of vital information as a result of easily accessible online medical records. This prompted HHS to also include a privacy rule and a security rule. "The Standards for Privacy of Individually Identifiable Health Information ('Privacy Rule') establishes, for the first time, a set of national standards for the protection of certain health information. HHS issued the Privacy Rule to implement the requirement of HIPAA. The Privacy Rule standards address the use and disclosure of individuals' health information—called protected health information (PHI) by organizations subject to the Privacy Rule, called covered entities—as well as standards for individuals' privacy rights to understand and control how their health information is used. Within HHS, the Office for Civil Rights (OCR) has responsibility for implementing and enforcing the Privacy Rule with respect to voluntary compliance activities and civil money penalties.

"A major goal of the Privacy Rule is to [ensure] that individuals' health information is properly protected while allowing the flow of health information needed to provide and promote high-quality health care and to protect the public's health and well-being. The Rule strikes a balance that permits important uses of information, while protecting the privacy of people who seek care and healing. Given that the health care marketplace is diverse, the Rule is designed to be flexible and comprehensive to cover the variety of uses and disclosures that need to be addressed."[8]

"While the Privacy Rule mandates policies and procedures to protect patient information in all forms, the purpose of the Security Rule is to adopt national standards to protect the confidentiality, integrity, and availability of electronic protected health information. This Rule is directed at the covered entities, which are health care providers, health care clearinghouses, and/or health plans, that transmit or maintain protected health information electronically [and] are required to implement reasonable and appropriate administrative, physical, and technical safeguards. The Security standards require that steps be taken to protect this information from reasonably anticipated threats or hazards. Built into the Security Rule, however, is some flexibility that allows covered entities to determine what is reasonable and appropriate based on their size, cost considerations, and their existing technical infrastructure. This built-in flexibility also makes allowances for the rapid changes in technology."[9]

"On July 27, 2009, Secretary of the Department of Health and Human Services Kathleen Sebelius delegated authority for the administration and enforcement of the Security Standards for the Protection of Electronic Protected Health Information (Security Rule) to [OCR]." This action will improve HHS's ability to protect individuals' health information by combining the authority for administration and enforcement of the federal standards for health information privacy and security called for in HIPAA. The HIPAA Privacy Rule is also administered and enforced by OCR.

"Congress mandated improved enforcement of the Privacy Rule and Security Rule in the Health Information Technology for Economic and Clinical Health (HITECH) Act, part of the American Recovery and Reinvestment Act of 2009. Privacy and Security are naturally intertwined, because they both address protected health information. Combining the enforcement authority in one agency within HHS will facilitate improvements by eliminating duplication and increasing the efficiency of investigations and resolutions of failures to comply with both rules. Moreover, combining the administration of the Security Rule and the Privacy Rule is consistent with the health care industry's increasing adoption of electronic health records and the electronic transmission of health information."[10]

The federal government is helping businesses to achieve the HIPAA-mandated goals of improved and efficient health care while protecting the privacy of the recipients and the security of their information. The well-being of a person is reflected not only in her or his treatment but also by the integrity of the system to keep personal information confidential. HIPAA and its consequences directly relate to documentation standards and handling of PHI.

Prospective Payment Systems

Years ago, people received therapy in hospitals, Medicare was billed, and the hospital was paid. Physical and occupational therapy departments were among the highest moneymakers in the hospital. This, unfortunately, led to excessive billing and resulted in the need for improved accounting. More recently, CMS has established stricter requirements in an effort to control spending and to have money available for future generations. These requirements also benefit patients today by accelerating the establishment of a medical diagnosis, allowing for faster implementation of therapeutic interventions and preventing billing or payment for unskilled services. Currently, under the prospective payment system (PPS), hospitals are paid a set amount per patient. The amount depends on the medical diagnosis and related morbidities. Payments are no longer related to the length of stay or procedures ordered. It is the hospital's responsibility to maximize its income by minimizing the patient's stay.

The Social Security Amendments of 1983 were responsible for the plan to save taxpayers money by creating incentives to improve efficiency in acute-care hospitals. This system applied to Part A Medicare beneficiaries and was designed to give the hospitals a lump sum for patients who fit into certain categories.

"Section 1886(d) of the Social Security Act (the Act) sets forth a system of payment for the operating costs of acute-care hospital inpatient stays under Medicare Part A (Hospital Insurance) based on prospectively set rates. This payment system is referred to as the inpatient prospective payment system (IPPS). Under the IPPS, each case is categorized into a diagnosis-related group (DRG). Each DRG has a payment weight assigned to it, based on the average resources used to treat Medicare patients in that DRG."[11]

Use of the IPPS and DRGs, in which Medicare payments are established in advance and determined by the medical diagnosis at discharge, created the opportunity to transform hospitals into more efficient and cost-effective organizations. It also became essential to accurately determine the discharge diagnosis of patients in the hospital. Appropriate "coding" of patients developed in the Health Information Management Departments of hospitals to determine the correct DRG and corresponding payment.

Although the DRG is associated with an average hospital cost per diagnosis and is calculated on a per-case-at-discharge basis, the actual payment is affected by many factors. There are two different paths that contribute to the final payment: the operating, or labor, expenses, and the capital, or nonlabor, expenses. On the operating expenses side, the wage index incorporates local labor costs. Cost of living adjustments are made on the capital side. Also taken into account is the geographical area (rural versus urban) where the hospital is located. To adjust for case mix, each DRG is weighted relative to its complexity against the other individual DRGs. There are several other possible factors contributing to the DRG payments. The indirect medical education adjustment is allocated when the hospital is an approved teaching hospital for graduate medical education. The new technology adjustment is granted if the hospital is using expensive new technology that significantly improves clinical outcomes. The disproportionate share of the hospital adjustment is provided to hospitals that treat a higher percentage of low-income patients. An outlier is an exceptionally expensive course of treatment that qualifies for additional funding. DRG payments may be reduced if the patient's length of stay is shortened by a transfer to another acute-care hospital or post–acute-care setting. Fiscal year 2009 completed the transition to MS-DRGs, which are based on secondary diagnosis codes and provide more specific information for resource allocation. Medicare Severity (MS) divides cases into three levels. MCC, major complications with comorbidities, is the most severe. CC refers to complications with comorbidities, and Non-CC, or no complications with comorbidities present, is the least likely to require additional hospital resources.

With the success of the IPPS in acute-care hospitals, additional legislation mandated extension into other settings with Medicare Part A beneficiaries. The BBA, the BBRA, and the Benefits Improvement Act of 2000 (BIPA) moved the PPS into skilled nursing and inpatient rehabilitation facilities (IRFs), HHAs, hospice, hospital outpatient, inpatient psychiatric facilities, and long-term care hospitals (LTCHs). Payments for each are based on different classification systems, although therapy services remain included in the lump sum. The basic payment in each facility may also be adjusted by the factors listed in the previous paragraph.

The initial PPS has encouraged the use of modified versions of this payment system by nongovernment third-party payers. Today, most inpatient services are covered by prospectively paid contracts with hospitals and health care facilities. Services not covered by prospective payment arrangements are often covered by per diem contract arrangements that pay a flat rate per day for inpatient services.

Outcome Measures

CMS has developed different methods of determining payment in the PPS for the various settings. In almost every case, the initial status of the patient determines the amount of money the facility will receive. Generally, the more complicated the patient's condition, the higher the reimbursement rate. The facility must then have a system to create a preliminary comprehensive "snapshot" of patients within days of their arrival at that particular setting. To ensure that patients receive the same standard of care and are treated equally, all patients are assessed by use of the Medicare preferred tools, even if they do not have Medicare coverage.

In the inpatient acute rehabilitation facility, the preferred tool is the Inpatient Rehabilitation Facility–Patient Assessment Instrument (IRF-PAI) to assist in determining the payment amount. The Resident Assessment Instrument (RAI) is the primary tool in subacute and skilled nursing facilities, and OASIS (Outcome and Assessment Information Set) is used in HHAs. These tools are discussed in more detail later in this chapter.

With each of these outcome measurement tools and in each setting, therapy documentation in the medical record must validate the tool's ratings. Each tool is completed when the patient is admitted to the program and also at the time of discharge. As the patient progresses, it is very important for therapy documentation to reflect improvement and goal achievement. Because of the relative insensitivity and ordinal scales of these comprehensive instruments, a significant amount of functional change is often required to document improvement from one level to the next.

It is expected that third-party payers will begin to use the outcome measurement tools as a way of assessing the performance of different facilities. With this information available for comparison, physicians and payers may choose to admit patients to those facilities that provide the best outcomes in the fewest number of days.

The IRF-PAI, RAI, and OASIS were developed with essentially the same goals in mind: (1) to measure patient outcomes and (2) to improve quality of care. These tools are each used in conjunction with the Medicare PPS to determine payments. However, the functional tools themselves are not related and therefore there is no one system available in the United States to provide "standardized, patient-centered outcome data that can provide policy officials and managers with outcome data across different diagnostic categories, over time, and across different settings where post-acute services are provided (p. 13)."[12] For the future, it is hoped that "functional outcome data that [are] applicable to patients treated across different clinical settings and applications, more efficient and less costly to administer, and sufficiently precise to detect clinically meaningful changes in functional outcomes (p. 23)"[12] will be developed.

Recent legislation instructed CMS to investigate this problem. By 2010, CMS had begun addressing the need for a standardized assessment tool that would be applied from the acute-care hospital to four possible post–acute-care settings (IRFs, skilled nursing facilities [SNFs], HHAs, and LTCHs). Named the Continuity Assessment Record and Evaluation, or CARE, tool, it was being used only in Demonstration Projects at the time of this writing. Similar to the other instruments discussed (IRF-PAI, Minimum Data Set 2.0 [MDS], and OASIS), the CARE tool is initiated at admission and completed at discharge. It incorporates demographics, medical status, cognitive status, and functional abilities. With the electronic medical record, a standardized assessment tool across the continuum of care, and Web-based technology, CMS will then be able to determine and compare specific case-mix outcomes and costs relative to the particular discharge status and setting. This will ultimately be able to guide payment policy.

Inpatient Rehabilitation Facility–Patient Assessment Instrument

In an IRF, the IRF-PAI is required by CMS as part of its PPS. On admission to the IRF, the patient is assigned an Impairment Group Code (IGC), which is the condition requiring a rehabilitation stay. "The IRF PPS uses data from the IRF-PAI to classify patients into distinct groups based on clinical characteristics and expected resource needs. These distinct groups are called 'case-mix groups' or 'CMGs.' To classify a 'typical patient,' one who has a length of stay of more than 3 days, receives a full course of inpatient rehabilitation care, and is discharged to the community, into a CMG, the admission IGC, the admission motor and cognitive scores from the FIM,* and the age at admission are required. The CMG and comorbidity tier determine the unadjusted federal prospective payment rate."[13]

The Patient Assessment Instrument is best known for having incorporated the Funct*ional Independence Measure (FIM)*[14] along with function modifiers, quality indicators, and addition*al patient information. "The FIM* instrument is a basic indicator of severity of disability . . . . The need for assistance (burden of care) translates to the time/energy that another person must expend to serve the dependent needs of the disabled individual so that the individual can achieve and maintain a certain quality of life. The FIM instrument is a measure of disability, not impairment. The FIM instrument is intended to measure what the person with the disability actually does, whatever the diagnosis or impairment, not what (s)he ought to be able to do, or might be able to do under different circumstances (p. III-1)."*[15]

Demographic, payer, medical, admission, and discharge information are included in the IRF-PAI. "The function modifiers assist in the scoring of related FIM items and provide explicit information as to how a FIM score has been determined."[15] These modifiers apply to bowel and bladder control, tub and shower transfers, and distances covered by walking or in a wheelchair. The FIM instrument specifically addresses the amount of assistance required for the functional activities of eating; grooming; bathing; upper body and lower body dressing; toileting; bladder and bowel management; bed, chair, and wheelchair transfers; toilet transfers; tub transfers; shower transfers; locomotion via walking or wheelchair; stairs; comprehension; expression; social interaction; problem solving, and memory. Each has its own algorithm to determine the FIM score. Quality indicators include respiratory status, pain, pressure ulcers, and safety (balance and falls).[15]

The FIM instrument has a total of seven levels of assistance. These are divided into two main categories, Independent—No Helper, and Dependent—Requires Helper. The two items in Independent—No Helper consist of Complete Independence—7 and Modified Independence—6. The highest score of 7 indicates that the patient completes the task safely, in a timely manner, and without any assistive devices. A score of 6 means that the patient requires a device or takes extra time or safety is an issue. The Dependent—Requires Helper category is further divided into two sections: the Modified Dependence—5, 4, and 3 scores, in which the patient provides 50% or more of the effort, and the Complete Dependence—2 and 1 scores, in which the patient's effort is less than 50%. Supervision or setup, 5, denotes no physical contact with the patient; the patient requires coaxing or someone standing by, or a helper may need to set up the equipment. Minimal contact assistance, 4, includes touching; the patient is doing 75% or more of the activity. Moderate assistance, 3, indicates that more than touching is required, with the patient giving 50% to 74% effort. Maximal assistance, 2, has the patient supplying 25% to 49% of the effort. In Total assistance, 1, the patient performs less than 25% of the workload. There is a training manual available to assist the clinician in completing this form.[15]

A similar data or documentation form is used in pediatrics: the WeeFIM II System. "The WeeFIM instrument was developed to measure the need for assistance and the severity of disability in children between the ages of 6 months and 7 years. The WeeFIM instrument may be used with children above the age of 7 years as long as their functional abilities, as measured by the WeeFIM instrument, are below those expected of children aged 7 who do not have disabilities. The WeeFIM instrument consists of a minimal data set of 18 items that measure functional performance in three domains: self-care, mobility, and cognition."[16]

Resident Assessment Instrument

In SNFs, the PPS is designed to cover the costs of providing care on a daily basis. This includes payment for ancillary services. The BBA required that the payments be adjusted for case mix. Case mix refers to the diversity of patients/residents on the basis of their complexity of medical problems or need for resources. This accounts for the increase in costs of complicated or involved cases. It ensures that facilities accept a variety of patients, rather than only those who require the least amount of services. In SNFs, a method of classifying each resident was developed to adjust the payments relative to the staff resources required to care for and to provide therapy to the residents. There is a higher cost associated with residents who require more resources or one-on-one care by staff. The facility should be reimbursed at a higher rate for these residents than for those who are more independent. Facilities are also reimbursed at a higher rate for residents who are receiving skilled services. All this information is acquired in the RAI, which is composed of three parts: the MDS, the Resident Assessment Protocols (RAPs), and the Utilization Guidelines. The RAI provides a structured method for the facility to create individualized care plans, to communicate on an internal and external basis, and to monitor quality performance. The MDS indicators are factored into the calculations for the Resource Utilization Groups, version III (RUG-III). RUG-III is the complex classification system used by CMS to determine the daily payment rate for the SNF PPS. RUG-III, in addition to many other categories, has a Rehabilitation category with five subcategories that describe the intensity of therapy received. The subcategories are determined by the number of minutes of therapy and the number of therapies each week.

The MDS is completed on a set schedule. After the initial 5-day, then 14-, 30-, 60-, and 90-day reports, the MDS is filed on a quarterly and annual basis. The MDS requires input from residents, their families, physicians, therapists, and dieticians. Facility staff from direct care, social services, activities, billing, and admissions is also consulted. The resident's performance over the entire 24-hour day is reviewed and recorded to create an individual picture of strengths and needs. The MDS includes a complete review of the resident's health, sensory systems, activity levels, behaviors, continence, activities of daily living (ADLs), physical and functional status, medications, procedures, and discharge plans. Although the MDS assesses activities similar to those of the FIM, the format is quite different. The Functional Status section is composed of Activities of Daily Living Assistance, Bathing, Balance during Transitions and Walking, Functional Limitations in Range of Motion, Mobility

*Copyright © 2001, 2002 UB Foundation Activities, Inc. (UBFA, Inc.) for compilation rights; no copyrights claimed in U.S. Government works included in Section I, portions of Section IV, Appendices I and K, and portions of Appendices B, C, E, G, H, and J. All other copyrights are reserved to their respective owners. Copyright © 1993-2001 UB Foundation Activities, Inc. for the FIM Data Set, Measurement Scale, Impairment Codes, and refinements thereto for the IRF-PAI, and for the Guide for the Uniform Data Set for Medical Rehabilitation, as incorporated or referenced herein. The FIM mark is owned by UBFA, Inc.

Devices, and Functional Rehabilitation Potential. The Activities of Daily Living Self-Performance subcategory of Activities of Daily Living Assistance includes bed mobility, transfers, walk in room, walk in corridor, locomotion on unit, locomotion off unit, dressing, eating, toilet use, and personal hygiene. The scoring system is based on an activity occurring three or more times. Use code 0 for Independent, no help or staff oversight; 1 for Supervision—oversight, encouragement, or cueing; 2 for Limited assistance if the resident is highly involved in the activity; 3 for Extensive assistance if the resident is involved in the activity and staff members provide weight-bearing support; and 4 for Total dependence if full staff performance is required every time. This section has a separate but related area to record the ADL Support Provided. In this case, the coding is 0 for no setup or physical help from staff; 1 for setup help only; 2 for one-person physical assistance; and 3 for physical assistance from two or more persons. The MDS has a training manual available to assist with completing the instrument.[17]

The RAPs are used to identify problems and to create individualized care plans. Certain responses from the RAPs initiate triggers, which identify potential or actual problems. From the triggers, areas of concern are further researched to determine complications and risk factors in addition to noting the need for referrals to appropriate health professionals. Utilization Guidelines are necessary to analyze the information gathered from the RAPs.

In response to providers, consumers, and others, CMS implemented the new and improved MDS Version 3.0 effective October 1, 2010. This redesigned version incorporated many significant changes. Based on a RAND/Harvard team effort, the MDS 3.0 is much easier to read and accomplishes several goals. These include improved resident input, improved accuracy and reliability, increased efficiency, and improved staff satisfaction and perception of clinical utility. A new development with MDS 3.0 is the addition of the Care Area Assessment (CAA) Process to assist with the interpretation of the information gathered from the MDS. As of October 2010, the RAI components are the MDS 3.0, the CAA process and the RAI utilization guidelines. An updated classification system, RUG-IV, was scheduled to be introduced at the same time as the MDS 3.0. However, while Section 10325 of the Affordable Care Act allowed CMS to implement the MDS 3.0 as scheduled, this same Section mandated a delay of the implementation of the RUG-IV classification system by one year. Portions of RUG-IV were implemented on an interim basis on October 1, 2010. The purpose of RUG-IV is to more accurately allocate payments. RUG-III bases payments on predicted therapy minutes from the MDS, causing inaccurate classifications and payments to SNFs in some instances. RUG-IV calculates the average daily number of therapy minutes based on the actual number of minutes provided to assign patients to Rehabilitation categories. The number of minutes of therapy received affects the reimbursement rate. This is why it is very important to correctly document the time spent treating the resident in addition to the resident's functional status.[18]

Outcome and Assessment Information Set

The home health PPS, introduced with the BBA, uses a similar system as do the acute-care facilities, IRFs, and SNFs. There is a standard base payment rate adjusted according to several variables, including geographical differences in wages, outliers, and the health condition and care needs of the patient. The latter, also referred to as the case mix, is determined by items in the Outcome and Assessment Information Set. On January 1, 2010, HHAs began using OASIS-C version 2.00 at the direction of CMS.

"The Outcome and Assessment Information Set (OASIS) is a group of data elements that represent core items of a comprehensive assessment for an adult home care patient and form the basis for measuring patient outcomes for purposes of outcome-based quality improvement. The OASIS is a key component of Medicare's partnership with the home care industry to foster and monitor improved home health care outcomes. The goal was not to produce a comprehensive assessment instrument, but to provide a set of data items necessary for measuring patient outcomes and essential for assessment—which home health agencies (HHAs) in turn could augment as they judge necessary. Overall, the OASIS items have utility for outcome monitoring, clinical assessment, care planning, and other internal agency-level applications."[19]

The OASIS includes sections on patient demographics, clinical record items, patient history and diagnoses, living arrangements, sensory status, integumentary status, respiratory status, cardiac status, elimination status, neuro/emotional/behavioral status, ADLs *and* instrumental activities of daily living (IADLs), medications, care management, and therapy need and POC. The ADL/IADL category is divided into grooming, upper body dressing, lower body dressing, bathing, toilet transferring, toileting hygiene, transferring, ambulation/locomotion, feeding or eating, ability to plan and prepare light meals, ability to use telephone, prior functioning ADL/IADL, and fall risk assessment. In the OASIS format, choices to describe patient function vary with the activity. Grooming, upper and lower body dressing, and toileting hygiene scales are 0 for independent; 1 for setup, no assistance; 2 if someone must help with the activity; and 3 if the patient is totally dependent. With bathing, the range is from 0, or independent, to 6, bathed totally by another person. For transfers, 0 is independent and 5 is bedfast, unable to move self. Ambulation/locomotion scores are from 0, able to independently walk on even and uneven surfaces, and negotiate stairs with or without railings and no device, to 6, bedfast, unable to ambulate or be up in a chair. Feeding or eating starts with 0 for able to independently feed self and extends to 5, unable to take in nutrients orally or by tube feeding. Ability to plan and prepare light meals (make cereal or sandwich or reheat delivered meals safely) ranges from 0 for independent or was able to but did not before this admission to 2 for unable. Ability to use telephone is 0 for able to dial numbers and answer calls appropriately and as desired to 5, totally unable to use the telephone. Prior functioning requests information about self-care, ambulation, transfer, and household tasks. Finally, the fall risk assessment asks if the patient is at risk for falls. A score of 0 means that no multifactor fall risk assessment was conducted, 1 indicates that the fall assessment was completed but does not indicate a risk for falls, and 2 indicates that the patient is at risk for falls. The care management section assesses the level of caregiver ability and willingness to provide assistance if needed in activities ranging from ADL assistance to patient advocacy. Note that although the OASIS is very precise, it also makes it difficult to measure progress. For example, in the ambulation category, a score of 4 indicates "chairfast, unable to ambulate but is able to wheel self independently"; 3 indicates "able to walk only with the supervision or assistance of another person at all times"; and 2 indicates "requires use of a two-handed device (e.g., walker or crutches) to walk alone on a level surface and/or requires human supervision or assistance to negotiate stairs or steps or uneven surfaces."[20] This is another example of the importance of documentation to report significant improvement in therapy.

DOCUMENTATION RECOMMENDATIONS

Documentation is communication of the professional judgment used to establish a patient's POC. Documentation should demonstrate the integration of the elements of patient management that determine the services that, in the professional opinion of the therapist, will provide the best possible outcome for the patient.

Medicare guidelines provide the minimum context standards required for adequate documentation. Satisfying minimum guidelines is not sufficient for the therapist who is thinking critically. This therapist should always be asking determinative questions (Box 10-1).

When the answer to whether therapy is necessary is "no," document the reason why services will not be rendered. This will explain the therapist's perspective. Generally this is an obvious decision because the therapist is unable to establish any goals.

When the answer is "yes," the therapist must be able to answer the additional questions in Box 10-1. These important questions justify treatment and payment. The patient may have insurance or may be receiving federal, state, or county aid. Either way, the therapist must not forget that someone is responsible for paying the bill and that someone deserves a meaningful and beneficial product in return.

The American Physical Therapy Association (APTA) has published Guidelines: Physical Therapy Documentation of Patient/Client Management.[21] These guidelines can be found on the APTA website (www.apta.org) under About Us—Policies and Bylaws—Board of Directors Positions and Policies, Section I—Practice. Although the general guidelines in Box 10-2 were written as part of an APTA document, they set a standard for therapists in the health care industry.

In addition to following APTA's Guidelines: Physical Therapy Documentation of Patient/Client Management, the medical record must follow requirements set forth by other agencies and regulating bodies. CMS sets minimum standards for documentation that are implemented on the local level by fiscal intermediaries or Medicare carriers, as appropriate. Fiscal intermediaries and Medicare carriers are responsible for acceptance or denial of claims made to them by the acknowledged provider of services. The standards pertaining to "reasonable and necessary" are available from individual fiscal intermediaries and Medicare carriers as local coverage determinations (LCDs).

The LCD standards and other helpful information are available through specific websites or through the Medicare Coverage page of the CMS website (www.cms.gov). Nongovernment third-party payers can follow guidelines of their own design. These may or may not be similar to Medicare guidelines. In general, when a therapist's documentation meets Medicare requirements, it satisfies the expectations of other third-party payers as well.

There are other regulating organizations, such as The Joint Commission, licensing boards, or state departments of health services, that set documentation standards to protect consumers of health care services. It is important that therapists be aware of all documentation required by the regulatory agencies associated with their patients when documenting in the medical record. Because of the unique requirements of payers at the various state, county, and local levels, this section of the chapter primarily addresses CMS guidelines for inpatient facilities.

Medicare requires specific information with bills that are submitted for payment. Following these rules will facilitate reimbursement for services because any deviation may be used as a reason for denial of payment. Proper documentation is always necessary for the appeals process when a claim has been denied. Medicare billing must include the following, which are appropriate for both inpatient and outpatient settings.

The patient must be eligible for therapy services on the basis of an active written POC. The POC must be ordered or certified by a physician or by another licensed independent practitioner. Time periods for certification and requirements for return physician visits may vary. These requirements may be different in states with direct access to physical therapy.

In addition, therapy must be a reasonable and necessary treatment for the particular illness or injury. Reasonable and necessary allows a broad interpretation, which is why documentation becomes so important. The following are components that establish medical necessity:

1. Intervention, as related to the specific profession, is an accepted standard of care for this diagnosis. There are specific and effective interventions (evidence-based practice) successfully used to treat the condition.
2. The treatments require the skilled services of a professional. Knowledge and judgment are required because of the complexity of the problem and sophistication of the therapist's unique body of knowledge.
3. Therapeutic intervention creates significant improvement, demonstrated by measurable gains in range of motion, strength, function, level of assistance, and so on.
4. The amount, frequency, and duration of treatment are reasonable. This is clarified by a POC with short- and long-term goals, predicted end of treatment, and reasonable potential to achieve the stated goals. Weekly reassessments or changes in the patient's condition will require the plan to be modified as necessary.

Reasonable and necessary are key words for therapists to synthesize as part of the critical thinking process. Two examples are given to assist the reader to further analyze the meaning of these words.

BOX 10-1 ■ DETERMINATIVE QUESTIONS

Is there any therapy-related skilled service that this patient requires?

If yes, what is the unique professional contribution to this person's rehabilitation?

Are therapy services medically reasonable and necessary and able to be correctly administered in a timely and beneficial way?

What are the therapy services and on what schedule will they be administered?

BOX 10-2 ■ GENERAL GUIDELINES

Documentation is required for every visit or encounter.

All documentation must comply with the applicable jurisdictional and regulatory requirements.

All handwritten entries shall be made in ink and will include original signatures. Electronic entries are made with appropriate security and confidentiality provisions.

Charting errors should be corrected by drawing a single line through the error and initialing and dating the chart or through the appropriate mechanism for electronic documentation that clearly indicates that a change was made without deletion of the original record.

All documentation must include adequate identification of the patient/client and the physical therapist (PT) or physical therapist assistant (PTA) (or occupational therapist or occupational therapist assistant):

- The patient's/client's full name and identification number, if applicable, must be included on all official documents.
- All entries must be dated and authenticated with the provider's full name and appropriate designation*:
- Documentation of examination, evaluation, diagnosis, prognosis, plan of care, and discharge summary must be authenticated by the PT who provided the service.
- Documentation of intervention in visit or encounter notes must be authenticated by the PT or PTA who provided the service.
- Documentation by PT or PTA graduates or other PTs and PTAs pending receipt of an unrestricted license shall be authenticated by a licensed PT, or, when permissible by law, documentation by PTA graduates may be authenticated by a PTA.
- Documentation by students in PT or PTA programs must be additionally authenticated by the PT, or, when permissible by law, documentation by PTA students may be authenticated by a PTA.

Documentation should include the referral mechanism by which physical therapy services are initiated. Examples include:

- Self-referral or direct access
- Request for consultation from another practitioner

Documentation should include indication of no shows and cancellations.[21]

*OT or occupational therapist assistant should use the same documentation system and protocol. Space prohibited using all professionals' initials.

CASE STUDY 10-1

A 60-year-old active, independent woman who falls and fractures her humerus may be, understandably, a little wobbly from the trauma, but she will not need therapy to achieve independent mobility. However, the situation changes completely when the same woman has an existing right hemiparesis, requires the use of a cane for balance, and then fractures her left humerus. Now therapy would be appropriate to address ADLs, safety, and gait to assist her in regaining her independence. Both physical and occupational therapists may be treating this patient, and each professional needs to be following similar processes for thorough documentation.

CASE STUDY 10-2

A patient who lives independently and is admitted to the hospital with a ruptured appendix would not usually require therapy services. The patient would need to spend time out of bed and to ambulate in the hallways to regain endurance, but this may be done with nursing staff or family. If the same patient had comorbidities such as multiple sclerosis or Parkinson disease that were exacerbated by the hospitalization, then therapy would be warranted. Therapy would establish a POC to address the issues that prevent a return to the prior level of function.

Recovery Audit Contractors

As part of the Medicare Modernization Act of 2003, Congress initiated a Recovery Audit Contractor (RAC) demonstration project to fight fraud, waste, and abuse in the Medicare system. "The demonstration resulted in over $900 million in overpayments being returned to the Medicare Trust Fund between 2005 and 2008 and nearly $38 million in underpayments returned to health care providers."[22] The RACs were so effective that Congressional legislation made them permanent in Section 302 of the Tax Relief and Health Care Act of 2006. This Act expanded the RAC program to cover all 50 states in January 1, 2010. These audits were designed with three purposes in mind: first, to protect Medicare beneficiaries; second, to protect taxpayer dollars used to make payments; and third, to ensure that claims were paid only for services that met Medicare requirements. The RAC teams, which are required to include nurses and therapists, are paid on a contingency fee basis in which the fee is returned if the provider wins at any level of appeal.

"The goal of the recovery audit program is to identify improper payments made on claims of health care services provided to Medicare beneficiaries. Improper payments may be overpayments or underpayments. Overpayments can occur when health care providers submit claims that do not meet Medicare's coding or medical necessity policies. Underpayments can occur when health care providers submit claims for a simple procedure but the medical record reveals that a more complicated procedure was actually performed. Health care providers that might be reviewed include hospitals, physician practices, nursing homes, home health agencies, durable medical equipment suppliers and any other provider or supplier that bills Medicare Parts A and B."[22] Because a complex review requires the medical record, documenting comprehensible reasonable and necessary skilled services is critical.

Skilled Services

People who have experienced trauma or a disease process that affects their ability to move or function would be readily labeled candidates for therapy services. Therapy intervention should be easy to justify. The challenge is twofold. The therapist must (1) be able to identify and then substantiate the need for skilled services and (2) be sure that the documentation allows other parties to follow and understand what has been provided. The following example of documentation compares two sentences that a reviewer might read: "Gait training to facilitate weight shifting onto the affected extremity with minimal assistance required for safety" versus "The patient ambulated down the hall." The first sentence conveys the need for the unique and necessary skills of a PT. The second fails to even suggest the presence of a therapist. Avoid referring to skilled physical or occupational therapy, which then infers that unskilled therapy is also available. Unskilled therapy, for which a reviewer should deny payment for services, could easily be represented by "The patient ambulated down the hall." Skilled services, on the other hand, reflect therapy provided by qualified therapists with clinical expertise and knowledge.

A list of the interventions provided does not demonstrate skilled care. A therapist must include the level and type of skilled assistance given, clinical decision making or problem solving involved, and continued analysis of patient progress. An explanation of why specific interventions are chosen and what makes them still necessary is *also required.* Documentation of the therapist's observations of the patient's movement and activity before, during, and after an intervention, the patient's specific response to the intervention, and the relationship of progress to goals are additional examples of skilled service.

Duplication of services is also a concern when there is collaboration across the disciplines. Many patients will benefit from treatments in which both OTs and PTs are present. However, if both therapists document, "Sat patient at edge of bed to work on balance," reviewers could easily question whether both therapists did the same thing at the same time. The reviewers might then have a problem approving payment for the care provided, with a possibility that both services would be denied payment. There are no questions of duplication when the medical record states that the PT treatment session included "instruction and demonstration of strategies for dynamic postural adjustments" and the OT treatment session was directed toward "ADL training with emphasis on dressing." The same is true for speech pathologists, OTs, and/or PTs in a multidisciplinary approach. A treatment session may have one therapist facilitating head control and midline orientation, another addressing upper extremity function and coordination, and a therapist from a third discipline focusing on the ability to swallow. Be sure the documentation reflects the specific skills and knowledge related to each therapy.

DOCUMENTATION: A LEGAL DOCUMENT

The medical record is a legal document that is read by many people who are not therapists. Patients have much greater access to and interest in their medical records today than ever before. The medical record is available to insurance case managers and medical reviewers who are outside the medical facility. Patients may share their records with their families, new physicians and therapists, or even attorneys. Because of the various interests and needs of these diverse groups, it is necessary to be concise, legible, objective, and professional when documenting. Remember that no documentation can be released to others without a patient's signed release of information form on file in the patient's medical record.

Therapists should realize that it is very possible that their notes may be subpoenaed in the future as part of a lawsuit. The person who is the keeper of the records at the time of the case may have to go to court and explain, via another's documentation, what was done for the patient, or it is possible that the therapist may be reading her own notes several years later while sitting in the witness box.

When documenting, be aware of the following important and sensitive areas. Remember that therapists receive a long and expensive education to enable them to write in the official legal record. Reviewers are basing their decision to pay for therapy on what has been recorded; be mindful of the need to meet criteria for skilled services. Patients and their entire medical team appreciate professional interventions and professional documentation.

Patient Advocacy

The therapist is the patient's advocate. As such, the therapist should champion the best care for the patient. This may mean consulting professionals in other disciplines or facilitating transfers to other facilities. It is the clinician's responsibility to ensure that the record reflects the patient's best interests. Do not let therapy notes hinder the patient's forward progress in any way. Patients with neurological conditions may have deficits that affect their orientation, judgment, initiation, ability to respond or comprehend, or insight. They may have visual-perceptual or other sensory problems that affect their ability to participate in therapy. Their ability to process information may be delayed. None of these components are reasons to withhold treatment, but they may affect the time required to achieve appropriate goals. These patients can and will progress with a creative, patient, and knowledgeable therapist.

Timeliness

Whenever possible, document immediately after seeing the patient. This ensures that the session is recorded accurately. It is better to report the results of consultations, test results, or phone calls rather than writing that the therapist intends to take action. The latter leaves the reader wondering if anything happened until the relevant findings are included in the medical record.

Motivation

A therapist should believe that a patient is motivated to improve. Sometimes there is damage to the brain that affects initiation, insight, or judgment; sometimes there is depression, pain, or another medical reason. It is the therapist's responsibility to find the key to unlock the patient's ability to participate. Do not record that the patient is unmotivated. The lack of motivation usually belongs to the therapist. (See Chapter 5 for additional information.)

Personal Opinion

The therapist's documentation must be absolutely objective. The PT or OT may provide direct quotations or accurately record an event that happened during a therapy session to allow the reader to make his or her own judgment. It is very important to never let personal feelings about the patient enter the medical record. Bias and antagonism on the part of the therapist may leave the medical record open to speculation and become a problem if litigation occurs. If the reader of the documentation senses animosity, certainly the patient will too! The validity of the comments and the therapy provided become questionable. Always keep personal opinions out of official documentation.

Abbreviations

Be careful with abbreviations because the individual documenting may be the only one who understands what is being stated. Most facilities have an approved abbreviations list; use it! The meaning of what has been written will change according to the reader's interpretation of the abbreviations used. It is possible that a reviewer will read the medical record and either find it incomprehensible or completely misunderstand the original intent. The purpose of documentation is to provide information. Claims may be denied because the reviewer does not understand the abbreviations used.

Pain

The Joint Commission has brought the patient's pain level to the forefront, making a patient's pain level the "fifth vital sign." It is required that a comprehensive pain assessment appropriate for the patient's age and condition be recorded at regular intervals. The most common pain scale is 0 to 10, with 0 signifying no pain and 10 signifying the worst pain the patient can imagine. To further explain the scale to the patient, the numbers 1 to 3 correspond to minimal pain, 4 to 7 to moderate pain, and 8 to 10 to severe pain. A score of 4 or higher requires immediate attention. It is important to explain to the patient that his or her pain scale response is accepted at face value and belongs only to the patient; the patient's numbers are not compared with those of anyone else. For children ages 3 years and older, the Wong-Baker FACES Pain Rating Scale[23] may be easier to understand. The purpose of a pain scale is to ascertain the effectiveness of pain medication or pain-reducing modalities. It is important to document the pain number at rest and during treatment, whether pain interferes with or prohibits participation in therapy, and what the therapist has done to remedy the painful situation. (See Chapters 5 and 32 for additional information.)

Reassessments

Reassessments are done on a weekly basis or sooner if short-term goals have been met or there has been a change in status. The reassessment should describe the patient's situation and address the short-term goals, either explaining why the goals have not been met or setting new goals when the previous ones have been achieved. In addition to addressing the short-term goals, the reassessment provides the opportunity to clarify the treatment plan, treatment frequency, and duration of treatment.

Patient, Family, and Caregiver Training

The education provided must be appropriate to the patient's abilities. It is important to assess the learning style and barriers to learning, then adjust the teaching accordingly. The patient or caregivers must be able to understand the information. For example, documenting that the patient is blind and that he was given written handouts would be inappropriate, unless it was also documented that the family was trained with the materials provided. With any teaching, it is important to record what was taught, the response, and how well the new information was comprehended, either by return demonstration or by correct responses to questioning. Indicate whether the patient will be safe alone or with the specified caregivers after the training or whether additional education is necessary.

Patient Rights

Patients have many rights, including the right to be treated with respect and dignity. Use terms that focus on the patient as a person; avoid labeling patients by their diagnosis. Informed consent, risks and benefits of treatment, and confidentiality are extremely important, both ethically and legally. Patients always have the right to refuse treatment. Therapy cannot be forced on individuals against their will. Therapists offer a service that medical and health care professionals know will be beneficial, but patients are responsible for paying for their health care and they must be given a choice.

Accountability

Whenever possible, include references to other health care team members in order to demonstrate an interdisciplinary approach to patient care. Perform a thorough review of the medical record. Information from other team members can aid therapists in their understanding of the patient's situation. Inquire about the patient's goals for therapy treatment to incorporate into the POC. Each case must be examined individually. No two cases should be assumed to have the same problems and the same plans for resolution. What appears to be a routine assessment may present subtle and intricate challenges to both the patient and the therapist. Be sure to take a critical look at what has already been entered into the medical record. Question any findings that do not make sense, especially if previous documentation does not correspond to all the information and clinical symptoms present. Take the initiative to solve problems and investigate inconsistencies. Patients depend on the skills and knowledge of their therapists. Therapists must be accountable for their own documentation.

CONTINUUM OF CARE

Acute Care

Different settings require a change in the focus of documentation. It is important for the therapist to understand this concept and to modify documentation as necessary. In the acute-care setting, discharge planning begins as soon as the patient is admitted. The primary role of the therapist is to assess the patient to determine the next level of care and to introduce therapeutic interventions to expedite that process. Time is of the essence; the therapist may have only one or two visits to make a discharge recommendation and fewer than five visits to achieve initial short-term goals.

Depending on various circumstances, patients may transfer from the acute-care hospital to home either directly or indirectly by way of acute inpatient rehabilitation or an SNF.

Although the primary goal is to return the patient home and continue therapy there or in an outpatient setting, some patients may never leave the SNF. The emphasis is on safety. The patient must be safe in her or his own environment. Caregivers, if necessary, must be capable of safely assisting the patient. It is important to realize that patients may not access every level of care, or they may require a combination of settings. In each location, the treatment techniques may vary and the short-term goals will be different, but the same documentation guidelines apply. The following paragraphs assume that the patient is initially admitted to an acute-care hospital and then describe the possible discharge options.

Subacute Care

A patient who is admitted to the hospital and then requires the use of both a ventilator and a feeding tube may benefit from a subacute setting before moving on to acute inpatient rehabilitation. In the subacute setting, respiratory therapists and the nursing staff have key roles. Patients who have had respiratory failure in addition to their neurological deficits require a much slower pace to achieve their rehabilitation goals (see Chapter 3). These patients, with extremely impaired endurance and low functional levels, may stay in subacute settings for several months before they develop sufficient strength to progress to acute inpatient rehabilitation or return home. Short-term goals are set month to month, in contrast to acute-care hospitals, where short-term goals may be met in a matter of visits or days.

Acute Inpatient Rehabilitation

The Commission on Accreditation of Rehabilitation Facilities (CARF) monitors quality standards for acute inpatient rehabilitation care and is respected at an international level. Patients admitted to rehabilitation facilities accredited by this commission must meet several requirements. First, the patient must be medically stable and able to participate in at least 3 hours of therapy throughout the day. The overall medical stability must still require 24-hour nursing care and physician monitoring for medical diagnoses such as hypertension or diabetes. Second, the physical disability is such that the patient must need at least two of the three rehabilitation disciplines of speech, occupational, and physical therapy. Finally, the patient must have a community discharge plan. The discharge plan is imperative because acute inpatient rehabilitation is a dynamic process and patients will be discharged from this setting. A patient who was living alone before hospitalization but whose long-term goals do not include independence may not be eligible for acute inpatient rehabilitation care.

Skilled Nursing Facility

If the patient does not meet the requirements for acute inpatient rehabilitation or if the patient does not have financial, family, or other resources to enable him or her to live at home with assistance, then an SNF may be a better option. The patient benefits by receiving rehabilitation services and having a place to live. The facility is able to bill the third-party payer at a higher rate than for someone who is not receiving therapy services. The patient is allowed to receive therapy at a slower pace for a longer period of time. As the patient improves, acute inpatient rehabilitation may then be considered.

Home Health

Patients who are discharged from hospitals and facilities may still require additional therapy. They may not have the ability or the endurance to travel to an outpatient setting and then also participate in the various therapies. In these cases, home health therapists provide the solution. To receive home therapy, a patient must be homebound. According to CMS, the definition of homebound is "Normally unable to leave home unassisted. To be homebound means that leaving home takes considerable and taxing effort. A person may leave home for medical treatment or short, infrequent absences for nonmedical reasons, such as a trip to the barber or to attend religious service. A need for adult day care doesn't keep you from getting home health care."[24] Documentation must explain why the patient is homebound. As the patient improves, this becomes more difficult and facilitates a decision for outpatient therapy or discontinuation of therapy services altogether.

Transitional Living Centers

Some communities are fortunate to have a transitional living center (TLC) available for clients to move beyond IRFs and into "real-world" situations. TLCs are community-based neurocognitive rehabilitation programs where the standard of care includes occupational, physical, and speech therapy; case management; and neuropsychology services. This treatment team pulls weekly documentation into a combined, goal-oriented individualized rehabilitation plan with summaries prepared for the payer source, physicians, family, and team. TLCs provide "custom-designed" life plans to facilitate reentry into home, school, or vocational settings. TLCs have been extremely successful as a way for older adolescents and young adults with neurological problems to progress from a rehabilitation center back into society.

Outpatient Therapy

Patients who have progressed to a level where they can easily leave home usually prefer to travel to therapy departments or offices for treatment. Once in outpatient therapy, patients receive the fine-tuning necessary to maximize their potential function. Usually these patients benefit from a gradually decreasing frequency with an increasing emphasis on independent home programs. Although the guidelines for outpatient and inpatient documentation are the same, the payment systems for outpatient services are quite different and will be covered in detail later in this chapter.

Therapy and Discharge Planning

Therapists in hospitals have the tremendous responsibility of seeing patients just a few times and making recommendations that may affect the patients for the rest of their lives. These decisions are not made in a vacuum; other members of the health care team are involved and initial plans may be amended. Often, however, the team looks to the therapists to determine the best discharge plan.

When discharge options are considered, there are questions a therapist should ask as part of the critical-thinking process (Box 10-3).

BOX 10-3 ■ CONSIDERING DISCHARGE OPTIONS

The questions a therapist should consider before making a discharge recommendation may include the following:

Is the patient capable of being successful at home, either alone or with selective assistance?

If selective assistance is still needed, is outpatient therapy appropriate or would home health care be a better choice?

Is the patient medically and physically stable enough to proceed to an acute inpatient rehabilitation facility?

Is the patient's medical condition at a level that warrants a skilled nursing facility?

BOX 10-4 ■ POINTS TO PONDER ABOUT DISCHARGING A PATIENT

TO HOME

Was the home environment safe before the patient entered the hospital?

Did the patient rely heavily on family, friends, or neighbors for assistance?

Does the patient have a history of falls? (Some patients know the paramedics by name.)

Are there stairs with rails or elevators available?

Are the rooms and halls wheelchair or walker accessible?

What kind of assistive equipment will need to be in the home?

Are there healthy and available family members willing to assist on a continuing basis?

Is there any money available to hire caregivers in the home, and will the patient consent to this?

Are there cultural factors in the family unit that may affect caregiving?

Does the patient need dialysis, and if so, how will this be accomplished?

How compliant will the patient be with an independent exercise program?

Will it be possible and easy for the patient to travel to an outpatient program?

TO A RETIREMENT COMMUNITY

How far must the patient walk to reach the dining area, or can meals be delivered to the room?

Are assistive devices allowed in public areas of this community?

If not, what options have been provided or recommended by this community?

There are no simple answers to any of these questions, but the questions need to be asked to arrive at the best discharge plan for the patient. When trying to ascertain the best solution, the therapist should remember that cognition is a major concern, as is the length of time expected for the patient to meet the long-term goals. The wishes of the patient and the family must always be involved in the decision-making process because sometimes they do not agree with each other or with the therapist's recommendations.

There are many aspects to consider. The patient's prior level of function is essential information, followed closely by the situation at home. The medical and surgical histories are also pertinent factors. Contemplate the questions listed in Box 10-4.

The therapist should consider the level of responsiveness, the ability to follow commands, the prior level of function, and the patient's support system before making a recommendation. To further challenge the therapist, insurance coverage may affect the discharge plans. There will be cases where particular insurance carriers will contractually mandate the patient's discharge disposition. In rare instances, patients must wait in an acute-care hospital until they become eligible for state or federal funding before moving on to the next level of care.

In situations such as multiple fractures with non–weight bearing on bilateral lower extremities, the patient only needs time to heal before being able to participate in a rehabilitation setting. Although the best-case scenario is for the patient to return home while recuperating, this is not always possible. The patient would then transfer to a facility for custodial care.

Another possible discharge option is that of a retirement housing community. This plan usually includes three levels of care: the independent living setting, assisted living, and a health center or SNF. People purchase a contract for a secure and predetermined health care future in the retirement community. The contract specifies receiving care at any and all of these levels. The members stay in independent living until they require medical intervention. They may slowly decline and move into assisted living for a few years before finally settling into the skilled nursing level of care, or they may have a medical emergency and be admitted to acute care. The hospital will then transfer them back to the community's health center for rehabilitation. These patients may stay in the assisted living facility temporarily before returning to their independent living setting.

Be careful! The therapist may adversely affect a patient's disposition on the basis of the POC. For example, a therapist in an acute-care hospital might routinely treat postoperative patients with orthopedic problems who elect to have surgery. These patients are expected to make major functional changes in just a few days. If a different patient arrives with a new subarachnoid hemorrhage and a maximum assist functional level, that same therapist may underestimate the amount of assistance and the duration of care that will be needed for this severely involved patient. The therapist's short-term goals might project independent mobility within a 2-week time frame. If the therapist does not amend the POC, then the discharge planner, insurance case manager, and physicians may decide that the patient is not making any progress at all. The patient is judged to have little to no rehabilitation potential, when, in reality, the therapist's POC was inappropriate. This kind of error could essentially end the patient's chances for acute inpatient rehabilitation and affect the patient's ultimate recovery level.

Less dramatic and possibly more common is the case of a patient who undergoes total hip arthroplasty for a hip fracture after an unwitnessed fall. The patient does not progress as quickly as the therapist would expect. The therapist must consider the possibility that this patient had a mild stroke and then fell and fractured the hip. The patient underwent workup for the obvious fracture, but the neurological symptoms went undetected by the orthopedic surgeon. Sometimes the patient's subtle medical problems are realized only during evaluations that identify mismatches between the medical diagnosis and the anticipated functional skills and limitations. Open and clear lines of communication must be established between individuals working within the medical disease or pathology model and therapists working on impairments, activity limitations, and participation restrictions. The therapists have the opportunity to assist the patient and influence the discharge plan by advocating for a facility that offers both orthopedic and neurological rehabilitation.

The third-party payer also has a say in the disposition of the case. Occasionally the discharge choice of the insurer, on the basis of the case manager's review of the medical records and the patient's coverage, is not the therapist's first choice for the patient. It may be possible to affect the decision regarding the patient's future only if the therapist has been a strong patient advocate and has consistently documented appropriately and thoroughly.

CASE STUDY 10-3

The following case illustrates the interaction of therapy on the continuum of care and the various assessment instruments used in different settings.

Ysabella D. is a 66-year-old woman, independent and healthy, who has been diagnosed with atypical Guillain-Barré syndrome. She is admitted to the acute-care hospital, and subsequently respiratory failure, flaccid quadriplegia, and cardiac arrhythmias develop.

Over the course of 5 months in the acute-care hospital, with more than one visit to intensive care, Ysabella undergoes tracheostomy and receives a feeding tube and a pacemaker. In the meantime, she also acquires pneumonia, dysphagia, and a decubitus ulcer. Although Ysabella receives occupational, physical, and speech therapy while in the acute-care hospital, she remains dependent in all areas. Because of the presence of the tracheostomy and percutaneous endoscopic gastrostomy tubes, Ysabella is transferred to a subacute setting, where she stays for another 8 months. Here she gradually improves in strength, endurance, and function.

After her tracheostomy and feeding tubes are removed, her skin has healed, and she has progressed to a regular diet, Ysabella is strong enough to meet the criteria for an acute inpatient rehabilitation facility and she is transferred there. She stays in the short-term rehabilitation facility for another 6 weeks before she reaches a minimal-assist level of care. At this point, she and her very supportive family have been trained and she is able to be discharged home. Because she lives in a second-story apartment, is still using a wheelchair, and continues to require occupational and physical therapy, Ysabella is eligible for home health therapy.

Ysabella has Medicare Part A and B insurance coverage. This enables the acute-care hospital to be reimbursed on the basis of her diagnosis-related group. In this case, her long and complicated stay would qualify her for the outlier adjustment, allowing the hospital to receive more money than it would have received for a patient with an uncomplicated Guillain-Barré diagnosis. At the subacute facility, the initial Resident Assessment Instrument Minimum Data Set (MDS)is completed after 5 days. The MDS is again completed after 14 days, 30 days, 60 days, 90 days, and then quarterly until her transfer to the short-term inpatient rehabilitation setting. Here the Inpatient Rehabilitation Facility–Patient Assessment Instrument (IRF-PAI), including the Functional Independence Measure (FIM) score, is completed after 3 days and at the time of discharge. When Ysabella finally returns home, the home health therapist opens the case using the Outcome and Assessment Information Set (OASIS). Each facility will be reimbursed after the submission of the appropriate information gathered from each assessment and outcome instrument, assuming these tools were completed correctly and there was no reason for payment to be denied. Proper documentation by the therapists would justify all her therapy if there were to be an appeals process.

MEDICAL AND FUNCTIONAL DIAGNOSIS AND INTERVENTION CODING: DIAGNOSIS CODING

Payment for rehabilitation services is dependent not only on the quality of the medical record produced during the course of care but also on the accuracy of the codes used to describe medical and functional diagnoses and therapeutic interventions used in treatment. Third-party payers and other health care system stakeholders rely on the accuracy of coding so that the appropriate payment policy can be applied during the claims adjudication process. This section will introduce the reader to the basics of diagnosis coding using ICD-9 codes and intervention coding using CPT codes.

The ICD-9-CM, or ICD-9 for short, is based on the official version of the World Health Organization's Ninth Revision of the International Classification of Diseases. ICD-9 classifies diagnosis, morbidity, and mortality information to allow systematic codification and standardized naming of diseases and injuries and allows indexing of data for outcome studies and for use in various payment, billing, and electronic information formats. Health care insurance companies and government agencies require the use of ICD-9 for billing and payment processes and for medical records as a result of HIPAA. To track outcomes, especially functional outcomes, standardized diagnosis nomenclature is absolutely essential. In rehabilitation settings the treating therapist is responsible for accurate identification of the physical therapy (treating) diagnosis and any comorbidities that could be factors during the course of care. Accurately identifying these diagnostic codes is an essential part of the advocacy role of the treating therapist because these coding decisions can have significant effects on third-party payer decisions for paying claims for patients and clients with potentially life-altering diseases and injuries.

Organization and Characteristics of ICD-9-CM

ICD-9-CM is organized into two volumes. Volume 1 is the tabular list of ICD-9 codes and five appendices. Codes from Volume 1 are not usually used for medical and functional diagnoses involved with rehabilitation. Volume 2 is an alphabetical list of ICD-9 codes. This listing contains a large number of medical and functional diagnoses that incorporate most of the diagnostic terms currently in use. A group composed of the American Hospital Association, CMS, National Center for Health Statistics, and American Health Information Management Association regularly updates ICD-9 codes, resulting in annual editions that are updated throughout each calendar year. When ICD-9 resources are consulted, it is important to always be sure that the most current edition is used.

ICD-9 codes can be up to five digits long: at least three digits are to the left of the decimal and up to two digits to the right of the decimal. The three digits to the left of the decimal define the diagnosis category, and the two available digits to the right of the decimal define more specific characteristics of the diagnosis by further defining site and location. We will look at several examples to illustrate the coding process (Box 10-5).

BOX 10-5 ■ ICD-9 CODING EXAMPLES

Following are two examples of common neurological conditions. You will need an ICD-9-CM book to do this exercise.

The name of the condition is the best place to begin. For example, code the diagnosis *complete paraplegia.*

- Go to Volume 2 (alphabetical index) and look up "Paraplegia, complete."
- Review the listings under 344 of Volume 2 under "Paraplegia." There is no listing that matches the term "complete."
- Go to "344.1 Paraplegia" in Volume 1 (tabular index). The main entry is "344 Quadriplegia and Paraplegia."
- Read the entries under 344 and find "344.1 Paraplegia." Note what conditions are included and excluded by the listed codes. Read the note under "344.1 Paraplegia" that says "paralysis of both limbs." This represents the closest match to "complete paraplegia."
- "344.1 Paraplegia" is the diagnostic code.

Coding *nonspecific encephalopathy:*

- Go to Volume 2 (alphabetical index) and look up "Encephalopathy."
- Review the listings under "Encephalopathy." There is no listing that matches the term "nonspecific."
- Go to Volume 1 (tabular index) and look up "348.30 Encephalopathy."
- Read the notes and descriptions under "348.3 Encephalopathy." Note what conditions are included and excluded by the listed codes.
- "348.30 Encephalopathy, unspecified" matches nonspecific encephalopathy most closely.
- "348.30 Encephalopathy, unspecified" is the diagnostic code.

Two terms need to be kept in mind when using ICD-9 codes. The first is Not Elsewhere Classified (NEC). This term is used when the ICD-9-CM does not provide a code that may be as specific as the diagnosis the therapist is trying to code, or when the clinician may not have enough information to code to a more specific diagnosis requiring the fourth-digit subcategory. The second term is Not Otherwise Specified (NOS). This term is used when the diagnosis is unspecified. Again, the reader will have an opportunity to look at examples of both abbreviations for illustration purposes.

Assigning ICD-9-CM Codes

In most cases the therapist will start with the name of a medical or functional diagnosis and will have to convert that name to the numerical ICD-9 code. In rare cases the opposite occurs; a diagnostic code is provided and the code will need to be converted to a name. For the purposes of this discussion it is assumed that a codebook is being used; however, readers will find that many software and Internet applications embed ICD-9 information within the application. When using embedded resources, it is important that the reader refer to the text included in the codebook because most of these applications use the "short language" form of the code and do not tell you whether fourth- or fifth-digit modification is required.

ICD-9 Coding Is a Five-Step Process

The following five-step process will guide the reader through the ICD-9 coding process:

Step 1: Start by consulting the alphabetical index (Volume 2) to identify the diagnostic category before using the tabular index (Volume 1). By identifying the correct name of the diagnostic category in the alphabetical index, therapists will avoid coding errors that will result in denied services.

Step 2: Identify the main medical or functional diagnostic term or category. The alphabetical index is arranged by condition. Conditions can be expressed as nouns, adjectives, and eponyms. Some conditions have multiple entries under their synonyms. Be sure to read any notes listed with the main term or category because these categories will help the reader identify the specific diagnostic code he or she is trying to identify.

Step 3: Interpret abbreviations, cross-references, and brackets. Cross-references used are "see," "see category," and "see also." The abbreviations NEC and NOS follow main terms or subterms. Identify a tentative code and locate it in the tabular index.

Step 4: By reading the entry in the tabular list, clinicians will be able to determine whether the code is at its highest level of specificity. Assign three-digit codes (category code) if there are no four-digit codes within the code category. Assign four-digit codes (subcategory codes) if there are no five-digit codes for that category. Assign five-digit codes (fifth-digit subclassification codes) for these categories where they are available.

Step 5: Assign the code.[25]

Box 10-5 provides two ICD-9 coding examples.

Depending on the treatment setting, patients/clients may come to the therapist with diagnoses that are already coded. In other situations, such as in acute-care facilities and IRFs, ICD-9 codes will be assigned by certified ICD-9 coders in the medical records department. In many outpatient settings the therapist will be required to "match" ICD-9 codes for Medicare patients with specific CPT codes to establish medical necessity for the rehabilitation interventions according to the Fiscal Intermediary or Carrier Local Coverage Decisions. In any case, the treating therapist should be absolutely clear in the medical record about the treating diagnoses and comorbidities that define the treatment program and POC of the patient or client.

The Future of Diagnosis Coding: ICD-10-CM

In 2013, changes in HIPAA regulations will replace ICD-9-CM with an updated diagnostic coding set: ICD-10-CM. This updated system will enhance accurate payment for services and facilitate evaluation and tracking of medical diagnoses and outcomes. ICD-10-CM will provide improvements through more detailed diagnostic information and increased specificity of location and pathologies and will have expanded ability to capture additional advancements in identification of pathology, diagnoses, and patient problems.

The ICD-10-CM classification system has been used in other countries since the mid-1990s; it has been adapted by the Centers for Disease Control and Prevention for use in the United States. The diagnostic coding under this system uses three to seven alphabetical and numerical characters and full code titles for each entry. Organization and format are very similar to those of ICD-9-CM.

Because of the impact this change will have on electronic data interchange and computer systems, the transitional plan for this significant change is already underway. Therapists and other health care providers should be aware of this impending change and participate in training opportunities as they become available.

INTERVENTION CODING

Just as ICD-9 codes allow therapists to communicate to payers and other health care stakeholders the conditions and injuries being treated, CPT codes allow therapists to identify and communicate the interventions being used in the course of patient care. In a world where most billing information is transmitted electronically, it is essential for therapists to use the most appropriate CPT codes to communicate the breadth, depth, and complexity of the treatment plans required in the care of patients/clients. Appropriate intervention coding is also essential to the billing and claims adjudication process and to maximize the health care benefits available to the patient with complex neurological conditions and injuries.

Current Procedural Terminology

Current Procedural Terminology,[26] Fourth Edition, is maintained, updated, and published by the AMA and is a registered trademark of the AMA. It is a code set designed to identify the interventions and other services performed by health care providers. Each intervention or service is described by a five-digit code. CPT is mandated by HIPAA as the appropriate code set for use in health care transactions in the United States.

CPT is used to report health care provider services to public and private or commercial insurance companies and payers. CPT codes are also used to report treatment encounter information to government agencies and private companies for the purposes of research, outcome tracking, and education.

The AMA first published the fourth edition of CPT in 1977. CPT is continually updated to keep the codes current with the community standard of practice by a process led by the AMA CPT Editorial Panel.[26] For the rehabilitation disciplines, the Health Care Professional Advisory Committee develops CPT coding changes and updates. The Committee consists of representatives from 16 nonphysician provider groups, including physical therapy, occupational therapy, and speech and language pathology.

The CPT code set is organized into six major sections: Evaluation and Management, Anesthesiology, Surgery, Radiology, Pathology/Laboratory, and Medicine. Each section is divided into subsections based on anatomical, procedural, condition, and descriptor headings as appropriate to that specialty section. The AMA, in publishing the CPT code set, recognizes that there may be significant overlap in the interventions, procedures, and services performed by health care providers and makes the following statement in the introduction:

> It is important to recognize that the listing of a service or procedure and its code number in a specific of this book does not restrict its use to a specific specialty group. Any procedure or service in any section of this book may be used to designate the services rendered by any qualified physician or other qualified health care professional.[26]

Typically, most codes used by rehabilitation professionals to describe treatment of neurological conditions are in the 97000 series of the CPT; however, any code that adequately represents the interventions or services performed by a provider with the appropriate qualifications may be used.

Using the CPT Codes

Selecting the correct CPT code that most adequately describes the intervention performed is often very challenging because most therapists have not had formal CPT training. Although in-depth coding training is beyond the scope of this text, this section will help the reader develop some basic skills in applying sound coding techniques to practice.

Most of the codes used to describe therapy interventions are found in the Physical Medicine section of the CPT code. Although therapists use these codes, so do a large number of other health care professionals and providers. For this reason it is important for therapists to be able to adequately describe their use of interventions using the correct CPT codes so the codes reflect the complex nature of the treatment plans implemented with their patients.

Physical Medicine CPT Codes

The Physical Medicine codes are located in a subsection of the Medicine section of the CPT code set. Some CPT codes in the Physical Medicine section represent interventions that occur in specified time intervals (e.g., 15 minutes) and are considered "timed" codes. Timed codes generally require constant attendance or direct (one-on-one) patient contact. Other codes are considered "occurrence" codes and do not have a time period associated with them. Some occurrence codes require direct contact, whereas others do not. Occurrence codes are billed only one time during a visit or treatment, but timed codes can be billed in multiple units as justified by the time it takes to provide the intervention. Consult a current CPT codebook for specific details, because these codes and their associated descriptions can change each year.

The Physical Medicine codes are organized into six groups of codes. The codes in these subsections have specific attributes.[26]

Evaluation/Reevaluation

Evaluation/Reevaluation codes are the evaluation and reevaluation codes for physical therapy, occupational therapy, and athletic training. These codes are occurrence codes requiring direct contact between the therapist and the patient.

Modalities

Modality codes are further divided into two groups: "Supervised" modalities (occurrence codes that do not require direct contact) and "Constant Attendance" modalities (timed codes that require direct contact).

Therapeutic Procedures

Therapeutic Procedure codes require direct patient contact by the therapist. All but one of these codes are timed, so if the time required for the intervention warrants, multiple units of a code can be charged.

Active Wound Care Management

Active Wound Care Management codes are occurrence codes that require direct contact.

Tests and Measures. Tests and Measures codes represent specific assessment and testing interventions that are separate and distinct from evaluations and reevaluations. These interventions require separate written reports.

Other Procedures

The Other Procedures section consists of a single code used to describe any "unlisted" physical medicine service or intervention.

Each year therapists should review the codes and sections commonly used for changes and additions that will better describe the interventions performed with their patients. All therapists should consult the CPT codes directly and avail themselves of training specifically designed to help them accurately describe their interventions. CPT coding resources are available from a number of sources, including the AMA and professional associations such as APTA.[27]

OUTPATIENT PAYMENT POLICY

The processes involved with billing, payment, and payment policy for outpatient services remains distinctly different compared with inpatient services. Although inpatient rehabilitation services are primarily paid on a prospective basis, outpatient rehabilitation services continue to be paid primarily on a retrospective basis. This means that, although services may have been authorized before delivery of care, the decision to pay for the services is made after care has been delivered and subject to reviews of medical necessity, appropriateness, and other policies. Financial class largely determines the types of policies and regulations that apply to any particular payer. There are four primary financial classes: Medicare, Medicaid, and government programs; commercial insurance and private coverage; automobile and accident insurance companies; and workers' compensation. To be effective advocates for patient care, therapists must be vigilant regarding regulations and payment policies that determine how care is approved, billed, and paid.

Medicare and Medicaid

Both the Medicare and Medicaid programs are overseen and regulated by CMS. Medicare, as a federal program, is heavily regulated. These regulations are readily available to providers through a number of resources, but the primary access to information is through the Internet at http://cms.gov. As previously discussed, Medicare pays for outpatient services through MACs. Each of these entities must maintain a website for beneficiaries and providers to allow for ready dissemination of pertinent information. MACs use Medicare's national policies to process and adjudicate claims. Although Medicare has national policies, MACs have some discretion in how these policies are implemented locally. Any MAC regulations or policies specific to particular services, interventions, or provider types are contained in LCDs that must go through a lengthy draft and approval process before they are made available to providers and implemented. Most MACs have LCDs specific to physical rehabilitation providers (physical therapy, occupational therapy, and speech and language pathology) as well as specific services or interventions such as wound care, biofeedback for incontinence, vestibular problems, and cardiac rehabilitation. Because MACs have defined geographic coverage areas, it is advisable for therapists to be sure they are familiar with Medicare's payment policies in the areas where they practice.

Medicaid, as discussed earlier, is a health program for the economically disadvantaged. Although it is partially funded with federal dollars, it is also funded at the state level. Because Medicaid is implemented at the state level, states have significant leeway in how their programs operate, approve care, and pay for services. Consequently there are large variations in the Medicaid program from state to state. Therapists should be aware within their individual work settings of the regulations and policies that may apply to them as a result of their employer's possible participation in the Medicaid program.

Medicare and other payers often attempt to mitigate their financial risk for costly episodes of rehabilitation by imposing arbitrary limits on care. These limits are often referred to as "caps." One example of such a limit is Medicare yearly cap on rehabilitation services. This cap was created as part of the BBA and went into effect in 1999. The cap was $1500 in payments per year for physical therapy and speech therapy and a separate $1500 cap for occupational therapy services. The cap applies in all outpatient settings except outpatient hospital rehabilitation units. The therapy cap is adjusted annually as a consequence of changes in the Medicare Economic Index that tracks health care costs and inflation.

Another way Medicare and Medicaid attempt to mitigate their financial risk is to use outpatient service programs that are prospectively paid. These programs operate by use of capitation, a system by which health care providers are paid in advance of rendering care to a defined group of beneficiaries. In this payment system the capitated health care providers provide care out of the prepaid pool of funds. These programs use contracted insurance companies, using large groups of health care providers representing a wide array of specialties, to provide the anticipated health care needs of the covered patients. Capitation agreements must be carefully negotiated. If the negotiated prospective payment is too low, or, if the therapist overtreats, the payment for services rendered will be inadequate to cover the cost of providing care to the covered patient population.

A number of smaller government programs also may have specific regulations and policies similar to those of Medicare. An example of such programs is CHAMPUS/TRICARE. This program provides health care insurance coverage for members of the military and their dependents and for military retirees. Other federal health care programs, such as the Veterans Administration, may vary significantly from Medicare and Medicaid in their policies.

Coverage programs for children with congenital or acquired conditions requiring extensive rehabilitation are financed through a number of federal, state, and local programs. Because of the huge diversity in the payment policies related to these programs, therapists should be aware of the particular program covering the care and should work closely with parents and agencies involved to ensure that proper coverage for services is achieved.

Commercial Insurance and Private Coverage

Commercial insurance coverage is financed by traditional health insurance companies, self-insured employers, and self-paying consumers. Commercial insurance companies are regulated at the state level, and self-insured companies are regulated at the federal level. Cash-paying consumers must rely on their own understanding and self-education to make their purchasing decisions regarding therapeutic care.

Commercial insurance companies operate by charging premiums to the beneficiaries (employers or individual consumers) and then paying for services delivered to their insured. Because these payers bear the risks associated with the health of their beneficiaries, they use a number of strategies to mitigate their risks in this delivery model. Many use preferred panels of health care providers to deliver services. These preferred providers agree to particular business processes, rates of payment, and utilization review and restrictions to have access to the beneficiaries of these payers. Some require the provider to obtain authorization before treatment is provided, whereas others provide strict review of care after delivery to decide whether payment is warranted. These companies also have a number of mechanisms to shift their financial risk to the patient and to the provider, including capitation and case-rate reimbursement. In case-rate reimbursement, a flat rate is paid for the entire course of care for a patient with a particular medical diagnosis.

Insurance companies often require the patient to pay different amounts toward their care on the basis of whether the patient sees a network provider (preferred provider) or an out-of-network provider (a provider who is not a contracted provider). These amounts can be based on a percentage of the charges, on a flat amount for each treatment (co-pay), or both. The required patient payment can have a significant effect on patients' and clients' financial abilities to participate in their respective treatments. By increasing co-pay amounts, payers know patients will have to make "harder" decisions regarding how much care they can afford. This can play an important factor when a therapist and his or her patient agree on a POC, how much therapy the patient can afford, and when the patient is discharged to a home program. For patients who pay cash for services, these decisions can be even more difficult and come far sooner in the POC. In other situations, especially in long-term management of an individual after central nervous system (CNS) injury, the therapist's role may become consultative. When the patient or family identifies functional changes, the therapist may be asked to establish new goal interventions as a home program to be carried out by the patient's support system.

Payers can also place limitations on the amount of services a patient can receive each year by limiting the number of visits, days, and dollars spent on therapy services. Therapists must be aware of these limitations and how these limitations may affect the potential interactions between long-term care and patient potential. With this understanding, a therapist can help identify the best use of patients' resources and facilitate those individuals' abilities to participate in their own care. The nearly infinite number of ways payers can shift risk and financial responsibility to patients and providers makes it imperative that systems be in place in each clinical setting to check for limitations and alert the patient and therapist to potential financial challenges that can have chilling effects on treatment and the potential for recovery.

Automobile and Accident Coverage and Third-Party Liability

When individuals are injured in automobile and other accidents, financial liability for care may become the responsibility of others who were involved in or responsible for the accidents. In the case of automobile accidents, people are generally required by state law to carry some minimum amount of public liability insurance to cover such costs. Health insurance companies usually have stipulations in their policies that allow them to recover any costs they incur as the result of the liability of others.

To further complicate matters related to accidents, many of these cases end up in lawsuits and litigation. This represents several challenges for the treating therapist. In terms of payment for services, it is not always entirely clear who will be paying for services and when they will pay. Many patients injured from the actions of others may feel that they are not responsible for paying for the care they receive, and they can be unaware of the cost of treatment as it mounts. This can be problematic if the party the patient believed was liable is exonerated or unable to pay.

Nearly all health care facilities have a policy that states that the patient, or his or her parent or guardian, is financially responsible for the treatment received, although the facility may be willing to bill other parties for those services.

Therapists should always be aware of the various possibilities that can occur during the course of care that can affect the ability of the patient to continue therapy. Therapists should also be aware that the medical records could end up being examined by a number of attorneys and end up in open court.

Workers' Compensation

Of all the insurance classes reviewed, workers' compensation has the highest degree of variability in regulation and payment policy. Each state legislates and regulates its treatment of injured workers independently of other states and federal involvement. This variability requires every facility treating workers' compensation patients to maintain a knowledge base of the laws and regulations governing the care of these patients as well as establishing procedures to ensure that they are followed. Many states use fee schedules that are based on CPT codes but are highly modified and have significant variations from "normal" coding. These types of fee schedules may require specific instruction to use so that the therapist can accurately describe the interventions used with patients covered by these fee schedules. In addition, the nature of work-related injuries produces other potential challenges for therapists.

Workers' compensation coverage is provided through purchased insurance or through self-insurance programs set up by employers. Workers' compensation cases are concurrently managed by insurance companies or by third-party administrators who manage self-insured employer programs. Concurrently managed care means that the payer requires the health care provider to preauthorize all proposed care and reviews documentation to ensure compliance with state-mandated fee schedules and use guidelines. Because of the assumed employer liability of work-related injuries, some of these cases progress to lawsuits and litigation as in the case of accidents. Therapists should remain aware, also, of the potential involvement of their patients' medical records in these legal proceedings. In the area of neurological rehabilitation, a workers' compensation package may become very complex. If the injury results in permanent CNS limitations, therapists are often asked to estimate the long-term needs of the patient to establish potential costs of long-term therapeutic management over the lifetime of the patient.

Evolving Health Care Reform Efforts and Effects on Payment Policy

In March 2010 President Barack Obama signed the Patient Protection and Affordability Act of 2010 (HR 3590) and its companion legislation the Health Care and Education Reconciliation Act of 2010, ushering in the most sweeping regulatory changes in health care payment policy since the Medicare Act of 1965, which established the Medicare program. The full effects of this legislation will not be fully implemented until 2016. The regulatory implications of this new law will be promulgated over the coming years. The reader should be forewarned that keeping current with major changes in health care policy is essential in providing proper advice and counsel to patients requiring long-term and intensive therapies to maximize their abilities to function. This legislation will allow many to access services who have been excluded by payer enrollment policies, inability to purchase health care coverage, or both. This new coverage burden will be shared largely by employers and by new state and federal programs financed through new taxes and efforts to curtail fraud and abuse in health care. Although the details of providing funding for this significant expansion in services are to be worked out, there will likely be significant downward pressure on payment for services as well as an increase in efforts to compensate health care providers on the quality of their clinical and financial outcomes. Implementation of evidence-based practice and keeping current in "best practices" will be essential for every therapist as compensation systems evolve to meet the needs of patients and clients and the rising costs of health care.

SUMMARY

Payment for rehabilitation services is a complex topic that involves many legal, regulatory, and contractual details. To completely explain the complexities involved in documentation of patient care, medical billing, and claims adjudication would fill a volume similar to the size of this text. We have attempted to provide the treating therapist with a basic understanding of the payment systems involved in inpatient and outpatient services and the importance of documentation to the billing and payment process, provided basic steps for inclusion of diagnosis and intervention coding, and provided an overview of payment policy for outpatient services. Therapists must keep in mind that the regulatory and legislative world of health care is in a continual state of flux and that there are a number of critical areas that affect payment for services that were not touched on in this chapter. These would include the areas of Medicare and corporate compliance, the HIPAA privacy and security rules, currently evolving issues related to the Medicare caps on therapy services, and individual state practice acts for various health care providers. The reader would be well served to get specific questions and concerns addressed by knowledgeable individuals or to consult source documents on these important areas. The increasing reliance on electronic data interchange will necessitate improvements in the ICD-9 coding system to ICD-10, requiring the reader to seek appropriate training. Emerging health care reform initiatives will create new opportunities for coverage of individuals with chronic conditions but will place additional financial strain on the system and our economy, with possible consequences on health care provider compensation and payment policies.

Acknowledgment

With sincere appreciation for editorial contributions by Bob Niklewicz, PT, DHSc.

References

To enhance this text and add value for the reader, all references are included on the companion Evolve site that accompanies this textbook. This online service will, when available, provide a link for the reader to a Medline abstract for the article cited. There are 27 cited references and other general references for this chapter, with the majority of those articles being evidence-based citations.

APPENDIX 10-A ■ Quick Reference Guide to Acronyms

ADLs = Activities of Daily Living
AFDC = Aid to Families with Dependent Children
AMA = American Medical Association
APTA = American Physical Therapy Association
ARRA = American Recovery and Reinvestment Act of 2009
BBA = Balanced Budget Act of 1997
BBRA = Balanced Budget Refinement Act of 1999
BIPA = Benefits Improvement Act of 2000
CAA = Care Area Assessment
CARE = Continuity Assessment Record and Evaluation
CARF = Commission on Accreditation of Rehabilitation Facilities
CAT = Care Area Trigger
CHIP = Children's Health Insurance Program
CHIPRA = Children's Health Insurance Program Reauthorization Act of 2009
CMG = Case-Mix Group
CMS = Centers for Medicare and Medicaid Services
COBRA = Consolidated Omnibus Budget Reconciliation Act of 1985
CPT = Current Procedural Terminology
DRG = Diagnosis-Related Group
DSH = Disproportionate Share Hospital
EPHI = Electronic Protected Health Information
ESEA = Elementary and Secondary Education Act of 1965
FI = Fiscal Intermediary
FIM* = Functional Independence Measure
HCFA = Health Care Financing Administration
HCPAC = Health Care Professional Advisory Committee
HCPCS = Healthcare Common Procedure Coding System
HEW = Department of Health, Education, and Welfare
HHA = Home Health Agency
HHS = Department of Health and Human Services
HIPAA = Health Insurance Portability and Accountability Act of 1996
HITECH = Health Information Technology for Economic and Clinical Health Act
HMO = Health Maintenance Organization
IADL = Instrumental Activities of Daily Living
ICD-9-CM = International Classification of Diseases, Ninth Revision, Clinical Modification
IDEA = Individuals with Disabilities Education Act
IGC = Impairment Group Code
IME = Indirect Medical Education
IPPS = Inpatient Prospective Payment System
IRF-PAI = Inpatient Rehabilitation Facility—Patient Assessment Instrument
LCD = Local Coverage Decisions
LTCH = Long-Term Care Hospital
MDS = Minimum Data Set
MS-DRG = Medicare Severity Diagnosis-Related Group
MSP = Medicare Savings Programs
NCLB = No Child Left Behind Act of 2001
NEC = Not Elsewhere Classified
NOS = Not Otherwise Specified
OASIS = Outcome and Assessment Information Set
OBQI = Outcome-Based Quality Improvement
OCR = Office for Civil Rights
PHI = Protected Health Information
POC = Plan of Care
PPS = Prospective Payment System
RAC = Recovery Audit Contractor
RAI = Resident Assessment Instrument
RAP = Resident Assessment Protocols
RUGs-III = Resource Utilization Groups, Version III
SCHIP = State Children's Health Insurance Program
SNF = Skilled Nursing Facility
SRS = Social and Rehabilitation Service
SSA = Social Security Administration
TLC = Transitional Living Center
WHO = World Health Organization

*Copyright © 2001, 2002 UB Foundation Activities, Inc. (UBFA, Inc.) for compilation rights; no copyrights claimed in U.S. Government works included in Section I, portions of Section IV, Appendices I and K, and portions of Appendices B, C, E, G, H, and J. All other copyrights are reserved to their respective owners. Copyright © 1993-2001 UB Foundation Activities, Inc. for the FIM Data Set, Measurement Scale, Impairment Codes, and refinements thereto for the IRF-PAI, and for the Guide for the Uniform Data Set for Medical Rehabilitation, as incorporated or referenced herein. The FIM mark is owned by UBFA, Inc.

SECTION II

Rehabilitation Management of Clients with Neurological System Pathology

CHAPTER 11 Neonates and Parents: Neurodevelopmental Perspectives in the Neonatal Intensive Care Unit and Follow-Up

JANE K. SWEENEY, PT, PhD, PCS, C/NDT, FAPTA, TERESA GUTIERREZ, PT, MS, PCS, C/NDT, and JOANNA C. BEACHY, MD, PhD, FAAP

KEY TERMS

high-risk clinical signs
medical complications of prematurity
neonatal intensive care unit environment
neuromotor assessment
neuromotor intervention
parent instruction
physiological and musculoskeletal risks
subspecialty training

OBJECTIVES

After reading this chapter the student or therapist will be able to:

1. Discuss three theoretical frameworks guiding neonatal therapy services in the neonatal intensive care unit.
2. Identify the physiological and structural vulnerabilities of preterm infants that predispose them to stress during neonatal therapy procedures.
3. Outline supervised clinical practicum components and pediatric clinical experiences to prepare for entry into neonatal intensive care unit practice.
4. Describe how the grief process may affect behavior and caregiving performance of parents of low–birth-weight neonates.
5. Differentiate the developmental course and neuromotor risk signs in infants with emerging neuromotor impairment from the clinical characteristics of infants with transient movement dysfunction.
6. Identify instruments for neuromotor examination of high-risk infants in neonatal intensive care units and in follow-up clinics and compare psychometric features of the tests.
7. Describe program plans and follow-up for low–birth-weight infants in neonatal intensive care unit and home settings.

Premature birth is associated with an increased prevalence of major and minor neurodevelopmental disability. Advancements in newborn resuscitation and neonatal intensive care have contributed to greatly improved survival of infants with low birth weight (LBW), but risk of neurodevelopmental sequelae remains high.[1,2]

Although brain injury can be documented by ultrasonography, computed tomography (CT), and magnetic resonance imaging (MRI) in infants, prediction of subsequent neurodevelopmental outcome is still relatively unreliable.[3-6] Serial clinical examinations and careful monitoring of neurodevelopmental status are therefore critical during the neonatal period and discharge from the neonatal intensive care unit (NICU) through the outpatient phase of care. Pediatric therapists with mentored, subspecialty training in neonatology and infant therapy approaches can serve these increasing numbers of surviving neonates at neurodevelopmental risk by (1) providing valuable diagnostic data through neurological and developmental examination, (2) participating in developmental and environmental interventions adapted to each infant's physiological, motor, and behavioral needs, (3) facilitating and coordinating interdisciplinary case management for infants and parents, and (4) reinforcing preventive aspects of health care through early intervention and long-term developmental monitoring.

Clinical management of neonates at developmental risk and their parents during the NICU and outpatient follow-up phases is the focus of this chapter. A theoretical framework for neonatal practice is presented, and an overview of neonatal complications associated with adverse outcomes is provided. In-depth discussion in the neonatal section includes indications for referral based on risk, neurodevelopmental examination instruments, high-risk profiles in the neonatal period, treatment planning, and therapy strategies in the NICU. The section on outpatient follow-up focuses on critical time periods for neuromotor and musculoskeletal reexamination, assessment tools, and clinical cases.

THEORETICAL FRAMEWORK

Concepts of dynamic systems, neonatal behavioral organization, and parental hope and empowerment provide a theoretical framework for neonatal therapy practice. In this section are three models that provide a theoretical structure for practitioners designing and implementing neuromotor and neurobehavioral programs for neonates and their parents.

Dynamic Systems

Dynamic systems theory applied to infants in the NICU refers first to the presence of multiple interacting structural and physiological systems within the infant to produce functional behaviors and second to the dynamic interactions between the infant and the environment. In Figure 11-1, neonatal movement and postural control are targeted as a core focus in neonatal therapy, with overlapping and interacting influences from the cardiopulmonary,[7] behavioral, neuromuscular, musculoskeletal, and integumentary systems. A change or intervention affecting one system may diminish or enhance stability in the other dynamic systems within the infant. Similarly, a change in the infant's environment may impair or improve the infant's functional performance.

This theory guides the neonatal practitioner to consider the many potential physiological and anatomical influences (dynamic systems within the infant) that make preterm infants vulnerable to stress during caregiving procedures, including neonatal therapy. In dynamic systems theory, emphasis is placed on the contributions of the interacting environments of the NICU, home, and community in constraining or facilitating the functional performance of the infant.[8]

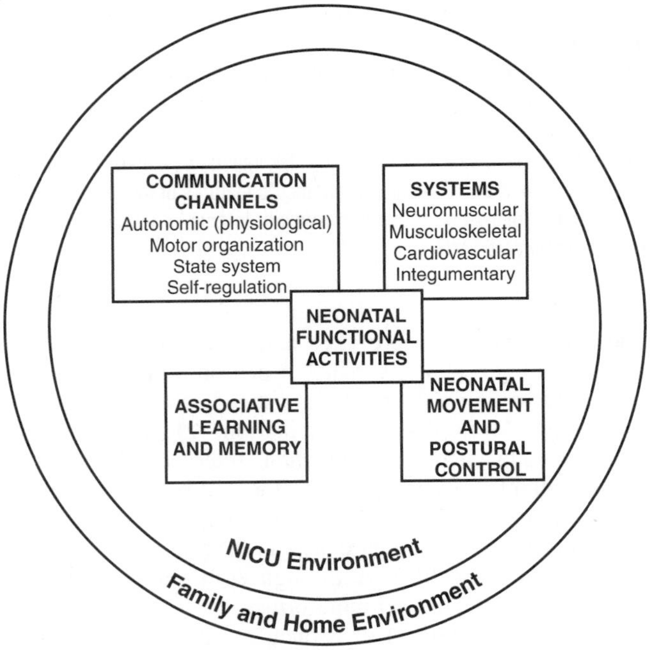

Figure 11-1 ■ Dynamic systems within neonates and interacting external influences on functional performance. (From Sweeney JK, Heriza CB, Blanchard Y, Dusing SC: Neonatal physical therapy. Part II: practice frameworks and evidence-based practice guidelines. *Pediatr Phys Ther* 22:3, 2010.)

Synactive Model of Infant Behavior

The synactive model of infant behavioral organization is a specific neonatal dynamic systems model for establishing physiological stability as the foundation for organization of motor, behavioral state, and attention or interactive behaviors in infants. Als and colleagues[9-11] described a "synactive" process of four subsystems interacting as the neonate responds to the stresses of the extrauterine environment. They theorized that the basic subsystem of physiological organization must first be stabilized for the other subsystems to emerge and allow the infant to maintain behavioral state control and then interact positively with the environment (Figure 11-2).

To evaluate infant behavior within the subsystems of function addressed in the synactive model, Als and colleagues[10,11] developed the Assessment of Preterm Infants' Behavior (APIB). With the development of this assessment instrument, a fifth subsystem of behavioral organization, self-regulation, was added to the synactive model. The self-regulation subsystem consists of physiological, motor, and behavioral state strategies used by the neonate to maintain balance within and between the subsystems. For example, many infants born preterm appear to regulate overstimulating environmental conditions with a behavioral state strategy of withdrawing into a drowsy or light sleep state, thereby shutting out sensory input. The withdrawal strategy is used more frequently than crying because it requires less energy and causes less physiological drain on immature, inefficient organ systems.

Fetters[12] placed the synactive model within a dynamic systems framework to demonstrate the effect of a therapeutic intervention on an infant's multiple subsystems (Figure 11-3). She explained that although a neonatal therapy intervention is offered to the infant at the level of the person, outcome is measured at the systems level, where many subsystems may be affected. For example, the motor outcome from neonatal therapy procedures is frequently influenced by "synaction," or simultaneous effects, of an infant's physiological stability and behavioral state. Physiological state and behavioral state are therefore probable

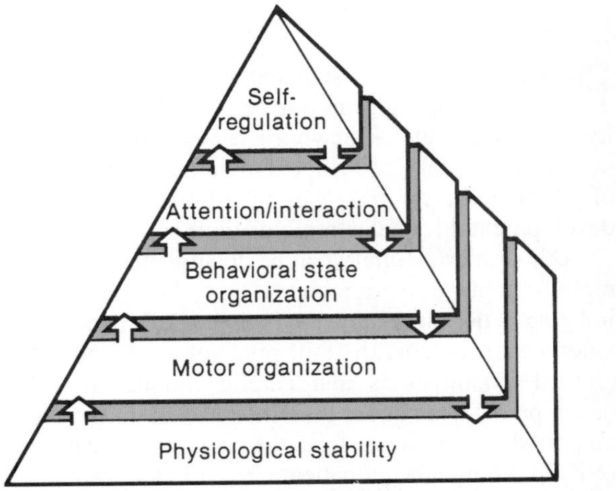

Figure 11-2 ■ Pyramid of synactive theory of infant behavioral organization with physiological stability at the foundation.

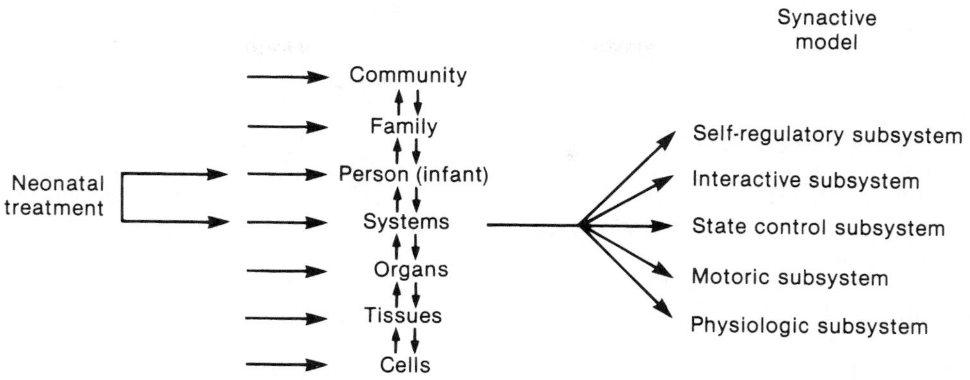

Figure 11-3 ■ Combined dynamic systems and synactive models. (Modified from Fetters L: Sensorimotor management of the high-risk neonate. *Phys Occup Ther Pediatr* 6:217, 1986.)

confounding variables during research on motor behavior in neonatal subjects. Neonatal therapists may find this combined dynamic systems and synactive framework helpful in conceptualizing and assessing changes in infants' multiple subsystems during and after therapy procedures.

Hope-Empowerment Model

A major component of the intervention process in neonatal therapy is the interpersonal helping relationship with the family. A hope-empowerment framework (Figure 11-4) may guide neonatal practitioners in building the therapeutic partnership with parents; facilitating adaptive coping; and empowering them to participate in caregiving, problem solving, and advocacy. The birth of an infant at risk for a disability, or the diagnosis of such a disability, may create both developmental and situational crises for the parents and the family system. The developmental crisis involves adapting to changing roles in the transition to parenthood and in expanding the family system. Although not occurring unexpectedly, this developmental transition for the parents brings lifestyle changes that may be stressful and cause conflict.[13] Because parents are experiencing (mourning) loss of the "wished for" baby they have been visualizing in the past 6 months, they often struggle with developing a bond with their "real" baby in the NICU.[14]

A situational crisis occurs from unexpected external events presenting a sudden, overwhelming threat or loss for which previous coping strategies either are not applicable or are immobilized.[15] The unfamiliar, high-technology, often chaotic NICU environment creates many situational stresses that challenge parenting efforts and destabilize the family system.[16] The language of the nursery is unfamiliar and intimidating. The sight of fragile, sick infants surrounded by medical equipment and the sound of monitor alarms are frightening. The high frequency of seemingly uncomfortable, but required, medical procedures for the infant are of financial and humanistic concern to parents. No previous experiences in everyday life have prepared parents for this unnatural, emergency-oriented environment. This emotional trauma of unexpected financial and ongoing psychological stresses during parenting and caregiving efforts in the NICU contributes to potential posttraumatic stress disorder in parents of infants requiring intensive care.[17,18]

The quality and orientation of the helping relationship in neonatal therapy affect the coping style of parents as they try to adapt to developmental and situational crises (see Figure 11-4). Although parents and neonatal therapists enter the

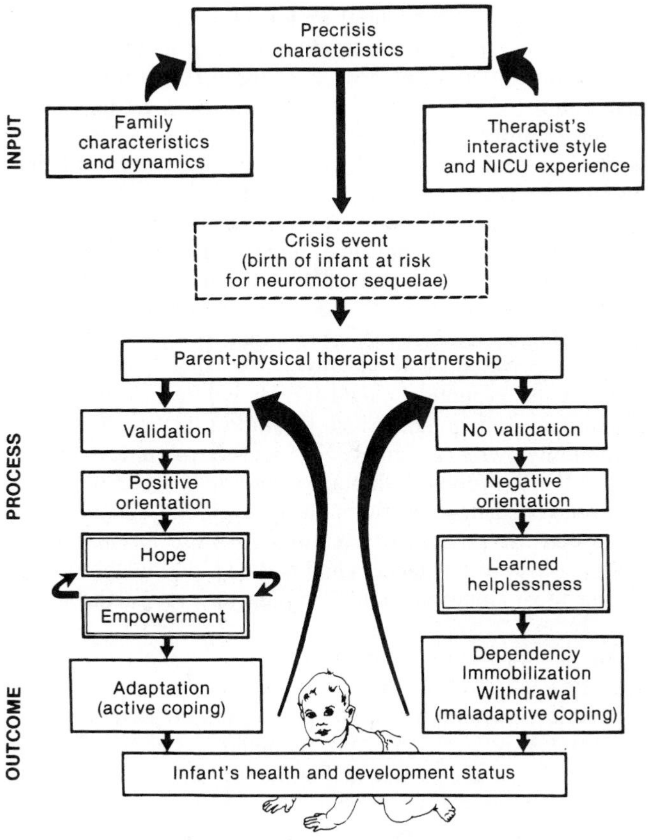

Figure 11-4 ■ Hope-empowerment *(left)* versus learned helplessness *(right)* processes of the therapeutic partnership between parents and the neonatal therapist.

partnership with established interactive styles and varying life and professional experiences, the initial contacts during assessment and program planning set the stage for either a positive or a negative orientation to the relationship.

Despite many uncertainties about the clinical course, prognosis, and quality of social support, a positive orientation is activated by validation or acknowledgment of parents' feelings and experiences. Validation then becomes a catalyst to a hope-empowerment process in which many crisis events, negative feelings, and insecurities are acknowledged in a positive, supportive, nonjudgmental context in which decision-making power is shared.[19] In contrast, a negative orientation may be inadvertently facilitated by information overloading without exploration and validation of parents' feelings, experiences, and learning styles. This may lead to magnified uncertainty, fear, and powerlessness with the misperception of excessive complexity in the proposed neuromotor intervention activities.

In a hope-empowerment framework, parent participation in neuromotor intervention allows sharing of power and responsibility and promotes continuous, mutual setting and revision of goals with reality grounding. Adaptive power can be generated by helping parents stabilize and focus energy and plans and by encouraging active participation in intervention and advocacy activities.[19] Exploring external power sources (e.g., Parent to Parent USA or other parent-to-parent support groups[20]) early in the therapeutic relationship may help parents focus and mobilize.[20-23]

Hope and empowerment are interactive processes. They are influenced by existential philosophy: the hope to adapt to what is and the hope to later find peace of mind and meaning for the situation, regardless of the infant's outcome. In describing the effect of a prematurely born infant on the parenting process, Mercer[24] related that "hope seems to be a motivational, emotional component that gives parents energy to cope, to continue to work, and to strive for the best outcome for a child." She viewed the destruction of hope as contributing to the physical and emotional withdrawal frequently observed in parents who attempt to protect themselves from additional pain and disappointment and then have difficulty reattaching to the infant.

Hope contributes to the resilience parents need to get through the arduous 1- to 4-month NICU hospitalization period and then begin to face the future in their home and community with an infant at neurodevelopmental risk. Groopman[25] proposed that hope provides the courage to confront obstacles and the capacity to surmount them. He described the process of creating a *middle ground* where truth (of the circumstances) and hope reside together as one of the most important and complex aspects in the art of caregiving.

In a hope-empowerment context, parental teaching activities are carefully selected to contribute to pleasurable interaction between infant and parent. Gradual participation in infant care activities and therapeutic handling in the NICU provide experience and build confidence for continuation in the home environment.

Conversely, if the parents' learning styles, goals, priorities, values, time constraints, energy levels, and emotional availability are not considered in the design of the developmental program, the parents may experience failure, loss of self-esteem, powerlessness, immobilization, or dependency. The neonatal therapist may recognize signs of learned helplessness in parents when they show nonattendance, noncompliance, negative interactions with infant and staff, or a hopeless outlook during bedside teaching sessions.

New events in the infant's health or developmental status may create new crises and destabilize the coping processes. In long-term follow-up many opportunities occur within the partnership to validate new fears and chronic uncertainties within a hopeful, positively oriented, helping relationship. The alleviation of hopelessness is a critical helping task in health care. This model provides a conceptual framework for sharing the gifts of hope and power with parents and caregivers.

NEONATAL COMPLICATIONS ASSOCIATED WITH ADVERSE OUTCOMES

Improvements in neonatal intensive care over the last 30 years have led to the increased survival of preterm and term infants. Specific obstetric advances include establishment of specialized tertiary care centers, earlier identification of high-risk pregnancies, improvements in prenatal diagnosis, and medications used to stabilize maternal medical conditions and enhance fetal well-being. Respiratory compromise in preterm infants has significantly decreased as a result of (1) maternal betamethasone administration to promote fetal lung maturity; (2) availability of commercial surfactant to improve pulmonary function; and (3) advances in ventilator design and capability, enhancing management of respiratory distress with significantly diminished pulmonary dysfunction. In addition, improvements in continuous monitoring of vital signs, radiological imaging techniques, delivery of medications, and maintenance of thermal stability have aided earlier identification of neonatal problems and enhanced improvements in care. Increased survival is most evident in the extremely low–birth-weight (ELBW) infant, that is, birth weight less than 1000 g. For infants born at 23 weeks of gestation, survival has increased from approximately 0% to more than 50%, and for infants born at 26 weeks of gestation, survival has increased from 25% to 85%.[26] It is important to note that the incidence of severe neurological injury has decreased over time in these extremely preterm infants. However, a significant number of preterm infants will exhibit long-term neurological impairment owing to increased survival.

The long-term effect of a neurological insult on the developing brain depends on the timing of the injury, the gestational age of the infant, and the nature and duration of the insult.[27] During the first month of gestation, the neural tube is formed. Neurological insult at this time leads to abnormal neural tube development, specifically anencephaly, encephalocele, or myelomeningocele. Neuronal proliferation is nearly complete by 5 months of gestation. All neurons and glial cells originate in the ventricular and subventricular zone (germinal matrix). Disorders of proliferation result in microcephaly, with either decreased size or decreased number of proliferating neuronal units or macrocephaly. Neuronal migration occurs at 3 to 6 months of gestation, and neurons are guided by glial cells to form neuronal columns. Subplate neurons, essential for correct organization of the brain, are formed at this time. Insults during this period of development result in marked disturbance of neurological structure and function with aberrations noted in gyral formation (lissencephaly, schizencephaly, and polymicrogyria) and/or absence of the corpus callosum.

Organization, consisting of elaboration of subplate neurons, orientation of cortical neurons, development of dendrites and axons, synaptogenesis and apoptosis, occurs from 5 months of gestation through several years after birth. Subplate neurons are present from 22 to 35 weeks of gestation; they form connections between neurons and guide axons and dendritic projections to the appropriate targets. Subplate neurons are sensitive to hypoxia and result in abnormal brain development and impaired long-term neurological outcome. Synaptogenesis before birth is experience independent. However, synaptic formation and elimination via apoptosis (programmed cell death) are most active after birth and are thought to be experience dependent. This process confers plasticity to the brain and is the basis of individuality. The presence and importance of subplate neurons as well as synaptogenesis coincide with the time that preterm infants are in the NICU and make the preterm brain especially vulnerable to perturbations such as hypoxia, medications, stress, and pain.

The final phase of brain organization is glial maturation to astrocytes and oligodendrocytes. Astrocytes help maintain the blood-brain barrier, provide nutrient support, regulate neurotransmitter and potassium concentration, and assist in neuronal repair after injury. Oligodendrocytes produce myelin, a protective fatty sheath that surrounds axons (white matter) and facilitates nerve transmission. Myelination starts in midgestation and continues through adulthood. Oligodendrocytes are especially sensitive to hypoxia and other insults. Disruption of normal myelination results in white matter hypoplasia and periventricular leukomalacia (PVL) (see later discussion) leading to impaired motor function.[27]

The most common neonatal problems associated with impaired neurological functioning and long-term developmental delay are listed in Table 11-1. In addition to descriptions of neonatal neurological conditions, a discussion is provided on the impact on neonatal development of maternal medication, such as drugs of abuse and psychotropic medications. The importance of developmental follow-up for healthy "late" preterm infants born at 34 to 36⁶⁄₇ weeks of gestation is also discussed in this section.

Intraventricular Hemorrhage

Intraventricular hemorrhage (IVH) is the most common brain injury in preterm infants born under 32 weeks of gestation and is a significant risk factor for the development of neurodevelopmental deficits. The incidence of IVH varies inversely with gestational age. Approximately 15% of infants born at 1000 g or less will have severe IVH. Although the incidence of severe IVH has decreased over time, an increased number of these infants survive owing to improvements in clinical care and technology, leading to an increase in the number of surviving preterm infants who are significantly affected by IVH.

IVH originates in the microcirculation or capillary network of the germinal matrix.[28] The germinal matrix is located adjacent to the ventricle and is a well vascularized area owing to the high metabolic demand from the rapidly proliferating neuronal stem cells. Vessels in the germinal matrix are thin walled and fragile, which predisposes them to rupture. In addition, preterm infants have impaired autoregulation—that is, the inability to maintain cerebral blood flow across a large range of blood pressures. Thus during labor, delivery, and the immediate postpartum transition period, changes in blood pressure can lead to cerebral hypoperfusion and ischemia as well as to hyperperfusion and vessel rupture. Alterations in CO_2 lead to either reduced cerebral blood flow from hypocarbia or increased flow from hypercarbia. Other risk factors for IVH include asphyxia, fluid bolus infusion (especially of hypertonic solutions), anemia, and pain.[29] Platelet and coagulation disturbances have been implicated as risk factors for the development of IVH. IVH is rarely seen in infants with gestational age greater than 32 weeks owing to the developmental involution of vessels in the germinal matrix.

Diagnosed by cranial ultrasound, IVH is graded in severity from 1 to 4,[28] with grade 1 IVH being the most mild because the hemorrhage is confined to the germinal matrix. In grade 2 IVH, the hemorrhage extends into the ventricle (Figure 11-5). Grade 3 IVH occurs when the hemorrhage fills more than 50% of the ventricle and causes ventricular distention. Grade 4 IVH, or periventricular hemorrhagic infarct (PVHI), is a complication of IVH caused by venous congestion of the terminal veins that border the lateral ventricles leading to white matter necrosis (see later).[30] It is important to note that IVH may not be apparent on cranial ultrasound in the first few days after birth. However, 90% of IVHs can be detected by day 4. In addition, the full extent of the hemorrhage may not be appreciated for several days after the initial diagnosis of IVH is made.[28] The evolution of grades 3 and 4 IVH over 10 days is shown in Figure 11-6, *A* and *B*.

Many researchers have investigated the relationship of IVH grades with severity of neurodevelopment delay. In general, grades 1 and 2 IVH are not associated with a significant increase in developmental abnormalities but do not ensure normalcy. Infants with severe IVH (grade 3 and/or 4) have increased mortality and are at markedly increased risk for developmental disabilities, specifically spastic hemiplegia or diplegia affecting the lower extremities. As can be seen in Figure 11-7, motor tracts innervating the lower extremities are in close proximity to the area of the germinal matrix and the site of the origin of IVH leading to lower-extremity spastic cerebral palsy (CP). However, abnormalities visible on cranial ultrasound are not able to absolutely predict long-term outcome because the amount of cortex damaged and the neuronal tracts affected by IVH cannot be identified by ultrasound. In addition, ultrasound may not be sensitive enough to identify PVL (see later).

TABLE 11-1 ■ NEONATAL COMPLICATIONS AFFECTING BRAIN DEVELOPMENT

AGE	SPECIFIC INSULT
Preterm	Intraventricular hemorrhage (IVH)
	Periventricular hemorrhagic infarct (PVHI)
	Posthemorrhagic ventricular dilatation (PHVD)
	Periventricular leukomalacia (PVL)
	Necrotizing enterocolitis (NEC)
Term	Hypoxic-ischemic encephalopathy (HIE)

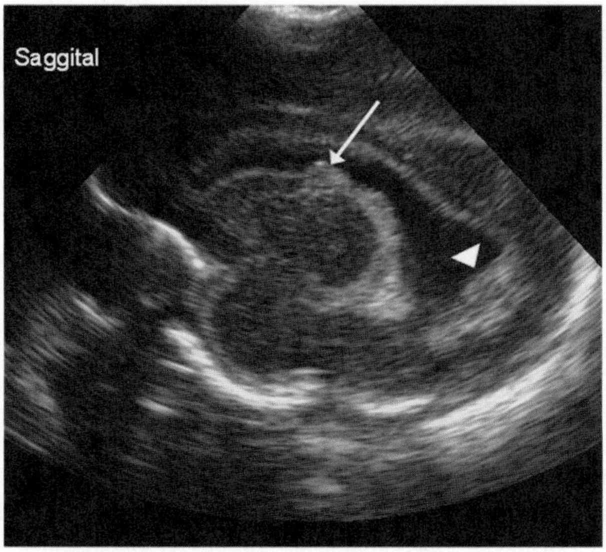

Figure 11-5 ■ Grade 2 intraventricular hemorrhage is illustrated by the *arrow* indicating the area of the germinal matrix bleed. The *arrowhead* points to blood layering in the posterior aspect of the lateral ventricle.

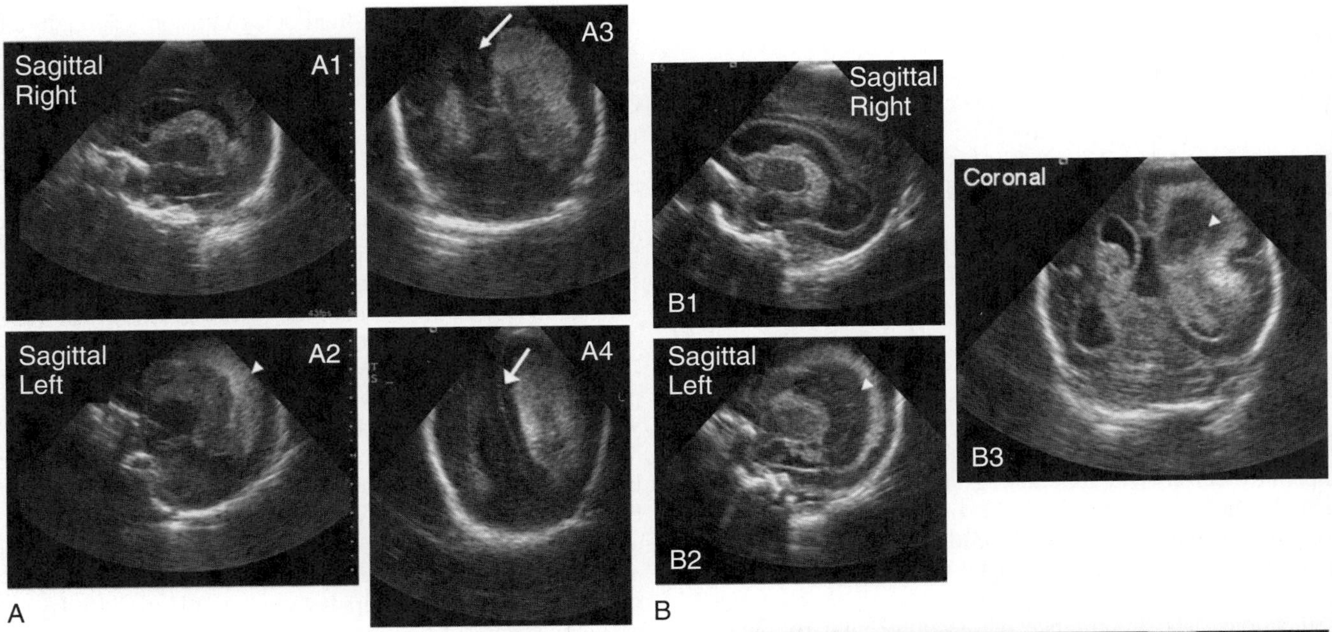

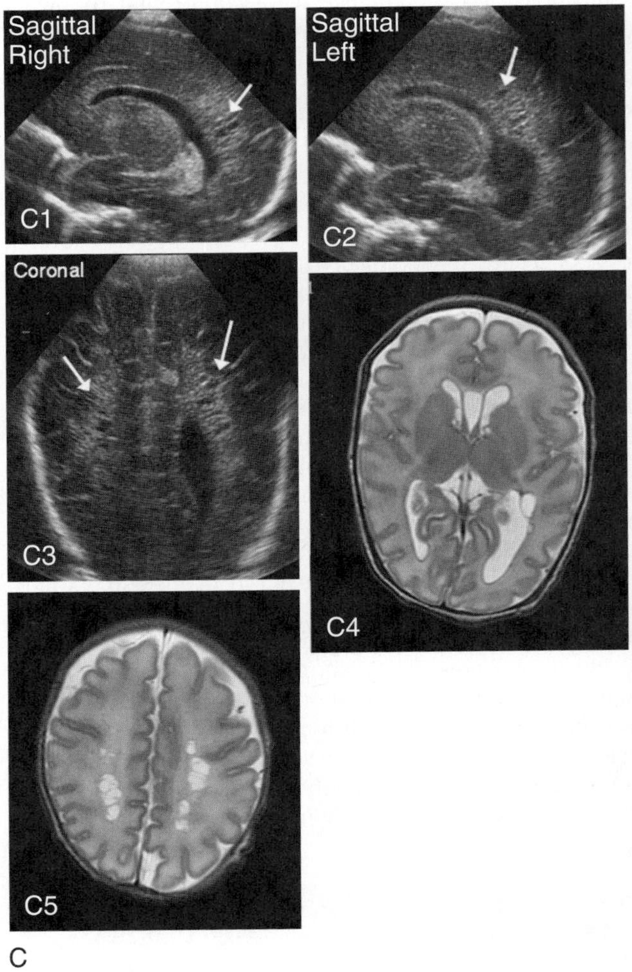

Figure 11-6 ■ **A,** Cranial ultrasound of right grade 3 intraventricular hemorrhage (IVH) and left grade 4 IVH (PVHI periventricular hemorrhagic infarct) on day 3 of life. *A1* and *A2* are taken in the sagittal plane with the arrowhead pointing to the area of PHVI. *A3* and *A4* are coronal views with the arrow pointing to midline shift caused by the left PVHI. **B,** Progression of right grade 3 IVH and left PHVI on day 13 of life. Note retraction of the clot with ventricular enlargement in *B1* and *B2*. There is marked expansion of PHVI *(arrowheads)* with dissolution of brain parenchyma in both *B2* and *B3*. **C,** Cystic periventricular leukomalacia (cystic PVL) is present on cranial ultrasound in both right (*C1* and *C2*) and left (*C2* and *C3*) sides of the brain as marked by arrows. Cysts in the same infant are more evident using MRI imaging (*C4* and *C5*).

Periventricular Hemorrhagic Infarct

Grade 4 IVH was originally thought to be an extension of IVH into the parenchyma but is actually a known complication of IVH.[30] PVHI is caused by venous compression of the terminal veins that border the lateral ventricles leading to impaired venous drainage and congestion and eventually hemorrhagic infarction. The usual initial distribution of PVHI seen on cranial ultrasound is fan-shaped echodensities in the periventricular location (see Figure 11-6, *A2-4*). Over time there is destruction of preoligodendrocytes and motor axons leading to white matter necrosis and the development of porencephalic cyst. PVHI is usually unilateral (approximately 70%),

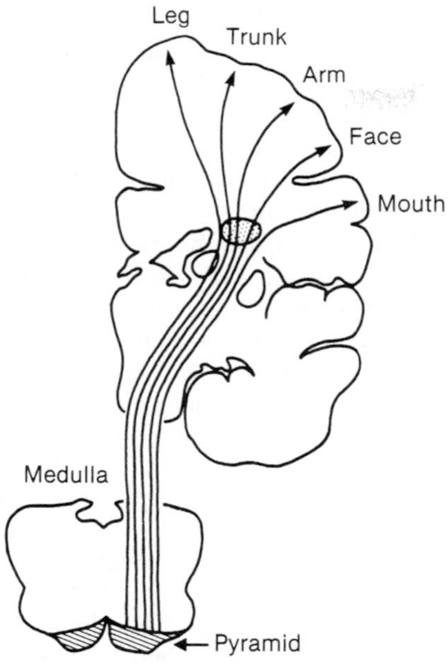

Figure 11-7 ■ Schematic diagram of corticospinal tract fibers that extend from the motor cortex through the periventricular region into the pyramid of the medulla. The lower motor neurons affected by intraventricular hemorrhage and periventricular hemorrhagic infarct are located in close proximity to the ventricle. Bulbar and upper motor neuron tracts are affected in term infants with hypoxic-ischemic encephalopathy and are parasylvian in location. (From Volpe JJ: Hypoxic ischemic encephalopathy: neuropathology and pathogenesis. In Volpe JJ: *Neurology of the neonate,* Philadelphia, 1995, WB Saunders.)

and approximately three quarters of cases are associated with severe IVH [grade 3 and 4]. Infants with small, unilateral PVHI have no increased risk of developmental delays compared with infants with grade 3 IVH. However, if the PVHI is bilateral or if multiple porencephalic cysts are present, the risk of severe motor impairment and CP is significantly increased. In addition, approximately 50% of infants with PVHI have visual field defects, probably secondary to damage to the axons of nerves carrying information to the visual cortex.[30]

Posthemorrhagic Ventricular Dilatation

Approximately 50% of infants with severe IVH will develop posthemorrhagic ventricular dilatation (PHVD) from either blockage of the normal flow of cerebrospinal fluid (CSF) or decreased absorption of CSF. Approximately 50% to 75% of these infants will develop *progressive* PHVD, resulting in need for treatment. The severity of ventricular dilatation can be measured via serial cranial ultrasound examinations.[31,32] Severe ventricular dilatation is usually evident by 2 to 3 weeks after birth. Rapid increase in head circumference does not occur until approximately 4 weeks after birth.[33] Posthemorrhagic ventricular dilatation is treated by serial removal of CSF by spinal tap, subgaleal shunt, or placement of an Ommaya reservoir. Removal of CSF has been shown to decrease intracranial pressure and improve cerebral perfusion[34] and also to increase cortical gray and white matter.[35] In addition, there is indirect evidence that ventricular distention itself may cause secondary brain injury through stretching and disruption of axons, gliosis, and loss of oligodendrocytes.

No consensus has been reached on the optimal management of PHVD. Ventriculoperitoneal (VP) shunt placement is necessary in infants with PHVD that does not resolve with serial removal of CSF. Significant complications of VP shunt include sepsis, specifically ventriculitis, or shunt malfunction such as blockage or failure. These complications necessitate shunt revisions, which further compromise these fragile infants. Researchers from a consortium of 17 tertiary NICUs recently published results on the neurodevelopmental outcome at 2 years of age of ELBW infants with grade 3 and 4 IVH who were born from 1993 to 2002.[36] Infants who required VP shunt placement had significantly worse outcomes than infants with grade 3 or 4 IVH alone (Table 11-2). Moreover, the number of infants who were untestable (MDI or PDI = 49) because of severe neurodevelopmental handicap was significantly increased in the group of infants who received a VP shunt. In addition, CP was significantly more prevalent in infants who had a VP shunt placed than in infants with only grade 3 or 4 IVH.

Recent retrospective studies from the Netherlands indicated that earlier intervention when the ventricles are moderately dilated significantly decreased the need for VP shunt from 62% to 16% and trended to improve long-term developmental outcome with a decreased incidence of moderate to severe handicap.[32,37] Thus, halting the progression of PHVD and decreasing the need for VP shunt is likely to improve long-term outcome in these infants. However, because PVHD can spontaneously resolve without intervention, identification of factors that can accurately predict which infant will develop persistent PHVD and consequently require VP shunt placement is needed.

Periventricular Leukomalacia

PVL is nonhemorrhagic cellular necrosis of periventricular white matter in the arterial watershed area and is present in less than 10% of preterm infants. Like IVH, PVL is inversely related to gestational age. PVL is the most common ischemic injury to the preterm infant and results from lack of cerebral autoregulation leading to decreased blood flow in the vulnerable watershed arterial vessels. Subplate neurons, critical for normal neuronal organization and interaction, are destroyed in PVL, leading to decreased white matter. In addition, preoligodendrocytes are exquisitely sensitive to oxygen and glucose deprivation leading to markedly abnormal myelination.

TABLE 11-2 ■ OUTCOME OF EXTREMELY LOW–BIRTH-WEIGHT INFANTS WITH GRADE 3 OR 4 INTRAVENTRICULAR HEMORRHAGE WITH OR WITHOUT VENTRICULOPERITONEAL (VP) SHUNT

	NO VP SHUNT	VP SHUNT	*P*
MDI <70	326/719 (45.3%)	146/214 (68.2%)	<.0001
MDI = 49	130/719 (18.1%)	87/214 (40.7%)	<.0001
PDI <70	263/711 (37.0%)	163/214 (76.2%)	<.0001
PDI = 49	149/711 (21.0%)	113/214 (52.8%)	<.0001
CP	217/767 (28.3%)	158/227 (69.6%)	<.0001

Modified from Adams-Chapman I, Hansen NI, Stoll BJ, et al: Neurodevelopmental outcome of extremely low birth weight infants with posthemorrhagic hydrocephalus requiring shunt insertion. *Pediatrics* 121:1167-1177, 2008.

CP, Cerebral palsy; MDI, Mental Developmental Index; PDI, Psychomotor Development Index.

PVL can be either cystic (see Figure 11-6, *C*) or global and may be difficult to identify on radiological images. Cystic PVL results from the focal dissolution of cellular tissue approximately 3 weeks after the insult and can be identified on ultrasound if greater than 0.5 cm in diameter.[27] However, cysts visualized by cranial ultrasound may disappear over time owing to fibrosis and gliosis. Thus the incidence of cystic PVL is felt to be underestimated by cranial ultrasound examination. Global PVL results from diffuse white matter injury and myelin loss. This finding can be subtle with moderate ventricular dilatation and/or a mild increase in extraaxial fluid on cranial imaging. Infants with severe PVL have marked ventricular dilatation, increased extraaxial fluid, and decreased head growth.

MRI obtained at term is more sensitive in identifying white matter injury than cranial ultrasound and is predictive of subsequent neurosensory impairment and cognitive delay present in up to 50% of extremely preterm infants.[38] Newer techniques, such as diffusion tensor imaging (DTI), functional connectivity MRI (fcMRI), and morphometry for analysis of cortical folding are being investigated as early markers of impaired neurodevelopmental outcome. Diffusion tension imaging measures the restriction of water diffusion in the myelin sheath surrounding axons and yields information at the microstructure level about axon caliber changes and aberrations in myelination. In addition, DTI allows for visualization of brain fiber tracks and neuronal connectivity. In research, fMRI is used to investigate interaction between areas of the brain at rest and during tasks by analyzing changes in blood flow. Morphometic analysis of sequential MRI scans has been used to create maps of cortical folding with quantification of surface area and degree of gyral formation. White matter injury results in delayed myelination and altered cortical folding.[38] Both fMRI and morphometric analysis of cortical folding are currently available only in research studies, not in clinical management.

Necrotizing Enterocolitis

Necrotizing enterocolitis (NEC) is the most common neonatal intestinal disease, with an incidence of 10% in extremely preterm infants. The hallmark of NEC is pneumatosis intestinalis. NEC is initially treated medically with antibiotic therapy and cessation of enteral feedings. Surgery for NEC refractory to medical treatment or for intestinal perforation occurs in up to 50% of cases and has increased mortality of 20% to 40% compared with infants who are able to be treated medically. The cause of NEC is not established, but risk factors include prematurity, umbilical artery catheterization, asphyxia, congenital heart disease, blood transfusion, and enteral feedings. Several viruses (adenovirus, enterovirus, and rotavirus) and bacteria have been implicated as causative agents for NEC. However, bacteremia may be a secondary finding because infants with NEC are frequently in a septic condition either at the time of presentation of NEC or after intestinal perforation.

Complications of NEC include sepsis, wound infection, and stricture formation (10% to 35%) requiring repeated surgery. Growth of infants with NEC can be impaired due to feeding intolerance, prolonged total parenteral nutrition (TPN), removal of significant amounts of intestine, and repeated surgeries and infections. Persistence of weight at less than 10% for age is correlated with poor neuromotor and neurodevelopmental outcome.[39] Failure to achieve normalization of head growth is associated with abnormal performance at 1 year and probably reflects significant white matter injury. Infants with surgically managed NEC have been shown to have significantly increased incidence of CP (24% versus 15%), deafness (4.1% versus 1.5%), and blindness (4.1% versus 1%).[39] Meta-analysis of seven studies investigating the impact of NEC on neurodevelopmental outcome showed that infants with surgically treated NEC have a statistically significant increase in cognitive, psychomotor, and neurodevelopmental impairment compared with age-matched preterm infants without NEC.[40] Impaired neurodevelopmental outcome in infants with NEC is further exacerbated by associated sepsis and the release of inflammatory cytokines and mediators in addition to hypoxia, all of which contribute to further insult to preoligodendrocytes, leading to white matter injury.

Cerebellar Injury

The cerebellum is essential for gross and fine motor control, coordination, and motor sequencing and plays an important role in attention and language.[36] The clinical hallmark of damage to the cerebellum is ataxia. However, recent advances in functional MRI (fMRI) have demonstrated that there are interactions between the cerebellum and nonmotor areas of the brain involved in language, attention, and mental imagery. Cerebellar injury can also be noted early in neonatal development from cranial ultrasound of the posterior fossa (mastoid view). The incidence of cerebellar injury may be as high as 20% in ELBW infants.[41] Although the mechanism for damage is unknown, IVH is present in more than 75% of infants with cerebellar injury, implying similar risk factors for both IVH and cerebellar hemorrhage or the possibility that IVH leads to cerebellar hemorrhage. The majority of cerebellar lesions (70%) are unilateral.

Preterm infants with isolated cerebellar hemorrhage exhibit significant neurological impairments: hypotonia (100%), abnormal gait (40%), ophthalmological abnormalities (approximately 40%), and microcephaly (17%).[42] Overall, preterm infants with cerebellar hemorrhage performed significantly lower on tests of gross and fine motor skills and have deficits in vision and expressive and receptive language. Infants with both cerebellar injury and IVH have greater motor impairment than infants with isolated cerebellar hemorrhage. Socially, infants with isolated cerebellar hemorrhage exhibit delayed communication skills, decreased social skills with more withdrawn behavior, and impaired ability to attend to tasks. Thus, cerebellar injury increases the risk for poor neurodevelopmental outcome in cognition, learning, and behavior in preterm infants.[42] For long-term effects of cerebellar damage, refer to Chapter 21.

Hypoxic-Ischemic Encephalopathy

Perinatal asphyxia, the result of a hypoxic-ischemic (HI) insult, affects three to five per 1000 live births and leads to hypoxic-ischemic encephalopathy (HIE) in 0.5 to one per 1000 live births. Impaired oxygen delivery to the fetus can result from maternal hypotension, placental abruption, placental insufficiency, cord prolapse, prolonged labor, and/or traumatic delivery. Approximately 15% to 20% of infants with HIE will die, and 25% of the surviving infants will exhibit permanent neurological sequelae. Clinical findings will vary depending on the timing and duration of the HI insult, preconditioning and fetal adaptive mechanisms, comorbidities, and resuscitative efforts. Infants who are intrauterine growth restricted are at increased risk of an HI insult due to decreased nutrient reserves.[43]

It is important to note that the injury from an HI insult is an evolving and progressive process that begins at the time of the insult and continues through the recovery period (Figure 11-8). The HI insult causes decreased oxygen and glucose delivery to the brain, causing a shift from aerobic to anaerobic metabolism. This causes a decrease in adenosine triphosphate (ATP) production, leading to failure of the membrane-bound Na^+-K^+-ATPase pump. Sodium enters the neuronal cell, causing depolarization and release of excitatory neurotransmitters, specifically glutamate. This initial phase can last several hours and is marked by significant acidosis, depletion of high-energy compounds (energy failure), cellular swelling caused by entry of sodium and water, and cellular necrosis, causing spillage of intracellular contents into the extracellular space. The degree of neuronal necrosis is directly related to the duration and severity of the HI insult. During the subsequent reperfusion phase, free radical production increases and activation of microglia from extruded intracellular contents occurs, causing release of inflammatory mediators. A second phase of energy failure ensues, but without acidosis. Calcium enters the cell and the mitochondria, which then turns on the apoptotic pathway (programmed cell death). During this second phase of energy failure, seizures are often present. Activation of the apoptotic pathway accounts for the majority of cellular death and is the target for treatment.[27,28] The specific timing of the initiation of the reperfusion phase and the second phase of energy failure is unclear in the clinical setting because the actual timing of the HI insult is not well defined. In animal studies, the latency between the first and second phases of energy failure is several hours.

In term infants with HIE the cerebral damage is located in the deep structures of the brain (basal ganglia, thalamus, and posterior limb of the internal capsule) as well as the subcortical and parasagittal white matter.[44] Diffusion-weighted MRI (DWI) is a very early diagnostic and sensitive technique to identify damage after the HI insult. As shown in Figure 11-8, a marked increase in signal in the subcortical and parasagittal white matter occurs as well as in the deep nuclear structures on DWI. MRI spectroscopy, localized to the basal ganglia or subcortical area, yields information about degree of secondary energy failure by analyzing for the depletion of the high-energy compound *N*-acetylaspartate and the presence of lactate.[44,45] The degree of secondary energy failure as noted on MRI spectroscopy is predictive of death and poor neurodevelopmental outcome at 1 and 4 years of age.

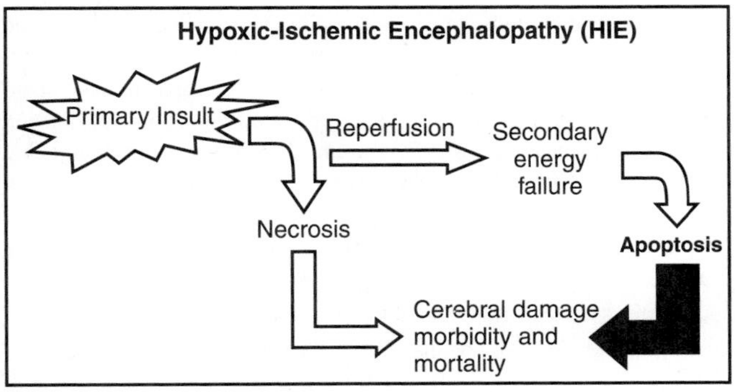

Figure 11-8 ■ Sequential events that occur after hypoxic-ischemic (HI) insult. Initial event leads to cellular necrosis and cerebral damage. Secondary energy failure and initiation of the apoptotic pathway lead to the majority of injury after HI insult. Degree of secondary energy failure as measured by magnetic resonance imaging spectroscopy is highly correlated with neurodevelopmental outcome. (From Adams-Chapman I, Hansen NI, Stoll BJ, et al: Neurodevelopmental outcome of extremely low birth weight infants with posthemorrhagic hydrocephalus requiring shunt insertion. *Pediatrics* 121:e1167–e1177, 2008.)

Classification of the clinical signs associated with HIE is shown in Table 11-3.[46] Infants with grade 1 HIE rarely have long-term sequelae. Infants with grade 2 or moderate HIE have abnormal tone and reflexes and decreased spontaneous activity, with seizures commonly present. Approximately 10% of infants with moderate HIE will die and up to 30% will have neurodevelopmental delay. Infants with severe HIE (grade 3) exhibit minimal or no spontaneous activity or reflexes. Clinically evident seizures are seldom present, but electrographically evident seizures are more common. Approximately 50% of these infants die, and of the survivors, more than 60% to 80% are profoundly impaired. Long-term consequences of HIE include bulbar palsies with difficulties in sucking, swallowing, and facial movement. These infants have difficulty with secretions and may require tube feeding owing to inability to protect the airway. Upper-extremity involvement is more prominent than lower-extremity deficits because the damage to the cerebral cortex is located in the parasagittal region (see Figure 11-7). The development of epilepsy occurs in about 30% of infants with HIE. Mental retardation and difficulties at school age occur frequently.

Mild hypothermia (33.5° C) from application of cooling blankets or caps is becoming the standard of care for infants ≥ 36 weeks' gestation who have an acute asphyxial event and moderate or severe HIE.[47] Hypothermia has been shown to decrease cerebral metabolic demand and thus help preserve high-energy compounds. Hypothermia also delays membrane depolarization and decreases neuronal excitotoxicity. Free radical production and microglial activation are decreased. Most important, the activation of the apoptotic pathway is diminished. Transient side effects of hypothermia, such as bradycardia, mild hypotension, thrombocytopenia, and persistent pulmonary hypertension, can be medically treated and are usually not significant.[48,49] A meta-analysis of published randomized studies comparing infants with moderate and severe HIE treated with either hypothermia or normothermia shows that hypothermic treatment significantly decreases mortality and morbidity (Table 11-4).[50] Hypothermia appears to more efficacious in ameliorating brain damage in infants with mild HIE than in infants with severe HIE. It is known that hypothermia is most effective when administered before the onset of the second phase of energy failure. Because the HI insult can occur before delivery, it is postulated that hypothermia should be initiated as quickly as possible after delivery to increase the likelihood that it will diminish the neuronal damage and improve neurodevelopmental outcome.

Maternal Medication

The impact of maternal medications on the developing fetal brain depends on the specific drug as well as on the timing and duration of the drug exposure. Whereas the insults

TABLE 11-3 ■ SARNET SCORING SCALE FOR ENCEPHALOPATHY

	STAGE 1 (MILD)	STAGE 2 (MODERATE)	STAGE 3 (SEVERE)
Level of consciousness	Hyperalert	Lethargy, obtunded	Stuporous
Neuromuscular signs			
Muscle tone	Normal	Mild hypotonia	Flaccid
Posture	Mild distal flexion	Distal flexion	Decerebrate
Movement	Spontaneous	Decreased to little	Noxious stimuli
Stretch reflexes	Overactive	Overactive	Decreased or absent
Primitive reflexes			
Suck	Weak	Weak or absent	Absent gag
Moro	Strong	Weak or incomplete	Absent
Autonomic function	Sympathetic Dilated pupils Tachycardia	Parasympathetic Constricted pupils Bradycardia Copious secretions Periodic breathing	Depressed Pupils nonreactive Variable heart rate Apnea Loss of temp regulation
Seizures	None	Common Focal or multifocal	Uncommon

Modified from Sarnat HB, Sarnat MS: Neonatal encephalopathy following fetal distress. A clinical and electroencephalographic study. *Arch Neurol* 33:696-705, 1976.

TABLE 11-4 ■ EFFECT OF MODERATE HYPOTHERMIA ON NEUROLOGICAL OUTCOMES AT 18 MONTHS COMPARED WITH CONTROLS

	RISK RATIO (95% CONFIDENCE INTERVAL [CI])	RISK DIFFERENCE (95% CI)	NUMBER NEEDED TO TREAT (95% CI)	*P* VALUE
Death or severe disability*	0.81 (0.71-0.93)	−0.11 (−0.18-−0.04)	9 (5-25)	.002
Survival with normal outcome†	1.53 (1.22-1.93)	0.12 (0.06-0.18)	8 (5-17)	<.001
Mortality	0.78 (0.66-0.93)	−0.07 (−0.12-−0.02)	14 (8-47)	.005
Severe disability in survivors*	0.71 (0.56-0.91)	− 0.11 (−0.20-−0.03)	9 (5-30)	.006
Cerebral palsy in survivors	0.69 (0.54-0.89)	−0.12 (−0.20-−0.04)	8 (5-24)	.004
Severe neuromotor delay in survivors‡	0.73 (0.56-0.95)	−0.10 (−0.18-−0.02)	10 (6-71)	.02
Severe neurodevelopmental delay in survivors§	0.71 (0.54-0.92)	−0.11 (−0.19-−0.03)	9 (5-39)	.01
Blindness in survivors	0.57 (0.33-0.96)	−0.06 (−0.11-0.00)	17 (9-232)	.03
Deafness in survivors	0.76 (0.36-1.62)	−0.01 (−0.05-0.03)	NA	.47

From Edwards AD, Brocklehurst P, Gunn AJ, et al: Neurological outcomes at 18 months of age after moderate hypothermia for perinatal hypoxic ischaemic encephalopathy: synthesis and meta-analysis of trial data. *BMJ* 340:c363, 2010.

*Severe disability was defined in the CoolCap and TOBY trials as the presence of at least one of the following impairments: Mental Development Index score of less than 70 (2 standard deviations below the standardized mean of 100) on the Bayley Scales of Infant Development; gross motor function classification system level 3 to 5 (where the scale is from 1 to 5, with 1 being the mildest impairment); or bilateral cortical visual impairment with no useful vision. The NICHD trial defined disability as a Mental Developmental Index score of 70 to 84 plus one or more of the following impairments: gross motor function classification system level 2; hearing impairment with no amplification; or a persistent seizure disorder.

†Survival with normal outcome was defined as survival without cerebral palsy and with a Mental Developmental Index score of more than 84, a Psychomotor Developmental Index score of more than 84, and normal vision and hearing.

‡Severe neuromotor delay was determined on the basis of a Psychomotor Developmental Index score of less than 70 in survivors.

§Severe neurodevelopmental delay was determined on the basis of a Mental Developmental Index score of less than 70 in survivors.

discussed previously cause predominantly cellular necrosis and apoptosis, medications given to the fetus and preterm infant cause alterations in the structure and function of genetic material as well as activation of the apoptotic pathway. The hypothesis that factors acting early in life have a long-lasting impact on development is called the *Barker hypothesis* or the *fetal origins of adult disease.* It is proposed that the biological value of this reprogramming is to prepare the fetus for maximal adaptation through methylation and deacetylation of histones, thereby determining the quantity of specific proteins that are produced. This topic is too extensive to be covered here and has been previously reviewed.[51,52] This section will focus on heroin, methadone, cocaine, methamphetamine, and selective serotonin reuptake inhibitors (SSRIs) used in the treatment of maternal depression.

Cocaine

It is difficult to ascertain the exact frequency of cocaine use during pregnancy, but reports indicate that 1% to 45% of females have used cocaine during their pregnancy.[28]

Cocaine is extracted from the leaves of the coca plant and can be smoked, inhaled, or injected into the bloodstream. Cocaine induces an intense and immediate euphoric state and can be very addictive. Unlike with opioids, physical dependence does not occur, but severe and intense cravings last for several months and can recur for years after cessation of cocaine use.

In the adult the actions of cocaine are mediated through several different neurotransmitter pathways in the brain. Cocaine may cause hypertension, tachycardia, and peripheral and coronary artery vasoconstriction via activation of adrenergic pathways. The sense of euphoria is mediated through dopamine pathways. Alterations in sleep-wake cycles are caused by the blocking of serotonin uptake. During pregnancy, cocaine causes decreased blood flow to the kidneys and is implicated in preterm labor, uterine irritability, premature rupture of membranes, and placental abruption.

Cocaine negatively affects neuronal proliferation, migration, growth, and connectivity, which distorts neuronal cortical architecture. However, the effects of intrauterine exposure to cocaine are difficult to determine because cocaine use is frequently associated with abuse of other illicit drugs, cigarettes, and alcohol. Other confounding variables include poor nutrition and limited prenatal care. In a large prospective blinded study, more infants exposed to cocaine in utero were delivered prematurely and exhibited decreased weight, length, and head circumference compared with matched controls.[53] However, cocaine exposure did not affect the incidence of congenital abnormalities.

The vasoconstrictive properties of cocaine increase the risk for HI injury and middle cerebral artery stroke. Neonates with prenatal cocaine exposure demonstrate tremors, hypertonia, irritability, and poor feeding ability. Cocaine-exposed infants have abnormal sleep patterns and are at a threefold to sevenfold increased risk of sudden infant death syndrome (SIDS). No difference was found in developmental testing[54] between cocaine-exposed infants and matched controls, but the tests did not effectively evaluate arousal, emotional control, and social interaction.[55] In utero cocaine exposure has been linked to increased incidence of behavioral problems and special education referrals in school-aged children. On fMRI, differences in the right frontal cortex and caudate nucleus are evident and indicate abnormalities in regulation of attention and cognitive abilities referred to as *executive function.*

Opioids

The opioids are used less frequently than cocaine during pregnancy, as less than 5% of pregnant woman test positive for opioids. Morphine, a naturally occurring opiate, and heroin, a synthetic opioid, readily cross the placenta and are highly addictive. Because heroin can be injected intravenously, there is an increased risk for infection, especially endocarditis, hepatitis, and human immunodeficiency virus (HIV) infection. Methadone, a synthetic opioid, is the standard for treatment of opioid dependence and has a significantly longer half-life than heroin and morphine. Over the past several years, a trend for increasing rather than decreasing methadone daily dose during pregnancy has helped to decrease maternal illicit drug abuse without increasing the incidence of withdrawal symptoms in the infant.

Opioid use during pregnancy has been associated with tubal pregnancies, premature rupture of membranes, uterine irritability, preterm labor, and preeclampsia. Infants exposed to opioids in utero are intrauterine growth retarded at birth, but methadone has a less severe impact on fetal growth. Infants exposed to opioids in utero are noted to have a decreased incidence of respiratory distress related to enhanced surfactant production[56] and decreased hyperbilirubinemia as a result of induction of the enzyme glucuronyl transferase used in the metabolism of bilirubin.

Withdrawal from narcotics occurs 2 to 3 days after delivery, but signs can be evident as long as 2 weeks after delivery. Methadone withdrawal usually occurs later than withdrawal from morphine or heroin related to its long half-life. Infants in withdrawal (neonatal abstinence syndrome [NAS]) exhibit gastrointestinal symptoms of vomiting and watery stools; neurological signs such as tremors; hypertonicity; high-pitched and incessant cry; hyperalert state; and sweating and fever. Infants with NAS have decreased ability to nipple feed despite excessive sucking on a pacifier. Seizures can be present in 2% to 11% of infants with NAS. Two commonly used scoring methods for severity of NAS are the Lipsitz[57] and the Finnegan[58] scales. The Lipsitz scale has 11 components that are scored from 0 to 3, with any score over 4 necessitating treatment.[57] The Finnegan scale is a more comprehensive assessment, with more than 30 elements, and treatment is recommended if the score is greater than 8.[58] A quiet, dimly lighted environment, decreased auditory stimulation, and swaddling or holding have been used to decrease neonatal irritability and pharmacotherapy. About 30% to 80% of in utero opioid-exposed infants will require medical treatment for NAS with morphine and either clonidine or phenobarbital. The goal of treatment is to decrease irritability, improve nippling efforts, and decrease vomiting and diarrhea.

Infants exposed to opioids in utero continue to demonstrate tremulousness, hypertonicity, irritability, and increased crying episodes. In addition, they are less able to interact with people, demonstrate decreased age-appropriate free play, and have delayed fine motor coordination. The incidence of apnea and SIDS is increased in opioid-exposed infants. An appropriate and nurturing home environment is essential after discharge from the hospital to maximize neurodevelopmental outcome.[59,60]

Selective Serotonin Reuptake Inhibitors

SSRI medications such as fluoxetine (Prozac, Fontex, Seromex, Seronil), sertraline (Zoloft, Lustral, Serlain, Asenta), paroxetine (Paxil, Seroxat, Sereupin, Paroxat), fluvoxamine (Luvox, Favoxil), escitalopram (Lexapro, Cipralex, Esertia), and citalopram (Celexa, Seropram, Citox, Cital) are commonly prescribed to treat depression and anxiety disorders. The SSRI drugs inhibit serotonin reuptake, potentiating serotonergic neurotransmitter signaling. At least 600,000 infants are born yearly to mothers who have a major depressive disorder during their pregnancy.[61] Medical therapy is the most common form of treatment for depression during pregnancy. Approximately 6% of pregnant woman use SSRIs during pregnancy, and almost 40% of depressed women have been reported to use antidepressants at some time during pregnancy.[62] The serotonergic system is present early in gestation and is important in brain development.

Perturbations in this system are associated with alterations in somatosensory processing and emotional responses.

The SSRI medications readily cross the placenta and are linked to an increased risk of spontaneous abortion but not an increased incidence of malformations.[61] A recently published meta-analysis found that maternal depression was significantly associated with an increased incidence of preterm labor and neonatal birth weight of less than 2500 g but not intrauterine growth retardation of the fetus.[63] Unfortunately, this study was unable to evaluate the effect of SSRI therapy on these outcomes. Infants exposed to SSRIs in the third trimester have symptoms similar to withdrawal from opioid exposure (irritability, tremors, jitteriness, agitation, and difficulty sleeping). Neonatal feeding difficulties are common, and seizures and abnormal posturing are occasionally present. These symptoms are transient, appearing 2 to 4 days after birth and disappearing by the second week of life.[64] It is difficult to identify any specific adverse neurodevelopmental outcomes in infants exposed prenatally to SSRIs from published studies because of the variability in the specific SSRI taken, the duration and timing of SSRI use, and the confounding factors of maternal depression and the use of multiple medications.[65]

Late Preterm Birth

Preterm births have increased over the last 10 years and now constitute about 13% of all births. Late preterm infants—that is, infants born at 34 to 36⁶⁄₇ weeks' gestation—make up approximately 70% of preterm births.[66] Many factors are implicated in the early delivery of late preterm infants, including preterm labor, preeclampsia, premature rupture of membranes, sepsis, and multiple gestation pregnancies. The late preterm infant is at increased risk of respiratory distress from insufficient surfactant production, transient tachypnea of the newborn from decreased pulmonary water absorption, persistent pulmonary hypertension, and complications of mechanical ventilation (pneumothorax). Hospital stay is prolonged in the late preterm infant compared with the infant born at term gestation owing to the increased difficulty with oral feeding, need for phototherapy for hyperbilirubinemia, and continuation of antibiotic therapy for suspected sepsis.

Recent evidence has supported the concept that even healthy late preterm infants are at higher risk for neurodevelopmental delay compared with infants at term gestation. The late preterm infant's brain is vulnerable to injury because a significant portion of brain development and maturation occurs during the last 2 months of pregnancy.[67] Recent studies have shown that late preterm infants tested lower in reading skills in kindergarten and first grade, but not in math skills, than infants born at term gestation.[68] However, kindergarten and first-grade teachers rated late preterm infants as not as competent as term infants in math and reading ability. Significantly more late preterm infants required special education in kindergarten and first grade compared with control infants. A trend toward increased enrollment in special education in the third and fourth grade was reported.[68] Late preterm infants were considered at increased risk for (1) developmental delay at 3 and 4 years of age, (2) retention in kindergarten, and (3) referral for special education.[69] However, maternal age and education were significantly decreased in late preterm infants compared with infants born at term gestation. In addition, the use of Medicaid, insufficient medical care, and maternal tobacco use were higher in the mothers of late preterm infants. These multiple factors, as well as the home environment, are significant risk factors in determining the effects of late preterm delivery on long-term outcome. Regardless of the specific insult, late preterm infants are at increased risk of neurodevelopmental disabilities and should receive timely developmental follow-up to identify potential underachievement and behavioral problems.

CLINICAL MANAGEMENT: NEONATAL PERIOD

Pediatric therapists with preceptor, subspecialty training in neonatology and infant therapy approaches can expand neonatal services by creating clinical protocols and pathways designed to optimize the development and interaction of neonates and parents. The therapeutic partnership between parents and neonatal therapists during developmental intervention in the NICU sets the stage for parental competency in caregiving and compliance with follow-up in the outpatient period. General aims of NICU clinical management of infants at risk for neurological dysfunction, developmental delay, or musculoskeletal complications are to (1) promote posture and movement appropriate to gestational age and medical stability; (2) support symmetry and biomechanical alignment of extremities, neck, and trunk while multiple infusion lines and respiratory equipment are required; (3) decrease potential skull and extremity musculoskeletal deformities and acquired joint-muscle contractures; (4) foster infant-parent attachment and interaction; (5) modulate sensory stimulation in the infant's NICU environment to promote behavioral organization and physiological stability; (6) provide consultation or direct intervention for neonatal feeding dysfunction and oral-motor deficits; (7) enhance parents' caregiving skills (feeding, dressing, bathing, positioning of infant for sleep, interaction and play, and transportation); and (8) prepare for hospital discharge and integration into home and community environments.

Educational Requirements for Therapists

Examination of and intervention for neonates are advanced-level, not entry-level, clinical competencies. Neonatology is a recognized subspecialty within the specialty areas of pediatric physical therapy[70] and pediatric occupational therapy.[71] No amount of literature review, self-study, or experience with other pediatric populations can substitute for competency-based, clinical training with a preceptor in an NICU. The potential for causing harm to medically fragile infants during well intentioned intervention is enormous.[72-74] The ongoing clinical decisions made by neonatal therapists in evaluating and managing physiological and musculoskeletal risks while handling small (2 or 3 lb), potentially unstable infants in the NICU should not be a trial-and-error experience at the infant's expense. Therapists with adult-oriented training and even those with general pediatric clinical training (excluding neonatal) are not qualified for neonatal practice without a supervised clinical practicum (2 to 6 months). The NICU is not an appropriate practice area for physical therapy assistants, occupational therapy assistants, or student therapists on affiliations for reasons outlined by Sweeney and colleagues[8]: "handling of vulnerable infants in the NICU requires ongoing examination, interpretation, and multiple adjustments of procedures, interventions, and sequences to minimize risk for infants who are physiologically, behaviorally, and motorically unstable or potentially unstable." The physical or occupational therapy assistant and student therapist are not prepared, even with supervision, to "provide moment-to-moment examination and evaluation of the infant and have the ability to modify or stop preplanned interventions when the infant's behavior, motor, or physiological organization begins to move outside the limits of stability with handling or feeding."[8] Appropriate nonhandling experiences for physical therapist or occupational therapist students in the NICU are delineated by Rapport and colleagues,[75] with a wide range of observational learning experiences with a preceptor recommended in this specialized practice environment. Refer to Box 11-1 for appropriate nonhandling experiences for entry-level students.

Delineation of advanced-level roles, competencies, and knowledge for the physical therapist[75-77] and the occupational therapist[71] in the NICU setting have been described separately by national task forces from the American Physical Therapy Association and the American Occupational Therapy Association. These practice guidelines provide a structure for assessing competence of individual therapists working in NICU settings and offer a framework for designing clinical paths for specific neonatal therapy services.

A gradual, sequential entry to neonatal practice is advised by building clinical experience with infants born at term gestation as well as with physiologically fragile older infants and children and their parents. The experience may include managing caseloads of hospitalized children on physiological monitoring equipment, external feeding lines, and supplemental oxygen or ventilators. Participating in discharge planning and in outpatient follow-up of high-risk neonates are other options for providing exposure to examination, intervention, and family issues when the infants and parents are more stable. This clinical experience and a competency-based, precepted practicum in the NICU offer the best preparation for appropriate, accountable, and ethical practice in neonatal therapy.[76-78] In-depth study of perinatal and neonatal medicine and related obstetrical, neonatal nursing, high-risk parenting, and neonatal therapy literature is recommended before pediatric therapy clinicians begin to participate on the intensive care nursery team.

BOX 11-1 ■ NEONATAL INTENSIVE CARE UNIT (NICU) OBSERVATIONAL EXPERIENCES FOR ENTRY-LEVEL STUDENTS[75]

- Reviewing neonatal literature and neonatal therapy clinical practice guidelines[71,75-77] before site visit to NICU
- "Shadowing" neonatal nurses to observe:
  - Neonatal equipment (refer to Table 11-6)
  - Caregiving routines
  - Teaching styles with parents and grandparents
  - Feeding procedures and equipment
  - Unique culture of the NICU compared with adult intensive care units
  - Skin-to-skin holding by parent
  - Environmental adaptations (light, sound, clustered handling)
- "Shadowing" neonatal therapist to observe:
  - Chart reviews
  - Interdisciplinary rounds
  - Discharge planning conferences
  - Behavioral and physiological baseline examinations
  - Examination and intervention procedures adapted for medically stable infants at varying gestational ages, acuity levels, and behavioral organization
  - Parental teaching
  - Collaboration with neonatal nurses for positioning, feeding, and parent instruction
- Observing and participating with neonatal therapist in NICU Follow-up Clinic

Indications for Referral

Research efforts in recent years have been directed toward determining which neonates will have adverse neurodevelopmental outcomes. Specific prenatal, perinatal, and neonatal conditions associated with an increased likelihood of long-term neuromotor disability have been identified as risk factors. However, the predictive value of these risk factors is compromised by the absence of uniform or consistent definitions, differences in the study samples and follow-up procedures, and lack of standard measures of neurodevelopmental outcome. In addition, ongoing changes in obstetrical and neonatal procedures limit the applicability of findings from longitudinal studies of infants born in earlier eras of NICU care.

Tjossem's[79] categories of biological, established, and social risk combined with risk factors for adverse neurodevelopmental outcome[80] provide a framework for categorizing indicators for neonatal therapy referral. An overview of developmental risk categories and risk factors for neonatal therapy referral is listed in Box 11-2 to assist clinicians in developing a referral mechanism for a clinical protocol based on risk categories.

Biological Risk

Biological risk refers to neurodevelopmental risk attributable to medical or physiological conditions in the prenatal, perinatal, or neonatal period.[79-81] Biological risks include placental abnormalities, labor and delivery complications, prenatal infection, and teratogenic factors. Examples of biological risk factors include asphyxia, neonatal seizures, prenatal exposure to drugs or alcohol, and the brain lesions previously described. Birth weight is a strong predictor of outcome; in general, lower birth weight is associated with greater risk of adverse developmental outcomes.[82,83]

Respiratory disease is generally considered an important risk factor for motor and cognitive disability in infants born preterm (Table 11-5).[84] Although the presence of respiratory disease alone does not appear to be predictive of neurodevelopmental outcome, severity of disease does appear to be related to long-term outcome.[82] Infants with chronic lung disease or bronchopulmonary dysplasia have been found to be at increased risk for CP and other neurodevelopmental abnormalities compared with preterm infants without bronchopulmonary dysplasia.[85,86] Prolonged mechanical ventilation and duration of supplemental oxygen were associated with increased risk of neurodevelopmental disability.[87] Administration of surfactant in the neonatal period has

BOX 11-2 ■ DEVELOPMENTAL RISK INDICATORS FOR NEONATAL THERAPY REFERRAL

BIOLOGICAL RISK

- Birth weight of 1500 g or less
- Gestational age of 32 weeks or less
- Small for gestational age (less than 10th percentile for weight)
- Prenatal exposure to drugs or alcohol
- Ventilator requirement for 36 hours or more
- Intracranial hemorrhage: grades 3 or 4
- Periventricular leukomalacia
- Muscle tone abnormalities (hypotonia, hypertonia, asymmetry of tone or movement)
- Recurrent neonatal seizures (three or more)
- Feeding dysfunction
- Symptomatic TORCH infections (*to*xoplasmosis, *r*ubella, *c*ytomegalovirus infection, *h*erpesvirus type 2 infection)
- Meningitis
- Asphyxia with Apgar score less than 4 at 5 minutes
- Multiple birth

ESTABLISHED RISK

- Hydrocephalus
- Microcephaly
- Chromosomal abnormalities
- Musculoskeletal abnormalities (congenitally dislocated hips, limb deficiencies, arthrogryposis, joint contractures, congenital torticollis)
- Brachial plexus injuries (Erb palsy, Klumpke paralysis)
- Myelodysplasia
- Congenital myopathies and myotonic dystrophy
- Inborn errors of metabolism
- Human immunodeficiency virus infection
- Down syndrome

ENVIRONMENTAL AND SOCIAL RISK

- High social risk (single parent, parental age younger than 17 years, poor-quality infant-parent attachment)
- Maternal drug or alcohol abuse
- Behavioral state abnormalities (lethargy, excessive irritability, behavioral state lability)

reduced the incidence and severity of respiratory disease in very low–birth-weight infants but has not been associated with a decline in neurodevelopmental disability.[85]

Established Risk

Established risk is the risk for neurodevelopmental deficits associated with a diagnosis that is clearly established in the neonatal period. Included in this category are congenital malformations, chromosomal abnormalities, central nervous system disorders, and metabolic diseases with known developmental sequelae.

Environmental and Social Risk

Environmental and social risk involves developmental risk related to competency in parenting roles and factors in family dynamics. Such risk may be heightened by prolonged hospitalization of infants with the following characteristics: (1) suboptimal levels of stimulation and interaction (overstimulation or deprivation) in the NICU environment, (2) inadequate infant-parent attachment, (3) insufficient educational preparation of parents for caregiving roles, (4) meager financial resources of parents, and (5) limited or absent family support to assist in taking care of and nurturing the infant in the home environment.

It is common for neonates born preterm to have a combination of risk factors from more than one major category. For example, an infant born prematurely to a single mother in a drug treatment program for heroin use during pregnancy is considered to be at both biological and environmental risk.

Pain, Gestational Age, and Neurological Examination

Multiple neonatal neurological and neurobehavioral examinations have been developed to assess the integrity and maturation of the nervous system[88-91] and to describe newborn behavior.[9,89] Most of these tests offer information on the quality of motor performance, attention, and interaction. Because these assessments are based on gestational age, an accurate calculation of gestational age is necessary at the time of the testing.[92,93]

TABLE 11-5 ■ FACTORS CONTRIBUTING TO PULMONARY DYSFUNCTION IN PRETERM NEONATES

Anatomical	Capillary beds not well developed before 26 weeks of gestation
	Type II alveolar cells and surfactant production not mature until 35 weeks of gestation
	Elastic properties of lung not well developed
	Lung space decreased by relative size of the heart and abdominal distention
	Type I, high-oxidative fibers compose only 10% to 20% of diaphragm muscle
	Highly vascular subependymal germinal matrix not resorbed until 35 weeks of gestation, increasing infant's vulnerability to hemorrhage
	Lack of fatty insulation and high surface area/body weight ratio
Physiological	Increased pulmonary vascular resistance leading to right-to-left shunting
	Decreased lung compliance
	Diaphragmatic fatigue; respiratory failure
	Decreased or absent cough and gag reflexes; apnea
	Hypothermia and increased oxygen consumption

Modified from Crane L: Physical therapy for the neonate with respiratory disease. In Irwin S, Tecklin JS, editors: *Cardiopulmonary physical therapy,* ed 2, St Louis, 1990, Mosby.

Pain Assessment

Despite immature myelinization, premature infants *definitely* perceive pain and retain the memory of painful experiences. Skin receptors are developed by 14 to 16 weeks' gestation. In addition, the density of pain receptors in the skin of neonates at 28 weeks of gestation is considered similar to and even exceeds adult density during maturation from birth to 2 years of age.[94-96] Blackburn[97] explained that although pain transmission in neonates occurs mainly through the slower, unmyelinated C fibers, the shorter distance in neonates that impulses travel to reach the brain compensates for the slower rate of transmission and creates substantial pain reception. Early pain experiences may create later increased sensitivity to pain and vulnerability to stress disorders.[98-100] If neonatal therapy assessment or intervention procedures immediately follow a noxious procedure in the NICU, handling techniques may need to be modified or therapy session rescheduled to avoid contributing to a cascade of aversive experiences for the infant.

Psychometric data and clinical use of the pain tools are described for infants as early as 28 weeks of gestation. Many elements in the pain assessments[101] have been identified by Als (the Neonatal Individualized Developmental Care and Assessment Program [NIDCAP]) as signs of excessive stimulation and stress in the preterm infant. Specific extremity movements, such as hand to face, elevated leg extension, salute, lateral extension of arms, finger splay, and fisting, have been proposed as indicators of stress and/or pain.[102]

In addition to practice guidelines on pain assessment developed primarily by neonatal nurses, numerous instruments are available to assess pain in infants. Pain scale data are integrated into NICU nursing assessments and can be a valuable adjunct to the neonatal therapist's baseline and posttherapy observations.

- The Premature Infant Pain Profile (PIPP)[103] assigns points for changes in three facial expressions (brow bulge, eye squeeze, and nasolabial fold), heart rate, and oxygen saturation. Gestational age and pre-procedural behavioral state are included in the assessment. The maximal PIPP score is 21; the higher the score, the greater the pain. A score of 0 to 6 points indicates minimal or no pain, whereas a score of 12 or more indicates moderate to severe pain.[103]
- The Face, Legs, Activity, Cry, and Consolability Behavioral tool (FLACC) uses grades of 0 to 2 for facial expression, leg activity, general activity, cry nature, and ability to be consoled and has been used in pediatric and adult settings. This test is capable of assessing pain in normal as well as cognitively impaired children, thus giving it a high degree of versatility and usefulness.[104] Change in FLACC score has been used to demonstrate that the use of sucrose and a pacifier during venipuncture is more effective in consoling infants younger than 3 months of age than infants older than 3 months of age.[105]
- The Neonatal Pain, Agitation, and Sedation Scale (N-PASS) uses five indicators: (1) cry and irritability, (2) behavioral state, (3) facial expression, (4) extremity movement and tone, and (5) vital signs. As with the PIPP scale, additional points are added for decreasing gestational age.[106] There was good correlation between the N-PASS and the PIPP assessments during routine heelstick in infants younger than 1 month old born at 23 to 42 weeks' gestation.[107]

Indicators of pain summarized across the instruments include the following categories: (1) physiological (heart rate, oxygen saturation, breathing pattern), (2) behavioral (eye squeeze, brow bulge, facial grimace, behavioral state including crying, sleeplessness), and (3) motor (tone and movement in extremities).

Clinical Assessment of Gestational Age in the Newborn Infant

A method for clinical assessment of gestational age in the newborn infant was developed by Dubowitz and colleagues[92] from data derived from a total of 167 preterm and term infants (28 to 42 weeks' gestation) tested within 5 days of birth. The tool focuses on criteria for calculation of gestational age from a composite of 10 neurological and 11 external (physical) characteristics.

This test rates criteria on a 4-point scale; it is commonly administered by nurses or physicians in the newborn nursery. The accuracy (95% confidence limit) of the gestational age score is determined within a variation of ±2 weeks on any single examination. This measurement error can be decreased to approximately ±1.4 weeks when two separate examinations are performed. From the analyses of multiple tests on 70 of the 167 infants, the age score was equally reliable in the first 24 hours of age as during the next 4 days of life. The behavioral state of the infant during the examination is not considered a significant variable in testing.

Calculation of gestational age is an important adjunct to all other neonatal assessment tools. It guides practitioners in interpreting neurological and behavioral findings relative to the expected performance of neonates at various gestational ages. Additional guidelines on gestational differences in neurological, physical, and neuromuscular maturation can be found in the work of French pediatric neurologist Amiel-Tison.[88,89,108]

Newborn Maturity Rating—Ballard Score

Ballard and colleagues[109-111] designed a simplified modification of the Dubowitz gestational age tool. It has been widely adopted because of the time efficiency (3 to 4 minutes versus 10 to 15 minutes) and the elimination of active tone items, which are difficult to evaluate reliably in physiologically unstable newborns. The Ballard instrument involves only six physical and six neurological criteria, with a 0 to 5 scale and a maturity rating. It is designed to be used for neonates (20 to 44 weeks gestation) from birth through 3 days of age and has demonstrated concurrent validity with the Dubowitz gestational age calculation tool. The gestational age of the infant is based on the obstetrical dating criteria unless the clinical assessment of the infant deviates more than 2 weeks from the obstetrical calculation.

Neurological Examination of the Full-Term Infant

The Neurological Examination of the Full-Term Infant was designed by Prechtl[112] to identify abnormal neurological signs in the newborn period. The examination was developed from an investigation of more than 1350 newborns and was standardized on infants born at the gestational age of 38 to 42 weeks. If the test is used in premature infants who

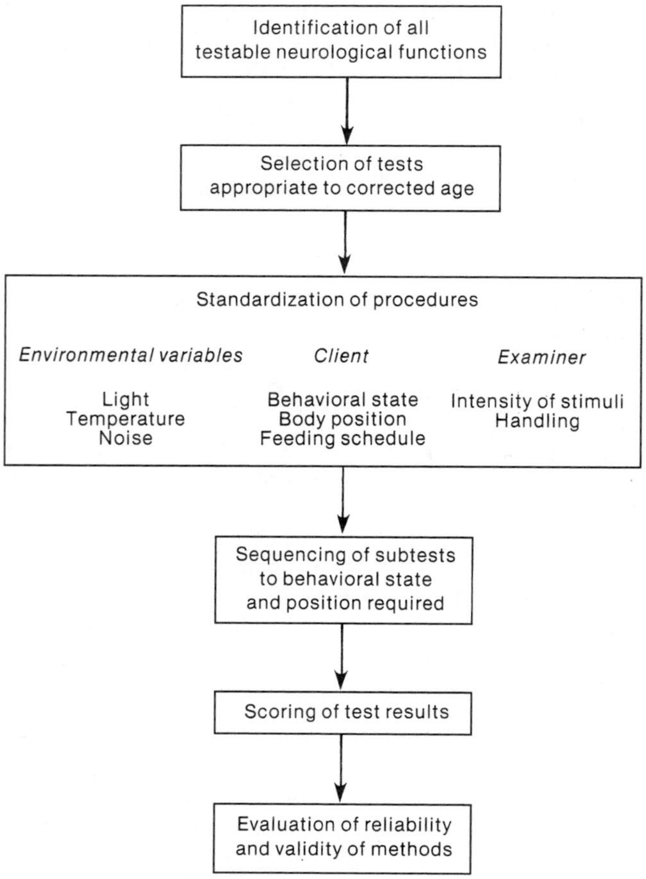

Figure 11-9 ■ Flow diagram illustrating decision steps in the neurological examination process.

have reached an age of 38 to 42 weeks of gestation, lower resistance to passive movements (lower tone) may be expected. Delay of testing until a minimum of 3 days of age is advised to maximize the stability of behavioral states and neuromotor responses for improved reliability and validity of results.

The pattern of examination includes periods of both observation and examination. A 10-minute screening test is offered to determine if the full 30-minute examination of posture, tone, reflexes, and spontaneous movement is required. Although specific requirements for examiner training are not addressed, Prechtl offers a flow diagram (Figure 11-9) to assist clinicians with organizing the neurological examination process. Significant findings from the examination are summarized in the following categories: (1) quality of posture, spontaneous movement, and muscle tone (consistency and resistance to passive movement); (2) presence of involuntary or pathological movements (clonus, tremor, athetoid postures or movements); (3) behavioral state changes and quality of cry; and (4) threshold or intensity of responses to stimulation. (Because of the transient pattern of neurological signs and rapid changes in the developing nervous system, Prechtl advised repeated examinations to monitor neurological status.)

Neonatal Behavioral Assessment Scale

To document individual behavioral and motor differences in infants at term gestation to 2 months of age, Brazelton and Nugent[113] developed a neonatal behavior scale to assess neuromotor responses within a behavioral state context. The 30- to 45-minute examination consists of observing, eliciting, and scoring 28 biobehavioral items on a 9-point scale and 18 reflex items on a 4-point scale. This is an interactive test and assesses the infant's ability to recover from stimuli and return to an alert state. The reflex items are derived from the neurological examination protocol of Prechtl and Beintema.[114]

The scale was designed to assess newborn behavior in healthy 3-day-old term (40 weeks of gestation) white infants whose mothers had minimal sedative medication during an uncomplicated labor and delivery. Use of this examination with infants born preterm requires modification of the examination procedure to the environmental constraints of an intensive care nursery and interpretation of findings relative to the gestational age and medical condition of the infant. For preterm infants approaching term gestation (minimum of 36 weeks of gestation), nine supplementary behavioral items are offered. Many of these items were developed by Als[9] for use with preterm and physiologically stressed infants (see discussion of the APIB, later). In the manual,[113] methods of adapting the Neonatal Behavioral Assessment Scale (NBAS) for preterm neonates with accompanying case scenarios are described to illustrate use of the findings to enhance parent-infant interaction and guide developmental interventions.

Six behavioral state categories are outlined in the NBAS: deep sleep, light sleep, drowsiness or semidozing, quiet alert, active alert, and crying. Behavioral state prerequisites are provided for each biobehavioral and reflex item to reduce the state-related variables in testing. During the assessment the examiner systematically maneuvers the infant from the sleep states to crying and back to the alert states to evaluate physiological, organizational, motor, and interactive capabilities during stimulation and physical handling. The scoring is based on the infant's best performance, with flexibility allowed in the order of testing, repetition of items encouraged, and scheduling of the assessment midway between feedings to give the infant every advantage to demonstrate the best possible responses.

Four dimensions of newborn behavior are analyzed in Brazelton's NBAS: interactive ability, motor behavior, behavioral state organization, and physiological organization. *Interactive ability* describes the infant's response to visual and auditory stimuli, consolability from the crying state with intervention by the examiner, and ability to maintain alertness and respond to social or environmental stimuli.

Motor behavior refers to the ability to modulate muscle tone and motor control for the performance of integrated motor skills, such as the hand-to-mouth maneuver, pull-to-sit maneuver, and defensive reaction (e.g., removal of cloth from face). In the assessment of *behavioral state organization,* the infant's ability to organize behavioral states when stimulated and the ability to shut out irritating environmental stimuli when sleeping are analyzed. *Physiological organization* is evaluated by observing the infant's ability to manage physiological stress (changes of skin color, frequency of tremulous movement in the chin and extremities, number of startle reactions during the assessment). For analysis, the information is divided into seven clusters: habituation, orientation, motor, range of state, regulation of state, autonomic stability, and reflexes. The cluster systems are highly useful for clinical interpretation and for data analysis in clinical research. Performance profiles of worrisome or deficient interactive-motor and organizational behavior are identified by clusters of behavior associated with potential developmental risk.[115]

Definite strengths of the NBAS are the well-defined indicators of autonomic stress, analysis of coping abilities of high-risk infants experiencing external stimuli and handling, and quality of infant-examiner interaction. These features generate specific findings to assist therapists in grading the intensity of assessment and treatment within each infant's physiological and behavioral tolerance and in guiding the development of parental teaching strategies to address the individual behavioral styles of infants. The NBAS has proved to be more sensitive to the detection of mild neurological dysfunction in the newborn period than have classic neurological examinations that omit the behavioral dimensions. This assessment is not predictive but gives a good analysis of the infant's strengths and weaknesses. Improved performance from repeat examinations over time is a better predictor of the infant's ability and potential.

Participation of the parent in the newborn assessment may yield long-term positive effects on infant-parent interaction and later on cognitive and fine motor development. Widmayer and Field[116]reported significantly better face-to-face interaction and fine motor-adaptive skills at 4 months of age and higher mental development scores at 12 months of age when teenage mothers of preterm infants (mean gestational age at birth, 35.1 weeks) were given demonstrations of the NBAS. These demonstrations were scheduled when the premature infants had reached an age equivalence of 37 weeks of gestation.

Nugent[117,118]developed parental teaching guidelines for using the NBAS as an intervention for infants and their families. Published by the March of Dimes birth defects foundation, the guidelines offer strategies for interpreting each item according to its adaptive and developmental significance, descriptions of the expected developmental course of the behavior (item) over several months, and recommendations for caregiving according to the infant's response to the items.

A three-step examiner training involving self-study, practice, and certification phases is coordinated through the Brazelton Institute, Children's Hospital, Boston, Massachusetts.[119,120] Wilhelm[115] recommended NBAS training for clinicians beginning to develop competence in examining at-risk infants. She explained that it provides a system for developing basic handling skills with healthy, term infants without concerns of stressing medically fragile preterm infants during the training period. Learning the NBAS in term infants before entering NICU practice provides familiarity with similar testing and scoring procedures for preterm infants.[115]

Newborn Behavioral Observations System

The Newborn Behavioral Observations (NBO) system, developed from the pioneering work and philosophy of Brazelton, is an interactive, observational tool for use with infants and parents in hospital, clinic, and home settings.[121] The focus is on prematurely born infants and at-risk infants, with emphasis on cultural competence, family-centered care, and infant development. The NBO system helps determine the behavioral profile of the infant and allows the practitioner to provide parents with individualized and unique information about their infant. This behavioral information promotes positive parent-infant interaction and also a positive partnership between parents and practitioners.

Certification in administering, interpreting, and scoring the 18-item NBO assessment is arranged through the Brazelton Institute in a 2-consecutive-day format. The training encompasses the following observation categories: (1) habituation to external light and sound; (2) muscle tone and motor activity level; (3) behavioral self-regulation (crying and consolability); and (4) visual, auditory, and social-interactive abilities.[119,120]

Neurological Assessment of the Preterm and Full-Term Newborn Infant

The Neurological Assessment of the Preterm and Full-Term Newborn Infant is a streamlined neurological and neurobehavioral assessment designed by Dubowitz and colleagues[122] to provide both a systematic, quickly administered newborn examination applicable to infants born preterm or at term gestation and a longer infant examination for children to 24 months of age. A distinct advantage of this tool is the minimal training or experience required by the examiner and the ease of adapting it to the infant and the environment. The adaptability of the test and use of the scoring form with stick figure diagrams have made it useful for implementation in developing countries where English is not widely spoken.

The test includes the six behavioral state categories of the NBAS and seven orientation and behavior items scored on a 5-point grading scale and sequenced according to the intensity of response. The orientation and behavior items consist of the following categories: (1) auditory and visual orientation responses; (2) quality and duration of alertness; (3) irritability (the frequency of crying to aversive stimuli during reflex testing and handling throughout the examination); (4) consolability (the ability after crying to reach a calm state independently or with intervention by the examiner); (5) cry (quality and pitch variations); and (6) eye appearance (absent, transient, or persistent appearance of sunset sign, strabismus, nystagmus, or roving eye movements).

The 15 items that assess movement and tone and the six reflex items evolved from clinical trials on 50 term infants using the clinical assessment of gestational age by Dubowitz and colleagues,[92] the neurological examination of the newborn by Parmelee and Michaelis,[123] and the neurological examination of the full-term newborn infant by Prechtl.[112] The examination format was then used during a 2-year period on more than 500 infants of varying gestational ages. After 15 years the authors revised the assessment in the second edition by eliminating seven items, expanding the tone pattern section, and developing an optimality score. Reliability data are not reported, but modification of examination procedures occurred during the pilot phase that promoted objectivity in scoring and a high interrater reliability among examiners, regardless of experience level.

The examination protocol is available in two formats: (1) Hammersmith Short Neonatal Neurological Examination and (2) Hammersmith Infant Neurological Examination (age range, 2 to 24 months). The examination forms are illustrated with stick figures and can accommodate both baseline and repeat assessments. For neonatal therapy examinations the forms can be effectively combined with a narrative impression, treatment goals, and plan of care. A numerical score for each item and a summary score are provided in the revised edition of the test. The authors advised that the scoring system was primarily intended for the purpose of research and for numerical charting of progress with sequential examinations. Because of the continued clinical emphasis on patterns of responses, selected parts of the protocol (without summary scoring) are appropriate for examining premature or acutely ill infants on ventilators, in incubators, or attached to monitoring or infusion equipment. Scheduling of examinations is recommended two thirds of the way between infant feeding sessions.

Evolution of neurological patterns in infants with IVH, PVL, and HIE is described in the test manual and correlated with brain imaging. Abnormal neonatal clinical signs associated with long-term neurological sequelae were persistent asymmetry, decreased lower-extremity movement, and increased tone. Infants with IVH had significantly higher incidence of abnormally tight popliteal angles, reduced mobility, decreased visual fixing and following, and roving eye movements. The authors cautioned that early signs of motor asymmetry in neonates with cerebral infarction may be associated with normal outcome, but normal neonatal neurological examinations after cerebral infarction do not exclude the possibility of later hemiplegia.[124]

Long-term follow-up data beyond 1 year have not been reported with this examination. Dubowitz and colleagues[125] reassessed 116 infants (27 to 34 weeks of gestation) at 1 year of age. Of 62 infants assessed as neurologically normal in the newborn period, 91% were also normal at 1 year of age. Of 39 infants assessed as neurologically abnormal in the newborn period, 35% were found to be normal at 1 year of age. According to Wilhelm,[115] the predictive value of a negative test result with this instrument was 92%, but the predictive value of a positive test result was only 64%.

Interpretations of evaluative findings from the Neurological Assessment for Preterm and Full-Term Newborn Infants for neonatal therapy practice are comprehensively described in a case study format by Heriza[126] and Campbell.[127] Dubowitz[128] discussed the clinical significance of neurological variations in infants and offered decision guidelines to clinicians on when to worry, reassure, or intervene with developmental referrals.

Assessment of Preterm Infants' Behavior

Als[9] designed the APIB to structure a comprehensive observation of a preterm infant's autonomic, adaptive, and interactive responses to graded handling and environmental stimuli. It involves six maneuvers with increasing challenging and complex interactions with a highly structured format. As previously described in the theoretical framework section of this chapter, this assessment is derived from synactive theory and is focused on assessing the organization and balance of the infant's physiological, motor, behavioral state, attention and interaction, and self-regulation subsystems. The APIB has testing sequences and a scoring format similar to those used in Brazelton's NBAS, with increased complexity and expansion for premature infants.

Administration and scoring of the APIB may require 2 to 3 hours per infant and often two or more sessions with the infant depending on examiner experience and infant stability. Although the APIB may be an instrument of choice for the clinical researcher, it is not usually practical (time efficient) for many neonatal clinicians with heavy caseloads in managed-care environments. Extensive training and reliability certification are required to safely administer and accurately score and interpret the test for clinical practice or research.

Neonatal Individualized Developmental Care and Assessment Program

Als[11] and Als and colleagues[11,129] developed NIDCAP to document the effects of the caregiving environment on the neurobehavioral stability of neonates. This naturalistic observation protocol includes continuous observation and documentation at 2-minute intervals of an infant's behavioral state and autonomic, motor, and attention signals, with simultaneous recording of vital signs and oxygen saturation. Documentation occurs before, during, and after routine caregiving procedures. The infant's strengths, weaknesses, and coping skills are identified. A narrative description of the infant's responses to the stress of handling by the primary nurse and to auditory and visual stimuli in the NICU environment is provided to assist caregivers and parents in identifying the infant's behavioral cues and providing appropriate interaction. Options are described in the care plans for reducing aversive environmental stimuli and modifying physical handling procedures. This clinical tool allows neonatal therapists to determine the infant's readiness for assessment and intervention by observing the baseline tolerance of the infant to routine nursing care before superimposing neonatal therapy procedures.[130] Sequential observations occur weekly or biweekly. Parental involvement is strongly encouraged and instrumental in facilitating a smooth transition to home. Examiner training in the NIDCAP may be coordinated through the National Training Center at Children's Hospital Boston, Massachusetts, where priority is now given to training NICU teams rather than individuals.[10]

NICU Network Neurobehavioral Scale

Lester and Tronick[131] developed a tool for preterm and drug-exposed infants from 30 weeks of gestation to 6 weeks post-term. The test includes items from the NBAS, APIB, Finnegan abstinence scale, and other neurological assessments and consists of 115 items in general categories of neurological and neuromotor integrity (tone, reflexes, and posture), behavioral state and interaction (self-regulatory competence), and physiological stress abstinence signs (drug-exposed infants). This test is state dependent and gives a comprehensive and integrated picture of the infant that is not divided into clusters. More than half[118] of the test items are infant observations, and 45 items require physical handling of the infant. Test-retest reliability of preterm infants indicated correlations of 0.30 to 0.44 at 34, 40, and 44 weeks of gestation. This test is useful for management of drug-exposed infants but may have limited predictive value. Training and certification in administration and scoring of the test are coordinated through Brookes Publishing Company and available in the United States and internationally with use of videoconferencing for lectures and demonstrations.

Test of Infant Motor Performance

Developed by Campbell and colleagues,[132] the 42-item Test of Infant Motor Performance (TIMP) is focused on evaluating postural control, spontaneous movement, and head control for neonates at 32 weeks of gestation to 16 weeks postterm. Functional motor performance is assessed through observation of infant movement and through responses to various body positions and to visual or auditory stimuli. Psychometric qualities of the test include (1) construct validity[133] and ecological validity,[134] (2) concurrent validity at 3 months of age with the Alberta Infant Motor Scale (AIMS),[135] and (3) predictive validity at 5 to 6 years of age with the Bruininks-Oseretsky Test of Motor Proficiency[136] and at 4 to 5 years of age with the Peabody Developmental Motor Scales and Home Observation for Measurement of the Environment: Early Childhood.[137] Training on test procedures is available through 2-day workshops or through a self-guided training method with a CD-ROM from the test developer.[138]

Neurobehavioral Assessment of the Preterm Infant

The Neurobehavioral Assessment of the Preterm Infant (NAPI) was developed by Korner as a developmental test to assess medically stable infants from 32 weeks to term gestation using a sequence of specific movements. This test focuses on tone, reflexes, movement, response to visual and auditory stimulation, and observation of cry and state. This tool does not require a specific preassessment state as is required by the previously mentioned tests, but starts with the infant asleep. It does not take as long to administer (less than ½ hour) than the previously described tests and is easy to analyze. The data are categorized into seven clusters and compared with standardized scores. With repeated examinations over time, persistent deviations from the normative scores indicate that the infant is at risk for developmental delays and is in need of close follow-up. In addition, the NAPI has been shown to be predictive of short-term and long-term neurodevelopmental outcomes.[139]

Qualitative Assessment of General Movements

The assessment tools reviewed so far in this chapter require direct handling of the infant. Infants born preterm are particularly vulnerable to developing physiological stress during the maneuvers required by most tools available for infant assessment. Instead, noninvasive, repeated longitudinal observation and assessment are needed to accommodate the concurrent motor variability, immature nervous system, and physiological vulnerability of the young, preterm infant.[140] Based on the pioneering work of Prechtl examining the continuity of prenatal to postnatal fetal movement,[141] this criterion-referenced test focuses on evaluating the quality of spontaneously generated movements in preterm, term, and young infants until 16 weeks postterm. A wide repertoire of endogenously generated spontaneous motility in the fetus including isolated limb movements, stretches, hiccups, yawning, and breathing movements can be identified as early as 9 weeks.[141-143]

General movements (GMs) are spontaneously generated complex movements involving the trunk, limbs, and neck. They vary in speed and intensity with a gradual onset, increase in speed and intensity, and a gradual end. These movements are among the number of movement patterns that emerge during fetal life and continue until approximately 16 weeks postterm, when goal-oriented and voluntary movements appear.[144] The quality of movement is assessed through observation and scoring of videotaped spontaneous movement of an infant in supine position without stimulation or handling.[144] A distinct difference occurs between the GMs in the preterm infant and those in the term and postterm infant. GMs in the term infant, and for the first 8 weeks, change in amplitude and speed, taking on a writhing quality. The writhing movements gradually give way to the fidgety movements, which are present in awake infants between 9 and 16 to 20 weeks postterm. Fidgety movements are small, circular movements of small amplitude and varying speed involving the neck, trunk, and extremities.[140] Other approaches to neurological assessment can be found in additional references.[140,144,145]

This neonatal and young infant assessment instrument has gained substantial attention in the past 20 years for its high reliability, sensitivity, and predictive validity. In a comprehensive review of the psychometric qualities of neuromotor assessments for infants, the GM assessment was rated among the tools with the highest reliability, averaging interrater and intrarater correlation coefficient, or *k*, greater than 0.85.[146] Multiple studies have corroborated the predictive validity and sensitivity of this method. The sensitivity is lower during the preterm period and during the writhing movements, improving during the fidgety movement period. Sensitivity as high as 95% has been reported.[140,147]

Testing Variables

Neuromuscular and behavioral findings in the newborn period may be influenced by several variables. Increased reliability in examination results and in clinical impressions may occur when these variables are recognized. Medication may produce side effects of low muscle tone, drowsiness, and lethargy. Such medications include anticonvulsants, sedatives for diagnostic procedures (CT scan, electroencephalography, electromyography), and medication for postsurgical pain management. Intermittent subtle seizures may produce changes in muscle tension and in the level of responsiveness. Mild, ongoing seizures may occur in the neonate as lip smacking or sucking, staring or horizontal gaze, apnea, and bradycardia. Stiffening of the extremities occurs in neonatal seizures more frequently than clonic movement. Fatigue from medical and nursing procedures can result in decreased tolerance to handling, decreased interaction, and magnified muscle tone abnormalities. Fatigue may also result when neurodevelopmental assessment is scheduled immediately after laboratory (hematologic) procedures, suctioning, ultrasonography, or respiratory (chest percussion) therapy. Tremulous movement in the extremities may be linked to conditions of metabolic imbalance (hypomagnesemia, hypocalcemia, hypoglycemia), and low muscle tone may be associated with hyperbilirubinemia, hypoglycemia, hypoxemia, and hypothermia.[148,149]

Summary

Practitioners must be aware of the normative and validation data and of the predictive characteristics of the test(s) administered to allow appropriate interpretation of the results. Specific clinical training with a preceptor is essential to administer, score, and interpret neonatal assessment instruments accurately; to establish interrater reliability; and to plan treatment based on the evaluative findings. Even low-risk, healthy preterm infants are vulnerable to becoming physiologically and behaviorally destabilized during neurological assessment procedures.[150-152] This risk is reduced with precepted, competency-based clinical training in the NICU.

Intervention Planning

Level of Stimulation

The issue of safe and therapeutic levels of sensory and neuromotor intervention is a high priority in the design of developmental intervention programs for infants who have been medically unstable. The concept of "infant stimulation," introduced by early childhood educators in the 1980s to describe general developmental stimulation programs for healthy infants, is highly inappropriate in an approach based on concepts of dynamic systems, infant behavioral organization, and individualized developmental care.

For intervention to be therapeutic in a special care nursery setting, the amount and type of touch and kinesthetic stimulation must be customized to each infant's physiological tolerance, movement patterns, unique temperament, and level of responsiveness. Rather than needing more stimulation, many infants, especially those with hypertonus or those with tremulous, disorganized movement, have difficulty adapting to the routine levels of noise, light, position changes, and handling in the nursery environment. General, nonindividualized stimulation can quickly magnify abnormal postural tone and movement, increase behavioral state lability and irritability, and stress fragile physiological homeostasis in preterm or chronically ill infants. Implementation of careful physiological monitoring and graded handling techniques are essential to prevent compromise in patient safety and to facilitate development. Infant modulation, rather than stimulation, is the aim of intervention. Techniques of sensory and neuromotor facilitation and inhibition developed for caseloads of healthy infants and children are inappropriate for the developmental needs and expectations of an infant with physiological fragility or premature birth history (less than 37 weeks of gestation).

Physiological and Musculoskeletal Risk Management

Many maturation-related anatomical and physiological factors predispose preterm infants to respiratory dysfunction (see Table 11-5). For this reason many preterm neonates require the use of a wide range of respiratory equipment and physiological monitors (Table 11-6). Pediatric therapists preparing to work in the NICU and those involved with designing risk management plans are referred to the neonatal nursing literature for evidence and perspectives on assessing and managing neonatal stressors during interventions in the NICU.[153-155] Because infants born prematurely or experiencing critical illness communicate via subtle behavioral cues, their understated language is "not easily interpreted unless caregivers understand how infants' ability to respond to stress reflects their maturation and neurodevelopment."[156] Their behavioral cues are considered more subtle and more likely to be disregarded than those of infants born at term gestation.

In this subspecialty area of pediatric practice, neonatal therapists are responsible for the prevention of physiological jeopardy in LBW infants while providing developmental services in the NICU. Before examination, discussion with the supervising neonatologist and clinical nurse are advised regarding specific precautions and the safe range of vital signs for each infant. Medical update and identification of new precautions before each intervention session are recommended because new events in the last few hours may not have been recorded or fully analyzed at the time therapy is scheduled. The nurse should be invited to maintain ongoing surveillance of the infant's medical stability and provide assistance in interpreting physiological and behavioral cues during neonatal therapy activities in case physiological complications occur. If medical complications develop during or after therapy, immediate, comprehensive co-documentation of the incident with the clinical nurse and discussion with the neonatology staff are essential to analyze the events, outline related clinical teaching issues, and minimize legal jeopardy.

Areas of particular concern during neonatal therapy activities include potential incidence of fracture, dislocation, or joint effusion during the management of limited joint motion; skin breakdown or vascular compromise during splinting or taping to reduce deformity; apnea or bradycardia during therapeutic neuromotor handling with potential deterioration to respiratory arrest; oxygen desaturation or regurgitation and aspiration during feeding assessment or oral-motor therapy; hypothermia from prolonged handling of the infant away from the neutral thermal environment of the incubator or overhead radiant warmer; and propagation of infection from inadequate compliance with infection control procedures in the nursery. Signs of overstimulation may include labored breathing with chest retractions, grunting, nostril flaring, color changes (skin mottling, paleness, gray-blue cyanotic appearance), frequent startles, irritability or drowsiness, sneezing, gaze aversion, bowel movement, and hiccups. Signals of overstimulation expressed through infants' motor systems are finger splay (extension and abduction posturing), arm salute (shoulder flexion with elbow extension), and trunk arching away from stimulation.[11] Harrison and colleagues[154] found that motor activity cues of preterm infants were correlated with low oxygen saturation and should be carefully monitored during caregiving procedures to minimize physiological instability.

Even a baseline neurological examination, usually presumed to be a benign clinical procedure, may be destabilizing to the newborn infant's cardiovascular and behavioral organization systems. The physiological and behavioral tolerance of low-risk preterm and term neonates to evaluative handling by a neonatal physical therapist was studied in 72 newborn subjects.[151] During and after administration of the Neurological Assessment of the Preterm and Full-Term Newborn Infant, preterm subjects (30 to 35 weeks of gestation) had significantly higher heart rates; greater increases in blood pressure; decreased peripheral oxygenation inferred from mottled skin color; and higher frequencies of finger splay, arm salute, hiccups, and yawns than in term subjects. Neonatal practitioners must examine the safety of even a neurological examination and weigh the risks and anticipated benefit of the procedure given the expected physiological and behavioral changes in low-risk, medically stable neonates.[150,151]

TABLE 11-6 ■ EQUIPMENT COMMONLY ENCOUNTERED IN THE NEONATAL INTENSIVE CARE UNIT (NICU)

EQUIPMENT	DESCRIPTION
Thermoregulation radiant warmer	Unit composed of mattress on an adjustable tabletop covered by a radiant heat source controlled manually and by servocontrol mode. Unit has adjustable side panels. *Advantage*: provides ready access to infant and increases area for equipment. *Disadvantage*: leads to convective heat loss, increases insensible fluid loss, and encourages stimulation (excessive).
Double-walled Isolette	Enclosed unit of transparent material providing a heated and humidified environment with a servocontrol incubator system of temperature monitoring. Access to infant through side portholes or opening side of unit. *Advantage*: barrier to tactile stimulation, decreased convective losses. *Disadvantage*: more difficult to get to infant, does not decrease noise from NICU, radiant heat loss if Isolette is single walled.
Thermal shield	Clear acrylic dome or plastic wrap placed over the trunk and legs of an infant in an Isolette to reduce radiant heat loss.
Respiratory assistance	
Conventional pressure	Delivers positive-pressure ventilation; pressure limited, with volume delivered dependent on the stiffness of the lung.
Volume ventilator	Delivers positive-pressure ventilation; volume limited, delivering same tidal volume with each breath, potentially decreasing barotraumas, as most use minimal pressure required to deliver a set tidal volume; common ventilator in use.
High frequency ventilator	Ventilator that delivers short bursts of air at high rates of flow (240-600 breaths/min).
Jet	Active inhalation with passive exhalation; requires conventional ventilator, noisy.
Oscillatory	Piston driven; active inhalation and exhalation.
Continuous positive airway pressure (CPAP) device	Nasal prongs of varying lengths provide CPAP and controlled oxygen delivery. Using *bubble* CPAP, positive pressure is adjusted by altering the depth of the expiratory tubing, which is under liquid. CPAP prongs can also be connected to a mechanical *ventilator* to deliver adjustable pressure and a breath rate if required.
Nasal cannula	Specific concentration of oxygen is delivered via soft nasal cannula, usually less than 1 L/min. *High-flow nasal cannula* delivers humidified oxygen at flows up to 6 L/min and a variable amount of distending pressure to help with alveolar inflation.
Oxyhood	Clear acrylic plastic hood fitting over the infant's head to provide an environment for delivering controlled oxygen and humidification delivery.
Monitors	
Cardiac, respiratory	One unit will display heart rate, respiratory rate, and blood pressure. High and low alarm limits can be set.
Oxygen saturation	Measures peripheral oxygen saturation and pulse from a light sensor secured to the infant's skin. Values can be displayed on the monitor.
Transcutaneous	Noninvasive method of monitoring partial pressure of O_2 and CO_2 from arterialized capillaries through the skin through the use of a heated sensor.
Cerebral oxygenation	Noninvasive method to measure regional oxygen saturation, usually cerebral and somatic, to ensure adequate oxygen delivery.
Amplitude-integrated electroencephalography (aEEG)	Continuous recording of cerebral electrical activity used to evaluate presence of seizures, baseline brain activity, and brain maturation.
Intravenous catheter	Used to deliver intravenous fluids, intralipids, and medications at a specific rate and to assist in obtaining blood for analysis. Specific catheters include arterial and venous umbilical lines, peripherally inserted central catheters (PICCs), surgically placed central catheter (Broviac, Cook), and peripheral intravenous catheter.
Extracorporeal membrane oxygenation (ECMO)	Heart-lung-kidney machine used for term infants with severe respiratory or cardiac failure.

High-Risk Profiles

Three general high-risk profiles are observed from a dynamic systems perspective. In these profiles movement abnormalities, related temperament or behavioral characteristics, and interactional styles associated with motor status are identified.

The first high-risk profile involves the irritable, hypertonic infant. These infants classically have a low tolerance level to handling and may frequently reach a state of overstimulation from routine nursing care, laboratory procedures, and the presence of respiratory and infusion equipment. They may express discomfort when given quick changes in body position by caregivers and when placed in any position for a prolonged time. Predominant extension patterns of posture and movement are associated with this category of infants. Quality of movement may appear tremulous or disorganized, with poor midline orientation and limited antigravity movement into flexion as a result of the imbalance of increased proximal extensor tone. Visual tracking and feeding may be difficult because of extension posturing or the presence of distracting, disorganized upper-extremity movement. In addition, increased tone with related decreased mobility in oral musculature may complicate feeding behavior. Hypertonic infants frequently demonstrate poor self-quieting abilities and may require consistent intervention by caregivers to tolerate movement and position changes. These temperament characteristics and the signs of neurological impairment previously discussed may place infants at considerable risk for child abuse or neglect as the stress and fatigue levels of parents rise and as coping strategies wear thin during the demanding care required by irritable, hypertonic infants.[7,157] Hypertonic, irritable infants constituted large percentages of neonatal therapy caseloads in the 1970s through the 1990s, but advances in neonatal pulmonary management have now decreased the numbers of infants matching this neurobehavioral profile.

Conversely, the lethargic, hypotonic infant excessively accommodates to the stimulation of the nursery environment and can be difficult to arouse to the awake states, even for feeding. The crying state is reached infrequently, even with vigorous stimulation. The cry is characteristically weak, with low volume and short duration, and related to hypotonic trunk, intercostal, and neck accessory musculature and decreased respiratory capacity. These infants are exceedingly comfortable in any position, and when held they easily mold themselves to the arms of the caregiver. Depression of normal neonatal movement patterns is common. To compensate for low muscle tone when in the supine position, some preterm infants appear to push into extension against the surface of the mattress in search of stability. Although potentially successful in generating a temporary increase in neck and trunk tone, the extension posturing from stabilizing against a surface in supine lying interferes with midline and antigravity movement of the extremities. Such infants dramatically respond to containment positioning in side-lying and prone positions. Drowsy behavior limits these infants' spontaneous approach to the environment and decreases their accessibility to selected interaction by caregivers. Feeding behavior is commonly marked by fatigue, difficulty remaining awake, weak sucking, and incoordination or inadequate rhythm in the suck-swallow process, with the need for supplementation of caloric intake by gavage (oral or nasogastric tube) feeding. The risk for sensory deprivation and failure to thrive is high for hypotonic infants because they infrequently seek interaction, place few if any demands on caregivers, and remain somnolent.

The third high-risk profile is the disorganized infant with fluctuating tone and movement who is easily overstimulated with routine handling but remains relatively passive when left alone. Disorganized infants usually respond well to swaddling or containment when handled. When calm, these infants frequently demonstrate high-quality social interaction and efficient feeding with coordinated suck-swallow sequence. When distracted and overstimulated, however, these infants appear hypertonic and irritable. Caregiving for intermittently hypertonic, disorganized, irritable infants can be frustrating for parents unskilled in reading the infant's cues, in implementing consolation and containment strategies, and in using pacing techniques during feeding. This profile of infant motor and behavioral disorganization represents a large proportion of infants in a typical neonatal therapy caseload.

Although these profiles address the extremes in motor and behavioral interaction, they suggest a need for identifying different tolerance levels of handling for neonates with abnormal tone and movement even though long-term developmental goals may be similar. Few neonates will demonstrate all behaviors described in the high-risk profile, but outpatient surveillance of neonates with worrisome or mildly abnormal motor and interactive behavior is advised to monitor the course of those behaviors and the developing styles of parenting.

Timing

The timing of neurodevelopmental examination and treatment for infants with high-risk histories or diagnoses is based on the medical stability of the infant and, in some centers, gestational age. All therapy activities need to be synchronized with the intensive care nursery schedule so that nursing care and medical procedures are not interrupted.

Neonatal therapists should not interrupt infants in a quiet, deep sleep state but instead wait approximately 15 minutes until the infant cycles into a light, active sleep or semiawake state. Higher peripheral oxygen saturation has been correlated with quiet rather than with active sleep in neonates. Preterm infants reportedly have a higher percentage of active sleep periods in contrast to the higher percentage of quiet sleep observed in term infants.[158] Allowing the preterm infant to maintain a deep, quiet sleep by not interrupting is a therapeutic strategy for enhancing physiological stability.

Timing of parental teaching sessions is most effective when readiness to participate in the care of the infant is expressed. Some parents need time and support to work through the acute grief process related to the birth of an imperfect child before participation in developmental activities is accepted. Other parents find the neonatal therapy program to be a way of contributing to the care of their infant that also helps them cope with overwhelming fears, stresses, and grief.

Treatment Strategies

This section addresses components of treatment for enhancing movement, minimizing contractures and deformity, promoting feeding behaviors appropriate to corrected age, developing social interaction behaviors, and fostering attachment to primary caregivers. Management approaches to body positioning, extremity taping, graded sensory and neuromotor intervention, neonatal hydrotherapy, and oral-motor and feeding therapy are presented; parental teaching is discussed here. Evidence-based practice recommendations for neonatal therapy are outlined in Table 11-7 and Box 11-3. In managing an intensive care unit caseload, the constant physiological monitoring; modification of techniques to adapt to the constraints of varying amounts of medical equipment; scheduling of interventions to coincide with visits of the parents and peak responsiveness of the infants; and ongoing coordination and reevaluation of goals, plans, and follow-up recommendations with the nursery staff create many interesting challenges and demand a high degree of adaptability and creativity from the

TABLE 11-7 ■ EVIDENCE-BASED RECOMMENDATIONS FOR NEONATAL PHYSICAL THERAPY

TYPE	RECOMMENDATIONS	LEVEL OF EVIDENCE	REFERENCES
Prevention	Collaborate with caregivers to reduce risk of skull deformity, torticollis, and extremity malalignment through diligent positioning for symmetry and neutral alignment	Level II Level II Level II	Van Vlimmeren et al, 2007[244] Vaivre-Douret et al, 2004[303] Monterosso et al, 2003[169]
Examination	Conduct baseline observation to determine physiological and behavioral stability (readiness) for evaluative handling	Level II	Sweeney, 1986[150]
	Provide continuous physiological and behavioral monitoring during and after evaluative handling to determine adaptation to evaluative handling and to signal the need for modification of pace and sequence, given expected physiological changes, particularly during neuromotor test procedures	Level II	Sweeney, 1989[151]
Intervention	Collaborate with caregivers to create a developmentally supportive environment with modulated stimulation from light, noise, and handling	Level I Level II Level I	Symington and Pinelli, 2006[304] Westrup et al, 2004[305] Peters et al, 2009[306]
	Support body position and extremity movement—(1) supine: semiflexed, midline alignment using blanket for swaddling containment or "nest" of positioning rolls; (2) prone: vertical roll under thorax; horizontal roll under hips	Level II Level II Level II Level II	Vaivre-Douret et al, 2004[303] Monterosso et al, 2003[169] Short et al, 1996[307] Ferrari et al, 2007[166]
	In selected neonates with movement impairment or disorganization consider therapeutic handling carefully graded in intensity and paced to facilitate head and trunk control, antigravity movement, and midline orientation	Level II	Girolami and Campbell, 1994[308]
	Consider gradual exposure to multimodal stimuli for stable neonates approaching hospital discharge	Level I	Symington and Pinelli, 2006[304]
	Provide opportunities for independent oral exploration through positioning with hands to face, and for nonnutritive sucking to improve state organization and readiness to feed	Level I	Pinelli and Symington, 2005[197]
	Determine readiness for and advancement of oral feeding trials using infant behavioral cues	Level II Level II	Kirk, Alder, and King, 2007[198] McGrath and Medoff-Cooper, 2002[309]
	Encourage parental involvement with feeding while providing interventions for physiological stability (pacing and slowed flow rate)	Level III Level II	Law-Morstatt et al, 2003[206] Chang et al, 2007[207]
	Consider hydrotherapy before feeding for stable infants with movement impairment	Level IV	Sweeney, 2003[191]
Education	Educate parents on behavioral cues and developmental status to mitigate parental stress and improve parental mental health outcomes	Level II Level I	Kaaresen et al, 2006[310] Melnyk et al, 2006[311]
	Implement multiple methods of instruction for parents and caregivers (demonstration, discussion, video, and written materials)	Level V	Dusing, Murray, and Stern, 2008[212]

From Sweeney JK, Heriza CB, Blanchard Y, Dusing SC: Neonatal physical therapy. Part II: Practice frameworks and evidence-based practice guidelines. *Ped Phys Ther* 22:2-16, 2010.

clinician. Willingness to change an established assessment plan, treatment strategy, or therapy schedule to meet the immediate needs of the infant, parents, or nursery staff is paramount. For some infants with prolonged periods of only borderline stability with handling, a discharge examination with recommendations for follow-up care may be the best practice. Productivity standards of billable hours used for other caseloads of stable pediatric or adult clients in the hospital are not appropriate for the NICU setting and necessitate negotiation and reinterpretation with rehabilitation or therapy department managers to protect both the infant and the neonatal therapist. Tolley[159] reported an expected mean productivity of 5.0 billable hours (range 4 to 6.5 hours) for hospital-based pediatric physical therapists among hospitals surveyed across 32 states and the District of Columbia.[93]

Positioning

A diligently administered positioning program can greatly assist infants on mechanical ventilators, receiving hood oxygen, or in incubators to simulate the flexed, midline postures of the neurologically intact term newborn swaddled in a bassinet. Preterm infants characteristically demonstrate low postural tone, with the amount of hypotonia varying with gestational age. Infants born prematurely do not have the neurological maturity or the prolonged positional advantage of the intrauterine environment to assist in the development of flexion. They are instead placed unexpectedly against gravity and presented with a dual challenge of compensating for maturation-related hypotonia and adapting to ventilatory and infusion equipment that frequently reinforces extension of the neck, trunk, and extremities.

BOX 11-3 ■ HIERARCHY OF EVIDENCE

LEVEL I
Randomized controlled trials (RCTs) or systematic reviews of RCTs

LEVEL II
Small RCTs, cohort studies, or systematic reviews of cohort studies

LEVEL III
Case-control studies or systematic reviews of case-control studies

LEVEL IV
Case series (no control group)

LEVEL V
Opinion of experts or authorities

Data from Oxford Centre for Evidence-Based Medicine, www.cebm.net, adapted with permission from Sweeney JK, Heriza CB, Blanchard Y, Dusing S: Neonatal physical therapy. Part II: practice frameworks and evidence-based guidelines. *Pediatr Phys Ther* 22:13, 2010.

Imbalance of excessive extension may occur in preterm infants with prolonged mechanical ventilation who appear to gain postural stability in the nonfluid extrauterine environment by leaning into or stabilizing against a firm mattress while in the supine position. De Groot[160] explained the postural behavior of preterm infants as an imbalance between low passive muscle tone and active muscle power. She theorized that because preterm neonates have prolonged periods of immobility (often in the supine position), exaggerated active muscle power may be observed in the extensor musculature, particularly in the trunk and hips. This imbalance of extension is viewed as nonoptimal muscle power regulation that may negatively influence postural stability, coordinated movement, and later hand and perceptual skills.[160]

Some neonates, especially those born at less than 30 weeks of gestation, may attempt to posturally stabilize by hyperextending the neck in supine or side-lying positions to compensate for maturation-related hypotonia.[161] Neck hyperextension posturing, without a balance of movement into flexion, may trigger later development of a host of related abnormal postural and mobility patterns to compensate for inadequate proximal stability.[160] In some infants, excessive postural stabilizing into neck hyperextension may contribute to sequential blocking of mobility in the shoulder, pelvis, and hip regions. The potential components of this high-risk, hypertonic postural profile appear in Box 11-4.

BOX 11-4 ■ POTENTIAL COMPONENTS OF HYPERTONIC POSTURAL PROFILE

Hyperextended neck
Elevated shoulders with adducted scapulae
Decreased midline arm movement (hand to mouth)
Excessively extended trunk
Immobile pelvis (anterior tilt)
Infrequent antigravity movement of legs
Weight bearing on toes in supported standing

Shaping of the musculoskeletal system occurs during each body position experienced by neonates in the NICU. A variety of positional deformities in the extremities and skull can result from inattention to alignment. In Table 11-8, common neonatal positional deformities, musculoskeletal consequences, and functional limitations are outlined. Supporting the skeletal integrity of infants born prematurely is challenging in the midst of numerous equipment obstacles, restricted physical handling because of physiological instability, and limited spontaneous movement. Infants with gastroesophageal reflux are frequently positioned on wedges that make symmetrical, midline postures difficult to maintain. Skull flattening may continue to evolve after NICU discharge from overuse of infant seats, reflux wedges, and limited prone play experiences. Plagiocephaly (asymmetrical occipital flattening) and a secondary torticollis may emerge when a strong head turn preference remains and parents do not vary the direction of head turn for sleeping and infant seat use.

Retracted shoulder posture (scapular adduction with shoulder elevation and external rotation) may accompany excessive neck and trunk extension posture in preterm infants. This abnormal posture can interfere with later reaching, shoulder stability in the prone position, and rolling during the first 18 months of life.[162,163] Excessive tibial torsion and out-toeing gait were reported in preterm infants at 3 to 8 years of age and traced to prolonged "frog leg" (excessive abduction and external rotation with foot eversion) in the NICU.[164,165]

Goals of neonatal positioning procedures include the following:

- Optimize alignment toward neutral neck-trunk position, semiflexed, midline extremity posture, and neutral foot position
- Support posture and alignment within "containment boundaries" of rolls, swaddling blanket, or other positioning aids; avoid creating a barrier to spontaneous movement, and allow space for controlled extremity movement
- Create positions that promote alert states for enhanced short-duration interaction and sleep states that promote comfort and physiological stability
- Offer positions that allow controlled, individualized exposure to proprioceptive, tactile, visual, or auditory stimuli while monitoring signs of behavioral and physiological stress from potential overstimulation

The use of blanket or cloth diaper rolls or customized foam inserts in a neonatal positioning program may modify increasing imbalance of extension in selected preterm or chronically ill infants and promote movement and postural stability from positions of flexion. After the infant is facilitated into a flexed posture in the side-lying position, posterior rolls behind the head, trunk, and thighs provide a surface against which the infant can posturally stabilize while a flexed midline posture is maintained (Figure 11-10). An additional anterior roll between the extremities and the use of a pacifier may promote further midline stabilization in flexion (Figure 11-11). Small neonates can be maintained in a flexed, symmetrical posture in a circular nest formed from a long blanket roll. Cloth buntings with circumferential body straps and a foot roll (Figure 11-12) provide positioning support and containment of extremity movement. Ferrari

TABLE 11-8 ■ MUSCULOSKELETAL MALALIGNMENT AND FUNCTIONAL LIMITATIONS IN NEONATES

POSITIONAL DEFORMITY	CONSEQUENCES	FUNCTIONAL LIMITATIONS
Plagiocephaly	Unilateral, flat occipital region; head turn preference; high risk for torticollis	Limited visual orientation from asymmetrical head position; delayed midline head control
Scaphocephaly	Bilateral, flat parietal and temporal regions	Difficulty developing active midline head control in supine position from narrowing of occipital region
Hyperextended neck and retracted shoulders	Shortened neck extensor muscles; overstretched neck flexor muscles; excessive cervical lordosis; shortened scapular adductor muscles	Interferes with head centering and midline arm movement in supine position; interferes with head control in prone and sitting positions; limits downward visual gaze
"Frog" legs	Shortened hip abductor muscles and iliotibial bands; increased external tibial torsion	Interferes with movement transitions into and out of sitting and prone positions; interferes with hip stability in four-point crawling; prolonged wide-based gait with excessive out-toeing
Everted feet	Overstretched ankle invertor muscles; altered foot alignment from muscle imbalance	Pronated foot position on standing; retained, immature foot-flat gait with potential delay in development of heel-to-toe gait pattern from excessive pronation

Adapted from Sweeney JK, Gutierrez T: The dynamic continuum of motor and musculoskeletal development: implications for neonatal care and discharge teaching. In Kenner C, McGrath JM, editors: *Developmental care of newborns and infants,* ed 2, Glenview, Ill., 2010, National Association of Neonatal Nurses.

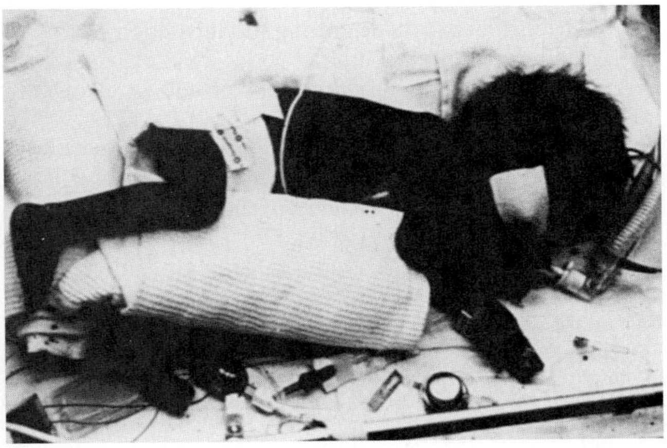

Figure 11-10 ■ Positioning with diaper rolls to reduce extension posturing.

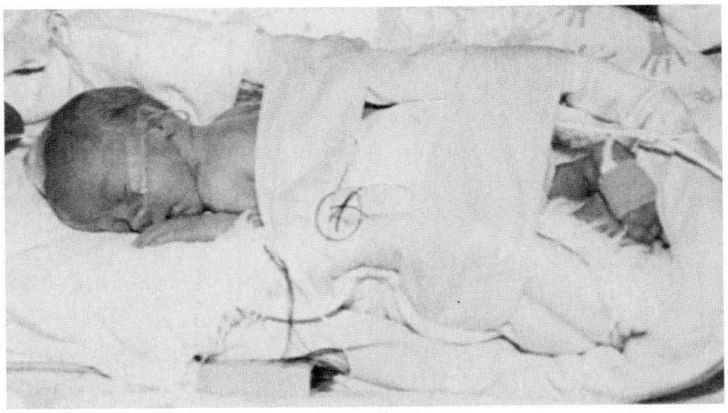

Figure 11-12 ■ Use of cloth bunting with circumferential straps, interior foot roll, lateral rolls, and sheepskin to promote body containment in prone flexion.

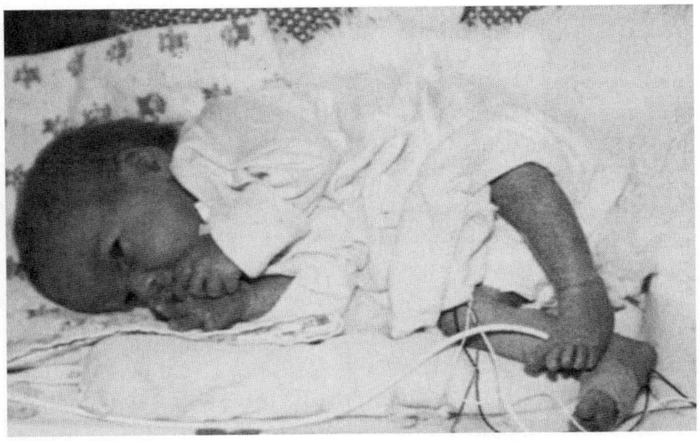

Figure 11-11 ■ Pacifier promotes flexion and long roll allows anterior and posterior containment of flexed side-lying position.

and colleagues[166] found increased frequency of extremity movements across midline and fewer stiff postures when neonates (25 to 31 weeks of gestation) were positioned in supine position in a circular nest compared with supine position without a nest.

Endotracheal tube placement frequently contributes to the neck hyperextension posture in infants who require mechanical ventilation (Figure 11-13). This iatrogenic component can be avoided by repositioning the ventilator hoses to allow enough mobility for slightly tucked chin and partially flexed trunk posture. For neurologically impaired infants with severe pulmonary disease necessitating prolonged ventilatory support, inattention to the alignment of the neck and shoulders may lead to the development of a contracture in the neck extensor muscles (Figure 11-14).

During the hospital stay, infants on ventilators (Figure 11-15) are now routinely positioned prone to enhance extremity and trunk flexion in the prone position, improve oxygenation, and decrease irritability.[167,168] Monterosso and

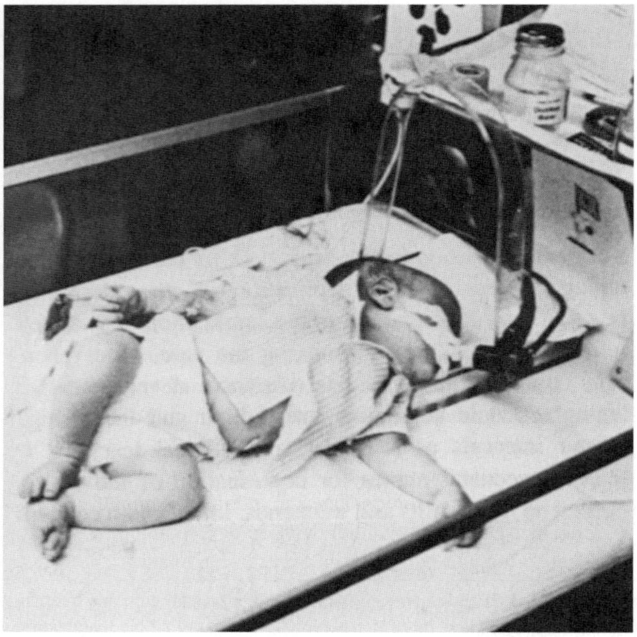

Figure 11-13 ■ Neck hyperextension posture magnified by the position of the endotracheal tube.

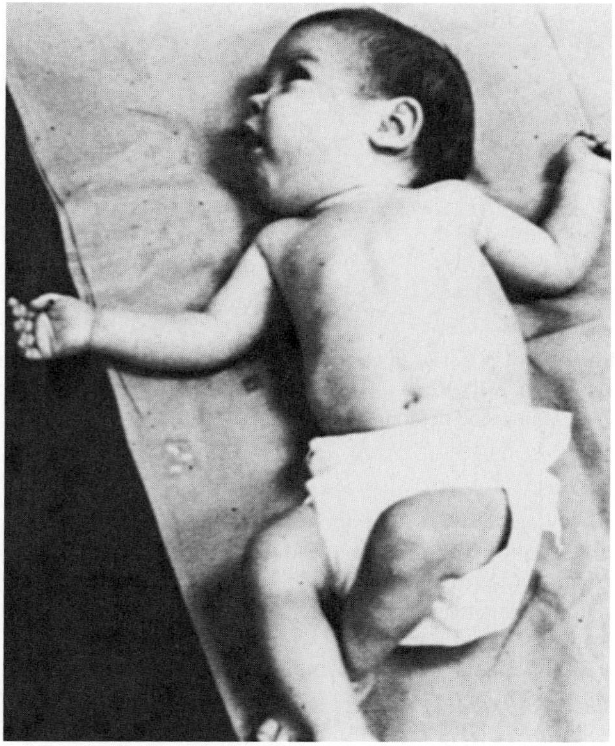

Figure 11-14 ■ Clinical presentation of contracture in neck extensor muscles related to hyperextension posture during prolonged mechanical ventilation.

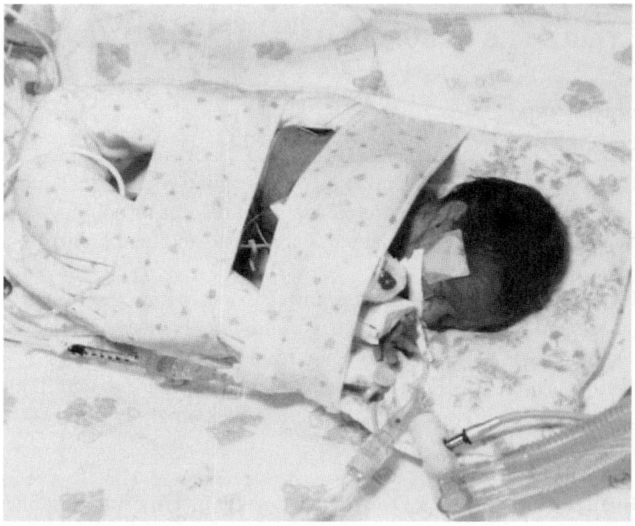

Figure 11-15 ■ Infant with endotracheal tube and ventilator positioned prone in nest with straps. (Reprinted from Hunter JG: Neonatal intensive care unit. In Case-Smith J, O'Brien JC: *Occupational therapy for children,* ed 6, St Louis, 2010, Mosby.)

colleagues[169] reported that using a small vertical roll along the torso (sternum to pubis) decreased scapular retraction in the prone position. Although placing infants on a sheepskin surface (see Figure 11-12) offers increased tactile input and has been correlated with increased weight gain in LBW infants compared with a matched group of infants on standard cotton sheets,[170] concern regarding the inhalation of microfibers from sheepskin has limited widespread use unless the sheepskin is covered by a thin blanket and used only to midchest level.[171]

After the infant has been moved from intensive care to intermediate care, transition to a standard mattress without positioning aids is recommended to allow time for adaptation to the type of mattress likely to be used at home. Infants are also transitioned to the supine sleeping position during the week before hospital discharge to reduce the risk of sudden infant death associated with the prone sleeping position and other factors.[171]

The neonatal therapist provides consultation on body alignment of infants in car seats when the LBW infant has not passed the peripheral oxygen saturation test in the car seat, which is usually conducted by the neonatal nurse before discharge. Some infants require the use of a car bed with body harness when they are unable to tolerate the semiupright position of a car seat without oxygen desaturation.

Preliminary evidence has been reported to support neonatal positioning programs emphasizing postures of extremities in flexion and head in midline.[166,172] Clinicians are referred to the work of Hunter[173,174] for detailed positioning techniques in the NICU. Continued research efforts are needed to measure effects of positioning and the risk-benefit effects of other neonatal therapy interventions to guide future directions of neonatal practice.

Extremity Taping

The presence of perinatal elasticity encourages early management of congenital musculoskeletal deformities in the neonatal period (birth to 28 days of age). A temporary ligamentous laxity is presumed to be present in the neonate because of transplacental transfer of relaxin and estrogen from the mother. In addition to the influence of maternal hormones, the rapid growth of the neonate can foster correction

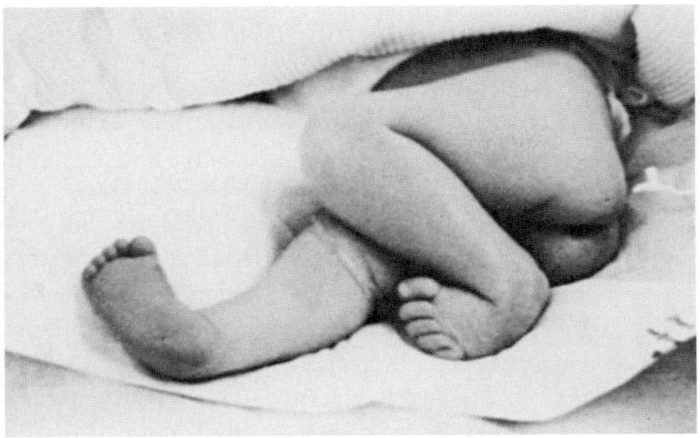

Figure 11-16 ■ Infant with lumbar meningomyelocele demonstrating marked varus foot deformities before taping.

of malalignment if the deforming forces are expeditiously managed. This peak period of hyperelasticity offers pediatric therapists with advanced orthopedic expertise many opportunities to manage congenital joint deformities.[175]

Intermittent taping of foot deformities (Figure 11-16) has been more adaptable to the nursery setting than either casts or splints and is more effective in achieving mobility than range-of-motion exercises. Access to the heel for drawing blood, inspection of skin and determination of vascular status, and placement of intravenous lines can be accomplished with the tape in place or by temporary removal of the tape as needed. Therapists without a sound knowledge of arthrokinematic principles and techniques should not attempt the taping procedure, which involves articulation of the joint(s) into a corrected position before taping. Other components of the taping process include application of an external skin protection solution under the tape, application of an adhesive removal solution when removing the tape, observance of skin condition and vascular tolerance, development of a taping schedule beginning with 1 hour and increasing by 1-hour intervals as tolerated, and clinical teaching with selected neonatal nurses for continuation of the taping if needed on night shifts and weekends. Infants with congenital foot deformities required shorter periods of casting in the outpatient period after taping of the extremity (Figure 11-17) was implemented during the inpatient phase. Taping is not appropriate for medically fragile infants on minimal handling protocols or for infants younger than 30 to 32 weeks of gestation because of potential epidermal stripping from tape removal or vascular compromise from inadvertent, excessive compression by either the tape or the underwrap layer.

The availability of thin, self-adherent foam material now allows taping on an underwrap (bandage) layer rather than on the infant's skin (Figure 11-18). Although this method creates a definite advantage in skin protection, it may cover the calcaneal region for blood drawing. Compromise in alignment may occur if the underwrap layer is applied loosely; conversely, restriction in circulation may be observed by edema or purple-blue color changes in the toes if the underwrap is excessively tight around the foot or ankle.

Infants with wrist drop from radial nerve compression related to intravenous line infiltration also benefit from the use of taping (Figure 11-19). The wrist is supported in a functional position of slight extension. As muscle function returns, the taping is used intermittently to reduce fatigue and overstretching of the emerging, but still weak, wrist extensor musculature.

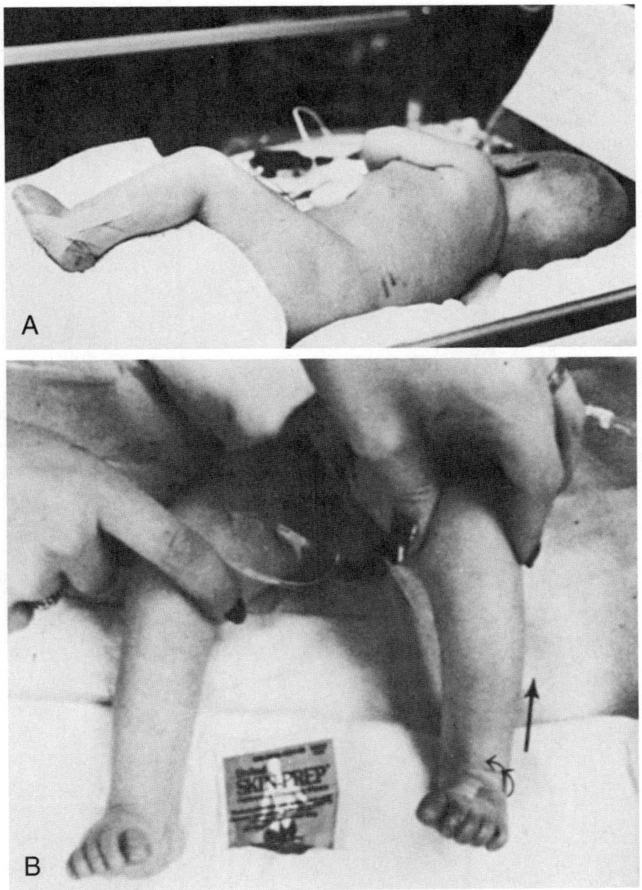

Figure 11-17 ■ Significant correction in alignment of varus foot deformities in neonate with a lumbar meningomyelocele. **A,** Lateral stirrup with open heel taping procedure. **B,** Moderate correction.

Soft Hand-Wrist Splint

Instead of using rigid, thermoplastic materials or taping, soft foam straps with Velcro closures provide an alternative method of support for wrist drop or hand-wrist malalignment (Figure 11-20). The splinting material is illustrated in Figure 11-21 with a small notch for the thumb on the longer strap placed across the palm and the shorter strap for the wrist band (longer strap attaches to posterior wrist band by Velcro). The wearing time is increased by 1-hour intervals to a 3-hour total wearing time and is often synchronized with nurse caregiving schedules (approximately 3-hour intervals) for alternate on-off application. Collaboration with neonatal nurses on wearing schedule, skin and vascular tolerance, alignment, and parental teaching is critical for successful integration of soft splints into the care plan.

Therapeutic Handling

Use of tactile, vestibular, proprioceptive, visual, and auditory stimuli to facilitate infant development has been reported and reviewed by many authors.[176-184] Selection and

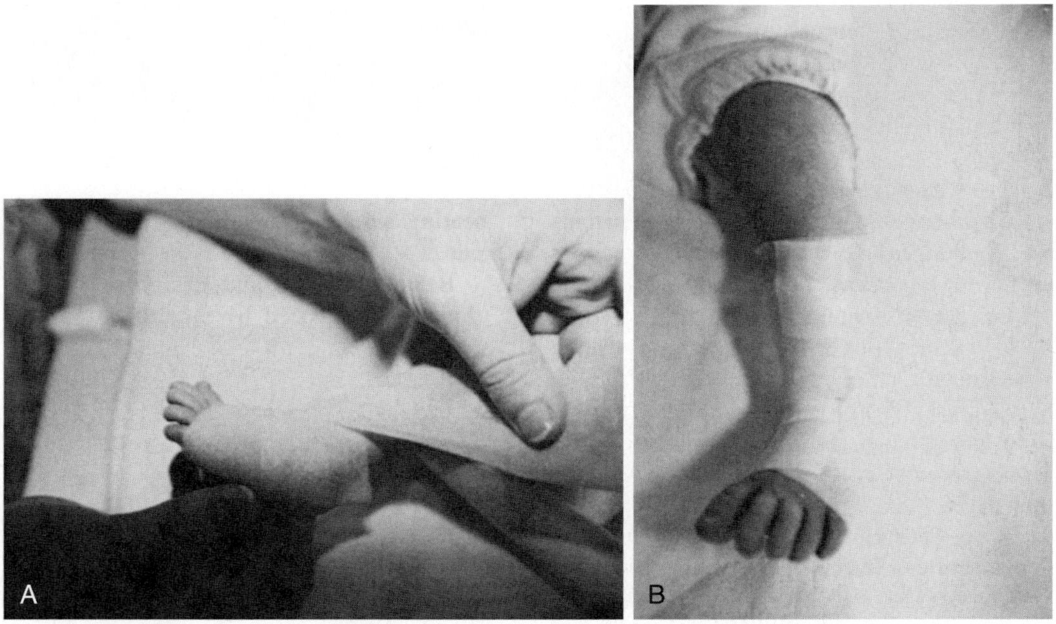

Figure 11-18 ■ Taping of varus foot deformity. **A,** Thin foam layer. **B,** Silk tape in lateral stirrup over foam layer.

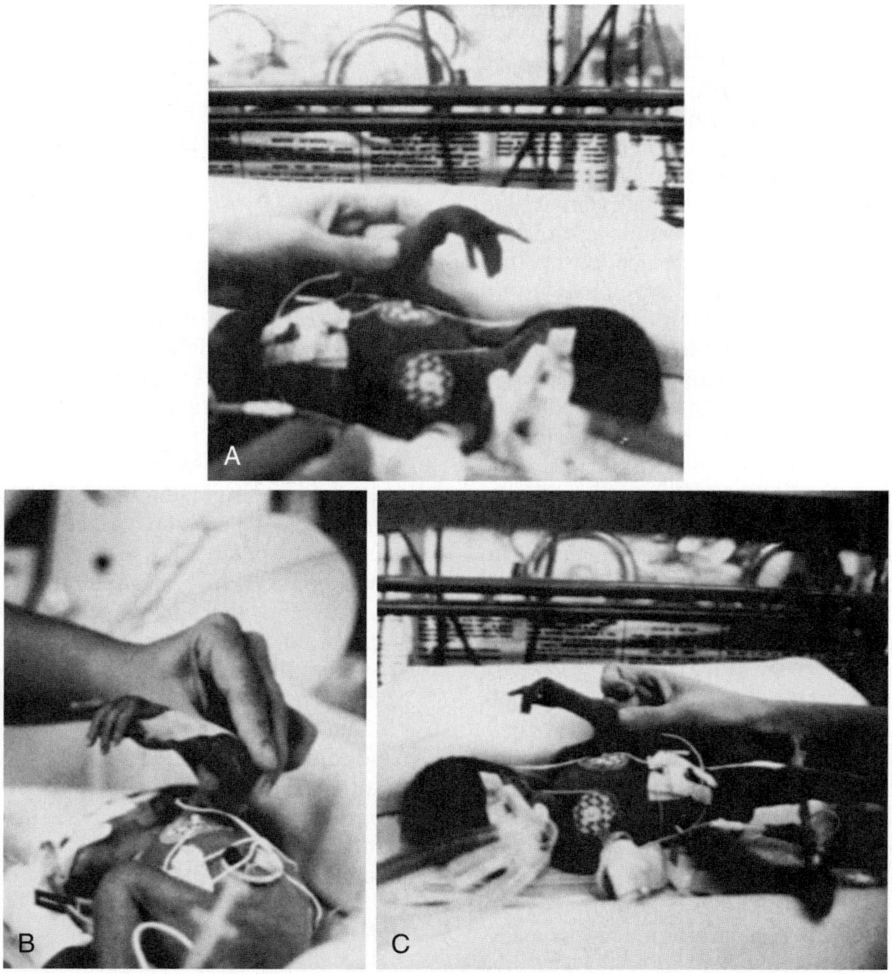

Figure 11-19 ■ Management of wrist drop in medically fragile neonate. **A,** Wrist drop before taping. **B,** Taping procedure. **C,** One week after taping.

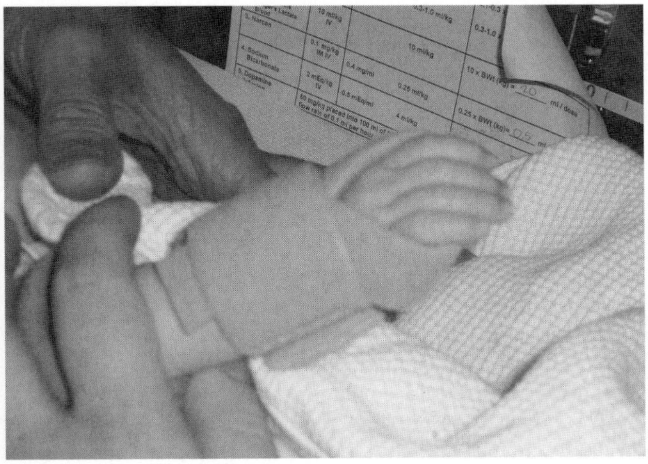

Figure 11-20 ■ Soft wrist extension splint.

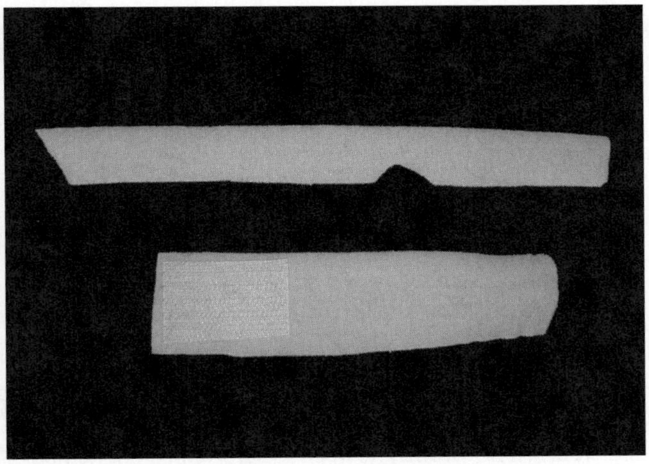

Figure 11-21 ■ Soft splint materials. The long strap is used across the palm with the notch for the thumb. The short strap wraps around the wrist to stabilize the long strap on the dorsum of the hand.

application of the sensory or neuromotor treatment options in neonatal therapy must occur with judicious attention to the prevention of sensory overload and related physiological consequences. Decision making on the type, intensity, duration, frequency, and sequencing of intervention within the context of infant physiological and behavioral stability can be learned only in a mentored clinical practicum in the NICU setting. The current general guidance on intervention is more observation, less handling, protection from bright lights and loud conversation, and readiness for handling determined on the basis of behavioral and physiological cues of the infant.[11,177,183,184]

Primary aims of therapeutic handling include assisting the newborn to achieve maximal interaction with parents and caregivers and facilitating the experience of postural and movement patterns appropriate to the infant's adjusted gestational age. Helping infants reach and maintain the quiet, alert behavioral state and age-appropriate postural tone appears to enhance opportunities for visual and auditory interaction and for antigravity movement experiences. The typical early movement experiences include hand-to-mouth movement, scapular abduction and adduction, anterior and posterior pelvic tilt, free movement of the extremities against gravity, and momentary holding of the head in midline.[127,185]

Behavioral state and some movement abnormalities can be modified by creative swaddling and gentle weight shifts and nesting in the caregiver's lap. Swaddling the infant in a blanket with flexed, midline extremity position appears to promote flexor tone, increase hand-to-mouth awareness, inhibit jittery or disorganized movement, and elicit quiet, alert behavior. These effects can also be accomplished in skin-to-skin holding of infants against the parent's chest, a procedure now commonly adopted in NICUs in North America.[186,187] Application of neonatal therapy techniques must be contingent on both the infant's readiness for interaction and the need for a recovery break in interaction because of sensory overload. Teaching parents and caregivers to read and respond to the infant's motor cues for interaction, feeding, change of body position, and rest breaks is a critical quality-of-life component of the infant's NICU therapy program.

A semi-inverted supine flexion position (Figure 11-22) with preterm neonates should be used with caution. This position may be used with older infants (6 months old) to facilitate elongation of neck extensor muscles and decrease the neck hyperextension posture, but with neonates the position may compromise breathing from positional compression of the chest and from potential airway occlusion associated with maximal flexion of the neck. The use of cardiorespiratory and oxygen saturation monitors during therapeutic handling activities is recommended for objective measurement of physiological tolerance. Although the peripheral oxygen saturation values from monitors may be intermittently unreliable because of motion artifacts from either the infant's spontaneous movement or the therapist's handling of the infant, reliable readings of oxygen saturation may be taken approximately 1 minute after the infant's body is not moved.

Easily overstimulated preterm infants may not tolerate multimodal sensory stimulation but may instead respond to a single sensory stimulus.[79,181] Implementation of a positioning program, oral-motor therapy, and environmental modifications and reinforcement of developmental activities with

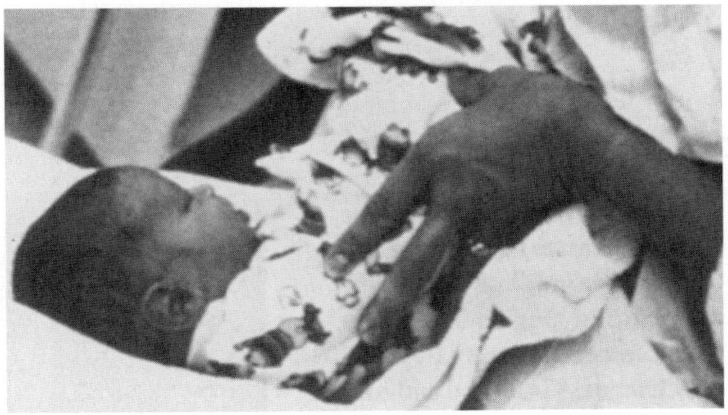

Figure 11-22 ■ Potential respiratory compromise to the infant from neck extensor muscle elongation in excessively flexed position while supine.

parents can be instituted only in collaboration with the shifts of bedside nurses who are in charge of the infant's 24-hour day in the NICU. Collaboration with nurses is a major component of precepted neonatal therapy training and requires integration into and valuing of the unique culture of the NICU.[130] Part of NICU culture is the unique ecology of environmental light and sound modifications, medical procedures, equipment, and caregiving patterns. Observing and analyzing the effects of the environment on an infant's behavior, physiological stability, postural control, and feeding function are critical elements to establish a prehandling baseline status before each neonatal therapy contact.[130]

Neonatal Hydrotherapy

Modified for use in an intensive care nursery setting, the traditional physical therapy modality of hydrotherapy has been adapted and implemented into neonatal therapy programs in some NICUs. Neonatal hydrotherapy was conceptualized in 1980 at Madigan Army Medical Center in Tacoma, Washington, and results of a pilot study of physiological effects were first reported in 1983.[188]

Indications for referral of medically stable infants to the hydrotherapy component of the neonatal therapy program include (1) muscle tone abnormalities (hypertonus or hypotonus) affecting the quality and quantity of spontaneous movement and contributing to the imbalance of extension in posture and movement (Figure 11-23); (2) limitation of motion in the extremities related to muscular or connective tissue factors; and (3) behavioral state abnormalities of marked irritability during graded neuromotor handling or, conversely, excessive drowsiness during handling that limits social interaction with caregivers and lethargy that contributes to feeding dysfunction.

Infants are considered medically stable for aquatic intervention when ventilatory equipment and intravenous lines are discontinued and when temperature instability and apnea or bradycardia are resolved. A standard plastic bassinet serves as the hydrotherapy tub, and the water temperature is prepared at 37.8° C to 38.3° C (100° F to 101° F). An overhead radiant heater is used to decrease temperature loss and enhance thermoregulation in the undressed infant. Agitation of the water is not included in the hydrotherapy protocol in the NICU.

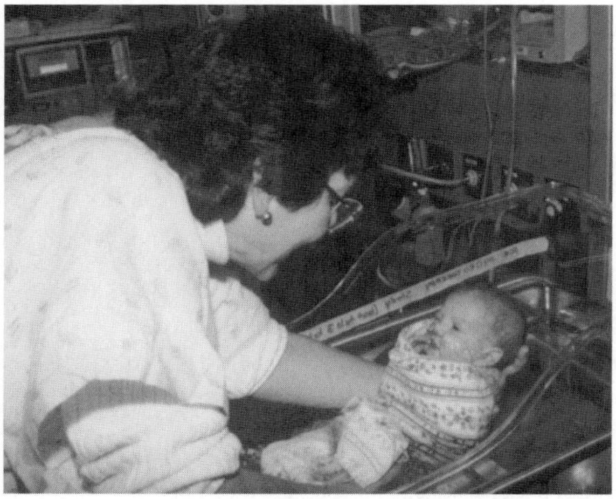

Figure 11-23 ■ Adjustment to water immersion before introduction of guided movement during neonatal hydrotherapy.

After medical clearance and individualized criteria for the maximum acceptable limits of heart rate, blood pressure, and color changes during hydrotherapy have been received from the neonatal staff, the baseline heart rate and blood pressure values are recorded and pretreatment posture and behavioral states are observed. The undressed infant is swaddled and moved into a semiflexed, supine position. The blood pressure cuff is placed around the distal tibial region to continuously measure heart rate and blood pressure at 2-minute intervals during the 10-minute water immersion period. After being lifted into the water, the swaddled infant is given a short period of quiet holding in the water without body movement or auditory stimulation to allow behavioral adaptation to the fluid environment (Figure 11-24). A second caregiver (e.g., nurse or parent) is recruited to stabilize the infant's head and shoulder girdle region while the neonatal therapist provides support at the pelvis (Figure 11-25).

Within the loosened boundaries of the swaddling blanket, the movement techniques involve midline positioning of the head and slow, graded movement incorporating slight flexion and rotation of the trunk, followed (if tolerated) by progression distally to the pelvic girdle region and finally to the shoulder girdle region. After guided trunk extensor flexion with partially dissociated movement at the shoulder or pelvic girdle, most infants will demonstrate active extremity movement in the water and the swaddling blanket is adjusted (or removed) to allow more movement or more stability depending on the response of the infant. The improved range and smoothness of spontaneous extremity movement is facilitated by the buoyancy and surface tension of the water. Movement experiences in the supine, sidelying, and prone positions are offered as tolerated. If the movement therapy becomes stressful, with agitation or crying by the infant, body movement is stopped immediately, and the infant is either consoled or removed from the water and held with warmed towels. Compromise in hemodynamic stability (increased heart rate, increased blood

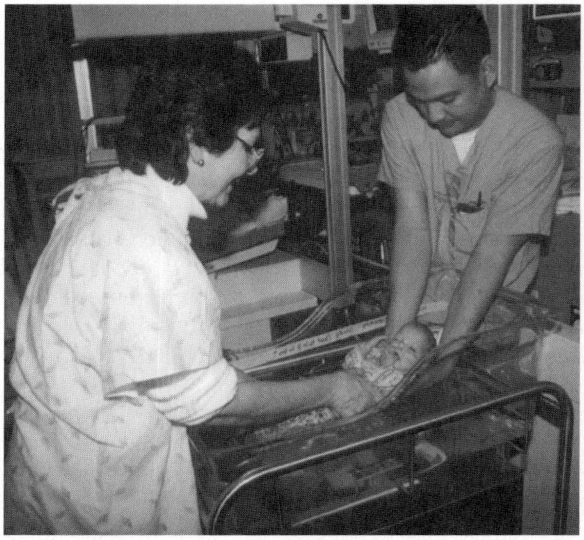

Figure 11-24 ■ Swaddled infant is supported in neonatal hydrotherapy tub by neonatal physical therapist and neonatal nurse. The blanket is gradually loosened to encourage spontaneous, midrange movement of the extremities.

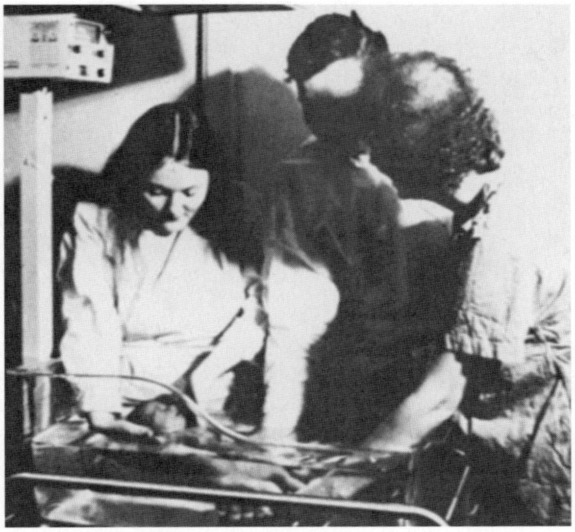

Figure 11-25 ■ Parents being trained in hydrotherapy techniques for later therapeutic bathing at home.

pressure, decreased respiratory rate) and decrease in arterial oxygen tension during crying have been well documented in neonates.[189] Careful monitoring of behavioral tolerance to hydrotherapy (with avoidance of crying) is considered critical for reducing physiological risk with hydrotherapy.

Multiple therapeutic benefits have been observed from the selective use of 10-minute aquatic intervention sessions. Improved postural tone with semiflexed posture is obtained with less time and effort by the therapist and with higher behavioral tolerance by the infant than when a similar therapeutic handling approach is used without the medium of water. Postural tone changes are frequently maintained for 2 to 3 hours when aquatic intervention is followed by flexed, midline body positioning in the side-lying or prone position on a water mattress or supported against rolls. Mild flexion contractures of knees and elbows and dynamic hip adduction contractures can be safely and quickly reduced by gentle muscle elongation techniques in warm water. Enhancement of visual and auditory orientation responses (e.g., visual fixing and tracking, auditory alerting, and localization to human voices), prolonged high-quality alertness, and longer periods of social interaction with caregivers are clinically observed during and after hydrotherapy sessions.

Improved sleep quality and behavioral organization were documented in 12 preterm infants (less than 36 weeks of gestation) after a 10-minute hydrotherapy session in a NICU in Brazil.[190] In this study the infants were used as their own controls, and responses were measured by a Neonatal Facial Coding System scale and by sleep-wake cycles from an adapted NBAS.

Feeding performance may improve when hydrotherapy is scheduled 30 minutes before feeding to prepare the infant for arousal to the quiet, alert state and for flexed, midline postural changes for optimal feeding. A sample of 31 preterm infants received both a 10-minute hydrotherapy session and a 10-minute rest period control condition (crossover design) before bottle feeding by a nurse blinded to the order of the treatment phase. Mean duration of feeding was significantly decreased ($P < .004$) after hydrotherapy compared with the rest condition. Mean daily weight gain after hydrotherapy was significantly higher ($P < .026$) than after the rest condition. All infants consumed 100% of the required feeding volume after the 10-minute hydrotherapy session, indicating that potential overstimulation or fatigue did not occur. On a short-term basis, weight gain was enhanced.[191]

Therapeutic bathing techniques are incorporated into the parental teaching program to foster early parental participation in child care and in specific neonatal therapy activities during the inpatient period to prepare for carryover into the home environment. This early pleasurable involvement of parent and child in hydrotherapy and therapeutic bathing may provide a strong base for future participation in aquatics as a family leisure sports activity and, if needed, as an adjunct to an outpatient therapy program.

When oriented to treatment goals and trained in specific hydrotherapy techniques for individual infants, the nursing staff can effectively carry on the hydrotherapy program established by the neonatal therapist. This release of the neonatal therapist's role to nurses allows additional use of hydrotherapy on evening and night shifts and continued teaching and supervision of parents during evening and weekend visits (see Figure 11-25).

An additional advantage of neonatal hydrotherapy is cost-effectiveness, with the use of equipment readily available in the newborn nursery and the short time (10 minutes) required for therapeutic bathing. Hydrotherapy becomes labor efficient for the neonatal therapist when it is incorporated into nursing care plans and conducted by nurses and parents, with the therapist assuming a supervisory role.

Although many clinical benefits may be obtained by judicious use of hydrotherapy in the newborn nursery, pilot study data obtained on physiological changes in high-risk infants during hydrotherapy clearly indicate a physiological risk.[188] This risk (7% increase in blood pressure and heart rate in the pilot sample) must be carefully evaluated relative to each infant's general medical stability and baseline heart rate and blood pressure status before hydrotherapy can be included safely in a neonatal therapy program. In collaboration with the neonatology and nursing staff, the therapist must use established criteria for general medical stability and the maximal limits during hydrotherapy for blood pressure, heart rate, and acceptable color changes; this step is essential for risk management. Physiological monitoring of mean blood pressure and heart rate with a neonatal vital signs monitor during aquatic intervention is recommended. The blood pressure cuff is a pneumatically driven device that is not electronically connected to the infant and can be safely immersed in water. Because hypothermia is a recognized risk with hydrotherapy, body temperature should be routinely measured before and after the hydrotherapy session by using a thermometer with a digital display. A risk-benefit analysis of the potential physiological risk to each infant and the expected therapeutic benefits is strongly advised before hydrotherapy techniques are incorporated into a neonatal therapy program.

Oral-Motor Therapy

Feeding difficulties in preterm neonates may be related to neurological immaturity, depressed oral reflexes, prolonged use of an endotracheal tube for mechanical ventilation and subsequent oral tactile hypersensitivity, or insufficient postural tone. Because behavioral state affects the quality of feeding behavior, feeding performance may be significantly improved by specific arousal or calming procedures before feeding. Other variables influencing feeding may include decreased tongue mobility, presence of tongue thrusting, decreased lip seal on nipple, nasal regurgitation, tactile hypersensitivity in the mouth, inefficient and uncoordinated respiratory patterns, insufficient proximal stability from hypotonic neck and trunk musculature, and hypertonic posturing of the neck and trunk in extension.[192,193]

Three instruments for assessing oral-motor and feeding behaviors in the nursery are the Neonatal Oral-Motor Assessment Scale (NOMAS),[194] the Nursing Child Assessment of Feeding Scale (NCAFS),[195] and the Early Feeding Skills (EFS) Assessment for preterm infants.[196] The NOMAS is used to evaluate the following oral-motor components during sucking: rate, rhythmicity, jaw excursion, tongue configuration, and tongue movement (timing, direction, and range). Tongue and jaw components are analyzed during nutritive and nonnutritive sucking activity. Cutoff scores were derived from a pilot study with the instrument: a combined score of 43 to 47 indicated "some oral-motor disorganization"; a score of 42 or less indicated oral-motor dysfunction.[194] The absence of a category to evaluate breathing pattern, work of breathing or respiratory exertion, and physiological variables during feeding limits the use of this instrument to low-risk, healthy neonates.

The NCAFS is used to analyze parent-infant interaction during feeding. It provides a method for evaluating the responsiveness of parents to infant cues, signs of distress, and social interaction opportunities during the feeding process. In concurrent validity studies, NCAFS scores were positively correlated with findings of the Home Observation for Measurement of the Environment inventory at 8 months ($r = 0.72$) and at 12 months ($r = 0.79$).[195]

The EFS Assessment is a 36-item observational measure of oral feeding readiness, feeding skill, and feeding recovery. The assessment tool includes examination of physiological and behavioral stability, behavioral feeding readiness cues, oral-motor coordination and endurance, coordination of breathing and swallowing, and postfeeding alertness, energy level, and physiological state. Preliminary content validity and intrarater and interrater reliability procedures were described as "stable and acceptable" (correlation data not reported) with predictive, concurrent, and construct validity testing in process.[196] This tool is specifically designed for feeding examinations in the NICU environment and with expanded psychometric testing will be a relevant instrument in managing neonates with feeding impairment.

General strategies during feeding may include semiflexed, upright positioning with light support under the chin (Figure 11-26). Techniques such as tactile facilitation of the facial muscles, use of a pacifier during gavage feedings, light manual support to the jaw or lip, and thickening of formula are frequent components of oral-motor therapy programs.[193,197] Scheduling of feeding based on the infant's readiness (behavioral cues of hunger and alertness) is usually implemented by neonatal nurses and shown to be effective in helping infants advance the frequency of oral (rather than gavage) feedings.[198,199]

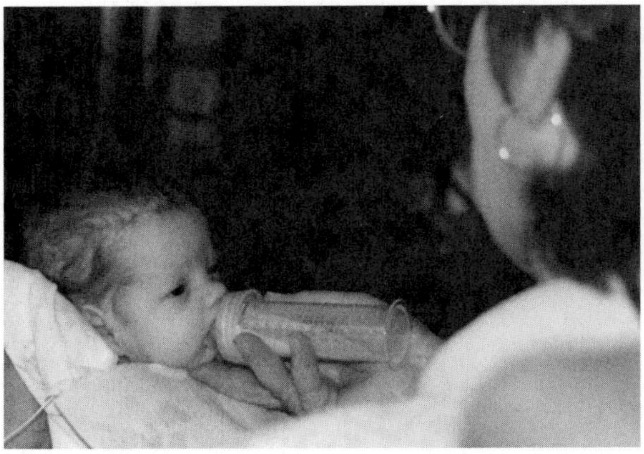

Figure 11-26 ■ Swaddled preterm infant fed in semiupright position with light support under chin.

For some infants, oral intake by bottle may be improved by individualizing nipple selection according to contour, length, hole size, texture, and compression resistance. Wolf and Glass[193,200] advised evaluation of the flow rate of liquid from various types of nipples and analysis of the effects of nipple size, shape, and consistency on an infant's sucking proficiency. Feeding infants in the side-lying position may improve tongue position, particularly if marked tongue retraction is present (Figure 11-27). The timing of movement therapy or neonatal hydrotherapy 30 minutes before feeding may improve performance by preparing postural tone, facilitating oral musculature, and enhancing alertness.

Infants with orofacial anomalies (e.g., cleft palate, hypoplastic mandible) often respond to bottle feeding with a Haberman feeding system (Medela, McHenry, Illinois), which allows control of the flow rate through a valve in the bottle and manual compression of the nipple. The Haberman feeder is an ideal option for infants with large bilateral cleft lip and palate because of the long, flexible nipple, which allows formula to be released from manual compression of the nipple by caregivers instead of requiring negative pressure for suction by the baby (Figure 11-28). Placement of the nipple on the middle of the tongue is advised regardless

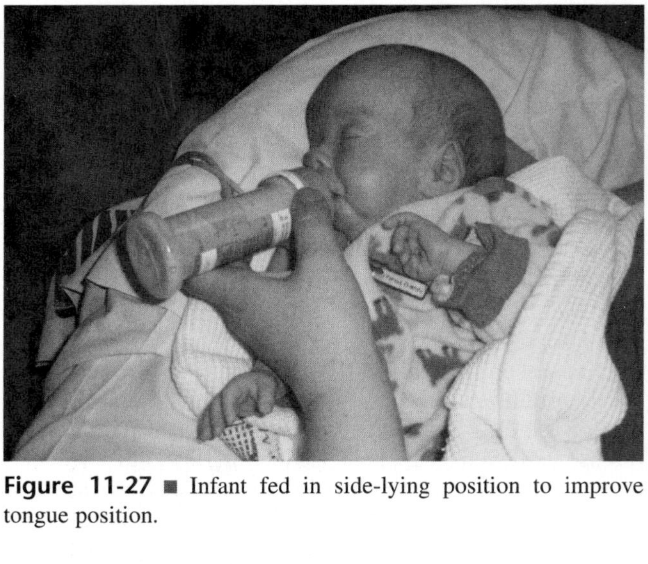

Figure 11-27 ■ Infant fed in side-lying position to improve tongue position.

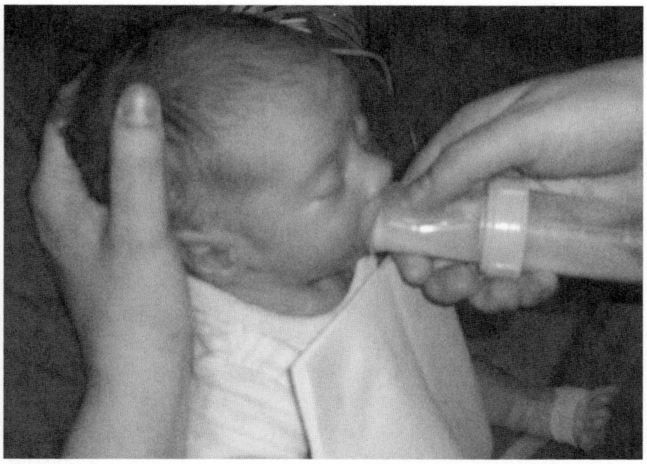

Figure 11-28 ■ Infant with cleft palate fed with specialized nipple (Haberman Feeding System).

of the location of the palate or lip defect.[201] The feeding performance of infants with severe cleft palate deformities may be improved by a dental obturator. This custom-fabricated prosthesis is inserted before feeding to cover the defect in the palate.

The increasing popularity of breast feeding has encouraged the development of breast-feeding aids (e.g., Lact-Aid, JJ Avery, Denver, Colorado). These devices allow supplementation of oral intake during breast feeding through a small tube that goes to the mouth from a sterilized bag containing infant formula.

Expected outcomes of oral-motor intervention supported by clinical research include (1) increased number of nutritive sucks after perioral stimulation,[202,203] (2) increased volume of fluid ingested during nipple feedings,[204] (3) decreased number of gavage feedings and earlier bottle feeding,[203,205] (4) accelerated weight gain,[205] and (5) earlier hospital discharge.[205] Research evidence has emerged on the benefits of interventions to assist pacing to allow breathing pauses[206] and to provide slower flow rate with specialized nipples[207] for preterm infants during the process of learning to bottle feed.

Monitoring the infant's physiological tolerance, breathing pattern, and work of breathing is critical during oral-motor examination, intervention, and feeding trials.[193] Heart rate values may be monitored from either the cardiorespirograph or with peripheral oxygen saturation from a pulse oximeter. Color changes, diminished tone in facial muscles, and behavioral stress cues (e.g., restlessness, trunk arching) must be carefully monitored to allow appropriate response to early signs of fatigue, overexertion, and potential airway difficulty. Regurgitation with aspiration of milk or formula into the lungs may occur during feeding trials, with complications of pneumonia, cardiopulmonary arrest, and associated asphyxia. Because of these risks, feeding trials should not be attempted by neonatal therapists untrained in managing the respiratory and general physiological monitoring components of neonatal feeding.[200]

Success during feeding activities enhances parent-infant interaction and perceived competency in parenting. Parents of infants with feeding dysfunction describe higher stress than that reported by parents of infants who are gaining weight and feeding satisfactorily. Oral-motor dysfunction has been reported as an early functional deficit in infants at high risk for later neuromotor sequelae[208]; early support for parents coping with a challenging feeding situation builds competence in caregiving and also commitment to continuity in outpatient developmental monitoring.

Parental Support

Grief Process

Strong, continuous support is essential to help parents through perhaps the most frightening crisis in their adult lives—the potential death or disability of their infant.[209,210] Although touching and holding infants contribute to infant-parent attachment,[211] parents may initially establish emotional and physical distance from the infant "s" as they cope with the knowledge that the infant may die. During this time of anticipatory grief, peer group support from other parents of prematurely born children can be of immeasurable value. Actively listening to the parents' feelings and concerns and providing support without judgment through their episodes of detachment and anger are critical. Although long-range plans include participation of parents in all aspects of the developmental program, the timing and amount of initial teaching must be individualized to the levels of stress and acute grief present.

When an infant dies, the neonatal therapist begins the important work of closure. This work includes attending memorial or funeral services to support the family, writing a note expressing sympathy to the family, and initiating a personal closure process. Neonatal therapists are advised to find a senior nurse mentor to guide them through the closure process of identifying and dealing with feelings of loss regarding the infant and family. Finding meaning and value in the process of caregiving rather than solely in functional outcomes is an important task in the work of closure and in preventing professional burnout.

Parent/Caregiver Teaching

Components of the parental/caregiver teaching process may include (1) discussion of the program goals and services in the NICU; (2) orientation to the interdisciplinary follow-up plan after discharge; (3) guidelines for recognizing and understanding the infant's temperament, stress, and stability cues; (4) methods of creating a calm environment with protection from aversive light and sound; and (5) specific instructions on selected corrected-age–appropriate developmental activities or therapeutic handling techniques. When used in conjunction with verbal instructions and demonstrations, a packet of written guidelines and pictures individualized to the infant's needs may improve parents' overall skills and understanding of the program.

Occasionally, when geographical distance prevents participation by parents in the neonatal therapy program, the infant's individualized developmental plan may be mailed and later reviewed at discharge or during outpatient follow-up. During times of separation, telephone contact with parents helps foster attachment to the infant and explain the purpose and content of the home developmental intervention program as well as providing opportunity to discuss the critical need for follow-up. Parents need this ongoing dialogue to make the infant seem real to them and to allow communication of their fears and concerns during the separation.

Teaching strategies are most effective when they are adapted to the learning style of the parents. This adaptation may involve more demonstrations and an increased opportunity for supervised practice for some parents, particularly those with reading or language difficulties that limit use of a written instructional packet. Parents have shown preference for combined educational methods including demonstration, video, and written materials rather than one single method.[212,213] Cultural caregiving practices of the family may necessitate elimination of common procedures such as use of pacifiers for nonnutritive sucking or hand-to-mouth engagement.

With consultation from and in collaboration with the neonatal therapist, neonatal nurses can incorporate recommendations to support skeletal and motor development into their routine discharge teaching activities. General considerations for discharge teaching by nurses may include the following[214]:

- Varying the direction of head turn for sleeping in the supine position to prevent plagiocephaly
- Placing the head in midline with lateral rolls extending along the side of the head and trunk for car seats and swings
- Limiting the use of infant seats and encouraging the use of prone play on the floor with a roll under the arms and upper chest to assist in head lifting and weight bearing on the arms
- Highlighting the importance of the prone play position for strengthening the neck, trunk, and arm musculature to prepare for sitting and rolling
- Reinforcing the value of interdisciplinary follow-up for musculoskeletal and neurodevelopmental monitoring
- Recommending expedient follow-up if parents notice signs of head flattening, persistent lateral head tilt, strong asymmetrical head turn preference, or asymmetrical arm use

In the neonatal period, the quality of infant-parent attachment and comfort level and proficiency in routine caregiving and therapeutic handling set the stage for later parenting styles. Helping parents find and appreciate a positive aspect of the neonate's motor or other developmental behaviors gives them a spark of hope from which emotional energy can be generated to help them through the marathon of the NICU experience. Empowering parents early in their parenting experience with the infant is crucial. In the life of the child, the effects of parent empowerment will last far longer than neonatal movement therapy and positioning strategies.

CLINICAL MANAGEMENT: OUTPATIENT FOLLOW-UP PERIOD

Purpose of Outpatient Follow-up for the at-Risk Infant

Systematic follow-up of the at-risk infant after discharge from the NICU is an essential component of the clinical management of high-risk infants. The purpose of this follow-up is threefold: (1) monitor and manage ongoing medical issues, such as respiratory problems and feeding difficulties; (2) provide support and guidance to parents and caregivers in care and nurturing of at-risk infants; and (3) assess the developmental progress of infants to ensure that neuromotor impairments and delays in motor development can be identified and intervention initiated as early as possible. Issues of assessment, intervention, and developmental profiles of the high-risk infant after discharge from the NICU are discussed in this section.

Medical Management

The routine medical care of preterm infants after discharge may be provided by a pediatrician, family practitioner, or health professional. Infants at neurodevelopmental risk are frequently followed by a number of additional professionals, including neurologists, ophthalmologists, cardiac or pulmonary specialists, nutritionists, public health nurses, physical and occupational therapists, and infant educators. Communication among these specialists is often minimal, especially when they are located at different facilities, and access to providers may be restricted by policies of varied hospital or managed-care systems. The parent or caregiver is often confronted with conflicting opinions, demands, and expectations of the family and the infant. The follow-up clinic can play a valuable role in this situation by providing case management to assist caregivers in coordinating necessary services, verify that all needs of the infant are being met, and help parents set realistic goals and priorities for themselves and their child.

Family Support

The stress that a vulnerable, premature, or at-risk infant brings to a family is well documented. Grief, anger, and depression are common reactions to the trauma and anxiety of an unanticipated premature birth.[209,215-217] The caregivers of high-risk infants are required to become knowledgeable about complex medical terminology and equipment. At discharge, they often become responsible for the administration of multiple medications of varying dosages, cardiopulmonary resuscitation procedures and equipment, and complicated feeding schedules requiring daily measurement and recording of nutritional intake and output. In addition, families are often faced with an unexpected, large financial obligation to the hospital and the confusion of dealing with different billing agencies and funding sources.

These stresses and demands are even more overwhelming for parents who are young, are single, or do not speak English. In contrast to the 1980s, a greater proportion of at-risk infants now seen in follow-up clinics are living with caregivers other than their biological mothers. These caregivers may include other relatives, such as single fathers, grandparents, aunts and uncles, foster care providers, or preadoptive parents. At the same time the changing demographics of American society are reflected in the increasing ethnic diversity of preterm infants. Whether they are recent immigrants to the United States, seasonal workers, or residents of an ethnic neighborhood, parents from minority ethnic groups are frequently overwhelmed by the complexities and procedures of a large medical institution. To serve this population adequately, a follow-up clinic team should have access to interpreters and include social workers who are knowledgeable about community resources outside the predominant culture. Cultural competence, defined as performing "one's professional work in a way that is congruent with the behavior and expectations that members of a distinctive culture recognize as appropriate among themselves," is an essential prerequisite for professionals working in a high-risk infant follow-up clinic.[218] For the physical therapist conducting an evaluation, cultural competence includes familiarity with differing cultural norms regarding personal interaction, child-rearing practices, and family dynamics.

Preterm or at-risk infants may be irritable, hypersensitive to stimulation, less responsive to the affective interactions of adults, and more irregular in sleeping and feeding schedules compared with the term infant.[219] The demands that such an infant place on caregivers can be extremely stressful, especially when other siblings in the home, financial concerns, and sleep deprivation are present. Although these stresses may resolve as the infant's schedule and temperament become more stable, some studies raise concerns about their long-term impact on the parent-infant relationship and the infant's social and affective development.[220,221]

The pediatric therapist in the follow-up clinic must be sensitive to these parent or caregiver stresses and concerns. Because social work and nursing services may not be routinely available, the therapist, within the context of the examination, needs to be alert to cues in the behavior of the infant or caregiver that may indicate problems in the home. Thoughtful questions regarding daily routines, feeding patterns, the sleep schedule of the caregiver as well as the infant, the caregiver's impression of the infant's temperament, and the availability of supportive resources can prompt a discussion of concerns that may not be readily communicated to a pediatrician or other professionals involved in the child's care.

Examination of Neurodevelopmental Status

Because preterm infants are at increased risk for neurodevelopmental disabilities, close follow-up is necessary during the first 6 to 8 years of life. Compared with term infants, the incidence of CP is greater in infants born preterm, and the rate of CP increases with decreasing birth weight levels.[82,222-225] CP is one of several major neurological conditions that are sequelae of prematurity; others include mental retardation, hydrocephalus, sensorineural hearing loss, visual impairment, and seizure disorder. When examined as a group, these major disabling conditions occur more frequently in LBW infants, and the incidence increases as the birth weight and gestational age of the infant decrease.[222,226-228]

Preterm infants are also at increased risk for more subtle neurodevelopmental disabilities, including visual-motor dysfunction, speech and language deficits, reading and math problems, balance and coordination impairment, and behavioral disorders such as attention deficit and hyperactivity.[83,228-232] Longitudinal studies indicate that by school age approximately half of all infants with LBW will have educational and learning deficits compared with a reported rate of 24% in the general population.[227,228] Overall 10% to 30% of preterm infants are estimated to eventually have "major" disabilities and another 40% to have "minor" disabilities.[227,228]

A primary objective of developmental follow-up in at-risk infants is the early identification of neurodevelopmental disabilities and the expedient referral to therapeutic intervention services. Preterm infants who participate in a follow-up clinic program have been shown to have advanced performance on cognitive measures and to receive more intervention services compared with unmonitored infants.[233,234] A confirmed or tentative diagnosis can direct the family toward intervention services, financial resources, and social supports. Systematic follow-up and recognition of developmental problems in a high-risk infant play a major role in supporting the relationship between an infant and the caregiver. The behavioral interaction of an infant with a developmental disability is often different from that of a typically developing infant, evoking negative maternal responses of anxiety, frustration, or withdrawal.[24,235] Diagnosis of a neurodevelopmental disability often facilitates dialogue about parental concerns and can assist caregivers in their process of accepting the disability and adjusting their expectations for the infant.

Follow-up Clinic Examination and Evaluation Processes

It is widely recognized that preterm infants are at risk for neurodevelopmental and musculoskeletal impairments that may lead to functional limitations.[6,236,237] Early assessment plays an important role for discharge teaching, follow-up planning, and identifying infants at the highest risk for developmental impairments so they can be appropriately referred for early intervention.

Although developmental assessment in the neonatal period is useful, it has been shown to have low predictive value for later outcome. The neonatal period and the first 2 to 3 months of life are characterized by variability in infant behavior and motor skills as well as instability of postural organization and control.[9,10] Longitudinal studies with sequential examinations indicate that neonatal examinations are less accurate in long-term prediction of neurodevelopmental outcome than examinations administered to older infants.[3-5] Ongoing repeated assessments to monitor developmental outcome are necessary to ensure early identification of potential functional activity limitations in infants.[6,146,238] Pediatric therapists are in a unique position as consultants to the multidisciplinary team to become involved in the process of identification of infants at risk, care coordination, and follow-up planning.[239] Critical examination periods and signs of neuromotor or musculoskeletal abnormality indicating a need for comprehensive examination by a pediatric physical therapist are described in the next sections.

Months 2 to 4

The American Academy of Pediatrics has established guidelines for the follow-up of high-risk infants[80] and has defined indicators for follow-up care.[240] No specific timelines or recommended schedules for follow-up visits are available, but general agreement exists that the lower the gestational age, the higher the risk for neurodevelopmental impairments. Although most early neonatal assessments have poor predictive value, it is recommended that infants at highest risk be followed closely to ensure early identification and referral.[6]

Important changes in postural control, movement, and behavioral organization occur at 2 to 4 months. Head control and balance reactions are emerging, and functional skills are present with orientation around the midline.[241] This is also the time when the transition from GMs to goal-directed movement begins to take place (Figure 11-29).[242] The pediatric therapist can perform an early developmental follow-up evaluation to monitor changes in posture and movement, development of head control, midline orientation, visual skills and provide parental education. A marked increase in the prevalence of positional plagiocephaly (also known in the literature as *nonsynostotic plagiocephaly, plagiocephaly without synostosis,* or *flat head syndrome*)[243,244] has occurred since 1992 when the American Academy of Pediatrics released a position paper recommending that all infants be positioned for sleeping on the back or side to minimize risk of SIDS.[245,246] Two to 4 months postterm is a critical window of time for identifying positional preferences in infants and providing parental education to prevent plagiocephaly.

Months 6 to 8

For most LBW infants, medical concerns have resolved at this age and caregivers are raising questions about developmental expectations. This is a period of great variability in the development of goal-directed behaviors and attainment of motor milestones that are dependent on postural control. General agreement exists that most typically developing infants achieve independent sitting in this time frame.[241] Definitive predictions on long-term prognosis are difficult for a preterm infant at this age. Tools measuring specific milestones have low clinical value owing to variability in the acquisition of motor skills and postural control.[242] A developmental assessment with emphasis on postural control at 6 to 8 months' adjusted age (e.g., Alberta Infant Motor Scale) can document an infant's current level of performance and provide a baseline for subsequent evaluations.

Months 10 to 14

During the first year of life, infants gain increasing levels of postural control and express neurological integrity and capabilities through movement and exploration. Lack of variability and variety in movement strategies may be an early indicator of atypical development. Learning to transition out of supine position and crawling are typically achieved at 10 to 12 months and by 12 to 14 months most infants have achieved the ability to walk independently.[241,242] By 12 months corrected or chronological age, infants demonstrate a wide repertoire of behaviors in other domains including cognitive and language intertwined with motor development. Multidisciplinary evaluation at 12 months is recommended for infants at risk, to create a more comprehensive developmental profile.[80]

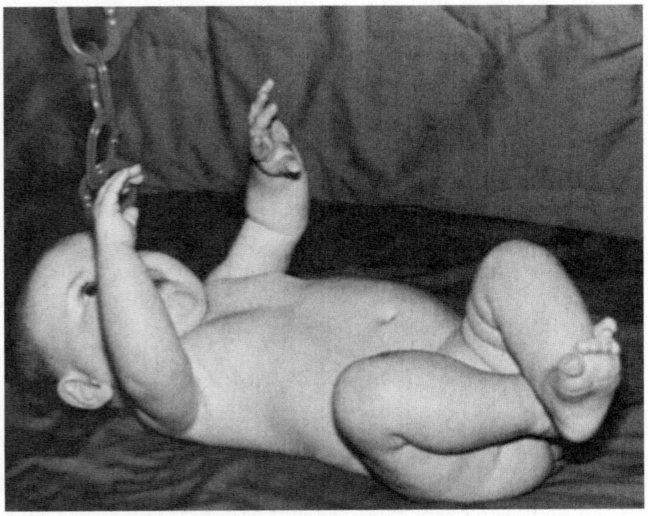

Figure 11-29 ■ Goal-directed reaching and symmetrical lower-extremity alignment in 4-month-old born at term gestation.

Months 18 to 24

With the foundation for gross motor skills well established by 18 months, identifying deficits in the fine motor, cognitive, social adaptive, and language domains that might interfere with school performance becomes the main focus of assessment during this period. High prevalence of positive screening for autism in infants born preterm has been described in the recent literature.[247] These data suggest that while the focus of most follow-up programs for high-risk infants is on motor and cognitive abilities, evidence now supports the inclusion of screening tools to identify early signs of social and behavioral dysfunction. Recent evidence also points to a high prevalence of cerebellar damage or dysgenesis in preterm infants. Cerebellar hemorrhage represents a high risk for cognitive and motor delays in these infants.[42,248] D'Amore and colleagues reported findings that assessment at 2 years of age can reliably identify developmental impairments.[249]

Comprehensive assessment at 24 months is recommended, including language, fine motor, adaptive, and cognitive skills. Most multidisciplinary follow-up programs stop at this time owing to cost and high rate of attrition.[80] Growing evidence is reported of higher rates of educational and behavioral challenges becoming apparent at school age among children with ELBW. Therefore, ongoing follow-up beyond 24 months is desirable.[249]

Age Correction

Premature infants are scheduled for evaluations in the follow-up clinic according to their corrected age (age adjusted for weeks of prematurity). The issue of whether to adjust for prematurity when assessing cognitive or motor development is an ongoing question. Several researchers have demonstrated that if chronological or unadjusted age is used for standardized testing, the premature infant who is developing appropriately will have a low developmental quotient and test scores indicative of motor delay.[250-254] If age is adjusted for prematurity, the performance of the premature infants is comparable to that of term infants at 1 year. Although some investigators caution that adjustment for prematurity tends to result in overcorrection, particularly for infants born at less than 33 weeks' gestation,[255] the general consensus is that infants born prematurely should be evaluated according to their corrected age.[255,256]

The decision regarding correction for gestational age in a follow-up clinic should be based on the objectives and testing protocol for that clinic. Consideration should be given to the following factors: (1) the testing instruments used, with attention to the competencies evaluated by the tool and the number of preterm infants in the normative sample, and (2) the overall purpose of the evaluation and whether the emphasis is on screening or diagnosis

Neuromotor Assessment of the at-Risk Infant

Neuromotor Assessment Tools: Purpose and Clinical Use

Evaluation of the at-risk infant with a quantitative, standard assessment tool serves two major purposes in a follow-up clinic:

1. Documentation of the infant's motor status relative to developmental norms or relative to the infant's performance on previous examinations. The information is used to determine the child's developmental progress, rate of change, or extent of motor delay. Achievement of this objective is determined by the scope and focus of the assessment tools used in the evaluation.
2. Identification of a neuromotor impairment to initiate appropriate intervention services. Early identification is not simply a task of detecting signs of neuromotor deviation. The challenge is to identify those infants who are most likely to have an abnormal neurodevelopmental outcome. Achievement of this objective is determined by the predictive validity of the assessment tools that are used.

Evaluation of Predictive Validity of Infant Assessment Tools

A primary goal of the neuromotor evaluation is prediction of the long-term developmental outcome of the child on the basis of a clinical examination of the infant. The ability to achieve this goal accurately depends on the clinical experience and expertise of the therapist as well as the predictive accuracy or validity of the assessment tool used. The predictive validity of a test is defined by sensitivity and specificity and positive and negative predictive values (Table 11-9).[257]

The *sensitivity* of a test evaluates how sensitive the test is in its ability to identify a defined developmental problem, such as CP. In the testing situation described here, sensitivity is calculated as the proportion of children with abnormal neurodevelopmental outcome who were correctly identified as "abnormal" when examined as infants. *Specificity* refers to how specific the test is in identifying *only* the defined developmental problem and not overdiagnosing by identifying children who do not have the problem. Specificity is calculated as the proportion of children with normal developmental outcome who were correctly identified as "normal" when examined as infants. The children with normal developmental outcome who were inaccurately classified as "abnormal" by the infant test are referred to as *false positives;* that is, they were falsely determined by the test to be positive for the developmental problem. On the other hand, children who were classified as "normal" when tested as infants but subsequently are diagnosed with CP are described as *false negatives* because the test falsely indicated that they were negative for the developmental problem.

The *positive predictive value* of a test refers to the accuracy of the infant test in its classification of infants as "abnormal." For example, of the infants who were identified as "abnormal" or "suspect" by the infant test, the proportion of infants who are actually diagnosed with CP represents the *positive predictive value.* The *negative predictive value* refers to the accuracy of the infant test in its classification of infants as "normal." It is calculated as the proportion of infants categorized as "normal" who actually have normal developmental outcome. To the therapist in a follow-up clinic, it may appear that the positive and negative predictive values of a given test would be most useful because they indicate the probability of a given outcome for an infant being tested. However, predictive value is not a stable measure of the predictive validity of a test because the predictive values vary according to the prevalence of the developmental problem within a group or population of infants. When a condition is common, the positive predictive value will be relatively high. When the outcome of interest is rare, the positive predictive value will be relatively low. Further discussion about test evaluation and measurement can be found in a number of excellent resources available to pediatric therapists.[257,258]

Examples of Infant Assessment Tools

In addition to the tools previously described for the assessment of the neonate, a number of testing instruments have been designed for evaluation of the infant. The choice of instrument for a particular clinical situation depends on the emphasis and purpose of the clinic as well as on the professional disciplines that are represented in the follow-up team. Neurological findings may be the most useful indicator of impairment in the neonate or young infant because this is a

TABLE 11-9 ■ PREDICTIVE VALIDITY OF AN INFANT ASSESSMENT TOOL

	OUTCOME (AT SPECIFIED AGE IN CHILDHOOD)		
INFANT TEST	NORMAL	ABNORMAL	
No risk	a Correct nonreferrals	b Incorrect nonreferrals (false negatives)	a + b = Total nonreferrals
Risk	c Incorrect referrals (false-positives)	d Correct referrals	c + d = Total referrals

a + c = Total normal at outcome.
b + d = Total abnormal at outcome.
Sensitivity = d/b, d × 100 = Percentage of abnormal children who were correctly identified as "no-risk" by the infant test.
Specificity = a/a, c × 100 = Percentage of normal children who were correctly identified as "risk" by the infant test.
Positive predictive value* = d/c, d × 100 = Percentage of infants identified as "risk" by the infant test who had abnormal outcome.
Negative predictive value* = a/a, b × 100 = Percentage of infants identified as "no risk" by the infant test who had normal outcome.

*Positive and negative predictive values will vary according to the prevalence of the abnormal outcome within the study population.

time when behavioral responses are influenced by the infant's affective state and when motor skills are rudimentary. As the infant matures, neuromotor integrity manifests with the acquisition of motor skills. For infants older than 3 months, longitudinal researchers indicated that observed neuromotor abnormalities were predictive of later CP only when accompanied by delay in one or more developmental milestones.[3,259] A brief review of the infant assessment tools commonly used in follow-up clinics is presented in the following sections.

Bayley Scales of Infant Development. The Bayley Scales of Infant Development (BSID) were first published in 1969 in a format used extensively in clinical and research settings throughout the United States. The BSID-II,[260] a revised version of the BSID, was published in 1993. The goals of the revision process included updating the normative data, extending the upper age level of the test from 30 to 42 months, and adding more relevant test items and materials. The revised test was standardized on 1700 young children representing a distribution of race, gender, geographical region, and level of parental education as an indicator of socioeconomic status. In addition, approximately 370 children with various clinical diagnoses, including autism, Down syndrome, developmental delay, preterm birth, and prenatal exposure to drugs, were tested with the BSID-II. Test scores from these children were not included in the normative data and are intended to provide a baseline of performance for children with these diagnostic conditions.[260]

The expanded age range and updated normative data offered by the BSID-II enhanced its overall use as an assessment tool. However, several areas of weakness have been identified in using the BSID-II, particularly with preterm infants.[261-263] Unlike the protocol of the original test, the administration of items and the scoring procedures for the BSID-II are based on item sets. The appropriate item set for an individual child is usually determined according to the child's chronological age, but the examiner is told to "select the item set that you feel is closest to the child's current level of functioning based on other information you might have."[260] The option to begin testing at different item sets, which can yield different raw scores for the same infant, introduces a level of variability in administration procedures and test results that is inconsistent with the purpose of a standardized test.[263] This problem is magnified for preterm infants because it places even greater importance on the decision of whether to test the infant according to chronological or corrected age.[260]

The third edition of the BSID (BSID-III), published in 2006, is the most recent update.[264] The goals for developing the current edition included updating the normative data, fulfilling the requirements set by the Individuals with Disabilities Education Improvement Act of 2004, strengthening psychometric measures, updating testing materials, simplifying test administration, and improving the test's clinical utility.[238,265] The BSID-III is a comprehensive assessment for children aged 1 to 42 months to be administered by experienced and trained professionals. This edition comprises five different subscales—cognitive, expressive, and receptive communication; gross and fine motor development; and parental report scales to assess social-emotional development and adaptive behaviors.

The cognitive scale of the BSID-III assesses sensorimotor development, object manipulation and relatedness, concept formation, memory, and simple problem solving. The expressive and receptive language subscales examine verbal comprehension, vocabulary, babbling, utterances, and gesturing. The fine motor subscale examines grasping, motor planning, speed, and visual motor activities, and the gross motor subscale includes sitting, locomotion, standing, and balance. Social-emotional and adaptive behaviors are tested using the parental report scales. Administration times vary depending on the age of the child but can range from approximately 50 minutes for children aged 12 months or younger to 90 minutes for children aged 13 months and older. The child's chronological age (adjusted for prematurity as needed) gives the examiner a starting point, designated by a letter *A* through *Q*. The rules for establishing basal and ceiling levels are the same for the cognitive, language, and motor scales. The child must pass three consecutive items in order to establish a ceiling, and the test is discontinued once the child fails five consecutive items. The BSID-III has expanded basal and ceiling levels with standardized scores ranging from 40 to 160. The mean for the standardized composite score for the cognitive, language, and motor skills is 100 with standard deviation of 15. The language and motor skills also yield scaled scores with a mean of 10 and standard deviation of 3. In addition, percentile rank, age equivalents, and growth scores can be derived.[264,265]

The BSID-III was standardized on a normative sample of 1700 children from the ages of 16 days to 43 months 15 days living in the United States in 2004. Stratification was based on age, gender, parental education level, ethnic background, and geographical area. Norms for the social-emotional and adaptive behavior scales were derived from smaller groups (456 and 1350 children, respectively) but the same stratification pattern was followed.[264] There are a total of 91 items in the new cognitive scale including 72 items from the BSID-II. Many items from the former cognitive scale were removed, modified, or moved to other subscales such as language and fine motor scales. The fine and gross motor scales contain a total of 66 items including 18 new items. The parental report scales are a new addition to assess social-emotional and adaptive behaviors.[264,266]

The psychometric attributes of the BSID-III are as strong as those of the earlier editions and are thoroughly described in the technical manual.[266,267] Reliability coefficients for the subscales and composite scores range from 0.86 to 0.93, with similar or higher coefficients obtained when the reliability was examined testing special groups. Test-retest reliability was examined in a sample of 197 children tested on two separate occasions with an average interval of 6 days. Reliability coefficients ranged from .67 to .94, with an average correlation score of .80. The technical manual describes in great detail the convergent and divergent validity, illustrating the correlation between the BSID-III and other relevant testing tools.[264,266]

The BSID-III is still relatively new, and many questions remain regarding its potential limitations and utility for clinical application. Administration of the full test is a lengthy procedure, and the composite scores are reported to be higher than those of the BSID-II.[267] Anderson and colleagues[268] recently examined the ability of the BSID-III to detect developmental delay in 2-year-old extremely preterm children and those born at term with normal birth weights. The study participants were former preterm infants born at less than 28 weeks or weighting less than 1000 g (n = 221). Two hundred and twenty healthy full-term infants with normal birth weight were randomly selected as a control group. Developmental assessment was conducted at 2 years (age corrected for prematurity) using the cognitive, language, and motor scales of the BSID-III. The social-emotional and adaptive behavior scales were not used. The authors observed a serious overestimation in the developmental progress of this sample. Questions were raised regarding the sensitivity of this test to detect developmental delay in children. More research is needed to examine this test's sensitivity and the interpretation of test results, especially for high-risk or premature infants. Continued use of the BSID-III should be conducted with caution in the absence of more data to establish the sensitivity of this tool.[266]

Alberta Infant Motor Scale. The AIMS[269] was designed to evaluate gross motor function in infants from birth to independent walking, or birth through 18 months. The stated purposes of the AIMS are (1) to identify infants who are delayed or deviant in motor development and (2) to evaluate motor maturation over time. The AIMS is described as an "observational assessment" that requires minimal handling of the infant by the examiner. The test includes 58 items, organized by the infant's position, designed to evaluate three aspects of motor performance: weight bearing, posture, and antigravity movements. The normative sample consisted of 2200 infants born in Alberta, Canada.

Raw scores obtained on the AIMS can be converted to percentile ranks for comparison with motor performance of the normative sample. Test-retest and interrater reliabilities, established on normally developing infants, ranged from 0.95 to 0.98 depending on the age of the child. The AIMS reportedly had high agreement with the Motor Scale of the BSID and the Gross Motor Scale of the Peabody Developmental Motor Scales (PDGMS) ($r = 0.93$ and $r = 0.98$, respectively).[5] An evaluation of concurrent validity between the AIMS and the Movement Assessment of Infants (MAI) at 4 and 8 months demonstrated acceptable agreement ($r = 0.70$ and $r = 0.84$, respectively).[270]

The Movement Assessment of Children. The Movement Assessment of Children (MAC) assesses functional gross motor and fine motor skills of children from age 2 months to 24 months.[271] The motor assessment is composed of three sections including head control, upper extremities and hands, and pelvis and lower extremities. In addition, there are four assessment sections (general observations, special senses, primitive reactions, and muscle tone) that contribute to the interpretation of MAC findings for any one child. These four sections assist therapists in making a therapy diagnosis, thus focusing the therapist's selection of treatment modalities. The MAC, on average, has five functional test items per month over 23 months of development. It is anticipated that this number of items will allow for accuracy in evaluative and discriminative measures, leading to effective clinical judgments. The MAC can be completed in less than 30 minutes (20 minutes for some children), and it takes 5 minutes to update during reevaluation.

Four hundred and seven assessments were completed on typically developing children aged 2 to 24 months in the greater Denver, Colorado area. The gestational ages of the children at birth were 37 to 42 weeks, and the majority were Caucasian (77%).

Construct validity of the MAC was established using Rasch analysis with the 407 assessments. In brief, 34 of the 37 super items fit the model based on fit statistics (infit and outfit mean square error values of 0.5 to 1.7). Unidimensionality of the MAC was also achieved: Rasch principal component analysis showed that the model explained 90.4 % of the variance. The Rasch analysis also indicated that the MAC has excellent person and item reliabilities. The person reliability index was .98, indicating that the person ability ordering would be stable if these children were assessed on another evaluation tool with the same construct as "the motor super items" of the MAC. Cronbach's alpha was .97, implying that the MAC super items were internally consistent with little redundancy. The item reliability index was 1.00, indicating that the difficulty hierarchy of these motor super items would be stable if another group of children with the same traits and sample size were tested.[272]

High-Risk Clinical Signs

Longitudinal studies of LBW infants have been used to identify specific clinical signs or conditions that are most predictive of abnormal neurodevelopmental outcome, such as CP. The conclusions among studies are inconsistent because of the lack of standard criteria for the risk variables, demographic and clinical variation in the study samples, and use of different outcome measures. Results from these studies are summarized in Table 11-10.

Neonatal Period

During the neonatal period through 1 to 2 months after term (40 weeks of gestation), clinical signs suggestive of neuromotor abnormality include stiff, jerky movements or a paucity of movement. Prechtl and colleagues[112] developed an assessment technique based on the recognition of GMs that occur at specific times during maturation. Abnormal GMs are characterized as movements with "reduced complexity and a reduced variation. They lack fluency and frequently have an abrupt onset with all parts of the body moving synchronously."[114] Persistence of these movements is considered to be predictive of CP or cognitive impairment.[273]

Infancy

At 4 months of age, hypertonicity of the trunk or extremities is recognized as a high-risk clinical sign.[89,259,274] Neck extensor hypertonicity has been reported to be highly predictive of CP.[3] This finding correlates with neck hyperextension and shoulder retraction associated with the tonic labyrinthine reflex in the supine position, which has been identified in other studies as a high-risk sign.[275] Although neck hypertonicity was the single item most predictive of CP in one study, the majority of infants (60%) who exhibited this clinical sign did not subsequently develop CP.[3]

The predictive value of primitive reflexes has been extensively debated. Reflexes and neurological signs, such as the asymmetrical tonic neck reflex (ATNR) and tremulousness, have been correlated with CP in some studies[3,276] but not in others.[275] Of the four sections in the MAI, primitive reflexes

TABLE 11-10 ■ MOTOR IMPAIRMENT "RED FLAGS" DURING NEONATAL INTENSIVE CARE UNIT FOLLOW-UP

2 months*	Persistent asymmetrical head position; risk for plagiocephaly and torticollis
	Absent midline orientation even when visual stimulation is present
	Jerky or stiff movements of extremities
	Excessive neck or trunk hyperextension in supine position
4 months*	Poor midline head control in supine position
	Difficulty engaging hands at midline and in reaching for dangling toy
	Persistent fisting of hands
	Difficulty lifting head and supporting weight on arms in prone position
	Trunk hypertonicity or hypotonicity
	Resistance to passive movement in extremities
	Persistent, dominant asymmetrical tonic neck reflex ("fencing" position of arms)
	Stiffly extended or "scissored" legs with weight bearing on toes in supported standing
8 months*	Inability to sit and roll independently
	Inability to transfer objects between hands
	Persistent asymmetry of extremities with differences in muscle tone and motor skill
	Hypertonicity of trunk or extremities
12 months*	Inability to pull to stand, four-point crawl, walk around furniture
	Movement between basic positions
	Persistent asymmetry of control in extremities

Reprinted with permission from Sweeney JK, Gutierrez T: The dynamic continuum of motor and musculoskeletal development: implications for neonatal care and discharge teaching. In Kenner C, McGrath JM, editors: *Developmental care of newborns and infants,* ed 2, Glenview, IL, 2010, National Association of Neonatal Nurses.

*Ages corrected for prematurity.

were found to be the least predictive of later outcome.[259,277] The positive support reflex, characterized by stiff extension of the lower extremities when the infant is held in supported standing, is frequently cited as a high-risk sign, but this posture is seen in both term and LBW infants and has not been consistently associated with adverse sequelae.[254,259,275] Persistent primitive reflex activity and asymmetry have been identified as early signs of athetoid CP, more common in infants born at term.[278] In Figure 11-30 a dominant ATNR posture is demonstrated by a 4-month-old infant with athetoid CP. Immature automatic reactions of balance and equilibrium at 4 months, including head righting and the Landau reaction, have been found to be a significant predictor of abnormal neurological outcome.[275]

Comparing an infant's spontaneous, active movements with reflex or passive responses is important in determining risk for neurodevelopmental disability. Systematic observation of kicking activity in LBW infants indicated that infants with neurological impairment demonstrated less alternate kicking movement compared with typically developing LBW infants.[279] Abnormal patterns of kicking, including simultaneous flexion and extension of the hips and knees, were associated with subsequent CP.[280] Abnormalities of kicking described by Prechtl as "cramped-synchronized," that is, limited in variety and characterized by "rigid movement with all limbs and the trunk contracting and relaxing almost simultaneously," were observed in 3-month-old infants who were subsequently diagnosed with CP.[281]

In addition to qualitative differences in motor function, delayed acquisition of motor milestones is an important indicator of neuromotor impairment. Several investigations of the predictive validity of the MAI found volitional movement (gross and fine motor skills) to be the most predictive MAI category at 4 and 8 months.[259,277] This finding is supported by other studies in which delayed developmental milestones were significant predictors of later CP (Figure 11-31).[3,282] In particular, delay in achieving upright, gross motor milestones, such as sitting without support, creeping on hands to knees, and pulling to stand, was found to be useful in identifying infants with neuromotor impairment.[282]

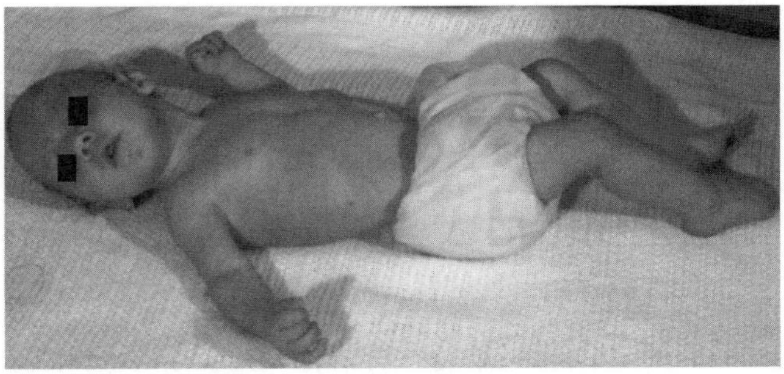

Figure 11-30 ■ Dominant asymmetrical tonic neck reflex in 4-month-old infant with athetoid cerebral palsy.

Challenges to Prediction of Neurodevelopmental Outcome

Accurate prediction of neurodevelopmental outcome of LBW infants on the basis of standard neuromotor tests is particularly challenging because of several complicating factors.

Impact of Medical Status on Test Performance

Infants with LBW often exhibit motor delay or neuromotor deviations because of their health or medical status, not because of neurological impairment. Two primary examples are residual influences from habitual positioning in the NICU and chronic medical conditions.

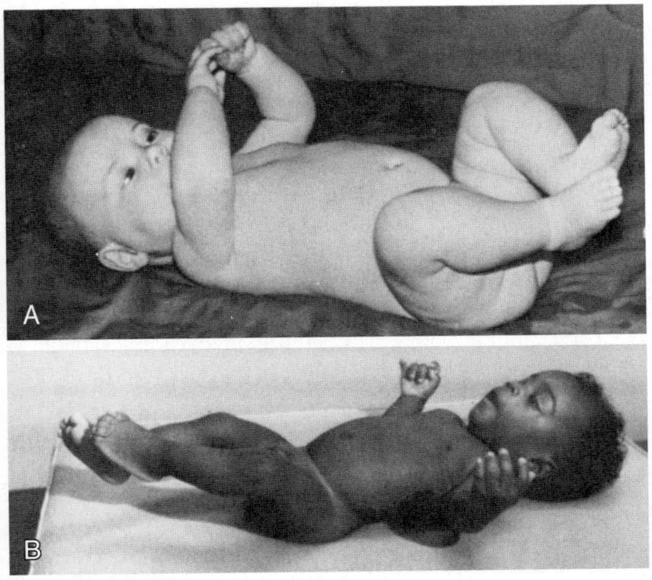

Figure 11-31 ■ **A,** Typically developing term infant at 4 months of age demonstrating ability to bring hands to midline and elevate legs with flexion and abduction of hips and dorsiflexion of ankles. **B,** Infant diagnosed with cerebral palsy at 5 months of age; note inability to bring hands to midline because of shoulder retraction, extension and adduction of hips with limited movement into flexion, and plantarflexion of ankles.

Variations in Posture and Movement Caused by Residual Influences from Time in the Neonatal Intensive Care Unit. Although current NICU positioning and handling procedures are increasingly sensitive to the developmental needs of the neonate, the application of life-sustaining interventions (e.g., mechanical ventilation) assumes priority in clinical management. On follow-up evaluation, these infants are typically delayed in reaching skills and in achieving antigravity postures.

LBW infants frequently exhibit asymmetry that may be related to intrauterine position or prolonged positioning in the NICU necessitated by surgical or medical intervention. On outpatient follow-up examinations, this asymmetry may appear as visual orientation to one side of the body, more mature upper-extremity skill on the same side, and asymmetry of primitive reflex activity. Physical deviations, such as tightness of neck musculature on the preferred side and relative weakness of the opposing muscles, or skull deformities (plagiocephaly) may also be present.[251,283] Asymmetrical motor function resulting from intrauterine or NICU positioning can usually be distinguished from early spastic hemiplegia or other hemisyndromes by clinical examination and by review of the infant's medical history.[251,259] Positional asymmetry is generally not associated with differences in muscle tone between the two sides of the body or with neuromotor abnormalities, such as fisting of the hand on the less-active side. Caregivers are advised to promote symmetrical posture through their physical handling of the infant, placement of the infant in relation to toys, social activity in the room, and use of cushions or rolls to maintain midline positioning for the infant's head and proximal musculature.

Prolonged Motor Delay from Chronic Medical Conditions. Infants with chronic lung disease typically exhibit low muscle tone, delayed gross motor function, and immature balance reactions. Motor skills are often delayed as long as the infant's pulmonary capacity is compromised, but the rate of developmental progress typically accelerates when the respiratory condition resolves.[233,284] Intervention for infants with persistent respiratory disease includes providing reassurance and support to the caregivers who are dealing with the demands and stresses of parenting a medically fragile child. Caregivers are advised to avoid aggressive physical activity and excessive sensory stimulation that could cause fatigue or tax the infant's limited respiratory capacity. At the same time, the child should be given opportunities to develop skills in nonmotor tasks. Adaptive positioning techniques reduce energy expenditure and fatigue while enabling the infant to be supported in age-appropriate postures (e.g., prone or upright sitting) for developing hand function, vestibular responses, and social skills.

Transient Dystonia

During the first year of life up to 60% of all LBW infants, as well as a number of term infants, exhibit abnormal neurological signs that subsequently resolve without evidence of major neurodevelopmental sequelae.[285-290] This phenomenon is referred to as "transient dystonia." The clinical characteristics of transient dystonia described most frequently are summarized in Table 11-11.

The presence of these findings on clinical examination poses a challenge to the physical therapist because they are often indistinguishable from clinical signs considered to represent early CP. From longitudinal studies researchers have suggested that infants with transient neuromotor abnormalities may be at increased risk for long-term neurodevelopmental problems. Infants who demonstrated abnormal neurological findings during the first 12 months, although considered to be developmentally normal at 1 year of age, reportedly had a higher incidence of mental, motor, and behavioral deficits in preschool and at school age.[88,287-289] However, a definite relationship between transient abnormalities in infancy and long-term developmental outcome has not been confirmed in other studies.[287,290,291]

TABLE 11-11 ■ CLINICAL CHARACTERISTICS OF TRANSIENT DYSTONIA

PERIOD	CLINICAL CHARACTERISTICS
Neonatal period	Neck extensor hypertonia Hypotonia Irritability; lethargy
Age 4 months	Increased muscle tone in extremities Truncal hypotonia Scapular adduction, shoulder retraction Persistent reflexes: asymmetrical tonic neck reflex; positive support reflex Asymmetry
Age 6-8 months	Increased muscle tone in lower extremities Truncal hypotonia; minimal trunk rotation Immature postural reactions Immaturity of fine motor skills

Abnormal neuromotor signs, even if they appear to be transient, should not be considered as clinically insignificant. These signs may indicate a child who is at risk for subtle neuromotor problems that will not be functionally evident until school age. Furthermore, neuromotor deviations, although transient, may interfere with the infant's ability to form attachments with caregivers. The infant who arches back into extension instead of cuddling, has poor head control and difficulty establishing eye contact, or stiffens when held may contribute to feelings of frustration, inadequacy, or resentment in caregivers. Instructing in handling techniques to minimize these postures, as well as informing caregivers that these behaviors reflect neurological instability commonly seen in LBW infants, are often valuable interventions during this transient period.

Differences between Preterm and Term Infant Neuromotor Function

Even when not compromised by chronic illness or neurological impairment, the motor development of preterm LBW infants differs from that of typical term infants. Compared with term infants, healthy preterm infants demonstrate variations in passive and active muscle tone and initially have greater joint mobility, such as increased popliteal angles and low muscle tone in the trunk.[283,292] In the older infant, increased extremity tone is often present, particularly in the hips and ankles.[253,283] Comparison studies have frequently noted that preterm infants tend to exhibit more neck hyperextension and scapular adduction and fewer antigravity movements in the supine position (Figure 11-32).*

Primitive reflexes such as the ATNR, Moro reflex, and positive support reflex persist longer in preterm infants, even when assessed at corrected age.[160,254,294] Gross and fine motor skills are frequently delayed in preterm infants, especially activities requiring active flexion, such as (1) bringing hands to midline and feet to hands, (2) trunk stability required for head control and upright sitting, and (3) trunk rotation for rolling and transitional movements.[283,293]

Preterm infants exhibit more asymmetry in active movement compared with infants born at term gestation, but asymmetry is usually not observed in passive tone or reflex activity.[251,283] One group of investigators concluded that "these findings convey an important clinical message: if motor asymmetries are only restricted to the facet of active muscle power, then they are unlikely to be of central origin and as such should not be seen as a sign of neurological impairment. In short, they constitute a typical feature of the post-term development of relatively healthy preterm infants."[251] For most premature infants, these early variations in movement and posture eventually resolve. However, in the first months of life neuromotor deviations may influence the infant's performance on a standard assessment of motor function or neurological status.

*References 163, 254, 274, 283, 289, 293.

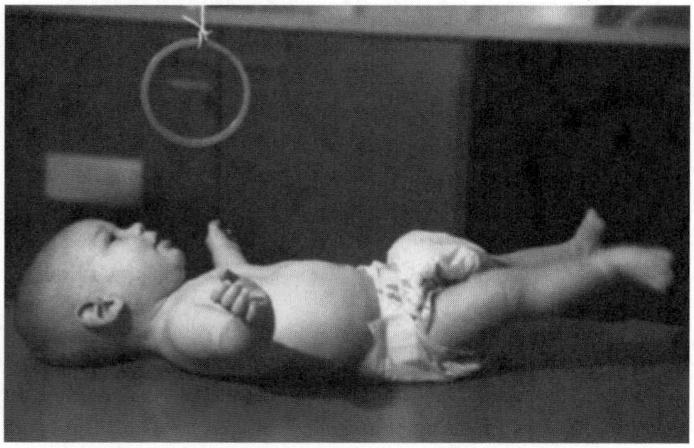

Figure 11-32 ■ Healthy preterm infant at 4 months of corrected age demonstrating neck hyperextension, scapular adduction and shoulder retraction, and limited antigravity movement into flexion.

NEUROMOTOR INTERVENTION

Levels of Intervention

Therapeutic intervention for the high-risk infant in the outpatient phase after discharge from the NICU occurs at multiple levels. Type and intensity of intervention depend on (1) the needs of the infant and family, (2) the structure and organization of the follow-up clinic, and (3) the availability of resources in a particular clinical and geographical setting.

Assessment as Intervention

The clinical assessment of an infant is a unique opportunity for intervention on behalf of the infant and family. For the full potential of this interaction to be realized, parents or caregivers must be informed and involved participants in the assessment process, not passive observers. The focus of intervention in this context is on parent or caregiver support with two primary components: education and positive reinforcement for parenting skills.

Education

The educational component of intervention includes enabling the parents of an at-risk infant to recognize their child's unique capabilities and strengths as well as his or her ability to respond to and influence the surrounding environment. Caregivers learn about their infant's individual responses to stimuli—for example, what causes their child to attend to a stimulus and what elicits stress reactions. Education of parents includes describing typical characteristics and common developmental patterns of the LBW or medically fragile infant that may differ from expectations that are based on observations or published descriptions of healthy, full-term infants. Parents of at-risk infants are informed about the appropriate sequence and pace of development for their child so they will be realistic in their expectations and interpretation of the child's progress. This anticipatory guidance enables parents to prepare for and maximize learning opportunities.

Reinforcement for Parenting Skills

During the follow-up examination, opportunities to provide positive reinforcement to caregivers need to be emphasized. Parents of a high-risk infant who responds inconsistently to affective cues should particularly be given positive feedback and affirmation for their investment of emotion and energy.[295] They should be reassured that they are providing appropriate and beneficial parenting and reminded that the infant's behavioral responses reflect neurobehavioral immaturity or instability rather than an unpleasant personality or negative affective feelings toward the caregiver.

Instruction in Home Management

A critical component of intervention is instruction in specific activities and handling techniques for home management. The recommendations are made on the basis of the therapist's knowledge of the infant's medical and neurological history, current health status, and findings from the neurodevelopmental assessment. The overall purpose may be to maximize a healthy child's growth potential or to promote developmental progress in an infant who demonstrates delay or neuromotor abnormality. In either case, the parent or caregiver must have a clear understanding of the purpose of the activity, what motor behavior it is intended to facilitate or counteract, the underlying neurodevelopmental process that the activity will support, and the desired response on the part of the infant. This enables the parent to participate more creatively in the process of intervention by adapting and modifying the recommendations according to the infant's responses and progress of the infant at home.

Although neuromotor handling recommendations are specific to the individual child, some intervention activities are applicable to many preterm infants.

Activities to Counteract Shoulder Retraction

Up to 50% of LBW infants reportedly demonstrate shoulder retraction.[163] This posture may inhibit the infant's ability to bring hands to midline and often results in delayed achievement of upper-extremity skills and rolling. To overcome shoulder retraction, play activities and carrying techniques that bring shoulders forward and hands to midline are encouraged.

Reaching

Most premature infants are immature in reaching skills, reducing their ability to interact with the environment. Activities to counteract shoulder retraction will promote reaching, but the infants should also be provided with other opportunities to practice this skill. Infants who are ready to initiate reaching at 3 to 4 months of age often have only a visually stimulating mobile suspended beyond their reach in the crib. Caregivers are advised to hang toys *within the child's reach* in the crib, playpen, infant seat, or other suitable places. Objects that are suspended, rather than handed to or placed in front of the infant, are preferred to promote the development of directed reach and grasp as well as shoulder stability (Figure 11-33). Commercially available, relatively inexpensive activity gyms that stand upright on the floor are highly recommended for infants at neurodevelopmental risk.

Head Centering and Symmetrical Orientation

Midline positioning of the head with symmetrical alignment of the trunk and extremities is encouraged to counteract the residual effects of asymmetrical positioning in utero or during hospitalization. Midline orientation will reduce the influence of the ATNR and promote symmetrical function of the right and left sides of the body. Asymmetry that is not caused by neurological dysfunction tends to resolve when positioning and environmental influences are modified.

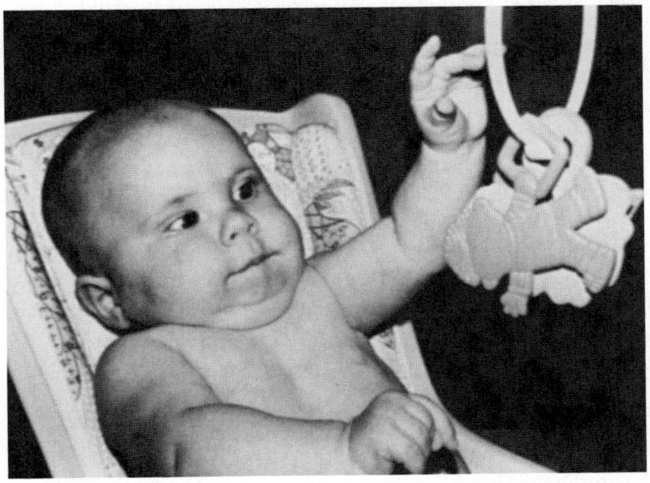

Figure 11-33 ■ Toys suspended directly in front of infant to encourage symmetrical reaching and midline orientation of head.

Prone Positioning

Active play time in the prone position with weight bearing on the arms is beneficial for the development of neck and trunk postural and shoulder girdle stability. The prone position also counteracts extension posturing tendencies because the influence of the tonic labyrinthine reflex in the prone position contributes to extremity flexion. However, parents of vulnerable premature infants are often hesitant to place their infants in the prone position for play. Many preterm infants demonstrate a low tolerance for prone positioning, particularly if they have relatively large heads and are visually attentive. Duration of the prone play position can be gradually increased; visually stimulating objects, including mirrors, musical toys, and the faces of siblings or caregivers, can be placed on the floor in front of the infant to encourage acceptance of the prone position. A roll or wedge positioned under the infant's axillae and upper chest will facilitate the ability to push up in prone, particularly for the infant with low muscle tone. An infant who is apprehensive or stressed when placed on the stomach may tolerate prone lying on the caregiver's chest, where reassuring eye contact can be maintained.

Head Balance

Balance activities to develop active head control are frequently recommended for preterm infants. Tilting responses are usually achieved most effectively with the infant in the parent's lap. Instruction to the caregivers often includes demonstration and practice using a doll before attempts with the infant. Emphasis is placed on the importance of (1) adequate trunk support; (2) movement through small ranges; (3) slow, graded motion; (4) desired head-righting response; and (5) sensitivity to indications of stress or fatigue.

Limited Use of Infant Jumper or Baby Walker

For infants with increased lower-extremity tone or a tendency for toe-standing, the use of baby walkers and jumpers is discouraged because of potential increased stiffness and extension posturing of the legs.[296] Mobile baby walkers are associated with a high risk of injury, including serious trauma such as burns, drowning, and severe head injuries resulting from falls down stairs.[297-300] However, baby walkers are usually enjoyable for infants and may provide caregivers with some needed moments of respite in stressed households. When recommending that time in a baby walker or jumper be restricted, the therapist should help the caregivers find alternative methods of positioning and amusement for the infant. Parents are often reluctant to discard a baby walker, believing that it promotes early ambulation and is beneficial for infants. Informing caregivers of the hazards of infant walkers and research findings indicating walker use may delay the acquisition of gross and fine motor skills enhances the likelihood of their cooperation to eliminate walkers and jumpers.[297,298,301,302] The lower-extremity tone and movement effects of semisitting activity centers that allow supported standing and some lateral steps have not been documented.

SUMMARY

This chapter on the NICU management and follow-up of at-risk neonates and infants has presented three theoretical models for NICU practice, reviewed neonatal neuropathological conditions related to movement disorders, and described expanded professional services for at-risk neonates and infants in a relatively new subspecialty within pediatric practice. Pediatric therapists participating in intensive care nursery and follow-up teams in the care of high-risk neonates and their parents are involved in an advanced-level practice area that requires heightened responsibility for accountability and for precepted clinical training (beyond general pediatric specialization) in neonatology and infant therapy techniques. Practice guidelines for the NICU from national task forces representing the American Physical Therapy Association and American Occupational Therapy Association indicate roles, proficiencies, and knowledge for neonatal therapy and designate the NICU as a restricted area of practice to therapy assistants, aides, and entry-level students on affiliation.

Inherent to this subspecialty practice is the challenge to design comprehensive neonatal therapy protocols and clinical paths that include standardized examination instruments, comprehensive risk-management plans, long-term follow-up strategies, and systematic documentation of outcome. Ongoing analyses of the physiological risk–therapeutic benefit relationship of neuromotor and neurobehavioral treatment for chronically ill and preterm infants must guide the NICU intervention process. The quality of collaboration between therapists and neonatal nurses largely determines the success of neonatal therapy implementation in the 24-hour care environment of the nursery.

Pediatric therapists working in neonatal units are encouraged to participate in follow-up clinics for NICU graduates to identify and analyze the development of movement dysfunction and behavioral sequelae that may, in the future, be minimized or prevented with creative neonatal treatment approaches. The important preventive aspect of neonatal treatment must be guided by careful analyses of neurodevelopmental and functional outcomes in the first year of life.

The preterm or medically fragile infant is at increased risk for major and minor neurodevelopmental problems that may manifest in infancy or not became evident until childhood. Prenatal and perinatal risk factors may identify infants who have a greater likelihood of neurological complications, but the relation between single factors and outcome is neither direct nor consistent. Abnormal neurological signs in the first year are also not reliably predictive of abnormal outcome. Attempts to identify factors that definitively indicate significant brain injury are complicated by changing NICU technology, management procedures, environmental variables, and variability among and within individual infants.

In deciding whether and when an infant requires regular intervention, consideration must be given both to the potential for abnormalities to resolve during the first year and to the time span that may elapse before definitive evidence of CP emerges. The pediatric therapist's long-term clinical management of the at-risk infant is guided by the developmental course of the individual infant over time, including behavioral and cognitive growth as well as neuromotor progress, considered within the context of the priorities and values of the family.

CASE STUDY 11-1 ■ HIGH-RISK INFANT A

Infant A was born prematurely at 29 weeks of gestation with a birth weight of 940 g. Her neonatal course was complicated by idiopathic respiratory distress syndrome, which was treated with surfactant.

She was first evaluated in the high-risk infant follow-up clinic at 4 months' corrected age (6 months' chronological age). Her mother stated that the infant had several respiratory illnesses after discharge from the NICU. She reported that her infant felt "tense" compared with her older child born at term and seemed to be "a little behind" in overall development. Performance on the BSID-II generated a Mental Development Index (MDI) of 94 and a Psychomotor Development Index (PDI) of 82. On the MAI this infant had a total risk score of 7. She had mildly increased lower-extremity muscle tone evident in mild resistance to passive range of motion of her hips and ankles. She demonstrated persistent primitive reflexes, including the ATNR, Moro reflex, and tonic labyrinthine reflex influence in the supine position. Head balance was immature, but emerging righting reactions were noted. When the infant was observed in the supine position her posture was extended, but she was beginning to bring her hands to midline. In prone, she had started to push up on elbows but posture was immature and unstable. Her parents were given recommendations for handling to include holding and carrying positions with shoulders forward to inhibit retraction, frequent play in the prone position, and increased opportunities for reaching in supine.

When the infant returned at 8 months' corrected age, her mother reported that progress had been made in the areas of rolling, talking, and sitting. She indicated that the body "stiffness" was less evident, but the infant still did not like to play on her "tummy" and instead preferred to use the baby walker. BSID-II scores at this time were MDI of 101 and PDI

CASE STUDY 11-1 ■ HIGH-RISK INFANT A—cont'd

of 81. The MAI total risk score was 9. Increased muscle tone observed previously was less evident and she had full hip mobility but some resistance to passive ankle movement. Muscle tone of the trunk was mildly hypotonic, but age-appropriate antigravity movements were demonstrated in all positions. Primitive reflexes were no longer evident except for the positive support reflex, characterized by toe-standing tendency during weight bearing. Balance reactions were present but immature in some areas, including head righting into flexion and protective extension reactions. In volitional skills, the infant was now sitting independently for up to 30 seconds, could roll from supine to prone, and could pivot sideways in the prone position. She could pick up a block with either hand and transfer objects. Immaturity was observed in sitting balance, inability to move out of sitting, and failure to move forward on the floor (i.e., low two-point crawl). She attempted to pick up a pellet but was unable to do so. Her parents were advised to discontinue using the baby walker and to maximize play time on the floor. Because the infant reportedly enjoyed watching her 4-year-old sibling, the therapist recommended that he play on the floor beside her. Her mother was also advised to provide the infant with tiny bits of food (e.g., Cheerios) to practice fine motor dexterity.

When seen at 12 months' corrected age, the infant had an MDI of 108 and a PDI of 88. Although not yet walking independently, she was cruising with good weight shift and balance. She was able to creep reciprocally on hands and knees and pulled to stand. She picked up a pellet with an inferior pincer grasp. No deviations of muscle tone or reflex development were observed during examination by the developmental pediatrician. The infant was developing normally and will return for follow-up at 2 years of age. Her parents were advised to call if she was not walking within 2 months or if they had any concerns regarding her pattern of independent walking.

In the management of this child who demonstrated abnormal signs, the primary responsibilities of the pediatric therapist were ongoing assessment and parental guidance and teaching. Although initial concerns about this infant's muscle tone and reflex deviations were present, diagnosing her with a particular condition would have been inappropriate. When followed up over time, the abnormalities resolved and proved to be transient. This child should continue to be followed up in the high-risk infant clinic because she remains at risk for other neurodevelopmental problems that may not become evident until school age.

CASE STUDY 11-2 ■ HIGH-RISK INFANT B

Infant B was born prematurely at 29 weeks of gestation with a birth weight of 1200 g. The neonatal course was complicated by idiopathic respiratory distress syndrome and persistent apnea and bradycardia. Cranial ultrasonography revealed a left subependymal hemorrhage with ventriculomegaly and left-sided PVL.

She was first seen in the high-risk infant follow-up clinic at 4 months' corrected age (6 months and 17 days' chronological age). The parents stated that they had no specific concerns regarding their daughter's development. On the BSID-II the infant received an MDI of 96 and a PDI of 87. On the MAI she received a total risk score of 14. Muscle tone was normal at rest but increased when she was active or agitated. Tone in the lower extremities was mildly increased with restricted passive movement in the hip adductor and gastrosoleus muscles bilaterally. In the supine position she was frequently in an extended posture and brought her hands to midline only once during the examination. In prone she was able to push up and elevate her head while kicking actively. In the prone suspended position, she showed good postural elevation but movements were stiff. Persistent primitive reflexes included the tonic labyrinthine reflex in supine, ATNR, neonatal positive support reflex, and bilateral ankle clonus. Plantar grasp with toe curling was observed on the right. Righting and equilibrium reactions were emerging. She showed a mature Landau reflex with full extension in prone suspension, which is atypical for her age. In volitional movement, mild asymmetry was evident because she had difficulty bringing her right arm forward when prone and brought her left arm to midline more frequently. Her kicking pattern when supine was low (close to the surface), and she did not elevate her hips. On the right side, hip extension was accompanied by knee extension and plantarflexion of the ankle. She was not yet reaching for objects, and her hands were frequently fisted, particularly on the right. Her parents were assisted with handling skills to reduce shoulder retraction and extension posturing and to facilitate symmetry in movements and posture.

When the family returned for a follow-up visit at 6 months they reported that their daughter was making good progress, but she continued to prefer use of her left hand in spite of their efforts to encourage use of the right hand. At this evaluation, Bayley Scale scores were an MDI of 94 and a PDI of 83; the MAI total risk score was 13. The infant had made the following developmental progress: (1) rolling from supine to prone (over the right side only), (2) beginning sitting balance, and (3) reaching out and grasping objects. She showed a preference for and greater skill and dexterity with her left hand. Occasional fisting was still observed on the right hand. She transferred objects only from right to left. Muscle tone continued to be increased in the lower extremities, with restricted passive mobility of the gastrosoleus muscles bilaterally. Toe clawing was observed on the right with minimal spontaneous dorsiflexion observed on this side. Primitive reflexes were integrated except for persistent neonatal positive support and ATNR to the right. Automatic reactions were improved, but balance responses were asymmetrical, with equilibrium reactions and protective extension reactions delayed on the right. Although the developmental progress was encouraging, the persistent asymmetry remained a major concern. The infant was referred to a developmental intervention program with the recommendation that she receive consistent pediatric therapy in her home at least once a week.

Continued

CASE STUDY 11-2 ■ HIGH-RISK INFANT B—cont'd

The infant was seen in the follow-up clinic at 12 months' corrected age (14 months' chronological age). On the BSID the MDI was 95 and the PDI was 82. She now was creeping reciprocally on hands and knees. When she pulled to stand she consistently brought the left foot up first. She cruised holding onto furniture with a tendency to stand on her toes on the right. She picked up cubes with either hand but showed partial palmar grasp on the right. She picked up a pellet with an inferior pincer grasp on the left but scooped it into the palm of the right hand. Muscle tone continued to be mildly increased in the lower extremities with Achilles tendon tightness, particularly on the right. She sat independently with a mildly flexed thoracic spine. When moving into and out of sitting, she lacked full trunk rotation, and weight was predominately over the left hip. Language development was considered appropriate for her age. The infant was diagnosed with mild right hemiplegic CP. It was recommended that she continue in the intervention therapy program and return for reevaluation at 2 years of age.

In the management of this child, the role of the pediatric therapist was assessment of neurodevelopmental status and referral to therapy when it became evident that the abnormalities of muscle tone were persisting and interfering with developmental progress. Of note, this child's MDI scores were in the normal range at both the 4- and 8-month examinations. Because the BSID-II does not require infants to perform tasks with both hands, a normal score can be obtained by using just one side of the body. This child should continue to be followed up in the high-risk infant clinic after 2 years of age to provide periodic reassessment and guidance to the family as they confront questions of school placement and program planning for their child.

Acknowledgement

We appreciate significant contributions to the case studies by Marcia Williams, PT, MPH, PhD.

References

To enhance this text and add value for the reader, all references are included on the companion Evolve site that accompanies this textbook. This online service will, when available, provide a link for the reader to a Medline abstract for the article cited. There are 311 cited references and other general references for this chapter, with the majority of those articles being evidence-based citations.

CHAPTER 12 Management of Clinical Problems of Children with Cerebral Palsy*

CLAUDIA R. SENESAC, PT, PhD, PCS

KEY TERMS

cerebral palsy
direct intervention
family
indirect intervention
postural and movement compensation
research
spasticity
treatment strategies

OBJECTIVES

After reading this chapter the student or therapist will be able to:

1. Identify the parameters of the diagnosis of cerebral palsy including motor, family, and psychosocial components.
2. Analyze the multifaceted aspects of the clinical problem and appreciate a multifaceted approach to evaluation and treatment.
3. Analyze treatment strategies and their application to clinical problems.
4. Identify and critique current research for the pediatric client with cerebral palsy.
5. Identify the therapist's role in the treatment of the child with cerebral palsy, with family involvement, in different settings, and with other health professionals.

OVERVIEW

Historical Perspective

Cerebral palsy is a misnomer at best. Little[1] suggested the name in the mid-1800s, but there is still no established direct relationship between the identifiable state of the brain and the distortions in posture and movement control that we are able to observe in the individual.[2,3] The condition is not always evident at birth, although the work of Prechtl[4] statistically supports the possibility of a link between the quality of spontaneous movements in the first months of life and later difficulties in coordinated movement expression. In only a small number of children has a specific lesion been identified that corresponds to the observed motor responses of the child, and this elite group includes children with porencephaly and other early developmental malformations of the brain. Whether there is a biochemical element in the brain of a child that distorts the actual motor learning process has not been established. There is a shocking variability in the age at which intervention is initiated for individual children and a wide variety of programs that do not necessarily take into account the current information available from clinical studies on efficient motor development and brain function. This confusion has led us astray in understanding the process of movement and postural distortion that characterizes children who carry the label of "cerebral palsy."

Historically, the evolution of diagnosis and treatment intervention or management is clear and relates to the recognition of the special needs of this minority of society. The British physician Little identified the condition on the basis of observable characteristics of movement and posture, or—in other words—the external features of the condition, so the initial efforts at remediation fell to orthopedists such as Deaver and Phelps.[3,5,6] Deaver placed importance on external bracing that was periodically reduced in the hope that the child would take over control of increasing parts of his or her own body.[5] Phelps used bracing and surgery and was a significant force in obtaining schooling for these children in the United States.[6] He pointed out that they did not belong in academic classes with children diagnosed as retarded or mentally handicapped and that children with cerebral palsy should be exposed to a traditional academic curriculum. In his Children's Rehabilitation Institute in Reisterstown, Maryland, he also advocated restriction of a more functional limb to encourage use of the one less used, particularly in work with the upper extremities.

In the 1950s and 1960s there simultaneously emerged new theories of neuromotor behavior that redefined the clinical characteristics of cerebral palsy and permitted clinicians to orient their intervention strategies to the principles of motor development and motor learning. Kabat in conjunction with Knott introduced proprioceptive neuromuscular facilitation (PNF), which was applied to children with movement disorders and to adults with a history of trauma.[7] The use of diagonal patterns of movement in this approach changed the customary postures of the child and introduced more functional movement patterns in logical learning sequences. Physical and occupational therapist Margaret Rood added the more specific sensory components of ice and light quick brushing of the skin surface to guide the desired motor response.[8] She spoke of the need to focus attention on both "heavy work" and "light work" during the early development of movement skills. These terms referred to the central body moving over limb support and limb movement with central stability. Bobath was working

*This chapter is dedicated to Christine Nelson—master clinician, true friend, and mentor. Her gifts as a clinician and artistic eclectic approach to the treatment of children were unmatched and often seemed beyond what one could comprehend. She ever changed those she touched and enlightened all those she taught. Christine will be forever missed and yet her *gift of touch* will be everlasting and live on in her patients, students, and friends.

in London at this same time and observed the need to have a dynamic interaction between stability and mobility, after finding that inhibition of the reflexive movements was not sufficient to change the functional outcome of the child with cerebral palsy.[9] They pointed out that the areas of the child's body that appeared to be spastic changed when the body was placed in a different relationship to gravity. This observation held up for reexamination the prevailing view of the time, namely, that spasticity existed in a tendon or muscle, a specific structure.

Cerebral palsy was identified in the mid-1900s as an incident that occurred shortly before, during, or shortly after the birth of the infant. Early intervention was recommended. This time line was extended to cover the first 2 years of life, which included early cases of meningitis, encephalitis, near-drowning accidents, and so forth. Although the clinicians mentioned tried to define cerebral palsy as a "disorder of posture and movement control," many of the children also had learning problems and inadequate general brain development. There was a general agreement on categories according to movement characteristics that included spasticity, athetosis, flaccidity, ataxia, and rigidity. Categorization according to the part of the body affected was added to identify hemiplegia, quadriplegia, diplegia, and even monoplegia, affecting one limb, and triplegia, affecting three limbs. It was noted that some children moved from one category to another as they matured, and therapists began to be aware that a child with high tone could have some low tone underneath when spasticity was inhibited. Fluctuating tone could be confused with ataxia, and the precise intervention strategy might be elusive.

The birth process is complex at many different levels. Sequential hormonal changes alert both the fetus and the mother that it is time for a separation. The infant moves into position for exiting the uterus through the birth canal while the mother's body prepares to participate in the work (labor) of the expulsion. When all goes smoothly, the head of the infant is molded by the passage through the birth canal, and the membranous-like cranial plates return to their balanced alignment and functional motion.

When the birth process is prolonged for any of many reasons, the physiological timing of these changes is interrupted. Unique combinations of pressure may make it difficult for the membranous structures to maintain their structural alignment. That lack of structural alignment may persist long after birth and affect future movement and development. Rapid changes of pressure, with minor misalignments of the head and body during the birth process, result in sufficient trauma to affect the nervous system and the delicate fascia and in a small percentage of infants to affect the expression of spontaneous movements. In the majority of healthy infants born at term the spontaneous movements seem to assist in the activation of the central body and the limbs so that physiological changes in the fascia are sufficient to permit a typical expression of developmental movement responses after birth. Body movement and respiration are coordinated with the infant's physiological rhythms in this initial adaptation to the world of gravity. With complications of the pregnancy or the birth process, these spontaneous movements that are so easily made by the healthy infant become laborious and sometimes impossible, affecting motor actions, postural mechanisms, and the basic physiological rhythms. Cerebral palsy is a heterogeneous collection of clinical syndromes, not a disease or pathological or etiological entity.[10] Little described cerebral palsy as "a persistent disorder of movement and posture appearing early in life and due to a developmental nonprogressive disorder of the brain."[3] Current definitions have reiterated that atypical execution of movement and interference with postural mechanisms are the key characteristics of this nonprogressive disorder affecting the developing brain.[10,11]

Cerebral palsy affects the total development of the child. The primary disorder is of motor execution, but common associated dysfunctions include sensory deficits (hearing or vision); epilepsy; learning disabilities; cognitive deficits; emotional, social, and behavioral problems; and speech and language disorders. The degree of severity varies greatly from mild to moderate to severe.[10-12]

Diagnostic Categorization of the Characteristics of Cerebral Palsy

In general, a diagnosis of cerebral palsy suggests that the individual has a lesion within the motor control system with a residual disorder of posture and movement control. Varying degrees of associated components are seen with this disorder that further define the category that a child may fall into: severity of motor abnormalities, anatomical and magnetic resonance imaging findings, extent of associated impairments, and the timing of the neurological injury. In addition, the labeling process often identifies the parts of the body that are primarily involved. Diplegia, hemiplegia, and quadriplegia, respectively, indicate that the lower extremities, one side of the body, or all four extremities are affected. This can be misleading to the therapist who is working with infants because these children often change their clinical signs and symptoms and their respective disabilities. The disorder is not progressive, but the presentation of involvement of body segments may manifest itself differently as the child grows and his or her structure and tonal distribution changes against gravity.

The clinician must be aware that the categorization of cerebral palsy is based on descriptions of observable characteristics; thus, it is a symptomatic description. The hypertonus of spasticity prevents a smooth exchange between mobility and stability of the body. Constriction of respiratory adaptability occurs with poor trunk control. Incrementation of postural tone occurs with an increase in the speed of even passive movement, and clonus may occur in response to sudden passive movement. Although diagnostic terms reflect the distribution of excessive postural tone, the entire body must be considered to be involved. Spasticity, by nature, involves reduced quantity of movement, which makes its distribution easier to identify. Recruitment of the corticomotor neuron pool is affected in the presence of spasticity, and therefore timing issues result in the poor grading of agonists and antagonists.[13,14] There is also a risk of reduction in the range of limb movements over time when therapy does not include active adaptation in end ranges and organization of postural transitions.[15] This category (spasticity) has the highest occurrence of cases of cerebral palsy.[16] There are several spastic types of cerebral palsy that require clarification. Spastic diplegia implies that the lower extremities are more involved than the upper extremities but could manifest with varying degrees of hand function, and often the involvement is asymmetrical.[14] Hemiplegia displays involvement of one side of the body and can manifest itself with the arm involved more than the leg or the leg involved as much as or more than the arm.[10] Quadriplegia, as the term implies, involves the entire body.[10]

Dyskinetic syndromes, which include athetosis and dystonic types of cerebral palsy, are characterized by involuntary movements. The term *dyskinetic* is commonly used with children who lack posture and axial and trunk coactivation. The excessive peripheral movement of the limbs occurs without central coactivation. Dystonic types of cerebral palsy are dominated by tension, and athetosis usually has a hypotonic base or underlying tone. Dyskinetic syndromes may occur with greater involvement in particular extremities, although the condition most often interferes with postural stability as a whole. When pathological or primitive reflexes are used to accomplish movement, there is a difficulty with midline orientation. Dyskinetic distribution of postural tone is changeable in force and velocity, particularly during attempted movement by the individual. Midrange control is limited if present at all, and frequently end ranges of motion are used to accomplish a motor task.[10] For these reasons, these children have a reduced risk for contractures over time.

Hypotonicity is another category of cerebral palsy, but it may also mask undiagnosed degenerative conditions (see Chapter 13). Recent reports suggest that "pure hypotonia" is not an attribute of cerebral palsy, and further testing to rule out other causation may be indicated.[16]

Hypotonia in a young infant may also be a precursor of a dyskinetic syndrome. Often, athetoid movements or spasticity are not noticed until the infant is attempting antigravity postures, although there may be some disorganization apparent to the careful observer. Generalized hypotonia often masks some specific areas of deep muscle tension with accompanying local immobility.

True ataxia is a cerebellar disorder that is seen more frequently as a sequela of tumor removal (see Chapters 21 and 25) than as a problem occurring from birth. Ataxic syndromes are more commonly found in term infants. This type of cerebral palsy is a diagnosis of exclusion. In a small number of patients there is congenital hypoplasia of the cerebellum. Most of these children are hypotonic at birth and display delays in motor acquisition and language skills.[10] Recruitment and timing issues remain problems in this population. Trajectory of the limbs, speed, distance, power, and precision are frequently documented as problems in this category. Midline is often achieved, but control of midrange movements of the extremities and control of trunk postural reactions are affected.

These classifications, even when accurately applied, give the therapist only a general idea of the treatment problem and must be supplemented by a specific analysis of posture and movement control during task performance, an interview for home care information, and assessment of treatment responses (see Chapters 7 and 8). The therapist is then ready to establish treatment priorities for the individual child.

Many of the characteristics described in the preceding paragraphs also apply to children who have had closed head traumas or brain infections. Further information can be obtained in Chapters 24 and 26. Some of the treatment suggestions that follow may also be applied in such cases. As with cerebral palsy, early positioning and handling after trauma may deter later problems.

EVALUATIVE ANALYSIS OF THE INDIVIDUAL CHILD

Initial Observations and Assessment

Examination of the individual child begins with careful observation of the interaction between parents and the child, including parental handling of the child that occurs spontaneously. Some additional insight can be gained about the relationship between parent and child by observing how the child is handled both physically and emotionally. Does the child receive and respond to verbal reassurance from the parent in the therapy situation? Are immediate bribes offered to the child? Does parent eye contact increase the child's confidence in responding? Does family communication convey the idea of negativity in the therapy situation or a difficult experience that will soon come to an end? The family orientation will affect the response of the child while working with the therapist. Making connections with the child and family is a critical component to a successful relationship that forms with ongoing treatment.

The therapist working as part of a team may have the advantage of a social worker or psychologist who will relate to the problems and motivations of the parents. Parental responses toward the disabled child arise from the parents' uncertainty, fear, concern for the future, disappointment, distress, and other typical reactions to this unforeseeable life experience. The therapist will observe positive changes in parental orientation to the child as the parents are educated as to what can be done to help the child move forward. They may be further assisted by opportunities to interact with well-adjusted parents of older children with a diagnosis of cerebral palsy. Assisting families to make connections with other families and children in the community provides them a supportive network of people who share similar experiences.

A problem-based approach to the assessment and management of the child with cerebral palsy includes the family as key members of the team.[17] While observing the child, the experienced therapist will want to periodically elicit from the parents their view of the problem. By listening carefully, the therapist will also be able to discern the emotional impressions that have surrounded previous experiences with professionals. Sometimes what is not said is more important than what is verbally offered immediately. Listening carefully and clarifying facts are more important than overwhelming the parents with excessive information and suppositions during early contacts. Observation of the family response to information will keep the therapist on track in developing a positive relationship with parents that deepens over time. The therapist's role is often as interpreter of medical information as parents attempt to make some sense of their child's diagnosis.

The next general step is to observe, in as much detail as possible, the spontaneous movement of the child when separated from the parent (Figure 12-1). Is the child very passive? Does he or she react to the supporting surface (Figure 12-2)? Are there atypical patterns of movement to

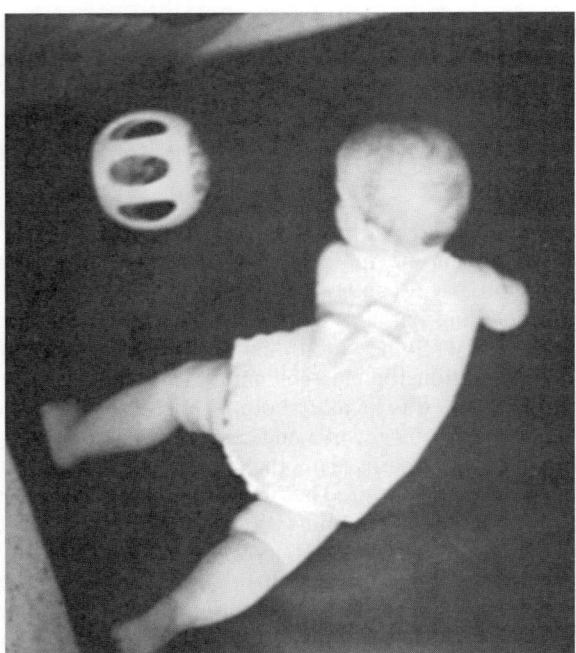

Figure 12-1 ■ Typical infants accumulate a multitude of experiences as they move smoothly in their environments.

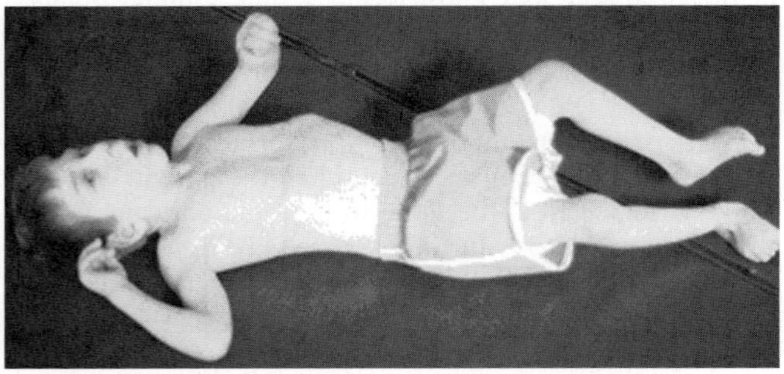

Figure 12-2 ■ Lack of support surface contact demonstrates difficulty conforming to and activating off of the supporting surface.

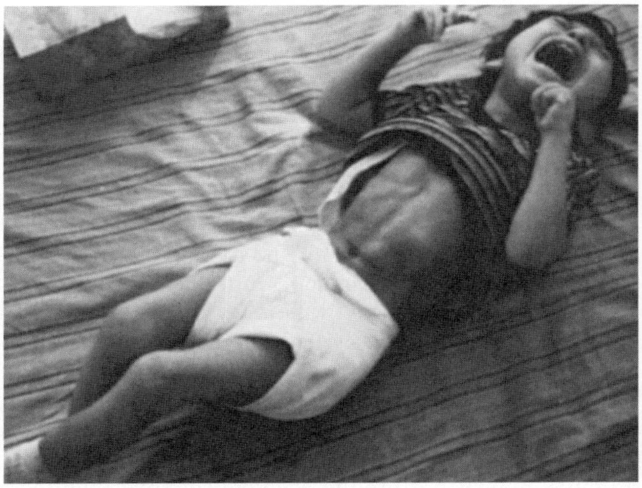

Figure 12-3 ■ Emotional reactions are also translated into stronger spastic reactions influencing respiratory adaptation (see Chapter 5 on the limbic system).

reach a toy? Are clearly typical responses occurring with specific interference by reflexive synergies or total patterns of movement? Does the child rely heavily on visual communication? Do the eyes focus on a presented object, or does the postural abnormality increase with an effort to focus the eyes? Does the child lead or follow hand activity? Does an effort to move result only in an increase of postural tone with abnormal distribution? Does respiration adapt to new postural adaptations (Figure 12-3)? Is the child able to speak as well while standing as while sitting?

This type of observation is valuable because movement patterns directly reflect the state of the central nervous system and can generally be seen while the parent is still handling the child.[18] Once the child is on the mat or treatment table, outer clothing can be removed to observe interactions of limbs and trunk. Movement responses of the child can gradually be influenced directly by the therapist. Many disabled children associate immediate undressing in a new environment with a doctor's office, and the chance to establish rapport is lost. In some instances it is preferable to have the parent gently remove some of the child's clothing or even to leave the child dressed during the first therapy session. Gaining the trust of the child and parent is crucial during the first few sessions.

Examination of the child's status is more likely to be adequate if the therapist follows the child's lead when possible. Notes can be organized later to conform to a specific format. It is often possible to jot down essential information while observing the child moving spontaneously or while the parent is holding the child. Reactions to the supporting surface will differ in these circumstances. After the session, the therapist may dictate the salient information into a tape recorder, or a videotape or digital tape can be made to capture the interactions and movement patterns. Attention should be given to the typical movements of the child and to those postures that the child spontaneously attempts to control. Building a treatment plan will be based on the strengths of the child noted in these first encounters. Eye alignment is important; the correspondence between visual and postural activity relates directly to the quality of movement control. It is important to note the interaction between the two sides of the body. In noting atypical reactions and compensatory movement patterns, the therapist must also indicate the position of the body with respect to the supporting surface. There is a tendency to compile more pertinent data by learning to cluster observations and relating one to the other. Children are vibrant beings. Their choices of position tell us something about their habits and how comfortable they are in this situation. To be the slave of a preformulated sequence destroys the decision-making initiative appropriate to the situation at hand. This is true for the therapist as well as for the child. Although it is important to see the child in every position, making smooth transitions from one to another will ensure that the child is secure and give the therapist a more accurate assessment of the child's abilities. Noting the "preferred" position or movement strategy can provide information about the ability to conform to a support surface, initiation of movement, muscle tightness, muscle tone distribution, and movement variety in the child's repertoire.

Standardized assessments are often used by facilities to document the developmental level of the functioning of a child with disability and to justify treatment. The Gross Motor Function Measure (GMFM) was developed to assess children with cerebral palsy and has good reliability and validity for children aged 5 months to 16 years.[19,20] The Gross Motor Function Classification System (GMFCS), developed in 1997, is often used in conjunction with the GMFM.[21,22] The GMFCS has five levels of classification for gross motor function, emphasizing movement initiation related to sitting, walking, and mode of mobility. Descriptors of motor function span an age range of 2 to 18 years, reflecting environmental and personal factors. The Pediatric Evaluation and Disability Inventory (PEDI) assesses children aged 6 months to 7.5 years in three domains: social, self-care, and mobility.[23] The Functional Independence Measure for Children was developed as a test of disability in children aged 6 months to 12 years. This assessment covers self-care, sphincter control, mobility, locomotion, communication, and social cognition.[24-26] This tool has been used to track outcomes over time. Although several instruments have been developed that meet psychometric criteria to document function in children with disabilities, the GMFM and the PEDI are thought to be the most responsive to change in this population of children because of their good reliability and validity.[27,28] Often the decision to use an instrument to assess development will be left up to the clinician or facility. To date, there is no one tool that will cover all the categories necessary to document change in a child with cerebral palsy, so the clinician will need to rely on observational skills to describe quality of movement and response to changes in position in space and handling.

Each child will differ in the ability to separate from her or his parents. Spontaneity of movement, interest in toys, general activity level, and communication skills will also vary from child to child.[29] Responding to the specific needs of the child enables the therapist to set priorities more effectively. If fatigue is likely to be a factor, it is important first to evaluate those reactions that present themselves spontaneously, followed by direct handling to determine the child's response and potential for more typical movements. Movements or abilities for which there is a major interference from spasticity, reflexive responses, or poor balance may be better checked at the termination of the assessment so that the child remains in a cooperative mood as long as possible. Information regarding favorite sleeping positions, self-care independence, and chair supports used at home can be requested as the session comes to a close.

Clinical reasoning involves taking information from the assessment, including observations, results from standardized tools, family input, and the therapist's handling of the child to formulate a treatment plan. Placing this information into a framework that makes sense to the therapist, the physician, other health professionals, and the family will assist in goal writing. The International Classification of Functioning, Disability and Health (ICF)[30] is well known in the field of health care and allows one to see the overall interaction of the person with his or her environment and activities in the presence of the health condition.[30]

Reactions to Placement in a Position

If the child totally avoids certain postures during spontaneous activity, these are likely to be the more important positions for the therapist to evaluate. Observing how the child conforms to the support surface and how much contact there is with the surface will provide information about the ability to initiate movement from the surface. Support surface contact is essential for weight bearing and weight shifting to occur; both are critical for movement. Placement of the child in the previously avoided position will permit the therapist to feel the resistance that prevents successful control by the child.[29] As mentioned previously, this may be held for the end of the assessment. The parent should play an active role in the assessment whenever possible. Continued dialog with the parents reveals factors such as the frequency of a poor sitting alignment at home or a habitual aversion to the prone position. Sitting close to the television set or tilting the head when looking at books should also be noted so that functional vision skills can be related to other therapy interventions.[31] These contributions by the parents establish the importance of good observation and the need for parents and the therapist to work cooperatively. Therapists of different specialties need to initiate continuing communication to coordinate therapy objectives.

According to the guide for typical development, infants should be able to maintain the posture in which they are placed before they acquire the ability to move into that position alone.[32,33] The problems presented by cerebral palsy occur to some extent as a reaction to the field of gravity in which the child moves.[32] Visual perceptions of spatial relationships motivate and determine movement patterns while the child must react at a somatic level to the support surface. It is helpful, therefore, to attempt placement of the infant or child into developmentally or functionally appropriate postures that are not assumed spontaneously (Figure 12-4). Resistance to placement indicates an increase in tone, a structural problem, or an inability to adapt to the constellation of sensory inputs for that alignment. A movement that resists control by the therapist will be even less possible for the child. What appears to be a passive posture may hide rapid increases in hypertonicity when movement is initiated or instability of a proximal joint when weight bearing is

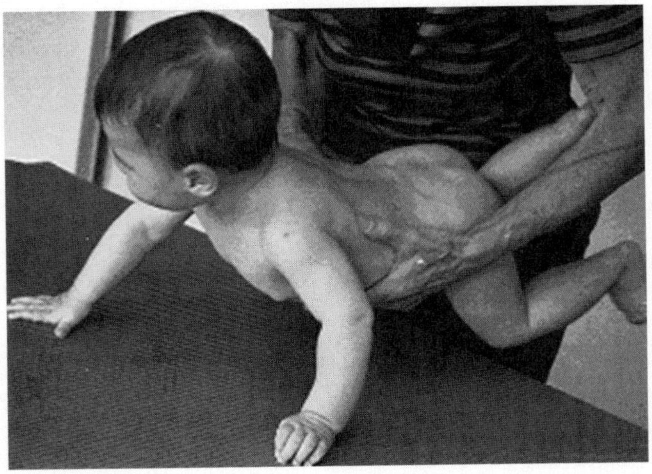

Figure 12-4 ■ Baby treatment must be dynamic and precisely oriented to individual needs.

initiated. A child may have learned to avoid excitation of the unwanted reactions and may fix the body position to avoid the alignment that cannot be controlled. Another child may enjoy the sensory experience of accelerated changes in postural tone and deliberately set them off as a means of receiving the resulting stimulation to his or her system.

VISUAL-MOTOR ASSESSMENT

It is the visual-motor aspect of performance function that is of primary concern to the therapist because spatial judgments are needed to control movement of the body in an upright alignment. The infant who is able to stand and walk along a support and then seems unable to let go of the support is often found to have functional vision interferences. The child with cerebral palsy most often demonstrates significant neuromotor delay in the developmental process, which often results in the inadequate establishment of matching of inputs from the postural and visual systems (Figure 12-5). Visual-motor learning experiences are filled with compensatory responses from both systems. Vision plays an important role in early motor development for learning about, manipulating, and exploring the environment. Therefore vision requires attention during the assessment of motor abilities. (Refer to Chapter 28.)

The visual system in its development has many parallels with the postural system.[34] Binocular control and freedom of movement are necessary for the system to function properly. Ambient visual processing must be integrated with central visual processing to take in information that relates to position in space and to focus on a particular target. A simple screening examination may check acuity at 20 feet on the E chart and declare vision to be normal. An ophthalmological examination is needed to determine the health of the eye structures, particularly in the case of infants born preterm. Equally important is a functional vision examination given by a behavioral or developmental optometrist to reveal the level of efficiency that the two eyes have achieved in working together and whether the ability to focus in far and near ranges is smoothly established. Strabismus dysfunctions commonly coexist with cerebral palsy and may cause the child to receive a double image of environmental objects. Judgments about space are related to a three-dimensional perception of the surrounding environment, which requires coordinated use of the two eyes. Conservative management of eye alignment problems is done with the use of lenses and prisms by the experienced optometrist, which permits the therapist to work for basic head control by the child before any irreversible changes are made to the eye muscles. Eye movement differentiates from head movement in much the same way that the hand differentiates from general arm movement, corresponding to general maturation of the central system.

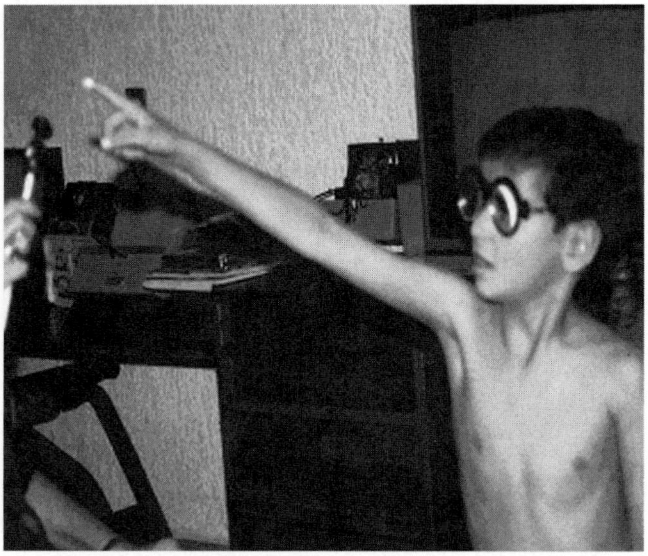

Figure 12-5 ■ Touching the target integrates the new visual perception with the motor response.

Because the visual system is first a motor system, children with cerebral palsy most often have difficulty separating eye movement from head movement and controlled convergence for focal changes. When their posture is supported, eye movement can proceed to evolve in accuracy and complexity. With inadequate alignment of the head in relation to the base of support, the visual system accumulates distortions and inconsistent input, which leads to the formation of an inadequate perceptual base for later motor learning (see Chapters 4 and 28). Even after improvement in the control of posture and movement, the visual system continues to adapt to the previous faulty visual-motor learning, resulting in perceptual confusion and inefficient organization of body movement in space. The therapist who is working for improved motor control may notice that such a child reacts with adequate postural adaptations when facing the therapist or a support and that the movement quality seems to disintegrate when the child faces an open space. This immediately jeopardizes the ability of the child to use her or his new responses after leaving the therapy environment. Visual orientation to the environment will dictate alignment against gravity, and the reverse is also true; poor alignment against gravity will affect visual orientation to the environment. Movement, postural stability, and muscle activation are closely related to vision.[35]

Padula, a behavioral optometrist specializing in neuro-optometric rehabilitation, has described a posttrauma vision syndrome in adults with acquired central dysfunction and has applied this information to children with cerebral palsy.[36] A perceptual distortion in the perceived midline of the body, known as *visual midline shift syndrome,* is corrected with the use of prescribed prism lenses, which then permits the child to step into the perceived space with more confidence (Figure 12-6). The observant therapist will begin to notice that the sudden increase in neuromuscular tension in a child taking steps in a walker is often accompanied by closing of the eyes. This seems to be a momentary inability of the central processing system to integrate the information arriving from different sources. With the use of prism correction, the child experiences the body as more coherent with visual-spatial perceptions. By incorporating an understanding of visual observations into intervention strategies, physical and occupational therapists are able to note compensatory adaptations by the complementary systems and use them to their advantage in effective treatment intervention.

Some children who walk on their forefeet or even on their toes and who have made little if any permanent gait change after the use of inhibitory casting or orthotics also fall into the population described previously. With prisms that

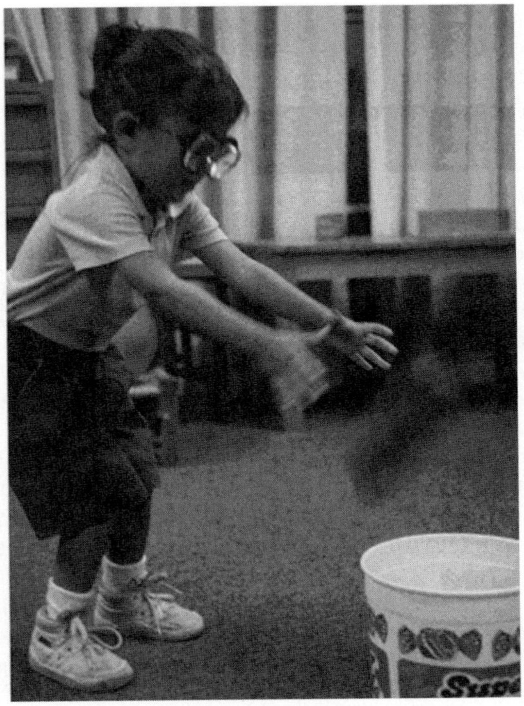

Figure 12-6 ■ This 3-year-old girl with diplegia takes her weight evenly over two feet with the help of prism lenses to shift her perception of space while engaged in a motor task.

correct the perception of forward space, the child places the entire foot in contact with the support. Such prism lenses are used during therapy handling as a perceptual learning experience for the child, with the optometrist and the therapist coordinating their efforts. Hand-coordination activities also require timing of reach and grasp that is based on feed-forward input from the visual system.[35] In some cases the therapist observes the visual system to overfocus in the moment that the child loses control of his or her postural stability. This suggests that the visual system may be attempting to compensate for the inadequacy of the postural control, much in the same way that we all adjust our head position to see better. Understanding the nature of the continuing dynamic interaction between these two functional subsystems of the central nervous system and attending to the needs of visual-postural orientation will increase the successful evolution of clients with cerebral palsy.

POSTURE AND MOVEMENT COMPENSATIONS

Compensatory patterns of movement arise from the motivation of the child to move in spite of various restrictions on the expression of that movement. Components in the developmental process that drive a person to right the head with the horizon and the body against gravity are met with interference from the central nervous system. Visual impressions of the environment motivate movement, and the infant attempts to influence nearby objects or confirm visual impressions by reaching into the environment and touching. As visual awareness enlarges to include more distant targets, the infant is motivated to move toward the object or person seen. With poor balance between flexion and extension and poor grading of agonist with antagonist, the resultant movements are influenced. When the child's body does not respond in a smooth way, the child begins to learn and perfect the uncoordinated reaction. Repetition of inadequate ranges of movement and limited variability of movement patterns begin to establish the atypical appearance of posture in the child with cerebral palsy.

The quality of a body posture or position in space determines the quality of the movement that is expressed. Lack of head control, poor midline organization, and deficient trunk strength begin the process of compensation. From a distorted starting position the movement initiated is one that is restricted (Figure 12-7). The lack of central "core" stability in the body restricts the full mobility of a limb. This limitation over time is increased by fascial and muscular restrictions on smooth coordinated muscle action. The child continues to learn the atypical responses because the movement patterns tend to be reinforced by either accomplishment or reinforcement of some kind from the environment. Compensatory movement patterns evolve because of necessity rather than any feedback as to efficiency or functional smoothness.

Habitual movement patterns are established on the basis of frequency of use, so the child with cerebral palsy tends to repeat the atypical responses that have been learned. In the therapy situation the child has the opportunity to learn new combinations of input to create the basis for a more stable postural control. Careful analysis of the postural adjustments and movement patterns of the child with cerebral palsy is crucial to initiate effective intervention strategies. There are many factors to be considered in the context of the continuing developmental changes in the child, which makes a simple solution impossible.

Active therapy intervention allows the sensorimotor learning of the child to be modified so that some part of the compensatory response becomes unnecessary and the movement becomes more typical (Figure 12-8). This relative

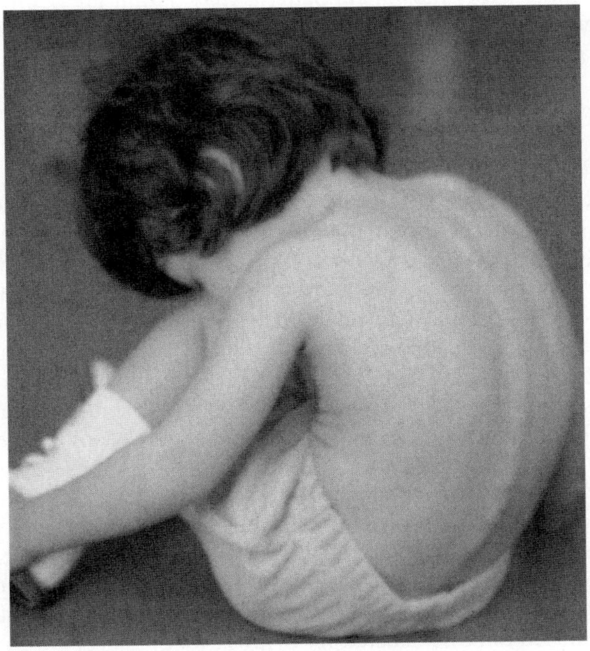

Figure 12-7 ■ Compensatory postures restrict movement initiation.

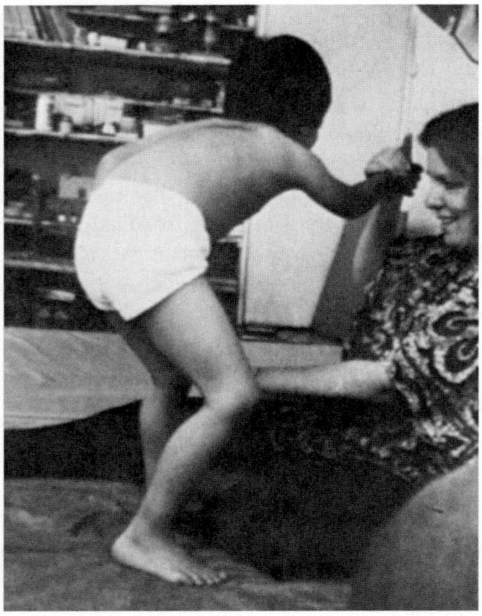

Figure 12-8 ■ The experience of coming to stand over the more affected side activates diagonal patterns of postural adjustment.

approximation of what is expected in a typical response may occur in the area of initiation, timing, strength, or ability to sustain an antigravity alignment. As movement expression and postural stability are better established, the compensatory patterns are used less often, and new motor learning occurs on a base of closer-to-normal experience.

Compensatory processes have their positive aspects.[37] The independence finally achieved by the older child reflects her or his intelligence and motivation and the family's attitude toward the child and the disability. The most debilitating handicap of cerebral palsy in an intelligent child may be social or psychological when the child is not accepted by the family and therefore cannot develop a positive self-image. Compensatory movement patterns may permit greater independence, if and when they do not limit or block the active learning of new motor strategies.

OTHER ASSESSMENT CONSIDERATIONS

Nutritional Aspects of Neuromotor Function

Nutrition is viewed as providing an important biochemical base for enhanced human performance. Williams,[38] author of the classic reference *Biochemical Individuality,* was one of the first to point out the existence of significant variability in the need for specific individualized nutrients because of differences in assimilation and other factors. Physicians Crook and Stevens,[39] Smith,[40] Pfeiffer,[41] and Cott[42] are a few of the leaders who have analyzed the link between nutrient intake and behavioral differences in children and adults. Many of these references address issues of attention and learning. To have efficient function of the transmitters at the myoneural junction and good health for the myelinated neurons of the nervous system, a variety of trace elements must be present.[41] Lack of dendritic proliferation is associated with malnutrition regardless of the cause.[43] The ambulatory child with cerebral palsy will need to be considered for a new level of energy expenditure to avoid short stature and poor nutritional status.[44]

Another body of work explains more about the direct link between food intake and muscle efficiency for high performance and normal function. The need for water is paramount for healthy fascia. In children with cerebral palsy and related disorders there is often from the beginning a difficulty in the smooth automatic sucking needed for nutritive intake. Uncoordinated patterns of mandibular and tongue motion persist when not addressed in early and precise intervention strategies. Even the digestive process is affected negatively by inadequate chewing, a higher-than-typical percentage of food allergies, and less-than-efficient physiological functions.[45]

It is likely that brain dysfunction in some of these children extends to the hypothalamus, thus influencing the entire digestive process. Duncan and colleagues[46] have documented the risk of osteopenia in nonambulatory children with cerebral palsy. This retrospective study showed that fewer than 75% of the calories needed were administered to 95% of the children with gastrostomy tubes. Nutrients were also deficient. This may explain part of the poor physical response level of such children. Sonis and colleagues[47] looked specifically at energy expenditure in children and adolescents with spastic quadriplegia in relation to food intake. They found dietary intake to be markedly overreported for this population and determined that nutrition-related growth failure was likely related to inadequate energy intake. Reflux is also common in infants with developmental problems. In some infants reflux subsides as the physical stress is reduced in the tissues bordering the upper thoracic and cervical spine, but it can be related to milk sensitivity or even susceptibility to environmental contaminants.

To supplement nutritional intake in the child with cerebral palsy, the individual child must be considered with regard to age, size, activity level, and growth factors.[48] Ideally, blood, urine, or hair analyses would be done to determine nutrient imbalances, and supplementation with specific nutrients would be guided by a specialist. Environmental medicine has taken the lead in this type of work. The rehabilitative process places increased demands on the entire system and requires fuel to set the stage for improved muscle function. Protein, carbohydrates, and adequate hydration are sources that build muscle and provide a foundation for strengthening and the advancement of motor skills in populations without disability.[49,50] A well-balanced diet will provide the requisite energy for exercise. However, little research has been done specifically on children with cerebral palsy and appropriate levels of protein during exercise. Therefore it is necessary to discuss these issues with the family using caution unless specifically trained to do so. A nutritional consultation is warranted when concerns arise in this area.

Consideration of Supplemental Oxygen

Oxygenation of muscle tissue is considered essential for smooth movement control, and it is generally accepted that respiratory support increases automatically to permit faster or stronger movement patterns in a typical subject. Therapists often note that children with cerebral palsy resist moving into new ranges of movement and that respiratory adaptation does not occur automatically. Supporting the child in the novel posture until a respiratory adaptation is noted results in acceptance of the new experience. Oxygen needs increase in children during growth spurts or when mastering more vertical postural alignments. Increased oxygen is also required for sustained activity such as continuous walking.

Shintani and colleagues[51] performed a careful study of 233 children with cerebral palsy to determine the presence of obstructive sleep apnea. In 10 children with cerebral palsy who were received at the hospital for treatment of severe obstructive sleep apnea, these authors determined that adenoidal or tonsillar hypertrophy were noted in only four children and that the main cause of sleep apnea in the other six children was pharyngeal collapse at the lingual base. Fukumizu and Kohyama[52] looked at central respiratory pauses, sighs, and gross body movement during sleep in 19 healthy children, ages 3 months to 7 years. Central pauses occurred more often during non–rapid-eye-movement sleep and increased with age. Developmental differences need further study.

Decreased oxygen levels have been associated with impaired cognitive and physical performance in the literature.[53] In the presence of inadequate peripheral oxygen saturation, low levels of oxygen can be administered during the night. This practice has been used with selected low-tone and athetoid children for improved energy during the day during growth changes, but formal study is needed on a larger group of children with cerebral palsy. Better oxygenation of the tissues can also result in increased food intake and consequently improved energy levels.

ROLES OF THE THERAPIST

Role of the Therapist in Direct Intervention

The primary role of the therapist is in direct treatment or physical handling of the child in situations that offer opportunities for new motor learning. This should precede and accompany the making of recommendations to parents, teachers, and others handling the child. Positioning for home and home handling recommendations should always be tried first by the therapist during a treatment session. As noted for the initial assessment, many interventions will cause a reaction unique to the particular youngster.[29,54] It is the role of the therapist to analyze the nature of the response that is accompanied by adaptation inadequacies, to analyze the movement problems, and to choose the most effective intervention (Figure 12-9). It will then be possible for other persons to manage play activities and supervise independent functioning that reinforce treatment goals.[55]

The therapist working with these children becomes an important and trusted resource to the family. At times the therapist who has had the more consistent contact with the child becomes the facilitator of better communication between the parents and medical or health care professionals. The child who starts early and continues with the same therapist may make of this person a confidant and share concerns that are difficult or uncomfortable for the child to explain to parents. It is a challenge for the therapist who follows the same child for an extended time to come up with appropriate goals and new activities to continue positive change. Part of direct intervention is to recognize when the amount of therapy can be reduced and replaced with recreational activities with peers.

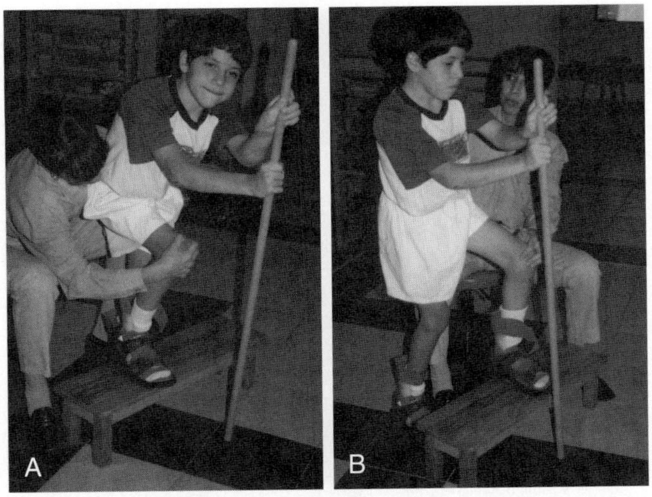

Figure 12-9 ■ The two sides of the body (**A** and **B**) often respond very differently to the same task, and therapy must be adapted accordingly.

Case Management and Direct Intervention

Simple documentation of observed changes in a child over a series of regular clinic visits is still too common for many children with cerebral palsy. Regular appointments, with periodic assignment of a new piece of apparatus, do not constitute active treatment. Although physical intervention in the form of direct handling of the child is considered a conservative treatment by most physicians, relatively few children receive sufficient physical treatment at an early age.[56,57] Therapists need to demonstrate their unique preparation and describe their interventions in ordinary language so that families as well as other health care professionals understand the importance of specific treatment versus general programs of early stimulation that are designed for neurologically intact infants.

The prognosis for change in cerebral palsy is too often based on records of case management rather than on the effect of direct and dynamic treatment by a well-prepared therapist. Bobath[32,58] documented accurately the developmental sequence expected in the presence of spasticity or athetosis. Her book consolidates some observations of older clients that help professionals understand the uninterrupted effects of the cerebral palsy condition. In any institution one can observe the tightly adducted and internally rotated legs, the shoulder retraction with flexion of the arms, and the chronic shortening of the neck so common as the long-term effects of cerebral palsy. The long-term influence of athetosis results in compensatory stiffness or limited movement patterns to create a semblance of the missing postural stability while a limited number of movement patterns with limited degrees of freedom are used to function (Figure 12-10).

Within the clinical community there is increasing evidence that soft tissue restrictions further limit spontaneous movement in children with cerebral palsy. The fact that these fascial restrictions are often found in infants suggests that they originate early rather than as a gradual result of limited ranges in movement. Because of the tendency of fascial tissue to change in response to any physical trauma or strong biochemical change, some of these characteristics might be originating with traumatic birth experiences, and they would

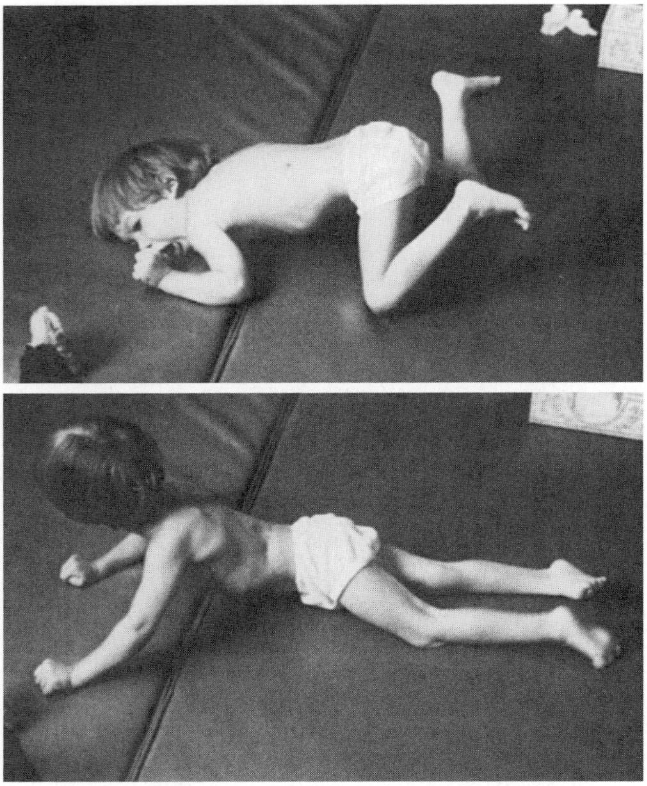

Figure 12-10 ■ Attempted movement activates atypical patterns and restrictions; restrictions are revealed with limited degrees of freedom available for function.

be exacerbated by daily use of limited patterns of movement. Tissue restrictions can also occur with immobilization or general infectious processes.[59-61] Soft tissue begins to change its physiological structure with the application of gentle sustained pressure, so it serves as documentation that there are changes caused by the therapist's simple hand contact. Some of the sensory information in the form of tapping or holding or application of pressure affects fascial meridians and muscle alignments.[62] A therapist must be prepared to defend his or her approach with a solid foundation, theory, and objective outcomes. Objective documentation is important when dealing with any population but essential for demonstrating therapeutic change.

Applying specific soft tissue treatment techniques to any person with a neuromotor disorder creates the need for immediate follow-up with practice of new skills using this improved range of motion. Creating excessive tissue mobility in a given area of the body can destroy the delicate patterns of coordination that permit synergic function in the person with cerebral palsy, so functional activation of the body after each specific mobilization is strongly recommended to integrate the tissue change. Well documented in the literature on current motor control and motor learning is the need to practice, practice, practice.[63] Practice time is related to skill performance; the amount and type of practice are determined by the stage of learning that an individual is in and the type of task to be learned[63-65] (see Chapter 4 on motor control and learning). Interestingly, most of what we know about motor control and motor learning is based on individuals who are "typicals," and it is yet to be determined whether the same principles that are considered important in healthy individuals apply to people with disability. However, it makes sense that practice would influence the use of any new or relearned skill.

An occupational therapist, Josephine Moore, stressed Bach-y-Rita's[66] works to emphasize some important points for therapists regarding the concept of increasing functional demands on the central system and the importance of the neck structures in developmental movement sequences. Children with spasticity often have a lack of developmental elongation of the neck, whereas children with athetoid or dystonic movement lack neck stability and consistent postural activation. Tone changes often originate with changes in the delicate postural interrelationship between head and body or with ambient visual processing.

By appreciating the abundance of polysynaptic neurons and parallel processing in the central nervous system, the therapist will become more optimistic regarding his or her role as facilitator and feedback organizer to guide new movement. Restak,[67] in his book *The New Brain,* confirms the continual reorganization of the brain in response to new input. Several animal and human studies on neuroplasticity have confirmed that the brain reorganizes after an injury and that this reorganization is shaped by rehabilitation and motor skill learning.[68-71] In the child with cerebral palsy, the therapist looks for subtle changes in the child's response to determine newly integrated sensorimotor learning. For example, excessive emphasis on extensor responses in the prone posture for the older child can jeopardize the quality of neck elongation in sitting, so it is essential to work on the components necessary for control of the new posture desired.

Therapy intervention is far from innocuous when it is responsibly applied. A truly eclectic treatment approach comes with clinical experience and personal consideration of observations of the functional problems presented by the complex issue of cerebral palsy at different ages. Priorities in intervention strategies have a practical aspect, and new developments in our knowledge lead us forward in clinical applications. The intricacies of typical development offer many new clues for new effective interventions. With high-quality treatment intervention the need for direct therapy service as a crucial aspect of case management for these children is confirmed. Clinical findings in individual case studies need to become part of the professional literature to strengthen the efficacy of intervention in this population.

Special Needs of Infants

The direct treatment of infants deserves special mention because there are significant differences in intervention strategies for the infant and the older child. Aside from the delicate situation of the new parents, the infant is less likely to have a diagnosis and presents a mixture of typical and atypical characteristics. It is essential that the clinician have a strong foundation in the nuances of typical developmental movement and early postural control.[4,72] Soft tissue issues must be addressed in detail. Direct intervention can be offered as a means of enhancing development and overcoming the effects of a difficult or preterm birth. It will be important, however, to pursue a diagnosis for the infant who reaches 8 or 9 months of age and continues to need therapy because third-party payers often require a diagnosis beyond developmental delay or prematurity.

Infants with early restrictions in motor control should be followed until they are walking independently, even if they no longer need weekly therapy. Infant responses can change rapidly as the therapist organizes the components of movement control. Soft tissue restrictions should be treated initially to have more success with facilitated movement responses. Careful observation is essential because all but the severely involved infant will change considerably between visits. The therapist should invest some time in training the parents to become skilled observers while appreciating the small gains made by their infant. Physiotherapist Mary Quinton[73] has written specific intervention strategies for babies (Figure 12-11). Infant massage is important to improve the bonding of mother and child and to improve physiological measures.[74,75]

Referral to other health care professionals is essential in the presence of possible allergies, new neurological signs, visual or auditory alterations, and persistent reflux or nutritional issues. There is always the possibility of convulsions when some brain dysfunction is present, and neurological evaluation should be recommended if this is a concern.

ORIENTATION TO TREATMENT STRATEGIES

The child whose movement is bound within the limitations of hypertonicity suffers first of all from a paucity of movement experience. Because early attempts to move have resulted in the expression of limited synergistic postural patterns, the child often experiences the body as heavy or awkward and loses incentive to attempt movement. The therapist will want to focus on the child's ability to sustain postural control in the trunk. Central "core" stability to support directed arm movement or weight shifts for stepping have not developed, so they need to be addressed during therapy intervention. Improved upper extremity control opens the possibility for new learning of more coordinated tasks. Specific work on hand preparation for reach and grasp follows use of the arm for directed movement and often results in improved balance in standing. Any freedom gained in upper body control results in more efficient balance in the upright posture.

Inhibiting or stopping the movement of one part of a movement range or even one limb must be done in a way that permits the child to activate the body in a functional way. The child who lies in the supine position with extreme pushing back against the surface is rarely seen when therapy intervention has started early. The therapist initially eliminates the supine position entirely but would incorporate into the treatment plan the activation of balanced flexion and extension in sitting with the ability to vary pelvic tilt for functional play and reaching (Figure 12-12). The child might later be reintroduced to a supine position with postural transitions that support balanced control of the body with more differentiated movement.

One of the primary considerations for the child with spasticity is adequate respiratory support for movement. Mobility of the thoracic cage and the midtrunk must be combined with trunk rotation during basic postural transitions (Figure 12-13). Consideration of age-appropriate movement velocity will guide the therapist in choosing activities that challenge better respiratory adaptability and prepare for speech breathing to support vocalization. The therapist will find it helpful to hum or sing or even make silly sounds that encourage sound production by the child during therapy. Movement of the child's body changes respiratory demands and frequently results in spontaneous sound production during therapy. Assessing the ability to sustain a breath to speak is easily done during a therapy session by counting the letters in the alphabet that can be said with one breath. This should be done with the child supine and in an upright position because trunk control required while sustaining a breath changes with the posture attained against gravity. Describing the chest shape and movement of the thorax observed can serve to assist the therapist in problem solving and prioritizing the treatment plan.

In some children respiratory patterns remain immature and superficial, which may be related to the causative factors of the impairment. A lack of postural control limits even the physiological shaping of the rib cage itself because the ribs do not have an opportunity to change their angle at the spine.

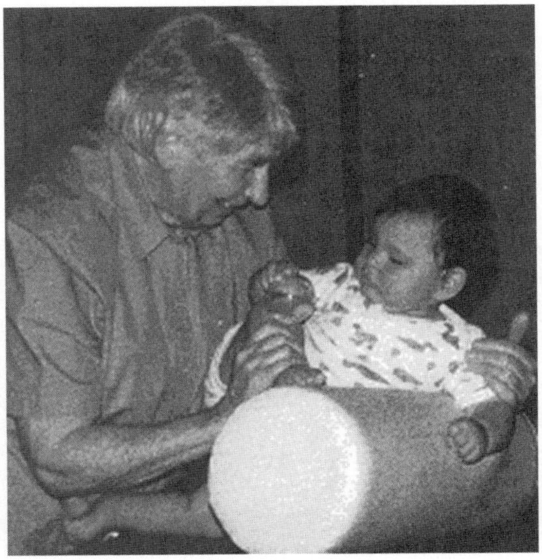

Figure 12-11 ■ Mary Quinton, British physiotherapist, is widely recognized as the originator of effective infant intervention.

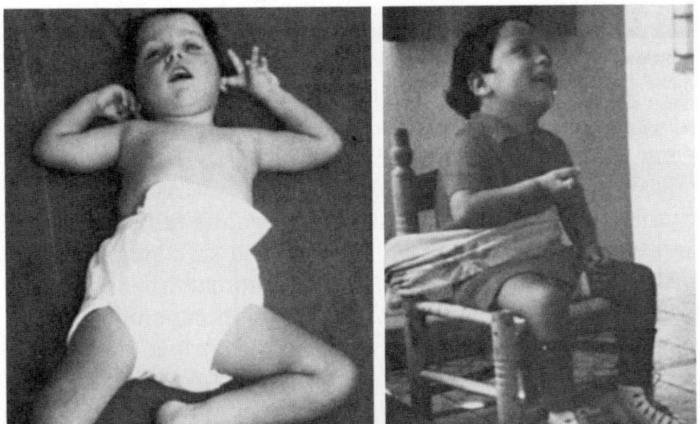

Figure 12-12 ■ **A,** Strong asymmetry and atypical tone in the supine position. **B,** Simple seating can inhibit strong asymmetry and make function a possibility.

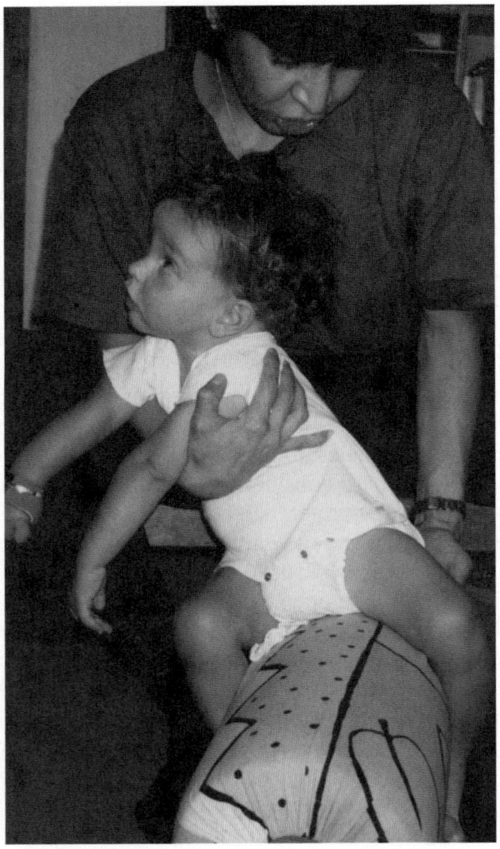

Figure 12-13 ■ Rotational patterns combined with transitional movements can be used to mobilize the thoracic cage.

The therapist must give careful support to sustain the transitional posture of the older child during transient respiratory change. An active respiratory adaptation will increase the variability of postural adaptation. Improved respiratory adaptation will improve trunk tone, just as dynamic trunk alignment facilitates better respiration.

Weight bearing changes postural tone. The trunk can be helped to experience weight bearing in a variety of alignments by using inflated balls or rolls that offer a contoured surface. The threshold of the original response is gradually altered so that the child begins to learn the new sensations and can follow guided postural transitions. When there are distinct differences between the two sides of the body, attention must be given to lateral weight shifts in sitting and standing. Changes near the vertical midline of the body seem to represent the more difficult input for the compromised system to integrate. It may be necessary to assist sustained weight over one side and then the other to initiate the change. It is important to assist the shoulders to align with the hips and that the visual orientation of the individual brings the head to a correct alignment. Young children need special help with segmental rotation of the trunk in the vertical alignment so that the weight-bearing side is relatively forward with dynamic balance of flexion and extension influences.

Children and adolescents with cerebral palsy often require a more intense or prolonged sensory cue for a desired movement response to be obtained. Weight bearing against the surface may need to be sustained for a prolonged period of time and a range of movement prepared beyond the essential range for the functional goal. The therapist is addressing a system that is deficient in its ability to receive, perceive, and use the available input. This makes careful analysis and functional orientation of the sensory input essential. If the microcosm of experience given the child during a therapy session is no more intense than an equal amount of time in her or his living environment, the therapist has failed to use this unique opportunity to deliver a meaningful message to encourage the learning of new motor behavior. Although therapists cannot provide during a treatment session every experience necessary for all movement scenarios, the therapist should provide the component parts necessary for motor skills to be transferred or generalized to other activities.

The therapist working with the child with cerebral palsy constantly monitors the quality of the child's motor response. These continuing observations guide the manipulation of the environment and the assistance given the child to move toward a functional goal. Is the body tolerating the position? Does the child adapt to the supporting surface and use the supporting surface contact for movement initiation (Figure 12-14)? Is the movement of a limb graded and without unwanted associated reactions in other parts of the body? By analyzing the answers to such questions, the therapist is guided to an appropriate sequence of the therapy session and is enabled to set functional treatment goals and realistically change prognoses.

The therapist makes constant judgments as to the child's responses during therapy, challenging the child's system while ensuring success and moving toward improved control. By using specific intervention strategies, the therapist works to introduce new somatosensory and motor learning. The therapist may introduce a slight modification of the child's response, such as an elongation of a limb as it is being moved. At other times the therapist augments sensory information that helps direct a movement. Weight bearing over the feet may be simulated with the young child's foot against the therapist's hand and pressure given through the knee. Visual-motor experiences can be altered with the child's use of prism lenses, prescribed by an optometrist for use during therapy.

To be meaningful, sensory input must be contextual and meaningful to the individual who is receiving it. Multiple sensory systems are simultaneously activated by most therapeutic input, and a variety of sights and sounds may be available in the immediate environment. Memory, previous

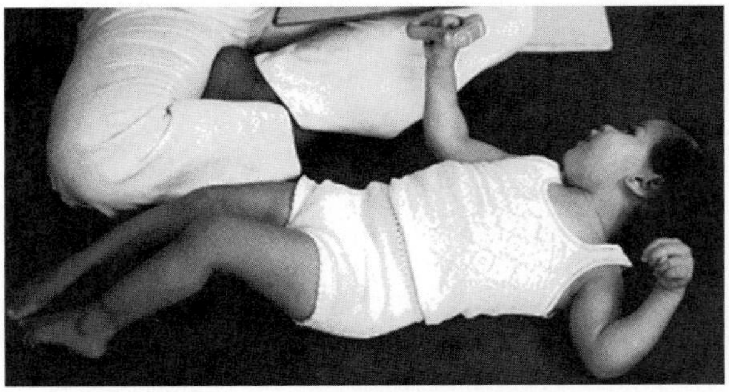

Figure 12-14 ■ This child has little contact with the supporting surface, resulting in poor movement initiation.

learning, and cognition are activated during the therapy interaction. The therapist makes a continuous reassessment of the child's experiential needs compared with the current input provided. When the therapist works with the child in a more upright alignment during at least part of the session, the central nervous system is alert and more receptive to the incoming information.

The developmental meaning attached to the sensation of typical movement is complex and starts with the ability to process contrasting stimuli. While several parts of the body are stable, another is moving. Stability of the proximal body permits a limb to extend forcefully or to be maintained in space. Each new level of developmental dissociation of movement increases the complexity of central nervous system processing. The process of self-feeding illustrates how internal and external stimuli impinge simultaneously on the central nervous system. The process of guiding a full spoon toward the mouth initially engages the child's attention. The arm is lifted at the shoulder to bring the fragrant food odor to the level of the mouth before elbow flexion takes the spoon to the face (Figure 12-15). Between 2 and 6 years of age the self-feeding pattern is modified and the elbow moves down beside the body. Now the motor aspect of the task has become procedural and more efficient, permitting the child to participate in social exchanges with the family at the same time that she or he manages independent self-feeding. The complexity of the task increases with the secondary task of social exchange.

A solid understanding of typical developmental sequences is essential for the clinician providing direct treatment intervention.[18,76] Early responses of the typical infant change from a self-orientation to an environmental orientation as new developmental competence emerges. More sophisticated balance in independent sitting occurs as the ability to pull to standing at a support begins to develop. Such knowledge of developmental details supports the therapist in introducing postural activities at a higher developmental level to integrate more basic abilities. The assisted self-dressing process is an effective way to introduce and integrate new movement and sensorimotor learning while using established movement skills. To sit well, the child needs practice moving over the base of support and coming in and out of sitting, and control of coming to stand from sitting. To walk well, the child may need to practice running to allow practice in changing rate, direction, range, and balance. Sitting is made more dynamic by using a gymnastic ball as a seat. Transitional adaptations of posture may be elaborated during therapy sessions to include more complex alignments. Specific techniques are reviewed in Chapter 9.

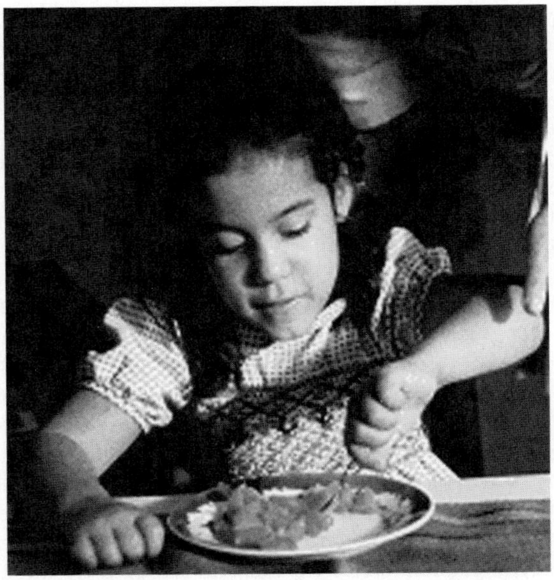

Figure 12-15 ■ Maintaining the child's elbow in this high position initially permits forearm pronation and activates the shoulder in the typical developmental pattern for improved motor learning.

With the child dominated by athetoid movement, the therapist's role relates primarily to organization and grading of seemingly erratic movement responses and establishing function around midline. These children have the ability to balance, but their balance reactions are often extreme in range and velocity. Their movements are rarely in the midline, asymmetrical, and frequently dominated by primitive reflexes, with poor midrange control of the trunk and extremities. Cognitively they are eager to participate and usually are responsive to working on specific goals that relate to functional success. By working to improve central control, the therapist gradually introduces taking of body weight over the limbs, with assistance to grade the postural control of the central body. By working closely with a behavioral optometrist the therapist can use visual input to improve the child's balance reactions. In these children the therapist may note that disruption of eye alignment or focusing results in a momentary disorganization of postural control (see Chapter 28).

Movement control must become procedural so that it is not interrupted by every environmental distraction. This is more likely to happen when balanced activity of the visual, vestibular, and proprioceptive systems has been achieved. Independent ambulation becomes practical when the individual is able to think of something else at the same time. The therapist begins this process by carrying on a conversation with the child to engage the cognitive attention so that the motor act becomes more automatic. The concept of graded stress is discussed in Chapters 5 and 6.

Direct intervention for the hemiplegic child takes into account the obvious difference in postural tone between one side of the body and the other. Treatment for children that addresses itself only to the more affected side of the body will not prove to be effective. The critical therapeutic experience seems to be that of integration of the two sides of the body and the establishment of midline (Figure 12-16). The child with hemiplegia differs from the adult stroke patient in that the adult had a clearly established midline and integration of both sides of the body by learning to cross midline before the stroke episode. The child with hemiplegia has not had that experience and will need emphasis on this during intervention. The integration of both sides of the body begins early for the typical infant, with lateral weight shifts in a variety of developmental patterns, and leads to postural organization that permits later reaching for a toy while the body weight is supported with the opposite side of the body. The child with a contrast in the sensorimotor function of the two sides of the body needs to experience developmental patterns that include rotation within the longitudinal body

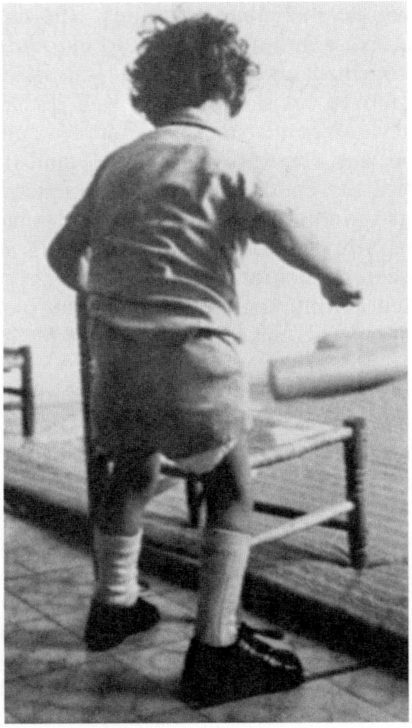

Figure 12-16 ■ This boy with hemiplegia tries to move a chair by orienting only his more active side to the task and bearing weight only briefly on the more affected side.

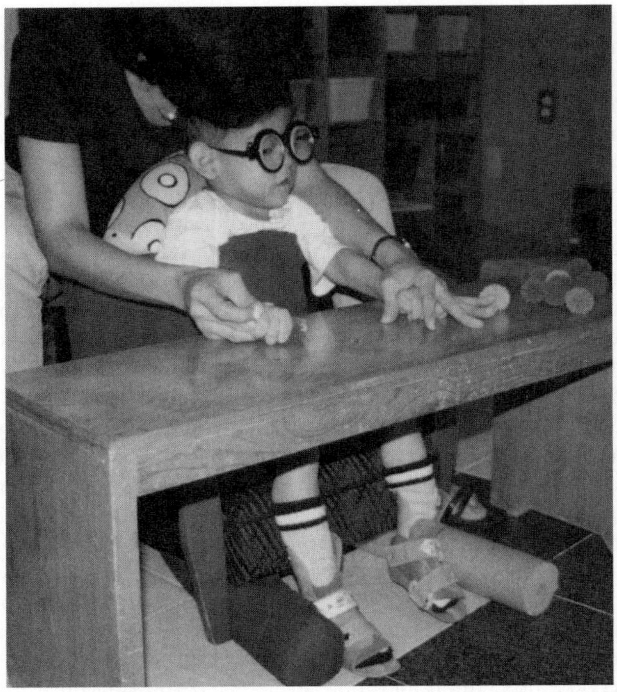

Figure 12-17 ■ Bilateral arm activity with visual regard that corresponds to hand motion incorporated into therapy.

axis and lateral flexion of the trunk, the more affected side forward. The more affected side needs the experience of supporting the body and the experience of initiating movement.

Development of hand use first focuses on bilateral arm activity while keeping the affected hand well within the functional visual field (Figure 12-17). The infant or young child works primarily in sitting until dynamic trunk flexion is activated. Pelvic mobility is essential to activate the necessary trunk responses. The therapist may find that true lateral flexion of the more affected side of the body is fully as difficult for some children as the initial active elongation of that side. There tends to be a high incidence of soft tissue restrictions in the shoulder and neck of the affected side. Children with hemiplegia have difficulty in sustaining a balanced posture against the influence of gravity, and some begin to struggle to do everything with the less affected side. This characteristic contrast in function may contribute to the development of seemingly hyperactive behavior that is related to the inability of the central nervous system to resolve contrasting incoming information. Hyperkinetic responses in one side of the body may compensate for relative inactivity in the opposite side. Leg length discrepancy, scoliosis, pelvic obliquity, and shortening between the ribs and pelvis may develop. One goal of treatment is to bring these divergent response levels closer together so that the child can experience more comfortable postural change and adapt to later school demands.

The limbs of the hemiplegic child will change in postural tone as the trunk reactions are brought under active control and lateral weight shifts more clearly to the more affected side. The two hands need the experience of sustaining the body weight simultaneously, as do the two feet. Although the more affected hand may not develop sensation adequate for skilled activity, an important treatment goal is sufficient shoulder mobility to move the arm across the body midline and to assume a relaxed alignment during ambulation. Early treatment increases the possibility that the more affected hand will be used as an assisting or helping hand. There are some children who have such severe sensory loss that active use is minimal, although considerable relaxation can be achieved.

The greater the discrepancy between the sensorimotor experience of the one side of the body and the other, the more tendency the system seems to have to reject one of the messages. This can lead to distortions in verticality and is a major interference in bilateral integration. Functional vision evaluation is important to avoid the midline shift problem that will distort postural control. As body weight is shifted to the more intact side, flexor withdrawal patterns of the limbs increase in frequency and strength in some children. These postural reactions are often associated with lack of full weight bearing on the more affected side. The presence of a lateral visual midline shift or some visual field loss may increase the avoidance of bearing weight on the more affected side.[72] One important therapy goal is the achievement of graded weight shift through the pelvis during ambulation (Figure 12-18).

Treatment strategies must incorporate a wide variety of more basic developmental alignments in which pelvic weight shift is a factor. The choice of prone, moving from sitting to four-point support, or a simple weight shift while sitting on a bench will depend on the movement characteristics observed by the therapist during the evaluative session. Diagonal adaptations are useful in the redistribution of tone for upright function. Careful attention must be given to pelvic alignment and mobility because the pelvis has a tendency to be rotated posteriorly on the more affected side in

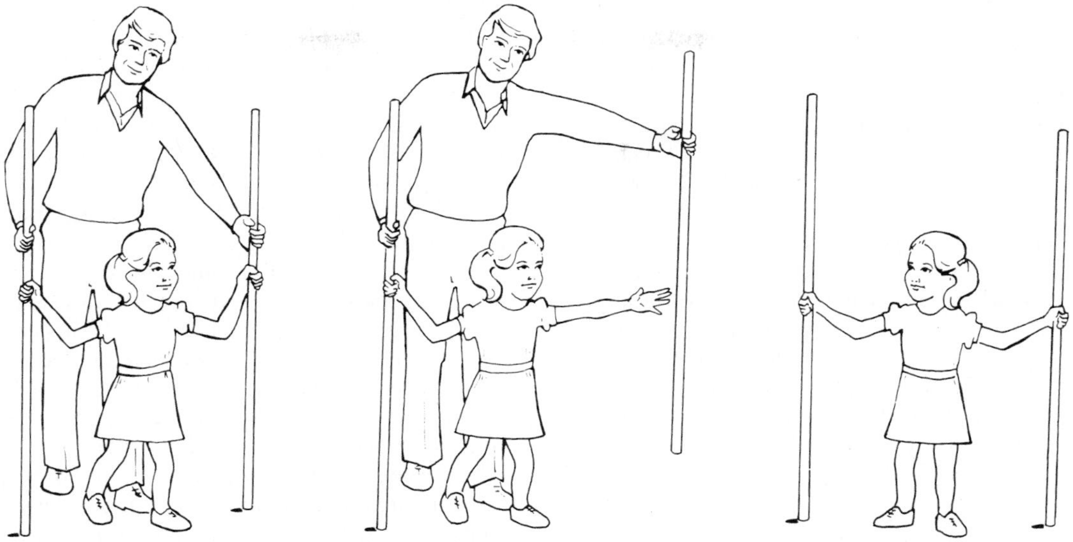

Figure 12-18 ■ The use of poles was introduced by the Bobaths as a way to achieve graded weight shift for increasingly complex postural adjustments in standing and walking.

children who have not had good early therapy. This can cause increased hip flexion and incomplete hip extension at terminal stance later if the child begins to walk with the more affected side held posteriorly, a characteristic that may be observed during analysis of leg position in gait. Dynamic foot supports will facilitate a more functional weight shift when the child is not in the treatment session. The goal of functional movement is best reached through a wide variety of weight-bearing postures, from the obvious developmental alignments to horizontal protective responses or reaching above the shoulders in sitting and standing to incorporate practical and commonly used adaptations.

The child with low muscle tone is perhaps the greatest challenge for both therapist and parent. Adequate developmental stimulation is difficult unless positioning can be varied. Placing the child in a more upright alignment, although it is achieved with complete support initially, seems to aid the incrementation of postural control. To prepare the low-tone body for function, it is helpful to review the articulations for possible soft tissue restrictions. However, equally important is not to take away muscle tightness that is providing a form of stability for the child without the ability to give him or her another form of stability for functional use. The neck and shoulder girdle are particularly vulnerable. Strong proprioceptive input while accurate postural alignment is ensured is an important part of the treatment session. A direct push-pull motion of the limbs, which is gentle traction alternated with approximation as described by Bobath,[77] also assists in maintaining antigravity positions and creates postural variance in the practice of antigravity postural reactions. Positioning at home may include a high table that supports the arms, allows for increased trunk extension in good alignment, and permits voluntary horizontal arm motion. The therapist must be cautious of the tendency to fixate in response to trunk instability and initial hypotonicity. This seemingly hypertonic response, which can be distributed in the deeper musculature, contributes to limited adaptability rather than differentiated postural control. It is difficult to ramp up the corticomotor neuron pool even though the child's motor output may remain limited; changes in positioning and opportunities for the child to have other sensory and visual experiences will often serve to motivate the child and contribute to motor learning. Home handling needs to include a variety of positions during each day for seating and play. Consistency in these practices is essential for the child with low tone to progress.

The process of undressing and dressing can be a dynamic part of the treatment program for any child (Figure 12-19).

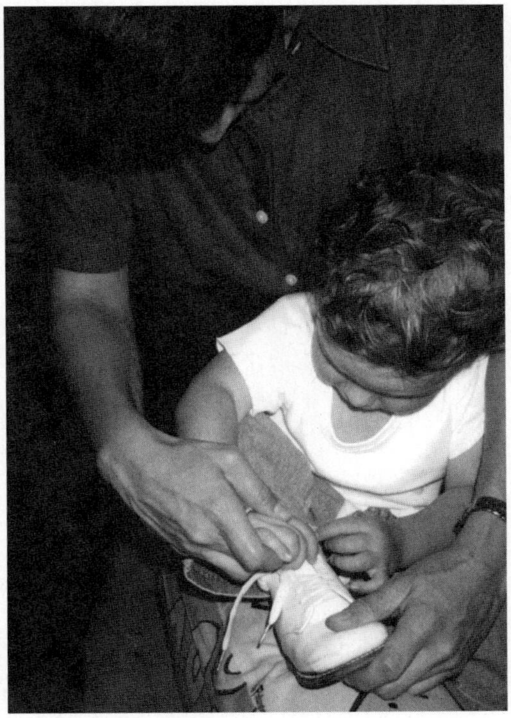

Figure 12-19 ■ With assistance, this boy with right hemiplegia is helped to improve his self-esteem by exploring dressing.

Diagonal patterns of movement that are incorporated into the removal of socks and shoes assist in the organization of midline orientation. Weight shifts and changes in stability-mobility distribution occur throughout the dressing process. Concepts of direction and spatial orientation are applied to the relationship of body parts and clothing. Directional vocabulary terms and names of clothing and body parts are learned with this experience. A bench is useful because it permits the adult to sit behind the child who is just beginning to participate actively. The older child with difficult balance reactions can use the bench in a straddle-sit alignment (Figure 12-20). Aside from the physical and perceptual benefits, this achievement of dressing independently is one that offers the child a feeling of pride and independence. It is also a very practical preparation for the future when it is introduced in keeping with individual developmental and emotional needs (Figure 12-21).

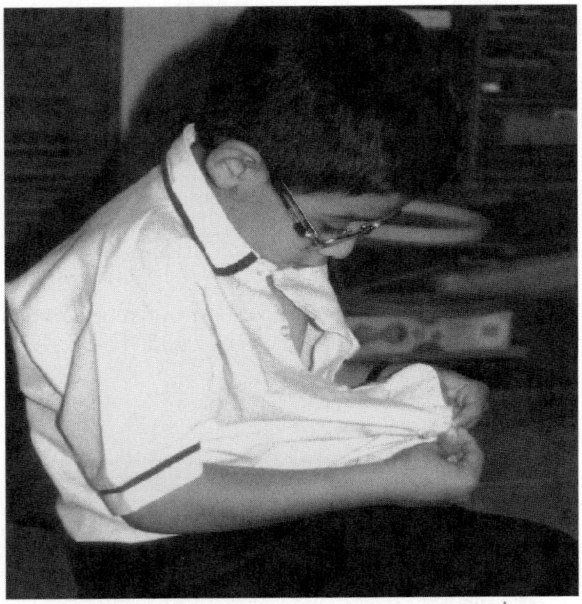

Figure 12-20 ■ Straddle-sitting on a bench gives this diplegic boy postural stability while he concentrates on the buttoning process.

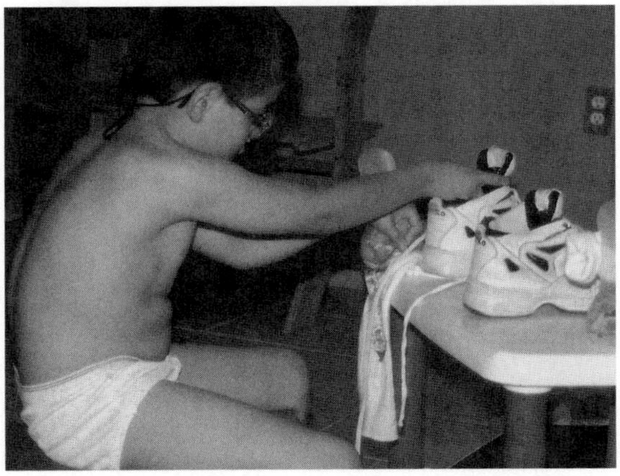

Figure 12-21 ■ Organization of clothing within reach is essential for success in independent dressing.

RESEARCH

Pediatric clinicians are faced with selecting treatments that are efficacious for children with cerebral palsy. Increasing pressure on clinicians to establish that treatments are effective in improving functional abilities is often dictated by third-party payers. In the past there was little research on pediatric treatment approaches and protocols that withstood the rigors of scientific investigation. Today, several methods that warrant mentioning are beginning to undergo systematic investigation.

Constraint-induced movement therapy (CIMT) was developed from basic science experiments on deafferenated monkeys to overcome learned nonuse of the upper extremity.[78,79] This forced use approach was adapted for adult patients after a stroke; the affected upper extremity is forced to participate in activities and the less involved upper extremity is constrained. Practice is intense, with 6 hours of mass practice for a 2-week period.[80-82] This protocol has been quite successful, with significant improvement in upper extremity movement and use of the affected limb. CIMT is very popular and is now beginning to appear in the clinical setting. The pediatric client has also demonstrated a favorable response to this treatment protocol in several single-case studies.[83-87] In a clinical randomized trial by Taub and colleagues,[88] children with hemiplegia or brain injury receiving CIMT for 21 consecutive days, 6 hours a day, demonstrated significant improvement in the amount of use, quality of movement, and spontaneous use of the affected upper extremity. These results were sustained at 6-month follow-up. Several studies from around the world are beginning to show up in the literature with varied methods. Most of these studies are promising; however, further investigation is necessary to establish the critical threshold, adequate dosage, and selection process for subjects who will benefit the most.[89-93] Clinicians are beginning to adapt these studies to their therapeutic settings and modify the protocols for clinical use and reimbursement potential.

Treadmill training has also been used in children with cerebral palsy.[94-101] The treadmill has been instrumental in rehabilitation for many years with a variety of purposes. This treatment began with animal studies on spinalized cats and rats and their responses to training on a treadmill in the recovery of a walking pattern.[102-105] Today this treatment is used in many populations, including those with spinal cord injury, traumatic brain injury, Parkinson disease, stroke, and cerebral palsy.[106] The use of the treadmill in children with cerebral palsy has shown promising results: improvement in gait pattern, increased walking speed, decreased coactivation in lower extremity musculature, overall gross motor skill improvement, and improved and stabilized energy expenditure.[94-101] Treadmill training interventions have taken on many different faces, including use of a regular treadmill, commercial equipment, and high-tech body-weight support systems (Figures 12-22 and 12-23). Commercial equipment is now available to assist with supporting the body weight of individuals who otherwise would not be candidates for such a treatment. Clinical adaptations have also been incorporated to accommodate smaller bodies on a treadmill, which allows the therapist to assist from behind or from the side. Setting goals for this treatment must be precise, with an understanding of the purpose intended for its use: improving endurance, changing the parameters of the gait pattern, strengthening, and gait training. Each goal must be based on a sound theoretical foundation, which is now available from the literature.

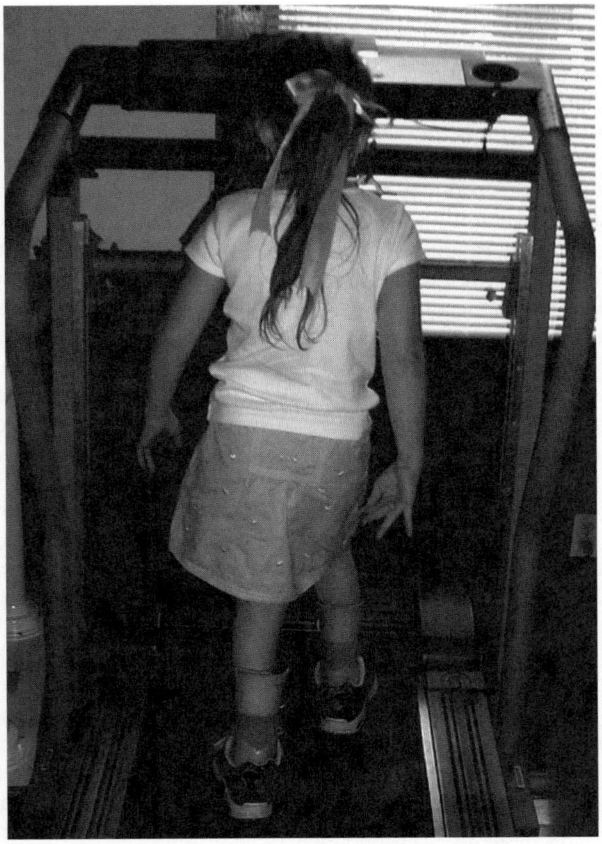

Figure 12-22 ■ This young girl is practicing walking on the treadmill without holding on and incorporating arm swing to improve her stride length.

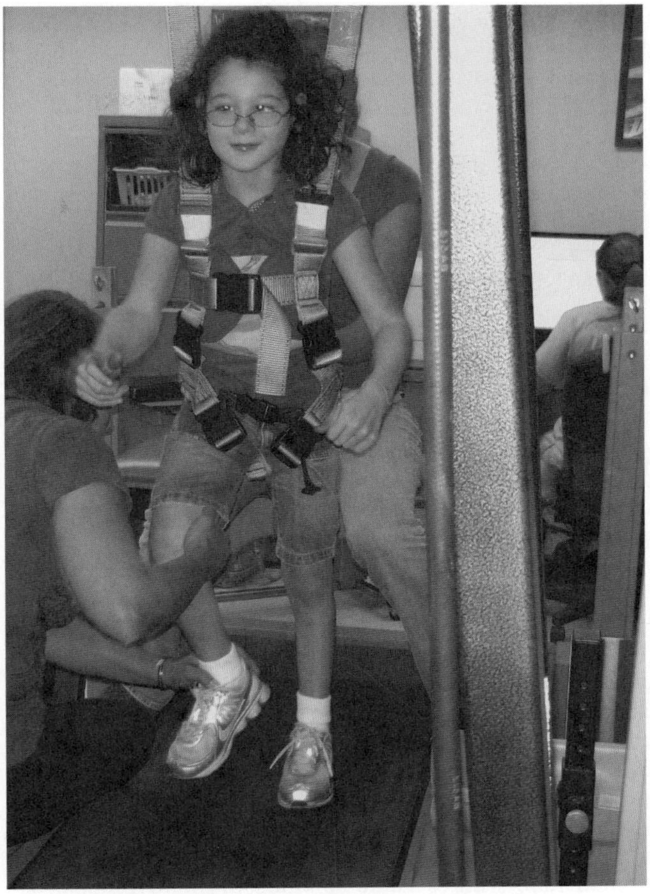

Figure 12-23 ■ This young girl, who is an independent ambulator with a rollator walker, is participating in partial body weight–supported locomotor training to improve her gait pattern.

Strength training was never thought possible in the presence of spasticity in children with cerebral palsy. Several studies have now shown that strength can improve in children with spastic cerebral palsy.[107-110] Circuit training was used in an afterschool training program for 4 weeks, two times a week for 1 hour of intense group training, resulting in improved strength and functional performance.[107] Strength was maintained in this group of individuals at an 8-week follow-up posttest. Dodd and colleagues[108] set up a home-based lower extremity strengthening program in a randomized clinical trial with 21 individuals with cerebral palsy. All subjects in the treatment group had improved lower extremity strength that was maintained at follow-up periods of 6 and 12 weeks. In a study focused on biofeedback and strength training to improve dorsiflexion and range of motion, Toner and co-workers[110] demonstrated significant changes in active range of motion and dorsiflexion strength.[110] Strength training in the presence of spasticity is also documented in adults as beneficial not only for conditioning, improved range of motion, and psychological well-being, but in some cases reduction of spasticity.[111-114] Strength training in children and adolescents with cerebral palsy has continued with investigations into the intensity, type of contractions to practice, and dosage.[115,116] Interestingly, a systematic review of common physical therapy interventions in school-aged children found that strength training demonstrated significant improvements in selected muscle groups but no meaningful change in function. Martin and colleagues[117] and Moreau and colleagues[118] studied muscle architecture as a predictor of maximum strength and its relationship to activity levels in cerebral palsy.[118] They found that ultrasound measures of the vastus lateralis muscle thickness adjusted for age and the GMFCS level were correlated and predictive of maximum torque in children with and without cerebral palsy. A variety of methods for strength training can be incorporated into a clinical treatment setting or home exercise program with anticipated improvement in muscle strength, which may also result in improved functional status for children with cerebral palsy. Strength training encompasses free weights, aerobic workouts, stretch bands or tubing, and machines that address resistive exercise (Figure 12-24).

Many adjuvant therapies that are popular in combination with other treatments are available to individuals with cerebral palsy. Electrical stimulation (ES) has been used in a variety of ways with children with cerebral palsy. In several case reports by Carmick,[119-121] neuromuscular ES used in conjunction with task-oriented practice was found to improve sensory awareness, strength, gait parameters, and passive and active range of motion. Neuromuscular ES was used as an adjunct therapy with upper and lower extremity practice protocols.[119-122] ES has been used in conjunction with 6 weeks of intensive therapy to improve sitting posture and trunk control for children with spastic cerebral palsy.

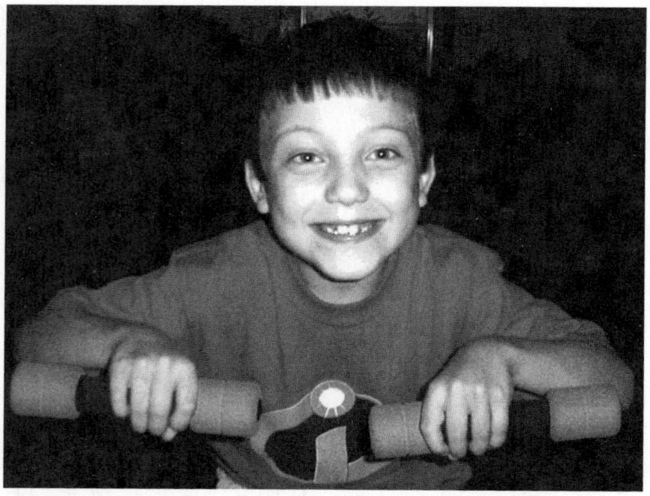

Figure 12-24 ■ Using free weights to strengthen the upper extremities while stabilizing the trunk while seated on an incline bolster.

Radiographic studies confirmed the statistical significance in decreasing the kyphotic angle of the spine and sitting score on the GMFM.[123] Two recent studies documented an improved gait pattern and reduced spasticity in 27 children with spastic diplegic cerebral palsy after use of transcutaneous electrical nerve stimulation on selected lower extremity musculature for 15 minutes, three times a day, for 1 week.[124,125] Neuromuscular ES was used successfully in combination with dynamic splinting to improve upper extremity range of motion at the elbow and wrist in 6 children with cerebral palsy.[126] ES has been in the therapy arena for many years, and its selective use with children who have cerebral palsy may supplement regular therapy sessions with enhanced results. (Therapeutic subthreshold ES at meridian points is discussed in the section on electroacupuncture treatments and in Chapter 39.)

Botulinum toxin A (BtxA) has been used to assist in decreasing spasticity because it provides a permissive condition that improves and increases range of motion and practice of new motor patterns without interference from increased muscle tone. Gait velocity, stride length, range of motion, and decreased spasticity were noted to be significant in 33 subjects with cerebral palsy after local injections of BtxA.[127] Several studies have shown a decrease in spasticity, successful treatment of foot deformities, and improved gait parameters with BtxA.[128-131] In a study by Galli and colleagues,[132] dynamic dorsiflexion improved during stance and swing phases of gait, with significant improvement in foot placement at initial contact. BtxA has been used with varying results as an adjunct treatment for the management of upper extremity spasticity.[133] Lukban and colleagues[134] reviewed six randomized clinical trials with a total of 115 children receiving BtxA in the upper extremities. Five of the six trials demonstrated a reduction in spasticity that was time limited, and four of the six trials documented improved hand function. Four systematic reviews concluded that there simply was not enough evidence to support or refute the effectiveness of BtxA for upper extremity use. It allows for the reduction of muscle tone and opens a window of practice opportunity, in combination with other treatments, to learn new movement possibilities. BtxA has a temporary effect, so the critical element is its combination with other treatment modalities. Park demonstrated improved range of motion and decreased spasticity in ambulatory children with cerebral palsy when BtxA was used in combination with serial casting.[135] It has also been used as an alternative to control the progression of hip dislocation and hip pain in children with cerebral palsy.[136]

Joint and trunk taping and strapping have been used to provide sensory input and alignment for posture, balance, and strengthening. To date, there is no evidence that these adjunctive treatments actually provide these benefits, but there is also no evidence that they do not. Further objective investigation will be necessary to address the issues presented by these additives to therapy. Both are considered noninvasive with few side effects other than those associated with adhesive allergy to tape and autonomic nervous system responses such as sweating and overheating. Several different types of tape (athletic, Leukotape P Patella Tape [Notoden, The Netherlands]; Kinesio Tape [Kinesio USA Corporation]) and strapping devices are available commercially.

Soft tissue mobilization is a method of stretching tight structures that have become restricted from overuse, spasticity, deformities, muscle shortening, surgeries, trauma, and poor nutrition. This type of stretching has strong roots in osteopathic medicine but is not limited to that area of expertise. Over the years, research investigating the cellular and tissue changes that occur with immobilization has revealed some interesting and shocking alterations in the muscle and collagen fibers. With immobilization, slow muscle fibers show greater atrophy than fast fibers do.[59] There is atrophy, a decrease in peak torque, an increase in fatigue resistance, loss of strength, and reduced central activation when the plantar flexors of the ankle are immobilized.[137,138] In a recent study of children with severe spasticity, muscle biopsies were performed on the vastus lateralis to determine collagen accumulation in the spastic muscle. An increased accumulation of collagen I fibers in the endomysium of the muscle was noted, with thickening and decreased muscle fiber content in the more severe cases.[139] This study, in combination with what we understand about healthy muscle, reinforces the need to keep the muscles flexible and active to help prevent this accumulation of collagen. Soft tissue mobilization and deep tissue stretching are methods that can improve the ability of the tissue to lengthen and fold, allowing for a more efficient activation of the muscle fibers, thus optimizing the formation of typical synergies during practice of motor skills.

As mentioned earlier, children with cerebral palsy often have visual difficulties that are not acuity problems and that are not correctable with a standard lens. Vision therapy has demonstrated good results when emphasis is placed on ocular motility and accommodation.[140] When children were given intense visuo-oculomotor training, improvement was noted in visuo-oculomotor control.[141] Improvement in the child's ability to execute smooth pursuit precision and maximum velocity, improvement of saccadic movement precision and stability, and shortening of the saccadic reaction time were significant after training.[141] Although many clinicians are not experts in the area of vision, vision is an important part of every therapy session. Incorporating vision as an integral part of a therapy session will not only improve the child's orientation in space but will address his or her ability to scan the environment while learning to move through space.

Many therapies become popular by purporting to be a "fix" for a particular problem associated with cerebral palsy. The clinician accepts responsibility for making sound judgments concerning treatment and outcomes for children with cerebral palsy. Not all the treatments used in therapy will be investigated rigorously in a scientific manner. However, when a treatment approach is presented as advantageous for many diagnoses and conditions, with claims of success beyond what is reasonable for those conditions, it is your duty to proceed with caution. Always stop and think what theory and frame of reference the approach will fit best. Does this "new" therapy make sense with the knowledge you have of anatomy, physiology, neurology, and motor learning? As clinicians we will always be tempted to try new approaches before the scientific community has investigated them thoroughly. Clinicians, because they are creative and innovative, have advanced our professions. It is essential to advance patient care with treatments that are safe and do no harm. Every environment affords research opportunities that contribute to the treatment of children with cerebral palsy. Single-case reports and single-case studies are the beginning of this process and, although descriptive in nature and with limited generalization, provide evidence for new therapeutic approaches and further systematic investigation.

MEDICAL INFLUENCES ON TREATMENT

Because the problems of cerebral palsy are so varied, the condition lends itself to diverse interventions, some of which have a longer life than others. Management of spasticity has always been an area of great concern and interest, and over the years several treatments have been offered to control this positive sign. Various medications have been used to control spasticity; baclofen, diazepam, and dantrolene remain the three most commonly used pharmacological agents in the treatment of spastic hypertonia.[142] (See Chapter 36 for additional information.) The baclofen pump has been used in children with excessive spasticity. This pump is implanted in the lower abdomen with a catheter leading to the intrathecal space for the administration of the drug. This treatment for spasticity has been effective for some types of cerebral palsy but led to complications in some patients with mixed cerebral palsy, low body weight, younger age, gastrostomy tubes, and nonambulatory status.[143-145]

The cerebellar implant so popular in the late 1970s offered the possibility of regulating tone by supplementing cerebellar inhibition.[146-149] As time passed, the procedure was used less often, and patients had difficulty getting repairs or replacement parts for the implant. The procedure that largely replaced the cerebellar implant was the placement of four electrodes in the cervical area to offer more control over postural tone.[150] These had the advantage of being adjustable so that the individual or a family member could make daily choices as to the optimal tone distribution. In some cases early success gave way to disappointment as the system adapted to the inputs. In some cases the child or adolescent had to make a decision whether movement or speech was more important on a given day. Therapy was always recommended after the procedure, although the nature of the specific program was left to the family to decide. The success of the cerebellar stimulator is considered moderate when used on a select group of individuals with cerebral palsy.[146-149] Other, more recent spasticity management programs are less invasive and are often considered before use of this invasive procedure.

In 1968 a posterior rhizotomy surgical intervention was developed, with some success reported in reducing spasticity.[151,152] It remained for Peacock and Arens[153] to apply the procedure more selectively and functionally and to bring it to the United States from South Africa. On the basis of their experience, Peacock and colleagues insisted on daily neurodevelopmental (Bobath) treatment for at least 1 year after the surgical intervention. Electromyographic testing before and during the surgery is used to determine which posterior nerve rootlets are creating the spasticity in the lower extremities.[154] The foundations for success are accurate selection of the child, an experienced surgeon, and careful analysis of therapy goals.

A more recent improvement in the selective dorsal rhizotomy (SDR) procedure was developed by Lazareff and colleagues,[155] who enter a limited number of levels rather than five levels of the spinal column and prefer to work close to the cauda equina, according to the technique of Fasano.[156] Several studies have documented improvement in function and strength and reduction of spasticity outcomes as far out as 3 to 5 years.[151,157] In a more recent longitudinal study by Nordmark and co-workers,[158] it was found that SDR was safe and effective in reducing spasticity without major complications. When combined with physical therapy and careful selection of candidates for the procedure, the functional outcomes over a period of 5 years were lasting. Trost and colleagues[159] reported on differences between preoperative and postoperative measures: the Ashworth scale for spasticity, the Gillette Gait Index, oxygen cost for gait efficiency, and the Gillette Functional Assessment Questionnaire for functional mobility. All outcome measures demonstrated improvement for the 136 subjects as a whole. Careful selection of the appropriate candidate for this surgery followed by intense therapy intervention is essential for the success of the procedure and for optimizing motor outcomes.

A new approach to controlling spasticity is percutaneous radiofrequency lesions of dorsal root ganglion (RF-DRG), a noninvasive procedure that has been reported in the literature recently. Vles and colleagues[160] performed a pilot study of 17 patients with a diagnosis of cerebral palsy. They reported that this new treatment is promising for reducing spasticity and improving function in children with cerebral palsy. Further investigation into this treatment is necessary to assess its effectiveness.

Alcohol (phenol) blocks and the use of botoxin (botulinum toxin) (BtxA) have been used locally to affect a change in the individual muscle or motor point injected.[142,161-167] Both orthopedists and neurologists have taken an interest in the use of botoxin to block selected muscle responses for a temporary period. BtxA has been reported to have fewer side effects than the phenol blocks and is now considered the drug of choice for this type of procedure.[130] These conservative interventions serve to delay surgery until the child is more capable of responding to postsurgical therapy programs. Botulinum toxin injection combined with serial casting has been shown to improve range of motion, muscle tone, and dynamic spasticity in ambulatory children with cerebral palsy.[135] Therapists should be involved in the decision-making process of determining interventions for reduction of spasticity because they often are the most familiar with the child's movement strategies and the postural changes that occur in muscle tone as the child moves against gravity.

Orthopedic surgical intervention continues to be effective in cerebral palsy when there are tendon contractures or specific structural limitations that are not accompanied by excessive levels of spasticity.[168,169] In any surgery the outcome is much improved by close coordination between therapist and surgeon, with a functional orientation toward goal setting for the child. Early standing after surgery and use of dynamic footplates inside the casts and orthotics after cast removal will generally improve functional outcomes. Bony surgeries that offer better joint stability are usually planned for the termination of growth. The orthopedist is also able to guide conservative positioning measures to prevent hip problems resulting from spasticity while direct treatment intervention continues. Bracing of the trunk, which is sometimes warranted for scoliosis or kyphosis, is prescribed by the orthopedist. Surgical intervention for spinal deformities is determined by the physician, with consideration of the child's age, condition, and health and the degree of curvature.

Children with cerebral palsy differ in their ability to relax completely during sleep, and a small number of these children can benefit from inhibitive casting or night bracing. More often this type of positioning is used during therapy sessions and independent ambulation to combine control with weight bearing.[170] The orthopedist should participate in any plan for prolonged immobilization or temporary casting that will be used on a 24-hour schedule, such as serial casting to improve range of motion.[171,172] A variety of lower-extremity bracing is available, and its selection is dependent on the segment to control and the outcomes sought in positioning or dynamic action, as in ambulation (Figure 12-25).

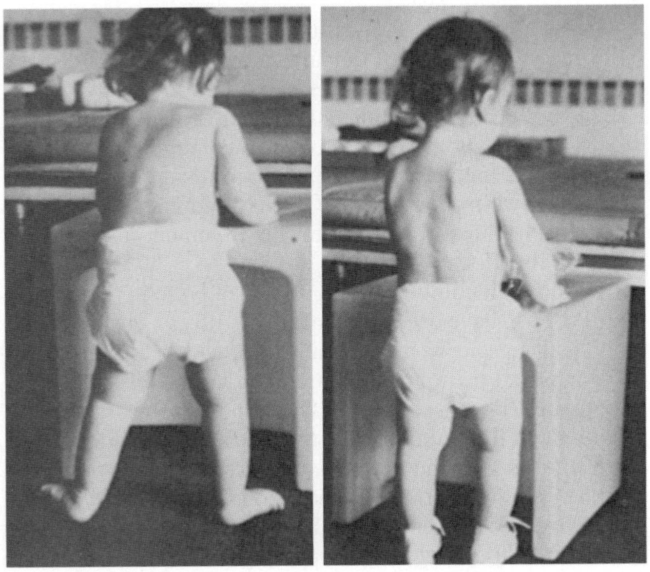

Figure 12-25 ■ A supportive shoe with footplates inside for this low-tone child facilitates more typical trunk reactions and permits use of the hands for play.

EQUIPMENT

Equipment recommendations must take into account the physical space in the home and the amount of direct treatment available to the child (Figure 12-26). Young children in particular can often use normal seating with slight adaptations. This not only is more socially and financially acceptable but also permits changes as required by the child's developmental progress. The portability of supportive seats or standers encourages the family to take the apparatus along for weekend outings or visits to relatives. Chair designs should place children at an age-appropriate level in their environments. This permits a better quality of visual exploration and facilitates social exchange with siblings and visiting peers. When planning the amount of physical support needed by the child, the therapist considers varying the structural control in relation to activity (Figure 12-27). The child who is merely watching the play of others or a television presentation may successfully control trunk and head balance independently with minimal support. However, concentration on hand skills or self-feeding may necessitate trunk control assistance via a chair insert to avoid the child's use of compensatory reactions. As postural reactions become more integrated and hence more automatic, support should be diminished. There are now several options available to the consumer on the internet. Families and therapists alike can search online for commercially available products and alternatives to commercially available products.

For the more severely disabled child, equipment should be easily and completely washable. Mothers should be able

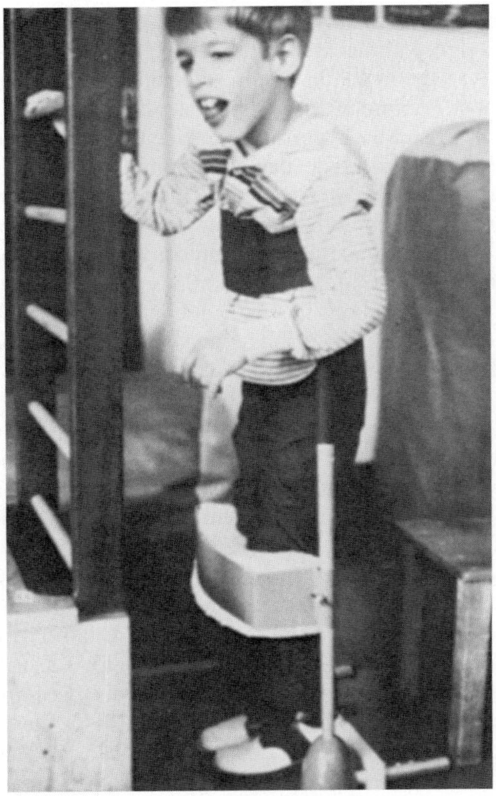

Figure 12-26 ■ An upright stander is easily incorporated into the home environment, providing the child with an upright position, stimulation, and an opportunity to participate in activities.

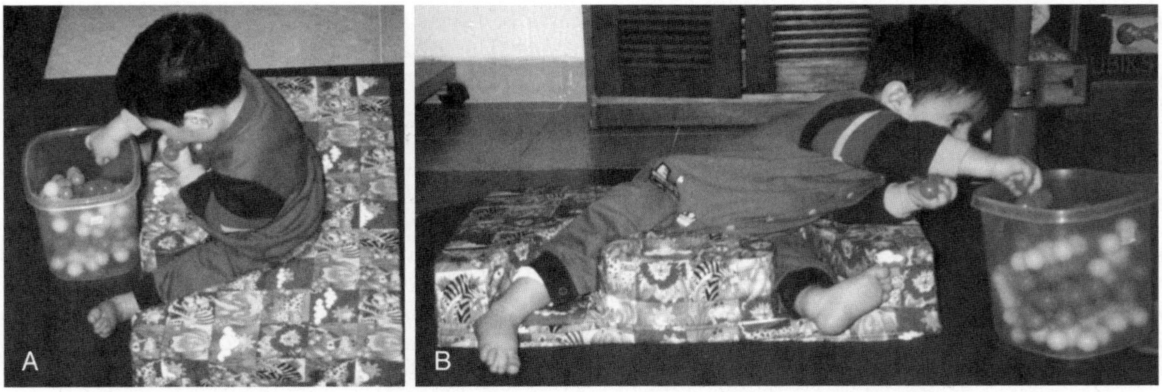

Figure 12-27 ■ Use of a simple cut-out space in 3-inch foam gives this 1-year-old child security while requiring more active trunk adaptation during play.

to place special seating inserts into wheelchairs or travel chairs with one hand while holding the child. Wheelchairs should be ordered with consideration for family needs and the child's environment. The most costly does not always offer the best solution. Control straps and seating should be adaptable and allow for future change on the basis of growth and improved function. The severely limited child needs seating changes at least once every hour during the day to prevent pressure and provide environment changes as in typical development. Pleasing color, good-quality upholstery, and professional finishing are important not only for the child but also for family members, who are accepting the equipment as part of their personal living environment.

As prices rise and the applicability of insurance changes, the therapist must consider cost-effectiveness more carefully. Parents are often desperate to do everything possible for the child and tend to be very susceptible to high-powered advertising and reassuring sales personnel. By providing a list of essential equipment features, the therapist will aid the parents in becoming informed consumers. Perusal of several catalogs permits some comparison of quality and prices. Adaptive equipment fairs are often open to parents and therapists and are great opportunities to actually try the equipment without the burden of the cost. Therapists can forge a relationship with a representative of a medical supply company and then access equipment on loan to try with their patients for short periods of time. Once the appropriate equipment has been purchased, periodic review of equipment used by the child can serve to encourage the family to pass along to someone else equipment items that are no longer needed. Investment in expensive equipment also has the hidden effect of influencing both parent and therapist to continue its use well beyond its effectiveness as a dynamic supplement to treatment. For this reason more than any other, large investments must be thoroughly researched with regard to their long-term applicability for the child.

Adaptive equipment is not the only type of equipment that the therapist must consider for clients. Conditioning and strengthening, now recognized as beneficial to children and adults with cerebral palsy, open the door for equipment that lends itself to these parameters.[107-114] Exercise bikes, treadmills (see Figure 12-22), light weights (see Figure 12-24), and balance equipment (Figure 12-28) are all valuable adjuncts to a home exercise program and should be considered, when appropriate, for a particular individual. Many of the commercially available items found at a sporting goods store can be well adapted to fit the needs of the higher functioning person with cerebral palsy. With more emphasis on working out, sports equipment can even be found in discount stores. Offering to adapt equipment for your clients can encourage and increase compliance with exercises given for home exercise programs.

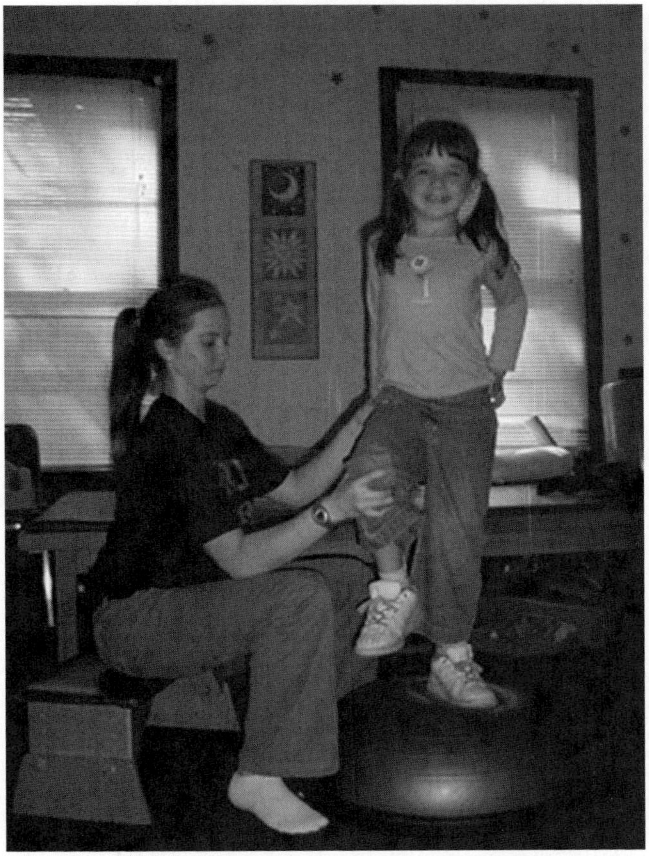

Figure 12-28 ■ Balance equipment allows for increased complexity in the therapy program with the refinement of balance reactions.

ALTERNATIVE THERAPIES

Hyperbaric oxygen treatment is gaining popularity as a treatment for cerebral palsy in children. Clinics are beginning to spring up worldwide for this type of therapy. Research on this treatment has been inconclusive, and scientific evidence for its efficacy is lacking.[173,174] Clinicians should keep abreast of the latest developments in the treatment of cerebral palsy and inform families about the pros and cons of designer treatments. Currently the Undersea and Hyperbaric Medicine Society (UHM) states that there is not enough evidence to recommend the use of hyperbaric oxygen therapy for cerebral palsy.[175,176] A systematic review by McDonagh and colleagues[177] found that there was no significant difference between pressurized air versus room air pressure and that the subjects in both groups made gains. This topic remains controversial even within the UHM. Several articles and editorials have been written with the overwhelming conclusion that randomized clinical trials should be carried out to determine the effectiveness of this treatment.

The Adeli suit is a compression garment with bungee cord–like elastic cords attached to the suit, along the trunk and extremities. This suit, once referred to as the *therapeutic space suit* or *treatment-loading suit,* was developed for Russian cosmonauts to counteract the adverse effect of long-term zero gravity on the skeletal muscles.[178] There are a few studies that suggest that there are benefits for children with cerebral palsy when they receive therapy in the suit.[175,178-181] The suit allows for controlled practice of activities with resistance, and assistance when necessary; the cords are attached in a variety of ways to give different types of practice repetitions. As is prescribed by the proponents of this approach, intense practice is warranted to reap the benefits. This therapy is expensive, and the suit, if bought to use at home, is also very expensive. Rosenbaum[175] has suggested that the benefits of this therapy vary with the type and severity of the involvement, the child's ability to participate in controlled movement, and the tolerance to wearing the suit for extended periods of time. In Australia the Upsuit, described by Blair et al as being made of a stretchy material, has been investigated for use with children with cerebral palsy.[182] Similar results have been noted by Chauvel et al that the type of cerebral palsy and the person's ability to participate in movement forecast the potential outcomes.[183] The Upsuit was also noted to compromise lung capacity, which interfered with the child's ability to participate.[182] As clinicians, it is important for us to stay abreast of the latest developments and to provide families with reasonable alternatives. Although intense practice is well known in the literature as being beneficial for motor learning, the addition of the suit brings in a component that "appears" to provide stability and graded control during practice. Caution when describing this approach to families is warranted because some evidence suggests that it may not be appropriate for every child with cerebral palsy. The long-term effects and measurable outcomes after the use of the Adeli suit and the Upsuit are not documented in the literature.[175,184,185] The following questions must be asked: What happens to the motor abilities of the child when the suit is removed? Has the suit actually prevented the development of postural antigravity coactivation of the trunk and proximal axial joints?

In the mid-1980s Pape[186] published a case series involving five children with cerebral palsy receiving therapeutic (subthreshold) ES. Reported from this case series was that overnight use of low-intensity ES in combination with standard therapy demonstrated significant improvement in gross motor, balance, and locomotor skills as measured by the Peabody Developmental Motor Scales in children with mild cerebral palsy.[186] Results reported were based on observations by individuals who were not blinded to the purpose of the study, and therefore the research design was biased. In a follow-up study Steinbok and colleagues[187] followed children who had undergone selected dorsal rhizotomy and received therapeutic ES for 1 year. Although this study reported improvement in gross motor function, no other measures were changed: range of motion, spasticity, or strength. Two well-controlled clinical trials investigating this method of threshold electrical stimulation (TES) delivery concluded that no objective effects on motor or ambulatory function or clinical benefit for children and youths with cerebral palsy were detected.[188,189] In two separate randomized placebo-controlled clinical trials using TES, the results indicated no significant clinical benefit observed when compared with neuromuscular ES.[188,190] (Refer to Chapter 9 for additional discussion.) Parents often report changes with this therapy, but the objective measures do not demonstrate significant results. Clinicians in the field have reported that overnight use of subthreshold ES builds muscle bulk, but unless combined with active participation of the musculature, overall improvement in movement may not be seen. This therapy, for children with cerebral palsy, requires a special stimulation unit that is subthreshold and capable of being used at night and has a shutoff setting that is activated if the electrodes become disconnected from the child. The unit is costly and further requires a clinician who is specially trained in its use to evaluate and periodically update the treatment protocol. Significant benefits for this type of ES have not been documented.

The Peto method or "conductive education" (CE), developed by Andres Peto in Budapest after World War II, has been used in children with disabilities.[191] This approach is an educational versus medical model, as the name implies, and the focus is on the many aspects of child development.[192] It is based on practice and repetition combined with verbal guidance of a trainer (conductor) and self-verbalization by the child as he or she performs the task or activity.[175] Most of the claims that promote its value have come from the Peto Institute in Budapest, Hungary. The institute has been very selective in choosing candidates for this approach on the basis of the child's potential for independent mobility and function with a good overall prognosis.[175,191,193] Research into this method of delivery of services to children with cerebral palsy has been sparse outside the Peto Institute's studies. In two studies in Australia, CE was found to have encouraging results in developmental changes.[194,195] In a randomized controlled study with children assigned to a CE group or a neurodevelopmental intervention group, no significant differences were noted in the two groups.[198] This approach advocates intense practice of all skills, motor and educational, with emphasis on self-doing regardless of whether a compensatory pattern is used. Various pieces of equipment are used to facilitate independent skills: wooden slatted beds to allow the child to pull and maneuver, and wooden ladders mounted on the wall to assist with dressing and transitions. The literature on CE does stress the concept of intense practice for motor learning. Similarly, promoting practice in the CE environment must transfer to home and community for carryover to everyday life situations.[63] To fully optimize the outcomes of CE, a commitment from the family is essential, as is the case in most therapeutic approaches. Further investigation into this approach is warranted before this philosophy is fully supported. For a selected group of individuals, CE research results seem hopeful, although transfer to unpracticed tasks and different environments may be minimal.[197-199]

The Feldenkrais method was developed by an Israeli engineer, Moshe Feldenkrais, while looking for a solution to his own knee problem. (Refer to Chapter 39 for additional discussion.) He started analyzing body alignment for more efficient movement.[200,201] This form of body work has been used to help dancers, gymnasts, and other skilled persons improve their performance. Some therapists have undertaken the long training necessary to understand typical movement in more detail and to improve the movement coordination of their clients with neuromotor challenges. There is no published research on this method, but several books and training courses exist that promote its use. In a review article by Liptak[184] on alternative interventions, the Feldenkrais method is described; however, no articles have been published examining its use with children who have cerebral palsy.

Ida Rolf, trained in physics, had a son with some postural disorganization.[202] She developed a structural approach, called the Rolfing technique, to improve body alignment; the technique uses specific release of deep soft tissue to restore effortless postural control against gravity.[203] She was able to make positive changes in the movement patterns of many children with cerebral palsy, but she never claimed to treat the disorder itself. This approach requires special training in the Rolfing technique, which is a type of deep tissue massage.

Dr. William Sutherland,[204] an osteopathic physician, developed direct treatment of the cranium, which is referred to commercially as *cranial therapy* or *cranial sacral treatment.* (Refer to Chapter 39 for additional information.) This type of therapy is believed to have wide application to many disabilities and conditions.[205] Today, there are persons trained at many different levels, so the family of a child with cerebral palsy seeking this treatment will need to be certain that the practitioner is a professional and that she or he has experience with small children.[206] Cranial treatment is purported to restore the physiological motion of the craniosacral system, improving circulation of fluids to the brain as well as respiratory function, to which it is believed to be closely linked. Research has been encouraged in this area to substantiate the claims of this approach.

DEVELOPING A PERSONAL PHILOSOPHY OF TREATMENT

The practicing therapist continues to learn much about the nuances of typical human development (see Chapter 3).[207] The dynamic interaction of developmental movement components becomes more significant as the therapist acquires greater clinical experience and recognizes developmental change as a reflection of central nervous system maturation. Increasing knowledge of the functional nature of sensory systems and central nervous system processing will influence the choice of treatment techniques. Direct intervention will have more depth and specificity to improve the child's control of posture and movement while the therapist appreciates the complex interaction of developmental factors in cerebral palsy. On the basis of individual experience, each therapist develops a personal philosophy of treatment that incorporates new research findings and evolving perceptions of the problem of central nervous system dysfunction. Without a philosophical or theoretical orientation for decision making, the therapist may succumb to following each promising treatment idea that is learned without having a clear image of the potential benefits for the specific client. "Commercial" programs may benefit the child whose needs match the program objectives. An "individualized" program adapts to the needs of the particular child and is shaped by the response of that child during therapy. Without an internalized treatment goal toward which independent techniques are applied, the result may remain ineffective and unconvincing. The therapist in a direct treatment situation must develop a concise visualization of what is to be achieved in each session with the individual child based on a sound foundation. The repetition and practice that are so critical for learning must often be carried out at home, and the therapist becomes responsible for family instruction. Home exercise programs must be tailored for both the child and the family situation and must be in alignment with the goals and expectations of the family. These programs need to be practical, fun ideas for practice that can be incorporated into the child's home life with reasonable assurance that the activities can and will be carried out regularly. Creative therapeutic ideas for playtime, dressing, grooming, mealtime, and relaxation time are best addressed in the home exercise program because these are everyday tasks that every family encounters and the family is likely to be compliant.[208] The time spent in therapy throughout the week cannot substitute for all the hours spent at home and school.

Specialized therapy, like typical development, is potentially a preparation for functional performance. Training in specific coordination skills may be necessary for the older child or adolescent and must begin with a thorough analysis of the whole person who happens to demonstrate the effects of cerebral palsy. Some children have learned self-care along with brothers and sisters. Others have needed therapy guidance for each achievement. Intelligent children with strong motivation may only need some assistance in avoiding use of atypical reactions, whereas others have poor spatial orientation and minimal motivation to achieve independence. The therapist most often needs to create a dialog with the individual who has the problem because parents are often fatigued and without energy to solve the issue of adolescent life skills. Perseverance is key to success with these individuals.

INVOLVING THE FAMILY

To be successful, therapy for the child with cerebral palsy includes active family participation. Variability of practice in different environments tends to promote more effective motor learning, and parents who learn to help their child early begin to understand the importance of their participation as well as the nature of their child's disability. Parents are in the process of healing their own self-image, which was so injured when they learned of their child's disability. They should not be expected to become therapists per se but should learn to observe small gains in treatment sessions that offer insight into the child's current strengths and weaknesses.[17]

Parents need to adapt their expectations in keeping with the child's continuing change and emotional maturity. Parenting a child with cerebral palsy is no easy task, and the therapist will do well to develop respect for this demanding role. No one provides more for the child with cerebral palsy than the nurturing parent who guides the child to self-acceptance of limitations without destroying personal initiative. This is the child who most often becomes an independent working adult (Figure 12-29).

The therapist must give serious thought to priorities in home recommendations. Therapists must consider the size of the family and whether there are siblings, outside employment of the mother and father, physical capabilities of the child, general health status of the child, and psychological acceptance of the problem within the family. The emotional needs of some parents demand a period of less, rather than more, direct involvement with the child. Other parents must be cautioned that repetition of an activity more times than recommended will not result in faster improvement. This impression is sometimes gained from wide advertising of commercial programs that offer the same activity sequence for every child and demand a large number of daily repetitions. Both parent and therapist must appreciate the need for the central nervous system to have some time to integrate new sensorimotor experiences and to perfect emerging control of postural adjustments. Excessive control of movement patterns and overprotection by an adult tends to reduce the child's initiation of postural change and decrease active sensorimotor learning. Health needs for good nutrition and adequate rest must also be considered by parents and professionals. The attitude of teachers in the first years is extremely important for the child with cerebral palsy. Advocating for a positive environment across the settings is advantageous for the child's achievement.

ROLE OF THE THERAPIST IN INDIRECT INTERVENTION

For many children with cerebral palsy, active treatment is not available. Geographical isolation, socioeconomic factors, poor or lack of insurance coverage, and lack of qualified therapists may interfere with the delivery of direct service. The therapist must then assume the role of teacher, counselor, or consultant. More often the new role emerges as one in which the therapist tries to meet a combination of needs and is frequently frustrated by lack of time, energy, and community resources. The therapist may be a member of a community team that includes a psychologist, a social worker, and a public health nurse. This sometimes creates more of a behavioral than a traditional medical orientation. Therapists can also be primarily responsible to the public school systems, introducing therapeutic positioning to classroom teachers. For these types of situations the clinician will find videotape a valuable adjunct to direct instruction. The individual child may be filmed with equipment, adequate positions, or therapeutic procedures. Useful topic-oriented videotapes are also available for professionals and families. Instruction of key personnel in these settings is critical to the success of the therapist's recommendations.

When children have no access to direct treatment, positioning is of paramount importance. The selected support is used to avoid contractures, scoliosis, and permanent limitations in range of movement. Even the most severely limited child should have a minimum of three positions that can be alternated during the day. In addition, the position selected should be as functional as possible for the individual child to allow access to the child's environment. In some cases this may mean encouraging eye contact. For another child, hand use becomes a possibility with proper trunk support. Each program should be individualized to maximize potential for the child in that environment.

Communication for the nonverbal client with cerebral palsy must be an integral part of the therapy or school program.[209] A simple start may be made with pictures to permit choices in food, clothing, and therapy activities. The parents need encouragement to begin the process of letting the child make some simple choices in food, clothing, or preferred activities. Although computers have their place, the child should have the communication device with him or her at all times. Language development in the young child is enhanced by having this type of alternative communication device available while articulation is still difficult. Use of head movement is a powerful influence on muscle tone changes that may cause negative regression in postural or visual control. Care and consideration should be taken when evaluating the body part to access the device. Postural and visual control is essential toward the goal of better function and communication. A solution that was successful with one 9-year-old athetoid girl was moving the elbow back to a switch mounted on the vertical bar of the wheelchair backrest to access her communication device. Any activity that is repeated on a daily basis should be examined in light of possible interference by atypical patterns.

Affordable electronic systems with voice recording, portability, and growth features are available. Communication, which can be achieved by coordinating efforts with the speech pathologist, can make the difference between passivity and active participation in the environment.[209] Play can be encouraged with the use of switch toys and touch-screen computers. Many new programs are being developed for computers and electronic interactive books.

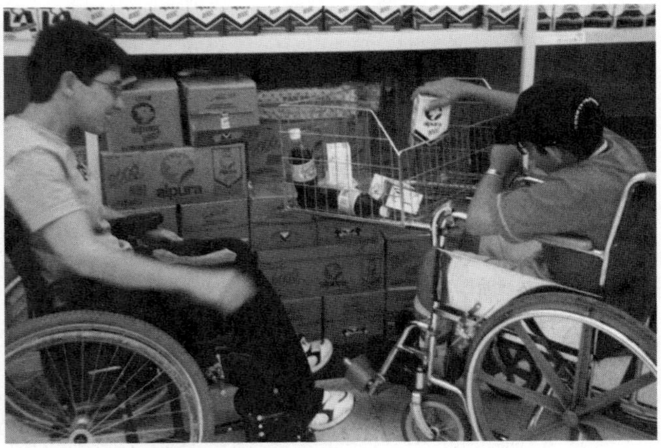

Figure 12-29 ■ Therapy goals must incorporate functional activities that lead to personal independence if they are to be pertinent for the older child and adolescent.

THERAPY IN THE COMMUNITY

Therapists are often concerned with body functions and structure and neglect to address participation in real-life activities such as school attendance, sports, employment, and involvement in the community.[210] Children with mild dysfunction as a result of cerebral palsy may be successfully incorporated into physical education (PE) classes if the teacher is prepared to make some small adaptations. Teachers generally appreciate the opportunity to discuss with the therapist specific limitations of the child and those movements that should be encouraged. Taking the opportunity to meet with the PE coach to establish adaptations and modifications or appropriate participation in activities is time well spent for the child's integration into the class. PE class is often rewarding for the child and important in establishing peer relationships. For better success the child with functional limitations can be incorporated into a class that follows the British form of movement education, which places much less emphasis on intragroup competition and encourages each child to progress at her or his own rate.

Classroom teachers who lack experience with children who have special needs are understandably reluctant to incorporate a child with movement limitations into the classroom until they know the child. A meeting with the therapist might be used to help the child demonstrate his or her strengths, physical independence, and ability to participate in classroom activities. The child may often play an active role in the problem-solving process necessary for a successful classroom experience. Children often have developed their own ways of managing the water fountain, the locker door, or personal care needs. Demonstrating these abilities reinforces strengths rather than limitations and empowers the child to receive positive responses from curious peers.

As programs that hire therapists move into the fields of prevention and early intervention, the therapist is dealing directly with a population that is not familiar with therapy per se nor aware of the need for this intervention. The therapist may discover a need to reorient previously accepted concepts of general rehabilitation. Clarification of one's own ideas is essential to establish effective communication with others. In some instances, active intervention to help the child will precede the labeling or diagnostic process, and referral to other specialists becomes part of the therapist's responsibility. Philosophically, early therapy becomes an enhancement of typical development rather than a remedial process, and it is advocated in the natural environment by federal funding agencies for children 0 to 3 years of age. This implies introducing new concepts of quality in early child development to the public. Day care programs are an example of new early childhood settings that incorporate children with impairments.

It is important to keep direct, active treatment available for older children, adolescents, and adults who are motivated to change. Now that more effective procedures are available for changing some of the basic neurophysiological movement characteristics observed in children with cerebral palsy, it is possible to achieve change with direct treatment of the older client. The adolescent often responds best to short-term, goal-oriented therapy programs that are patient centered. Motor learning concepts are better understood by both the therapist and the client and can be incorporated in activities after mobilizing tissues that have been unused for so many years (see Chapters 4 and 9). With current program directions, many older clients may not have had the opportunity for direct treatment over time by a qualified therapist. For the minimally involved teenager, young adult, and adult with cerebral palsy the local gym offers an alternative to direct therapy. General conditioning is very popular in community programs including weight training, endurance training, water exercises, yoga, and walking programs. A therapist can be consulted to establish an appropriate program for the individual who wants to work out at the gym on equipment, attend special classes that are offered, or work out in the pool. When asked, it is the therapist's area of expertise to help identify and make recommendations regarding functional movement and activity participation for adults with developmental disabilities such as cerebral palsy. (See the section in Chapter 35 on adults with developmental disabilities.) The movement toward a health orientation as opposed to crisis intervention for illness will also affect services for children and adults with cerebral palsy. This population does not have an illness or an active disease process, and they strive to lead as normal a life as possible. Many adults with neuromotor disabilities express their preference to participate in the decisions that are made for them regarding their ultimate lifestyle and participation in the community. The therapist who works with this population should familiarize himself or herself with the patient's living situation—family home, group home, or independent living—as well as the support system and work environment if applicable. These factors should be considered when establishing a viable program. Many opportunities for employment and volunteerism exist in communities for individuals with disabilities. This may require that the therapist venture into the workplace to assess accessibility and modifications that can be done in that environment to make for successful integration of the individual into the community. Optimal health for the adult with cerebral palsy has yet to be described, and much more data must be collected. However, it is an exciting time as our society moves forward in its views and acknowledgment of disability (see Chapter 35).

PSYCHOSOCIAL FACTORS IN CEREBRAL PALSY

We have defined cerebral palsy as a condition existing from the time of birth or infancy. The developing child has no memory of life in a different body. Movement limitations circumscribe the horizon of the child's world unless the family is able to provide enriching experiences. The development of both intelligence and personality relies heavily on developmental experiences and the opportunity for self-expression.

The child with spastic diplegia or spastic quadriplegia may be hesitant in making decisions or reaching out for a new opportunity because the world may seem overwhelming and threatening. The child may find it easier to withdraw toward social isolation. Parents and professionals can help children, adolescents, and adults with cerebral palsy avoid these reactions by encouraging independence in thought and in physical tasks. Early choices can be made by the child regarding which clothes to wear or which task to do first. Understanding the child's limitations helps build successes rather than failures. To function in spite of the constraints of spasticity or other movement problems demands considerable effort on the part of the child.

Athetoid children, in contrast, have adapted to failures as a transient part of life. However disorganized their movements, they repeatedly attempt tasks and eventually succeed. Their social interactions reflect this life experience. Most people will sooner or later succumb to the positive smiling approach without analyzing the deeper communication offered by the child. These children are difficult for parents to discipline and structure during their early years. Early treatment with concomitant guidance for young parents ameliorates some of the problems by making the developmental expectations for the child more appropriate. The words of professionals who are in contact with the parents at the time of the diagnosis echo through time to influence future decision making for the child.

Intelligent children with low tone demand that the world be brought to them. Mentally limited children may fail to receive sufficient stimulation for optimal development at their functional levels. Many of these children need visual or auditory evaluations and intervention, and some of them need a special educational approach. Whatever the learning potential of the child with cerebral palsy, it is not always evident early in the child's life. Parents find it difficult to know how to guide a child when they are not certain that an assigned task or calm explanation is understood by the child.

Parental guidance of the child with functional limitations is also influenced by the adults' adaptation to their offspring's problem. Parents need to resolve in their own way the emotional impact of the child's disability. Parents need time to grieve the loss of dreams they had for their child, and each person will approach this in his or her own way and time. Each major milestone anticipated in a typical child's life may bring on the grieving process again. Most parents feel inadequate, ignorant, and relatively helpless at being unable to remedy the situation for their child. They need help in feeling good about themselves before they can effectively guide the child toward self-acceptance as an adequate human being. Parents need guidance to provide themselves with opportunities to rest and renew their energies. Therapists can be instrumental during this process by remaining nonjudgmental. (Refer to Chapter 6 for additional information.)

The therapist plays an important role in the psychosocial development of children who receive regular treatment. The child may perceive the therapist as a confidant, disciplinarian, counselor, or friend at various stages of development. Some children accept the therapist as a member of their extended family. This is natural, considering the extent to which therapists influence clients' own self-awareness through changes in their physical bodies. However, it also places a personal responsibility on the therapist to be aware of the continuing interaction and its effect on the maturational process of the child. Long-term relationships with patients and their families must remain professional for the therapist to be effective.

Any evaluation of personality characteristics in a disabled child must take into account the unnatural lifestyle that is imposed by the need for therapy, medical appointments, limited environmental exploration, and hospitalization. The child is expected to separate from parents earlier than the average child and usually confronts many more novel situations. There is little time or physical opportunity for free play. Continuous demands are placed on children to prove their intellectual potential in evaluations of various types. Adults most often monitor their social interaction while they assume a dependent role. Nonetheless, these children's social acceptance frequently rests on their skill in interacting with persons in their environments. It is not fair to the child to evaluate the evolution of personality without considering these experiential factors.

DOCUMENTATION

Developing a plan of care (POC) with objective measurable goals is required for documentation of progress in intervention and reimbursement from third-party payers. (Refer to Chapter 10 for additional recommendations.) Carefully extracting a child's strengths and weaknesses from the assessment should drive the POC. Using timed measures, distance, number of repetitions, standardized tools, and other measurable outcomes provides a source of encouragement for families and justification for continued intervention.

Data collection is an important task in the treatment of cerebral palsy. Change occurs at variable rates, but it is important to document the cause and effect of change whenever possible. Slides or videotapes are useful in recording functional comparisons over time. Digital video now allows a specific analysis of movement sequences. A motor drive unit or automatic advance on a 35-mm single-lens reflex camera can record a sample of movement five or more times per second. Placing the subject against a spaced grid in a specific alignment to perform a movement task allows for measurement of efficiency of movement. These ideas may be applied to documentation of treatment effectiveness or analyzed for an understanding of similar movement problems in other clients. When attempting to document using photographs or filming, consistency in the environment is critical to the outcome and analysis. Reliable comparisons made between one time point and another require the same testing environment, time of day, and conditions.

Methods of intervention or treatment are measurable for research and applicable to the functional problems presented by a diagnosis of cerebral palsy. Once a specific research question has been formulated, systematic recordings of appropriate data can be gathered over time to accumulate data for a viable study. There is value in longitudinal reporting of a single case or a small group of individuals who have some characteristics in common because this aids our understanding of what we need to prevent in the young child to permit optimal function later. (See Chapters 8 and 10 for suggestions of impairment and disability measurements to be used as objective measures for functional outcome studies and record keeping.) Clinicians have a difficult time putting into words exactly what takes place during intervention, which further complicates research investigation into the efficacy of treatment. Descriptive analysis of treatment is essential to document and begin to understand what a therapist does during a therapy session. Understanding what takes place in therapy will help identify questions that could be investigated more closely.

The way in which therapists learn to view a problem determines, to a large extent, the potential range of solutions available to them. Cerebral palsy is a complex of motor and movement inabilities that cluster about the inadequacy of central nervous system control, visual and soft tissue restrictions, and the amazing ability of the human body to compensate. Therapists need to look critically at developmental processes, qualities of movement, postural adjustments, timing and limitations of movements, and the range of dynamic functional movement. New areas of motor learning and systems and chaos theories offer the researcher novel approaches to the challenge of cerebral palsy and the resultant disorder of posture control and movement learning. Environmental factors may have as much influence as specific central nervous system limitations. Early intervention should be analytical, specific, and based on a theoretical foundation. Posture and movement control begins to change with direct treatment. Analysis of the postural components and movement characteristics of children with cerebral palsy will lead to meaningful research more quickly than will professional reliance on the traditional definitions of the medical condition. Thorough documentation of therapy progress using objective measures is critical for development of more effective intervention strategies in the future (see Chapter 10).

CASE STUDIES

To understand the problems of children with cerebral palsy, it is essential to follow some children over time to capture the evolution of family problems. Functional treatment must change according to the developmental level, chronological age, and neuromotor responses of the child. Intervention must be specific to the presenting problem of the moment while the missing aspects of complete motor development are considered. The case study comparison of two boys illustrates the typical lack of clinical correlation between history and manifested characteristics of cerebral palsy.

References

To enhance this text and add value for the reader, all references are included on the companion Evolve site that accompanies this textbook. This online service will, when available, provide a link for the reader to a Medline abstract for the article cited. There are 210 cited references and other general references for this chapter, with the majority of those articles being evidence-based citations.

CASE STUDY 12-1

A young woman was pregnant with her first child. She was middle class, was well nourished, and had no identified risk factors. In the seventh month of pregnancy, her older sister died, causing considerable emotional upheaval. The much-anticipated infant was born, small for gestational age, at the correct date. It was theorized that there had been inadequate intrauterine nourishment during the first 6 to 7 months. The child, L. P., weighed 3 pounds, 8 ounces (1587 g) and was fed initially by nasogastric tube. Her movements were quick, and eye movement was very active for a newborn infant. She was seen for therapy at 17 days of age, immediately after hospital discharge.

The initial therapy focus was on the practical task of adequate nutritional intake so that the nasogastric tube could be removed before scarring occurred from repeated passage of the tube. Swaddling was suggested to calm the infant and assist her organization of body movement. Simple handling was oriented toward moving the trunk over midline to let the head follow and assisting the infant to assume age-appropriate antigravity postures.

At 3 years of age L. P. continued to have difficulty with control of her head position in space and was unable to initiate postural changes with her head. The clinical picture was one of low tone with athetoid movement. She could not speak, communicated with looks and a few word approximations, and hitched along the floor in a seated position with one supporting hand.

By 5 years of age L. P. was still receiving therapy three times per week and could walk in a hesitating way with her hands held. At this stage she was evaluated by a behavioral optometrist and started vision therapy to prepare her to participate in preschool activities. As a secondary benefit her balance in walking improved markedly. L. P. began walking up and down 27 steps daily in her new home.

Now, at 7 years of age, L. P. can walk independently on level surfaces. She has physical therapy once a week and vision therapy once a week to maintain her control of posture and movement. Her school performance is adequate to keep her with her age peers and she attends a regular school.

CASE STUDY 12-2

D. D. and E. D. were born within 6 months of each other at 6 months 1 week of gestation. Both were first-born infants for their respective mothers. D. D.'s mother was discovered to have a double uterus when she had a miscarriage early in the pregnancy. E. D. had malnutrition during his intrauterine development. D. D. started therapy just before he was 5 months old, and E. D. began therapy at almost 7 months old.

At 6 years of age D. D. walks alone with very mild athetotic "overflow." He wears corrective lenses that were fit at 2 years of age, and he returns for follow-up examinations with the behavioral optometrist once a year. Vision therapy was an important adjunct to physical handling because it introduced changes in spatial perception on the basis of specific sessions with prism lenses. At age 4 years D. D. was discovered to have a mild to moderate hearing loss; he still uses a hearing aid in one ear. He speaks English and Spanish, as do his parents, and he understands the French spoken to him by his grandparents. He functions in a regular school with his age peers and is a well-adapted, active child.

At 6 years of age E. D. has moderately severe diplegia, with some immaturity of hand use and trunk control. He speaks English and Spanish well, although he demonstrates some emotional instability and difficulty in dealing with his disability. He is creative in storytelling and offers to tell original stories for other children in therapy. He is just beginning to walk with a walker within interior environments and with low resistance.

CHAPTER 13 Genetic Disorders: A Pediatric Perspective

SANDRA G. BELLAMY, PT, MS, DPT, PCS, and EUNICE YU CHIU SHEN, PT, PhD, DPT, PCS

KEY TERMS

evaluation
functional skills
genetic disorders
natural environments
occupational therapist
physical therapist

OBJECTIVES

After reading this chapter the student or therapist will be able to:

1. Describe the main types of genetic disorders and give examples of each type.
2. Differentiate between genetic disorders diagnosed with clinical versus laboratory methods.
3. Describe three modes of inheritance for single-gene disorders.
4. Recognize key impairments that are common to many genetic conditions in pediatric clients.
5. Explain the physical or occupational therapist's role in the recognition, referral, and multidisciplinary management of genetic conditions in pediatric clients.
6. Identify resources and strategies for accessing information and increasing knowledge about genetic disorders for use in clinical decision making.
7. Explain why it is important to include family members in the planning and development of therapy programs for children with genetic disorders.
8. Describe and give examples of three types of assessment tools, and state the intended purpose of each.
9. Describe the importance of developing therapy programs for children that are outcome focused on functional skills in natural environments.

Genetic disorders in children can result in a wide variety of movement impairments and disabilities. The resultant impact of certain genetic conditions on the child may be evident before or immediately after birth, whereas other conditions may not be diagnosed until later in life when problems manifest. In this chapter we discuss disorders of known genetic origin that physical and occupational therapists are most likely to encounter in therapy programs for children.

The Human Genome Project, completed in 2003,[1] expanded knowledge about the genetic basis for disease and congenital malformations. The impact of this project is just being realized, with new research into diagnostic techniques and treatment options for genetic disorders. Pediatric health care professionals will be faced with questions from families who, in seeking diagnostic and prognostic information, are accessing the wealth of information both in the lay scientific press and on the World Wide Web (Box 13-1 and Table 13-1).

An accurate diagnosis of a specific genetic disorder (syndrome or disease) is necessary for a prognosis to be provided, for eligibility for therapy and education services to be determined, and as a basis for genetic counseling for the child's family.[2] The diagnostic process for genetic disorders includes a combination of clinical assessments by the physician who collects the child's medical history and a clinical geneticist who may construct a family history or "pedigree" to recognize disorders with familiar inheritance patterns. Molecular studies may confirm a clinical diagnosis, differentiate between diagnoses with similar clinical presentation, and identify the genetic cause of the disorder. Some genetic disorders are not easily identified, and laboratory testing can be extensive, prolonged, and often inconclusive; therefore pediatricians may refer children to occupational and physical therapy before the nature of their condition is fully known.[2,3] Although sometimes far removed from the hospitals and specialized centers that perform genetic testing and diagnosis, the pediatric therapist is often able to contribute clinical evidence that will assist the diagnostic process.[4-6] Furthermore, many genetic diseases and syndromes are increasingly survivable into adulthood; thus it is vital that physical and occupational therapists achieve competence in genetics and genomics in order to deliver care throughout the patient's life span.[6,7] An overview of the general categories and subtypes of genetic disorders is presented first. Specific examples of each type are given, along with a brief description of key diagnostic features and issues commonly addressed with medical and therapeutic intervention. A summary of impairments common to many pediatric genetic disorders is presented in the second section. The third section includes a discussion of the medical management of genetic disorders, genetic counseling, and the ethical implications of genetic screening and testing. The final section focuses on the physical or occupational therapist's role in the clinical management of children with genetic disorders. The therapist's role and responsibilities in developing competence in recognition, referral, and clinical practice when working with patients and families affected by a genetic disorder are discussed. Evaluation procedures, treatment goals and objectives, and general treatment principles and strategies are discussed from a family-centered perspective. A list of educational resources for clinicians and families is provided.

BOX 13-1 ■ RESOURCES ON TOPICS IN GENETICS FOR CLINICIANS AND FAMILIES

TEXTBOOK

Jorde LB, Carey JC, Bamshad MC, et al: *Medical genetics,* ed 2, St Louis, 2000, Mosby.

Review for clinicians of basic genetic science; helpful illustrations.

WORLD WIDE WEB

1. *Understanding Genetics*
   http://geneticalliance.org/sites/default/files/ksc_assets/pdfs/manual_all2.pdf
   Free pdf-format primer on basics of human genetics for health professionals and families.
2. *Human Genome Project Information*
   www.ornl.gov/sci/techresources/Human_Genome/home.shtml
   Links to research; teacher and student tools; gene testing; summary of current scientific knowledge in genomics; and fundamentals of genetics including interactive map of each human chromosome and associated diseases and disorders.
3. *Genetics Fact Sheets, Centre for Genetics Education*
   www.genetics.com/au/pdf/factsheets/fs01.pdf
   Consumer-friendly pdf-format modules on basic genetics with simple illustrations for difficult-to-understand scientific concepts.
4. *Genetics Home Reference, National Library of Medicine (Bethesda, Md), 1993-2008*
   http://ghr.nlm.nih.gov
   Consumer-friendly genetics glossary and encyclopedia of genetic conditions.
5. *Family Village*
   www.familyvillage.wisc.edu
   Website for children and adults with disabilities and their families, friends, and allies.
   Covers various diagnoses, assistive technology, legal rights and legislation, special education, and leisure activities.
6. *Making Sense of Your Genes: A Guide to Genetic Counseling*
   www.nsgc.org/client_files/GuidetoGeneticCounseling.pdf
7. *American College of Medical Genetics*
   www.acmg.net
   Information about educational courses in genetics for health care professionals.
8. *Genetics and Public Policy Center*
   www.dnapolicy.org
   Information on currently available genetics testing and family planning.
9. *National Newborn Screening and Genetics Resource Center*
   http://genes-r-us.uthscsa.edu/resources/newborn/00chapters.html
   Lists what genetic screening tests are being performed in the 50 U.S. states. Gives definitions of various genetic disorders.

AN OVERVIEW: CLINICAL DIAGNOSIS AND TYPES OF GENETIC DISORDERS WITH REPRESENTATIVE CLINICAL EXAMPLES

Genetic disorders are typically divided into four categories: chromosomal, single-gene, mitochondrial, and multifactorial. Chromosomal disorders arise when there is an alteration in either the number or structure of chromosomes that exist in either autosomal or sex (X, Y) chromosomes.[8] Numerical or large structural chromosomal abnormalities can be seen through a microscope; therefore a sample of the patient's peripheral blood can be used in detection of disorders such as Down syndrome. When there is a suspicion of a clinical spectrum associated with some of the known chromosomal microdeletions, translocations, or inversions, direct deoxyribonucleic acid (DNA) analysis techniques such as fluorescence in situ hybridization (FISH) with use of specific sequence DNA probes can confirm a specific suspected diagnosis. Indirect DNA analysis techniques such as linkage analysis can be performed to confirm single-gene disorders when the gene or genomic region associated with the disorder is unknown.[9]

Of our 20,000 to 25,000 protein-coding genes,[1] a single gene may be responsible for approximately 6000 known genetic traits. Approximately 4000 of these known traits are diseases or disorders.[10] Single-gene disorders may be transmitted through three different patterns: autosomal dominant, autosomal recessive, and sex linked. *Dominant* refers to the case in which a mutated gene from one parent is sufficient to produce the disorder in offspring. *Recessive* refers to the case in which the disorder will not be expressed unless offspring inherited a mutated copy of that gene from both parents. It is incorrect to say that a *gene* is recessive or dominant; rather the *trait,* or disorder, is dominant or recessive.[7]

Inheritance is usually a term reserved for the transmission of a previously recognized family trait to subsequent offspring. However, many genetic disorders arise from new, spontaneous mutations in a *gamete,* the single egg cell from the mother or a sperm cell from the father. The remainder of the gametes from either parent are most likely normal. In this case their offspring will be the first in the family to display the *sporadic* disorder, and the faulty gene can then be passed onto subsequent generations. A disorder that results from a single copy of a mutated gene is referred to as a *dominant* disorder, even if it is acquired by a spontaneous mutation. Not all literature sources will include spontaneous mutations in the description of *inherited* disorders.

It is important to understand how a disorder was acquired, because the relative risks to other offspring for the disorder vary according to mode of transmission. For example, the risk of having another child with the same genetic disorder that occurred as a result of a spontaneous mutation is low. However, when one parent is affected by an inherited dominant mutation, the risk of passing that faulty gene onto each child is 50%.[8]

Most congenital malformations and many serious diseases that have an onset in childhood or adulthood are not caused by single genes or chromosomal defects; these are called *multifactorial disorders.*[7,8]

Mitochondrial disorders are caused by alterations in maternally inherited cytoplasmic mitochondrial DNA (mtDNA). The clinical manifestations of mtDNA-related disorders are extremely variable,[11] and the occurrence is reportedly rare

TABLE 13-1 ■ ASSISTIVE TECHNOLOGY

RESOURCE	WEBSITE	INFORMATION
AbleData	www.abledata.com	Information about assistive technology (AT) products and rehabilitation equipment
AccessIT	www.washington.edu/accessit	National Center on Accessible Information Technology in Education
Alliance for Technology Access	www.ataccess.org	Public education, information, referral; network of technology resources
Assistive Technology Industry Association	www.atia.org/i4a/pages/index.cfm	Information on products and services
Assistive Technology Partners	www.assistivetechnologypartners.com	Information to assist persons with cognitive, sensory, and/or physical disabilities
Assistive Technology Training Online Project	http://atto.buffalo.edu	AT applications that help students with disabilities learn in elementary classrooms
Family Center on Technology and Disability	www.fctd.info	Provides guide to AT and transition planning
National Public Website on Assistive Technology	www.assistivetech.net	Features products by related functional area or disability, by activity, and by vendor
Protection and Advocacy for Assistive Technology Program	www.workworld.org/wwwebhelp/protection_and_advocacy_systems_overview.htm	Provides protection and advocacy services to help individuals with disabilities of all ages acquire, use, and maintain AT services or devices; website identifies each state's program
Rehabtool.com	www.rehabtool.com	Information on AT products by categories
National Institute of Standards and Technology (Standards.gov)	http://standards.gov/standards_gov/index.cfm	Authoritative information and guidance on measurement and standards for all industry sectors

(5.0 per 100,000)[8,12]; however, collectively as a group of neuromuscular disorders, they account for substantial use of health care resources.[12]

Currently there are over 1000 genetic tests available in the United States.[1] Specific DNA testing may soon be able to identify nearly all human genetic disorders. This not only allows for accurate and more complete diagnosis but should pave the way for the development of mechanisms for treatment, cure, and prevention of certain genetic conditions.[4,5,8,9] Table 13-2 lists examples of specific disorders in categories of the most common pattern of inheritance by which each occurs.

Chromosomal Disorders

Cytogenics is the study of chromosomal abnormalities. A karyotype is prepared that displays the 46 chromosomes—22 pairs of autosomes arranged according to length, and then the two sex chromosomes that determine male or female sex. Modern methods of staining karyotypes enable analysis of the various numerical and structural abnormalities that can occur. Most chromosomal abnormalities appear as numerical abnormalities (aneuploidy) such as one missing chromosome (monosomy) or an additional chromosome, as in trisomy 21 (Down syndrome).[8] Structural abnormalities occur in many forms. They include a missing or "extra portion" of a chromosome or a translocation error, which is an interchange of genetic material between nonhomologous chromosomes. The incidence of chromosomal abnormalities among spontaneously aborted fetuses may be as high as 60%.[8,13] About one in 150 live-born infants have a detectable chromosomal abnormality; and in about half of these cases the chromosomal abnormality is accompanied by congenital anomalies, intellectual disability, or phenotypical changes that manifest later in life.[8] Of the fetuses with abnormal chromosomes that survive to term, about half have sex chromosome abnormalities and the other half have autosomal trisomies.[8]

The following section provides a brief overview of common genetic disorders seen by physical and occupational therapists working with children.

Autosomal Trisomies

Trisomy is the condition of a single extranuclear chromosome. Trisomies occur frequently among live births, usually as a result of the failure of the parental chromosomes to disjoin normally during meiosis. Trisomy can occur in autosomal or sex cells. Trisomies 21, 18, and 13 are the most frequently occurring trisomies; however, few children with trisomy 18 and 13 survive beyond 1 year of age.[1]

Trisomy 21 (Down Syndrome). Trisomy 21 occurs in approximately one in every 740 live births,[14] and its incidence is distributed equally between the sexes.[10] The pathophysiological features of Down syndrome are caused by an overexpression of genes on human chromosome 21. Ninety-five percent of individuals have an extra copy in all of their body's cells. The remaining 5% have the mosaic and translocation forms.[15] In the United States the incidence of Down syndrome increases with advanced maternal age.[10] Detection of Down syndrome is possible with various prenatal tests, and the diagnosis is confirmed by the presence of characteristic physical features present in the infant at birth.[16] Down syndrome is the most common chromosomal cause of moderate to severe intellectual disability.[15] The typical phenotypical features observable from birth are hypotonia,

TABLE 13-2 ■ PARTIAL LISTING OF PEDIATRIC GENETIC CONDITIONS

SYNDROME OR DISEASE	APPROXIMATE INCIDENCE (UNITED STATES)
CHROMOSOMAL ABNORMALITIES	
Autosomal Trisomy	
Trisomy 21	1:740
Trisomy 18	1:5000
Trisomy 13	1:16,000
Sex Chromosome Aneuploidy	
Turner syndrome	1:2500 females
Klinefelter syndrome	1:500-1000 males
Partial Deletion	
Prader-Willi syndrome	1:10,000-30,000
Angelman Syndrome	1:12,000-20,000
Cri-du-chat syndrome	1:20,000-50,000
SINGLE-GENE ABNORMALITIES	
Autosomal Dominant	
Neurofibromatosis type 1	1:3500
Tuberous sclerosis	1:5800
Osteogenesis imperfecta	6-7:100,000
Autosomal Recessive	
Cystic fibrosis	1:2500-3500 Caucasians (highest ethnic incidence)
Spinal muscle atrophy	1:6000-10,000
Phenylketonuria	1:10,000-15,000
Hurler syndrome	1:100,000
Sex-Linked	
Duchenne muscular dystrophy	1:3500
Fragile X syndrome	1:4000 males, 1:8000 females
Hemophilia A	1:4000-5000 males
Rett syndrome	1:10,000-22,000 females
MULTIFACTORIAL ABNORMALITIES	
Cleft lip with or without cleft palate	1:1000
Clubfoot (talipes equinovarus)	1:1000
Spina bifida	7:10,000
MITOCHONDRIAL ABNORMALITIES	
Mitochondrial myopathy	Rare
Kearns-Sayre disease	Rare

epicanthic folds, flat nasal bridge, upward slanting palpebral fissures, small mouth, excessive skin at the nape of the neck, and a single transverse palmar crease (Figure 13-1).

Information compiled by the Centers for Disease Control and Prevention for years 1968 through 1997 indicates that the median survival age of individuals with Down syndrome is 49 years, compared with 1 year in 1968. Improvements in the median survival age were less in races other than white, although the reasons for this remain unclear.[14] Half of all children with Down syndrome have congenital heart defects.[16] Congenital heart problems, respiratory infection, and leukemia are the most common factors associated with morbidity and mortality in childhood,[17] whereas a possible increased tendency for premature cellular aging and Alzheimer disease may account for higher mortality rates later in life.[18]

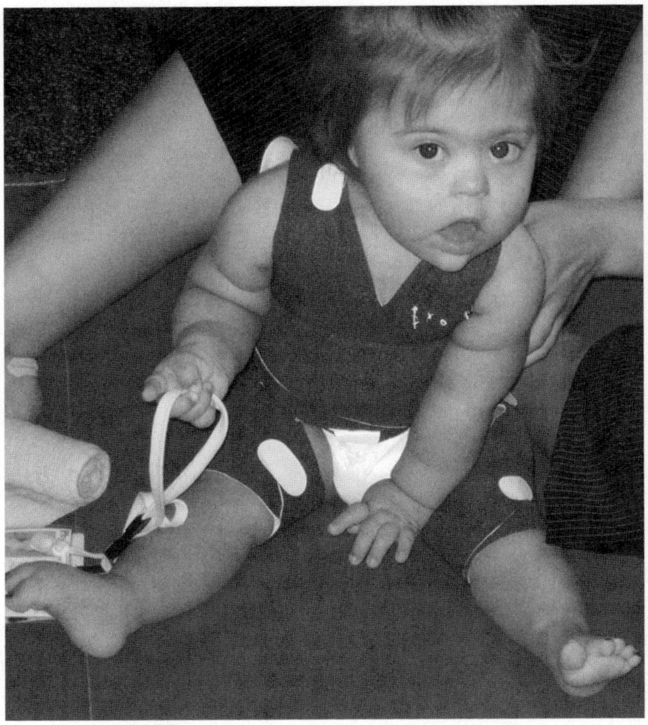

Figure 13-1 ■ Ten-month-old girl with Down syndrome.

Impairments of visual and sensory systems are also common in individuals with Down syndrome. As many as 77% of children with Down syndrome have a refractive error (myopia, hyperopia), astigmatism, or problems in accommodation.[19] Hearing losses that interfere with language development are reportedly present in 80% of children with Down syndrome. In most cases the hearing loss is conductive; in up to 20% of cases the loss is sensorineural or mixed.[16,20] Obstructive sleep apnea has been reported to exist frequently in young children[21,22] and adults with Down syndrome.[23] Craniofacial impairments such as a shortened palate and midface hypoplasia, along with oral hypotonia, tongue thrusting, and poor lip closure, frequently result in feeding difficulties at birth.[24] Bell and colleagues studied the prevalence of obesity in adults with Down syndrome and reported it in 70% of male subjects and 95% of female subjects.[25] Children with Down syndrome also appear to have a higher risk of being overweight or obese,[26-28] which may be, in part, a result of the retarded growth and endocrine and metabolic disorders associated with trisomy 21.[28] In a small population study of children with Down syndrome, Dyken and co-workers[29] reported that there was a high prevalence of obstructive sleep apnea associated with a higher body mass index.

Children with Down syndrome may have musculoskeletal anomalies such as metatarsus primus varus, pes planus, thoracolumbar scoliosis, and patellar instability and have an increased risk for atlantoaxial dislocation,[30-32] which has been observed through radiography in up to 10% to 30% of individuals with this syndrome[30,31] with and without neurological compromise.[33] There is some controversy in the medical community as to the necessity and efficacy of radiographic screening for the instability.[31,32] Proponents of radiographic screening argue that neurological symptoms of atlantoaxial instability may often go undetected in this population because symptoms are often masked by the wide-based gait and motor dysfunction already associated with the disorder. If the child is unable to verbalize complaints or the child is uncooperative with physical and neurological examinations, symptoms may be missed. There is particular concern about cervical instability if these children undergo surgical procedures requiring general anesthesia[32] and participate in recreational sports such as the Special Olympics.[31] Symptomatic instability can result in spinal cord compression leading to myelopathy with leg weakness, decreased walking ability,[33] spasticity, or incontinence. Although reportedly rare, there have been cases where atlantoaxial dislocation has resulted in quadriplegia.[30]

Several researchers have explored the neuropathology associated with Down syndrome. Changes in brain shape, size, weight, and function occur during prenatal and infant development of babies with Down syndrome, with important differences apparent by 6 months of age.[34] The relatively small size of the cerebellum and brain stem was reported by Crome and Stern in the 1970s.[35] Marin-Padilla[36] studied the neuronal organization of the motor cortex of a 19-month-old child with Down syndrome and found various structural abnormalities in the dendritic spines of the pyramidal neurons of the motor cortex. He suggested that these structural differences may underlie the motor incoordination and intellectual disability characteristic of individuals with Down syndrome. Loesch-Mdzewska[37] also found neurological abnormalities of the corticospinal system (in addition to reduced brain weight) in his neuropathological study of 123 individuals with Down syndrome aged 3 to 62 years. Crome[38] reported lesser brain weight in comparison with normal persons. Finally, Benda[39] noted a lack of myelinization of the nerve fibers in the precentral area, frontal lobe, and cerebellum of infants with Down syndrome. As McGraw[40] has pointed out, the amount of myelin in the brain reflects the stage of developmental maturation. The delayed myelinization characteristic of neonates and infants with Down syndrome is thought to be a contributing factor to the generalized hypotonicity and persistence of primitive reflexes characteristic of this syndrome.[41]

Trisomy 18. Trisomy 18, or Edwards syndrome, is the second most common of the trisomic syndromes to occur in term deliveries, although it is far less prevalent than Down syndrome. It occurs in one in 5000 newborns, and approximately 80% of affected infants are female.[42] As with Down syndrome, advanced maternal age is positively correlated with trisomy 18. Most cases of Edwards syndrome occur as random events during the formation of reproductive cells; fewer cases occur as errors in cell division during early fetal development; and inherited, translocation forms rarely occur.[42] Only 10% of infants born with trisomy 18 survive past the first year of life; female and non-Caucasian children survive longest.[43] The survival of girls averages 7 months; the survival of boys averages 2 months.[43] Individuals surviving past infancy most often have the mosaic form, and there is high variance in phenotype (Figure 13-2).[44]

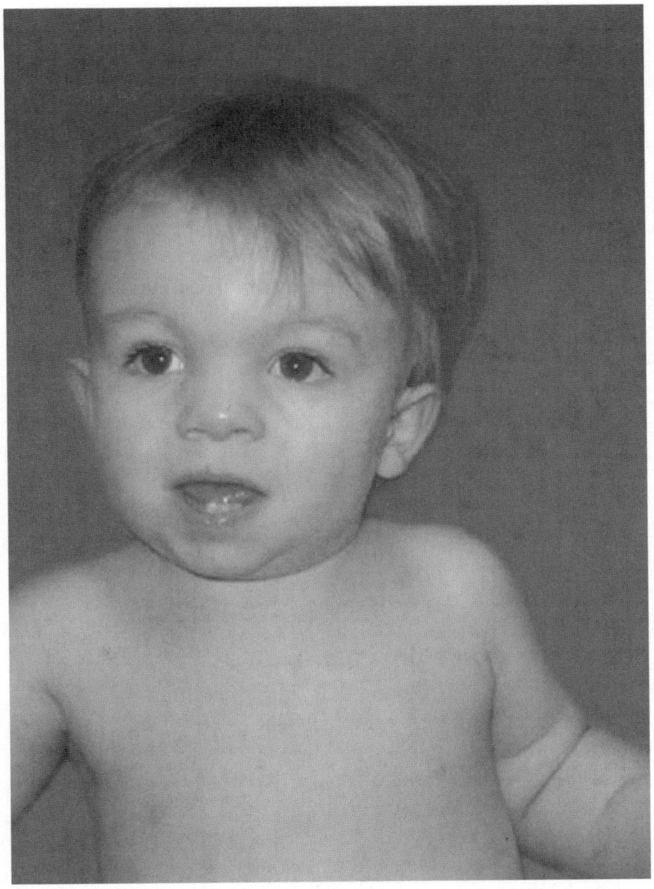

Figure 13-2 ■ Twenty-one–month-old male with mosaic form of trisomy 18. (Reprinted with permission of Tucker ME, Garringer HJ, Weaver DD: Phenotypic spectrum of mosaic trisomy 18: two new patients, a literature review, and counseling issues. *Am J Med Genet A* 143:505–517, 2007.)

Individuals with trisomy 18 generally have far more serious organic malformations than seen in those with Down syndrome.[45] Typical malformations affect the cardiovascular, gastrointestinal, urogenital, and skeletal systems. Infants with trisomy 18 have low birth weight and small stature, with a long narrow skull, low-set ears, flexion deformities of the fingers, and rocker-bottom feet. Muscle tone is initially hypotonic, but it becomes hypertonic in children with longer than typical life span.[45] The period of hypertonicity in the early years may change to low tone and joint hyperextensibility by preschool and school age. Microcephaly, abnormal gyri, cerebellar anomalies, myelomeningocele, hydrocephaly, and corpus callosum defects have been reported in individuals with trisomy 18.[46]

Common skeletal malformations that may warrant attention from the developmental physical or occupational therapist include scoliosis,[46] limited hip abduction, flexion contractures of the fingers, rocker-bottom feet, and talipes equinovarus.[45] Infants with trisomy 18 may also have feeding difficulties as a result of a poor suck.[47] Profound intellectual disability is another clinical factor that will affect the developmental therapy programs for children with trisomy 18.[46,47]

Trisomy 13. Trisomy 13, also commonly called *Patau syndrome,* is the least common of the three major autosomal trisomies, with an incidence of one in 10,000 to 20,000 live births.[8,42] As in the other trisomic syndromes, advanced maternal age is correlated with the incidence of trisomy 13.[48] Fewer than 10% of individuals with trisomy 13 survive past the first year of life[42,43]; girls and non-Caucasian infants appear to survive longer.[42,43] Individuals surviving past infancy most often have the mosaic form, and there is high variance in phenotype.[43] As with Edwards syndrome, most cases of Patau syndrome occur as random events during the formation of eggs and sperm, such as nondisjunction errors during cell division.[48]

Trisomy 13 is characterized by microcephaly, deafness, anophthalmia or microphthalmia, coloboma, and cleft lip and palate.[48] As in trisomy 18, infants with trisomy 13 frequently have serious cardiovascular and urogenital malformations and typically have severe to profound intellectual disability.[49] Skeletal deformities and anomalies include flexion contractures of the fingers and polydactyly of the hands and feet.[10] Rocker-bottom feet also have been reported, although less frequently than in individuals with trisomy 18. Reported central nervous system (CNS) malformations include arhinencephalia, cerebellar anomalies, defects of the corpus callosum, and hydrocephaly.[50]

Sex Chromosome Aneuploidy

The human X chromosome is large, containing approximately 5% of a human's nuclear DNA. The Y chromosome, much smaller, contains few known genes.[8] Females, with genotype XX, are mosaic for the X chromosome, meaning that one copy of their X chromosome is inactive in a given cell; some cell types will have a paternally derived active chromosome, and others a maternally derived X chromosome. Males, genotype XY, have only one copy of the X chromosome; therefore diseases caused by genes on the X chromosome, called *X-linked diseases* (see section on sex-linked disorders), can be devastating to males and less severe in females.[8] In the presence of abnormal numbers of sex chromosomes, neither male nor female individuals will be phenotypically normal.[8] Two of the most prevalent sex chromosome anomalies are Turner syndrome and Klinefelter syndrome.

Turner Syndrome. Turner syndrome affects females with monosomy of the X chromosome. The syndrome, also known as *gonadal dysgenesis,* occurs in one in 2500 live female births.[51,52] Turner syndrome is the most common chromosomal anomaly among spontaneous abortions.[53,54] Most infants who survive to term have the mosaic form of this syndrome, with a mix of cell karyotypes, 45,X and 46,XX. The *SHOX* gene, found on both the X and Y chromosomes, codes for proteins essential to skeletal development. Deficiency of the *SHOX* gene in females accounts for most of the characteristic abnormalities of this disorder.[52,55] Three characteristic impairments of the syndrome are sexual infantilism, a congenital webbed neck, and cubitus valgus.[56] Other clinical characteristics noted at birth include dorsal edema of hands and feet, hypertelorism, epicanthal folds, ptosis of the upper eyelids, elongated ears, and shortening of all the hand bones.[51,57] Growth retardation is particularly noticeable after the age of 5 or 6 years, and sexual infantilism, characterized by primary amenorrhea, lack of breast development, and scanty pubic and axillary hair, is apparent during the pubertal years. Ovarian development is severely deficient, as is estrogen production.[10,58] Congenital heart disease is present in 20% to 30% of individuals with Turner syndrome,[57] with a fewer number of cardiovascular malformations in individuals with the mosaic form[59]; 33% to 60% of individuals with Turner syndrome have kidney malformations.[51] Hypertension is common even in the absence of cardiac or renal malformations.[57,60]

There are numerous incidences of skeletal anomalies, some of which may be significant enough to require the attention of a pediatric therapist. Included among these are hip dislocation, pes planus and pes equinovarus, dislocated patella,[51] deformity of the medial tibial condyles,[46] idiopathic scoliosis,[57] and deformities resulting from osteoporosis.[10,57]

Sensory impairments include decrease in gustatory and olfactory sensitivity[61,62] and deficits in spatial perception and orientation,[61] and up to 90% of adult females have moderate sensorineural hearing loss. Recurrent ear infections are common and may result in future conductive hearing loss.[60] Although the average intellect of individuals with Turner syndrome is within normal limits, the incidence of intellectual disability is higher than in the general population.[45] Noonan syndrome, once thought to be a variant of Turner syndrome, has several common clinical characteristics; however, advancements in genetics research have shown that the syndromes have different genetic causes.[63,64]

Klinefelter Syndrome. Klinefelter syndrome is an example of aneuploidy with an excessive number of chromosomes that occurs in males. The most common type, 47,XXY, is usually not clinically apparent until puberty, when the testes fail to enlarge and gynecomastia occurs.[65] Nearly 90% of males with Klinefelter syndrome possess a karyotype of 47,XXY, and the other 10% of patients are variants.[66] The incidence of Klinefelter syndrome (XXY) is about one in 500 to 1000 males, and an estimated half of 47,XXY conceptions are spontaneously aborted.[8] The extra X chromosome(s) can be derived from either the mother or the father, with nearly equal occurrence.[67] Advanced maternal age is widely accepted as a causal factor.[8,66] FISH analysis of spermatozoa from fathers of boys with Klinefelter syndrome suggests that advanced paternal age increases the frequency of aneuploid offspring.[68-70]

Most individuals with karyotype XXY have normal intelligence, a somewhat passive personality, and a reduced libido. Eighty-five percent of individuals having the nonmosaic karyotype are sterile. Individuals with the karyotypes 48,XXXY and 49,XXXXY tend to display a more severe clinical picture. Individuals with 48,XXXY usually have severe intellectual disability, with multiple congenital anomalies, including microcephaly, hypertelorism, strabismus, and cleft palate.[10,65] Skeletal anomalies include radioulnar synostosis, genu valgum, malformed cervical vertebrae, and pes planus.[10] A 2010 systematic review of literature[71] on neurocognitive outcomes of persons with Klinefelter syndrome concluded that problems of delayed walking in children and persistent deficits in fine and gross motor development, and problems in motor planning.[71,72] Giedd and co-workers published the results of a case-control study examining brain magnetic resonance imaging (MRI) scans of 42 males with Klinefelter syndrome and reported cortical thinning in the motor strip associated with impaired control of the upper trunk, shoulders, and muscles involved in speech production.[73]

Partial Deletion Disorders

Deletions are one example of mutations that cause changes in the sequence of DNA in human cells. A sequence change that affects a gene's function can cause the final protein product to be altered or not produced at all.

Cri-du-Chat Syndrome. Cri-du-chat syndrome, also referred to as *cat-cry syndrome,* and *5p minus syndrome* results from a partial deletion of the short arm of chromosome 5. Example nomenclature for a female with this syndrome is (46,XX,del[5p]). The incidence of the syndrome is estimated to be one case per 20,000 to 50,000 live births.[10,74] Although approximately 70% of individuals with cri-du-chat syndrome are female, there is an unexplained higher prevalence of older males with this disorder.[75] Advanced parental age is not a causal factor. A study completed in 1978 indicated that life expectancy was 1 year for 90% of infants born with this disorder,[76] but now life expectancy is nearly normal with routine medical care.[77]

Primary identifying characteristics at birth include a definitive high-pitched catlike cry, microcephaly, evidence of intrauterine growth retardation, and subsequent low birth weight.[10,76,78] Abnormal laryngeal development accounts for the characteristic cry, which is present in most individuals and disappears in the first few years of life.[76] Other features of individuals with this syndrome include hypertelorism, strabismus, "moon face," and low-set ears.[10,76,78] Associated musculoskeletal deformities include scoliosis, hip dislocations, clubfeet, and hyperextensibility of fingers and toes. Muscular hypotonicity is associated with this syndrome, although cases with hypertonicity have also been noted.[79] Severe respiratory and feeding problems have also been reported.[77] Postnatal growth retardation has been documented, with the median near the 5th percentile of the normal growth curve.[80]

Although intellectual disability and physical deformities are more severe with larger deletions,[74] there is evidence that with early developmental intervention these children can develop language, functional ambulation, and self-care skills.[81,82]

Prader-Willi Syndrome and Angelman Syndrome. Prader-Willi syndrome (PWS) and Angelman syndrome (AS) are discussed together because they result from a structural or functional loss of the PWS and AS region of chromosome 15 (15q11-13), which can occur by one of several genetic mechanisms.[83,84] PWS has an incidence of one in 15,000 to 30,000[83] and AS has an incidence of one in 12,000 to 20,000.[83,84] These two syndromes illustrate the effect of *genomic imprinting,* which is the differential activation of genes of the same chromosome and location, depending on the sex of the parent of origin (Figure 13-3).[8]

PWS results from a failure of expression of paternally inherited genes in the PWS region of chromosome 15.[83] Conversely, AS results when the maternal contribution in the 15q11.2-q13 region is lost.[84] *OCA2* is a gene located within the PWS and AS region of chromosome 15 that codes for the protein involved in melanin production. With loss of one copy of this gene, individuals with PWS or AS will have light hair and fair skin. In the rare case that both copies of the gene are lost, these individuals may have a condition called *oculocutaneous albinism,* type 2, which causes severe vision problems.[84]

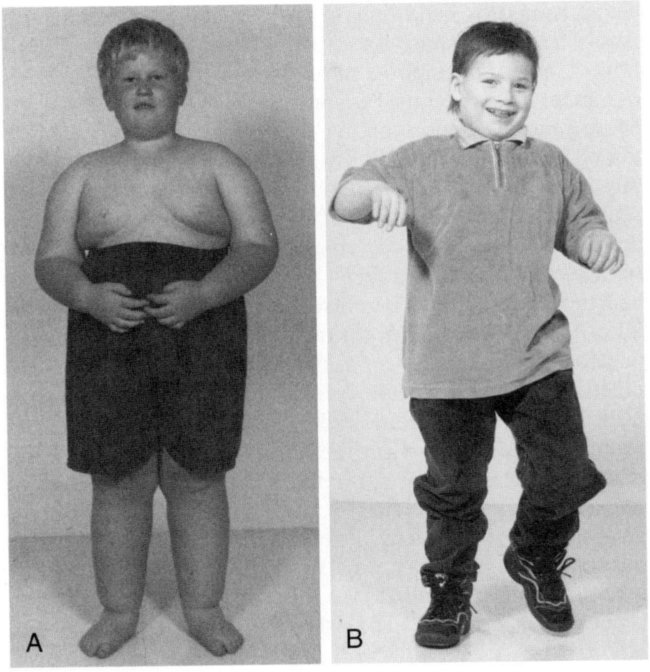

Figure 13-3 ■ Illustration of the effect of imprinting on chromosome 15 deletions. **A,** Inheritance of the deletion from the father produces Prader-Willi syndrome. **B,** Inheritance of the deletion from the mother produces Angelman syndrome. (From Jorde L, Carey J, Bamshad M, White R: *Medical genetics,* ed 3, St Louis, 2005, Mosby.)

Characteristics of PWS in infancy include hypotonia, poor feeding, lethargy, and hypogonadism.[85,86] Developmental milestones in the first 2 years of life are not acquired until approximately twice the normal age.[87,88] Between 1 and 4 years of age, hyperphagia is apparent and if uncontrolled will lead to morbid obesity and its associated health complications.[86,87,89] Most individuals with PWS have mild to moderate intellectual disability, although some individuals have IQ scores within normal limits.[90] Maladaptive behaviors such as temper tantrums, aggression, self-abuse, and emotional lability have been reported.[91] As a result of extreme obesity, many individuals with PWS have impaired breathing that can produce sleepiness, cyanosis, cor pulmonale, and heart failure.[91] Scoliosis is common but does not appear to be related to obesity.[92]

Clinical diagnosis is confirmed by laboratory genetic testing techniques including DNA-based methylation testing, FISH probe, and pyrosequencing assays.[86,93] Most cases of PWS are caused by random mutations in parental reproductive cells.[87] Other cases may result from translocation errors.[86,94] Parental studies are important in translocation cases because 20% of cases cited in the literature involved familial rearrangements, which may significantly increase the risk of recurrence.[95]

Angelman syndrome, named after Dr. Harry Angelman, who first described children with AS in 1965, is characterized by developmental delay or intellectual disability, seizures, ataxia, progressive microcephaly, and severe speech impairments. Tongue thrusting, drooling, and sucking and swallowing disorders occur in 20% to 80% of children. Individuals often display spontaneous bouts of laughter accompanied by hand-flapping movements and a characteristic walking posture of arms overhead and flexed elbows.[8,84,96] Infants appear normal at birth, but severe developmental delay becomes apparent by 6 to 12 months of age. More unique features of the disorder do not appear until after 1 year of age. Children with AS typically have structurally normal brains on MRI and computed tomography (CT) scans, but electroencephalogram (EEG) findings are often abnormal, showing a characteristic pattern that may assist with diagnosis before other clinical symptoms emerge,[84,97] and molecular studies can also confirm the disorder before all of the clinical criteria for this diagnosis are met.[84]

Most cases of AS occur as a result of mutations involving deletion or deficient function of the maternally inherited *UBE3A* gene. This gene codes for an enzyme, ubiquitin protein ligase, involved in the normal process of removing damaged or unnecessary proteins in healthy cells. In most of the body's tissues except the brain, both copies (maternal and paternal) of the *UBE3A* gene are active. Only the maternal copy of the gene is normally active in the brain, so if this copy is absent or deficient, the normal cellular housekeeping process breaks down.[84] The risk of having another child with AS can vary from 1% to 50% depending on which of the six known genetic mechanisms is responsible for the disorder.

Translocation Disorders

Translocation errors have been identified in many childhood hematologic cancers and sarcomas.[98,99] Translocation errors are also commonly seen in couples with infertility.[100] Translocation abnormalities occur when genetic material is exchanged and rearranged between two nonhomologous chromosomes (those not in the same numbered pair). The structural abnormality can result in the loss or gain of chromosomal material (an unbalanced arrangement) or no loss or gain of material (a balanced arrangement). Unbalanced arrangements can produce serious disease or deformity in individuals or their offspring. Carriers of balanced arrangements—estimated at one in 500 individuals—often have a normal phenotype, but their offspring may have an abnormal phenotype.[8] There are two basic types of translocations: reciprocal translocation and robertsonian translocation. Reciprocal translocations occur when two different chromosomes break and the genetic material is mutually exchanged. A robertsonian translocation occurs when there is a break in a portion of two different chromosomes, with the longest remaining portions of both chromosomes forming a single chromosome. The shorter portions that broke away usually do not contain vital genetic information; therefore the individual may be phenotypically normal.[8] An example notation of a reciprocal translocation is 46,XY,t(7;9)(q36;q34). This individual is male with a normal number of chromosomes but with a translocation of genetic material on chromosomes 7 and 9; "q" refers to the short arm of these chromosomes, and the numbers "36" and "34" refer to the location.

Translocations occur in children seen in therapy settings, including about 3% to 5% of children with Down syndrome,[10] and translocations are found in 40% of all cases of acute lymphoblastic leukemia (ALL).[101]

Acute Lymphoblastic Leukemia. ALL accounts for one fourth of all childhood cancers, and it is the most common type of childhood cancer.[102-104] ALL occurs when the DNA of immature lymphoblasts is altered and they reproduce in abnormal numbers, crowding out the formation of normal cells in the bone marrow.[102,105] Sixty percent of cases of ALL occur in children, with the peak incidence in the first 5 years of life. A rise in the incidence of ALL has been reported during major periods of industrialization worldwide[105,106] and is hypothesized to be associated with exposure to radiation[107] and other environmental teratogens[108,109] in the preconception, gestational, and postpregnancy periods.[103,106]

With advancements in medical treatment protocols for pediatric patients, 5-year survival rates have improved to 80%.[104] Children aged 1 to 9 years at diagnosis have a better prognosis than infants, adolescents, or adults diagnosed with ALL.[103] There are numerous forms of translocation mutations associated with ALL. Some translocation forms of ALL do not respond well to combination chemotherapy treatment; an example is the translocation that occurs between chromosomes 9 and 22, known as the "Philadelphia chromosome."[104,110] Other translocations that result in hyperdiploidy (more than 50 chromosomes), in particular within chromosomes 4, 10, and 17, may confer a more favorable outcome.[111]

Frequently, diagnosis is made when a physician relates the child's history of a persistent viral respiratory infection with other characteristic clinical signs and symptoms consistent with hematopoietic leukemia. The key symptoms of ALL are pallor, poor appetite, lethargy, easy fatigue and bruising, fever, mucosal bleeding, and bone pain.[99] A complete blood count will show a shortage of all types of blood cells, including red, white, and platelets. Diagnosis is confirmed by the presence of lymphoblasts in bone marrow. Radiographs may be necessary to determine metastases, and cerebrospinal fluid will be examined because early involvement of the CNS has important prognostic implications.[106] Cytogenetic studies will be performed to aid in selection of treatment protocols and prognosis.[104]

Referral to physical and occupational therapists is made for other common problems such as muscle cramps, muscle weakness, impaired gross and fine motor performance, decreased energy expenditure, osteopenia, and osteoporosis.[112]

Single-Gene Disorders

The previous section described genetic disorders that occur because of chromosomal abnormalities involving more than one specific gene. Other genetic disorders commonly seen among children in a therapy setting include those that result from specific gene defects. The inheritance patterns of single-gene traits were described by Gregor Mendel in the nineteenth century. These patterns, autosomal dominant, autosomal recessive, and sex linked, are discussed separately, and specific examples of syndromes or disorders associated with each type are presented.

Autosomal Dominant Disorders

Mutations on one of the 22 numbered pairs of autosomes may result in isolated anomalies that occur in otherwise normal individuals, such as extra digits or short fingers. Each child of a parent with an autosomal dominant trait has a 50:50 chance of inheriting that trait.[8] Other autosomal dominant disorders include syndromes characterized by profound musculoskeletal and neurological impairments that may require intervention from a physical or an occupational therapist. Three examples of autosomal dominant disorders are osteogenesis imperfecta (OI), tuberous sclerosis, and neurofibromatosis (NFM).

Osteogenesis Imperfecta. OI is a spectrum of diseases that results from deficits in collagen synthesis associated with single-gene defects, most commonly of *COL1A1* and *COL1A2,* located on chromosomes 17 and 7, respectively.[10,113] OI is characterized by brittle bones resulting from impaired quality, quantity, and geometry of bone material and hyperextensible ligaments.[114,115] Deafness, resulting from otosclerosis, is found in 35% of individuals by the third decade of life.[45] New knowledge about this disease from molecular genetic studies and bone histomorphometry has expanded the classification subtypes of OI into types I through VII.[113,116] These classifications are helpful in determining prognosis and management, although there is a continuum of severity of clinical features and much overlap in the features among the different classifications.[116] Types I, IV, V, and VI occur in the autosomal dominant pattern; whereas type VII occurs as a recessive trait, and types II and III can occur as either dominant or recessive traits.[113] OI types V and VI account for only 5% of cases, and type VII has been found to date only in a Native Canadian population.[116] This section will compare and contrast only types I through IV.

The overall incidence of OI is one in 10,000 live births in the United States, with types I and IV accounting for almost 95% of all patients with OI.[113] Ninety percent of dominant forms of OI can be confirmed by DNA analysis.[117] Type I is the least severe form, followed by types IV and III, with type II being the most severe.

Type I is characterized by blue sclera, mild to moderate bone fragility, joint hyperextensibility, and hearing loss in young adulthood.[117] There are no significant deformities; individuals with this type may not sustain fracture until ambulatory, and incidence of fractures decreases with age.[117] Type IV OI is characterized by more severe bone fragility and joint hyperextensibility than is type I. Bowing of long bones, scoliosis, dentinogenesis imperfecta, and short stature are common.[114,116,118]

Children with type IV OI are often ambulatory but may require splinting or crutches.[114]

Children with type III OI have severe bone fragility and osteoporosis; often there are fractures in utero. Type III occurs primarily in autosomal dominant inheritance in North Americans and Europeans.[116] The less frequent, autosomal recessive form of OI, type III is characterized by progressive skeletal deformity, scoliosis, triangular facies, large skull, normal cognitive ability, short stature, and limited ambulatory ability.[114,116,119] The long bones of the lower extremities are most susceptible to fractures, particularly between the ages of 2 to 3 years and 10 to 15 years,[45] with the frequency of fractures diminishing with age. Intramedullary rods inserted in the tibia or femur may minimize recurrent fractures.[36]

Type II, the most severe form, is most often lethal before or shortly after birth, although there are a few cases of children living to 3 years.[116,119] Infants with type II OI have multiple fractures, often in utero, and underdeveloped lungs and thorax; therefore many die from respiratory complications after birth. Most type II cases are the result of spontaneous mutations; because only one copy of the gene is sufficient to cause the disorder, it is still commonly classified as an autosomal dominant condition. There are fewer cases of autosomal recessive inheritance.[8]

Prevention of fractures is an important goal in working with individuals with OI, but fear of handling and overprotection by caregivers may limit a child's optimal functional independence. Caregiver education in careful handling and positioning should begin in the patient's early infancy, and training in the use of protective orthoses and assistive devices is appropriate from the period of crawling through ambulation.[115,120,121] Aquatic therapy can be a valuable treatment strategy for children with OI.[120,121]

Tuberous Sclerosis Complex. Tuberous sclerosis complex (TSC) is characterized by a triad of impairments: seizures, intellectual disability, and sebaceous adenomas; however, there is wide variability in expression, with some individuals displaying skin lesions only.[122] Infants are frequently normal in appearance at birth, but 70% of those who go on to show the complete triad of symptoms display seizures during the first year of life. Although tuberous sclerosis is inherited as an autosomal dominant trait, 86% of cases occur as spontaneous mutations, with older paternal age a contributing factor. TSC affects both sexes equally, with a frequency of one in 5800 births.[123] Mutations in the *TSC1* and *TSC2* genes are known to cause tuberous sclerosis.[10] The normal function of these genes is to regulate cell growth; if these genes are defective, cellular overgrowth and noncancerous tumor formation can occur.[123] Tumor formation in the CNS is responsible for most of the morbidity and mortality with TSC,[123] followed by renal disease associated with formation of benign angiomyolipomas.[122] Diagnostic criteria for TSC have been established, and the determination can be made clinically; results of genetic testing are currently viewed as corroborative.[122] Hypopigmented macules are often the initial finding. These lesions vary in number and are small and ovoid. Larger lesions, known as *leaf spots,* may have jagged edges.[123] Sebaceous adenomas first appear at age 4 to 5 years, with early individual brown, yellow, or red lesions of firm consistency in the nose and upper lips. These isolated lesions may later coalesce to form a characteristic butterfly pattern on the cheeks. Known also as hamartomas (tumor-like nodules of superfluous tissue), the skin lesions are present in 83% of individuals with tuberous sclerosis.[45]

Delayed development is another characteristic during infancy,[124] particularly in the achievement of motor and speech milestones. Cerebral cortical tubers are present in over 80% of patients and account for cognitive disability including autism.[122] Ultimately, 93% of individuals who are severely affected will have seizures, usually of the myoclonic type, in early life, progressing in later life to grand mal seizures. Seizure development is the result of formation of nodular lesions in the cerebral cortex and white matter.[45] Tumors are also found in the walls of the ventricles. Neurocytological examination reveals a decreased number of neurons and an increased number of glial cells and enlarged nerve cells with abnormally shaped cell bodies.[10] Surgical excision of seizure-producing tumors has been successful in some cases.[122]

Other associated impairments include retinal tumors and hemorrhages, glaucoma, and corneal opacities.[123] Cyst formation in the long bones and in the bones of the fingers and toes contributes to osteoporosis. Cardiac and lung tissues are also affected by TSC, and these effects are included in the major diagnostic criteria.[122]

Neurofibromatosis. There are two recognized forms of NFM: neurofibromatosis 1 (NFM1) and neurofibromatosis 2 (NFM2).[125-127] Neurofibromas, or connective tissue tumors of the nerve fiber fasciculus, impede the development and growth of neural cell tissues[126,127] and are the hallmark feature of NFM1. Neurofibromas are noncancerous, and malignant changes are rare in children[128] but an increased risk of malignancy has been observed in adult patients with NFM1 and is a major contributor to decreased life expectancy by approximately 15 years.[129] Tumors typically increase in number with increasing age. About half of all cases of NFM are caused by sporadic mutation in parental germ cells or during fetal development.[125-127] Schwannomas are the main tumor type of NFM2 and classically appear bilaterally on the vestibular nerves.[127,130] NFM1 is also known as *von Recklinghausen disease.* Compared with type II, type I is more common (one per 3000 births)[10,126] and usually identified in younger children. It is associated with mutations in the *NF1* gene, which produces a protein, neurofibromin, the complete function of which is not yet understood but which is suspected to be a tumor suppressor. Diagnostic criteria for NFM1 include the presence of two of the following features: six or more café-au-lait spots, two or more fibromas, freckling in the axillary or inguinal region, optic pathway glioma, two or more Lisch nodules, specific osseous lesions, and a first-degree relative with NFM1.[126] Infants usually appear normal at birth, but initial café-au-lait spots appear by age 3 years in 95% of individuals (Figure 13-4).[131] Cognitive impairment is the most common neurological complication of NFM1[131] and is postulated to be caused by altered expression of neurofibromin in the brain and/or hyperintense lesions in the brain seen on MRI.[131] These focal areas of high signal intensity on T2-weighted MRI, known as *unidentified bright objects* (UBOs), are seen in 60% of children and young adults with NFM1. The lesions, commonly found in the basal ganglia, internal capsule, thalamus, cerebellum, and brain stem,[128,132] tend to disappear in adulthood and often do not cause other overt neurological symptoms.[128] Fewer than 10% of individuals are mentally retarded, but about 30% to 60% of affected children have learning disabilities that are mild and nonprogressive.[128,133] Poorer social skills and differences in personality, behavior, and quality-of-life perception have been reported in children with NFM1 compared with children without the disorder.[126]

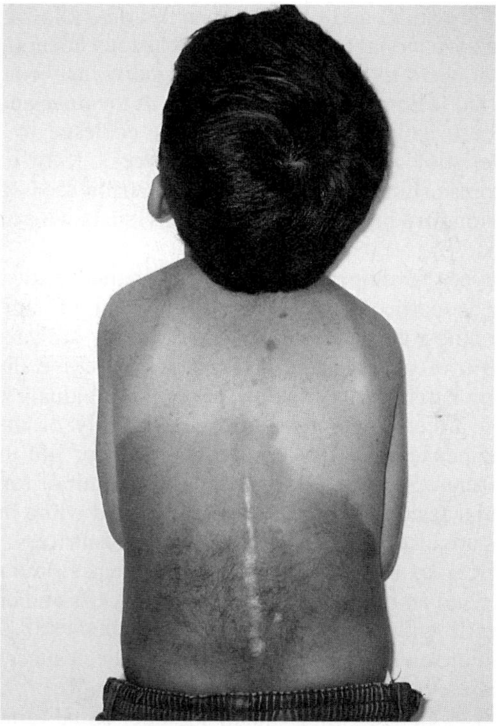

Figure 13-4 ■ Four-year-old boy with neurofibromatosis and characteristic café-au-lait spots on trunk.

In older children and adolescents, pain, itching, and stinging can occur from cutaneous neurofibromas, and in approximately half of all patients, neurological motor deficits occur from plexiform neurofibromas when the growth puts pressure on peripheral nerves, spinal nerve roots, and the spinal cord.[131] One percent to 5% of children aged 0 to 6 years develop symptoms associated with optic pathway glioma.[126,128] Neurofibromatous vasculopathy interferes with arterial and venous circulation in the brain.[126,131,134] Hydrocephalus occurs in some individuals.[126,128] Hypertension is common and may develop at any age,[126] and cardiovascular disease is a major cause of premature death.[129,131,135] Headaches are a commonly reported symptom in children, adolescents, and adults.[126,128,136,137]

Scoliosis may develop in 10% of patients and is rapidly progressive from ages 6 to 10 years, or it may manifest in a milder form without vertebral anomalies during adolescence.[126] Other skeletal deformities include pseudarthrosis of the tibia and fibula, tibial bowing, craniofacial and vertebral dysplasia, rib fusion, and dislocation of the radius and ulna.[126] Differences in leg length[126] also have been noted and may contribute to scoliosis. NFM2 occurs less frequently than type I (one in 25,000 to 40,000 births)[10] and is caused by a mutation in the gene encoding the protein neurofibromin 2, also called *Merlin.*[10] Merlin is produced in the nervous system, particularly in Schwann cells that surround and insulate the nerve cells of the brain and spinal cord. Although type II shares characteristics with type I, it is commonly characterized by tumors of the eighth cranial nerve (usually bilateral), meningiomas of the brain, and schwannomas of the dorsal roots of the spinal cord.[10] Contrary to first descriptions of NFM1 and NFM2, café-au-lait spots are seldom a singular feature of NFM2[127]; rather, signs and symptoms of tinnitus, hearing loss, and balance dysfunction usually appear during adolescence or in the person's early 20s.[125,127] Problems with visual acuity caused by strabismus and refractive errors are common in young children.[138] NFM2 may be underrecognized in children up to 10 years old because early hearing loss and tinnitus are present in only 20% of cases and otherwise only singular features of the condition are observed. Infants may have cataracts, and children may demonstrate unilateral facial paralysis, eye squinting, mononeuropathy (foot or hand drop), meningioma, spinal tumor, or cutaneous tumor. It is recommended that children of parents with NFM2 should be considered to be at 50% risk for NFM2 and screened from birth.[130]

Autosomal Recessive Disorders

An unaffected carrier of a disease-causing trait is *heterozygous* for the abnormal gene (possessing one normal and one mutated copy of the gene). If both parents are unaffected carriers of the gene, each of their offspring has a 25% risk of exhibiting the disorder.[8] Consanguinity involving close relatives increases the chance of passing on autosomal recessive traits.[8] Certain types of limb defects, familial microcephaly, and a variety of syndromes are passed on through autosomal recessive genes. Four examples of autosomal recessive disorders affecting children in therapy settings are presented in this section: cystic fibrosis (CF), Hurler syndrome, phenylketonuria (PKU), and spinal muscle atrophy (SMA).

Cystic Fibrosis. CF is one of the most common autosomal recessive disorders and is more common in Caucasians, affecting one in 2000 to 4000.[10] The CF gene has been mapped to chromosome 7, and its protein product, CF transmembrane regulator (CFTR).[8] CFTR is involved in the regulation of chloride channels of the bowel and lung, which is dysfunctional in patients with CF. Although CF has markedly variable expression, the overall median survival time has improved from about 6 years of age in the 1940s to an average of 36 years of age in 2006.[139] In addition to the phenotypical features of CF, diagnosis of CF is made when two or more disease-causing mutations exist on the CTFR gene.[139] Newborn screening tests for CF are required in all states in the United States.[140]

Fibrotic lesions of the pancreas cause pancreatic insufficiency in the majority of patients, which leads to chronic malnutrition. Ten percent to 20% of newborn infants with CF also have intestinal tract involvement with a meconium ileus. The sweat glands are commonly affected; high levels of chloride found in the sweat is the basis for the sweat chloride test used in diagnosis. The most serious impairment in CF is the obstruction of the lungs by thick mucus, which leads to chronic pulmonary obstruction, infection that destroys lung tissue, and eventual death from pulmonary disease in 90% of individuals.[8]

Improved survival rate in recent decades is a result of improved antibiotic management, aggressive chest physical therapy, and pancreatic replacement therapy. Postural drainage, percussion, vibration, and breathing exercises are key components of the management program provided by the therapist and caregivers.[141] Modern and less labor-intensive devices such as those that provide positive expiratory pressure may not be as effective at clearing secretions as conventional chest physiotherapy,[141] but patient and caregiver compliance with a regular program may be improved with them.[142] Attention to diet is important, and every attempt should be made to maintain a routine exercise program with a goal of helping the children be more active to improve their respiratory status and to prevent secondary impairments of adolescence and adulthood such as stress incontinence in young women caused by excessive coughing,[143,144] chronic back pain, and osteopenia and osteoporosis.[145]

Massery[143] describes the relationship among respiration, postural control, and secondary impairments that develop in individuals with CF in the musculoskeletal and neuromuscular systems. She addresses the threefold problem faced by individuals with CF: (1) lung dysfunction leading to increased respiratory demand; (2) increased workload of respiration as a deforming force on the immature musculoskeletal frame; and (3) resultant impaired motor strategies for postural control during physical activity. Patients were once widely cautioned to avoid overexertion and fatigue with exercise, but as patients are living longer, more evidence supports the benefits of regular, even vigorous exercise for children and adults with CF. Guidelines for exercise frequency and intensity have been published by the Association of Chartered Physiotherapists in Cystic Fibrosis.[146]

Hurler Syndrome (Mucopolysaccharidosis I, Severe Type). Hurler syndrome is an inborn error of metabolism that results in abnormal storage of mucopolysaccharides in many different tissues of the body.[97] The incidence is estimated to be one in 100,000 live births for the severe forms[10] and one in 500,000 for milder forms.[147] *IDUA* is the only gene currently known to be associated with this multisystem disorder.[147]

Infants born with Hurler syndrome are usually normal in appearance at birth, may have inguinal or umbilical hernias,[147] and may have higher birth weights than their siblings. Symptoms of this progressively deteriorating disease usually appear during the latter half of the first year of life,[147] with the full disease picture apparent by 2 to 3 years of age.[10,147] Diagnosis is made by identification of deficiency in lysosomal enzymes.[147,148] Premature death, usually from cardiorespiratory failure, occurs within the first 10 years of life.[147]

Characteristic physical features are caused by storage of glycosaminoglycans (GAGs)[147] and include a large skull with frontal bossing, heavy eyebrows, edematous eyelids, corneal clouding, a small upturned nose with a flat nasal bridge, thick lips, low-set ears, hirsutism, and gargoyle-like facial features. Growth retardation results in characteristic dwarfism.[147] Some individuals with the physical characteristics of Hurler syndrome have normal intelligence, but most have progressive and profound intellectual disability.[10,147]

Spastic paraparesis or paraplegia and ataxia have been observed in individuals with Hurler syndrome.[8] Commonly reported orthopedic deformities include flexion contractures of the extremities, thoracolumbar kyphosis, genu valgum, pes cavus, hip dislocation, and claw hands as a result of joint deformities.[45] Defective ossification centers of the vertebral bodies results in spinal deformity, complications of nerve entrapment, atlanto-occipital instability, and restricted cervical range of motion.[147] Conductive and sensorineural hearing loss is common.[147] Delayed motor milestones have been noted as early as 10 months of age,[148] with severe disabilities occurring with increasing age. Adaptive equipment often is needed, and most children with Hurler syndrome become wheelchair users in their later years.[148]

Phenylketonuria. PKU is the result of one of the more common inborn errors of metabolism. Mutations of the *PAH* gene located on chromosome 12 cause a deficiency in the production of phenylalanine hydroxylase.[149] Without this enzyme, there is no conversion of phenylalanine to tyrosine, resulting in an abnormally excessive accumulation of phenylalanine in the blood and other body fluids.[149,150] If untreated, this metabolic error results in mental and growth retardation, seizures, and pigment deficiency of hair and skin.[151] PKU is most prevalent among individuals of northern European ancestry, with a frequency of one in 10,000 to

15,000 births in the United States.[149] It is estimated that one of every 50 individuals is heterozygous for PKU.[8]

Children born with PKU are usually normal in appearance, with microcephaly and delayed development becoming apparent toward the end of the first year. Parents usually become concerned with the child's slow development during the preschool years.[151] If PKU is untreated, the affected child may go on to develop hypertonicity (75%), hyperactive reflexes (66%), hyperkinesis (50%), or tremors (30%),[152] in addition to intellectual disability. IQ levels generally fall between 10 and 50, although there have been reported rare cases of untreated individuals with normal intelligence.[151]

A simple blood plasma analysis, which is mandatory for newborn infants in all 50 U.S. states,[140] can detect the presence of elevated phenylalanine levels in nearly 100% of cases.[150] This test is ideally performed when the infant is at least 72 hours old. If elevated phenylalanine levels are found, the test is repeated, and further diagnostic procedures are performed. Placing the infant on a low phenylalanine diet (low protein) can prevent the intellectual disability and other neurological sequelae characteristic of this disorder.[151] Follow-up management by an interdisciplinary team consisting of a nutritionist, psychologist, and appropriate medical personnel is advised in addition to the special diet. Individuals with poor compliance with the recommended diet have a greater risk of osteopenia in adulthood.[150]

Spinal Muscle Atrophy. SMA (5q SMA) is characterized by progressive muscle weakness because of degeneration and loss of the anterior horn cells in the spinal cord and brain stem nuclei.[153,154] Diagnosis of SMA is based on molecular genetic testing for deletion of the *SMN1* gene (named for "survival of motor neuron 1"), location 5q13. Another gene, *SMA2,* can modify the course of SMA. Individuals with multiple copies of *SMA2* can have less severe symptoms or symptoms that appear later in life as the number of copies of the *SMN2* gene increases.[155] The overall disease incidence of SMA is five in 100,000 live births.[155]

The clinical classifications of SMA are still evolving.[153,154,156] At present, four subtypes (types I to IV) are well accepted, and a fifth, type 0, is being explored. The subtypes are based on age at symptom onset and expectations for maximum physical function, the latter being more closely related to life expectancy.[156]

SMA type 0 is characterized by extreme muscle weakness apparent before 6 months of age that likely had a prenatal onset.[153,154] Some infants have a prenatal history of decreased fetal movements during the third trimester.[153]

SMA I, otherwise known as *Werdnig-Hoffmann disease* or *acute infantile SMA,*[10] has an onset before 6 months of age.[153,156] Incidence is estimated to be one in 20,000 live births.[10] It is characterized clinically by severe hypotonicity, generalized symmetrical muscle weakness, absent deep tendon reflexes, and markedly delayed motor development. Intellect, sensation, and sphincter functioning, however, are normal.[153] Children usually cannot sit without support and have poor head control.[156] They have a weak cry and cough and problems with swallowing, feeding, and handling oral secretions.[154] The diaphragm is spared, but combined with weakness in intercostal muscles, infants exhibit paradoxical breathing, abdominal protrusion, and a bell-shaped trunk with chest wall collapse.[154] Overall, this pattern of chest wall weakness and poor respiratory function contributes to the greatly increased susceptibility to pulmonary infection, which usually results in death before the age of 2 years.[10,154,155]

SMA II, otherwise known as *intermediate* or *chronic infantile SMA*, has an onset at age 6 to 18 months and is associated with delayed motor milestones.[156] Seventy percent of children diagnosed with SMA II are alive at 25 years of age.[153]

Children with SMA II can usually sit independently if placed but never stand unsupported.[154] Bulbar weakness with swallowing difficulties, poor weight gain, and diaphragmatic breathing are common.[155] Finger trembling is almost always present.[153,154] Joint contractures are present in most individuals. Kyphoscoliosis of severity to require bracing and/or surgery often develops, but patients are at risk of postanesthesia complications.[154] Respiratory failure is the major cause of morbidity and mortality. Nocturnal oxygen desaturation and hypoventilation occur before daytime hypercarbia and are early indications of need for ventilator support.[154]

SMA III is characterized by onset of symptoms in childhood after 18 months.[153] It is also known as *juvenile SMA* or *Kugelberg-Welander syndrome.*[10] These individuals have a normal life span and usually attain independent ambulation and maintain it until the third or fourth decade of life.[153] Lower extremities are often more severely affected than the arms. Strength is often not sufficient for stair climbing, and balance problems are common.[153] Muscle aches and joint overuse symptoms are frequently reported.[154]

SMA IV typically has an onset at older than 10 years of age and is associated with a normal life expectancy and no respiratory complications.[154,156] Individuals maintain ambulation during the adult years.[154]

Variants of SMA occur in individuals with similar phenotypes and clinical diagnostic features of electromyography (EMG) that are not associated with deletion of *SMN1.*[156] Genetic testing for *SMN* gene deletion achieves up to 95% sensitivity and nearly 100% specificity.[154] For cases that remain unclear, a clinical diagnosis may be accomplished through EMG and muscle biopsy, which reveal neurogenic atrophy. Key physical signs are common: symmetrical weakness in the more proximal musculature versus distal, and lower extremity weakness that is greater than in the arms.[154] Traditional strength measurements are not practical for children with SMA. The Gross Motor Function Measure[157] has excellent reliability in studies of gross motor evaluation in this population.[154,158] Consensus guidelines on pulmonary care including assessment, monitoring, and treatment; feeding and swallowing, gastrointestinal dysfunction and nutrition; and orthopedic management have been published by the Standard of Care Committee for Spinal Muscle Atrophy.[154] Currently there are no efficacious drugs to effectively treat the symptoms of SMA.[160,161]

Sex-Linked Disorders

The third mechanism for transmission of specific gene defects is through sex-linked inheritance. In most sex-linked disorders, the abnormal gene is carried on the X chromosome. Female individuals carrying one abnormal gene usually do not display the trait because of the presence of a normal copy on the other X chromosome. Each son born to a carrier mother, however, has a 50:50 chance of inheriting the abnormal gene and thus exhibiting the disorder. Each daughter of a carrier mother has a 50:50 chance of becoming a carrier of the trait.[8] Four syndromes that result in disability are discussed in this section: hemophilia, fragile X syndrome (FXS), Lesch-Nyhan syndrome (LNS), and Rett syndrome (RS).

Hemophilia. Hemophilia is a bleeding disorder caused by a deficient clotting process. Affected individuals will have hemorrhage into joints and muscles, easy bruising, and prolonged bleeding from wounds. The term *hemophilia* refers to hemophilia A (coagulation factor VIII deficiency) and hemophilia B or Christmas disease (coagulation factor IX deficiency). There are numerous other clotting diseases, and some that were once referred to as hemophilia are now genomically distinguished. For example, von Willebrand disease has a distinctly different genetic basis from hemophilia; it follows an autosomal recessive or autosomal dominant pattern and involves mutation of the von Willebrand factor (VWF) gene, located on chromosome 12. VWF plays a role in stabilizing blood coagulation factor VIII.[162] Hemophilia A and B occur as X-linked recessive traits owing to mutations of genes *F8* and *F9,* respectively, both of which are located on the X chromosome.[163,164]

Hemophilia A is reported to affect one in 4000 to 5000 males worldwide.[163] Hemophilia B is less common, affecting one in 20,000 males worldwide.[164] Hemophilia can affect females, though in milder form. The severity and frequency of bleeding in hemophilia A are inversely related to the amount of residual factor VIII (less than 1%, severe; 2% to 5%, moderate; and 6% to 35%, mild).[163] The proportions of cases that are severe, moderate, and mild are about 50%, 10%, and 40%, respectively.[165] The joints (ankles, knees, hips, and elbows) are frequently affected, causing swelling, pain, decreased function, and degenerative arthritis. Similarly, muscle hemorrhage can cause necrosis, contractures, and neuropathy by entrapment. Hematuria and intracranial hemorrhage, although uncommon, can occur after even mild trauma. Bleeding from tongue or lip lacerations is often persistent.[8]

Hemophilia is usually diagnosed during childhood, with the most severe cases diagnosed in the first year of life: bleeding from minor mouth injuries and large "goose eggs" from minor head bumps are the most frequent presenting signs in untreated children.[163] Children are especially vulnerable to bleeding episodes owing to the nature of their physical activity combined with periods of rapid growth.[163]

Treatment includes guarding against trauma and replacement with factor VIII derived from human plasma or recombinant techniques.[8] In the late 1970s to mid 1980s it was estimated that half of the affected individuals in the United States contracted hepatitis B or C or human immunodeficiency virus (HIV) infection when treated with donor-derived factor VIII. The initiation of donor blood screening and use of heat treatment of donor-derived factor VIII has almost completely eliminated the threat of infection.[8] Although replacement therapy is effective in most cases, 30% of treated individuals with hemophilia A and 3% of individuals with hemophilia B have neutralizing antibodies that decrease its effectiveness.[163,164] Before treatment with clotting factor concentrates was available, the average life expectancy was 11 years[163]; currently, excluding death from HIV, life expectancy for those with severe hemophilia who receive adequate treatment is 63 years.[163] Factor replacement therapy is credited for increasing the ease and safety of vigorous exercise and sports participation for individuals.[166] The benefits of regular exercise are the same as for unaffected individuals and outweigh the risks in treated persons.[167] A 2002 pilot study by Tiktinsky and colleagues[167] found decreased episodes of bleeding in a population of young adults with a long-term history of resistance training that began in adolescence.

Fragile X Syndrome. FXS is the most common sex-linked inherited cause of intellectual disability, affecting one in 4000 males and one in 8000 females.[168] Males manifest a more severe form than females. A fragile site on the long arm of an X chromosome is present, with breaks or gaps shown on chromosome analysis. A region of the X chromosome, named *FMR1,* normally codes for proteins that may play a role in the development of synapses in the brain. Mutations of this region are errors of trinucleotide repeats, in which the number of CGG triplets at this region is expanded, thereby making the gene segment unable to produce the necessary protein.[168]

Developmental milestones are slightly delayed in affected males.[168] Eighty percent of males are reported to have intellectual disability, with IQs of 30 to 50 being common but ranging up to the mildly retarded to borderline range.[168] *Penetrance* (the proportion of individuals with a mutation that actually exhibit clinical symptoms) in the female is reported to be only 30%.[8] Other impairments include epilepsy, emotional lability, attention-deficit/hyperactivity disorder (ADHD), and clinical autistic disorder in 30% of males.[168,169] Life span is normal for individuals with this condition.[168]

Lesch-Nyhan Syndrome. Also known as *hereditary choreoathetosis,*[170] LNS leads to profound neurological deterioration. First described in 1964 by Lesch and Nyhan,[171] it is associated with a mutation in the *HPRT1* gene on the X chromosome. This gene codes for an enzyme, hypoxanthine guanine phosphoribosyltransferase, which allows cells to recycle purines, some of the building blocks of DNA and ribonucleic acid (RNA).[172] Without this gene's normal function, there is an overproduction of uric acid (hyperuricemia),[172] which accumulates in the body. High uric acid levels are thought to cause neurological damage.[170,172]

The prevalence of LNS is one in 380,000 individuals.[172] Females born to carrier mothers have a 25% chance of inheriting the mutation. There are rare reports of females demonstrating this syndrome as a result of X chromosome inactivation. Most female carriers are considered to be asymptomatic, but some may have symptoms of hyperuricemia in adulthood.[172]

LNS is detectable through amniocentesis, and genetic counseling is advisable for parents who have already given birth to an affected son.[173]

The prenatal and perinatal course is typical for affected individuals. Hypotonia and delayed motor skills are noticeable by age 3 to 6 months.[172] Dystonia, choreoathetosis, and opisthotonus indicative of extrapyramidal involvement emerge during the first few years of life.[172] Many children are initially diagnosed with athetoid cerebral palsy when pyramidal signs such as spasticity, hyperreflexia, and abnormal plantar reflexes emerge.[172] Most children never walk. A hallmark of the disease is severe and frequent self-injurious behaviors such as lip and finger biting, which emerge in almost all affected children by their third birthday.[172] Because of the extreme self-mutilation that characterizes this disorder, it has been questioned whether these children have normal pain perception.[174] Although these children have the abnormal catecholamine metabolism seen in other patients with congenital pain insensitivity,[175] behaviors documented in children with LNS suggest that they do sense pain, demonstrated by their apparent relief when they are restrained from hurting themselves. Children may actually request the restraining device[176] even when the device may be one that would not physically prevent biting, such as a glove or bandaid.[172] A reported survey of parents of children with LNS indicated that parents often find behavioral programming techniques helpful in modifying aggression toward self or others.[176] However, there is no consensus on the best kind of behavioral treatments, as any reward, either positive or negative, may increase the frequency of self-injury.[177] Some parents have reported that they elected tooth extraction as a means to prevent biting. Other impairments in children with LNS include severe dysarthria and dysphagia. Bilateral dislocation of the hips may occur as a result of the spasticity.[172] Growth retardation is also apparent, as well as moderate to severe intellectual disability.[10] Individuals may have gouty arthritis and kidney and bladder stones.

Blood and urine levels of uric acid have been decreased successfully through the administration of allopurinol, with a resultant decrease in kidney damage. With current management techniques, most individuals survive into their second or third decade of life.[172]

Rett Syndrome. RS is inherited in an X-linked pattern and it affects females almost exclusively, as it is most often lethal in boys before age 2 years. Males may inherit RS with an extra X chromosome in many or all of the body's cells.[178-181] The estimated incidence is one in 15,000 to 20,000 females.[10,182] It has been reported that 99% of all cases of RS are the result of sporadic mutations.[181,183] Most cases of RS, called *classic RS,* are caused by mutations in the *MECP2* gene, which is responsible for directing proteins critical for normal synaptic development; however, it is unclear how these mutations lead to all the signs and symptoms of the syndrome.[181,184] Several variants of RS exist; they have overlapping features with classic RS but may have a much milder or more severe course.[181]

Classic RS is characterized by apparently normal development during the first 6 months of life, followed by a short period of developmental plateau, and then rapid deterioration of language and motor skills typically occurring at 6 to 18 months of age.[181,185] Most girls survive into adulthood.[181] The hallmark of the syndrome is that during the period of regression, previously acquired purposeful hand skills are also lost and replaced by stereotypical hand movements. These nonspecific hand movements have been described as hand wringing, clapping, waving, or mouthing. Virtually all language ability is lost, although some children may produce echolalic sounds and learn simple manual signing. Evidence of minimal receptive language skills may be observed. Autistic behaviors, inconsolable crying and screaming, and bruxism are common features of individuals with RS.[181] Almost all individuals with RS function in the range of severe to profound intellectual disabilities.

Head circumference is normal at birth, and its increase may decelerate in early childhood, but microcephaly is not a consistent feature of RS.[181] Retarded growth and muscle wasting are observed in most girls, likely associated with poor food intake and gastrointestinal problems.[181]

Almost one fourth of girls with RS never develop independent ambulation skills; otherwise the onset of walking is usually delayed until about 19 months of age.[186] Initially hypotonia may be evident, but with advancing age, spasticity of the extremities develops.[187] Increased muscle tone is usually observed first in the lower extremities, with continued greater involvement than in the upper extremities. Peripheral vasomotor disturbances, especially in the lower limbs, are often noted.[181]

Scoliosis, which is often severe enough to require surgical correction, occurs in most girls by adolescence, characterized by a long C-shaped thoracolumbar curve, kyphoscoliosis, and an early onset of posterior pelvic tilt and abducted shoulder girdles.[186,188-192] Heel cord tightening, and hip instability have also been identified as areas of potential concern.[188] Abnormal EEG and seizures occur in 70% of individuals with RS in the first 5 years of life. Cranial CT results are normal or show mild generalized atrophy. Breathing dysfunction, including wake apnea and intermittent hyperventilation,[186] is also associated with RS. Interventions reported in the literature have focused on splinting,[193] behavioral modification techniques to teach self-feeding skills,[194] aquatic therapy,[195] occupational therapy,[196] music therapy,[197] physical therapy,[181,190,191,197] and the first two combined in a dual-intervention approach.[198]

Mitochondrial DNA Disorders

In addition to the nuclear genome, humans have another set of genetic information within their mitochondria. Nuclear genes exist in pairs of one maternal and one paternal allele. In contrast, there are hundreds or thousands of copies of mtDNA in every cell. mtDNA is small, circular, and double stranded. It has been well studied and was mapped long before the human nuclear genome. mtDNA contains 37 genes responsible for normal function of the mitochondria in all body cells.[198a] Humans inherit mtDNA maternally. mtDNA is highly susceptible to mutation, and the molecule has limited ability to repair itself. Tissues that have a high demand for oxidative energy metabolism, such as brain and muscle, appear to be most vulnerable to mtDNA mutations.[11] Normal and mutated versions of mtDNA can coexist within a patient's body, but when a certain critical number of mutations exist, the body's tissues will show clinical signs of dysfunction. These disorders affect the metabolic functions of the mitochondria, such as the generation of the body's energy currency, adenosine triphosphate. Many patients with point mutations of mtDNA exhibit symptoms in early childhood; these mutations may be the most frequent cause of metabolic abnormality in children.[11] The minimum birth prevalence of childhood mitochondrial respiratory chain disorders is reported to be 6.2 per 100,000.[12,199-201] Medical intervention for mitochondrial encephalomyopathies cannot treat the underlying disease, but the value of rehabilitative therapies has been reported.[202,203] An example of a childhood disorder that can result from an mtDNA mutation is Leigh syndrome.

Leigh Syndrome

Leigh syndrome, or subacute necrotizing encephalomyopathy, may also be transmitted by X-linked recessive and autosomal recessive inheritance. Approximately 20% of all cases of Leigh syndrome are caused by mitochondrial mutations.[204] The discussion in this section will focus on characteristics of mtDNA-associated Leigh syndrome.

Leigh syndrome has an onset in infancy, typically at 3 to 12 months of age. Initial features may be nonspecific, such as a failure to thrive and persistent vomiting.[204,205] It is a progressive disorder caused by lesions that can occur in the brain stem, thalamus, basal ganglia, cerebellum, and spinal cord. Common clinical features include seizures, epilepsy, muscle weakness, peripheral neuropathy, speech and feeding difficulties, gastrointestinal and digestive problems, and heart problems. Most affected children have hypotonia, movement disorders such as chorea, and ataxia. Life expectancy is 2 to 3 years; death most often results from respiratory or cardiac failure.[204]

Multifactorial Disorders

Multifactorial disorders are believed to be a result of the combined effects of mutations in multiple genes and environmental factors.[8] Environmental factors may be those that have an impact on a developing fetus, such as prenatal diet, or those that have an impact on humans as we age, such as cigarette smoking. Disorders in this category can result in congenital malformations such as spina bifida and clubfoot. An in-depth discussion of spina bifida can be found in Chapter 15. Management information on clubfoot can be found in pediatric textbooks that include orthopedic information.[206-209]

Many diseases such as cancer can result when the environment interacts with genetic variations that exist in all humans.[8] Scientists are exploring genetic contributions to premature births.[210,211] Premature birth is the leading cause of infant mortality and morbidity,[212,213] and it most likely is a result of multiple genetic and environmental determinants that tend to run in families.[210,211] Premature infants are at higher risk of neurological, musculoskeletal, and respiratory problems than term infants are. Management of infants with low birth weight is discussed in Chapter 11 of this text.

BODY STRUCTURE AND FUNCTION PROBLEMS COMMON TO MANY PEDIATRIC GENETIC DISORDERS

Specific examples of genetic disorders in children were presented in the foregoing section. Although there are many disorders that physical and occupational therapists may see often, others are rare and may only be suspected based on clustered problems of body structure, function, and activity limitations. Decisions about which interventions to implement and the expected outcomes will be largely influenced by the diagnosis of the specific disorder, once attained. Many genetic conditions share in common a short list of primary problems that will negatively affect the child's physical movement and daily activities and participation, both immediately and in the long term. Table 13-3 summarizes the problems common to many genetic disorders that are most relevant for physical or occupational therapists.

Hypertonicity

Abnormalities of tone may result from dysgenesis or injury to developing motor pathways. Hypertonia is common to many motor disorders and is defined as "abnormally increased resistance to externally imposed movement about a joint."[214] Examples of externally imposed movement are passive movement by the therapist or changes in ankle and knee position resulting from ground reaction forces during ambulation. Children with hypertonus generally display stiff or jerky movements that are limited in variety, speed, and coordination. Controlled, voluntary movements tend to be limited to the middle ranges of a joint. Total patterns of flexion or extension may dominate, with limited ability for selective joint movements. Motor development of children with hypertonicity may be further complicated by the retention of primitive reflexes, which can result in stereotyped movements associated with sensory input.[214]

Sanger and colleagues[214] proposed a classification system to objectively define and distinguish different types of hypertonicity. Three general types of hypertonicity—spasticity, dystonia, and rigidity—may occur alone or in combination. Spasticity is a velocity-dependent, increased resistance to muscle stretch that may occur above a given threshold of speed and/or joint angle and may depend on the direction of joint movement. Dystonia is also an involuntary alteration in the pattern of muscle activation during voluntary movement or maintenance of posture. The observable disorder is demonstrated by intermittent muscle contractions causing twisting or repetitive movement, postures, or both.[214] Dystonia may be triggered by attempts at voluntary movement or to prevent the movement of a joint (e.g., to prevent knee buckling in stance). The pattern and magnitude of the abnormal muscle activity may change with the child's arousal, emotional state, and tactile contact.[214] Rigidity is a form of hypertonus in which the speed of movement and joint angle do not affect the movement quality. Stiffness caused by diminished tissue length and extensibility of muscles and connective tissue is not included in the recent definitions of hypertonus (but may exist alongside hypertonicity).[214,215]

Children may learn to use stereotypical patterns of movement and hypertonus to achieve functional goals by activating the muscle synergies of a reflex without sensory feedback.[216] If a goal of therapy is to facilitate functional movement that is not dominated by persistent reflexes, it is critical to practice new motor patterns to accomplish the functional activity for which that reflex is being used. The focus of therapy activities needs to be on active movement of the child and not on passive inhibition techniques of abnormal reflexes for the sake of "normalization" of tone and movement.[216-219]

Hypotonicity

In contrast to hypertonia, low tone or hypotonia is not clearly defined. The "floppy" infant or child is commonly characterized as having hypermobility of joints that lack resistance to passive movement, with diminished antigravity movement and postural stability. Hypotonia may occur because of central or peripheral nervous system dysfunction,

TABLE 13-3 ■ CHARACTERISTIC FEATURES OF SELECTED GENETIC CONDITIONS

GENETIC CONDITION	TYPICAL AGE AT DIAGNOSIS	CRANIOFACIAL DYSMORPHISM	MUSCULOSKELETAL INVOLVEMENT	NEUROMUSCULAR SYSTEM INVOLVEMENT AND TONE	CARDIO-PULMONARY INVOLVEMENT
Trisomy 21	Prenatal or infancy	Yes	Joint laxity and instability	Hypotonia	Yes
Trisomy 18	Prenatal, neonatal	Yes	Yes	Hypotonia	Yes
Turner syndrome	Infancy, adolescence; girls	Yes	Short stature, hip dislocation, scoliosis		Yes
Klinefelter syndrome	Adolescence; adulthood; males	Yes	Yes	Varies with age	
Cri-du-chat syndrome	Infancy	Yes	Yes	Hypotonia	Yes
Prader-Willi syndrome	Infancy	Yes	Scoliosis	Hypotonia	Secondary to obesity
Angelman syndrome	Infancy	Microcephaly		Hypotonia and seizures, ataxia	
Acute lymphoblastic leukemia	Childhood		Bone pain and muscle cramps		
Osteogenesis imperfecta	Varies with type and severity		Multiple fractures and muscle weakness		Yes
Tuberous sclerosis complex	Infancy, early childhood		Yes, cyst formation	Hypertonia; seizures	Yes, cyst formation
Neurofibromatosis type 1	Infancy, childhood		Yes		
Cystic fibrosis	Infancy		Chest wall deformity, muscle and bone pain		Yes
Hurler syndrome	Infancy	Yes	Yes	Yes	Yes
Spinal muscle atrophy type II	Infancy		Yes	Hypotonia	Yes
Hemophilia type A	Childhood or earlier if severe		Joint pain and hemarthroses		
Fragile X syndrome	Childhood	Yes	Joint laxity		Yes
Lesch-Nyhan syndrome	Infancy		Gouty arthritis	Varies	
Rett syndrome	Late infancy to early childhood		Scoliosis	Hypotonia, ataxia, seizures	

as is the case in newborns with PWS and toddlers with SMA type II, respectively. Many genetic disorders are revealed in newborns based on the common features of severe, global hypotonia and low Apgar scores.[220] Retrospective studies of newborns report key features of absence of antigravity movements and decreased reflexes. The presence of fetal hypokinesia and/or polyhydramnios is reported to be predictive of neonatal hypotonia in many cases.[221] In full-term neonates with hypotonia, studies report that 30% to 60% of cases are associated with a genetic disorder. A clinical neurological examination such as described by Dubowitz and the use of dysmorphic data bases can identify the majority of cases.[221,222] First-line genetic testing is indicated in neonates with hypotonia plus facial dysmorphism or signs of peripheral hypotonia (e.g., as seen in SMA).[221]

Martin and colleagues[223] surveyed physical and occupational pediatric therapists and reported that the majority of therapists do not use formal examination methods to quantify hypotonia directly, but rather use measurements for various expressions of hypotonia, most often muscle strength and developmental milestones. This study also confirmed that most therapists agree that children with hypotonicity have diminished postural control and thus tend to lean on supports to maintain a position. Examples of this behavior

OTHER SYSTEM INVOLVEMENT	OTHER DISEASE PROCESSES	SENSORY DYSFUNCTION	MOTOR DELAY	COGNITIVE DELAY	HALLMARK FEATURE(S)
	Alzheimer disease, sleep apnea, obesity	Vision, hearing	Yes	Yes	Facial features, simian crease
Yes		Yes	Yes	Yes	Life span < 1 year
Distal lymphedema; reproductive system		Hearing			Webbed neck appearance and short stature
Endocrine and reproductive system			Yes	Yes	Intellectual disability; course of gonadal development
		Vision			"Cat cry"
Reproductive system	Morbid obesity	Vision	Yes	Yes	Hypotonia, obesity
			Yes	Yes	Happy demeanor, sleep disorders
	Osteopenia, osteoporosis				Lethargy, fever, respiratory infections
	Dentinogenesis	Hearing (type I)			Multiple fractures
Skin lesions, adenomas; renal disease		Vision	Yes	Yes	Sebaceous adenomas, seizures
Café-au-lait spots and cutaneous neurofibromas; vasculopathy		Vision			Café-au-lait spots, neurofibromas
Gastrointestinal system; urinary stress incontinence in females	Osteoporosis, osteopenia				Lung and digestive dysfunction
Yes		Vision, hearing	Yes	Yes	Progressive craniofacial abnormalities and developmental deterioration
Yes			Yes		Progressive loss of peripheral motor function
Skin bruising					Bleeding, bruising, joint pain, and loss of motion
		Yes		Yes	Intellectual disability, autism
Urogenital system		Yes	Yes	Yes	Self-injurious behavior, gouty arthritis
		Yes	Yes	Yes	Regressive developmental delay; stereotypical, purposeless hand movements

are locking out weight-bearing joints and assuming positions that provide a broad base of support to maximize their stability (Figure 13-5). Although retention of primitive reflexes is less likely in children with hypotonia compared with those with hypertonia, delays in the development of postural reactions are a major concern. Limited strength and lack of endurance are often concerns with children who have hypotonicity. Hypotonicity and joint laxity are often associated with motor delay; however, therapists should not assume that hypotonia and joint laxity are absolutely predicative of persistent motor delay.[224] For example, many premature infants, with or without a genetic disorder, have global hypotonia at birth that resolves and does not cause long-term functional impairment.[224,225] Hypotonicity is a persistent problem in many children with developmental delay. Therapists may address hypotonia and problems of postural control with a variety of treatment modalities and techniques including aquatic therapy,[226] hippotherapy,[227] and neurodevelopmental therapy.[228]

Hyperextensible Joints

Hyperextensible joints are commonly observed in children with hypotonicity and are noted in many children with a variety of genetic disorders, representing different

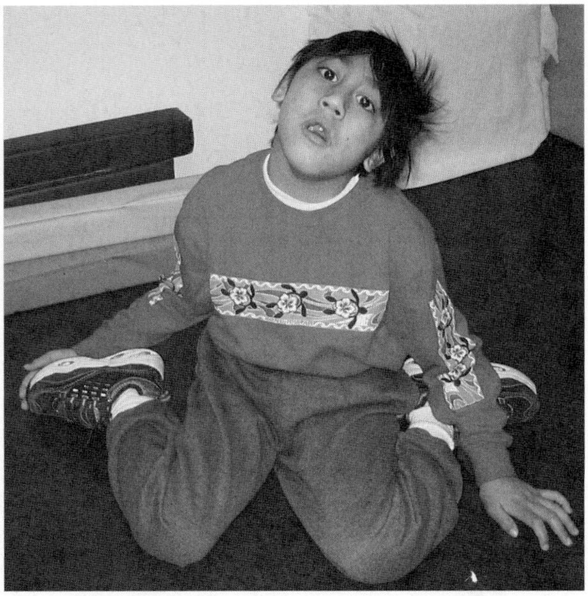

Figure 13-5 ■ Eight-year-old boy with hypotonia associated with a chromosomal translocation error. Note the broad base of support in this "W" sitting position.

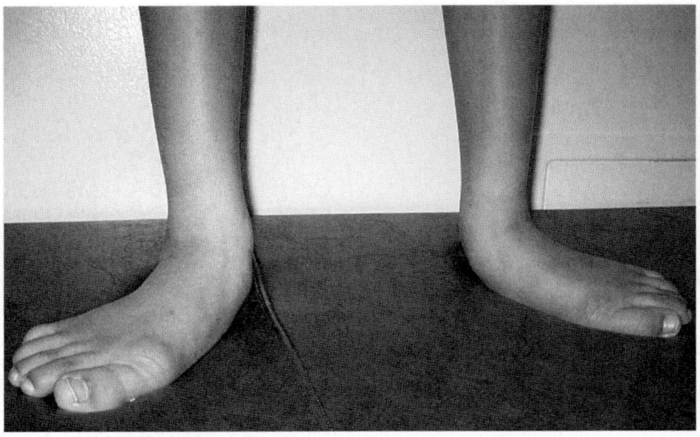

Figure 13-6 ■ Excessive bilateral pronation and flat feet associated with hyperextensibility in 8-year-old boy with global hypotonia.

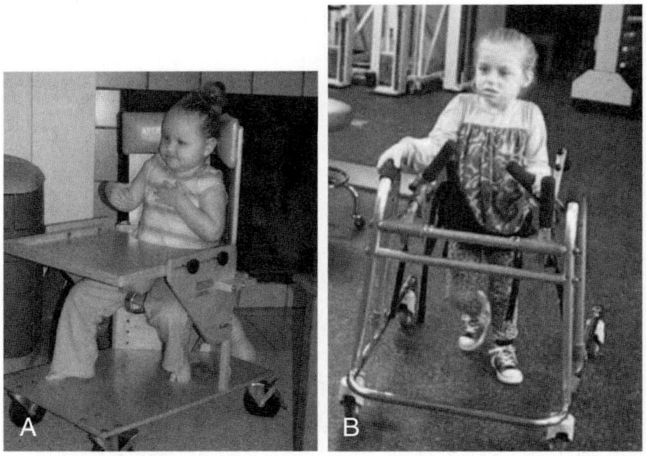

Figure 13-7 ■ Adapted equipment to promote participation in upright activities for children with trunk weakness and poor postural control. **A,** The corner chair provides this child with Rett syndrome the proper back support, and toys can be placed within her reach on the tray. **B,** This particular gait trainer allows appropriate patterns of weight-shifting to occur while providing her with stability in the pelvis and lower trunk.

underlying organ structure problems. Activities should be modified to avoid undue stress to these joints and the surrounding ligaments, tendons, and fascia. For example, positions that allow the knee or elbow joints to lock into extension should be modified so that weight bearing occurs through more neutral alignment. Varying the placement of toys and support surfaces, providing physical assistance, and using adaptive equipment can help modify weight-bearing forces to achieve more neutral alignment.[229] For example, if hyperextensibility of ligaments leads to excessive pronation in stance (Figure 13-6), the use of ankle-foot orthoses may provide enough support to the structures to allow functional activities in standing (see the discussion of orthotics in Chapter 34). For a child who stands with knee hyperextension, a vertical stander may allow that child to stand and play at a water table with her or his classmates for extended periods with the knees in a more neutral position. Rather than restricting a child's repertoire of upright positions, it is preferable to modify an activity or provide external support to enable a child to participate fully (Figure 13-7).[230]

Contractures and Musculoskeletal Deformities

Skeletal anomalies and deformities are associated with many genetic disorders. The therapist should be aware of factors that can contribute to the development of deformities to prevent or minimize such problems. The physical or occupational therapist may work with orthopedists, prosthetists, and orthotists to detect and prevent the progression of a variety of conditions.

Conditions that cause hypertonicity or spasticity are well known to place children at risk for joint contracture.[231] Children with hemophilia are at great risk of joint contractures associated with hemarthroses and intramuscular hemorrhages.[232] Spinal deformities, such as lumbar lordosis and thoracic kyphosis and scoliosis, are also common concerns in children with hypertonia or hypotonia. Although joint contractures are less likely to occur in a child with hypotonicity, habitual positioning may lead to soft tissue restrictions. For example, children with hypotonia often adopt a constant position of wide abduction, external rotation, and flexion at the hips ("frog" or "reverse W" position)[233]; in these children, soft tissue contractures can develop at the hips and knees. Children whose hips are maintained in a position of adduction, flexion, and internal rotation are at risk for hip subluxation or dislocation.[233]

Deformation of the anterior chest wall and shoulder girdles may result from primary problems in the cardiopulmonary system such as in children with CF. When coupled with hypotonicity and poor postural control, the anterior chest wall muscles tighten as a result of the long-term rounded, internally rotated shoulders and protracted scapulae, in which case therapeutic interventions should target improving chest wall and scapulothoracic mobility as well as strengthening postural muscles (Figure 13-8).[234-236] In general, contractures and deformities are a concern for most children who display a limited variety of postures and

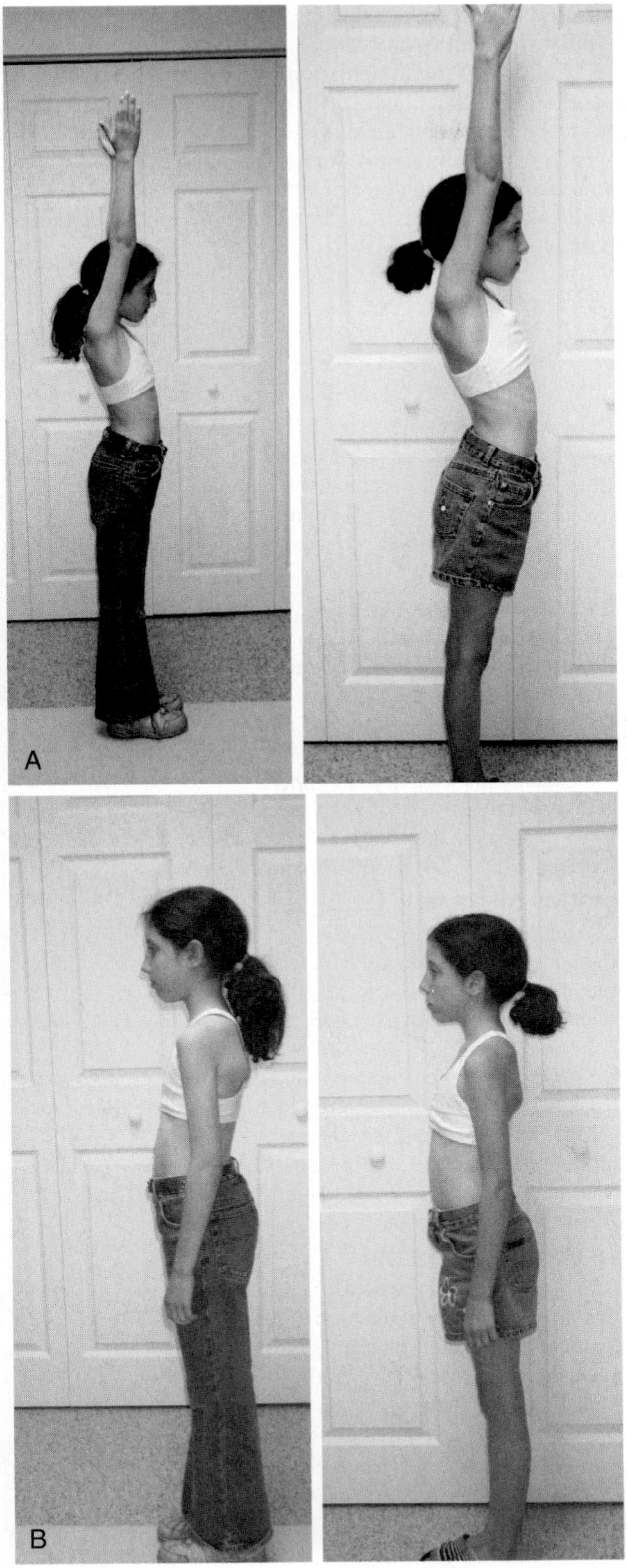

Figure 13-8 ■ Postural changes after therapeutic intervention to improve mobility in chest wall and shoulder girdles and strengthen postural muscles in a child with cystic fibrosis. (Before intervention on left, after intervention on right.)

movements. Therapists should consider the nature of the disorder that places the child at risk for contractures when choosing treatment techniques; disorder-specific techniques can be found in pediatric occupational and physical therapy textbooks.[206,237]

Respiratory Problems

A genetic risk for respiratory distress in infancy has been suggested by reports of family clusters.[238] Furthermore, comparison of short- and long-term respiratory function in infants with respiratory distress syndrome suggests that if all other factors of nutrition, previous mechanical ventilation, and gestational development are comparable, genetic risk may account for cases of chronic and potentially irreversible respiratory failure.[238]

Respiratory problems are often observed in children with limited mobility. If the mobility impairments are the result of hypotonicity or hypertonicity, impaired respiration may be a result of chest and skeletal deformities. Many infants with genetic disorders are born prematurely and are more susceptible to respiratory problems than infants born at full term.[210,211,233] Prolonged mechanical ventilation and other medical procedures may increase the time neonates spend in the supine position, thus increasing the risk of gravity-induced deformity of the rib cage and inefficiency of the respiratory musculature.[234,239,240]

Some children may find it difficult to tolerate one position for an extended time owing to respiratory difficulties. For these children, frequent changes of position and use of adapted positioning devices may be necessary. Premature infants in the neonatal intensive care unit may benefit from regular prone positioning to facilitate restorative sleep,[240-242] improved arterial oxygen saturation,[243] and improved respiratory synchrony.[244] Children with respiratory problems may require mobilization techniques, deep breathing, chest expansion exercises, and postural drainage. In the case of children with CF, a comprehensive program of respiratory care is the primary therapy goal.[245]

Developmental Delay

Genetic disorders that affect neuromuscular, somatosensory, and cognitive function are frequently associated with developmental delays in children. The genetic basis for multisystem syndromes such as Down syndrome or LNS can be identified by cytogenetic and molecular techniques. Congenital malformations, hearing impairment, and mental or growth retardation are examples of common components of developmental delay that often have a genetic basis.

Developmental delay is typified by the failure to meet expected age-related milestones in one or more of five areas: physical, social and emotional, intellectual, speech and language, and adaptive life skills. Developmental milestones that are typically assessed in the first 5 years of life can be found in Box 13-2.

Physical and occupational therapists can observe the interaction among each of the five areas of development in an infant or child. For example, a child with severe hypotonia who has limited movement experiences will not develop a well adapted sensory system. Children with problems processing sensory information often withdraw from social interaction through which they would otherwise find opportunities to develop speech, language, and social skills. Dynamical systems theory[246] explains this relationship among all of the developing components in a child; language does not develop independently of gross motor skills, and the ability to feed or dress oneself is as related to social, emotional, and intellectual development as it is to fine motor skills.

Suspicion of developmental delay often leads to physician referral. An accurate medical diagnosis is important in that it facilitates knowledgeable surveillance for potentially associated health problems. A delayed diagnosis can preclude timely implementation of beneficial medical, therapeutic, and educational services. Children who are identified to be at risk for developmental delay may be referred to early intervention programs. Examples of assessment techniques and interventions for children with developmental delay can be found in pediatric physical therapy textbooks.[247,248]

BOX 13-2 ■ DEVELOPMENTAL MILESTONES

BY 1 MONTH

Sucks poorly and feeds slowly
Lower jaw trembles constantly even when infant is not crying or excited
Does not respond to loud sounds or bright light
Does not focus on and follow a nearby object moving side to side
Rarely moves
Extremities seem loose and floppy or very stiff

BY END OF THIRD MONTH

No Moro reflex
Does not notice own hands by 2 months
Does not grasp and hold objects
Eyes cross most of the time or eyes do not track well together
Does not coo or babble

BY END OF FOURTH MONTH

Head flops back when infant is pulled up to sitting by his or her hands
Does not turn head to locate sounds
Does not bring object to mouth
Does not smile spontaneously
Inconsolable at night

BY END OF FIFTH MONTH

Persistent tonic neck reflexes
Cannot maintain head up when placed on stomach or in supported sitting position
Does not reach for objects
Does not roll in both directions

BY END OF SEVENTH MONTH

Reaches with one hand only
Cannot sit with help by 6 months
Does not follow objects at a distance
Does not bear some weight on legs
Does not laugh; does not try to attract attention through actions
Refuses to cuddle; shows no affection for caregiver

BY END OF TWELFTH MONTH

Does not creep on all fours
Cannot stand when supported
Does not search for toy hidden while he or she watches
Says no single words (e.g., "mama" or "dada")
Does not use gestures such as waving hand or shaking head; does not point to objects or pictures

BY END OF SECOND YEAR

Cannot walk by 18 months
Failure to develop heel-toe walking pattern after several months of walking
Does not speak at least 15 words by 18 months
Does not use two-word sentences by 2 years
Does not know the function of common objects (brush, telephone, spoon) by 15 months
Does not imitate actions or words; does not follow simple instructions

BY END OF THIRD YEAR

Frequent falling and difficulty with stairs
Persistent drooling or unclear speech
Inability to build a tower of more than four blocks
Difficulty manipulating small objects
Cannot copy a circle
Cannot communicate in short phrases
No pretend play
Little interest in other children
Extreme difficulty separating from caregiver

BY END OF FOURTH YEAR

Cannot throw a ball overhand
Cannot jump in place with both feet
Cannot ride a tricycle
Cannot grasp a crayon between thumb and fingers; cannot scribble
Resists dressing, sleeping, using the toilet
Does not use sentences of more than three words; does not use "me" and "you" appropriately
Ignores other children or people outside the family
Does not pretend in play; no interest in interactive games
Persistent poor self-control when angry or upset

BY END OF FIFTH YEAR

Does not engage in a variety of physical activities
Has trouble eating, sleeping, using the toilet
Cannot differentiate between fantasy and reality
Seems unusually passive or aloof with others
Cannot correctly give her or his first and last names
Does not use plurals or past tense when speaking
Does not talk about daily experiences
Does not understand two-part commands
Cannot brush teeth efficiently
Cannot take off clothing
Cannot wash and dry hands
Cannot build a tower of six to eight blocks
Does not express a wide range of emotions
Seems uncomfortable holding a crayon

Behavioral Phenotypes in Genetic Syndromes

Study into the cognitive and behavioral aspects of individuals with certain genetic syndromes has given rise to the term *behavioral phenotype*. Certain clusters of behavior that characterize a given syndrome can aid in the early recognition and diagnosis of a syndrome and can guide intervention choices. Example aspects of behavioral phenotypes include social interaction, sleeping patterns, mood, attention, motivation, adaptive and maladaptive strategies, intellect, and memory.[249-253]

Down syndrome, PWS, AS, FXS, and LNS are examples of genetic disorders discussed in this chapter with delineated behavioral phenotypes.[250,251] Compulsive overeating in children with PWS, sleep disturbances in children with AS, and self-injury in children with LNS are behavioral problems that can have significant negative impact on quality of life for children and their families. Although children with Down syndrome have fewer maladaptive behaviors than most children with intellectual disabilities,[249,251,253] they have been shown to abandon challenging tasks sooner than other children at similar developmental levels in exchange for peer social interaction.[252] Furthermore, this strength of sociability in children with Down syndrome contributes to the child's learning through modeling and peer collaboration. A knowledgeable, observant therapist can use peer groups to motivate and model for a child with Down syndrome but should also recognize that the child may be distracted by other children and default to a social strategy and avoid the task at hand.[252]

MEDICAL MANAGEMENT AND GENETIC COUNSELING

The physical or occupational therapist should have general knowledge of both medical management of children with genetic disorders and genetic counseling for family members. This information allows the therapist to answer the family's general questions and to refer family members to the appropriate persons for more specific information.

Medical Management

Early detection of genetic disorders has improved the health and survival of individuals with certain genetic disorders such as PKU, hemophilia, and CF. Medical treatment for the other disorders is not curative but rather palliative or directed at specific associated anomalies.

Surgical Intervention

The congenital heart defects present in many individuals with Down syndrome can in most instances be corrected by cardiac surgery.[20] Orthopedic surgery in the form of insertion of intramedullary rods in the tibia or femur may minimize the recurrence of repeated fractures associated with OI.[115,253] Surgical correction of dystrophic scoliosis may be warranted in individuals with NFM,[131] RS,[186,189,191,192,197] or Werdnig-Hoffmann disease[154] if the deformity is severe and bracing is not successful. Radiographic screening for atlantoaxial instability in children with Down syndrome can be initiated beginning at age 2 years.[16] If atlantoaxial instability is excessive or results in a neurological deficit, a posterior fusion of the cervical vertebrae is recommended.[33] Surgical removal of obstructive or malignant tumors is advisable in certain cases of NFM, as is removal of cerebral nodular growths for the control of seizures in individuals with tuberous sclerosis.[122] Surgical interventions such as gastric bypass, small intestinal bypass, and jaw wiring have been attempted for weight control in children with PWS but have had limited success.[83,90]

Pharmaceutics

Second-generation bisphosphonates can reduce fracture frequency, improve bone quality, and improve outcomes after orthopedic surgery in children and lessen the severity of osteoporosis in adults.[115] Antibiotics and pneumoeustachian tubes to lessen the frequency and severity of otitis media can reduce the incidence of hearing loss in individuals with Down syndrome[20] and Turner syndrome.[57] The use of appetite-regulating drugs for individuals with PWS has had equivocal results. Reproductive hormone therapy can promote pubertal development in girls with Turner syndrome[57,60] and boys with Klinefelter syndrome.[67,254] Growth hormone has been shown to improve stature in girls with Turner syndrome.[57] The use of anticonvulsants is an important part of seizure management for individuals with RS[186,190] and tuberous sclerosis.[123] Allopurinol has been used for individuals with LNS to prevent urological complications, although it has no effect on the progressive neurological symptoms.[172] The use of large, potentially toxic amounts of vitamins and minerals (the orthomolecular hypothesis) has been proposed for children with many different types of developmental disabilities. This approach has been rejected for children with Down syndrome on the basis of the results of several investigations. In addition, supplementation of individual metabolites such as 5-hydroxytryptophan or pyridoxine for children with Down syndrome is ineffective.[255]

Pharmacogenetics is a new field of scientific research that helps provide a biochemical explanation for why some patients respond well to a medication and others with the same condition being treated do not. "Personalized medicine" is the concept in which doctors may make decisions regarding which medications, dosages, and combinations with other drugs to prescribe based on the analysis of selected genes in their patients.[15]

Cell Therapy

Hematopoietic stem cell transplantation and enzyme replacement therapy can increase survival in children with Hurler syndrome.[147] Gene therapy could potentially correct defective genes responsible for disease, but there has not yet been much success in clinical trials. The purpose of gene therapy is to replace missing or mutated genes, change gene regulation, or enhance the "visibility" of disease genes to improve the body's immune response. Gene therapy trials have been approved for use in humans only on somatic cells. A vector carries the gene product to the person's cells; vectors may be either an altered virus, stem cells, or liposomes.[256] Gene therapy is still only experimental and is moving along cautiously in the United States. In 1999 and again in 2003, individuals died while participating in gene therapy trials.[1]

The oversight of gene therapy falls under the U.S. Department of Health and Human Services, which oversees agencies that in turn are responsible for establishing research protocols (National Institutes of Health [NIH]), evaluating investigational gene products (Food and Drug

Administration), monitoring ethics (Recombinant DNA Advisory Committee), and educating human subjects (Office for Human Research Protections).[257] The clinical development of a gene product that could be widely dispensed must include four phases: phase 1 consists of regulatory approval of the protocol and then human pharmacology focusing on safety and tolerability and pharmacokinetics; phase 2 examines the effectiveness in terms of dose and regimen and target populations; phase 3 determines a basis for licensure and marketing of the product; and phase 4 establishes therapeutic use in a wider population.[257] As of November 2011 the U.S. Food and Drug Administration had not approved any human gene therapy products for sale,[212] but the United States led all others in the numbers of initiated protocols.[258,259] Approximately 600 gene therapy protocols have been initiated in the United States, most in the area of cancer research.[1] In the United States about 50 therapy protocols have focused on treating nine different single-gene disorders including CF, Duchenne muscular dystrophy, hemophilia B, and mucopolysaccharidosis.[258] To date, a gene therapy protocol is underway for Duchenne muscular dystrophy but not for any of the disorders described in this chapter. The interested reader can obtain an up-to-date listing of current gene therapy protocols from the NIH's Genetic Modification Clinical Research Information System (GeMCRIS) on the World Wide Web at www.gemcris.od.nih.gov/Contents/GC_HOME.asp.

In light of the limited medical treatment strategies available for children with genetic disorders, the physical or occupational therapist must be concerned with maximizing the child's developmental or functional potential within the limitations imposed by the lack of possible cures and the prospect of the shortened life span that characterizes many of these disorders. When deterioration of skills is expected, therapy must be directed at maintaining current functioning levels, minimizing decline, and minimizing caregiver support as much as possible.

Genetic Counseling

Developmental physical or occupational therapists must have an understanding of the modes of inheritance of the various genetic disorders and information about the services that can be offered through genetic counseling. Although the physician has primary responsibility for informing the parents of a child with a genetic disorder about the availability of genetic counseling, the close professional and personal relationships that therapists often develop with families may prompt family members to seek this type of information from the therapist.

Although a physical or occupational therapist cannot fill the role of a qualified genetic counselor, it is important that therapists be aware of the availability and location of genetic counseling services so that they may be assured that parents of a child with a genetic disorder have this information. Most major university-affiliated medical centers provide genetic counseling.

Process of Genetic Counseling

Six steps or procedures in genetic counseling were introduced in the 1970s by Novitski; they included descriptions of various genetic tests and a clinical interview.[260] The desired outcome of genetic counseling is to make an accurate medical diagnosis of the child's disorder. In the case of a suspected chromosome abnormality, this usually involves determining the karyotype of the child and possibly the karyotypes of the parents. Other diagnostic procedures may include a medical examination, FISH, DNA studies, biochemical studies, muscle biopsy, and other laboratory tests.

A pedigree or family tree is constructed of all known relatives and ancestors of both parents.[260] Pedigree information includes the age at death and cause of death of ancestors, a history of stillbirths and spontaneous abortions, and a history of appearance of any other genetic defects or unknown causes of intellectual disability. The country of origin of ancestors is also important because certain genetic defects, such as PKU, are far more prevalent in families of a particular ethnic origin. Once the defect has been identified and a pedigree constructed, Novitski[260] advises that further information be obtained from one of the comprehensive resource texts on genetic disorders. Informing family members about the characteristics of the disorder and its natural history may diminish fears of the unknown.

The third procedure in genetic counseling is to estimate the risk of recurrence of the disorder.[261] In specific gene defects, the probability of recurrence is fairly straightforward, with a risk of 25% for autosomal recessive disorders and a 50% risk for each male child in sex-linked disorders. These percentages, however, do not hold true in cases of spontaneous mutations. In cases of chromosomal abnormalities, such as Down syndrome, karyotyping is mandated to determine whether the child has the translocation type of Down syndrome. In that case the risk of recurrence is much greater than with a history of standard trisomy 21 Down syndrome.

Informing parents of the probability of recurrence is the next procedure. Novitski[260] points out the common misunderstanding that if a risk is one in four for a child to be affected, as in an autosomal recessive disorder, many parents assume that if they have just given birth to a child with the disorder, the next three children should be normal. It is important to explain that each subsequent child faces a one in four risk of inheriting the disorder regardless of how many siblings with the disorder have already been born. Estimating the risk of multifactorial disorders is a complex process. Although these conditions tend to cluster in families, there is no clear-cut pedigree pattern. The risk of recurrence of a multifactorial disorder is typically low, but if a couple has had two children with the same condition, the recurrence risk is presumed higher, with either a high genetic susceptibility or a chronic environmental insult suspected.

The fifth step in genetic counseling is for the parents to decide on the course of action they will take for future pregnancies once the counselor has presented all available facts to them.[261] Some parents may choose not to have any more children; others may elect to undergo prenatal diagnostic procedures for subsequent pregnancies. These decisions rest entirely with the parents and may be influenced by their individual religious or ethical preferences.

Follow-up counseling and review of the most recent advances in medical genetics are the final steps in the genetic counseling procedure.[260] Genetic counseling can play an important role in opening channels of communication among parents, other family members, and their friends;

connecting parents and siblings to support groups; and helping families to address their grief, sadness, or anger.[262] The effect of a child's disability on the family may modify the parents' earlier decision to have or not to have more children. Recent medical advances may allow a more certain prenatal diagnosis of specific genetic disorders.[263,264]

Early Detection of Genetic Conditions

Diagnosis of many genetic disorders is made clinically, as in observation of a congenital malformation; however, many serious conditions are not immediately apparent after birth. Detection of genetic conditions is performed through various screening procedures, followed by specific diagnostic testing to confirm a suspected disorder. With technological advancements in genetics, these procedures have been expanded for the unborn and the newborn. Couples planning to have children can be tested for specific genetic disorders before conception or embryonic implantation.[265] Health care professionals and parents should be informed about both the positive and the negative aspects of using this new knowledge and technology. The American College of Medical Genetics has published lists of the more common reasons for genetics referral as guidelines for health care providers working with infants, children, or couples planning to have children.[266]

Newborn Screening

Routine newborn screening is required practice in the United States. Screening is performed on whole populations for common disorders. The purpose of screening is the early identification of infants who are affected by a certain condition for which early treatment is warranted and available. Of the 4 million newborn infants screened each year, approximately 3000 have detectable disorders.[267] Currently all 50 states require screening for three disorders: PKU, congenital hypothyroidism, and galactosemia.[140] Some populations known to be at higher risk of certain disorders may be screened automatically, or individuals may elect state-specific screening.[267] Most states screen for eight or fewer disorders.[268] Tandem mass spectrometry (MS/MS) is a laboratory technique that allows for the identification of several metabolic disorders using a single analysis of a small blood sample drawn from the neonate. Many states use MS/MS for newborn screening for various disorders and have expanded their list of those that are mandated and those that are part of limited pilot programs.[269] Some genetic screening is performed primarily for research purposes when the disorder is not preventable, for example, type I diabetes. Screening for type I diabetes is available in some states, and early reports are that 90% of parents consent to the test.[270]

Benefits of newborn screening are earlier definitive diagnosis and medical intervention for the affected child. Concerns about expanded newborn screening include hasty medical decisions before conclusive evidence is available, and parental stress because of a lag time between screening and definitive results. A study by Waisbren and colleagues[271] conducted on parents of children screened for biochemical genetic disorders recognized that parents generally reported less stress the earlier a diagnosis could be made. However, in the same study, in cases in which the test yielded a false-positive result, parents reported a higher stress index and their children were twice as likely to experience hospitalization (usually the emergency department) than in mothers of children with normal screening results.[271] In the case of a positive screening result, infants will typically undergo more definitive genetic testing.

Genetic Testing in Infants and Children

Many genetic disorders can be diagnosed by clinical criteria specific to that disorder. If a diagnosis cannot be made on the basis of the patient's clinical presentation, then genetic testing may be warranted. There are currently about 900 genetic tests that can be offered by diagnostic laboratories; specific information can be found at www.genetests.org. In the United States, the standards and methods of all laboratories performing clinical genetic tests are governed at the federal level.[265]

Prenatal Testing

Tests to diagnose a genetic disorder in a developing fetus can be placed into two broad categories: invasive and noninvasive procedures. Currently, in contrast to the most common invasive procedures, noninvasive methods typically cannot permit a definitive diagnosis, but they can be performed with less risk to the fetus. Invasive procedures are recommended in cases of high risk for a serious disorder, when definitive diagnosis could lead to treatment, and to allow parents to make decisions about the pregnancy.[272] The ethical implications for prenatal testing are many. Parents are often given information that requires a sophisticated understanding of biology and medicine to fully understand the implications and results of a diagnostic procedure. For example, amniocentesis can detect many chromosomal abnormalities, but the functional outcome of some disorders can have great variety.[273]

Invasive Procedures. The most common prenatal diagnostic procedure is amniocentesis, which is used to detect early genetic disorders in the fetus at 11 to 20 weeks' gestation.[272] This method involves inserting a long, slender needle through the mother's abdominal wall and into the placenta to extract a small amount of amniotic fluid.[274] Laboratory tests of amniotic fluid reveal all types of chromosome abnormalities and a number of specific gene defects, including LNS, and some disorders of multifactorial inheritance, such as neural tube defects. This procedure carries a risk of miscarriage of about 0.5% to 1.7%,[275] and the risk increases the earlier that it is performed.[272]

Chorionic villus sampling involves extracting and examining a portion of the placental tissue. It has nearly a 99% detection rate for chromosomal abnormalities,[272] and it can be definitive earlier than amniocentesis; however, the risk of severe limb defects (amniotic band syndrome) increases the earlier that it is performed. The miscarriage rate with this procedure is estimated to be 0.5%.[272]

Noninvasive Procedures. Ultrasonographic examination of a fetus has been used to identify congenital malformations since 1956. It is currently offered to most women in the United States. It is currently believed that there is no inherent risk from this procedure. First-semester sonography is performed mainly to confirm the gestational age, to identify multiple pregnancy, and to measure nuchal thickness (NT). NT is a measure of the subcutaneous space between the skin and the cervical spine in the fetus; increased NT is often associated with trisomies. Second-trimester ultrasonography can detect problems in the quantity of amniotic fluid, large fetal structural defects, and certain smaller defects associated with a genetic disorder. A definitive diagnosis is not made on the basis of the presence of small defects alone, but the findings are considered along with the other risk factors present.[276] Again, there are ethical questions about the risk to the parents (emotional stress and uncertainty) versus the benefits of early detection.

Tests of maternal serum screening done at about 15 to 20 weeks' gestation can detect chromosomal abnormalities, but the accuracy depends on many factors, such as gestational age, maternal weight, ethnicity, multiple pregnancy, maternal type I diabetes, and maternal smoking.[272] Finally, it is possible to perform cytogenic analysis of fetal blood cells that can be isolated from a sample of the mother's blood, but this requires expensive equipment and expertise.[272]

Assisted Reproductive Technology and Preimplantation Genetic Diagnosis

Couples who want to conceive often seek genetic counseling if one or more parents is aware of a familial genetic condition, if they are having difficulty conceiving, and commonly in cases of advanced maternal or paternal age. More than 1 million babies have been born worldwide as a result of in vitro fertilization (IVF).[277] IVF has enabled couples with fertility problems to conceive and more recently is used to diagnose a genetic disease or condition in an embryo when it has differentiated into just eight cells.[278] Chromosomal abnormalities are the most common detected abnormality, and approximately 100 single-gene disorders have been diagnosed.[278] The ultimate purpose of preimplantation genetic diagnosis is to implant only mutation-free embryos into the mother's uterus; however, infants conceived with assisted reproductive technology (ART) are two to four times more likely to have certain types of birth defects than children conceived naturally.[277] The reasons for the increased risk of birth defects is unknown, but it may be that ART results more often in multiple births, which are at higher risk regardless of use of ART.[277] Intracytoplasmic sperm injection (ICSI) is another form of ART used often in cases of paternal infertility. Male infertility caused by azoospermia or oligozoospermia is associated with several genetic factors such as paternal sex chromosome aneuploidy in the case of Klinefelter syndrome.[70,279] Preimplantation genetic testing is optional in the United States but recommended in cases of family history and in men with nonobstructive azoospermia.[279]

Ethical, Social, and Legal Issues in Genetics

Advancements in genetics have led to important ethical questions about testing and screening for genetic disorders during the course of a couple's family planning and after the birth of the child. Ethical debates about genetic testing are inevitable. The persistent ethical issue in newborn screening surrounds mandatory or voluntary approaches taken by the states.[2] All states require newborn screening, usually without parental consent for the tests. Thirty-three states have newborn screening statutes or regulations that allow exemptions from screening for religious reasons, and 13 additional states have newborn screening statutes or regulations that allow exemptions for any reason. The majority of states have statutes that contain confidentiality provisions, but these provisions are often subject to exceptions.[268]

Traditionally in pediatric medicine, parents are presumed to be best suited to make the decision whether to pursue genetic testing. Organizations such as the American Academy of Pediatrics (AAP) have argued that parental autonomy should not be absolute in cases of life-threatening situations coupled with clear medical treatment benefit, but the AAP supports efforts to make informed parental consent a standard in the United States. Furthermore, the AAP does not support the broad use of carrier screening in children or adolescents or the position that newborn screening should be used to identify carrier status in parents of newborns identified as having disorders through newborn testing.[2] The American Society of Human Genetics has recommended that family members not be informed of misattributed paternity revealed through testing for the purpose of screening for disorders and that informed consent should include cautions regarding the unexpected finding of a different disease.[280]

Pediatricians and other health care professionals should be prepared to equip families with the appropriate information to use in the decision-making process about genetic testing. From a medical standpoint, Ross and Moon[281] propose a decision algorithm that weighs the risks and benefits of genetic testing. A decision to pursue genetic testing would be advised if the child was symptomatic, had a suspected genetic condition, or was from a high-risk family; if early diagnosis would decrease morbidity or mortality; and if the testing method was considered ethical and the testing would lead to a beneficial treatment. Lastly, practitioners and researchers should be prepared to educate families on the protections and limitations of the Genetic Information Nondiscrimination Act of 2008 (GINA). This federal law, which sets a nationwide level of protection for U.S. citizens, does not preempt state law, which usually provides broader safeguards. GINA prohibits health insurers from using the results of *predictive* genetic testing done for an individual to determine policy rates for that individual or for persons in a similar population; this includes information discovered in the course of medical testing and research. However, it does not protect a person's right to insurance for a genetic illness that is diagnosed. GINA prohibits insurers from requesting or requiring that person undergo a genetic test. It prohibits employers from requesting, requiring, or using a person's genetic information in making employment decisions, including information about the employee's family's genetic information. GINA does not apply to decisions about life, disability, or long-term care insurance, nor does it apply to members of the military.[282]

INTEGRATING GENETICS INFORMATION FOR PRACTICAL USE IN PEDIATRIC CLINICAL SETTINGS

Therapists in all settings frequently find it challenging to keep up with practice issues and the growing body of knowledge and evidence in rehabilitative medicine. In clinical settings where most of a therapist's day is spent in actual hands-on treatment, the wealth of information that is available may seem burdensome and practically inaccessible. Patients and their families will present the therapist with many questions about medical interventions, diagnostic procedures, and research. Although therapists know that a working knowledge of all of these areas is important, often time and access to resources are limited.

Pediatric therapists know the importance of collaboration with other professionals, including a type of collective knowledge about the child and his or her diagnosis, impairments, functional limitations, and quality-of-life issues identified by the family. A 1998 survey of individuals from six different health professions, including physical therapists, revealed that most professionals are not confident in their education and working knowledge in the field of genetics.[283] Additional studies have indicated that there are not enough genetic counselors[271,281] to meet the growing needs of patients and families and that patients often express the most stress and dissatisfaction because their primary care physician does not appear to be informed about their child's disorder.[271,284] See Case Study 13-1, Part 1.

CASE STUDY 13-1, PART 1 ■ THERAPISTS' ROLE IN EARLY RECOGNITION AND CLINICAL DIAGNOSIS OF GENETIC DISORDERS

This case study series portrays how basic knowledge and skills competence in genetics are essential for therapists in the delivery of services for pediatric patients with genetic disorders. Two female patients with presenting signs of developmental delay received physical therapy services before and after receiving a definitive diagnosis.

SCREENING FOR GENETIC DISORDERS AT INITIAL VISIT

Developmental delay is a common classification for infants and young children entering into physical therapy services before a definitive diagnosis of a particular genetic disorder has been made. Family history and course of pregnancy are key areas for the physical therapists to consider during ongoing assessment. The sensitive nature of this information requires that appropriate trust and rapport have been established between practitioner and family.

For the female patients discussed in this case, no remarkable information was revealed to indicate that a genetic disorder was suspect: Each of the girls was the first-born child and lived with her biological parents, in whom there was no previous family history of a genetic disorder. This was the first pregnancy for the mothers of both girls. The mothers each became pregnant in their late 20s without the assistance of reproductive technology, and they received the recommended course of prenatal care without specialized prenatal testing. The course of the mothers' pregnancies and deliveries were unremarkable, as was the neonatal period for the children.

Both girls were Caucasian with blond hair, blue eyes, and absence of notable dysmorphism. Figure 13-9, *A* and *B* shows 2 females. The first child was 16 months and the second was 14 months before given a medical diagnosis.

MEDICAL RECORDS REVIEW

	DYLEN: CONTRASTING FEATURES	DANIKA: CONTRASTING FEATURES	FEATURES OF BOTH GIRLS
0-6 MONTHS OF AGE			
Parental concerns	Vomiting and abnormal eye movements		Low muscle tone and slow motor development.
Tests and measures	Normal brain MRI scan and EEG at 3 months	No tests	
Development			Normal head control. Purposeful reach, grasp, and object release. Good eye contact and "happy" disposition. Some babbling and one-syllable sounds.
6-8 MONTHS OF AGE			
Parental concerns	Tongue thrusting and episodic nystagmus; parents suspect seizures	Sleep disturbances Visual disturbance suspected	Both girls are slow to achieve independent sitting and crawling.
Tests and measures			
Development	Pivots in prone position at 8 months. Sits without support at 8 months.	Not yet sitting.	Delayed trunk control. Both girls roll over by 7 months.

EEG, Electroencephalogram; *MRI,* magnetic resonance imaging.

Pediatric therapists should recognize that marked developmental delay and global hypotonia are two features common to many genetic disorders. However, in the case of both girls, the urgency of a genetics referral was lessened by the following factors: no dysmorphic features, healthy neonatal development, absence of family history of genetic disorders, and no other major presenting risk factors (e.g., no prior loss of pregnancies, young maternal age, and normal course of pregnancy).

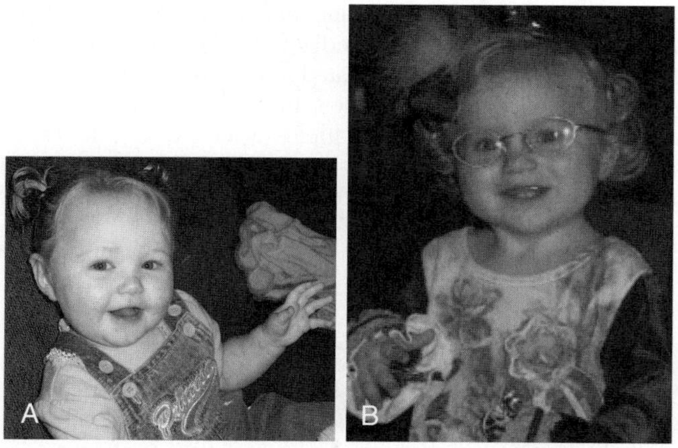

Figure 13-9 ■ **A,** Dylen at 16 months of age. **B,** Danika at 14 months of age.

Basic Knowledge and Skills Competence for Physical and Occupational Therapists

The National Coalition for Health Professional Education in Genetics (NCHPEG) is an organization of individuals from approximately 120 health profession. They have proposed basic competencies for all health care professionals.[7] With a working knowledge about genetics, therapists can develop competence in eliciting and accessing genetic information from subjective interviews with proper patient consent, can learn how to protect patient privacy while making appropriate recommendations to genetics professionals, and can understand the social and psychological implications of genetic services.[283,285]

Professional education for physical therapists[3] and occupational therapists[286] faces challenges to prepare practitioners who meet the minimum competencies set forth by NCHPEG.[7] Most physical therapists responding to the survey by Long and colleagues[283] reported that they received most of their information through nonscientific media and that they had limited or no education in genetics. Some of the barriers to implementation of genetics content in professional programs include lack of faculty qualified to teach the content and time limitations within a didactic program.[3] Continuing education courses for practicing clinicians are in short supply. Physical therapists have identified needs for continuing education in genetics to include topics such as the role of genetics in common disorders such as cancer and heart disease, an overview of human genetics, what treatments were available, and how to direct clients to information resources. Although occupational therapists were not part of Long's study, it is felt that colleagues would stress similar needs.[283]

Service Delivery for Children with Genetic Disorders and Their Families

For therapists to be supportive of families they are working with, they must acknowledge the importance of family priorities, respect the family's cultural values and beliefs,[287-289] include families as integral team members, and promote and deliver services that build on family and community resources.

This section includes strategies for supporting families of children with genetic disorders, assessment strategies, construction of therapeutic goals and objectives, and guiding principles for pediatric interventions.

Family-Centered Service

Family-centered service is both a philosophy and an approach to service delivery that is considered to be a best practice in early intervention and pediatric rehabilitation.[290-292] Children with genetic disorders have complex, long-term needs that can be addressed by a family-centered service delivery model. At the core of this model is the manner in which therapists interact with the children and their families—the therapists' mindfulness, attentiveness, and respectfulness, elements that are as important as the actual interventions delivered.[293,294] Therapists educated in the family-centered approach are also able to understand the impact of disability on a family as well as the value of support systems such as family and community.[262]

Bailey and colleagues[262] highlight the particular needs of families who have children diagnosed with genetic disorders to have productive partnerships with health care providers. Therapists should not be reluctant to learn about a rare condition from parents, as many are not "passive recipients of information" but rather "co-producers" of what and how information available may be used in their child's care.[262,295] Parents can be trusted to be a reliable source in the recognition of their child's condition and needs,[296] but in some instances the therapist's role may be to steer families to accurate information or assist with interpreting information which they have discovered. For example, the term "untreatable condition" may be misinterpreted by parents to mean that there are no reasonable interventions that may benefit their child (see Case 13, Part 4).

The *Relational Goal-Oriented Model* (RGM) of service delivery links the "what" with a more in-depth consideration of the "how" (how service providers and organizations can optimize both the process and outcomes of service delivery).[297] The role of the family in the child's life and the importance of the insights of parents into their child's abilities and needs[298] are crucial. Three important aspects of caregiving—information exchange, respectful and supportive care, and partnership or enabling—are foundational to family-centered care.[299] Family-centered service recognizes that each family is unique, that the family is the constant in the child's life, and that the family members are experts in the child's abilities and needs. The family works together with service providers to make informed decisions about the services and supports the child and family receive. The strengths and needs of all family members are considered in family-centered service.[300] In the interactional exchange between the child and family and the therapists, understandings occur, commitments and decision are made, the child and family receive affirmation and support, and information is translated into meaningful, usable knowledge through the process of communication.[301,302] Developing mutual trust and open communication among the child, the family, and the physical and occupational therapists as well as other practitioners is at the core of clinical practice.

Therapists working with children need to recognize and acknowledge the multitude of tasks that all families work to accomplish. In addition to tasks specifically related to caring for a child with a disability, families must perform functions to address the economic, daily care, recreational, social, and educational and vocational needs of both individual members and the family as a whole.

As Turnbull and Turnbull[303] have cautioned, each time professionals intervene with families and children, they can potentially enhance or hinder the family's ability to meet important family functions. For example, intervention that promotes a child's social skills can be an important support to positive family functioning. On the other hand, intervention that focuses on the child's deficits can have a negative impact on how the family perceives that child and the place of the child in the family. The RGM emphasizes the importance for therapists to join with parents to provide responsive and flexible therapy services in accordance with changing family needs and circumstances.[304]

The *Life Needs Model*[292,297] acknowledges the need for therapists to work collaboratively with service providers in other disciplines to improve community participation and quality of life for children and youth with disabilities, based on the expressed needs of the child and his or her family members. Assisting the family in identification of a support group is often helpful for adjustment and continuing encouragement in coping with issues. Support groups can be found at www.geneticalliance.org, a comprehensive website provided by the Alliance of Genetic Support Groups. Family empowerment mediates relationships between family-centered care and improvements in children's behaviors[305] and directly affects families' satisfaction with services for their children and their well-being.[306]

Assessment Strategies

Knowledge of a child's diagnosis can aid in the selection of appropriate assessment tools and can alert the therapist to any potential medical problems or contraindications associated with the specific syndrome that might affect the assessment procedures (tests and measures). Therapists must be careful, however, not to develop preconceived opinions about a child's capabilities on the basis of how other children with similar diagnoses have performed. It is critical to remember that there is wide behavioral and performance variability among children within each genetic disorder. For example, wide variability in the achievement of developmental milestones has been reported among children with Down syndrome.[307]

The assessment process includes many components that in certain areas are specific to the practice of either physical or occupational therapy. For the physical therapist, use of the *Guide to Physical Therapist Practice*[308] is recommended as a framework to identify appropriate tests and measures for impairments or disabilities. For the occupational therapist a useful reference is the assessment section of the textbook *Occupational Therapy for Children*.[237]

Typically a therapist's assessment begins with movement observation and analysis followed by testing of the neuromuscular status of the child, such as primitive reflexes, automatic reactions, and muscle tone. For children with orthopedic involvement, assessment of muscle strength, joint range of motion, joint play, and soft tissue mobility is also important. An assessment of the child's developmental level and functional ability should be completed. Such assessments can be used to discriminate between typical and delayed development, to identify the constraints interfering with the achievement of functional skills, and to guide the development of treatment goals and strategies. Most developmental assessment tools fall into one of the following categories: (1) discriminative, (2) predictive, and (3) evaluative measures.[309] Each of these three types of developmental assessment tools yields a different type of information. It is important to understand these differences and the intended purpose for each type of assessment to ensure that evaluation tools are used appropriately. A list of tests and measures commonly used by pediatric physical therapists is summarized in Table 13-4.

Discriminative Assessment

A discriminative assessment is used to compare the ability of an individual with the ability of members of a peer group or with a criterion selected by the test author.[309] Such instruments provide information necessary to document children's eligibility for special services but rarely provide information useful for planning or evaluating therapy programs.[310] Norm-referenced tests such as the Alberta Infant Motor Scale,[311] the Bayley Scales of Infant Development (motor and mental scales),[312] and the Peabody Developmental Motor Scales[313] are examples of tests used with infants and young children to verify developmental delay or to assign age levels. The Test of Infant Motor Performance is used to identify the risk of developmental delay in infants from 32 weeks postconception to 16 weeks after term.[314] An example of a norm-referenced assessment tool for older children is the Bruininks-Oseretsky Test of Motor Proficiency.[315]

It may be possible to detect improved motor performance by administering a developmental test used to identify children who have motor delays. Such tests, however, usually cannot detect small increments of improvement because there are relatively few test items at each age level and developmental gaps between items are often large. In assessing whether intervention has been effective, the use of most discriminative tools does not examine a child's performance of functional activities in natural environments.[310]

Predictive Assessments

Predictive measures are used to classify individuals according to a set of established categories and to verify whether an individual has been classified correctly.[309] Measures designed to predict future performance are often used to detect early signs of motor impairment in infants who are at risk for neuromotor dysfunction.[310] Knowledge of developmental milestones and the ability to identify typical and atypical movement at various ages is paramount to the therapist's competency in administering a structured assessment such as those used to predict future disability in children. Prechtl and others[316] have described how assessment of "general movements" in infants can be used to identify children with cerebral palsy.[317] The Movement Assessment of Infants[318] was designed to assess muscle tone, reflex development, automatic reactions, and volitional movement and has value in predicting future neurodevelopmental problems in high-risk infants when administered during the first year of life.[319,320] The Test of Infant Motor Performance[314] and the Alberta Infant Motor Scale[311] are other instruments commonly used to predict poor motor outcomes.

Evaluative Assessments

An evaluative measure is used to document change within an individual over time or change occurring as the result of intervention.[309] Helping Babies Learn[321] is a curriculum-referenced test that provides information about a child's developmental progress relative to a prespecified curriculum sequence.

TABLE 13-4 ■ TESTS AND MEASURES COMMONLY USED IN PEDIATRIC PHYSICAL THERAPY

TESTS AND MEASURES	AGE RANGE	PURPOSE
Alberta Infant Motor Scale (AIMS)[311]	Birth to 18 months	Identifies motor delays and measures changes in motor performance over time
Batelle Developmental Inventory[359]	Birth to 8 years	Identifies developmental level and monitors changes over time
Canadian Occupational Performance Measure (COPM)[360]	Any age	Identifies changes in parent's perception or child's self-perception of performance over time
Bayley Scales of Infant Development, ed 2 (BSID-II)[312,361]	1 to 42 months	Identifies developmental delay in gross motor, fine motor, and cognitive domains; monitors progress over time
Berg Balance Scale[362]	5 years and older	Performance-based measure of balance during specific movement tasks
Bruininks-Oseretsky Test of Motor Proficiency (BOTMP)[315]	4.5 to 14.5 years	Identifies motor abilities and can be used for program planning; monitors change over long periods of time for child with mild disabilities
Childhood Health Assessment Questionnaire (CHAQ)[363]	Any age	Measures quality of life from patient's or parents' perspective
Child Health Questionnaire[364]	2 months to 15 years	Measures quality of life from patient's or parents' perspective
Denver Developmental Screening Test II[365]	2 weeks to 6.5 years	Screening tool for developmental delay
Early Intervention Developmental Profile[366]	Birth to 3 years	Measures development of gross and fine motor, language, perception, social, and self-care skills
Energy Expenditure Index (EEI)[367]	3 years and older	Measures endurance level for activity; monitors changes over time
Functional Independence Measure (FIM)[323]	7 years and older	Measures changes in mobility and activities of daily living skills; used for program evaluation and rehabilitation outcomes assessment
Functional Independence Measure for Children (WeeFIM II)[324]	6 months to 7 years	Measures changes in mobility and activities of daily living skills; used for program evaluation and rehabilitation outcomes assessment
Functional Reach Test (FRT)[368]	4 years and older	Measures anticipatory standing balance during reach
Goal Attainment Scale[369]	Any age	Individualized goal-setting format to detect small, patient-relevant changes over time
Gross Motor Function Measure (GMFM)[157]	5 months to 16 years	Measures change in gross motor function over time
Harris Infant Neuromotor Test (HINT)[370]	Birth to 12 months	Screening tool to detect early signs of cognitive and neuromotor delay
Health Utilities Index Mark 3[371]	Any age	Measures child's functional health status; computes cardinal utility value that represents health-related quality of life
Modified Ashworth Scale (MAS)[372]	4 years and older	Qualitative measurement of spasticity through resistance to passive joint movement
Modified Tardieu Scale[373,374]	4 years and older	Qualitative measurement of spasticity through resistance to passive joint movement
Movement Assessment of Infants (MAI)[318]	Birth to 12 months	Identifies motor abilities or dysfunction
Peabody Developmental Motor Scales (PDMS-2)[313]	Birth to 5 years	Identifies gross and fine motor delays; used to monitor progress
Pediatric Clinical Test of Sensory Integration for Balance (P-CTSIB)[375]	4 to 10 years	Measures sensory system contributions to standing balance and postural control
Pediatric Evaluation of Disability Inventory (PEDI)[325]	6 months to 7.5 years	Measures self-care and mobility performance in the home and community; monitors progress over time
Pediatric Outcomes Data Collection Instruments (PODCI)[376]	0 to 19 years	Assesses overall health, pain, quality-of-life components, and participation in ADLs (and sports in older children)
Pediatric Quality of Life Inventory (PedsQL)[377]	2 to 18 years	Parent report and/or child self-report measuring health-related quality of life (HRQOL) in healthy children, adolescents, and those with acute and chronic health conditions
School Function Assessment (SFA)[326]	Kindergarten to 6th grade	Measures function in the school environment
Sensory Integration and Praxis Test[378]	4 to 9 years	Measures sensory systems' contribution to balance and motor coordination
Sensory Profile[379]	3 to 10 years	Determines which sensory processes contribute to child's performance of activities of daily living
6-Minute Walk Test[380]	5 years and older	Measures walking endurance; monitors progress over time
Test of Infant Motor Performance (TIMP)[314]	32 weeks to 4 months	Provides early identification of motor delay; assesses posture for early skills acquisition
Test of Sensory Function in Infants[381]	4 to 18 months	Identifies sensory processing dysfunction and those at risk for developmental delay or learning problems
Timed Up and Go (TUG)[382]	4 years and older	Performance-based measure of anticipatory standing balance, gait, and motor function
Toddler and Infant Motor Evaluation (TIME)[383]	4 months to 3.5 years	Identifies children with mild to severe motor problems; measures sensory development; monitors progress over time

ADLs, Activities of daily living.

To determine whether a child's ability to perform meaningful skills in everyday environments has improved, a functional assessment should be used. Functional assessments focus on the accomplishment of specific daily activities rather than on the achievement of developmental milestones. Emphasis is placed on the end result in terms of the achievement of a functional task, although the form or quality of the movement should never be ignored by the therapist. Assistance in the form of people or devices is incorporated into the assessment of progress, with the measurement of progress focusing on the achievement of independence.[322] Qualitative aspects of movement that have important functional implications, such as accuracy, speed, endurance, and adaptability, are also considered.

Functional assessments can be used to screen, diagnose, or describe functional deficits and to determine the resources needed to allow the child to function optimally in specific environments (e.g., school, home). Another use of functional assessments is to evaluate the nature of the problem and the specific task requirements limiting function to develop educational plans and teaching strategies.[322] A final use of functional assessments is to examine and monitor for changes in functional status. Such assessments can be used for program evaluation and for determining the cost-effectiveness of services or programs. (See Chapter 8 for additional information regarding evaluation tools.)

The Functional Independence Measure (FIM) is an example of a functional assessment. The FIM assesses the effectiveness of therapy on functional dependence in the areas of self-care, sphincter control, mobility, locomotion, communication, and social cognition.[323] Seven levels of functional dependence ranging from needing total assistance to complete independence are used to determine an individual's status. An adaptation of the FIM places greater emphasis on functional gains as opposed to the level of care. The WeeFIM[324] has been developed for use with children through the age of 6 years.

The Pediatric Evaluation of Disability Inventory (PEDI) is a functional assessment that focuses on the domains of self-care, mobility, and social cognition.[325] The PEDI incorporates three measurement scales: (1) the capability to perform selected functional skills, (2) the level of caregiver assistance that is required, and (3) identification of environmental modifications or equipment needed to perform a particular activity. The PEDI has been standardized and normed and is intended for use with children whose abilities are in the range of a typical 6-month-old to 7-year-old child.

The final example of a functional assessment is the School Function Assessment (SFA).[326] The SFA is designed to measure a student's performance in accomplishing functional tasks in the school environment. It is composed of three sections that focus on (1) the student's participation in major school activities, (2) the task supports needed by the student for participation, and (3) the student's activity performance. The SFA is standardized and was conceptually developed to be reflective of the functional requirements of a student in elementary school. See Case Study 13-1, Part 2.

CASE STUDY 13-1, PART 2 ■ ASSESSMENT STRATEGIES

	DYLEN: CONTRASTING FEATURES	DANIKA: CONTRASTING FEATURES	FEATURES OF BOTH GIRLS
9-13 MONTHS OF AGE			
Tests and measures			Both girls have abnormal EEG findings Alberta Infant Motor Scale score: below 5th percentile PEDI: Composite independence in functional skills less than 12% with total caregiver assistance
Development	Regression in motor skills: sitting, rolling, and fine motor Babbling vocalization Emergence of truncal and extremity ataxia	Sits alone at 11 months	Dylen demonstrates skill regression; Danika slowly attains motor skills.
Other objective findings	Cold feet with reddened appearance; normal BP and HR	Emergence of hand-flapping behaviors	Both girls have small head circumference.

BP, Blood pressure; *EEG,* electroencephalogram; *HR,* heart rate; *PEDI,* Pediatric Evaluation of Disability Inventory.

Another role of the therapist is to use assessment instruments that will help establish a baseline of motor and self-help skills and to monitor for progress or regression; the Alberta Infant Motor Scale and the PEDI, respectively, were initially used for these purposes. Lastly, the results of these tests and outcomes of intervention are interpreted and conveyed to the family and the child's pediatricians. In the case of both girls, delays in motor, language, and self-help skills persisted, and ultimately both girls and their families were referred for genetic evaluation. Both girls received 1 to 2 hours of physical therapy weekly in their natural environment. The Peabody Developmental Motor Scales were added to monitor progress, guide goal development, and justify the need for continued early intervention services.

Family-Driven Goals and Objectives

Therapy Goal Orientation

Goal orientation is a second fundamental feature of effective service. The earlier section on relation-based practice described how relationships among child, family, and therapists are fundamental in providing effective intervention. Goal orientation encompasses both joint goal setting by (1) parents, caregivers, and families and (2) therapists and other service providers[327] and the pursuit of meaningful child-, parent-, and family-selected goals.[328] Goals of parents and families are to create a supportive environment for their child, provide opportunities for growth and belonging, and assist their child to live as adaptive and independent a life as possible.[297] Family-centered care incorporates trusting relationships in which the therapist demonstrates respect for the family's values, beliefs, and goals rather than imposing a plan of care on the child and family that aims to correct "deficiencies."

After a child's strengths and needs have been evaluated and the family's objectives identified, therapy goals and objectives can be developed. In the past, establishment of these goals has primarily been the responsibility of professionals and often did not incorporate the needs and desires of the family. More recently, however, professionals have recognized the value of having families guide the process of establishing intervention goals and objectives.[329,330] This shift toward collaborative goal setting and family-centered care has occurred largely as a result of the belief that families should determine their vision of the future for their children and that professionals should act as consultants and resources to assist families in achieving that vision. The stress that caregivers experience with the everyday care of a child can reduce compliance with a home therapeutic program,[331] which further supports the notion that parents should be jointly involved with therapists to determine goals and the means by which to attain identified outcomes.[332] When parents and families contribute to the planning process, they are more likely to believe in goals that are set and to play a role in ensuring that relevant strategies are implemented.[297] They gain a sense of control over their child's services, supports, and resources that contributes to their personal and family's well-being.[333] For children living in the United States, these goals are developed within the context of individualized service plans.

Individualized Service Plans

In the United States, the Individuals with Disabilities Education Act (IDEA) requires public schools to develop an Individualized Education Plan (IEP) for every student with disability. An IEP is designed to meet the unique educational needs of a student with disability as defined by federal regulation 34 CFR 300.320.[334] Under IDEA 2004, a free appropriate public education (FAPE) is provided that is individualized to a specific student with a disability and that emphasizes special education and related services to prepare the student for further education, employment, and independent living [20 U.S.C. 1400 et seq, 20 U.S.C. 1400 © (5)(A)(i)].

Beginning with the enactment of United States Public Law 94-142 in 1975[335] and several important legislative revisions in 1990 (IDEA),[335-337] 1991 (PL 102-119), 1997 (PL 105-17), and 2004 (PL 108-446, Individuals with Disabilities Education Improvement Act of 2004),[338] physical and occupational therapists working in public school settings are required to establish long-term annual goals and short-term therapy objectives within the framework of each child's educational needs. The document that defines a child's educational needs, including therapy services, from preschool to twelfth grade is the IEP. Similar requirements are in effect for infants to preschool-age children, documented in the individualized family service plan (IFSP). An IFSP must be written after a multidisciplinary assessment of the strengths and needs of the child has been completed. This assessment must include a family-directed assessment of the supports and services necessary to enhance the family's capacity to meet the needs of their child with a disability.[337,338] A comparative table of the components of an IEP and IFSP is found in Table 13-5.

Functional Objectives

The development of behaviorally written, measurable therapy objectives is crucial for monitoring the effects of intervention in a child with a genetic disorder. Many of the clinical symptoms listed in the descriptions of genetic disorders described earlier in the chapter may be monitored through systematic, periodic, data-keeping procedures. One example is the monitoring of functional hand skills in girls with RS (see Case Study 13-1, Part 2). Periodic vital capacity measures for a child with OI or a child with Werdnig-Hoffmann disease can reflect progress toward a goal of maintaining respiratory function.

Typically, in the past, therapy objectives focused on a child's deficits. For example, delays in achieving motor milestones are often used to identify gaps in development, and therapy objectives are written and programs established to address these deficits. When the child meets an objective, new deficits are identified and new objectives are developed. A different model for goal development that is consistent with a family-centered intervention philosophy is the "top-down" approach, described by Campbell[339] and later by McEwen[340] and Effgren.[208] In this model, the child and family identify a desired functional outcome that is the driving factor for the therapeutic intervention plan. An example of this approach is seen in goal attainment scales. Goal attainment scaling (GAS) is an individualized, criterion-referenced measure of small, clinically important changes in a child's functional performance over time.[341,342] Similar to behavioral objectives, GAS requires (1) identification of observable goals, (2) reproducibility of conditions under which performance is measured, (3) measurable criteria for success, and (4) a time frame for goal achievement. In contrast to behavioral objectives, however, GAS identifies five possible outcomes with accompanying score values. By using five possible levels of attainment, it can be determined whether a child has made progress despite not having achieved the expected outcome or whether progress has exceeded the expected outcome. Case Study 13-1, Part 3 is an example of use of a goal attainment scale to assess a parent and child functional objective of sitting up on the floor to play with toys.

CASE STUDY 13-1, PART 3 ■ FAMILY-DIRECTED GOALS AND OBJECTIVES

Both girls had poor postural control with muscular weakness and hypotonia that limited the activity of sitting. The parents of both girls expressed a desire that their daughters would be able to sit up and play with toys on the family-room floor. The table illustrates the use of GAS for the goal of seated play with toys. In the course of care, Danika made good progress toward the goal depicted in this goal attainment scale; however, Dylen did not, and in fact demonstrated regression. Dylen's poorer outcome was indicative of the diagnosis of Rett syndrome (RS) that was revealed later. The family's goals for Dylen were revised, and the GAS was still a suitable framework.

SCORE	ATTAINMENT LEVEL IN TIME FRAME (INSERT) ______	CRITERION-REFERENCED GOALS WITHIN EACH RANGE (TIME FRAME: 3 MONTHS)
−2	Much less than expected outcome with therapy	(Child name) ring-sits on the floor supported on one or two hands plus 25% physical assistance for balance support and guided reach and grasp of toys placed near her lap.
−1	Less than expected outcome with therapy	(Child name) ring-sits on the floor with standby assistance and uses both hands to play with toys placed near her lap.
0	Expected outcome with therapy	(Child name) ring-sits on the floor with supervision, reaches and retrieves toys placed in front of her at arm's length away.
+1	Greater than expected outcome with therapy	(Child name) sits on floor independently and plays with toys placed at arm's length in front and to sides of her.
+2	Much greater than expected outcome with therapy	(Child name) sits on floor independently and retrieves toys placed slightly out of reach in front, to sides, and 45 degrees behind her and returns to upright for play.

TABLE 13-5 ■ COMPARISON OF REQUIRED COMPONENTS OF THE INDIVIDUALIZED EDUCATION PLAN (IEP) AND INDIVIDUALIZED FAMILY SERVICE PLAN (IFSP)

CONTENT	IFSP IDEA PART C (34CFR303.344)	IEP IDEA PART B (34CFR300.320 THROUGH 300.324)
Information about child's status	A statement of child's present levels of physical, cognitive, communication, social or emotional, and adaptive development (physical development includes vision, hearing, and health status)	A statement on child's present levels of academic and functional performance
Family information	Statement of family's resources, priorities, and concerns related to enhancing the child's development	Information regarding parent's concerns can be documented in the present information about the child's status
Outcomes	Statement of measurable outcomes expected to be achieved for child and family and the criteria, procedures, and timelines used to determine the degree of progress toward outcomes and whether modification or revisions of outcomes or services were necessary	Statement of measurable annual goals, including academic and functional goals Include a description of how child's progress toward annual goals will be measured and process to report child's progress to parents
Services	Statement of specific Early Intervention (EI) services necessary to meet child's needs; include frequency, intensity, method of service delivery, location of services and natural environments	Statement of specific special education and related services to be provided, modifications, and supplementary aids to be provided to child
Schedule of services	Projected dates for initiation of services, anticipated duration	Projected date for beginning and ending date of service; any modification needed; frequency, location, and duration of services
Service coordinator	Identification of the service coordinator	No comparable requirement
Transition plan	Procedures and steps for transition from EI to preschool services under Part B Establish transition plan: 90 days to 9 months before third birthday	Procedures needed for postsecondary goals related to training, education, employment, and, where appropriate, independent living skills To be in effect when child turns 16 yr of age
Transfer of rights	n/a	Must include statement that child has been informed about reaching the age of majority
Other		Explanation of any time the child will not participate along with nondisabled children

IDEA, Individuals with Disabilities Education Act.

Rather than focusing on a child's deficits, such outcome-focused objectives provide a more positive and supportive context for therapy and at the same time address the family's needs and priorities. This approach to developing therapy goals and objectives in ways that support positive family functioning is also an important aspect of delivering therapy services to children and their families.

General Intervention Principles

Several general treatment principles guide the delivery of therapy services to children with genetic disorders and are detailed in this section. Special considerations for treatment of a child with a specific genetic condition may be found in the preceding section. The reader is also referred to Chapter 9 for information on interventions in neurological rehabilitation.

Focus on Activities and Participation

The goal of any therapeutic program for children should be to improve the quality and quantity of their participation in society. Achievement of basic motor skills such as sitting, standing, and walking is an outcome that can be measured with commonly used clinical tools, but whether or not children actually apply new skills on a regular basis (participation) is more difficult to capture objectively.[343] Therapists need to possess knowledge, skills, and tools if they are to assess and treat children in all domains defined by the World Health Organization (see Case Study 13-1, Part 1). With the purpose of improving participation in the end, pediatric therapists employ a variety of intervention strategies to increase opportunities for children to achieve independence and enjoyment of activities at home and school and in the community

Many of the classic therapeutic approaches for children with neurological disorders incorporate techniques targeting impairments of body structure and function, such as abnormal muscle tone or joint alignment, to improve movement quality.[228] Motor learning science and task-oriented models of neurological rehabilitation are based on the rationale that control of movement arises from appropriate practice of skills within the context of functional activities and enriched environments.[343-346] Intervention, therefore, is aimed at teaching motor problem solving (adaptability to varied contexts),[347] developing effective compensations that are maximally efficient, and providing practice of new motor skills in functional situations. Rather than teaching individuals to perform movement patterns in a controlled therapy setting, this approach focuses on the learning that must take place for an individual to function independently of a therapist's guidance.[343,345] Environmental adaptations can take many forms and include assistive technology that aids in the attainment of functional outcomes such as independence in self-help skills, communication, and mobility.[348] For example, children with Down syndrome commonly have hypotonia, joint laxity, and delayed walking. Orthotics such as supramalleolar orthoses may be used to improve underlying joint and postural instability,[349] and treadmill training has been shown to diminish delays in walking.[350]

Modern neurophysiologic approaches use hands-on physical guidance with the child during movement practice of functional skills and activities. The inhibition of certain movements and facilitation of others are based on the rationale that less used movements will be eliminated in the pruning process of the developing brain and frequently used movement patterns will be reinforced[228,343,351]; therefore approaches of this nature may be beneficial for infants and very young children with movement disorders.

Learning and performance of an activity seldom require just one component of function (e.g., mobility, language, cognition); therefore it should be understood and expected that improvements in one domain may indirectly, but significantly, have a positive impact on another. For example, Damiano[351] stresses the benefits of a lifetime of regular movement activity, with or without adaptations, on the overall development of children. Regardless of treatment techniques, it is a widely accepted principle that children learn new skills best when they are taught and practiced within the context in which they will be used.[352]

Delivery of Services in Natural Environments

The term "natural environment" refers to places and settings in which infants and children typically spend their day.[337] The movement toward integrating therapy into classroom settings is one example of providing services in a natural environment.[353-355] In an integrated model of service delivery, therapists work in the classroom with teachers, rather than removing students to an isolated therapy room to provide services. Therapists work closely with the teacher to establish common goals for the student and to devise programs that will allow therapeutic activities to be interwoven into a variety of activities throughout the day in a natural manner.

Another example of providing therapy in a natural environment is providing home-based services for infants and young children. Home-based programs are "normal" options for young children because the natural environment for most infants and toddlers is the home—either their own or that of a day care provider.[353-355] For children who are medically fragile, it is the preferred option for therapy.[356,357] For other families, transportation to a center-based program may be difficult because of the expense or length of travel required.

Incorporating Therapy Activities into Daily Routines

Therapists need to work collaboratively with families to develop activities that incorporate therapeutic activities into the family's daily routine (e.g., during play, dressing, bathing, meals). Rather than practicing narrowly defined tasks in a controlled clinic environment, therapy activities should be interwoven into a variety of activities throughout the day in a natural manner. Practicing skills in the context of daily routines allows the child to learn to adapt to the real-life contingencies that arise during a functional task.[345] In addition, activities become more meaningful to both the child and the family (Figure 13-10).

Use of Assistive Technology Devices

The Assistive Technology Act of 2004 defines an assistive technology device as any item, piece of equipment, or product system, whether acquired commercially, modified, or customized, that is used to increase, maintain, or improve functional capabilities of individuals with disabilities (29 U.S.C. Sec 2202[2]).[358] Information for clinicians and families can be found in Table 13-1.

As noted previously, an important aspect of providing developmental therapy services is the use of assistive technology devices to maximize a child's functional abilities, level of independence, and inclusion in school and community activities with peers. Examples of assistive technology include mobility devices, augmentative communication devices, and adapted computer keyboards. Assistive technology also includes adaptive devices such as splints, bath chairs, prone standers, and other positioning equipment that can be used to provide optimal body alignment and minimize the risk for contractures or deformities while encouraging a greater variety of movement patterns. Such devices can be constructed from readily available materials or obtained commercially. The developmental physical or occupational therapist works with the family and other team members to select, construct, or order assistive devices and to assist caregivers in the use of the devices.

Case Example 13-1, Part 4 demonstrates how these general treatment principles are applied to a particular child receiving therapy services. The case example also shows how the family's priorities and needs are considered and supported in the planning and delivery of services.

CASE STUDY 13-1, PART 4 ■ FOCUS ON ACTIVITIES AND PARTICIPATION IN MEANINGFUL ENVIRONMENTS AND ROUTINES

Both families were referred by their respective physicians for genetic counseling and evaluation on the suspicion of AS based on cluster of developmental delay, features of blue eyes and blonde hair, head circumference, and abnormal EEG findings. Danika received an earlier referral to a geneticist at 14 months of age; subsequent test results confirmed the diagnosis of AS by the time she was 16 months old. The course of medical diagnosis for Dylen was confounded by her presenting signs of frequent, intense vomiting coinciding with suspicion of seizure activity. Dylen did not receive genetic testing until she was 30 months of age. In the cases of both girls, their documented response to therapy and course of motor development were weighed by their respective physicians in their course of care and referral for genetics evaluation. AS was ruled out first for Dylen, and subsequent testing confirmed a diagnosis of RS.

During the period immediately after their child's diagnosis, the parents in each family shared many questions and newfound knowledge with the treating therapist. Both families accessed local and national family support groups and were encouraged to learn of activities that their children would likely enjoy. The partnership between the therapists and the families was strengthened by clarifying that "untreatable condition" means that neither condition can be remedied by medical intervention and by focusing on the families' values and priorities.

Both girls had limited postural endurance in sitting and standing that was anticipated to persist for several months. Adaptive equipment for these activities was employed for both girls to allow them to participate in functional upright activities (see Figure 13-7). Danika enjoyed aquatic activities and tricycling more than she tolerated hippotherapy. Dylen was found to enjoy movement activities more when music was employed during treatment.

	DYLEN: CONTRASTING FEATURES	DANIKA: CONTRASTING FEATURES	FEATURES OF BOTH GIRLS
14-36 MONTHS OF AGE			
Diagnosis; body organ or structure and function	Rett syndrome; gastroesophageal reflux	Angelman syndrome; sleep disorder	Global developmental delay, seizures, hypotonia
Activities, limitations, and development	Motor skills plateaued at 9 months' chronological age, followed by period of skills regression to 6 months' developmental level	Ambulatory with assistive devices Persistent absence of expressive language but learns to respond to her name Expresses pleasure with giggles and subtle, jerky motions Uses raking motion to pick up small foods	Attends special education preschool
Physical therapy interventions	Movement-oriented activities with music	Aquatic therapy	Postural strengthening, sensorimotor activities
Assistive and adaptive equipment	Adaptive seating provides best opportunities to interact with others in learning environment	Walks indoors and outdoors with a gait trainer (see Figure 13-7, *B*) and shorter distances with a conventional posterior four-wheeled walker	Gait trainer Adaptive tricycle Bilateral ankle-foot orthoses
Participation of child and family			Support group events: walk, ride, stroll

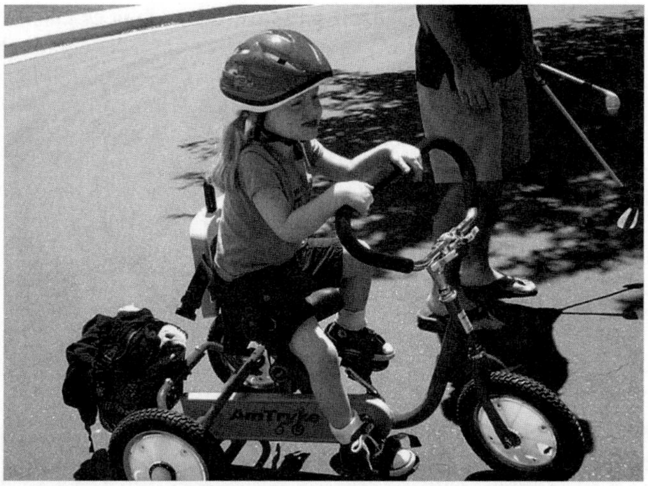

Figure 13-10 ■ This child with Angelman syndrome enjoys riding her adaptive tricycle to the park with her family.

SUMMARY

This chapter has addressed several chromosomal abnormalities and specific gene defects that are most likely to be seen in children in a typical developmental therapy setting. The inclusion of family members in all aspects of therapy has been stressed, along with the need to consider family goals, priorities, and resources in the development and implementation of therapy services. The importance of developing functional goals and delivering services in natural environments has also been emphasized. Finally, many diseases or conditions have a genetic component that must be considered in the course of medical management. Physical and occupational therapists should expand their working knowledge of genetics to appropriately refer patients for genetic services. Readers are encouraged to consult Box 13-1 for a list of resources about genetic disorders, education, testing, and interventions not described in this chapter.

References

To enhance this text and add value for the reader, all references are included on the companion Evolve site that accompanies this textbook. This online service will, when available, provide a link for the reader to a Medline abstract for the article cited. There are 383 cited references and other general references for this chapter, with the majority of those articles being evidence-based citations..

CHAPTER 14 Learning Disabilities and Developmental Coordination Disorder

STACEY E. SZKLUT, MS, OTR/L, and DARBI BREATH PHILIBERT, MHS, OTR/L

KEY TERMS

developmental coordination disorder
learning disabilities
life span disability
model of disablement
motor learning
neurodevelopmental treatment
nonverbal learning disabilities
praxis
sensory integration
verbal learning impairments

OBJECTIVES

After reading this chapter the student or therapist will be able to:

1. Be aware of characteristics that typically identify a child with learning disabilities.
2. Become familiar with accepted definitions and terminology used in the field of learning disabilities.
3. Investigate the proposed causes of learning disabilities.
4. Understand the clinical presentation of subgroups within the learning-disabled population.
5. Become familiar with members of the specialist team and service provision types for children with learning disabilities.
6. Recognize the characteristics of the child with developmental coordination disorder.
7. Identify areas of evaluation to assess motor deficits effectively in the child with a learning disability.
8. Become familiar with theoretical development and intervention techniques applicable to children with learning disabilities and motor deficits.
9. Understand the lifelong ramifications for the individual with learning disabilities.

AN OVERVIEW OF LEARNING DISABILITIES

Clinical Presentation

Learning disabilities are not a singular disorder but a group of varied and often multidimensional disorders.[1] Difficulties in learning may manifest themselves in various combinations of impairments in language, memory, visual-spatial organization, motor function, and the control of attention and impulses.[2,3] The characteristics of a child with a learning disability are often diverse and complex. Each child presents a different composite of system problems/impairments, functional deficits, preventing participation in activities and societal limitations.

The most commonly recognized performance difficulties in learning are associated with academic success. Fletcher and colleagues[4] argued that learning disabilities should be characterized as "unexpected" because the child is not learning up to expectations despite adequate instruction. Typically the areas of deficits are observed in verbal learning, including difficulties with reading, the acquisition of spoken and written language, and arithmetic. Impairments in nonverbal learning are equally important and more recently recognized. The three primary areas affected by nonverbal learning disorders include visual-spatial organization, social-emotional development, and sensorimotor performance.[5] Accompanying behavioral manifestations may include problems with self-regulatory behaviors, such as lack of attention, hyperactivity, and poor impulse control. Difficulties in social perception and social interactions may also be observed.[5,6] These learning and behavioral difficulties may be isolated (e.g., academic, motor, or behavioral), combined (e.g., academic and motor), or global (academic, motor, and behavioral).[7] In addition to verbal and nonverbal disabilities, specific motor impairments also can be present and affect academic achievement or daily life tasks.[8,9]

Definition

The heterogeneity of persons with learning disabilities has made consensus on a single definition difficult. Many disciplines describe learning disabilities according to their own frames of reference. Medical professionals tend to relate the deficit to its cause, particularly to cerebral dysfunction. Terms historically used include *brain injured,*[10] *minimal brain dysfunction,*[2] and *psychoneurological disorder,*[11] all implying a neurological cause for the deviation in development. Educational professionals, however, prefer to describe the child's difficulties in behavioral or functional terms. Educators view children with learning disabilities as "children who fail to learn despite an apparently normal capacity for learning."[12] Current terminology within the academic environment includes *reading disorder, mathematics disorder, disorder of written expression,* and *intellectual disabilities* (formerly called *mental retardation*).[13,14] The lack of consensus for one accepted definition continues to affect consistency in diagnosis, research, and intervention for persons with learning disabilities.

After multiple revisions, the National Joint Committee on Learning Disabilities (NJCLD), which represents several professional organizations, proposed the following definition:

Learning disability is a general term [for a condition] that:

- Is intrinsic to the individual . . . [the term] refers to a heterogeneous group. (Each individual with learning disabilities presents with a unique profile of strengths and weakness.)
- Results in significant difficulties in the acquisition and use of listening, speaking, reading, writing, reasoning, or mathematical abilities. (These difficulties are evident when appropriate levels of effort by the student do not result in expected performance, even when provided with effective instruction.)
- Is presumed to be due to central nervous system dysfunction and may occur across the life span. (They persist throughout life and may change in their presentation and severity at different stages of life.)
- May occur concomitantly with other impairments or other diagnoses. (For example, difficulties in self regulation and social interaction may exist separately or result from the learning disability. Individuals with attention-deficit disorders, emotional disturbances or intellectual disabilities may experience learning difficulties but these diagnoses do not cause or constitute them.)
- Is not due to extrinsic factors. (Such as insufficient or inappropriate instruction, or cultural differences.)[15]

This definition identifies a proposed cause but does not provide a clear exclusion statement regarding what learning disabilities may not result from. A positive component of this definition is the lifelong nature of the condition. Also, by including the behavioral manifestations of regulatory and social difficulties, a more complete picture of functional problems for the individual with learning disabilities is presented. This could assist in the creation of more comprehensive and life-spanning programs of service and ultimately help in the recognition and remediation of functional and societal limitations.

The definition used in educational settings was initially passed in Public Law 94-142 and later incorporated into the Individuals with Disabilities Education Act (IDEA) (Section 602.26).

Children with learning disabilities are defined by IDEA as follows:

- Individuals with a disorder in one or more of the basic psychological processes involved in understanding or using spoken or written language. (This emphasizes the receptive and expressive difficulties a student may demonstrate.)
- Those who are experiencing difficulties in the ability to listen, think, speak, read, write, spell, or do mathematical calculations. (These highlight the academic difficulties the student may experience.)
- Those who may have conditions such as perceptual disabilities, brain injury, minimal brain dysfunction, dyslexia, and developmental aphasia.
- Those who have a learning problem that does not result from other disabilities such as motor deficits, emotional disturbances, or environmental, cultural, or economic differences.

This description does not specifically address cause but does highlight psychological processes versus neurological impairments. The primary disability focus is on language, which may exclude difficulties in learning that involve nonverbal reasoning. This definition does not mention regulatory, reasoning, and social perception difficulties that may contribute to understanding the student's complete profile. On a foundational level this definition formed the basis for creating academic programs and delineating appropriate services for children with learning disabilities.

IDEA mandates that all children will have free and appropriate education and authorizes aid for special education and educationally relevant services for children with disabilities. IDEA influences how children with learning disabilities are identified and classified. The 1997 amendments of IDEA, by promoting the early identification and provision of services, redirected the focus of special education services by adding provisions that would enable children with disabilities to make greater progress and achieve higher levels of functional performance.[16]

The IDEA 2004 amendments eliminate a previous requirement that students must exhibit a severe discrepancy between intellectual ability and achievement for eligibility. This "severe discrepancy" policy often mandated that children would have to experience failure for several years to demonstrate the requisite degree of discrepancy.[17] The current goal is to identify ways of serving students more quickly and efficiently once they begin to show signs of difficulty.[17] Congress also indicated specifically that (1) IQ tests could not be required for the identification of students for special education in the learning disabilities category, and (2) states had to allow districts to implement identification models that used Response to Instruction (RTI).[18] The RTI models suggest that the learning difficulty may be intrinsic to the child, inherent in the instruction, or a combination of both. The models propose systematically altering the quality of instruction and repeatedly measuring the child's response to that instruction. Inferences can then be made about the child's deficits contributing to learning difficulties.[19]

IDEA 2004 also limits the schools from finding a student eligible for special education services if the learning problems are determined to be caused by a lack of appropriate instruction. The law now encourages schools to use scientific, research-based interventions to maximize a student's opportunity for success in the general education setting (least restrictive environment [LRE]) before being placed in special education. IDEA encourages educators to stress the importance of identifying individual differences and patterns of ability within each child and adjust the educational methods accordingly. Academic achievement relies heavily on the effectiveness of the teacher and the instructional techniques. Studies indicate that learning disabilities do not fall evenly across racial and ethnic groups, with a higher incidence of special education services needed for black, non-Hispanic children.[20] The No Child Left Behind Act challenges states and school districts to become more accountable for improving educational standards by intensifying their efforts to close the achievement gap between underachieving students and their peers.

Classifications

The two most widely used classification systems are those of the American Psychiatric Association (*Diagnostic and Statistical Manual of Mental Disorders* [DSM])[21] and the World Health Organization (WHO) (International Classification of Diseases [ICD]).[22] Educational professionals prefer the DSM classification for its academic relevance. A variety of specific academically related disorders are outlined in the DSM. The latest edition, DSM-IV-TR, classifies learning disabilities under "disorders usually first diagnosed in infancy, childhood, or adolescence." It subclassifies disorders into the following categories:

Learning Disorders

- Reading disorder
- Mathematics disorder
- Disorder of written expression

Motor Skills

- Developmental coordination disorder

Communication Disorders

- Expressive language disorder
- Mixed receptive-expressive disorder
- Phonological disorder
- Stuttering

The classification system commonly used by therapists is the ICD. The ICD codes are state mandated diagnostic codes used for billing and information purposes. In the recently revised ICD-10 the category "specific delays in development," which included "other specific learning difficulties," was changed to "disorders of psychological development." The term "learning" is no longer part of this classification. This updated classification is as follows:

Disorders of Psychological Development

- Including specific developmental disorders (SDD) of speech and language (including acquired aphasia with epilepsy)
- SDD of scholastic skills
- SDD of motor function
- Pervasive developmental disorder

Model of Disablement

Beyond classifying learning disabilities as a diagnosis, the National Center for Medical Rehabilitation Research (NCMRR)[23] and WHO have integrated related approaches to classify functional performance. This conceptual approach, the Model of Disablement, describes the multiple dimensions of disability and identifies various internal and external factors that affect the way a disability manifests. The purpose of this model is to shift classification of a disability to include assessment of functional performance and societal participation as opposed to solely identifying component deficit areas.

Five dimensions are outlined in the Model of Disablement. They include pathophysiology, impairments, functional limitations, disabilities, and societal limitations. *Pathophysiology* refers to the underlying disease or injury processes at the tissue or cellular level. Proposed causative factors related to learning disabilities at this level include brain damage, biochemical abnormalities, genetics, and metabolic disorders. The challenge for interventionists is to recognize the signs and symptoms that confirm the diagnosis.[24]

The second dimension, impairment, includes the organ and system dysfunction that potentially has a negative effect on functional performance. Children with learning disabilities may demonstrate impaired balance, endurance, and coordination of movements. Impairments that occur in one or more systems may lead to functional limitations, the third dimension. The challenge for the clinician is to treat impairments within the context of daily functional performance because impairments do not always result in functional limitation.

Functional limitations involve whole-body functions that are typically assessed but may or may not receive remediation.[24] For a child with learning disabilities this may include poor hand function in the performance of manipulation activities involved in dressing and handwriting. When persistent functional limitations are not remediable and cannot be adequately compensated for with assistive technology or other supports, disabilities in daily life occur. The child then fails to be an active participant in life roles, such as activities of daily living and school tasks. Emotional difficulties, such as depression and decreased self-esteem, which may result from learning difficulties, can ultimately impair social interactions.

Community and environmental barriers, called *societal limitations,* also can lead to restriction in social participation. An example of structural or attitudinal barriers that prevent optimal participation in society is a child who cannot use playground equipment because of lack of accessibility. The ultimate goal for the clinician is to facilitate functional abilities and performance as well as provide necessary supports so the child can become an active participant in society.

The Model of Disablement proposes that the environment, purpose, and level of participation should all be considered when evaluating performance. Determination of the presence, severity, or kind of disability should be made on the basis of a combination of these factors. Within this framework, a clinician does not assume that a handicap exists because of an impairment but rather considers levels of functional and societal abilities. This allows the therapist to determine intervention needs based on functional performance in relevant environments rather than being driven purely by diagnosis. A 9-year-old child with learning disabilities, for example, might have impairments in motor components of muscle strength and balance. Although these impairments can be identified on assessment, the Model of Disablement suggests that a disability does not exist unless these deficits affect functional performance (e.g., ascending and descending stairs) and limit societal participation (e.g., child cannot leave house independently to go to school or play). The identified impairments, based on assessment in an academic setting, would have to affect participation within the educational environment (be educationally relevant) to warrant intervention.

Incidence and Prevalence

Current data indicate that 15 million children nationwide have been diagnosed with some kind of learning disability.[25] According to a 2007 report to Congress on the implementation of IDEA, nearly 2.6 million students aged 6 to 21 years are receiving special education services for specific learning disabilities. As of 2007, this represents 44%

of students with disabilities nationwide.[25] Children with specific learning disabilities represent the highest incidence (number of new cases identified in a given period) among 13 disability categories, representing 44% of the total population of children receiving special education. Overall, the estimated prevalence (total number of cases in a population at a given time) of learning disabilities is approximately 15% of the U.S. population, which translates to one out of seven people.[9] In children under age 18 years, 8% to 10% of the population have some type of learning disability.[26] Boys are more likely than girls to be identified as having a learning disability. According to Child Trends, 10% of boys and 6% of girls aged 3 to 17 years had a learning disability in 2004.[27]

Perspectives on the Causes of Learning Disabilities

Learning disability is a diverse diagnosis with varied manifestations; therefore searching for a single cause would be inadequate. Historically, researchers have studied causative factors including (1) brain damage or dysfunction caused by birth injury, perinatal anoxia, head injury, fetal malnutrition, encephalitis, and lead poisoning; (2) allergies; (3) biochemical abnormalities or metabolic disorders; (4) genetics; (5) maturational lag; and (6) environmental factors, such as neglect and abuse, a disorganized home, and inadequate stimulation.[28-30]

Current sources agree that possible causes of learning disabilities can include problems with pregnancy and birth (e.g., drug and alcohol use, low birth weight, anoxia, and premature or prolonged labor), and incidents occurring after birth (e.g., head injuries, nutritional deprivation, and exposure to toxic substances such as lead).[31-34] Genetic and hereditary links also have been observed, with learning difficulties often seen across generations within families.[34] The emotional and social environment have also been considered as a contributing factor to learning disabilities.[14]

Children with learning disabilities frequently display a composite of neuropsychological symptoms that interfere with the ability to store, process, or produce information. These symptoms typically include disorders of speech, spatial orientation, perception, motor coordination, and activity level. Researchers have attempted to identify areas of the brain that may be responsible for these functional limitations. Tools being used include empirical measures of physiological function such as electroencephalography, event-related potentials (ERPs), brain electrical activity mapping (BEAM), regional cerebral blood flow (rCBF), positron emission tomography (PET), and functional magnetic resonance imaging (fMRI). These measures expand the understanding of brain functioning but are best used in conjunction with data on functional and behavioral manifestations.

Research findings on brain structure have documented that certain functions are specialized within each hemisphere and this specialization is optimal for efficient learning.[35,36] The left hemisphere processes information in a sequential, linear fashion and is more proficient at analyzing details. Academically, this hemisphere is responsible for recognizing words and comprehending material read, performing mathematical calculations, and processing and producing language.

The right hemisphere processes input in a more holistic manner, grasping the overall organization or the "gestalt" of a pattern.[37,38] This type of organization is advantageous for spatial processing and visual perception. Functionally, the right hemisphere synthesizes nonverbal stimuli, such as environmental sounds and voice intonation, recognizes and interprets facial expressions, and contributes to mathematical reasoning and judgment. Over time these differences in left and right brain processing have become accepted and are commonly labels of cognitive style (i.e., left-brained versus right-brained learner).

A strict left-right dichotomy is oversimplified because it does not take into account many aspects of functional brain organization.[37,39] Both hemispheres must work together for a variety of specific academic outcomes such as reading and mathematical concepts. In addition to the communication that occurs between the hemispheres via the corpus callosum, essential communication within the hemispheres is also present. Intrahemispheric communication is critical for developing higher level cognitive functions such as memory, language, visual-spatial perception, and praxis.[40] Research suggests that children with learning disabilities show different patterns of cerebral organization than normal children.[37,39] However, brain plasticity is the basis for designing and implementing a variety of intervention techniques aimed at improving processing.

Subgroups

In early attempts to classify learning disabilities, Denckla and Rudel[41] determined that approximately 30% of the 190 children they assessed by neurological examination could be classified into three recognizable subgroups. The other 70% exhibited an unclassifiable mixture of signs. Of the 30%, the first subgroup was classified as children having a *specific language disability.* These children, who were failing reading and spelling, showed a pattern of inadequacy in repetition, sequencing, memory, language, motor, and other tasks, all of which require rote functioning. The second group had a specific *visual-spatial disability.* These children had average performance in reading and spelling with delayed arithmetic, writing, and copying skills. The children in this subgroup all had social and/or emotional difficulties. The third group manifested a *dyscontrol* syndrome. These children had decreased motor and impulse control, were behaviorally immature, and were average in language and perceptual functioning.

Grouping children with learning disabilities based on patterns of academic strengths and weakness is as important as grouping them based on neuropsychological or cognitive measures. With an academic classification the heterogeneity of learning disabilities can be more clearly recognized and learning modalities can be adjusted to the individual child. A child with a specific reading difficulty, for example, could be experiencing deficits in word recognition, fluency, or comprehension. Through identification of the specific areas of weakness in reading, intervention can be individualized to improve academic performance.[4]

Based on historical and current trends the following general subgroups will be explored: verbal learning impairments, nonverbal learning disabilities (NVLDs), motor coordination deficits, and social and emotional challenges.

Verbal Learning Impairments

Verbal learning impairments typically include dyslexia, dyscalculia, and dysgraphia. Harris[13] classifies these deficits in functional terms, with dyslexia including disorders of reading and spelling, dyscalculia denoting a mathematics disorder, and dysgraphia describing a disorder of written expression. These learning disorders may occur individually or concurrently. Each of these verbal learning impairments will significantly influence academic performance.

Dyslexia (Developmental Reading Disorder). Dyslexia is a learning impairment in which the ability to read with accuracy and comprehension is substantially less than expected for age, intelligence, and education and that impairs academic achievement or daily living.[21] The International Dyslexia Association adopted the following definition in 2002: "Dyslexia is a specific learning disability that is neurological in origin. It is characterized by difficulties with accurate and/or fluent word recognition and by poor spelling and decoding abilities. These difficulties typically result from a deficit in the phonological component of language that is often unexpected in relation to other cognitive abilities and the provision of effective classroom instruction. Secondary consequences may include problems in reading comprehension and reduced reading experience that can impede the growth of vocabulary and background knowledge."[42]

Characteristics of dyslexia include the following[43,44]:

- Difficulty learning to recognize written words
- An inability to sound out the pronunciation of an unfamiliar word
- Seeing letters or words in reverse (*b* for *d* or *saw* for *was*)—although seeing words or letters in reverse is common for children younger than 8 who do not have dyslexia, children with dyslexia will continue to see reversals past that age
- Difficulty comprehending rapid instructions or following more than one command at a time
- Problems remembering the sequence of things, such as learning the order of the alphabet or spelling
- Difficulty distinguishing between similar sounds in words; mixing up sounds in multisyllable words (auditory discrimination) (e.g., *aminal* for *animal, bisghetti* for *spaghetti*)
- Slow or inaccurate reading, with difficulty reading out loud
- Difficulty rhyming

Dyslexia is the most common learning disorder, affecting as many as 80% of individuals identified as learning disabled.[45] Prevalence rates range from 10% to 15% of the school-aged population,[46] with the highest noted estimate of 17.4%.[47] Historically, dyslexia was considered more common in boys than in girls, but data indicate an equal distribution between the sexes.[48] Boys are more likely to act out as a result of having a reading difficulty and are therefore more likely to be identified early. Girls, on the other hand, are more likely to try to "hide" their difficulty, becoming quiet and reserved.[18]

Causes of dyslexia can be both genetic and neurobiological.[14,18,42] Genetic causation has been linked to chromosomes 1, 2, 3, 6, 11, 13, 15, and 18.[49] There is a strong inheritability of the genetic links for dyslexia. Statistics suggest that 30% to 50% of children with dyslexia have a parent with the disorder.[50] Neuroanatomical abnormalities, atypical brain symmetry, and disruptions in neural processing have been observed in children with reading disorders.[14,18,48,51] Anatomically, the measurements that best discriminate between children with and without dyslexia are the right anterior lobe of the cerebellum and the area involving the inferior frontal gyrus of both hemispheres.[18] Dynamic investigations using functional brain imagining techniques (PET, fMRI, and the newer ultrafast echo planar imaging [EPI]) are providing significant information on brain functioning during cognitive tasks such as reading and picture naming.[14,48]

Reading skills consist of a combination of visually perceiving whole words and phonetically decoding letters, morphemes, and words.[52] Individuals with reading disorders exhibit brain activation patterns that provide evidence of an imperfectly functioning system for segmenting words into phonological (language) parts and linking the visual representations of letters to the sounds they represent.[47] These disruptions of the posterior reading system result in increased reliance on ancillary systems during reading tasks, including the frontal lobe and right hemisphere posterior circuitry. This suggests that the child with dyslexia may be compensating for poor phonological skills with other perceptual processes, helping to explain why individuals with dyslexia can develop reading skills, although they often remain slow and nonautomatic.[48]

Dyscalculia (Mathematics Disorder). Dyscalculia is a learning impairment in which mathematical ability is substantially less than expected for age, intelligence, and education and that impairs academic achievement or daily living.[21] Difficulties occur with comprehending a variety of math concepts, including number quantities, money, time, and measurement. This disorder also involves difficulties with computations and problem solving of specific math functions, which affects the ability to understand, remember, or manipulate numbers or number facts.[18] This heterogeneous disorder may involve both intrinsic and extrinsic factors.[53] Intrinsic factors are hypothesized to include deficits in visual-spatial skill, quantitative reasoning, sequencing, memory, or intelligence. Extrinsic factors can be a combination of poor instruction in the mastery of prerequisite skills as well as attitude, interest, and confidence in the subject.

Characteristics of dyscalculia include the following[54]:

- Confusing numbers and math symbols (+, −, ×, ÷)
- Inconsistent ability in addition, subtraction, multiplication, and division
- Problems sequencing numbers, or transposing them when repeated
- Difficulty with abstract concepts of time and direction
- Poor mental math ability
- Difficulty with money, budgeting, balancing checkbooks, and financial thinking (e.g., checking change or estimating the cost of items in a shopping basket)
- Problem reading analog clocks
- Trouble keeping score during games and playing games with flexible rules of scoring such as poker

Prevalence of dyscalculia is 5% to 6% in the school-aged population, with a nearly equal male-to-female ratio.[14,55] Geary[56] concludes that individuals with arithmetic disabilities currently appear to constitute at least two subgroups: those with only mathematic disorders and those with concomitant reading disorders and/or attention-deficit disorder.

Although there is evidence that this disorder is familial and heritable, much less research on its cause is provided than on the causes of most other learning disorders. Dyscalculia shares genetic influences with reading and language measures. The association between dyslexia and dyscalculia seems to be largely genetically mediated.[14,55] Other risk factors for development of dyscalculia include prematurity and low birth weight. In addition, environmental deprivation, poor teaching, classroom diversity, and untested curricula have been linked to cause.[55]

The neurological cause of dyscalculia was initially hypothesized to be right hemisphere dysfunction because of the strong relation of visual-spatial skills to numerical computation.[57] Additional research supports the involvement of both hemispheres because mathematics computation involves a complex relation of spatial problem solving, sequential analysis, language processing, and memory.[55] Specifically involved are portions of the parietal and frontal lobes.[14] In an effort to compensate, individuals with dyscalculia can recruit alternate brain areas, but this substitution often results in inefficient cognitive functioning.[55]

Dysgraphia (Disorder of Written Expression). Dysgraphia is a learning impairment in which writing ability is substantially less than expected for age, intelligence, and education that impairs academic achievement or daily living.[21] The DSM, fourth edition (DSM-IV) diagnosis of "disorder of written expression" depends on recognition of "writing skills substantially below those expected given the person's chronological age, measured intelligence, and age appropriate education" that "significantly interferes with academic achievement or activities of daily living that require composition of written texts."[21] Children with dysgraphia have specific difficulties in the ability to write, regardless of the ability to read. This may include problems using words appropriately, putting thoughts into words, or mastering the mechanics of writing. Classifications of dysgraphia can include penmanship-related aspects of writing (e.g., motor control and execution), linguistic aspects of writing (e.g., spelling and composing), or a combination.[58] This heterogeneous disorder is frequently found in combination with other academic, learning, and attention disorders.[13,18]

Characteristics of dysgraphia include the following[59]:

- Poor legibility: irregular letter size and shapes, poor spacing
- Mixing uppercase and lowercase letters; unfinished letters
- Spelling difficulties
- Fatigues quickly or complains of pain when writing
- Decreased or increased speed of copying or writing
- Needs to say words out loud while writing
- Struggles with organizing thoughts on paper
- Difficulty writing grammatically correct sentences and organized paragraphs
- Large gap between knowledge base and ability to express ideas in writing
- Awkward pencil grip

Limited data are available on the prevalence of dysgraphia. Although 10% to 30% of school-aged children struggle with handwriting, we cannot assume they have been diagnosed with dysgraphia.[60] Difficulties in written expression are frequently underidentified and can be masked by reading disorders or considered to be attributable to poor motivation. Studies have suggested that dysgraphia may be as common as reading disorders and may occur in 3% to 4% of the population.[13,58]

Dysgraphia has been suggested to be a neurological processing disorder that seldom occurs in isolation and can result from a number of other dysfunctions, including attention deficit, auditory or visual processing weakness, and sequencing problems.[14,61] The complex nature of written expression makes finding the cause difficult. Writing involves integration of spatial and linguistic functions, planning, memory, and motor output. This suggests involvement of both the left and right hemispheres for skill in decoding, spelling, formulating and sequencing ideas, and producing work in correct spatial orientation, all coupled with rules of punctuation and capitalization.

Nonverbal Learning Disability

NVLDs (or NLDs) are considered by some to be a neuropsychological disability. Although this condition has been identified for more than 30 years, it has not yet been included as a diagnostic category in the DSM.[62] The pioneer in the field, Dr. Byron P. Rourke, first identified in 1985 this separate and distinct learning disability. In 1995 he defined nonverbal disability as "a dysfunction of the brain's right hemisphere—that part of the brain which processes nonverbal, performance-based information, including visual-spatial, intuitive, organizational and evaluative processing functions."[63] Nonverbal learning disorders affect both academic performance and social interactions in children. Three primary areas affected by NVLDs include visual-spatial organization, sensory-motor integration, and social-emotional development. The social and emotional difficulties for individuals with nonverbal learning disorders are paramount, leading some researchers to label this a *social-emotional learning disability*.[13,64] NVLDs are generally identified by a distinct pattern of strengths and deficits, with excellent verbal and rote memory skills and poorly developed sensory-motor and graphomotor ability, executive functioning, and social interactions.[13,65,66]

Characteristics of NVLDs include the following[14,62,67]:

- Higher verbal IQ compared with performance (nonverbal) on the Wechsler Intelligence Scale for Children (WISC)
- Develops speech, language, and reading skills early
- Strong vocabulary and spelling
- Ability to memorize and repeat a massive amount of information provided it is in spoken form
- Learns better and faster through hearing information rather than seeing it
- Difficulties with constructional and spatial planning tasks
- Fine and gross motor difficulties affecting printing and cursive writing, physical coordination, and balance

- May exhibit limited facial expression, flat affect, unchanging voice intonation, and robotic speech
- Poor interpretation of emotional responses made by others
- Trouble reading and understanding facial expressions, gestures, and voice intonations
- Nuances of spoken language, such as hidden meanings, figures of speech, jokes, and metaphors are interpreted on a concrete level
- Struggles with conversation skills, dealing with new situations, and changing performance in response to interactional cues
- Difficulties in problem solving and understanding cause-effect relationships
- Poor awareness of social space
- Can be intrusive and disruptive

NVLDs make up 5% to 10% of all individuals with learning disabilities.[68] NVLD is frequently overlooked in the educational arena because children with this disorder are highly verbal and develop an extensive vocabulary at a young age. Well-developed memory for rote verbal information positively influences early academic learning of reading and spelling. Yet these students will have difficulty performing in situations where adaptability and speed are necessary, and their written output will be slow and laborious.[65] Nonverbal learning disorders are therefore challenging to identify at younger ages but become progressively more apparent and debilitating by adolescence and adulthood. The challenges in early identification, the absence from the DSM-IV, and the different views held by psychological and educational disciplines often result in lack of awareness of, accurate diagnosis of, and appropriate service provision for these students.

Little is known about possible genetic or environmental causes of NVLD. There are no family, twin, adoption, segregation, or linkage studies available.[14] Pennington[14] proposes that both Turner syndrome and fragile X syndrome in females appear to be possible genetic causes of NVLD. Similarities include deficits in executive functions, increased difficulties in math versus reading and spelling, functional structural language but impaired pragmatic language, and social anxiety and shyness.[14] Differential diagnosis is essential because NVLD can occur in conjunction with dyscalculia, attention deficit, adjustment disorder, anxiety and depression, emotional disturbances, and obsessive-compulsive tendencies.

Motor Coordination Deficits

Children with learning disabilities may or may not manifest motor coordination problems. Conversely, some children have motor and coordination problems but do not experience learning difficulties. Children with motor deficits typically have difficulty acquiring age-appropriate motor skills and move in an awkward and clumsy manner. Difficulties in daily functional tasks and performance areas (e.g., school and leisure skills) are common. Motor deficits can result from a wide variety of neurological, physiological, developmental, and environmental factors. These impairments can manifest in diverse ways depending on the severity of the disorder and the areas of motor and social performance affected. This will be discussed at length in the next section.

Social and Emotional Challenges

Behavioral patterns or disorders associated with learning disabilities include frustration, anxiety, depression, attention deficits, conduct problems, and global behavior problems. Ames[69] stressed that no single behavior pattern is prevalent in children with learning disabilities. Children with learning disabilities not only struggle in the classroom, but experience difficulties in the social arena as well.[70] Issues in learning and related behaviors affect one another in a complex manner, leaving us to wonder which is the cause and which is the symptom.

Frustration, deflated self-esteem, and other social and emotional difficulties tend to emerge when instruction does not match learning styles.[71] This frustration mounts as the child notices classmates surpassing them, and this often results in exasperation with trying to keep up. The pressure then becomes for the child to "try harder," when ironically most do not understand just how hard the child is trying. The dissatisfaction in not meeting the teacher's expectations is often overshadowed by the inability to succeed in personal goals and a lack of self-worth. This can result in the development of internal perfectionism to deal with the lack of competence, with the belief of the child that he or she should not make mistakes.[72]

Anxiety is another response that may occur with persistent difficulties in understanding and successfully completing schoolwork. This occurs when the child feels out of control and lacks the ability to plan and execute strategies for success.[71] The mismatch between ability, expectations, and outcomes can cause frustration, disappointment, and stress, triggering a range of emotions and behaviors that interfere with everyday functioning in multiple environments.[71]

Other emotional difficulties are noted in attention. When a lesson is taught in a manner that is too complex, the child may become inattentive. Attention problems can influence behavior, often relating to difficulties with impulse control, restlessness, and irritability, affecting learning and peer interactions. These issues frequently coincide with frustration, anger, and resentment, which may manifest as a conduct problem (e.g., verbal and nonverbal aggression, destructiveness, and significant difficulties interacting with peers). Children with learning disabilities often become discouraged and fearful, are less motivated, and develop negative and defensive attitudes. These patterns of behavior can worsen with age, contributing to juvenile deliquency.[3] Low self-esteem and depression are common during school years and tend to escalate around age 10 years.[73]

Poor academic progress, additional prompting needed from teachers, and negative attention for disruptive behaviors can cause children with learning disabilities to perceive themselves as being "different."[74] Lack of success in school experiences can influence the development of positive self-perception and can have powerfully negative effects on self-esteem.[71] A self-defeating cycle may be established: the child experiences learning problems, school and home environments become increasingly tense, and disruptive behaviors become more pronounced. These responses, in turn, further affect the child's ability to learn. Lack of success generates more failure until the child anticipates defeat in almost every situation.

Assessment and Intervention

Specialists

Evaluation and intervention for children with learning disabilities should involve an interdisciplinary team owing to the varied nature of presenting problems. Most children with learning disabilities are seen by a group of professionals, the makeup of which depends on the purpose, location, philosophical orientation, or availability of resources of a particular program. Box 14-1 lists the different professionals and specialists who might participate in assessment or remediation of children with learning disabilities. The types of professionals are grouped into the four categories of education, medicine and nursing, psychology, and special services; they have been listed only once, although some professions could be categorized in multiple ways.

Therapists should be familiar with the roles of the various medical specialists and of primary care physicians. Psychologists have two distinct and often separate roles in the care of children with learning disorders. The first role is in identification of learning strengths and weaknesses. Psychological testing is often essential in the recognition of specific learning problems and may be done by clinical psychologists, school psychologists, or clinical neuropsychologists who specialize in diagnosis of learning disorders. The second role of psychologists is to provide mental health services and support systems to address academic, social-emotional, and behavioral issues. Counseling and behavior management can also be provided by a psychiatrist, behavioral specialist, or social worker. School adjustment or guidance counselors offer support and advice on specific academic difficulties, social conflicts, and affective issues.

Physical educators, adaptive physical educators, physical therapists (PTs), occupational therapists (OTs), and speech therapists also may be involved in the assessment of motor deficits and related areas. Overlap in the areas assessed may occur. The unique training of each professional influences both the selection of tests and the qualitative aspects of assessment on the basis of observations of a child's performance. Although the evaluations may appear similar, differences among professions are apparent in orientation and rationale when interpreting dysfunction.

Planning an assessment protocol can prevent unnecessary duplication of testing and provide comprehensive information related to the referral concerns. The assessment is driven by the referral concerns and the functional difficulties the child is experiencing. Communication of information between professionals and the parents will generate a comprehensive picture of the child's areas of strength and weakness, necessary for effective intervention planning.

Coordinating Multiple Interventions

As the number of disciplines involved in the assessment and therapeutic management of children with learning disabilities has steadily increased, communication for effective programming has become more challenging. Despite the benefits of specific skills brought to the case by each professional, the huge variety of well-meaning recommendations can result in service delivery overkill. Case Study 14-1 provides an example of the negative impact of overabundant specialized intervention on the child and family. In this case, if all the interventionists had communicated, a more realistic and effective plan could have been developed.

BOX 14-1 ■ TYPES OF SPECIALISTS WORKING WITH CHILDREN WITH LEARNING DISABILITIES

EDUCATION
- Classroom teacher
- Special educator
- Guidance counselor
- Learning disability specialist
- Educational diagnostician
- Reading specialist
- Physical educator
- Adaptive physical educator

MEDICINE AND NURSING
- Family physician
- Pediatrician
- Pediatric neurologist
- Psychiatrist
- School nurse
- Biochemist
- Geneticist
- Endocrinologist
- Nutritionist
- Ophthalmologist or optometrist
- Otologist or ear, nose, and throat (ENT) specialist

PSYCHOLOGY
- Clinical psychologist
- Neuropsychologist
- School psychologist
- Child psychologist

SPECIAL SERVICES
- Occupational therapist
- Physical therapist
- Speech and language pathologist
- Audiologist
- Vision specialist
- Social worker
- Recreational therapist
- Music therapist
- Vocational education specialist

CASE STUDY 14-1 ■ MATT

Matt is an 8-year-old boy who was referred for clinic-based physical therapy intervention for 1 hour per week for remediation of severe motor coordination and planning problems that accompanied his learning disability. In addition to Matt's weekly treatment sessions, suggestions were made to his mother for a home program to be accomplished three times a week for 15 to 30 minutes each time. Meanwhile, Matt also received other services. Although he was mainstreamed into a regular classroom in accordance with the special education law, he was seen by the resource teacher on a daily basis and by the adaptive physical education teacher twice a week to meet his specialized needs. The classroom teacher told Matt's mother that Matt must read at least one book a night because he needed additional reading practice. A reading tutor came to Matt's house on Saturday mornings. Ocular motor problems were identified, so he was evaluated by an optometrist, who recommended weekly visits plus ocular exercises for 30 minutes a day. Matt developed secondary emotional problems, partly because he was bright yet aware of his learning disability and frustrated by it. Thus Matt also saw a psychotherapist on a weekly basis. The psychotherapist recommended participation in weekly group sessions, in addition to Matt's individual sessions, to help improve peer relationships. Thus Matt's therapists had developed a 12-hour-a-day program for him and his family. It was no wonder that Matt had difficulty in developing peer relationships; he never had time. Matt's schedule also affected interaction in his own family. His mother believed that being a "therapist" to Matt interfered with her role as his mother. She felt unable to carry out the home program and felt guilty for not doing it.

What became apparent with Matt's case was that although each professional involved with him made an important contribution to evaluation and intervention, the massive input, to some extent, had a detrimental effect on Matt and his family. Coordinating interventions and providing additional support at home can create a drain on the family and limit time for family activities and extracurricular participation.

Effective coordination of intervention services presents a dilemma because no single discipline is specifically trained for that role.[75] Kenny and Burka[75] stress the need for a person to act as a coordinator for the management and integration of the interventions received by the child. Unfortunately, this role does not exist; therefore the parent must assume this responsibility.

School-Based Service Delivery Models

The model of service delivery for each individual child should be developed to facilitate the student's ability to be successful in the learning environment. A continuum of services exists to enable interventionists to be responsive to all children's needs. The continuum includes consultation, integrated or supervised therapy, and direct service.[76] Unfortunately, a lack of available resources can influence what type and frequency of services are provided. In creating a plan that truly addresses the issues hindering a child's learning within the academic setting, the team must work together to fabricate relevant and inclusive goals.

IDEA currently requires that all children in special education be educated in the least restrictive environment. The law requires that students with disabilities be educated to the extent appropriate with their peers, within the inclusion classroom. Removing the child from the classroom for special education and intervention is discouraged unless it is absolutely necessary for the student to learn effectively. Although the model of inclusion can be effective for many children, it requires members of the team to work closely together with the regular education teacher. This collaborative effort ensures an understanding of the child's special learning needs and incorporation of therapeutic procedures into the regular classroom to facilitate the best learning environment.

Bricker[77] contends that adhering strictly to this model can be detrimental to certain students, and each case must be looked at individually. The least restrictive environment should be determined after assessing the specific needs of the child. If services in a regular classroom, coupled with supplemental aids and services, do not meet the needs of the child, an alternate environment should be considered. The first adaptation might be to have the child participate for the majority of the day in the regular classroom and leave for special instruction for part of the day. In some educational settings, children with learning disabilities are given full-time instruction in a special classroom with a small group of other children with learning disabilities. A special education teacher or a learning disability specialist is in charge of the classroom. The most specialized environment would be a private school only for children with learning disabilities.

LEARNING DISABILITIES AND MOTOR DEFICITS OR DEVELOPMENTAL COORDINATION DISORDER

Approximately half of children with learning disabilities have motor coordination problems.[78] Motor deficits are often the most overt sign of difficulty for the child with learning disabilities. Lowered academic achievement within any or all areas of learning (reading, spelling, writing) is also seen in children with developmental coordination disorder (DCD).[8,21] A study by Jongmans and colleagues[78] indicates that children with concomitant perceptual-motor and learning problems are more severely affected in motor difficulties than those with only DCD or who are only learning disabled. At times, extreme discrepancy in competence over a range of motor skills exists, with strengths in some motor areas and significant weaknesses in others. Presentation of difficulties may change over time depending on developmental maturation, environmental demands, and interventions received.

An International Consensus Meeting on Children and Clumsiness was held in 1994 with expert educators, kinesiologists, OTs, PTs, psychologists, and parents. These experts discussed a common name to identify "clumsy" children with movement, coordination, and motor planning difficulties. The term *developmental coordination disorder* (DCD), as first described in DSM-III,[21] was identified to distinguish these children from those with severe motor impairments (such as those with cerebral palsy or paraplegia) and children with normal motor movements. A child with DCD often exhibits difficulty with motoric academic tasks such as handwriting and gym class, self-care skills such as dressing and using utensils, and leisure activities including playground games and social interactions.[79]

Definition

As described in the DSM-IV-TR[21] as one of the motor skill disorders, DCD has the following criteria:

- A marked impairment in the development of motor coordination (criterion A)
- An impairment that significantly interferes with academic achievement or activities of daily living (criterion B)
- The presence of coordination difficulties that are not the result of a general medical condition (e.g., cerebral palsy, hemiplegia, or muscular dystrophy); the criteria for pervasive developmental disorder are not met (criterion C)
- If mental retardation is present, the motor difficulties are in excess of those usually associated with it (criterion D)

Clinical Presentation

DCD is a childhood disorder characterized by poor coordination and clumsiness. Typically, there is no easily identifiable neurological disorder accompanying this lack of motor skills required for everyday life.[80] Characteristics can be seen in developmental areas such as gross motor, fine motor, visual motor, self-care, and social-emotional areas. Children tend to develop at a slower rate and require more effort and practice to accomplish age-level tasks. The salient features are coordination difficulties that include decreased anticipation, speed, reaction time, and quality and grading of movement.[81,82] These children often have difficulties analyzing the task demands of an activity, interpreting cues from the environment, using knowledge of past performance, and transferring and generalizing skills.[83]

Coordination difficulties are most apparent when complex motor activities are attempted. Physical education class often presents major problems. For example, a 9-year-old boy described his motor problems as follows: "When the gym teacher tells us to do something, I understand exactly what he means. I even know how to do it, I think. But my body never seems to do the job."[84] Case Study 14-2 describes the motor difficulties frequently encountered in children with DCD.

CASE STUDY 14-2 ■ PAUL

The following is a mother's description of her child, Paul, who had motor coordination problems and learning disabilities: "I think when Paul was first born I tried to ignore the problem. Paul is a child who never climbed or ran or drew pictures the way other kids did. But until he went to nursery school, I didn't pay much attention to it. Maybe I didn't want to pay attention to it. Maybe I knew it was there and I didn't want to know about it. I'm not sure. But Paul was always a verbal child and a creative and imaginative child. He and I had something special because I used to enjoy that kind of creative imaginative play. We used to have our own world of various fantasies, heroes, and places.

"Paul sat up at about 7 months; he crawled and crept on time. He didn't learn to walk until he was about 15 months old. He walked cautiously, holding on and not letting go. He walked late, but he talked early. He said his first clear word, "cat," at 6 months. He knew what a cat was and could relate to it. My husband and I were so enthusiastic about his sounds. In those days they said that if you stimulated your child and talked to him and got him ready to talk, he could read early. I was concerned that Paul would be able to talk and have a marvelous vocabulary and read because I had a reading disability and a spelling disability.

"When Paul was 4 years old and in nursery school, at my first conference the teacher said, 'Look out the window, Mrs. B.—see Paul sitting at the bottom? All the other kids are climbing on top of the jungle gym.' And then she showed me some art work. Paul couldn't cut, he couldn't paste, he couldn't do any of it. We could definitely, at the age of 3 or 4, see his problems. He was bright, but he couldn't cut, paste, or draw, he couldn't climb, and he really didn't know how to run. That was where his handicaps were first being noticed, more by other teachers and professionals than by my husband and myself.

"When we had to make the decision as to whether to put Paul into kindergarten or hold him back, we were frustrated because Paul was very bright and very alert. He has always known everything that was going on in the world.

"Now, the kids Paul knows and the kids who know Paul know that he can't do motor tasks and they'll come over and play rocket ships with him. But there will come a time, as the kids are getting older, that they won't want to do this."

Paul's mother, who also had learning and motor difficulties, described her own disability as follows:

"The hardest course for me was gym. I was unfortunate enough to have the same gym teacher throughout high school. The teacher always used to think I was a lazy kid, that I just never wanted to try to do the exercises. Although I tried, I couldn't do the stunts and tumbling for anything. The other girls would do a somersault and I would still do it like a 4-year-old. I'd just about get over.

"I took dance a couple of times. I never could figure out as a kid why I couldn't point my toes. The teacher would say, 'Point your toes,' and it never made any sense to me. I always curled my toes up. Only when somebody sat down with me and actually showed me did I know that that was how you were supposed to point your toes. With other kids, they just did what the teacher did. Nobody had to stop and tell them. I was the klutzy kid. I never could do the nice leaps across the floor. But I would try. After two or three sessions my mother stopped giving me lessons. She was probably embarrassed.

CASE STUDY 14-2 ■ PAUL—cont'd

"As a girl, it wasn't as traumatic not being athletic. As I got older, the need for a woman to be athletic tended to decrease, whereas for a boy, the need to be athletic and competitive tends to increase. I foresee this as one of the major problems for Paul.

"Most of my life my friendships have always relied on other people. I met most of my friends through other friends because I've gone along to things. I think it goes back to being teased as a child about the things I couldn't do or the way I looked. If you looked at me, I probably looked like a lot of the learning-disabled kids that you see: my clothes were not put together properly, my shoelaces were untied, and my hair was never quite combed properly.

"It was very difficult for me to learn how to put on makeup and use a hairdryer. It would take many hours of trying to learn. For a long time, my fingernails were cut very short because I didn't know how to file them. It is still very hard for me to put on eye makeup and look in the mirror and try to figure it out. I still don't feel as though I am completely put together. And I put a lot of effort and energy into looking good."

Development of gross and fine motor skills, coupled with the child's ability to master body movements, enhances feelings of self-esteem and confidence. Through persistence in mastering the varied challenges of motor exploration the child builds self-reliance. The frustrations and accomplishments enhance confidence and the ability to take risks. By engaging in group activities children develop essential social skills, including how to compromise, work as a team, and deal with conflicts and different personality styles.

Poor motor coordination often results in significant social and emotional consequences. When a child is poorly coordinated she or he is often teased and shunned from group play. This may lead to anxiety and avoidance of participation in games, as children frequently judge themselves to be both physically and socially less competent.[85] Anxiety may be more prevalent in adolescence, most notably in boys.[86] Because they are often unsuccessful in group participation, difficulties with navigating the changing demands of cooperative play and negotiating with others and reluctance to advocate for themselves often result. Boys with learning and motor coordination problems have been found to demonstrate significantly less effective coping strategies in all domains of functioning compared with a normative sample.[87] Feelings of incompetence, depression, or frustration are common and can be lifelong problems.[88,89] The impact of motor coordination difficulties on social behavior is exemplified by this statement from a child with learning disabilities and motor deficits:

> "They always pick me last. This morning they were all fighting over which team had to have me. One guy was shouting about it. He said it wasn't fair because his team had me twice last week. Another kid said they would only take me if his team could be spotted four runs. Later, on the bus, they were all making fun of me, calling me a "fag" and a "spaz." There are a few good kids, I mean kids who aren't mean, but they don't want to play with me. I guess it could hurt their reputation."[84]

Gross motor characteristics of DCD include the following:

- Diminished core strength and postural control
- Delayed balance reactions
- Often falling, tripping, and bumping into things; acquiring more than the usual number of bruises
- Motor movements that are performed at a slower rate despite practice and repetition[82]
- Motor milestones that may be achieved in the later range of normal development
- Poor anticipation (do not use knowledge of past performance to prepare)
- Notably different quality of running and ball skills from typical peers
- Difficulty learning bilateral tasks such as riding a bicycle, catching a ball, and jumping rope
- Possible hesitance with and avoidance of new or complex motor tasks (e.g., playground equipment, gym class)
- Possibly poor safety awareness
- Inability to smoothly turn and position body when going up ladder to a slide or to get into a chair
- Possible sedentary activity level; may prefer to engage in solitary play
- Tendency to not play games by the rules
- Often, avoidance of team sports such as T-ball and soccer

Fine motor characteristics of DCD include the following:

- Diminished wrist and hand strength
- Maladaptive or immature grasp patterns
- Possible use of excess or not enough pressure
- Poor refinement of small motor movements with hands (qualitatively, the child looks like he or she is wearing a pair of gloves when trying to manipulate small objects)
- Often dropping or breaking of items
- Delayed dressing skills (buttons, zippers, fasteners, shoelaces)
- Trouble with eating utensils (scooping, piercing)
- Difficulty with tool use (e.g., scissors, pencils, stapler, hole punches)
- Writing that is laborious and often illegible
- Impaired drawing ability characterized by poor motor control, with wobbly lines, inaccurate junctures, and difficulty coloring within the lines.
- Decreased ability with pasting, gluing, manipulating stickers and other art materials
- Difficulty with constructive, manipulative play (e.g., block building, Tinkertoys, Legos)
- Often the presence of associated articulation deficits, possibly because of the fine motor nature demanded for articulation

Visual motor characteristics of DCD include the following:

- Difficulty with visually guided motor actions (i.e., eye-hand and eye-foot coordination)
- Hesitancy or decreased safety on stairs

- Trouble with timing needed for kicking, hitting, and catching ball
- Difficulty with hopscotch and four squares
- Poor judgment of spatial relationships (knowing where the body is in space)
- Delayed development of prepositional and directional concepts
- Difficulty with spatial planning tasks such as puzzles, building models, and constructional toys
- Handwriting that is often labored, with spacing and sizing problems evident; letters may be irregular, illegible, and poorly organized on the page

Self-care characteristics of DCD include the following:

- Slowness to develop independence in activities of daily living
- Overreliance on parents to help with self-care skills
- Clothes that are often on backward or crooked
- Struggles with cutting fingernails, putting on makeup, tying necktie, using a hair dryer
- Difficulty blowing nose with tissue, putting on Band-Aid
- Trouble putting toothpaste on toothbrush
- Messy eater, spills often, does not recognize food on face
- Difficulty pouring from a container, opening lunch box, unwrapping sandwich, opening containers, peeling fruit
- Trouble packing a bag, backpack, or suitcase
- Difficulty sequencing daily routines

Social and emotional characteristics of DCD include the following:

- Often emotionally immature
- May exhibit behavioral difficulties such as acting out or becoming class clown
- May be more introverted and anxious
- Can appear fiercely competitive, hating to lose, complaining that rules are unfair
- Can be self-deprecating, calls self "stupid"
- Often easily frustrated
- May experience depression and feelings of incompetence
- Has difficulty making and maintaining friendships, plays alone
- Has feelings of low self-worth, poor self-esteem[90]
- Perceived by others as lazy, overprotected, or immature[91]
- Adolescents may have fewer social pasttimes and hobbies than peers

Prevalence

Estimating the prevalence of children with DCD is challenging. Great variety exists in the clinical presentation, with some children exhibiting motor deficits in all areas and others having only isolated concerns. Among professionals there is a lack of clarity on the definition and diagnostic criteria.[91] Overlap of symptoms associated with other conditions such as attention-deficit/hyperactivity disorder (ADHD), autism spectrum disorders, perceptual-motor problems, and speech and language impairments further complicates differential diagnosis.[14,80,92] In addition, there is no single test or screening measure that can be used to confidently identify the problem.[93] Other factors influencing prevalence rates include the criteria used to delineate a child with DCD from a typical peer, differences in terminology, types and methods of testing, reliability of the tests used, and heterogeneity of the test sample.[79,93,94]

An estimated 5% to 10% of children aged 5 to 11 years had DCD.[21] Boys diagnosed with DCD outnumber girls by two to one. This difference may reflect higher referral rates for boys as a result of increased behavioral difficulties of boys with motor incoordination.[95]

Perspectives on the Causes of Developmental Coordination Disorder

There is no single explanation for the cause of DCD. Neurological dysfunction, physiological factors, genetic predisposition, and prenatal and perinatal birth factors have been proposed to explain the basis of DCD.[91,96] It is recognized that DCD is heritable and is genetically distinct from ADHD, although the comorbidity rate is up to 50%.[14] Comorbidity is high with other diagnoses, including autism spectrum disorders,[80] as well as a variety of developmental learning problems such as math disability, reading disability, specific language disabilities, spelling and writing disabilities, and so on. Correlation has also been noted between preterm infancy and low birth weight with characteristics of DCD. The heterogeneity of DCD makes finding a unitary cause difficult. Children with DCD present wide variability in both locus of specific problems and functional disabilities. Further complicating an understanding of the cause is that the intervention for the child with DCD is driven by competing treatments.[97]

Few studies have been conducted to look at brain images in children with DCD, with no particular patterns of abnormality observed.[91] Hadders-Algra[98] has suggested that DCD is a result of damage at the cellular level in the neurotransmitter and receptor systems, rather than a specific region of the brain. Resulting coordination difficulties can be from a combination of one or more impairments in proprioception, motor programming, timing, or sequencing of muscle activity.

Possible physiological origins of motor coordination deficits have highlighted multisensory processing. Ayres,[99] in her theory of sensory integration, suggested that the integration among sensory systems is imperative for refined motor performance in children. She proposed that normal development depends on intrasensory integration, particularly from the somatosensory and vestibular systems. Lane[100] outlines the role of vision, combined with vestibular and proprioceptive inputs, as a foundation to motor performance. In combination, these systems sustain postural tone and equilibrium, provide awareness and coordination of head movements, and stabilize the eyes during movement in space.

More recently, Piek and Dyck[101] found support for the correlations between DCD and deficits in kinesthetic perception, visual-spatial processing, and multisensory integration.[101] In general, it is thought that reduced rates of processing information and deficits in handling spatial information may underlie the deficits in motor control.[80] Obviously more work is needed on the cause of DCD.

Subtypes of Developmental Coordination Disorder

Various approaches have been used to investigate subtypes of DCD, including classification by underlying causes, clinical and descriptive approaches, and statistical clustering.[94] Initial attempts at classifying subtypes within DCD support the heterogeneity of this group of children.[102] Work by

Dewey and Kaplan[103] suggests that children with DCD may be classified into subgroups based on distinctions in motor planning and motor execution deficits. They identified three subgroups: children who exhibited deficits in motor execution alone, those whose primary deficits were in motor planning, and children who exhibited a generalized impairment in both areas.

Macnab, Miller, and Polatajko[104] identified five different profiles of children with DCD. They used measures of kinesthetic acuity, gross motor skill, static balance, visual perception, and visual motor integration. Two distinct groups emerged, with children exhibiting generalized visual deficits and generalized dysfunction in all areas. Generalized gross motor deficits did not emerge as a distinct subgroup, as the third group demonstrated a discrepancy between static balance and complex gross motor tasks, and the fourth group had poor performance on running but performed well on kinesthetic acuity. Other groups included children with deficits in visual motor and fine motor problems. These results suggest that a subtype based on motor execution or planning problems alone may be too general.

Assessment of Motor Impairments

A variety of professionals may be involved in a comprehensive assessment of motor deficits. Pediatric OTs and PTs are often the core team assessing functional motor concerns. Areas assessed by pediatric OTs and PTs often overlap, so communication is essential to ensure that testing is not replicated. Ideally, performance will be evaluated in multiple environments and include components of skill, functional performance areas, and social and societal participation. Specific recommendations should include activities to enhance performance in the environments in which the child functions on a daily basis.

Clinical judgment of the therapist is important in designing an assessment protocol and synthesizing information to create a complete profile of the child. A variety of standardized and nonstandardized evaluation tools should accompany structured clinical observations and caretaker interviews. Observations of the child can yield more readily usable information than a standardized score,[105] enabling the therapist to view the child in natural routines, self-directed activities, and unstructured play. The interview process is essential to gather information about the child's interactions and participation. This process paints a verbal picture of the child to help us to understand levels of functioning and participation in a variety of environments. Other crucial information obtained is how the child's difficulties are affecting the ability to parent or teach the student.[105]

Before choosing an evaluation tool the therapist should be aware of the intended purpose of this measure. Tools used to assess children with DCD are used for distinct purposes: identify impairments, describe severity of impairments, or explore activity or participation limitations.[83] The choice of evaluations may also be determined by the setting, frame of reference of the therapist, and functional concerns of the child. A therapist should be familiar with all aspects of test administration and scoring for evaluation tools and should comply with the training requirements described in the test manual. Test construction, reliability, and validity for assessing DCD should be considered. Appendix 14-A provides an overview of standardized tests available for the assessment of motor dysfunction in children with learning disabilities. Uses and limitations of the individual tests and test batteries are listed.

Identification of subtle motor difficulties is critical and challenging. These subtle motor difficulties initially can be undetected, leading to unrealistic expectations of age-level motor performance. The child's difficulty with skilled, purposeful manipulative tasks or with finely tuned balance activities may not be readily apparent in the classroom or may be perceived as lack of effort. Children with DCD may be able to perform certain motor tasks with a level of strength, flexibility, and coordination that is qualitatively average but must use increased effort and cognitive control for sustained success.

Levels of performance in gross and fine motor testing may fall in the borderline range. Careful observations are of paramount importance, because the child's deficits are often qualitative rather than quantitative. A child might have age-appropriate balance on testing but lack ability in weight shifting and making quick directional changes, which affects the ability to participate in extracurricular activities such as soccer or baseball. When assessing children with subtle motor deficits, it is important to realize that many evaluation tools have been developed for children with moderate to severe neurological impairments.

Children with DCD do not exhibit obvious evidence of neuropathological disease (i.e., "hard" neurological signs such as a cerebral lesion). Subtle abnormalities of the central nervous system are frequently noted by the presence of "soft" neurological signs. Deficits associated with soft neurological signs include abnormal movements and reflexes, sensory deficits, and coordination difficulties. Evaluation of soft neurological signs is typically part of an examination by a pediatric neurologist, although therapists can assess these areas in conjunction with standardized testing. Box 14-2 lists soft neurological signs frequently used to assess this population.

Researchers suggest that a high percentage of children with learning disabilities exhibit certain soft neurological signs. An early study reported that 75% of 2300 children with positive total "neurological soft sign" ratings had the symptom of poor coordination.[106] More recently, 169 children aged 8 to 13 years were assessed for a relation between soft neurological signs and cognitive functioning, motor skills, and behavior. Those children with a high index for soft neurological signs were found to have significantly worse scores in each domain.[107] The relationship between neurological soft signs and DCD is difficult to validate without more current systematic research; however, they are indicators that intervention may be needed.[108]

In general, a composite of soft neurological signs is more predictive of dysfunction than single signs. Children without notable motor difficulties can frequently exhibit one or more soft signs; therefore identification of a single sign must be interpreted cautiously. Neurological signs involving complex processes were found to be the most predictive. The clinician needs to be familiar with typical developmental patterns, as certain soft neurological signs such as motor overflow, right-left confusion, visual tracking difficulties, and articulatory substitution are expected at younger ages and mature in quality over time.

BOX 14-2 ■ COMMON SOFT NEUROLOGICAL SIGNS USED IN ASSESSMENT OF CHILDREN WITH LEARNING DISABILITIES AND MOTOR DEFICITS

MINOR NEUROLOGICAL INDICATORS
Left-right discrimination
Finger agnosia
Visual tracking
Extinction of simultaneous stimuli
Choreiform movement
Tremor
Exaggerated associated movements
Reflex asymmetries

COORDINATION
Finger-to-nose touching
Sequential thumb-finger touching
Diadochokinesia
Heel to shin
Slow controlled motions
Postural-motor measures
Muscle tone
Schilder's arm extension posture
Standing with eyes closed (Romberg test)
Walking a line
Tandem walking (forward and backward)
Hopping, jumping, skipping
Ball throw and catch
Imitation of tongue movements
Pencil and paper tasks
Fine motor tasks (stringing beads, building block towers)

SENSORY INDICATORS
Graphesthesia
Stereognosis
Localization of touch input

Assessment measures of soft neurological signs vary considerably for children with learning disabilities, both in what signs are included in the assessment and how they are grouped. This list represents a compilation of possible soft neurological signs.

Compiling a complete picture of motor deficits in children with learning disabilities involves assessing the following complex skills: (1) postural control and gross motor performance, (2) fine motor and visual motor performance, (3) sensory integration and sensory processing, (4) praxis and motor planning, and (5) physical fitness. Each of these interrelated functions is described in this chapter as an area of clinical assessment.

Postural Control and Gross Motor Performance

Muscle Tone and Strength. Low muscle tone and poor joint stability have been identified as characteristic of some children with learning disabilities. On observation, the child with low tone may look "floppy" and may have an open-mouth posture, lordotic back, sagging belly, and knees positioned closely together. Muscles may be poorly defined and feel "mushy" or soft on palpation, and joints may be hyperextensible. A common method for assessing muscle tone and proximal joint stability involves placing the child in a quadruped position and observing the ability to maintain the position without locking of the elbows, winging of the scapula, or sagging (lordosis) of the trunk. The therapist can determine joint stability by asking the child to "freeze like a statue." The therapist then provides intermittent pushes to the trunk, assessing the child's ability to remain in a static position.

Children with low tone may develop patterns of compensation called *fixing patterns.* These patterns often include elevated and internally rotated shoulders, internally rotated hips, and pronated feet. The child compensates for low tone by using the stable joint positions and holding himself or herself stiffly for increased stability. These patterns may resemble those of children with slightly increased tone. Careful observation and palpation of muscles will help to differentiate fixing patterns from increased muscle tone. Judgments of muscle tone are primarily made through clinical observations and felt in a hands-on assessment.

Manual muscle testing can provide detailed information about impairment in strength of individual muscles but is not regularly used in assessing children with learning disabilities, unless concerns of a possible degenerative disease exist. More appropriately, strength should be assessed by the child's functional ability to move against gravity during activities. Within developmental assessments, the therapist is observing range of motion against gravity in skills such as reaching, climbing, throwing, and kicking. The therapist also can have the child hold positions against gravity to assess strength and endurance (e.g., prone extension and supine flexion).

Early Postural Reflexes. Early reflexes are essential for the development of normal patterns of motor development. These reflexes facilitate movement patterns that become integrated into purposeful motions. If they are not fully integrated, qualitative differences in muscle tone, postural asymmetries, transitional movement patterns, bilateral coordination, and smooth timing and sequencing of motor tasks may be observed. Residual reactions (e.g., asymmetrical tonic neck reflex [ATNR] and symmetrical tonic neck reflex [STNR]) that might be noted in children with DCD are generally subtle and most often are seen in stressful, nonautomatic tasks. McPhillips and Sheehy looked at incidence of primitive reflex patterns and motor coordination difficulties in children with reading disorders.[109] The group with the lowest reading scores had a significantly higher rate of ATNR and motor impairments when compared with good readers. Assessment for persistence of primitive reflex patterns in children with learning disabilities should emphasize impact on functional aspects of performance.

The effect of lack of integration can be observed during tasks such as writing at a table or gross motor activities such as using ball skills and jumping rope. Persistence of these primitive reflexes may be seen in the child's inability to sit straight forward at the table. The ATNR influence might be observed by a sideways position at the table with the arm on the face side used in extension. During ball games the child may have diminished ability to throw with directional control because head movements will influence extension of the face-side arm. If the STNR is not fully integrated the child is often unable to flex the legs while sitting at a desk looking down at his or her work (neck flexion). Although residual reflex involvement may affect performance of these tasks, many other components are involved that require consideration.

Righting, Equilibrium, and Balance. Righting and equilibrium are dynamic reactions essential for the development of upright posture and smooth transitional movements. Righting reactions help maintain the head in an upright alignment during movement in all directions. Equilibrium reactions occur in response to a change in body position or surface support to maintain body alignment. In simpler terms, equilibrium reactions get us into a position, and righting reactions keep us in that position. Together these reactions provide continuous automatic adjustments that maintain the center of gravity over the base of support and keep the head in an upright position.

Righting and equilibrium reactions are best assessed on an unsteady surface such as a tilt board or large therapy ball. These reactions occur in all developmental positions, and complete assessment will consider a range of positions during functional performance in gross and fine motor activities. To test equilibrium, the child's center of gravity is quickly tipped off balance. The equilibrium response is one of phasic extension and abduction of the downhill limbs for protection and of flexion of the uphill body side for realignment. In daily actions, most of the righting reactions are subtle and occur continuously to relatively small changes in body position. Subtle shifts of the support surface can be made to assess the child's ability to maintain the head and trunk in a continuous upright position. Righting and equilibrium reactions are the basis for functional balance and postural control.

To balance effectively, we use visual information (about the body and external environment), proprioceptive information (about limb and body position), and vestibular information (about head position and movement), in order to initiate an appropriate corrective response.[110] Balance reactions occur as a response to changes in the center of gravity that stimulate the vestibular receptors (utricles and semicircular canals). This stimulation causes muscles to activate, allowing balance to be maintained in static and dynamic activities (e.g., sitting in a chair, walking, standing on a bus). When the vestibular system works in conjunction with vision and information from the muscles (proprioception), balance is easier and more refined. Considering the impact of these sensory systems working together is important during assessment. The therapist should test the child's balance with the child's eyes open and closed and observe differences in ease and quality of performance. Standing with eyes closed relies more on vestibular and proprioceptive input, and difficulty may indicate that the child depends heavily on the visual system for balance. To further assess this sensory interaction, balance should also be observed on steady and unsteady surfaces (e.g., dense foam or a tilt board) with and without visual orientation. Traditional tests of balance include (1) the Romberg position—standing with feet together and eyes closed, (2) Mann position—standing with feet in tandem with eyes closed, and (3) standing on one leg with eyes open and eyes closed. The Bruininks-Oseretsky Test of Motor Proficiency, second edition (BOT-2)[111] and the Sensory Integration and Praxis Tests[112] have comprehensive balance subtests (see Appendix 14-A).

Postural Control. Postural control is dependent on muscle tone, strength, and endurance of the trunk musculature, as well as automatic postural reactions required to maintain a dynamic upright position. A child has adequate postural control when he or she can maintain upright positions, shift weight in all directions, rotate, and move smoothly between positions. These areas are often deficient in children with DCD, affecting both gross and fine motor performance.

The child may fatigue quickly and fall often during gross motor play. Other body parts may be used for additional support because of weak postural musculature—for example, placing the head on the ground when crawling up an incline or sticking out the tongue when climbing or pumping a swing. In sitting, a child with diminished postural control will fatigue quickly, either leaning on his or her hands for additional support or moving frequently in and out of the chair. These compensations affect the child's ability to perform fine motor tasks or maintain attention for cognitive learning because so much effort is exerted on sitting up. Observing the effects of fatigue is important because both sitting and standing postures may deteriorate over the course of a day. Generally the problem stems from motor programming problems versus muscle power.

Gross Motor Skills. *Gross motor coordination* refers to motor behaviors related to posture and locomotion, from early developmental milestones to finely tuned balance. Children with learning disabilities and DCD may attain reasonably high degrees of motor skill in specific activities. Motor accomplishments frequently remain highly specific to particular motor sequences or tasks and do not necessarily generalize to other activities, regardless of their similarities. When variation in the motor response is required, the response often becomes inaccurate and disorganized.

Although children with DCD can sit, stand, and walk with apparent ease, they may be awkward or slow in rolling, transitioning to standing, running, hopping, and climbing. Skilled tasks such as skipping may be accomplished with increased effort, decreased sequencing and endurance, and associated movements.

Evaluation of gross motor skills should include both novel motor activities and age-appropriate skills. The child, for example, can be asked to imitate a hopping sequence or maneuver around a variety of obstacles. Skills that have been accomplished can be varied slightly (e.g., hopping over a small box). Age-appropriate social participation tasks, such as tag and dodge ball, can be observed for qualitative difficulties in timing and spatial body awareness. Developmentally earlier skills also should be observed to assess the quality of performance. BOT-2[111] and the Peabody Developmental Motor Scales[113] are examples of tools for standardized assessment of gross motor skills (see Appendix 14-A).

Fine Motor and Visual Motor Performance

Fine Motor Skills. Fine motor coordination involves motor behavior such as discrete finger movements, manipulation, and eye-hand coordination. A child with DCD often demonstrates multiple fine motor concerns. Areas of difficulty typically include grasp and manipulation of small objects and dexterous hand skills, such as buttoning or putting coins into a vending machine. Assessment should include both standardized assessments and structured observations of functional performance.

A complete fine motor assessment should include observations of proximal trunk control to distal finger movements. Trunk control and shoulder stability affect the accuracy and control of reaching patterns and create a stable base from which both hands can be used to perform bilateral skills. The assessment of distal control considers wrist stability, development of hand arches, and separation of the two sides of the hand, all providing a foundation for the control of distal movement. Qualitative observations of distal fingertip control include finger motions to move objects into and out of the palm of the hand and rotate an object within the hand.

Although standardized assessments such as BOT-2[111] and the Peabody Developmental Motor Scales[113] have fine motor sections, they do not adequately measure manipulative components described previously. Combining qualitative observations during a variety of fine motor tasks with knowledge of typical development is important. Soft neurological signs, including diadochokinesia (rapid alternation of forearm supination and pronation), sequential thumb-to-finger touching, and stereognosis (identifying objects and shapes without visual input) can provide further qualitative information.

Eye-Hand Coordination, Visual Motor Integration. Eye-hand coordination is the ability to use the eyes and hands together to guide reaching, grasping, and release of objects. This can include larger motions such as catching and throwing a ball to more refined tasks such as putting pennies in a bank or buttoning a shirt. Coordination of the eyes and the feet (eye-foot coordination) is important for skills such as ascending and descending stairs and kicking a ball. Children with DCD often exhibit difficulties in one or more of these areas. Qualitatively, they demonstrate poor coordination in the timing and sequencing of their actions. Evaluations such as BOT-2,[111] Movement Assessment Battery for Children, second edition (Movement ABC-2),[114] and the Motor Accuracy Test of the Sensory Integration and Praxis Tests[112] have subtests that assess eye-hand coordination in a standardized way. Supplemental clinical observations include the assessment of ball skills, fine motor tasks such as stringing beads and building block towers, and written accuracy tasks of drawing or coloring within a boundary.

Visual motor tasks involve the ability to reproduce shapes, figures, or other visual stimuli in written form. This skill is multidimensional, involving perceiving a visual image, remembering it, and integrating it to a written response. Visual motor integration is the foundational skill needed for handwriting. In addition, handwriting involves combination of fine motor control, motor planning, and sensory feedback to be accurate and legible. Children who have difficulties with handwriting commonly produce sloppy work with incorrect letter formations or reversals, inconsistent size and height of letters, variable slant, and irregular spacing between words and letters.

Assessment of visual motor skills can be completed through standardized measures such as the Developmental Test of Visual Motor Integration (BEERY VMI, Fifth Revision),[115] the Test of Visual Motor Skills,[116] and the Spatial Awareness Skills Program (SASP).[117] The production of handwritten work can be assessed by using the Evaluation Tool of Children's Handwriting (ETCH),[118] the Test of Handwriting Skills (THS),[119] and Handwriting Without Tears: The Print Tool.[120] Handwriting and drawing samples provide important information regarding functional abilities in written production.

Sensory Integration and Sensory Processing

Ayres[99] originally defined sensory integration as "the ability to organize sensory information for use." Information is received through the senses and organized throughout the nervous system to help us participate effectively in social, motor, and academic learning. Integration of sensory input underlies basic functions such as arousal state, attention, regulation, and postural and ocular control. Skills such as eye-hand coordination, bilateral coordination, projecting body movements in space (projected action sequences), motor planning, and skilled motor execution are end products of efficient sensory processing. More recently, it has been proposed that the term *sensory processing* be used for the assessment and diagnosis of sensory challenges impairing daily routines.[121]

The process begins with *registration* or recognition of incoming sensory input *("What is it?")*. The incoming information is quickly scanned for relevance in a process called *sensory modulation ("Is it important?")*. Sensory modulation determines the appropriate action for a situation and regulates arousal. Our system needs to respond strongly and quickly if our hand moves near a hot stove, but should not respond as strongly if we are unexpectedly bumped. *Discrimination* of sensory input involves discerning subtle differences in sensation to learn about the qualities of objects and refine body movements within space. When we are receiving clear information from our sensory receptors we can understand and label what is happening (e.g., sour-sweet, hot-cold, soft-firm, heavy-light, up-down, fast-slow). Efficient sensory registration, modulation, and discrimination result in organized social and motor behavior.

Children with DCD often experience sensory processing difficulties. Diminished registration of sensation can result in poor body and environmental awareness, low arousal levels, and delayed postural reactions and motor coordination. These children may be sedentary or seek out strong sensation. *Sensory modulation* difficulties manifest primarily in emotional and behavioral responses. Behaviors often include oversensitivity, with aversive or exaggerated responses to sensation. These children struggle to remain regulated during typical daily events, and may avoid uncomfortable sensations, demonstrate behavioral disorganization, seek strong, potentially unsafe input, become aggressive, or have tantrums. They often have difficulty performing in situations involving integration of multiple inputs (e.g., cafeteria, gym class, playground, team sports). Sensitivity to movement input can also cause the child to avoid playground equipment or become nauseated during car rides. Delayed *sensory discrimination* typically results in poor body awareness that may underlie qualitative motor difficulties observed in children with DCD. They often exhibit poor motor coordination and planning, deficient safety awareness, and poor grading of force, as well as timing and sequencing difficulties. These children may avoid complex motor challenges, team sports, and playground activities. Discrimination difficulties can also affect the acquisition of prepositional concepts (up, down, left, right, in front of, behind, next to). The child who has difficulty discriminating information from the body typically exhibits deficits in skilled actions involving balance, timing movements in space, bilateral and eye-hand coordination, fine motor control, and handwriting.

Clinical observation of a child's responses to a variety of sensory inputs and the ability to organize multiple inputs provides essential information regarding the integration of sensory input. Sensory modulation dysfunction is not easily identified with standardized, skill-based measures because of its physiological basis. Caregiver questionnaires, such as the Sensory Processing Measure[122,123] and the Sensory Profile[124,125] can provide valuable information on modulation and regulation.

Gross and fine motor tasks that involve postural and ocular responses, bilateral motor coordination, planning, and sequencing reflect efficient sensory processing. Soft neurological signs, coupled with observations of play (e.g., playground, gym class, recess) can provide qualitative information on sensory discrimination and planning. The Clinical Observations of Motor and Postural Skills (COMPS) assessment tool[126] is a set of six standardized clinical observations and soft signs that can be useful in identifying motor deficit with a postural component. The Sensory Integration and Praxis Tests,[112] the Miller Assessment for Preschoolers,[127] and the Toddler and Infant Motor Evaluation (TIME)[128] are used most commonly to assess various aspects of sensory integration function. Other tests, such as BOT-2[111] and the Movement ABC-2,[114] can provide qualitative observations in addition to quantitative measures of motor skill.

Praxis and Motor Planning

Praxis involves the ability to plan and carry out a new or unusual action when adequate cognitive and motor skills are present. The components of praxis include *ideation* or generating an idea of how one might act in the environment, *planning* or organizing a program of action, and *execution* of the action sequence. Motor planning involves the same components relative to a novel motor task.

Children with praxis difficulties, or dyspraxia, may exhibit a paucity of ideas. The child may enter a room filled with toys or equipment and have limited capacity to experiment and play. Other children with dyspraxia may move from one activity to the next without generating effective plans for participating in or completing tasks. Lack of variation and adaptation in play can be another indication of planning problems. Observations of typically developing children show continuous modifications in play, with spontaneous adaptations to motor sequences, making explorations varied and increasingly successful. Children with dyspraxia often have difficulties in situations characterized by changing demands, such as unstructured group play. Transitions also may be difficult because they involve the creation or adaptation of a plan. Frustration and difficulties with peer interactions frequently are part of the composite.

Observations of motor planning deficits may include trouble figuring out new motor activities, disorganized approaches, resistance or inability to vary performance when a task is not successful, and awkward motor execution. Poor planning abilities can lead to the child being adult dependent, hesitant, or resistant to trying new activities. At times, children with dyspraxia also may exhibit poor anticipation of their actions. They can quickly engage in play with the equipment but demonstrate little regard for safety (e.g., kicking a large ball across the room where other children are playing). Movements are often performed with an excessive expenditure of energy and with inaccurate judgment of the required force, tempo, and amplitude.[129] Such children typically require more practice and repetition to master more complex, sequential movements. Frequently, children with planning problems recognize the differences between their performance and that of other children the same age, which significantly affects their self-esteem.

Manifestations of poor motor planning ability are apparent in many daily tasks. Dressing is often difficult. Children are not able to plan where or how to move their limbs to put on clothes. Problems are often demonstrated in constructive manipulatory play, such as building with toys, cutting, and pasting. Similarly, learning how to use utensils, such as a knife, fork, pencil, or scissors, is difficult. The child with dyspraxia often also has problems with handwriting.

Standardized assessments of praxis include the tests of Postural Praxis, Sequencing Praxis, Praxis on Verbal Command, Oral Praxis, Constructional Praxis, and Design Copy of the Sensory Integration and Praxis Tests.[112] The First-STEP[130] is a preschool screening tool with a section assessing motor planning abilities. Clinical observations can add valuable information regarding the child's ability to see the potential for action, organize and sequence motor actions for success, and anticipate the outcome of an action.

Physical Fitness

Physical fitness involves a person's ability to perform physical activities that require aerobic fitness, endurance, strength, or flexibility. Factors influencing fitness include motor competency, frequency of exercise, physical health, and genetically inherited ability. Physical fitness can encompass health-related and skill-related fitness.[131] Cardiorespiratory endurance, muscular strength and endurance, flexibility, and body composition are components of health-related fitness and important to monitor. Agility, speed, and power are the skill-related fitness components and are needed for the acquisition of motor skills and sports and recreational activities.[132]

Children with DCD often have performance difficulties in games and athletic activities. They are often less active than typical peers and withdraw from physical activity. As a result, the level of physical fitness, strength, muscular endurance, flexibility, and cardiorespiratory endurance may be poorly developed. Hands and Larkin[131] found that body mass index (BMI) in children with motor difficulties was higher than in a control group of typical peers.[131] The percentage of overweight and obese 10- to 12-year-olds was found to be significantly higher in a DCD group than in typically developing peers.[133] This increased weight may further increase their movement difficulties.

In a study of 52 children aged 5 to 8 years with DCD, Hands and Larkin[131] revealed significantly lower scores on tests for cardiorespiratory endurance, flexibility, abdominal strength, speed, and power than the age- and gender-matched controls. Another study of 261 children aged 4 to 12 years found similar disparities for children with DCD, with poor performance in fitness tests, with the exception of flexibility.[133] These disparities in fitness were found to increase with age between the two groups.[133]

One task of the PT is to differentiate between poor physical fitness, resulting from low motor activity as opposed to problems of low muscle tone, joint limitations, decreased strength, and reduced endurance. The low motor activity is a neurologic sign and leads to a developmental lag or deviation in motor function. Collaboration among the physical educator, the adaptive physical educator, and the PT is critical. The President's Challenge is a physical fitness test administered twice a year in schools across the country. Children complete five events that assess their level of physical fitness in strength, speed, endurance, and flexibility. The test was founded in 1956 by Dwight Eisenhower to encourage American children to be healthy and active, after a study indicating that American youths are less physically fit than European children.[134] Standardized assessments of gross motor functioning, such as BOT-2,[111] that assess strength, speed, and endurance can provide information related to a child's fitness level.

INTERVENTION FOR THE CHILD WITH LEARNING DISABILITIES AND MOTOR DEFICITS OR DEVELOPMENTAL COORDINATION DISORDER

Creating an Intervention Plan

Using the information gathered throughout the assessment process, the therapist synthesizes areas of strength and weakness to develop an intervention plan. If impairments, activity limitations, and participation restrictions exist that affect the child's successful performance, intervention may be warranted. Children with DCD, for example, might demonstrate impairments in coordination or balance that underlie activity limitations in catching or throwing a ball, which create participation restrictions in playing baseball with peers.[135] Determining the child's functional difficulties and identifying the severity of the impairment will be important to justify service and guide the service delivery model and type of intervention. For children with DCD who have greater impairment and activity limitations, individualized treatment may be more beneficial, whereas those with less involvement may thrive with group intervention.[136]

Interpreting test data, integrating findings, identifying functional limitations, and creating goals is a complex process. Initial impressions of the child's areas of difficulty may result in the recommendation for further examination before outlining refined goals relevant to functional performance. Collecting additional assessment information may involve observations in other environments or during functional daily tasks, and/or formal testing. The end product is the creation of statements that delineate the type and quality of behavior desired as a result of remediation. In other words, the therapist must set treatment goals to be achieved through intervention.

Setting goals for the child with learning disabilities with motor deficits must be done by considering a variety of factors:

1. Referral information and age of the child
2. Medical, developmental, and sensory processing history
3. Parents' and teachers' perception of the child's strengths and concerns about functional impairments
4. Educational information
   a. Major difficulties experienced in school
   b. How motor problems are interfering with the child's daily participation
   c. Current services being received
5. Child's peer relationships, play and leisure activities, and self-esteem
6. Therapists' observations and assessment of the child through informal and formal evaluation, both standardized and nonstandardized
7. Functional expectations and abilities at home and school

Goals for the child should be stated in terms of long-term and short-term objectives. Goal setting ideally involves establishing specific, measurable, attainable, realistic, and time-targeted objectives. Short-term objectives are generally composed of three parts: (1) the *behavioral statement* is what will be accomplished by the child; (2) the *condition statement* provides details regarding how the skill or behavior will be accomplished; and (3) the *performance statement* denotes how the skill or behavior will be measured for success. The most important consideration is ensuring that the goals and objectives chosen are relevant to the child's functional daily performance and are meaningful to the team, including the family, working with the child. Case Study 14-3 provides an example of functional objectives.

CASE STUDY 14-3 ■ JONATHAN

Jonathan was a 6-year-old referred for an occupational therapy evaluation by his parents and teacher because of concerns regarding motor skill development. Assessment results revealed several areas of impairment, including poor discrimination of his body position and movement in space, diminished postural control and balance reactions, motor planning deficits, delayed eye-hand coordination, qualitative fine motor deficits, and delayed visual-motor integration affecting his handwriting. Jonathan's mother reported that he was clumsy and seemed to bump into things constantly. Of greater concern was that Jonathan seemed fearful of activities that his peers found pleasurable, such as climbing the jungle gym and coming down the slide at the neighborhood playground. Jonathan tended to play on the outskirts of groups. When he did attempt to interact he became angry because the children would not play the game by his rules. At home, Jonathan often was frustrated by tasks of daily living such as putting on his coat, snapping his pants, and tying his shoes. His mother reported that Jonathan frequently called himself "stupid" when he could not independently complete self-care skills.

When determining appropriate behavioral objectives for Jonathan, looking at the areas of functional relevance such as pleasure and safety in gross motor play, peer interactions, and

CASE STUDY 14-3 ■ JONATHAN—cont'd

independence in age-appropriate activities of daily living is critical. These areas of concern for Jonathan were consistent with those of his parents. His parents wanted him to feel more competent and less frustrated in play, at home, and at school. Jonathan's goal was to "not be so stupid that kids won't play with me." The OT believed that through remediation of sensory discrimination and motor deficits Jonathan could develop improved motor competence and planning abilities. This would lead to greater success in peer interactions and improved feelings of self-confidence. Based on these common desires the following goals and objectives were made.

One of the long-term goals was *Improve Jonathan's planning and coordination abilities to increase his confidence and success in gross motor activities.* Jonathan was interested in learning to ride a bicycle without training wheels, and his parents were hopeful that he could become more confident at the neighborhood playground. These behavioral objectives would measure the development of improved proficiency in discrimination of his body in space, postural control balance reactions, and motor planning. The following objectives were written:

1. Jonathan will independently climb the ladder and come down the slide without exhibiting fear, bumping into other children, or falling.
2. Jonathan will develop the ability to ride his bicycle without training wheels in straight lines and will learn to turn corners. (*Note:* Successfully riding the bicycle becomes the performance measure of behavior in this objective.)

To address improvement in independence for self-care:

1. Jonathan will put on his coat independently in correct orientation and successfully zip it four out of five times.
2. Jonathan will successfully tie his shoes without assistance in a timely manner.

To address greater success in peer interactions:

1. Jonathan will participate in a structured game, following the rules, for 10 minutes.
2. Jonathan will play outside with the children in the neighborhood without conflict for at least 1 hour.

Although impairment level objectives could have been written to address the same areas, they would have been of limited relevance to Jonathan and the team working with him. Balance and postural control also could be addressed by an objective stating that Jonathan would stand on one foot for 10 seconds. The functional implications of this objective would not have been clear, and Jonathan and his parents would be without an outcome measure that was measurable and meaningful to them. Thus it would have negated the effects of working as a cohesive team toward a common goal.

If the OT or PT is working as a member of a team within the school, behavioral objectives will have implications for the child's performance in the school environment. Within the school system, statements of goals and specific objectives are included in the Individualized Educational Plan (IEP). In Jonathan's case, specific objectives that were meaningful to the classroom situation included the ability to sit in the chair to complete written assignments for 15 minutes and increase accuracy of letter formation, size, and spacing on written assignments. Other areas related to gross and fine motor skills and peer interactions also were influential to Jonathan's success at school. Specific objectives written pertaining to school would have functional outcome measures chosen from tasks within the school environment such as gym class, playground interactions, and classroom expectations.

Models of Intervention

Improvements in motor deficits can be achieved through a variety of models of intervention, both indirect and direct. Indirect intervention involves working with key people in the child's life to help them facilitate the child's delineated goals. An indirect model can occur through consultation, specialized instruction, and coaching. Direct intervention involves the therapist working directly with the child on specific goal areas or skills.

Mild deficits, subtly affecting participation in activities, may be addressed through a consultative (indirect) approach. This model of service provision incorporates the use of another team member's expertise to be responsible for the outcome of the child.[76,137] The therapist may suggest environmental or task adaptations to facilitate more successful participation. Consultation with parents would be appropriate for the goal of riding a bicycle without training wheels. Parents may not understand the complexity of the task and may be focused only on the end product, which can cause frustration for all involved. To facilitate confidence and success, the therapist might recommend environmental modifications such as beginning on an open stretch of grass or dirt, with no other people around to decrease the child's anxiety. Breaking the task down into incremental steps for the parent and child (i.e., practicing getting on and off bike, balancing on still bike, gliding, braking, steering, pedaling) can allow success at each step.

Within a school setting, environmental adaptations might include changing the height or position of the desk or decreasing extraneous visual and auditory distracters. Task accommodations could include using a special grip to facilitate more refined pencil grasp or allowing more time for written work. In these instances the teacher would be responsible for carrying out the program and determining its effectiveness. Communication between the therapist and teacher encourages problem solving and changing action plans over time. Kemmis and Dunn[138] demonstrated positive outcomes on a variety of functional classroom goals when an OT and teacher met weekly throughout the school year in what they called a "collaborative consultation approach." Using this model they achieved 63% (134 of 213) of their outlined goals. This collaborative effort supports the shared responsibility for identifying the problem or weakness of the child, creating possible solutions, implementing the intervention as the solution, and altering the plan as necessary for increased effectiveness.[76]

Another model of indirect therapy involves teaching members of the team to implement treatment strategies.

Specialized instruction or coaching allows the therapist to support a child within the natural environment by working with care providers who are with the child every day. The aim is to educate key people in the child's life to coach the child within the context of teachable moments.[139] These moments, when a child is interested and working on acquiring a new skill, occur throughout the day and in many different environments.[140] This allows for therapeutic consistency and repeated practice, thereby increasing the chances for skill acquisition within the context of daily routines.

With this model, the therapist observes children and adults doing familiar routines and collaborates with the adults to enhance those routines in varied environments.[141] When implementing an intervention strategy, the therapist might teach another adult to guide specific, developmentally appropriate skill sets with the child, or problem solve to create strategies for greater success. Over time parents and other caregivers are empowered to look at a toy, an activity, or an experience and find ways to adapt it to increase successful involvement and skill development. Successful coaching can enhance parent-child relationships indirectly by helping parents to feel more comfortable and competent in their abilities to meet their child's needs.[142]

Direct intervention involves designing individualized treatment plans and carrying them out with the child individually or in a small group. This approach can focus on developing the foundations that underlie motor performance such as sensory processing, postural control, and motor planning. Specific skills, such as shoe tying or bike riding, can be practiced with the therapist as well, breaking these tasks down into component skills. Through combining approaches, adapting methods over the course of therapy, and responding to the changing needs of the child over time, progress is achieved more effectively.[97] Best practice dictates that direct therapy should always be provided in conjunction with one of the other service models to ensure generalization of skills to natural settings.[76] Without the use of other models, therapists cannot be confident that changes observed in the isolated setting are affecting the child's overall performance.

Intervention Approaches

According to the International Classification of Functioning, Disability and Health (ICF),[143] interventions should be directed toward several distinct goals:

- To remediate impairment
- To reduce activity limitations
- To improve participation

Interventions focused on remediating impairments generally target the improvement of processing abilities (e.g., visual, proprioceptive, and vestibular) or performance components (e.g., balance and strength). The tenet is that by strengthening these foundational skills the child will develop greater success in appropriate activities and participation. This type of intervention is referred to as a "bottom-up" approach and is based on neuromaturational or hierarchical theories. Ayres's sensory integration therapy is an example of bottom-up intervention. Missiuna, Rivard, and Bartlett[83] suggest that addressing secondary, preventable impairments, such as loss of strength and endurance, may be an appropriate focus of intervention for children with DCD.

Typically, skill-based interventions are used to address activity limitations. These interventions emphasize the development of specific skills, rather than underlying components alone. This is referred to as a "top-down" approach, using cognitive strategies and problem solving. The therapist, family, and child identify specific functional activities to work on. Breaking the activity into smaller, incremental steps can facilitate the ease of learning by encouraging success. Shoe tying is a good example of a skill best taught in steps.

At times, skill-based intervention and practice occur outside the context where the child will typically perform that task. Certain skills may not be easily generalized and would be best taught in the context where the child would do the skill, such as tooth brushing. Progress is seen more rapidly when a task-related behavior that is meaningful to the child is used. Eye-hand coordination tasks, for example, become more meaningful within the context of a game of hot potato or baseball. Barnhart[95] suggests an integrated approach to facilitating development in the child with DCD, including both bottom-up, physiological interventions, and top-down, cognitive strategies.

Recently, emphasis has shifted to models of treatment that highlight participation. Intervention focuses on increasing the child's ability to take part in the typical activities of childhood.[83] These treatment methods assume that skill acquisition emerges from interaction among the child, the task, and the environment.[97] Intervention is contextually based, occurring in everyday situations and focusing on the activities and tasks inherent to that situation. Problem solving, preparatory activities, and skill training may be used together to increase successful participation. This type of approach may minimize the challenges of learning new skills for a child who cannot easily generalize learning to new situations.

The intervention methods presented in this chapter for remediation of motor deficits in the child with learning disabilities include Ayres sensory integration; neurodevelopmental treatment (NDT); motor learning approaches (e.g., Cognitive Orientation to Daily Occupational Performance [CO-OP])[144]; sensorimotor treatment techniques; motor skill training approaches (e.g., Ecological Intervention[145]); and physical fitness. None are mutually exclusive, and each requires a level of training and practice for competence as well as experience in normal development. Most therapists synthesize information from different intervention techniques and use an eclectic approach, pulling relevant pieces from a variety of intervention modalities to best meet the needs of each child.

Ayres Sensory Integration

The sensory integration theory and treatment were developed by A. Jean Ayres,[99,112] with concepts drawn from neurophysiology, neuropsychology, and development. Her purpose in theoretical development was to explain the observed relationship between difficulties organizing sensory input and deficits in academic and neuromotor "learning" observed in some children with learning disabilities and motor deficits.[146] The theory proposes that "learning is dependent on the ability of normal individuals to take in sensory information derived from the environment and from movement of their bodies, to process and integrate these sensory inputs within the central nervous system, and to use this sensory information to plan and organize behavior."[146] Ayres[112] used "learning" in a broad sense to include the development of concepts, adaptive motor responses, and behavioral change.

The goal of sensory integration intervention is to elicit responses that result in better organization of sensory input for enhanced participation and generalization of functional skills. Sensory integration treatment is based on the belief that active involvement in individually designed, meaningful activities that are rich in sensory input will enhance the nervous system's organization and integration of sensation.[147] Active exploration and variation in the context of play results in adaptive responses,[148] which positively affect the child's ability to participate in daily life activities. During intervention, sensory input is provided in a planned and organized manner while eliciting progressively harder adaptive behavioral and motor responses. The therapist strives to find activities that are motivating and tap the child's inner drive to encourage adaptation. "Evincing an adaptive behavior promotes sensory integration, and, in turn, the ability to produce an adaptive behavior reflects sensory integration."[99] Effective intervention requires melding the science of a neurophysiological theory with the art of "playing" with the child.

A sensory integration treatment session for a child with postural difficulties might involve having the child riding a swing pretending to be a fisherman while keeping a lookout for whales that might bump his boat. This "pretend play" scenario taps the child's motivation and inner drive to be productive (fishing), while challenging him with a potential "out of my control" situation (whales). The therapist will adapt this activity in a variety of ways to maintain an appropriate level of challenge and adaptation (adaptive response). The type and amount of sensory input, postural demands, bilateral control, timing, and planning requirements are all considered and can be adapted to an easier or harder level to maintain adaptation and learning. Sensory input can be controlled through the speed and direction the boat moves and the amount of work the child must do with his arms to propel the boat and catch fish. Additional sensory input can be provided through "rocky seas" and "whales crashing the side of the boat." The boat can facilitate more or less postural adaptation by the amount of support it provides and the speed of its movement. The child can pull a rope to propel the swing, or the therapist can provide the movement to decrease the bilateral coordination and postural demands. A more demanding bilateral response could include pulling a rope and catching a fish simultaneously. Unexpected movements of the boat, fish, and whales will require greater timing and planning for success.

For this intervention technique to be appropriate, the motor and planning difficulties observed in a child with learning disabilities need to be a result of deficits in processing sensory information. Each child's intervention plan should be individualized based on the results of a comprehensive evaluation and responses to sensory input within therapy. Contributions of sensory registration, modulation, and discrimination should be considered for their impact on functional performance including social, emotional, and motor development. Children with sensory processing difficulties will exhibit problems that limit their occupational performance in a variety of environments.[149]

Vestibular, proprioceptive, and tactile sensory inputs used in therapy are powerful and must be applied with caution. The autonomic and behavioral responses of the child must be monitored carefully. The therapist should be knowledgeable about sensory integration theory and intervention before using these procedures. Monitoring behavioral responses after the therapy session also is suggested through parent or teacher consultation. Intervention precautions are elaborated by Ayres,[99] Koomar and Bundy,[150] and Bundy.[151]

Research on the Effects of Sensory Integration Procedures. Sensory integration is an evolving theory, based on developments in the fields of neuroscience, research, and clinical practice.[152] The current neuroscience literature supports the basic tenets of sensory integration including neuroplasticity, and positive changes in behavior and learning as a result of enriched environmental conditions, dynamic participation in meaningful activities, and developmentally appropriate sensory motor experiences.[147] Within the field of occupational therapy, sensory integration is the most extensively researched intervention procedure, with over 80 research studies that measure some aspect of treatment effectiveness.[153] Clinically, sensory integration principles are estimated to be used by approximately 90% of American OTs working in the school system for children with learning disabilities and motor deficits.[154] Despite over 35 years of theoretical development, research, and intervention practice, the value and effectiveness of this therapeutic modality continues to be questioned and critiqued.[155-158] The complexity of sensory integration theory, the individualized approaches that treatment warrants, and the difficulty finding sensitive outcome measures create many challenges in designing appropriate and valid research studies.

Clinicians using sensory integration procedures attest to the effectiveness of this treatment approach in making important functional changes. Testimonials from parents of children who have received occupational therapy with sensory integration procedures are frequently heard. In Cohn's research, parents identified two important outcome measures for intervention.[159] The first included change in the child, such as improved self-regulation, perceived competence, and social participation. The second was related to parents developing the ability to understand their child's behavior in a new way and having their experiences validated to better support and advocate for the child.

Accurate analysis of the efficacy of sensory integration is complicated by a wide variety of methodological design flaws in the available research. The majority of the studies include heterogeneous samples, small sample sizes, and inconsistencies in the frequency, length, and duration of treatment. Schaaf and Miller[153] note that a major challenge in interpreting the existing research is related to the outcome measures used. Researchers have not consistently used a theoretical base to explain how treatment techniques influence the outcomes chosen.[153] In addition, the dependent variables measured were often not related to the expected outcomes of treatment, were too many in number, or were poor measures of change over time.[153,156] Many studies include outcome measures that are not sensitive to small increments of change or meaningful to parents as treatment priorities.[159]

Perhaps the most challenging aspect of developing strong research studies is the variability of sensory integration intervention. Treatment is individualized and adapted frequently in response to the child's changing needs and successes.[160] Many of the studies that claim to be using sensory integration therapy do not adhere to the core theoretical principles, or they violate them.[161] Developing standardized and replicable treatment is a major challenge for future research studies. Researchers and clinicians have focused extensively on improving the quality of efficacy research, resulting in the development of improved functional outcome measures (goal attainment scaling)[162] and treatment fidelity (fidelity measure).[161] Significant progress has also been made in defining homogeneous subgroups for analysis, describing replicable treatments, and choosing valid outcome measures.[153]

Schaaf and Miller[153] note that diverse findings are not surprising given the current level of research. The knowledge base in sensory integration research is still in its infancy, with the need for substantial work to generate more rigorous empirical data to support the efficacy of this intervention approach.[153] Increased emphasis on high-quality, randomized controlled studies is essential.[163]

Approximately half of the research studies conducted to date show some positive effects, with sensory integration treatment being more effective than or equally as effective as other approaches used.[153] In a recent systematic review of 27 research studies, May-Benson and Koomar[164] concluded that the synthesis of evidence indicates that sensory integration may result in a variety of positive outcomes. Specific areas identified included sensory-motor skills, motor planning, social skills, attention, behavioral regulation, and reading and reading-related activities, as well as functional outcomes as measured by individually designed goal attainment scales (e.g., improved sleep patterns, increased food repertoire, pumping a swing, and manipulating fasteners). Positive gains in motor performance were found in 10 of 14 studies reviewed, with the implication that the gains were maintained after the cessation of treatment. Arbesman and Lieberman[149] identified that the positive development of motor skills as a result of sensory integration intervention was most consistently noted in their review of 198 articles. Other recent, well designed studies have demonstrated positive effects on behavioral outcomes including significant gains in attention, cognitive and social skills,[163] and socialization[165] and increased engagement, with decreased aggression.[166] May-Benson and Koomar[164] suggest that given the current level of positive results, OTs can begin to use this information to support the use of sensory integration treatment, particularly for sensory motor outcomes and client-centered functional goals.

Neurodevelopmental Treatment

NDT is a treatment technique formulated by Karel and Berta Bobath[167,168] to enhance the development of gross motor skills, balance, quality of movement, hand skills, and daily tasks such as mobility and self-care for individuals with movement disorders.[169,170] These techniques were originally designed for use with children with cerebral palsy in whom the underlying problem was a lesion in the central nervous system that produced abnormal muscle tone and deficits in coordination of posture and movement, affecting functional performance.[168] The original framework was based on hierarchical levels of reflex integration in the nervous system and the normal developmental sequence. Abnormal postural responses were lower-level hierarchical reactions that did not integrate in a typical time frame (e.g., ATNR, STNR), thereby inhibiting the development of mature postural mechanisms and voluntary movements. The NDT approach emphasized specific ways to inhibit abnormal reactions and facilitate more normal muscle tone and movement.[171,172] The assumption was that encouraging more normalized automatic movement patterns would lead to functional carryover.[172]

The original hierarchical "impairment-based" model of reflex integration has been replaced with a more dynamic "interactive systems" model that emphasizes both internal and external factors of motor control. Currently, NDT therapists view the execution of movement as a complex interaction of the neural and body systems, organized by the specific task requirements and constrained by physical laws of the environment.[170] The nervous system is viewed as dynamic and adaptable, capable of initiating, anticipating, and controlling movements with ongoing sensory feedforward information and feedback.[170,173] Many body factors are recognized as contributing to dysfunctional movement patterns, including abnormal muscle tone, primitive reflex patterns, delayed development of righting and equilibrium reactions, specific muscle weakness, body biomechanics, cardiovascular or respiratory weakness, lack of fitness, and sensory, cognitive, or perceptual impairments.[170,173,174] As NDT's theoretical and clinical development progressed, there was acknowledgement that intervention had not automatically carried over into functional performance as had been anticipated. As a result, treatment strategies began to shift, with preparation for specific functional tasks done in settings where children typically participate.[175] The focus on normalizing muscle tone and altering movement patterns as a foundation for performance was replaced with emphasis on activity-related impairments and client-directed functional outcomes.[170,172,173] Ecological, family-centered intervention was identified as essential to target key environments, activities, and functional outcomes.[170] This dynamic treatment approach now emphasizes active involvement in meaningful tasks to enhance independent participation in various environments. The goal of NDT intervention is for the child to use more efficient movement strategies to complete life skills with greater success. Over the life span these strategies will minimize secondary impairments that can create additional functional limitations or disability.[170,174]

NDT uses physical handling techniques directed toward developing the components of movement necessary for functional motor performance. Movement components of postural alignment and stability, mobility skills, weight bearing, weight shifting, and balance are all foundations for smoothly executed movements in space.[169] Assessment and analysis of posture and movement components are ongoing, using a problem-solving approach that identifies and builds on the child's strengths and limitations.[170]

Therapists employ a combination of handling techniques and encouragement of active movements targeted toward the specific functional skills on which the child is working.[98] Feedback involves both tactile-proprioceptive ("hands-on") and verbal cues, which are graded back or changed according to the needs and emerging skills of the individual child.[172] The therapist's hands guide the reactions, with the child actively participating in problem solving and adapting performance. Practice of more effective postural reactions and reduction of abnormal movement patterns are embedded into meaningful activities. A skilled therapist balances the quality of movement patterns with the importance of active involvement in learning new motor tasks.[173] At times, participation and independent task completion are more important than qualitatively normal movement patterns.

Although NDT was developed for children with central nervous system insults resulting in deficient postural and movement control for daily skills, it lends its use to children with more minimal motor involvement. Of particular relevance to the child with learning disabilities and DCD is facilitation of improved righting and equilibrium responses, automatic postural adjustments, and balance reactions. Handling techniques can help develop improved qualitative control, as well as encouraging active problem solving and task adaptation by the child.

Research on the Effects of Neurodevelopmental Treatment. NDT is an evolving theoretical and treatment approach, based on principles derived from research in neural plasticity, motor development, motor control, and motor learning.[170] It is the most commonly used treatment framework for children with cerebral palsy.[176] Despite this, relatively few studies are available on the efficacy of NDT to date.[172] Those that are available have not definitively shown NDT to be effective as a treatment modality or more valuable than other therapies.[175,177] One of the major problems confounding interpretation of the current state of research has been the significant change in theoretical development and clinical application over time. The revised practice model of NDT is better reflected in the current research, which shows more promise.[170,178] It has been suggested by Bain[172] that studies conducted before 2000, when NDT was defined with outdated operational definitions, should not be considered as evidence that current practice is ineffective.

Methodological concerns in many of the available studies make interpretation of efficacy more challenging. In a review of older treatment studies, Royeen and DeGangi[169] noted significant methodological problems that were attributable to the lack of conclusive evidence regarding NDT. These included poorly defined objective outcome measures, overreliance on subjective clinical observations, and small sample sizes. In addition, sample populations varied greatly, including adults and children with cerebral palsy and Down syndrome as well as high-risk infants. More recently Sharkey and colleagues[178] highlighted difficulties in developing well designed treatment studies, including the heterogeneity of children with cerebral palsy, both in functional limitations and goals, small sample sizes, and ineffectiveness of standardized outcome measures to assess qualitative and functional changes. Butler and Darrah[175] cautioned interpretation of efficacy from the 21 studies they reviewed owing to unclear population definitions, unclear treatment protocols and goals, and lack of clarity regarding therapist skill levels.

Several current research studies have demonstrated positive changes in gross motor performance as a result of intensive NDT intervention.[176,179,180] Arndt and colleagues[179] used an operational definition of NDT based on trunk coactivation for treating infants with posture and movement difficulties. After 10 hours of treatment over 15 days, the infants who received the NDT protocol significantly improved in gross motor function compared with infants in the control play group. These skills were maintained at a 3-week follow-up evaluation. Bar-Haim and colleagues[176] used a randomized controlled trial for 24 children with cerebral palsy, with 40 hours of treatment over a period of 4 weeks. They compared intensive NDT treatment with the use of the Adeli suit (AST), which stabilizes the trunk and extremities of the wearer to help normalize motor actions. Although there was no superiority noted between these two intensive treatment modalities, both groups made significant gains in gross motor function that were sustained after nine months. Tsorlakis and colleagues[180] further assessed the variable of intensity of services in their 16-week treatment study. The efficacy of NDT for children with spastic cerebral palsy was supported by this study, as both groups of children who received NDT intervention demonstrated statistically significant gains in gross motor function. Increased intensity of services was also supported, as motor gains were statistically greater for the group that received intervention five times a week compared with two times a week.

Brown and Burns[177] completed the only systematic review that was identified as high quality by colleagues.[181] They selected 17 studies to include on the basis of use of NDT as the treatment modality, reported clinical outcomes, and random group assignment. Their analysis did not provide definitive evidence that NDT is beneficial for children with neurological dysfunction. The authors suggest that available research did not reveal either efficacy or inefficacy of NDT as a treatment approach. Butler and Darrah[175] suggest that absence of evidence on the effectiveness of NDT should not be construed as proof that the treatment is not effective, but certainly reflects areas in which more meaningful research is needed. Sharkey and colleagues[178] suggest that recognition of these limitations will encourage practitioners to implement "second-generation" research that is characterized by well designed studies that systematically evaluate operationally defined intervention techniques and determine what works for specific ages and diagnoses of children.

Motor Learning Theories

Motor learning refers to the process of acquiring, expanding, and improving skilled motor actions. The basic treatment premise of motor learning theories is that improvement in movement skills is elicited through appropriate practice and timely feedback. Motor learning has taken place when a permanent change in the child's ability to respond to a movement problem or achieve a movement goal has occurred, regardless of the environment.[182] Therefore therapists measure learning through tests that measure retention and transfer of skills.[183]

The closed-loop theory of Adams[184] is recognized as the first comprehensive explanation for motor learning. Adams believed that the central nervous system, based on sensory feedback, controls the execution of movement. He proposed that once a movement has occurred, errors are detected and compared with existing "memory traces." With practice, these memory traces become stronger and the accuracy of the movement increases, thus emphasizing learning through feedback.

In 1975 Schmidt contributed the idea of "open loop" motor learning, which emphasized the ability to produce rapid action sequences in the absence of sensory feedback (e.g., hitting a baseball). He proposed that new movements were created from previously stored motor programs (schemas) of similar movements, as opposed to feedback from individual motor actions.[185] Schemas comprise general rules for a specific group of actions that can be applied to a variety of situations.[186] When a motor action occurs, the initial movement conditions, parameters used, outcomes, and sensory consequences of the action are stored in memory. With each goal-directed movement, specific parameters are used (e.g., force needed to pour juice into a glass), and consequences occur (e.g., spillage or not). Repeated actions using different parameters and creating different outcomes create data sets that help refine the motor program, reducing errors and improving anticipation or feed-forward information.[186] Schmidt's[185] schema theory contributed to current theories of motor learning principles regarding practice schedules and feedback about outcome of movements, known as *knowledge of results.*

Based on the knowledge of motor skill development in children with DCD, four key variables are important to consider in targeted intervention. They include stage of the learner, type of task, scheduling of practice, and type of feedback.

Three stages of the learner have been proposed[187,188]: the *cognitive stage,* the *associative stage,* and the *autonomous stage.* As a child learns and develops new motor actions, he or she progresses through the various stages at different rates, depending on the complexity of the skill. The *cognitive stage* is the initial phase of learning in which there is large variability as the child gets the general idea of the movement.[135] Awkward body postures are observed, errors are often made, and awareness of what needs to be improved or changed does not exist. (Consider when a young child attempts to throw a ball; the throw is a gross movement, the projection of the ball varies, and the movement appears uncoordinated.) As practice continues, the degree of accuracy increases, which is characteristic of the *associative stage.* Fewer errors are made and error information is used to correct the movement patterns. (As the child continues to throw the ball, the ball may get closer to the target with improved coordination observed.) During the *autonomous stage,* the skill is performed fluently and automatically, without as much effort or thought. Improvements in accuracy continue and errors are detected, with corrections made automatically. (The child can now throw a ball at a target and hit the target with coordinated, accurate movements, such as pitching; however, if a child were introduced to throwing a curve ball, the stages would start over.)

The type of task is a mechanism to classify motor skills in a dimensional fashion. Task components contribute to intervention decisions. The types of tasks are *gross motor* or *fine motor; simple* or *complex; discrete, serial,* or *continuous;* and *environment changing* or *stationary.* Gross and fine motor tasks are classified according to the type of muscle groups required.[189] *Gross motor skills* use large muscles and tend to be fundamental skills (e.g., walking and running). *Fine motor skills* tend to require greater control of small muscles and usually have to be taught (e.g., handwriting, cutting). Task complexity refers to the level of difficulty and amount of feedback required. *Simple* tasks, such as reaching, require a decision followed by a response. A *complex* task, such as cutting out a picture, requires continual monitoring and feedback until completion. Tasks can require simple single actions or the coordination of sequential motions for completion. A single *discrete* movement has a clear beginning and ending, such as activating a button. *Serial* movements require a series of distinct movements combined to achieve the outcome, such as writing a sentence. *Continuous* movements, such as running, contain movements that are repetitive. Tasks that are discrete or serial can be practiced in parts, but continuous tasks usually need to be practiced as a continuous segment.

Environmental variations can greatly increase the complexity of the task, requiring higher levels of feed-forward information and feedback. In an unstable or *changing* environment, the child has to learn the movement and monitor the environment to adapt to changes—for example, running on an uneven surface. The more predictable and stable the task and environments are, the easier it is to learn and replicate motor skills. Tooth brushing is an example of a task that generally occurs in a *stationary* environment. Home and classrooms can be stable, in that many elements within these settings are fixed and do not change. The size and shape of chairs, location of toys on the floor, and movements of other children are considered "variable features" within these stable environments. These variable features require a greater amount of motor control because the child must adjust movements and actions to the changing demands. Therapists generally practice in stable environments and therefore must ensure that the children are able to function under varied circumstances encountered in daily life situations.

Practice is believed to increase learning of a skill or movement. Variations in practice can occur in the order tasks are performed, in the environment where the tasks are practiced, and by changing aspects of the task. Practice schedules can be developed based on the practice techniques (*blocked* or *random*), or how task learning is approached (*component* or *whole task*). *Blocked* practice means the task is repeatedly rehearsed, sometimes focusing on one aspect of a technique or a specific motor sequence (e.g., hitting a golf ball off a tee with the same club). Repetitive, blocked practice often leads to improved immediate performance, particularly in situations that are stable. *Random* practice involves performing a number of different tasks in varied order or employing several different aspects of technique (e.g., hitting golf balls from a tee, sand trap, and rough with the appropriate club). Random practice encourages learners to compare and contrast strategies used in performing the task, which positively influences performance in changeable environments.

If a task is discrete or contains multiple parts, breaking it down into *components* for blocked practice may be beneficial. For success in changeable situations in which the task component is integrated into skilled action, *whole-task* practice is essential—for example, practicing shooting basketballs, then practicing while moving or running toward the basket. When generalization is the goal, practice sessions can progress from stable (shooting from specific positions on the court) to a changeable environment (such as shooting basketballs with a person trying to block the shot). Opportunity and variety in practice appear to improve motor learning, particularly when skills are practiced in a random manner. Practice should therefore be varied and occur in multiple environments (e.g., home and school) to maximize motor learning.

Different types of feedback also affect the process of learning. *Intrinsic* feedback is received from any of the child's internal sensory systems and is usually not perceived consciously unless external direction draws attention to it (e.g., when a child performs a task with his or her tongue sticking out). *Extrinsic* feedback is received from an outside source observing the results of an action and can be provided in the form of knowledge of performance (KP) or knowledge of results (KR). KP focuses on movements used to achieve the goal, whereas KR focuses on the outcome.

Therapists tend to provide excessive feedback, especially when task performance is below what is expected. Low frequency and fading feedback, progressively decreasing the rate at which feedback is provided, appear to be most effective in facilitating learning.[129] One proposed reason is that with less feedback the individual can more readily engage in the processes that enable learning versus focusing on external cues. During intervention, feedback should not be provided for every movement or task execution. It is more beneficial to offer children the opportunity to self-evaluate and correct their own performance. The therapist can provide feedback as necessary to encourage successful task completion and reduce frustration. Verbal feedback can be general—"Did that work?"—or specific—"Do you need to throw it harder or softer to reach the target?"

Children with DCD often lack the skills required to analyze task demands, interpret environmental cues, use knowledge of performance to alter movements, or adapt to situational demands.[190] They therefore do not interpret and use sensory or performance feedback as well as children who are developing typically.[183] Motor observations of the child with DCD often reveal clumsiness, difficulty judging force, timing, and amplitude of motions, and deficits in anticipating the results of a motor action. Reactions, movements, and response times are typically slower.[191] With this in mind, the type of task and the method of teaching should be considered when recommending participation in sports and leisure activities.[135] Children with DCD can become successful in repetitive sports, such as swimming, skating, skiing, and bicycling. Ball-related sports, however, such as hockey, baseball, tennis, football, and basketball, tend to be more difficult and frustrating owing to the high level of unpredictability and frequent changes in the direction, force, speed, and distance of the movement.[135]

When using the motor learning model of practice, the therapist should incorporate a variety of teaching techniques including verbal instructions, positioning, and handling, as well as observational learning (demonstrations).[183] The task and environment should be structured with extrinsic and intrinsic feedback provided, using a practice schedule that is optimal for the type of task.[192] Children with DCD benefit from experiential and guided learning when practice is performed so that each repetition of the action becomes a new problem-solving experience. To test whether motor learning has occurred, the therapist must create opportunities for demonstration of retention (repeating what was learned in a previous session), transfer (perform a different but closely related task), and generalization (perform a learned task in a new environment).

One method of intervention based on the principles of motor learning is the CO-OP, a frame of reference developed as a treatment approach specifically for children with DCD.[144] In this cognitive-based approach, the therapist focuses on the movement goal and facilitates the child's identification of the important aspects of the task, examines the child's performance during the task, identifies where the child is having the most difficulty, and problem solves alternative solutions.[192] Rather than using verbal instructions, this approach uses guided questions to help the child discover the problems, generate solutions, and evaluate his or her attempts in a supportive environment. Furthermore, the therapist solicits verbal strategies from the child that can help guide the motor behavior, such as typical verbal cues that the therapist tends to provide during intervention.

To benefit from the CO-OP approach, the child must have sufficient cognitive and language ability to rate the level of his or her performance and satisfaction of self-identified goals using the Canadian Occupational Performance Measure (COPM).[193] The basic objectives of this approach include skill acquisition, cognitive strategy development, and generalization or transfer of skills into daily performance. CO-OP is delivered over 12 one-on-one sessions, each lasting approximately 1 hour. The therapy process is divided into five phases: preparation, assessment, introduction, acquisition, and consolidation. Children are taught to talk themselves through performance issues using an approach of Goal-Plan-Do-Check. Domain-specific strategies are used to enhance performance, with the purpose of helping the child to see how he or she can set goals, plan actions, talk through doing, and check outcomes. Using this frame of reference, therapists help the child acquire occupational performance skills using a metacognitive problem-solving process.[144]

Research on the CO-OP Model of Motor Learning. Current beliefs regarding the nature of motor learning for children with DCD suggest that assessment of participation, versus impairments, should be used to determine change over time.[183] By increasing the child's ability to participate in childhood activities, secondary deficits such as loss of strength and endurance might be prevented. Relatively new intervention strategies that employ contemporary motor learning principles emphasize the role of cognitive processes (top down) in development of specific skills. The CO-OP model uses this approach to help children achieve their functional goals.[144]

Research on the effectiveness of this approach to improve motor skills and functional performance is limited but shows promise. Polatajko and Cantin[194] reviewed three articles describing four studies and concluded that there was convergent evidence for the effectiveness of the CO-OP approach for children with DCD.

An exploratory study completed in 1994 by Wilcox as part of his graduate work was discussed by Polatajko and colleagues.[195] This initial single case study included 10 children aged 7 to 12 years who were referred to occupational therapy for motor problems. Using a global problem-solving approach to intervention, this study sought to identify whether children with DCD could use these strategies to acquire skills of their choice, and, once learned, whether the skills were maintained and performance in other areas enhanced. Children selected skills that were challenging and meaningful for them, such as shuffling playing cards, applying nail polish, making a bed, and writing legibly. Each of the 10 children made gains in the chosen activity, with 29 of the 30 targeted skills showing improvement.

A pilot study compared the CO-OP model to a traditional treatment approach with a group of 20 children aged 7 to 12 years. Findings indicated that the CO-OP model of intervention produced larger gains on client-selected goals. Improvements in self-ratings of performance and satisfaction were greater than in the comparative group. Although informal, the follow-up data suggested that children maintained their acquired skills and applied strategies to other motor goals.

Limitations in making conclusions regarding the effectiveness of this treatment are mandated by the small number of research studies, primarily carried out by the same research group. Mandich and colleagues[97] suggest that larger studies with control groups are needed. Suggestions for future research include identification of the salient features of this treatment approach, as well as determining the generalization and skill transfer to other settings.

Sensorimotor Intervention

Sensorimotor activities provide the foundation for the development of play in children.[196] The first level of play (i.e., sensorimotor) is pleasurable, intrinsically motivated activity that involves the exploration of sensation and movement.[196] As children react with adaptive motor responses to the array of sensations from their bodies and the environment, central nervous system organization occurs. The assumption that the organization of sensory and motor experiences is essential to effective motor performance is the premise of sensorimotor intervention.[197] Treatment encourages the child to actively engage in a variety of sensory-rich, motor-based activities, to enhance functional motor performance.[195] Evolution of sensorimotor intervention has not revolved around a single, unified theory but has incorporated a variety of theoretical foundations.[198]

The goals of sensorimotor intervention are outcome based, with emphasis on the development of age-appropriate perceptual-motor and gross motor skills. The therapist chooses activities that meet the child's developmental levels, promote sensory and motor foundations, and encourage practice of appropriate motor skills. For the child having difficulty keeping up with the skilled activities in gym class such as rope jumping, components of these activities will be encouraged, with emphasis on sequencing and timing. The therapist may use a heavier jump rope or wrist and ankle weights to provide more sensory information for improved task performance.

In sensorimotor intervention, tasks are chosen for their innate sensory and motor components. The child is directed to activities that encourage the use of the body in space to complete a structured motor sequence. Activities incorporate sensory components such as movement (vestibular), touch (tactile), and heavy work for the muscles and joints (proprioception). Play interactions are considered important to encourage sensorimotor integration within the context of meaningful interactions with persons and objects.[196] Children may propel themselves prone on a scooter board through an "obstacle maze" while looking for matching shapes, for example. This activity provides tactile, proprioceptive, and vestibular sensory input and encourages the development of postural strength and endurance while addressing perceptual skill development.

Research on Sensorimotor Intervention. Sensorimotor intervention is a widely accepted modality, used by 92% of school-based therapists as a foundation for improving handwriting.[199] The activities used and goals addressed in treatment are extremely varied, as all functional motor skills involve some level of sensory and motor organization. Activities can range from horseback riding to using a vibrating pen when learning how to write letters. Owing to the enormous variation in intervention strategies and outcome measures, operationalizing treatment to make comparisons between research studies can be difficult. In a recent systematic review Polatajko and Cantin[194] found five studies that met their criteria for using sensorimotor intervention. In those five studies both the techniques used (e.g., therapeutic riding, movement therapy, educational kinesiology) and the populations addressed (autism, sensory modulation disorder, DCD) varied greatly. This review suggested that evidence for the effectiveness of sensorimotor intervention was "inconclusive," with the heterogeneity of diagnoses and functional problems limiting the ability to interpret efficacy.[194]

Overall, relatively few studies have investigated the efficacy of sensorimotor integration. In an early comparison study, DeGangi and colleagues[200] found that children provided with structured sensorimotor therapy made greater gains in sensory integrative foundations, gross motor skills, and performance areas such as self-care than children who engaged in child-centered activity. More recently, Chia and Chua[201] used sensorimotor intervention in a random controlled study of 14 children with learning disabilities and DCD. Intervention consisted of providing sensory stimuli and facilitating a normal motor response while remediating impairments in posture and muscle weakness. Positive results in neuromotor functioning were noted. In a second study, Inder and Sullivan[202] used educational kinesiology techniques in four single-subject design experiments. Positive gains were documented in some aspects of sensory organization and in an overall decrease in the number of falls children had.

Four studies have explored the effects of sensorimotor remediation on handwriting. Those programs that used sensorimotor interventions over only a short period of time did not yield positive results. Sudsawad and colleagues[203] compared the effects of kinesthetic-based intervention with handwriting practice with 45 first graders over a 4-week period. They found neither group to make significant improvements in handwriting, and suggest that there is no support that kinesthetic training improves handwriting legibility for this age. In 2006, Denton and colleagues[204] compared sensorimotor intervention with therapeutic practice in 38 school-age children with handwriting difficulties over 5 weeks. These authors noted moderate improvements in handwriting with therapeutic practice and a decline in ability in the sensorimotor group. They suggest that although sensorimotor foundations did improve with sensorimotor intervention, there is no indication that these foundations affect the development of handwriting. Their findings suggest that structured therapeutic practice using motor learning principles has a much stronger impact on the development of handwriting.

Two studies that investigated the combined effects of sensorimotor intervention and higher-level teaching strategies did demonstrate a positive impact on handwriting.[205,206] Peterson and Nelson[205] found that low socioeconomic first graders who received 20 sessions of occupational therapy combining sensorimotor, biomechanical, and teaching-learning strategies made significant gains over those receiving academic instruction alone. Weintraub and colleagues[206] compared a control group with two treatment conditions (task-oriented approach versus combination of sensorimotor and task orientation). Immediately after treatment, and at a 4-month follow-up, significant gains in handwriting were observed in both treatment groups compared with the control group. The authors support the use of "higher-level" teaching strategies to improve the skill of handwriting.

Motor Skill Training

Motor skill training involves learning skills and subskills functionally relevant to the child's daily performance. Tasks are taught in a sequential manner by developmental ages or by steps from simple to complex. Skill training can occur for a wide variety of gross, fine, and visual motor tasks, as well as activities of daily living. An assortment of theoretical models and techniques may be used based on the child's impairment and activity and participation deficits.

Motor skill training can involve both indirect and direct facilitation of specific motor tasks. Activities that include balance, locomotion, body awareness, and hand-eye coordination can improve functional skills such as being able to sit at a desk within the classroom and complete written work, as well as success in recess games such as basketball. Specific skills such as dribbling and foul shooting can also be specifically taught and practiced. The goal is to provide a great variety of motor activities at the child's developmental motor level to promote motor generalizations for more successful participation.

An example of this approach is Sugden and Henderson's[145] "ecological intervention," which is a method of skill training for children with DCD. In this model the therapist, called a *movement coach,* provides instruction to many individuals who interact with the child on how to develop specific targeted skills. All caregivers are actively involved in goal development and achievement. By having a variety of individuals work together across daily life environments, children more quickly become skilled.[145] This approach also develops the caregivers' ability to understand the demands of specific tasks and to help facilitate the child's performance in all settings.

Physical Fitness Training

As previously reviewed, children with DCD are at great risk of low levels of physical fitness. The benefits of fitness and physical activity in minimizing disease and maximizing overall wellness are well documented. Deleterious effects resulting from DCD or factors associated with it include but are not limited to fatigue, hypoactivity, poor muscle strength and endurance, decreased flexibility, poor speed and agility, and diminished power.

Specific muscular training may be needed to undo the effects of reduced activity.[207] Poor muscle strength, especially in the abdominal area, can lead to musculoskeletal issues such as back pain because posture and pelvic alignment require adequate muscle strength. Children with DCD often require specific instruction to perform muscle strengthening activities (e.g., sit-ups, push-ups) with appropriate form. Decreased flexibility and muscle tightness in the lower extremities can contribute to difficulties in running, jumping, and hopping. Flexibility can be encouraged with a regimen of stretches specific to the areas of tightness. Gentle and regular stretching can be incorporated into warmups during sessions or physical activities.

Fitness can improve and be maintained when children participate in regular, preferably daily, physical activity. These activities often require more structure and direction for children with movement difficulties. As therapists, our overall goal should be to educate children about the value and enjoyment of regular activity.[207] Hands and Larkin[207] suggest the following plan to ensure children with DCD learn or rediscover the joy of movement:

- Educate children to understand and monitor their bodies' responses to exercising (e.g., heart rate increases when they run).
- Assist them in finding developmentally appropriate activities they will enjoy with some success.
- Encourage them to maintain a healthy, active lifestyle by encouraging participation in lifelong activities such as swimming, cycling, golf, sailing, yoga, or weight training.

In sports and leisure activities, the emphasis should be on participation and fitness rather than competition. Encourage activities that do not require constant adaptation, as children with DCD tend to be more successful in sports that have a repetitive nature to the movements (e.g., swimming, running, skating, skiing).[135,207] Sports that have a high degree of spatial challenge or unpredictability, such as baseball, hockey, football, and basketball, are less likely to be successful for children with DCD.[208] Activities that are taught through sequential verbal guidance, such as karate, may be easier to learn.[135]

PTs and OTs can have a positive impact on participation in fitness activities for children with DCD. A summary of key suggestions,[83] including the following, can assist with encouraging involvement in community sports and leisure activities:

- Provide frequent encouragement and reward effort.
- Encourage participation, rather than competition; emphasize fun, fitness, and skill building.
- Use a variety of teaching methods to demonstrate new skills (one-on-one instruction, verbal cues, demonstration).
- Provide hand-over-hand instruction during the early acquisition phase.
- Break down skills into smaller, meaningful parts.
- Keep the environment as predictable as possible.
- Modify or adapt equipment for safety (e.g., use foam balls instead of hard balls).
- Focus on the enjoyment, not the product.
- Encourage multiple roles in some activities (e.g., referee, scorekeeper, time keeper).
- Recognize the child's strengths, and reinforce social interaction.

Encouraging and facilitating participation in a healthy lifestyle can aid in ending the vicious cycle of withdrawal, diminished opportunities for physical development, and decreased fitness and strength over time, a pattern very commonly seen in children with DCD.[83]

LEARNING DISABILITIES AND DEVELOPMENTAL COORDINATION DISORDER ACROSS THE LIFE SPAN

Learning disabilities persist into adulthood and present lifelong challenges. Continuing issues with attention, cognition, emotional adjustment, and interpersonal skills can affect education, employment, family life, and daily routines. Adolescents and adults with learning disabilities frequently struggle with the concentration and organization needed to effectively manage daily routines and finances, vocational education or training, job procurement and retention, and finances.[209,210]

A recent longitudinal study[211] demonstrated that IQ scores remain stable from childhood to adulthood, as do deficit areas. Therefore, poor readers remain poor readers, poor spellers remain poor spellers, and delayed math skills persist. In addition, adults who had affective illness or mood disorders as children have a significant risk of recurrent episodes (e.g., depression, bipolar disorder). An early 20-year longitudinal study of individuals with learning disabilities cited a rate of 42% for adult psychological disturbance (e.g., depression, alcohol abuse, anxiety disorders), compared with 10% in the general population.[212]

More recently, Seo and colleagues[213] found more optimistic results in their comparison of outcomes for individuals age 21 and 24, with and without documented learning disabilities. No significant differences were found in postsecondary school achievement or employment rates and earned income, although the 21-year-olds with learning disabilities did receive significantly more public aid, such as food stamps, social security, and unemployment. The learning-disabled group did not have increased incidence of committing crimes or feeling victimized as young adults. Emotional health[211] and strong social relationships[214] are crucial for success; therefore children should be supported to develop healthy social connections and personal talents.

Several attributes have been identified as predictors of success for adults with learning disabilities.[212,215] A combination of internal and external factors supports the individual in the belief that he or she can take control, evaluate needs, and develop appropriate coping strategies, while knowing when to seek additional help.[215] The ability to be proactive, set goals, and persevere is a key internal element to attaining success. Having an understanding of one's learning disability, with recognition of strengths and limitations, affords more thoughtful choices in life roles. Self-esteem and confidence are promoted with external emotional support and positive feedback from family, friends, teachers, work colleagues, and employers.

The persistent motor coordination difficulties attributed to DCD further affect perceptions of competence[89,216] and successful accomplishment of daily life skills.[217] Raskind and colleagues[212] found that physical status, including motor impairment, was an important variable in determining success in adulthood. Slowness and variability in movement continue to be a pervasive feature, causing difficulties in tasks that require sequencing and dual-task performance, such as driving a car.[217] Adults with DCD report higher levels of difficulty with motor-related tasks such as self-care and handwriting.[218] Compared with adults with dyslexia, a greater number of adults with DCD continue to live at home with their parents, have fewer spare-time activities, and are more socially isolated.[218,219]

Learning disabilities with motor impairments appear to have a persistent effect on a sense of competence and self-concept.[8,219] Many individuals develop negative perceptions of themselves as they experience frustration and ineffectiveness. They set lower aspirations, further reinforcing the cycle of failure. A combination of ADHD and DCD was found to be the most important predictor of poor psychosocial functioning in early adulthood.[220] Higher incidence of drug and alcohol abuse, affective disorders, crime conviction, and unemployment have been documented. Without adequate support, adults with DCD have difficulties reaching their potential. They may benefit from counseling about their condition, vocational assessment and guidance to assist with finding a suitable work environment, time management and organizational strategies, workplace and academic accommodations, and behavioral management.

These cycles of ineptitude, frustration, and poor self-concept are highlighted in Case Study 14-2. Paul's mother, Mrs. B., was not diagnosed with learning disabilities until age 20 years. Nevertheless, she completed both bachelor's and master's degrees in counseling. Although the academic frustrations are no longer an issue, the learning disability continues to interfere with her work and home performance. Mrs. B. describes her organizational difficulties and identifies a continuous need to make lists to function in her job. She concentrates on not looking "clumsy" and is fearful she will trip over things and look foolish. Learning and accomplishing tasks continue to require increased effort compared with her peers. Thus even in adulthood the learning disability continues to present difficulty in functional performance.

A letter from a woman with learning disabilities, motor coordination impairments, and sensory integration problems is included in Box 14-3. She describes how her learning disability affects her current functioning and how it affected her when she was a child.

BOX 14-3 ■ A LETTER FROM AN ADULT WITH A LEARNING DISABILITY

I am 26 years old, a professional bassoonist with a master's degree in music performance. My name is Wendy. Through Jane, an occupational therapist, I discovered when I was 24 years old that I had learning problems and sensory integration problems.

I invert letters and especially numbers. When people speak English to me, I feel it's a foreign language. There's translation lag time. When learning new things, I either understand intuitively or never. I can't seem to go through step-by-step learning processes.

Physically, I'm extremely sensitive to motion. When I was little, we moved every year. I spent the first 5 years of my life feeling sick. It seems that I feel everything more strongly than most people. I have an extremely low threshold of pain, and even pleasure tends to overload me. If I am touched unexpectedly it hurts, it's so jarring. This causes a lot of problems with interpersonal relationships. I can't stand to have people close to me; it produces an adrenalin reaction.

Motor activities are also a problem; my muscles don't seem to remember past motions. Despite the many times I've walked down steps and through doors, I still have to think about how high to lift my foot and about planning my movements. When eating, I have to think about chewing or I bite my tongue or mouth. I don't think other people think about these things. I'm physically inept; I can bump into the same table 10 times running. I'm always bruised, and as a child people constantly labeled me as clumsy. Physical education courses were hell as a child, especially gymnastics, where you are forced to leave the ground and swing or walk on balance beams or uneven bars. I cannot begin to explain the terror or disorientation.

Academically, I was labeled stupid or, more frequently, lazy. I was told that I was not trying. Actually, my IQ is high and my coping mechanisms are complex. If they only knew how hard I was trying. I was lucky because I taught myself to read at an early age. I would never have learned to read otherwise. Even so, my first grade teacher wouldn't believe that I could read so far past my age. She called me a liar when I said that I had finished each "Dick and Jane" book. I was forced to read each one 50 times before she would give me a new one.

Not all teachers were so insensitive. My fourth grade teacher made every effort to let me go at my own pace, letting me read on a college level and do 2 years of math on my own. Left to my own devices, I can learn and love to do so. My fifth grade teacher forced me to do math the long way with steps. I just know the answer by looking at multiplication or division problems, even algebra problems, but to this day I cannot understand how one does it in steps. If a teacher didn't accept this, I was in for a year of hell. I cried a lot in school, from frustration mostly, and I pretended to be sick a lot.

I never had friends until college. I guess I was too different to be acceptable. I grew up in a rigid, repressive, religious community, which made it especially difficult to be accepted. My differences were labeled evil, or, at best, I was ignored. I left high school at age 16 for college, where at least I could structure what I wanted to learn. It's never been easy for me to make friends, although it's better now. Music circles tend to be a bit crazy so I fit in more easily.

My learning disabilities still are problems. My motor and learning problems get in the way of my music, but my coping mechanisms are strong. I deal better with my clumsiness now. Just being diagnosed by Jane has made a big difference. To have things labeled, to be told and realize that it's not my fault, has given me a sense of peace. It's also allowed me to turn from inward depression to outward anger at those who labeled me stupid and clumsy. Just being able to admit anger allows one to let it go.

Other than my testing and subsequent conversations with Jane, I have not received treatment for my problems. I believe that adults with my problems can be helped. I wish programs were available in all areas of the country. At age 26, I feel much better about myself than I did even at age 24. It's a matter of growth and coping with major differences.

The greatest advice I would give to educators and therapists working with problem children is to accept. Accept what they can do well; don't make an issue of what they can't do. We all have our strengths and weaknesses. If a child can't do math, so what! Buy the child a calculator and the child will do a lot better with it than with a label of stupidity following her through life.

SUMMARY

Learning disabilities are heterogeneous and multidimensional in their presentation. Research continues to work on identifying the causes and the associated functional deficits of learning disabilities, as well as developing effective intervention techniques. The variability of the group suggests a spectrum of neurological processing difficulties. As physiological measures of brain function improve, our theoretical understanding increases.

Assessment and teaching methods continue to be refined to identify underlying deficits and effective remediation strategies. The current trend is to recognize issues inherent in the child (i.e., a true learning disability) versus issues from inadequate or ineffective instruction. Early identification of difficulties and systematic alteration of instruction methods are advocated to serve students more quickly and efficiently. The challenge for the clinician is to recognize the multitude of components that interact to impede functional abilities and social participation for the child with learning disabilities.

Children with learning disabilities frequently manifest motor coordination problems. These motor deficits may be subtle and difficult to identify in a neurological evaluation or standardized testing. With better awareness and assessment measures, more children are being identified and diagnosed with DCD. Many theoretical models have been developed in an attempt to explain the qualitative motor deficits observed in children with learning disabilities as well as provide constructs to develop intervention programs. Continued formal research and careful documentation of clinical outcomes are needed to synthesize therapeutic approaches that best meet the individual needs of the child.

Identification, advocacy, teaching, and remediation are important aspects of the OT's and PT's roles. The goal is to formulate an intervention program that best addresses the underlying deficits in foundation skills and the functional weaknesses in daily life tasks. The experienced interventionist will combine knowledge from many areas of theoretical development and remediation to facilitate the best performance in each child.

It is clear that learning disabilities and DCD both persist across the life span and can have a multitude of detrimental effects. All areas of daily life performance can be affected, including social and emotional functioning, self-care, education, vocation, and interpersonal relationships. Both intrinsic factors (perseverance, insight, sense of control) and extrinsic factors (emotional support, mentoring, positive feedback) play a role in the ultimate success of the individual with learning and motor challenges. Our role as a pediatric therapist is to provide the necessary extrinsic support and effective intervention to alleviate the deleterious effects of living with a disability.

References

To enhance this text and add value for the reader, all references are included on the companion Evolve site that accompanies this textbook. This online service will, when available, provide a link for the reader to a Medline abstract for the article cited. There are 234 cited references and other general references for this chapter, with the majority of those articles being evidence-based citations.

APPENDIX 14-A ■ A Summary of Standardized Motor Tests

Bruininks-Oseretsky Test of Motor Proficiency, Second Edition (BOT-2) (2005)[111]

Authors

Robert H. Bruininks, PhD and Brett D. Bruininks, PhD

Source

American Guidance Service, Inc., Circle Pines, MN 55014

Ages

4 to 21 years

Administration

Individual. Complete form: 45 minutes to 1 hour. Short form: 15 to 20 minutes.

Equipment

Test kit needed

Description

The Bruininks-Oseretsky Test of Motor Proficiency–2 is the most recent revision of the Oseretsky Tests of Motor Proficiency, first published in Russia in 1923. The Bruininks-Oseretsky Test is designed to provide information on a wide range of motor skills and is sensitive enough to identify mild to moderate motor control problems. In this revision the authors worked to improve the test item presentation, quality of the test kit, and functional relevance of test content. They also expanded the norms through age 21 and improved the test items for 4- to 5-year-olds. The BOT-2 yields standard scores, scaled scores, and percentile ranks, separately for males and females, and combined. Age equivalency scores are also available. The test assesses motor functioning in eight areas:

1. Fine Motor Precision: Functionally relevant drawing, paper folding, and cutting item that focuses on assessment of precise finger control. These items are untimed and they focus on qualitative refinement.
2. Fine Motor Integration: Copying geometric shapes of increasing complexity as accurately as possible. These items are untimed, as they focus on precision.
3. Manual Dexterity: Goal-directed activities that involve reaching, grasping, and bimanual coordination with small objects (pennies, pegboard, card sorting, and stringing beads). Emphasis is placed on speed and accuracy (dexterity), and all items are timed.
4. Bilateral Coordination: Items that measure skill in sequential and simultaneous coordination of the upper and lower extremities. Includes both familiar tasks (e.g., jumping jacks and finger pivots ["itsy-bitsy spider"]), as well as novel tasks (e.g., tapping feet and fingers with opposite sides of the body).
5. Balance: Static and dynamic balance items measure motor control for maintaining posture when standing, walking, and making transitional movements in space (e.g., reaching for a plate on a shelf). Assesses three areas that affect balance: trunk stability, static and dynamic postural control, and use of visual cues.
6. Running Speed and Agility: Four activities to assess speed and agility (shuttle run, hopping on one and both feet, stepping over balance beam).
7. Upper-Limb Coordination: Items that involve visual tracking and coordinated hand and arm movements (eye-hand coordination). Tasks include catching, throwing, and dribbling, with one or both hands together.
8. Strength: Assesses trunk and upper and lower extremity strength necessary for effective gross motor performance in daily activities.

Construction and Reliability

The Bruininks-Oseretsky Test has been carefully standardized on 1520 subjects from 38 states, stratified across sex, ethnicity, socioeconomic, and disability status. Sample sizes were larger in the younger age ranges, as children develop more rapidly than adolescents. Three measures of reliability were determined for subtests, composites, short form, and complete form: internal consistency, test-retest, and interrater. In general all were high, with best reliability shown when the complete form was used.

Comment

The Bruininks-Oseretsky Test of Motor Proficiency–2 appears to be one of the better standardized tests of motor performance. The 1978 version has been one of the most widely used tests to assess motor proficiency and has been used in research to identify motor deficits in individuals with DCD.[221,222] It offers various levels of testing and screening with a comprehensive "complete form" that provides the most reliable measure of overall motor proficiency. The short form can be used for screening, to determine if further evaluation is necessary. In addition, only those single subtests or composites that are relevant to the child's areas of difficulty can be administered. When qualifying a student for special education, it is suggested that this thorough assessment be used. In this revision the authors focused on including a variety of tasks that are engaging and goal directed, assessing both quantitative and qualitative aspects of motor performance. When testing children with motor dysfunction, careful attention must be paid to qualitative performance on individual items. A child may demonstrate the ability to complete a test item, but qualitatively it is accomplished with increased effort, decreased refinement, and speed.

Movement Assessment Battery for Children (Movement ABC-2) (2007)[114]

Authors

Sheila E. Henderson, David A. Sugden, and Anna L. Barnett

Source

Harcourt Assessment, Proctor House, 1 Proctor Street, London, WC1V6EU

Ages

3 to 16 years

Administration

Individual; 20 to 30 minutes

Equipment

Test kit required

Description

The Movement ABC-2 is a recent revision of the M-ABC, which was originally developed from the Test of Motor Impairment (TOMI)–Henderson Revision. The Movement ABC-2 is a norm-based assessment of gross and fine motor performance whose main intent is to identify and describe children with movement difficulties. The test was also designed for intervention planning, program evaluation, and research. There are three components of the Movement ABC-2: the standardized evaluation, a checklist of competency in specific daily motor behaviors, and a companion manual for program planning (Ecological Approach to Intervention).[145] The evaluation tool yields standard and percentile scores, with two determined cut-off points delineating definite movement difficulties and children at risk. The age ranges have been expanded, and the test is divided into three age brackets: children aged 3 to 6 years, 7 to 10 years, and 11 to 16 years. The test items vary in each age range, with increased complexity and skill required in the older age

Continued

APPENDIX 14-A ■ A Summary of Standardized Motor Tests—cont'd

bands. There are eight tasks assessing three areas of coordination: manual dexterity, ball skills, and static and dynamic balance.

1. Manual Dexterity: Speed and dexterity with the preferred hand. Includes two manipulative tasks such as coins in a bank, stringing beads, pegs in a pegboard, threading lace, and turning pegs and nuts and bolts, as well as a written maze.
2. Ball Skills: Eye-hand coordination is assessed with two beanbag and ball tasks emphasizing aiming at a target and catching.
3. Static and Dynamic Balance: One task of static balance with eyes open, and two tasks of dynamic balance that emphasize spatial precision and control of momentum.

Construction and Reliability

The standardization sample included 1172 children in the United Kingdom. A stratified sampling was done to ensure that representative proportions of age, gender, race and ethnicity, and parent educational level were included. Before the main study, testing was done around the world and revealed no culture-specific problems. The researchers consider this revision to be similar enough to the M-ABC that the studies employed with that test remain relevant. Test-retest reliability for consistency of individual item scores fell within a range deemed acceptable, from 0.64 to 0.86. The mean of 0.77 was achieved for the test as a whole. Interrater reliability was excellent, exceeding 0.95.

Comment

This revision is the culmination of a lengthy program of research and development begun in 1966 by two groups of researchers. The Movement ABC-2 offers some additional advantages: (1) the checklist helps teachers identify children with movement problems; (2) information is provided for a cognitive-motor approach to intervention across environments. The test items are easy to administer and score. Although the manual provides a clear picture of what the task looks like, there are no standardized verbal instructions given in this revision. Scoring is based on a traffic light system, with the red zone (at or below 5th percentile) indicating significant movement difficulty, amber zone (6th to 15th percentile) delineating children at risk, and the green zone (above 15th percentile) indicating the absence of movement difficulties. Percentile scores are useful for parents and teachers because they are easily understood, but therapists should recognize that they do not form an equal interval scale, tending to cluster near the median of the normal curve. Therefore for subtest raw scores near the median, a change of 1 point to the raw score could result in an increase of 8 percentile points, whereas at either end of the normal curve this might only translate to 2 percentile points.

Peabody Developmental Motor Scales, Second Edition (PDMS-2) (2000)[113]

Authors

M. Rhonda Folio and Rebecca R. Fewell

Source

Pro-Ed, 8700 Shoal Creek Boulevard, Austin, TX 78757

Ages

Birth to 5 years

Administration

40 to 60 minutes (test items may be scored by direct observation or by parent or teacher report)

Description

An early childhood motor development program that provides, in one package, both in-depth assessment and training or remediation of gross and fine motor skills. The assessment is composed of six subtests that measure interrelated motor abilities that develop early in life. The PDMS-2 can be used by OTs, PTs, diagnosticians, early intervention specialists, adapted physical education teachers, psychologists, and others who are interested in examining the motor abilities of young children. The PDMS was designed for use with children who show delay or disability in fine and gross motor skills. Test items are similar to those on other developmental scales, but only motor items are included. Items are scored on a 3-point scale: 0 for unsuccessful, 1 for partial, and 2 for successful performance. Age-equivalent scores, motor quotients, percentile rankings, and standard scores are provided. Scoring software for the PDMS-2 is available to convert the PDMS-2 scores into standard scores, percentile ranks, and age equivalents and generate composite quotients. The software also can be used to compare PDMS-2 subtest performances and composite performances to identify intraindividual differences and provide a printed report of the student information, including treatment goals and objectives.

Subtests

1. Reflexes: This eight-item subtest measures a child's ability to automatically react to environmental events. Because reflexes typically become integrated by the time a child is 12 months old, this subtest is given only to children from birth through 11 months.
2. Stationary: This 30-item subtest measures a child's ability to sustain control of his or her body within its center of gravity and retain equilibrium.
3. Locomotion: This 89-item subtest measures a child's ability to move from one place to another. The actions measured include crawling, walking, running, hopping, and jumping forward.
4. Object manipulation: This 24-item subtest measures a child's ability to manipulate balls. Examples of the actions measured include catching, throwing, and kicking. Because these skills are not apparent until a child has reached the age of 11 months, this subtest is given only to children aged 12 months and older.
5. Grasping: This 26-item subtest measures a child's ability to use his or her hands. It begins with the ability to hold an object with one hand and progresses up to actions involving the controlled use of the fingers of both hands.
6. Visual-motor integration: This 72-item subtest measures a child's ability to use his or her visual perceptual skills to perform complex eye-hand coordination tasks such as reaching and grasping for an object, building with blocks, and copying designs.

Composites

1. Gross Motor Quotient: This composite is a combination of results on the subtests that measure the use of the large muscle systems:
   - Reflexes (birth to 11 months only)
   - Stationary (all ages)
   - Locomotion (all ages)
   - Object manipulation (12 months and older)
2. Fine Motor Quotient: This composite is a combination of results on the subtests that measure the use of the small muscle systems:
   - Grasping (all ages)
   - Visual-motor integration (all ages)
3. Total Motor Quotient: This composite is formed by a combination of results on the gross and fine motor subtests. Because of this, it is the best estimate of overall motor abilities.

APPENDIX 14-A ■ A Summary of Standardized Motor Tests—cont'd

Construction and Reliability

Reliability coefficients were computed for subgroups of the normative sample (e.g., individuals with motor disabilities, African Americans, Hispanic Americans, girls, and boys) as well as for the entire normative sample. The normative sample consisted of 2003 persons residing in 46 states and was collected in the winter of 1997 and spring of 1998. Normative samples relative to geography, sex, race, and other critical variables are therefore representative of the current U.S. population.

A test-retest reliability of 0.84 for the Gross Motor Scale and of 0.73 for the Fine Motor Scale (0.89 Total Motor) was reported based on a sample of 30 children from Austin, Texas, in the age range of 2 to 11 months. A second group of 30 children from Nacogdoches, Texas, ages 12 to 17 months, were tested with a test-retest reliability of 0.93 for the Gross Motor Scale and 0.94 for the Fine Motor Scale (0.96 Total Motor). These values are of sufficient magnitude for a tester's confidence in the test scores' stability over a period of time. The correlation coefficients between the PDMS and the PDMS-2 for criterion-prediction validity in the Gross and Fine Motor Quotients exceed 0.80, which supports the equivalency of the tests.

The PDMS-2 scores were correlated with those of the Mullen Scales of Early Learning: AGS Edition (MSEL:A) when both tests were administered on the same day to 29 children, aged 2 months to 66 months, in Evansville, Indiana. The relations of the PDMS-2 and MSEL:A demonstrated that Gross and Fine Motor Quotients exceed 0.80, high enough to support the equivalency of the tests. When the concurrent validity of the age equivalent and standard scores of the Bayley Scales of Infant Development II (BSID-II) Motor Scale and PDMS-2 were calculated, the standard scores show poor agreement and had low concurrent validity, particularly the BSID-II Motor Scale and the PDMS-2 Locomotion Subscale.[223] The differences in the scores of these two tests warrant concern when using one test to make clinical decisions for service eligibility.

Comment

The PDMS-2 is primarily useful for children with mild to moderate motor deficits, such as a child with learning disabilities or a child with developmental delay. The test does not discriminate among children with moderate to severe motor disability because they fall far below the standard scores given. The skill categories are unevenly distributed and have too few items at some age levels to be meaningful. Despite the drawbacks, the PDMS-2 is probably the most valuable motor scale test currently available for preschool children.

Clinical Observations of Motor and Postural Skills, Second Edition (COMPS) (2000)[126]

Authors

Brenda N. Wilson, MS, OT(C), Nancy Pollock, MSc, OT(C), Brenda Kaplan, PhD, and Mary Law, PhD, OT(C)

Source

Therapro Inc., 225 Arlington Street, Framingham, MA 01702

Ages

5 to 11 years

Administration

Individual; 15 to 20 minutes

Equipment

Test kit required for ATNR measurement tools. Stopwatch and mat needed for certain items.

Description

The COMPS is a standardized screening tool using six clinical observations suggested by Ayres[99,224] of "soft neurological signs" to identify motor problems with a postural component. Historically, the clinical observations used by therapists have not had standardized administration or objective scoring and they have not taken into account the child's age and changes in abilities as the child matures. The authors felt it was important to objectify these observations and relate performance to age, as neuromotor maturation is very rapid in this age group. The test is designed to measure cerebellar function, postural control (stability), and motor coordination (mobility). Motor planning and sequencing are not intended to be measured directly, and repetition of directions, therapist prompting, and item practice are meant to separate motor performance from the cognitive aspects of planning. The test has six test items:

1. Slow Movements: Assesses the ability to move arms in a slow and symmetrical manner. Scoring is based on quality of performance, speed, and symmetry.
2. Rapid Forearm Rotation: A test of diadochokinesis; score is based on the number of forearm rotations accurately completed in 10 seconds.
3. Finger-Nose Touching: Measures proprioceptive mechanisms of motor control by switching midtask from eyes open to eyes closed. Scoring is based on accuracy, fluidity of motion, and force of touch.
4. Prone Extension Posture: The child holds a position of extension against gravity. Scoring is based on the duration of ability to hold position, quality of extension, and effort.
5. Asymmetrical Tonic Neck Reflex: The degree of inhibition of this reflex is looked at by measuring elbow flexion with manual head turn in a quadruped position. This test is also useful for identifying poor postural stability through observations including needing a wide base of support to sustain the position and locking elbows for stability.
6. Supine Flexion Posture: The child holds a position of flexion against gravity. Scoring is based on the duration of ability to hold position, quality of extension, and effort.

Construction and Reliability

Standardization of the test was done in two cities (Calgary and Hamilton) on a sample of 123 children, 67 who demonstrated DCD and 56 with no known motor problem. Test-retest reliability, interrater reliability, internal consistency, and construct validity were completed with a sample of 132 children with and without DCD. Test-retest reliability over 2 weeks was 0.98, and interrater reliability for pediatric OTs was 0.87. The internal consistency was high, indicating that the test discriminates well between children with and without motor problems, although the sample size was small.

Comment

The COMPS is a useful standardized tool for identifying subtle motor problems in children and was designed for and tested on children with DCD. The COMPS was not designed for children with known neurological or neuromotor problems such as intellectual delay, cerebral palsy, or epilepsy. It can be used as a screening tool for motor dysfunction, to assist in determining intervention approaches that would be beneficial for the child, and possibly to measure change over time. Children with motor performance problems can score within normal limits on the COMPS, and children who demonstrate low scores may not be exhibiting functional difficulties. The association between these clinical observations and functional performance is not always clear; therefore it is essential to gather information regarding the child's current functioning from observation and interview.

Continued

APPENDIX 14-A ■ A Summary of Standardized Motor Tests—cont'd

Miller Assessment for Preschoolers (MAP) (1988)[127]

Author

Lucy Jane Miller, PhD

Source

Psychological Corporation, 555 Academic Court, San Antonio, TX 78204-0952

Ages

2 years, 9 months to 5 years, 8 months

Administration

Individual; 20 to 30 minutes, including scoring

Equipment

The MAP Test Kit

Description

The MAP was designed to identify preschool children who exhibit mild to moderate developmental delays. The MAP is a developmental assessment intended for use by educational and clinical personnel to identify children in need of further evaluation and remediation. It can also be used to provide a comprehensive, clinical framework that would be helpful in defining a child's strengths and weaknesses and that would indicate possible avenues of remediation. The test is composed of 27 items and a series of structured observations. The test items are divided into five performance indexes:

1. Foundations: Items generally found on standard neurological examinations and sensory integrative and neurodevelopmental tests
2. Coordination: Gross, fine, and oral motor abilities and articulation
3. Verbal: Cognitive language abilities, including memory, sequencing, comprehension, association, following directions, and expression
4. Nonverbal: Cognitive abilities such as visual figure-ground, puzzles, memory, and sequencing
5. Complex Tasks: Tasks requiring an interaction of sensory, motor, and cognitive abilities

Construction and Reliability

The MAP has been well standardized on a random sample of 1200 preschool children. The sample was stratified by age, race, sex, size of residence, community, and socioeconomic factors. Data were collected nationwide in each of nine U.S. Census Bureau regions. Reported reliabilities are good. In a test-retest on 90 children, 81% of the children's scores remained stable. The coefficient of internal consistency on the total sample was 0.798. Interrater reliability on 40 children was reported as 0.98.

Comment

The MAP was developed by an OT and provides information that is of particular relevance to therapists. It is carefully standardized and fills a need for early identification of learning and motor deficits in children. Several articles have been published supporting the validity of this test as a screening instrument.[225-228] Reviews of the MAP in the *Ninth Mental Measurements Yearbook* have described it as "the best available screening test for identifying preschool children with moderate preacademic problems"[229] and "an extremely promising instrument which should find wide use among clinical psychologists, school psychologists, and OTs in assessing mild to moderate learning disabilities in preschool children."[230] A more complete review of this test is provided by King-Thomas and Hacker.[231]

FirstSTEP (Screening Test for Evaluating Preschoolers) (1993)[130]

Author

Lucy J. Miller, PhD

Source

Psychological Corporation, 555 Academic Court, San Antonio, TX 78204-0952

Ages

2 years, 9 months to 6 years, 2 months

Administration

Individual; 15 minutes

Equipment

Test kit

Description

The FirstSTEP is a quick screening test for identifying developmental delays in all five areas defined by IDEA and mandated by PL 99-457: cognition, communication, physical, social-emotional, and adaptive functioning. Twelve subtests assess cognitive, communication, and motor domains. An optional Social-Emotional Scale includes 25 items from five areas (task confidence, cooperative mood, temperament and emotionality, uncooperative antisocial behavior, and attention communication difficulties) that are scored on the basis of behaviors observed by the examiner during the test session. The Adaptive Behavior Checklist is an optional measure completed by parent interview to assess the child's self-help and adaptive living skills. The Parent/Teacher Scale provides additional information about the child's typical behavior.

Cognitive Domain

1. Money Game (quantitative reasoning): The child is asked a series of questions about coins, regarding quantity, amount, comparisons, size, and numeration. This subtest requires cognitive understanding of simple arithmetic concepts.
2. What's Missing? Game (picture completion): The child is asked to identify what is missing from the pictures of common objects or events by naming or pointing. This subtest measures visual figure-ground as well as gestalt closure abilities.
3. Which Way? Game (visual position in space): The child is asked to look at a stimulus figure that is turned in a specific direction. The child then selects the response figure that matches. This subtest measures visual discrimination and the ability to perceive directionality visually.
4. Put Together Game (problem solving): The child is asked to select the pieces that best fit a certain space. The subtest requires abstract thinking.

Language Domain

1. Listen Game (auditory discrimination): This two-part activity requires the child to listen as the examiner names and points to three similar-sounding pictures. Then the child chooses the pictures that represent the words. The second part requires the child to discriminate between words that are the same and words that are different. This task taps phoneme discrimination and requires good auditory processing skills.
2. How Many Can You Say? Game (word retrieval): The child's linguistic fluency and word-finding skills are measured by asking the child to count, recall animals, and recite rhyming words.
3. Finish Up Game (association): The child is asked to complete a phrase that is initiated by the examiner. The subtest requires the child to demonstrate an understanding of the association between concepts (e.g., big and little).
4. Copy Me Game (sentence and digit repetition): The child is asked to repeat a series of meaningful verbal stimuli and then a series of numbers. This subtest measures verbal memory, grammatical abilities, and verbal expression skills.

APPENDIX 14-A ■ A Summary of Standardized Motor Tests—cont'd

Motor Domain

1. Drawing Game (visual-motor integration): The child is presented with paper and pencil tasks. This subtest requires the integration of fine motor and visual-perceptual abilities.
2. Things with Strings Game (fine motor planning): The child is asked to perform a series of motor movements with the upper extremities with a wooden cube and a string. These items tap the ability to plan and execute a series of motor actions and measure fine motor planning or praxis.
3. Statue Game (balance): The child is asked to assume a series of increasingly more difficult positions that require the child to balance with eyes open and vision occluded. The subtest taps the abilities needed to maintain equilibrium and screens for proprioception, vestibular perception, and visual processing difficulties.
4. Jumping Game (gross motor planning): The child is asked to imitate the examiner through a series of increasingly more difficult tasks that involve jumping in specific patterns. Gross motor and motor planning abilities are measured.

Construction and Reliability

The FirstSTEP is norm referenced and was standardized on 1433 children. Norms are provided in 6-month intervals for each of seven age groups. The standardization sample closely matches demographic characteristics provided by the U.S. Census Bureau. Scores are reported in standard scores as well as a three-category, color-coded risk status to indicate whether the child is functioning in the normal or delayed range. The FirstSTEP is a highly reliable instrument. Overall test reliability (split half) is 0.90, with individual domains ranging from 0.71 to 0.87. Test-retest reliability indicated a high degree of consistency in the classification of a child's performance across two test sessions (90% agreement for composite score; 85% to 93% for individual domain scores). Results also indicated a high level of interrater agreement ($r = 0.94$ on composite scores).

Validity studies of the FirstSTEP indicate that the FirstSTEP has good construct, content, and discriminant validity. Therefore it can effectively identify children with developmental delays. A study of 900 children demonstrated that children with delays perform 1.5 to 2 standard deviations below the mean in all domains. The results of a concurrent validity study suggest that the motor domain of the FirstSTEP measures constructs similar to those measured by the Bruininks-Oseretsky Test of Motor Proficiency and support the use of the motor domain of the FirstSTEP as an indicator of the child's motor functioning.

Comment

The FirstSTEP is an easy-to-administer test that is highly effective as a screening instrument. The FirstSTEP was developed by the OT who also developed the MAP (the Miller Assessment for Preschoolers), and like the MAP the test provides information that is of particular relevance to therapists. Although individual items on the FirstSTEP differ from the MAP, many are derived from the MAP, and the test is based on the same theoretical framework as the MAP. Area domains, social-emotional scales, and the adaptive behavior checklist from this tool can also be used in conjunction with other tests to provide additional information on the child's areas of strengths and weakness. A Spanish version, Primer Paso, is also available for use.

School Function Assessment (SFA) 1998[232]

Authors

Wendy Coster, PhD, OTR/L, Theresa Deeney, EdD, Jane Haltiwanger, PhD, and Stephen Haley, PhD, PT

Source

Pro-Ed, 8700 Shoal Creek Boulevard, Austin, TX 78757-6897
Website: www.proedinc.com

Ages

5 to 12 years

Administration

Individual; untimed. Individual scales may be completed in 5 to 10 minutes.

Equipment

Record form; rating scale guides

Description

The SFA is a judgment-based, criterion-referenced assessment to evaluate and monitor a student's performance on functional tasks that support school participation. This measure was designed to facilitate collaborative program planning for students with a variety of physical and cognitive disabilities. The SFA measures a student's ability to perform activities within the school setting that support participation in the academic and social aspects of an elementary program (grades K-6). Functional skills such as moving around the school, using classroom materials, interacting with peers, and caring for personal needs are included. The instrument is best completed by school professionals who are familiar with the student's typical performance. Task items are written in measurable, behavioral terms that can be used directly in the student's IEP. Criterion cut-off scores are provided for use in determining eligibility for special services. The SFA contains three parts:

1. Participation: Rates the student's involvement in six major school activity settings: regular or special education classroom, playground or recess, transportation, bathroom and toileting activities, transitions to and from class, and mealtime or snack time.
2. Task Supports: Identifies and rates the assistance and adaptations currently provided to the student for both physical and cognitive and behavioral tasks. Two types of task supports are examined separately: assistance (adult help) and adaptations (modifications to the environment or program, such as specialized equipment or adapted materials).
3. Activity Performance: Examines the student's performance of specific school-related functional activities. Physical Tasks include travel, maintaining and changing positions, recreational movement, manipulation with movement, using materials, setup and cleanup, eating and drinking, hygiene, clothing management, going up and down stairs, written work, and computer and equipment use. Cognitive/Behavioral Tasks include functional communication, memory and understanding, following social conventions, compliance with adult directives and school rules, task behavior and completion, positive interaction, behavior regulation, personal care awareness, and safety.

Construction and Reliability

A sample of 678 students in two groups participated in the standardization of SFA. One group included children with special needs (363 students). These students had a variety of disabilities, including motor impairment, communication impairment, emotional or behavioral difficulties, and cognitive limitations. The second group included 315 students in regular education programs. Internal consistency was excellent at 0.92 to 0.98, indicating that items in a scale relate to one another and measure the same construct. Test-retest reliability was 0.82 to 0.98.

Continued

APPENDIX 14-A ■ A Summary of Standardized Motor Tests—cont'd

Comment

This assessment is unique in its focus on activity and participation levels, versus identifying impairments. It helps school personnel recognize and ameliorate functional limitations that are affecting successful school participation. The comprehensiveness of assessment and functional IEP-ready goals makes it a useful tool to qualify and develop programs for children in need of special education services. Complete instructions are contained in the assessment booklet. Therefore the respondent does not need to refer to a manual to complete items, easing data collection. The manual is then used to compute transformed scores and interpret results.

The Sensory Integration and Praxis Tests (SIPT) (1989)[112]

Author

A. Jean Ayres

Source

Western Psychological Services, 12031 Wilshire Boulevard, Los Angeles, CA 90025

Ages

4 years to 8 years, 11 months

Administration

Individual; 2 hours; examiner certification required

Equipment

SIPT Test Kit

Description

The SIPT is a major revision and restandardization of the Southern California Sensory Integration Tests.[239] Four new tests of praxis were added, five tests underwent major revisions, eight tests underwent minor revisions, and four tests were deleted. The tests are designed to identify sensory integration and praxis deficits in children with learning disabilities. The 17 tests are described as follows:

1. Space Visualization: Select from two blocks the one that will fit into a form board. Mentally manipulating the forms is required to arrive at the correct choice on the more difficult test items.
2. Figure-Ground Perception: The child selects from six pictures the three that are superimposed or embedded with other forms on the test plates.
3. Manual Form Perception: Part I—A geometric form is held in the hand and the counterpart is selected from a visual display. Part II—A geometric form is felt with one hand while its match is selected from several choices with the other hand.
4. Kinesthesia: With vision occluded, the child attempts to place his or her finger on a point at which this finger had been placed previously by the examiner; a separate recording sheet is provided for each child.
5. Finger Identification: With hands screened from view, the examiner touches the child's finger, the shield is removed, and the child then points to the finger touched.
6. Graphesthesia: The examiner uses his or her finger to draw a design on the back of the child's hand without the child looking; the child then reproduces the design.
7. Localization of Tactile Stimuli: With vision occluded, the child touches the spot on his or her hand or arm that was touched by the examiner with a specially designed pen.
8. Praxis on Verbal Command: The examiner verbally describes a series of body movements, and the child executes them.
9. Design Copying: Part I—The child copies a design by connecting dots on a dot grid. Part II—The child copies a design without the use of a dot grid; both process and product are scored.
10. Constructional Praxis: Working with blocks, the child attempts to duplicate two different block structures. In the first structure, the child observes the examiner building the model; the second structure is preassembled.
11. Postural Praxis: The child imitates unusual body positions demonstrated by the examiner.
12. Oral Praxis: The child imitates movements of the tongue, lips, and jaw demonstrated by the examiner.
13. Sequencing Praxis: The child imitates a series of simple arm and hand movements demonstrated by the examiner.
14. Bilateral Motor Coordination: The child imitates a series of bilateral arm and foot movements demonstrated by the examiner.
15. Standing and Walking Balance: This subtest consists of 15 items in which the child assumes various standing and walking postures.
16. Motor Accuracy: The child traces a printed, curved black line with a red, nylon-tipped pen, first with the preferred hand and then with the nonpreferred hand.
17. Postrotatory Nystagmus: The child is rotated first counterclockwise and then clockwise on a rotation board; the duration of postrotatory nystagmus, a vestibulo-ocular reflex, is observed.

In addition to these 17 tests, a series of clinical observations aids in interpreting the SIPT. These clinical observations include the following:

- Eye dominance
- Eye movements
- Muscle tone
- Co-contraction
- Postural background movements
- Postural security
- Equilibrium reactions and protective extension
- Schilder's arm extension posture
- Supine flexion
- Prone extension
- Asymmetrical tonic neck reflex
- Hyperactivity, distractibility
- Tactile defensiveness
- Ability to perform slow motions
- Thumb-finger touching
- Diadochokinesis
- Tongue-to-lip movements
- Hopping, jumping, skipping

Construction and Reliability

The construction of the SIPT was based on a theoretical model developed from observation of children with learning disabilities and supported by factor analytical and cluster analysis studies. Interpretation follows a clinical model based on patterns of scores rather than a poor score on any one test.

The SIPT was nationally standardized on 1997 children from across the United States and Canada. Sex, geographical location, ethnicity, and type of community are represented in proportion to the 1980 U.S. Census. Test-retest reliability was evaluated in a sample of 41 dysfunctional children and 10 normally functioning children with ranges from moderate to high. As a group, the praxis

APPENDIX 14-A ■ A Summary of Standardized Motor Tests—cont'd

tests had the highest reliabilities. Interrater reliability is excellent, with most correlations between raters at 0.90 or higher.

Comment

The SIPT is computer scored and interpreted, and a full eight-color profile (WPS Chronograph) is provided that summarizes major SIPT testing and statistical results in a clear manner. Initial validity studies of the SIPT indicate a good ability to discriminate between normal and dysfunctional groups and across ages. The SIPT is the most comprehensive assessment of sensory integration and praxis; however, it requires specialized training for administration and interpretation, and the test kit and scoring of protocols are expensive.

Beery-Buktenica Developmental Test of Visual-Motor Integration (BEERY VMI), Fifth Revision (2010)[115]

Authors

Keith E. Beery, PhD, Norman A. Buktenica, and Natasha A. Beery

Source

Multi-Health Systems, Inc., 3770 Victoria Park Ave,Toronto, Ontario, Canada M2H 3M6 Email: customerservice@mhs.com; website: www.mhs.com

Ages

2 to 18 years

Administration

Individual or group; 5 to 15 minutes

Equipment

Protocol booklets (test forms), No. 2 pencil

Description

The BEERY VMI was developed for early screening and intervention of visual-motor deficits. It tests the ability to integrate visual and motor abilities by presenting 30 geometric forms of increasing difficulty to copy. A booklet is provided; below the design is a blank space in which the child replicates the form. A shorter format including the first 21 items is best suited for children aged 2 to 7 years. Items are judged pass or fail on criteria given in the manual, and scores are reported in standard scores and percentiles. Age equivalents are also available. If the child has significant difficulty completing the test or scores below the average range, this may be indicative of a visual-motor integration delay. To further assess where the difficulties lie, two additional tests are available to assess visual perception and motor coordination separately.

1. Visual Perception: Visual perception is assessed by limiting the motor response to pointing. The child matches geometric forms to a stimulus. Administration takes approximately 3 minutes.
2. Motor Coordination: Motor accuracy is assessed on a task of drawing within a double-lined path. Administration takes approximately 5 minutes.

Construction and Reliability

The Beery VMI is based on a significant amount of research on visual-motor integration, coordination, and development. The test has been normed five times between 1964 and 2003, with a total of more than 11,000 children. For this revision the Visual Perception and Motor tests were standardized on the same sample of 2512 children. This test has an extensive range of age-specific norms, with 600 children for the age range of 2 to 6 years. Test-retest reliability is high for the three test components, ranging from 0.90 to 0.92. Various studies of interrater reliability, internal consistency, and concurrent and construct validity are reported in the manual. Comparisons to other tests assessing visual-motor integration supported the validity the Beery VMI.

Comment

The VMI provides a quick and easy method to assess the development of a child's ability to copy geometric forms. The uses are varied, including identification of significant difficulties with visual-motor integration and determination of an effective intervention program, as well as use as a research tool. For complete assessment of the child with learning disabilities and DCD, it is best used in conjunction with other tests of gross motor, fine motor, visual perception, and eye-hand coordination. This culture-free, nonverbal assessment is suitable for children with diverse educational, environmental, and language backgrounds. New to this addition are teaching materials to promote visual-motor integration for children from birth through elementary school. These include *My Book of Letters and Numbers; My Book of Shapes;* a laminated wall chart of basic gross motor, fine motor, and visual developmental milestones; and a checklist for parents of over 200 developmental "stepping stones" to help parents observe skill development and track progress.

Test of Visual-Motor Skills Revised (TVMS-R) (1995)[116]

Author

Morrison F. Gardner

Source

Children's Hospital of San Francisco, Publication Department OPR-110, PO Box 3805, San Francisco, CA 94119

Ages

3 to 13 years

Administration

Individual or group; three to six children

Equipment

Protocol booklet, No. 2 pencil

Description

The TVMS-R consists of a series of 23 forms to be copied by the child. Each form is on a separate page of the booklet. The booklet contains some forms commonly used in visual-motor tests (e.g., lines and circles), but many forms are unique to this test. Care was taken to avoid forms that resemble language symbols. The revision of the TVMS has updated norms, standardization, and scoring criteria.

Two different scoring methods are now available. Modifications in scoring the TVMS-R include a classification system to characterize errors in one of eight categories. The eight classifications are closure, angles, intersecting and overlapping lines, size of design, rotation or reversals, line length, overpenetration or underpenetration, and modification of design. Scoring of each design is completed by following a definitive criterion, with errors and strengths identified. The examiner can identify specific areas of strength and weakness in visual-motor integration on the basis of the number of errors and accuracies recorded. Standard scores, scaled scores, percentile ranks, and stanines are available for both weaknesses and strengths. An alternative scoring method (ASM) was also designed to allow a straight point system designation for each form. The forms are scored on a 0- to 3-point scale. A score of 0 indicates that the child is unable to copy the form with any degree of motor accuracy. Scores of 1 and 2 indicate various visual-motor errors for which criteria are both written and illustrated. A score of 3 demonstrates precision in execution. Age equivalents, standard scores, scaled scores, percentile ranks, and stanines are provided.

Continued

APPENDIX 14-A ■ A Summary of Standardized Motor Tests—cont'd

Construction and Reliability

The TVMS-R was administered to 1484 children in the San Francisco Bay area aged 3 years to 13 years, 11 months. The overall sample was 51.9% male and 48.1% female. Cronbach's coefficient alpha was used to determine the internal consistency of the test. These reliability coefficients ranged from 0.72 to 0.84 over the age ranges, with a value of 0.90 for the sample as a whole. Test-retest reliability was not reported in the manual, but the author noted the need for research in that area.

Comment

The TVMS-R is a companion test to the Test of Visual-Perceptual Skills (TVPS), which is a motor-free test of form perception. Using the tests together can determine whether the child's form reproduction reflects incorrect visual perception or whether the problem is in motor execution. The TVMS-R places greater expectations on motor precision than do other visual-motor tests. For example, a line must touch an intersecting line without crossing over it. Therefore this test should be used only when motor control and constructive abilities are important.

Spatial Awareness Skills Program (SASP) (1999)[117]

Author

Jerome Rosner

Source

Pro-Ed, 8700 Shoal Creek Boulevard, Austin, TX 78757

Ages

4 to 10 years

Administration

Individual; 5 minutes to administer

Equipment

Protocol booklet, test booklet, No. 2 pencil, and transparent scoring guide

Description

The SASP test and curriculum was developed and revised from two earlier programs by the same author called *Perceptual Skills Curriculum* (PSC) and *Preparation for Learning* (PREP). These programs focused on teaching analytical abilities to improve visual and auditory perceptual skills that are important for academic learning. The SASP test is designed to assess spatial analysis and organizational skills through copying progressively harder spatial figures. Items are judged pass or fail on criteria given in the manual and through use of a scoring transparency. Raw scores are converted to age equivalents and used to determine the child's placement level within the SASP curriculum. The assessment and curriculum are designed to address the visual motor deficits exhibited by children with often hard-to-explain learning problems.

Spatial awareness refers to the ability to recognize what one can see, as well as understand space and time concepts that cannot be seen. It is a critical precursor to elementary school achievement as a foundation to spatial concepts such as decoding words and performing mathematical calculations. The SASP curriculum teaches spatial analysis skills with activities that show children how to break patterns into their structural elements, paying attention to features such as absolute and relative qualities, position, and magnitude. This type of organization enhances the ability to chunk information into larger units for more efficient processing of information. Spatial reasoning forms the logic of coding systems used for spelling, reading, writing, and math.

Construction and Reliability

The SASP was field tested on a sample of 322 children aged 4 to 11 years attending two schools in Houston, Texas. These schools were selected for their demographic diversity. The small sample size was deemed appropriate given the nature of the test. The internal consistency reliability was examined using Cronbach's coefficient analysis, yielding an average score of 0.76, indicating overall reliability of the SASP across ages. Interrater reliability was 0.96. Content description and content identification were found to be valid for the limited purpose of this assessment, indicating that examiners can use the SASP test with confidence to determine entry points for the SASP curriculum.

Comment

Spatial awareness skills are considered to develop both hierarchically and cyclically, with the child developing a more complex understanding of global and part relationships over time. By the age of 10 the foundational spatial skills assessed by the SASP are thought to be fully developed. Therefore a maximum score is expected for children aged 10 or older. Although the SASP was normed for children aged 4 through 10, it is possible to use it with individuals above this age. If an older child does not perform appropriately on testing, and academic achievement is consistent with this substandard score, then the remedial program can be used to encourage spatial awareness skills. The author cautions that the remedial program will not eliminate academic deficits but will provide strategies to assist in learning.

Evaluation Tool of Children's Handwriting (ETCH) (1995)[118]

Author

Susan J. Amundson

Source

O.T. Kids, PO Box 1118, Homer, AK 99603

Ages

First through sixth grades (6 to 11 years)

Administration

Individual

Equipment

Protocol booklet, task sheets and wall charts, stopwatch, No. 2 pencil

Description

The ETCH is designed to evaluate manuscript and cursive writing for components of legibility and speed. Specific components of the child's handwriting, including letter formation, spacing, size, and alignment, are included for assessment. The following tasks are presented in order:

1. Lowercase alphabet letters (from memory)
2. Uppercase alphabet letters (from memory)
3. Numeral writing (from memory)
4. Near point copying (visual model)
5. Far point copying (visual model)
6. Dictation (verbal)
7. Sentence composition (independent)

A quick reference card is included with standardized directions and timing criteria. Written and illustrated scoring criteria have been designed to assist the evaluator in determining the legibility of letters and numbers. The primary focus of scoring is whether the written material is readable.

Construction and Reliability

Based on the efforts of numerous occupational therapy practitioners, students, and professors, the ETCH itself has evolved through scientific investigation. Pilots of the ETCH were designed by using

APPENDIX 14-A ■ A Summary of Standardized Motor Tests—cont'd

adaptations of written tasks from existing tools. Three editions of the ETCH have been sampled by practitioners working in school systems, with feedback given on the examiner's manual, ease of administration and scoring, item selection, scoring procedures, and face validity of the instrument. When the ETCH was published, it lacked normative and psychometric information. Since that time, test reliability, validity, and normative data of the ETCH are being compiled through various research studies. Eight studies of handwriting speed are included for reference in the manual. The most recent examination of test-retest reliability studies[234] identified adequate stability of total word (0.95), letter (0.88), and number (0.84) scores. Individual letter, word, and number subtests were not as stable and should be used cautiously in interpretation of problems. Interrater reliability ranged from 0.63 to 0.94 for individual manuscript items and 0.64 to 0.97 for cursive. Overall, the total word reliability is more stable than task scores, ranging from 0.90 to 0.98.

Comment

The ETCH assesses functional writing skills that are relevant to academic performance. The varied tasks allow the examiner to identify areas of strength and weakness in written performance, including legibility components, speed, and composition models (visual, verbal, and memory). Information received from the ETCH is qualitative at this point because of the lack of normative samples. The author suggests that the ETCH be used in conjunction with observations of the child's writing activity in natural environments, such as classroom and home, as a determination of difficulties in functional written performance.

Test of Handwriting Skills (THS)[119]

Author

Morrison F. Gardner

Source

Psychological and Educational Publications, Inc., PO Box 520, Hydesville, CA, 95547

Ages

5 through 11 years; manuscript norms 5 to 8 years, cursive norms 9 to 11 years

Administration

Individual or group administration; 15 to 20 minutes

Equipment

THS manual, manuscript or cursive test booklet, No. 2 pencil, and stopwatch

Description

The purpose of the THS is to assess a child's neurosensory integration ability in handwriting, with focus on uppercase and lowercase letter formation as well as numbers. It is designed to assess strengths and weaknesses in the motoric aspects of handwriting, including legibility and speed. Varied aspects of written performance are assessed, including the following:

1. Spontaneously writing, from memory, uppercase and lowercase letters of the alphabet in sequence
2. Writing, from dictation, uppercase and lowercase letters of the alphabet out of alphabetical sequence
3. Writing, from dictation, numbers out of numerical order
4. Copying selected letters of the alphabet
5. Copying selected words
6. Copying selected sentences
7. Writing selected words from dictation

Scoring criteria are well delineated in the manual. Sample visual representations are given to illustrate the quality needed to achieve each score and provide information on typical developmental performance and error types. Possible errors include overextended or underextended lines, broken lines, overlapping or reworked lines, parts missing, distortion of shape, or omitted dots or line crossings. Additional scoring looks at the speed of performance as well as reversed letters, case substitutions, and touching letters.

Construction and Reliability

The THS was standardized with children from various parts of the United States. Approximately equal numbers of boys and girls were tested, with representation for both right and left handedness. The manuscript version was administered to 494 children with a median age of 6 years, 11 months; 406 were right handed and 61 were left handed. The cursive version was administered to 345 children with a median age of 9 years, 8 months; 309 were righted handed and 36 were left handed. Norms were derived for each of the 10 subtests as well as the additional scores. Cronbach's alpha was used to calculate the internal consistency of the test at each age level. These reliability coefficients ranged from 0.51 to 0.78 for the manuscript version and 0.29 to 0.87 for the cursive version. Two items on each version had low reliabilities (writing eight numbers and copying 10 letters), probably a result of the small number of items in the subtest. Scores on the manuscript version correlated positively with scores on the TVMS-R, indicating that the handwriting skills being tested involve a visual-motor component.

Comment

This test was developed primarily as a means for various professionals to measure children's handwriting skills. The THS can be administered by OTs, teachers, psychologists, resource specialists, educational diagnosticians, learning specialists, and optometrists. While gathering pertinent information for test development, the author arranged two conferences with teachers from kindergarten to fifth grade and obtained information from various professionals throughout the United States. In designing this test he recognized that three main methods of handwriting were being taught (D'Nealian, Palmer, and Zaner-Bloser) and that children, in general, have better accuracy for copied letters and words versus dictation that involves holding symbols in memory.

This test is functional and relevant to academic performance. The varied tasks and additional scoring allow the clinician to identify areas of strength and weakness in written performance. This can provide the foundation for recommendations within the classroom and/or guide intervention.

The Print Tool[120]

Authors

Jan Olsen, OTR and Emily Knapton, OTR/L

Source

Handwriting Without Tears, 8001 Mac Arthur Boulevard, Cabin John, MD 20818

Email: janolson@hwtears.com; website: www.hwtears.com

Ages

6 years old and older

Administration

Individual; administration for handwriting sample takes 15 minutes, scoring about 30 minutes

Equipment

Student booklet and pencil, or a writing sample can be collected from school; evaluation score sheet; transparent measuring tool for accurate scoring; comprehensive scoring overview; handwriting

Continued

APPENDIX 14-A ■ A Summary of Standardized Motor Tests—cont'd

remediation plan forms to develop goals; and strategies for remediation

Description

The Print Tool is a formal printing assessment to use in evidence-based remediation programs. The Print Tool is used to evaluate handwriting skills, plan intervention, and measure progress in students experiencing handwriting difficulty. A student's ability to print dictated letters and numbers is assessed. Evaluation scores for each specific skill area assessed help identify the student's strengths and needs. The Print Tool provides general remediation suggestions and specific strategies to be carried out with the author's remedial Handwriting Without Tears curriculum. This tool can be used in all school and therapy settings and with all curricula. Eight handwriting components for capitals, lowercase letters, and numbers are considered:

1. Memory: remembering and writing dictated letters and numbers
2. Orientation: Facing letters and numbers in the correct direction
3. Placement: Putting letters and numbers on the baseline
4. Size: How big or small a child chooses to write
5. Start: Where each letter or number begins
6. Sequence: Order and stroke direction of the letter or number parts
7. Control: Neatness and proportion of letters and numbers
8. Spacing: Amount of space between letters in words and between words in sentences

Construction and Reliability

The Print Tool has been recently released. Standardization has not been completed; however, suggested age-related expectations are provided in the manual. Data collection is in process for standardization in the future.

Continuing education is recommended to understand the complete process of observing, scoring, and compiling a remediation plan with The Print Tool. A Level 1 Certification is offered by the Handwriting Without Tears organization. Both the assessment and the award-winning Handwriting Without Tears curriculum were developed based on the authors' many years of successful practice in evaluating and remediating handwriting problems. The Handwriting Without Tears program is a structured remedial program geared toward different age and skill levels. It is multisensory, developmentally based, and easy to implement. Support is provided via the Handwriting Without Tears website.

CHAPTER 15 Spina Bifida: A Congenital Spinal Cord Injury

KRISTIN J. KROSSCHELL, PT, MA, PCS, and MARI JO PESAVENTO, PT, PCS

KEY TERMS

Chiari malformation
crouch-control ankle-foot orthosis
diastematomyelia
hydrocephalus
lipomeningocele
myelodysplasia
myelomeningocele
reciprocating gait orthosis
sacral agenesis
spina bifida cystica
spina bifida occulta
standing A-frame
tethered spinal cord

OBJECTIVES

After reading this chapter the student or therapist will be able to:

1. Identify the various types of spina bifida.
2. Recognize the incidence and etiology of spina bifida.
3. Identify the clinical manifestations of myelomeningocele, including neurological, orthopedic, and urological sequelae.
4. Comprehend medical management in the newborn period and beyond.
5. Determine physical and occupational therapy evaluations, including manual muscle testing, range of motion, sensory testing, reflex testing, developmental and functional and mobility assessments, and perceptual and cognitive evaluations.
6. List the major physical and occupational therapy goals and appropriate therapeutic management for each of the following stages: (a) before surgical closure of sac, (b) after surgery during hospitalization, (c) preambulatory, (d) toddler through preschool age, (e) primary school age through adolescence, and (f) transition to adulthood.
7. Identify psychological adjustment to congenital spinal cord injury.

A spinal cord injury is a complex disability. When a spinal cord lesion exists from birth, additional complexity is added. This congenital condition predisposes many areas of the central nervous system (CNS) to not develop or function adequately. In addition, all areas of development (physical, cognitive, and psychosocial) that depend heavily on central functioning will likely be impaired. The clinician therefore must be aware of the significant impact this neurological defect has on motor function as well as a variety of related human capacities.

A developmental framework, the *Guide to Physical Therapist Practice,*[1] and the International Classification of Functioning, Disability and Health (ICF) have been used to aid in understanding the sequential problems of the child with spina bifida. The developmental model, however, must always stay in line with the functional model for adult trauma because the problems of the congenitally involved child grow quickly into limitations in functional activities and participation in life of the injured adult. With concentration on the present but with an eye to the future, appropriate management goals can be achieved.

OVERVIEW OF CONGENITAL SPINAL CORD INJURY

A congenital spinal cord lesion occurs in utero and is present at the time of birth. Understanding how this malformation develops requires an appreciation of normal nervous system maturation. The nervous system develops from a portion of embryonic ectoderm called the *neural plate.* During gestation, the neural plate develops folds that begin to close, forming the neural tube (Figure 15-1). The neural tube differentiates into the CNS, which is composed of brain and spinal cord tissue. In the normal embryo, neural tube closure begins in the cervical region and proceeds cranially and caudally. Closure is generally complete by the twenty-sixth day.

Types of Spina Bifida

Spina bifida involves a defect in the neural tube closure and the overlying posterior vertebral arches. The extent of the defect may result in one of two types of spina bifida: occulta or cystica. Spina bifida occulta is characterized by a failure of one or more of the vertebral arches to meet and fuse in the third month of development. The spinal cord and meninges are unharmed and remain within the vertebral canal (Figure 15-2, *A*). The bony defect is covered with skin that may be marked by a dimple, pigmentation, or patch of hair.[2] The common site for this defect is the lumbosacral area, and it is usually associated with no disturbance of neurological or musculoskeletal functioning. Spina bifida cystica results when the neural and overlying vertebral arches fail to close appropriately. Cystic protrusion of the meninges or the spinal cord and meninges is present through the defective vertebral arches.

The milder form of spina bifida cystica, called *meningocele,* involves protrusion of the meninges and cerebrospinal fluid (CSF) only into the cystic sac (see Figure 15-2, *B*). The spinal cord remains within the vertebral canal, but it may exhibit abnormalities.[3] Clinical signs vary (according to spinal cord anomalies) or may not be apparent. This is a relatively uncommon form of spina bifida cystica.

A more severe form of spina bifida cystica, called *myelocele* or *myelocystocele,* is present when the central canal of the spinal cord is dilated, producing a large, skin-covered

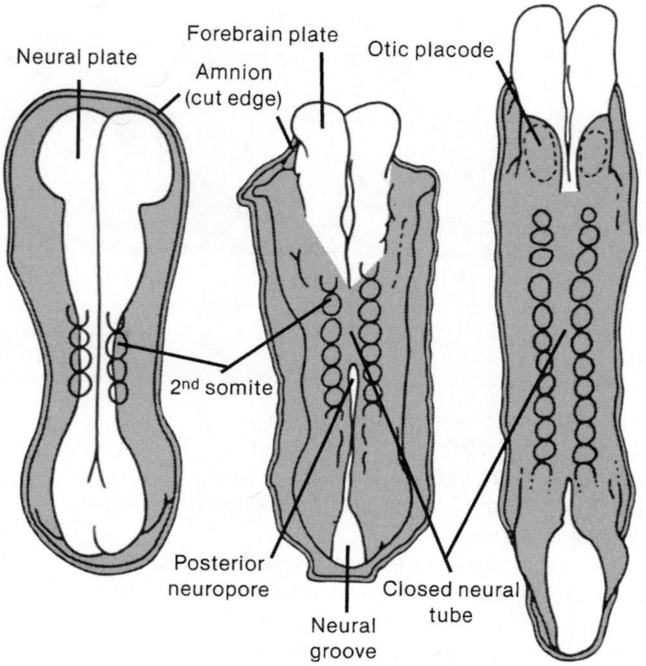

Figure 15-1 ■ Neural tube forming. (From Stark GD: *Spina bifida: problems and management*, London, 1977, Blackwell Scientific.)

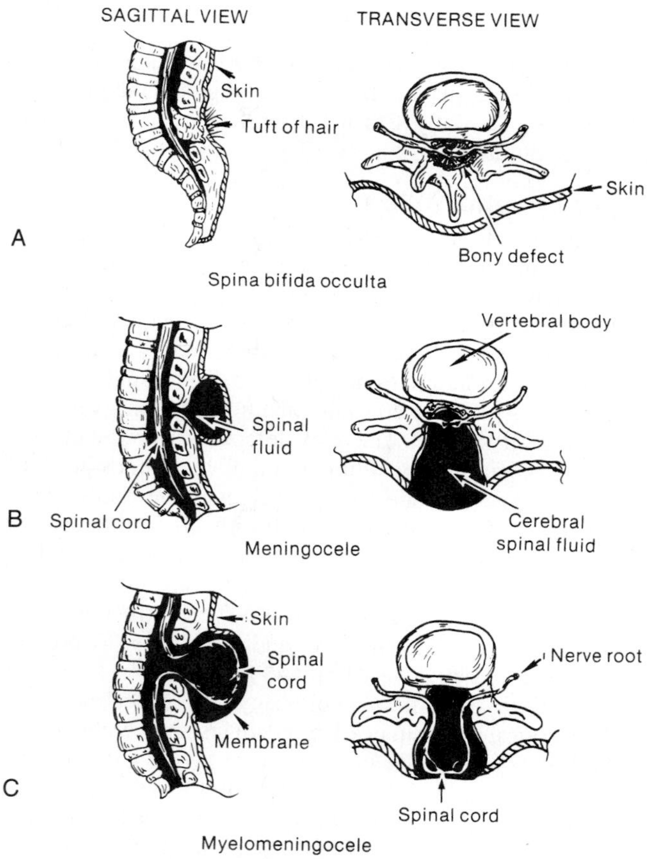

Figure 15-2 ■ Types of spina bifida. **A,** Spina bifida occulta. **B,** Meningocele. **C,** Myelomeningocele. (From McLone DG: *An introduction to spina bifida,* Chicago, 1980, Northwestern University.)

cyst. The neural tube appears to close normally but is distended from the cystic swelling. The CSF may ceaselessly expand the neural canal. Prompt medical attention is mandatory. This form of spina bifida is also rare.[4]

The more common and severe form of the defect is known as *myelomeningocele,* in which both spinal cord and meninges are contained in the cystic sac (see Figure 15-2, *C*). Within the sac the spinal cord and associated neural tissue show extensive abnormalities. In incomplete closure of the neural tube (dysraphism), abnormal growth of the cord and a tortuous pathway of neural elements make normal transmission of nervous impulses abnormal. The result is a variable sensory and motor impairment at the level of the lesion and below.[2] In an open myelomeningocele, nerve roots and spinal cord may be exposed, with dura and skin evident at the margin of the lesion. Exposure of the open neural tube to the amniotic fluid environment leads to neuroepithelial degeneration, with massive loss of neural tissue by the end of pregnancy.[5]

Although spina bifida cystica can occur at any level of the spinal cord, myelomeningoceles are most common in the thoracic and lumbosacral regions. Myelomeningocele occurs in 94% of the cases of spina bifida cystica, and two thirds of open lesions involve the thoracolumbar junction.[2] The terms *spina bifida, myelodysplasia,* and *myelomeningocele* are frequently used interchangeably.

Other forms of spinal dysraphism include diastematomyelia, lipomeningocele, and sacral agenesis. Diastematomyelia is present in 30% to 40% of patients with myelomeningocele and is secondary to partial or complete clefting of the spinal cord.[6] Lipomeningocele, another form of spina bifida cystica, is usually caused by a vertebral defect associated with a superficial fatty mass (lipoma or fatty tumor) that merges with the lower level of the spinal cord. No associated hydrocephalus is present, and neurological deficit is generally minimal; however, problems with urinary control and motor control of the lower extremities may be noted.[7] Neurological tissue invasion may be caused by a tethered spinal cord; therefore early lipoma resection is indicated for cosmesis and to minimize neurological sequelae. Lumbosacral or sacral agenesis may occur and is caused by an absence of the caudal part of the spine and sacrum. Children with this form of dysraphism may have narrow, flattened buttocks, weak gluteal muscles, and a shortened intergluteal cleft. The normal lumbar lordosis is absent, although the lower lumbar spine may be prominent. Calf muscles may be atrophic or absent. The pelvic ring is completed with either direct opposition of the iliac bones or with interposition of the lumbar spine replacing the absent sacrum. These children may have scoliosis, motor and sensory loss, and visceral abnormalities including anal atresia, fused kidneys, and congenital heart malformations. Management is started early and is symptomatic for each system.[8]

Failure of fusion of the cranial end of the neural tube results in a condition known as *anencephaly.* In this condition some brain tissue may be evident, but forebrain development is usually absent.[9] Sustained life is not possible with this neural tube defect; therefore this condition is not discussed further.

Incidence, Etiology, and Economic Impact

Statistics about the incidence of spina bifida vary considerably in different parts of the world. Spina bifida and anencephaly, the most common forms of neural tube defects, affect about 300,000 newborns each year worldwide.[10] In the United States the incidence is currently 2.48 per 10,000, down from approximately 7.23 per 10,000 births from 1974 through 1979 (before the folic acid mandate).[11,12] Current worldwide folic acid fortification programs have resulted in decreased incidence of spina bifida,[13,14] with annual decreases of 6600 folic acid–preventable spina bifida and anencephaly births reported since 2006.[15] There was a 31% decline in spina bifida prevalence rates in the immediate postfortification period (October 1998 through December 1999).[13] There was a continued decline in spina bifida prevalence rates from 1999 to 2004 of 10%.[16] Studies have also demonstrated that decline varied by ethnicity and race from prefortification to optional fortification to mandatory fortification in the United States.[16,17] Initially after fortification, the largest decline in prevalence was noted in Hispanic and non-Hispanic white races or ethnicities. Despite this initial decline, postfortification prevalence rates remain highest in infants born to Hispanic mothers, and less in infants born to non-Hispanic white and non-Hispanic black mothers.[16] In addition to periconceptual folate supplementation, it is thought that incidence has decreased subsequent to food fortification in several countries, decreased exposure to environmental teratogens, and increased and more accurate prenatal screening for fetal anomalies.[10]

Spina bifida is thought to be more common in females than in males, although some studies suggest no real sex difference.[3] A study of the association of race and sex with different neurological levels of myelomeningocele found the proportions of whites and females to be significantly higher in patients with thoracic-level spina bifida.[4] A significant relation also has been noted between social class and spina bifida: the lower the social class, the higher the incidence.[18,19]

A multifactorial genetic inheritance has been proposed as the cause of spina bifida, coupled with environmental factors, of which nutrition, including folic acid intake, are key. Cytoplasmic factors, polygenic or oligogenic inheritance, chromosomal aberrations, and environmental influences (e.g., teratogens) have all been considered as possible causes.[5,15] Genetic factors seem to influence the occurrence of spina bifida. The chances of having a second affected child are between 1% and 2%, whereas in the general population the percentage drops to one fifth of 1%.[20,21] Although these factors are related to the incidence of spina bifida, the cause of this defect remains in question. Environmental conditions, such as hyperthermia in the first weeks of pregnancy, or dietary factors, such as eating canned meats or potatoes or drinking tea, have been implicated but not substantiated.[22,23] In addition, historically, nutritional deficiencies, such as of folic acid and vitamin A, have been implicated as a cause of primary neural tube defects.[24-27] Approximately 50% to 70% of neural tube defects can be prevented if a woman of childbearing age consumes sufficient folic acid daily before conception and throughout the first trimester of pregnancy. As a result of research findings in support of folic acid implementation, the U.S. Public Health Service has mandated folic acid fortification since 1998 as a public health strategy. Prenatal vitamins, especially folic acid, are recommended to discourage the condition's development. Current fortification programs are preventing about 22,000 cases, or 9% of the estimated folic acid–preventable spina bifida and anencephaly cases.[15] Genetic considerations, such as an Rh blood type, a specific gene type (HLA-B27), an X-linked gene, and variations in the many folate pathway genes have been implicated, but not conclusively.[28,29] Malformations are attributed to abnormal interaction of several regulating and modifying genes in early fetal development.[30] Disturbance of any of the sequential events of embryonic neurulation produces neural tube defects (NTDs), with the phenotype (i.e., spina bifida, anencephaly) varying depending on the region of the neural tube that remains exposed.[5] Environmental factors combined with genetic predisposition appear to trigger the development of spina bifida, although definitive evidence is not available to support this claim.[31]

The incidence of spina bifida has declined since the advent of amniocentesis and the use of ultrasonography for prenatal screening. The presence of significant levels of alpha fetoprotein in the amniotic fluid has led to the detection of large numbers of affected fetuses.[32] Currently, maternal serum alpha-fetoprotein levels have been effective in detecting approximately 80% of neural tube defects.[33] Prenatal screening can be most effective when a combination of serum levels, amniocentesis or amniography, and ultrasonography is used.[34-36] Although this screening is not yet performed routinely, it is suggested for those at risk for the defect. Knowledge of the defect allows for preparation for cesarean birth and immediate postnatal care. This includes mobilization of the interdisciplinary team that will continue to care for the child. For parents who decide to carry an involved fetus to term, adjustment to their child's disability can begin before birth, which includes mobilizing their own support system. Education from an integrated team regarding what will follow after delivery and neurosurgical closure is imperative to aid families in decision making and to allow families to assess and understand the child's disability and future care options.

Other advances in the field of prenatal medicine that affect spina bifida management and outcome include in utero treatment of hydrocephalus and in utero surgical repair to close the myelomeningocele. This challenging surgical procedure is practiced in only a few specialty centers and so far has been shown to offer palliation of the defect at best.[37] Treatment such as this, in conjunction with prenatal diagnosis, has been shown to have a positive impact on the incidence and severity of complications associated with spina bifida.[38-45] Limitations of current postnatal treatment strategies and considerations of prenatal treatment options continue to be explored. Ethics, timing of repair, and surgical procedures are all being investigated. In addition, continued assessment of outcomes from those who have undergone presurgical management requires continued exploration. The Management of Myelomeningocele Study (MOMS) was initiated in 2003 as a large randomized, clinical trial designed to compare the two approaches to the treatment of infants with spina bifida (prenatal or fetal surgery versus postnatal surgery) to determine if one approach was better than the other. The primary end point of this trial was the need for a shunt at one year, and secondary end points included neurologic function, cognitive outcome, and maternal morbidity after prenatal repair. This study had 112 patients enrolled in 2007 with a projected enrollment of 200.[46-49] The trial was stopped for efficacy of prenatal surgery after enrollment of just 183 infants. Results demonstrated that prenatal surgery significantly reduced the need for shunting and improved mental and motor function at 30 months. Reduced incidence of hindbrain herniation at 12 months and successful ambulation by 30 months were also reported. While prenatal surgery was associated with improved function and reduced need for shunting, maternal and fetal risks, including preterm delivery and uterine dehiscense at delivery were reported.[49a]

In 1996 the lifetime cost to society per affected person with spina bifida was estimated to be $635,000.[50,51] More recent estimates have not been reported; however, with an economy in flux it is likely that this value underassesses costs to society today. In addition to medical management costs per child, there are additional costs that affect both the family and society across the life span that are variable and often related to differential market forces and social welfare policies.[50]

In 2007, Ouyang[52] reported that average medical expenditures during the first year of life for those with spina bifida during 2002 and 2003 averaged $50,000 (using MarketScan 2003 database). The majority of expenditures during infancy were from inpatient admissions secondary to surgeries being concentrated during this time period for those with spina bifida. After infancy, average medical care expenditures during 2003 ranged from $15,000 to $16,000 per year among different age groups of persons with spina bifida. Incremental expenditures associated with medical care were not stable, but decreased with increasing age, from $14,000 per year for children to $10,000 per year for adults 45 to 64 years of age.[52]

Clinical Manifestations

The most obvious clinical manifestation of myelomeningocele is the loss of sensory and motor functions in the lower limbs. The extent of loss, while primarily dependent on the degree of the spinal cord abnormality, is secondarily dependent on a number of factors. These include the amount of traction or stretch resulting from the abnormally tethered spinal cord, the trauma to exposed neural tissue during delivery, and postnatal damage resulting from drying or infection of the neural plate.[2] Specific clinical impairments that commonly lead to functional limitations for the child with spina bifida are addressed in this section.

Sensory Impairment

Children with spina bifida have impaired sensation below the level of the lesion. The loss often does not match exactly the level of the lesion and needs to be carefully assessed. Sensory loss includes kinesthetic, proprioceptive, and somatosensory information. Because of this, children will often have to rely heavily on vision and other sensory systems to substitute for this loss.

Musculoskeletal Impairment

Weakness and Paralysis. Determining neurological involvement is not as straightforward as assumed. At birth, two main types of motor dysfunction in the lower extremities have been identified. The first type involves a complete loss of function below the level of the lesion, resulting in a flaccid paralysis, loss of sensation, and absent reflexes. The extent of involvement can be determined by comparing the level of the lesion with a chart delineating the segmental innervation of the lower limb muscles. Orthopedic deformities may result from the unopposed action of muscles above the level of the lesion. This unopposed pull commonly leads to hip flexion, knee extension, and ankle dorsiflexion contractures.

When the spinal cord remains intact below the level of the lesion, the effect is an area of flaccid paralysis immediately below the lesion and possible hyperactive spinal reflexes distal to that area. This condition is quite similar to the neurological state of the severed cord seen in traumatic injury. This second type of neurological involvement again results in orthopedic deformities, depending on the level of the lesion, the spasticity present, and the muscle groups involved.

Orthopedic Deformities. The orthopedic problems that occur with myelomeningocele may be the result of (1) the imbalance between muscle groups; (2) the effects of stress, posture, and gravity; and (3) associated congenital malformations. Decreased sensation and neurological complications also may lead to orthopedic abnormalities.[53]

Besides the obvious malformation of vertebrae at the site of the lesion, hemivertebrae and deformities of other vertebral bodies and their corresponding ribs also may be present.[53,54] Lumbar kyphosis may be present as a result of the original deformity. In addition, as a result of the bifid vertebral bodies, the misaligned pull of the extensor muscles surrounding the deformity, as well as the unopposed flexor muscles, contributes further to the lumbar kyphosis. As the child grows, the weight of the trunk in the upright position also may be a contributing factor.[54] Scoliosis may be present at birth because of vertebral abnormalities or may become evident as the child grows older. The incidence of scoliosis is lower in low lumbar or sacral level deformities.[54,55] Scoliosis may also be neurogenic, secondary to weakness or asymmetrical spasticity of paraspinal muscles, tethered cord syndrome (TCS), or hydromyelia.[55] Lordosis or lordoscoliosis is often found in the adolescent and is usually associated with hip flexion deformities and a large spinal defect.[3,54] Many of these trunk and postural deformities exist at birth but are exacerbated by the effects of gravity as the child grows. They can compromise vital functions (cardiac and respiratory) and therefore should be closely monitored by the therapist and the family.

As has been alluded to previously, the type and extent of deformity in the lower extremities depend on the muscles that are active or inactive. In total flaccid paralysis, in utero deformities may be present at birth, resulting from passive positioning within the womb. Equinovarus (clubfoot) and "rocker-bottom" deformity are two of the most common foot abnormalities. Knee flexion and extension contractures also may be present at birth. Other common deformities are hip flexion, adduction, and internal rotation, usually leading to a subluxed or dislocated hip. Although many of these problems may be present at birth, preventing positional deformity (such as the frog-leg position), which may result from improper positioning of flaccid extremities, is of the utmost importance. Orthopedic care varies throughout the course of the child's life. Changes in clinical orthopedic management have evolved to establish evidence-based interventions.[56]

Osteoporosis. Because the paralyzed limbs of the child with spina bifida have increased amounts of unmineralized osteoid tissue, they are prone to fractures, particularly after periods of immobilization.[57,58] Early mobilization and weight bearing can aid in decreasing osteoporosis.[54,59] Fortunately, these fractures heal quickly with appropriate medical management.

Neurological Impairment

Hydrocephalus. Hydrocephalus develops in 80% to 90% of children with myelomeningocele.[21,60] Hydrocephalus results from a blockage of the normal flow of CSF between the ventricles and spinal canal. The most obvious effect of the buildup of CSF is abnormal increase in head size, which may be present at birth because of the great compliance of the cranial sutures in the fetus, or it may develop postnatally.[61] Other signs of hydrocephalus include bulging fontanels and irritability. Internally, a concomitant dilation of the lateral ventricles and thinning of the cerebral white matter are usually present. Without reduction of the buildup of CSF, increased brain damage and death may result.

Chiari Malformation. Patients with myelomeningocele have a 99% chance of having an associated Chiari II malformation.[6] Cardinal features of the Chiari II malformation include myelomeningocele in the thoracolumbar spine, venting of the intracranial CSF through the central canal, hypoplasia of the posterior fossa, herniation of the hindbrain into the cervical spinal canal, and compressive damage to cranial nerves. This malformation is a congenital anomaly of the hindbrain that involves herniation of the medulla and at times the pons, fourth ventricle, and inferior aspect of the cerebellum into the upper cervical canal. The herniation usually occurs between C1 and C4 but may extend down to T1.[6,62,63] In those with Chiari II malformations and spina bifida there is a significant reduction in cerebellar volume, and within the cerebellum the anterior lobe is enlarged and the posterior lobe is reduced.[64] Not all Chiari II malformations are symptomatic. As a result of a symptomatic Chiari malformation, problems with respiratory and bulbar function may be evident in the child with spina bifida.[2] Paralysis of the vocal cords occurs in a small percentage of patients and is associated with respiratory stridor. Apneic episodes also may be evident, although their direct cause remains in question. Children with spina bifida also may exhibit difficulty in swallowing and have an abnormal gag reflex.[2] Problems with aspiration, weakness and cry, and upper-extremity weakness also may be present in children with a symptomatic Chiari II malformation.[65,66] Thus, depending on the orthopedic deformities present and the neurological involvement, severe respiratory involvement is possible in the affected child. These symptoms may be caused by significant compression of the hindbrain structures or dysplasia of posterior fossa contents, which can also occur in patients with Chiari II malformation.[6,67] This complex hindbrain malformation is a common cause of death in children with myelomeningocele despite surgical intervention and aggressive medical management.[68]

Association Pathways. Diffusion tensor tractography studies of association pathways in children with spina bifida have revealed characteristics of abnormal development, impairment in myelination, and abnormalities in intrinsic axonal characteristics and extraaxonal or extracellular space. These changes in diffusion metrics observed in children with spina bifida are suggestive of abnormal white matter development and persistent degeneration with increased age.[69]

Hydromyelia. Twenty percent to 80% of patients with myelomeningocele have hydromyelia.[6,70,71] Hydromyelia signifies dilation of the center canal of the spinal cord as hydrocephalus signifies dilation of the ventricles of the brain. The area of hydromyelia may be focal, multiple, or diffuse, extending throughout the spinal cord. The hydromyelia may be a consequence of untreated or inadequately treated hydrocephalus with resultant transmission of CSF through the obex into the central canal, with distention a result of increased hydrostatic pressure from above.[6] The increased collection of fluid may cause pressure necrosis of the spinal cord, leading to muscle weakness and scoliosis. Common symptoms of hydromyelia include rapidly progressive scoliosis, upper-extremity weakness, spasticity, and ascending motor loss in the lower extremities.[6,72] Aggressive treatment of hydromyelia at the onset of clinical signs of increasing scoliosis is mandatory and may lead to improvement in or stabilization of the curve in 80% of cases. Surgical interventions may include revision of a CSF shunt, posterior cervical decompression, or a central canal to pleural cavity shunt with a flushing device.[6,67]

Tethered Cord. *Tethered spinal cord* is defined as a pathological fixation of the spinal cord in an abnormal caudal location (Figure 15-3). This fixation produces mechanical stretch, distortion, and ischemia with daily activities, growth, and development.[73] Ischemic injury from traction of the conus directly correlates with degree of oxidative metabolism and degree of neurologic compromise. In addition to ischemic injury, traction of the conus by the filum may also mechanically alter the neuronal membranes, resulting in altered electrical activity.[74-78] The presence of tethered cord syndrome (TCS) should be suspected in any patient with abnormal neurulation (including patients with myelomeningocele, lipomeningocele, dermal sinus, diastematomyelia, myelocystocele, tight filum terminale, and lumbosacral agenesis). Presenting symptoms may include decreased strength (often asymmetrical), development of lower-extremity spasticity, back pain at the site of sac closure, early development of or increasing degree of scoliosis (especially in the low lumbar or sacral level),[79,80] or change in urological function.[68,81-83] Approximately 10% to 30% of children will develop TCS after repair of a myelomeningocele. Because essentially all children with repaired myelomeningocele will have a tethered spinal cord, as demonstrated on magnetic resonance imaging (MRI), the

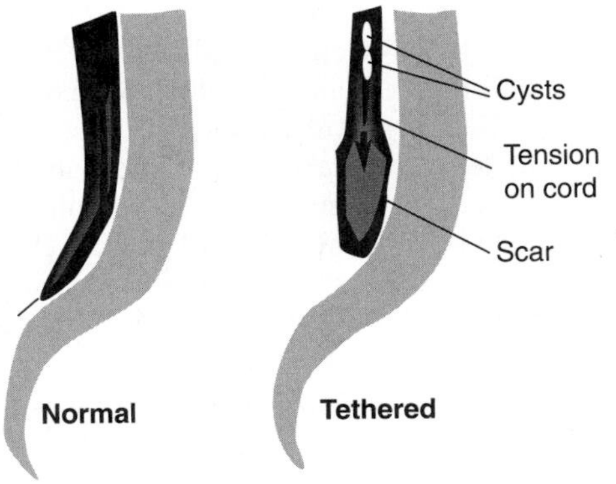

Figure 15-3 ■ Tethered cord in myelodysplasia. (From Staheli LT: *Practice of pediatric orthopedics,* Philadelphia, 2001, Lippincott Williams & Wilkins.)

diagnosis of TCS is made based on clinical criteria. The six common clinical presentations of TCS are increased weakness (55%), worsening gait (54%), scoliosis (51%), pain (32%), orthopedic deformity (11%), and urological dysfunction (6%).[84] This clinical spectrum may be primarily associated with these dysraphic lesions or may be caused by spinal surgical procedures.[73] The cord may be tethered by scar tissue or by an inclusion epidermoid or lipoma at the repair site.[6] The primary goal of surgery is to detach the spinal cord where it is adherent to the thecal sac, relieving the stretch on the terminal portion of the cord. Surgery to untether the spinal cord (tethered cord release [TCR]) is performed to prevent further loss of muscle function, decrease the spasticity, help control the scoliosis,[80,85] or relieve back pain.[86,87]

The effectiveness of a TCR may be demonstrated by an increase in muscle function, relief of back pain, and stabilization or reversal of scoliosis.[80,85,87] It has been reported that scoliosis response to untethering and progression of scoliosis after untethering vary with location of tethering[80,87] as well as Risser grade[88] and Cobb angle.[89] Those with Risser grade 3 to 5 and Cobb angle less than 40 degrees are less likely to experience curve progression after untethering. Those with Risser grades 0 to 2 and Cobb angle greater than 40 degrees are at higher risk of recurrence.[74,89] Spasticity, however, is not always alleviated in all patients.[90] Selective posterior rhizotomy has been advocated for patients whose persistent or progressive spastic status after tethered cord repair continues to interfere with their mobility and functional independence.[68,70]

Bowel and Bladder Dysfunction. Because of the usual involvement of the sacral plexus, the child with spina bifida commonly deals with some form of bowel and bladder dysfunction. Besides various forms of incontinence, incomplete emptying of the bladder remains a constant concern because infection of the urinary tract and possible kidney damage may result.[91] Regulation of bowel evacuation must be established so that neither constipation nor diarrhea occurs. Negative social aspects of incontinence can be minimized by instituting intervention that emphasizes patient and family education and a regular, consistently timed, reflex-triggered bowel evacuation.[92]

Cognitive Impairment and Learning Issues. The last major clinical manifestation resulting from the neurological involvement of myelomeningocele is impaired intellectual function. Although children with spina bifida without hydrocephalus may have normal intellectual potential, children with hydrocephalus, particularly those who have shunt infections, are likely to have below-average intelligence.[93-95] These children often demonstrate learning disabilities and poor academic achievement.[96] Even those with a normal IQ show moderate to severe visual-motor perceptual deficits.[97] The inability to coordinate eye and hand movements affects learning and may interfere with activities of daily living (ADLs), such as buttoning a shirt or opening a lunchbox.[98] Difficulties with spatial relations, body image, and development of hand dominance may also be evident.[2,98] Children with myelomeningocele demonstrate poorer hand function than age-matched peers. This decreased hand function appears to be caused by cerebellar and cervical cord abnormalities rather than hydrocephalus or a cortical pathological condition (see Chapter 21).[99]

Prenatal studies have shown that the CNS as a whole is abnormally developed in fetuses with myelomeningocele.[100-103] The impairment of intellectual and perceptual abilities has been linked to damage to the white matter caused by ventricular enlargement.[2] This damage to association tracts, particularly in the frontal, occipital, and parietal areas, could account for the often severe perceptual-cognitive deficits noted in the child with spina bifida.[69,104] Lesser involvement of the temporal areas may account for the preservation of speech, whereas the semantics of speech, which depends on association areas, is impaired. The "cocktail party speech" of children with spina bifida can be deceptive because they generally use well-constructed sentences and precocious vocabulary. A closer look, however, reveals a repetitive, inappropriate, and often meaningless use of language not associated with higher intellectual functioning. Research on learning difficulties in children with spina bifida and hydrocephalus suggests that many of these children experience difficulties. Tasks and skills affected include memory, reasoning, math, handwriting, organization, problem solving, attention, sensory integration, auditory processing, visual perception, and sequencing.[101-103]

Integumentary Impairment

Latex allergy and sensitivity have been noted with increasing frequency in children with myelomeningocele, with frequent reports of intraoperative anaphylaxis.[105-109] These children have also been reported to have a higher than expected prevalence of atopic disease.[110] A 1991 Food and Drug Administration Medical Bulletin estimated that 18% to 40% of patients with spina bifida demonstrate latex sensitivity,[105,111] with others reporting an incidence of 20% to 67%.[112,113] Within latex is 2% to 3% of a residual-free protein material that is thought to be the antigenic agent.[107] Frequent exposure to this material results in the development of the immunoglobulin E antibody. Children with spina bifida are more likely to develop the immunoglobulin E sensitivity because of repeated parental or mucosal exposure to the latex antigen.[114] Because of the risk of an anaphylactic reaction, exposure to any latex-containing products such as rubber gloves, therapy balls, pacifiers, spandex, dental dams, elastic or rubber bands, balloons, adhesive bandages, or exercise bands should be avoided. Latex-free gloves, therapy balls, treatment mats, and exercise bands are now widely available and should be considered for standard use in all clinics treating children with spina bifida. Spina bifida, even in the absence of multiple surgical interventions, may be an independent risk factor for latex sensitivity. Foods reported to be highly associated with latex allergy include avocado, banana, chestnut, and kiwi.[115] Latex-free precautions from birth are more effective in preventing latex sensitization than are similar precautions instituted later in life.[115-117] Latex sensitization decreased from 26.7% to 4.5% in children treated in a latex-free environment from birth.[117]

The presence of paralysis and lack of sensation on the skin places the child with spina bifida at major risk for pressure sores and decreased skin integrity. Various types of skin breakdown have occurred in 85% to 95% of all children with spina bifida by the time they reach young adulthood.[118] Common areas at risk for pressure sores include the lower back, kyphotic or scoliotic prominences, heels, feet, toes, and perineum. A pressure sore may result from excessive skin pressure that can cause reduced capillary flow, tissue anoxia, and eventual skin necrosis. Excessive pressure may manifest itself early as reactive hyperemia, a blister, and later as an open sore or overt necrosis. Chronic, untreated sores may lead to osteomyelitis and eventual sepsis.[110] Pressure sores often result in loss of time from school and work and can lead to financial hardship from medical treatment and hospitalizations. These negative consequences can largely be prevented with attention to education and instruction of the child and family. The goal of such education is to foster an understanding of the causes of skin breakdown and the necessary meticulous attention to skin care that must be carried out on a regular basis.

Growth and Nutrition

Nutritional intake and weight gain and loss have been found to be problematic in children with myelomeningocele. Early on, infants with spina bifida may have feeding issues as a result of an impaired gag reflex, swallowing difficulties, and a high incidence of aspiration.[2,66] Altered oral-motor function has been attributed to the Chiari II malformation.[119] These impairments may lead to nutritional issues and delayed growth and weight gain. Speech, physical, and occupational therapists as a team are often needed to address these issues.

Conversely, obesity can be a significant issue for children with spina bifida. This problem is complex and multifactorial.[120] Mobility limitations and decreased energy expenditure result in lower physical activity levels. In addition, decreased lower limb mass diminishes the ability to burn calories, which leads to weight gain. Decreased caloric intake as well as a lifelong engagement in rewarding and physically challenging physical activities are both necessary to enhance weight control and control obesity.

Children with myelomeningocele are short in stature. Growth in these children may be influenced by growth-retarding factors as a result of a neurological deficit such as tethered cord.[121] Endocrine disorders and growth hormone deficiency have also been found to contribute to short stature in this population.[122] As a result of complex CNS anomalies (midline defects, hydrocephalus, Arnold-Chiari malformation), these children are at risk for hypothalamopituitary dysfunction leading to growth hormone deficiency.[123,124] Treatment with recombinant human growth hormone has proven successful in fostering growth acceleration in these children.[123,125,126]

Psychosocial Issues

Considering all the clinical manifestations resulting from this congenital neurological defect, social and emotional difficulties will arise for these children and their families. These will be considered as appropriate when discussing the stages of recovery and rehabilitation from birth through adolescence.

The preceding discussion concerning the clinical problems of the child with spina bifida is intended to inform, not overwhelm, the clinician. With a firm understanding of the difficulties to be faced, evaluation and intervention can be more efficient and effective.

Medical Management

At or before birth, the myelomeningocele sac presents a dynamic rather than a static disability. The residual neurological damage will be contingent on the early medical management that the fetus or newborn receives.

Neurosurgical Management

Since the early 1960s the presence of a myelomeningocele has been treated as a life-threatening situation, and sac closure most often takes place within the first 24 to 48 hours of life.[2,127] Recent advances in treatment have led to investigational treatment in utero to repair the defect before birth.[38] The aim of either surgery is to replace the nervous tissue into the vertebral canal, cover the spinal defect, and achieve a watertight sac closure.[128] This early management has decreased the possibility of infection and further injury to the exposed neural cord.[24,128,129]

Progressive hydrocephalus may be evident at birth in a small percentage of children born with myelomeningocele. A greater majority, however, have hydrocephalus 5 to 10 days after the back lesion has been closed.[128,130-132] With the advent of computed tomography (CT), early diagnosis of hydrocephalus can be made in the newborn without the need for clinical examination.

Although clinical signs are not always definitive, hydrocephalus may be suspected if (1) the fontanels become full, bulging, or tense; (2) the head circumference increases rapidly; (3) a separation of the coronal and sagittal sutures is palpable; (4) the infant's eyes appear to look downward only, with the cornea prominent over the iris ("sunsetting sign"); and (5) the infant becomes irritable or lethargic and has a high-pitched cry, persistent vomiting, difficult feeding, or seizures (Table 15-1).[21,61,133]

If the results of CT confirm hydrocephalus, a ventricular shunt is indicated. This procedure involves diverting the excess CSF from the ventricles to some site for absorption. In general, two types of procedures—the ventriculoatrial (VA) and ventriculoperitoneal (VP) shunt—are currently used, the latter being the most common (Figure 15-4). The shunt apparatus is constructed from Silastic tubing and consists of three parts: a proximal catheter, a distal catheter, and

TABLE 15-1 ■ SIGNS AND SYMPTOMS OF SHUNT MALFUNCTION

Infants	Bulging fontanel
	Swelling along the shunt tract
	Prominent veins on scalp
	Downward eye deviation ("sunsetting")
	Vomiting or change in appetite
	Irritability or drowsiness
	Seizures
	High-pitched cry
Toddler	Headache
	Vomiting or change in appetite
	Lethargy or irritability
	Swelling along the shunt tract
	Seizures
	Onset of or increased strabismus
Older child	All the above, plus:
	Deterioration in school performance
	Neck pain or pain over myelomeningocele site
	Personality change
	Decrease in sensory or motor functions
	Incontinence that begins or worsens
	Onset of or increased spasticity

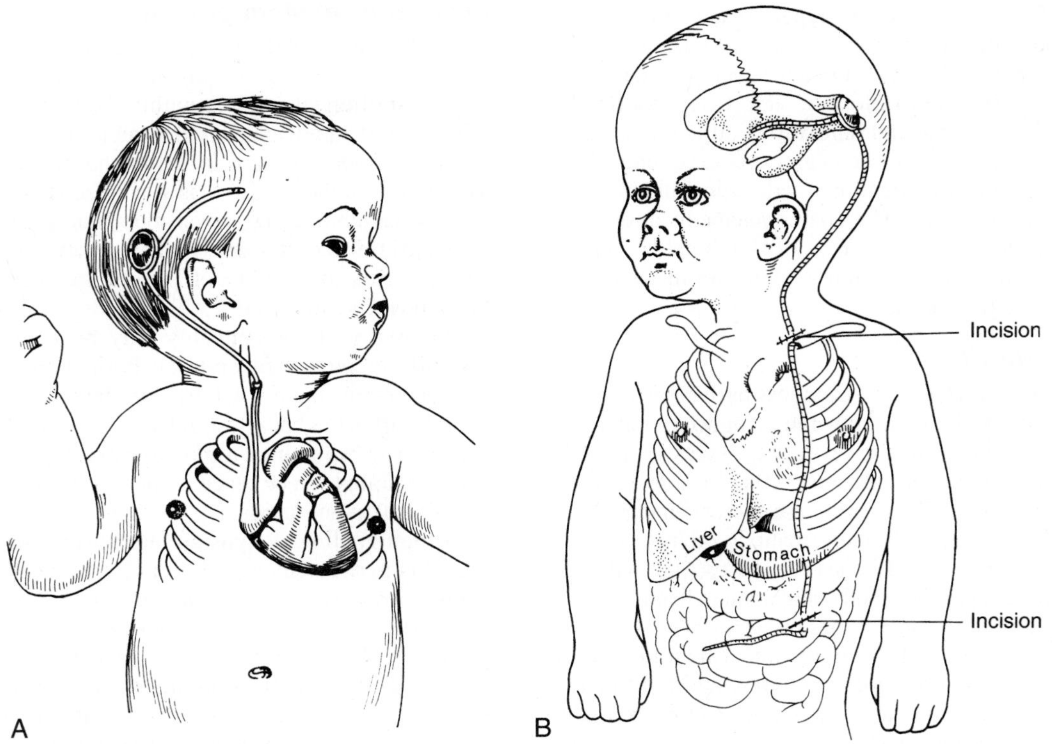

Figure 15-4 ■ **A,** Ventriculoatrial shunt. **B,** Ventriculoperitoneal shunt. (From Stark GD: *Spina bifida: problems and management,* London, 1977, Blackwell Scientific.)

a one-way valve. As CSF is pumped from the ventricles toward its final destination, backflow is prevented by the valve system. In this manner intracranial pressure is controlled, CSF is regulated, and hydrocephalus is prevented from causing damage to brain structures. An alternate means of controlling hydrocephalus may be the use of endoscopic third ventriculostomy (EVT). EVT is a procedure that, in selected patients with obstructive hydrocephalus, allows egress of CSF from the ventricles to the subarachnoid space. This can decompress the ventricles and allow normal intracranial pressures and brain growth. This procedure is typically reserved for last resort.[134]

Unfortunately for children with spina bifida, their problems do not end after the back is surgically closed and a shunt is in place. Management strategies in the care of shunted hydrocephalus vary.[135] Shunt complications occur frequently and require an average of two revisions before age 10 years.[60] The most common causes of complications are shunt obstruction and infection.[2,136] Revising the blocked end of the shunt can clear obstructions. Infections may be handled by external ventricular drainage and courses of antibiotic therapy followed by insertion of a new shunting system.[2] The problem of separation of shunt components has been largely overcome by the use of a one-piece shunting system. The single-piece shunt decreases the complications of shunting procedures.

Prophylactic antibiotic therapy 6 to 12 hours before surgery and 1 to 2 days postoperatively is effective in controlling infection for both sac repair and shunt insertion.[71] This brief course of antibiotics has not led to resistant organisms. The main cause of death in children with myelomeningocele remains increased intracranial pressure and infections of the CNS. With the use of antibiotics, shunting, and early sac closure, the survival rate has increased from 20% to 85%.[61,94,137]

Urological Management

Initial newborn workup should include a urological assessment. The urology team aims to preserve renal function and promote efficient bladder management. An early start to therapy helps to preserve renal function for children with spina bifida.[138] Initially, a renal and bladder ultrasound is performed to assess those structures.[100] Urodynamic testing can be performed to determine any blockage in the lower urinary tract. Functioning of the bladder outlet and sphincters, as well as ureteric reflux, also can be evaluated. These tests, plus clinical observations of voiding patterns, help the urologist classify the infant's bladder function. If the bladder has neither sensory nor motor supply, a constant flow of urine is present. In this case infection is rare because the bladder does not store urine and the sphincters are always open.[139]

If no sensation but some involuntary muscle control of the sphincter exists, the bladder will fill, but emptying will not occur properly. Overflow or stress incontinence results in dribbling urine until the pressure is relieved. Because of constant residual urine, infection is a potential problem and kidney damage may result.[139] When some voluntary muscle control but no sensation is present, the bladder will fill and empty automatically. The child can eventually be taught to empty the bladder at regular intervals to avoid unnecessary accidents.

Regardless of the type of bladder functioning, urine specimens are taken to check for infection, and blood samples are taken to determine the kidney's ability to filter the body's fluids. On the basis of clinical findings, the urologist will suggest the appropriate intervention.

A program of clean intermittent catheterization (CIC) done every 3 to 4 hours prevents infection and maintains the urological system.[140-143] Parents are taught this method and can then begin to take on this aspect of their child's care. At the age of 4 or 5 years, children with spina bifida can be taught CIC; thus they become independent in bladder care at a young age. Achieving this form of independence adds to the normal psychological development of these children. Some children may require urinary diversion through the abdominal wall (ileal conduit) or through the appendix (Mitrofanoff principle appendicovesicotomy)[144-146] or other, less common methods, such as intravesical transurethral bladder stimulation, to handle their urinary condition.[140,147] Although CIC is not possible for all children with spina bifida, it remains the method of choice for bladder management.

Bowel management and training programs should be started early. Medications, enemas, and attention to fiber content in the diet are all of value in establishing a bowel management program. The Malone antegrade continence enema (ACE) procedure is an important adjunct in the case of adults and children with problems of fecal elimination in whom standard medical therapies have failed.[148,149]

Orthopedic Management

Orthopedic management of the newborn with a myelomeningocele will generally concentrate on the feet and hips. Soft tissue releases of the feet may take place during surgery for sac closure. Casting the feet (Figure 15-5) and performing early aggressive taping are also effective in the management of clubfoot deformities.[150,151] Short-leg posterior splints (ankle-foot orthoses [AFOs]) may be used to maintain range and prevent foot deformities.

The orthopedist also will evaluate the stability of the hips. In children with lower-level lesions, attempts to prevent dislocation are made by using a hip abductor brace (Figure 15-6, *A*) or a total-body splint (Figure 15-6, *B*) for a few months after birth. With higher-level lesions, dislocated hips are no longer treated because they do not appear to have an effect on later rehabilitation efforts.[133,152-154]

Orthopedic management needs to be ongoing throughout the child's lifetime, with continued assessment of orthopedic

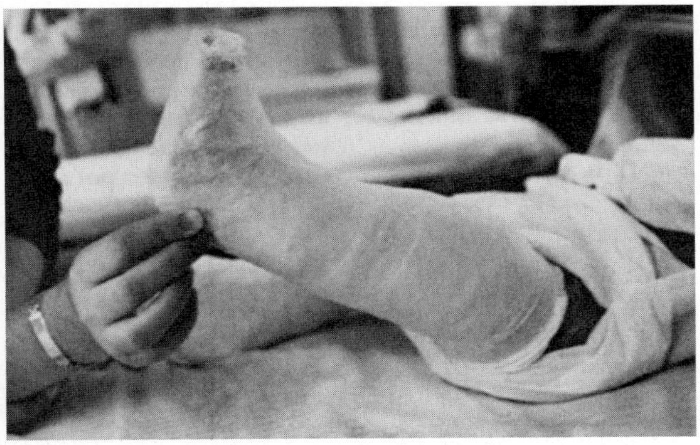

Figure 15-5 ■ Plaster cast of the foot and ankle to reduce clubfoot deformities.

deformities and need for surgical intervention. Important management issues relevant to function that the physical therapist (PT) should be aware of may include hip dislocation, knee valgus stress, scoliosis, foot deformities, fractures, osteoporosis, and postoperative management.

Hip Dislocation. Hip dislocations may occur at any level of neurologic deficit.[155] The goal of treatment for those with hip dislocation should be maximum function, not radiographic realignment. The most important factor in determining ability to walk is the level of neural involvement and not the status of the hip.[153,156-159] A level pelvis and good hip range of motion (ROM) are more important than hip relocation. In those with lower lumbar lesions and asymmetry caused by contracture, treatment will be directed at releasing the contracture and no attempts will be made to reduce the hip. Hip dislocations in those with sacral level lesions should be considered as lever-arm dysfunction, and surgical hip relocation is indicated.[56,155,157,158] Immobilization after hip dislocation may lead to a frozen immobile joint from an open reduction procedure, redislocation from a lack of significant dynamic forces available for joint stability around the hip joint, and an increased fracture risk. Recently a questionnaire, the Spina Bifida Hips Questionnaire (SBHQ), to evaluate the ADLs that are important to children with spina bifida and dislocated hips and their families has been developed and has demonstrated construct validity as well as reliability.[160]

Knee Valgus Stress. Many children with spina bifida who walk have excessive trunk and pelvic movement, knee flexion contractures, and rotational malalignment that may lead to excessive knee valgus stress. The most common deformities leading to this problem are rotational malalignment of the femur and femoral anteversion in association with excessive anterior tibial torsion. These deformities should be addressed via surgical correction as excessive knee valgus stress can lead to knee pain and arthritis in adult life.[56,159,161,162] In addition, the PT may need to reassess the child's gait pattern and use of assistive aids and bracing to minimize stress and maintain long-term joint viability for those with spina bifida over the life span.

Scoliosis. The prevalence of scoliosis in spina bifida is estimated to be as high as 50%. Increasing scoliosis can lead to loss of trunk stability when curves are greater than 40 degrees and when associated pelvic obliquity becomes 25 degrees or more. Surgical intervention, often recommended to prevent further progression, may improve or further impair sitting balance, ambulation, and performance of ADLs.[163] Various authors have reported that although surgery can improve curves by up to 50%, surgical morbidity must be considered and complications may be as high as 40% to 50%. Functional benefits are largely unsubstantiated owing to poorly constructed studies.[164-166] Wai[166] suggests that spinal deformity may not affect overall physical function or self-perception. After surgical correction it may take up to 18 months to appreciate functional improvement, and walking may be difficult for those who were just exercise ambulators before correction. Although surgical repair of scoliosis does improve quality of life in patients with cerebral palsy and muscular dystrophy, this has not been demonstrated in those with spina bifida.[167] Interventions such as chair modifications to shift the trunk to improve balance in the coronal plane and reduce pelvic obliquity and truncal

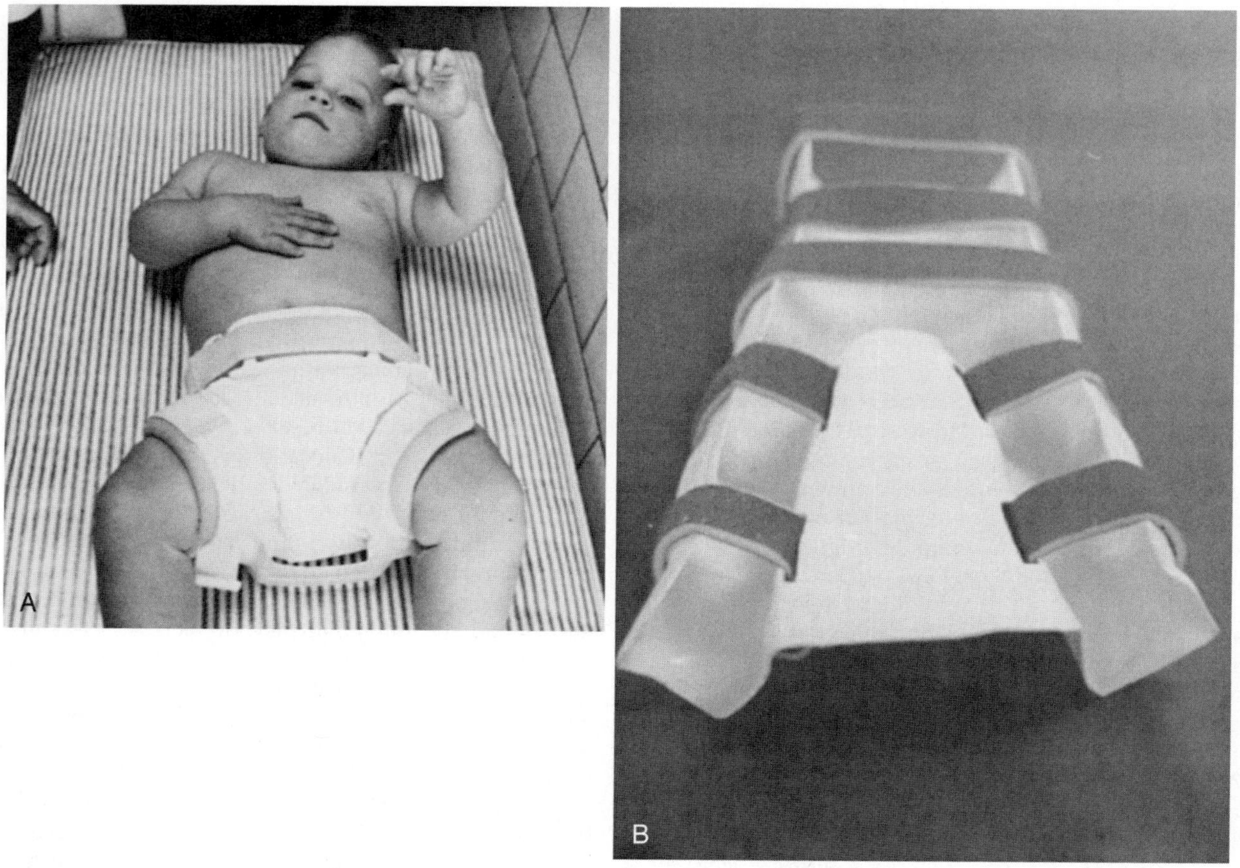

Figure 15-6 ■ **A,** Hip abductor brace. **B,** Total body splint.

asymmetry should be considered as a first option, before surgical correction.[163,167]

Back Pain. Back pain needs to be efficaciously evaluated in those with spina bifida who report back pain. Knowing when the patient experiences pain, what increases pain, what positions exacerbate pain, and what region of the body is affected can help lead to appropriate referral, testing, and management. Knowing if your patient has a shunt, spinal rods, and/or a Chiari malformation will also be important to your assessment and management. Pain in the neck, shoulders, and upper back with associated weakness and/or abnormal sensory findings should be evaluated by the treating neurosurgeon to rule out shunt malfunction. Spinal rods that have broken or that are breaking through the skin may also be a source of pain in this area. Pain not caused by rods, a shunt, Chiari issues, or a syrinx may have a mechanical cause and could be a result of poor posture, tension, or weight gain. A patient who reports low back pain may have a symptomatic tethered cord if the patient is also reporting changes in gait, increased tripping or falling, bladder changes, and/or pain shooting down the legs. Manual muscle testing (MMT) and urodynamic testing (refer to Chapter 29) are appropriate at this point and should be compared with baseline testing findings. Mechanical low back pain may be a result of abnormal gait mechanics, asymmetrical strength, and use of older orthotics that no longer fit. Assessment of seating and support systems, including cushions, and gait mechanics and use of orthotics and ambulatory aids are mandatory to increase stability and redistribute balance over stressed joints and to maximize reduction of the patient's pain and discomfort. Strengthening, particularly of the gluteal muscles, for those who are ambulatory may also be indicated. In addition, programs aimed at weight reduction may be necessary to alleviate stress and pain to preserve long-term viability of tissues. In addition, for women the chest may cause tension on the upper back, and breast reduction has been advocated for some to relieve this tension.[168-170]

Foot Deformity. The goal of treatment of the foot in spina bifida should be a flexible and supple foot. An insensate flail foot often becomes rigid over time, and foot management can become complicated by pressure sores. Up to 95% of patients will use an orthosis, and a supple flail foot will be easier to manage over time. Surgeries that are extraarticular with avoidance of arthrodesis, as well as simple tenotomies versus tendon releases and lengthenings, may best manage outcomes for bracing and ambulation.[56] Equinovarus deformities may be managed with early and intensive taping in the newborn period, known as the *French method,*[171,172] stretching and casting, and surgical intervention. The Ponsetti method, advocated by some, also has been reported to have positive outcomes; however, the significant investment in time and commitment by the family for frequent cast changes may affect the ability to carry out other ADLs without disruption.[155] In those with lipomas, foot deformity that may be acquired over time is best managed in a similar manner. Maintaining a supple and plantigrade foot with adequate muscle balance with use of soft tissue correction through tendon lengthening, tendon transfer, and plantar fascial release is recommended until 8 years of age. After that time, deformities may become more rigid and may necessitate more bony procedures.[173]

Osteoporosis, Osteopenia, and Fracture. Osteoporosis (thinning of the bone) and osteopenia (low bone mineral density [BMD]) in the legs and spine have been described in children and teens with spina bifida. These conditions increase the risk of fracture, increase the time for healing after fracture, and may lead to back pain. A study by Valtonen and colleagues in 2006 documented the occurrence of osteoporosis in adults with spina bifida. This condition often is not recognized.[174] Medical factors such as physical inactivity, decreased vitamin D, diminished exposure to sunlight, urinary diversion, renal insufficiency, hypercalciuria, medication for epilepsy, and oral cortisone treatment for more than 3 months increase the risk of osteoporosis.[59,175,176] It can be assumed that patients with meningomyelocele are at potential risk to develop osteoporosis at a younger age because of impaired walking ability and subsequent low physical loading of the lower limbs. Older age and higher levels have been associated with increased numbers of fractures in spina bifida.[174] The optimal strategies for prevention and treatment of osteoporosis in this population have not been established. Further research is required to see if the methods used to prevent and treat osteoporosis in individuals without spina bifida also work for teens and adults who have spina bifida. Considering the effects of prolonged immobilization on independence in daily activities and quality of life, there should be no disagreement that all efforts are necessary to prevent these fractures. Furthermore, osteoporotic fracture may lead to a vicious cycle of immobilization, decreased bone density, and repeated fractures.[174] Annual incidence of fracture is 0.029% in adolescents and 0.018% in adults.[177] Studies have shown promising results of regular functional electric stimulation–assisted training, but this is often nearly impossible to carry out in daily life.[178] The effects of standing programs on bone density are unclear.[179,180] The prevention of fractures should be among the major goals in the rehabilitation of people with meningomyelocele. The assessment of BMD is worthwhile in patients with risk factors for osteoporosis, because low BMD is a known risk factor for fractures.[175]

Postoperative Management. Care should be taken to avoid postoperative complications such as skin breakdown and postimmobilization fractures in the postoperative period. To decrease the risk of nonunion and allow for early mobilization and weight bearing, one should consider rigid internal fixation versus Kirschner wire fixation. After surgery, immobilization in a custom-molded body splint rather than a hip spica cast is preferred. Postoperative physical therapy should begin as soon as wounds are stable and healing is occurring. Therapy should focus on ROM (active and passive) and early weight bearing. Crawling should be strictly forbidden for a minimum of 3 to 4 weeks postimmobilization to reduce the risk of fracture.[159]

EVALUATIONS

In attempting to evaluate the child with spina bifida, a number of evaluations can be chosen, each designed to test specific yet perhaps unrelated components of function. The following section discusses those test procedures or specific standardized tests that would best define the complexity of the problem.

Manual Muscle Testing

The first and most obvious request for evaluation may be to determine the extent of motor paralysis. In the newborn, testing may be done in the first 24 to 48 hours before the back is surgically closed. In this case, care must be taken not to injure the exposed neural tissue during testing. Prone and side lying to either side are the most convenient and safe positions for evaluation during this time. Subsequent testing is done soon after the back has been closed and as indicated throughout childhood. The traditional form of MMT is not appropriate or possible for the infant or young child. Following is a discussion of how muscle testing can and must be adapted for this age group.

In evaluating the newborn, the importance of alertness is paramount. A sleeping or drowsy infant will not respond appropriately during the evaluation. The infant must be in the alert or crying state to elicit the appropriate movement responses. Testing hungry or crying infants provides an advantage because they are likely to demonstrate more spontaneous movements in these behavioral states.

The cumulative effect of a variety of sensory stimuli may be more effective in bringing the infant to alertness than using one stimulus in isolation. For example, the infant may be picked up and rocked vertically to allow maximum stimulation to the vestibular system and to help bring the child to an alert state. In addition, the therapist may talk to the child to help him or her fixate visually on the therapist's face. Tactile stimuli above the level of the lesion further add to the child's level of arousal, thus contributing to more conclusive test results. In this way the CNS receives an accumulation of information from a variety of sensory systems rather than relying on transmission from one system that may be weak or inefficient.

As the child is aroused, spontaneous movements can be observed and muscle groups palpated. Additional methods to stimulate movement may be necessary. For example, tickling the infant generally produces a variety of spontaneous movements in the upper and lower extremities. Passive positioning of children in adverse positions may stimulate them to move. For example, if the legs are held in marked hip and knee flexion, the infant may attempt to use extensor musculature to move out of that position. If the legs are held in adduction, the child may abduct to get free. Holding a limb in an antigravity position may elicit an automatic "holding" response from a muscle group when spontaneous movements cannot be obtained in any other way.

In grading muscle strength, differentiation between spontaneous, voluntary movement and reflexive movement is important. After severing of a spinal cord, distal segments of the cord may respond to stimuli in a reflexive manner. This results from the preservation of the spinal reflex arc and is known as *distal sparing.* If distal sparing of the spinal cord is present, the muscles may respond to stimulation or muscular stretch with reflexive, stereotypical movement patterns. The quality of this reflexive movement will be different from that of spontaneous movement and must be distinguished when testing for level of voluntary muscle functioning.

Muscle strength is generally graded for groups of muscles and can be graded by using either a numerical (1 to 5) or an alphabetical designation (Figure 15-7) or simply by noting presence or absence of muscular contraction by a

THE CHILDREN'S MEMORIAL HOSPITAL
PHYSICAL / OCCUPATIONAL THERAPY

MUSCLE EXAM - MM

PATIENT NAME ______________________ M.R. # ____________

ATTENDING M.D. ______________________ PT. D.O.B. ____________

DIAGNOSIS ____

DATE: ____________________

P.T. NAME: ______________________________

	*	LEFT	RIGHT	*	COMMENTS: (Include ROM limitations, spasticity, reflexive movements, etc.)
ILIOPSOAS (L_1 - 2)					
SARTORIUS (L_1 - 3)					
HIP ADDUCTORS (L_2 - 4)					
TENSOR FASCIA LATA					
GLUTEUS MEDIUS (L_4 - S_1)					
GLUTEUS MAXIMUS (L_5 - S_1)					
QUADRICEPS (L_2 - 4)					
MEDIAL HAMSTRINGS (L_4 - S_2)					
LATERAL HAMSTRINGS (L_4 - S_1)					
ANTERIOR TIBIALIS (L_4 - L_5)					
POSTERIOR TIBIALIS (L_4 - L_5)					
PERONEUS LONGUS (L_5 - S_1)					
PERONEUS BREVIS (L_5 - S_1)					
GASTROC - SOLEUS (S_1 - S_2)					
EXT. HALLUCIS LONGUS (L_5 - S_1)					
FLEX. HALLUCIS LONGUS (S_1 - S_2)					
EXT. DIGITORUM LONGUS (L_4 - S_1)					
EXT. DIG. B. (L_4 - S_1)					
FLEX. DIGITORUM LONGUS (L_4 - S_1)					
FLEX. DIG. B. (L_4 - S_1)					
LUMBRICALES					

*INDICATE INCREASE (↑) OR DECREASE (↓) IN STRENGTH IN COMPARISON TO PREVIOUS TEST DATED ____________

PLEASE NOTE ANY SIGNIFICANT INFORMATION ON OTHER MUSCLE GROUPS UNLISTED ABOVE (i.e., EHB; Flex. HB; Internal or External Rotators)

X	PRESENT	UNABLE TO BE GRADED
N	NORMAL	COMPLETE RANGE OF MOTION AGAINST GRAVITY WITH FULL RESISTANCE
G	GOOD	COMPLETE RANGE OF MOTION AGAINST GRAVITY WITH MODERATE RESISTANCE
G-	GOOD MINUS	COMPLETE RANGE OF MOTION AGAINST GRAVITY WITH SOME RESISTANCE
F+	FAIR PLUS	COMPLETE RANGE OF MOTION AGAINST GRAVITY WITH SLIGHT RESISTANCE
F	FAIR	COMPLETE RANGE OF MOTION AGAINST GRAVITY
F-	FAIR MINUS	INCOMPLETE (GREATER THAN 1/2 WAY) RANGE OF MOTION AGAINST GRAVITY
P+	POOR PLUS	LESS THAN 1/2 WAY AGAINST GRAVITY OR FULL ROM GRAVITY ELIMINATED PLUS SL RESISTANCE
P	POOR	COMPLETE RANGE OF MOTION WITH GRAVITY ELIMINATED
P-	POOR MINUS	INCOMPLETE RANGE OF MOTION WITH GRAVITY ELIMINATED
T	TRACE	CONTRACTION IS FELT BUT THERE IS NO VISIBLE JOINT MOVEMENT
O	ZERO	NO CONTRACTION FELT IN THE MUSCLE

FORM 354042790

Figure 15-7 ■ Muscle examination form using alphabetical designation. (Courtesy Josefina Briceno, PT, Children's Memorial Hospital, Chicago.)

plus or a minus on the muscle test form. The last method may be sufficient initially, but as the child matures a more definitive muscle grade should be determined.

By use of a MMT form that lists the spinal segmental level for each muscle group, an approximate level of lesion can be determined from the test results (see Figure 15-7). Because the spinal cord is often damaged asymmetrically, MMT does not always accurately reflect the level of the lesion. If reflex activity is also noted on the form, the presence of distal sparing of the spinal cord can be determined. Muscle testing of the newborn gives the clinician an appreciation of muscle function and possible potential for later ambulation as well as an awareness of possible deforming forces. For example, if hip extensors or abductors are not functioning, then the action of hip flexors and adductors must be countered to prevent future deformities.

Muscle testing of the toddler or young child may require some of the techniques previously described. In addition, developmental positions can be used to assess muscle strength in an uncooperative youngster. For example, strength of hip extensors and abductors can be assessed as a child attempts to creep up steps or onto a low mat table. With addition of resistance to movements, fairly accurate muscle grades can be determined. To elicit hip flexor action in sitting, if an interesting toy or object is placed on the child's ankle or between the toes, the child will often lift the leg spontaneously to reach for it. Ingenuity and creativity are prerequisites for muscle testing in the young child. Reliability of MMT in children with spina bifida younger than 5 years is difficult but has been demonstrated in a clinic setting where all therapists were trained in specific MMT technique to ascertain consistency in testing.[181] By the age of 4 or 5 years, muscle grades can generally be determined by traditional testing techniques, although the reliability of the test results will increase with the age of the child.[182] In most clinics MMT is used to assess strength and changes in strength over time. Reliability of MMT may be called into question when trying to assess meaningful detectable changes in power against gravity. If that is the case, one can use hand-held dynamometry (HHD) to test muscles with a grade of 3 or greater. Excellent intertester reliability of HHD for children with spina bifida has been demonstrated.[183]

Muscle testing is indicated before and after any surgical procedure and at periodic intervals of 6 months to 1 year to detect any change in muscle function. Timely detection of any loss in strength is critical, as the child may encounter increased weakness resulting from tethering of the spinal cord or shunt malfunction as he or she grows. The level of innervation should not decrease throughout the life of the child with spina bifida. In the growing child or adolescent, an increasing weakness resulting from shunt malfunction, tethering of the spinal cord, or hydromyelia frequently can be substantiated by a muscle test of the lower extremities. The MMT is also valuable in determining the motor level so that potential future functional level can be determined (Figure 15-8).

Sensory Testing

Sensory testing of the infant and young child is simplified to determine the level of sensation as accurately as possible with a minimal amount of testing. Full sensory tests are not possible until the child has acquired sufficient cognitive and language abilities to respond appropriately to testing.

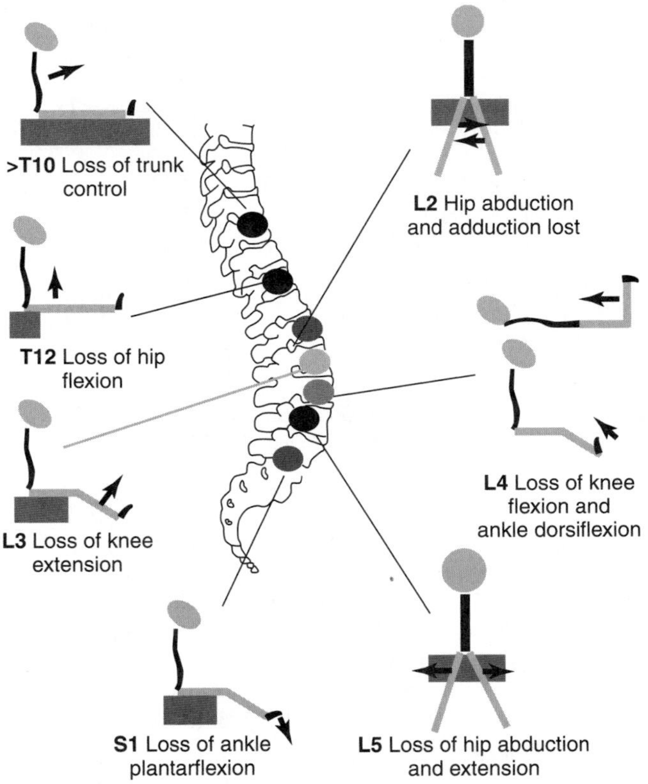

Figure 15-8 ■ Weakness related to level of spinal defect. (From Staheli LT: *Practice of pediatric orthopedics,* Philadelphia, 2001, Lippincott Williams & Wilkins.)

In the newborn, sensory testing can best be done if the child is in a quiet state. Beginning at the lowest level of sacral innervation, the skin is stroked with a pin or other sharp object until a reaction to pain is noted. Although none of these methods is fail-safe, they may be helpful in adapting a muscle test to a newborn or young infant. Repeated evaluation may be necessary to get an accurate picture of muscle function.

Because of dermatome innervation the pin is usually drawn from the anal area across the buttocks, down the posterior thigh and leg, then to the anterior surface of the leg and thigh, and finally across the abdominal muscles. Reactions to be noted are a facial grimace or cry, which indicates that the painful sensation has reached a cortical level. Care must be taken to see that each sensory dermatome has been evaluated. Results can be recorded by shading in the dermatomes where sensation is present (Figure 15-9).

The therapist may be called on to evaluate the newborn before surgical closure of the spinal meningocele. Although sensory and motor levels can be determined as previously described, the infant's general condition should be considered in interpreting test findings. Any medication taken by the mother during labor and delivery may influence the neonate's performance and thus should be noted. In addition, the physiological disorganization normally seen in all infants during the first few days after birth may also affect testing.[184] At best, this presurgical evaluation establishes a tentative baseline, but significant changes in the infant's neurological status in the first few weeks of life should not be surprising to the clinician.

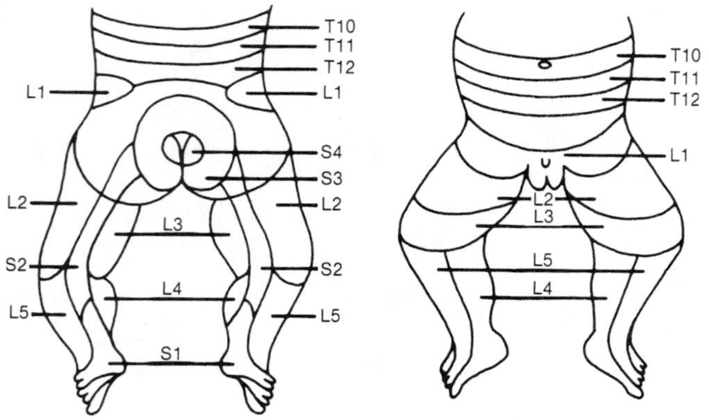

Figure 15-9 ■ Lower-limb dermatomes. (From Brocklehurst G: Spina bifida for the clinician. *Clin Dev Med* 57:53, 1976.)

In the young child from 2 to 7 years of age, light touch sensation and position sense can be tested in addition to pain sensation. Again, to elicit an appropriate response and reliable test results, the ingenuity of the therapist will be required. Using games such as "Tell me when the puppet touches you" may be more effective for the young child than traditional testing methods. Sensory dermatome mapping using the chart in Figure 15-9, or a similar form such as the WeeSTeP once the child with spina bifida gets older, can aid in establishing sensory level as well as insensate areas that may be at high risk of injury.[185]

From age 7 years through adolescence, additional sensory tests of temperature and two-point discrimination may be added. Traditional methods are usually sufficient to ensure reliable testing, but a more behavioral approach may be indicated depending on the individual's cognitive functioning.

After testing, a survey of the sensory dermatome chart should indicate whether sensation is normal, absent, or impaired. MMT and sensory testing (dermatomes) can assist in determining spinal level of function (Figure 15-10).

Range-of-Motion Evaluation

A complete ROM evaluation of the lower extremities is indicated for the newborn with spina bifida. The therapist must be aware of normal physiological flexion that is greatest at the hip and knees. In the normal newborn these apparent "contractures" of up to 35 degrees are eliminated as the child gains more control of extensor musculature and kicks more frequently into extension.

In the child with spina bifida, contractures may be evident at multiple joints at birth because of unopposed musculature (Figure 15-11). Hip adduction should not be tested beyond the neutral position to avoid dislocation of hips, which are often unstable. Range should be done slowly and without excessive force to avoid fractures so often experienced in paralytic lower extremities. ROM should be checked with the same frequency as MMT. Active ROM of the upper extremities can be assessed by observation and handling the infant. A formal ROM evaluation for the upper extremities is not usually indicated. A baseline ROM and tone assessment of the upper extremities should be completed.

Reflex Testing

The purpose of reflex testing is twofold: to check for the presence of normal reflex activity and to check for the integration of primitive reflexes and the establishment of more mature reactions. In the newborn, for example, strong rooting and sucking reflexes are expected. In the child with spina bifida, because of possible involvement of the CNS as previously described, these reflexes may be depressed or absent. Because these reflexes play an integral part in obtaining nutrients for the infant, their value is obvious. On the other hand, primitive reflexes that persist past their expected span also may indicate abnormality. For example, if the asymmetrical tonic neck reflex persists past 4 months, it will limit the infant's ability to bring the hands to midline for visual and tactile exploration.

As the primitive reflexes (initially needed for survival and to experience movement) become integrated, they are

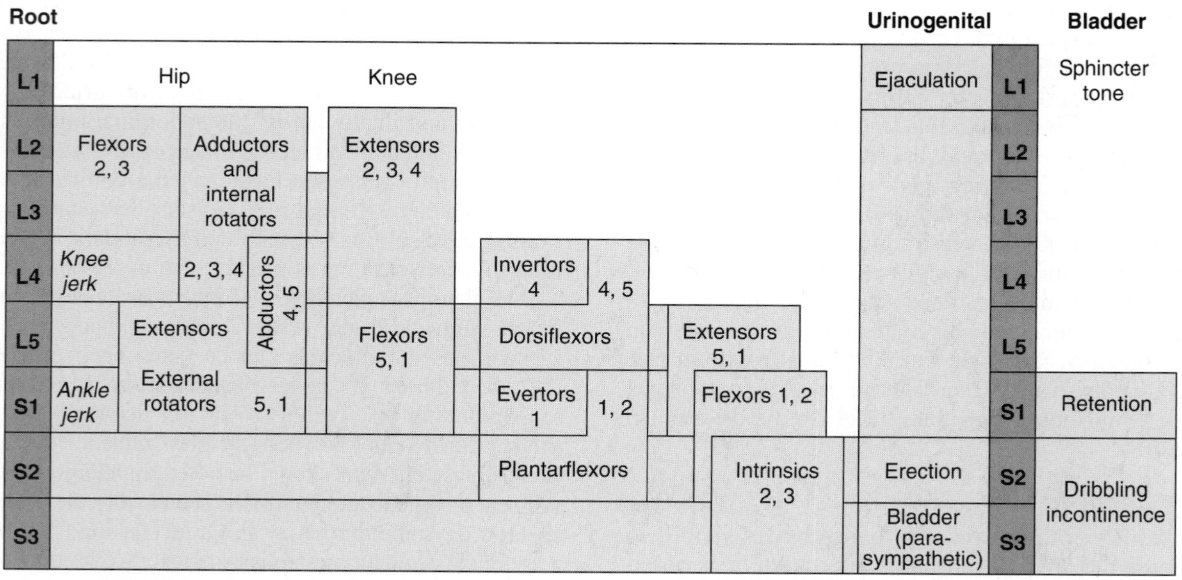

Figure 15-10 ■ Segmental nerve supply of the lower extremities. (From Stokes M: *Physical management in neurological rehabilitation,* London, 2004, Elsevier.)

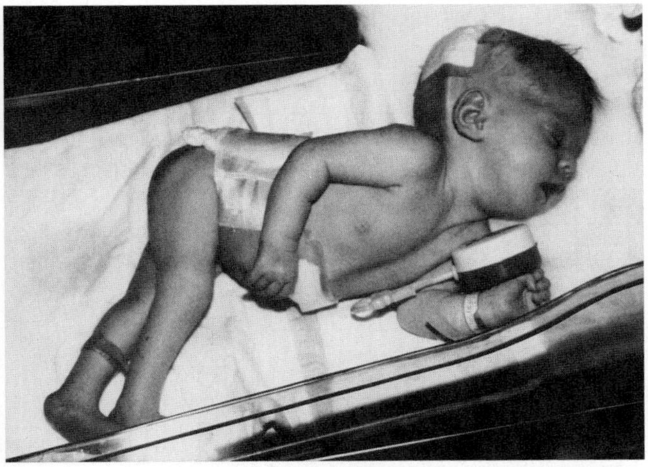

Figure 15-11 ■ Infant with myelomeningocele with contractures. (From Molnar GE, Alexander MA: *Pediatric rehabilitation,* Philadelphia, 1999, Hanley & Belfus.)

replaced by more mature and functional reactions. The righting and equilibrium reactions help the child attain the erect position and counteract changes in the center of gravity. Because these reactions depend on an intact CNS as well as a certain level of postural control, they may be delayed, incomplete, or absent in the child with spina bifida. For example, a child with a low thoracic spinal cord lesion may show an incomplete equilibrium reaction in sitting. This may be caused by the lack of a stable postural base or by lack of initiation of the reaction centrally. Both the neurological and muscular components of these reactions must be considered. Reflex testing for the child with spina bifida may not be as intensive as that for a child with cerebral palsy. It may, however, provide a check on the progress of normal development and as such reflect the integrity of the CNS (see Chapters 3 and 16).

Developmental and Functional Evaluations

Besides being aware of a child's sensory and motor levels, assessing the functional level is also important. Two important questions need to be asked: "Does the child show normal components of posture and movement synergies?" and "What is the child's level of function and mobility?" Several developmental and functional evaluations can be used with the child with spina bifida. The following are some suggestions for evaluation approaches or specifically designed tests to assist in assessment of this area.

Initially, a developmental sequence may be used to assess how a child is functioning. In each position used, both posture and movement are evaluated. The goals in using this type of assessment are to determine what a child can and cannot do, the quality of the action, and what is limiting the child. The progression begins in the supine position, rolling to prone, prone on elbows, prone on hands, up to sitting, on hands and knees, kneeling, half-kneeling, standing, and walking. Both the ability to attain and the ability to maintain the positions should be assessed.

The way in which a task is accomplished is as important to evaluate as the accomplishment itself. For example, in rolling, is head righting sufficient to keep the head off the supporting surface? From the hands-knees position, can reciprocal crawling be initiated without the lower extremities being held in wide abduction? Can the child pull to stand easily by using trunk rotation? Assessing the quality of the child's abilities will assist the clinician in determining where therapeutic measures should begin and what the goals of such intervention will be. Standardized assessments may provide the families with guidelines and a record of motor skills over time (see Chapter 3).

There are no standardized functional or motor assessments specific to those with spina bifida. Some assessments look at development relative to standardized norms and may guide the family and therapist in determining treatment goals and challenges. This information may be invaluable in determining bracing needs and other equipment needs as well as timing of various interventions. If a standardized assessment were desired to use with the infant with spina bifida, the Alberta Infant Motor Scale (AIMS) might be appropriate. The AIMS[186] is designed to measure motor development from birth to 18 months of age. It is a 58-item observational test of infants in supine, prone, sitting, and standing positions. Each item includes detailed descriptions of the weight-bearing surface, the infant's posture, and antigravity movements expected of the infant in that position. The AIMS requires minimal handling of the infant and can be completed in 20 to 30 minutes. The test was normed on a cross-sectional sample of 2200 infants in Alberta, Canada. Interrater and test-retest reliability are high (0.95 to 0.99), as is concurrent validity with the Peabody Developmental Motor Scales (PDMS) (0.99) and the Bayley Scales of Infant Development (0.97). Predictive validity of the AIMS appears to be fair.[187] For the child with spina bifida the AIMS could be used to assess current motor development and track progress in motor development over time.

The Milani-Comparetti Motor Development Screening Test for Infants and Young Children may also be useful in assessing the functional level of the child with spina bifida. This screening examination is designed to evaluate motor development from birth to 2 years of age (Figure 15-12).[188] It requires no special equipment and can be administered in 4 to 8 minutes. The test evaluates both spontaneous behavior and evoked responses. Spontaneous behavior includes postural control of the head and body in various positions as well as a sequence of active movement patterns. Primitive reflexes, righting, and equilibrium reactions constitute the evoked responses. The Milani-Comparetti test was normed on a sample of 312 children from Omaha, Nebraska. Interrater reliability percent of agreement was 89% to 95%. Test-retest reliability percent agreement was 82% to 100%. Predictive validity of the test has not been well established.[188] The Milani-Comparetti test should assist the clinician in evaluating each child's underlying postural mechanisms and his or her ability to attain the erect position. The test manual provides information on special examination procedures and scoring.

The Ages and Stages Questionnaire (ASQ) is a screening assessment that assesses developmental and social-emotional delays during crucial early ages of life. This test is available in English and Spanish and can be completed in 10 to 15 minutes.[189] It was developed and validated on 15,138 children in all 50 states and several U.S. territories. The test-retest reliability (0.92), interrater reliability (0.93), validity (0.82 to 0.88),

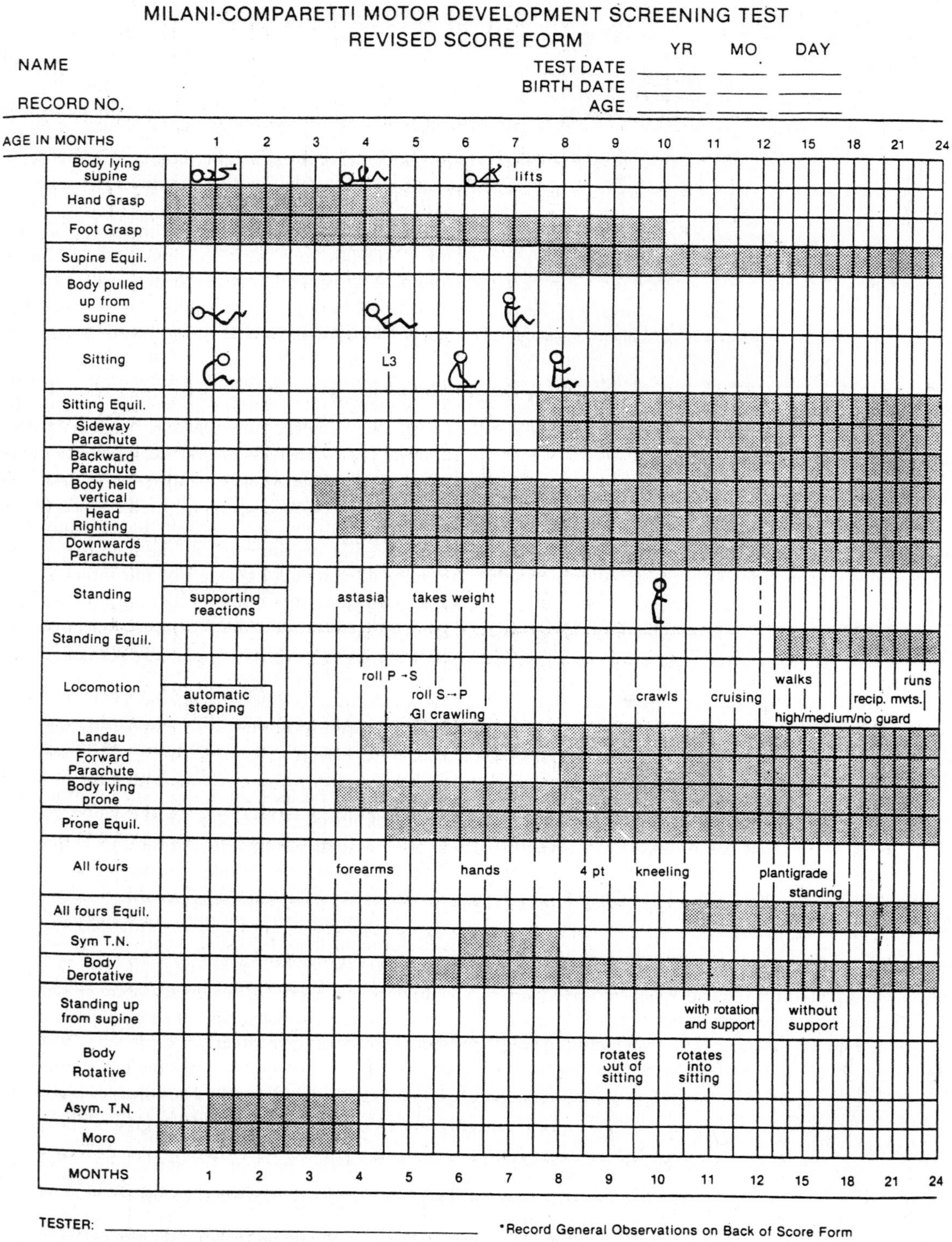
MILANI-COMPARETTI MOTOR DEVELOPMENT SCREENING TEST
REVISED SCORE FORM
NAME
RECORD NO.
YR MO DAY
TEST DATE
BIRTH DATE
AGE
AGE IN MONTHS
1 2 3 4 5 6 7 8 9 10 11 12 15 18 21 24
Body lying supine
lifts
Hand Grasp
Foot Grasp
Supine Equil.
Body pulled up from supine
Sitting
L3
Sitting Equil.
Sideway Parachute
Backward Parachute
Body held vertical
Head Righting
Downwards Parachute
Standing
supporting reactions
astasia
takes weight
Standing Equil.
Locomotion
automatic stepping
roll P→S
roll S→P
GI crawling
crawls
cruising
walks
runs
recip. mvts.
high/medium/no guard
Landau
Forward Parachute
Body lying prone
Prone Equil.
All fours
forearms
hands
4 pt
kneeling
plantigrade
standing
All fours Equil.
Sym T.N.
Body Derotative
Standing up from supine
with rotation and support
without support
Body Rotative
rotates out of sitting
rotates into sitting
Asym. T.N.
Moro
MONTHS
1 2 3 4 5 6 7 8 9 10 11 12 15 18 21 24
TESTER:
*Record General Observations on Back of Score Form

Figure 15-12 ■ Milani-Comparetti Motor Development Screening Test revised score form.

sensitivity (0.86), and specificity (0.85) have been well documented.[189] This test provides parents and providers with a checklist to easily assess change over time.

The PDMS-2 is another standardized assessment that may prove helpful in evaluating a child with congenital spinal cord injury.[190] The PDMS-2 was developed using item response theory (IRT) and consists of six gross and fine motor subtests from birth through 6 years of age. The test takes 45 to 60 minutes to complete or 20 to 30 minutes per subtest. The two scales allow a comparison of the child's motor performance with a normative sample of children at various age levels. A stratified sample of 2003 children from 46 states in the United States was used to develop PDMS-2 test norms. Test-retest and interrater reliability are high. Content, construct, and concurrent validity have been well established. Although the child with activity limitations would not be expected to succeed on many of the gross motor items at the later age levels, the scale still serves as a reminder of expected gross motor performance at each age. The fine motor scale offers a chance to assess fine motor performance of children with congenital spinal cord injury. This area has been frequently overlooked in children with myelomeningocele. Fine motor development, however, may be affected because of congenital abnormalities in brain development associated with myelomeningocele or related to tethering of the spinal cord that can result in fine motor paresis. In addition, the PDMS-2 offers guidelines for administering the test to children with various activity limitations.[190]

The Bruininks-Oseretsky Test of Motor Proficiency, second edition (BOT-2) can be used to evaluate the higher functioning ambulatory child with lower lumbar or sacral level spina bifida.[191] Fine manual control, manual coordination, body coordination, and strength and agility subtests can be used to assist in evaluating areas of fine motor control, balance, and coordination difficulties. This test has been standardized on a sample of 1520 subjects from age 4 through 21 years.[191]

The Movement Assessment Battery for Children, second edition (Movement ABC-2), can be used to identify children who are significantly behind their peers in motor development, assist in planning an intervention program in either a school or a clinical setting, and measure change as a result of intervention or can serve as a measurement instrument in research involving motor development. This tool may be useful to assess children with lower lumbar and sacral level myelomeningocele, as well as children with lipomeningocele. The Movement ABC identifies and evaluates the movement problems that can determine a child's participation and social adjustment at home or school. The Movement ABC Checklist provides classroom assessment of movement difficulties, screening for "at risk" children (ages 5 to 12 years), and systematic monitoring of treatment programs. It provides a comprehensive assessment for those identified as "at risk" (3 to 16 years, 11 months), yielding both normative and qualitative measures of movement competence, manual dexterity, ball skills, and static and dynamic balance.[192]

Finally, the Pediatric Evaluation of Disability Inventory (PEDI) is a comprehensive assessment of function in children aged 6 months to 7 years.[193] The PEDI measures both capability and performance of functional activities in three areas: self-care, mobility, and social function. Capability is a measure of the functional skills for which the child has demonstrated mastery. Functional performance is measured by the level of caregiver assistance needed to accomplish a task. A modifications scale provides a measure of environmental modifications and equipment needed in daily functioning. The PEDI has been standardized on a normative sample of 412 children from New England. Some data from clinical samples (N = 102) are also available. Interrater reliability of the PEDI is high as demonstrated by high intraclass correlation coefficients (ICCs = 0.96 to 0.99). Concurrent validity of the PEDI with the WeeFIM (child's version of the Functional Independence Measure) was also high (r = .80 to 0.97).[193] The PEDI can be administered in approximately 45 minutes by clinicians or educators familiar with the child or by structured interview of the parent. The PEDI should provide a descriptive measure of the functional level of the child with myelomeningocele as well as a method for tracking change over time. The PEDI has had a rich tradition in helping to document functional development, and new methods proposed for the next generation of the PEDI include using item banks and computer adaptive testing. The computer adaptive testing feature and the revised and expanded content of the new PEDI will enable therapists to more efficiently assess children's functioning to a broader age group of children.[194,195]

Another assessment of motor performance that may be commonly used with the school-age child with spina bifida is the School Function Assessment (SFA). The SFA is standardized and was conceptually developed to reflect the functional abilities and needs of a student in elementary school. The three areas assessed include the student's participation in school activities, task supports required by the student for participation, and the student's activity performance.[196,197] It was designed to facilitate collaborative program planning for students with a variety of disabling conditions. The instrument is a judgment-based (questionnaire) assessment that is completed by one or more school professionals who know the student well and have observed his or her typical performance on the school-related tasks and activities being assessed. Items have been written in measurable, behavioral terms that can be used directly in the student's Individualized Educational Plan (IEP).[196]

Gait Analysis

Formal computerized gait analysis was initially used to evaluate children with cerebral palsy. Increasingly it is being used to evaluate children with meningomyelocele once they have established a gait pattern to determine factors leading to changes in gait, including changes in alignment, muscle length, muscle torque, and symmetry. The gait analysis may aid in decision making regarding orthotic and orthopedic interventions. Whether it is useful to do formal gait analyses in all children with spina bifida remains to be determined.[198] Gait analyses have also been useful in establishing a database of trends in kinetics and kinematics for various levels of spina bifida.

Perceptual and Cognitive Evaluations

When evaluating a child with spina bifida, some assessment of perceptual and cognitive status is important to include. The appropriate assessment depends largely on the age of the child. The assessment may be performed by the physical, occupational, or speech therapist, depending on the setting.

For the newborn from 3 to 30 days old, the Brazelton Neonatal Behavioral Assessment scale may be adapted to assess the infant's organization in terms of physiological response to stress, state control, motoric control, and social interaction.[184] Ideally the infant should be medically stable and free from CNS-depressant drugs before evaluation. Generally this evaluation will occur after the back lesion has been closed and a shunt has been positioned to relieve the hydrocephalic condition.

Although test results may not have prognostic value because of the plasticity of the nervous system at this young age, they supply the clinician with information concerning the current status of the child. This information can be conveyed to the infant's caregivers—both medical personnel and parents—so that strengths can be appreciated and weaknesses anticipated and handled appropriately. Helping parents identify that their infant has his or her own unique characteristics and assisting them in dealing with these characteristics does a great deal to strengthen already precarious parent-infant bonding.

Repeated administration of the Brazelton Neonatal Behavioral Assessment scale in the first month of life may help monitor the infant's progress in organization and reflect the curve of recovery. Although the manual for this behavioral assessment is complete, proper administration, scoring, and interpretation require direct training with someone already proficient in using the scale.[199] Excellent training videos for the Brazelton Neonatal Behavioral Assessment scale are available through the Brazelton Institute for purchase or through the local university's learning resource centers.[200]

A full developmental evaluation appropriate for the infant and toddler with spina bifida is the Bayley Scales of Infant and Toddler Development, Third Edition (BSID-III).[201] The Bayley Scales, consisting of a mental and motor scale and a behavioral rating scale, can be used to test children from age 1 month to 42 months. The test provides information on gross motor, fine motor, language, social-emotional, adaptive, and cognitive development.

The BSID-III is well standardized and reliable and takes approximately 45 minutes to administer. It is not an easy test to learn and initially requires supervision of an experienced tester. This edition provides new normative data, extended age range, expanded content coverage, and improved psychometric qualities.

The BSID-III provides the clinician with a broader view of the child's total development. The gross motor information from this developmental assessment will not be specific enough for a therapist evaluating a child with spina bifida. The additional information on fine motor, language, personal-social, and cognitive development, however, is sufficient and will be important in planning a comprehensive intervention program.[201]

Various tests are available as screening tools to test visual-motor integration and perception. The Beery-Buktenica Developmental Test of Visual-Motor Integration, 6th Edition (Beery VMI) is an early screening tool to aid in diagnosis of learning problems in children. It assesses integration of visual perception and motor control of children from age 2 years through 18 years. The test takes 10 to 15 minutes to complete and requires the child to be able to copy designs. The Beery VMI is norm referenced and was standardized on a large sample of children chosen from throughout the United States. There is also an adult version that can be used with individuals 19 to 100 years of age that facilitates identification of neurological and related problems in the adult.[202]

Children with spina bifida often exhibit upper-extremity weakness in addition to probable sensory dysfunction. As a result, fine motor skills in children with spina bifida are often impeded by slowness and inadequate adjustment of manipulative forces, and a non–motor-perceptual test is often desired.[203-205] The Motor-Free Visual Perception Test, Third Edition (MVPT-3)[206] and the Test of Visual Perceptual Skills, Non-Motor, Third Edition (TVPS-3)[207] can be used to determine the child's visual perceptual processing skills on the basis of a non–motor assessment of these skills. Both tests evaluate visual discrimination, visual memory, spatial relations, figure-ground, and visual closure. The TVPS-3 also evaluates form constancy and sequential memory. The MVPT-3 can be used with individuals from 4 to 70 years of age, and the TVPS-3 can be used with children from 4 to 18 years of age. The TVPS-3 has two levels; the lower level tests children from ages 4 to 12 years, and the upper level tests children from ages 12 years to 17 years, 11 months. Both tests are easy and quick to administer (less than 15 minutes) and, based on the examiner's experience and training, interpretations can be made with prescription for remediation. The MVPT-3 was standardized on a nationally representative sample. The test-retest reliability of the MVPT-3 was 0.81.[206] Performance on the motor-free test has been shown to be independent of the degree of motor involvement when compared with other tests of visual perception.[206] The TVPS-3 was standardized on a nationally stratified sample of 2000 children across the United States.

With a firm database provided by a thorough physical and occupational therapy evaluation with referrals to other professionals as appropriate, a reasonable treatment plan can be developed and updated as necessary.

TREATMENT PLANNING AND REHABILITATION RELATED TO SIGNIFICANT STAGES OF DEVELOPMENT

Newborn to Toddler (Preambulatory Phase)

Stage 1: Before Closure of Myelomeningocele—Early Newborn Period

Physical therapy management of the infant in stage 1 is limited by his or her medical condition (Table 15-2). Therapists are called on a regular basis in large tertiary care centers to carry out preoperative MMT to help to ascertain functional motor level. Physicians (neurosurgeons and orthopedic surgeons) on the spina bifida care team rely on this assessment to guide their discussion with the families regarding care and prognosis. When carrying out the preoperative MMT, great care must be taken to avoid contaminating an open sac, which is usually covered with a Telfa nonadherent dressing or a wet sterile dressing that must be kept moist with a saline solution.

Stage 2: After Surgery, during Hospitalization, and Transition to Home—Newborn through Early Infancy

Therapeutic intervention after surgical back closure during stage 2 is often limited by the infant's neurological and orthopedic status. A major goal during this stage is to prevent contractures and maintain ROM while giving stimulation to provide as normal an environment as possible. Traditional ROM exercises can be taught to nursing staff and family. They also can be carried out while the child is being held at the adult's shoulder or prone over the adult's lap. These positions allow closeness between the caregiver and infant, thus encouraging maximal relaxation and interaction between them. ROM movements and positioning in prone or side lying may be initiated to prevent or decrease contractures in the lower extremities. If clubfeet are present, soft tissue stretching may be indicated. Stretching begins distally on the soft tissue of the forefoot and proceeds proximally toward the calcaneus. This is done to take advantage of the pliability of soft tissue structures and to minimize fixed deformity later. In addition, taping may be used to maintain optimal ROM and alignment between periods of

TABLE 15-2 ■ SUMMARY OF TREATMENT PLANNING AND REHABILITATION RELATED TO SIGNIFICANT STAGES OF DEVELOPMENT

STAGE OF RECOVERY	MAJOR PHYSICAL THERAPY GOALS	PHYSICAL THERAPY MANAGEMENT
NEWBORN TO TODDLER (PREAMBULATORY PHASE)		
Stage 1: before surgical closure of myelomeningocele—newborn	Determine functional motor level	Preoperative manual muscle testing
Stage 2: after surgery, during hospitalization—newborn to infant	Confirm functional motor level Prevent contracture and deformity Encourage normal sensorimotor development	Postoperative manual muscle testing ROM exercises taught to hospital personnel and family Positioning in prone and side lying Provide toys of various colors, textures, and shapes Graded auditory and visual stimuli: music boxes, squeaky toys, brightly colored objects Therapeutic handling to encourage good head and trunk control
Stage 3: condition stabilized—infant to toddler	Confirm functional motor level Encourage normal development sequence	Manual muscle testing once or twice per year Work in sitting on head righting and equilibrium reactions Eye-hand coordination activities Early weight bearing on lower extremities Encourage prone progression Weight shifting in standing frame Comprehensive home program
TODDLER THROUGH ADOLESCENT (AMBULATORY PHASE)		
Stage 4: toddler through preschool	Confirm functional motor level Begin ambulation Continue development in cognitive and psychosocial areas Collaborate on goals with other team members	Manual muscle testing once or twice per year Choose appropriate orthotic device Gait training Development and strengthening of righting and equilibrium reactions Consider referral to EI program Public preschool program Continue home program Open communication with other team members
Stage 5: primary school through adolescence	Confirm functional motor level Reevaluate ambulation potential Maintain present level of functioning Prevent skin breakdown as child becomes more sedentary Promote independence in self-care skills Remediate any perceptual-motor problems Provide appropriate adaptive devices Promote self-esteem and social-sexual adjustment	Postoperative manual muscle testing Replace orthotic device as necessary Wheelchair prescriptions as necessary Teach locomotion activities Maintain strength in trunk and extremities Teach skin care Work with team members to teach dressing, feeding, hygiene, and bowel and bladder care Provide program and activities for sensorimotor integration Check for fit and proper use of adaptive devices Collaborate with other team members in counseling efforts

EI, Early intervention; *ROM,* range of motion.

stretching.[150] In treating the newborn after surgery, great care must be taken to avoid contaminating the surgical dressing, which is usually covered with Xeroform Petrolatum Gauze (3% bismuth tribromophenate in a special petrolatum blend on fine mesh gauze). This dressing is nonadherent and clings and conforms to all body contours. The Xeroform dressing is covered with Telfa. This postoperative dressing remains on for 2 weeks.

Because of their medical conditions, hospitalized infants often experience early separation from their parents. Teaching the family to handle the child as described may enhance parent-infant bonding. Adequate bonding is essential for normal psychosocial development to occur.

When the child is not being handled, resting positions can be used to maintain ROM and enhance development. The prone position is the most advantageous because it prevents hip flexion contractures and encourages development of extensor musculature as the child lifts his or her head. Side lying, which allows the hands to come to midline and generally encourages symmetrical posture, can be used for alternate positioning. As much as possible, the supine position should be avoided because the child is most dominated by primitive reflexes and the effects of gravity in this position. For example, for the child with spina bifida with CNS involvement, the effects of the tonic labyrinthine reflex combined with paralytic lower extremities may make movement from the supine position extremely difficult. Before initiating activities in the supine position, the therapist should obtain medical clearance.

A normal sensory experience should be presented to the child in spite of the hospital setting. Toys of various colors, textures, and shapes should be available. Musical mobiles held low enough for the child to reach provide a variety of sensory experiences. Stimuli such as squeaky toys or the human face and voice can be used to encourage visual and auditory tracking. Controlled stimulation relevant to the infant's neurological state, rather than overstimulation, should be the rule. Depending on the age of the child, appropriate learning situations must be presented to provide the child with as normal an environment as possible for perceptual and cognitive growth.

A major therapeutic goal is to guide the child through the developmental sequence, ultimately preparing him or her to assume the upright posture. In this immediate postsurgical stage, the primary emphasis should be on attaining good head and trunk control and eliciting appropriate righting reactions. For example, the child can be seated on the therapist's lap, facing the therapist, and alternately lowered slowly backward and side to side. This action helps stimulate head righting and strengthen neck and abdominal muscles. Weight shifting in various positions and through therapeutic handling is important to enhance development of early head and trunk control. Developmental handling may be limited by surgical interventions that limit mobility.

This second stage ends as the child is discharged from the hospital. After discharge the child should be monitored closely by the spina bifida team, which may include a neurosurgeon, an orthopedist, a urologist, a nurse clinician, a PT, an occupational therapist (OT), an orthotist, and a social worker. Before discharge, a definitive home program as well as referral to the local Early Intervention (EI) program should be given to the family because the child will most likely require ongoing therapy, including both PT and OT. Other professionals who may be involved in the child's EI program may include speech and language pathologists (SLPs), developmental therapists (DTs), social workers, and psychologists.

Stage 3: Condition Stabilized—Infant to Toddler (Preambulatory)

In the third stage of rehabilitation, the major emphasis is on preparing the child mentally and physically for upright standing and mobility. In addition, routine MMT should be performed every 6 to 12 months to reassess functional motor level and to ascertain that no change in status has occurred. Goals of preventing contractures and maintaining ROM will remain throughout the child's life. Unless this is done, standing and ambulation become more difficult and often impossible. If possible, prone positioning during play and sleeping assists greatly in stretching tight musculature. Resting splints for the lower extremities or a total-body splint can be used as necessary to position and maintain ROM and alignment.

Developmental strategies should be aimed at facilitating movement and motor control. Assuming that the child has previously gained good head and trunk control, the next step is development of sitting equilibrium reactions. As sitting balance improves, fine motor and eye-hand coordination activities should be introduced. Upper-extremity functioning is often overlooked in the child with spina bifida, whose problems appear to be concentrated in the lower extremities. However, most children with spina bifida show decreased fine motor coordination, and this problem should be addressed as developmentally appropriate. The normal infant begins to reach and grasp by 6 months of age; therefore the child with spina bifida must be given ample opportunities to practice and perfect these same skills at an early age. Because many children with spina bifida may be receiving PT as their primary service through EI in these early months, referral to and consultation with an OT at this age are highly recommended.

Following a normal developmental sequence, the child with spina bifida will usually begin some form of prone progression as trunk and upper-extremity stability improve. This is a significant phase of development because it allows for the development of a sensorimotor base as the child expands environmental horizons. During this phase of high mobility, insensate skin must be checked for injury frequently and often must be protected by heavier clothing. This may help prevent any major skin breakdown, which could significantly delay the rehabilitation process. For some children with high-level lesions in whom prone mobility is not safe or practical for long distances, a Star Car (Tash) (Figure 15-13), the Ready Racer (Tumble Forms), or the PlasmaCar may be used. These provide the child with a means of exploring the environment safely but independently.

Emphasis on head and trunk control and strengthening exercises in a variety of sitting postures is quite important in this early preambulatory phase. Development of adequate strength and motor control for trunk righting, equilibrium reactions, and protective reactions will ultimately lead to improved sitting balance. Hands-free sitting with good balance is the optimal goal in this stage to allow for

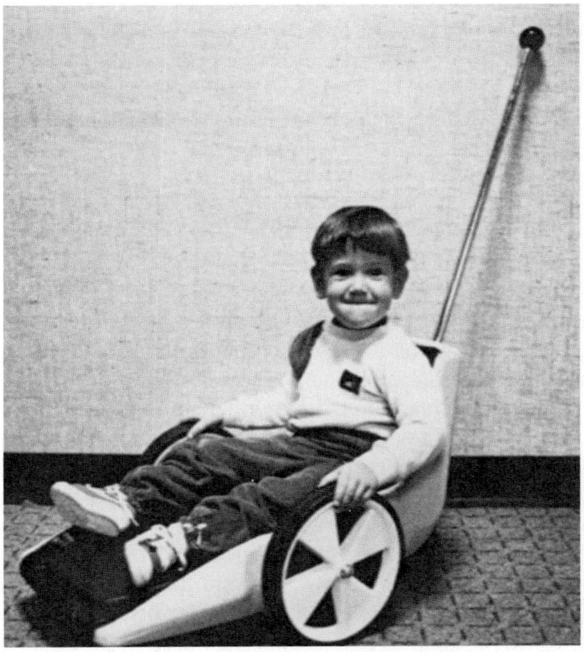

Figure 15-13 ■ Caster cart used for independent mobility.

independence and freedom in play skills. In addition, hands-free sitting is a necessary precursor to ambulation with lower-extremity bracing and often is the determinant in deciding if a child will use a standing frame or will become a functional ambulator.

Early weight bearing is also of utmost importance, both physiologically and psychologically. The upright position has beneficial effects on circulation and renal and bladder functioning as well as on the promotion of bone growth and density.[59,176,208,209] Psychologically, weight bearing in an upright posture allows a normal view of the world and contributes to more normal perceptual, cognitive, and emotional growth. One way to achieve this weight bearing is in the kneeling position. This is developmentally appropriate because children 8 to 10 months old frequently use kneeling as a transition from all fours to standing.

Because young infants are frequently held in the standing position and bounced on their parents' laps, this form of weight bearing on the lower extremities is appropriate from birth onward. Failure to promote weight bearing in this manner may deprive the child with spina bifida of the normal experience of standing at a very early age. When standing these children, however, care must be taken to see that the lower extremities are in good alignment and that undue pressure is not exerted on them (Figure 15-14). In this way the risk of fractures is minimized and a normal weight-bearing experience is provided.

Also in this phase of preambulation, transitions from one position to another should be assessed and facilitated. Teaching the child strategies for transitions will enhance his or her optimal functional independence. Compensations may be taught to substitute for weakened musculature. In addition, adaptive equipment and mobility devices may be recommended to enhance acquisition of age-appropriate milestones. Providing appropriate facilitation of mobility at a level similar to that of a child's peers is important for psychosocial growth and development (Figure 15-15).

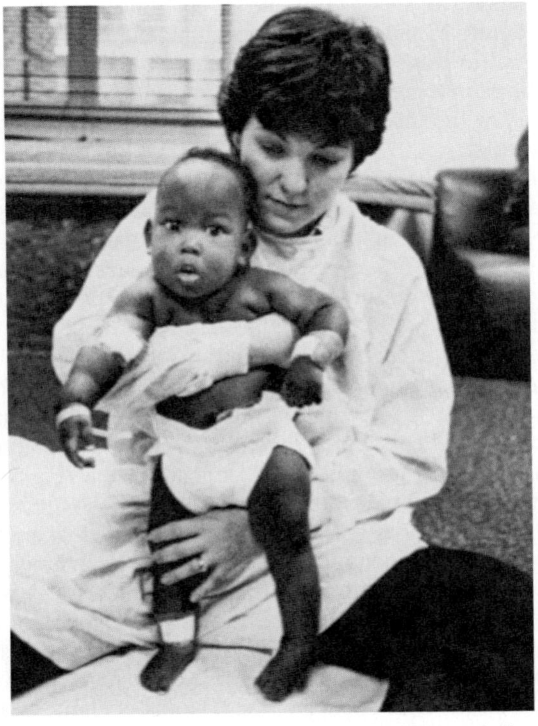

Figure 15-14 ■ Assisted standing with normal postural alignment.

When the child attempts to pull to a standing position or would be expected to do so normally (at 10 to 12 months of age), the use of a standing device is indicated. Generally a standing frame is the first orthosis chosen. This is a relatively inexpensive tubular frame to which adjustable parts are attached (Figure 15-16). Because it is not custom made, it can be fitted fairly quickly, although adjustments may be necessary to accommodate spinal deformities. This standing device offers support of the trunk, hips, and knees and leaves the hands free for other activities. Time spent in the standing frame should be increased gradually. This allows the child to adjust to the upright position in terms of muscle strength, endurance, blood pressure, and pressure on skin surfaces.

After children have built up a tolerance for standing, they may be taught to move in the device by shifting their weight from side to side. Initial shifting of weight onto one side of the body is necessary to allow the other side to move forward. This preliminary weight shift is also a prerequisite for developing equilibrium reactions in the standing position and thus will prepare the child for later ambulation. As the child shifts weight, the trunk musculature on the weight-bearing side should elongate and on the non–weight-bearing side should shorten as muscle strength allows. This normal reaction to weight shifting also includes righting of the head and should be closely monitored by the therapist for completeness.

A therapy program must be designed to meet the individual's needs in each area. Age alone does not determine the appropriate therapeutic goals. Goals that are not suited for the child's cognitive and emotional needs, in addition to physical needs, will not facilitate best outcomes. For example, an 18-month-old may have the physical capabilities to ambulate independently with crutches and braces. The child may not, however, have the cognitive skills necessary to learn a four-point gait or be ready emotionally to separate from his or her mother for intensive therapy sessions. A more realistic goal may be to let the child walk holding onto furniture (cruising) while a wheeled walker for more independent ambulation is slowly introduced. Another alternative to using a conventional walker is to encourage the child to play with push toys such as grocery carts and baby buggies.

During this preambulatory stage, therapy goals may be accomplished through a comprehensive home program, with frequent checks to note progress or problems and to change the program accordingly. For the more involved child, increased frequency of direct intervention may be indicated to achieve optimal developmental progress.

The program often must be reevaluated and goals changed if conditions such as shunt malfunctions or fractures occur. The warning signs for shunt dysfunctions are generally those previously described for suspected hydrocephalus. In addition, swelling along the shunt site may indicate a malfunction. Swelling and local heat or redness of a limb are the usual signs of a fracture. The limb may also look misaligned. Fever may accompany a fracture. As previously mentioned, these fractures generally heal quickly with proper medical intervention and minimally interrupt rehabilitation efforts.

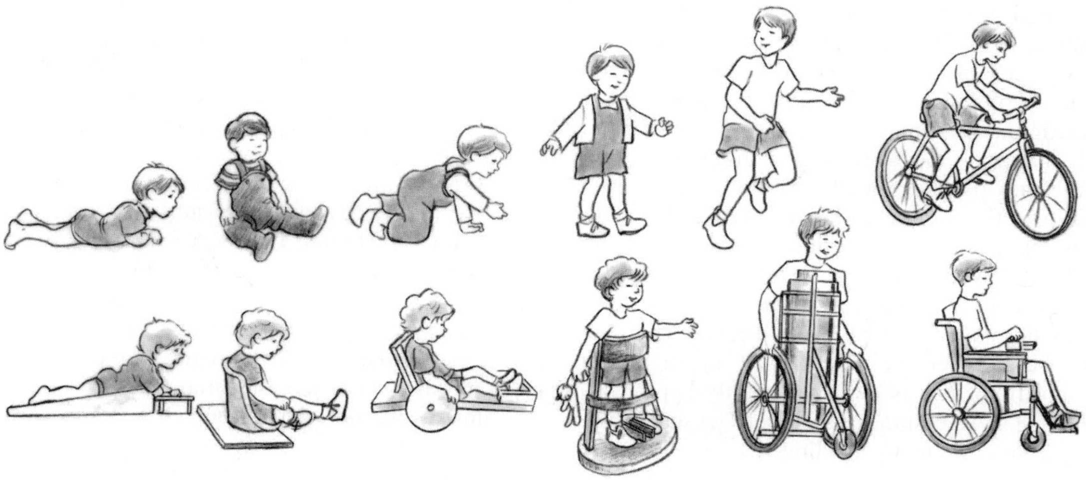

Figure 15-15 ■ Adaptive devices can help the young child with spina bifida reach major milestones at the same time as peers. (From Ratcliffe KT: *Clinical pediatric physical therapy,* St Louis, 1998, Mosby.)

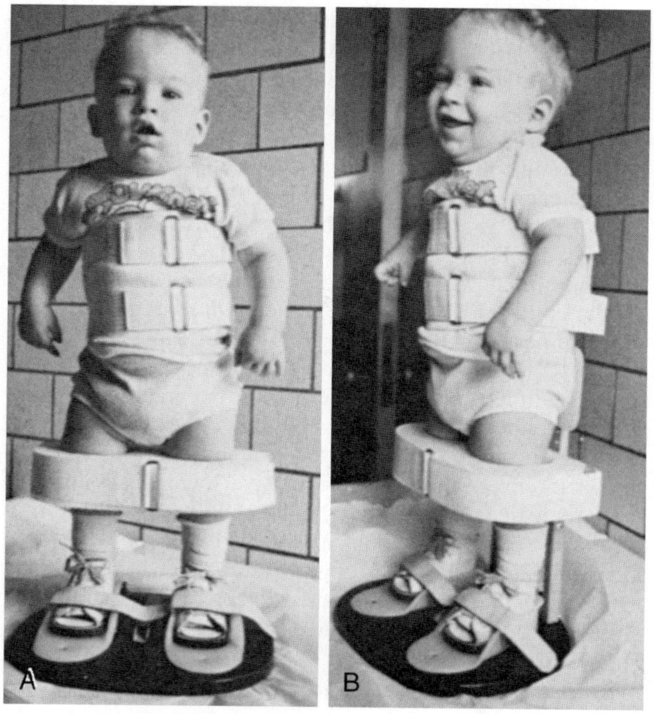

Figure 15-16 ■ Standing frame. **A,** Anterior view. **B,** Lateral view.

Toddler through Adolescent (Ambulatory Phase)

Stage 4: Toddler through Preschool

The fourth period in development marks the end of infancy and the beginning of childhood. For the typically developing child who has developed a strong sensorimotor foundation, physical development is marked by increased coordination and refinement of movement patterns. In addition, a great variety of motor skills will be achieved as the typically developing child learns to throw, catch, run, hop, and jump. This is also a period of great cognitive growth, as children's use of mental imagery and physical knowledge of their environments expand. Concepts of size, number, color, form, and space are all developing. Emotionally, most children are becoming more independent and begin to break away from the sheltered environment of the home. They are now more interested in interacting with others and become social beings to a greater extent.

All these changes in physical, cognitive, and emotional development will be evident in the child with spina bifida, although the degree depends on the extent of the functional limitations and their effect on the child's ability to participate in life. The characteristics of normal development must be understood so that cognitive, emotional, and motor behaviors can be nurtured and enhanced in the child with spina bifida.

Goals for this as for any other stage must address physical, cognitive, and emotional development. The most obvious goal at this stage is to help the child who is already standing to progress to an ambulatory status. Even the child with a low thoracic lesion can usually manage some form of ambulation.

Thus far, the child has learned to shift weight in the standing frame. By rotating the trunk toward the weighted side, the non–weight-bearing side can be shifted forward (Figure 15-17). By reversing the weight shift, the opposite side can be moved forward and a type of "pivoting forward" progression can be accomplished. To maintain balance while shifting, the child may initially use a two-wheeled walker. The therapist may help initiate weight shift and trunk rotation by alternately pulling the arms forward.[210] Once the child has gained this form of mobility, the type of permanent bracing chosen will depend on the level of the lesion and a variety of other factors.

The overall goal for ambulatory training is to promote efficient, independent mobility with the least amount of bracing while maintaining optimal joint integrity. Ambulatory potential as well as choice of bracing depends on many factors, including neurosegmental level of the lesion, motor power at the neurosegmental level, extent and degree of orthopedic deformity, balance, age, height, weight, sex, motivation, spasticity, design and effectiveness of the orthosis,

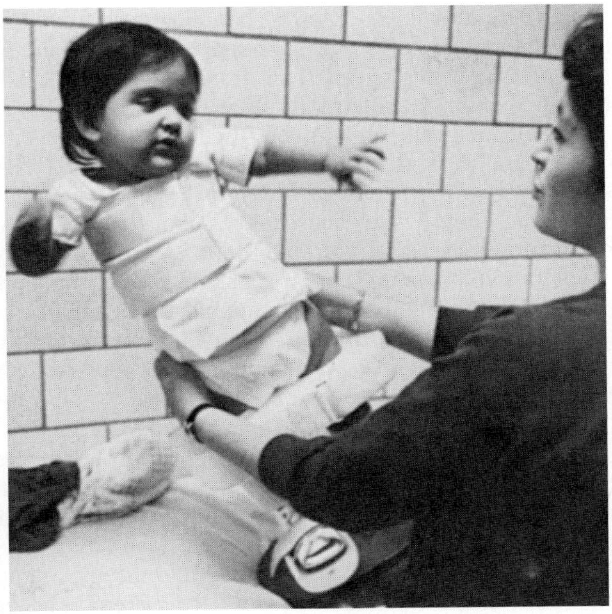

Figure 15-17 ■ Weight shift and forward rotation in standing frame.

effectiveness of PT intervention, environmental factors, upper-extremity strength and control, and cognitive level.[163,211] The best prognosis for ambulation is most often seen in the child who is not shunted and has good cognition, good quadriceps power, no deformity, a stable neurological condition, and hands-free sitting balance. Factors that may limit potential for ambulation include hydrocephalus, high-level lesions, kyphosis or kyphoscoliosis, and unstable neurology.

Developmental progression preceding ambulation in spina bifida shows a high degree of variability.[212] A study by Bartonek in 2010[212] confirmed that those with greater muscle power of the lower limb muscles ambulated earlier and more frequently. Those engaged in physical therapy programs aimed at achieving the specific goal of walking are also likely to make earlier strides toward ambulation, although this has not been formally studied. Those who have been enrolled in early treadmill body-weight support training (BWST) programs as infants have demonstrated early stepping responsiveness, and it has been suggested that BWST training intervention could promote muscle strengthening and take advantage of neural plasticity to promote development of the neuromuscular patterns necessary to support the onset of gait. There is also potential to improve bone density, cardiovascular function, and the integrity of lower spinal sensorimotor function. Infants with spina bifida demonstrate developmental delay as early as 3 months of age, and BWST intervention during the first postnatal year has the potential to reduce this delay and promote earlier onset of gait in the population with spina bifida.[213] Efficacy of enhanced sensory inputs during treadmill stepping in children with spina bifida has also been examined. Increasing friction by using Dycem matting and enhancing visual flow by using a checkerboard pattern on the treadmill belt both appear to be more effective than the standard black treadmill belt in eliciting stepping.[214] Teulier and colleagues[215] studied stepping responses in infants with spina bifida. They reported a decrease in number of steps per minute compared with typically developing peers (14.4 versus 40.8 steps per minute) and a decrease in frequency of alternating steps. In contrast to these interlimb coordination differences, they reported that within-limb step parameters in infants with spina bifida were quite similar to those in children who were typically developing.

For thoracic and high-level lumbar lesions, a parapodium is often chosen. The parapodium was developed by the Ontario Crippled Children's Centre in 1970 and is similar to the standing frame except that hinges at the hips and knees allow for sitting and standing.[210] It also can be adjusted for growth and can accommodate orthopedic deformities. As with the standing frame, proper alignment of the parapodium is critical. The therapist, in conjunction with the orthotist, should check for correct standing alignment. The prevention of additional orthopedic deformities, development of good muscular control, and normal body image depend on a well fitting orthosis.

After a pivoting gait has been learned with the parapodium, a swing-to or swing-through gait can be attempted. By 4 to 5 years of age, a swing-through gait, with the child using Lofstrand crutches, can usually be accomplished. Variations of the parapodium allow for easier locking and unlocking of hip and knee joints. A swivel or pivot walker also may be attached to the footplate to allow for crutchless walking.

Another type of orthosis for the child with a thoracic or high lumbar lesion is the Orthotic Research and Locomotion Assessment Unit (ORLAU) swivel walker. It consists of modular design similar to that of the standing frame, with a chest strap and knee blocks attached to swiveling footplates.[216] Rather than the whole base moving forward, as when weight is shifted in the parapodium, in the swivel walker each footplate is spring-loaded and is able to swivel forward independently. This allows for independent balance on one foot and therefore crutchless ambulation. The ORLAU swivel walker is manufactured in the United Kingdom, and assembly kits may be ordered; however, availability is limited (Appendix 15-A).[217] Another parapodium in use is the Rochester parapodium. Separate hip and knee joints allow a variety of free movement for sitting and bending down. The lower portion remains rigid and supportive when hips are flexed. Therefore a child can bend and pick up objects from the floor, and the unlockable hip and knee joints will relock automatically on extension.[218]

There is a perception that although children with myelomeningocele use orthoses effectively, very few continue ambulation into adulthood. Two studies of patients with thoracic-level myelomeningocele[219] demonstrated that the ORLAU can be used effectively into the adult years. Both studies noted a 58% to 59.4% compliance rate. Patients in the studies who started using the ORLAU after 11 years of age continued use for 3 to 24 years. Mazur and colleagues[219] noted that those with myelomeningocele who did not ambulate had a fivefold increase in pressure sores and twice the number of fractures compared who those who did ambulate. Vigorous walking programs should be considered to assist long-term health.

Both the parapodium and swivel walker have had some problems with instability, ease of application, and cosmesis. New designs attempt to correct these problems.[220] Nevertheless, existing limitations in the parapodium and swivel walker, particularly energy cost of walking, slow rate of locomotion, and cosmesis, have limited their use, primarily to the younger child. These devices, however, remain an effective means of preventing musculoskeletal deformities caused by long-term sitting, wheelchair positioning, and general immobility. They also enhance social-emotional development gained from the upright position.[216,221] Another option for the child with a higher-level lesion and good sitting balance is the reciprocating gait orthosis (RGO). This brace consists of bilateral long-leg braces with a pelvic band and thoracic extension, if necessary. The hip joints are connected by a cable system that can work in two ways: If the child has active hip flexors, he or she can activate the cable system by shifting weight and flexing the non–weight-bearing extremity. This brings the weight-bearing extremity into relative extension in preparation for the next step. Without hip flexors, the child extends his or her trunk over one extremity, thus positioning it in relative extension. By virtue of the cable system, the non–weight-bearing extremity moves into flexion, thus initiating a step. Several types of the RGO are in use, including the dual-cable LSU[222] and the horizontal-cable type.[223]

Most recently the Isocentric Reciprocating Gait Orthosis (I-RGO) (Center for Orthotics Design, Campbell, California) has been used for children with high-level spina bifida. It has a more cosmetic and efficient design compared with the dual-cable LSU or horizontal-cable–type RGO. This cableless brace has two to three times less friction and therefore is more energy efficient. The brace stabilizes the hip, knee, and ankle joints and balances the person, enabling him or her to stand hands free without the use of crutches or a walker (Figure 15-18).[223] Leg advancement for walking occurs through use of hip flexor or lower abdominal muscle contraction or through use of active or passive trunk extension. In a study of 15 patients with lesions from T10-L3, use of the RGO produced favorable results. It was used effectively by 13 of the 15 patients. Initial use of the RGO was initiated at 5 years, and eight of the 15 discontinued use at 10 years of age. During the period of use, four became community ambulators, nine were household ambulators, and two remained nonfunctional (standing only). Average daily use ranged from 6 hours for those ambulating in the community to 30 minutes for those who were nonfunctional ambulators. Six of the 15 had no quadriceps power yet were able to functionally use the RGO for ambulation. Strong motivation and realistic goals are important to successful use.[224]

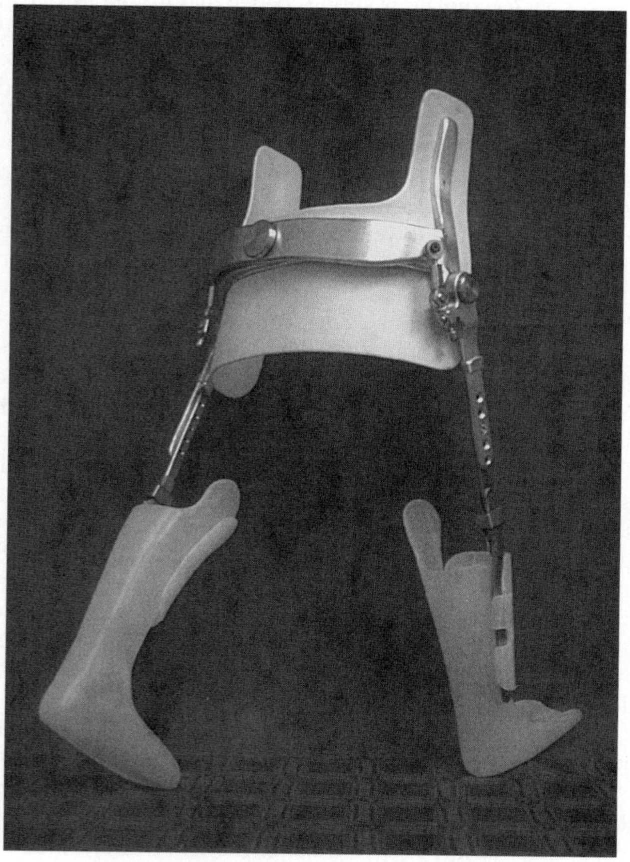

Figure 15-18 ■ Reciprocating gait orthosis.

A more common means of maintaining the upright position has been through the use of long- or short-leg braces. Polypropylene braces and carbon-reinforced braces are considerably lighter than metal bracing and therefore reduce the energy cost of walking for the child with spina bifida. They allow close contact and can be slipped into the shoe rather than worn externally, thus affording the patient a better-fitting, more cosmetic orthosis.

The type of orthosis chosen (long-leg, with or without pelvic band, or short-leg) depends on the level of the myelomeningocele and the muscle power within that level (Table 15-3). Because lesions are frequently incomplete, muscle strength must be accurately assessed before bracing is prescribed. Independent sitting balance with hands free also is a prerequisite for use of long- or short-leg braces. Even children with L3 to L4 lesions who demonstrate incomplete knee extension may be able to use a short-leg brace with an anterior shell rather than requiring long-leg bracing.[225] This crouch-control AFO (CCAFO) will prevent a crouching gait pattern by improving knee extension during gait (Figure 15-19).[226] Another alternative to a standard solid ankle AFO may be the carbon fiber spring AFO. This brace provides dynamic assist, supports the patient through the entire stance phase, and increases the energy return during the third rocker phase of push-off, simulating the natural push-off action.[227] For children demonstrating excessive knee valgus caused by hip adduction, use of a Ferrari KAFO (FKAFO) may be considered.[228] The PT must work in conjunction with the orthopedist and orthotist to have each child fitted with the minimal amount of bracing that allows for joint stability and a good gait pattern (see Chapter 34).

Children with lower-level lesions (L5-S1) who use below-knee bracing often develop the ability to or choose to ambulate without assistive devices. However, recent studies have shown that crutch use may decrease excessive pelvic motion, which results in reducing abnormal joint forces.[162,229] Use of crutches may prevent abnormal joint forces, maintain joint integrity, and decrease the risk of additional orthopedic complications.

Literature has suggested that crutch-assisted ambulation may result in long-term pathology. In patients with higher lumbar lesions (L3-L4) who use Lofstrand crutches, the dynamics and kinematics of upper-extremity function were explored during swing-through and four-point reciprocal modes of gait. Although there were better joint kinematics in the shoulder and other upper-extremity joints during swing-through gait, kinetics were more problematic with increased force and torque in shoulder and wrist joints in

TABLE 15-3 ■ COMMON GAIT PATTERNS AND LEVELS OF ASSISTANCE REQUIRED IN MYELOMENINGOCELE

LEVEL OF LESION	MUSCLE PERFORMANCE	RECOMMENDED LEVEL OF ASSISTANCE AND BRACING	AMBULATORY PROGRESSION
T8-L1 and above	Flaccid LEs with fair to poor trunk	Parapodium: ORLAU, Toronto, Rochester Assistive devices often unnecessary with ORLAU but may improve function with Toronto or Rochester braces.	
L1-L2	Flaccid LEs with hip flexors present	Parapodium with progression to RGO RGO, ambulating with hips locked.	Begin ambulating with a walker, progress to forearm crutches. Four-point or swing-through gait.
L3-L4	Fair quadriceps with weak or absent hamstrings	HKAFOs may be used with severe lordosis because of weak or absent gluteal musculature and decreased trunk control or to control rotation and abduction and adduction. If quadriceps are less than fair strength, KAFOs may be needed. As the patient progresses he or she may be cut down from KAFOs to AFOs; AFOs may be used with or without twister cables.	Begin ambulating with a walker, progress to forearm crutches. Four-point gait. Begin ambulating with a walker and progress to forearm crutches. In some rare cases the patient may progress to no assistive device at all depending on the gait pattern. With increased use of trunk reversal the patient should be returned to forearm crutches to allow for a pattern that is more cosmetic and energy efficient. Four-point gait pattern.
L5	Good hip flexors and quadriceps; fair anterior tibialis; weak gluteus medius and maximus, toe extensors and gastrocsoleus	AFOs with or without twisters depending on gluteal strength. AFO is used to prevent a crouch gait pattern from weak gastrocsoleus.	Forearm crutches or no assistive devices. Four-point gait.
S1	Good hip flexors, quadriceps, gluteus medius, and toe extensors; weak gluteus maximus and gastrocsoleus	AFO	Generally no assistive device is used unless decreased balance reactions or excessive lateral trunk flexion is present.
S2-S3	Good hip flexors, quadriceps, gluteus medius and maximus, and gastrocsoleus	Often no bracing needed.	Often no assistive devices needed.

AFO, Ankle-foot-orthosis; *HKAFO,* hip-knee-ankle-foot orthosis; *KAFO,* knee-ankle-foot orthosis; *LE,* lower extremity; *RGO,* reciprocating gait orthosis.

those using a swing-through gait. Whereas the swing-through gait allows a potentially faster mode of ambulation, long-term use of this pattern may lead to increased upper-extremity pathology. Careful monitoring of all joints, including upper-extremity joints, during gait reassessment should be considered in order to deter and manage these potential issues that may compromise overall joint integrity and function.[230]

The excessive femoral torsion present in all newborns at birth does not decrease with growth and development in the child with spina bifida because of abnormal gait and activity.[159] Children ambulating with AFOs often show excessive rotation at the knee because of the lack of functioning lateral hamstrings. Rather than going to a higher level of bracing, a twister cable can be added, which often decreases the rotary component during gait.[159] Twister cables can be heavy-duty torsion or more flexible elastic webbing, depending on function. Typically, the young child who is just beginning to pull to stand and remains reliant on floor mobility as the primary means of mobility should have elastic twisters prescribed to allow for ease of creeping and transitions. The older and more active child will require heavy-duty torsion cables. Rotational stresses may eventually lead to onset of late degenerative changes around the knee. A tibial derotation osteotomy may be indicated to prevent these changes from occurring.[159,231,232]

For children with low lumbar or sacral lesions who have at least fair strength in their dorsiflexors and plantar flexors, often a University of California Biomechanics Laboratory (UCBL) or polypropylene shoe insert to control foot position is the only bracing needed. These inserts fit snuggly inside the shoe and help control calcaneal and forefoot instabilities. A supramalleolar orthosis (SMO) will also fit easily inside the shoe but will provide additional medial and lateral support and stability that an insert would not provide. Even though a child may be able to ambulate without an assistive device or bracing, consideration must be given to the stresses that occur at the joints that over time may lead to

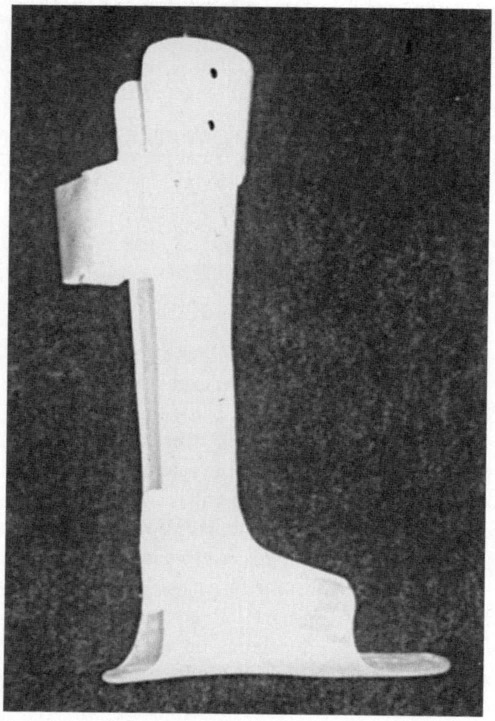

Figure 15-19 ■ Crouch control ankle-foot orthosis.

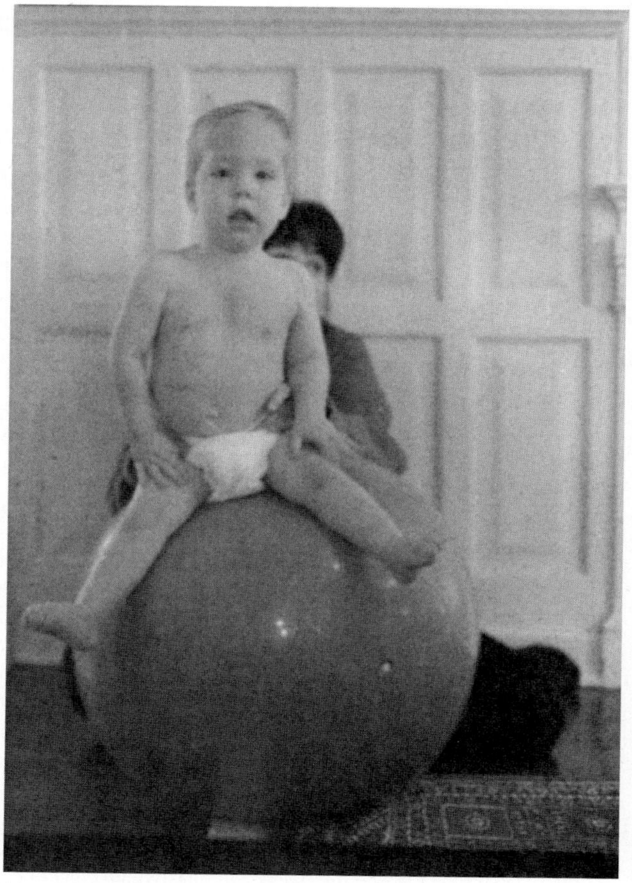

Figure 15-20 ■ Balance and strengthening exercises done on a movable surface.

orthopedic deformity. The greatest risk of joint instability often occurs at the knee. Barefoot walking versus use of an AFO has shown increased instability, joint stress, and pain at the hip and knee as well as increased energy expenditure.[233-235] Even though children may be able to ambulate without the use of crutches, comparison of gait kinetics and kinematics of walking with crutches has shown a significant decrease of valgus forces at the knee and better overall alignment of the lower extremities.[229] Treatment aimed at strengthening the gluteus medius and maximus to aid in increasing pelvic stability and reducing kinematic compensations can also be important in the management of patients with lesions at this level to enhance their efficiency during ambulation.[236,237]

Gait training, begun as the child first starts to stand, can now continue in a more formalized manner. By using the appropriate orthosis and assistive devices (walker, crutches, or cane), each child must be helped to achieve the most efficient and effective gait pattern possible (see Table 15-3). As a part of gait training, the child should be taken out of the bracing and "challenged" so that righting and equilibrium reactions can be developed to their maximum. For example, having a child maintain balance while sitting on a ball or other movable surface (tilt board, trampoline) requires the participation of all available musculature, especially abdominal and trunk extensor muscles (Figure 15-20). Strengthening available musculature is a primary objective in this phase of treatment. Slow gains in muscle strength are often the result of continued emphasis on strengthening during physical therapy. In addition to trunk muscles, the gluteus medius, gluteus maximus, and quadriceps are often targeted. Prone activities such as picking up toys while over a Swiss ball or moving around while prone on a scooter board require use of these muscles while providing an enjoyable exercise for the child. Participation in hippotherapy and aquatherapy programs at this age can also be beneficial. These treatment approaches can be used to improve muscle strength in general and the gait pattern when bracing is reapplied. Regardless of the strengthening activities chosen, the pediatric therapist has the special task of using creativity to involve the child in therapeutic play activities. The ideas for creative activities are limitless but essential for combining therapy with age-appropriate cognitive abilities.

Studies examining the effects of strength and endurance training in those with spina bifida[238-240] have demonstrated enhanced functional outcomes. These studies included individuals in wheelchairs as well as ambulators. Interventions aimed at strengthening those with spina bifida, including electrical stimulation,[241,242] behavioral treatment,[243,244] and motor skills training[243] have been reported. The evidence supporting strengthening, using exercise, electrical stimulation, and motor skills training was recently examined by Dagenais and colleagues in a systemic review.[245] This review synthesized six studies supporting interventions in strengthening.[240-246] The level of evidence for the studies was determined using the American Academy of Cerebral Palsy and Developmental Medicine Levels of evidence.[247] Levels of evaluated studies were graded and noted to be II (smaller randomized controlled trials with wider confidence intervals, n <100), IV (case series or cohort study without concurrent control, case-control study) or V (case study).

The total number of subjects in all of the studies was 26, with 50% of those subjects in the Andrade and colleagues[246] study. All six studies reported improvements in strength; however, only three noted statistically significant results. Although the evidence suggests the possibility of being able to increase muscle strength using these modalities, in this population one must interpret the results with caution owing to lack of rigor, small subject populations, and variability across studies.

Spina bifida is a congenital-onset condition that requires intervention by the PT from infancy through adolescence. Most of the impairments and functional deficits described throughout this chapter last throughout a lifetime. Health providers familiar with the complexity of the secondary impairments should follow individuals with spina bifida on a regular basis. The PT plays an important role in screening for potential problems and providing recommendations for maintenance of mobility and health-related fitness as well as promoting activity and participation for children with spina bifida. OTs within the school systems often provide interventions within the area of integration of perceptual function. However, additional research needs to be done to guide "best practice," as there is little support for those interventions that expert clinicians deem beneficial in the habilitation of these patients.

Obesity affects ability for interaction and participation at multiple levels across the life span of those with spina bifida. Obesity may affect independence in transfers and ambulation, self-care and mobility, as well as personal social interactions at all ages. Often the child with spina bifida may be the last to be asked to participate and/or the child's inability may affect his or her ability or willingness to participate in physical games and activities with peers. Equipment and orthotic needs can also be complicated by increases in weight gain and obesity as the child ages.

Studies using dual-emission x-ray absorptiometry (DEXA) have shown that those with spina bifida have significantly decreased lean body mass as compared with controls.[248] Children with spina bifida likely have lower metabolic rates secondary to decreased muscle mass and decreased ability to burn calories. Those with higher-level lesions often have greater issues with obesity owing to decreased lower-extremity muscle activity, decreased physical activity, and decreased overall muscle mass. Adult wheelchair users have been shown to require 1500 fewer calories per day, and overall nutritional intake should be lower for those with spina bifida than their typically developing peers.[249-251] Interventions to address physical inactivity and obesity may include increased physical activity, regular exercise, behavioral modifications, nutrition education programs, and attention to weight control. Exercise programs targeting upper-extremity resistance combined with aerobic activities such as swimming and arm-cycling using arm-ergometry can be helpful in addressing obesity in those with spina bifida. Adolescents with spina bifida who used an upper-extremity cycling program that was integrated with video gaming three times per week for 16 weeks improved oxygen uptake and maximum work capability.[248,252,253]

Sensory limitations may impede progress during early ambulation training. Because of limited kinesthesia and proprioception, available sensory systems must be augmented and the child taught to substitute with nonimpaired sensory systems. Impaired kinesthesia in children with myelomeningocele impedes their ability to anticipate changes in terrain and poses a safety problem. Vision may be the most relevant system to allow them to scan and preplan for changes in their walking environment.

Gait training and muscle strengthening are not the only consideration of the therapist. How cognitive and psychosocial development can be enhanced during this stage of the child's development is also important. One appropriate solution is to place the child in a center-based EI program. Although these programs may vary in the services they provide, most usually include age-appropriate play activities and some type of parental counseling. In addition, many offer therapeutic intervention from physical, occupational, and speech therapists. This intervention may occur in groups or individually and typically occurs in the child's natural environment.

In addition to the socialization that center-based EI programs provide for the child with myelomeningocele, they also teach the child age-appropriate ADLs, such as dressing and undressing. At this age ADL skills are more appropriately taught in a group setting than individually. For many children the EI program, along with individualized therapy, is sufficient to enhance development in the physical, cognitive, and psychosocial realms.

Presently, when children reach age 3 years, public school education becomes available to them. The preschool or early childhood (EC) program continues to offer the same fundamental benefits as the EI program. It is the role of the EI therapist to communicate the specific needs of each child entering the public school system. In this way continuity in the child's rehabilitation program is preserved.

The spina bifida team, usually headed by a pediatrician or clinical nurse specialist, continues to follow the child closely during this stage. The neurosurgeon checks shunt functioning and performs revisions as necessary. The orthopedist supervises bracing efforts to prevent and correct deformities in the spine and lower extremities. Well-child care and general medical treatment are the responsibility of the pediatrician on the team. The urologist continues to monitor renal functioning while keeping the child dry and free of infection. At this stage the clinical nurse specialist will usually teach bowel and bladder training to the child and family. This clinician generally initiates this training according to age-appropriate developmental guidelines.

Bladder training usually consists of transferring the job of CIC from the parents to the child. Children as young as 3 years, but certainly by the age of 5 years, can learn CIC in a short period.[254] Children may first practice on dolls with male and female genitalia. Next, using mirrors to understand their own genital anatomy, they are able to accomplish the technique on themselves. CIC in conjunction with pharmacotherapy is useful in achieving continence in children with spina bifida.[140] Another method of bladder training recently being used in the United States is intravesical transurethral bladder stimulation. This technique has allowed children with neurogenic bladder to rehabilitate their bladder function so that they can detect bladder fullness and generate effective detrusor contractions, leading to improved continence.[100,255]

Bowel training can be achieved through proper diet, regular evacuation times, and appropriate use of stool softeners and suppositories.[100] Constipation (and resulting bypass diarrhea) can be prevented by proper habit training and use of fiber supplements. Stool softeners (not laxatives and enemas) and suppositories should be used to keep the stools soft and help stimulate evacuation. Finally, toilet training, which amounts to scheduled toileting in time with the stool stimulants, usually achieves bowel continence. Surgical procedures, such as the Malone ACE procedure,[91] may be necessary when other interventions have failed. The Malone ACE procedure, performed in conjunction with a Mitrofanoff procedure to gain urinary continence, can help these patients attain a better quality of life. Consistency at each step along the way is the key to successful bowel training. A therapist may be called on to assist the parents and child in achieving independence in this ADL.

Other members of the team, such as the psychologist, social worker, and dietician, continue to function in their appropriate roles, interacting with the child and family as necessary. PTs and OTs, as members of the team, must collaborate with the efforts of other team members in the creation of their treatment plans.

Mobility and bladder and bowel dysfunction in toddlers and school-age children represent ongoing stressors for parents of children with spina bifida. It has been noted by many that spina bifida represents a considerable challenge to all family members, particularly mothers. Family climate, parents' partner relationships, and social support networks play a considerable role in balancing stress and psychological adjustment for parents. Awareness of available systems of support for the patient and family as well as resources to which parents and their children can be referred for psychological and social support as needed is important for all health care practitioners.[256,257]

Stage 5: Primary School through Adolescence

The fifth stage of development is marked by less rapid growth than earlier childhood but ends with a period of rapid physiological growth. Children in the 6- to 10-year age group are interested in a wider variety of physical activities as they challenge their bodies to perform. The adolescent, however, is going through a period of great sexual differentiation as primary and secondary sexual characteristics develop more fully.

Cognitively, children are able to solve problems in a more sophisticated manner, although they revert to illogical thinking with complex problems. As they reach adolescence, they become capable of hypothetical reasoning and their thought processes approach those of adults.

Emotionally, the 6- to 10-year-old is in a period of relative calm. Children are interested in schoolwork and are eager to produce. This is a period during which they are developing relationships outside of the family and beginning to assume an identity and autonomy. Problem-solving and decision-making skills are at the crux of this time period. However, it is also challenging to promote independence and minimize self-reliant behaviors. Social passivity may ensue as "learned helplessness" behaviors emerge. Therefore professionals, including both PTs and OTs, should begin targeting independent function early, and before adolescence.[258] Relevant family education regarding this issue should be inherent in all care plans, and independent behaviors should be promoted from very early on. Engagement in family decision making and opportunities for active problem solving have been linked to increased positive self-esteem and ego development.[259] During this time period, children with spina bifida are at risk for developmental delays in social functioning.[258]

During this period, they are building the skills of the future, preparing them for adult work. This is a prime time to introduce and teach new skills while fostering increased autonomy and independence. Autonomy is difficult for the youngster with spina bifida. Motor skills impeding progress toward autonomy vary for each child and are dependent on the level of spina bifida as well as any cognitive impairment. However, it has been observed that the motor skills hardest to attain are those that involve motor planning and that the process skills hardest to attain are related to adaptation of performance and initiation of new steps. Thus guidance to learn not only how to do things but how to get things done is important.[260] Interventions targeting independence have been embedded into several camp programs throughout the country geared specifically toward those with spina bifida. O'Mahar and colleagues[261] report on one such camp program focused on campers 7 to 14 years of age in northern Illinois. Camp Ability emphasized individualized collaborative (i.e., parent and camper) goal setting, group sessions with psychoeducation and cognitive tools, and goal monitoring by the camp counselor. Campers reported significant gains in individual goals, management of spina bifida responsibilities, and independence. Medium effect sizes in goal attainment and progress from the start to the end of the camp session were noted.[261] It appears that these camps may have significant benefit in addressing management of one's disability as well as independence in self-care skills. An added benefit is the social interaction and physical activity that the camp participants engaged in while working toward their goals.

As the energy cost of walking becomes too high, use of a wheelchair for locomotion often becomes appropriate. To a teenager whose emotional needs include a strong peer identity, transitioning to a wheelchair may foster increased independence owing to improved ability to participate and engage with peers. Appropriate alternatives may be to delay the decision to use a wheelchair full time or limit ambulation to short distances or to those places most important to the child. Again, goals must be tailored to the child's needs and encompass his or her whole being.

In accordance with the child's growth spurts, frequent adjustment or reordering of bracing will be necessary. Continual reevaluation of orthotic needs may reveal that the level of bracing may decrease as the child grows and becomes stronger; the opposite development is also a possibility.

Usually during this stage, if it has not occurred previously, the evaluation of future ambulation potential occurs. The child whose larger size and limited abilities make ambulation more difficult each day frequently requests this evaluation. Strength does not increase in the same proportion as body weight.[127] Ambulation, although possible for the young child, may be impossible for that same person as a young adult.

Although no guidelines include every patient, generally children with thoracic-level lesions are rarely ambulators by the late teens.[152,262,263] Those with upper lumbar lesions may be household ambulators with long-leg bracing but will require wheelchairs for quick and efficient mobility as adults. With low lumbar lesions, most adults can become community ambulators. Patients with sacral-level lesions are usually able to ambulate freely within the community. Many require minimal bracing and ambulate without assistive devices.[152,159] It must be remembered that ambulatory status is not determined by level of the lesion alone. The muscle power available; degree of orthopedic deformity; age, height, and weight of the patient; and, of course, motivation are also determining factors.[82,154,159,264]

Because a large number of older children with spina bifida will become wheelchair dependent, potential problems connected with a sedentary existence must be explored. Skin care, always a concern for the child with spina bifida, becomes a priority for the constant sitter. Mirrors may be used for self-inspection of the skin twice daily. Well-constructed foam, gel, or air-cell seat cushions are essential for distributing pressure evenly. Children should be taught frequent weight shifting within the chair to relieve pressure areas. Clothing should not be constricting but should be heavy enough to protect sensitive skin from wheelchair parts. Children must also be taught to avoid extremes of temperature and environmental hazards, such as radiators, sharp objects, and abrasive surfaces. The therapist must reinforce the importance of skin care to prevent setbacks in the rehabilitation process that may result when skin breakdown develops.

Children with higher-level lesions may need spinal support to prevent deformities. A polyethylene body jacket or thoracolumbar-sacral orthosis (TLSO) can be used to provide this support and, it is hoped, prevent the progression of any paralytic deformities. Whatever type of device or wheelchair padding is used, the therapist must check to see that weight is distributed equally through both buttocks and that the spine is supported as needed. Part of the therapeutic intervention is to provide strengthening exercises or activities to be done out of the supporting orthosis. This is necessary to maintain existing trunk strength and to preserve the child's present level of function.

Generally, in late childhood or early adolescence, orthopedic deformities that have been gradually developing require surgical intervention. Progressive scoliosis or kyphosis may require internal fixation when conservative methods fail.[265] Sectioning of tight or contracted muscles at the hip and knee is often required.[152] The iliopsoas, adductors, and hamstrings are frequently the offending muscles. These surgeries, followed by strengthening exercises and gait training, often add to the ambulatory life of the child with spina bifida. For example, in a child who displays an extreme lordotic posture, hip flexion contractures may be present and surgical lengthening of the tight muscles may be required to allow improved biomechanical alignment for standing and balance. Strengthening of the hip extensors and abdominals also helps prevent future muscle imbalances that may lead to contractures and tightness. A postoperative therapeutic program might include periods of prone lying to prevent future contractures and strengthening of hip extensors and abdominals that were previously overstretched by the lordotic position.

Of primary importance during this stage is preparing the child for independence in ADLs, which may be broken down into self-care, locomotion-related, and social interaction activities. In conjunction with the nurse, PT, and OT, self-care skills of dressing, eating, and food preparation; general hygiene; and bowel and bladder care can be addressed. Because the adolescent is so concerned with achieving independence, he or she is more likely to comply with a regimen of strengthening exercises if shown how they relate to functional independence. A creative therapist may, for example, incorporate trunk stability and upper-extremity strengthening work in activities such as making popcorn or getting ready for a dance. In addition, fostering social and recreational independence through adaptive sports and fitness programs and leisure activities should not be overlooked. Participation in adaptive sports can aid immensely in improving strength, endurance, and self-esteem. Community adaptive recreational programs may include T-ball, martial arts, swimming, tennis, basketball, skiing, bowling, and many other common sports and leisure activities (Figures 15-21 through 15-23).

Locomotion activities should include all gait-related skills, such as falling down, getting up, and ambulation on various terrains and stairs. Transfers of all types should also be included in locomotion activities. Again, a creative therapeutic program helps make achievement of skills more palatable. For example, school-aged children may enjoy a competitive relay race situation in which each child falls, gets up, walks across the room, and sits down in a chair safely. This type of activity combines gait-training activities with group socialization and may meet a variety of goals (motor and psychosocial) at the same time.

Achievement of independence in ADLs for the child and adult with spina bifida does not depend solely on the level of paralysis. Also important are psychosocial and environmental factors. Mean ages for the achievement of various ADL activities have been developed and may assist the therapist in establishing realistic therapeutic goals in this area.[266]

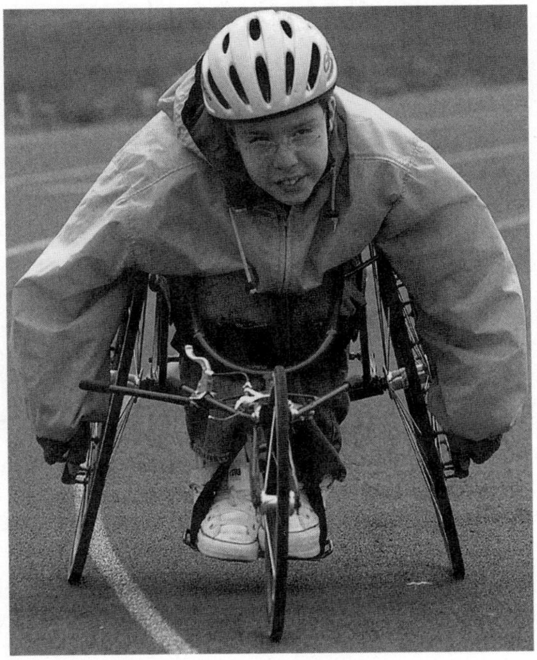

Figure 15-21 ■ Participation in wheelchair racing. (Courtesy Su Metzel.)

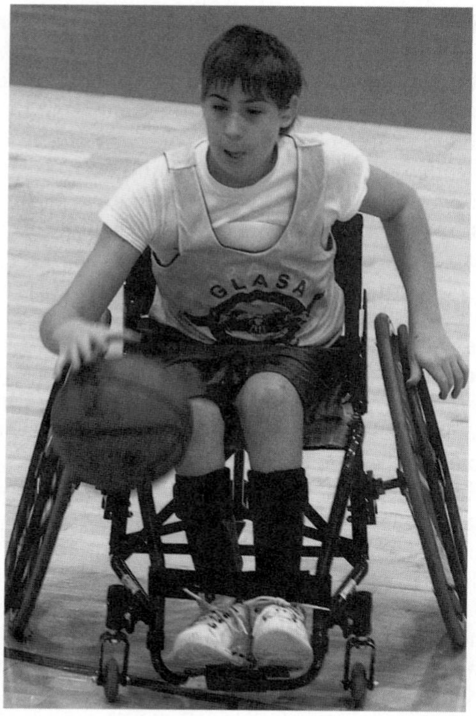

Figure 15-22 ■ Participation in wheelchair basketball. (Courtesy Su Metzel.)

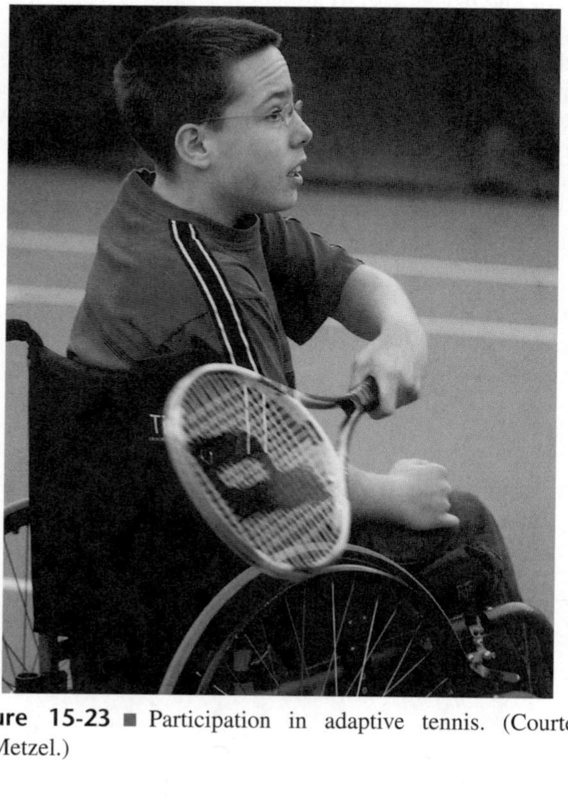

Figure 15-23 ■ Participation in adaptive tennis. (Courtesy Su Metzel.)

Often during this stage of rehabilitation the therapist is asked to assist in assessing cognitive function. The perceptual and cognitive evaluations previously discussed may be administered and the results interpreted for parents and school personnel.

Also as previously discussed, children with spina bifida have a general perceptual deficit that can manifest itself in a variety of ways. First, the child may have difficulty recognizing objects and the relations that they have to one another. He or she may therefore perceive the world in a distorted manner and have reactions that are unstable and unpredictable. These perceptual difficulties will most likely affect academic learning, and the child may associate failure with the learning process. Difficulties in attaining independence in ADLs are also linked to perceptual problems. Finally, emotional disturbances may be attributed in part to the perceptual difficulties of the child with spina bifida.[98]

Remedial programs, such as the Frostig Program for the Development of Visual Perception, have been effective in improving the visual perception of children with spina bifida.[98] Programs of this type are most effective when remediation begins early—preferably at or before the time the child enters school. Developmental optometry examination and remediation programs focusing on vision training may also be of benefit.

Children with spina bifida may also have difficulties with tasks requiring sensorimotor integration. Children requiring programs for sensorimotor integration should be referred to a therapist certified in this area. If one is not available, many appropriate activities for sensorimotor integration may be adapted from Ayres[267] or Montgomery and Richter.[268]

Regardless of the school setting chosen for the child, the therapist should be able to serve the classroom teacher as a consultant. Advice on adaptive seating and therapeutic goals appropriate for the classroom help ensure that the rehabilitation process will continue in the classroom as well as promote optimal conditions for learning.

When a child is moving from the preschool to the elementary school setting, the support of the therapeutic team is essential and invaluable. The teacher's expectations, as created by the therapist, regarding the child's special needs and abilities often spell the difference between success and failure of complete academic and psychosocial integration within the school setting. Even though the child may no longer require direct therapeutic intervention, periodic consultation, including site classroom visits, is recommended to prevent minor problems from developing into major ones. For example, bowel and bladder accidents can be avoided by scheduling regular times for toileting. The teacher may be able to make minor adjustments in the teaching schedule to accommodate this scheduling. Also, full-control braces (from hip to ankles) may seem overwhelming to the layperson. If the teacher is shown how the braces lock and unlock to allow the child to sit or stand to walk, he or she may feel more at ease if ever called on to assist the child.

The psychological perspective of the child colors therapeutic goals in this stage. As the child nears adolescence, these psychosocial aspects become of paramount importance. Although the therapist should not take on the role of the psychologist, collaborative efforts in the area of counseling will be necessary. Questions will arise many times during physical and occupational therapy sessions, requiring factual answers that the therapist can and should provide.

TRANSITIONS: ADOLESCENCE

The consequences of the physical, medical, and cognitive effects of spina bifida extend into young adulthood and have an impact on quality of life.[269] Adolescence is a stormy emotional period. Adolescents remain in turmoil as they seek their identities through sexual, social, and vocational activities. As their value systems develop, they feel less ambivalence between remaining as children and striving for independence. For the child with myelomeningocele, adolescence is not an optimal time to introduce new skills leading toward self-care and independence.

TRANSITION TO ADULTHOOD

Eighty-five percent of infants born with spina bifida will reach their adult years.[169] For the adolescent with spina bifida the transition to adulthood includes a new set of expectations. Independent mobility expands to driving or arranging public transportation and getting to the correct destination in unfamiliar surroundings, including accessibility to the community for leisure and recreation, continued education, or job opportunities. Self-care includes performing ADLs but expands to household management and financial responsibilities. Social relationships expand to a larger arena including long-term partnerships with friends and business contacts and encounters with equipment vendors, insurance professionals, and medical providers and may include hiring, firing, and directing personal health care assistants. Recent information from the *American Journal of Public Health* indicates that 50% to 70% of adults with spina bifida live with family or in an assisted-living arrangement.[270] For some adults with spina bifida, living independently in our society is a difficult goal to reach.

The individual with spina bifida continues to require assistance with management of and resources related to medical, rehabilitative, and social-emotional needs through adulthood.[169,270-272] Secondary impairments span a wide range of domains, but management of secondary health conditions is a priority in reducing mortality, deterioration of general health, and further impairments through the adult years. Renal, respiratory, and cardiac complications have been identified as frequent causes of death.[169] Living with the long-term consequences of spina bifida places increased demands on the musculoskeletal system, and the effects of aging can appear earlier than usual. Osteoporosis, increased risk of fractures, risk of osteoarthritis, and muscular pain from overuse of the upper extremities with use of crutches, longer-distance wheelchair propulsion over all terrains, increased transitions for self-care management and routines, and abnormal stresses placed on the knee from weak hip abductors and calf muscles can lead to degenerative changes and joint pain. Obesity and weight gain resulting from a more sedentary lifestyle and hypertension, heart disease, and diabetes are common problems with aging.[273] Thinner and less elastic skin that is susceptible to breakdown, insufficient pressure relief and poor tissue perfusion, incontinence and perspiration, wound infections after surgical procedures, burns and bumps that occur to insensate limbs, and long-term immobilization during hospitalizations have been major sources of decreased skin integrity.[169,273,274]

Muscular strength, flexibility, balance, and endurance decrease during the aging process. Changes in the CNS affect memory, reaction time, and attention span. An increased risk of depression and anxiety has been documented in several studies that measure quality of life in the adult with spina bifida.[169,272,275] Secondary conditions in adults with spina bifida have been linked to admission rates to hospitals that are nine times higher than in the nondisabled population. Adults with spina bifida have medical expenditures that are three to six times greater than those of adults without spina bifida.[169]

Although there are few standard protocols to follow in the medical management of adults with spina bifida, the coordinated interdisciplinary approach shown to be effective in the care of children and adolescents is not available to most adults with spina bifida. A recent study from the Netherlands that reviewed life span issues of people with childhood-onset disabilities reported that more than 50% requested more information on their specific medical condition and the consequences of this condition on adulthood recreation.[275] In a 2009 study from the University of Pittsburgh that surveyed 179 adults from 19 to 64 years of age, 75% could not name their primary care physician and had not seen a medical professional in over a year.[169]

Dicianno and colleagues[169] identified five key elements necessary for the successful transition from pediatric to adult medical care. These included early preparation and education of the individual and family, flexible timing of the transition, introduction to the transition clinic, interested adult center providers, and a coordinated transfer of care approach among the individual, family, pediatric primary care providers, and adult specialists. The barriers included child health care providers refusing to "let go," reluctance to leave a family-centered care program, and adult care providers having limited knowledge about or interest in caring for these individuals. Finding a primary care physician or physiatrist who can assist with identifying a team of health care specialists for referrals as needed is a major concern for this adult population. The Spina Bifida Association of America publishes a health guide for adults living with spina bifida, based on feedback from adults across the United States. The *Health Guide* was sponsored by a grant from the National Center for Birth Defects and Developmental Disabilities and the Centers for Disease Control and Prevention.

Additional unmet needs reported by adults surveyed were related to functional mobility, household management, and active recreation. Being independent with regard to mobility was the most important determinant in quality-of-life surveys.[16,275] A review of the literature of the past few years has indicated high unemployment rates for people with disabilities. For those with spina bifida, 47% of adults were in competitive employment, 15% were in sheltered or supported employment, and 38% were unemployed or had never been employed.[276] Limited mobility accounts for only part of the high unemployment rate. Accessibility into public buildings is another factor that limits employment opportunities. Tight doorways, steep ramped entrances and exits, inefficient workstations, and unreliable public transportation all play a role in a lower employment rate. Universal design (broad-spectrum solutions that produce products and environments that are usable and effective for everyone), construction of newer buildings with attention to adjustable work tables for computers and equipment access for people with different body proportions, wider doorways, lower counters, doors that open electrically, and bathroom modifications (for both manual and power wheelchair users) with Americans with Disabilities Act (ADA) specifications for building modifications will improve universal access for all people with and without disabilities. Modifications of bathrooms that accommodate wheelchair and crutch users including different height grab bars and roll-in shower arrangements, sloping landscape for entrances and exits, and room modification with lower counters and closet access, to name a few considerations, may enhance travel and leisure time and recreational opportunities.

According to the *American Journal of Public Health,* most adults with spina bifida use some form of assistive technology (AT) that plays a significant role in increasing independence at home and in the community.[272] Thirty-five percent use bracing, 23% use walking devices, and 57% to 65% use lightweight wheelchairs (both manual and power assisted). PTs and OTs have extensive knowledge in the field of rehabilitation. Mobility equipment needs change as people age. Therapists have expertise in adaption and modification and can recommend solutions for decreased mobility. Physical changes in the workplace and home to decrease excessive stress on joints while maintaining flexibility and musculoskeletal alignment for efficiency without pain may also be required. Evaluating the individual needs of the client and locating and selecting the types of technology that may enhance the adult's personal care management and improve efficiency in household tasks may make the difference in helping the client have a more satisfying quality of life. Cell phones, computer access, and watch timers for pressure relief and personal care routines can all assist memory and organizational skills.[272]

AFOs with carbon springs that store energy, crutch tips that can be changed to accommodate different surfaces (e.g., with spikes attached for snow and ice), forearm crutches with hand grips and forearm cuffs that distribute weight and reduce joint stress to shoulders and wrists, powered add-on devices for manual wheelchairs to reduce stress on painful shoulders, adjustable furniture, and wrist rests, footrests, and arm supports to ensure correct posture and reduce cervical and lumbar strain are examples of current and experimental AT that may promote greater independence. Specific devices are supported by the individual needs assessment of the patient by the therapist and education in the device's maintenance for appropriate use and durability. It is beyond the scope of this chapter to discuss specific equipment items.

Spina bifida is a congenital-onset condition that requires intervention by the therapists from infancy through adolescence. Most of the impairments and functional deficits described throughout this chapter last throughout a lifetime. Health providers familiar with the complexity of the secondary impairments should follow individuals with spina bifida on a regular basis. Both PTs and OTs play an important role in screening for potential problems and providing recommendations for maintenance of mobility and health-related fitness.

Adolescents with spina bifida show great concern about self-esteem and social-sexual adjustment.[277] These concerns appear directly related to efficient bowel and bladder management.[278] Strategies to cope with bowel and bladder difficulties, as previously outlined, combined with appropriate emotional support from family and medical personnel help alleviate this concern.

Although great advances in medical management of children with myelomeningocele have occurred, a contrasting lack of improvement related to sexual function and reproductive issues exists. Five factors have contributed to delayed social and sexual growth in these adolescents: (1) severity of the mental handicap, (2) poor manual dexterity, (3) lack of education, (4) overprotective parents, and (5) limitations in health care personnel's ability to address sexuality with physically disabled patients and their families.[279] Either the parents or the child may bring up questions about sexuality. Parents of children with spina bifida realize the need to teach their children about sexuality, but they often feel inadequate about doing so and are reluctant to bring up questions to health care professionals.[280] The therapist must be open, informed, and able to provide resources to both parents and children.

Generally, the sexual capacity of the female with spina bifida is near normal—that is, she has potential for a normal orgasmic response, is fertile, and can bear children.[281] The pregnancy, however, may be considered high risk, depending on existing orthopedic abnormalities. Affected males are frequently sterile and have small testicles and penises. Their potential for erection and ejaculation depends on the level of the lesion. In many cases psychological problems may be a primary cause of sexual failure. Sexuality is not merely a process involving the genitalia; it also depends on a positive body image and a feeling of self-esteem that is nurtured from birth.[282]

PSYCHOSOCIAL ADJUSTMENT TO CONGENITAL CORD LESIONS

The previous sections on goal setting and rehabilitation of the child with spina bifida covered birth through adolescence. After adolescence, rehabilitation can be handled in much the same manner as an adult spinal cord injury. Keeping in mind the global effects of spina bifida on the growing child as he or she approaches adulthood is important, however.

Because of the congenital nature of spina bifida, psychological adjustment is somewhat different from adjustment to a traumatic spinal cord injury. The psychological adjustment to this congenital disability must be considered from the perspective of the parents, the family, and, of course, the child.[283]

A longitudinal study concerning the psychological aspects of spina bifida showed that the parents go through a series of steps in the adjustment process. From birth to approximately 6 months of age, the parents experience shock and bewilderment. Information given during this time may be rejected or misinterpreted. Health care professionals therefore must be ready to repeat the same information to parents on several occasions during the first few years of the rehabilitation process. The period of 6 to 18 months of the child's life may be the most stressful on parents. Frequent hospitalizations during this time place increased pressure on the whole family. Parents are now able to comprehend fully the implications of their child's functional limitations and inability to participate in life. They begin to worry about the future and the impact of the disability on the rest of the family structure. The period from age 2 years through the preschool years is relatively peaceful. The parents are more concerned with toilet training, social acceptability, and general information on child rearing. They seem less aware of their child's cognitive limitations as he or she continues to develop into a relatively happy, well-adjusted child.

By the age of 6 years, children are becoming more aware of their limitations and parents are concerned about problems that may arise as their children enter elementary school. The child's psychological adjustment depends on the severity of the motor problems but primarily on the attitude of the parents and family and on the environmental conditions to which he or she is exposed.[284,285]

Because of their disabilities, children with spina bifida are often denied small tasks or chores that promote a sense of responsibility in the growing child. To promote emotional growth and psychological well-being, caregivers must be persuaded to let go. Children with spina bifida must develop responsibility and independence by being given the chance to interact and even compete with their peers. During adolescence, concerns regarding independent living situations and vocational placement must be addressed. With a foundation of strong support systems fostering emotional maturity, the future can be bright for the child with a congenital spinal cord injury (Case Study 15-1).

CASE STUDY 15-1 ■ MICHAEL

This case study focuses on the physical therapy management of Michael, a teenage boy with myelomeningocele, a congenital spinal cord injury. Michael is now 16 years old and a sophomore in high school.

A spinal cord injury is a complex disability. When a spinal cord lesion exists from birth, an additional level of complexity is added. This congenital condition predisposes the CNS to have many areas that may not develop or function adequately. In addition, all areas of development—physical, cognitive, and psychosocial—that depend heavily on central functioning will likely be impaired. The clinician therefore must be aware of the significant impact this neurological defect has on motor function as well as a variety of related human capacities. Management can best be organized by using the *Guide to Physical Therapist Practice.* The following case study uses the concepts in the *Guide* to discuss several episodes of care throughout Michael's life.

The *Guide to Physical Therapist Practice* is designed to provide a framework for the PT to assist in client management.[1] During the infant to adolescent period of life, Michael's specific PT needs will change. Michael's presentation of congenital spinal cord dysfunction may be best represented through the life span by preferred practice patterns, which may include the following[1]:

- 4F: Impaired joint mobility, motor function, muscle performance, range of motion, and reflex integrity associated with spinal disorders
- 5C: Impaired motor function and sensory integrity associated with nonprogressive disorders of the central nervous system—congenital origin or acquired in infancy or childhood
- 6E: Impaired ventilation and respiration or gas exchange associated with ventilatory pump dysfunction or failure
- 7A: Primary prevention and risk reduction for integumentary disorders

Examination (evaluation) is a comprehensive screening and specific testing process that leads to a diagnostic classification required before intervention and is performed for all clients. It consists of three components: client history, systems review, and tests and measures. The PT may identify impairments, functional limitations and disability, and changes in physical function or overall health status. The PT synthesizes the findings to establish a working diagnosis (ICD-9 code 741.0). Results from the evaluation are established, and interventions with anticipated outcomes are made.[1] Refer to Tables 15-4 to 15-10 for a detailed synopsis of Michael's episodes of physical therapy during his 16 years. The OT should go through a similar process of screening and testing to develop a conceptual model for case management within the scope of occupational therapy. Many of the examination tools and intervention strategies may be the same, although the objective outcome may focus on different expectations.

NEWBORN EPISODE OF CARE

Michael was a term baby delivered by planned cesarean section with a prenatal diagnosis of myelomeningocele. The diagnosis was made during the second trimester after fetal ultrasound evaluation and amniocentesis. The family met with the neurosurgeon before delivery. Michael was delivered at 38 weeks of gestation and was transferred at 1 day of age to the local children's hospital for a planned surgical closure of his spina bifida. An orthopedic, urological, neurosurgical, and physical therapy assessment occurred at 1 day of age before back closure. Michael was the second child for this family. His mother was diagnosed with breast cancer at his birth. His sister is 2 years older and lives at home. Both parents are professional working parents; they have a nanny to assist with child care.

Presurgical MMT showed the presence of hip and knee musculature (L2-L4). Three days after the back closure, Michael required VP shunt insertion to control hydrocephalus. Postoperative MMT findings at 7 days of age were identical to preoperative results. Before discharge at 8 days of age, the parents were instructed in ROM exercises, positioning, and developmental handling. Michael would be monitored in a myelomeningocele clinic twice a year for an MMT and functional assessment with a team of health care providers (see Table 15-4).

EPISODE OF CARE: 6-MONTH FOLLOW-UP

At the age of 6 months Michael was readmitted to the hospital because of a shunt malfunction that necessitated VP shunt revision. After 2 weeks at home Michael returned to the clinic for postoperative follow-up. No medical concerns were present, but clinicians discovered that Michael had not yet begun to roll over. An evaluation with a standardized test was conducted. The AIMS was administered as well as additional tests of ROM, strength (by observation), reflexes, muscle tone, and endurance to establish a developmental baseline. At this visit a total-body night splint was fabricated to maintain hip alignment and prevent contractures of the lower extremities. Family education in latex precautions was provided. The need for assistive and adaptive devices was also assessed.

At this point, Michael had not received physical therapy because of the mother's health issues. Because of this situation, physical therapy that could be provided at home was recommended. The family was given a referral to their local EI system and a list of local pediatric physical therapy providers to obtain services (see Table 15-5).

Continued

CASE STUDY 15-1 ■ MICHAEL—cont'd

EPISODE OF CARE: EARLY INTERVENTION

The family contacted their local EI program after the previous clinic visit. An evaluation and assessment determined Michael was eligible for services. A variety of appropriate developmental assessments were used to determine eligibility (see Table 15-6). At the individual family service plan meeting, physical therapy intervention was determined to be the primary service at this time. Occupational, developmental, and speech therapies were not recommended. Michael received weekly physical therapy from age 6 months through 3 years. Therapy focused on developmental exercises to promote mobility, sitting and standing balance activities, strengthening available lower-extremity musculature, and orthotic assessment and gait training. The EI PT instructed the family in activities to complement the weekly physical therapy program. Michael began crawling at 1 year. At 10 months he used a vertical stander to initiate an upright stand position and began gait training at 15 months. Michael began walking with AFOs and a forward walker at 30 months (see Table 15-6).

EPISODE OF CARE: EARLY CHILDHOOD

At age 3 years, Michael transitioned into an EC program at his local school. Physical therapy was a related service that was included as part of his IEP. The transition meeting from EI to EC programming provided continuity of care unique to his needs. A global assessment tool to assess his mobility and self-care skills was administered. This test, the PEDI, was administered by the PT. Physical therapy management included ROM, strengthening, and gait training as it affected his ability to function in the preschool classroom and surrounding play areas. The school he attended was environmentally appropriate for his needs. It was one level, with wide doorways that allowed the use of his walker and then progressive use of forearm crutches with AFOs to advance his mobility skills. At the suggestion of his PT in the outpatient myelomeningocele clinic, Michael became involved in a toddler swimming program at the park district. A tricycle was adapted at the recommendation of the same therapist to assist with strengthening his lower extremities and to allow him to efficiently keep pace with his peers (see Table 15-7).

Another framework that can organize the management of Michael's interventions is the ICF. The ICF identifies components of health and contextual factors that are important for achievement of desired outcomes.[286] Relationships between components of health and contextual factors change over time. An example is given for one episode of care in EC (Figure 15-24).

At age 5.5 years, an IEP meeting was conducted before Michael entered kindergarten. The family and school team decided that no resources or special adaptations were necessary to enhance his education. The school he was to attend was determined to be environmentally appropriate to meet his needs.

EPISODE OF CARE: TETHERED CORD EPISODE (AGE 6 YEARS)

At his semiannual visit to the myelomeningocele clinic, the parents mentioned that Michael was falling frequently while using his forearm crutches and AFOs. Reddened areas at the left lateral calcaneus were noted. Routine MMT showed decreased strength in his left leg with an increase in muscle tone through his left leg. An MRI revealed a tethered spinal cord. A neurosurgical TCR was performed and his AFOs were revised. Two months after TCR Michael was again independent in ambulation and had progressed to stair climbing with one rail. His next routine 6-month MMT showed a return of strength to the level that preceded his tethered cord episode (see Table 15-8).

EPISODE OF CARE: PREADOLESCENCE (7 TO 10 YEARS OF AGE)

Michael's physical conditioning continued to progress, and from ages 7 to 10 years he participated in adaptive sports and activities in his community. Swimming had become a favorite activity. He had been swimming to increase strength and endurance since he was a toddler at the suggestion of his PT. Because of his activity level and independence in most functional activities, routine physical therapy had been discontinued, with only biannual clinic visits remaining. Michael and his family continued intensive stretching and a prone positioning program that they had been performing since Michael was a toddler. At his 10-year clinic visit, the therapist administered formal MMT and ROM assessment and also carried out the PEDI. Scaled scores on the PEDI were used because he was above the age of normed standards for the test. An area of skin breakdown was noted on the left malleolus and decreased weight bearing was noted during gait. MMT and orthopedic examinations showed no changes. A brace check noted the AFO was too small and needed to be replaced. The brace was replaced and the PT reviewed skin care and brace fit with Michael and his family (see Table 15-9).

EPISODE OF CARE: ADOLESCENCE (AGE 13 YEARS)

At age 13 years Michael had gained a significant amount of weight that was limiting endurance for long-distance ambulation. Michael was referred to a nutritionist for counseling. The PT in conjunction with the physician discussed with Michael and his parents the possibility of using a wheelchair for long-distance travel. After much discussion and initial resistance from Michael, Michael and his family decided to try a wheelchair. At age 16 years, Michael continues to be an independent ambulator and uses a wheelchair for long distances only. He continues to be monitored on an annual basis or as needed as problems arise. Michael's physical therapy has encouraged and continued to motivate him to maintain his participation in sports activities during his teenage years (see Table 15-10).

EPISODE OF CARE: ADULTHOOD

Michael has graduated from high school and has been attending college on a large campus the past few years as a graduate student majoring in history. He works part time as a tour guide at the Museum of Natural History. As he drives to work, he is required to transfer to and from his car on a regular basis. He needs to disassemble his chair to get it in and out of his car efficiently. Increased frequency of transfers to and from the car, as well as the need to disassemble and reassemble his chair on a regular basis, has led to an increase in shoulder pain and discomfort. He continues to use his crutches for short distances (150 feet) at work using a swing-through gait. He uses an ultralight manual wheelchair for all other mobility throughout the day. His wheelchair is equipped with carrying loops for his crutches at the back of his chair. Michael returned to his primary care physician because of his new episode of pain. He was referred to PT to address his issues with pain. The PT has evaluated his gait and recommended that to minimize stress on his shoulders he should switch from a swing-through to a four-point gait pattern (Table 15-11). He has also been referred to OT for further assessment of efficient transfer techniques to and from the car. In addition, a referral to an AT team has been recommended to evaluate the need for assisted power wheels as well as an additional means of transportation to reduce stress on his shoulders.

TABLE 15-4 ■ NEWBORN EPISODE OF CARE FOR CHILD WITH SPINA BIFIDA

PRACTICE PATTERNS	SYSTEMS TO REVIEW	TESTS AND RESULTS	INTERVENTIONS	ANTICIPATED GOALS AND EXPECTED OUTCOMES
4F 7A 6E 5C	Musculoskeletal Integumentary Cardiopulmonary Neuromuscular Cognition and communication	MMT: No innervation below L4 Muscle length: WFL ROM: WFL Skin integrity: WFL HR/RR/CE: WFL Reflexes: Absent DTRs below knee (+) Suck/swallow (+) Galant Muscle tone: Flaccid below L4; low in trunk; UEs WFL Motor skills: On informal testing turns head, kicks, clears head in prone Observation: Decreased pain in LEs	Collaborate and coordinate systems review evaluation results with health care team. Document impairments, functional limitations, and strengths. Prepare a plan of treatment. Therapeutic exercises to improve balance, muscle strength, and mobility. Family training: instruction in ROM; developmental positioning for function and enhancement of performance; instruction regarding sensory impairment and skin integrity and areas of pressure; and instruction in signs of VP shunt malfunction.	Joint integrity and mobility improves. Postural control and muscle performance improves. Sensory awareness develops appropriately. Risk prevention: parents understand signs and symptoms of VP shunt malfunction. Caregivers understand importance of checking skin for irritation and breakdown. Cognition and language develops appropriately. Improved infant and family sense of well-being. Stressors decrease.

CE, Cardiorespiratory endurance; *DTR,* deep tendon reflex; *HR,* heart rate; *LE,* lower extremity; *MMT,* manual muscle testing; *ROM,* range of motion; *RR,* respiratory rate; *UE,* upper extremity; *VP,* ventriculoperitoneal; *WFL,* within functional limits.

TABLE 15-5 ■ SIX-MONTH FOLLOW-UP EPISODE OF CARE FOR CHILD WITH SPINA BIFIDA

PRACTICE PATTERNS	SYSTEMS TO REVIEW	TESTS AND RESULTS	INTERVENTIONS	ANTICIPATED GOALS AND EXPECTED OUTCOMES
4F 7A 6E 5C	Musculoskeletal Integumentary Cardiopulmonary Neuromuscular Cognition and communication	MMT: No innervation below L4 Muscle length: WFL ROM: WFL Skin integrity: WFL HR/RR/CE: WFL Reflexes: Absent DTRs below knee (+) Suck/swallow (+) Galant Muscle tone: Flaccid below L4; low in trunk; UEs WFL Motor skills: AIMS completed; could not roll over, head righting emerging in prone and supported sitting Observation: Decreased pain in LEs VP shunt malfunction	Revised shunt: neurosurgery. Collaborate and coordinate systems review evaluation results with health care team. Document impairments, functional limitations, and strengths. Prepare a plan of treatment. Therapeutic exercises to improve balance and mobility. Family training: review instruction in ROM, positioning for function, signs of shunt malfunction, and latex precautions. Refer to EI program. Fabricate night splint for LE alignment. Transition to vertical stander at 10 months of age.	Joint integrity and mobility improve. Motor control and muscle performance improve. Established in physical therapy program. Risk prevention: parents understand signs and symptoms of VP shunt malfunction and importance of checking skin for irritation and breakdown. Latex precautions understood. Sensory awareness develops appropriately. Cognition and communication develop appropriately. Improved infant and family sense of well-being. Infant and family stressors decrease.

AIMS, Alberta Infant Motor Scale; *CE,* cardiorespiratory endurance; *DTR,* deep tendon reflex; *EI,* Early Intervention; *HR,* heart rate; *LE,* lower extremity; *MMT,* manual muscle testing; *ROM,* range of motion; *RR,* respiratory rate; *UE,* upper extremity; *VP,* ventriculoperitoneal; *WFL,* within functional limits.

TABLE 15-6 ■ EARLY INTERVENTION EPISODE OF CARE FOR CHILD WITH SPINA BIFIDA

PRACTICE PATTERNS	SYSTEMS TO REVIEW	TESTS AND RESULTS	INTERVENTIONS	ANTICIPATED GOALS AND EXPECTED OUTCOMES
4F 7A 6E 5C	Musculoskeletal Integumentary Cardiopulmonary Neuromuscular Cognition and Communication	MMT: No innervation below L4 Muscle length: WFL ROM: WFL Skin integrity: WFL HR/RR/CE: WFL Reflexes: Absent DTRs below knee Emerging head and trunk righting Muscle tone: Flaccid below L4 low in trunk; UEs WFL Motor skills: BSID-2 administered by PT with a 30% delay noted; fine motor domains of PDMS-2 administered by OT with no delays noted Observation: Decreased pain in LEs Hawaii Early Learning Profile (HELP) administered; WFL for age Oral-motor, language: WFL	Collaborate and coordinate systems review evaluation results with health care team. Document impairments, functional limitations, and strengths. Prepare IFSP; case manager established physical therapy as primary service by collaboration with developmental, occupational, and speech therapists. Therapeutic exercises to improve balance, mobility, and strength. Standing with vertical stander at 10 months, gait training with vertical stander and walker at 15 months, and progression to ambulation with AFOs and forward walker at 30 months. Family training: instruction in ROM and developmental activities to improve performance; sensory stimulation and body awareness activities; skin integrity; and assessment of adaptive equipment needs (vertical stander at 10 months, AFOs to position feet in standing, adjustment of stroller to provide leg support, and walker for progression of gait).	Joint integrity and mobility improves. Postural control and muscle performance improves. Risk prevention: parents understand developmental exercises, appropriate equipment use, and importance of checking for skin irritation and breakdown. Sensory awareness develops appropriately. Cognition and language develop appropriately. Improved infant and family sense of well-being. Infant and family stressors decrease. Developmental, occupational, and speech therapists will reassess at 6-month intervals and intervene if needed.

AFOs, Ankle-foot orthoses; *BSID-2,* Bayley Scales of Infant Development, Second Edition; *CE,* cardiorespiratory endurance; *DTR,* deep tendon reflex; *HR,* heart rate; *IFSP,* Individual Family Service Plan; *LE,* lower extremity; *MMT,* manual muscle testing; *OT,* occupational therapist; *PDMS-2,* Peabody Developmental Motor Scales, second edition; *PT,* physical therapist; *ROM,* range of motion; *RR,* respiratory rate; *UE,* upper extremity; *WFL,* within functional limits.

TABLE 15-7 ■ EARLY CHILDHOOD EPISODE (3 TO 5 YEARS) OF CARE FOR CHILD WITH SPINA BIFIDA

PRACTICE PATTERNS	SYSTEMS TO REVIEW	TESTS AND RESULTS	INTERVENTIONS	ANTICIPATED GOALS AND EXPECTED OUTCOMES
4F 7A 6E 5C	Musculoskeletal Integumentary Cardiopulmonary Neuromuscular Cognition and communication	MMT: No innervation below L4 Muscle length: WFL ROM: WFL Gait: ambulates with AFOs and walker Skin integrity: WFL HR/RR/CE: WFL Established baseline walking distance and time with 6-minute walk test Reflexes: Absent DTRs below knee Muscle tone: Flaccid below L4; low in trunk; UEs WFL Motor skills: PEDI carried out Independent walking with walker and AFOs ADLs are age appropriate with assist School Function Assessment (SFA) completed at 5 years of age Cognition: WFL PEDI social function section: WFL	Collaborate and coordinate systems review evaluation results with health care team. Document impairments, functional limitations, and strengths. Improve mobility in school environment through therapeutic exercise and progressive gait training with crutches. Family training: instruction in gait with crutches. Health and wellness: swimming and biking in community setting. Tricycle adapted. Educate family and Michael regarding latex precautions.	Joint and skin integrity maintained. Postural control and muscle performance improves. Mobility improves. Risk prevention: parents understand progression with crutches. Parents understand latex precautions in community environment and home. Sensory awareness develops appropriately. Improved child and family sense of well-being. Child and family stressors decrease.

ADLs, Activities of daily living; *AFOs,* ankle-foot orthoses; *CE,* cardiorespiratory endurance; *DTR,* deep tendon reflex; *HR,* heart rate; *MMT,* manual muscle testing; *PEDI,* Pediatric Evaluation of Disability Inventory; *RR,* respiratory rate; *UE,* upper extremity; *WFL,* within functional limits.

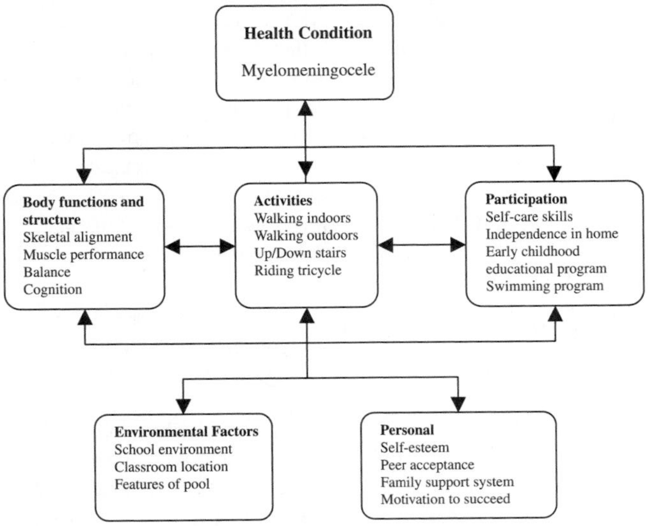

Figure 15-24 ■ Michael's early childhood episode of care as illustrated by the International Classification of Functioning, Disability and Health model.

TABLE 15-8 ■ TETHERED CORD EPISODE OF CARE FOR CHILD WITH SPINA BIFIDA (AGE 6 YEARS)

PRACTICE PATTERNS	SYSTEMS TO REVIEW	TESTS AND RESULTS	INTERVENTIONS	ANTICIPATED GOALS AND EXPECTED OUTCOMES
4F 7A 6E 5C	Musculoskeletal Integumentary Cardiopulmonary Neuromuscular Cognition and communication	MMT: decreased strength left leg Muscle length: WFL ROM: not WFL Gait: changed; weakness left side Skin integrity: redness lateral border of calcaneus HR/RR/CE: 6-minute walk test exhibits decreased pace Reflexes: Hyperreflexive DTRs below L3 on left Absent DTRs below knee on right Muscle tone: increased through left leg, flaccid below L4 on right, low in trunk UEs WFL Motor skills: falling more often Decreased ability to stand and walk; weight shifted toward right Status: unchanged	Collaborate and coordinate systems review evaluation results with physician. Physician ordered MRI, surgery for release of tethered spinal cord. Document impairments, functional limitations, and strengths. Prepare a plan of treatment. Increase therapeutic exercises, neuromuscular rehabilitation, and gait training to restore balance and gait with crutches. Family training: instruction in stretching for muscle length and developmental activity to progress, enhance performance. Refer to orthotist for brace adjustments.	Joint integrity, strength, and mobility are restored. Gait performance improves. Risk prevention: parents understand signs and symptoms of tethered cord. Skin integrity is maintained. Sensory awareness develops appropriately. Cognition and language skills develop appropriately. Improved child and family sense of well-being. Stressors decrease.

CE, Cardiorespiratory endurance; *DTR,* deep tendon reflex; *HR,* heart rate; *MMT,* manual muscle testing; *MRI,* magnetic resonance imaging; *ROM,* range of motion; *RR,* respiratory rate; *UE,* upper extremity; *WFL,* within functional limits.

TABLE 15-9 ■ PREADOLESCENT EPISODE OF CARE FOR CHILD WITH SPINA BIFIDA (AGE 10 YEARS)

PRACTICE PATTERNS	SYSTEMS TO REVIEW	TESTS AND RESULTS	INTERVENTIONS	ANTICIPATED GOALS AND EXPECTED OUTCOMES
4F 7A 6E 5C	Musculoskeletal Integumentary Cardiopulmonary Neuromuscular Cognition and communication	MMT: Back to baseline; no innervation below L4 Muscle length: WFL ROM: WFL Skin integrity: WFL HR/RR/CE: WFL Reflexes: Absent DTRs below knee Balance and equilibrium appropriate for L4 spinal level Muscle tone: Flaccid below L4, low in trunk; UEs WFL Motor skills: PEDI conducted; maximal score of 100 achieved Measured self-care, mobility, and social function Observation: WFL	Collaborate and coordinate systems review evaluation results with health care team. Document impairments, functional limitations, and strengths. Discharge from formal PT. Home program to continue and include intensive stretching and prone activities. Continue health and wellness programs, including swimming and community recreational programs. Continue to educate Michael on importance of skin integrity, latex sensitivity, and brace fit. Referred to orthotist for brace replacement.	Postural control and muscle performance are maintained. Joint integrity and mobility are maintained. Michael understands the importance of checking skin for irritation and breakdown and appropriate brace fit. Michael becomes active in the community adapted sports programs. Improved child and family sense of well-being. Client satisfaction.

CE, Cardiorespiratory endurance; *DTR,* deep tendon reflex; *HR,* heart rate; *MMT,* manual muscle testing; *PEDI,* Pediatric Evaluation of Disability Inventory; *PT,* physical therapy; *ROM,* range of motion; *RR,* respiratory rate; *UE,* upper extremity; *WFL,* within functional limits.

TABLE 15-10 ■ ADOLESCENT EPISODE OF CARE FOR CHILD WITH SPINA BIFIDA (AGE 13 YEARS)

PRACTICE PATTERNS	SYSTEMS TO REVIEW	TESTS AND RESULTS	INTERVENTIONS	ANTICIPATED GOALS AND EXPECTED OUTCOMES
4F 7A 6E 5C	Musculoskeletal Integumentary Cardiopulmonary Neuromuscular Cognition and communication	MMT: No innervation below L4 Muscle length: WFL ROM: WFL Skin integrity: WFL Anthropometric: Increase in height and weight HR/RR/CE: Increased HR and decreased distance traveled in 6-minute walk test; increased fatigue during long-distance ambulation Reflexes: Absent DTRs below knee Muscle tone: LEs no change; UEs WFL Motor skills: Decreased ability to keep pace with peers Observation: Increased social abilities	Collaborate and coordinate systems review evaluation results with health care team. Document impairments, functional limitations, and strengths. Prepare a plan of treatment. Assistive equipment, wheelchair evaluation; to be used for long distances. Short-distance ambulation with forearm crutches to continue at home and school. Client education: weight shifts every hour while using wheelchair for skin integrity. Refer to nutritionist. Design a plan to incorporate driver's education through high school as well as rehabilitation resources.	Joint integrity and walking mobility are maintained. Risk prevention: Michael understands signs and symptoms of decubitus pressure areas. Michael's long-distance mobility increases independence. Social and recreational opportunities increase. Improved client sense of well-being. Stressors decrease.

CE, Cardiorespiratory endurance; *DTR,* deep tendon reflex; *HR,* heart rate; *LE,* lower extremity; *MMT,* manual muscle testing; *ROM,* range of motion; *RR,* respiratory rate; *UE,* upper extremity; *WFL,* within functional limits.

TABLE 15-11 ■ EPISODE OF CARE FOR ADULT WITH SPINA BIFIDA (AGE 25 YEARS)

PRACTICE PATTERNS	SYSTEMS TO REVIEW	TESTS AND RESULTS	INTERVENTIONS	ANTICIPATED GOALS AND EXPECTED OUTCOMES
4F 7A 6E 5C	Musculoskeletal Integumentary Cardiopulmonary Neuromuscular Cognition and communication	MMT: No innervation below L4 Muscle length: WFL ROM: decreased in shoulder WFL LE Skin integrity: WFL Anthropometrics: Increase in height and weight HR/RR/CE: Increased HR and decreased distance traveled in 6-minute walk test; shoulder pain during short distance ambulation, fatigue with longer distances Reflexes: Absent DTRs below knee Muscle tone: LEs, no change; UEs WFL Motor skills: Decreased ability to keep pace with peers Observation: Painful right shoulder during walking and transfer of wheelchair into vehicle for transport	Collaborate and coordinate systems review evaluation results with health care team. Document impairments, functional limitations, and strengths. Prepare a plan of treatment. Assistive equipment, wheelchair modification to decrease shoulder stress for long distances. Short-distance gait training four-point with forearm crutches to continue home and community ambulation. Incorporate flexibility and strength training. Client education: reduce shoulder stress with efficient body mechanics. Refer to occupational therapy. Design a plan to incorporate efficient transfer of wheelchair to car and rehabilitation resources.	Joint integrity and walking mobility are maintained. Risk prevention: Michael understands signs and symptoms of joint overuse. Michael decreases stressful walking and increases independence. Social and recreational opportunities increase. Improved client sense of well-being. Stressors decrease.

CE, Cardiorespiratory endurance; *DTR,* deep tendon reflex; *HR,* heart rate; *LE,* lower extremity; *MMT,* manual muscle testing; *ROM,* range of motion; *RR,* respiratory rate; *UE,* upper extremity; *WFL,* within functional limits.

Acknowledgment

We dedicate this chapter to Jane W. Schneider and all the children who have taught us so much.

References

To enhance this text and add value for the reader, all references are included on the companion Evolve site that accompanies this textbook. This online service will, when available, provide a link for the reader to a Medline abstract for the article cited. There are 286 cited references and other general references for this chapter, with the majority of those articles being evidence-based citations.

APPENDIX 15-A ■ ORLAU Swivel Walker Distributors

United States
Mopac Ltd
206 Chestnut Street
Eau Claire, WI 54703
(715) 832-1685

United Kingdom
J. Stallard, Technical Director
Oswestry Orthopaedic Hospital
Shropshire, SY107AG
UK

CHAPTER 16 Traumatic Spinal Cord Injury

MYRTICE B. ATRICE, PT, BS, SARAH A. MORRISON, PT, BS, SHARI L. McDOWELL, PT, BS, PAULA M. ACKERMAN, MS, OTR/L, TERESA A. FOY, OT, BS, and CANDY TEFERTILLER, DPT, ATP, NCS

KEY TERMS

American Spinal Injury Association (ASIA)
autonomic dysfunction
autonomic dysreflexia
body-weight–supported treadmill (BWST)
bulbocavernosus reflex
complete lesion
deep vein thrombosis (DVT)
discomplete
Functional Independence Measure (FIM)
incomplete lesion
intermittent catheterization
locomotor training
lower motor neuron
mobile arm support (MAS)
neuroprosthetics
offset feeder
orthostatic hypotension
paraplegia
pressure ulcer
pulmonary embolism (PE)
spinal cord injury (SCI)
spinal shock
tenodesis
tetraplegia
upper motor neuron

OBJECTIVES

After reading this chapter the student or therapist will be able to:

1. Describe the demographics, etiology, and mechanism of injury of spinal cord injury.
2. Discuss the acute medical management of person with spinal cord injury.
3. Describe the secondary complications of spinal cord injury, the appropriate interventions, and the impact of complications on the rehabilitation process.
4. Identify the basic components of the examination process.
5. Identify patient problems based on the examination, establish appropriate goals, and plan individualized treatment programs for patients with a spinal cord injury.
6. Describe adaptive equipment available to increase function.
7. Discuss progression of each individual and the process of discharge planning throughout the rehabilitation process.
8. Describe functional expectations for individuals with complete spinal cord injuries.
9. Identify equipment needs for a given spinal cord injury lesion.
10. Describe various aspects of activity-based therapies to promote recovery after spinal cord injury.

Spinal cord injury (SCI) is a catastrophic condition that, depending on its severity, may cause dramatic changes in a person's life. SCI usually happens to active, independent people who at one moment are in control of their lives and in the next moment are paralyzed, with loss of sensation and loss of bodily functions, which can lead to dependence on others for even the most basic needs. To reduce negative impact, individuals with SCI need a well-coordinated, specialized rehabilitation program to assist them in maximizing the development of skills necessary to live a satisfying and productive postinjury life.[1,2]

A successful rehabilitation program requires a team of health care professionals who work in unison to address alterations in body function, increase the individual's independence in all daily activities, and return the individual to the highest level of community participation specific to that individual's life situations. Minimally, the team should include a physician, case manager, occupational therapist, physical therapist, therapeutic recreation specialist, prosthetist or orthotist, nurse, speech-language pathologist, dietician, assistive technologist, respiratory care practitioner, psychologist, social worker, vocational counselor, rehabilitation engineer, and chaplain.[3-5] The most important element determining success in any rehabilitation program is the patient's and family's active participation throughout the rehabilitation process.

This chapter provides a general overview for the management of individuals with SCI throughout inpatient and postacute phases of the rehabilitation continuum. The information is intended to aid health care professionals in the treatment of individuals with SCI by providing guidelines to maximize each individual's return to their preinjury lifestyle.

SPINAL CORD LESIONS

SCI occurs when the spinal cord is damaged as a result of trauma, disease processes, vascular compromise, or congenital neural tube defect. The clinical manifestations of the injury vary depending on the extent and location of the damage to the spinal cord.

Tetraplegia

Tetraplegia (preferred to *quadriplegia*) refers to impairment or loss of motor and/or sensory function as a result of damage to the cervical segments of the spinal cord. Function in the upper extremities, lower extremities, and trunk is affected. It does not include brachial plexus lesions or injury to peripheral nerves outside the neural canal.[6]

Paraplegia

Paraplegia refers to impairment or loss of motor or sensory function as a result of damage to the thoracic, lumbar, or sacral segments of the spinal cord. Depending on the level of the damage, function may be impaired in the trunk and/or lower extremities. This term is used to refer to cauda equina and conus medullaris injuries but not to lumbosacral plexus lesions or injury to peripheral nerves, which are considered outside of the central nervous system.[6]

Complete, Discomplete, and Incomplete Lesions

In a complete lesion, sensory and motor function in the lowest sacral segments (S4-S5) is absent postinjury.[6] The American Spinal Injury Association (ASIA) classification for this type of injury is ASIA Impairment Scale (AIS) A. Complete injuries to the spinal cord are usually the result of extensive trauma or disease and are often segmentally associated with damage to the nerve roots in the intervertebral foramina.[7] Function of the roots originating from the more cranial portion of the intact cord can be expected to return within 6 months.[7]

Discomplete injury is a relatively new term in SCI research and practice. It is defined as a lesion that is "clinically complete but which is accompanied by neurophysiological evidence of residual brain influence on spinal cord function below the level of the lesion."[8] Studies of persons whose spinal cord injuries were considered complete under ASIA standards have shown that in a large percentage (84%) there was residual brain influence on the spinal cord below the level of the lesion.[8,9] The current gold standard for testing, the AIS, is unable to detect this residual function, which suggests that AIS testing may be providing an inaccurate picture of the patients' neurological plasticity and recovery potential. The Brain Motor Control Assessment (BMCA) is emerging as a desirable adjunct to the standard ASIA testing.[9] In the BMCA, surface electromyography (EMG) is used to quantify the motor unit activity of the lower extremities in response to a standard testing protocol including active and passive movement of the lower extremities, reinforcement maneuvers (e.g., Jendrassik or Valsalva) performed above the level of injury, tendon taps and vibration, and elicitation and suppression of reflex activity. The motor unit responses are quantified and compared with normative data to establish a voluntary response index and a similarity index. In other words, the results of the BMCA help to determine how different the subjects' motor responses are from those of persons with intact neurological systems.[8-11] This testing requires specialty equipment but can easily be administered by physical therapists once they have received the appropriate training.

With incomplete lesions there is detectable residual sensory or motor function below the neurological level and specifically in the lowest sacral segment. According to ASIA standards, any sensation in the anal mucocutaneous junction, or deep anal sensation, indicates that the lesion is incomplete. If only sensation is preserved, the injury is classified as AIS B. If motor function in key muscles is maintained to some degree, patients may achieve level C, D, or E classification. This testing will be reviewed further in this chapter.[6,12]

DEMOGRAPHICS

The incidence of traumatic SCI in the United States is approximately 12,000 new cases per year.[13] Approximately 3000 new cases of spinal cord impairment resulting from disease and congenital anomalies occur each year. The number of people living in the United States today with SCI is between 231,000 and 311,000.[13] Fifty-three percent of traumatic SCIs occur in persons aged 16 to 30 years. However, the median age of the general population of the United States has increased by 8 years since the mid 1970s, and the average age of the SCI population has steadily increased. Since 2005, the mean age at the time of injury is 40.2 years.[13,14] Persons older than 60 years of age at injury have increased from 4.7% before 1980 to 11.5% for injuries occurring since 2000. This trend explains the increase in the median age during this same time period from 27.9 years to 35.3 years. Table 16-1 lists additional demographics.

In 2005 the average length of inpatient stay was 50 days (12 days in an acute-care facility and 38 days in rehabilitation). The average yearly health care and living expenses

TABLE 16-1 ■ SPINAL CORD INJURY DEMOGRAPHICS

Mean age at injury	40.2 years
Most common age at injury	19.0 years
SEX	
Male	80.9%
Female	19.1%
CAUSES OF INJURY	
Motor vehicle accident	41.3%
Falls	27.3%
Violent acts	15.0%
Sports injuries	7.9%
Other	8.5%
NEUROLOGICAL CATEGORIES AT DISCHARGE	
Incomplete tetraplegia	38.3%
Complete paraplegia	22.9%
Incomplete paraplegia	21.5%
Complete tetraplegia	16.9%
No deficits	0.7%
COMMON INJURY SITES[64]	
C5	14.9%
C4	13.6%
C6	10.8%
T12	6.7%
C7	5.3%

Data from National Spinal Cord Injury Statistical Center: *Spinal cord injury: facts and figures at a glance,* February 2010, Birmingham, AL, 2010, University of Alabama, National Spinal Cord Injury Statistical Center. Available at www.uab.edu/NSCICSC.

vary according to severity of injury. In the first year, individuals with high tetraplegia spend $829,843, whereas individuals with paraplegia spend an average of $303,220.[13] Today 87.7% of persons with SCI are discharged to a noninstitutional residence. Life expectancies for patients with SCI continue to increase but are still below the national average of persons without SCI. Mortality rates are significantly higher during the first year after injury, especially for severely injured persons. According to the National SCI Database, the leading causes of death after an SCI are pneumonia, pulmonary emboli, and septicemia.[13]

Statistics suggest a high incidence of multiple trauma associated with a traumatic SCI (55.2%).[15] The most common injuries are fractures (29.3%) and loss of consciousness (28.2%).[15] Traumatic pneumothorax or hemothorax are reported in 17.8% of persons with SCI. Traumatic head injuries of sufficient severity to affect cognitive or emotional functioning are reported in 11.5% of all cases.[15] Skull and facial fractures, along with traumatic head injuries and vertebral artery and esophageal disruptions, are common in cervical injuries.[16] Limb fractures and intrathoracic injuries (rib fractures and hemopneumothorax) are frequent in thoracic injuries, whereas intraabdominal injuries to the liver, spleen, and kidneys are associated with lumbar and cauda equina injuries.[16]

SEQUELAE OF TRAUMATIC SPINAL CORD INJURY

As stated previously, most spinal cord injuries occur as a result of trauma, be it motor vehicle accidents, falls, violence, or sports-related injury. The degree and type of forces that are exerted on the spine at the time of the trauma determine the location and severity of damage to the spinal cord.[17] Injuries to the vertebral column can be classified biomechanically as flexion or flexion-rotation injuries, hyperextension injuries, and compression injuries.[18] Penetrating injuries to the cord are usually the result of gunshot or knife wounds.[18]

Spinal cord damage can also be caused by nontraumatic mechanisms. Circulatory compromise to the spinal cord resulting in ischemia causes neurological damage at and below the involved cord level. This can be caused by a thrombus, swelling, compression, or vascular malformations and dysfunction. Degenerative bone diseases can cause compression of the spinal cord by creating a stenosis of the spinal canal and intervertebral foramina. Stenosis can also result from the prolapse of the intervertebral disc into the neural canal. The encroachment of tumors or abscesses within the spinal cord, the spinal canal, or the surrounding tissues can also lead to SCI. Congenital malformation of the spinal structures, as in spina bifida, can also compromise the spinal cord and its protective layers of connective tissue. Some of the more common diseases and conditions that result in compromise of the spinal cord include Guillain-Barré syndrome, transverse myelitis, amyotrophic lateral sclerosis, and multiple sclerosis.[12]

After the spinal cord has sustained damage, cellular events occur in response to the injury and are classified in three phases of progression: acute, secondary, and chronic responses. The acute process begins on occurrence of an injury and continues for 3 to 5 days.[19] Abrupt necrosis or cell death can result from both mechanical and ischemic events. The impact of an SCI often causes direct mechanical damage to neural and other soft tissues as well as severe hemorrhaging in the surrounding gray and white matter, resulting in immediate cell death.[20,21] In the next few minutes after the insult, injured nerve cells respond with trauma-induced action potentials, which lead to increased levels of intracellular sodium. The result of this influx is an increase in osmotic pressure movement of water into the area. Edema generally develops in up to three levels above and below the original insult and leads to further tissue deconstruction.[19,21,22] Increased levels of extracellular potassium and intracellular concentrations of calcium also result in an electrolyte imbalance that contributes to a toxic environment.[23-25] Abnormal concentrations of calcium within the damaged cells disrupt their functioning and cause breakdown of protein and phospholipids, leading to demyelination and destruction of the cell membrane.[25] The cascade of these events consequentially contributes to a dysfunctional nervous system.

During this acute phase, evidence of spinal shock may be present. Spinal shock occurs 30 to 60 minutes after spinal trauma and is characterized by flaccid paralysis and absence of all spinal cord reflex activity below the level of the spinal cord lesion.[26,27] This condition lasts for about 24 hours after injury, represents a generalized failure of circuitry in the spinal neural network, and is thought to be directly related to a conduction block resulting from leakage of potassium into the extracellular matrix.[28] The completeness of the lesion cannot be determined until spinal shock is resolved. The signs of spinal shock resolution are controversial; however, the return of reflexes may be a good indication.

The secondary phase of the injury occurs within the course of minutes to weeks after the acute process and is characterized by the continuation of ischemic cellular death, electrolytic shifts, and edema. Extracellular concentrations of glutamate and other excitatory amino acids reach concentrations that are six to eight times greater than normal within the first 15 minutes after an injury.[24] In addition, lipid peroxidation and free radical production also occur.[29] Apoptosis (a secondary programmable cell death) occurs and involves reactive gliosis. There is also an important immune response that adds to the secondary damage that may be a result of a damaged blood-brain barrier, microglial activation, and increased local concentrations of cytokines and chemokines.[30] The lesion enlarges from the initial core of cell death, expanding from the perilesional region to a larger region of cell loss.

In the chronic phase, which occurs over a period of days to years, apoptosis continues both rostrally and caudally. Receptors and ion channels are altered, and with penetrating injuries scarring and tethering of the cord occurs. Conduction deficits persist owing to demyelination, and permanent hyperexcitability develops with consequential chronic pain syndromes and spasticity in many SCI patients.[26] Changes in neural circuits result from alterations in excitatory and inhibitory inputs, and axons may exhibit regenerative and sprouting responses but go no farther than 1 mm.[24]

Medical interventions are evolving to limit the impact of the acute SCI and the subsequent progression that follows. Growing interest in protection and repair of the injured nervous system has led to an improved understanding of the pathophysiology associated with SCI and has resulted in the implementation of several therapeutic strategies that are currently being investigated in phase 1 and 2 clinical trials. The effects of methylprednisolone sodium succinate, tirilizad mesylate, monosialotetrahexosylganglioside, thyrotropin-releasing hormone, gacyclidine, naloxone, and nimodipine have all been examined in randomized controlled trials over the last few years. Although the primary outcomes in these studies did not demonstrate statistically significant effects, a secondary analysis demonstrated that methylprednisolone sodium succinate given within 8 hours of injury was associated with modest clinical benefits.[17] Phase 2 trials with monosialotetrahexosylganglioside and thyrotropin-releasing hormone also yielded some therapeutic benefits, but further studies need to be completed to determine efficacy. Several current or planned studies exist to evaluate the potential benefits of early surgical decompression and electrical field stimulation, neuroprotective strategies such as riluzole and minocycline, the inactivation of myelin inhibition by blocking Nogo and Rho, and the transplantation of various substrates into the injured spinal cord.[17] Promising clinical trials are also underway to minimize the secondary phase of injury and to promote healing and neuronal regeneration (Table 16-2). If medical interventions can bridge the central lesion or limit the secondary progression, the functional loss that follows SCI will be minimized and chances of recovery improved.

TABLE 16-2 ■ PHASES OF INJURY TABLE

PHASE	DESCRIPTION
Acute	Systemic hypotension and spinal shock
	Hemorrhage
	Cell death from direct insult or ischemia
	Edema
	Vasospasm
	Shifts in electrolytes
	Accumulation of neurotransmitters
	Induced hypothermic treatment
Secondary	Continued cell death
	Continued edema
	Continued shifts in electrolytes
	Free-radical production
	Lipid peroxidation
	Neutrophil and lymphocyte invasion and release of cytokines
	Apoptosis
	Calcium entry into cells
Chronic	Continued apoptosis radiating from site of injury
	Alteration of ion channels and receptors
	Formation of fluid-filled cavity
	Scarring of spinal cord by glial cells
	Demyelination
	Regenerative processes, including sprouting by neurons
	Altered neurocircuits
	Syringomyelia

Data from Hulsebosch CE: Recent advances in pathophysiology and treatment of spinal cord injury. *Adv Physiol Educ* 26:238–255, 2002; and Sekhon LH, Fehlings MG: Epidemiology, demographics, and pathophysiology of acute spinal cord injury. *Spine* 26(24 suppl):S2–S12, 2001.

CLINICAL SYNDROMES

Some incomplete lesions have a distinct clinical picture with specific signs and symptoms. An understanding of the various syndromes can be helpful to the patient's team in planning the rehabilitation program. Figure 16-1 depicts the anatomy of the spinal cord.[30,31] This basic anatomy of the spinal cord can be referred to as the various syndromes are described.

Central Cord Syndrome

Hyperextension injuries usually result in a central cord syndrome.[31] This injury causes bleeding into the central gray matter of the spinal cord, resulting in more impairment of function in the upper extremities than in the lower extremities.[31] Most incomplete lesions result in this syndrome, especially in elderly individuals when cervical stenosis is present.[30] Although the prognosis for functional recovery is good for individuals with central cord syndrome, the pattern of recovery is such that intrinsic hand function is the last thing to return. Approximately 77% of clients with central cord syndrome will attain some level of ambulatory function, 53% bowel and bladder control, and 42% hand function.[12,32,33]

Anterior Spinal Artery Syndrome

Anterior spinal artery syndrome is usually caused by flexion injuries in which bone or cartilage spicules compromise the anterior spinal artery.[31] Motor function and pain and temperature sensation are lost bilaterally below the injured segment.[31] The prognosis is extremely poor for return of bowel and bladder function, hand function, and ambulation.[12,33]

Brown-Séquard Syndrome

Occasionally, as a result of penetrating injuries (gunshot or stab wounds), only one half of the spinal cord is damaged. The Brown-Séquard syndrome is characterized by ipsilateral loss of motor function and position sense and contralateral loss of pain sensation several levels below the lesion.[31] The prognosis for recovery is good. Nearly all clients attain some level of ambulatory function, 80% regain hand function, 100% have bladder control, and 80% have bowel control.[12,33]

Posterior Cord Syndrome

Posterior cord syndrome is rare, resulting from compression by tumor or infarction of the posterior spinal artery. Clinically, proprioception, stereognosis, two-point discrimination, and vibration sense are lost below the level of the lesion.[31]

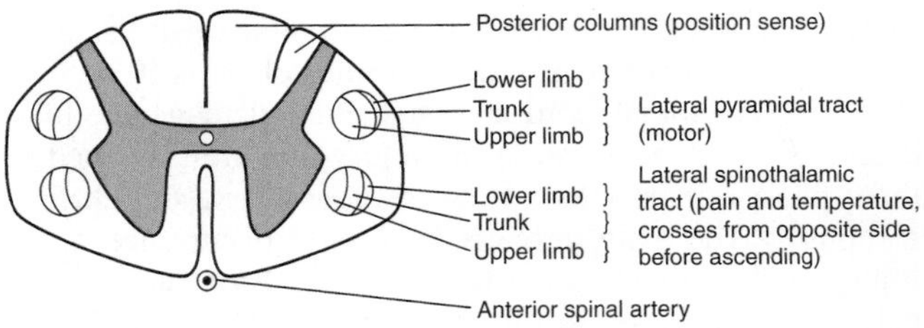

Figure 16-1 ■ Cross-sectional anatomy of the spinal cord.

Cauda Equina Syndrome

Damage to the cauda equina occurs with injuries at or below the L1 vertebral level. This syndrome results in a lower motor neuron lesion that is usually incomplete. This lesion results in flaccid paralysis with no spinal reflex activity present.[12,26]

Conus Medullaris Syndrome

Injury of the sacral cord and lumbar nerve roots within the neural canal results in a clinical picture of lower-extremity motor and sensory loss and areflexic bladder and bowel.[12,31]

MEDICAL MANAGEMENT

Short-term medical treatment includes anatomical realignment and stabilization interventions and pharmacological management to prevent further neurological trauma and enhance neural recovery.

Surgical Stabilization

One of the first interventions after acute traumatic SCI is to stabilize the spine to prevent further cord or nerve root damage. In the emergency department, diagnostic studies reveal the severity of the spinal injury and the type and degree of the instability. On the basis of these findings, the physician, client, and family decide on treatment. Many options must be considered regarding the optimal operative strategy. Indications for surgical intervention include, but are not limited to, signs of progressive neurological involvement, type and extent of bony lesions, and degree of spinal cord damage.[34] The following discussion describes nonsurgical and surgical interventions.

Cervical Spine

At the scene of the accident, emergency medical professionals exercise extreme caution to immobilize the injured patient and prevent excessive movement. If there is compression of neurological tissue, vertebral fracture, or dislocation, reduction must occur to minimize ischemia and edema formation.[35] In the emergency department, reduction is accomplished by cervical traction with the goal of immediate and proper alignment of bone fragments and decompression of the spinal cord until further stabilization.[34,36,37] The most widely used traction method is the Gardner-Wells tongs (Figure 16-2), which are inserted into the skull. Weights are added at approximately 5 pounds of traction per level of injury to achieve reduction of the dislocation and to maintain alignment.[36]

Precautions must be taken during therapy to prevent unnecessary movement at the injury site. The traction rope must be kept in alignment with the long axis of the cervical spine, and the weights must be allowed to hang freely. Cervical rotation must be prevented. In addition, continued traction should be maintained at all times.

When surgical stabilization is indicated, common surgical protocols include posterior and anterior approaches. Figure 16-3 shows radiographs of a person who had an anterior and lateral cervical fusion at C3-C4. Unstable compression injuries are usually managed by a posterior procedure except when there is a deficient anterior column. Anterior approaches are indicated for patients with evidence of residual anterior spinal cord or nerve root compression and persistent neurological deficits.[34]

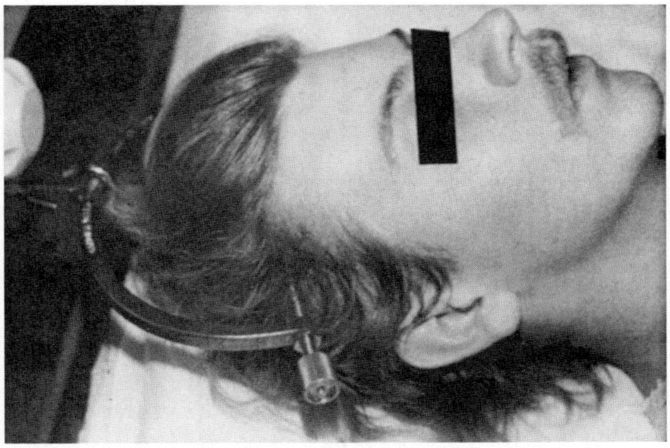

Figure 16-2 ■ Gardner-Wells tongs. Reduction is accomplished through weights attached to the traction rope. (Courtesy Dr. H. Herndon Murray, Assistant Medical Director, Shepherd Spinal Center, Atlanta, Georgia.)

After cervical surgical stabilization, a hard collar such as a Philadelphia collar (Figure 16-4) or sternal-occipital-mandibular immobilizer (SOMI) brace is used until solid bony fusion has developed. The Aspen collar also provides this stability (Figure 16-5). The solid bony fusion usually takes 6 to 8 weeks. Postoperatively, care must be taken to protect the bony fusion.

When surgery is not indicated, or when more postoperative stabilization is required, halo traction may be indicated. The halo device restricts more movement in the upper cervical spine compared with the lower cervical spine.[38] The halo traction device consists of three parts: the ring, the uprights, and the jacket (Figure 16-6). The ring fits around the skull, just above the ears. It is held in place by four pins that are inserted into the skull. The uprights are attached to the ring and jacket by bolts. The jacket is usually made of polypropylene and lined with sheepskin. This equipment is left in place for 6 to 12 weeks until bony healing is satisfactory.[5] The advantage of using the halo device is the ability to mobilize the client as soon as the device has been applied without compromising spinal alignment. This allows the rehabilitation program to commence more rapidly. It also allows for delayed decision making regarding the need for surgery.

The disadvantage of the halo device is that pressure and friction from the vest or jacket may lead to altered skin integrity.[7] Special attention must be given to ensure the skin remains intact. During more active phases of the rehabilitation process, the halo device may slow functional progress because of added weight and interference with the middle to end range of upper-extremity movement. In a small percentage of patients, there are complications of dysphagia and temporomandibular joint dysfunctions associated with wearing the halo device.[7]

Thoracolumbar Spine

Internal fixation of the thoracolumbar region is necessary when stability and distraction cannot be maintained by other means.[39] Common thoracic stabilization procedures include transpedicular screws (Figure 16-7) and a hybrid type of instrumentation.

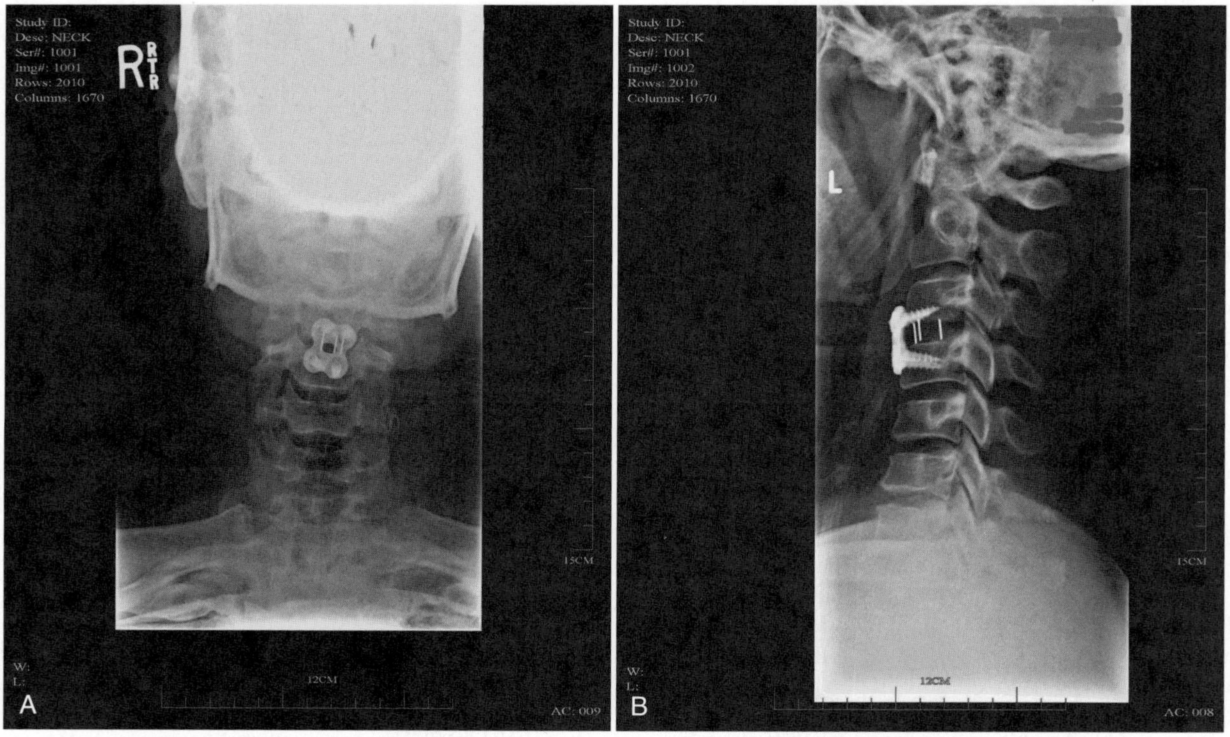

Figure 16-3 ■ **A,** Radiograph of person who had an anterior cervical fusion at C3-C4. **B,** Lateral radiologic view of anterior fusion C3-C4.

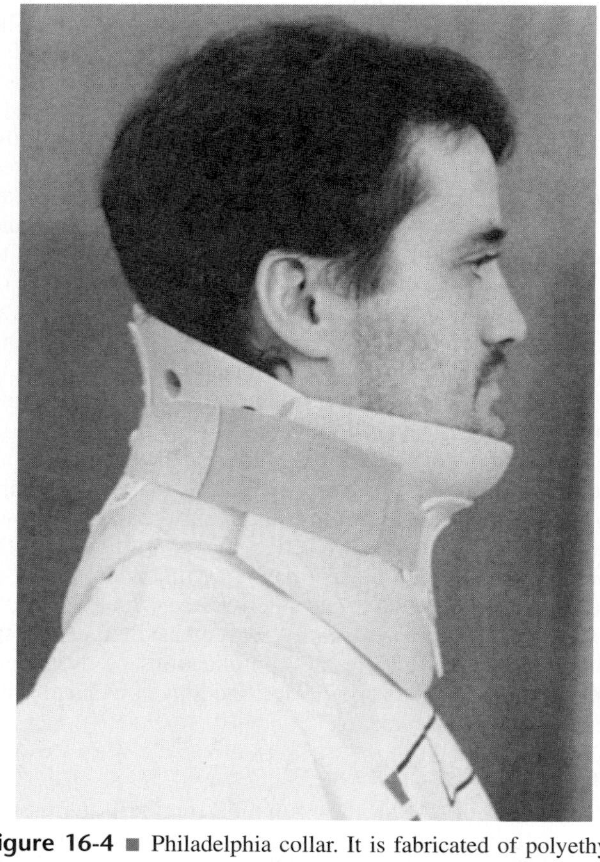

Figure 16-4 ■ Philadelphia collar. It is fabricated of polyethylene foam with rigid anterior and posterior plastic strips, it is easily applied via Velcro closures, and it limits flexion, extension, and rotary movements of the cervical spine.

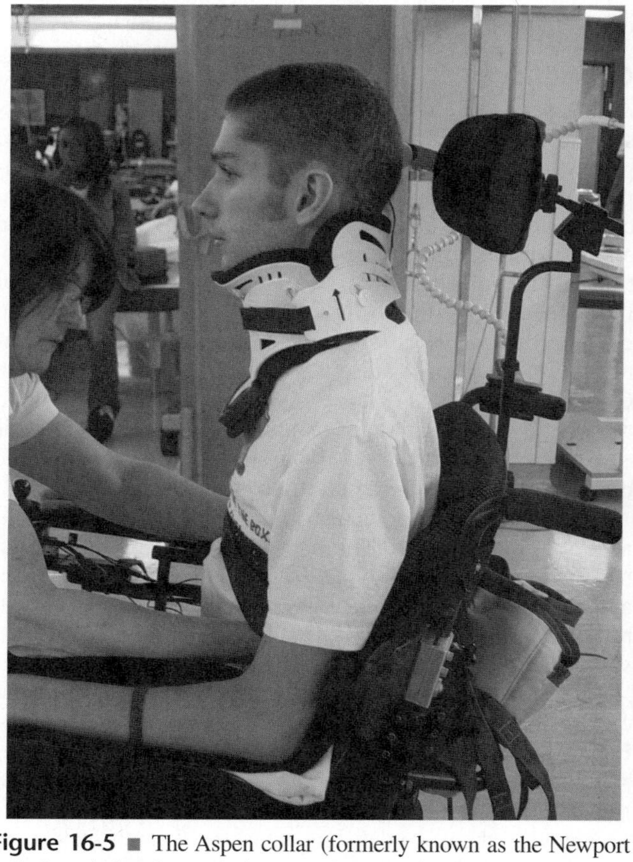

Figure 16-5 ■ The Aspen collar (formerly known as the Newport collar) encircles the neck, is somewhat open, and provides cervical motion restriction. It is rigid yet flexible at its edges to conform to each patient's anatomy. Pads and shells are removable and washable.

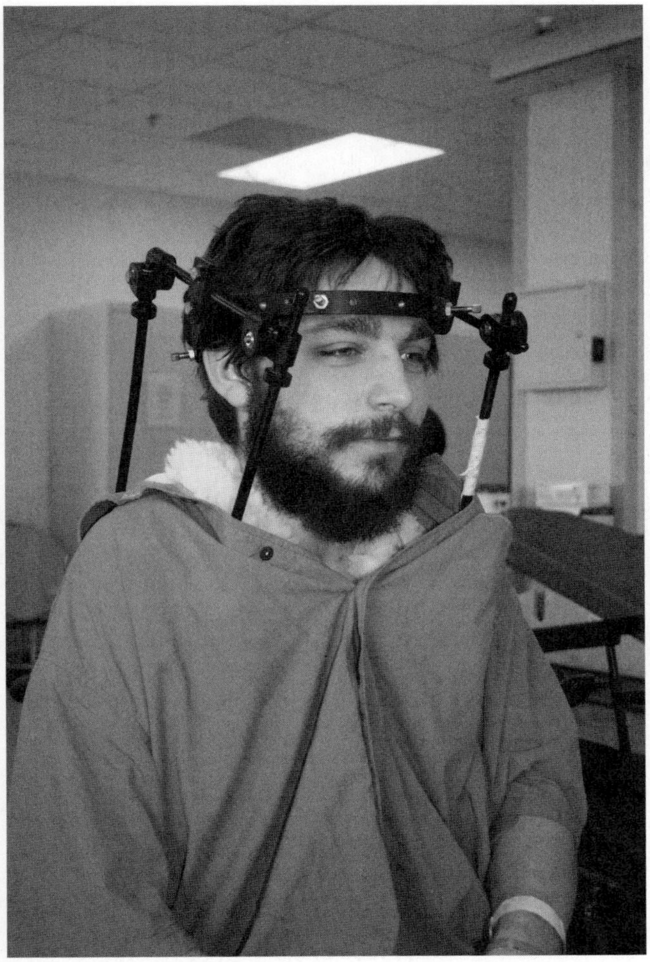

Figure 16-6 ■ Halo vest. Basic components are the halo ring, distraction rods, and jacket (jacket not pictured).

Postoperatively, an external trunk support may be necessary to limit excessive vertebral motion and to maintain proper thoracic and lumbar alignment.[39] This may be achieved by a custom thoracolumbosacral orthosis (Figure 16-8) or a Jewett brace (Figure 16-9). Initially the client's activity may be limited to allow for a complete fusion to take place and to minimize the possibility of rod displacement. All spinal limitations should be discussed with the surgeon postoperatively.

The goals of the operative procedures at any spinal level discussed are to reverse the deforming forces, to restore proper spinal alignment, and to stabilize the spine.[40] All these procedures have advantages and disadvantages. The surgeon, client, and family must be involved in the decision-making process to select the most appropriate method of treatment. This will allow the therapeutic rehabilitation process to begin.

Pharmacological Management Immediately after Traumatic Spinal Cord Injury

Neurological damage from SCI may be a result of (1) physical disruption of axons traversing the injury site, or (2) as described earlier, cellular events that follow the primary injury. Investigators believe that secondary injuries to surrounding tissues can be lessened by pharmacological agents, specifically methylprednisolone and monosialotetrahexosylganglioside

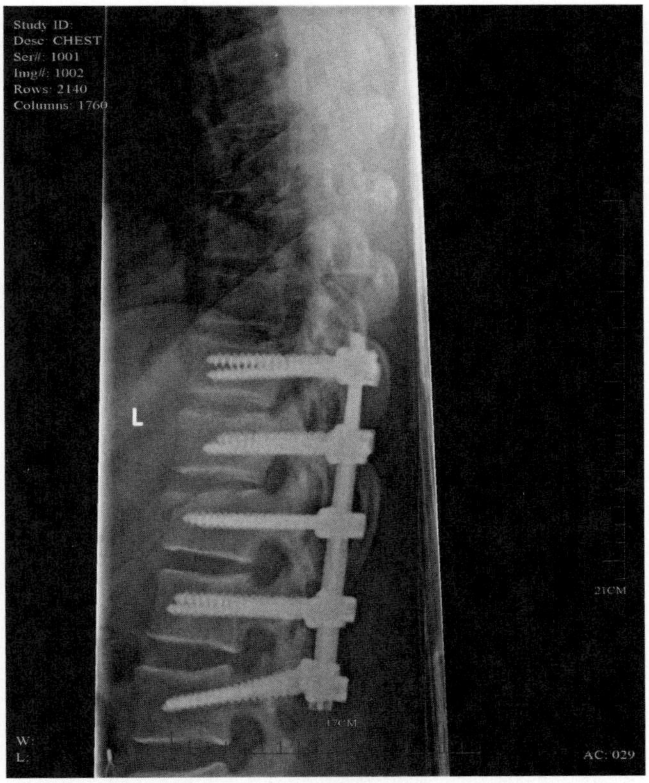

Figure 16-7 ■ Radiograph of transpedicular screws. (Courtesy Dr. H. Herndon Murray, Assistant Medical Director, Shepherd Spinal Center, Atlanta, Georgia.)

(GM1). To date, two major pharmacological clinical trials have been completed.

The National Acute Spinal Cord Injury Study[41] (NASCIS-2) used high doses of methylprednisolone and showed significant improvements in sensory and motor function 6 months after injury.[42] Young and Flamm[43] showed that methylprednisolone enhanced the flow of blood to the injured spinal cord, preventing the typical decline in white matter, extracellular calcium levels, and evoked potentials, thus preventing progressive posttraumatic ischemia.[44-47] The dosage recommended by the NASCIS-2 study is 30 mg/kg of methylprednisolone followed by an infusion of 5.4 mg/kg/hr for 23 hours.[41] The therapist must be aware of side effects that may occur with such high doses of steroids, including gastric ulcers, decreased wound-healing time, hypertension, cardiac arrhythmias, and alteration in mental status.[42]

THERAPEUTIC REHABILITATION CONTINUUM OF CARE

Therapeutic rehabilitation can be effectively delivered beginning in an acute-care setting at the time of injury and continuing on through a lifetime of care. Rehabilitation teams may use one of three models: multidisciplinary, interdisciplinary, and transdisciplinary.[3] The standards set forth by the Commission on Accreditation of Rehabilitation Facilities (CARF) suggest that the interdisciplinary model of team structure is optimal in the rehabilitation setting.[31]

The continuum of care may be divided into several phases that include medical management (previously described),

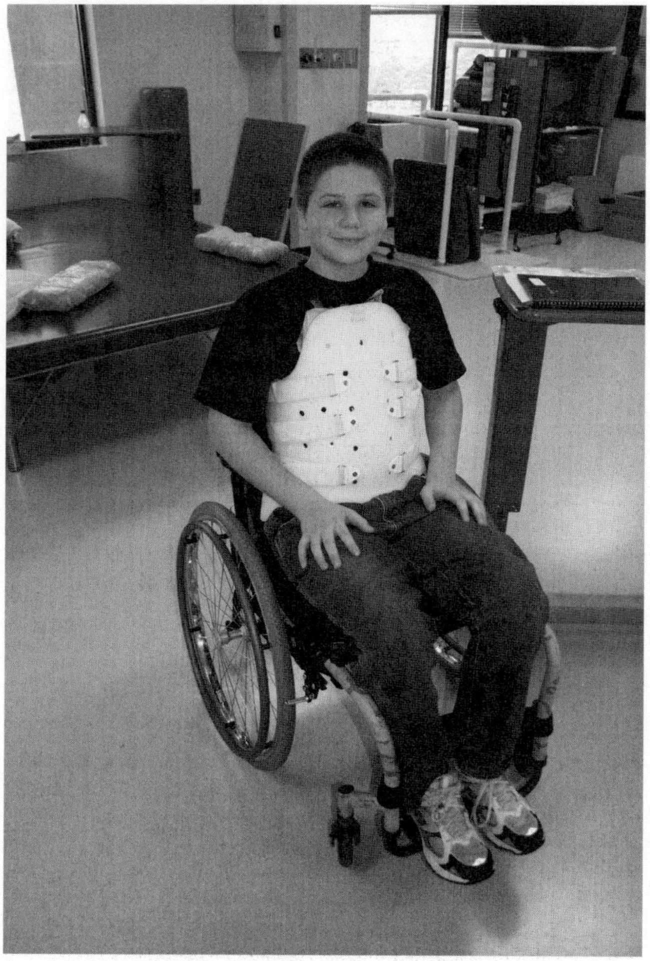

Figure 16-8 ■ Custom thoracolumbosacral orthosis. This molded plastic body orthosis has a soft lining. It controls flexion, extension, and rotary movements until healing of the bone has occurred.

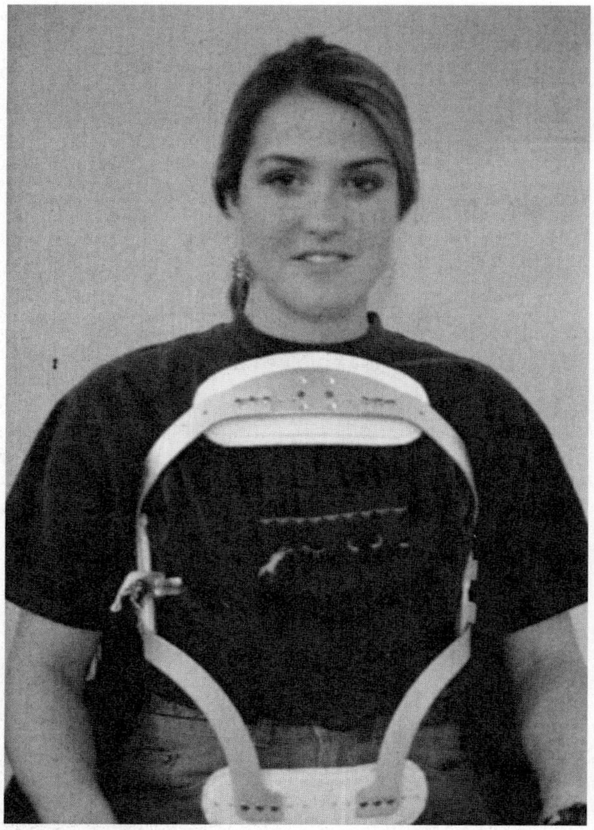

Figure 16-9 ■ Jewett hyperextension brace. A single three-point force system is provided by sternal pad, suprapubic pad, and thoracolumbar pad. Forward flexion is restricted in the thoracolumbar area.

inpatient rehabilitation, outpatient rehabilitation, and home health. The continuum also includes returning the patient into wellness programs and community reentry outreach programs. The progression of a patient through the rehabilitation process will vary greatly from one person to the next. The patient may also move back and forth throughout the continuum of care.

Inpatient Rehabilitation

Inpatient rehabilitation begins during the critical and acute-care stages after an SCI. The primary emphasis of early rehabilitation is to lessen the adverse effects of neurotrauma and immobilization. This focus may last from a few days to several weeks, depending on the severity and level of injury and other associated injuries. Although therapeutic intensity may be limited, clients may begin participating in early therapy that should include, but should not be limited to, out-of-bed activities, gaining upright tolerance, range-of-motion (ROM) exercises, early strength training, and skin-management education. Goals during this phase should focus on prevention of secondary complications and preparing the client for full rehabilitation participation. The treatment team must begin discharge planning and family training in this phase.

As the acute phase progresses, out-of-bed activities are tolerated for longer periods of time and the patient begins to work toward specific long-term goals. In accordance with Medicare guidelines for inpatient rehabilitation, the client is able to participate in therapeutic programs a minimum of 3 hours a day.[48,49] The intensity of therapy may continue to be limited according to unresolved medical issues.

As medical issues resolve and endurance improves, the patient will progress to a higher and more active level of participation. During inpatient rehabilitation, the patient gains varying levels of independence in specific skills. The patient may be taught advanced skills to perform activities of daily living (ADLs), transfers, and mobility. Community outings may be scheduled to refine advanced skills, identify further needs, and foster community reintegration and participation. In addition, the following will be completed unless otherwise indicated by the rehabilitation team: (1) family training, (2) home and school or work evaluation, (3) delivery and fitting of discharge equipment, (4) instruction in home management, (5) instruction in home exercise programs, (6) dependent passenger driving evaluations, (7) assistive technology (AT) referrals for devices to enable computer access and other electronic aids to daily living (EADLs), (8) referrals for continued services, and (9) driving evaluation. Discharge planning largely encompasses activities aimed at a smooth transition back into the community whenever possible.

Outpatient Rehabilitation and Community Reentry

Discharge from an inpatient rehabilitation program marks only the beginning of the lifelong process of adjustment to changes in physical abilities, community reintegration, and participation in life activities. Inpatient rehabilitation provides an environment best suited for learning self-care skills, yet "the implications of living in the community with SCI can scarcely be anticipated accurately by the newly injured individual or the able-bodied staff."[50] Because of the shortened lengths of hospitalization, services provided after discharge are becoming increasingly important. A direct consequence of this shift results in outpatient treatment of patients who have more acuity, greater care needs, and fewer skills attained in the inpatient rehabilitation program before entry into the outpatient arena. Common outpatient therapy treatment programs have included advanced transfer training, advanced wheelchair mobility training, locomotor training, upgraded ADL training, and upgraded home exercise program instruction. This is a shift in the typical program structure because these skills were traditionally a part of the inpatient rehabilitation.

Services provided after inpatient discharge may include day programs, single-service outpatient visits, wellness programs, and routine follow-up visits and services. The "day program" concept has emerged to meet the demand for more comprehensive rehabilitation services. The primary purpose of these services is to provide a coordinated effort for the client to return to full reintegration into the community. There is a variety of day program options for individuals, with each program offering various levels of care that range from two coordinated disciplines to services like those of an inpatient rehabilitation program. One common thread for virtually all day program settings is that the clients are medically stable, do not require skilled nursing services during the night, and need a coordinated approach for two or more services with the focus on performance of functional skills and on the transference of these skills into the community.

EXAMINATION AND EVALUATION OF BODY FUNCTION AND STRUCTURE

Regardless of where the patient begins the rehabilitation process, an examination is completed on admission. The examination and evaluation will assist in establishing the diagnosis and the prognosis of each patient as well as determining the appropriate therapeutic interventions. The client and caregivers participate by reporting activity performance and functional ability.[51] Any pertinent additions to the history stated by the client should be described. The client's statement of goals, problems, and concerns should be included. The main areas of the examination are outlined here.

History

A review of the medical record is the first step toward the examination because it provides the background information and identifies medical precautions. The history should include general demographics, social history, occupation or employment, pertinent growth and development, living environment, history of current condition, functional status and activity level, completed tests and measures, medications, history of current condition if applicable, medical and surgical history, family history, reported patient and family health status, and social habits.[52] If the history suggests a loss of consciousness or brain injury, the clinician should consider the possibility of compromised cognition and should include tests and measures during the examination and assessment appropriate to that impairment.

Systems Review

The physiological and anatomical status should be reviewed for the cardiopulmonary, integumentary, musculoskeletal, and neuromuscular systems. In addition, communication, affect, cognition, language, and learning style should be reviewed.[51]

Tests and Measures

Depending on the data generated during the history and systems review, the clinician performs tests and measures to help identify impairments, activity limitations, and participation restrictions and to establish the diagnosis and prognosis of each client. Tests and measures that are often used for persons with SCI are included in Box 16-1. For more detail related to specific tools, refer to the *Guide to Physical Therapist Practice.*[52]

Neurological Examination

American Spinal Cord Injury Association Examination

It is recommended that the international standards of ASIA be used for the specific neurological examination after an SCI.[53] See Figure 16-10 for the ASIA motor and sensory examination form. Assessment of muscle performance allows for specific diagnosis of the level and completeness of injury. The examination of muscle performance includes each specific muscle and identifies substitutions from other muscles.

BOX 16-1 ■ TESTS AND MEASURES[52]

Aerobic capacity and endurance
Anthropometric characteristics
Assistive and adaptive devices assessment
Community and work integration or reintegration
Environmental home and work barriers examination
Gait, locomotion, and balance
Integumentary integrity
Joint integrity and mobility
Motor function
Muscle performance
Orthotic, protective, and supportive devices
Pain
Posture
Range of motion
Reflex integrity
Self-care and home management
Sensory integrity
Ventilation, respiration, and circulation
Diagnosis of impairment and disabilities

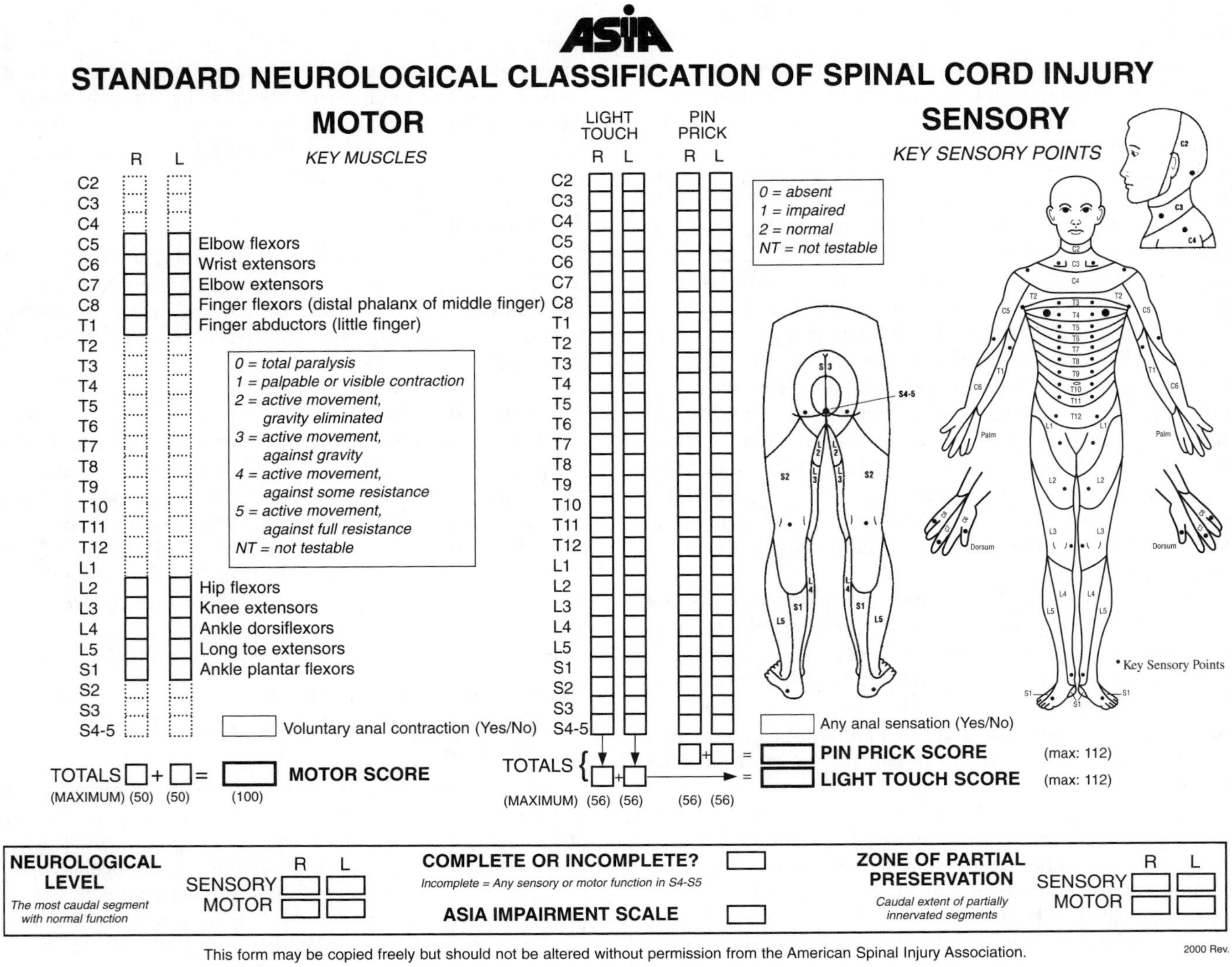

ASIA
STANDARD NEUROLOGICAL CLASSIFICATION OF SPINAL CORD INJURY
MOTOR
KEY MUSCLES
R L
C2
C3
C4
C5 Elbow flexors
C6 Wrist extensors
C7 Elbow extensors
C8 Finger flexors (distal phalanx of middle finger)
T1 Finger abductors (little finger)
T2
T3
T4
T5
T6
T7
T8
T9
T10
T11
T12
L1
L2 Hip flexors
L3 Knee extensors
L4 Ankle dorsiflexors
L5 Long toe extensors
S1 Ankle plantar flexors
S2
S3
S4-5
0 = total paralysis
1 = palpable or visible contraction
2 = active movement, gravity eliminated
3 = active movement, against gravity
4 = active movement, against some resistance
5 = active movement, against full resistance
NT = not testable
Voluntary anal contraction (Yes/No)
TOTALS + = MOTOR SCORE
(MAXIMUM) (50) (50) (100)
SENSORY
KEY SENSORY POINTS
LIGHT TOUCH
PIN PRICK
R L R L
0 = absent
1 = impaired
2 = normal
NT = not testable
Any anal sensation (Yes/No)
TOTALS
PIN PRICK SCORE (max: 112)
LIGHT TOUCH SCORE (max: 112)
(MAXIMUM) (56) (56) (56) (56)
• Key Sensory Points
NEUROLOGICAL LEVEL
The most caudal segment with normal function
SENSORY
MOTOR
COMPLETE OR INCOMPLETE?
Incomplete = Any sensory or motor function in S4-S5
ASIA IMPAIRMENT SCALE
ZONE OF PARTIAL PRESERVATION
Caudal extent of partially innervated segments
This form may be copied freely but should not be altered without permission from the American Spinal Injury Association.
2000 Rev.

Figure 16-10 ■ American Spinal Injury Association motor and sensory evaluation form. (Courtesy American Spinal Injury Association, Atlanta, Georgia.)

Along with the strength of each muscle, the presence, absence, and location of muscle tone should be described. The Modified Ashworth Scale is a common tool used to describe hypertonicity.[54] The client's sensation is described by dermatome. The recommended tests include (1) sharp-dull discrimination or temperature sensitivity to test the lateral spinothalamic tract, (2) light touch to test the anterior spinothalamic tract, and (3) proprioception or vibration to test the posterior columns of the spinal cord. Sensation is indicated as intact, impaired, or absent per dermatome. A dermatomal map is helpful and recommended for ease of documentation.

Functional Examination

It is recommended that a complete functional assessment be performed on initial examination and thereafter as appropriate. Myriad tools exist to assess functional skills. Many institutions develop functional assessments that address home, community, and institutional mobility and ADL functional skills. The Functional Independence Measure (FIM) is one of the more commonly used tools that is currently applied for many impairment diagnostic groups, including SCI.[55] Another tool that is recognized as a primary outcome measure to assess functional recovery for the client with SCI is the Spinal Cord Injury Independence Measure III (SCIM III).[56] This tool was specifically designed for the functional assessment of individuals with SCI. The SCIM III has been shown to be valid, reliable, and easily administered.[57-59] Other tools, such as the Quadriplegia Index of Function (QIF)[60] and the Craig Handicap Assessment and Reporting Technique (CHART),[61] are options. Additional assessments for patients with SCI are described in Table 16-3.

GOAL SETTING FOR ACTIVITY AND PARTICIPATION SKILLS

Goal setting is a dynamic process that directly follows the examination. Each activity limitation identified should be addressed with specific short- and long-term goals. The clinician must interpret new information continuously, which leads to continuing reevaluation and revision of goals.[62] Goals are always individualized and should be established in collaboration with the treatment team, the client, and the caregiver, and with realistic consideration of anticipated

TABLE 16-3 ■ ASSESSMENT OF FUNCTION SUMMARY TABLE

OVERALL FUNCTIONAL ASSESSMENTS	DESCRIPTION
SPINAL CORD INJURY (SCI) FUNCTIONAL ASSESSMENTS	
Spinal Cord Injury Independence Measure (SCIM)[239]	Designed for the functional assessment of individuals with spinal cord injury in the categories of self-care, respiratory, sphincter management, and mobility skills
Quadriplegia Index of Function (QIF)[60]	Assesses function for individuals with tetraplegia in the categories of transfers, grooming, bathing, feeding, dressing, wheelchair mobility, bed activities, bowel, bladder, and knowledge of personal care
Capabilities of Upper Extremity (CUE) instrument[240]	Assesses the action of grasp, release, and reaching in individuals with tetraplegia by measuring reaching and lifting, pulling and pushing, wrist action, hand and finger actions, and bilateral action
WALKING FUNCTION ASSESSMENTS	
Spinal Cord Injury Functional Ambulation Inventory (SCI-FAI)[241]	Observational gait assessment that assesses gait, assistive device use, and walking mobility
Walking Index for Spinal Cord Injury (WISCI)[242]	An ordinal scale describing walking function that takes into consideration level of independence, assistive device use, and lower-extremity orthotic use
Six-minute walk test[243]	An endurance walking test that measures the distance walked over a 6-min period of time
Ten-meter walk test[244]	Measures walking speed by measuring how fast an individual walks a distance of 10 m
Timed Up-and-Go Test[244]	Assesses standing, walking, turning, and sitting
WHEELCHAIR FUNCTION ASSESSMENTS	
Wheelchair Circuit[245]	Assesses the performance of various wheelchair propulsion skills by measuring ability, performance time, and physical strain for eight standardized skills
Wheelchair Assessment Tool[246]	Measures the ability and time to perform six mobility and wheelchair skills for individuals with paraplegia
Wheelchair Skills Test[247]	Assesses the ability to perform 50 separate skills in the areas of wheelchair handling, transfers, maneuvering the wheelchair, and negotiating obstacles
Obstacle Course Assessment of Wheelchair User Performance[248]	Assesses the wheelchair user's performance in 10 difficult environmental situations
Wheelchair Users Functional Assessment (WUFA)[249]	A 13-item assessment of wheelchair skills in individuals who primarily use a manual wheelchair for their mobility
Wheelchair Physical Functional Performance (WC-PFP)[250]	Assesses the ability to complete various tasks from the wheelchair by measuring upper body strength, upper body flexibility, balance, coordination, and endurance
Functional Evaluation in a Wheelchair[251]	Assesses functional performance from a manual and/or power wheelchair via a self-administered questionnaire

needs on return to the home environment. Factors to consider in the goal-setting process include age, body type, associated injuries, premorbid medical conditions, additional orthopedic injury, cognitive ability, psychosocial issues, spasticity, endurance, strength, ROM, funding sources, and motivation.

Long-term goals for the rehabilitation of patients with SCI reflect functional outcomes and are based on the strength of the remaining innervated or partially innervated musculature. Short-term goals identify components that interfere with functional ability and are designed to "address these limiting factors while building component skills"[7] of the desired long-term goals.[63]

Functionally based goals are established in the following areas: bathing, bed mobility, bladder and bowel control, communication, environmental control and access, feeding, dressing, gait, grooming, home management, ROM and positioning, skin care management, transfers, transportation and driving, wheelchair management, and wheelchair mobility. Refer to Table 16-4 for anticipated goals for each level of injury. Information presented in this table should be recognized as general guidelines because variability exists. These guidelines are most usefully applied to patients with complete SCI. Goal setting for individuals with incomplete SCI is often more challenging, given the greater variability of client presentations and the uncertainty of neurological recovery. As with any patient, continual reevaluations provide additional insight into functional limitations or progression and potential and thereby direct the goal-setting process. In addition to specific functional goals and expectations, family training; home, work, or school modifications; and community reentry should be considered.

Rehabilitation teams may elect to hold a goal-setting or interim conference for each patient, during which team

Text continues on page 475

TABLE 16-4 ■ FUNCTIONAL EXPECTATIONS FOR COMPLETE SPINAL CORD INJURY LESIONS

FUNCTIONAL COMPONENT	OUTCOME POTENTIAL	ANTICIPATED EQUIPMENT TO ACHIEVE OUTCOMES
C1-4		
Sitting tolerance	80-90 degrees for 10-12 hours per day	Power wheelchair with power tilt, recline Wheelchair cushion
Communication		
Mouth stick writing	Minimal assistance	Mouth sticks and docking station
ECU	Setup	ECU
Page turning	Minimal assistance to setup	Book holder
Computer operation	Minimal assistance to setup	Computer
Call-system use	Setup	Call system or speaker phone
Cuff-leak speech (ventilator dependent)	Up to 6 hours	
Feeding	Dependent, but verbalizes care	
Grooming	Dependent, but verbalizes care	
Bathing	Dependent, but verbalizes care	Reclining shower chair
Dressing	Dependent, but verbalizes care	
Bowel management	Dependent, but verbalizes care	
Bladder management	Dependent, but verbalizes care	
Bed mobility		
Rolling side to side	Dependent, but verbalizes care	Four-way adjustable hospital bed to assist caregiver with task
Rolling		
Supine, prone		
Supine to and from sitting		
Scooting		
Leg management		
Transfers		
Bed	Dependent, but verbalizes care	Overhead lift system
Tub, toilet		Hydraulic lift
Car		Slings
Floor		
Power wheelchair mobility		
Smooth surfaces	Modified independent	Power wheelchair with power recline or tilt system
Ramps	Modified independent	
Rough terrain	Modified independent	Lap tray
Curbs	Dependent, but verbalizes	Armrests, shoulder supports, and lateral trunk supports
Manual wheelchair mobility		
Smooth surfaces	Dependent, but verbalizes	Manual reclining or tilt wheelchair with same options as power wheelchair
Ramps		
Rough terrain		
Curbs		
Stairs		
Skin		
Weight shift	Modified independent with power wheelchair	Recline or tilt wheelchair
Padding, positioning	Dependent, but verbalizes	Wheelchair cushion
Skin checks	Dependent, but verbalizes	Pillow splints, resting splints Mirror
Community: ADL-dependent passenger evaluation	Dependent, but verbalizes	Modified van
ROM exercises to scapula, upper extremity, lower extremity, and trunk	Dependent, but verbalizes	
Exercise program	Independent for respiratory and neck exercises	Portable or bedside ventilator (C1-3 only)

TABLE 16-4 ■ FUNCTIONAL EXPECTATIONS FOR COMPLETE SPINAL CORD INJURY LESIONS—cont'd

FUNCTIONAL COMPONENT	OUTCOME POTENTIAL	ANTICIPATED EQUIPMENT TO ACHIEVE OUTCOMES
C5		
Sitting tolerance	90 degrees for 10-12 hours per day	Power recline or tilt wheelchair Wheelchair cushion
Communication		
Telephone use	Modified independent	Telephone adaptations
ECU	Setup	ECU
Page turning	Setup	Book holder, wrist support with cuff
Computer operation	Supervision	Computer
Writing, typing	Setup	Long Wanchik brace
Feeding	Minimal assist to setup	Mobile arm support or offset feeder Adaptive ADL equipment
Grooming		
Wash face	Minimal assistance to setup	Mobile arm support or offset feeder
Comb or brush hair	Minimal assistance	Wrist support with adapted cuff
Oral care	Minimal assistance to setup	Adaptive ADL equipment
Bathing	Dependent, but verbalizes care	Upright or tilt shower chair
Dressing	Dependent, but verbalizes care	
Bowel management	Dependent, but verbalizes care	
Bladder management	Dependent, but verbalizes care	Automatic leg bag emptier
Bed mobility		
Rolling side to side	Dependent to maximal assistance	4-way adjustable hospital bed to assist caregiver with care
Rolling		
Supine, prone		
Supine to and from sitting		
Scooting		
Leg management		
Transfers		
Bed	Dependent to maximal assistance for level transfers, verbalizes unlevel transfers	Overhead or hydraulic lift and slings
Tub, toilet		Possible transfer board
Car		
Floor		
Power wheelchair mobility	Recommended mode of locomotion	Power wheelchair with power recline or tilt system
Smooth surfaces	Modified independent	
Ramps	Modified independent	Recommend lap tray
Rough terrain	Modified independent	Armrests, shoulder supports, lateral trunk supports
Curbs	Dependent, but verbalizes	
Manual wheelchair mobility		
Smooth surfaces	Dependent to minimal assistance for short distances on smooth surface	Upright or reclining wheelchair with special back and trunk supports
Ramps	Dependent, but verbalizes care	
Rough terrain	Dependent, but verbalizes care	Consider manual wheelchair with power assist pushrims
Curbs	Dependent, but verbalizes care	
Stairs	Dependent, but verbalizes care	
Skin		
Weight shift	Modified independent with power wheelchair Maximal assistance to dependent with manual wheelchair	Recline or tilt wheelchair and wheelchair cushion
Padding, positioning	Dependent, but verbalizes	Pillow splints or resting splints
Skin checks	Dependent, but verbalizes	Mirror
Home management		
Prepare snack	Maximal to moderate assistance	Wrist support with cuffs Adaptive ADL equipment

Continued

TABLE 16-4 ■ FUNCTIONAL EXPECTATIONS FOR COMPLETE SPINAL CORD INJURY LESIONS—cont'd

FUNCTIONAL COMPONENT	OUTCOME POTENTIAL	ANTICIPATED EQUIPMENT TO ACHIEVE OUTCOMES
Community ADL		
Drive van	Independent	Highly adapted vehicle
Dependent passenger evaluation	Dependent	Modified van
ROM exercises to scapula, upper extremity, lower extremity, and trunk	Dependent, but verbalizes	
Exercise program		Airsplints or light cuff weights
Upper extremity and neck	Minimal assistance	E-stim unit
C6		
Sitting tolerance	90 degrees for 10-12 hours per day	
Communication		
Telephone use	Modified independent	Adaptive ADL equipment
Page turning		Tenodesis splint
Writing, typing, keyboard		Short opponens splint
Feeding	Modified independent	Adaptive ADL equipment
Grooming	Minimum assistance to modified independent	Adaptive ADL equipment Tenodesis splint
Bathing		
Upper body	Minimal to modified independent assistance	Upright shower chair
Lower body	Moderate assistance	Various bathing equipment
Dressing		
Upper body	Modified independent	Adaptive ADL equipment
Lower body (bed)	Maximum to minimal assistance	
Bowel management	Maximum to modified independent	Dil stick Adaptive ADL equipment
Bladder management	Male: moderate assistance to modified independent Female: moderate assistance to dependent	Tenodesis Adaptive ADL equipment
Bed mobility		
Rolling side to side	Independent to minimal assistance	Four-way adjustable hospital bed or regular bed with loops or straps; or no equipment
Rolling		
Supine, prone		
Supine to and from sitting		
Scooting		
Leg management	Minimum assistance to dependent	
Transfers		
Bed	Minimal assistance	Transfer board
Tub, toilet	Moderate assistance	
Car	Maximal to moderate assistance	
Floor	Dependent, but verbalizes procedure	
Power wheelchair mobility	Recommended mode of locomotion	Power upright wheelchair for weak C6
Smooth surfaces	Modified independent	
Ramps	Modified independent	
Rough terrain	Modified independent	
Curbs	Dependent, but verbalizes	
Manual wheelchair mobility		Ultralight upright wheelchair (recommended as primary only if scapulae grades are 3 or better)
Smooth surfaces	Modified independent	May need adaptations to facilitate more efficient propulsion (i.e., push pegs, plastic-coated handrims)
Ramps	Modified independent	
Rough terrain	Moderate to minimal assistance	
Curbs	Dependent, but verbalizes procedure	Consider manual wheelchair with power assist pushrims
Stairs	Dependent, but verbalizes procedure	

TABLE 16-4 ■ FUNCTIONAL EXPECTATIONS FOR COMPLETE SPINAL CORD INJURY LESIONS—cont'd

FUNCTIONAL COMPONENT	OUTCOME POTENTIAL	ANTICIPATED EQUIPMENT TO ACHIEVE OUTCOMES
Skin		
Weight shift	Modified independent	Upright wheelchair with push handles
Pad, positioning	Moderate to minimal assistance	Mirror
Skin checks	Moderate to minimal assistance	
Home management		
Light home management	Minimal assistance	Various adaptive ADL equipment
Heavy home management	Dependent to moderate assistance	
Community ADL		
Driving vehicle	Modified independent	Modified vehicle
ROM exercises to scapula, upper extremity, lower extremity, and trunk	Minimal assistance	Leg lifter to assist with lower-extremity ROM
Exercise program	Minimal assistance	Cuff weights Air splints E-stim unit
C7-8		
Sitting tolerance	90 degrees for 10-12 hours per day	
Communication		
Telephone use	Modified independent	Adaptive ADL equipment
Page turning		
Writing, typing, keyboard		
Feeding	Modified independent	Adaptive ADL equipment
Grooming	Modified independent	Adaptive ADL equipment
Bathing		
Upper body	Modified independent	Upright shower chair
Lower body	Modified independent	Various bathing equipment
Dressing (upper and lower body)	Modified independent for upper-body dressing	Adaptive ADL equipment
In bed	Minimal assistance to modified independent for lower-body dressing	
In wheelchair		
Bowel management	Modified independent	Dil stick
Bladder management		
Bed	Male: modified independent	Various bladder management or adaptive ADL equipment
Wheelchair	Female: moderate assistance to modified independent Male: modified independent	
Bed mobility		
Rolling side to side	Modified independent	Leg lifter
Rolling		
Supine, prone		
Supine to and from sitting		
Scooting		
Leg management		
Transfers		
Bed	Modified independent	Transfer board
Tub, toilet	Modified independent	May not need transfer board for even surfaces
Car	Minimal assistance for loading wheelchair	
Floor	Maximal assistance	
Power wheelchair mobility		
Smooth surfaces	Modified independent	Power upright wheelchair
Ramps	Modified independent	
Rough terrain	Modified independent	
Curbs	Dependent, but verbalizes	

Continued

TABLE 16-4 ■ FUNCTIONAL EXPECTATIONS FOR COMPLETE SPINAL CORD INJURY LESIONS—cont'd

FUNCTIONAL COMPONENT	OUTCOME POTENTIAL	ANTICIPATED EQUIPMENT TO ACHIEVE OUTCOMES
Manual wheelchair mobility		
Smooth surfaces	Modified independent	Upright wheelchair
Ramps	Modified independent	
Rough terrain	Modified independent	
Curbs	Minimal to moderate assistance	
Stairs	Maximal assistance	
Skin		
Weight shift	Modified independent	Upright wheelchair with push handles
Pad, positioning	Minimal assistance to modified independent	
Skin checks	Minimal assistance to modified independent	Mirror
Home management		
Light home management	Modified independent	Various ADL equipment
Heavy home management	Moderate assistance	
Community ADL		
Driving vehicle	Modified independent	Modified vehicle
ROM exercises to scapula, upper extremity, lower extremity, and trunk	Modified independent	Leg lifter to assist with lower-extremity ROM
Exercise program	Modified independent	Cuff weights or e-stim unit
PARAPLEGIA		
Sitting tolerance	90 degrees for 10-12 hours per day	
Communication	Independent	
Feeding	Independent	
Grooming	Independent	
Bathing		
Upper body	Independent	Upright tub chair
Lower body	Modified independent	Long-handled sponge and hand-held shower hose
Dressing (upper and lower body)	Adaptive ADL equipment	
In bed	Modified independent	
In wheelchair	Modified independent	
Bowel management	Modified independent	Dil stick if positive bulbocavernous reflex Suppositories if negative bulbocavernous reflex
Bladder management	Modified independent	
Bed mobility		
Rolling side to side	Modified independent	
Rolling		
Supine, prone		
Supine to and from sitting		
Scooting		
Leg management		
Transfers		
Bed	Modified independent	May need a transfer board
Tub, toilet		
Car		
Floor		
Upright wheelchair		
Manual wheelchair mobility		Upright wheelchair
Smooth surfaces	Modified independent	
Ramps		
Rough terrain		
Curbs	Moderate assistance to modified independent	
Stairs (three or four)		

TABLE 16-4 ■ FUNCTIONAL EXPECTATIONS FOR COMPLETE SPINAL CORD INJURY LESIONS—cont'd

FUNCTIONAL COMPONENT	OUTCOME POTENTIAL	ANTICIPATED EQUIPMENT TO ACHIEVE OUTCOMES
Ambulation	Depends on level of injury	
Smooth surfaces	Modified independent for T12 injuries and below Will vary with higher thoracic injuries	Appropriate orthotics and assistive device(s)
Ramps		
Rough terrain		
Curbs		
Stairs		
Skin		
Weight shift	Modified independent	
Pad, positioning		
Skin checks		Mirror
Home management		
Light home management	Modified independent	
Heavy home management	Modified independent	Various adaptive ADL equipment
Community ADL		
Driving vehicle	Modified independent	Hand controls for vehicle
ROM exercises to left extremity and trunk	Modified independent	Leg lifter to assist with lower-extremity ROM
Exercise program	Modified independent	Cuff weights, e-stim if any weakened lower-extremity muscles

ADL, Activity of daily living; *ECU,* enviornmental control unit; *ROM,* range of motion.

members, including the client, have the opportunity to discuss the long-term goals that have been established. It may be useful to request that the patient sign a statement acknowledging understanding of, and agreement to, all long-term goals.

EARLY REHABILITATION AND COMPLICATION PREVENTION

Early rehabilitation of the patient with SCI begins with prevention. Preventing secondary complications speeds entry into the rehabilitation phase and improves the possibility that the patient will become a productive member of society.

Table 16-5 describes an overview of the primary complications that can arise after an SCI. In this table, known causes and common management activities are reviewed. Tests and measures commonly used to determine the complication and the recommended medical and/or therapeutic interventions are listed in the table. Although various reports of incidences are published, the largest database is the Model Spinal Cord Injury Care Systems report.[41,64] Because of their high incidence and potential effect on long-term outcomes, the following complications require further discussion: skin compromise, loss of ROM or joint contractures, and respiratory compromise after SCI.

Preventing and Managing Pressure Ulcers and Skin Compromise

After SCI and during the period of spinal shock, patients are at greater risk for development of pressure ulcers.[65,66] The use of backboards at the emergency scene and during radiographic procedures contributes to potential skin compromise; therefore, immediate concern for tissue death, especially at the sacrum, should be taken into account. Recently, padded spine boards have become available and are recommended to reduce the risk of skin complications.

Preventive skin care begins with careful inspection. Soft tissue areas over a bony prominence are at greatest risk for acquiring a pressure sore.[67] Key areas to evaluate include the sacrum, ischia, greater trochanters, heels, malleoli, knees, occiput, scapulae, elbows, and prominent spinous processes. A turning schedule should be initiated immediately. Even if the patient has unstable fractures or is in traction, he or she can be turned and positioned with flat pillows using the logroll technique. Even small changes off the sacrum and coccyx are helpful. The patient's position in bed should be initially established for turns to occur every 2 to 3 hours.[66] This interval can be gradually increased to 6 hours with careful monitoring for evidence of skin compromise. A reddened round area over the bone that does not disappear after 15 to 30 minutes is the hallmark start of a pressure sore, and action to avoid or minimize pressure in the area must be taken immediately to avoid progression. Turning positions include prone, supine, right and left side-lying, semiprone, and semisupine positions.[68,69] Secondary injuries such as fractures and the presence of vital equipment, such as ventilator tubing, chest tubes, and arterial lines, should be considered when choosing turning positions. The prone position is the safest position for maintaining skin integrity but may not always be feasible.

Pillows or rectangular foam pads may be used to bridge off the bony prominences and relieve potential pressure. This is especially helpful above the heels. Padding directly over a prominent area with a firm pillow or pad may only increase pressure and should be avoided. Great care should

TABLE 16-5 ■ COMPLICATIONS AFTER SPINAL CORD INJURY

COMPLICATION	CAUSE	DIAGNOSTIC TESTS AND MEASURES	MEDICAL TREATMENT OR INTERVENTION	THERAPEUTIC INTERVENTION
CARDIOPULMONARY				
Pneumonia Atelectasis	Bacterial or viral infection, prolonged immobilization, prolonged artificial ventilation, general anesthesia	Radiographic studies, diagnostic bronchoscopy	Antibiotics, bronchodilator therapy, therapeutic bronchoscopy, suctioning	Chest physical therapy: percussion, vibration, postural drainage, mobilization, inspiratory breathing exercises
Ventilatory failure	Weakness or paralysis of the inspiratory muscles, unchecked bronchospasm	Pulmonary function tests (PFTs), arterial blood gases (ABGs), end-tidal CO_2 monitoring, pulse oximetry	Artificial ventilation and supportive therapy, management of underlying cause (e.g., pneumonia), oxygen therapy	Airway and secretion management treatment as above, early mobilization once stabilized, biofeedback to assist with ventilator weaning as appropriate
Deep vein thrombosis (DVT)*	Venous status, activation of blood coagulation, pressure on immobilized lower extremity, and endothelial damage[65-67]	Doppler studies, leg measurements, extremity visual observation and palpation, low-grade fever of unknown origin	Subcutaneous heparin[3,252] Prophylactic anticoagulation can decrease incidence to 1.3%[5] Vena cava filter for failed anticoagulant prophylaxis	Early mobilization and range of motion (ROM) for prevention, centripetal massage for prevention, compression garments, education about smoking cessation, weight loss, and exercise; avoid constricting garments and monitor overly tight leg bag straps and pressure garments (Paralyzed Veterans of America DVT guidelines)
Pulmonary embolus	Dislodging of DVT	Ventilation-perfusion lung scan, signs and symptoms including chest pain, breathlessness, apprehension, fever, and cough	Vena cava filter Anticoagulation therapy	None
Orthostatic hypotension	Vasodilation and decreased venous return, loss of muscle pump action in dependent lower extremities and trunk[253]	Monitor blood pressure with activity and changes in position, observation for signs and symptoms	Medications to increase blood pressure, fluids in the presence of hypovolemia	Gradient compression garments: Ace wraps, abdominal binders, appropriate wheelchair selection to prevent rapid changes in position early in rehabilitation
Apneic bradycardia	True origin unknown; believed to be caused by sympathetic disruption resulting in vagal dominance in response to a noxious stimulus or hypoxia[254]	Electrocardiogram Heart rate Respiratory rate	Hyperventilation	Remove noxious stimulus
INTEGUMENTARY SYSTEM				
Pressure ulcers	Prolonged external skin pressure exceeding the average arterial or capillary pressure[255]	Wound measurements, staging classification, nutritional assessment[71]	Nutritional support as needed, surgical or enzymatic debridement, surgical closure, muscle flap, skin flap or graft, antibiotics as appropriate	Irrigation and hydrotherapy, dressing management, electrotherapy[71]
Shearing	Stretching and tearing of the blood vessels that pass between the layers of the skin[7]	See pressure ulcers	See pressure ulcers	Add protective padding during functional activities, skill perfection, correct handling techniques
Moisture	Excessive sweating below the level of injury, urinary and bowel incontinence, poor hygiene	See pressure ulcers	See pressure ulcers, treat possible urinary tract infection, medications for bladder incontinence	Protective barrier ointments and powders, establish effective bowel and bladder programs, educate for improved hygiene, and refine activity of daily living (ADL) skills

TABLE 16-5 ■ COMPLICATIONS AFTER SPINAL CORD INJURY—cont'd

COMPLICATION	CAUSE	DIAGNOSTIC TESTS AND MEASURES	MEDICAL TREATMENT OR INTERVENTION	THERAPEUTIC INTERVENTION
NEUROMUSCULAR				
Spasticity	Upper motor neuron lesion[73] Deep tendon reflex spasticity scale evaluation	Ashworth or Modified Ashworth Scale Baclofen pump insertion[75]	Antispastic pharmacological agents: baclofen, diazepam (Valium), dantrolene Surgical intervention: myelotomy, rhizotomy, peripheral neurotomy[73] Botox injection	Prolonged stretching; inhibitive positioning or casting Cryotherapy, weight-bearing exercise, and aquatic therapy
Flaccidity	Lower motor neuron lesion[7,256] Most often in injuries at L1 level and below	Deep tendon reflexes (would be absent)	None	None for treating flaccidity; however, secondary treatments that need to be considered include positioning to improve postural support, education for skin protection, and bracing and splinting to maintain joint integrity
Neurogenic bowel[†]	Refer to bowel management	Positive bulbocavernosus reflex: indicates reflexic bowel	Oral laxative, suppositories, and enemas	Establish comprehensive bowel program
Autonomic dysreflexia	Triggering of an uncontrolled hyperactive response from the sympathetic nervous system by a noxious stimulus[7]; noxious stimuli may include bowel or bladder distention, urinary tract infection, ingrown toenail, tight clothing, and pressure sore	Sudden rise in systolic blood pressure of 20-40 mm Hg above baseline[254] Observation of signs and symptoms: Sweating above level of injury Goose bumps Severe headache Flushing of skin from vasodilation above level of injury[254]	Catheterization of the bladder, irrigation of indwelling catheter, pharmacological management if systolic blood pressure is greater than 150 mm Hg Remove ingrown toenail if present	Immediately position the client in upright position, identify and remove noxious stimuli, check clothing and catheter tubing for constriction, and perform bowel program if fecal impaction is suspected
Ulcers, gastrointestinal	Venous status, activation of blood	Radiographic studies, diagnostic	Medications to increase blood pressure	Gradient compression garments; Ace wrap
OTHER				
Thermoregulation problems	Interruption between communication with autonomic nervous system and hypothalamus Lack of vasoconstriction and inability to shiver or perspire[254]	Body temperature	Cooling or warming blanket if extreme	Education about risk and proper protection from elements; behavior modification, education for proper hydration and appropriate clothing
Pain	Radicular pain originating from the injury,[7,257,258] kinematic or mechanical pain, direct trauma, referred pain[258,259]	Pain scales, functional assessment,[260] taxonomy	Immobilization and rest, pain medications, injections for pain or antiinflammatory measures	Restore ideal alignment and posture; thermal modalities and electromodalities; manual therapy, improve movement patterns
Urinary tract infections	Presence of excessive bacteria in urine	Urinalysis, urine culture and sensitivity, temperature	Antibiotics	Monitor fluid intake and educate for proper technique during bladder care
Contractures	Muscle imbalance around joint; prolonged immobilization, unchecked spasticity, pain	Goniometric measurements	Tendon release; Botox injection for isolated spasticity	ROM functional use of extremity, casting or splinting, achieving and maintaining optimal postural alignment

Continued

TABLE 16-5 ■ COMPLICATIONS AFTER SPINAL CORD INJURY—cont'd

COMPLICATION	CAUSE	DIAGNOSTIC TESTS AND MEASURES	MEDICAL TREATMENT OR INTERVENTION	THERAPEUTIC INTERVENTION
Heterotopic ossification (HO)	Unknown	Alkaline phosphatase levels (increase after 6 weeks)[261,262]; observation for sudden loss of ROM, local edema, heat, erythema, nonseptic fever	Etidronate disodium (Didronel): use prophylactically or during inflammatory stage Surgical resection	Maintain available ROM; avoid vigorous stretching during inflammatory stage; achieve and maintain optimal wheelchair positioning
Osteoporosis and joint changes degenerative	Bone demineralization[263]	Bone scan	None; calcium supplement for prevention	Weight-bearing techniques: amount and type unknown, specific to spinal cord injury
Spinal deformities	Muscle imbalance or weakness around spinal column; poor postural support, asymmetrical functional activities	Posture evaluation, seating evaluation	If severe: surgical fixation, thoracic orthosis	Restore postural alignment, avoid repetitive asymmetrical activities, control spasticity
Gastroduodenal ulcers, gastrointestinal bleeding	Acute: disruption of central nervous system, abdominal trauma or stress response to neuroendocrine system[264] Chronic: impairment of autonomic nervous system[7]	Hematocrit and hemoglobin; observation of gastrointestinal fluids	Surgical intervention; restore normal gastrointestinal function	Establish effective bowel program, establish high-fiber diet, provide education and stress management
Metabolic, endocrine	Impairment of autonomic nervous system	Observe for fatigue, malaise; undesirable weight gain[62]	None known	Education, exercise, and weight control

*Consortium for Spinal Cord Medicine Clinical Practice Guidelines: *Prevention of thromboembolism in spinal cord injury,* Washington, D.C., February 1997, Paralyzed Veterans of America.

†Consortium for Spinal Cord Medicine Clinical Practice Guidelines: *Neurogenic bowel management in adults with spinal cord injury*, Washington, D.C., March 1998, Paralyzed Veterans of America.

be taken for regular checks if this bridging technique is used in the trunk or buttocks region while the patient is in bed, owing to eventual shifting of the foam.

Keeping the head of the bed as low as tolerated minimizes the risk for shearing and excessive sacral pressure. For patients who are not appropriate for rigorous turning schedules (e.g., patients with unstabilized fractures), specialty alternating pressure mattresses are available. Low air loss, alternating pressure, or even air-fluidized mattresses are available for those who require the head of the bed to be elevated more than 30 degrees for prolonged periods and also have other extenuating conditions such as respiratory distress, diabetes, and/or low prealbumin.[70]

While the patient is sitting, an appropriate pressure redistribution (relief) cushion is recommended and a pressure relief (weight shift) schedule is established and strictly enforced.

Although pressure is one of the most prevalent causes of skin compromise, other forces may lead to problems, including friction, shearing, excessive moisture or dryness, infection, and bruising or bumping during activities. This is especially true of clients with SCI because of altered thermoregulation, changes in mobility, decreased or absent sensation, and incontinence of bowel and bladder. In addition, as patients begin to learn functional skills, they may have poor motor control and impaired balance and must be carefully monitored to avoid injury.

Should skin compromise occur, the first intervention is to identify and remove the source of the compromise. Modifications to the seating system or changing to a more pressure-reducing mattress system or cushion may be necessary. Examination and treatment will then need to focus on healing the wound and preventing other secondary complications that may occur as a result of potential immobility and delayed physical rehabilitation. The reader is encouraged to refer to *Pressure Ulcer Treatment: Clinical Practice Guideline,* developed by the Agency for Health Care Research and Quality, for examination tools, including the classification of pressure ulcers.[71,72]

Treatment interventions may include hydrotherapy, specialty wound dressings, electro-modalities, and thermal modalities to increase circulation.[71] Mechanical, autolytic, enzymatic, or surgical debridement may be necessary to obtain and maintain a viable wound bed. If the wound does not heal, surgical interventions with myocutaneous or muscle flaps may be necessary for closure. Coordinated return-to-sit programs or protocols after such medical interventions are necessary to prevent opening of the surgical site. Such surgical procedures are costly and significantly delay functional rehabilitation.

After closure and healing of the wound, education becomes a priority to maintain skin integrity. The client must adhere to a more rigorous skin check program as rehabilitation continues, giving special attention to the affected area. Teaching patients to advocate for themselves and to problem solve equipment and lifestyle issues that may affect their skin condition will reduce the recurrence rate. Alcohol, tobacco, and drug use (both recreational and prescription) should be managed for long-term success. Prevention of skin compromise is critical and cannot be stressed enough to health care providers, patients, and caregivers.

Prevention and Management of Joint Contractures

The development of a contracture may result in postural misalignment or impede potential function. Daily ROM exercises, proper positioning, and adequate spasticity control may help prevent contractures.[66] Contracture prevention includes the use of splints for proper joint alignment, techniques such as weight bearing, ADLs, and functional exercises. Patients exhibiting spasticity may require more frequent ROM intervention.[66,73]

Adaptive Shortening or Adaptive Lengthening of Muscles

Although isolated joint ROM should be normal for all patients, allowing adaptive shortening or adaptive lengthening of particular muscles is recommended to enhance the achievement of certain functional skills.[69,74] Likewise, unwanted shortening or lengthening of muscles should be prevented. The following section reviews a few examples of these concepts as they relate to SCI.

Tenodesis is described as the passive shortening of the two-joint finger flexors as the wrist is extended. This action creates a grasp, which assists performance of ADLs (Figure 16-11).[69,75] A patient with mid to low tetraplegia may rely on adaptive shortening of these long finger flexors to replace active grip.[69] If the finger flexors are stretched across all joints during ROM exercises, the achievement of some functional goals may be limited. ROM to the finger flexors should be applied only while the wrist is in a neutral position. There is controversy over shortening of the flexor tendons. Some clinicians argue that the client can develop a fixed flexion contracture of the proximal interphalangeal joints, interfering with future surgical attempts to restore finger function.[38] It is recommended to promote tenodesis functioning via adaptive shortening while maintaining joint suppleness.

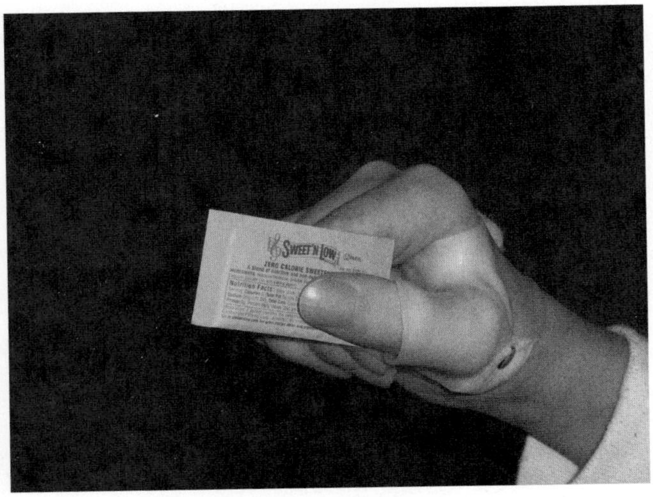

Figure 16-11 ■ Tenodesis grasp.

In the presence of weakened or paralyzed elbow extensors, shortening of the elbow flexors should be prevented because it will impair ADL function and transfer skills.[7,69] Contracted elbow flexors or pronator muscles in a client with an SCI level of C6 can cost this client his or her independence. Likewise, the rotator cuff and the other scapular muscles should be assessed for their length-tension relationships and their ability to generate force. Normal length of these muscles should be maintained. For example, achieving external rotation of the shoulder (active and passive) is critical for clients with low-level tetraplegia. Shortening of the subscapularis and other structures can quickly result in a decrease in motion, limiting bed mobility, transfers, feeding, and grooming skills. Patients with complete paraplegia who are candidates for ambulation require normal ROM in the lower extremities. If the hip flexors or knee flexors are allowed to shorten, achieving standing and ambulation goals will be more difficult.

The combination of lengthened hamstrings and tight back extensor muscles provides stability for balance in the short- and long-sitting positions. This aids in the efficiency of transfers and bowel and bladder management. Balance in long sitting assists with lower-extremity dressing and other ADLs. Hamstrings should be lengthened to allow 110 to 120 degrees of straight leg raising without overstretching back extensor muscles.

Splinting to Prevent Joint Deformity

Deformity prevention is the first goal of splinting.[76] Patients with cervical spinal cord injuries may have lost normal neural input to musculature in their wrists and hands. Other clients may have partial motor control, which may lead to muscle imbalances and loss of ROM. In the absence or weakness of elbow extensors, a bivalve cast or an elbow extension splint at night may be beneficial to prevent joint contractures. At the wrists, a volar wrist support is commonly used initially and may be progressed to a longer-term option of a definitive wrist orthosis. Other splints often used for deformity prevention of the hands include resting hand splints with proper positioning to maintain the support of the wrist and web space (Figure 16-12, *A*).[77] Another hand-based option is the intrinsic plus splint (Figure 16-12, *B*), which places the metacarpophalangeal joints closer to 90 degrees of flexion and decreases intrinsic hand muscle tightness.

Another goal of splinting in the SCI population is to increase function. Patients with tetraplegia at the C5 level rely on an orthosis to be independent with communication, feeding, and hygiene. They must have joint stability and support at the wrist and the hand to perform these skills. The splint is often adapted with a utensil slot or cuff so that the client can effectively perform the skills mentioned previously.

Patients who are not strong enough to use their wrists for tenodesis may require splinting to support their wrists until they can perform wrist extension against gravity. Long opponens splints can be used to position the thumb for

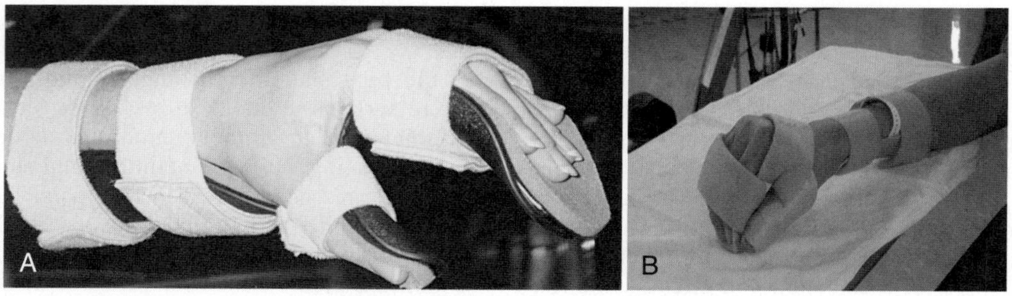

Figure 16-12 ■ **A,** Resting hand splint. **B,** Volar intrinsic plus splint maintains alignment of the wrist and fingers to promote metacarpophalangeal flexion for tenodesis grasp.

function but support the weak wrist (Figure 16-13). Once the wrist muscles strengthen, the long opponens splint can be cut down to a hand-based short opponens to maintain proper web space and thumb positioning while maximizing tenodesis.

As mentioned previously, clients with injuries at the C6 level can use their wrists for a tenodesis grasp.[75,78,79] Critical components of the splint assessment for these clients are the positioning of the thumb, web space, and index finger observed during the grasp. It is recommended that the client's hand be positioned with the thumb in a lateral pinch position because this is the most commonly used prehension pattern to pick up objects. Clients who are not splinted may not have the proper positioning to pick up objects because their tenodesis is "too tight" or "too loose."

Clients with C8 to T1 injuries or clients who have incomplete injuries may have "clawing" or hyperextension of the metacarpophalangeal joints. This is caused by finger extensor musculature that is stronger than finger flexor musculature.[75,80] To prevent this, a splint can be made to block the metacarpophalangeal joints and promote weak intrinsic muscle function. Depending on the extent of the imbalance, these splints can be used during function or worn only at night. Cost, time, material, and clinician experience are important considerations when deciding between custom and prefabricated splints. A well fitting, prefabricated splint can be as effective as a custom-fabricated splint in certain situations. Custom splints require additional resources and clinician expertise. One way to minimize time spent in fabrication of splints is to use a good pattern and premade straps. Finally, educating the client on the splint-wearing schedule, skin checks, and splint care is important for preventing skin breakdown.

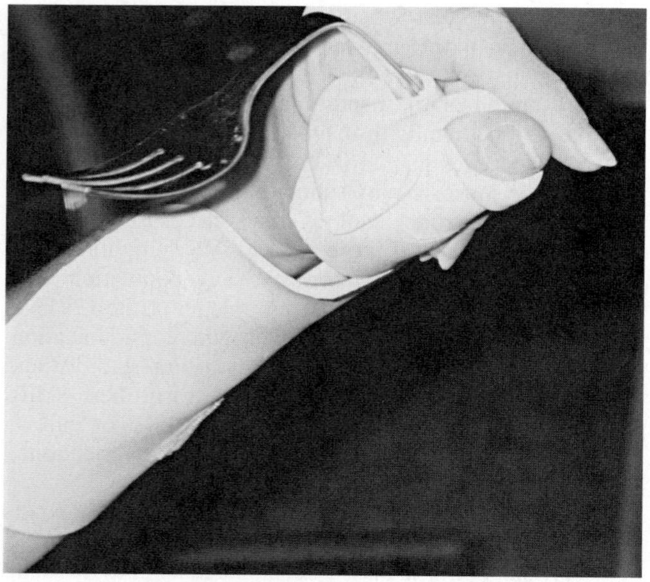

Figure 16-13 ■ Long opponens splint with fabricated utensil holder.

Treatment for Joint Deformity

If a joint contracture occurs despite preventive measures, more aggressive treatments are necessary. This may include more aggressive use of splinting, plaster or fiberglass casting techniques, or botulinum toxin type A (Botox) injections.[81-83] When splinting is not effective, fabrication of serial or bivalve casts may be indicated. The client with minimal ROM limitations may require only one cast. Most commonly, the client has a significant limitation and requires serial casts, in which several casts are applied and then removed over a period of weeks to increase extensibility in the soft tissues surrounding the casted joint.[84] The involved joint is placed at submaximal ROM.[85] Once the cast is removed, the joint should have an increase of approximately 7 degrees of ROM.[85] This process continues until the deformity is minimized or resolved. The final cast is a bivalve so that the cast can act as a positioning device that can be easily removed. Casting contraindications are skin compromise over the area to be casted, heterotopic ossification, edema, decreased circulation, severe fluctuating tone, and inconsistent monitoring systems. The elbow, wrist and hand, and finger joints are the most common joints casted for clients with SCI. Casting for most of these clients may be the last resort to regain increased ROM before a client can begin using feeding, grooming, or communication skills. Long-arm casts are used when elbow and wrist contractures must be managed simultaneously. If evaluation of the upper extremity reveals a pronation or supination contracture, a long-arm cast would also be the cast of choice. Dropout casts are used with severe elbow flexor or extensor contractures, but the patient should be in a position in which gravity can assist. Wrist-hand and finger casts are indicated for contractures that prevent distal upper-extremity function. Most commonly, a client will have a wrist flexion-extension contracture or have finger flexor-extensor tone and will require a cast to use the tenodesis or individual fingers for fine motor skills. Sometimes wrist casts with finger shells or resting hand extensions on casts are needed to ensure that the hand, fingers, and web space are maintained in a position of optimal function. Casting is an expensive and labor-intensive treatment modality, but if indicated and used appropriately it can assist a client in regaining lost joint ROM needed for increased independence and function.

Botox may be used in conjunction with casting. In a study conducted by Corry and colleagues[83] tone reduction was evident when botulinum toxin type A was used; however, ROM and functional improvement varied among subjects. Pierson and co-workers[82] found that, with careful selection, subjects who received botulinum toxin type A had significant improvements in active and passive ROM. Research indicates that patients who have flexor spasticity without fixed contracture will benefit the most.

Surgical intervention may be recommended by an orthopedic physician in severe cases of joint contracture.[86] Some of the more commonly used surgical options include joint manipulation under anesthesia, arthroscopic surgical releases, open surgical releases, and rotational osteotomy.

Prevention and Management of Respiratory Complications

Early management must focus heavily on preventing pulmonary complications and maximizing pulmonary function so the patient may perform physical activities. The clinician should first determine which ventilatory muscles are impaired. The primary ventilatory muscles of inspiration are the diaphragm and the intercostals. The diaphragm is innervated by the phrenic nerve at C3 through C5. The intercostals are innervated by the intercostal nerves positioned between the ribs. If the diaphragm is weak or paralyzed, its descent will be lessened, reducing the patient's ability to ventilate.[87-90]

Accessory muscles of ventilation are primarily located in the cervical region.[91] The accessory muscles are used to augment ventilation when the demand for oxygen increases, as during exercise. Accessory muscles may also be recruited to generate an improved cough effort.[66] The most commonly cited accessory muscles are the sternocleidomastoids, the scalenes, the levatores scapulae, and the trapezius muscles.[88,89] The erector spinae group may also assist by extending the spine, thus improving the potential depth of inspiration.[89]

The abdominals are the primary muscles used for forced expiration in such maneuvers as coughing or sneezing. The latissimus dorsi, the teres major, and the clavicular portion of the pectoralis major are also active during forced expiration and cough in the client with tetraplegia.[92] Alterations in the function of these muscles will have an impact on the patient's ability to clear secretions and produce loud vocalization. Gravity plays a crucial role in the function of all ventilatory muscles.[89] Neural input to the diaphragm increases in the upright position in persons with intact nervous systems. As one moves into an upright position, the resting position of the diaphragm drops as the abdominal contents fall.[89] The diaphragm is effectively shortened, which makes generating a strong contraction more difficult. With intact abdominal musculature, however, a counter pressure is produced and adequate intraabdominal pressure is maintained, allowing the diaphragm to perform work. If weakness or paralysis of the abdominal wall is present, the client may need a binder or corset to maintain the normal pressure relationship.[69,87,93-95] Unless the SCI has affected only the lowest sacral and lumbar areas, some degree of ventilatory impairment is present and should be addressed in therapeutic sessions.

Many treatment techniques are available to address the myriad causes of ventilatory impairment. Decreased chest wall mobility and the inability to clear secretions should always be addressed. Interventions may include inspiratory muscle training, chest wall mobility exercises, and chest physical therapy.[69,74,90,96,97]

Inspiratory Muscle Training

Inspiratory muscle training may be used to train the diaphragm and the accessory muscles that are weakened by partial paralysis, disuse from prolonged artificial ventilation, or prolonged bed rest. In the presence of significant impairments, it is generally recommended that training be initiated in the supine or side-lying position and progressed to the sitting position when tolerated. When training a moderately weak diaphragm, gentle pressure during inspiration may be used to facilitate the muscle (Figure 16-14). Accessory muscle training may be facilitated with the client in the

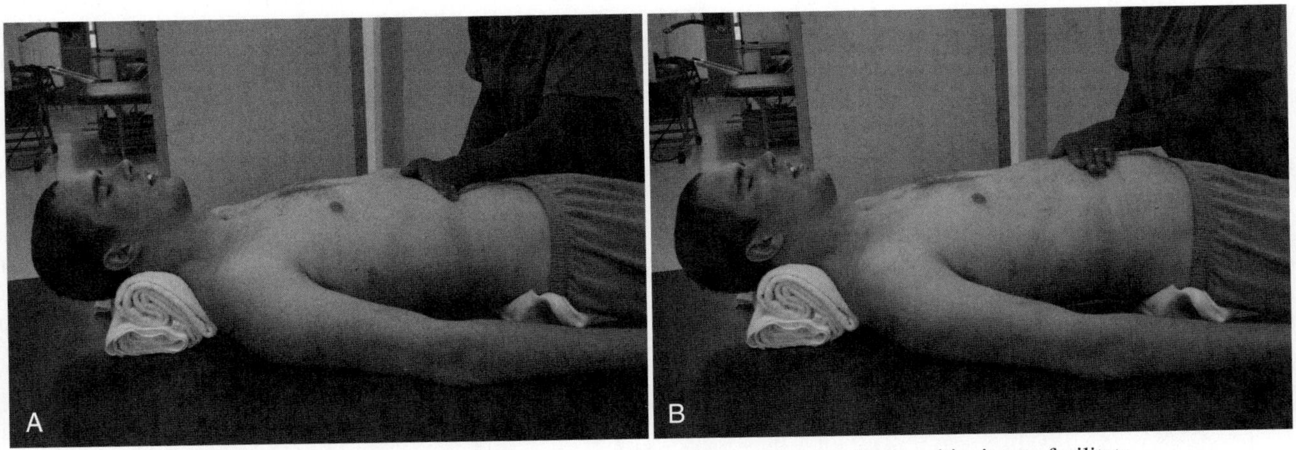

Figure 16-14 ■ Diaphragm facilitation. **A,** Hand placement and patient positioning to facilitate the diaphragm and inhibit accessory muscle activity. **B,** Firm contact is maintained throughout inspiration. The lower extremities are placed over a pillow in flexion to prevent stretching of the abdominal wall.

supine position while a slight stretch is placed on these muscles.[74] The stretch is accomplished by shoulder abduction and external rotation, elbow extension, forearm supination, and neutral alignment of the head and neck. A more challenging position incorporates upper thoracic extension. The clinician's hands are placed directly over the muscle to be facilitated. The patient is instructed to breathe into the upper chest (Figure 16-15). As the treatment progresses, the diaphragm may be inhibited for short training periods by applying pressure over the abdomen in an upward direction. Care must be taken to avoid excessive pressure to prevent occlusion of vital arteries.

As the inspiratory muscles strengthen, resistive inspiratory devices may be used. Inspiratory devices are relatively inexpensive and most function similarly. Most devices have a one-way valve that closes when the patient inspires, forcing him or her to breathe either through a small aperture or against a spring-loaded resistance. Although evidence fully supporting this intervention remains inconclusive,[98] some researchers have shown improvements in total lung capacity[99] and improved endurance measures.[100] The diaphragm may also be trained by using weights on the abdominal wall with the client positioned supine. Derrickson and colleagues[101] concluded that both inspiratory muscle training devices and abdominal weights are effective in improving ventilatory mechanics. Muscle trainers, however, appear to promote more of an endurance effect than the use of abdominal weights.

Diaphragm and Phrenic Nerve Pacing

When the primary inspiratory muscles are no longer volitionally active as a result of SCI, diaphragm or phrenic nerve pacing may be used to cause the diaphragm to contract. These interventions are most commonly indicated when the lesion is at or above the C3 level.[101-106] Electrical stimulation may be applied directly or indirectly through a vein wall or the skin or directly to the phrenic nerve via thoracotomy. Transdiaphragmatic pacing, in which electrodes are placed laparoscopically on the diaphragm, is also an option.[107] Transdiaphragmatic pacing is less invasive than direct phrenic nerve pacing, may be implanted and initiated on an outpatient basis, and may result in improved outcomes. Both of these procedures require a reconditioning program that involves extensive caregiver and client training. Many clients

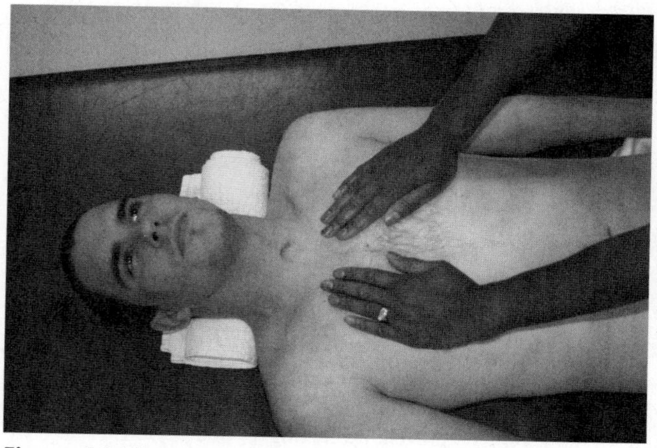

Figure 16-15 ■ Accessory muscle facilitation. Hand placement and patient positioning.

require some residual use of mechanical ventilation even after maximal tolerance has been achieved so as not to overfatigue the phrenic nerve. Other researchers are considering also pacing intercostal muscles[108] or using a combination of diaphragmatic and intercostal pacing. There is limited evidence comparing the outcomes associated with these devices in isolation or in combination therapies.

Glossopharyngeal Breathing

Glossopharyngeal breathing is another way of increasing vital capacity in the presence of weak inspiratory muscles.[90,94,97] Moving the jaw forward and upward in a circular opening and closing manner traps air in the buccal cavity. A series of swallowing-like maneuvers forces air into the lungs, increasing the vital capacity. This technique has been reported to increase vital capacity by as much as 1 L.[74] Although this technique is rarely used to sustain ventilation for long periods of time,[109] it may be used in emergency situations and to enhance cough function. The client with high tetraplegia should attempt to master this skill.

Secretion Clearance

Ventilatory impairment occurs when the client is unable to clear secretions.[87,110] Factors such as artificial ventilation and general anesthesia hamper secretion mobilization. With artificial ventilation, clients may require an artificial airway.[110,111] The presence of this airway in the trachea is an irritant, and the client subsequently produces more secretions.[87] A description of various types and parameters of ventilation is beyond the scope of this chapter. Clinicians working with clients requiring artificial ventilation are referred to other publications.[110,112]

Secretions are most commonly removed by tracheal suctioning, unassisted coughing, or assisted coughing. Recently there has been a resurgence of previously used technologies that provide rapidly alternating pressures through a mouthpiece or an endotracheal tube to remove secretions. This is commonly referred to as insufflation-exsufflation.[113] To date, conclusive research determining which single technique or combination of techniques achieves the best outcome is not available. Insufflation-exsufflation may result in fewer complications and is reported to be more comfortable to the client. Barriers to implementation of these techniques may include expense of the equipment and competency barriers in that training is required. Postural drainage, percussion or clapping, and shaking or vibration are used to assist with moving secretions toward larger airways for expectoration.[17,69,79]

Assisted coughing is typically used with people who are unable to generate sufficient effort.[97] The assistant places both hands firmly on the abdominal wall. After a maximal inspiratory effort, the patient coughs and the assistant simply supports the weakened wall. A gentle upward and inward force may be used to increase the intraabdominal pressure, yielding a more forceful cough (Figure 16-16).[84,97] Excessive pressure over the xiphoid process should be avoided to prevent severe injury.

Patients may learn independent coughing techniques. In preparation for a cough, the patient positions an arm around the push handle of the wheelchair, opening the chest wall to enhance inspiratory effort. The other arm is raised over the head and chest during inspiration. This procedure is followed by a breath hold, strong trunk flexion, and then a

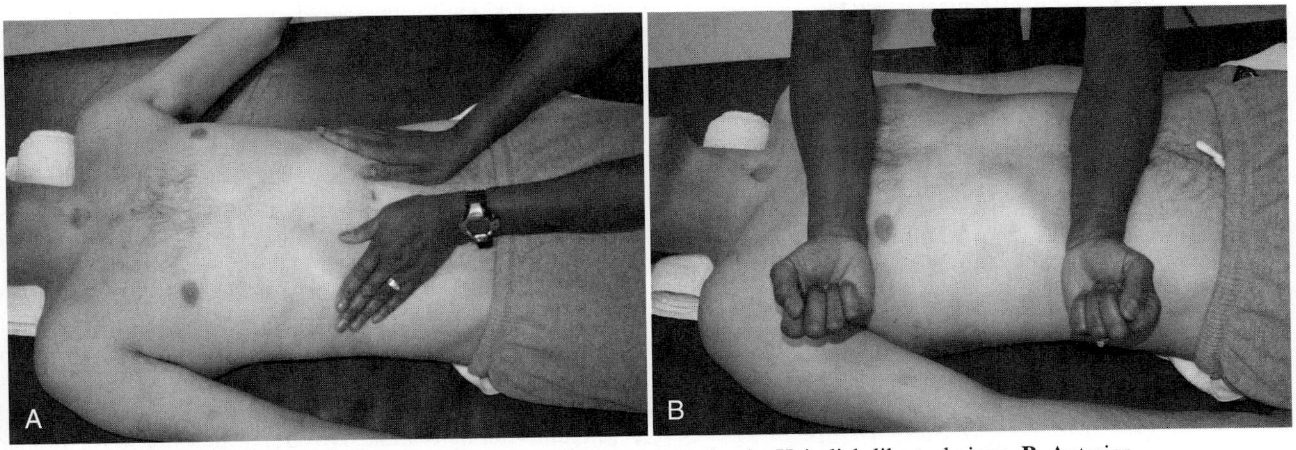

Figure 16-16 ■ Quad coughing. **A,** Hand placement for the Heimlich-like technique. **B,** Anterior chest wall quad coughing. The inferior forearm supination promotes an upward and inward force during the cough.

cough (Figure 16-17).[97] Another technique for independent coughing is accomplished by placing the forearms over the abdomen and delivering a manual thrust during cough. This technique is more difficult and may not provide an inspiratory advantage.

Early Mobilization

Getting the patient upright as soon as possible promotes self-mobility and should be planned carefully. An appropriate seating system for pressure relief and support should be chosen. Most patients require a reclining wheelchair with elevating footrests or tilt-in-space wheelchairs when they are first acclimating to the upright position.[69,74,97]

The client is transferred initially to a reclining or tilting back position and progressed to an upright position as signs and symptoms of medical stability allow. The client should be monitored for evidence of orthostatic hypotension. Dizziness or lightheadedness is most common. Ringing in the ears and visual changes also may occur. Changes in mental function may indicate more serious hypotension, and the client should be reclined immediately. Assessing blood pressure before and during

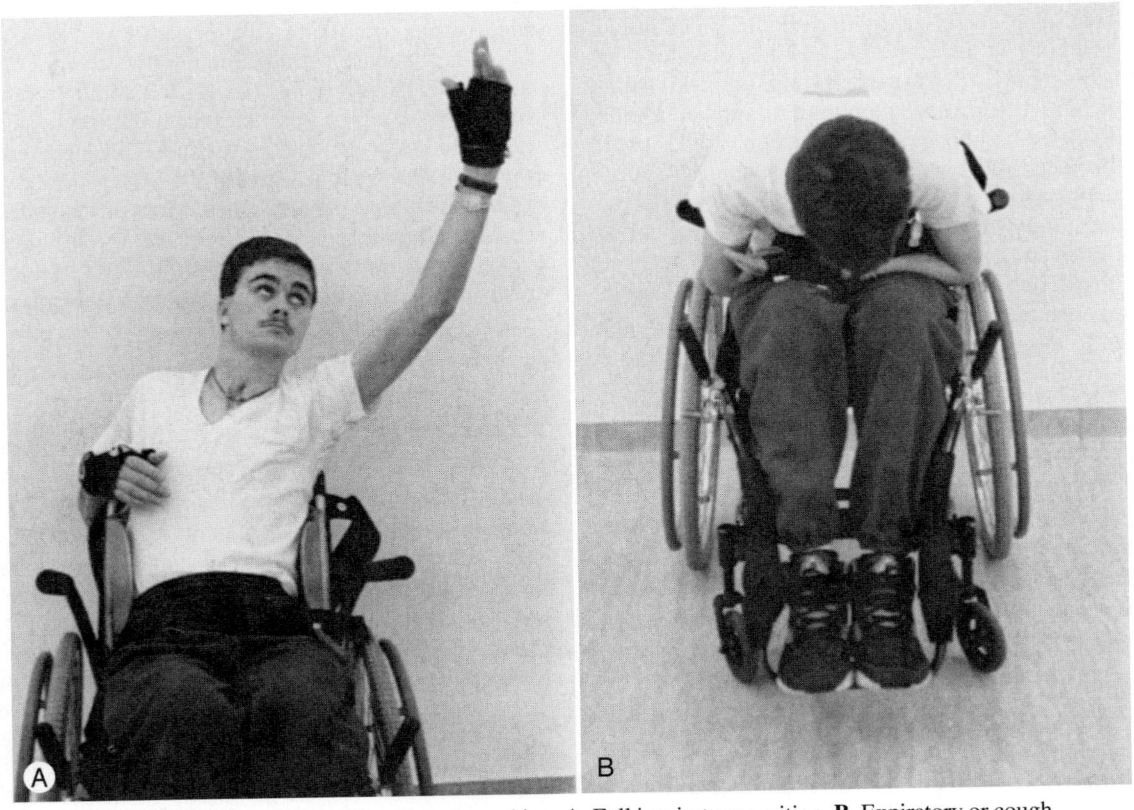

Figure 16-17 ■ Self-produced quad coughing. **A,** Full inspiratory position. **B,** Expiratory or cough position.

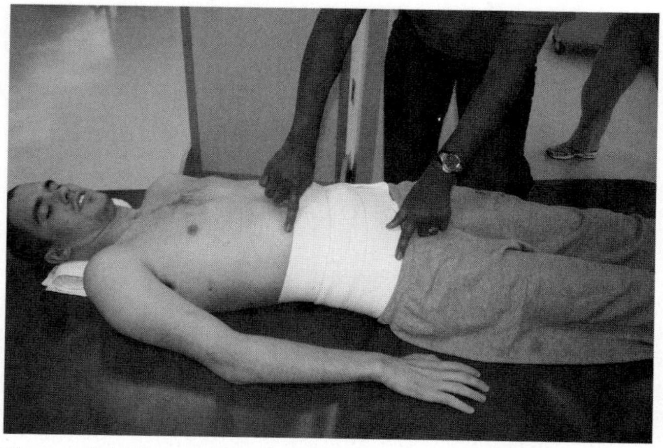

Figure 16-18 ■ Abdominal binder. Correct placement is over the anterior-superior iliac spine and at the level of lower rib cage. Custom corsets may be used if an elastic binder does not provide adequate support to enhance vital capacity.

activities provides an objective measurement of the client's status.

Because of paralysis, the abdominal wall may not support the internal organs and viscera. In these cases an abdominal binder or corset should be applied to all clients with lesions above T12 to assist in venous return[74,95,97]; as discussed, this will enhance ventilatory function. If the client has a history of vascular insufficiency or prolonged bed rest, wrapping the lower extremities with elastic bandages while applying the greatest pressure distally may be beneficial.

Abdominal binders and corsets are fitted so that the top of the corset lies just over the lower two ribs.[95] The bottom portion is placed over the anterior iliac spine and iliac crest (Figure 16-18). The corset or binder should be adjusted slightly more tightly at the bottom to assist in elevating the abdominal contents.[69,74,97] Properly fitting the abdominal binder is essential. If it is placed too high or allowed to ride up, ventilation may be impaired by restriction of chest wall excursion. If placed too low, it will not provide the necessary abdominal support.

The client can be transferred initially with a manual or mechanical lift. Lift systems may be advantageous because they allow total control of the client and give the assistant more time to ensure that monitoring devices, lines, or tubes attached to the client remain intact. Lift systems may be freestanding hydraulic lifts or electronic devices or may be mounted on the ceiling.

Once the client is out of bed, a weight shift or pressure relief schedule is immediately established. Initially, weight shifts are performed at 30-minute intervals and modified according to skin tolerance.[67] A timer may be issued to ensure reminders for weight shifts. This is particularly important if the client has cognitive deficits. The skin is inspected thoroughly before and immediately after out-of-bed activities. Total sitting time is progressed according to tolerance.

REHABILITATION: ACHIEVING FUNCTIONAL OUTCOMES

Once secondary complications are managed and the client is able to tolerate out-of-bed activities, more aggressive functional training begins. The following information will address special considerations for functional progression related to SCI.

Optimal neck, shoulder, and upper-extremity strength and ROM are important factors to consider in order to maximize functional outcomes. Neck musculature is typically painful and restricted in cervical injuries, especially after surgical procedures. Most clients will have a cervical orthosis in place postoperatively to prevent rotation and flexion and extension. Cervical spine mobility may be so limited that correcting a forward head posture is the first goal. Soft tissue massage, manual therapy, and other modalities may be beneficial. When cleared by the physician, the client can begin more aggressive neck exercises.

Key muscle groups in the shoulder to consider are the scapular stabilizers and movers, which allow for humeral flexion, adduction and abduction, shoulder internal and external rotation, and scapular movements. Clients with high cervical injuries have the potential for development of tight upper trapezius muscles. Upper trapezius inhibitory or scapular taping to relax the tight muscles and facilitate the weak scapular musculature is often beneficial. In the injury levels above C7, the scapular musculature may not be fully innervated, and thus positioning in the proper alignment and strengthening the innervated musculature are essential. The clinician will use findings from manual muscle testing and the goniometric examination to determine the appropriate stretching and strengthening programs. Patients may need to begin with gravity-eliminated exercises using air splints, bilateral slings, skateboards, and functional electrical stimulation (FES).

Activities of Daily Living and Instrumental Activities of Daily Living

ADLs include skills such as communication, feeding, grooming, bathing, dressing, bladder and bowel management, home management, and community reentry. Instrumental activities of daily living (IADLs) encompass multistep activities to care for self and others,[114] such as parenting, household management, and financial management. Depending on the level and severity of the SCI, patients will achieve varying levels of independence. Most of the ADL areas discussed in this section will address skill levels with a complete injury. Activities should be graded differently for an incomplete injury after completion of ASIA and manual muscle testing. For purposes of this discussion we will use terms used in the FIM.

Patients with high-level tetraplegia (C1 to C4) will be dependent in most ADLs as well as IADLs but will be able to verbalize how to safely perform all skills. Patients with low-level tetraplegia (C5 to C8) may achieve some level of independence, but this will vary according to the amount of intact musculature and the patient's body shape and weight, age, and motivation level. The ability of these patients to achieve maximum independence in all areas of ADLs may be accomplished only through the use of appropriate orthoses or adaptive equipment. See Table 16-4 for functional expectations and Table 16-6 for orthotic indications.

Patients with injuries at the C5 or C6 level are especially challenging in this area of rehabilitation. These patients must have biceps function and adequate elbow ROM before any ADL goals can be achieved. To achieve these goals, patients also need to work toward supporting their body

TABLE 16-6 ■ UPPER-EXTREMITY ORTHOTICS

SPLINT	LEVEL OF SPINAL CORD INJURY	RATIONALE
DYNAMIC ORTHOTICS		
Mobile arm support (ball-bearing feeder)	Weak C5 Incomplete injuries Also indicated with shoulder weakness (internal-external rotator muscle grades 2− to 3/5; bicep-supinator muscle grades 2−/5)	Function Assists in reaching in horizontal and vertical planes Increases functional ROM and strength Independence with feeding and hygiene after setup Provides support to allow correct movement patterns
Overhead rod and sling	Weak C5 Incomplete injuries Also indicated with shoulder weakness (internal-external rotator muscle grades 3 to 3+/5; bicep/supinator muscle grades 3/5)	Function Increases functional ROM and strength Independence with wheelchair driving after setup Independence with feeding and hygiene after setup Provides support to allow correct movement patterns
STATIC SPLINTS, CASTS, AND ORTHOTICS		
Resting hand splint	C1-C7	Position Prevent joint deformity Preserves web space Preserves balance with intrinsic and extrinsic musculature
Intrinsic plus splint	C1-C7	Position Same as resting hand splint but places finger MP joint in more flexion Long term, allows better tenodesis alignment of first digit and thumb
Elbow extension splints, bivalve cast	C5-C6	Position Prevents elbow contracture from muscle imbalance and/or hypertonicity
Rolyan TAP splint (prefabricated)	C5-C6	Position Provides constant low stretch Use with muscle imbalance and/or mild hypertonicity
Dorsal wrist support splints	C5	Function (e.g., slot for utensils) and position Prevents severe wrist drop and ulnar deviation If positioning is needed long term, may consider permanent splint fabricated by orthotist
Long opponens splint	C5	Position and function Can be dorsal or volar Prevents wrist drop and ulnar deviation Preserves web space and supports thumb, reducing subluxation Slot may be fabricated for function
Wrist cock-up splint	C5 Incomplete injuries	Position and function Supports wrist in slight extension Allows finger movement for incomplete injuries
Short opponens splint	C6-C7	Position and function Supports thumb to prevent subluxation Improves tenodesis and prehension
Tenodesis brace or splint	C6-C7	Function Enhances natural tenodesis in either tip-pinch or lateral pinch May consider permanent splint fabricated by orthotist
MP block splint	C8-T1	Position Prevents "claw hand" or hyperextension of the MP joints Protects weak intrinsic musculature

MP, Metacarpophalangeal; *ROM,* range of motion.

weight with simultaneous extension of the shoulder, elbow, and wrist, otherwise known as *propping* (see Figure 16-35, *A* to *C*). Elbow positioning devices such as pillow splints, casts, or resting splints enhance alignment. Other orthotics to consider for maximizing function include definitive wrist supports and mobile arm supports (MASs)[115] or short opponens splints if the patient has wrist extension. Appropriate wheelchair positioning with lap trays, armrests, wedges, or lateral trunk supports is important to maximize function for persons with C5 or C6 injuries.

Patients with a C7 or C8 level of injury generally will not prove to be as challenging for the rehabilitation therapist. With the presence of triceps, the ADL skills are easier to achieve. Most patients, given the right body type, will be able to achieve these goals with only minimal assistance from a caregiver.

Patients with paraplegia usually achieve total independence with communication, feeding, and grooming. These patients may need adaptive equipment to perform some of these IADL and ADL skills; however, they should be able to be performed without assistance from another person. Endurance is a major concern for the patient's independence while performing ADLs. Some skills require a considerable amount of time and effort. If endurance becomes a factor, patients should choose to perform some activities while receiving assistance for other skills that are too challenging or time-consuming.

Feeding

Patients with C1 to C4 tetraplegia are dependent in feeding but can verbalize this skill. Patients with C5 SCI with weak shoulders and biceps musculature require a dynamic orthosis to support the upper extremity during feeding. The most common orthoses used are the MAS[115,116] (Figure 16-19) and the offset feeder (Figure 16-20). Patients with low-level tetraplegia may not have weakness in the shoulder that would affect feeding, but they may have weak wrist function. Some of the dorsal wrist supports have a cuff built in that can be functional. The patient with no finger function can use a wrist-driven tenodesis brace for managing objects or to hold a feeding utensil (Figure 16-21). A universal cuff can be worn on the hand to hold feeding utensils (Figure 16-22, *A*). The patient with weak finger function can use built-up handles on the utensils. There are also commercially available and esthetically pleasing utensils such as those in Figure 16-22, *B*. Cutting can be difficult for patients without finger function.

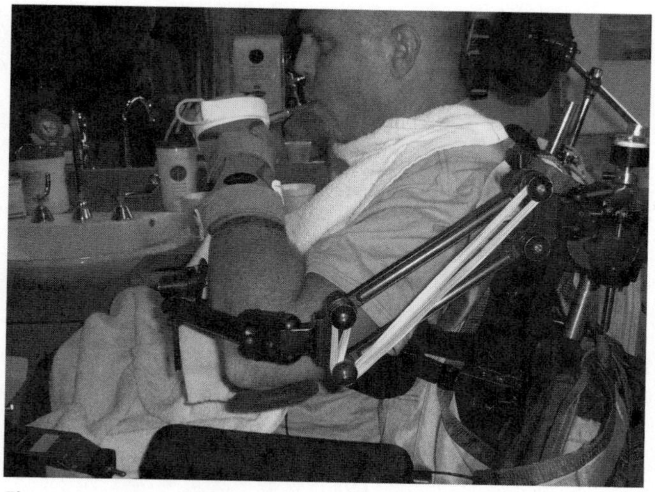

Figure 16-19 ■ Mobile arm support (MAS) used during feeding.

Grooming

The basic components of grooming are washing the face, combing or brushing the hair, performing oral care, shaving, and applying makeup. More advanced grooming activities may include nail care, donning and doffing of contact lenses, or other hygiene tasks specific to the individual. Individuals with C1 to C4 tetraplegia are dependent but can verbalize these skills. Patients with C5 injuries perform these skills with some assistance but may require orthotic devices, such as an MAS or offset feeder for shoulder support and a splint for wrist support. Patients with low-level tetraplegia may need cuffs or built-up grips on razors, brushes, and toothpaste to be independent (Figure 16-23). A proper bathroom setup for optimal wheelchair positioning is important for all patients. Patients with tetraplegia often rely on the support of the elbows as an assist, so sink height should be considered. The proper positioning and adaptive equipment will be the difference between independence and dependence in these skills (Figures 16-24 and 16-25).

Bathing

Bathing includes washing and rinsing the upper and lower extremities and the trunk. Patients with C1 to C4 tetraplegia are dependent in bathing but are instructed to verbalize this skill. Patients with C5 injury can range from requiring maximal assistance to being dependent in bathing. Patients with low-level tetraplegia bathe with moderate assistance to total independence with use of adaptive devices. Patients with paraplegia are typically independent in bathing but may need

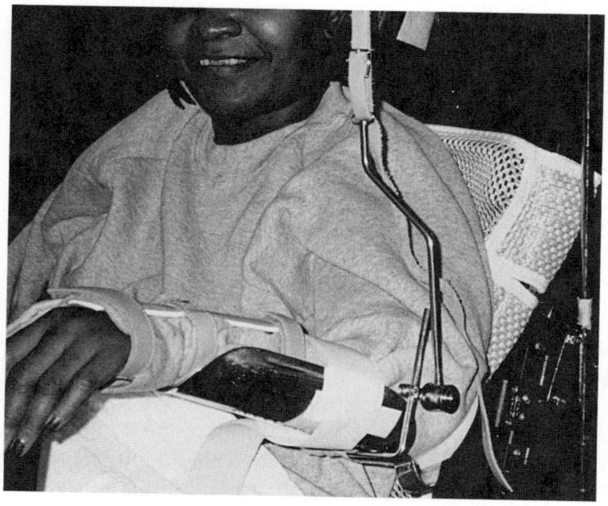

Figure 16-20 ■ Offset feeder orthosis.

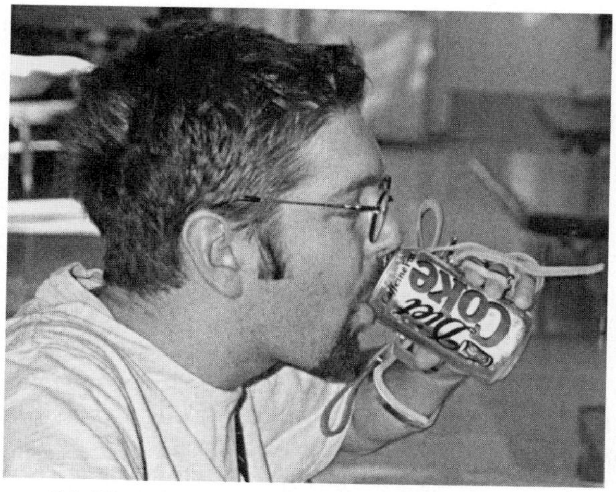

Figure 16-21 ■ Tenodesis braces have varying grasps. The largest grasp position allows the client to hold a soft drink can.

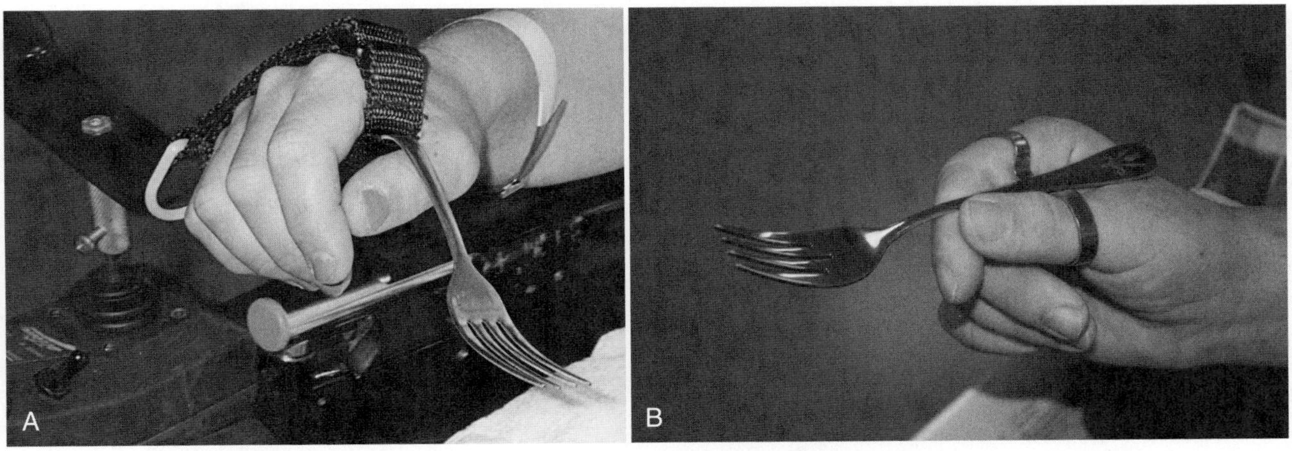

Figure 16-22 ■ **A,**Universal cuff used for feeding. **B,** Dining with Dignity is one commercially available type of flatware for individuals with impaired grip.

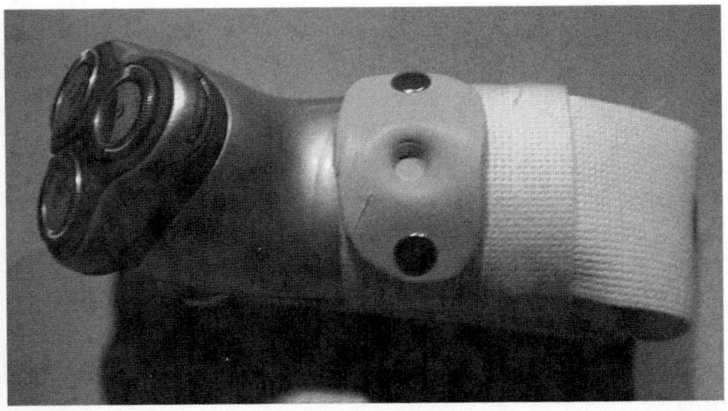

Figure 16-23 ■ Simple razor adaptation that helps turn razor on and off with a grosser motor movement.

adaptive devices. After examination of the patient's upper-extremity strength, balance, spasticity, body type, endurance, and home accessibility, the therapy team can determine the appropriate bathing equipment and setup for the patient (Figure 16-26). Patients with limited upper-extremity and trunk strength may need straps to assist with trunk support and adaptive cuffs to control the hand-held shower head. Basic bathing safety should be taught to all patients. Bathing safety includes checking the water temperature with a known area of intact sensation, skin checks before and after bathing, and skin protection during the transfers. These precautions are necessary to prevent burns and skin breakdown during the bathing process.

Dressing

Dressing includes dressing and undressing the upper and lower extremities with clothing that fits the patient's premorbid lifestyle. Patients with C1 to C5 tetraplegia are dependent,

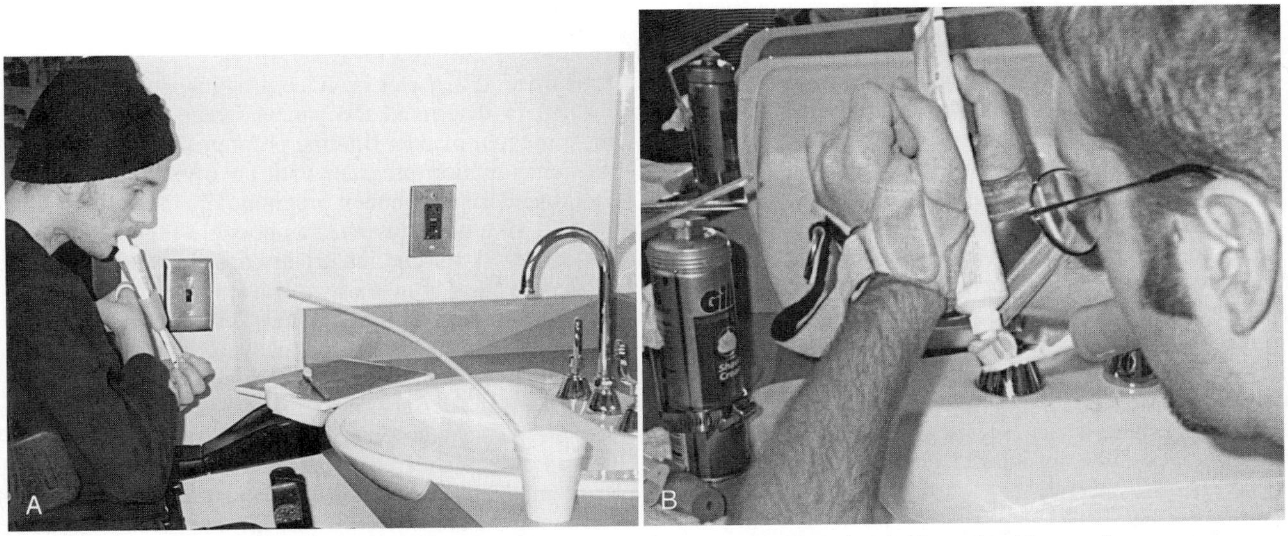

Figure 16-24 ■ **A,** A client with a C5 spinal cord injury is able to brush his teeth with use of a cuff, adapted long straw, and proper wheelchair positioning at the sink. **B,** Client with C6 spinal cord injury uses bilateral tenodesis to support toothpaste while holding a toothbrush in his mouth.

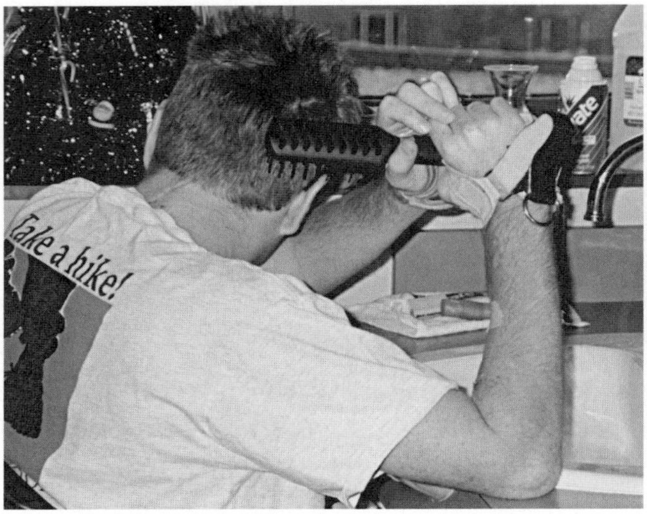

Figure 16-25 ■ Sink height can be important in assisting this client with C6 spinal cord injury to brush his hair.

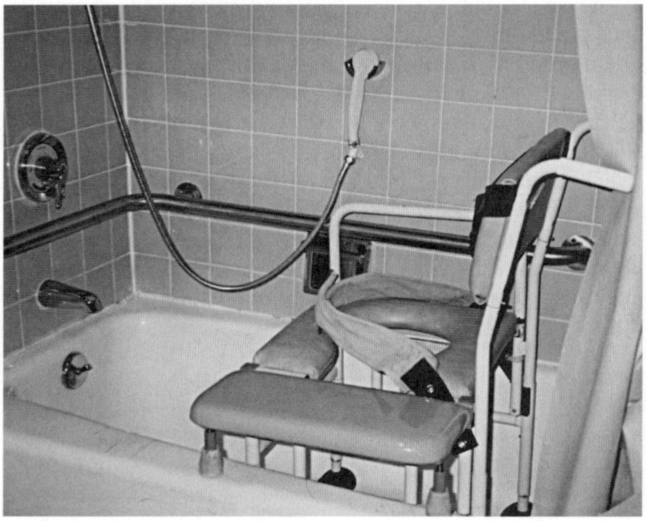

Figure 16-26 ■ Bathroom setup with shower or commode chair and hand-held shower head.

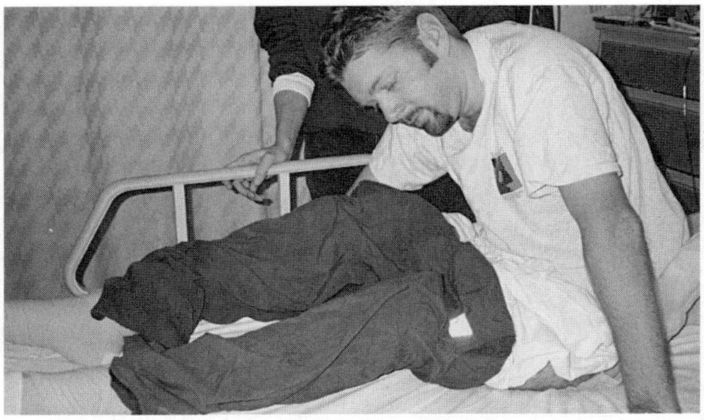

Figure 16-27 ■ Client with low-level tetraplegia maintains balance while performing lower-extremity dressing in bed.

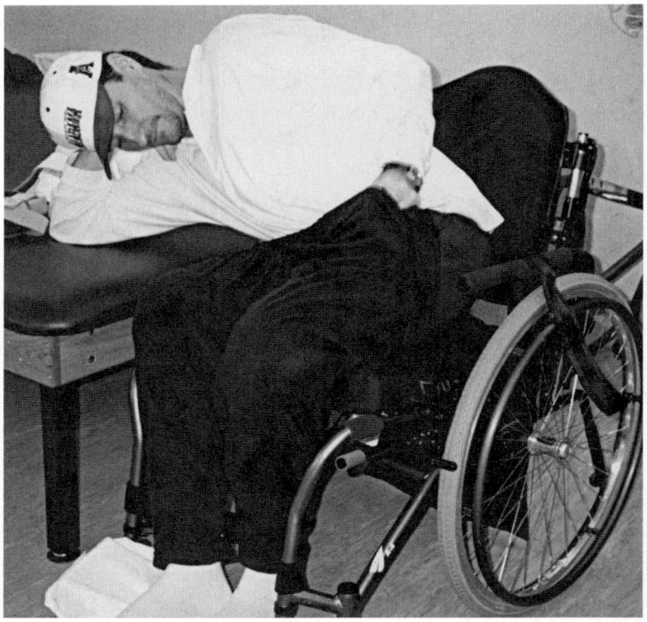

Figure 16-28 ■ Early practice when dressing in the wheelchair may involve leaning on a surface to assist with this skill.

but they can verbalize safe techniques to perform all the dressing skills. Independence in this skill for patients with low tetraplegic and paraplegic injuries may depend on where the skill is performed (e.g., mat, bed, or wheelchair). Patients with low-level tetraplegia can perform upper body dressing and undressing independently with equipment such as a button hook, hook and loop fasteners (Velcro), or adapted loops. Lower-body dressing is usually performed in bed (Figure 16-27) versus the wheelchair because of endurance, strength, and body type issues. Patients with paraplegia are expected to dress with total independence in the bed, but they may need equipment such as a leg lifter or a long-handled shoehorn for dressing in the wheelchair (Figure 16-28). This should be encouraged, if possible, for independence in the community.

Bladder Management

Bladder management includes determining and performing the bladder program, clothing management, body positioning, setup and cleanup of equipment, disposal of urine, and cleanup of self. Water or video urodynamic studies are performed to determine the patient's bladder status and the most optimal bladder training program. Patients often enter the rehabilitation program with an indwelling catheter as their bladder management program. The indwelling catheter should be removed as soon as possible because it puts the patient at risk for chronic urinary tract infections.[117]

On the basis of injury level, patients have either a reflexive bladder (upper motor neuron lesions) or an areflexive bladder (lower motor neuron lesions).[69] The reflexive bladder reflexively empties when the bladder is full. The therapeutic goals for managing the reflexive bladder include low-pressure voiding and low residual urine volumes. The nonreflexive bladder will not empty reflexively and needs to be manually emptied at regular intervals. The goals for managing the areflexive bladder include establishing a regular emptying schedule and continence between emptying. Management of an areflexive bladder includes performance of intermittent catheterizations.

Patients with C1 to C5 tetraplegia are typically dependent in their bladder programs. An automatic leg-bag emptier can assist with just the elimination component of the bladder skill; however, the patient will still be dependent in all of the other components of bladder management. Male patients with injuries at C6 level and below may be able to complete portions of the bladder management. Patients with limited hand function may need adaptive devices such as orthoses to assist with catheter insertion, adaptive scissors to open bladder packages, leg bags with flip-top openers, and leg bag loops (Figure 16-29). Female patients with paraplegia will most likely need to begin their training in bed with a mirror to obtain the most ideal position. Touch technique can be taught so they will not be reliant on a mirror if they have good finger sensation and use, and they may progress to using the touch technique in a wheelchair. Some people with SCI may decide to have a suprapubic catheter placed or a bladder augmentation procedure as a lifestyle choice.

Bowel Management

The goal of bowel management is to have the patient able to predictably induce regular elimination. As described under bladder management, the level of injury will assist in telling if the patient will have either a reflexive bowel or a nonreflexive bowel.[69] The bulbocavernosus reflex (BCR) is elicited by pinching the dorsal glans penis or by pressing the clitoris and palpating for bulbocavernosus and external anal sphincter contraction.[118] If the patient has a positive BCR, this is indicative of a reflexive bowel. With a reflexive bowel, tone of the internal and external anal sphincter is present although the patient will not feel the need to have a bowel movement. Voluntary anal contraction and relaxation are not possible, but the nerve connection between the colon and the spinal cord are still intact, allowing the patient to reflexively eliminate stool. This can be done with chemical or mechanical stimulation.[118]

Flaccid bowel programs are much more difficult to regulate because there is no internal or external anal sphincter tone. Timing and diet are critical for the success of this program. A suppository may be required to assist with the process, and in this situation the rectum should be emptied before suppository insertion.[119] If the established bowel program is not followed consistently, involuntary bowel movements or impaction may occur.

Bowel management training must begin as soon as the patient is medically stable. The components of bowel management include clothing management, body positioning, setup and cleanup of equipment, performance of the bowel program, disposal of feces, and cleanup of self. To establish the most effective bowel training program, the interdisciplinary team must work together. The team will need to discuss patient medications that may affect the bowels, the time of day when the patient plans to perform the program, the physical appropriateness related to scapular strength and endurance, and all equipment that will be used.

Patients with injury above the C6 level will be dependent in performing the bowel program; however, they should be independent in the verbalization of the technique. Patients with limited hand function (C6 to C7) may require a digital bowel stimulator and a suppository inserter with an adapted cuff or splint (Figure 16-30). In addition, a roll-in shower chair or upright shower or commode chair with a padded cutout in the seat will allow the patient to reach the buttock area to perform the stimulation. For this level of injury, it may be advantageous to perform the bowel program in conjunction with the shower to conserve energy with transfers. For individuals with paraplegia, full independence is expected for completion of all bowel management skills. These programs are typically performed on appropriate bathroom equipment or the bed.

To increase the effectiveness of the bowel program the patient should follow the guidelines identified in Box 16-2.

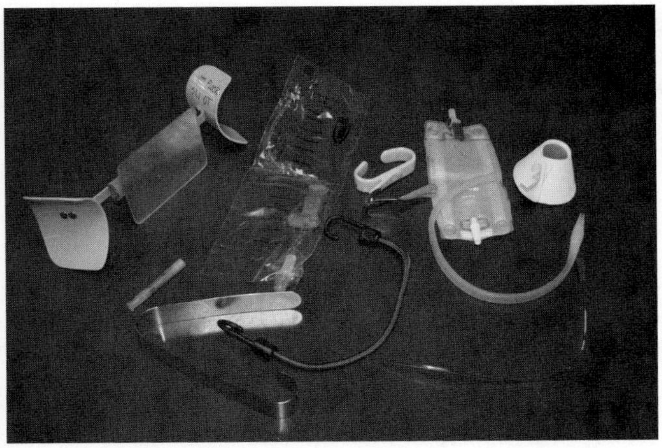

Figure 16-29 ■ Bladder management supplies may include knee spreader with mirror, sterile catheter kit, catheter inserter, leg bag with tubing and adapter, catheter, "HouseHold" for positioning, bungee cord to hold pants, pants holder, small prelubricated female catheter.

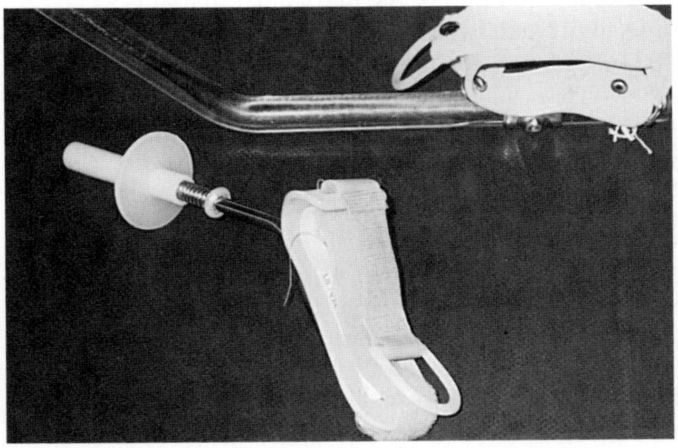

Figure 16-30 ■ Dil stick and suppository inserter with adaptive cuffs.

BOX 16-2 ■ GUIDELINES FOR BOWEL PROGRAM

1. Perform the bowel program at the same time each day.
2. Follow a diet high in fiber (25 to 35 g recommended).
3. Drink at least eight glasses of water per day.
4. Drink a hot liquid 30 minutes before initiating the bowel program.
5. Perform the bowel program in an upright position.
6. Consider premorbid bowel schedule.

Home Management

Home management may be divided into two components: light home management and heavy home management. Light home management includes managing money, preparing a snack in the kitchen, doing laundry, and making the bed. Heavy home management includes shopping for groceries, preparing a complex meal in the kitchen, dusting, and vacuuming. The clinician should discuss the role the patient would like to assume at home. The patient may want to resume previous home management roles or may want to discuss changing roles with a family member or caregiver to have energy for other skills.

Patients with C1 to C5 tetraplegia will be dependent in home management. Patients with limited or no hand function will need adaptive kitchen devices, adapted utensils, and adapted cleaning equipment. Preplanning activities may be essential for independent function with patients at all levels of injury. Patients with hand function may require extended handles on equipment and must incorporate energy conservation techniques.

Parenting

Research has shown the importance of parenting behavior and attitude on children's ability to adjust to various circumstances. This adjustment is not, however, affected by the disability status of a parent.[120,121] Patients with C1 to C5 tetraplegia may be dependent in the physical aspects of parenting. Patients with low-level tetraplegia may be able to participate in the more physical aspects of parenting with some level of adaptations such as a wheelchair-accessible table with sides to change an infant.[122] Parenting skills for a patient with paraplegia would depend on the environment and the specific activity being performed as well as the mobility of the individual. Therapists can provide advice and ideas to assist with selection of parenting and baby equipment as well as be a resource in discussing and adapting equipment options such as slide-down cribs, adjustable-height high chairs, carrying slings or supports, and baby strollers that can be more easily pushed with one hand.[122,123]

Assistive Technology

AT can be helpful in letting people resume more independent lives in areas of self-care, work, and recreation. AT is defined by the 1998 Technology-Related Assistance for Individuals with Disabilities Act (Public Law 105-394). It defines AT devices as "any item, piece of equipment, or product system, whether acquired commercially, modified, or customized, that is used to increase, maintain, or improve functional capabilities of individuals with disabilities." Hedrick and colleagues[124] found that in both civilians and veterans the most frequently used AT devices were (1) manual mobility and independent living devices (e.g., manual wheelchairs, manual exercise equipment, manual motor vehicle control devices such as a steering knob, walkers, reachers); (2) powered mobility and independent living devices (e.g., power lifts, power doors, motorized wheelchairs, power-assisted motor vehicle operation devices); (3) prosthetics and orthotics (static and dynamic, such as splints, mentioned earlier); (4) alternative computer access devices, which may be as simple as a typing splint to as complex as brain control; and (5) speech-generating devices (SGDs) formerly known as *augmentative and alternative communication devices.*

Many specialty facilities that treat large numbers of SCI patients will have specialized therapists called Assistive Technology Practitioners (ATPs) and/or AT departments to specifically assess, select, and train in the use of device(s)—specifically seating, driving, and electronic access. Seating departments will evaluate and prescribe customized manual or powered mobility seating systems. This is essential as professionals struggle to assist the patient with reimbursement for the mobility devices as well as the always-changing technology. Not everyone has access to someone with this specialized certification; thus consideration should be given by the therapist in the evaluation phase to include where the patient will use the chair and how it will get there, looking at the "big picture" rather than only the mobility device. For example, how will the wheelchair be transported? Can the wheelchair be locked down so the patient may drive in a van or be a dependent passenger? Can the patient load the manual chair into his or her car (Figure 16-31)? There are specially trained practitioners called *driving rehabilitation specialists* who specialize in recommending equipment and transportation of the patient as a passenger in addition to providing driver education and driver training. They help to evaluate and to assist with making correct vehicle modifications and adaptive equipment choices for the patient as a driver. There are over 600 specialists in the United States represented in each of the 50 states. A professional can be found on the Association for Driver Rehabilitation Specialists (ADED) website (www.drivers-ed.org).[125] When considering a sedan, these specialists will evaluate the patient to see how he or she operates primary and secondary vehicle controls, opens and closes the door, transfers into the vehicle, and stores, secures, and retrieves the wheelchair. If the patient is unable to perform any of those tasks then a van may be an option. Modifications can allow a person to transfer to the van's driver seat or to drive from the wheelchair. The driving control technology that is available to compensate for reduced strength or ROM includes steering systems, hand controls, and reduced effort and zero effort steering and braking. The rehabilitation specialist will provide a comprehensive evaluation to determine the patient's ability to drive. That evaluation will consider visual, perceptual, and functional abilities as well as reaction time and behind-the-wheel assessment. In both sedan and van selection, it is always best to recommend that the patient consult the driving rehabilitation specialist before purchasing and modifying the vehicle.

In this day of ever-changing technology, the patient may need assistance to access many electronic devices, such as computers, televisions, lights, call systems, personal digital assistants (PDAs), cell phones, music systems, or digital readers or the not-yet-invented device that will be coming on the market in the future. Dexterity is required to operate many standard devices such as computers. There are many "off-the-shelf" adaptations using universal designs to enable persons with limited dexterity to use a computer. A person with a higher tetraplegic level of injury can use alternative methods to access a computer, such as a microphone with speech recognition software, pneumatic controls (sip-and-puff devices), or an eye gaze system. The most popular and inexpensive way to access a computer is speech recognition

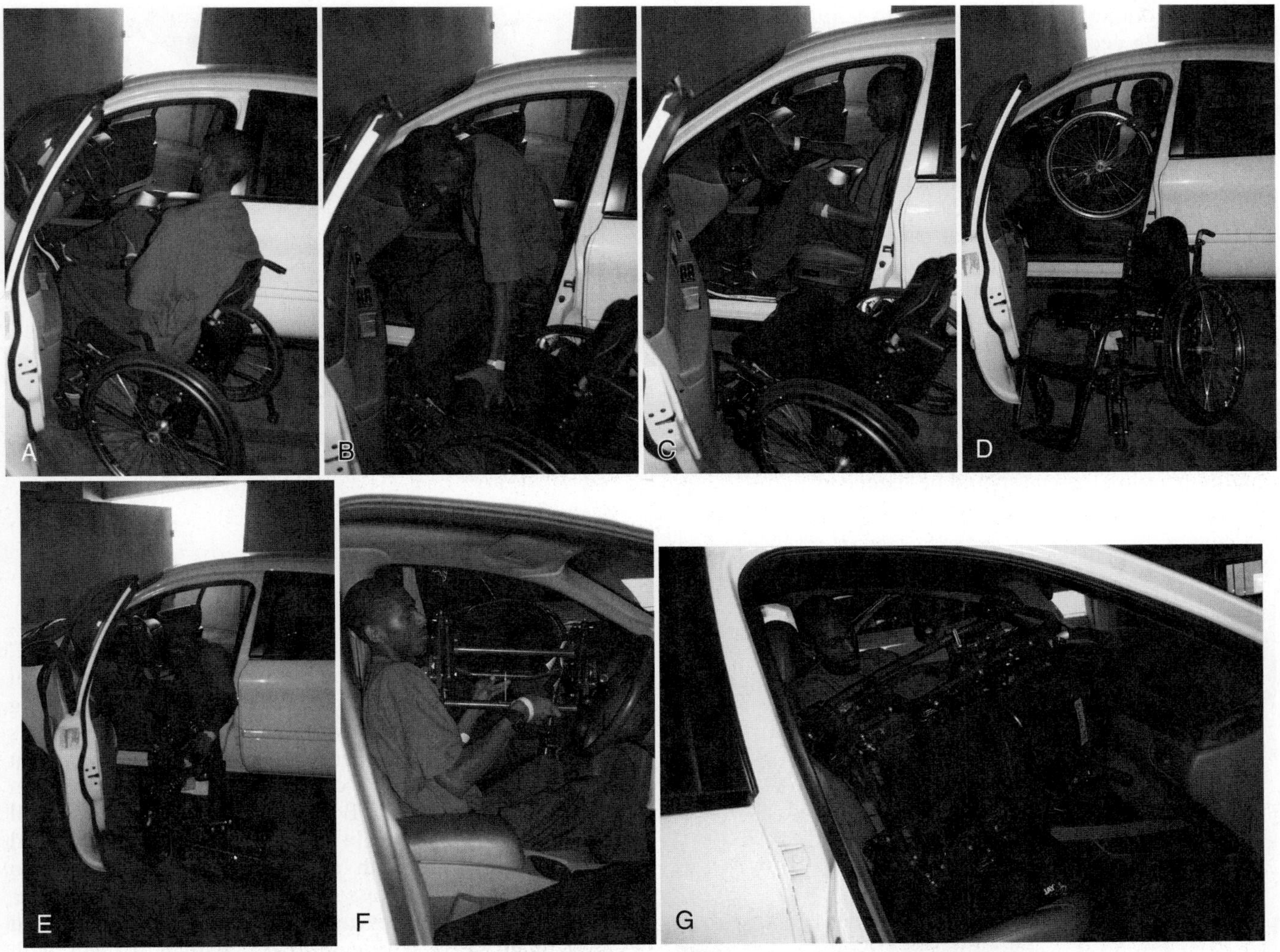

Figure 16-31 ■ Car transfer. Most patients with a paraplegic level of injury are modified independent (FIM level 6) in the performance of a car transfer. The patient approaches the car on the driver's side and opens the door. **A,** After stabilizing the wheelchair, he may place his foot or feet into the car or leave them on the footrest or the ground. **B,** He performs a depression-style transfer onto the seat of the car; **C,** positions his lower extremities appropriately inside the car; and **D,** prepares to get the wheelchair into the car by removing the wheels (quick release) and cushion and placing these on the floor in the front passenger area or in the back seat. **E** to **G,** The rigid model of wheelchair is folded and transferred across the patient onto the passenger seat. Transferring out of the car is the reverse process, beginning with getting the wheelchair out of the car and reassembling it.

software. However, the computer-brain interface is a newer technology currently in clinical trials and uses intact brain function to address these needs. In recent years computer companies have been more sensitive to the population with disabilities. The operating systems have adjustments that make the keyboard easier to use, referred to as *Ease of Access* or *Universal Access features.* These are very helpful for someone who may be entering commands with a single point such as a mouth stick or a pointer on only one hand. This adjustment can change how the keyboard works or can provide an on-screen keyboard. There are shortcuts that allow the patient to do everything with the keyboard, thus eliminating a mouse, which may be difficult for a mouth stick user. Many of these keyboard commands are not needed if the individual uses an already built-in speech recognition program or purchases one. There are detailed tutorials on both the Microsoft and the Apple websites. Manufacturers do not always consider how persons needing adaptations will access their device. Cell phones and all commercial Bluetooth technology still requires some touch to activate; however, some vendors have made modifications available, although they are expensive. Surface touch screens are not disability friendly, and many phones and music systems use that technology. The therapist's role is to help assess, decide, and adapt how the access should be achieved for the patient, taking advantage of whatever the patient has to use. EADLs such as call systems or computer systems can be adapted using pneumatic controls (sip-and-puff devices) or voice-activated controls for independence from the bed and the wheelchair. There are switches that can be activated with head or eye control, allowing patients with little movement the ability to communicate. Patients with C3 to C4 injuries, depending on neck strength and ROM, can use lower-tech equipment such as mouth sticks for pushing cell phone buttons from the wheelchair in addition to the head rest buttons or a sip-and-puff switch (Figure 16-32). Patients with C5 injuries begin to use their biceps, deltoids, and internal and external rotator strength to interact with their environment. Positioning of the buttons, devices, or mounts for devices is important for these patients, who may or may not be using an MAS. Adaptive splinting for support at the wrist can allow these patients to use their upper arms in writing, typing, turning pages, and using computers (Figure 16-33). Patients with wrist function but no finger function can use utensil holders with a pointer to "dial" a phone number, for example, or can use their natural tenodesis to grasp and manipulate objects (Figure 16-34). For injuries at the T1 level and below, interaction with the environment in all areas should be independent.

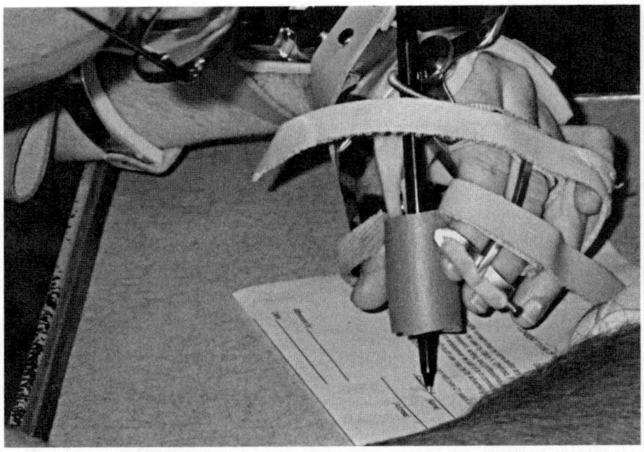

Figure 16-34 ■ Tenodesis brace writing by use of a pen with a built-up grip.

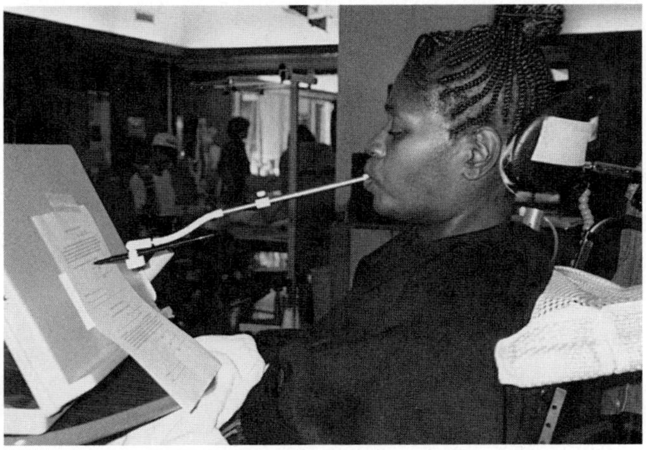

Figure 16-32 ■ Mouth stick writing can be accomplished with the client upright in the wheelchair and with the support of a bedside table and bookstand.

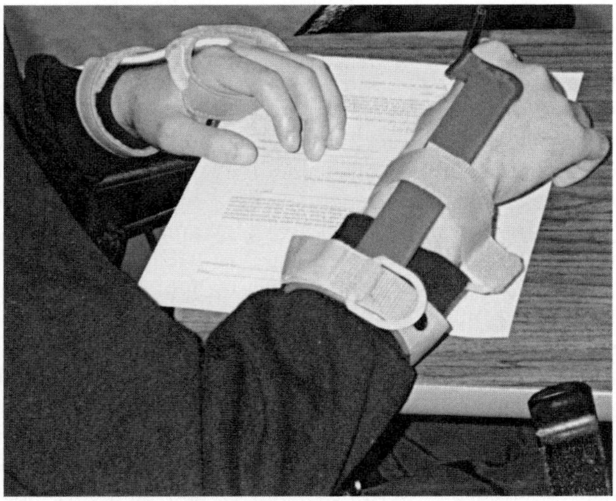

Figure 16-33 ■ Long Wanchick writing device.

Mobility

Bed Mobility and Coming to Sit

The components of bed mobility include rolling side to side, rolling supine to prone, coming to sit, and scooting in all directions while either long or short sitting. Initial training for bed mobility is usually conducted on the mat, as it is easier to learn on the firmer surface. When skills on the mat are mastered, the patient can be progressed to a less firm surface, such as the bed. Bed mobility is a challenging skill for clients with tetraplegia to learn because of their limited upper-extremity strength (Figure 16-35, *A* to *C*).[7,62] To accommodate for the loss of upper-extremity musculature, compensatory strategies and assistive devices, such as bed loops, may be used (Figure 16-35, *F* to *I*). Clients with paraplegia often master bed mobility skills quickly and much more easily than clients with tetraplegia because of their intact upper-extremity musculature.

Pressure Relief in the Upright Position

The client with high tetraplegia achieves independent pressure relief in the wheelchair through appropriately prescribed specialty controls. For example, a pneumatic control switch may be used to activate the recline mode of a power wheelchair (Figure 16-36). When the client is unable to operate a specialty switch, an attendant control may be used. When powered options are not feasible because of cognitive deficits, financial limitations, or other reasons, a manual recliner (Figure 16-37) or tilt wheelchair is used. When clients are dependent in performing pressure relief, they can be taught to instruct others in this skill. Clients with mid- and low-level tetraplegia are taught to perform a side or forward lean technique for pressure relief if the strength of the shoulder musculature is appropriate (Figure 16-38). The client with paraplegia is usually taught to perform a pushup (depression) for pressure relief (Figure 16-39).

The appropriate time to maintain the change in position is usually 60 seconds at intervals of 30 to 60 minutes. The treatment plan should include instructing the client in ways to ensure that the schedule for pressure relief is maintained in all settings. The use of watches, clocks, timers, and attendant care may be necessary.

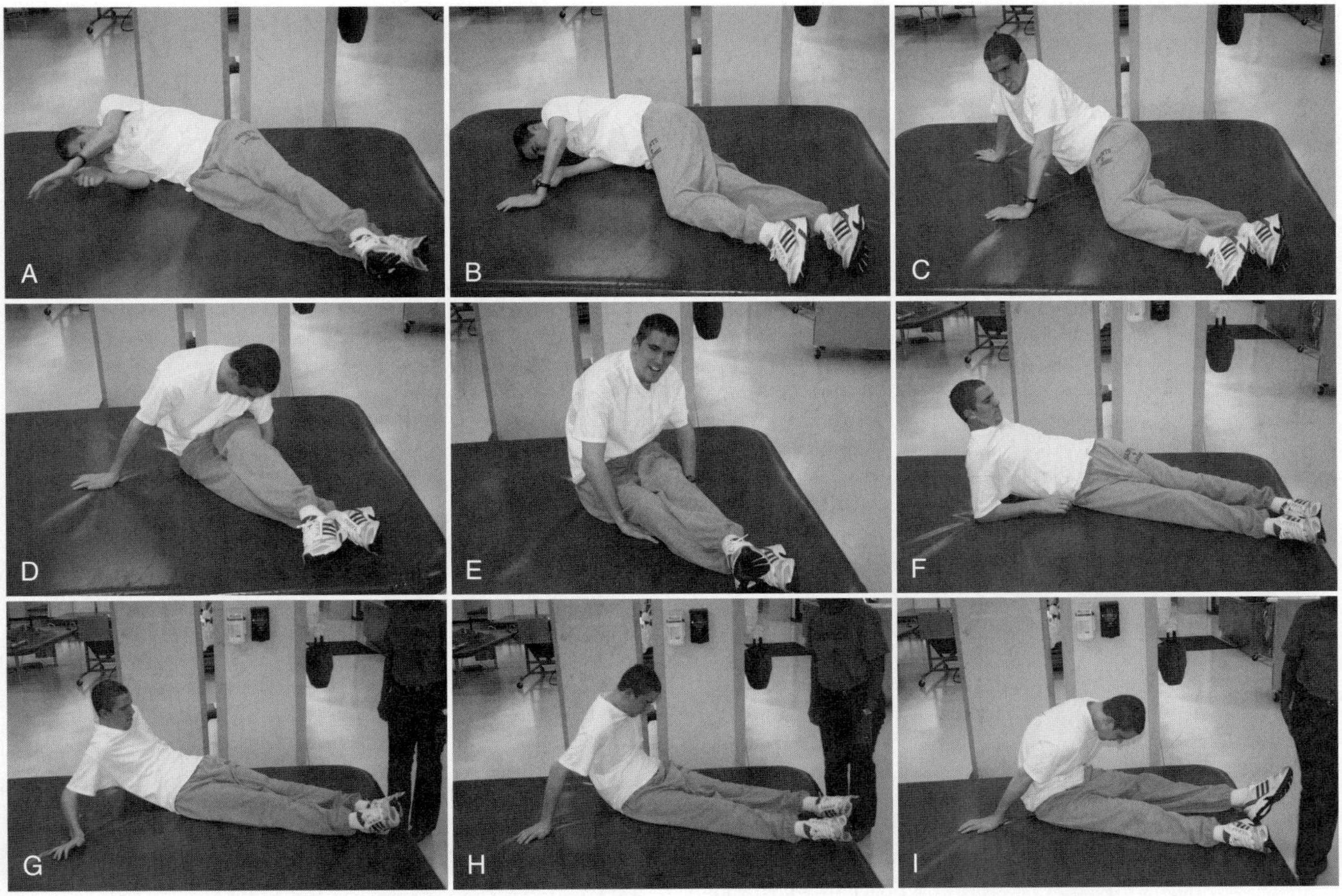

Figure 16-35 ■ Bed mobility and coming to sit. **A,** The patient rolls from supine to side-lying position. **B,** He progresses to supporting his weight through the downside elbow and shoulder. **C,** He pushes up onto extended arms. **D,** While shifting his weight onto the left arm, he unweights the right arm and hooks his right hand behind his right knee, gaining enough leverage to push and pull himself toward upright in a long sitting position. **E,** He continues to shift his weight to the right until he gains a balanced sitting position with his weight forward over his extended legs. Supine to sitting: **F** and **G,** Starting from a supine position on a bed or a mat, the arms are extended and the hands positioned under the buttock or in the curve of the back (lumbar spine); the head is lifted; and leverage is used to pull up until the upper body weight is supported on bilateral elbows. **H,** The weight is shifted from right to left or vice versa, and the elbows are extended to support the upper body weight. **I,** While the elbows are kept extended, the hands are carefully walked forward until balanced long sitting has been achieved.

Wheelchair Transfers

The physical act of moving oneself from one surface to another is described as a *transfer.* Wheelchair transfers may be accomplished in many different ways. The type of transfer used by a client is determined by the injury level, assistance needed, client preference, and safety of the transfer. When performing transfers, both the client and the person assisting must give attention to the use of appropriate body mechanics.

Dependent transfers may be accomplished with an electric (power) lift, hydraulic lift, manual pivot, transfer board, or manual lifts, which may require two or three people. A transfer with an overhead power lift is the least physically challenging on the part of the caregiver; however, these lifts are costly and are not easily transportable. The use of a hydraulic lift may be desirable if funding is not available for a power lift or the transfer needs to be done in an outdoor environment (i.e., car transfer). However, the hydraulic lift may not be the method of choice because the lift is bulky, difficult to store, and awkward to transport. Pivot transfers or manual lifts may be used because of client or caregiver preference or when clients are smaller in stature and when other, more costly lift systems are not available to the individuals.

Transfers can be performed with the use of a transfer board, depression-style, or via the stand or squat and pivot method. The mechanics of teaching an assisted transfer to a client with C7 tetraplegia is depicted in Figure 16-40. The client is taught to position the wheelchair, position the transfer board, use correct body mechanics to get the best leverage to effect movement in the desired direction, remove the board, and position his or her body appropriately.[7,62]

Wheelchair transfers are performed on many different surfaces. The training procedure begins with the easiest transfer and progresses to the more difficult transfer. Instructions

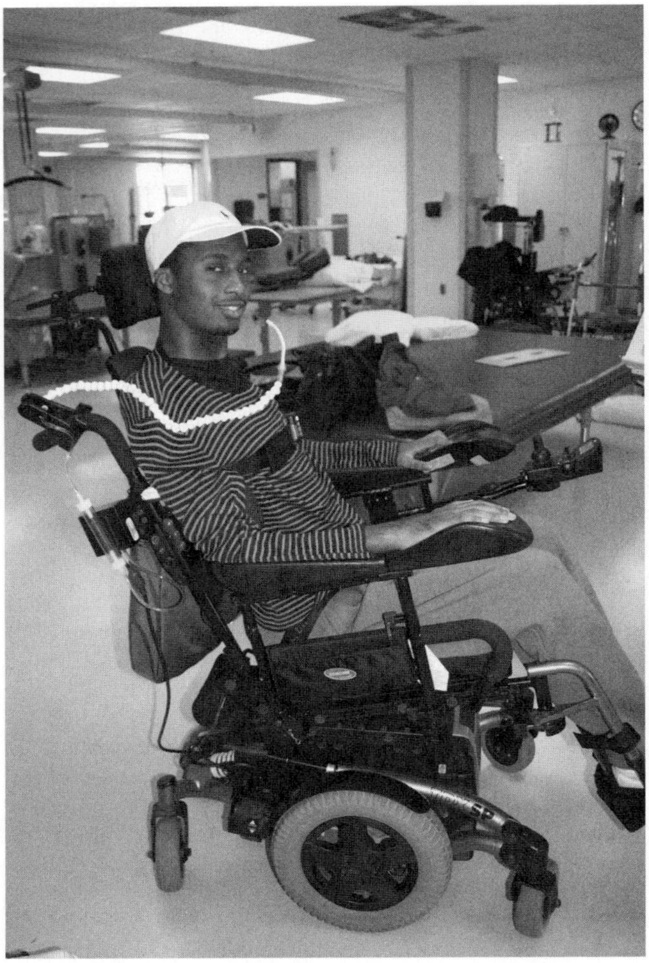

Figure 16-36 ■ The pneumatic control (sip-and-puff straw) is usually ordered on a power reclining or tilt-in-space wheelchair for patients with injury levels above C6. The straw is removable, and several are supplied with the wheelchair. The straw is attached to a flexible arm, and it is adjustable to different heights and angles to fit the needs of the patient.

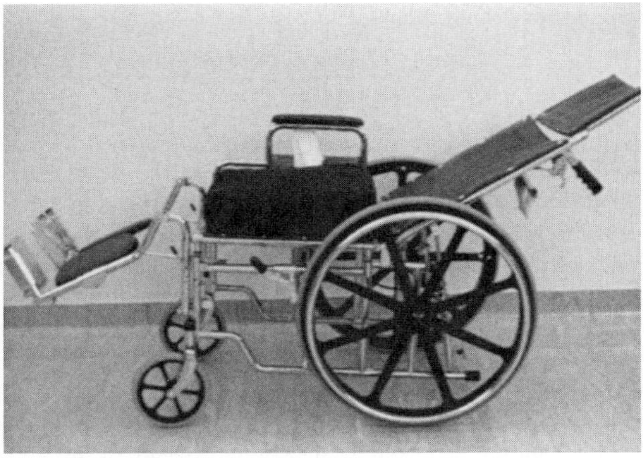

Figure 16-37 ■ The manual reclining wheelchair is a piece of durable medical equipment that is prescribed on a temporary or a permanent basis. The back of the wheelchair fully reclines, and the legrests elevate to allow for effective pressure relief while the client is out of bed. Other features of the wheelchair are desk armrests, which may be adjustable in height; a removable headrest; and removable legrests. The wheelchair folds and may be transported in a vehicle.

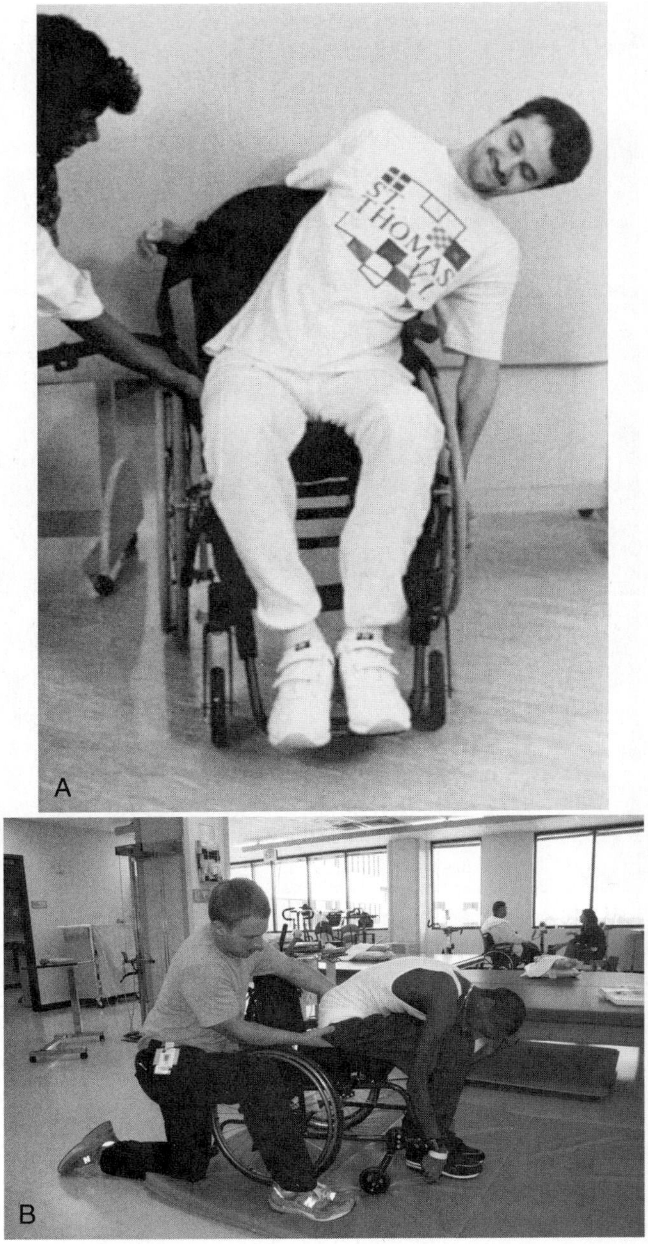

Figure 16-38 ■ **A,** Pressure relief: side lean. The tetraplegic patient with C6- to C7-level injury may use a side lean to achieve pressure relief over the ischial tuberosities. The patient hooks one upper extremity around the push handle of the wheelchair on one side and leans away from the hooked upper extremity until the ischium on the hooked side is clear of the wheelchair cushion. The position is maintained for 1 minute and repeated on the other side. **B,** Pressure relief: forward lean. The forward lean method of pressure relief is used for many different injury levels. The subject must have adequate range of motion at the hips and in the lumbosacral spine to allow the ischia to clear the wheelchair cushion at the end range position.

for wheelchair transfers usually begin on level surfaces and progress to uneven surfaces as individual strength and skill allow.[7,62] Given these two principles, the following list is an example of how one might proceed with transfer training:

1. Mat transfer (see Figure 16-40)
2. Bed transfer

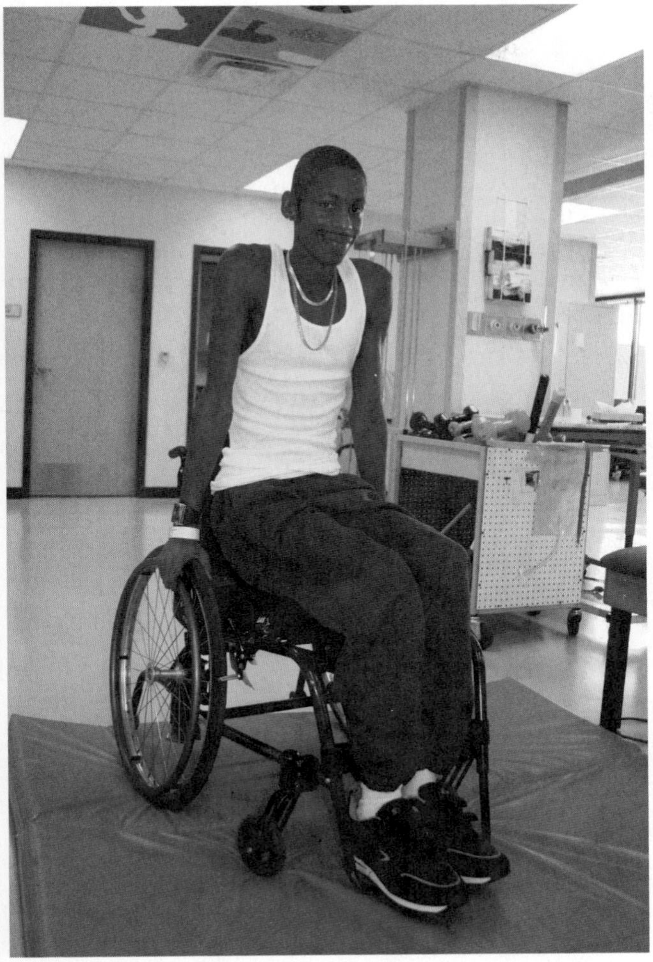

Figure 16-39 ■ Pressure relief: depression. This method of pressure relief is consistent with a full pushup in the wheelchair. Most patients with a paraplegic level of injury and some patients with a low tetraplegic injury level are able to perform this method of pressure relief.

3. Toilet transfer
4. Bath transfer
5. Car transfer (see Figure 16-31)
6. Floor transfer (Figures 16-41 to 16-43)
7. Other surfaces (e.g., armchair, sofa, theater seat, pool)

Wheelchair Mobility Skills

Instructions in the safe and appropriate use of the wheelchair may begin before getting the client out of bed by orienting the client to the wheelchair and its component parts.

Ideally, a power reclining or tilt wheelchair is supplied for clients with C1 to C5 tetraplegia to promote maximal independence. The most common drive-system options available for these clients include, but is not limited to, chin drive, pneumatic systems (see Figure 16-36), and head control (Figure 16-44). A client with mid- to low-level tetraplegia may be instructed in the use of both power and manual upright wheelchairs. The client with paraplegia is instructed in the use of a manual upright wheelchair unless there are extenuating circumstances. For example, a power wheelchair is appropriate for a client who is 50 years old and has severe rheumatoid arthritis.

A newer wheelchair that combines the benefits of a manual wheelchair with a power wheelchair is the pushrim-assisted power assist wheelchair (Figure 16-45).[126] This wheelchair may be best suited for clients who have some upper-extremity weakness, joint degeneration, upper-extremity pain from propelling a manual wheelchair, or reduced exercise capacity or endurance. This type of wheelchair could potentially delay secondary injuries of manual wheelchair users.[127] Both power and manual wheelchair mobility training begins on level surfaces. When a client is instructed on how to propel a manual wheelchair, it is suggested that a semicircular pattern be used to reduce the trauma to the upper extremities.[127] Wheelchair gloves are beneficial in reducing friction over the palms of the hands during propulsion (Figure 16-46). Research evidence is available that demonstrates the safety and superior efficacy of a formal approach to wheelchair skills training of wheelchair users and their caregivers. The Wheelchair Skills Program (WSP) is one example of such a program and is available free on the Internet.[128] This program includes useful evaluation and training tools to help practitioners translate this research evidence into clinical practice.[129]

Training progresses toward more difficult skills as follows:

1. Mobility on level surfaces in open areas
2. Setup for transfers
3. Mobility in tight spaces
4. Mobility in crowded areas
5. On and off elevators
6. Up and down ramps
7. Through doors
8. Wheelies (Figure 16-47)
9. Negotiation of rough terrain
10. Up and down curbs and steps (Figures 16-48 and 16-49)

Ambulation Considerations—Orthotic Disposition

"Will I ever walk again?" is a question often asked during SCI rehabilitation. The team must be empathetic toward and acknowledge the client's goals for ambulation, and the subject should be discussed openly. The professionals involved in the care of the patient must be careful not to take hope away from the client. Hope is important to maintain positive survival skills in SCI rehabilitation.

When ambulation is an appropriate goal, the treatment program may be short and relatively uncomplicated for some and extremely laborious for others. Treatment techniques may include therapeutic exercise, biofeedback, neuromuscular stimulation, locomotor training (discussed later in this chapter), balance training, standing, and various other pregait and gait activities. The clinician must consider the postdischarge environment and include those surfaces in training.

The walking disposition of patients with incomplete SCI is challenging owing to the complexity of problems and varying degrees of impairment. These patients may have pain, ROM limitations, ventilator pump dysfunction, weakness, and spasticity, as well as sensory and balance dysfunction. In addition, their premorbid physical condition must be considered. Musculoskeletal asymmetries, such as muscle shortening on the stronger side and lengthening on the weaker side, may lead to pelvic obliquity and scoliosis. A team approach to orthotic prescription is desirable to meet the needs of patients with incomplete SCI. Even if

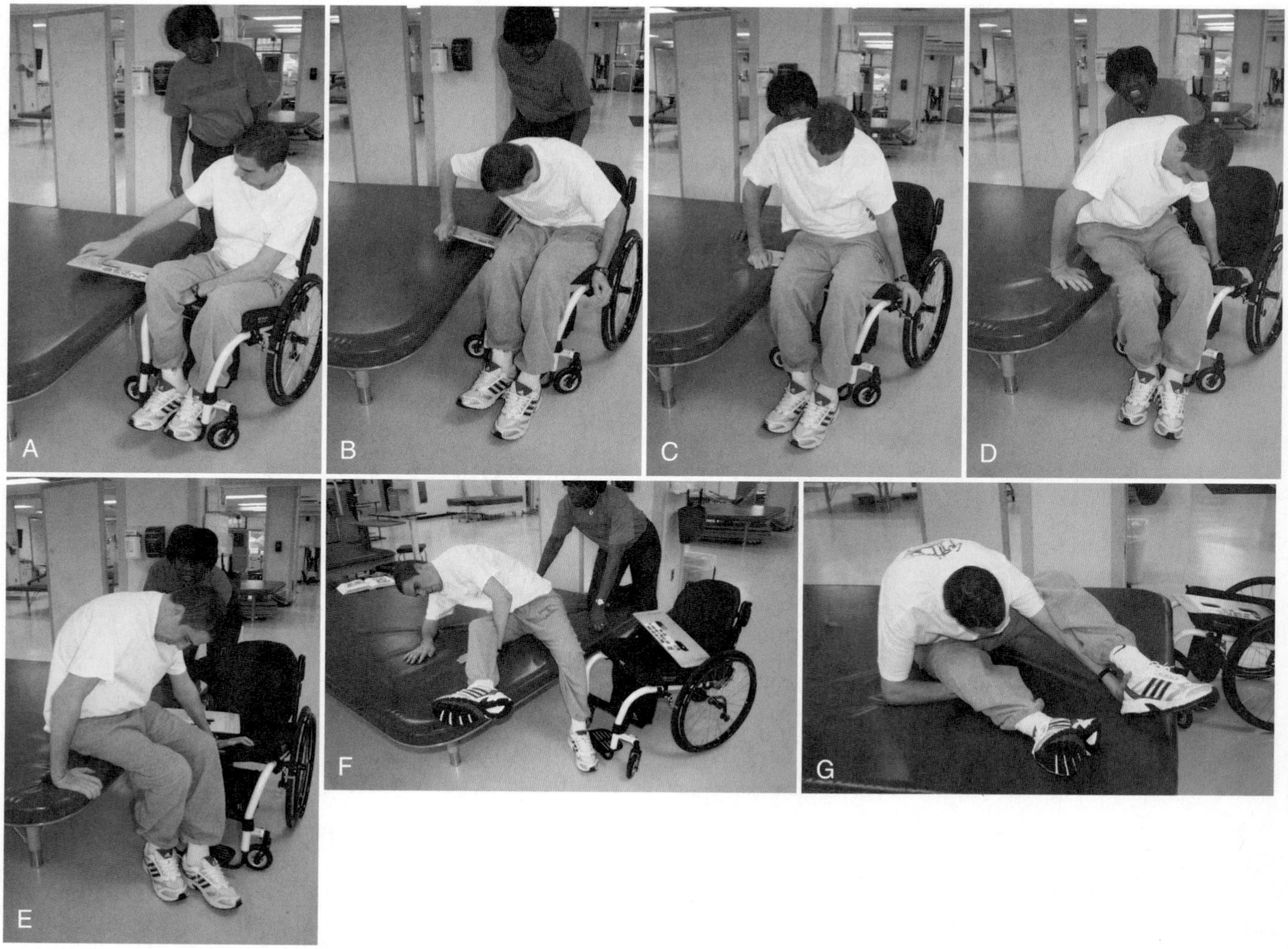

Figure 16-40 ■ Wheelchair to mat transfer using a transfer board. **A,** The patient positions the wheelchair at a 20- to 30-degree angle to the surface to which he is transferring and positions the board with or without assistance. **B,** The patient moves forward in the wheelchair to clear the tire in preparation for lateral movement on the transfer board. **C,** To achieve the appropriate mechanical leverage, the patient is instructed to twist the upper body and look over the trailing shoulder (**D**). He pushes and lifts to effect movement across the board. **E,** When the client has achieved a safe position on the transferring surface, the transfer board is removed. **F** and **G,** The patient is helped to get his feet onto the surface.

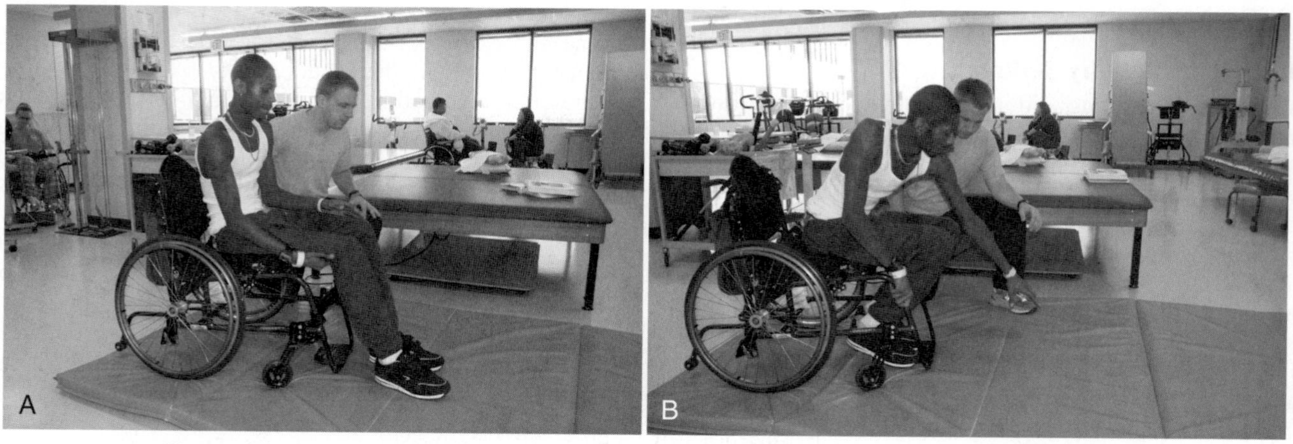

Figure 16-41 ■ Floor transfer. The independent performance of a floor transfer is a goal for most patients who have a paraplegic level of injury. The patient may use different techniques to get onto the floor. Forward floor transfer: **A,** The patient positions his feet off the footrest and moves forward onto the front edge of his cushion. **B,** He reaches for the floor, first with one hand then with both, and

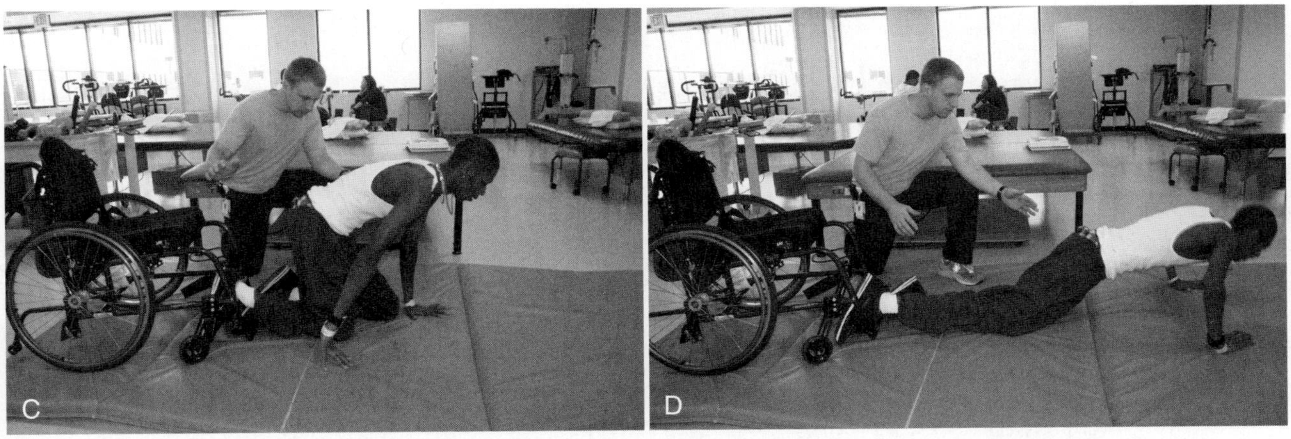

Figure 16-41, cont'd **C,** lowers his knees to the floor. **D,** He advances his hands forward until his body is clear of the wheelchair.

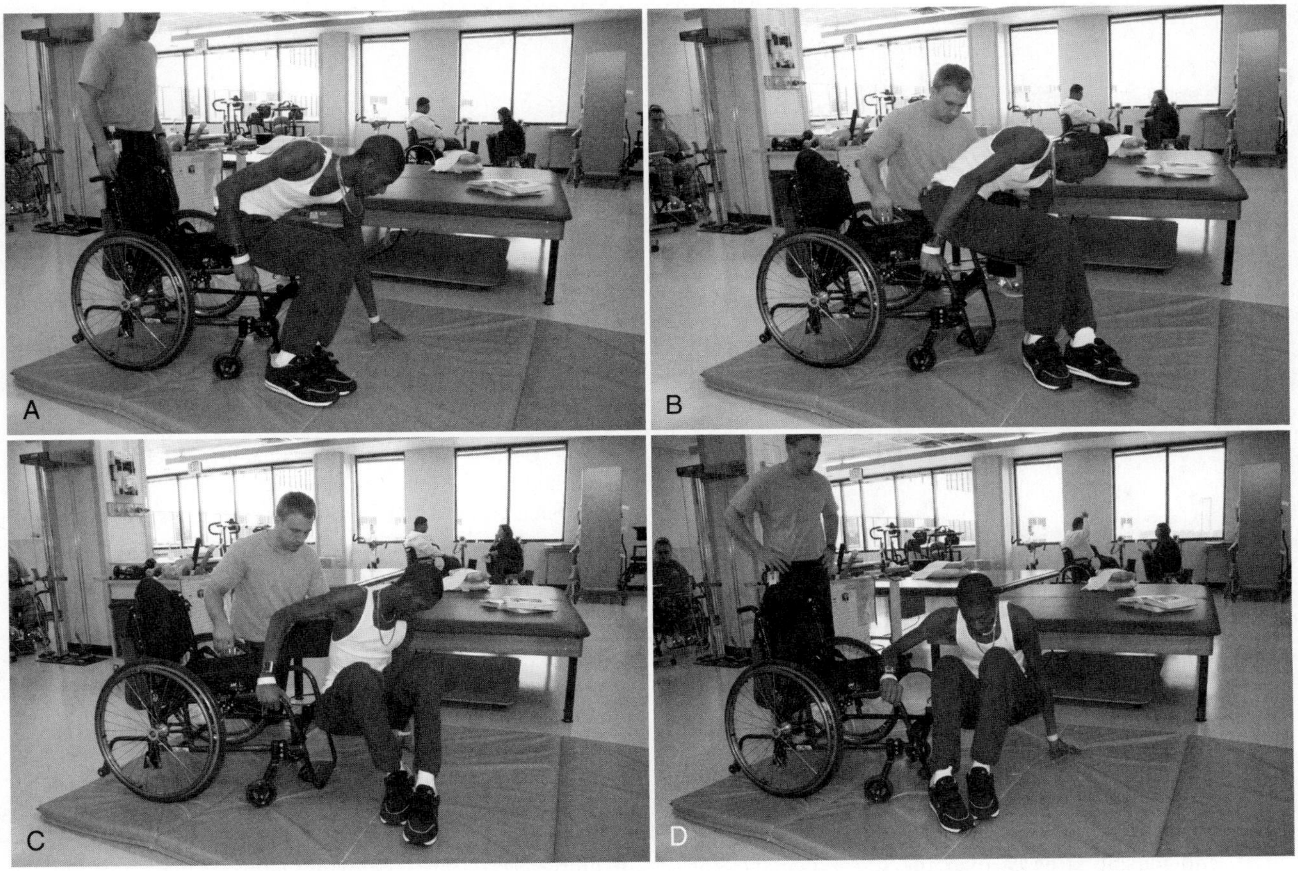

Figure 16-42 ■ Floor transfer sideways. After moving to the front of the wheelchair seat, **(A)** the patient leans to the left and reaches for the floor and **(B)** shifts his weight toward the left arm. **C** and **D,** He balances his weight between both arms and in a very controlled manner lowers his body to the floor.

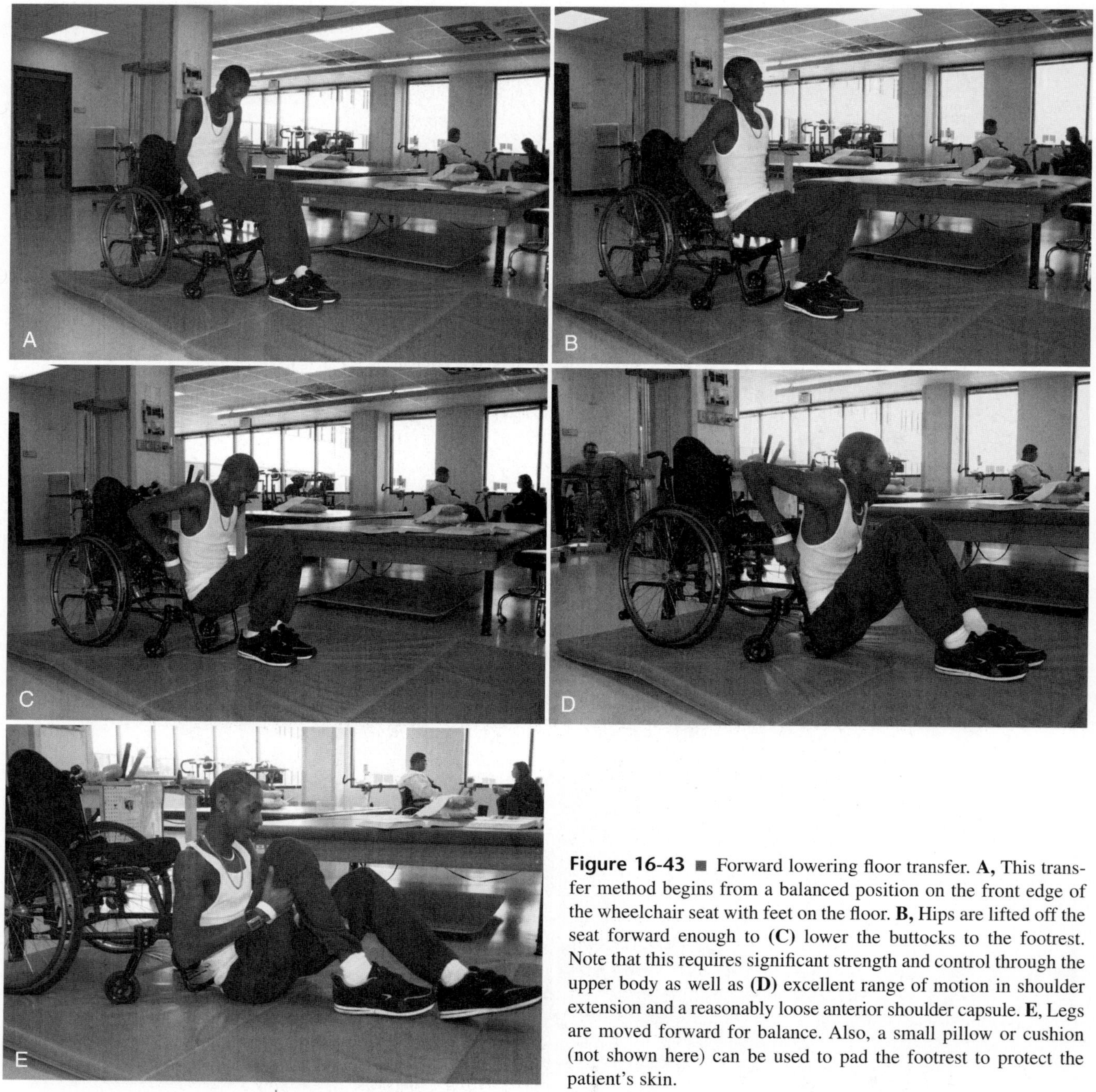

Figure 16-43 ■ Forward lowering floor transfer. **A,** This transfer method begins from a balanced position on the front edge of the wheelchair seat with feet on the floor. **B,** Hips are lifted off the seat forward enough to **(C)** lower the buttocks to the footrest. Note that this requires significant strength and control through the upper body as well as **(D)** excellent range of motion in shoulder extension and a reasonably loose anterior shoulder capsule. **E,** Legs are moved forward for balance. Also, a small pillow or cushion (not shown here) can be used to pad the footrest to protect the patient's skin.

orthotic devices enable these patients to become independent with standing or walking, the energy costs, joint deterioration, and muscle stresses over the life expectancy of each individual need to be considered. Orthotic prescription should be approached systematically. The patient's goals, funding, premorbid and current health status, social support, and the environment to which they are returning should be considered. A basic clinical algorithm for the selection of orthoses for persons with neurological impairment has been proposed by researchers at Rancho Los Amigos Medical Center. This algorithm is referred to as the Rancho ROADMAP (Recommendations for Orthotic Assessment, Decision-Making, and Prescription).[130] Successful brace prescription uses the minimum amount of bracing to achieve the maximum amount of function. It also anticipates changes in each patient's clinical picture. For example, braces may be manufactured with joints built into the plastic, or joints that begin as fixed, and are later cut to allow articulation. Some models of knee-ankle-foot orthoses (KAFOs) can be altered to become ankle-foot orthoses (AFOs).[131]

The philosophy regarding the use of orthoses for ambulation for individuals with complete paraplegia varies greatly among rehabilitation centers. Some facilities encourage ambulation for these individuals, whereas others strongly discourage it, given that only a small percentage of these clients continue to use orthotics after training has been completed.[132,133]

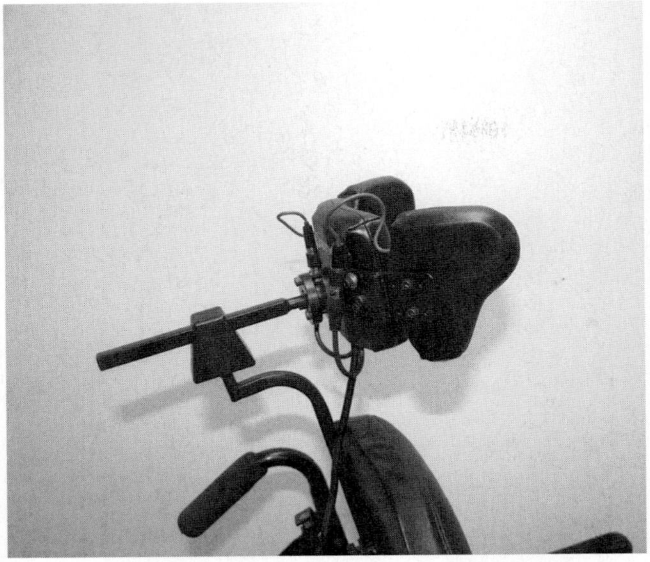

Figure 16-44 ■ Head array is a headrest and head control for driving wherein the position of the head activates the drive control of the wheelchair. It is appropriate for persons with high cervical injuries. The head array switches can be adjusted to the individual's specific needs relative to their active range of motion and control of their head. The switches are embedded in the headrest panels and not only control driving but can also control activation of other devices for environmental control. The side panels of the headrest can be straight or curbed depending on the needs of the patient. Additionally, the head array can be sized for either adult or pediatric patient.

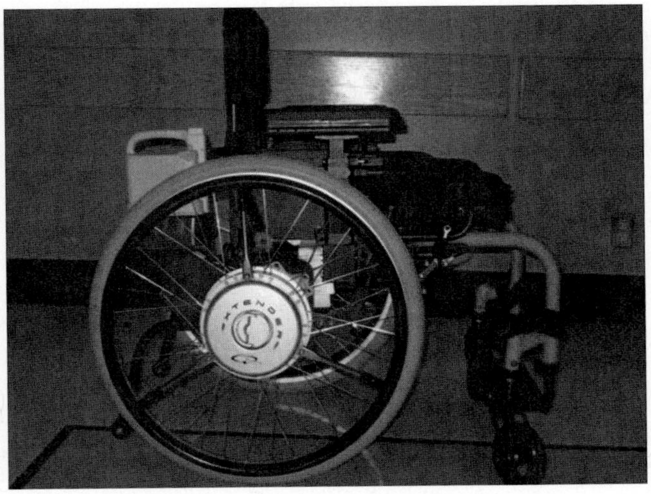

Figure 16-45 ■ Power assist system. The Xtender by Sunrise Medical is one of three power assist systems available. The motors are in the wheels. The battery extends off the back of the wheelchair. There is a connection between the motors in the wheels. The system is added to a manual wheelchair. There are two power assist levels.

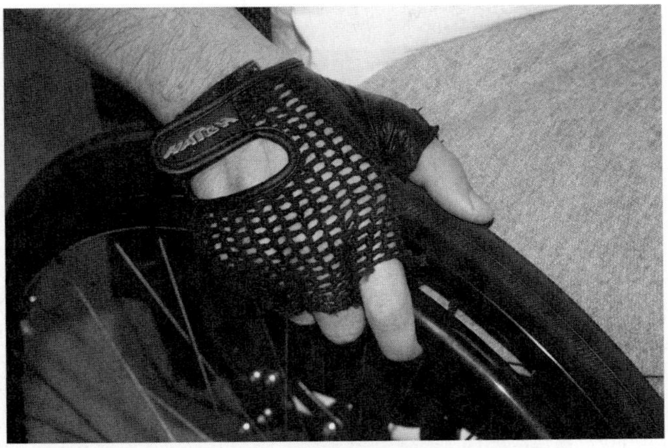

Figure 16-46 ■ Para Push gloves. Wheelchair gloves, mesh back, open fingers, and leather-padded palm. Usually appropriate for patients with paraplegia-level injuries. Available from multiple suppliers.

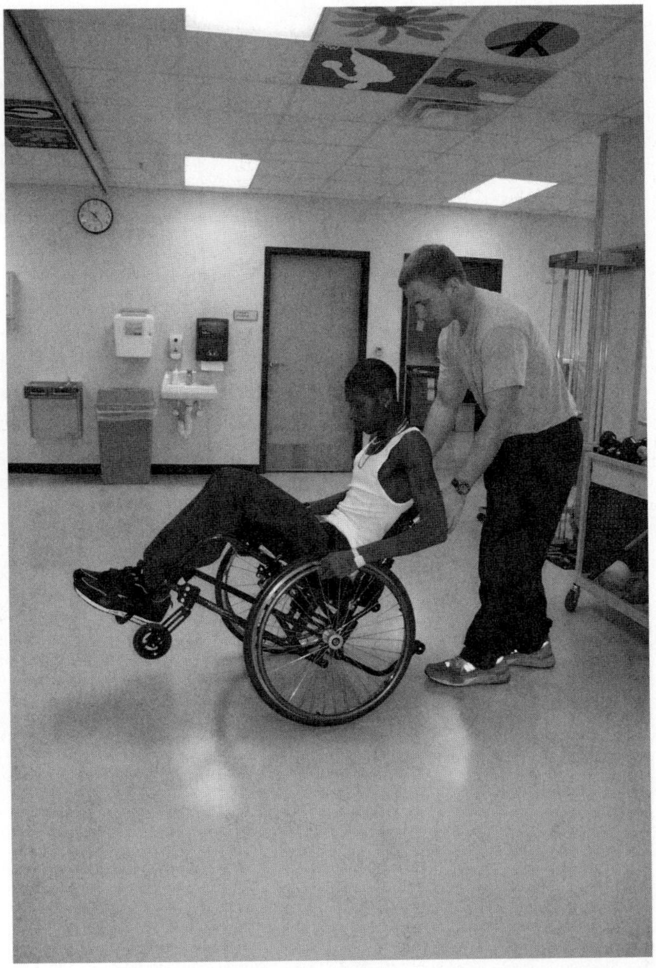

Figure 16-47 ■ A wheelie is a functional mobility skill that enhances functional independence. The performance of a wheelie is a precursor to negotiating steep ramps, curbs, steps, and rough terrain.

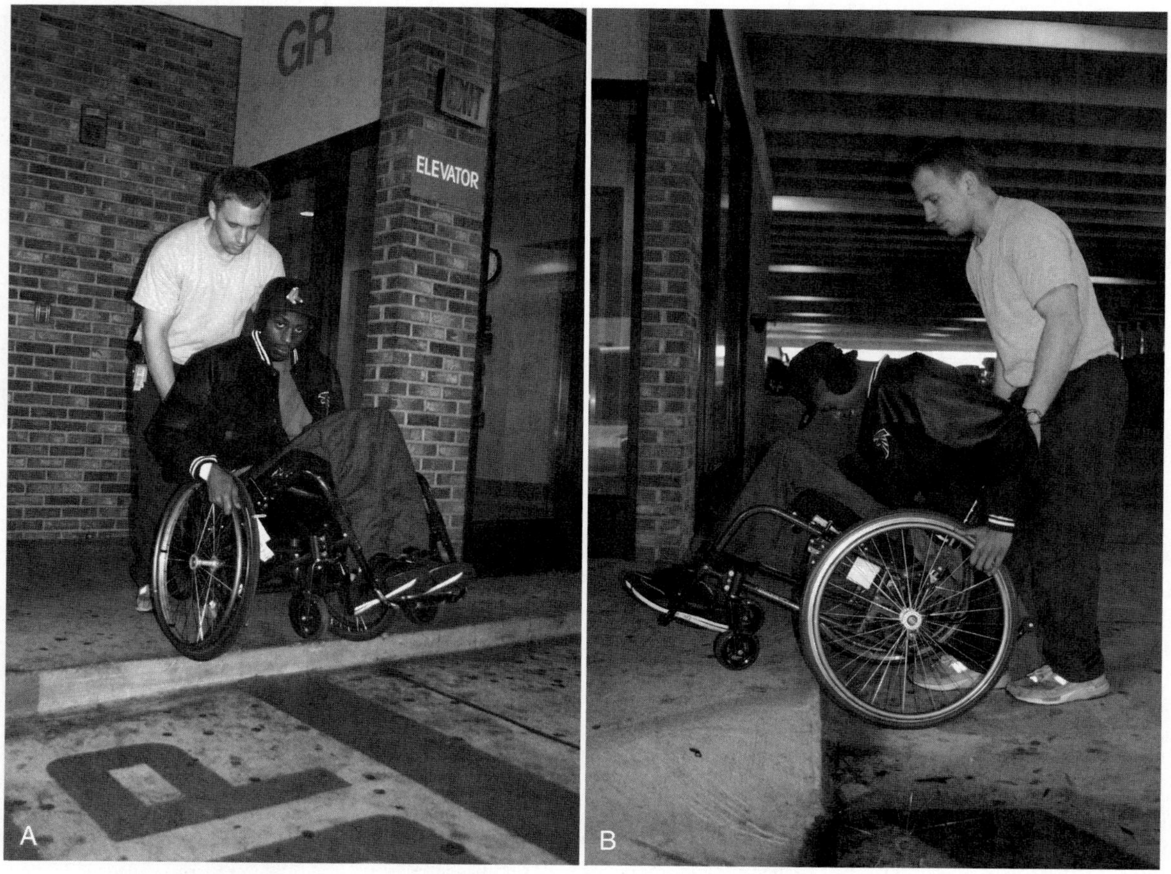

Figure 16-48 ■ **A,** Descending a curb is an advanced wheelchair mobility skill. This man with AIS A, T12 paraplegia assumes the balanced wheelie position and approaches the curb in a forward position. The wheelie position is maintained as he rolls off the curb. **B,** Climbing a curb with assistance is also an advanced skill. This is the same man as in **A.** He "pops" into a wheelie and advances his wheelchair to move his casters up onto the curb. He then reaches back to his wheel, leans forward, and pushes as the helper assists by lifting the back of the chair. A more advanced skill would be to perform this activity by approaching the curb with speeds fast enough to gain momentum, "pop" a wheelie, and advance up and over the curb in one continuous movement (not shown). The curb height, strength, level of injury, and body composition of the patient are determining factors for speed requirements.

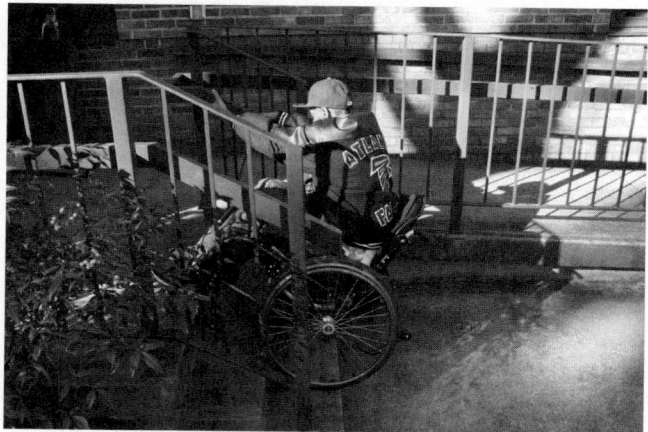

Figure 16-49 ■ Descending steps using one handrail. This patient with AIS A, level T12 approaches the steps backward, using the handrail on his right with both hands, and lowers himself down three steps. This is one of several methods that may be used to negotiate steps.

When the philosophy of the rehabilitation center is to use orthoses for clients who do not have functional motor control below their level of injury, criteria should be established so that both the client and the professional staff are consistent in their approach to ambulation. This gives the client specific information and clarifies goals to be attained, ensuring the most positive outcome (Box 16-3).

The ambulation trial gives the client and the team an opportunity to simulate orthotic use. If the decision is made to order orthoses, specific goals should be set. Goals range from standing and exercise ambulation to community ambulation. Most persons with complete injuries above the L2 level achieve only exercise ambulation because of the energy necessary for functional ambulation.

Research has demonstrated that the energy cost of ambulation for individuals with complete lesions at T12 or higher is above the anaerobic threshold and cannot be maintained over time. This study also concluded that ambulation for these individuals using a swing-through gait pattern is equivalent to "heavy work" or a variety of recreational and

BOX 16-3 ■ CRITERIA FOR AMBULATION TRIAL FOR COMPLETE INJURIES

Expressed desire for ambulation with appropriate goals
Body weight not to exceed 10% of ideal
Range of motion: Hip extension 5 degrees, full knee extension, ankle dorsiflexion 5 to 15 degrees, passive straight leg raise 110 degrees
Intact skin
Stable cardiovascular system
Controlled spasticity
Independent function at the wheelchair level

sporting activities.[132-136] Consequently, it is easy to understand why lower-extremity orthoses may end up in the closet unused.

The energy cost for ambulation is highest for persons with complete paraplegia who use a swing-through gait pattern and lowest for persons who use bilateral AFOs or a combination of an AFO and a KAFO. Even individuals requiring only bilateral AFOs have a gait efficiency of less than 50% of normal, underscoring the importance of the hip extensor and abductor muscles required for normal ambulation. These muscles are severely or completely paralyzed in this population.[134,135]

Assuming that a patient has upper extremities with intact function, the energy cost of ambulation is progressively reduced when more residual motor function is present in the lower extremities. Conversely, the person with incomplete tetraplegia has higher energy costs for ambulation despite spared lower-extremity function because of upper- and lower-extremity weakness (Boxes 16-4 and 16-5 and Figures 16-50 to 16-54).[132-136]

Factors that affect orthotic selection are cost, injury level, residual motor function, experience bias of the clinician, patient's medical status, skin and cardiovascular integrity, and patient's acceptance. Generally, the hip, knee, ankle, and foot orthosis (HKAFO) is used when selected motions of the hip need control or the benefits of the reciprocating gait orthosis (RGO) are desired, as is the case with the pediatric population. The use of a KAFO is indicated when the quadriceps muscle strength is less than 3/5. AFOs are indicated in the presence of ankle instability and weakness and to control hyperextension of the knee joint.[134-137]

Materials and components of bracing continue to evolve. Carbon fiber is becoming more common in bracing, including in low-profile AFOs, either customized or off the shelf.

BOX 16-4 ■ FOUR CATEGORIES OF AMBULATION[131]

1. Standing only
2. Exercise—ambulates short distances
3. Household—ambulates inside home or work, uses wheelchair much of the time
4. Community-independent on all surfaces; does not use wheelchair

BOX 16-5 ■ LOWER-EXTREMITY ORTHOSES[137]

HIP-KNEE-ANKLE-FOOT ORTHOSES
Reciprocating gait orthosis (RGO) (see Figure 16-50)
Bilateral knee-ankle-foot orthoses (KAFOs) with pelvic band

KNEE-ANKLE-FOOT ORTHOSES
Scott-Craig KAFOs (see Figure 16-51)
Conventional KAFOs (metal uprights)
Polypropylene KAFOs (see Figure 16-52)
Hybrid KAFOs (see Figure 16-52)

ANKLE-FOOT ORTHOSES
Conventional ankle-foot orthoses (AFOs) (metal)
Custom polypropylene AFOs
Solid ankle AFOsyes (see Figure 16-53, *A*)
Custom polypropylene AFOs, articulated ankle (see Figure 16-53, *B*)
University of California Biomechanics Lab (UCBL) orthotic (see Figure 16-54)

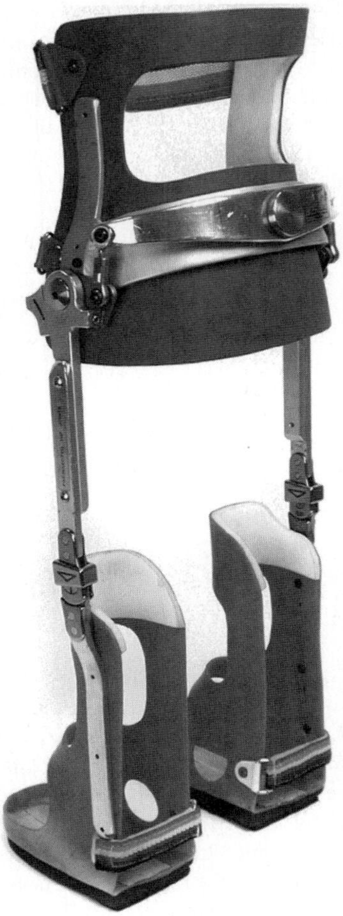

Figure 16-50 ■ The reciprocating gait orthosis (RGO), although generally used with children, is also used with adults. Its main components are a molded pelvic band, thoracic extensions, bilateral hip and knee joints, and lower limb segments that may be of polypropylene construction with a solid ankle. The RGO uses a dual cable system to couple flexion of one hip with extension of the other.

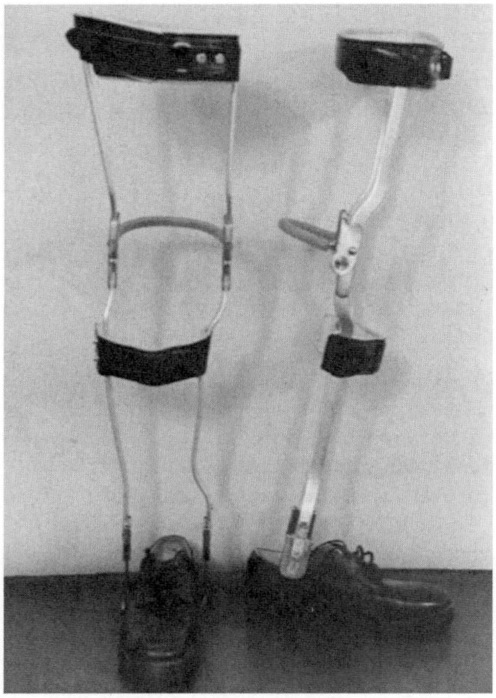

Figure 16-51 ■ Scott-Craig knee-ankle-foot orthosis (KAFO) is a special design for spinal cord injury. The orthosis consists of double uprights, offset knee joints with pawl locks and bail control, one posterior thigh band, a hinged anterior tibial band, an ankle joint with anterior and posterior adjustable pin stops, a cushion heel, and specially designed longitudinal and transverse foot plates made of steel.

There is a trade-off with carbon fiber, however. The benefits of using carbon fiber are that it is lightweight and rigid. However, it is not easily modified after it is manufactured (Figure 16-55, *A*).

Components have advanced quickly in the last 10 years. A recently introduced new joint, Sensor Walk, allows persons with no quadriceps function to stand with control from the joint and then swing the limb freely. Multiple sensors in the footplate of this KAFO signal to the knee joint the position and weight-bearing status of the leg. The joint does not require full knee extension for position of the knee to be maintained, an advantage over other types of stance-control mechanisms. If the patient has gluteal function, this device also allows the individual to ascend and descend stairs using a step-over-step gait pattern (Sensor Walk Electronic KAFO).[138] Other, similar joints in the category of stance-control knee joints are now available from several different manufacturers and include the E-MAG and Horton knee joints. These devices use a knee locking mechanism that is either mechanically or electronically controlled and is triggered by heel contact. During stance the knee is locked and with unweighting the limb is allowed to swing through in a normal reciprocal pattern. The advantages of this technology are obvious from a functional perspective. However, the experience of orthotists and clinicians are that these devices are costly and insurance companies are hesitant to cover the additional expense.[139-141]

A new system for ambulation that has undergone clinical trials in the United States is the ReWalk system. This exoskeleton uses motion sensors, onboard computers, and robotics to assist persons with paraplegia in walking and ascending

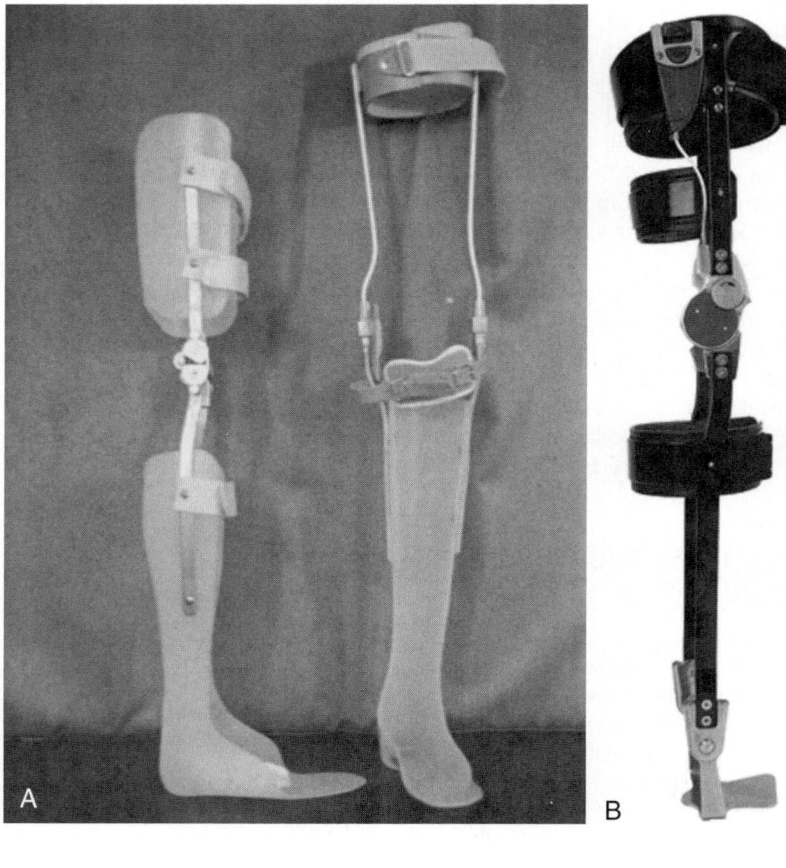

Figure 16-52 ■ **A,** Polypropylene knee-ankle-foot orthosis (KAFO) and combination plastic and metal KAFO. **B,** Stance-control KAFO knee joint. This joint combines the stability of a locked knee during the stance phase of walking but allows flexion of the limb for the swing phase of gait. A locked knee makes it much harder to clear the leg over the ground. Some long leg brace users are perfect candidates for the stance-control KAFOs. These devices, through a few different types of joint mechanisms, create a locked knee when the leg is supporting the weight of the body but unlock when the leg is lifted to allow for easy advancement of the leg as it is allowed to bend. For the right patients, this allows them as much mobility to get around as it does stability.

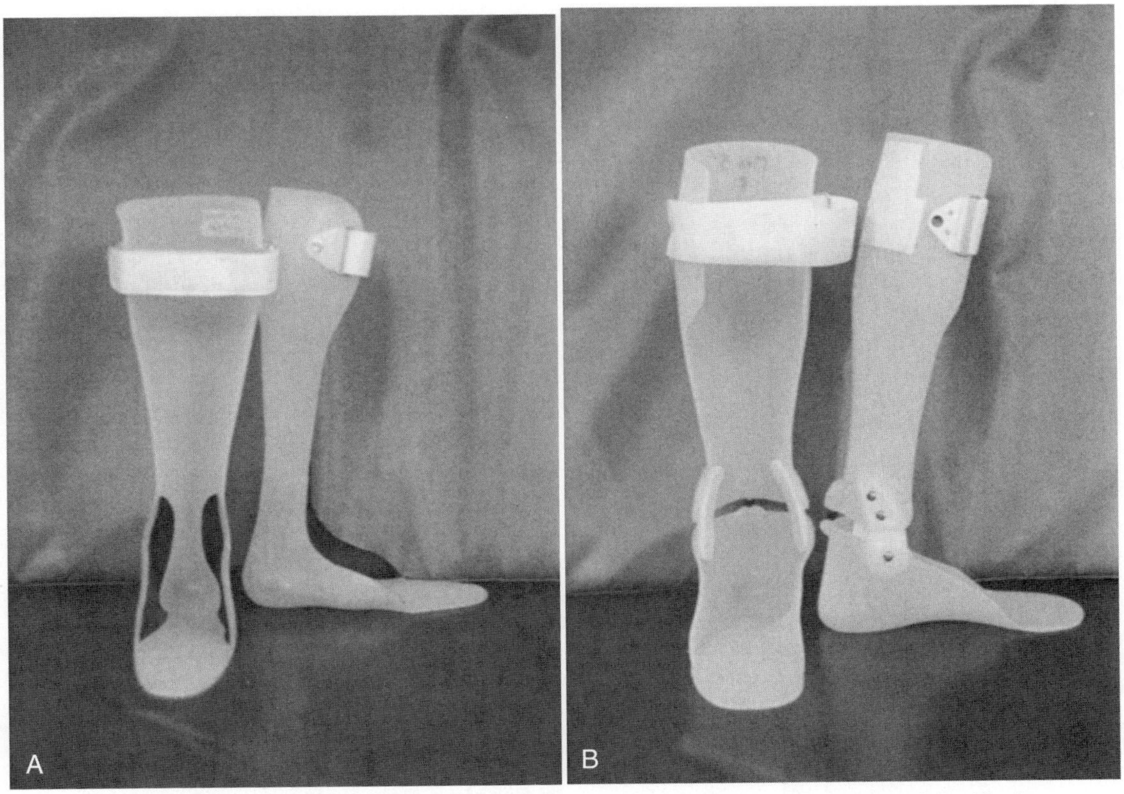

Figure 16-53 ■ **A,** Custom-made solid ankle-foot orthoses (AFOs) in 5 degrees of dorsiflexion with full footplates. **B,** Custom-articulated AFOs with adjustable Oklahoma ankle joints.

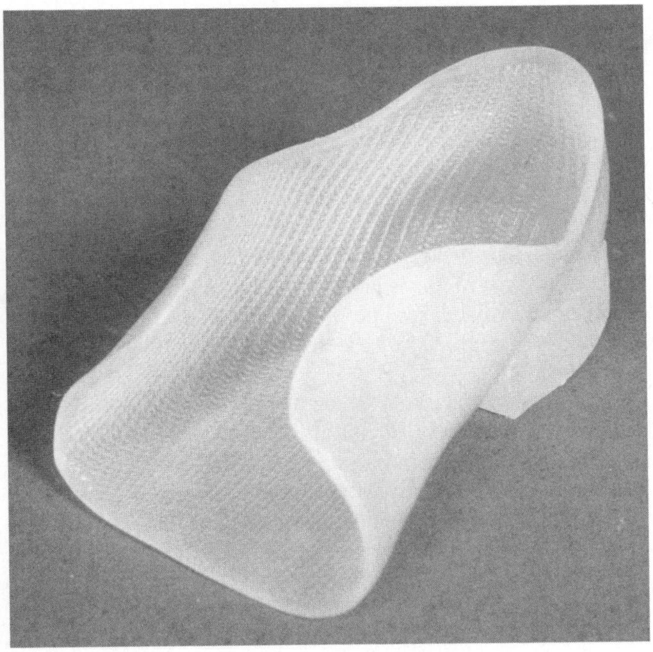

Figure 16-54 ■ University of California Biomechanics Laboratory (UCBL) orthosis. This orthosis is designed with a deep heel cup that holds the calcaneus securely. In addition, the high medial and lateral trimlines support the joints of the midfoot and allow more optimal subtalar joint function. The orthosis also supports the longitudinal arch of the foot. (From Lusardi MM, Nielsen CC: *Orthotics and prosthetics in rehabilitation,* Woburn, MA, 2000, Butterworth Heinemann.)

and descending curbs, ramps, and stairs. Individuals wearing this exoskeleton have reportedly been able to come from sitting to standing, to ambulate using forearm crutches, to walk community distances, as well as negotiating environmental obstacles. Clinical trials have been performed at MossRehab in Philadelphia as well as internationally. The parent company, Argo Medical Technologies, began full production and distribution in early 2011 (Figure 16-55, *B*). Other companies are now in the developmental stages and performing clinical trials with similar exoskeletal devices in preparation for Food and Drug Administration (FDA) approval. Among these are Ekso Bionics, Berkeley, California, and Vanderbilt University research department, Nashville, Tennessee.

Ideally, each patient's neurological recovery potential is maximized before or while brace prescription takes place. Advances in rehabilitation strategies that facilitate neural plasticity and recovery of function (i.e., walking) include the use of body-weight support during locomotor training. This technique of training may employ aquatics, a robot to assist with movement of the extremities, or manual facilitation of stepping performed by physical therapists and their rehabilitation teams using a body-weight suspension system. The principles of locomotor training are discussed later in this chapter.

Equipment

In SCI rehabilitation, the use of equipment is necessary to achieve the expected outcomes. Clinicians work closely with the physician and other team members, including the rehabilitation technology supplier, to determine the most

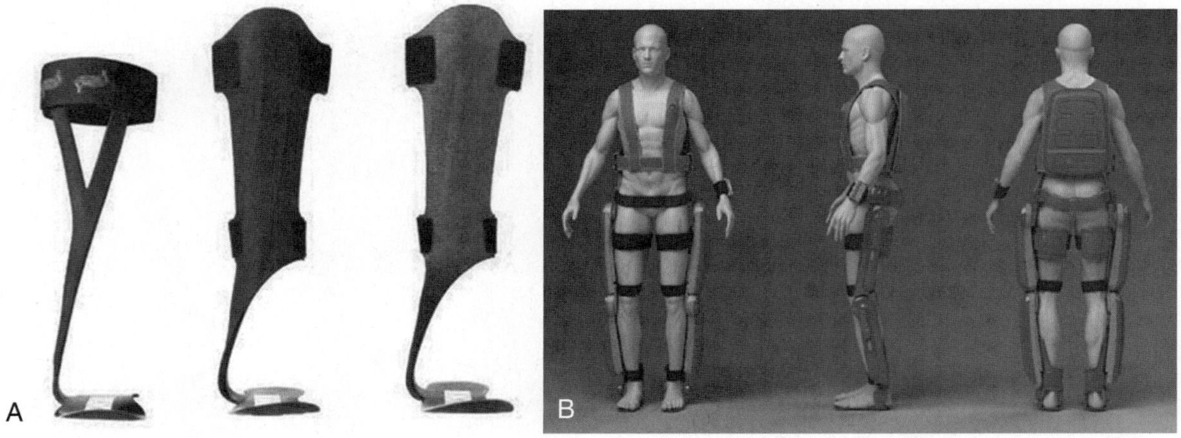

Figure 16-55 ■ **A,** Allard braces. The Allard family of ankle-foot orthoses (AFOs) include a prefabricated shell that can be customized by the trained orthotist to the specific needs of the patients. These dynamic orthoses are constructed of carbon composites, which accounts for their strength as well as their light weight. There are three different AFOs in the series: Ypsilon, ToeOFF, and BlueRocker. The AFOs are intended to be used with a custom foot orthotic. **B,** ReWalk is a wearable, motorized, quasi-robotic suit. Partially concealable under clothing, ReWalk provides user-initiated mobility-leveraging advanced motion sensors, sophisticated robotic control algorithms, on-board computers, real-time software, actuation motors, tailored rechargeable batteries, and composite materials.

appropriate equipment to meet individual needs. It is important to have access to trial equipment so the client has the opportunity to practice with equipment similar to what will be prescribed. Ideally the rehabilitation technology supplier should be accessible to the rehabilitation team to allow for necessary adjustments to the equipment. In addition, rehabilitation technology suppliers should be knowledgeable and responsible for educating rehabilitation professionals regarding new products. When possible, all equipment should be ordered from a single supplier to reduce confusion when the need for repairs arises. To ensure that the most appropriate piece of equipment is prescribed, the following must be considered: durability, function, transportability, comfort, cost, safety, cosmesis, and acceptance by the user.[62] Generally, the higher the injury level, the more costly the equipment owing to the technology involved. Table 16-7 lists equipment according to injury level.

Ideally, equipment should be ordered as soon as possible so the client can be fitted before discharge. Shorter lengths of stay make early equipment ordering difficult. For example, a client may not have 3/5 wrist extension to be fitted with a tenodesis brace but with strengthening over time would be an excellent candidate. Clinicians need to negotiate with the funding source so that equipment may be ordered in the outpatient setting. Equipment required for the SCI population is costly, requiring extensive review by third-party payers before funding is approved or denied. Many health care policies do not cover the funding of needed equipment. As a result of these factors, many clients are discharged without the equipment they need. Lack of appropriate equipment may result in (1) a feeling of loss of control, (2) contractures and postural deformities, (3) skin breakdown, (4) a loss of skills learned in rehabilitation, (5) poor self-image, and (6) increased dependence on others.

Seating Principles

Many individuals spend 8 hours or more per day in their wheelchairs after an SCI. Consequently, proper seating of these clients may be the most important intervention clinicians provide. The seating process should be addressed on admission, continually throughout the rehabilitation program, and regularly after discharge to help prevent and minimize complications.[77,142] The wheelchair is an integral part of the client's self-image and in many ways will help define personal lifestyle.[62] Goals for seating the client with an SCI are identified in Box 16-6.

Every seating session begins with a thorough examination, as described earlier. Trial simulations are essential to determine how the patient will function and maintain posture over time in the seating system. Simulations help to avoid costly mistakes. The patient must be involved in the decision-making process to ensure that the seating system will work.

Individuals with SCI are at high risk of pressure ulcers owing to lack of mobility and impaired sensation. Great care must be taken to reduce pressure over bony prominences and to distribute pressure over as large an area as possible.[143] Pressure-distributing cushions should be evaluated clinically and with pressure-sensing devices to determine the optimal wheelchair cushion for each individual.[142,144] Many patients with muscle paralysis of the trunk find that the effects of gravity in a sitting position pull the head and upper torso forward and over the pelvis, resulting in a long kyphosis or a C-curved posture (Figure 16-56).[144] Two resulting problems are increased weight bearing on the sacrum and development of a thoracic kyphosis, leading to neck hyperextension in an effort to maintain a horizontal gaze.[142] This position is also assumed by patients to improve their balance. This occurs when the seat-to-back angle is closed and the client feels as if he or she is falling forward. Unfortunately, this poor seating posture is

TABLE 16-7 ■ EQUIPMENT NEEDS CORRELATED TO INJURY LEVEL

INJURY LEVEL	EQUIPMENT	COST (IN DOLLARS)	INJURY LEVEL	EQUIPMENT	COST (IN DOLLARS)
C1 to C3	Ventilator (bedside)	14,700		Wheelchair cushion	450-600
	Ventilator (portable for wheelchair)	14,700		Bedside table	225
	Power tilt or recline wheelchair	17,000-26,000		ECU	250-7000
	Manual recline wheelchair for transport	2100-4200		Electric hospital bed	2000-4000
	Wheelchair cushion	450-600		Specialized mattress	800-10,000
	Reclining commode or shower chair	1800-3000		Commode or shower chair	1500
	ECU	1900-9000		ADL equipment	900-1500
	Call system	1025-1500		Tenodesis splint	1700
	Bedside table	225		Transfer board	100-200
	Fully electric hospital bed	2000-4000		Hand control for car	300-1500
	Specialized mattress	800-10,000		Bowel-bladder equipment	125-250
	Adapted computer	2000-4000	C7 to C8	Power upright wheelchair	7500-15,000
	Communication devices	400-11,000		Manual wheelchair	2000-6500
	Overhead power lift	4000-15,000		Wheelchair cushion	450-600
	Hydraulic lift for transfers	1400-2000		Bedside table	225
C4 to C5	Power tilt or recline wheelchair	17,000-26,000		ECU	250-1000
	Manual wheelchair for transport	2100-4200		Electric hospital bed	2000-3000
	Lap tray	250-700		Specialized mattress	600-10,000
	Wheelchair cushion	450-600		Commode or shower chair	1500
	Bedside table	225		Hand controls for car	300-1500
	ECU	1500-10,000		ADL equipment	300-1000
	Fully electric hospital bed	2000-4000		Transfer board	100-200
	Specialized mattress	800-10,000		Bowel and bladder equipment	125-250
	Commode or shower chair	1500-3000	Paraplegia	Manual upright wheelchair	2000-5500
	Communication devices	300-1500		Wheelchair cushion	450-600
	ADL equipment	400-1400		Raised or padded commode seat (cutout)	210
	Hydraulic lift for transfers	1400-2000		Tub bench	220
	Overhead power lift	4000-15,000		Hand controls for car	400-700
	Mobile arm support	500-1000		ADL equipment	100-300
	Upper-extremity orthotics	700-1200		Bowel and bladder equipment	50-250
C6	Power upright wheelchair	7500-20,000		Lower-extremity orthotics (if ambulation is a goal)	4000-6000
	Manual wheelchair	2000-4500			
	Power assist wheels	9000			

ADL, Activity of daily living; *ECU,* environmental control unit.

Based on 2009-2010 Atlanta, Georgia, retail prices.

quickly learned and difficult to correct.[142] This posture can often be prevented by tilting the wheelchair slightly backward while maintaining a fixed seat-to-back angle (Figure 16-57).[142] In this position, the effects of gravity augment sitting balance and facilitate good spinal alignment. Education regarding proper positioning, the use of a sacral block, a firm wheelchair seat and back, and properly applied pelvic positioning devices also aid in preventing the kyphotic posture.[142]

Asymmetrical muscle strength, asymmetrical spasticity, and preferential use of one upper extremity over another often result in poor trunk alignment. The use of lateral trunk supports, lateral pelvic supports, and properly applied seat belts may aid in maintaining symmetrical trunk posture.

Strong muscle spasms, combined with the effects of gravity, may cause the person with severely impaired mobility to slide down in the wheelchair, resulting in increased pressure on the sacrum and shearing of the skin. For these patients, a manual wheelchair with adjustable seat and back angles can be used to improve stability. Power wheelchairs with power tilt systems allow users to reposition themselves and use the power tilt for improved stability.

Optimal pressure distribution is achieved by maximizing the surface area, allowing immersion into the seat cushion, and promoting a symmetrical posture. The width of the seat should be slightly more than that of the widest body part. The seat depth should come to approximately within 1 to 2 inches of the popliteal fossae, except when it interferes with lower extremity (LE) management. The height of the back should reflect the client's motor function and seated stability. If the back is too high, it can restrict functional activities such as wheelchair propulsion and wheelies. Patients with tetraplegia who use the push handles of the wheelchair to hook while

BOX 16-6 ■ GOALS FOR SEATING THE CLIENT WITH SPINAL CORD INJURY

1. Maximize functional independence
2. Improve pressure distribution and relief of pressure
3. Optimize comfort
4. Enhance the quality of life
5. Optimize good postural alignment and sitting balance
6. Compensate for fixed deformities
7. Allow for transportation of the mobility system

The following are basic seating concepts of proper postural alignment:

- Neutral pelvic alignment
- Symmetrical alignment of the trunk and neck
- Neutral head positioning over the pelvis
- Maintenance of a horizontal gaze
- Maintenance of ankle in neutral alignment with full support of the foot
- Maintenance of the thighs in neutral abduction and adduction with full contact with the cushion
- Neutral shoulder positioning to avoid shoulder elevation, protraction, or retraction and to provide adequate upper-extremity support[142,144]
- Elbow angle that approximates 100 to 120 degrees when the hand is resting at the top of the wheel or pushrim[126]

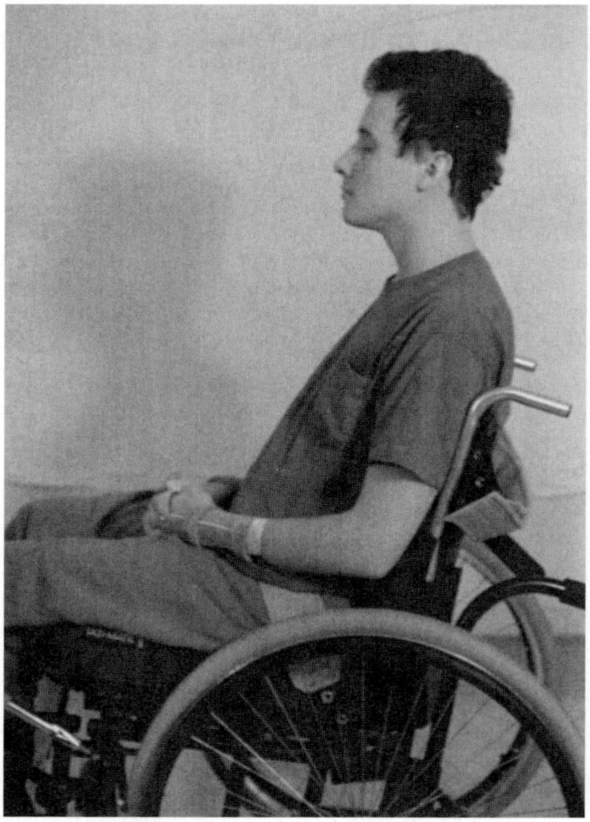

Figure 16-57 ■ Example of corrected C-curve posture.

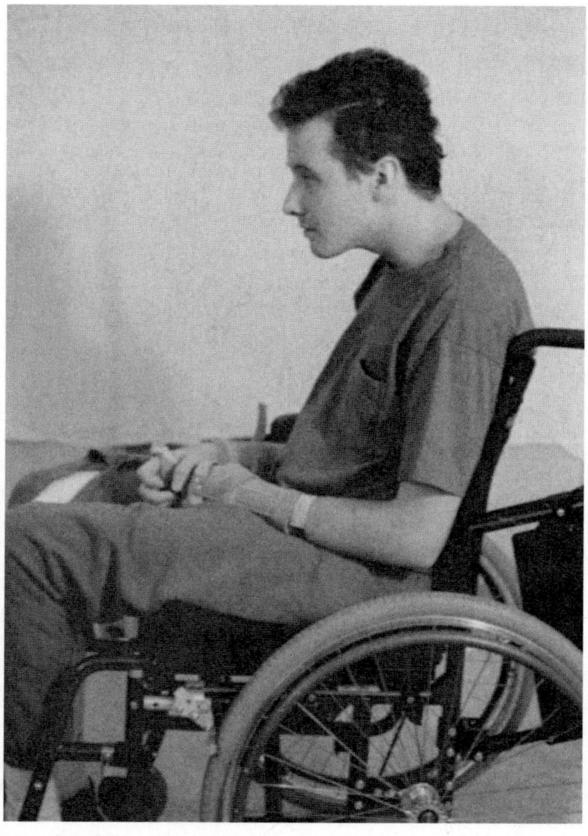

Figure 16-56 ■ Example of typical kyphotic C-curve posture in the patient with tetraplegia.

performing functional activities may require custom modification of the wheelchair back (Figure 16-58).

The size, weight, and portability of the wheelchair seating system affect the individual's lifestyle. The client's home or work environment must be evaluated closely for accessibility so that the wheelchair seating system can be used effectively in those environments. The buildings must be structurally sound and spacious to accommodate heavy-power wheelchair systems. The means of transportation of the wheelchair (car versus van) may determine whether a rigid or folding wheelchair frame is indicated. Transit options and tie-down systems must be considered for safe transportation. The wheelchair must be adjusted to make it as efficient as possible to propel to reduce stress on upper-extremity joints. Many manual wheelchairs are lightweight (less than 35 pounds) and have multiple adjustments and choices of tires and casters that make manual wheelchair propulsion more efficient. Reducing rolling resistance, positioning the rear axle for maximum propulsion stroke efficiency, and teaching efficient propulsion techniques reduce shoulder musculature fatigue and upper-extremity injury. Rear wheel size should be selected so that when the wheelchair user is seated, he or she is able to touch the rear axle with the middle finger. This position increases the range of contact during propulsion. In addition, shifting the distribution of the user's weight back over the rear axle (usually accomplished by moving the rear wheel axle forward) reduces the percentage of weight on the front casters, making propulsion more efficient.[145] This adjustment reduces the rear stability of the wheelchair, so the use of

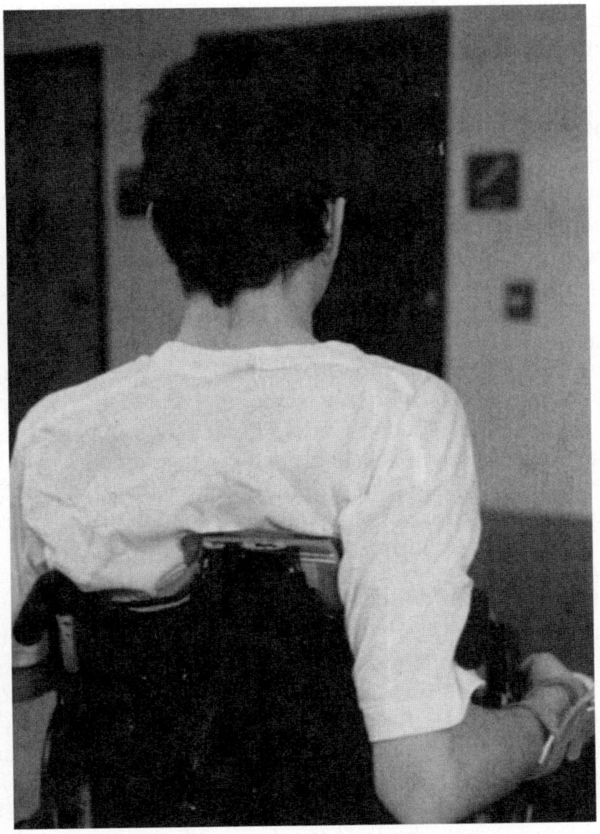

Figure 16-58 ■ Example of custom modification of a wheelchair back to allow a patient with tetraplegia to hook the push handle with one upper extremity.

anti-tip bars and/or training in wheelie maneuvers is essential. Finally, along with wheelchair fit, the esthetics of the wheelchair can affect the individual's self-image and therefore the community reentry. This should be considered when assisting the patient to make wheelchair seating decisions.

Education

Education of the client and caregivers is an integral part of the rehabilitation process. Formal education includes group and individual instruction and family and caregiver training. Clients and caregivers are taught preventive skin care, bowel and bladder programs, safe ways to perform all ADL tasks, nutritional guidelines, thermoregulation precautions, pulmonary management, cardiopulmonary resuscitation, management of autonomic dysreflexia, equipment management and maintenance, transfer techniques, wheelchair mobility, ambulation, proper body positioning, ROM exercises, ADL basics, and leisure skills. Home programs are taught to maintain or increase strength, endurance, ROM, and function. Energy conservation techniques and proper body mechanics are incorporated into all aspects of training.

Clients are formally tested on their knowledge, and remedial instruction should be provided in deficient areas. During family training, caregivers are formally evaluated on their abilities to safely provide care to the client. Supervised therapeutic outings and passes allow the client, caregivers, and the team to identify problem areas and provide additional education in those areas.

Psychosocial Issues

The immediate reaction to the onset of SCI is physical shock accompanied by anxiety, pain, and fear of dying. The response to such an injury varies greatly and depends on the extent of the injury, the premorbid activity level, the style of coping with stress, and family and financial resources. There may be great sensory deprivation from immobilization, neurological impairment, and the monotony of the hospital routine. Several psychological theories have been proposed to describe responses and coping mechanisms.[65] The process of coping with these changes is referred to as *adjustment* (see Chapter 6)

Rehabilitation personnel are becoming more aware of the need not only to teach functional skills but also to teach psychosocial and coping skills to the client and significant others. Education in the following areas facilitates the adjustment process: creative recreation, financial planning, negotiating community barriers, social skills, managing an attendant, creative problem solving, accessing community resources, fertility and child care options, assertiveness, sexual expression, vocational planning and training, and the use of community transportation. These skills may be introduced in the inpatient rehabilitation setting but will be developed further in the home and community environments. True adjustment and adaptation begin after discharge from rehabilitation.[146,147]

Sexual Issues

Sexuality is how people experience and express themselves as sexual beings and is a normal part of being human,[148] so it is not surprising that persons with SCI place a high priority on resuming sexual functions after their injury.[149] After SCI, men may experience impairments in penile erection, ejaculation, orgasm, and fertility. Women with SCI may experience impairments in the ability to become aroused or achieve orgasm and/or may have decreased vaginal lubrication.[150] Improving sexual functions is a high priority for both men and women after SCI.[149] Table 16-8 lists the relationship of the level of spinal injury to sexual function. Treatment of sexual dysfunction should be a coordinated effort among the patient, significant other, and appropriate health care professionals. Sexual counseling, educational programs, and medical management provide opportunities to address the areas of sexual dysfunction, alternative behaviors, precautions, and other related areas.[150]

Depending on the level and completeness of the SCI, most men can attain an erection either through psychogenic (via T11 to L2 pathways) or reflexogenic pathways (S2 to S4)[151]; however, these erections are often not reliable or adequate for sexual intercourse. The first-line treatment for erectile dysfunction after SCI is the use of phosphodiesterase type V inhibitors such as sildenafil (Viagra), tadalafil (Cialis), and vardenafil (Levitra). Other treatments include intracavernosal (penile injectable) medications, mechanical methods such as vacuum devices and penile rings, and, as a last resort, surgical penile implants.[148]

Male orgasm and ejaculation are likely to occur together; however, after SCI an orgasm may not always lead to ejaculation, or there may be retrograde ejaculation into the bladder.[152] A study by Sipski and colleagues showed that 78.9%

TABLE 16-8 ■ RELATION OF LEVEL OF SPINAL INJURY TO SEXUAL FUNCTION

INJURY LEVEL	SEXUAL FUNCTION
Cauda equina/conus	***Males***
	Usually no reflex erections
	Rare psychogenic erection
	Ejaculation occasionally occurs
	Females
	Vaginal secretions often absent
	Patients generally fertile
Thoracic/cervical	***Males***
	Reflex erections predominate (usually short duration)
	Psychogenic erections generally absent
	Ejaculation occasional
	Females
	Vaginal secretions present as part of genital reflex
	Fertility preserved
	Sensation of labor pain absent

of men with incomplete upper motor neuron SCI achieved orgasm as compared with 28% of men with complete upper motor neuron injuries ($P < .001$), whereas 0% of men with lower motor neuron injuries affecting their sacral cord achieved orgasm.[152]

"Will I ever be able to become a father?" is a common question of men after SCI. Pregnancy rates in partners of men with SCI are lower than in the general population, but there is a good chance (greater than 50%) that men with SCI can become biological fathers with advances in reproductive assisted technology. Roughly 2 weeks after an SCI, semen quality declines[153] to levels approaching those observed in males with chronic SCI.[154] There is evidence that bladder management with clean intermittent catheterization may improve semen quality over other methods of bladder management.[155] The two most common methods of sperm retrieval are vibrostimulation (less invasive) and electroejaculation. These methods are successful for persons with lesions above T10. If these methods are not successful, there is an option of surgical aspiration. Depending on the semen quality, a progression from intravaginal insemination, intrauterine insemination, in vitro fertilization (IVF), to IVF plus intracytoplasmic sperm injection is recommended.[148]

Women with SCI may have impairment in arousal and orgasm. The vagus nerves are thought to facilitate the presence of vaginal-cervical perception of orgasm. Preservation of T11 to L2 sensory dermatomes is associated with psychogenically mediated genital vasocongestion and lubrication.[156] There is some evidence that supports the use of sildenafil in women to partially reverse subjective sexual arousal difficulties.[148] For women who have a lower motor neuron lesion, vaginal secretions are often absent, and an artificial lubricant is recommended.

Amenorrhea may occur immediately after SCI and last up to 4 to 5 months. Despite this delay, it is believed that fertility in women is unaffected by SCI.[157] Women are able to conceive; however, there are increased risks to pregnancy, which may include bladder problems, spasticity, pressure sores, autonomic dysreflexia, and problems with mobility.[158]

Discharge Planning

Discharge planning begins from the time the client is being considered for admission and continues through the rehabilitation program. It is a continuous process that includes the client, family, treatment team, and community resources, with the goal being successful community reintegration and a perceived good quality of life. The rehabilitation team must identify the specific needs of the client and must structure the program to enhance the chance of success. Lengths of stay are getting shorter in response to pressure from third-party payers to contain costs. This requires the discharge planning process to be expedited so that procurement of needed equipment, completion of architectural modifications, and referrals to outpatient and community resources occur in a timely manner.

Architectural Modifications

Architectural barriers in the home, transportation system, workplace, or school may prevent access to opportunities. The architectural changes required by the person with SCI for independence in the home and community depend on the degree of impairment, financial resources, and client and family acceptance of modifications or equipment. The clinician should discuss equipment options with the client and family on the basis of the degree of modification they plan to make to their home. Thinking creatively about low-tech adaptations should be considered part of the therapist's role. Problem solving with and by the client is vital to the process of identifying alternatives as ideas for the future (Figure 16-59).

Many available resources describe the dimensions of the basic wheelchair and specifications for making homes and facilities accessible to wheelchair users. See Appendix 16-A at the end of this chapter for resources on architectural modification.

Return to Work or School

Successful community reintegration after SCI includes returning to preinjury social roles and, more specifically, returning to work, school, and/or leisure interests. Public school systems have a legal obligation to provide an appropriate school setting for a child with a disability. Rehabilitation teams may assist with school reentry by adding school visitations and education for faculty or peers. School accessibility can be assessed and the patient and therapists can have an opportunity to share appropriate information about the new impairments before reentry into the school system. Also, rehabilitation programs that are CARF accredited must offer academic programs. School reentry programs may enhance communication between academic rehabilitation faculty and school, bridging the gap for return. Students returning to college may need assistance developing problem-solving skills related to campus accessibility, Americans with Disabilities Act (ADA) rights, campus transportation options, and self-advocacy for sports adaptations.

Rehabilitation programs must also emphasize returning to work throughout the process. For patients who have

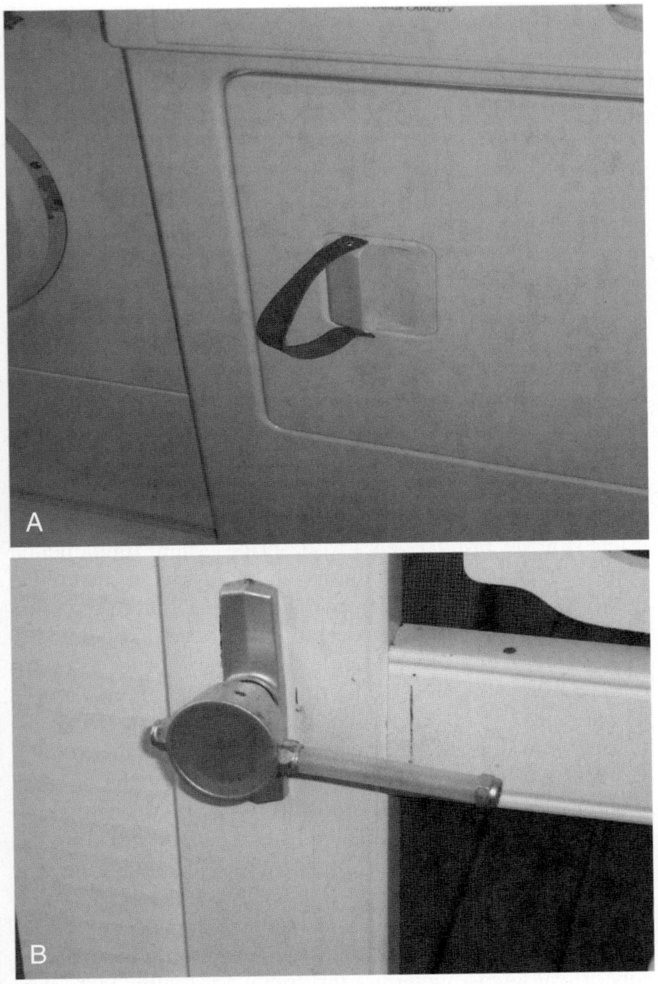

Figure 16-59 ■ Low-tech home adaptations. **A,** A strap is added to make a clothes dryer door accessible. **B,** A hole is drilled and a handle added to a screen door knob.

sustained a traumatic SCI and are included in SCI model systems data,[13] 57.5% report being employed at the time of the accident. Only 11.6% are employed at the 1-year anniversary, but by year 20 35.4% are employed. At year 10 after injury, people with paraplegia (31.7%) have a slightly better employment outcome versus those with tetraplegia, of whom 26.4% are employed.[41] Many individuals can return to their previous jobs after SCI.[159,160] The Americans with Disabilities Act of 1990 (PL 101-336) prohibits businesses with 15 or more employees from discriminating against "qualified individuals with disabilities" with respect to the terms, conditions, or privileges of employment.[161] Job site and job responsibilities may need to change to accommodate the new impairments, allowing the patient to fully participate. For those who are unable to perform previous jobs or who were unemployed before injury, many programs exist for training in vocational skills. The Department of Rehabilitation Services (DRS) evaluates clients for skills and functional abilities and provides funding for those qualifying for job training, job site modification, and the purchase of essential equipment that may include transportation. Services offered by the DRS vary from state to state. Each state agency has a list of resources available in the community, such as rehabilitation technology, independent living centers, and job training and placement programs. Individuals should refer to their state DRS for assistance with employment.

Engaging in sports and other leisure skills can open doors for patients returning to the community. Participating in sports and leisure, whether learning a new skill or adapting something previously enjoyed, may boost physical capacity and enhance self-worth. Adapted sporting activities found in the United States include power soccer, quad rugby, wheelchair basketball, tennis, swimming, and snow skiing, to name a few. The Paralympics provide competitive venues for elite athletes, and many road races across the United States have opened the roads for wheelchair athletes to compete alongside able-bodied runners. A handful of colleges and universities have developed adapted sports teams and are beginning to offer student scholarships.

Health Promotion and Wellness

Individuals with spinal cord injuries are living longer owing to improvements in medical management, but this has also led to increased incidence of chronic diseases, such as cardiovascular disease (CVD) and diabetes mellitus, in this population.[162-164] The Surgeon General's Report on Physical Activity and Health identifies persons with disabilities as among the most inactive subgroup in the United States.[165] Cardiopulmonary disease has been identified as a primary source of morbidity for persons with aging spinal cord injuries,[32,166] and nearly all cardiovascular risk factors are increased in individuals with SCI. Increased rates of diabetes, impaired glucose tolerance, metabolic syndrome, and obesity—all conditions that are exacerbated by physical inactivity—contribute to the development of CVD.[167] Muscle atrophy is common in people with complete and incomplete SCIs, with an associated increase in fat mass resulting from the imposed immobility caused by the neurological impairment. These are all key factors when considering the impact of resting energy expenditure (REE) on metabolism in people with SCIs[168] and in evaluating the risk of obesity in this population.

Key components of a health and wellness program for persons with SCI are exercise, prevention of secondary complications, injury prevention, good nutrition, and good psychological support. Physical activity after SCI has been shown to improve muscle strength, endurance, mobility, the ability to fall asleep, self-image, and blood lipid profiles and decrease the risk of premature death. In addition, exercise has been shown to decrease anxiety, loneliness, depression, stress, heart disease, blood pressure, respiratory illness, diabetes, obesity, and other medical complications.[169]

Exercise programs for individuals with SCIs must take into consideration the musculoskeletal, respiratory, cardiovascular, and autonomic nervous system changes that occur after SCI. Components of an exercise program should include flexibility, muscular strength, and cardiovascular endurance, and an appropriate exercise prescription should address exercise mode, intensity, duration, and frequency. It is important to find a type of exercise that is enjoyable for each individual so that it can be easily integrated into his or her lifestyle. Required exercise intensity to improve cardiovascular fitness and reduce the risk of CVD is 50% to 80% of peak oxygen uptake.[170] American College of Sports

Medicine (ACSM) guidelines suggest that able-bodied individuals exercise 30 to 60 minutes most days of the week, and these guidelines are often extrapolated to the disabled population as well.[171] However, they do not take into account that individuals with SCIs are also using their upper extremities to complete many of their ADLs and mobility tasks, so 30 minutes of exercise two or three times per week may be sufficient for them to maintain their fitness.[170] Circuit resistance training programs using alternating resistance maneuvers and high-speed, low-resistance arm exercise have been shown to be beneficial in improving muscle strength, endurance, and anaerobic power of middle-aged men with paraplegia while also significantly reducing their shoulder pain.[172] Circuit resistance training has also been shown to increase peak oxygen consumption and cardiorespiratory endurance in patients with chronic paraplegia.[173,174]

Exercise programs, both in the clinic and home, may incorporate specialized equipment. The types of equipment available for exercise testing or training in persons with SCI are well documented in the literature. Arm crank ergometers, wheelchair ergometers, wheelchair treadmills, lower-extremity cycling with FES, suspended ambulation protocols, and field test protocols are among the more widely used equipment in the clinic.[175,176] Exercise equipment varies in expense, and each clinic must choose the method that best fits its treatment setting and budget. Home exercise programs may be established with equipment such as weights and cuff weights, elastic bands and tubing, and hand cycles.

Overuse syndromes are common among long-term wheelchair users. When any type of exercise program is established, factors that are specific to SCI should be considered.[172] Long-term wheelchair use can lead to an increased incidence of carpal tunnel syndrome, elbow or shoulder tendonitis, early onset of osteoarthritis, and rotator cuff injuries. The motion and resistance of the upper-extremity muscles during wheelchair propulsion can lead to an overdevelopment of anterior shoulder muscles, scapular protraction, and posterior shoulder weakness. This musculature imbalance may lead to elevation and internal rotation of the humeral head that may cause pain as a result of impingement. Injuries can be prevented or slowed if clients perform a proper warmup with stretching and flexibility exercises, wear protective equipment (e.g., helmet and padded gloves), alternate modes of exercise, and get proper rest between exercise sessions.

Through an established health and wellness program, a person with SCI has the potential to increase quality of life, improve ADLs, decrease secondary complications, decrease depression, and decrease the number of related hospitalizations. It is a goal that integration to wellness programs for individuals with SCIs will become a standard in all facilities.

RESTORATION AND RECOVERY

Upper-Extremity Restoration

Improving hand and upper-extremity function plays a critical role in achieving independence with ADLs.[177,178] Surgical restoration of hand grasp, lateral pinch, or elbow extension in a patient with tetraplegia can be an option through tendon transfers.[179,180] Typically, before individuals are considered for surgery, their neurological function has reached a plateau, they are psychologically stable, and they have functional goals.[180] Individuals seeking restorative surgery to the upper extremity undergo a preoperative evaluation using the International Classification for Surgery of the Hand in Tetraplegia (ICSHT).[181] Before any surgical interventions, therapy may be recommended to ensure that the individual is a candidate for tendon transfer procedures.[180] Postoperative rehabilitation varies on the basis of specific procedures and may consist of 2 months or more, with strength improvements continuing for up to 1 year postoperatively.[182,183] Tendon transfer procedures may be an option to improve upper-extremity function.[183]

Activity-Based Therapy

The terms *activity-based restorative therapies, activity-based therapies,* and *activity-based rehabilitation* have been coined in the last 10 years to describe a new fundamental approach for treating deficits induced by neurological paralysis. The goal of this approach is to achieve activation of the neurological levels located both above and below the injury level using rehabilitation therapies in order to facilitate recovery after a debilitating neurological incident.[184] The theory behind the achievement of recovery from participation in intense therapy programs, often called *activity-based therapy programs,* involves plasticity of the nervous system. Dunlop defines *plasticity* as the ability of neurons to rearrange their anatomical and functional connectivity in response to environmental input, thereby achieving new or modified outputs.[185] Several lines of evidence suggest that the central nervous system is capable of synaptic plasticity and anatomical reorganization occurring at both cortical and subcortical levels, including the spinal cord, after SCI.[186-188] Facilitating reorganization of the injured nervous system is the goal of these types of intensive therapy programs, and rehabilitative interventions are thought to affect plasticity in several ways, including behaviorally, physiologically, structurally or neuroanatomically, cellularly, and molecularly.[189]

For clinicians, this "emerging paradigm shift" in the practice of SCI rehabilitation has recently been described as a transfer from therapy that focuses on teaching compensatory strategies such as learning to use the upper extremities for mobility when the lower extremities are impaired, toward intensive recovery programs specifically designed to improve locomotor abilities in people with incomplete spinal cord injuries.[190] Traditional therapy for the treatment of these types of injuries is designed to improve a client's independence using techniques that promote the use of assistive devices to compensate for lost function, such as using a wheelchair for mobility. In contrast, intensive therapy programs for people with SCI focus on recovering the ability to use their trunk and limbs to stand and walk as they did before their injury along with promoting lifelong health and wellness in this population. Although not clearly defined, activity-based therapy often involves intensive practice and repetition of task-specific mobility training to promote recovery and facilitates revitalization of the central nervous system. (Refer to Chapter 4 for additional discussion.)

Specialized rehabilitation technology is often used in this type of therapy approach, including but not limited to body-weight–supported treadmill (BWST) systems, robotic BWST systems, FES bikes, and LE FES systems designed to improve overground walking ability. (Refer to Chapters 9 and 38 for further discussion of rehabilitation technologies.)

Improving Walking Function

Research on locomotor training through the use of BWST systems first began with spinalized cats in the 1980s[191-195] and then progressed to human subjects with increasing popularity in the 1990s and 2000s (Figure 16-60, *A*).[190,196-200] Much of the theory behind this rehabilitation approach is based on activating intrinsic connections of spinal cord circuitry to elicit the appropriate patterns of muscle activation for walking called *central pattern generators* (CPGs).[201] Research involving the cat model has provided the most conclusive and descriptive evidence for the presence and activity of CPGs,[202] including the ability to produce locomotor output in spinalized animals.[203] However, the evidence in humans has been less conclusive and is mainly based on the presence of alternating flexor and extensor activity seen in fetuses in utero and the presence of "locomotor-type patterns" seen in patients with complete SCIs through tonic epidural stimulation.[204]

Although many locomotor training studies have demonstrated improved walking function in response to training in patients with incomplete SCIs, questions remain regarding the efficacy of this type of training over more traditional gait training approaches. However, as interest in locomotor training interventions continued to grow, so did concern over the amount and intensity of labor required by therapists to complete this rehabilitation technique. The advent of robotic-assisted locomotor training devices offered a less burdensome alternative to facilitate walking in persons with incomplete SCIs while reducing therapist strain (Figure 16-60, *B*).[198,205,206] Over the last several years various types of locomotor training approaches have been studied with regard to incomplete SCIs; however, many questions still remain regarding efficacy of specific intervention choices and timing for this population. In a randomized controlled trial, Dobkin and colleagues reported that after 12 weeks of equal administration of locomotor training using manual assistance and conventional overground gait training, no differences in walking abilities were reported in patients with incomplete SCIs with either intervention.[197] Field-Fote and co-workers[198] randomly assigned 27 patients with motor incomplete SCIs into one of four different stepping groups using body-weight support including treadmill training with manual assistance, treadmill training with electrical stimulation, overground training with stimulation, and treadmill training with robotic assistance. After 12 weeks of training, all subject groups demonstrated a significant effect of training on walking speed, but differences among the four groups

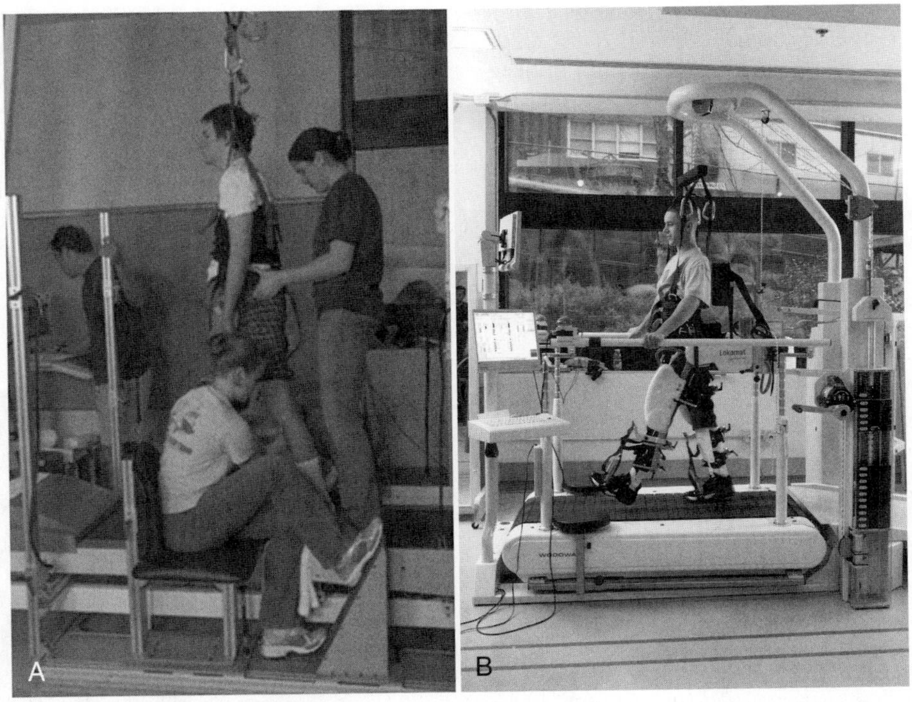

Figure 16-60 ■ **A,** Manual treadmill. Treadmill training with body-weight–supported and manual assistance is being completed on the TheraStride Innoventor, which combines a treadmill and support harness system with software that measures variables of gait training, including speed, weight supported, and amount of time walked. Two or three therapists are needed to provide assistance at the trunk and lower limbs to facilitate an appropriate gait pattern. **B,** Robotic treadmill. The Lokomat by Hocoma is a robotic-assisted treadmill that provides adjustable body-weight support and gives clinicians the ability to adjust gait-specific parameters when completing training with patients who have mobility deficits.

were not statistically significant.[198] Finally, two systematic reviews have also concluded that there is insufficient evidence at this time to conclude that any one locomotor training strategy is superior to any other to improve walking function in people with incomplete SCIs.[207,208] However, Lam and colleagues did suggest that patients with chronic SCIs might benefit more from the combined approach of locomotor training with electrical stimulation.[207]

Upper-Extremity Neuroprosthetics

The first developments in upper-extremity FES began in the 1960s with use of a flexor hinge orthosis, much like a tenodesis brace.[210] Later developments focused on improving hand function, primarily palmar grasp and lateral pinch.[211] The use of surface electrodes then led to the development of implantable FES systems. The NeuroControl Freehand System is an implanted medical device that uses electrical stimulation electrodes that are attached to muscles in the hands and forearms and a pacemaker-type stimulator that is surgically implanted in the chest. Signals come from the external controller to the electrodes and cause muscles to contract and the hand to open and close. The system was approved by the FDA in 1997, but marketing was stopped in 2001. The future of upper-extremity implantable neuroprosthetics is currently uncertain, with no systems having been made commercially available since the NeuroControl Freehand.

More recent development of upper-extremity neuroprosthetics has been focused around external neuroprosthetics with products such as the Bioness H200 (Handmaster) or the bionic glove by Hanger Orthopedic. The Bioness H200 system enables appropriately selected clients with midcervical injuries to flex and extend the thumb and fingers, allowing a useful pinch and grasp, by hitting a switch or a trigger (Figure 16-61). The bionic glove uses three channels to activate and flex the thumb and extend or flex the fingers by using wrist extensors or flexors to control the neuroprosthesis.[212]

Lower-Extremity Neuroprosthetics

The first system for standing and stepping to gain FDA approval was the Parastep II system, developed by Sigmedics (Northfield, Illinois).[213] This type of system generally uses two to 12 channels of stimulation. The system in its simplest form uses one set of electrodes placed over the quadriceps muscle and another set over the sural, saphenous, or peroneal nerve. This system consists of a computer control box, lead wire, electrodes, and a cable connected to a walking device that houses the command switch(es) for step function. Other walking systems that use implanted electrodes are being investigated at this time, but none are FDA approved. Both FES systems, the surface electrode system and the implanted system, in their present state show promise for the future. However, these systems currently do not present a viable alternative to wheelchair use because of the high energy requirement.[214,215] In addition, there is limited research in the use of epidural spinal cord stimulation to facilitate ambulation.[143,216]

Hybrid FES orthosis systems are orthotic systems that incorporate FES. Usually the FES is a simple configuration of approximately four channels and uses surface stimulation. One such system, used with the RGO, was developed by Douglass and colleagues at Louisiana State University Medical School. Systems such as this offer the advantage of increased energy efficiency compared with the use of only orthoses or only FES. Conversely, the bulkiness of the systems impedes the completion of some ADLs, and donning and doffing is more difficult.[80,217,218]

FES devices have also been designed to address foot drop dysfunction to improve overground locomotion in patients with incomplete SCIs. Promising results have been demonstrated in all outcome measures of walking, such as functional mobility, speed, spatiotemporal parameters, and the physiological cost of walking.[219-221] Improvements in walking function could be associated with plasticity in central nervous system organization, as seen by the modification of the stretch reflex and modifications

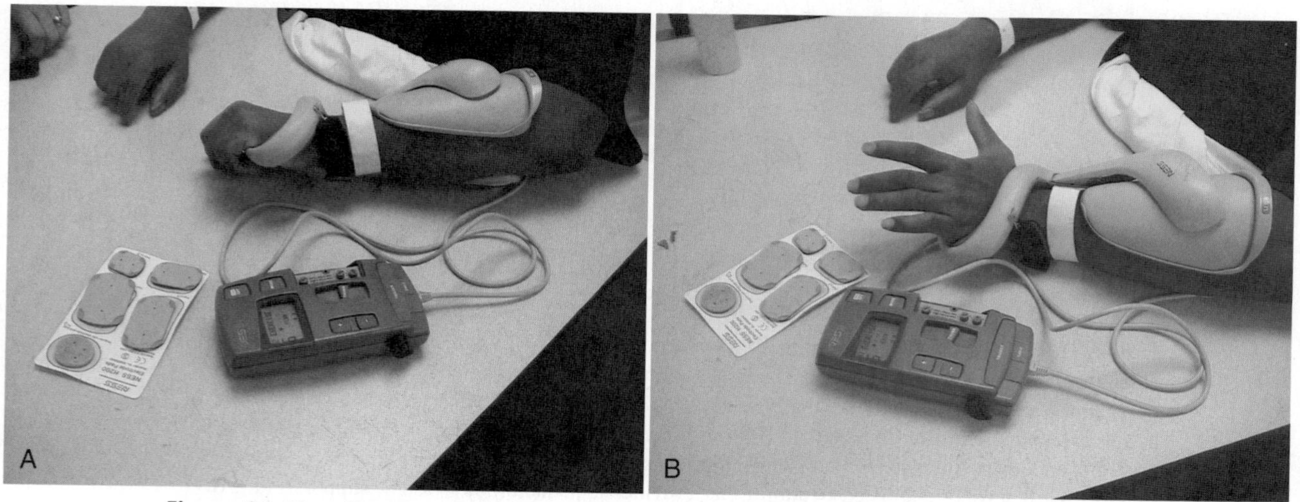

Figure 16-61 ■ The Bioness H200 system enables appropriately selected patients with midcervical injuries to flex **(A)** and extend **(B)** the thumb and fingers, allowing a useful pinch and grasp, by hitting a switch or a trigger.

in the corticospinal activation of lower leg muscles.[222] Commercially available products designed to improve overground walking in people with neurological injuries with foot drop include the Bioness L300 (Figure 16-62) and the WalkAide by Innovative Neurotronics (Figure 16-63). Both devices are single-channel foot drop stimulators that synchronize the electrical impulses to the dorsiflexors with gait. Overcoming many of the technical shortcomings of conventional FES units, these units have increased compliance and community use of this technology. Several studies have reported the immediate effects and short-term gains; however, long-term benefit of foot drop stimulation for people with SCI is yet to be sufficiently established in the literature.[219-221,223]

Functional Electrical Stimulation Cycling

FES cycling has gained acceptance in recent years in treatment of patients with spinal cord injuries. Many authors have reported significant health and wellness benefits that are both physiological and psychological when treating patients with SCIs with this technology.[209] During this intervention, electrodes are applied to various muscle groups of the lower extremities including the quadriceps, hamstrings, gluteal muscles, tibialis anterior, and gastrocnemius and soleus. The bike then electrically stimulates the selected muscle groups at the appropriate intervals to produce the torque that turns the ergometer at a preset speed. The FES-driven workload can be supplemented by an internal motor within the ergometer. Currently there are three commercially available products, including the RT300 by Restorative Therapies (Figure 16-64), ERGYS 2 by Therapeutic

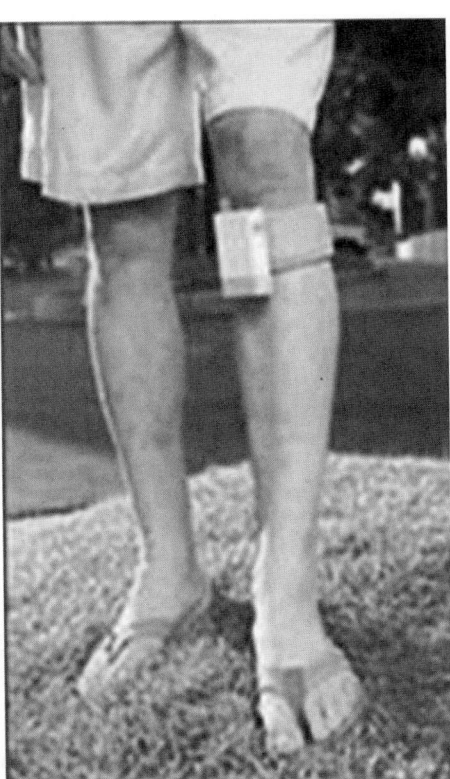

Figure 16-63 ■ The WalkAide System is a neuroprosthetic device that contains an orthotic cuff and electrodes. It fits just below the knee to supply functional electrical stimulation (FES) to the lower leg, stimulating the appropriate muscles and causing dorsiflexion. It is activated by a tilt sensor mechanism and relies on the angle of the tibia for appropriate timing of the FES to assist with foot drop.

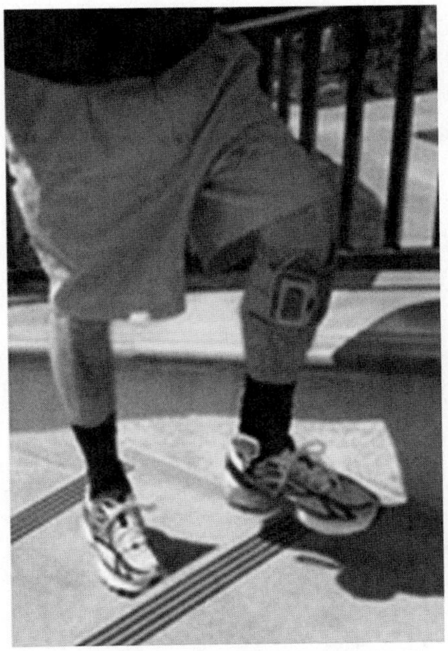

Figure 16-62 ■ Bioness L300 system is a neuroprosthetic device that contains an orthotic cuff and electrodes. It fits just below the knee to supply functional electrical stimulation (FES) to the lower leg, stimulating the appropriate muscles and causing dorsiflexion. A gait sensor is placed in the client's shoe, and as he or she shifts weight off of the affected limb, FES is triggered to assist with foot drop.

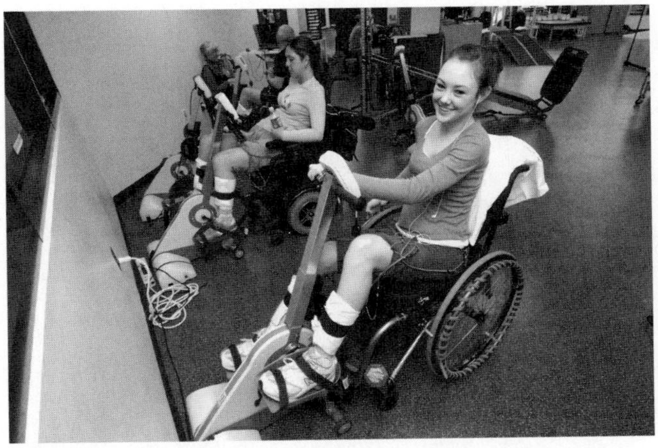

Figure 16-64 ■ RT300-SL leg FES system is a portable functional electrical stimulation (FES) bike that can be easily accessed from the patient's wheelchair. Adhesive electrodes can be applied to a variety of lower-extremity muscles including the quadriceps, hamstrings, gluteals, tibialis anterior, and gastrocnemius. These muscles are stimulated at the appropriate time to facilitate a cycling motion using a lower-extremity ergometer. FES bike software has the capability to store patient-specific parameters between sessions and patients.

Alliances, and the RehaMove by Hasomed. The following benefits from FES cycling have been reported in patients with spinal cord injuries: improved cardiorespiratory fitness, increased leg circulation, increased metabolic enzymes or hormones, greater muscle volume and fiber size, enhanced functional exercise capacity, decreased spasticity, decreased blood glucose and insulin levels, and improved bone mineral density.[209,224-230]

Newer technology also may include upper-extremity FES (Figure 16-65) cycling in which the electrodes may be applied to various muscle groups of the arm and scapula. The most commonly used muscle groups are the anterior deltoids, biceps, and triceps. Use caution in the presence of unresolved glenohumeral subluxation. There has been less research directly looking at the benefits of the upper-extremity FES cycle systems, but clinicians in the field suggest that it may yield many of the same benefits as lower-extremity FES cycling.

Whole Body Vibration

Whole body vibration (WBV) training has become increasingly accessible and popular for training individuals with and without disabilities in recent years. Vibration is used as a mechanical stimulus to increase motor unit recruitment through the feet when standing on a vibration platform (vertical or oscillating) or via the tendon of a muscle belly when a hand-held unit is used.[231] In a meta-analysis looking at the effects of vibration on muscular development in the able-bodied population, Pedro and Rhea determined that vibration exercise can be effective at eliciting chronic muscle strength adaptations and can be used by professionals to improve muscular strength in individuals. It was also determined that vertical platforms elicit a significantly larger effect for chronic adaptations than oscillating platforms, but oscillating platforms elicit a greater treatment effect for acute effects than vertical platforms.[232] A variety of literature has recently been published demonstrating the benefits of using this modality in people with a variety of clinical conditions including cerebral palsy,[233] Parkinson disease,[234] stroke,[235] and SCI.[236] However, there is still only a small body of evidence describing the effects of WBV on individuals with SCIs.[237] Ness and colleague[237] found a statistically significant improvement in cadence when treating individuals with chronic SCIs with WBV that was comparable to improvements seen in individuals who have undergone locomotor training. In a follow-up study[236] these authors also reported a decrease in quadriceps spasticity after individuals with chronic SCIs completed 12 sessions of WBV training. Overall, further research needs to be completed on this intervention to determine the most efficacious use of parameters with patients who have sustained SCIs, but early research supports that this may be a useful intervention to improve walking speed and decrease spasticity in individuals with chronic SCIs (Figure 16-66).

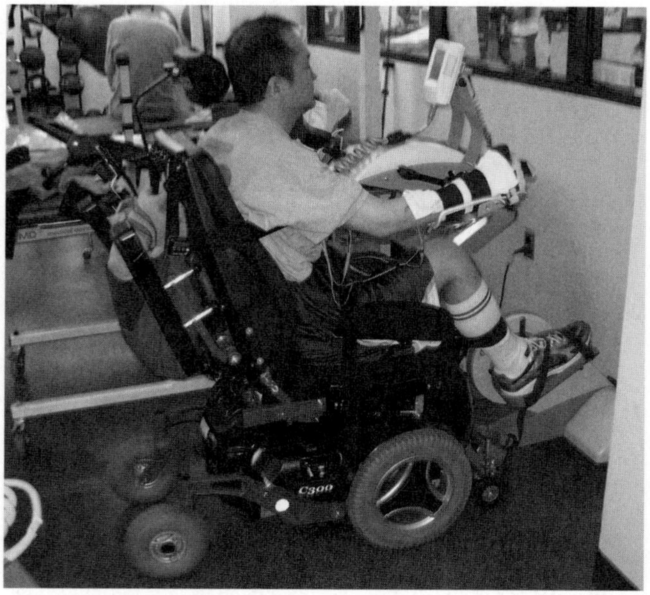

Figure 16-65 ■ RT300 SA Arm system is a functional electrical stimulation (FES) upper body ergometer designed to stimulate muscles of the upper extremities. Adhesive electrodes can be applied to a variety of muscle groups over the trunk, shoulders, and arm muscles and are stimulated at the appropriate time to facilitate a cycling motion using the upper-extremity ergometer. FES bike software has the capability to store patient-specific parameters between sessions and clients.

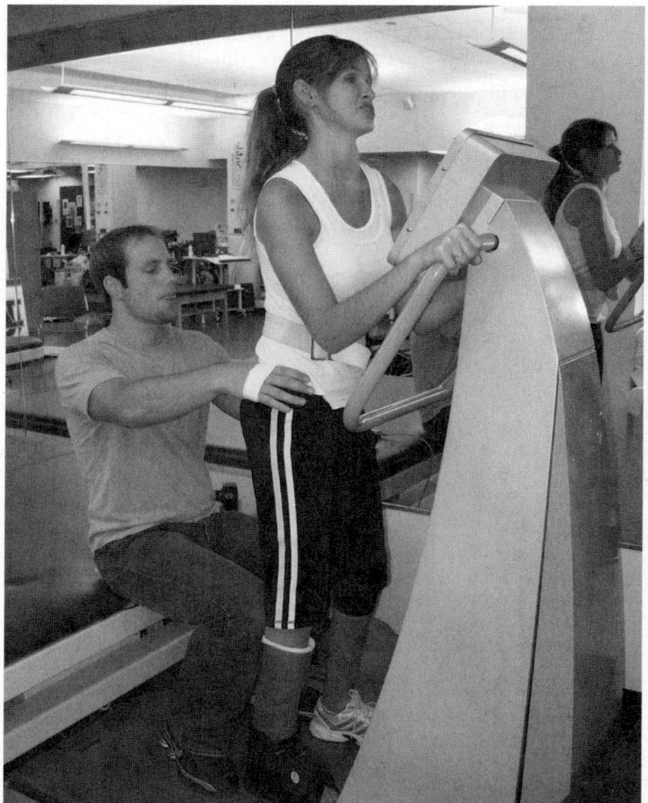

Figure 16-66 ■ The Wave vibration plate is used in the clinical setting to facilitate upright standing posture and can also be used to facilitate upper- and lower-extremity strengthening exercises.

In conclusion, recovery of walking is an increasing possibility for a large number of people with SCI. New modalities of treatment have become available for this population, but most still need to be evaluated for their efficacy.

CONCLUSION

Comprehensive treatment of the individual with SCI can be very challenging. Health care reform issues force the rehabilitation team to explore new cost-efficient options to continue to provide high-quality rehabilitation. New medical and rehabilitation interventions provide the clinician with a plethora of interventions to improve functional recovery as well as promote neurological recovery after SCI (Table 16-9). Scientists continue to research ways to prevent and/or cure paralysis and loss of function after SCI; however, until those goals have been achieved the best defense against SCI is to prevent the injury from occurring. Programs such as ThinkFirst are aimed at helping individuals of all ages learn to reduce their risk of SCI by educating them to make safe choices. Key concepts include "Buckle up. Drive safe and sober. Avoid violent situations. Lower your risk to fall. Wear a helmet. Check the water before you dive."[238]

References

To enhance this text and add value for the reader, all references are included on the companion Evolve site that accompanies this textbook. This online service will, when available, provide a link for the reader to a Medline abstract for the article cited. There are 264 cited references and other general references for this chapter, with the majority of those articles being evidence-based citations.

TABLE 16-9 ■ SUMMARY OF SPINAL CORD REGENERATION EFFORTS

AGENT/ INTERVENTION	MECHANISM	SPONSOR	TRIAL STATUS/RESULTS
Methylprednisolone (MP)	Antiinflammatory, blocks glutamate receptors, reduces accumulation of free radicals.	Pharmacia	Standard trauma protocol; effective in high dosages if given 1st 48 hours post-injury. Celebrex may be as effective.
Monosialiac ganglioside (GM-1)	Neurotrophic factor limits cell death by buffering excitotoxicity and preventing apoptosis	Sygen	May accelerate recovery in 1st 6 weeks but no difference @ 6-12 mos.
Activated macrophages	Bolsters immune response, introduces nerve growth factors.	Proneuron	Phase II 2003-06; early termination due to $$; results not released.
Cell matrix modifiers - Cordaneurin (acute) CordaChron (chronic)	Modify inhibitory glial scar matrix, allowing axon sprouting, growth, and functional plasticity.	Neuraxo	Preclinical studies completed; no Phase I announced at present.
Minocycline	Synthetic tetracycline antibiotic that inhibits activity of inflammatory cytokines, free radicals, etc. causing excitotoxicity.	NACTN	Promising preclinical work and human trials likely in Canada.
Decorin	Naturally occurring protein molecule that suppresses scar tissue formation.	Baylor College of Medicine and Integra Lifesciences	Preclinical
4-Aminopyridine (Fampridine or 4-AP)	Potassium channel blocker restores action potential conduction in de- or poorly-myelinated nerves; enhances synaptic transmission.	Acorda	Chronic SCI; Two Phase II studies (spasticity, bladder control) 2003-05; moderately effective. FDA may approve in 2010 for MS.
HP-184	Synthetic protein that functions as a potassium channel blocker to improve nerve conduction.	Aventis	Chronic SCI; Phase II completed; limited efficacy; no further development planned.
Riluzole	Sodium channel blocker and antiexcitotoxic drug marketed for treatment of ALS.	NACTN	Phase II trial in acute SCI likely to be funded by NACTN.
Glial growth factors (Neuregulin)	NGF stimulates myelin production from remaining oligodendrocytes.	Acorda	Preclinical; may initiate Phase I in MS; no date projected.
Monoclonal antibodies	Several antibodies have been identified with potential to repair CNS myelin and restore neurological function in MS and SCI.	Acorda, Biogen Idec, Amgen	Preclinical studies
AIT-082 (Neotrofin)	NGF promotes axonal sprouting.	Neurotherapeutics	Clinical trial completed but no results released.
Inosine + Axiogenesis Factor (AF-1)	NGFs that promote axon growth in the corticospinal tract.	Boston Life Science	Phase I trial pending with stroke patients.
Glial derived neurotrophic factor (GDNF)	Neurotrophic effect on sensory neurons superior to other nerve growth factors (NGF, NT-3, NT-4/5)	Amgen	Phase II trial with advanced Parkinson's; teminated early due to lack of efficacy.
Oscillating Field Stimulator (OFS) Andara	Implanted electrodes above and below lesion deliver OFS, which promotes axonal growth.	Cyberkinetics	Small Phase I in acute SCI; humanitarian device exemption requested.

PREVENT SECONDARY INJURY EFFECTS				COMPENSATE FOR LOSS OF MYELIN		ENCOURAGE AXONS TO GROW			REPLACE DEAD CELLS	
BLOCK EXCITOTOXICITY	LIMIT APOPTOSIS	BOLSTER IMMUNE RESPONSE	PREVENT GLIAL SCARRING	STIMULATE MYELIN PRODUCTION	PREVENT DISSIPATION OF NERVE IMPULSES	INTRODUCE TROPHIC FACTORS	BLOCK GROWTH INHIBITORY FACTORS	GUIDE AXON GROWTH	IMPLANT REPLACEMENT NERVE CELLS	INDUCE DIFFERENTIATION OF PROGENITOR CELLS
X										
X	X									
	X	X				X				
			X							
X	X		?							
			X							
					X					
					X					
					X					
				X			X			
				X			X			
						X				
						X				
						X				
							X	X		

Continued

TABLE 16-9 ■ SUMMARY OF SPINAL CORD REGENERATION EFFORTS—cont'd

AGENT/ INTERVENTION	MECHANISM	SPONSOR	TRIAL STATUS/RESULTS
Neurotrophic factor (NT-3)	NGF improves bowel function in chronic SCI.	Regenereon	Phase II trial completed; no further development planned.
IN-1 antibody	Binds to Nogo, a myelin-growth inhibitor, thereby stimulating axonal growth and remyelinization.	Novartis	Phase I in Europe; Phase II in US considered but no estimated start date.
Nogo-66 nogo receptor blocker	anti-NgR1 antibody that blocks uptake of Nogo.	Biogen Idec	Preclinical studies in MS and SCI.
Chondroitinase ABC	Enzyme that breaks down chondroitin-6-sulfate proteoglycans (CSPG), a growth inhibitor, to promote axonal growth.	Acorda	Preclinical studies
Recombinant C3 toxin (Cethrin)	Blocks rho signaling protein, which mediates inhibitory Nogo and may be responsible for apoptosis; stimulates axon regeneration.	Alseres	Phase I/IIa completed in '07; promising results; Phase IIb trials pending but funding appears to be an issue.
Schwann cell transplants	Myelin producers in peripheral nerves cross into CNS at dorsal root; may be used to deliver trophic factors and as bridges to support axonal growth.		Clinical evaluation.
Olfactory ensheathing glial (OEG) cells	Cells may function in 3 ways: encourage cell migration, guide direction of axon growth, provide a bridge or scaffold over cord damage.	Portugal, China, Russia, Australia	Several uncontrolled treatments offered overseas - one safety review article; no published efficacy findings.
Fetal spinal cord transplants	Experimental procedure for treatment of syringomyelia.	Univ. of Florida	Phase I trial completed; cells survived and filled syrinx. No further studies - Replaced by hESC studies (Geron).
Fetal pig neural stem cells	Replace neural cells and promote differentiation.	Diacrin	Appears to be safe in Phase I trial; no effectiveness results released.
Bone marrow stromal stem cells	Autologous bone marrow-derived cells differentiate into neuron and glial cells and improve functioning in preclinical studies.	Brazil, Ukraine	No US trials planned.
Fetal neural stem cells	Cultured neural stem cells derived from a single 8-week fetus.	NeuralStem	US Phase I trial for ALS at Emory in 2010.
Human embryonic neural stem cells	Embryonic stem cells that have been differentiated into precursors of neuron-support cells. Source is H1 cell line "approved" human embryonic stem cell line.	Geron	Phase I trial on FDA hold as of August 2009. Expect restart in late 2010.
Umbilical cord blood stem cells	Cells used in treatment of leukemia, autoimmune diseases (lupus), and sickle cell anemia.	Stemcyte, China, India	China conducting CB + Lithium trial. Possibility of US trial in >2011?

PREVENT SECONDARY INJURY EFFECTS				COMPENSATE FOR LOSS OF MYELIN		ENCOURAGE AXONS TO GROW			REPLACE DEAD CELLS	
BLOCK EXCITOTOXICITY	LIMIT APOPTOSIS	BOLSTER IMMUNE RESPONSE	PREVENT GLIAL SCARRING	STIMULATE MYELIN PRODUCTION	PREVENT DISSIPATION OF NERVE IMPULSES	INTRODUCE TROPHIC FACTORS	BLOCK GROWTH INHIBITORY FACTORS	GUIDE AXON GROWTH	IMPLANT REPLACEMENT NERVE CELLS	INDUCE DIFFERENTIATION OF PROGENITOR CELLS
				X			X			
				X			X			
				X			X			
			X				X			
	?			X		X	X			
				X		X		X	X	X
						X		X	X	X
							X		X	
									X	X
									X	X
				?					X	X
									X	X

APPENDIX 16-A ■ Selected References: Architectural Modification

Accessibility in Georgia: a technical and policy guide to access in Georgia, Raleigh, NC, 1986, Georgia Council on Developmental Disabilities.

An accessible bathroom, Madison, WI, 1980, Design Coalition.

An accessible entrance: ramps, Madison, WI, 1979, Design Coalition.

Handbook for design: specially adapted housing, Veterans Administration pamphlet 26-13, Washington, DC, 1978, Department of Veterans Benefits, Veterans Administration.

Harber L, Mae R, Orleans P, et al: *UFAS retrofit guide: accessibility modifications for existing buildings,* New York, 1993, Van Nostrand Reinhold.

Lebrock C, Behar S: *Beautiful barrier-free: a visual guide to accessibility,* New York, 1993, Van Nostrand Reinhold.

Mace RL: *The accessible housing design file,* New York, 1991, Van Nostrand Reinhold.

CHAPTER 17 Neuromuscular Diseases

ANN HALLUM, PT, PhD, and DIANE D. ALLEN, PT, PhD

KEY TERMS

amyotrophic lateral sclerosis
disuse atrophy
Duchenne muscular dystrophy
Guillain-Barré syndrome
overwork damage
polyradiculoneuropathy

OBJECTIVES

After reviewing this chapter the student or therapist will be able to:

1. Describe the basic pathology and medical treatment of amyotrophic lateral sclerosis, Guillain-Barré syndrome, and Duchenne muscular dystrophy.
2. Describe the current goals and interventions for each condition.
3. Describe the "safe" exercise windows related to disuse atrophy and exercise (overwork) damage.
4. Be able to apply intervention concepts discussed in this chapter to other neuromuscular diseases.

Neuromuscular diseases encompass disorders of upper or lower motor nerves or the muscles they innervate. This chapter traces the connections among the central nervous system (CNS), peripheral nervous system (PNS), and musculoskeletal system through the disordered functioning associated with three neuromuscular diseases: amyotrophic lateral sclerosis (ALS), which damages upper and lower motor neurons; Guillain-Barré syndrome (GBS), which compromises lower motor neurons and the PNS; and Duchenne muscular dystrophy (DMD), which affects the muscles themselves. To review the normal connections, upper motor neurons originate in the motor cortex of the brain (Betz cells). Axons from these upper motor neurons descend by means of the corticobulbar and corticospinal tracts to synapse with lower motor neurons in the brain stem (neurons of the cranial nerves with motor functions) and spinal cord (anterior horn cells or alpha motor neurons). Simultaneously, corticobulbar tract fibers innervate neurons originating within the brain stem and descending through the spinal cord to provide additional input to lower (alpha) motor neurons. Axons from the lower motor neurons within both the brain stem and spinal cord run within the peripheral nerves, which include motor and sensory fibers, to synapse with muscle fibers. The muscle fibers respond to excitation by contracting. Depending on the site of the pathology, neuromuscular diseases can be classified as neurogenic or myopathic. ALS and GBS are neurogenic disorders; DMD is a primary myopathy (Figure 17-1).

In considering the movement dysfunction associated with these diseases, strength and endurance are most affected, with flexibility deficits resulting from these.[1] All three disorders decrease a person's ability to generate force in the affected muscles, with weakness as a primary symptom. Loss of muscle strength can lead to speech, swallowing, and respiratory difficulties along with functional limitations. Fatigue is another primary deficit, although the neurogenic disorders tend to result in central fatigue (deficit in ability to recruit motor units) as opposed to the peripheral fatigue of the myopathies (deficit in ability of muscle fibers to contract forcefully).[2] Secondary movement problems include loss of range of motion (ROM) in immobile muscles and joints, and pain or muscle spasms. Adaptability, the ability to sense obstacles or changes in the environment and change the course of a movement in response,[1] may be affected with the sensory loss in GBS but is not typically a problem in ALS or DMD.

AMYOTROPHIC LATERAL SCLEROSIS

Pathology and Medical Diagnosis

ALS, commonly known in the United States as *Lou Gehrig disease,* is a relentless, degenerative, terminal disease affecting both upper and lower motor neurons. Massive loss of anterior horn cells of the spinal cord and the motor cranial nerve nuclei in the lower brain stem results in muscle atrophy and weakness (amyotrophy). Demyelination and gliosis of the corticospinal tracts and corticobulbar tracts caused by degeneration of the Betz cells in the motor cortex result in upper motor neuron symptoms (lateral sclerosis).

The cause of ALS is unknown; however, numerous theories have been proposed. Ninety percent of the cases of ALS are sporadic without a known genetic component; however, most neurodegenerative diseases are now thought to be related to complex protein misfolding disorders. The latest research suggests that ALS and other neurodegenerative disorders are related to TDP-43 proteinopathy.[3] Approximately 5% to 10% of the cases seem to have a complex genetic basis coded on *ALS1* through *ALS8* and other mutations that are associated with frontal lobe dementias. Twenty percent of genetic causes of ALS are thought to be related to mendelian mutations in the superoxide dismutase–1 (SOD1) gene *(ALS1).* Other factors considered in the genesis of ALS are vascular endothelial growth factors, toxicity leading to motor neuron death, oxidative stress and mitochondrial dysfunction related to microglial inflammation,[4,5] and environmental factors.[6]

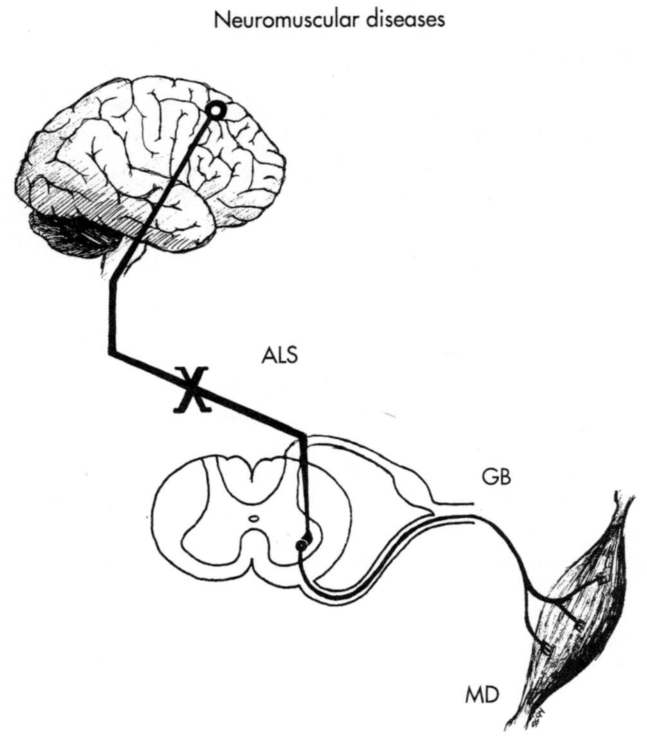

Figure 17-1 ■ Primary sites of pathological features of amyotrophic lateral sclerosis (AMLS), Guillain-Barré syndrome (GBS), and Duchenne muscular dystrophy (DMD).

The differential diagnosis for ALS is extensive. The possibility of cervical or lumbar spondylosis, syringomyelia, multiple sclerosis, primary lateral sclerosis, and diseases associated with lower motor neuron pathology, among other diagnoses, needs to be excluded before the diagnosis of ALS is made.[7] Currently, no single laboratory test is available to confirm a diagnosis of ALS, although creatine phosphokinase levels are elevated in approximately 70% of patients and tend to be higher in patients with limb onset ALS rather than bulbar onset.[8] Genetic testing to identify the mutations in the Cu,Zn SOD1 gene is available when a family history of ALS is present. Other laboratory tests, such as identification of biochemical markers in the blood and cerebrospinal fluid, are used to exclude other neurological diseases. Electromyography (EMG) and nerve conduction studies can be helpful to confirm the presence of widespread lower motor neuron disease without peripheral neuropathy or polyradiculopathy. Neuroimaging studies are used to rule out conditions that may have clinical signs similar to those of ALS.[9]

Because of the absence of clear laboratory markers of ALS, the clinical diagnosis must be made on the basis of recognition of a pattern of observed and reported symptoms of both upper and lower motor neuron disease and persistent declines in physical functions supported by inclusionary and exclusionary diagnostic testing. Because of the overlap of symptoms with other neuromuscular disorders, misdiagnosis is not uncommon.[10]

ALS is the most common form of motor neuron disease, with an incidence of approximately three to five cases per 100,000 persons. Mean age at onset is 57 years, with two thirds of patients aged 50 to 70 years old at time of onset.[11] Men are affected approximately 1.3 to two times more frequently than are women, although the differences are less with late onset of disease (ages 70+).[12]

Clinical Presentation

The World Federation of Neurology (WFN) has developed suggested diagnostic criteria (suspected, possible, probable, and definite) for patients with ALS entering clinical research trials. Essentially, a patient with "definite" ALS must show concomitant upper motor neuron and lower motor neuron signs in three spinal regions or in two spinal regions with bulbar signs. Either upper or lower motor signs must also be evident in other regions of the body.[13] Exclusionary criteria are oculomotor nerve pathway abnormalities (the oculomotor nerve is spared in ALS), significant movement disorder patterns, sphincter control problems, the presence of sensory and autonomic nervous system (ANS) dysfunction, and cognitive deterioration.[14] (Refer to the WFN ALS website [www.wfnals.org] section on ALS education for up-to-date criteria used for clinical studies.)

Although a consistent diagnostic criterion for ALS has been the absence of sensory involvement, some evidence exists that there is a progressive functional deficit in sensation, perhaps related to ongoing immobility.[15]

Similarly, cognitive deficits are considered exclusionary criteria for an ALS diagnosis. However, a small subgroup of patients with both familial and sporadic forms of ALS has been identified as having concomitant evidence of frontotemporal dementia (FTD), showing lower scores on executive cognitive functions, word finding, and phrase length.[16] A combination of ALS and FTD suggests a common cause may be possible.[17] Because of these findings, therapists should be aware of the possibility of cognitive deficits in their patients with ALS, manifested as a decrement in executive skills such as planning and organization and language problems. Such patients may have more difficulty following through on medication and therapeutic recommendations, and their families may need more support. Unassociated with overall cognitive impairment, some deficits in action knowledge as opposed to object knowledge have been noted in patients with ALS, correlating with atrophy in the motor and premotor cortex.[18] Specific cognitive deficits, therefore, may be more common than previously noted.

The earliest clinical markers heralding ALS are fasciculations (especially unequivocal fasciculation in the tongue), muscle cramps, fatigue, weakness, and atrophy.[13,19] During initial diagnostic visits, patients frequently report to their physicians a profound sense of fatigue or the loss of exercise tolerance.[19] Ninety percent of patients report weakness occurring in a striated muscle or group of muscles. Because the onset of ALS is insidious, most patients are not aware of the strength changes, or they have adjusted to the changes until they have difficulty with a functional activity such as tying shoes or climbing stairs. Physical examination usually demonstrates more widespread weakness and atrophy than reported by the patient. By the time most patients report weakness, they have lost approximately 80% of their motor neurons in the areas of weakness. This demonstrates the plasticity of the nervous system and its drive to adapt to meet functional goals. The weakness spreads over time to include musculature throughout the body. Succeeding symptoms of weakness in other muscles depends on the continued loss of motor neurons to the 20% threshold needed for perception of weakness.[20,21] A typical, but not absolute, pattern of motor progression is early distal involvement followed by proximal limb involvement. In some cases bulbar symptoms herald the onset of ALS, but bulbar symptoms more commonly occur later in the disease. Flexor muscles tend to be weaker than extensor muscles.[22]

Although the atrophy and weakness component of ALS is most obvious, 80% or more of patients show early clinical evidence of pyramidal tract dysfunction (e.g., hyperreflexia in the presence of weakness and atrophy, spasticity, and Babinski and Hoffmann reflexes).[13] Although in some cases the upper motor neuron signs may be absent clinically, Chou[23] has shown on autopsy that significant involvement may be present despite the lack of clinical evidence.

The pattern of ALS onset is highly varied, with several patterns identified by primary area of onset. Lower-extremity onset is slightly more common than upper-extremity onset, which is more common than bulbar onset. Some patients show initial symptoms in distal musculature of upper and lower extremities. A significant diagnostic feature of the pattern of disease is the asymmetry of the weakness and the sparing of some muscle fibers even in highly atrophied muscles. For example, a patient may have weakness of the right intrinsics and shoulder musculature or weakness of the left anterior tibial muscles. Bulbar symptoms are presaged by tongue fasciculations and weakness, facial and palatal weakness, and swallowing difficulties, which result in dysphagia and dysarthria. Pseudobulbar palsy is sometimes present in ALS, manifested by spontaneous laughing or crying unrelated to the situation.[24] Despite the pattern of onset, however, the eventual course of the illness is similar in most patients, with an unremitting spread of weakness to other muscle groups leading to total paralysis of spinal musculature and muscles innervated by the cranial nerves. Death is usually related to respiratory failure.[25]

In a longitudinal study using monthly questionnaires, direct patient interviews, record reviews, physician interviews, and family member interviews, Brooks and colleagues[20] followed 702 patients with ALS. Their findings suggest that spread of neuronal degeneration occurred more quickly to adjacent areas than to noncontiguous areas. The spread to adjacent areas was more rapid at the brain stem, cervical, and lumbar regions. Limb involvement after bulbar onset was more aggressive in men than in women.[20]

One study focused on developing methods to assess the natural history of the progression of ALS so that medical and supportive treatment planning and interventions could be instituted.[26] Hillel and colleagues[27] have developed the ALS severity scale for rapid functional assessment of disease stage. Their 10-point ordinal scale allows clinicians and therapists to score patients in four categories: speech, swallowing, and lower-extremity and upper-extremity function (Box 17-1).

A five-point scale of severity is currently being used in ALS clinical drug trials. Patients in stage 1 (mild disease) have a recent diagnosis and are functionally independent in ambulation, activities of daily living (ADLs), and speech. Stage 2 (moderate) identifies patients with mild deficits in function in three regions or a moderate to severe deficit in one region and mild or normal function in two other regions. Stage 3 (severe) defines patients who need assistance because of deficits in two or three regions; for example, the patient needs assistance to walk or transfer, needs help with upper-extremity activities, and/or is dysarthric or dysphasic. Stage 4 identifies patients with nonfunctional movement of at least two regions and moderate or nonfunctional movement of a third area. Stage 5 is death.[22] (See Brooks and colleagues[14] and Pradas and colleagues[28] for information on the natural history of ALS and its importance in the design of clinical treatment trials.)

Along with the primary impairments of weakness and fatigue affecting body structure and function in ALS, patients also have progressive limitations in activity and participation.[29] Activity limitations result in gradual loss of independence in community and then household tasks. Mechanical and electronic adaptive devices can help extend independence in some ADLs past the initial strength losses. Participation limitations result in progressive isolation from the community and family unless extraordinary efforts persist to retain a communication system at home and through electronic media.

Medical Prognosis

In almost all cases ALS progresses relentlessly and leads to death from respiratory failure. The rate of progression seems to be consistent for each patient but varies considerably among patients. Patients with an initial onset of bulbar weakness (dysarthria, dysphagia) and respiratory weakness (dyspnea) tend to have a more rapid progression to death than patients whose weakness begins in the distal extremities.[30] Death usually follows within 2 to 4 years after diagnosis, with a small number of patients living for 15 to 20 years.[10]

Years of survival after diagnosis may change as drug therapies are developed.[31] In addition, increasing numbers of patients are electing to prolong life with home-based mechanical ventilation as opposed to palliative or comfort care only.

Medical Management

ALS has no known cure and minimal effective disease-slowing treatments. Mitchell and Borasio[24] have created a table (see Table 2 in their study) that summarizes the results of trials of the many putative ALS-modifying pharmaceuticals. Only riluzole has been approved for treatment of ALS. Riluzole provides very modest improvement over a placebo in both bulbar and limb function, but not in actual strength of muscles.[32] The drug extended lifespan an average of 2 to 3 months. The side effects were minimal in some studies, but fatigue and weakness have been noted in 26% and 18% of patients taking riluzole compared with a placebo.[33]

The popular press has reported on nutritional cures for ALS, including regular use of vitamin E. However, Orrell and colleagues[34] found insufficient evidence to support clinical use of vitamin E supplements in ALS as an additive to riluzole treatment or as adjunctive therapy, although no apparent contraindication was found to taking the supplement. Other nutritional and nonpharmaceutical supplements have had some success in animal models of ALS, but this has not yet been confirmed in humans.[35]

Cannabis has been studied for its effect on spasticity in patients with multiple sclerosis and spinal cord injury. In a study of 131 people with ALS, 13 used cannabis, with reports of reduction in spasticity, pain, and depression.[36] Because of the apparent hopelessness of the diagnosis, many physicians,

BOX 17-1 ■ AMYOTROPHIC LATERAL SCLEROSIS SEVERITY SCALE: LOWER EXTREMITY, UPPER EXTREMITY, SPEECH, SWALLOWING

LOWER EXTREMITIES (WALKING)

Normal		
10	Normal ambulation	Patient denies any weakness or fatigue; examination reveals no abnormality.
9	Fatigue suspected	Patient experiences sense of weakness or fatigue in lower extremities during exertion.
Early Ambulation Difficulties		
8	Difficulty with uneven terrain	Difficulty and fatigue when walking long distances, climbing stairs, and walking over uneven ground (even thick carpet).
7	Observed changes in gait	Noticeable change in gait; pulls on railings when climbing stairs; may use leg brace.
Walks with Assistance		
6	Walks with mechanical device	Needs or uses cane, walker, or assistant to walk; probably uses wheelchair away from home.
5	Walks with mechanical device and assistant	Does not attempt to walk without attendant; ambulation limited to less than 50 ft; avoids stairs.
Functional Movement Only		
4	Able to support	At best, can shuffle a few steps with the help of an attendant for transfers.
3	Purposeful leg movements	Unable to take steps but can position legs to assist attendant in transfers; moves legs purposefully to maintain mobility in bed.
No Purposeful Leg Movement		
2	Minimal movement	Minimal movement of one or both legs; cannot reposition legs independently.
1	Paralysis	Flaccid paralysis; cannot move lower extremities (except, perhaps, to close inspection).

UPPER EXTREMITIES (DRESSING AND HYGIENE)

Normal Function		
10	Normal function	Patient denies any weakness or unusual fatigue of upper extremities; examination demonstrates no abnormality.
9	Suspected fatigue	Patient experiences sense of fatigue in upper extremities during exertion; cannot sustain work for as long as normal; atrophy not evident on examination.
Independent and Complete Self-Care		
8	Slow self-care	Dressing and hygiene performed more slowly than usual.
7	Effortful self-care performance	Requires significantly more time (usually double or more) and effort to accomplish self-care; weakness is apparent on examination.
Intermittent Assistance		
6	Mostly independent	Handles most aspects of dressing and hygiene alone; adapts by resting, modifying (e.g., use of electric razor), or avoiding some tasks; requires assistance for fine motor tasks (e.g., buttons, ties).
5	Partial independence	Handles some aspects of dressing and hygiene alone; however, routinely requires assistance for many tasks such as applying makeup, combing, and shaving.
Needs Attendant for Self-Care		
4	Attendant assists patient	Attendant must be present for dressing and hygiene; patient performs the majority of each task with the assistance of the attendant.
3	Patient assists attendant	The attendant directs the patient for almost all tasks; the patient moves in a purposeful manner to assist the attendant; does not initiate self-care.
Total Dependence		
2	Minimal movement	Minimal movement of one or both arms; cannot reposition arms.
1	Paralysis	Flaccid paralysis; unable to move upper extremities (except, perhaps, to close inspection).

SPEECH

Normal Speech Processes		
10	Normal speech	Patient denies any difficulty speaking; examination demonstrates no abnormality.
9	Nominal speech abnormalities	Only the patient or spouse notices speech has changed; maintains normal rate and volume.
Detectable Speech Disturbance		
8	Perceived speech changes	Speech changes are noted by others, especially during fatigue or stress; rate of speech remains essentially normal.
7	Obvious speech abnormalities	Speech is consistently impaired; rate, articulation, and resonance are affected; remains easily understood.

BOX 17-1 ■ AMYOTROPHIC LATERAL SCLEROSIS SEVERITY SCALE: LOWER EXTREMITY, UPPER EXTREMITY, SPEECH, SWALLOWING—cont'd

Intelligible with Repeating		
6	Repeats message on occasion	Rate is much slower, repeats specific words in adverse listening situation; does not limit complexity or length of messages.
5	Frequent repeating required	Speech is slow and labored; extensive repetition or a "translator" is commonly used; patient probably limits the complexity or length of messages.
Speech Combined with Nonvocal Communication		
4	Speech plus nonverbal communication	Speech is used in response to questions; intelligibility problems need to be resolved by writing or a spokesperson.
3	Limits speech to one-word responses	Vocalizes one-word responses beyond yes and no; otherwise writes or uses a spokesperson; initiates communication nonvocally.
Loss of Useful Speech		
2	Vocalizes for emotional expression	Uses vocal inflection to express emotion, affirmation, and negation.
1	Nonvocal	Vocalization is effortful, limited in duration, and rarely attempted; may vocalize for crying or pain.
X	Tracheostomy	
SWALLOWING		
Normal Eating Habits		
10	Normal swallowing	Patient denies any difficulty chewing or swallowing; examination demonstrates no abnormality.
9	Nominal abnormality	Only patient notices slight indicators such as food lodging in the recesses of the mouth or sticking in the throat.
Early Eating Problems		
8	Minor swallowing problems	Reports some swallowing difficulties; maintains essentially a regular diet; isolated choking episodes.
7	Prolonged times, smaller bite size	Meal time has significantly increased and smaller bite sizes are necessary; must concentrate on swallowing thin liquids.
Dietary Consistency Changes		
6	Soft diet	Diet is limited primarily to soft foods; requires some special meal preparation.
5	Liquefied diet	Oral intake adequate; nutrition limited primarily to liquefied diet; adequate thin liquid intake usually a problem; may force self to eat.
Needs Tube Feeding		
4	Supplemental tube feedings	Oral intake alone no longer adequate; patient uses or needs a tube to supplement intake; patient continues to take significant (greater than 50%) nutrition orally.
3	Tube feeding with occasional oral nutrition	Primary nutrition and hydration accomplished by tube; receives less than 50% of nutrition orally.
No Oral Feeding		
2	Secretions managed with aspirator and/or medications	Cannot safely manage any oral intake; secretions managed with aspirator and/or medications; swallows reflexively.
1	Aspiration of secretions	Secretions cannot be managed noninvasively; rarely swallows.

Adapted with permission from Hillel AD, Miller RM, Yorkston K, et al: Amyotrophic lateral sclerosis severity scale. *Neuroepidemiology* 8:142, 1989.

especially those not associated with major medical centers having neuromuscular disease units, do not refer patients with ALS for services, yet few primary care physicians or neurologists have extensive experience in the care of patients and families coping with ALS because of the low incidence of the disease. Yet, referral of patients with ALS to a multidisciplinary clinic typically extends the patient's lifespan, especially patients with bulbar onset of ALS.[25,37]

Muscle Spasms and Pain

Some patients experience muscle cramps and spasms related to upper motor neuron pathology, and up to 73% of patients complain of pain, typically in the later stages.[24] Although most spasms can be relieved with stretching or increased movement, some patients require medications such as quinine or baclofen to relieve symptoms (see Chapter 36 for information on drug therapies). In a review of studies on the treatment of spasticity in ALS, Ashworth and colleagues[38] found only one randomized study addressing spasticity: a moderate-endurance exercise regimen decreased spasticity at 3 months after initiation of the program. Stretching and massage may prove helpful for nocturnal muscle cramps.[25] Kesiktas and colleagues[39] report that in a controlled study of spasticity in patients after spinal cord injury, adding hydrotherapy to a program of medication and exercise decreased severity of spasms and decreased the amount of medication required. A similar response could be hypothesized in patients with ALS. In addition to muscle spasms, patients report nonspecific aching and muscle soreness, probably related to immobility and trauma to paralyzed muscles during caregiving procedures. However, many patients do not receive adequate pain medication, or the pain is not controlled by the medication taken.[40] A Cochrane review in 2008 found no randomized or quasi-randomized controlled trials of drug therapy for pain in ALS, although several case series reported the use of acetaminophen, nonsteroidal antiinflammatory drugs (NSAIDs), or opioids.[41] Careful administration of medications such as baclofen, tizanidine, dantrolene sodium, and diazepam is useful for some patients with spasticity. Because each has a different action and side effects, the medications may have to be adjusted to find the right dosage and combination. In some patients with severe cramping, botulinum toxin injections might be helpful, but they must be carefully administered to prevent further weakness. Because many patients have compromised respiratory function, the physician must take great care when prescribing pain medication, especially opiates, which are often used when antispasmodics or antiinflammatory pain medications no longer work.[25] Patients should be instructed to keep a daily reporting log of the effectiveness of the medication so that the dosage can be adjusted if necessary.

Dysphagia

Dysphagia, a difficulty swallowing liquids, foods, or saliva, accounts for considerable misery in the patient with advanced ALS, and it must be dealt with aggressively. Patients with dysphagia have both nutritional and swallowing problems associated with weakness of the lips, tongue, palate, and mastication muscles.[42] As the progressive loss of swallowing develops, patients are also at extreme risk for aspiration. Most patients with dysphagia also have severe problems with management of their saliva (sialorrhea). If a patient has difficulty transporting saliva back to the oropharynx for swallowing, choking and drooling are common.[43] This condition is disconcerting to the affected person, who must constantly wipe the mouth or have someone do it for him or her.

In addition, secretions are often thickened because of dehydration. With pooling of the thickened saliva, the possibility of aspiration is increased. Viscosity of saliva can best be treated by hydration and, in some cases, pharmaceuticals. Drugs, such as decongestants, antidepressant drugs with anticholinergic side effects, and atropine-type drugs, can help control the amount of saliva, provided the patient is well hydrated.[44] In extreme cases, various surgical procedures such as ligation of the salivary gland ducts, severing the parasympathetic supply to the salivary glands, and excision of the salivary glands have been used effectively.[45] Newer treatments to decrease excessive secretions are radiotherapy and botulinum A toxin injections into salivary glands.[46]

Although dietary treatment is not known to be effective in changing the course of the disease, a nutritious diet to meet caloric, fluid, vitamin, and mineral needs must be maintained. Seventy-three percent of patients with ALS have difficulty bringing food to the mouth, making them dependent on others for their dietary needs. Because of the time it takes to be fed, many patients decrease their intake. All patients with dysphagia should be referred for a dietary consultation to determine the choice and progression of solid and liquid foods and supplements.[47] Appel and colleagues[47] describe nutritional plans to maintain nutrition and hydration in patients with motor neuron diseases. Patients with bulbar symptoms and severe dysphagia who are no longer able to consume nutrients orally because of motor control problems and recurrent aspiration may need a percutaneous endoscopic gastrostomy (PEG) for feeding, depending on the patient's wishes for long-term care. Some evidence exists that the PEG should be performed early in the disease process to prevent severe weight loss and aspiration.[48] Although a PEG does not appreciably lengthen survival time,[49] patients may have less fear of choking or aspiration. Receiving nourishment from a PEG does not prevent the person from taking food orally if desired.

Dysarthria

Dysarthria, impairment in speech production, is the result of abnormal function of the muscles and nerves associated with coordinated functions of the tongue and lips, larynx, soft palate, and respiratory system. Speech impairments are the initial symptom in most patients with bulbar involvement. Speech intelligibility is compromised by hypernasality, abnormalities of speed and cadence of speech, and reduced vocal volume. Speech is further compromised by inadequate breath volumes for normal phrasing. A possible option to help patients with severe hypernasality is a palatal lift prosthesis to augment velopharyngeal function.[50,51] Because little can be done medically to delay the loss of speech control, early referral to a speech therapist is essential. Numerous augmentative and alternative communication systems are now available, the simplest being voice amplification systems or homemade point boards and computer-based head or eye tracking text-to-speech systems that can be modified as the patient status changes. The type of communication system should be chosen with awareness of the patient-caregiver environment.[52]

Respiratory Management

Progressive respiratory failure is the primary cause of death in ALS patients. Respiratory failure is related to primary diaphragmatic, intercostal, and accessory respiratory muscle weakness.[53] Respiratory failure should be anticipated and discussed early following the diagnosis of ALS so that patients and their caregivers can express their wishes and develop an advanced directive for care in the terminal phase of the disease.[54]

Physiological tests used to indicate respiratory dysfunction include vital capacity, sniff nasal pressure, and nocturnal oximetry.[10] Clinical signs of increased respiratory dysfunction are dyspnea with exertion or lying supine; hypoventilation; weak or ineffective cough; increased use of auxiliary respiratory muscles; tachycardia (also a sign of pulmonary infection with fever and tachypnea); changes in sleep pattern; daytime sleepiness and concentration problems; mood changes; and morning headaches.[55]

In early stages of patient care, physical therapists (PTs) may help manage respiratory dysfunction by providing postural drainage with cough facilitation (suctioning if necessary), especially during acute respiratory illnesses. The patient and care providers should also be taught breathing exercises, chest stretching, and incentive spirometry techniques, as well as postural drainage techniques if the caregivers are prepared to provide such support. Although breathing exercises consisting of resisted inspiratory muscle training can facilitate functional respiration, even practicing unresisted breathing for 10 minutes three times a day has been shown to result in improved function.[56] An assessment of the home environment is imperative to identify sleeping positions and energy conservation techniques that can be incorporated into the patient's daily life.

As respiratory symptoms increase, oxygen at 2 L/min or less can be used intermittently at home. When hypoventilation with a decline in oxygen saturation becomes common during sleep, resulting in morning confusion and irritability, patients have the option to initiate noninvasive, positive-pressure ventilation (NIV) such as bilevel positive airway pressure (BiPAP). BiPAP, which provides greater inspiratory pressure than expiratory pressure to decrease the effort of breathing, can be administered by either mask or contoured nasal delivery systems. Some evidence indicates that early use of NIV can increase survival time by several months and increase quality of life.[57] When a patient can no longer benefit from NIV, a decision must be made about initiating ventilation by tracheostomy or palliative care.[58] (See also Miller and colleagues[59] for an excellent discussion of practice parameters in the decision-making process related to ventilatory support.) Although in the initial stages of ALS most patients indicate they would not want prolonged respirator dependence at home, patients may change their minds as they adapt to the disease restrictions.[60] A small study of patients who started tracheostomy intermittent positive-pressure ventilation (TIPPV) demonstrated increased long-term survival (2 to 64 months).[54] In another series of 70 patients on long-term TIPPV, 50% of the patients were living after 5 years; however, 11.4% of these patients had entered a "locked-in state in which they were unable to communicate in any manner."[61] Decisions about long-term respirator use should be made by the patient and involved family members or partners, with input from the interdisciplinary team caring for the patient. Discussions of preferred long-term care options should be revisited as the patient's condition changes.

If a patient decides that home ventilation is a reasonable option, those involved in the decision should visit another patient who is using in-home mechanical ventilation, if possible. Because the decision for home mechanical ventilation (HMV, NIV, or TIPPV) also affects the life of the patient's spouse, children, and extended family who may be responsible for some aspects of home care, or whose lives may be affected by the presence of in-home nurses or attendants, the decision for HMV should not be taken lightly. Extensive preparation, ongoing support, and respite options for caregivers are necessary if HMV is to be successful. Success of HMV also depends on such variables as third-party payment for home care equipment and nurse or attendant staffing, working status of the partner or spouse, age and physical fitness of the spouse and children, pre-ALS family psychosocial interactions, and financial factors. HMV should be viewed as long term, often extending for more than 1 year. Initiation of HMV results in a reasonable perceived quality of life for the patient, yet caregivers report that their quality of life may be lower than the patient's because of the burden of care that must be provided.[62]

With chronic respiratory insufficiency, the patient and family must be involved in the long-term care decisions related to instituting mechanical assistance under either emergency situations or in response to gradual deterioration. This discussion should occur before the patient develops respiratory failure. Acute respiratory failure can be frightening, and few patients or family members are prepared to forego intubation and artificial ventilation during the emergency. Patients and caregivers should understand that not making a decision about mechanical ventilation, noninvasive or invasive, is a decision to support mechanical ventilation.[63]

Physicians and health care workers who work with the patient and family must be aware of their own feelings and beliefs about prolonging life. For example, a healthy physician or therapist who values control and an active lifestyle may envision a life on a ventilator as intolerable and pass that value on to the patient, who may or may not have the same needs. The patient's decision, or change in decision, must be respected by the medical team involved in care.[64] In medical centers that use a team approach, patients and families may find support by meeting with counselors or peers with ALS who are making or have made decisions about long-term ventilator care.

Therapeutic Management of Movement Dysfunction Associated with ALS

Perhaps because of the multitude of issues to consider when managing the impairments and limitations associated with ALS, evidence suggests that patients treated by a specialized ALS multidisciplinary team fare better than do those treated by single-source providers,[65] or in general neurology clinics.[33] A Cochrane review of the evidence for multidisciplinary care advantages in this population concluded that the evidence is of low quality, so far, with no controlled trials identified.[66] Whether administered through an ALS-specific team or not, therapeutic management will necessitate examination of the patient's current status, evaluation of the deficits in relation to patient preferences and needs, and establishment of a plan based on mutually determined and realistic goals. The rate of the patient's disease progression, the areas and extent of involvement, and the stage of illness must be considered. A patient at the initial stages will have different needs than a patient at later stages who has chosen NIV or tracheostomy ventilation that may extend life span at a markedly reduced mobility level. The goal at all stages is to optimize health and increase the quality of life. With guidance and environmental adaptations, patients with slowly progressing weakness may be able to continue many of their ADLs for an extended number of years. In the final stages of the disease, when the patient is bedridden, programs to increase strength or endurance are not appropriate, and interventions such as stretching may not effectively control contracture development. However, patients may still benefit from positioning and range-of-motion (ROM) exercises to decrease muscle and joint pain related to immobility. The prescription of assistive devices and training of caregivers will also be needed. The efficacy of therapeutic interventions will be related to the timing of interventions, the motivation and persistence of the patient in carrying out the program, and support from family members or caregivers.[67] Objective documentation of outcome measures will help justify the usefulness of therapeutic interventions at all stages of this disease.

Examination

The extent of the therapeutic examination of a patient with ALS will depend on whether the therapist is working as a member of a rehabilitative team or as an independent or clinic-based therapist receiving a referral to evaluate and treat. PTs and OTs working as team members may have a more circumscribed role related to gross motor function and ADLs, with other consultants focusing on bulbar, respiratory, and environmental adjustments. The therapist working in a facility without a neuromuscular disease clinic or in a community or rural environment, however, should be aware of the need to carry out a broad-based assessment. In addition to the standard neuromuscular, musculoskeletal, and functional-level examinations, the therapist should also evaluate the patient's stated or observed functional problems relative to bulbar and respiratory impairments, environmental blocks to independence, and caregiving demands.

If possible, before the patient's initial visit, the therapist should contact the patient and request that he or she keep an activity log for several days. If an early contact is not possible, the therapist can assign that task during the initial session. The log should include 15-minute time increments in which the patient or caregiver can record what she or he was doing during a specific period. The log should also indicate whether the patient was experiencing fatigue or pain during the activity and how the patient perceived her or his respiratory status. An example of an activity log and how it is used is shown in Figure 17-2. The sense of fatigue with repetitive muscle activity or functional activity should be specifically tracked by the patient.

Weakness will be the primary deficit, with other problems following depending on the location of strength loss. Muscle weakness and the experience of fatigue may be independent measures of ALS pathology, however.[68] Although weakness may affect balance during gait, patients with ALS have not shown deficits in postural control during quiet stance despite significant paresis or tone changes, possibly because sensation is relatively preserved.[69]

The therapist's examination will vary depending on the patient's situation[29]; however, a typical initial assessment may include the following:

- Review of the patient's medical and activity records, especially time since diagnosis, time course of disease progression to date, current medications, concurrent medical issues, current activities and participation and tolerance for them.
- History should focus on current and recent activities and participation signifying patient's lifestyle, ADL tasks, hobbies or interests, and work focus; primary complaints, including weakness, fatigue, pain, respiratory status, safety, or speech and swallowing issues; psychosocial support issues (family, caregivers, and agencies); patient's and family members' understanding of ALS and the likely progression and prognosis; and patient's current concerns and goals.
- Screening for multisystem involvement should include checking vital signs at rest, skin integrity, bony abnormalities, sensory integrity, communication ability, and ability to follow multistep commands. More extensive examination of systems showing deficits may be indicated, or the patient may be referred to appropriate health care professionals.
- Baseline testing of muscle strength (manual muscle testing [MMT] or electronic handheld dynamometer testing if standards are clear and can be replicated), ROM, spasticity, and endurance; documentation of any areas of atrophy.
- Assessment of functional activity level (using a standardized test or assessment tool whenever possible) to include, as appropriate: transfers, gait, upper-extremity function, postural control, and assistive devices; suggested tools include the ALS functional rating scale (ALSFRS),[70] the ALS severity scale (ALSSS),[27] timed walk test, or Purdue Pegboard.[70]
- Documentation of pain (type, site, and intensity; use body chart and subjective pain scale); identify what makes pain worse or better.
- Assessment of bulbar and respiratory function. (For an in-depth evaluation of bulbar function, the patient should be referred to an ear, nose, and throat clinic or communications disorders clinic unless full evaluation is available in a comprehensive ALS clinic. See Table 17-1 for bulbar and respiratory evaluation suggestions.)
- Environmental assessment with a focus on energy conservation and safety at current and future functional capabilities.

Brinkmann and colleagues[70] identify standards for assessment of patients with ALS in clinical trials. The review and description of standardized methods for performing recommended tests and measurements is extremely valuable for any therapist assessing and treating patients with ALS.

In evaluating the results of the examination, the therapist should synthesize data to define the following, all of which are necessary for developing goals with the patient.

- Rate of the patient's disease progression
- Distribution of weakness and spasticity, respiratory factors leading to hypoxemia, and ease of fatigability and bulbar involvement
- Phase of the disease
- Any preexisting impairments and/or activity limitations (see Chapter 8)

Goals of Therapeutic Intervention

Intervention goals and the recommended exercise and activity program designed by PTs or OTs must be based on the patient's personal goals. Goals are often a difficult area for therapists to discuss with the patient because the disease is progressive despite intervention. Patients, therapists, and physicians commonly assume that because nothing can be done to "cure" the disease, not making additional demands on a patient who is already coping with daily loss is somehow kinder. Some believe that exercise programs may create false hopes that exercise will delay progression. Others believe that exercise will hasten progression.[71] The literature on rehabilitation in neuromuscular disorders, however, suggests that patients with ALS can benefit from carefully designed exercise and activity programs. Active participation in determining goals for therapy can provide the patient and the family with some sense of control over a difficult situation.[7]

The general, broad goals for both patient and therapist are related to maintaining maximal independence in daily living and a positive quality of life for as long as possible.

Name: J. Costello

DATE: 5-10-00
DAY: Saturday

DAILY ACTIVITY LOG

Instructions:

1) In column I write in what you are doing during the 24 hour period. You may draw a line or an arrow to indicate when the activity occurs for more than one 15 minute time period.

2) In column II indicate whether you are lying down, sitting, standing, or moving actively (walking, etc.) during the activity.

3) In column III on a 10 point scale, indicate how fatigued you feel while performing the activity (No fatigue = 0, extreme fatigue = 10.)

4) In column IV indicate where you feel pain if any and score the intensity on a 10 point scale (No pain = 0, extreme pain = 10.)

Try to fill out your log three or four times a day so you don't forget what you have been doing. An example is shown below.

	I	II	III	IV	
	What are you doing? Type of activity	What position are you in (lying, sitting, standing, moving)	Fatigue level 0 – 10	Pain	
				Location	Intensity 0 – 10
5:30 AM	Sleep	lying	0		
45					
6:00					
15					
30	Bathroom	standing	2	neck	3
45	Shave, etc				
7:00					
15	Breakfast	sitting	3	neck	3
30					
45					
8:00	Reading	sitting	3	neck	3
15				shoulder	
30					
45	walk	standing, walking	4	neck	2
9:00					
15	nap				
30		lying	2	neck	4
45				hips	
10:00	Reading/TV	sitting	4	neck	3
15				hips	
30					
45	walk	standing, walking	5	hips	3
11:00					

Figure 17-2 ■ Example of a log for monitoring activity level of patients with amyotrophic lateral sclerosis.

TABLE 17-1 ■ COMMON PHYSICAL FINDINGS IN BULBAR AMYOTROPHIC LATERAL SCLEROSIS

ANATOMICAL SITE	INNERVATION	METHOD OF EVALUATION	PROGRESSION OF FINDINGS	PROGRESSION OF SYMPTOMS
GROUP I				
Tongue	XII	Inspect for fasciculations at rest	Fasciculations evident	Dysarthria (disturbance of lingual-alveolar consonants *t, d, l,* and so on)
		Range of motion	Slow, incomplete lateral movements Loss of lateral force Unable to reach palate with mouth open	Inability to clear buccal sulcus of food Marked dysarthria (slow rate and slurring of consonants)
		Protrusion	Unable to protrude beyond lips	Oral transport difficulties Dietary changes
		Perform rapid lateral motion	Unable to protrude beyond incisors Atrophy evident Paralysis	Speech intelligibility problems
Lips	VII	Suck on gloved finger Smile or curl lips over teeth Hold seal and blow out cheeks	Lack of suction Inability to complete a seal Inability to purse lips	Inability to whistle Inability to use a straw Dysarthria (loss of bilabial consonants *p* and *b*) Drooling
GROUP 2				
Palate	V, X, XI	Visual examination during phonation and stimulation of gag Puff out cheeks to check for nasal air leak (hold lips closed if necessary)	Unsustained or slow palatal elevation Soft palate fails to reach Passavant ridge Absence of palatal movement	Dysarthria (hypernasal speech) Inability to use a straw Nasal air emission during speech Nasopharyngeal reflex on swallowing
Muscles of mastication Masseter, temporalis	V	Palpate during bite Visual inspection for wasting	Noticeable wasting Unable to palpate contraction	Chewing fatigue Elimination of specific, tough foods from diet Dietary changes (soft foods and liquids) Mouth breathing and drying of secretions
Pterygoids		Move jaw from side to side	No observable lateral jaw movement	Unable to use dentures
GROUP 3				
Neck and shoulder	XI			
Trapezius		Hold arm in coronal plane, hand externally rotated, as patient elevates arm against resistance while the trapezius is palpated	Progressive inability to raise the arm (often asymmetrical weakness)	Inability to comb hair Inability to perform facial grooming
Sternocleidomastoid or mounted head support		Turn the head against resistance applied to opposite side of patient's chin	Progressive weakness in turning the head against resistance (often asymmetrical)	Inability to lift head when supine Inability to support head while sitting; wears neck collar, has weakness
Vocal cords	X	Mirror or fiberoptic laryngoscopy	Progressive loss of abduction of vocal cords: mild abductor weakness, near-midline paralysis Paradoxical vocal cord movement	Strained or strangled voice Short of breath (stridor usually not present because of impaired respiratory function)

TABLE 17-1 ■ COMMON PHYSICAL FINDINGS IN BULBAR AMYOTROPHIC LATERAL SCLEROSIS—cont'd

ANATOMICAL SITE	INNERVATION	METHOD OF EVALUATION	PROGRESSION OF FINDINGS	PROGRESSION OF SYMPTOMS
GROUP 4				
Extraocular muscles	III, IV, VI	Assessment of extraocular movements	Limitation of extraocular movement	Limitation of gaze
Respiratory group				
Diaphragm	C3-5	Pulmonary function test or handheld respirometer for vital capacity	Diminishing vital capacity: 1.5-2.0 L	Shortness of breath during exertion if patient has remained active
Intercostal	C7-L3			
Accessory muscles of respiration	VII, XI, XII, C5-8	Cough Sustain a vowel Blow against a tissue	1.0-1.5 L	Weak cough Change in speech phrasing (5-10 syllables per breath)
			0.5-1.0 L	Speech produced in syllable-by-syllable fashion (if vocal) Shortness of breath on swallowing

Modified with permission from Hillel AD, Miller RM: Bulbar amyotrophic lateral sclerosis: patterns of progression and clinical management. *Head Neck* 11:51–59, 1989. Copyright 1989. Reprinted by permission of John Wiley & Sons, Inc.

More specific therapeutic goals are (1) maintenance of mobility and independent functioning, to include safe mobility for patient and caregiver; (2) maintenance of maximal muscle strength and endurance within limits imposed by ALS; (3) prevention and minimization of secondary consequences of the disease, such as contractures, thrombophlebitis, decubitus ulcers, and respiratory infections[7,67]; (4) management of energy conservation techniques and respiratory comfort; (5) determination of adaptive equipment needs to include mobility, self-help and feeding devices, augmentative communication units, and hygiene equipment that supports both patient and caregiver[7]; and (6) eliminating or preventing pain.[72]

Therapeutic Considerations

To prevent more rapid functional loss than expected from the natural history of the disease, both the patient and therapist must delicately balance the level of activity between the extremes of inadequate exercise and excessive exercise. Exercise has been recommended for the general public for its many benefits.[73] Inadequate exercise may result in loss of strength and endurance from disuse, as well as secondary problems such as loss of ROM, muscle cramping, and pain. Excessive exercise may result in excessive fatigue and consequent inability to perform ADLs during recovery periods. Overuse injury with excessive strengthening exercise may also lead to unnecessary pain and loss of strength. The next two sections review the evidence for the optimum amount of activity or exercise.

Disuse Atrophy. Because ALS is a disease of older adults, patients may not have maintained their aerobic fitness or muscle strength before the onset of their neuromuscular problem. Newly diagnosed patients also commonly report that they had markedly decreased their activity level in the months before diagnosis because of a sense of fatigue or increasing clumsiness from increasing weakness. If the patient had led a sedentary lifestyle before diagnosis, the additional decrease in activity level after the onset of ALS can lead quickly to marked cardiovascular deconditioning and disuse weakness. The disuse weakness lowers muscle force production and reduces muscle endurance.[74]

Exercise or Overwork Damage. Anecdotal evidence that muscle activity or overwork exercise can lead to a loss of muscle strength has been reported since the poliomyelitis epidemic of the 1940s and 1950s.[75] During that epidemic, physicians and therapists noted that patients with poor- and fair-grade muscles who exercised repeatedly or with heavy resistance after reinnervation often lost the ability to contract the muscle at all[76] (see Chapter 35). Controlled testing of this observation suggests that overwork damage occurs in mostly denervated muscles, not in all muscles. Reitsma[77] noted that vigorous exercise damaged muscles in rats if less than one third of motor units were functional. If more than one third of the motor units remained, exercise led to hypertrophy. An additional mechanism of potential overwork damage is inhibition of the collateral sprouting of intact axons to innervate "orphaned" muscle fibers when other axons degenerate. Yuen and Olney[78] provided evidence that collateral sprouting of intact axons can partially reinnervate orphaned muscle fibers in ALS. In a rat model, highly intensive activity reduced the ability of adjacent axons to sprout after fewer than 20% of intact motor units remained.[79] In contrast, vigorous exercise in a mouse model had no adverse effect on the course of ALS.[80] Lui and Byl[81] systematically reviewed the literature reporting exercise effects in animal models of ALS and calculated an effective size of 1.39 (where numbers over 0.8 are considered large) in favor of exercise. The few negative effects they noted were associated with either very-high–intensity exercise or a slow rate of exercise (slower than usual activity for animals when unrestricted in activity). In addition to generic overwork, evidence exists that repeated maximal eccentric contractions may specifically damage even normal muscle fibers, resulting in muscle weakness of several weeks' duration.[82] Although normal muscle eventually adapts to repeated eccentric exercise, whether the reparative effect is possible in patients with neuromuscular diseases is uncertain. Aboussouan[55] reviews some of the specific mechanisms of exercise intolerance in neuromuscular diseases, including mitochondrial dysfunction, abnormal muscle metabolism, impaired muscle activation, and central activation failure.

Many researchers have expressed concern about the possible relation between high-resistance exercise and muscle fiber degeneration in humans with motor neuron disease.[83,84] Because of the concerns about damage from stressing substantially denervated muscles, Sinaki and Mulder[85] published recommendations in 1978 that patients with ALS not engage in any vigorous exercise and focus instead on exercise associated with walking and daily activities. On the other hand, McCrate and Kaspar[86] review the possible mechanisms by which exercise protects nerves from more rapid degeneration. Evidence regarding the positive benefits of exercise in ALS has been accumulating, with fewer adverse effects than some expected.

Sanjak and colleagues[87] reported that muscle damage does not necessarily result from resistance exercise testing or training, although fatigue occurs more easily during both anaerobic and aerobic exercise. Milner-Brown and Miller[88] found that mild progressive resistance exercise was helpful in neuromuscular disorders if the patient had muscle strength in the good (4/5) to normal (5/5) range. They determined that patients should begin their exercise program early because strength training of muscles with less than 10% of normal function was generally not effective. Aitkens and colleagues[89] noted strength gains of 4% to 20% without deleterious effects after a 12-week program of moderate-resistance (30% of maximum isometric force) exercises in patients with slowly progressive neuromuscular diseases. Kilmer and colleagues,[90] in the same population, found no additional advantage to high-resistance training (12 weeks of exercise using the maximum isometric force the individual was able to lift 12 times) and noted evidence of overwork in some subjects. In a case report of a patient with ALS, strengthening 6 days a week for 10 weeks with proprioceptive neuromuscular facilitation (PNF) patterns using maximal resistance applied manually or with tubing resulted in strengthening of 14 muscle groups out of 18 with no adverse effects.[91] Aksu and colleagues[92] compared a supervised versus home exercise protocol in 26 ambulatory ALS patients. They noted that supervised breathing exercises, stretching, manually applied resistance exercise with PNF, and functional mobility training 3 days a week for 8 weeks resulted in small gains in function in the first 4 weeks and a slower decline over the subsequent 10 months compared with home-based breathing, stretching, and active ROM exercises. The groups were not randomly allocated but were not significantly different in the measured variables at baseline.[92] In a randomized controlled trial, Drory and colleagues[93] assigned 25 patients with ALS to a group continuing their normal daily activities or a group participating in a moderate daily program of exercise individualized for each patient. The primary exercise focus was to have muscles of the trunk and limbs work against "modest" loads while undergoing significant shortening (not lengthening or eccentric contractions). The exercises were completed twice daily for 15 minutes at home with phone contact by the treating therapist every 14 days. Data were evaluated for 3 and 6 months after initial assessment. All patients showed continued disease progression; however, in all cases, at the 6-month assessment patients who exercised showed positive effects in maintenance of muscle strength, less fatigue, less spasticity, less pain, and higher functional ratings.[93] In another randomized controlled trial, moderate load and moderate-intensity resistance exercises prescribed individually to patients with ALS in the early stages resulted in significantly less decline in function, small improvements in strength, and no reported adverse effects, compared with patients who performed stretching exercises alone.[94] A Cochrane review designated the quality of the Drory and colleagues (2001) study as "fair" and the Dal Bello-Haas and colleagues[94] study as "adequate."[95] Table 17-2 summarizes some of the studies of strength training in neuromuscular diseases.

Fewer researchers have considered endurance in neuromuscular disorders.[73] Sanjak and colleagues[87] noted that exercise energy requirements during bicycle ergometry testing were greater than expected, possibly because of motor inefficiency caused by weakness. Work capacity and maximal oxygen consumption were decreased, but heart rate, respiratory responses, and blood pressure were within normal limits. Wright and colleagues[96] found small positive physiological effects from an aerobic walking program in patients with slowly progressive neuromuscular disorders. Pinto and colleagues[97] provided eight ALS patients with NIV during exercise to compensate for respiratory insufficiency. Patients walked on a treadmill for 10 to 15 minutes to the point of subjective fatigue, leg pain, heart rate above 75% of resting value, or desaturation of oxygen not correctable with NIV. In comparison to a nonexercising control group, the exercising group had a significant reduction in the rate of decline of respiratory function test results, strength, and function over the 1-year training period.[97]

Endurance training for longer than 10 to 15 minutes in patients with ALS may be restricted by central fatigue, the decreased ability to recruit all motor units or develop high discharge rates,[98] and not merely respiratory function. Sharma and colleagues[99] explored the mechanism of fatigue in ALS. Both maximum voluntary contraction and tetanic force decreased in patients with ALS compared with controls following a 25-minute low-intensity intermittent exercise, but with similar recovery. Fatigue may thus be a consequence of chronic denervation resulting in secondary muscle changes such as altered muscle metabolism and impaired calcium kinetics along with the loss of motor unit activation.[99]

In addition to strength and endurance gains from exercise, ongoing, gentle exercise programs may also help decrease persistent pain and muscle stiffness that often accompany weakened, overtaxed muscle groups.[100] A case study of a patient with ALS undergoing a focused exercise program revealed a positive psychological effect on the patient's coping strategies.[101] Besides exercise programs, some preliminary evidence exists to suggest that creatine supplementation may increase isometric power in patients with ALS over the short term.[102] Modafinil has been noted to have potential in helping with severe fatigue in ALS.[103]

Many studies focus on the impact of exercise on muscle strength; however, knowledge of impairments does not necessarily correlate directly with functional status.

TABLE 17-2 ■ SUMMARY OF STRENGTH TRAINING STUDIES IN NEUROMUSCULAR DISEASES

AUTHOR	STUDY POPULATION AND SAMPLE SIZE	DURATION OF TRAINING	TRAINING MODALITY	TRAINING PROTOCOL	RESPONSE(S)
Vignos and Watkins, 1966[291]	Various neuromuscular diseases (NMDs) (24)	12 months	Weight training (multiple muscle groups)	Unspecified, but based on 10-repetition maximum (RM)	Strength increased; percentage increase correlated with initial strength
Milner-Brown and Miller, 1988[88]	Various NMDs (12)	>12 months (variable)	Weight training (elbow flexion and knee extension)	Initially one set of 10 reps based on 15 RM performed on alternate days; gradually increased to a maximum of five sets 4 days/week; protocol individualized	Strength increased significantly when the initial degree of strength loss was not severe (<10%)
McCartney et al, 1988[297]	Various NMDs (12)	9 weeks	Weight training (arm curl and leg press)	3 days/week; initially two sets of 10-12 reps at 40% of 1 RM; gradually progressed to three sets of 10-12 reps (one set at 50%, 60%, and 70% of 1 RM); contralateral arm control	Strength and muscular endurance increased; considerable inter-subject variability
Aitkens et al, 1993[89]	Slowly progressive NMD (27) and able-bodied controls (14)	12 weeks	Weight training (elbow flexion, knee extension, grip one side only)	3 days/week; resistance at 30% of 1 RM; work increased commensurate with ability	Significant improvement in most isokinetic strength measures (not grip) in both groups; cross-training effect
Kilmer et al, 1994[90]	Slowly progressive NMD (10) and able-bodied controls (6)	12 weeks	Weight training (elbow flexion, knee extension, one side only)	3-4 days/week; high-resistance exercise (resistance based on 12 RM; progressed from one to five sets of 10 reps)	Results mixed; increase in leg strength but decrease in arm strength in NMD
Lindeman et al, 1995[325]	MD (33) and HMSN (29); nonexercise control group	24 weeks	Weight training (knee extension and flexion, hip extension and flexion)	3 days/week; initially three sets of 25 reps at 60% of 1 RM; progressed to three sets of 10 reps at 80% of 1 RM	In MD group, no change in strength In HMSN group, increased strength of knee extensors; no adverse effects
Drory et al, 2001[93]	ALS (25): randomly assigned to treatment or control groups	24 weeks	Moderate load, trunk and limbs, concentric contractions	Twice daily, 15 min per session	Treatment group: maintenance of strength, less fatigue, less spasticity, less pain, higher function
Aksu et al, 2002[92]	ALS (26): convenience assignment to treatment and control groups	8 weeks	Breathing exercises, PNF, stretching, vs stretching and ROM and breathing exercises	3 days/week supervised vs home	Increased ROM, strength in treatment group; function sustained better in treatment group
Dawes et al, 2006[326]	Various NMDs: 11 randomly allocated to control group, nine to treatment group	8 weeks	Walking and strengthening exercises	Walking for 20 min at light to moderate intensity alternating days with progressive resistance and repetitions in strength	Treatment group had increase in leg muscle strength; no change either group in 2-min walk test

Continued

TABLE 17-2 ■ SUMMARY OF STRENGTH TRAINING STUDIES IN NEUROMUSCULAR DISEASES—cont'd

AUTHOR	STUDY POPULATION AND SAMPLE SIZE	DURATION OF TRAINING	TRAINING MODALITY	TRAINING PROTOCOL	RESPONSE(S)
Dal Bello-Haas et al., 2007[94]	ALS (27 early stage): randomly allocated to resistance exercises plus stretch or just stretch groups	24 weeks	PT-prescribed resistance exercises performed at home to patient tolerance	3 days/week resisted exercise plus stretch vs just stretch group	Slowed decline in treatment group and small strength gains

HMSN, Hereditary motor and sensory neuropathy; *MD,* myotonic dystrophy; *PNF,* proprioceptive neuromuscular facilitation; *PT,* physical therapist; *ROM,* range of motion.

Although some research has shown improvements in muscle force production with strengthening and endurance training, associated functional improvements were evident in some studies[92] but not others.[104] Jette and colleagues[82] calculated the percentage of predicted normal maximal isometric force (%PMF) relative to four walking levels in patients with ALS: unable to walk, walking within the home only, walking in the community with assistance, and independent walking in the community. Although they found great variation in muscle force production between and within the different levels of walking for each patient, they demonstrated that relatively small changes in force production were associated with losses of functional levels. For example, on average, when an independent ambulator began to need assistance in the community, the lower-extremity strength dropped to less than 54%PMF. When the patient became an in-home ambulator only, the average strength dropped to approximately 37%PMF, and it was approximately 19%PMF when the patient was no longer able to walk. Jette and colleagues[82] acknowledge that many factors need to be considered when interpreting their work; however, their study relates functional skills to isometric muscle force production in a concrete way. Factors such as spasticity, age at onset of ALS, prior levels of fitness and activity, and psychological factors, including past responses to extremely challenging situations and satisfaction with social support, must also be considered.

Based on the evidence and current practice, exercise prescription in the early stages of ALS should address the following[72]:

1. To improve compliance, include both a formal exercise program and enjoyable physical activities.
2. Include activities with opportunities for social development and personal accomplishment.
3. Strengthening programs should emphasize concentric rather than eccentric muscle contractions; use moderate resistance rather than high resistance; and focus on muscles that have at least antigravity strength.
4. Endurance programs should be monitored for signs of fatigue, more so when continuous activity lasts longer than about 15 minutes. Activity programs should include rest periods.
5. Patients should ensure that they have adequate oxygenation, aeration, and carbohydrate loads[73] as well as adequate fluids before exercising.
6. Muscle strength must be monitored to assess for possible overwork weakness; in unsupervised programs, patients must be instructed about signs and symptoms that indicate overwork, including feeling weaker within 30 minutes after exercise, having excessive soreness 24 to 48 hours after exercise, and experiencing severe muscle cramping, heaviness in the extremities, or prolonged shortness of breath[105]; and therapists should check with an independently exercising patient regularly to assess whether any deterioration in strength may be from progression of the disease or overwork weakness.

If a patient shows evidence of significant, persistent weakness after institution of an exercise program or persistent morning fatigue after exercise on the previous day, the therapist must carefully redesign the patient's exercise program and activity level and increase the frequency of monitoring the patient's program. The program must be adjusted as the disease progresses. Figure 17-3 is a diagram showing the appropriate exercise "window" for use in working with a patient with a neuromuscular disorder.

Therapeutic Interventions

Maintenance of strength and endurance requires daily activity and repetitive muscle contractions. In normal persons, absence of muscle contraction can result in decreases of 3% to 5% in muscle strength per day. If the patient's exercise level requires less than 20% of the maximal voluntary contraction of the muscles, a decrease in strength will occur; yet overwork must be avoided.[106]

Sinaki[107] has described three phases and six substages of ALS with recommended exercise levels (Box 17-2). Although therapists should not assume that all patients will fit precisely within the stages as described, the stages do provide sugges-

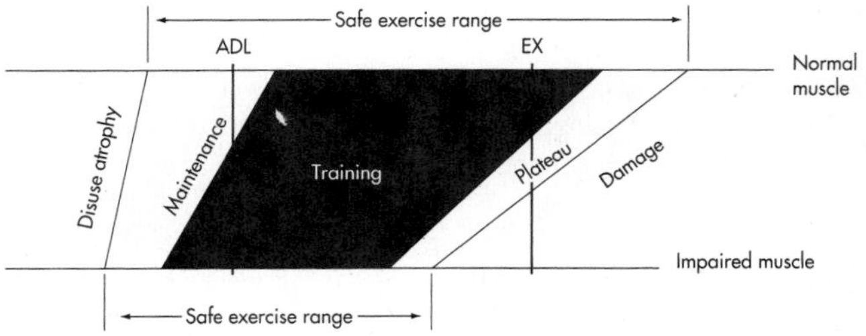

Figure 17-3 ■ Exercise window for normal and damaged or denervated muscles. (From Coble NO, Maloney FP: Effects of exercise on neuromuscular disease. In Maloney FP, Burks JS, Ringel SP, editors: *Interdisciplinary rehabilitation of multiple sclerosis and neuromuscular disorders,* New York, 1985, JB Lippincott.)

BOX 17-2 ■ EXERCISE AND REHABILITATION PROGRAMS FOR PATIENTS WITH AMYOTROPHIC LATERAL SCLEROSIS ACCORDING TO STAGE OF DISEASE

PHASE I (INDEPENDENT)

Stage 1

Patient Characteristics

Mild weakness
Clumsiness
Ambulatory
Independent in activities of daily living (ADLs)

Treatment

Continue normal activities or increase activities if sedentary to prevent disuse atrophy
Begin program of range-of-motion (ROM) exercises (stretching, yoga, tai chi)
Add strengthening program of gentle resistance exercises to all musculature with caution not to cause overwork fatigue
Provide psychological support as needed

Stage 2

Patient Characteristics

Moderate, selective weakness
Slightly decreased independence in ADLs, such as:

- difficulty climbing stairs
- difficulty raising arms
- difficulty buttoning clothing

Ambulatory

Treatment

Continue stretching to avoid contractures
Continue cautious strengthening of muscles with manual muscle testing (MMT) grades above F+ (3+); monitor for overwork fatigue
Consider orthotic support (e.g., ankle-foot, wrist, thumb splints)
Use adaptive equipment to facilitate ADLs

Stage 3

Patient Characteristics

Severe selective weakness in ankles, wrists, and hands
Moderately decreased independence in ADLs
Easily fatigability with long-distance ambulation
Ambulatory
Slightly increased respiratory effort

Treatment

Continue stage 2 program as tolerated; use caution not to fatigue to point of decreasing patient's ADL independence
Keep patient physically independent as long as possible through pleasurable activities such as walking
Encourage deep breathing exercises, chest stretching, postural drainage if needed
Prescribe wheelchair, standard or motorized, with modifications to allow eventual reclining back with head rest, elevating legs

PHASE II (PARTIALLY INDEPENDENT)

Stage 4

Patient Characteristics

Hanging-arm syndrome with shoulder pain and sometimes edema in the hand
Wheelchair dependent
Severe lower-extremity weakness (with or without spasticity)
Able to perform ADLs but fatigues easily

Treatment

Heat, massage as indicated to control spasm
Preventive antiedema measures
Active assisted passive ROM exercises to the weakly supported joints; caution to support, rotate shoulder during abduction and joint accessory motions
Encourage isometric contractions of all musculature to tolerance
Try arm slings, overhead slings, or wheelchair arm supports
Motorized chair if patient wants to be independently mobile; adapt controls as needed

Stage 5

Patient Characteristics

Severe lower-extremity weakness
Moderate to severe upper-extremity weakness
Wheelchair dependent
Increasingly dependent in ADLs
Possible skin breakdown as a result of poor mobility

Treatment

Encourage family to learn proper transfer, positioning principles, and turning techniques
Encourage modifications at home to aid patient's mobility and independence
Electric hospital bed with antipressure mattress
If patient elects home mechanical ventilation (HMV), adapt chair to hold respirator unit

PHASE III (DEPENDENT)

Stage 6

Patient Characteristics

Bedridden
Completely dependent in ADLs

Treatment

For dysphagia: soft diet, long spoons, tube feeding, percutaneous gastrostomy
To decrease flow of accumulated saliva: medication, suction, surgery
For dysarthria: palatal lifts, electronic speech amplification, eye-pointing electronics
For breathing difficulty: clear airway, tracheostomy, respirator if patient elects HMV
Medications to decrease impact of dyspnea

Modified with permission from Sinaki M: Exercise and rehabilitation measures in amyotrophic lateral sclerosis. In Yase Y, Tsubaki T, editors: *Amyotrophic lateral sclerosis: recent advances in research and treatment,* Amsterdam, 1988, Elsevier Science.

tions for interventions on the basis of degree of impairment, functional limitations, and level of disability. In the following section, staging patterns are used as the framework for therapy interventions. Staging information is particularly helpful to therapists who do not have the opportunity to work with large numbers of patients with ALS.

Most patients need specific guidance about what type of activities and exercises they should do.[61] Although many physicians may suggest to patients that they increase their activity level, their suggestions are seldom specific. Examples of exercise advice that patients have recalled are "Try to move around as much as possible," "Walk some more," and "Be active, but don't overdo it." Because changing their typical exercise pattern is difficult for most patients, even when they know doing so is important, referral for a physical therapy consultation can be helpful.[108]

Phase I (Independent): Stages 1 to 3. A program to increase activity must be specifically designed, with input from the patient about willingness to participate and knowledge of the patient's environmental situations and social support systems. In the early stages of the disease, patients should be encouraged to continue as many prediagnosis activities as tolerated. For example, a golfer should continue to golf for as long as possible. Walking the course should be encouraged if it is not too fatiguing. When walking or balance becomes difficult on uneven terrain, the golfer can use a golf cart, decrease the number of holes played, move to a par 3 course, or hit balls at a driving range. If upper-extremity weakness is a major problem that interferes with swinging the club for distance shots, the player can continue playing the greens or on putting courses. Some golfers may need adaptations to club handles with nonskid material such as Dycem (Dycem Non-Slip products, www.dycem.com) or Scoot-Gard (Vantage Industries Product) to prevent the club from rotating on impact.

Patients with newly diagnosed ALS who had a sedentary lifestyle before diagnosis should be encouraged to increase their activity level. This may include activities that require muscular effort within or around the home, such as sharing household and gardening tasks or beginning a walking program around the neighborhood. After diagnosis, some patients begin searching for in-home exercise devices such as bicycles and rowing machines. As with healthy persons who start an exercise program after the purchase of exercise equipment, patients with ALS are not likely to use the equipment consistently if they did not before a diagnosis. The search for a "perfect" exercise machine may reflect the patient's desperation to do something tangible. Without taking away the patient's motivation to exercise, therapists can encourage participation in exercise programs that do not require expensive equipment, such as walking or working out to specific exercise routines. A clever therapist can make a video for each patient that includes stretching and gentle exercise programs that elicit muscle contractions from all functional muscle groups (by using inexpensive elastic bands or small weights) with follow-up breathing, "warm down," and relaxation exercises. Patients could follow a program of six maximal isometric contractions held for 6 seconds and isotonic elastic band exercises at submaximal levels to maintain and improve muscle strength.[109] Patients should exercise for short periods several times a day rather than attempting to exercise all muscle groups in one session.

For most patients in the early stages of ALS, pleasurable, natural activities such as swimming, bowling (can gradually decrease weight of ball if shoulder strength is a problem), walking, bicycling (three-wheeler may be needed or in-home stationary bicycle, either of which must be evaluated for easy mounting and dismounting), or tai chi should be recommended. Some patients prefer to exercise alone, whereas others will gain confidence and companionship by joining a group activity. Listening to the patient's desires related to group activities is important. The dropout rate is high among those who have been pressured to participate. Some spouses or family members are supportive of the patient's activity needs and will join the patient in his or her regimen. If possible, the spouse and family members should be engaged in the treatment planning process.[110]

The therapist must observe the patient completing her or his entire recommended activity program. The patient's response to the program must be monitored because fatigue from exercise sessions can interfere with the ability to carry out other normal daily activities. If the patient becomes too exhausted at the end of a session, he or she may learn to fear exercise and may become depressed about the decreased activity status. This depression may lead to decreased activity and further deconditioning (see Chapter 6).

Phase II (Partially Independent): Stages 4 and 5. During phase II, the goal of physical and occupational therapy intervention should be to help the patient adapt to limitations imposed by weakness and spasticity, an increasingly compromised cardiorespiratory status, and possible pain from stress related to weakness or muscle imbalance. This transition stage is often frightening for patients because the decrease in function and independence becomes clear; therapists should accentuate what the person can do and how accommodations can be made to help maintain independence. After a full physical assessment of the patient's motor status similar to the initial evaluation, the patient, family members, and therapists (including PT, OT, and speech therapist if a team approach is possible) should discuss treatment options and adaptive devices that can help the patient remain as independent as possible.

During late phase I and through phase II, many patients show significant weakness of both upper- and lower-extremity musculature, but each patient has his or her own pattern and rate of progression of weakness and onset of spasticity, bulbar, and respiratory symptoms. A typical patient at this time may have marked weakness of the intrinsic muscles, shoulder muscle weakness (in some cases "hanging arm" syndrome) with shoulder pain, and generalized lower-extremity weakness (in some cases more severe distally). Patients may be able to walk within the home environment, but many patients have precarious balance and fall easily because of muscle weakness. At this stage, most patients report fatigue with minimal work and have to rest frequently when carrying out ADLs. ROM can deteriorate quickly in this phase of the disease, requiring daily stretching to end range for the calf, quadriceps, hip adductors, trunk lateral flexors, and long finger flexors.[29] Moderate exercise can have a modest effect in reducing spasticity.[93]

Patients at this point, even if ambulatory, should consider using a wheelchair outside the home to conserve energy.[72] Factors to consider in choosing a wheelchair include extent of insurance coverage or financial assistance programs for purchase of wheelchair (some policies or programs may provide only one type of wheelchair or only one wheelchair, either motorized or manual); transportability of motorized chair from home to community and work (few motorized wheelchair brands fold for stowing in car trunk, and few families can afford to purchase a van that will allow the patient to drive or be driven while in a motor chair); reclining potential of chair back and headrest (preferably electric) to allow the patient to shift weight and rest while in the chair during later stages of the disease; removable arm rests for ease of transfer; potential for headrest attachment or extension; potential mounting area for portable respirator equipment if needed; and ease with which caregiver can help patient with chair mobility transfers.[72] Chairs should have lumbar support and appropriate cushioning to prevent pressure ulcers.[105]

At this stage, patients with more advanced bulbar symptoms begin to experience dysarthria and may need guidance in dealing with communication issues. Murphy[111] indicated four major reasons for communication: to identify needs or request help, share information, respond politely in social situations, and maintain social closeness. The primary focus of communication for the study participants was to maintain social closeness. Although few patients had any instruction in ways to deal with communication problems, most patients and caregivers created ways to make themselves understood, such as giving cues about the topic and context, creating a "shorthand" language, and checking with the dysarthric speaker to ensure that the listener understands the patient correctly. A number of patients in the study who had significant dysarthria commented that attempting to communicate socially was extremely tiring. Therapists who are guiding patients with energy conservation techniques should be aware of the exhaustion that can be associated with communication. A number of strategies recommended by the American Speech-Language-Hearing Association[112] can be used by the person with ALS to deal with the effects of dysarthria, including the following:

- Reduce background noise in the room.
- Face the person while talking.
- Use short, simple phrases rather than long, complicated ones.
- Take the time to say what needs to be said; do not allow people to rush conversation.
- Make extra use of body language, such as gestures and facial expressions, and use writing to supplement speech, if possible.
- Do not worry about saying things correctly; if the basic message being conveyed is understood, then that is enough.

Also in this stage, some patients and families may need support to identify adapted feeding systems (special utensils, adapted plates, adjustable tables) and hygiene equipment if transfers within the family bathroom are problematic.[113]

Because Mr. Turner in Case Study 17-1 was cared for in a neuromuscular disease clinic, he benefited from input from multiple specialists working as a team to help him maintain his independence. Unfortunately, many patients do not have the benefit of such a coordinated treatment environment. Therefore, when necessary, the therapist must be in a position to provide input on adaptive and safety devices and bulbar issues if other specialist input is not available. Therapists working in smaller communities and rural areas most likely need to be chameleon-like to play many therapeutic roles when working with the patient with ALS.

CASE STUDY 17-1 ■ MR. TURNER

Mr. Turner is a 45-year-old man diagnosed 2 years ago with ALS. He lives at home with his wife, who works full time, and two teenaged children. Mr. Turner is a computer programmer for an engineering firm in the area. Since his diagnosis, Mr. Turner has been able to continue his full-time work schedule, although he states that he is no longer able to touch type and can type with the index fingers only. He has noticed that his shoulders and neck hurt (4 out of 10 on a numerical pain rating scale) after an hour at the computer. In the last 2 weeks he has found it fatiguing to walk to the cafeteria for lunch (approximately 100 meters), and he fears that he will be knocked down when walking in crowds. He dropped his tray last week, which was embarrassing, so he decided to eat in his office even though he misses the socialization and opportunity to discuss work issues with his colleagues.

Mr. Turner has been able to continue most of his nonwork activities, although he is no longer able to operate his sailboat independently and is having trouble maintaining his balance when golfing. Also when golfing, he now uses a cart and plays only nine holes. He states that his wife and children are supportive and that they have made some changes in the home environment to accommodate his increasing weakness. He also revealed, however, that his children seem frustrated with him because he is so much slower than he was before the illness.

On assessment, Mr. Turner showed marked wasting of hand intrinsics. He was unable to abduct or flex either shoulder past 90 degrees. His right shoulder showed considerable atrophy, especially of the deltoid and supraspinatus muscles. All other upper-extremity movements were weakened but in the G− (4−) range. His neck posture was forward: neck extension is F+ (3+), neck flexion is G− (4−). Scapular winging was noted bilaterally. No spasticity or loss of passive ROM was evident in the upper extremities. Lower-extremity musculature showed generalized weakness at the F (3) to F+ (3+) range, with left musculature weaker than right, marked wasting of the foot intrinsics, and a cavus foot position bilaterally. Spasticity of the hip adductors and hamstrings was noted (Modified Ashworth Scale grade 2), but no passive ROM loss was detected in the lower extremities. Most obvious during gait was inadequate dorsiflexion for heel strike and no propulsion during heel-off. He showed a bilateral corrected gluteus medius pattern on weight bearing. He needed to pause to lock each knee during weight bearing and at times he pushed his knee into extension with his hand. He had great difficulty ascending and descending the four steps to enter his home. There were no stairs to negotiate at work.

Until this appointment, Mr. Turner had not been willing to discuss the use of adaptive equipment or a wheelchair. During

Continued

CASE STUDY 17-1 ■ MR. TURNER—cont'd

prior clinic visits his decisions were supported and he was told that when he was ready, therapists would work with him and his family to help with equipment decisions.

Mr. Turner also showed some early bulbar signs. He noted that he sometimes had to catch drool when working intensely, and that his pillow was moist in the morning. Food sometimes got stuck in his cheek area and he could not move it out with his tongue. Swallowing was still adequate for eating all foods; however, he had had a few coughing episodes when drinking coffee and wine. He showed increased use of accessory musculature when breathing but had no reports of respiratory distress. His cough was adequate to clear secretions.

With input from the therapist, Mr. Turner and his wife identified the following general goals:

1. Increase mobility while conserving energy
2. Control fatigue and pain of upper extremities and neck during computer work
3. Maintain maximal muscle strength and ROM (patient reported that he felt stiff)
4. Identify safety issues within the home and work environment and adjust household and work environment to prepare for the time when Mr. Turner could not ascend and descend stairs safely

A treatment plan was discussed to achieve the following:

1. Increase mobility. Because of his increased walking difficulties, Mr. Turner decided to use a front-wheeled walker with a seat attachment at home. Because of his hand grip weakness, he felt most stable using attached forearm troughs. For his worksite, he selected a motorized wheelchair so that he could maintain his independence at work. Although he found that he could push an ultralight manual chair, his upper-extremity strength was clearly decreasing. Mr. Turner decided that he preferred the motorized chair to an electric scooter because of the financial cost of switching devices when the scooter no longer provided adequate postural support.

   Because Mr. Turner's insurance and Medicare would not fund an additional manual chair and because the family had no way to transport the electric wheelchair, the ALS Society loaned the family a manual wheelchair for home use. Although not ideal, it was functional. Mr. Turner's son made some inexpensive adjustments to adapt the chair for a headrest, and his daughter and grandchildren repainted the chair to his specifications.

   Because Mr. Turner wanted to keep as active as possible and use his walker within the home, he was fitted with bilateral ankle-foot orthoses (AFOs) with a flexible ankle joint and pretibial shell to facilitate knee extension. Straps were simple overlap style because Mr. Turner had poor thumb and grasp control.
2. Decrease fatigue and pain of upper extremities. Mr. Turner was taught some simple ROM exercises of the neck and arms to perform every half hour while working at the computer. In a simulated work environment the therapist noted that Mr. Turner had a forward head position when working at a computer similar to his workstation. The height of the computer was adjusted to decrease his neck strain, and the desk height was adjusted to allow his wheelchair to fit under the desk so that his arms could rest fully on the surface. He felt immediate relief with the adaptations. He was also fitted for a soft neck collar to wear when he felt he needed more neck support. (As his condition worsened, he learned to rest his head on the headrest of his chair and recline slightly for a few minutes every 15 minutes.)
3. Maintain maximal muscle strength and ROM. Mr. Turner was taught as many self-ranging maneuvers as possible, which he was encouraged to do in small segments frequently throughout the day. For example, his series of motions included neck rotations, side bends, and flexion and extension within strength limits; upper-extremity motions with the exception of shoulder flexion and abduction past 90 degrees; hip flexion, abduction, and rotations; full knee extension; and all ankle motions. When using the walker, Mr. Turner was encouraged to extend each hip fully and to stretch his heel cords. Mrs. Turner and their adult children were taught to administer full ROM exercises, including trunk rotations, with special attention to ranging of the shoulder to prevent impingement. Simple massage techniques were also taught to all family members who felt comfortable with the task.

   Mr. Turner had been active before the onset of ALS and he liked to exercise. He rented a portable pedaling unit to attach to a chair at home. He pedaled two to four times a day, with no additional resistance, to the point at which he felt fatigue (usually 3 to 5 minutes at this stage). He carefully monitored his soreness and fatigue level after exercise and increased and decreased his pedaling depending on how he felt immediately and several days after exercise. Mr. Turner felt invigorated by this exercise, which he usually did while watching television. He was also taught a series of simple elastic band exercises, with tensile strength adjusted according to his ability to contract his muscles without fatigue. Mr. Turner was also shown a series of isometric exercises for all muscle groups to do throughout the work day. Because he had some foot and ankle edema, he was encouraged to wear lightweight pressure stockings while sitting. Mr. Turner also had access to a swimming pool, and he was encouraged to carry out walking and upper-extremity exercises as long as another adult was with him in the water at all times.
4. Assess environment of home and work. Occupational therapy input was requested to help with ADL aids such as reachers, utensil adaptors to facilitate grip, rubber pen grippers, key adaptors to permit turning, and thumb abduction splints to assist in pincer grasp. Mr. Turner's OT made several visits to his worksite and home to identify adaptations of the environment for safety and independence. His wheelchair was eventually adapted with universal joint arm troughs to decrease his effort during self-feeding and basic upper-body hygiene. Ramps were recommended for home entry, and nonpermanent safety rails were placed in the bathroom. Mr. Turner was able to assist with transfer to a shower chair, and the shower head was replaced with a handheld unit.

A speech pathology consultation was also requested. Using information from the PT's manual muscle testing, the speech pathologist carried out a thorough bulbar evaluation and provided information about swallowing

CASE STUDY 17-1 ■ MR. TURNER—cont'd

techniques. The speech therapist focused on ways to decrease drooling and ways to cope with food pocketing (tongue mobility was impaired) by using techniques such as hand pressure on the cheek to push food back to the center of the mouth. The therapist also instructed Mr. Turner and his wife how to prepare foods with textures that were easily swallowed and manipulated. Mr. Turner had lost 5 pounds during the last 6 months, so he was also referred to the dietician for information about how to maintain nutritious calorie intake.

PROGRESSION OF THE DISEASE

Within 3 to 4 months after initial examination, Mr. Turner was no longer able to continue working despite workplace adaptations. At home, he became more dependent. Mr. Turner had great difficulty adjusting to his physical dependence. Because of his slow onset of dysphagia and his augmented communication system, he was able to continue control over his expressive, cognitive, and emotional life for another few months. Initially Mr. Turner angrily resisted his wife's attempts to help him with eating and dressing tasks. This began to alienate her and the children until a family meeting was held with their medical social worker and PTs and OTs. All family members had the opportunity to express their frustrations. A major irritation to the children was what they perceived to be their constant waiting for their father to complete a task. Mrs. Turner was most irritated when Mr. Turner yelled at her when she attempted to help even though he frequently expressed anger about his clumsiness. Mr. Turner sadly admitted that he was having increasing difficulty with his ADLs and was sometimes too tired after dressing to participate in family activities. At the end of the meeting, the family had worked out a compromise plan. Mr. Turner would continue to do as much as possible for himself. He would specifically ask for help from Mrs. Turner when he wanted it so she did not get caught in his anger about needing help. He preferred that the children not have to take any role in his care at this point but realized that he might need their help later. Visiting nurse support was requested twice a week to help with bathing, and the OT was requested to make another home visit to help with toileting needs. Mr. Turner felt comfortable with his wife and children carrying out ROM exercises. A therapy home visit was arranged to review the exercise and positioning program as well as respiratory exercises and postural drainage techniques.

As Mr. Turner became totally dependent, he needed 24-hour care. Professional nurses were provided through his insurance contract 14 hours a day from 6:30 AM to 8:30 PM. Family members provided care until midnight. Initially Mr. Turner was able to activate a bell at night to call for help. His wife and children followed a schedule to turn him every 3 hours throughout the night. When Mr. Turner became respirator dependent and was no longer able to call for help, it became clear that the nighttime responsibilities were taking a heavy toll on his wife, who worked full time, and the children, who were in high school and college. Fortunately the family was able to pay for a nurse assistant to remain at Mr. Turner's bedside throughout the night, although the family members all felt that they had no privacy. Although the family was committed to having Mr. Turner remain at home until his death, all agreed that they needed respite. Thus several week-long hospitalizations were made to give the family a break in the constant care needs.

Although Mr. Turner had elected HMV, he also had signed a durable power of attorney for health care, indicating that he did not want treatment for infections and that palliative care for comfort should direct his treatment. He had a strong lust for life, but he had come to accept his impending death. He did not have strong religious views, but he had talked with all his caregivers and therapists about his concerns related to death. He freely expressed his fear of "nonbeing." Because his caregivers and therapists were willing to talk about his and their own feelings, Mr. Turner came to believe that he would live on in the minds, hearts, and behaviors of those he had known. This idea seemed to give him great comfort. He particularly liked to talk to others about special times they had had together and how their interactions had affected each other. To help Mr. Turner process his death, his family, friends, and medical team put together an album of pictures and statements about their time together. Mr. Turner frequently liked to have his wife read through the book with him. His family continued to carry out his ROM exercises and massage because Mr. Turner had indicated that the treatments provided him physical comfort and the spiritual closeness he needed with his family. His primary treatment during the last few days consisted of morphine to decrease his respiratory discomfort. After 5 to 6 months of being totally dependent for all care and respiratory function, Mr. Turner died at home in his sleep after a respiratory illness.

Phase III (Dependent): Stage 6. PTs and OTs are usually less involved in the care of the patient in phase III, and nursing personnel become more active. During this phase, therapists make home visits to support caregivers and respond to questions about pain control, bed mobility, positioning to prevent pressure ulcers, ROM, and equipment adaptations.[29,72,105] Therapists should be sure to teach all caregivers some basic body mechanics to use during lifting and patient care activities. If possible, caregivers should be taught how to safely move the person with ALS from the bed to a reclining wheelchair or other reclining chair during specific times of the day so that the person can continue to be part of the family activities. However, the ease of caregivers in transferring and caring for the person in the wheelchair must also be considered. Although some patients want to be in the midst of family activities even when dependent on HMV, other patients feel uncomfortable with their dependency and appearance and are reasonably content to stay in their room with television and visits from family members. This highly personal decision by patients must be respected. The therapist should review ROM procedures with family and professional caregivers and provide splinting or positioning devices if spasticity or paralysis leads to caregiving difficulties (e.g., excessive adductor tone and contractures interfering with hygiene and bowel care) or tissue damage and pain. If nursing care providers do not give advice on pressure relief beds or mattresses of air or foam,[105] therapists should be prepared to do so. Unfortunately, many insurance providers and Medicare may not fund special mattresses, and they can be costly. Therapists may also need to review postural drainage techniques with caregivers.

Of greatest importance in phase III, and sometimes in earlier stages, is the patient's ability to communicate. In the earliest manifestation of dysarthria, therapists train patients to slow the speech rate and cadence, exaggerate lip and tongue movements, and manage phrasing through breath control.[83] Although spouses and caregivers can often interpret their partner's or patient's severely dysarthric speech (see earlier discussion of phase II), most patients who use NIV or invasive ventilation for a prolonged period need to find nonverbal methods to communicate. If severe bulbar impairments precede extremity paralysis, paper and pencil, alphabet and word boards, and adapted computer keyboards can be used with minimal upper-extremity or finger strength for pointing. The American Speech-Language-Hearing Association provides suggestions for developing communication boards with the specific language most appropriate for the patient's situation.[112] For example, the board may be designed with commonly needed sentences, words used in the person's daily life, and the alphabet. As the person's ability to finger point decreases, the language board can be redesigned. When no extremity movement is possible, subtle neck movements or pressures, eye gaze, eye blink, upper facial movements, and electroencephalographic activity can be harnessed to operate communication devices.[114,115] Learning to use electroencephalographic interfaces, however, takes months of intense training and may not provide a reasonable system for communication for most patients with ALS.[116]

Some patients with hypernasality benefit from using an orthodontic palatal appliance. Patients with a tracheostomy may benefit from use of a Passy-Muir (Irvine, Calif) speaking valve tracheostomy tube. These devices require recommendation by communication specialists. As speech quality deteriorates and sound projection wanes, the spouse or caregiver can use an electronic speech amplifier to magnify the patient's speech. Speech pathologists and therapists have information on commercially available amplifying devices that are often used by persons with hearing problems but can be used by hearing people to amplify the speech of a person with severe weakness of phonation.

When selecting a communication device, therapists must work closely with the patient and family members to ensure that the system is compatible with patient skills and communication needs and preferences. Expensive systems commonly lie unused because of simple factors such as lack of proximity to the patient, interference of the unit with personal care, increased caregiver workload to manage the unit, and slowness of communication processing. The best systems are tailored to the precise needs of the patient; however, many patients do not have the financial or insurance support to purchase the device, and many patients in the end stages of ALS do not have the time to wait for systems designed for their specific needs. Therefore commercially manufactured systems may be most appropriate. (See Cook and Hussey[114] for a comprehensive list of communication devices and control interfaces.)

Some patients and caregivers learn to communicate effectively with simple eye gaze, eye blinking, and clicking techniques with Morse code or self-developed codes. At minimum, patients with no ability to communicate or move and their caregivers must have some system to communicate emergency needs; for example, looking to the right means "help" and looking to the left means "pain." Therapists should help patients develop alternative modes of communication before intelligible speech becomes impossible. (See also Cobble[117] for information on language impairments.)

In addition to communication systems, environmental control systems can be programmed to turn on and off television, lights, and other electronic units with the same type of switching units used for communication (e.g., eye blink, infrared beam, head movement pressure). Unfortunately, these devices are often expensive and may not be available to all patients. (See Cook and Hussey[114] for a comprehensive review of environmental control systems.) Financial support is often not extended for high-tech equipment by third-party payers because of the patient's limited life expectancy. The ability to communicate and call for help, however, is of paramount importance with completely dependent patients.

By phase III most patients have significant problems eating and maintaining nutrition, although these problems may manifest in earlier stages. Patients often report choking or coughing after swallowing liquids or problems moving food around in the mouth or to the back of the throat for swallowing. These problems are best handled medically and can be assessed with videofluoroscopy or videoendoscopy. The aggressiveness of treatment intervention depends on the patient's preference and whether she or he still wants to attempt any oral feeding (e.g., syringe feeding, oral gastric tubes) or wishes to have a PEG or another alternative to oral feedings implemented. Therapists, however, can help patients and caregivers develop strategies that improve eating and nutrition, such as adjusting eating position, changing head and neck alignments, adding thickeners to liquids, and adjusting portion sizes and texture of foods.[7]

Psychosocial Issues

Giving the bad news of a terminal diagnosis is difficult for even the most experienced clinician. In dealing with the diagnosis of ALS, most physicians now believe that the diagnosis, prognosis, and possible patterns of progression should be shared with the patient and family or partners and caregiving friends. Only by knowing the truth can patients and families deal openly with one another and make plans for the future.[118] McCluskey and colleagues[119] suggest that those giving the medical or therapeutic diagnosis should attend to good practice parameters when giving bad news, such as creating the appropriate setting, identifying patient and caregiver needs, asking what patients and caregivers want to know, providing knowledge, exploring feelings of the patients and caregivers, and formulating a strategy for dealing with the situation. Patients and family members seldom remember what they are told when first given a terminal diagnosis. They do, however, remember how the information was given. Therefore information should be given honestly but with a sense of hope. All information need not be given at the time of diagnosis. Rather, the patient and family can be exposed to more in-depth information over a number of sessions when they have the opportunity to ask questions that occur during the assimilation process. Therapists, especially those working in isolation from a comprehensive clinic, should also follow these guidelines by providing information, helping the patient and family identify goals, and establishing a plan for intervention. Patients should know that the goals will have to be adjusted and plans reset as the disease process continues. If patients and families know that they can contact the therapist for support and advice, many of the negative aspects of the illness can be confronted in a positive manner. Preferably, an appointment for a follow-up visit will be set so patients and family members feel that contact with the care provider is expected.

Information about transitions related to nutrition, communication, and respiratory functions should be delivered to patients and families in time to make thoughtful decisions rather than just before a time of crisis, such as after a choking episode or during a respiratory arrest. Care should also be taken to respect the cultural and spiritual views of the patient and family.[58] Preferably, patients and family members will prepare an advance medical directive that should be reviewed with the physician at least every 6 months.[120]

Therapists treating patients who do not have access to a multidisciplinary ALS clinic should remember that they are often the person who works most closely with the patient, and they should plan on spending enough time with the family to respond to concerns and help with problem solving. Patients will progress through the diagnostic process with different responses and at different rates on a continuum from taking a cognitive approach by asking many questions and reviewing the most current research to the extreme of marked denial and disinterest in participating in any medical or therapeutic recommendations.

Purtilo and Haddad[121] identified four major fears of the patient who has a terminal condition: fear of isolation, fear of pain, fear of dependence, and fear of death itself. Patients with progressive diseases often see their social contacts decrease. Mr. Turner in Case Study 17-1 was concerned when he was no longer able to join his colleagues in the company cafeteria. After he received his motorized wheelchair he was able to continue his social contacts until his bulbar symptoms progressed to a point that he chose not to eat in public. When Mr. Turner lost the ability to speak and had to use his computerized speech system, he noticed that fewer colleagues stopped by his office to talk because of the slowness of the communication process. Although he understood the problem, Mr. Turner mourned the loss of friendship and his loss of standing as a competent computer expert. Because of his need for social contact, Mr. Turner continued to work until he could no longer tolerate the sitting position. His fear of isolation increased when he became homebound. Although colleagues came for visits regularly at first, as Mr. Turner progressed to a near locked-in state only a few close friends came by for brief visits. Mr. Turner's greatest fear was being separated from his family and abandoned to hospital care with inconsistent staffing patterns. Fortunately, in his community, Mrs. Turner was able to set up visitations from several church members, clerics, and hospice volunteers.

Fear of uncontrolled pain is common among people with terminal diseases. Patients need assurance that their pain will be controlled. Fortunately, today pain medications can be administered in many forms, dosages, and frequencies that can be tailored to the patient's specific needs. In a study of the final month of life with ALS, caregivers reported that a major emphasis of care was to eliminate as much pain and discomfort as possible, even if it shortened the patient's life.[122] Keeping a pain log of intensity, type, location, and time of pain may provide the physician with information necessary to best prescribe dosages. Many patients with ALS do experience significant pain from musculoskeletal sources, persistent spasms, or spasticity and pressure sores. Most of these problems can be handled with appropriate pain medications, muscle relaxants, careful positioning, frequent ROM exercises, and tissue massage. Undertreated and uncontrolled pain is associated with a patient's seeking information on assisted suicide.[123] Some patients who expressed interest in assisted suicide options did not follow up because of religious beliefs and concerns about possible loss of life insurance coverage for surviving family members.[124]

A major concern of patients with ALS is the dependence necessary for ADLs associated with late phase II and phase III of the disease. Because the process is gradual, most patients have the opportunity to make adjustments. The dependency issues and resulting privacy issues are more uncomfortable for some patients than for others, especially for the person who has always valued self-control and independence. Some patients are concerned about their increasing dependence because of the consequences of increasing burden of care on spouses or other caregivers.[125] That concern for others sometimes causes patients to choose hospital, nursing home, or in-patient hospice care over home care during the terminal stage of the disease. Not all patients with terminal illness react the same way during the dying process. Throughout the process, patients and family members may cycle back and forth through a range of different emotional and coping reactions: depression, anger, hostility, bargaining, and acceptance and adaptation (order is not implied).[121] How the patient coped with life's difficulties before the illness and her or his prior relationship patterns often direct how the patient will deal with the terminal illness. In one study, patients adjusted most successfully to the changes in their functional status if they did not look back to the past and compare their losses to their future.[126]

Health care providers and family members often have great difficulty coping with a patient who is depressed; they may make repeated efforts to "talk the person out of" the depression. Medical professions must be able to distinguish between depression that can be destructive and the mourning or grieving that is a necessary and vital response to dealing with loss. In both states the person may feel a level of withdrawal, sadness, apathy, loss of interest in activities, and cognitive distortions. In a depressive state, however, the patient experiences an accompanying loss of self-esteem. A person in mourning rarely experiences that loss of self-esteem essential to a diagnosis of depression. The grieving person's feelings are congruent with the degree of loss experienced.[127] A person who grieves for what is lost but who has adapted to the prognosis may make plans for the impending death. Such behaviors are positive coping strategies. However, depressive symptoms related to hopelessness, uncontrolled suffering, and perceived burden on caregivers are more related to a choice for treatment discontinuance of feeding or ventilatory support.[124]

The issue of depression is complicated by the pseudobulbar effect of emotional lability (inappropriate laughing and crying), which is manifested by approximately 50% of patients with ALS. This emotional lability is not under complete control of the patient and is often misunderstood by family members and caregivers. Although current treatment is antidepressant medications, underlying clinical depression may or may not be present that would respond to higher doses of antidepressant medication and counseling.[120]

Yet, pressuring a patient who appears depressed to see a mental health clinician can lead to loss of trust if the patient is not comfortable talking about feelings or confiding in a counselor. Therefore, OTs and PTs and other persons involved in the direct care of a dying patient may find that their patients feel safer talking with nonprofessional counselors or psychotherapists about the burden of their care on family members or their own impending death. Rehabilitation personnel should, therefore, be aware of local options for in-home support services, palliative care, and end-of-life options and services and be prepared to listen to the patient's concerns if the patient expresses the need for emotional support.

Caregiver Issues

Often in the concern for the patient's needs, health care professionals pay little attention to the effect a person's degenerative illness has on other members of the family. ALS significantly affects the person's extended family because the patient gradually becomes increasingly dependent on family members, partners, or caregiving friends for physical care, social arrangements, cognitive stimulation, and emotional support. For some families, the spouse may have to take on additional work, return to work, or, in the case of some older women, join the workforce for the first time to deal with the financial stresses that occur when chronic illness invades the family unit. Family members must absorb the former family duties of the dependent person. For example, a spouse or child may have to handle all the cooking, cleaning, or other household chores or work to help support the family. Once the patient becomes dependent, the caregiver may need to reduce or discontinue employment to take care of the patient. All family members may have to become involved in the physical care of the increasingly dependent person with ALS.

Children of patients with ALS also have to deal with major changes in their lifestyle. Although they may love their parent who is sick, at some level most are frustrated with factors such as the need to provide physical care to parents. This is a difficult problem for children who have not had a positive relationship with that parent. Children living in the home of a parent who is dying of ALS also express frustration about the lack of privacy in their home when nursing personnel and attendants are present, interruptions in family and personal life plans, embarrassment because of the parent's appearance and dependency, lack of attention from the caregiving and working parent, and fear of financial crises (e.g., possible loss of home, no financial support for college).

The entire family is affected by the sick person's increasing dependency and impending death. In a small study of 11 family caregivers, many caregivers felt frustrated and resentful because their lives were consumed with the caregiving responsibilities. Most caregivers had adjusted to some degree after 2 to 4 years. Caregivers who adjusted most successfully learned to take time for themselves without guilt and to tap their social support systems for help.[126,128] Similarly, 40 caregivers of young adults with severe disabilities reported being overwhelmed by the physical requirements of daily care and felt a severe loss of spontaneity in their lives.[129] They also reported a sense of isolation from everyday social interactions. Although they highly valued their social support systems, they expressed frustration that few people offered instrumental or direct service support, such as respite care or help with medical appointments, housekeeping, or shopping. Despite the stresses of caregiving, the caregivers felt positive about their roles in helping the dependent adult by finding meaning in their acts of caregiving.[129] Fortunately, most families manage to cope with the process—the major contributing factor being the coping ability of families before the illness. To be really effective, the therapist working with the patient with ALS must be prepared to help families and caregivers find appropriate ways of coping with the emotional, social, and physical stress of caregiving. For example, therapists should present, without pressing, adaptive equipment options to patients when they first start to show impairment in functional ability. If shown how the equipment will help them maintain independence, most patients are receptive to its use. Even when presented in a positive way, however, a wheelchair or adaptive devices may be resisted long after the adaptations would facilitate mobility and ADLs. Therapists must be attentive to patients' feelings and fears at this time because use of a wheelchair heralds to many patients the beginning of the end.

Other factors that affect the family of a patient with ALS include medical insurance and differing levels of long-term care coverage. Some families are fortunate to have excellent coverage that provides extensive home nursing support, whereas other families are unable to cope with the financial stresses and must accept public assistance during the final stages of the disease. As opposed to Germany and Japan, which provide long-term nursing care insurance, in the United States financial stress on patients with ALS can reach more than $150,000 per year for ventilation support at home.[63] Financial burden significantly impacts patient and caregiver decisions. (See Case Study 17-1 and end-of-life issues resources at www.nlm.nih.gov/medlineplus/endoflifeissues.html#cat1.)

GUILLAIN-BARRÉ Syndrome

Pathology and Medical Diagnosis

In the past 15 years a broad spectrum of inflammatory demyelinating polyradiculoneuropathies has been identified. GBS, or acute inflammatory demyelinating immune-mediated polyneuropathy, is the most common form of the disease. GBS affects nerve roots and peripheral nerves, leading to motor neuropathy and flaccid paralysis with possible sensory and ANS effects.[130] Purely motor forms and mixed motor and sensory forms of GBS have been identified.[131] Unlike ALS, GBS usually has a good prognosis, with most patients returning to their prior functional status by 1 year after onset.

The incidence of GBS is approximately one to four cases per 100,000 persons. A variant form is acute motor axonal neuropathy, which, like GBS, has a good prognosis. Less common forms are acute motor and sensory axonal neuropathy, which has a less positive prognosis (and which some consider to be a distinct type of peripheral neuropathy); Miller-Fisher syndrome, with primarily cranial nerve symptoms, ataxia, and areflexia[132]; and chronic inflammatory demyelinating polyradiculoneuropathy (CIDP), which causes progressive or relapsing and remitting numbness and weakness.[133] Epidemiological studies show that males are affected by GBS twice as often as are females.[134]

Approximately 27% of patients with GBS have no identified preceding illness; however, more than two thirds had symptoms of an infectious disease 2 weeks before the onset of GBS symptoms. Although no consistent predisposing factors are known, evidence exists to support connections with *Campylobacter jejuni, Mycoplasma pneumoniae,* cytomegalovirus, and Epstein-Barr virus. In GBS the spinal roots and peripheral nerves are infiltrated with macrophages and T lymphocytes. Macrophages then attack and strip the myelin sheaths. In milder cases of GBS the axons are left intact and the nerves are remyelinated, typically in a matter of weeks.[135] However, in some cases, the axons also degenerate, with recovery dependent on axonal regeneration from intact elements, which takes months and may be incomplete.[135] In acute axonal motor neuropathy, macrophages invade the axon directly, leaving the myelin intact.[136] Some evidence exists in a substantial number of patients with GBS that axonal loss is related to long-lasting or permanent muscle weakness.[137,138]

Because of damage to the myelin sheath, saltatory propagation of the action potential is disturbed, resulting in slowed conduction velocity, dyssynchrony of conduction, disturbed conduction of higher frequency impulses, or complete conduction block.[139] Partial conduction block is most often seen in the early stages of GBS, and the conduction block increases as the patient reaches a plateau. The most common conduction block findings are in the peroneal nerve, followed by the tibial nerve. Proximal conduction block is evident more often than distal conduction block. In axonal neuropathy, conduction block is more severe, and the number of functional motor units is decreased (Figure 17-4).[140] The diagnostic criteria for GBS are detailed in Box 17-3.

Clinical Presentation

GBS in both children and adults is characterized by a rapidly evolving, relatively symmetrical ascending weakness or flaccid paralysis. Motor impairment may vary from mild weakness of distal lower-extremity musculature to total paralysis of the peripheral, axial, facial, and extraocular musculature. Severe fatigue is present in 38% to 86% of patients with GBS, depending on the cutoff point used to define severity and the age of the sample, with a positive correlation between severe fatigue and age.[141] Tendon reflexes are usually diminished or absent. Twenty percent to 38% of patients may require assisted ventilation because of paralysis or weakness of the intercostal and diaphragm musculature.[142,143] Impaired respiratory muscle strength may lead to an inability to cough or handle secretions and to decreased vital capacity, tidal volume, and oxygen saturation. Secondary complications such as infections or organ system failure lead to death in approximately 5% of patients with GBS.[144] Approximately 35% to 50% of patients develop some cranial nerve involvement, primarily facial muscle weakness, although patients may also develop oropharyngeal and oculomotor involvement.[143,145]

ANS symptoms are noted in approximately 50% of patients. Low cardiac output, cardiac dysrhythmias, and marked fluctuations in blood pressure may compromise management of respiratory function and can lead to sudden death. Other typical ANS symptoms may result in peripheral pooling of blood, poor venous return, ileus, and urinary retention.[146]

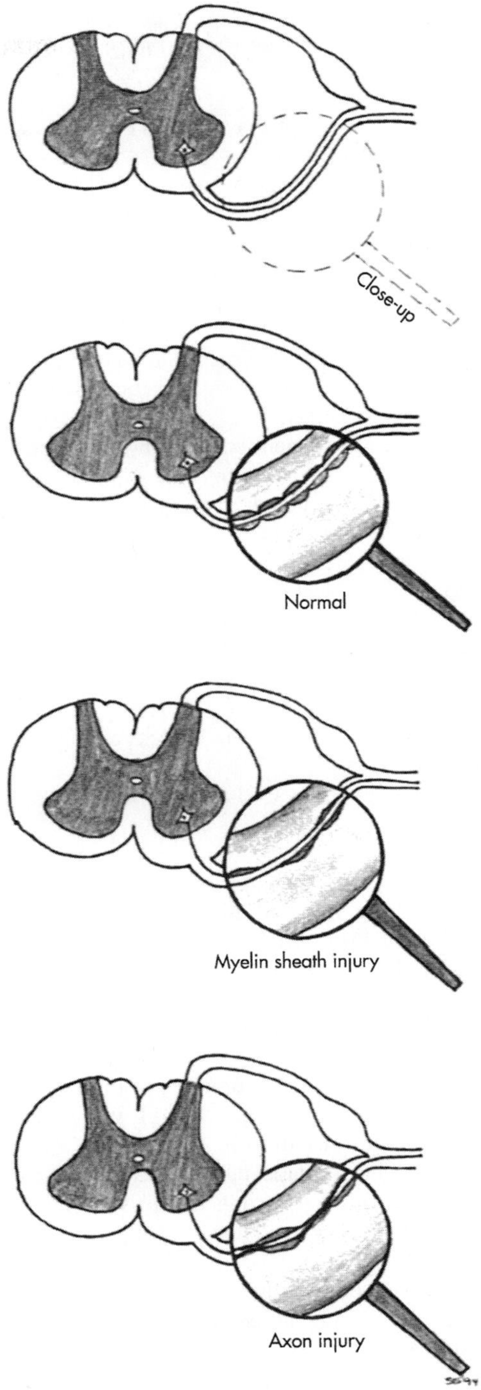

Figure 17-4 ■ Peripheral nerve showing axonal degeneration and demyelination.

Sensory symptoms such as distal hyperesthesias, paresthesias (tingling, burning), numbness, and decreased vibratory or position sense are common. The sensory disturbances often have a stocking-and-glove pattern rather than the dermatomal distribution of loss. Although the sensory problems are seldom disabling, they can be disconcerting and upsetting to patients, especially during the acute stage.[147,148]

Pain was identified as a significant presenting symptom reported in the original articles describing GBS. When

BOX 17-3 ■ COMMON DIAGNOSTIC FEATURES OF GUILLAIN-BARRÉ SYNDROME

A. Motor weakness
   1. Progressive symptoms and signs of motor weakness that develop rapidly
      a. Relative symmetry of motor involvement
      b. Usual progression of weakness from distal to proximal; self-limiting to distal limbs of upper and/or lower extremities or may extend to full quadriplegia with respiratory and cranial nerve involvement
   2. Areflexia of at least distal tendon responses

B. Mild sensory symptoms or signs, particularly paresthesias and hypesthesias

C. Autonomic dysfunction such as tachycardia and arrhythmias, vasomotor symptoms

D. Absence of fever at onset of symptoms; history of flulike illness common

E. Laboratory test results nonspecific but may show elevation of cerebrospinal fluid protein; cerebrospinal fluid cells at 10 or fewer mononuclear leukocytes per cubic millimeter of cerebrospinal fluid

F. Electrodiagnostic testing, nerve conduction velocities usually abnormal

G. Recovery usually begins 2 to 4 weeks after plateau of disease process

pain was prominent, patients spontaneously revealed its presence during a medical history. Therefore therapists who may be working with patients with an onset of low back pain not associated with known injury or stress and reports of paresthesias (pins and needles) and vibratory or decreased tendon reflexes should evaluate or monitor for possible GBS.[149,150]

The most common description of presenting pain was of muscle aching typically associated with vigorous or excessive exercise. Pain was usually symmetrical and reported most frequently in the large-bulk muscles such as the gluteals, quadriceps, and hamstrings and less often in the lower leg and upper-extremity muscles. Some pain reported during late stages of the illness was described as "stiffness." Pain was consistently more disturbing at night.[150] As the disease progresses, some patients experience severe burning or hypersensitivity to touch or even air movement, which can interfere with nursing care and limit therapy interventions. The types of pain reported include paresthesias, dysesthesias, axial and radicular pain, joint pain, and myalgias.[151] Dysautonomia (orthostatic hypotension, blood pressure instability, cardiac arrhythmias and sometimes bowel and bladder dysfunction) is relatively common in patients with GBS requiring ventilatory support; in one prospective study of 297 patients, cardiac arrest associated with dysautonomia was the leading cause of death.[137] In patients with paraplegia or quadriplegia, approximately one fourth had problems with urinary retention caused by detrusor areflexia or overactivity, overactive urethral sphincter, and disturbed bladder sensation.[134] The possibility of deep vein thrombosis (DVT) and pulmonary embolus must also be monitored and prophylactic treatment used.[152]

Medical Prognosis

Although some patients have a fulminating course of progress with maximal paralysis within 1 to 2 days of onset, 50% of patients reach the nadir (the point of greatest severity) of the disease within 1 week, 70% by 2 weeks, and 80% by 3 weeks.[145] In some cases the process of increasing weakness continues for 1 to 2 months. Onset of recovery is varied, with most patients showing gradual recovery of muscle strength 2 to 4 weeks after progression has stopped or the condition has plateaued. Although 50% of the patients may show minor neurological deficits (e.g., diminished or absent tendon reflexes) and 15% may show persistent residual deficits in function, approximately 80% become ambulatory within 6 months of onset of symptoms. The most common long-term deficits are weakness of the anterior tibial musculature and, less often, weakness of the foot and hand intrinsics, quadriceps, and gluteal musculature. Three percent to 5% of patients die of secondary cardiac, respiratory, or other systemic organ failure.[134,151] Fatigue or poor endurance was also noted as a long-term consequence of GBS, possibly attributable to deconditioning and peripheral fatigue related to muscle fatigue during the healing process.[141,153] Vasjar and colleagues[154] also report that fatigue and poor exercise tolerance were common persisting symptoms in children who appeared to have fully recovered from acute GBS.

Although often not the focus of most studies on the long-term impact of GBS, sensory deficits (impaired response to pinprick, light touch, and vibration and proprioception in combination with other sensory losses) are an ongoing problem for patients 3 to 6 years after recovery from acute GBS. In a study of 122 subjects, 38% showed sensory deficits in the upper extremities[155] and 66% had ongoing sensory deficits of the lower extremities.[151] The muscle aches and cramps experienced by some of these patients appeared to be related to sensory rather than persistent motor dysfunctions as usually thought.

Overall, factors associated with a poor prognosis are severity of muscle weakness (especially quadriplegia), the need for respiratory support, cranial nerve involvement associated with loss of eye movement and swallowing, rapid rate of progression from onset, length of time to nadir, older age at onset, history of gastrointestinal illness, and recent cytomegalovirus infections.[134,142] In a prospective study of 297 patients with GBS in Italy, disease severity was not associated with time to clinical recovery, but it did predict ultimate outcome, along with shorter length of time to nadir, older age at onset, evidence of axon damage, and recent gastroenteritis.[137]

Medical Management

Medical treatment depends on the rate and degree of ascending paralysis. Because most patients return to their prior functional status, excellent supportive care during the acute stage is imperative. Respiratory compromise should be expected, and all patients, including those with limited paralysis and sensory dysfunction, must be closely monitored for the rapid onset of pulmonary and cardiac decompensation or cardiac arrhythmias, paroxysmal or orthostatic hypotension, urinary retention, and paralytic ileus caused by dysautonomia.[152] Because of the possibility of sudden respiratory failure, patients with evidence of GBS must be hospitalized so that immediate cardiorespiratory support can be given if functional vital capacity (FVC) falls below 20 mL/kg or oxygen saturation falls below 75%.[144] Patients who progress to respiratory paralysis must be treated in an intensive care environment where adequate respiratory function can be maintained, secondary infections can be prevented or limited, and metabolic functions can be carefully monitored. The patient should be intubated if the FVC falls below 12 mL/kg or if the patient is increasingly dyspneic even if FVC is above the cutoff level.[145,156] Twenty-five percent of patients who experience respiratory failure will develop pneumonia.[151] Even if daytime respiration seems adequate, night-time respiratory insufficiency (sleep-disordered breathing) should be ruled out if patients have persistent sleepiness or fatigue.[141]

Patients with GBS in the intensive care unit (ICU) on ventilation and with varying levels of paralysis and sensory dysfunction feel trapped and out of control because they cannot express their needs. These patients can usually hear well and most can see what is happening around them. They benefit from being oriented to time, having the personnel explain all procedures, and having some means of obtaining help. Therapists can work with the ICU staff to provide the patient with alternative forms of communication, such as eye blink, clicking, and communication boards designed for their needs. Having some form of communication and knowing that they will not be left alone will help prevent traumatic stress reactions.[152]

In addition to the intensive monitoring of progression and supportive care required for patients with GBS, two specific immunotherapy-based treatments—plasma exchange (removal of plasma from withdrawn blood with retransfusion of the formed elements back into the blood) and intravenous immunoglobulin (IVIg) (taking blood from a vein, separating plasma, and returning the blood cells with a plasma substitute)—have been under investigation for their ability to decrease the duration of respirator dependence and the time to onset of improvement. Systematic reviews of these interventions as of 2010 have found that plasma exchange decreases recovery time and is most beneficial if begun within the first week of diagnosis and can be beneficial up to 30 days after diagnosis.[157] Plasma exchange is also cost-effective as used in patients with mild, moderate, or severe courses of GBS.[158] IVIg is somewhat safer and easier to administer than plasma exchange; IVIg speeds recovery by the same amount of time as plasma exchange and is more effective than supportive care only. Adding IVIg to plasma exchange did not improve time to recovery any more than either treatment alone.[159] High-quality evidence is available to support IVIg use in adults with GBS; the quality of evidence is slightly less high to support its use in children with GBS.[160]

Although corticosteroids have been used to decrease the inflammatory process in GBS since the 1960s, a review of clinical studies of corticosteroid effectiveness showed that corticosteroid treatment alone does not hasten recovery from GBS.[161] Hughes and colleagues have developed practice parameters associated with these findings.[162]

Therapeutic Management of Movement Dysfunction Associated with Guillain-Barré Syndrome

Therapeutic management of the movement deficits associated with GBS includes supportive management during the acute phase, prevention of long-term medical comorbidities during the acute through early recovery stages, and rehabilitation throughout recovery.[163] With the assumption that the patient will have significant return of function within months, therapists must help maintain the integrity of functioning systems, address pain, teach compensatory strategies, and appropriately promote increasing activity after the plateau. The immediate needs of the patient will change as the patient moves through the acute stage, the plateau at the nadir, and the recovery stage of GBS before and after muscles attain antigravity strength. Transitioning between the changes in immediate therapeutic goals necessitates careful examination of the current status, progression of disease, and needs of the patient.

Examination

A comprehensive examination of the patient's movement and function includes factors shown in Box 17-4. The extent of the examination in any one session depends on the patient's condition and ability to participate. History taking should include the course of the disease, along with any recent illness, preexisting neuromotor or other medical conditions, current concerns, and the patient's immediate goals. Screening tests can help determine whether sensory and autonomic systems are involved along with motor systems. Checking vital signs at rest and immediately after activity, assessing skin integrity especially in immobile patients, screening cranial nerve performance, and noting communication ability are all important components. Additional testing of sensation (and documentation on a body chart, for example) or autonomic systems may be required if the screening tests indicate.

In GBS, assessment of muscle strength and ROM as specifically as possible is important so the patient's course of progression or improvement can be tracked, possible patterns leading to contractures can be predicted and prevented, and the appropriate level of exercise can be implemented. MMT, dynamometry, or isokinetic testing could be useful in various stages; goniometry is typically used for ROM testing. Full MMT and joint ROM may require several sessions in the initial stages, and a few specific muscles and joints may be selected (e.g., sternocleidomastoids, deltoids, triceps, flexor carpi ulnaris, lumbricals, iliopsoas, gluteus medius, anterior tibialis, flexor hallucis longus; shoulders, fingers, ankles) to test for changes weekly.

Several factors may interfere with complete assessment in the initial stage. Patients who report considerable pain during handling or active movement may not tolerate or may be unwilling or unable to cooperate with testing. The therapist should track the patient's level of pain, for example, on a numerical rating of pain scale, to help distinguish between weakness and loss of ROM related to pathological condition, immobility, or pain.

Fatigue and respiratory difficulties may also preclude complete strength assessment in a single session. Fatigue may result from deconditioning, increased effort required to perform similarly with weakened muscles, and inability to recruit sufficient motor units to maintain contractions.[164] Fatigue can be documented in relation to amount of activity tolerated (with specific symptoms noted before rest is required) or with a questionnaire such as the Fatigue Severity Scale (FSS), Fatigue Impact Scale (FIS), or the Visual Analogue Scale for Fatigue (VAS-F).[141] Functional tests may include standardized scales of independence in ADLs or balance, tests of manual dexterity, and temporal measures

BOX 17-4 ■ FACTORS TO CONSIDER IN THE EXAMINATION OF PATIENTS WITH GUILLAIN-BARRÉ SYNDROME

HISTORY

Patterns and sequence of symptom onset

Recent illness or injury, prior episodes of sensorimotor problems

MOTOR FUNCTION

Visual inspection to identify symmetry of muscle bulk and function

Myotatic reflexes, rule out tonic reflexes

Manual muscle testing, carefully identifying pattern of weakness (testing should be as muscle specific as possible rather than assessing muscle groups only; use form for serial recording)

Presence of muscle fasciculations

Cranial nerves

Range of motion (use form for serial recording)

Equilibrium reactions sitting and standing (if testable)

Current functional status (activities of daily living, including bowel and bladder function, ambulation)

Endurance and experienced fatigue

SENSORY SYSTEM

Identify pattern of sensory loss or changes (use body chart)

Identify specific type of sensory change (e.g., paresthesias, anesthesia, hypesthesias) (use body chart)

Identify pain type and location (use body chart): what makes it better, what makes it worse?

Identify pressure points or areas that might lead to pressure sores

AUTONOMIC SYSTEM

Blood pressure resting and immediately after activity (prone, sitting, standing, if possible)

Heart rate resting and immediately after activity, dysrhythmias

Body temperature stability

Bowel and bladder control

PSYCHOSOCIAL SYSTEMS

Identify patient and family concerns in acute circumstances and concerns about long-term issues that may affect patient and family. Assessment need not be extensive if referral can be made for social service evaluation of patient and family financial concerns, day-to-day living problems (e.g., transportation, child care), support systems, and coping strategies.

ELECTRODIAGNOSTIC TESTING

Nerve conduction velocity. (Physician will order these studies to be performed by a clinician skilled in the procedures. This may be a physical therapist, physician, or technician depending on facility.)

of gait. Chehebar and colleagues[163] review some of the pros and cons of standardized tests such as the Barthel Index, modified Hughes scale of GBS disability, and the Functional Independence Measure. Health-related quality-of-life measures used in related populations include the Nottingham Health Profile and the SF-36.[164] Forsberg and colleagues[165] provide a comprehensive list of tests they administered in a prospective study of 42 patients followed for 2 years after the onset of GBS. At 2 weeks postonset, 40 of 42 patients had submaximal scores on total muscle strength, grip strength, balance, and gait speed testing. At 2 months, total muscle strength was still most affected, whereas 25% of the patients had regained maximal grip strength, balance, and gait speed (designated as 1.4 to 1.5 m/sec). By 2 years, over half of the subjects still lacked the maximum total muscle score, and 40% claimed fatigue. Sensory deficits were claimed by up to 36% of patients at 2 years.[165]

Changes in the patient's condition should be monitored with serial MMT, ROM assessments, sensory testing, and functional status examinations. See Karni and colleagues[166] for suggestions on serial functional assessments. Before the patient is discharged from the hospital or rehabilitation unit, therapists should complete an assessment of the patient's home environment so that appropriate safety and adaptive equipment can be in place in time for the patient's return home.

Respiratory and Dysphagia Examination

Therapists are usually involved early in the care of patients with GBS. For patients with respiratory or bulbar paralysis, the therapist's initial contact may be in the ICU. Although most hospitals have fully equipped ICUs, a therapist working in a rural or smaller community hospital may be the first person to note a patient's changing respiratory status during an evaluation and treatment session for muscle weakness or back pain. Therefore the therapist must be prepared to advise nursing and medical staff about the need to test oxygen saturation levels and FVC. Therapist attention to respiratory complications is particularly important in the managed care environment, which discourages hospitalization if presenting symptoms are not life endangering.[145] A simple estimate of FVC can be done at bedside. If after taking a large breath the patient can count out loud only to 10, the forced vital capacity is approximately 1 L and intubation should be considered. Complete information on the PT's evaluation of patients in acute respiratory failure is provided by Irwin and Tecklin.[167]

Patients who have been intubated or who have cranial nerve involvement with oral motor weakness commonly have a high incidence of aspiration. Patients with severe oral-motor problems and dysphagia should be evaluated thoroughly and treated by a therapist skilled in oral-motor dysfunction and feeding. This may be a speech therapist, OT, or PT depending on the facility. Patients with a feeding tube (PEG) should receive their feedings in a relatively upright position and should remain in that position for 30 to 60 minutes after feeding to decrease the chance of aspiration. According to Logemann,[168] approximately 40% of patients receiving bedside swallowing assessments have undetected aspiration. Therefore the bedside evaluation should be considered only a preliminary step in the diagnostic process. In addition to careful assessment of oral-motor control, some clinicians recommend cervical auscultation to listen to swallowing sounds, particularly during the acute phase of the illness.

With evidence of swallowing difficulties and possible aspiration, the patient should be referred for comprehensive testing with videofluoroscopy. Swallowing also can be assessed by techniques such as fiberoptic endoscopy, ultrasound, electroglottography to determine laryngeal movement, and scintigraphy, which involves scanning a radioactive bolus during swallowing.[169] (Refer to section on medical management of ALS for suggestions for dealing with dysphagia.)

Intervention Goals

General goals for the care of the patient with GBS, to be specified with reference to the patient's preferences, include the following:

- Facilitate resolution of respiratory problems and dysphagia
- Minimize pain
- Prevent contractures, decubitus ulcers, and injury to weakened or denervated muscles
- Introduce a graduated program of active exercise while monitoring overuse and fatigue
- Resume psychosocial roles and improve quality of life

Therapeutic Interventions

In a Cochrane review of exercise in people with peripheral neuropathies, no randomized or quasi-randomized controlled trials were identified for patients with GBS as of September 2009.[135] However, some treatment programs used for patients with other neuromotor dysfunctions can be adapted for use with patients with GBS.

Respiratory and Cranial Nerve Dysfunction

Depending on the facility, PTs may be involved in the respiratory care of patients with GBS. PTs may conduct chest percussion, breathing exercises, resistive inspiratory training, or strict protocols to prevent overfatigue of respiratory muscles while weaning patients from mechanical ventilation.[170] Goals of treatment are related to increasing ventilation or oxygenation, decreasing oxygen consumption, controlling secretions, and improving exercise tolerance. See Irwin and Tecklin[167] for coverage of treatment programs and techniques appropriate for the GBS patient with acute or residual respiratory dysfunction.

When patients are placed on mechanical ventilators, communication can be difficult and frustrating.[171] The rehabilitation team can help develop and execute alternative means of communication.

In the more severe cases of GBS, cranial nerve involvement can lead to multiple complications such as dysphagia and vocal cord paralysis. In many facilities, speech pathologists or OTs are responsible for establishing a dysphagia treatment program. Therapists responsible for treatment of patients with dysphagia and swallowing problems should refer to Logemann's classic text on the evaluation and treatment of swallowing disorders.[168] Therapeutic goals are the prevention of choking and aspiration and the stimulation of effective swallowing and eating. The act of chewing and swallowing is complex and requires coordinated reflexive and conscious action. Intervention is focused on positioning (upright with head tilted slightly forward),[171] head control, and oral-motor coordination (e.g., sucking an ice cube, stimulating the gag response, facilitating swallowing with quick pressure on the neck and thyroid notch timed with intent to swallow). A conscious swallowing technique is introduced with thick liquids and progressed to thinner liquids after the patient's oral-motor coordination response is enough to control movement of fluids. Once the patient has good lip closure, fluids should be introduced one sip at a time from a straw cut to a short length to minimize effort. Semisoft, moist foods are gradually introduced (pasta, mashed potatoes, squash, gelatin). Any crumbly or stringy foods (coffee cakes, cookies, snack chips, celery, cheeses) should be avoided, and the patient should not attempt to talk or be interrupted during eating until choking does not occur and swallowing is comfortable and consistent.[172] Feeding training should occur during frequent, short sessions to prevent fatigue. Therapists should be prepared to use the Heimlich maneuver if choking occurs or have a suction machine available at bedside.

Pain

If pain seems to be a major factor limiting the patient's passive or active motion, the treatment team should determine the best approach to alleviate pain. According to one study, patients with GBS did not seem to show a consistent response to any specific pain medication, although six of the 13 patients seemed to have a positive response to codeine, oxycodone plus acetaminophen (Percocet), and oxycodone plus aspirin (Percodan).[147] Some patients may find relief with medications used to treat neurogenic pain, such as the tricyclic antidepressants, carbamazepine, or gabapentin (anticonvulsants).[151] For patients who do not respond to conventional analgesics or tricyclic antidepressants, a short course of high-dose corticosteroids can lead to pain relief.[144]

Some patients with neuropathy have noted decreased pain after using transcutaneous electrical nerve stimulation (TENS).[173,174] Although no study has examined the effect of TENS specifically on pain associated with GBS, it might be a treatment option to help with desensitization in patients whose pain is not controlled with passive movement or pain medications.

Another option is capsaicin, the active ingredient in chili peppers, which when applied topically interacts with the sensory neurons to relieve pain from peripheral neuropathies.[151] Therapists, wearing gloves, apply a topical anesthetic until the area is numb. The capsaicin is then applied topically. The capsaicin remains on the skin until the patient starts to feel the heat, at which point it is promptly removed. Because the nerves are overstimulated by the burning sensation, the sensory gateway is unable to report pain for an extended period.[175]

Some patients who experience extreme sensitivity to light touch, such as from movement of sheets, air flow, and intermittent touch contact, benefit from a "cradle" that holds sheets away from the body. Some find relief if the limbs are wrapped snuggly with elastic bandages, which provide continuous low pressure while warding off light and intermittent stimuli. Alternatively, the patient's pain response can be desensitized through methodical stimulation with frequent, consistent stimuli to the affected area for short durations to allow acclimatization.[170]

Contractures, Decubitus Ulcers, and Injury to Weakened or Denervated Muscles

Positioning. In the acute stage of GBS, rehabilitation will focus on positioning and passive ROM to prevent contractures and decubitus ulcers.[176] Preventing pressure sores starts within the first few days of hospitalization, especially for the patient who has complete or nearly complete paralysis. A positioning program for the dependent patient is the first line of defense, with turning at least every 2 hours for both pressure relief and lung drainage.[171] In addition, the patient should have a special mattress or unit that constantly changes the pressure within the mattress to shift the patient's position or is designed to spread pressure over wide surfaces. Patients who are slender or who have lost significant muscle mass from GBS-induced atrophy will have prominent bony surfaces; the therapist may need to fashion foam "doughnuts" or pads or use sheepskin-type protection for pressure relief. Patients who have muscle pain may prefer to have their hips and knees flexed. If so, the patient must be taken out of the flexed position for part of each hour to avoid muscle shortening.

As part of a complete positioning program, therapists should consider how best to maintain the physiological position of the hands and feet. Research has shown that mild continuous stretch maintained for at least 20 minutes is more beneficial than stronger, brief stretching exercises.[177] Thus the use of splints for prolonged positioning is superior to the use of short bursts of intermittent, manually applied passive stretching for maintaining functional range. Although some facilities still use a footboard to control passive ankle plantarflexion, most therapists now use moldable plastic splints that can be worn when the patient is in any position. Because ankle-foot splints often prevent visual inspection of the heel position, care must be taken to ensure that the heel is firmly down in the orthosis and that the strapping pattern is adequate to secure the foot. The strap system must be simple enough to be positioned properly by all staff and family members caring for the patient. The ankle-foot splint should extend slightly beyond the end of the toes to prevent toe flexion and skin breakdown from the toes rubbing on sheeting. Care should be taken not to compress the peroneal nerve with the splint as it crosses the fibula,[148] a particularly vulnerable area after the loss of muscle mass in the lower legs from the GBS.[139] Wrist and hand splints may be prefabricated, resting-style splints, or molded to meet the patient's specific needs. Because spasticity is not a problem in the patient with GBS, a simple cone or rolled cloth may be adequate to maintain good wrist, thumb, and finger alignment for short-term immobility.

Range of Motion. To be effective, the ROM program must start within the first couple of days of hospitalization and include both accessory and physiological motions to increase circulation; provide lubrication of the joints; and maintain extensibility of capsular, muscle, and tendon tissue. Passive ROM exercises to the ends of normal range for all extremity joints, fingers and toes, neck, and trunk should be performed twice daily—more frequently if the patient has no active movement. Patients can be instructed to perform the ROM exercises themselves if they can move actively without pain or fatigue; during the acute stage of declining strength, they should be observed during ROM activities to ensure adequacy of the range and any changes in quality of movement. If the patient cannot complete movement through full range independently, a therapist or well-instructed and monitored caregiver can assist the patient in moving to the end of range. This may not be easy if the patient has pain with motion. Knowing whether to "push through the pain" or stay within the limits of pain is often a great dilemma for the therapist. The therapist needs to find a balance between working for full joint range and reacting to the patient's reports of pain. If the ends of ranges start to become stiff, stretch should be slow and sustained at the end point for 10 to 30 seconds.

Denervated or weakened muscles can be injured easily; therefore the therapist is responsible for ensuring that joint structures are not damaged and that ROM activities are done with appropriate support of the limb to prevent sudden overstretching. Instruction to caregivers regarding passive ROM activities must include details such as externally rotating the shoulder during abduction to prevent impingement and ensuring that the subtalar joint is in the neutral position during dorsiflexion to avoid overstretching of the midfoot. In hospitals where the patient is treated by a changing therapy or nursing staff or by family members, a positioning schedule with diagrams, a splinting plan, and ROM recommendations should be presented in poster format at the patient's bedside to facilitate consistent treatment.

ROM can usually be maintained with standard positioning and ROM programs. Nevertheless, some patients, especially those who have reported severe extremity and axial pain early during the disease process and those who have been quadriplegic and respirator dependent for prolonged periods, may develop significant joint contractures despite preventive interventions. As with patients with spinal cord or severe head injuries, heterotopic ossification has been reported in patients with GBS.[178] Meythaler and colleagues[179] note that early mobilization was related to therapeutic decreases in serum calcium levels and suggest that aggressive ROM (but not hard or abrupt movements that may injure the muscle) may impede the effects of heterotopic bone overgrowth, which can have a severe impact on ROM. Once heterotopic ossification has been identified, treatment includes modification of ROM exercise to use only active and passive motion within the pain-free arc.[170]

Soryal and colleagues[180] reported on three patients with GBS who had marked residual contractures that limited function after strength improved. None of the patients had radiological signs of erosive arthropathy or inflammatory joint disease. Soryal hypothesized a number of possible mechanisms for the limitations in ROM: (1) therapists and nurses may have been reluctant to take patients who reported marked pain during passive movement through the full ROM; (2) the contractures may have been a result of pain or damage caused by inappropriate excessive passive movement of hypotonic and sensory-impaired joints and muscles (often caused by poor movement of the patient in bed or by poorly trained staff or family members moving limbs); (3) the paralysis may have resulted in lymphatic stasis with accumulation of fluid in tissue spaces and nutritional disturbances; and (4) vasomotor disturbances resulting from autonomic neuropathy may have led to adhesions and fibrosis. Although the authors found few reports describing contractures as a significant residual problem, they suggested that ROM programs must be defined precisely as to frequency and duration, particularly for patients reporting early joint pain.[180]

Some patients will prefer to position their limbs so muscle and tendons are in the shortened range in an attempt to decrease muscle pain. This may lead to capsular contractures. The therapist should be aware of changes in "end feel" over time when testing ROM of each joint to determine if capsular and ligamentous structures are also becoming more restricted as the muscle and tendon tissue shortens. Patients who have intact sensation of pain and temperature may respond positively to the use of heat (up to approximately 45° C or 113° F) before stretching to decrease muscle pain and facilitate tissue elongation before stretching. Several basic studies of rat tail tendon and the relation between load and heat have shown that attaining permanent length increases in collagenous tissue is possible with a combination of heat and stretch.[181-184] (Caution: Heat should not be used on a patient with a sensory deficit that inhibits ability to distinguish differences in temperature.)

On the basis of evidence that continuous passive motion (CPM) is effective in maintaining joint range in both rabbits and human beings,[185] Mays[186] described a case study of a patient with GBS (quadriplegia with 7 days of mechanical ventilation) who had persistent pain and stiffness of the upper extremities and fingers approximately 3 months after the onset of GBS. CPM of the hands and fingers was added to a program of occupational therapy that included ROM, splinting, and ADLs. The author reported an increase in the rate of recovery of finger range and a decrease in pain after use of CPM. Numerous other studies have reported the value of CPM in maintaining or increasing ROM after hip and knee surgery. It may be a useful adjunct to traditional therapy for patients with GBS, especially those who continue to develop contractures with standard, intermittent ROM programs. Patients with severe paresthesias or dysesthesias may not be able to tolerate CPM equipment.

Massage also may play a positive role in maintaining muscle tissue mobility and tissue nutrition while limiting the amount of intramuscular fibrosis development. The use of massage in patients with GBS has not been reported; however, it makes intuitive sense that it may be a useful adjunct to ROM exercises in patients who do not have marked hypersensitivity to touch, significant muscle pain, or a history of DVT. Patients with or without a history of DVT who are immobile for long periods or who have concomitant cardiac illnesses may have marked swelling of the distal limbs. After medical clearance, edema-specific massage and limb-elevation techniques may be useful if tolerated by the patient. Early active ROM exercises creating "muscle pumping" contractions in muscles with at least fair strength can help prevent uncomfortable edema.

Progressive Program of Active Exercise while Monitoring for Overuse and Fatigue

Although most patients with GBS recover from the paralysis, the course and rate of recovery may vary significantly among patients. The decline of strength may take 2 days to 4 weeks, with a plateau of a few days to a few weeks after the nadir. Strength returns over the course of weeks to months, depending on whether the disease process affected only myelin or the axons themselves. Strength usually returns in a descending pattern—opposite to the pattern noted during onset of the disease. No evidence exists to indicate that active exercise can change the rate of progression of the disease or regrowth of myelin or axons, although it may improve function through increased strength and aerobic capacity once muscles are reinnervated. The major goal of therapeutic management throughout the course of GBS must be to maintain the patient's musculoskeletal system in an optimal ready state, prevent overwork, enhance circulation and cardiorespiratory endurance within the limits of active movement, and pace the recovery process to obtain maximal function as reinnervation occurs.

In the acute stage of GBS, active exercise is limited to whatever the patient can move without pain or excessive fatigue. Slings or adaptive devices may help support the weight of a limb to continue active movement in a gravity-eliminated plane for those muscles that have lost antigravity strength. As the disease reaches its nadir, activity remains limited. Once weakness stops progressing, passive maintenance of ROM may be the only activity possible for immobile patients. As strength begins to return after the plateau, therapists must prescribe limited amounts of low-resistance activities, with strict avoidance of antigravity strain on the muscles until strength reaches the 3/5 (Fair) range of MMT. Active exercise can be added very slowly, with frequent rest periods and monitoring to avoid fatigue.[177,187] Activity should be halted at the first point of fatigue or muscle ache; abnormal sensations (tingling, paresthesias) that persist for prolonged periods after exercise may also indicate that the exercise or activity level was excessive. Any progression of resistance or repetitions of strengthening exercises should be monitored for 3 to 7 days for increase in weakness, muscle spasms, or soreness before exercises are progressed further.[188] If additional weakness or soreness ensues, the additional activity must be eliminated for several days, with reinitiation at a lower level of resistance or number of repetitions and more gradual increase. Work simplification and energy conservation strategies may be useful to improve function in the recovery stage of GBS.[170] As strength increases, additional resistance may be applied to those muscles showing good recovery while avoiding strain on muscles that have not yet reached the same level, frequently the most distal musculature. Even when strength has returned throughout, rehabilitation and exercise may need to continue to address fatigue that may persist at each of the International Classification of Functioning, Disability and Health (ICF) levels: body function and structure, activity, and participation.[141] For an example of treatment progression during the acute stage from week 1 through week 12, see Table 17-3.

In the initial stages of upright activity after any period of bed rest, therapists must progress patients with GBS very carefully because 19% to 50% of this population show orthostatic hypotension along with dysautonomia.[139,146] A program to improve tolerance to upright position can be started in the ICU if the patient is on a circle electric or Nelson standing bed. If a standing bed is not available, a sitting program can be initiated as soon as it is tolerated. A progressive standing program can be instituted when the patient's respiratory system and ANS are no longer unstable and the patient can be moved to a tilt table. Caution should be taken to stabilize the patient fully to maintain alignment and to limit activity in muscles having strength below the fair range. When beginning training, some patients benefit from using an abdominal binder or foot-to-thigh compression stockings if tolerated. Because of the relation between poor hydration and hypotension, therapists must ensure the patient is well hydrated before beginning upright or standing tolerance programs.[139]

As was discussed in the section on therapeutic considerations for patients with ALS, a muscle that has significant denervation is more likely to respond to exercise with overwork fatigue (see Figure 17-3 for the therapeutic window for exercise). Studying the effect of exercise on rat muscle after nerve injury, Herbison and colleagues[187] identified a loss of contractile proteins during initial reinnervation. After reinnervation the same amount of exercise resulted in muscle

TABLE 17-3 ■ MEDICAL STATUS OF PATIENTS WITH GUILLAIN-BARRÉ SYNDROME AND POSSIBLE TREATMENT OUTLINE

MEDICAL STATUS	TREATMENT*
Tracheostomy Respirator dependent Complete cranial nerve paralysis Quadriplegia	Week 1: Postural drainage every 3 hours around the clock Passive ROM exercises to all joints Splinting (molded plastic) of hands and feet to maintain functional position Positioning, splinting, and ROM program schedule posted at bedside
	Weeks 2-5: Postural drainage decreased to two times each shift (every 8 hours) Passive ROM exercises, physiological and accessory motions, gentle stretching of intercostal musculature, trunk rotations Continue splinting and positioning program Family education: family members taught gentle physiological ROM techniques, with attention to correct shoulder patterns and simple massage techniques
Respirator set on intermittent mandatory ventilation Weaning to respirator at night by end of week 7 No active muscle contractions except eye opening and lip movements Dysphagia	Weeks 6-7: Postural drainage two times each shift (every 8 hours) Continue ROM program, splinting, and positioning Begin to build tolerance of upright sitting with good trunk alignment Begin facilitation of active facial and tongue muscle activity in patterns necessary for swallowing, eating, and speaking; speech pathology, occupational therapy consultation for dysphagia training Family members active in care, helping with ROM, splinting, and positioning schedule as they choose
Palpable muscle activity in neck, trunk, proximal musculature of upper and lower extremities	Weeks 8-12: Postural drainage one time each shift Chest stretching, breathing exercises Dysphagia program in collaboration with speech consultant Muscle reeducation program with electromyographic biofeedback progressing to gravity-eliminated exercises using suspension slings attached to bed Tilt-table standing program to increase tolerance to upright (wearing positioning splints if necessary) Collaborate with occupational therapist for treatment in wheelchair with suspension slings to facilitate active arm motion in gravity-limited position Exercise, rest, positioning schedule posted Family, patient educated about stimulating activity level to prevent fatigue, overuse of reinnervating muscles

ROM, Range of motion.

*Treatment depends on rate of recovery.

hypertrophy. Bensman[188] reported on eight patients who had stabilized after acute polyradiculoneuritis (among them patients with GBS). All eight patients had a temporary loss of function after strenuous physical exercise. Three patients apparently had significant decreases in strength. All patients were then placed on a program of passive ROM exercises, and an increase in muscle strength was noted. Recurring episodes of a temporary loss of function appeared to be related to strenuous exercise and fatigue. The current position for patients with GBS, then, is that excessive exercise during early reinnervation when only a few functioning motor units are present can lead to further damage rather than to the expected exercise-induced hypertrophy of muscle.

During the initial stages of exercise, the repetitions per exercise period should be low and the frequency of short periods of exercise should be high.[177] As reinnervation occurs and motor units become responsive, the early process of muscle reeducation exercise used by the therapist may be similar to that used after polio. To encourage active contraction of the muscle the therapist should carefully demonstrate to the patient the expected movement. The therapist then passively moves the patient's limb while the patient observes. After gaining a clear picture of what movement is expected, the patient is encouraged to contract muscles. Facilitatory techniques such as skin stroking, brushing, vibration, icing, and tapping may be used in conjunction with the muscle reeducation process if the sensory and pain status of the patient permits. The patient is taught to reassess his or her movements and make corrective responses. As the patient gains strength, the movements are translated into functional activities.[187]

Functional activities should be appropriate for the muscle grade of that muscle or muscle group. For example, if the patient's deltoid muscle has a poor (2/5) grade on MMT (full ROM with gravity eliminated), the patient should be cautioned not to attempt to elevate her or his arm against gravity (e.g., to shave or do one's hair). Patients may exercise when the limb weight is supported (using overhead slings, powder boards, pool exercises) to allow the patient to move actively through a full range until he or she can take resistance in the gravity-eliminated position. Children, teenagers, or adults with impaired judgment often need a strict schedule of rest and activity. Patients and staff also need to be reminded that prolonged sitting in bed or in a wheelchair, even when supported, may tax the axial musculature. A program of gradual sitting should be instituted, with the final goal being independent, unsupported sitting with functional equilibrium reactions. In busy hospitals a schedule of sitting and activity should be posted in clear view at the patient's bedside.

As reinnervation progresses and strength and exercise tolerance increases, the therapist may choose to use facilitative exercise techniques such as neurodevelopmental sequencing[189] or PNF[190,191] to recruit maximal desired contraction of specific muscle groups. Although PNF techniques are excellent for eliciting maximal contraction, care must be taken not to overwork the weaker components of the movement pattern. A positive aspect of PNF techniques is that they can be tied in with functional patterns such as rolling, which is necessary for bed mobility, transitions to quadruped, kneeling, sitting, standing, and gait.

Because patients with GBS are transferred from acute care facilities to rehabilitation, skilled nursing, or home environments more quickly than in the past, therapists must be careful to document any serial negative changes or plateaus in motor, sensory, or respiratory impairments or functional status that may herald a relapse.[139] Although 65% to 75% or more of patients with GBS show a return to clinically normal motor function, 2% to 5% of patients have a recurrence of symptoms similar in onset and pattern to the original illness.[192] Recurrence of symptoms should trigger immediate cessation of activity and possibly medical reassessment in case of respiratory insufficiency.

Anecdotal and empirical evidence shows that patients with GBS can continue to show deficits during strenuous exercises that require maximal endurance. Four soldiers who were considered clinically recovered from GBS (normal motor power with or without reappearance of reflexes and the absence of sensory impairment) were unable to pass the Army Physical Fitness Test (APFT), which is designed to measure a minimal acceptable age-related level of physical fitness for military duty (maximal effort to challenge respiratory and muscular endurance, strength, and flexibility). Before onset of GBS, the four patients had all exceeded the APFT standards. None was able to pass the APFT as long as 4 years after the illness, indicating that the persistent deficit interfered with their ability to continue their military careers.[193] The possibility of long-term endurance deficits should be considered when patients appear to have reached full recovery but report difficulty when returning to work or activities that require sustained maximal effort.[194,195]

So far, no pharmaceutical agents have been helpful in alleviating fatigue in this population. In a study of the use of amantadine to relieve severe fatigue in 74 patients with GBS randomly allocated to treatment or placebo groups, the groups showed no difference in any of the primary or secondary measures recorded.[196] Determining the effectiveness of interventions to affect fatigue may be complicated by differences in measures of experienced fatigue (subjectively reported) versus physiological fatigue (central or peripheral reduction in voluntary muscle force production) and the weak relationship between these in many neuromuscular disorders.[197]

Cardiovascular fitness may also be compromised after recovery from GBS. This may be caused by altered muscle function, but it is also related to deconditioning from an imposed sedentary lifestyle.[154] Several studies have reported the effect of endurance exercise training after GBS. In one case study a 23-year-old woman with a chronic-relapsing form of GBS with onset at age 15 years was placed on a walking and cycling program at 45% or less of her predicted maximal heart rate reserve. The low-intensity exercise program was selected to prevent possible fatigue-related relapse. After the program, the subject had improved her walking time 37%, walking distance approximately 88%, and cycle ride time more than 100%. Although no standardized or formalized recording of functional level was recorded before and after the exercise program, the patient reported that her energy level for ADLs was a "little higher" and that stair walking was easier.[194] In another single-subject study of a 54-year-old man 3 years after onset of GBS with residual weakness, the authors demonstrated similar improvements in cardiopulmonary and work capacities as well as leg strength after a 16-week course of a thrice-weekly aerobic exercise program. The subject also reported expanded ADL capabilities. The authors suggested that their training regimen may disrupt the cycle of inactivity after recovery from GBS that leads to disuse atrophy and further deconditioning in patients with mild residual weakness.[198] Fehlings and colleagues[199] tested muscle strength and endurance in a group of children at least 2 years after acute onset of GBS. Although the children appeared essentially recovered, endurance of the arm muscles was lower than that of the lower extremities. They hypothesize that the typical walking, running, and cycling activities that the children participated in were sufficient to improve strength and endurance of lower-extremity muscles, and they recommended that children be encouraged to participate in activities such as swimming to improve upper-extremity endurance. Controlled tetherball and volleyball activities are also appropriate. Tuckey and Greenwood[200] reported positive results of treatment with partial body-weight support (PBWS) treadmill exercise for a patient with severe GBS. Garssen and colleagues[201] reported a 20% reduction in fatigue levels, along with improved physical condition and strength, after a 12-week intensive bicycling exercise program for patients several years after the onset of GBS.

Improvements in strength and endurance after GBS may continue for months to years. A prospective study following 6 patients for 18 months after onset of GBS recorded continuing improvement of muscle strength on average throughout the assessment period, and yet the average strength of major muscle groups had not yet reached that of healthy controls.[202] Although the traditional thought has been that little clinical improvement occurs after 2 to 3 years, Bernsen and colleagues[203] found that 21% of the patients in a study of 150 patients after recovery from acute GBS reported improvement after 2.5 to 6.5 years, although the authors thought the perception of improvement was related to improved sensory function. Of future research and clinical interest are the long-term consequences of GBS and how the normal aging process will affect patients who have some mild residual effects—for example, whether some patients will develop increasing weakness over time similar to persons with postpolio syndrome.[139]

For those patients who experience significant losses in proprioception after GBS, sensory reintegration activities and high repetitions of task practice may help to redevelop motor engrams that are based on the altered sensory perception.[139]

Patients with GBS have a significantly reduced health-related quality of life compared with control subjects at approximately 1 year after onset, associated with decreased functional scores and changes in work status.[204] Although physical training may be expected to improve functional scores and work capabilities, Bussmann and colleagues[205] found little correlation between physical fitness and other domains. They hypothesized that training has psychological components, such as positive effect on mood and self-confidence, that influence quality of life in addition to physical changes.

Adaptive Equipment and Orthoses

Judicious use of orthotic devices and adaptive equipment should be considered an integral part of the rehabilitation process. The purpose of the orthotic and adaptive devices is twofold: (1) to protect weakened structures from overstretch and overuse and (2) to facilitate ADLs within the limits of the patient's current ability. Orthotic devices and adaptive equipment should be introduced and discontinued on the basis of serial evaluations of strength, ROM, and functional needs. For example, a hospitalized patient who has poor (2/5) middle deltoid strength may practice upper-extremity activities such as eating while using suspension slings. A thumb position splint may be used temporarily to aid thumb control in grasping tasks.

Most patients will need a wheelchair for several months until strength and endurance improve. As strength returns, patients recovering from severe paralysis may need to change from use of a wheelchair with a high, reclining back with a head rest to use of a lightweight, easily maneuverable chair. A quandary for the therapist is to predict how long a wheelchair will be necessary and whether it should be rented or purchased as the patient progresses through different stages of recovery. While moving from wheelchair mobility to independent ambulation, patients will usually progress from parallel bars to a walker with a seat to allow frequent resting, and then to crutches or a cane. Because wheelchairs, walkers, crutches, and canes, especially custom appliances, are expensive and not always covered by insurance, the therapist should carefully consider the cost to the patient during the recovery process.

Although most patients with GBS are able to walk within 8 months of onset, many show a prolonged residual weakness of calf and, most commonly, anterior compartment musculature, requiring the use of an AFO. The decision whether to use a prefabricated orthosis or custom appliance is not always simple. Several temporary orthotic measures can be considered. For example, if the patient shows good gastrocnemius-soleus strength with mild weakness of the dorsiflexors, a simple elastic strap attached to the shoelaces and a calf band may be sufficient to prevent overuse of the anterior compartment muscles. An old-fashioned, relatively inexpensive spring wire brace, which can be attached to the patient's shoes to facilitate dorsiflexion, is a good choice for patients who report sensory hypersensitivity when wearing a plastic orthosis.

Most therapy units today have access to varied sizes of plastic, fixed-ankle AFOs that can be used until a decision is made to have the patient fitted with custom AFOs. A newer system of prefabricated AFOs with adjustable ankle motion cams has been developed that allows the therapist to limit plantar flexion and dorsiflexion to the specific needs of the patient. For patients with reasonable control of plantar flexion and dorsiflexion but with lateral instability because of peroneal weakness, a simple ankle stirrup device such as the AirCast Air-Stirrup Ankle Brace (AirCast, Summit, NJ) can be used temporarily to provide lateral ankle stability. Although few patients with GBS need knee-ankle-foot orthoses (KAFOs) on a long-term basis, inexpensive air splints or adjustable long-leg metal splints to control knee position are sometimes helpful when working on standing weight bearing and during initial gait training. See Chapter 34 for additional information on orthotics.

Psychosocial Issues

Although most patients with GBS have a good recovery over a period of 2 or more years, the acute stage of the disease can be frightening, especially to patients who progress to complete paralysis and respiratory failure. Nancy, in Case Study 17-2, reported that she was terrified during the time she was totally paralyzed (including eyelid movement) and on a respirator. She said that nurses, doctors, and hospital staff seemed to assume she could not hear because she was unable to respond in any manner. In her words,

> *"They acted like I was already dead, and I thought I would be from the way they were talking. The thing I hated the most was when the night nurses from the registry would come in and ask how to make the ventilator work! I felt panicked. Can you imagine having your life depend on a machine and knowing that the person who was supposed to make it work had no idea what to do if a tube came unconnected? They were always worried about my blood pressure. Who wouldn't have high blood pressure in that situation! The thing I liked about my therapists was that they told me what they were going to do even when I couldn't respond. They didn't just start doing things or pulling on me like other people did."*

CASE STUDY 17-2 ■ NANCY

Nancy, a 16-year-old girl with a history of repeated hospitalizations for asthma, was admitted to the hospital with tingling in the hands and feet and mild respiratory distress. Because staff thought her asthma attacks had a significant emotional component, her repeated complaints of paresthesias, muscle pain, and weakness were largely ignored or attributed to anxiety attacks. The day after admission, Nancy began staggering while walking and became extremely agitated and hysterical, screaming that she was dying and could not breathe. A medical assessment showed evidence of wheezing with a normal chest radiograph and decreased FVC. She was uncooperative during strength testing, although strength was estimated to be within normal limits except for approximately Fair (3/5) strength of the dorsiflexors and everters and Good (4/5) strength of the plantar flexors. She became extremely upset when her feet were touched.

Because of her psychological history, she was referred for psychiatric assessment and was placed on an anxiolytic medication. Two hours later she had a full respiratory arrest and was intubated and maintained on mechanical ventilation. Over the

CASE STUDY 17-2 ■ NANCY—cont'd

next 3 days she developed flaccid quadriplegia and within 5 days she had complete cranial nerve involvement. She was weaned from the respirator after 29 days after several episodes of pneumonia. After extubation, she had swallowing and speech problems that resolved by discharge at 3 months after onset. During the acute stage, she was catheterized because of urinary retention and was treated for a bowel obstruction. Sensation was normal for perception of temperature changes and deep pressure.

Proprioception was diminished at the ankle, knee, and fingers. Paresthesias and hypesthesias, aggravated by light touch, were present in a glovelike pattern in both hands and a stocking pattern in both feet.

Nancy's physical therapy treatment began in the ICU. Formal strength testing was inappropriate; passive ROM was full but felt stiff at ends of ranges in the wrist, fingers, and ankles. The goals were to assist in respiratory care, prevent joint contractures, and prevent stasis ulcers during the period of immobility. Although her postural drainage treatment was performed by using respiratory therapy techniques in conjunction with aerosol medication by intermittent positive-pressure ventilation (IPPV), PTs began a course of chest stretching techniques in coordination with a fastidious ROM program performed twice a day by a therapist and on the evening and night shifts by a nurse. A pressure relief mattress was ordered for her bed. To prevent contracture development, an OT fabricated bilateral wrist and finger splints; a PT molded ankle splints to maintain 90 degrees of dorsiflexion with neutral eversion-inversion. A positioning and ROM schedule in poster form with pictures of positions and ROM patterns was posted at Nancy's bedside.

Because Nancy reported severe hypersensitivity to light touch or to any passive movement of her limbs, a cradle was placed on the bed to prevent sheets from touching her and to prevent air flow changes from irritating her skin. She was fitted for above-knee light pressure stockings, which seemed to decrease her sensitivity to light touch.

Progression of the GBS process seemed to plateau at approximately 15 days after onset with a gradual return of respiratory function complicated by infections. Weaning from the respirator was difficult, and the PT played a major role in instructing Nancy, the staff, and her family in appropriate breathing exercises to be performed every 1 or 2 hours. Because her parents wanted to be involved with her care, they were taught ROM techniques with special attention to correct shoulder ROM techniques. The PTs continued to follow Nancy twice a day to ensure that accessory motions were completed with the physiological motions. Moist hot packs were used effectively before ROM exercises for 1 week to minimize severe muscle pain.

As part of her positioning program, Nancy was placed in a supported semisitting position while on the respirator. As muscle control returned, a muscle reeducation program was initiated that focused initially on the head and trunk and then on the upper and lower extremities. Exercise periods were limited to 15 minutes twice a day. She would have benefited from more frequent short sessions; however, this was not possible. Her parents were shown how to guide her active exercise program cautiously so that she was able to exercise more frequently at low repetitions. When each muscle group reached an MMT grade of Fair (3) or greater, Nancy was allowed to use the muscles in functional activities with specified limitations in activity duration. When she was able to tolerate upright sitting and had some bed mobility, Nancy was transferred to a Nelson bed in which she could begin a gradual standing weight-bearing program.

A speech therapist worked with Nancy in the ICU to help her relearn safe swallowing patterns and to reintroduce her to different-textured foods. A dietician had been working with Nancy throughout her hospitalization to ensure adequate nutrition while intubated, and she worked closely with the speech therapist to progress Nancy's diet as she became able to handle liquids and solids.

After being weaned from the respirator and transferred to the general floor, Nancy was brought to the physical therapy department for treatment, which was frequently done in conjunction with occupational therapy. As strength increased, she began a program of resisted exercise. Trunk and upper- and lower-extremity PNF patterns were used as the primary exercise technique; however, great caution was used to avoid overworking weak muscle groups evoked during use of the PNF pattern. A full mat program with rolling and coming to sitting was also instituted. OTs focused on graduated use of Nancy's upper extremities, first using overhead slings attached to a wheelchair and later using a lap board to support her weakened shoulder musculature while practicing hand activities.

After 2 months of hospitalization, Nancy was discharged home to return for daily outpatient rehabilitation. Because Nancy appeared to be regaining strength well, she was provided with an ultralight rental wheelchair through her insurance for use until a final determination was made for long-term need. Nancy was also fitted with prefabricated adjustable AFOs, which were purchased through the physical therapy department. After 4 to 6 months a determination would be made about expected recovery of her persistently weakened dorsiflexors. If Nancy appeared to need AFOs for a prolonged period, a set of specifically molded AFOs would be ordered. At discharge, both the PT and OT made a home visit with the hospital social worker and parents to determine what home adaptations and support services would be necessary.

Follow-up of Nancy's outpatient therapy showed that she continued to make gradual recovery over the next 1.5 years. She returned to school 3 months after rehabilitation discharge using a wheelchair. She graduated to a walker, then to forearm crutches, and finally to independent ambulation. She refused to be seen using a walker at school, so she continued to use the wheelchair at school until she was independent on crutches. She continued to wear bilateral AFOs but was weaned from full-time use approximately 14 months after discharge. During the weaning process, Nancy wore her AFOs at school while walking and for any walking distance over four city blocks or if she heard her feet begin to slap from fatigued dorsiflexors. By 14 months, Nancy showed no evidence of overuse weakness after her regular activities, although she had difficulty with endurance activities in her physical education classes. When hiking, she carried her AFOs to use when she expected a long downhill trek to prevent overwork from eccentric muscle activity. By age 19 years—3 years postonset—Nancy had returned fully to her normal activity level.

Skirrow and colleagues[206] remind clinicians that the "intensive care patient is plunged into a world of machines that flash and beep; of tubes and wires that seem to spring from almost every orifice; and of mind-numbing sedative and analgesic medications." Needless to say, evidence is increasing that patients treated in acute trauma rooms or ICUs can have posttraumatic stress disorder (PTSD). Particularly vulnerable are patients who have had previous traumatic experiences. PTSD places patients at marked risk for increased startle responses, extreme vigilance or anticipation of painful events, sleep disorders, terrifying dreams, and dissociative flashbacks after leaving the ICU; sometimes these symptoms are left untreated for years after the experience.[152,207] Patients discharged from prolonged ICU experiences, especially those who had respiratory failure, have an increased incidence of anxiety, depression, and panic disorders years after discharge.

In a nursing study of patient experiences in the ICU, researchers found that patients often felt anxious, apprehensive, and fearful. The patients expected ICU nurses to be experienced and technically adept, but those who felt most secure despite the traumatic ICU experiences felt that the nurses were vigilant to their needs and offered personalized care,[152,208] a point clearly made by Nancy in the case study. Although one might expect ICU staff to be carefully tuned in to patient needs, the highly technical nature of modern ICUs may attract personnel less focused on individual patient care, or it may prevent caring staff from attending to the little kindnesses that are so comforting to critically ill patients. Baxter[207] suggests that caregivers in the ICU try to orient patients to what is being done, to approach the patients within their field of vision, and to minimize unexpected noises and sudden touching.

Although most patients recover well from GBS, 3 to 6 years after onset of GBS 38% of patients in a Dutch study had to make a job change to accommodate their physical status, 44% had to alter their leisure activities, and nearly 50% described ongoing psychosocial changes.[203] Similar findings were reported in a study of Japanese patients recovering from GBS.[209,210]

In summary, the rehabilitation program for a person with GBS must be graded carefully according to the stage of illness. In the acute care environment when respiratory deficits are present, the initial emphasis is directed toward support of maximal respiratory status through postural drainage, chest stretching, and breathing exercises. Because of prolonged bed rest and immobility related to weakness, accessory and physiological ROM must be maintained with around-the-clock efforts. Splinting or positioning devices are recommended to maintain functional positions during prolonged periods of immobility. A gradual program to increase upright tolerance is begun when respiratory and autonomic functions have stabilized. Therapists must keep in mind the potential to damage denervated muscles with aggressive strengthening programs when developing a rehabilitation plan and a home-based conditioning program. Perhaps as a result of cautious exercise programs, cardiovascular conditioning appears to lag significantly behind strengthening, so endurance training should specifically follow the return of strength. Adaptive equipment and orthoses should be used as needed to protect weakened muscles, facilitate normal movement, and prevent fatigue during the reinnervation process. Although a rehabilitation program has been found to make a measurable difference in patient long-term recovery, many patients are being discharged without follow-up care.[211] Therefore therapists should be assertive in ensuring that their patients with GBS have ongoing contact with rehabilitation specialists who can guide the recovery process (see Case Study 17-2).

DUCHENNE MUSCULAR DYSTROPHY

Pathology and Medical Diagnosis

Muscular dystrophy refers to forms of hereditary myopathy characterized by progressive muscle weakness associated with deterioration, destruction, and regeneration of muscle fibers. During the process, muscle fibers are gradually replaced with fibrous and fatty tissue. Each of the inherited forms of myopathy (e.g., Becker dystrophy, myotonic dystrophy, limb-girdle dystrophy, and facioscapulohumeral dystrophy) has its own unique genetic and phenotypic characteristics. (For a comprehensive review of the forms of muscular dystrophy and myopathy, see Dubowitz.[212]) Because Duchenne (pseudohypertrophic) muscular dystrophy (DMD) is one of the most commonly known forms of muscular dystrophy, it is used as a model for discussion of treatment implications for therapists. DMD is a disease of progressive muscle weakness leading to total paralysis and early death in the late teens or young adulthood. It has an incidence of 13 to 33 cases per 100,000 live births and a new mutation rate of approximately 1 in 10,000 (i.e., one third or more of cases occur in families without a history of DMD). The abnormal gene for DMD has been detected on the X chromosome at band Xp21.2, which encodes for dystrophin, a 427-kD cytoskeleton protein in the membrane. Because it has an X-linked recessive pattern, the disease affects males almost exclusively.[213] However, in nearly one third of DMD cases, DNA analysis is normal and diagnosis must be confirmed by protein analysis or immunohistology tests.[214]

In almost 100% of patients with DMD there is a complete absence of dystrophin from muscle tissue. This loss of dystrophin results in a weakened cell membrane that is easily damaged in muscle contraction.[213] However, loss of dystrophin alone is not considered the sole explanation of the severity and lethality of muscular dystrophy.[215]

Laboratory studies show serum creatine kinase (CK) elevated more than 100 times normal in early stages of the disease. These CK levels decrease over time with loss of muscle mass. Elevated CK level is evident at birth long before symptoms are evident. Muscle biopsy specimens show degeneration with gradual loss of fiber, variation in fiber size, and a proliferation of connective and adipose tissue. Histochemical studies indicate loss of subdivision into fiber types, with a tendency toward type I fiber predominance. Electromyographic studies show patterns of low-amplitude, short-duration, polyphasic motor unit action potentials.

Although the absence of dystrophin is usually discussed relative to skeletal muscle, dystrophin is also evident on the membrane surfaces of the cardiac Purkinje fibers and is thought to contribute to the cardiac conduction problems seen in DMD. Cardiac involvement is present in more than 60% of boys with DMD across all ages; however, the common electrocardiogram and electrocardiographic abnormalities are reflected early in clinical complications in 30% of boys until late stages of the disease, when more than 95% of boys have significant cardiomyopathy. Because of the increased life span secondary to in-home ventilation for respiratory failure, nearly 20% to 30% of deaths can be attributed to cardiac disease.[216]

The average IQ of boys with DMD is approximately 85, with one third of the boys testing below 75, as reflected in delayed developmental milestones. A specific deficit in verbal intelligence and verbal memory that leads to significant impairment in later cognitive development has been identified.[217,218]

Clinical Presentation

Although histological studies have indicated that DMD may be identified in the fetus as early as the first trimester, symptoms are seldom noted until the child is 2 to 5 years of age. When recalling the child's early development, parents often state that the affected child was more placid and less physically active than expected.[219] The earliest obvious manifestations of DMD, however, may be the delay of early developmental milestones, particularly crawling and walking. In many cases the onset is gradual. Parents or teachers may first identify a problem because the boy is noted to have difficulty keeping up with peers during normal play activities and to be somewhat clumsy, with frequent falling when attempting to run, jump, climb structures, or negotiate uneven terrain. By age 5 years, symmetrical muscle weakness can usually be clearly identified by MMT. Deep tendon reflexes may be absent by 8 to 10 years or earlier. Sensation is normal.[220]

The typical progression of weakness is symmetrical from proximal to distal, with marked weakness of the pelvic and shoulder girdle musculature preceding weakness of the trunk and more distal extremity muscles. Bowel and bladder function is usually spared. Progression of weakness is slow but persistent. Weakness of trunk and lower-extremity musculature typically leads to changes in gait at 3 to 6 years of age. Muscle mass continues to decline, with increasing weakness of the trunk, anterior neck, and upper-extremity musculature affecting functional activities. A typical child will continue walking until about age 12 or 13 years, at which time the process of transition to a wheelchair becomes imperative. A rapid decrease in strength may occur after prolonged periods of immobilization caused by illness, injury, or surgery.[221]

Progression of Lower-Extremity Weakness

Before age 5 years, hypertrophy of the calf muscles is frequently noted. Pseudohypertrophy is evident as the muscle tissue is replaced by fat and fibrous tissue. Even in the early stages of the disease, few boys with DMD walk with a normal gait pattern. Because of early pelvic girdle muscle weakness, most young boys retain a developmentally immature, wide-based gait pattern. An early distinctive feature of DMD is the Gowers maneuver, in which the child gets up from the floor by using his arms to crawl up his own legs (Figure 17-5).[219]

Muscle imbalance occurs in typical patterns as a result of weakness and contractures. As the posterior hip muscles weaken, the child must arch his back when standing and retract his shoulder girdle to maintain the center of gravity behind the hip joint. This creates a pattern of lumbar lordosis with protrusion of the abdomen. As the quadriceps weaken, the child must maintain his knees in hyperextension to place the axis of rotation posterior to the line of gravity. At this point, mild equinus contractures caused by a muscle imbalance between the plantar and dorsiflexors may help the child maintain knee control because the gastrocnemius-soleus group provides a torque that opposes knee flexion. If plantar flexion contractures become severe, however, the child will not be able to maintain standing balance because his base of support is too small and his ankle adaptive strategies are nonfunctional.

Once the child stops weight bearing, development of severe equinovarus deformities is common. Figure 17-6 shows a pattern of progression of muscle imbalance affecting the trunk and lower extremities in stance. Note the increasing lordosis and plantar flexion as the boys attempt to maintain their center of gravity posterior to the hip joint and anterior to the knee joint.

Progression of Gait Pattern Changes

The typical changes in gait pattern over time are identified in Figure 17-7; however, age alone is not an adequate index of predicted gait pattern. Many factors influence how long a child will be able to ambulate. Contributing factors are rate of progression of weakness; severity of contractures (hip flexion, external rotation, abduction, knee flexion, and plantar flexion—inversion contractures occur as disease progresses); influence of body weight; degree of respiratory compromise; type of treatment interventions such as bracing, surgery, and exercise; extent of family support; and the child's personal motivation to ambulate. When the child can no longer ambulate functionally, a wheelchair must be ordered to fit the specific needs of that child within his home and community environment. (For an extensive analysis of changes in gait pattern see Sutherland and colleagues.[222])

Progression of Upper-Extremity Weakness

The upper-extremity pattern of weakness is similar to that in the lower extremities, with proximal musculature being affected before distal musculature. Functional changes related to weakness of upper-extremity musculature, however, usually lag behind those in the lower extremities by 2 to 3 years. The early weakness of the scapular stabilization muscles interferes with controlled movement of the arms and hands during reaching. The child gradually loses biceps and brachioradialis function, followed by continued deterioration of triceps and more distal musculature. The marked instability of scapular musculature is clearly evident when the child tries to elevate his trunk with his arms (e.g., when attempting to use crutches) or when he is lifted from under the shoulders.[220,223] A classic test of scapular stability is the test for the Meryon sign, in which the child slips from the examiner's grip as the child is being lifted from under the arms (Figure 17-8). Typical progression of upper-extremity weakness is shown by use of the reaching test (Figure 17-9).

By the time the child reaches stage 3 of the reaching test, he needs considerable help with eating, hair care, and oral hygiene. Because of major trunk involvement and marked lower-extremity weakness, the child will also be dependent for most ADLs, such as hygiene, dressing, and transferring. Weakness of the respiratory muscles (diaphragm, chest wall, and abdominal musculature) is usually evident by the tenth or twelfth year, although the diaphragm remains functional

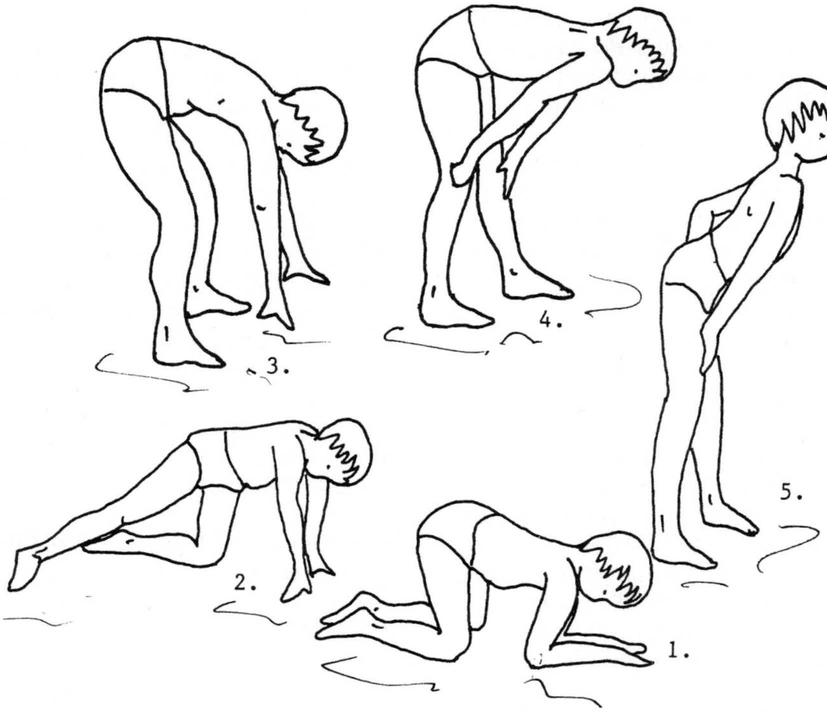

Figure 17-5 ■ Child demonstrating Gowers maneuver necessary to achieve upright posture because of pelvic and trunk weakness caused by Duchenne muscular dystrophy.

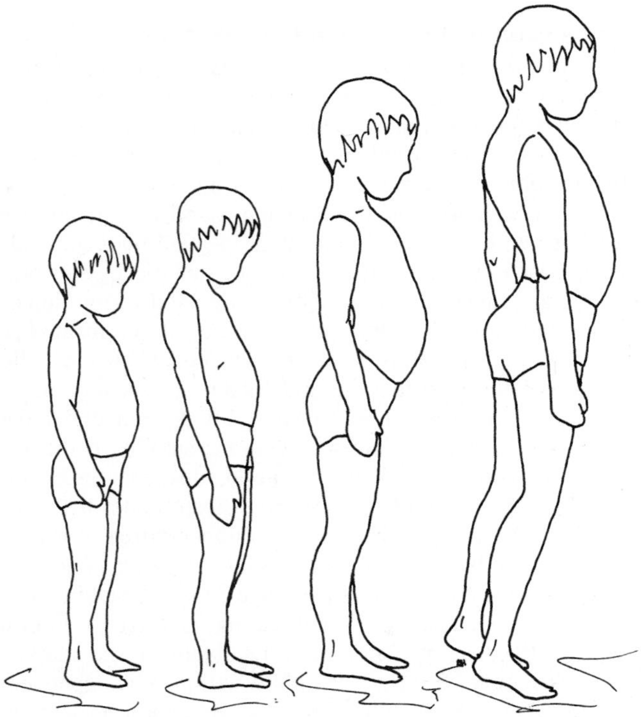

Figure 17-6 ■ Pattern of progression of muscle imbalance affecting trunk and lower extremities in Duchenne muscular dystrophy.

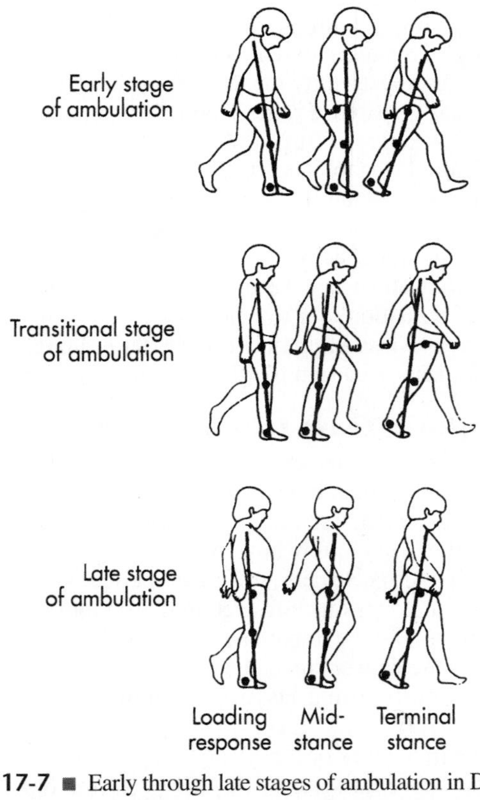

Figure 17-7 ■ Early through late stages of ambulation in Duchenne muscular dystrophy demonstrating changes in alignment at loading response, midstance, and terminal stance phases of gait. (From Hsu JD, Furumasu J: Gait and posture changes in the Duchenne muscular dystrophy child. *Clin Orthop Relat Res* 288:122–125, 1993.)

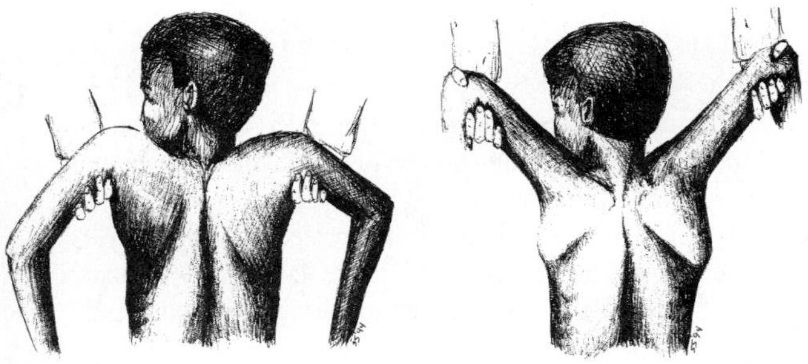

Figure 17-8 ■ Meryon sign shows lack of scapular stability as the child slips from the examiner's grip when lifted from under the arms.

longer than do the intercostal and accessory muscles. A progressive, sometimes severe scoliosis may contribute to respiratory compromise. Pure respiratory failure, restrictive lung disease, or respiratory failure caused by infection is the usual cause of death, most commonly at age 18 to 25 years.[224] Typical functional stages in DMD are identified in Box 17-5. See Emery and Muntoni[213] for a comprehensive review of the clinical process of DMD.

Medical Intervention

Treatment of Primary Pathology

DMD has no cure. Some clinicians suggest that until an effective treatment can be found, the best way to decrease the number of children with DMD is through genetic counseling. Serum CK is elevated in the female carriers, and genetic molecular probes of possible carriers are now available to identify deletions within the Xp21 region (the short arm of the X chromosome) at a 95% accuracy level. Of course, some families may have belief systems that do not allow consideration of pregnancy termination to prevent having a boy with possible DMD. Those views must be respected. Prenatal diagnosis of DMD for women without a family history of the disease is not yet practical.[225]

Despite much effort, an effective pharmaceutical agent has not been identified to treat DMD. In a Cochrane review, Manzur and colleagues[226] concluded that glucocorticoid corticosteroid therapy improves muscle strength in the short term of 6 months to 2 years; however, adverse effects such as weight gain, excessive hair growth, osteoporosis, and behavioral problems were noted. Researchers have also attempted to implant the normal precursor muscle cells or myoblasts directly into dystrophic mice and, in several cases, into children with DMD to precipitate the proliferation of normal donor muscle cells into the host muscles of dystrophic subjects, but results have not led to significant improvement.[227] Animal studies using helper-dependent adenoviral vectors for dystrophin gene transfer to muscles in dystrophic mice show promise for patients with DMD.[228]

Although no cure for DMD is on the horizon despite the positive research on gene transfer, the functional status of the patient, quality of life, and life expectancy can be influenced with thoughtful, functionally based treatment and supportive care. Figure 17-10 provides an overall scheme for the management of DMD.

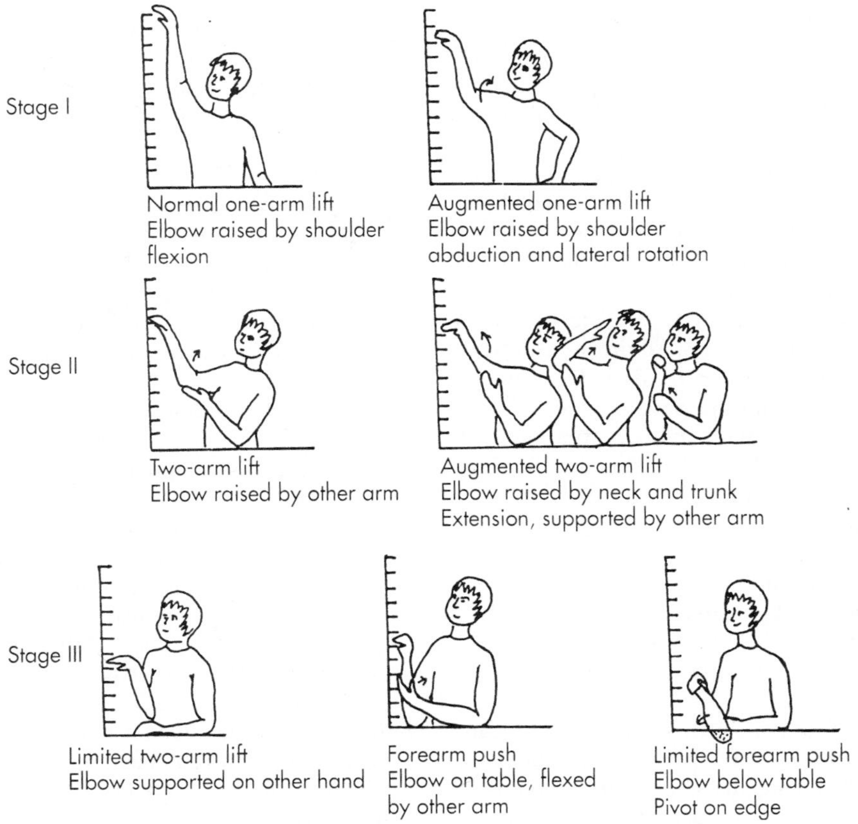

Figure 17-9 ■ Method of evaluating the working hand as demonstrated by the reaching test.

BOX 17-5 ■ FUNCTIONAL TRANSITIONS IN PATIENTS WITH MUSCULAR DYSTROPHY

1. Ambulates with mild waddling gait and lordosis. Can run with marked effort, gait problems magnified. Can ascend, descend steps, curbs.
2. Ambulates with moderate waddling gait and lordosis. Cannot run. Difficulty with stairs and curbs. Rises from floor using Gowers maneuver. Rises from chair independently.
3. Ambulates with moderately severe waddling gait and lordosis. Rises from chair independently but cannot ascend or descend curbs or stairs or rise from floor independently.
4. Ambulates with assistance or in some cases with bilateral knee-ankle-foot orthoses. May have had surgical release of contractures. May need assistance with balance. Needs wheelchair for community mobility. Propels manual chair slowly. Independent in bed and self-care, although may need help with some aspects of dressing and bathing because of time constraints.
5. Transfers independently from wheelchair. Unable to walk independently but can bear and shift weight to walk with orthoses if supported. Can propel self in manual chair but has limited endurance. Motorized chair more functional. Independent in self-care with transfer assist for bath or shower.
6. Wheelchair independence in motorized chair. May need trunk support or orthosis. Needs assistance in bed and with major dressing. Can perform self-grooming but is dependent for toileting and bathing. May need alternating pressure relief mattress.
7. Wheelchair independence in motorized chair but may need to recline intermittently while in chair. Dependent in hygiene and most self-care requiring proximal upper-extremity control.
8. As previous stages; will also use two hands for single-hand activities—one hand supports working arm. May perform simple table-level hand activities, some self-feeding with arm support.
9. Sits in wheelchair only with trunk support and intermittent reclining or transfer to a supine position. Boys attending school may need to be on gurney for part of day. May benefit from nighttime ventilatory support or intermittent daytime positive-pressure ventilation. (Some patients may have had an elective tracheostomy and need ventilatory support unit attached to wheelchair.) May have some hand control if arms supported. Will need help with turning at night.
10. Totally dependent. Unable to tolerate upright position, may elect home ventilatory support. Tracheostomy necessary for prolonged ventilation. Tracheostomy may be adapted for speech if oral musculature adequate. Needs 24-hour care. If around-the-clock home care cannot be arranged, patient must be hospitalized.

Treatment of Cardiopulmonary Factors

Respiratory failure is the cause of death in 70% to 80% of patients with DMD. Cardiac and other causes account for the remaining deaths. Although cardiac involvement is evident early, because of limited physical activity the clinical impact of heart disease is not a significant problem until the adolescent years. Even while ambulatory, children with DMD have a lower exercise performance than age-matched healthy children, with higher resting heart rates and diminished cardiopulmonary response to submaximal and maximal exercise.[229] Once the child becomes wheelchair dependent, his cardiorespiratory fitness deteriorates markedly. With increasing weakness of the respiratory musculature and the development of scoliosis, physicians must be vigilant in their treatment of respiratory infections.[230] The American Thoracic Society consensus statement on the respiratory care of boys with DMD suggests the following:

- A child should be seen at age 4 to 6 years for baseline pulmonary function testing.
- Patients should be seen by a pediatric respiratory physician twice a year after becoming wheelchair dependent if the FVC falls below 80% or the child is older than 12 years.
- Patients who need mechanically assisted airway clearance or mechanically assisted ventilation should be seen by a pulmonary specialist every 3 to 6 months.
- All patients should undergo cardiac and pulmonary assessments before any surgery.[214]

Assistance in respiration progresses in steps.[221] In the first step, a self-inflating manual ventilation bag may be sufficient. Step two is associated with manual and mechanically assisted cough techniques. Steps three and four consist of the institution of nocturnal and daytime ventilation, respectively. Step five consists of tracheostomy, if the patient and family prefer.

Sleep-disordered breathing and hypoventilation are common in the later stages of DMD, and the onset is often subtle. Early symptoms include repeated nighttime awakenings, early morning headache, and daytime sleepiness. Inexpensive oximetry can be used in the home to identify nighttime oxygen desaturation if polysomnography with continuous carbon dioxide monitoring is not available.[231]

Because sleep hypoxia is common in the later stages of DMD, IPPV or noninvasive ventilation by nasal mask or mouthpiece is recommended to control oxygen desaturation at night. Eventually most boys with DMD enter a stage of constant hypoventilation throughout the day and night, and a decision needs to be made about the use of 24-hour ventilation support. Daytime ventilation should be considered when waking P_{CO_2} exceeds 50 mm Hg or hemoglobin saturation is lower than 92% while awake.[214] Motorized wheelchairs can be adapted to handle ventilator systems so that the boys can remain active and mobile.

Once a patient with DMD requires daytime and nighttime ventilation and has severe bulbar muscle weakness, a decision must be made to elect ventilation by tracheostomy

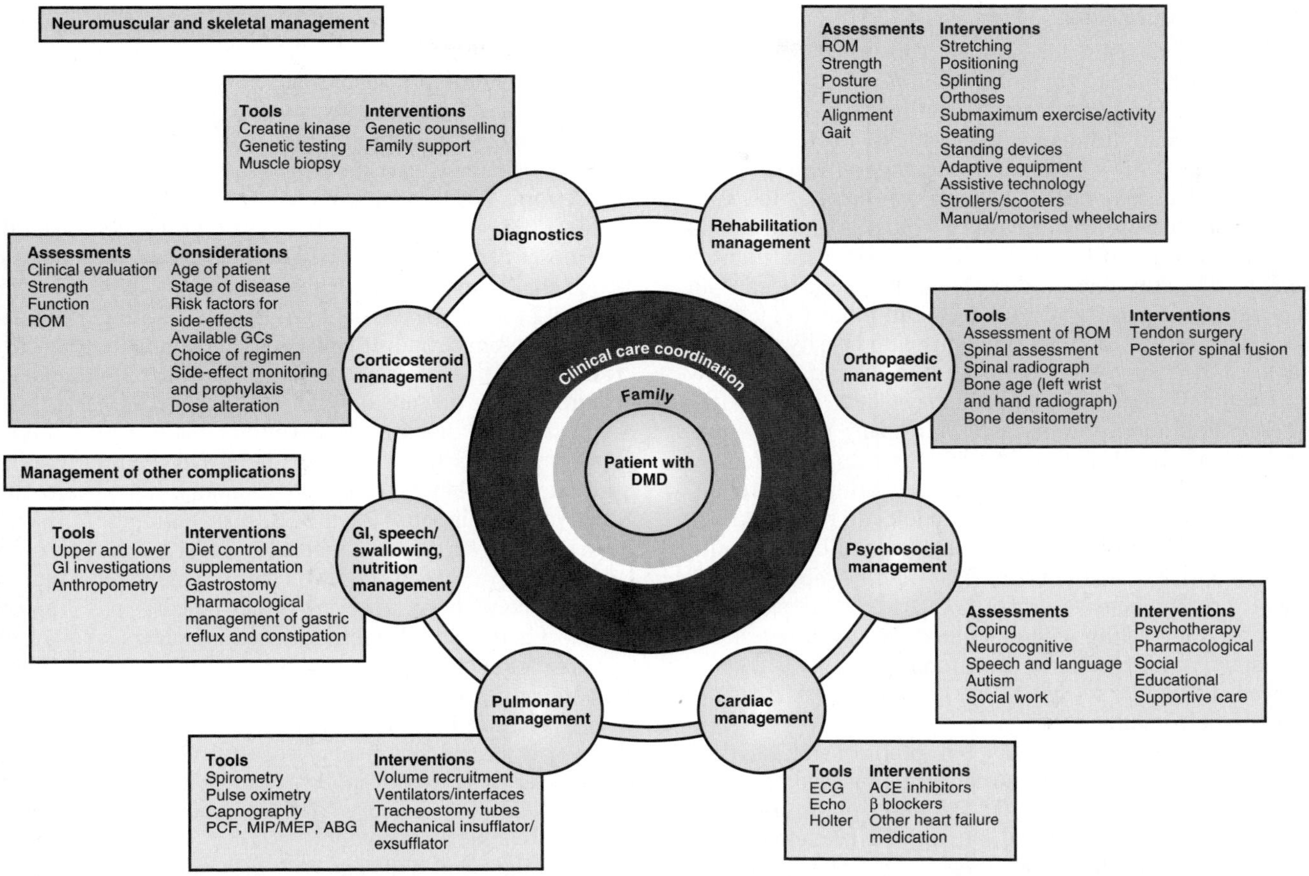

Figure 17-10 ■ Management of Duchenne muscular dystrophy (DMD). Coordination of clinical care is a crucial component of the management of DMD. This care is best provided in a multidisciplinary care setting in which an individual and family can access expertise for the required multisystem management of DMD in a collaborative effort. A coordinated clinical care role can be provided by a wide range of health care professionals depending on local services, including (but not limited to) neurologists or pediatric neurologists, rehabilitation specialists, neurogeneticists, pediatricians, and primary care physicians. It is crucial that the person responsible for the coordination of clinical care be aware of the available assessments, tools, and interventions to proactively manage all potential issues involving DMD. *ABG,* Arterial blood gas; *ACE,* angiotensin-converting enzyme; *DMD,* Duchenne muscular dystrophy; *ECG,* electrocardiogram; *Echo,* echocardiogram; *GC,* glucocorticoids; *GI,* gastrointestinal; *MEP,* maximum expiratory pressure; *MIP,* maximum inspiratory pressure; *PCF,* peak cough flow; *ROM,* range of motion. (From Bushby K, Finkel R, Birnkrant DJ, et al: Diagnosis and management of Duchenne muscular dystrophy, part 1: diagnosis, and pharmacological and psychosocial management. *Lancet Neurol* 9:77–93, 2010.)

or palliative care. Ventilation by tracheostomy allows higher ventilation pressures and a better patient-ventilator interface.[232] However, use of a tracheostomy requires careful stoma hygiene to prevent infections and mucus plugs and requires 24-hour caregiver vigilance.[233] Although many patients and families adapt well to tracheostomy use, the ability to speak audibly may be affected. Consideration must be given to use of a speaking valve system.[214] Several cases of pneumothorax have been reported with long-term IPPV.[234] Also, as increasing numbers of patients use long-term tracheostomy-based ventilation, the potential for tracheal erosion or tracheobronchomalacia, which must be monitored to prevent hemorrhaging, is increasing.[235] As with patients with ALS, many significant treatment and ethical decisions must be made by the patient, family, and health care providers when submitting to prolonged HMV.[236] Patient autonomy and family input after adequate patient education about prolongation of life by tracheostomy ventilation must be respected.[214]

Cardiomyopathy is present in 59% of children with DMD by 10 years of age, but the cardiac problems seldom become symptomatic until the end stages of DMD because the child's decreased activity level does not stress the weakened heart muscle. In later stages of the disease, however, cor pulmonale with right-sided heart failure may occur. Medical treatment of any cardiac symptoms generally follows the conventional interventions. Some boys with severe scoliosis that creates cardiac compression may require correction by spinal fixation.[237,238] Retrospective data suggest that children treated before ventricular dysfunction with corticosteroids have a lower incidence of cardiac involvement.[214]

Nutritional Concerns

Excessive weight gain that impairs functional ability is a frequent and difficult problem for children with DMD and their families. The typical active child needs approximately 2400 calories daily to maintain weight and grow; however, the child with DMD who is more sedentary or who is wheelchair dependent may need 1200 or fewer calories to maintain weight. Because of decreased esophageal and intestinal motility, exacerbated by weak or absent abdominal muscle strength, a healthy low-fat diet should be encouraged with adequate bulk foods, stool softeners, and fluids to facilitate bowel function and motility. Problems with obesity are often related to the family's typical pattern of eating and nurturing. The child and family members may "feed" their anxiety or depression about the disease.[225] In many cases, family members and friends feel that the child's only pleasure may be eating. Although this may seem true, caring for a totally dependent obese teenager or young adult can become problematic for both the child and the caregivers. Before obesity becomes an issue, the child and his family should be referred for comprehensive nutritional advice from a specialist experienced in dealing with childhood obesity. Suggestions for adapting eating behavior and food choices will not be followed if they are too restrictive or unreasonable for the child's social situation.[239,240]

Although obesity is a common problem for children with DMD (greater than 54%), malnutrition is also common. Malnutrition usually occurs in the late stages of the disease as a result of dysphagia.[214] Special care must be taken to provide adequate nutrition after spinal surgery. One review showed that postsurgical weight loss was related to the inability to self-feed; therefore the investigators suggest that before surgery a feeding evaluation should be done and an appropriate plan should be put in place to prevent postsurgical malnutrition.[241]

As the disease progresses, some children develop problems swallowing, and then weight loss and malnutrition can become an issue. To decrease the possibility of aspiration, careful attention must be paid to food textures and chewing and swallowing functions (see page 537 for information on dealing with bulbar symptoms). Depending on the patient's and family's decisions about prolongation of life, some patients now elect to have a permanent PEG placed once self-feeding and swallowing become a problem rather than a pleasure. Even if the patient can still swallow and enjoys eating in the late stages of DMD, the patient may not be able to physically take in adequate calories; the PEG allows the delivery of needed calories and fluids beyond what the patient can take orally (see page 563 for information on dysphagia and eating issues).[242] Consensus is that body weight and body mass index should be reviewed regularly and family education on nutrition should be an ongoing process. Evaluation of swallowing should be assessed by taking a history of choking episodes and observing the child eat different foods and fluids. Videofluoroscopy should be used to determine if aspiration is a problem, and appropriate adjustments in feeding should be instituted under the supervision of the appropriate therapist.[214] (See also Bushby and colleagues.[221])

Treatment of Scoliosis

Scoliosis is a frequent complication of DMD, with a reported incidence of nearly 90%. Consequences of severe scoliosis are increased respiratory problems in boys with respiratory compromise, chronic pain related to musculoskeletal problems, sitting tolerance difficulties, and caregiving issues. Figure 17-11 presents an example of a boy with moderate scoliosis that affects sitting posture. Note the pelvic asymmetry that would seriously affect sitting alignment.

Scoliosis tends to occur in two basic patterns: the early-onset form (seen in approximately 23%), which becomes evident before the child begins to use a wheelchair, and the late-onset form, which develops, on average, 4 years after wheelchair dependency. In the early-onset form the curve usually becomes severe and progressive, leading to pulmonary compromise and structural-based pain. In the late-onset form the course is usually mild. Unfortunately, attempts to control sitting posture through the use of a spinal orthosis and wheelchair seating inserts (inserts that place the child in lumbar lordosis to lock facets, thereby preventing rotation and lateral collapse, or, more commonly, lumbar and thoracic lateral supports) have been disappointing.[243] Bach[244] states that thoracolumbar bracing is never indicated to slow scoliosis development in DMD and it cannot substitute for surgical correction; however, spinal bracing may improve comfort and postural stability in some patients who are not eligible for surgical correction because of severe respiratory or cardiac involvement.[242]

Efforts have been made to delay the time of onset of scoliosis with steroid treatment protocols. Evidence supports the hypothesis that onset of scoliosis can be delayed; however, a longer follow-up period would be required to determine if scoliosis can be prevented.[245]

Cervellati and colleagues[246] reported on a study of 20 boys treated from 1985 to 1995 and concluded that early surgery significantly reduces the risk factors associated with severe spinal deformities. The period after spinal surgery requires careful coordination of medical, respiratory, and physical therapy services. Depending on the hospital culture, PTs may be responsible for the pulmonary drainage and breathing exercise programs as well as typical passive and active exercise programs while the child is in ICU and postsurgical care environments. Preferably, therapists should introduce postural drainage and breathing techniques as well as exercise expectations to the child before surgery to gain better cooperation after surgery.

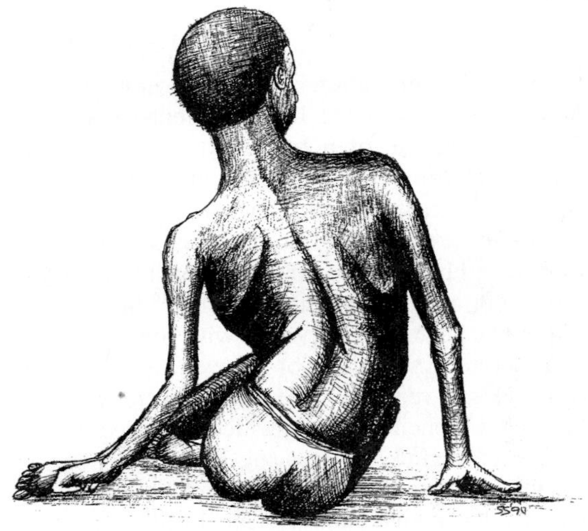

Figure 17-11 ■ Moderate scoliosis affecting sitting stability.

Treatment of Other Musculoskeletal Dysfunctions

The primary effect of progressive weakness in DMD generally results in secondary effects such as decreases in muscle extensibility, joint contractures, and bone demineralization. Strength loss diminishes the ability to move actively through full range, shift out of static positions, balance muscle forces around a joint, and avoid fibrotic changes in muscle tissue.[221] Loss of ROM from muscle shortening and joint stiffening will occur if not aggressively prevented. Once present, contractures can severely complicate function. Long bone fractures in children with DMD are a serious problem that can have a significant long-term impact on ambulation. In a study of 378 patients, 21% had incurred fractures, primarily from falling. Leg fractures predominate in independent ambulators and wheelchair users, whereas upper-extremity fractures more often occurred in boys using KAFOs. Twenty percent of those who had fractures lost the ability to ambulate.[247]

In standard treatment protocols for children with DMD who have impending loss of ability to walk independently, bilateral KAFOs are used in conjunction with surgical release of contractures.[248] At the point of surgery, a pattern of contractures has magnified the effect of weakness from the loss of approximately 60% of muscle mass.[249] Surgery is typically followed by an aggressive therapy program. Bach and McKeon[250] studied 13 boys with DMD who had surgery to release lower-extremity contractures. Seven boys were ambulating independently before surgery (early surgery group), and six boys were preparing to use or had begun to use a wheelchair before surgery (late surgery group). Depending on the contracture patterns, the boys underwent surgical procedures that typically included subcutaneous release of the Achilles tendons and hamstring muscles and fasciotomy of the iliotibial bands. Four patients had rerouting of the posterior tibialis to the dorsal surface of the second or third cuneiform to balance the foot and prevent the often severe varus position of the foot. Boys in the late surgical group required more extensive inpatient rehabilitation, whereas boys in the early surgical group were treated as outpatients after a short hospitalization. Physical therapy was started on the second postoperative day. The program consisted of general conditioning exercises of the trunk and extremities (e.g., rolling, trunk stabilization, neck and head control), stretching exercises, and intensive weight bearing in standing while wearing bilateral long-leg casts or below-knee casts, depending on the surgery. One child participated in a pool therapy program. Bach and McKeon[250] suggest that early surgery for contractures followed by intensive physical therapy can prolong brace-free ambulation. The number of falls experienced by the boys decreased markedly after the surgery and rehabilitation period. Boys in the early intervention groups benefited from the surgical interventions more than the boys in the later intervention groups. All patients and their families in the early surgery group thought that the procedures were helpful. Boys in the late surgery group, however, stated either that they would not have had the surgery if they had a chance to decide again or that they had no opinion. Roposch and colleagues[251] reviewed the records of 91 boys with the typical equinovarus deformity in DMD and strongly recommended surgical intervention, including a posterior tibialis transfer, over conservative, nonsurgical treatment to maintain foot position and lengthen time of ambulation.

Manzur and colleagues[252] carried out a randomized, controlled trial of 20 boys with DMD (ages 4 to 6 years) to study the effect of early release of contractures versus conservative (stretching) programs. The boys were followed for 12 months or more. Surgery corrected the contractions and improved the speed of gait and transfers over conservative treatment as measured at 12 months, but a 2-year follow-up of six of the boys who had surgery revealed a recurrence of ankle contractures. In addition, some of the boys in the operated group showed more rapid deterioration. The authors did not recommend routine early surgery to relieve contractures.

Therapeutic Management of Movement Dysfunction Associated with Duchenne Muscular Dystrophy

Like ALS, DMD has a relentless and incurable progression toward total dependence and eventual early death. The differences are the population (children rather than adults) and time course, with DMD taking 15 to 25 years rather than the 3 to 5 years typical of adults with ALS. As in ALS and GBS, strength and endurance remain the primary impairments of DMD, with secondary problems such as contractures and respiratory problems following from immobility. Unlike in the other neuromuscular disorders, the endurance problems in DMD are related to peripheral fatigue, fatigue stemming from the muscles themselves rather than from the lack of ability to recruit additional motor units.[253] As in ALS and GBS, therapeutic management in DMD will involve evolution of the intensity and frequency of exercise to correspond to changes in the strength and endurance of the patient. In all three disorders, the general therapeutic goals are to maximize function, manage discomfort, and promote optimal quality of life. The differences among the disorders mean that the actual form of the exercises and interventions in DMD may require adaptation to suit a child or adolescent. Ideally, a team of specialists should be involved in the long-term care of a child with DMD and his family. The therapist's primary role is twofold: to perform serial examinations of the child's movement capabilities and to adjust the child's intervention program as the disease progresses. Even with relentlessly progressive diseases, rehabilitation programs can have potential psychological benefits, such as more positive coping strategies, while physical activity continues to decline.[254]

Examination

A typical therapy examination should include a history, systems review, and tests and measures to assess muscle strength, endurance, and ROM impairments along with levels of activity and participation. In some facilities the therapist also collects data on the child's pulmonary status.[167] History taking should include the course of the disease, any recent illnesses or losses of function, coexisting neuromotor or other medical conditions, current concerns, and the goals of the patient and family. Screening tests can help rule out sensory deficits, identify cardiac and respiratory issues, and determine skin integrity, especially in immobile patients. Checking vital signs at rest and immediately after activity, noting communication ability, and assessing ability to follow multistep commands are all important components. When screening tests indicate a deficit, follow-up should occur with additional testing or referral to the appropriate professional. The tests and measures appropriate for assessing the movement dysfunction of patients with DMD include measures of strength, ROM, function, activity, and quality of life. Palmieri and colleagues[255] review many of the measures reported in the literature for use in this population.

Manual Muscle Testing. MMT is used extensively for measuring muscle strength of children with DMD[255,256] and is relatively reliable if consecutive examinations are made by the same rater. Intrarater reliability of scores in the gravity-eliminated position have been shown to be highest in this population.[257] DMD shows a linear pattern of decreased muscle strength (loss of about 0.25 MMT unit per year from ages 6 to 13, and 0.06 MMT unit per year from age 13 on)[258] without marked increases in the rate of deterioration in strength over time. Thus, marked, precipitous changes in muscle strength noted in a few months with initiation of bracing or wheelchair use,[223] for example, or immobilization after fracture, generally reflect disuse atrophy rather than disease progression. Such transitory weakness may respond to increased activity and exercise. The history and medical records can help differentiate weakness stemming from various sources and thus determine the potential for strengthening. Cable and strain-gauge tensiometers, handheld myometers and dynamometers, and isokinetic dynamometers may also be useful for a more discriminating documentation of muscle strength.[255,256]

Range of Motion. ROM is assessed with goniometry in most cases of DMD.[256] As with MMT, serial ROM evaluations should be completed by the same therapist because intrarater reliability is higher than interrater reliability in this population.[259] The two-joint muscles are most prone to developing shortness, so the positioning of limbs for testing of ROM must be considered. The lack of upright weight bearing and reliance on a wheelchair for mobility tend to accelerate contracture development in DMD; therapists should be particularly vigilant about monitoring lower-extremity ROM as the child becomes more sedentary.[260] Some boys with significant shoulder girdle weakness begin to develop contractures even before they become wheelchair dependent. Early attention should be paid to possible subluxation of the shoulder.[261]

Particular attention should be given to the accuracy of measuring hip ROM. Rideau and colleagues[262] recommend the "dangling leg" test, in which the child is placed supine with his lower legs hanging over the end of the table. An inability to bring the thighs to midline indicates shortening of the iliotibial band and hip abductors. One can quantify the shortening by measuring the distance of the thigh from the midline and from the surface of the table. In addition, the therapist should note pelvic obliquity, preferably with serial photographs taken with the child in the sitting and supine positions. Ideally, the patient can be photographed from the back in sitting position against a simple clear, framed plastic sheet with grid squares to allow easy, nonradiographic tracking of scoliosis.

Functional Status. The child's functional status continues to be relatively stable for some time even when MMT indicates that the child is losing strength. Because the weakness is gradual, many children develop remarkably adaptive adjustments in movement patterns to remain functional even with marked strength loss. Lue and colleagues[263] developed the Muscular Dystrophy Functional Rating Scale (MDFRS) to standardize assessment of the functional impact of muscular dystrophy, including people with DMD—more than half of those tested. The MDFRS consists of 33 items covering mobility, basic ADLs, arm function, and impairment (including contractures, strength of the trunk and neck, scoliosis, and respiratory issues). The developers reported test-retest and interrater reliabilities of 0.98 to 0.99 and good evidence of validity. Brooke and colleagues[264] and Vignos and colleagues[265] have described previous functional scales for use in DMD; the MDFRS compares favorably with each of these, with some advantages for determining the child's status and for predicting appropriate care, perhaps because it is longer.[263] As part of any functional assessment in DMD, adaptive behaviors should be noted. For example, a child may not be able to lift his arm overhead, but he may use his fingers (strength often remains intact even after respiratory support is necessary) to "crawl" up his chest to reach his head or he may lean forward to approximate his chest to his hand or use his other arm or a lever system to assist with activities.[244]

For ambulatory patients, gait velocity can help predict how long the patient has before transitioning to a wheelchair. In a longitudinal study of 51 boys with DMD, 100% of those who took 9 seconds or more to walk 30 feet were wheelchair bound within 2 years.[258] McDonald and colleagues[266] also recommend the use of the 6-Minute Walk test as a standardized and functional measure of endurance for this population. Slight modifications may be necessary to keep younger children on-task for this test.[266] Observational gait analysis can help to identify adaptive behaviors and use of compensatory strategies during locomotion.[256]

Respiratory Function. The PT's role in evaluating respiratory status in children with DMD will vary depending on the facility and area of the country in which the therapist works. For more in-depth information regarding evaluating pulmonary status, refer to Chapter 30 or see Irwin and Tecklin.[167] At a minimum the therapist should evaluate bulbar function, cough effectiveness, and FVC (a simple spirometer available in most clinics is adequate). For more sophisticated testing, the child should be seen by a pulmonary function specialist. In addition, the therapist may monitor activity levels via armbands or pedometers or may assess metabolic equivalents or caloric consumption to design the optimal activity program for children with DMD and obesity.[255] One method of testing a child's energy cost during ambulation is the energy expenditure index,[267] which divides walking heart rate (WHR) minus resting heart rate (RHR) by walking speed (distance [D] divided by time [T]):(EEI = [WHR − RHR]/[D/T]). Determinations of energy expenditure while walking may factor into the decision to transition to a wheelchair, at least for longer distances.

In late stages the therapist may need to assess the child's bulbar function to prevent swallowing and aspiration problems caused by tongue and oral-facial muscle weakness.

Therapeutic Goals. The basic goals for a therapeutic program are straightforward: (1) to prevent contractures that can lead to further disability and pain, (2) to maintain maximal strength and endurance and prevent disuse atrophy, (3) to facilitate maximal functional abilities by using appropriate adaptive equipment, (4) to maintain maximal respiratory muscle strength and movement of secretions, and (5) to foster realistic child and family expectations within the context of the environment. These are broad-based goals; the therapist will need to write more specific, time-oriented goals for a particular episode of care.

Therapeutic Interventions

Younger children with disabilities are usually eligible for school-based therapy services. However, therapists increasingly act primarily in the role of consultant rather than direct service provider, especially for older children. Much of the child's exercise program must be carried out at home by parents or caregivers. When both parents work outside the home or when the child lives in a single-parent home with a working parent, compliance with home programs can be problematic. As many exercise activities as possible should be encouraged within the child's school day so that parents can focus on parenting, nurturing, general caregiving, and simple positioning and bedtime exercises. Under the supervision of a consulting therapist, the child's therapy often can be provided in some form at the child's school if on-site therapists, personal attendants, or adaptive physical education teachers are available.

Respiratory and Dysphagia Care. In the school therapy environment, where most children with DMD are monitored, the therapist should be prepared to provide the child and family with methods to improve breathing efficiency. In the early stages of the disease, the child and family can be taught simple breathing exercises stressing diaphragmatic breathing, full chest expansion, air shifts, and rib cage stretching. Most children enjoy playing with handheld incentive spirometer units and playing blowing games (e.g., bubbles, pinwheels). Respiratory exercise in different studies has resulted in improvement in respiratory endurance,[268] ventilatory muscle endurance but not respiratory muscle strength,[269,270] and both respiratory muscle strength and endurance.[271] In the last study, two thirds of the 27 subjects had DMD, with percent predicted vital capacities of 27% to 96% that had decreased over the 6 months immediately preceding the exercise protocol. The exercise protocol, monitored via a visual feedback system, consisted of twice-daily sessions of 10 cycles of resisted inspiratory breaths at 70% to 80% of the patient's maximum inspiratory pressure, plus 10 maximal static inspiratory efforts that reached at least 90% of the maximally generated inspiratory pressure. The intervention lasted for 2 years, with increases noted in the first 10 months and a plateau maintained through the end of the training period. Winkler and colleagues[272] noted similar effects in a 9-month training protocol, somewhat dependent on the rapidity of respiratory function decline in the year preceding the training. In the 6-month training period of another study, subjects training with resisted inspiratory and expiratory breathing had significantly greater benefit than subjects randomly allocated to the group performing the same breathing exercises without resistance. The static inspiratory and expiratory pressures returned to baseline within 3 months after training ceased, but improvements in perceived exertion persisted for up to 1 year postintervention.[273]

Respiratory exercise cannot reverse the process of respiratory failure; however, attention to pulmonary hygiene can help the child cope more effectively with respiratory infections and the discomfort accompanying respiratory compromise. Although inspiratory exercises tend to be the focus of interventions, expiratory inefficiency may play a major role in the inability to clear secretions.[274] Once the child begins to have difficulty clearing secretions, the family should be taught manual or mechanically assisted postural drainage techniques as long as the patient has an adequate cough. Patients who need support with coughing can be taught "air stacking" techniques (taking a series of breaths without exhaling between breaths) to increase intrathoracic pressure needed to cough effectively. Some patients respond well to manual coughing assistance. Increasingly patients and caregivers are being taught to use a mechanical insufflator-exsufflator (positive pressure followed by negative pressure) to stimulate coughing.[275,276] These techniques should be reviewed and used aggressively whenever the child is bed bound for more than 1 or 2 days and before and after all surgical procedures.[214] Physical therapy interventions, such as postural drainage and breathing exercises, are invaluable in preventing early death from respiratory failure. The Muscular Dystrophy Association continually updates its information on breathing and respiratory care.[277,278]

In end stages of DMD when the child is dependent, dealing with oral-motor problems that may interfere with eating and swallowing is imperative. Techniques such as positioning, increased sensory input (texture, temperature), and volume changes in foods may improve the child's swallowing and allow the child to continue taking food orally.[279] The interventions are similar to those described for ALS. The Muscular Dystrophy Association also publishes informational manuals dealing with dysphagia problems (see www.mdausa.org).

Prevention of Contractures. Diligent ROM exercises for the whole body will require cooperative efforts of the rehabilitation team and the patient and family. Stretching may progress as weakness dictates, from active to active-assisted to passive to prolonged elongation phases using positioning, splinting, orthoses, and standing devices.[221] During the ambulatory phase of the disease, focus should be on the hips, knees, and ankles. Later, focus will shift to the shoulders and the elbow, wrist, and finger flexors. At the first sign of loss of end ROM, the therapist should adjust the child's program to include specific stretches.[261,280]

Evidence provides a protocol for stretching in people with normal muscles to increase ROM: stretches performed 2 to 5 days a week, once per day, held for 10 to 30 seconds for three or four repetitions over a 6-week time frame.[281,282] Unfortunately, no such evidence exists for the best stretching protocols in DMD to maintain ROM. Palmieri and colleagues recommend that stretching be performed a minimum of 4 to 6 days per week for any joint or muscle group.[255] The stretch should be slow to avoid muscle reflex contractions, and sustained at the end point for 10 to 30 seconds. To increase muscle extensibility, dry or wet heating, electromagnetic stimulation, or a warm bath may help; for best effect, follow a bath by drying with prewarmed towels to avoid shivering and muscle stiffening.[255]

In a 2010 Cochrane review[283] of the best methods for increasing ankle ROM in patients with neuromuscular disease, only two studies of DMD were noted, with interventions of early surgery[252] or prednisone use.[284] Surgery eliminated the contractures, but in most cases the contractures had recurred by the 2-year follow-up.[252] Prednisone had no significant effect on ROM in comparison to a placebo or when comparing two different doses.[284] Hyde and colleagues[285] noted an annual delay of 23% in the development of contractures at the Achilles in boys with DMD randomly allocated to a group receiving both stretching and night splints compared with boys who had stretching alone. Brooke and colleagues[220] reported similar findings, and Scott and colleagues[286] noted that boys who had both AFOs and stretching were able to continue walking longer than boys who did not. This evidence indicates that multiple simultaneous strategies may be most beneficial in preventing shortening and maximizing function. Patient and family preferences must be considered for any plan to be effective, however. Some young patients do not tolerate night splinting well. In such cases, AFOs to control plantarflexion contractures may be preferred over long-leg orthotics that prevent knee flexion contractures or align hips (using an additional bar between legs to control rotations).

Early in the course of the disease process, both parents and the child must be educated about the expected changes in muscle balance and how they can play an active role in preventing or limiting the impact of contractures caused by muscle imbalance. Because contractures at the hip, knee, and ankle interfere with the mechanical alignment necessary to stand erect and walk, each day the child should be encouraged to move his own limbs to end ranges through normal play activities to slow development of contractures related to sedentary positioning. Some research supports the view that the combination of positioning, stretching, and splinting should begin before contractures exist. For example, the child can be encouraged to watch television or play video games while lying prone with legs aligned out of the common "frog leg" (hip abduction and external rotation) pattern. Once a child has significant hip flexor or iliotibial band contractures, stretching techniques must be specific because simple prone positioning can force the lumbar spine into excessive lordosis. Although difficult to accomplish in some mainstreamed school environments, positioning the child in a standing frame during several class periods helps provide prolonged stretch to hip, knee, and ankle musculature. Later in the course of the disease, resting hand splints are appropriate to control shortening of the long finger flexors.[221]

Although development of contractures of the hip, knee, and ankle from muscle imbalances has been thought the cause of early loss of ambulation instead of weakness,[287] others believe that weakness causes the loss of ambulation instead.[280] Some authors note that loss of ambulation can occur from either case.[255] Limiting contracture development facilitates mobility and handling throughout the course of the disease, however, and the best approach to contractures is to prevent them.[260]

Exercise and the Maintenance of Maximal Functional Level. Because DMD affects muscles throughout childhood and adolescence, when strength and endurance are generally developing, effectiveness of strengthening and aerobic exercise has been difficult to assess.[267] Training programs may maximize muscle and cardiorespiratory function, but they have also led to reports of weakness after physical exertion.[288] The debate over the value of exercise in DMD and the relative lack of controlled trials have limited the ability of clinicians to provide evidence-based therapy. No definitive protocols can be provided at this time. In general, however, both strengthening and aerobic exercises should be considered, the frequency and intensity of which should be appropriately prescribed based on the disease course and the patient's abilities and goals.

Strengthening exercises have had mixed support in the past.[289] de Lateur and Giaconi[290] noted small gains in strength of the exercised compared with the unexercised quadriceps muscle of four boys with DMD during and for 18 months after a 6-month exercise program of submaximal isokinetic contractions, 30 repetitions, 4 to 5 days per week. No postexercise weakness or increases in deterioration were noted in the exercised muscles. Vignos and Watkins[291] instituted a home program of maximal resistance exercises for 1 year; the 14 patients with DMD in the exercised group improved in strength for the first 4 months and then reached a plateau, compared with declines in strength of the control group. Scott and colleagues[292] noted diminished strength after a strengthening home-exercise program for 18 boys, although with no control group, possible reductions in disease progression could not be confirmed.

Evidence for the effectiveness of strengthening exercises in other muscle disorders is insufficient[293] and cannot thus be generalized to DMD. Elder[294] reviewed animal studies suggesting that dystrophic mice trained on a treadmill showed increased damage to muscle tissue, whereas forced swimming in dystrophic mice had no adverse effect. In a case review of three generations of patients with facioscapulohumeral muscular dystrophy (seven cases and one suspected case), Johnson and Braddom[295] noted asymmetrical weakness of the upper extremities. They related the weakness to patterns of overuse (dominant side or side used most often in work activities). On the basis of their information and additional evidence that muscle-derived enzymes (CK and myoglobin concentrations in blood) were markedly elevated in patients with DMD after prolonged exercise,[296] repetitive exercise may be contraindicated.[297] In contrast, Cup and colleagues[293] reported that in their review of 33 studies of exercise therapy for neuromuscular diseases, they found absent or negligible adverse effects; one study reported that "3 of 20 patients decreased their training for 1 or 2 sessions due to delayed-onset soreness."

Given the evidence to date, Hasson[298] concluded that exercise consisting of brief periods of low- or high-intensity activity can improve strength for patients with minimal to moderate weakness. The increased recruitment of motor units from training effects also may improve muscle coordination and reduce disuse atrophy. However, exercise programs have minimal effect on strength of muscles already severely weakened.

In addition to active and resistive exercise programs, Scott and colleagues[286] completed a small study of the effect of intermittent, long-term, low-frequency electrical stimulation on dystrophic anterior tibialis muscles. They demonstrated a significant increase in mean voluntary contraction force and suggested that electrical stimulation can have a beneficial effect if used with children whose muscles are not already markedly weakened. Zupan[299] supports this finding, but children under treatment were unable to maintain strength beyond 4 to 5 months.

Evidence for the effect of aerobic training in DMD is sparse.[300] Hasson,[298] in a review of exercise studies of patients with muscular dystrophy, reports that oxygen consumption improved with endurance training, although whether repetitive endurance training at moderate or high intensity (70% of $\dot{V}O_2max$) causes muscle damage is unknown. Muscle biopsies in DMD have revealed reduced or missing nitric oxide synthase, necessary for sufficient nitric oxide levels.[55] Nitric oxide normally limits vasoconstriction in muscles during and after exercise and also provides cytoprotection and antiinflammation in muscle tissue. Muscle fatigue in DMD may thus be exacerbated by ischemic exercise.[55] However, aerobic training in other muscular diseases has shown indications of positive effect on aerobic capacity as well as measures of activities and participation,[293] so generalization to DMD has a possible rationale. In addition, strengthening exercises in combination with aerobic exercises in other muscle disorders have been shown to have a likely positive effect.[293]

Overall, the data from animal and human studies suggest that submaximal exercise is not harmful and it may be helpful in maintaining maximal function if the patient does not exercise into marked fatigue. Because muscle endurance and peak power are diminished in addition to muscle strength, a focus on program design related to functional exercises individualized to each child's functional requirements is recommended.[274]

Ideally, the child's exercise can be incorporated into pleasurable activities adapted for children with movement and weakness-related balance problems. Many ambulatory children enjoy ball activities, walking-based simple obstacle courses, parachute games, table tennis, cycling (preferably tandem), and especially swimming. Swimming is an excellent exercise for children with DMD because they often are quite buoyant because of their increased fat/muscle ratio. Many children can continue to float or swim independently on their backs even when nonambulatory (if supervised) and able to move only distal musculature. The Muscular Dystrophy Association has an excellent guide to water-based exercises: "No Sweat Exercise: Aquatics."[301]

A safe indicator of extent and intensity of exercise is that the patient should recover from exercise fatigue after a night's rest. When designing an active play program, therapists should review the types of muscle contractions that the activity requires, considering that possible muscle damage occurs when muscles are active and functioning in an eccentric manner.[302] Concerns about damage from eccentric muscle contractions were supported in animal studies in which dystrophic muscles were found to be more susceptible to stretch-induced muscle damage.[303] Figure 17-12 shows responses of normal and impaired muscle to exercise. (See Eagle's report on exercise in neuromuscular diseases.[304]) In a summary of findings on effects of physical exercise on conditioning in muscular dystrophy, Ansved[305] found that the scientific basis for clear recommendations on exercise prescription is poor, but evidence does show the importance of maintaining an active lifestyle with limitations on high-resistance and eccentric training activities.[305]

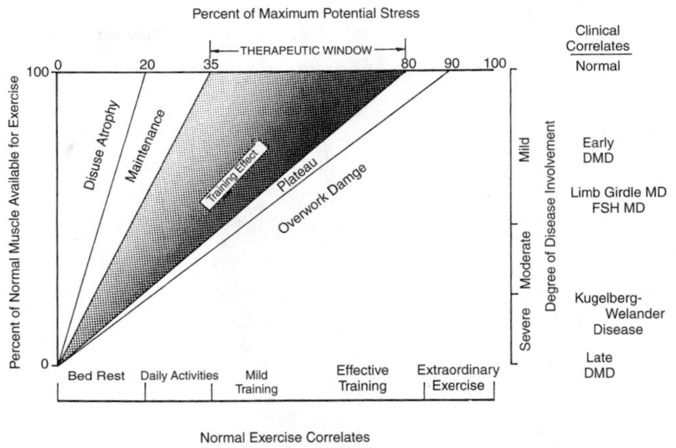

Figure 17-12 ■ Idealized response of normal and impaired muscle to exercise. The therapeutic window of safe exercise narrows progressively. Activities (lower X axis) causing normal exercise effects in normal muscle (upper X axis) correlate with different effects in impaired muscle. (From Coble NO, Maloney FP: Effects of exercise on neuromuscular disease. In Maloney FP, Burks JS, Ringel SP, editors: *Interdisciplinary rehabilitation of multiple sclerosis and neuromuscular disorders,* New York, 1985, JB Lippincott.)

Maintenance of Ambulation. As DMD progresses, the child's posture (a result of both weakness and contracture) and gait pattern abnormalities become extreme and he must work harder to maintain balance while walking. Most children gradually discontinue walking about a year after they lose their ability to deal with stairs or when daily ambulation time decreases to less than 30 minutes per day.[212] Toward the end of the child's independent walking stage, he has a marked anterior pelvic tilt with lordosis and a protuberant abdomen. His shoulders are retracted and he may hold his hands behind his hips or elevated in a mid-guard position to stabilize his hips. He has a severe waddling gait with a shortened stride, and he must carefully lock his knees at each step. He falls frequently, which may result in fractures of the lower or upper extremities.

If the child and his family have followed an aggressive ROM, positioning, and activity program, the child's walking time may be extended by months. In most cases, however, the contractures from muscle imbalance continue relentlessly and the child begins to need support when walking.[262] When contractures at the hip, knee, and ankle show evidence of interfering with the child's ability to stabilize each joint during stance, most children are referred for surgery to restore functional joint motion. Figure 17-13 shows the typical walking pattern of a boy with DMD who is being considered for release of contractures and bracing.

Bracing either before or after surgery may be indicated to assist with positioning and stabilizing joints for function. Ideally, bilateral KAFOs should be measured and fitted in final form before surgery to release contractures so the child can begin upright weight bearing in the KAFO the day after surgery. KAFOs are commonly fabricated of molded plastic thigh units (ischial weight-bearing quadrilateral socket) with metal joints at the knee (drop locks) and ankle (or a flexible plastic ankle component) (Figure 17-14).[306] If the orthoses are not immediately available, the child can begin the standing program in long-leg casts. Casting must be kept to a minimum because of the risk of disuse atrophy in immobilized muscles. (See Grossman and colleagues[307] for a review

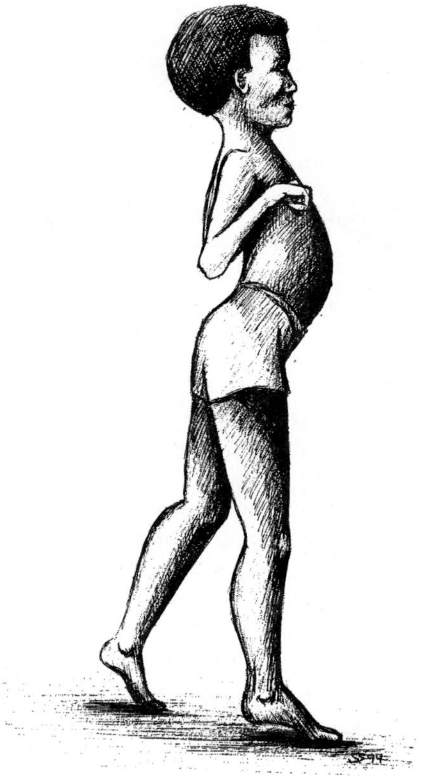

Figure 17-13 ■ Typical walking pattern of a boy with Duchenne muscular dystrophy who is being considered for release of contractures and bracing.

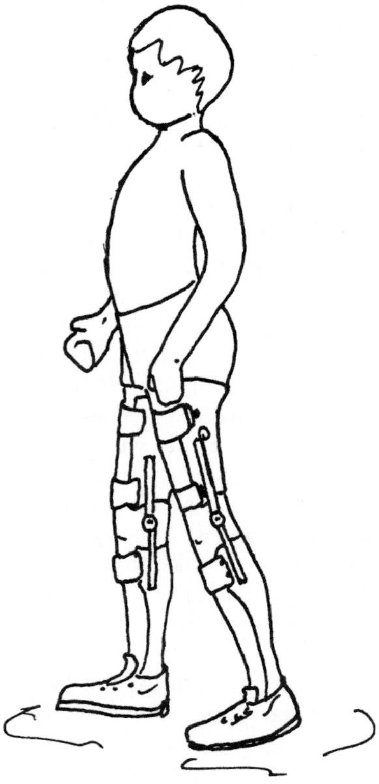

Figure 17-14 ■ Example of boy walking in knee-ankle-foot orthoses showing ischial weight-bearing quadrilateral socket, knee drop locks, and plastic ankle component.

of the effect of immobilization on normal muscle and appropriate therapy interventions.)

In the hospital, standing in bilateral KAFOs can be initiated on a tilt table. Most children are fearful after surgery and report significant pain when their legs are moved or if they are placed upright. For therapy to be successful during this early standing stage and during passive ROM exercises, the child must have adequate pain medication. If the child is not properly medicated in the first few days after surgery, the therapist may have to deal with difficult, resistant behaviors of the child that persist long after the pain should have subsided. Pain protocols must be discussed before the child's surgical procedures. The child should be medicated at least 30 minutes before the therapist's visit.

Gait training is usually begun within 48 hours after surgery. Initial work focuses on helping the child regain his sense of standing balance because his old patterns of equinus, lordosis, and shoulder retraction may no longer be adaptive. The child should be allowed to find his own best center of balance, and he should be allowed to use compensatory gait deviations necessary to allow the best mobility and stability. Depending on the child's upper-extremity strength and control, he may progress from parallel bars for balance assist, to pushing a wheelchair or weighted walker, to balance assist from a therapist with a safety strap to prevent falls. Some children who seem to need a walker for balance transition do best if they use a walker with forearm rests and vertical hand grips, which seem to help them stabilize their arms more effectively than a standard walker. Fortunately, most children do learn to walk independently without support again after surgery, although they are unable to negotiate steps or inclines or rise from the floor independently.[308] Hyde and colleagues[306] report that 24 of 30 boys treated with KAFOs were able to achieve functional ambulation again. Vignos and colleagues[309] report in a review of long-term treatment of DMD that a combination of operative procedures, orthotics, stretching, and a program of standing and walking resulted in extended walking until a mean age of 13.6 years and standing for 2 years after that. With the early use of surgery and bracing procedures to maintain ambulation, the expected deterioration in muscle strength and function as a result of becoming sedentary in a wheelchair is deferred.[310]

Because most children with DMD are discharged home within a few days of surgery, PTs must provide options for continuing standing within the home. Standing frames are often available through the child's school district or therapy unit. If they are not, the therapist can help the family build a simple standing frame for home. This frame often can be made from a piece of plywood, or a gluteal strap system can be attached to a table at home. If possible the child should be positioned just forward of the line of gravity to encourage back extension with facet stability and to allow the child better head control in the presence of weak anterior neck muscles. Use of swivel walkers has been recommended by some therapists and physicians because the child does not need upper-extremity control for support. Although the concept of hands-free walking seems logical, boys with DMD had more difficulty using the walkers compared with children with paraplegia because of the more delicate postural adjustments needed by children with dystrophy and their greater sensitivity to the motion restriction of the swivel walker. In addition, older children with DMD are seldom willing to wear externally visible bracing outside the home or school system. Some therapists have reported success with the ORLAU variable center of gravity swivel walker (Mopac Ltd., Eau Claire, Wisconsin)[311]; however, support for its use is not widespread.

Bakker and colleagues[312] reviewed the literature on the effectiveness of treatment with surgery and KAFOs. They found that the scientific strength of the studies was poor. Although the treatment approach seemed to prolong the walking time, whether it extended functional walking was not clear. The children who benefited most were highly motivated and had slower rates of deterioration.

Transition to Wheelchair. Although surgical and orthotic interventions may prolong ambulation within the home and classroom past the predicted time for cessation of independent walking (8 to 12 years), most children begin to use a wheelchair for community mobility and long distances before this time. When children begin to spend more time in their chair, the rate of development of contractures, disuse weakness, and obesity increases.[249,306] Because of this more rapid deterioration in the child's functional skills, professionals and parents often discourage the child from using a chair for mobility. Children, however, tend to welcome use of the chair because they have more energy for their social interactions and learning tasks.[306]

Selection of the appropriate wheelchair is often difficult for the patient and family because of the multiple decisions that must be made. Few children with DMD can propel a manual wheelchair for more than a few years because of their increasing upper-extremity weakness. In addition, their propulsion speed in their manual chair is seldom adequate to keep up with their peers. Eventually, the child will need a motorized chair. Although this provides tremendous freedom for the child, a motorized chair presents problems to many families because transporting the chair requires a van and lift unit, which is seldom funded by insurance. Ideally, the child should have both a manual and a motorized chair; however, in today's health policy climate, parents or advocates often must engage in protracted efforts to obtain adaptive equipment for the patient.

An important consideration when purchasing a wheelchair is the trunk support system. Traditionally, boys with DMD are thought to develop a gravity collapse of the spine related to their functional sitting posture. To control the collapsing spine, spinal orthoses and seat inserts to lock the spine in extension (to prevent lateral bending and rotation) are frequently recommended. Unfortunately, the effectiveness of positioning devices to control the development of scoliosis has been disappointing.[243,244] The therapist therefore should work with the child, the family, and the orthopedist to determine the best system to maintain optimal spinal alignment and trunk stability as the child weakens. In addition, as the child becomes more physically dependent, the chair may need to be fitted with a pressure-relief molded seat and trunk cushions, elevating leg rests, and a reclining back with a head rest.[313] The Tilt-in-Space chair (LABAC Systems, Denver) is a good example of a chair that can be motorized to allow mobility as well as maximal adjustment of seat position by using mouth control systems. It can also be adapted for a respirator attachment. The decision about the type of power chair necessary in the later stages of disease progression takes considerable thought. Therapists, the patient, and the parents or caregivers must review environmental constraints, access issues, social goals, and work and recreational needs.

Because of the problems associated with increased wheelchair use, the therapist must work closely with the family and any school-based personnel to design a realistic plan to prevent rapid deterioration in strength and independent function. If possible, the child's standing program in KAFOs should be continued at school and at home as long as possible, with a goal of 3 to 5 hours of standing per day. With mainstreaming, however, continuing a standing program at school is sometimes difficult because attendants and equipment are not available, the child may need to move from room to room for different classes, and the child may not like being singled out for special treatment. It is helpful to caregivers if the child continues to wear his KAFOs when using the chair until he is totally dependent for transfers and can no longer be pivoted from the chair to another surface.

If the child uses a motorized wheelchair, directional control systems must be adapted to each child's needs. Most young people with advanced DMD do well for years with a standard joystick hand control system; however, because of extended survival times relative to the long-term use of mechanical ventilation, many patients must have their control systems adjusted frequently to minimize the need for muscle control, such as pinch strength. The need for ventilation support while using the wheelchair does not seem to interfere with the ability to drive.[314] (See Cooper[315] for a comprehensive manual on wheelchair selection. This information is equally valuable for patients with ALS and GBS.)

When the child can no longer tolerate the sitting position, some children have continued to attend school on a gurney. Once the person with DMD is no longer able to attend school or work, the home environment will need to be adapted for maximal self-direction despite significant physical dependence. Both low- and high-tech environmental control systems are more readily available today than they were 10 years ago. Television control units, voice-activated telephones, switch-activated bed controls, and page turners are among the low-tech systems. Sip-and-puff, blink-operated, and voice-activated control units can be adapted to operate most electronic devices. OTs and PTs can provide invaluable support to the person with DMD and the caregivers by making several home visits to suggest modifications and adaptive devices and systems. (See Cook and Hussey[114] for detailed information on assistive technology systems. Also see an excellent website for home automation, environmental control, and electronic aids for daily living [EADLs]: www.makoa.org/ecu.htm.)

Psychosocial Issues

Psychosocial issues related to DMD are family issues. At the time of the child's diagnosis, the parents are often emotionally devastated and cycle back and forth through many phases of denial, anger, sadness, and active coping, especially if they feel guilt that they "caused" their child's disease. This process tends to recur when the child does not meet expected normal physical and social milestones or when he reaches predicted stages of deterioration, such as the transition to a wheelchair. Because children with DMD have concomitant developmental and cognitive delays or issues, educational and social interactions can be compromised in addition to the physical changes. Because DMD is a multisystem multiprocess disease, early in the child's life the family should be guided to encourage the child's independence and to discourage overprotection.[316] Therapists can play an important role in helping the child and family identify realistic goals for independence. In addition, therapists can be instrumental in extending independence and a sense of self-direction by anticipating patient needs for adaptive equipment and identifying appropriate assistive devices and environmental control systems that empower the person with DMD and provide relief for caregivers from the constant attention required by a completely dependent person. Key to family support is access to a multidisciplinary clinic with specialists in neurology, pulmonology, orthopedics, rehabilitation services, psychology, social work, and dietetics. Only through comprehensive clinics do families of children and adults with DMD receive the level of education and support necessary to deal with the changing levels of function and demands on family systems.[214]

Psychosocial support should be made available to the child and family during predictable times of crisis. Major times of crisis occur around the age of 5 years when the child begins to realize his differences, at age 8 to 12 years when the child loses the ability to walk independently, during the adolescent years when social interactions become restricted, and around the time of high school graduation when the child and family must face vocational limitations and almost certain death within the next decade.[317] Transition times are often accompanied by depression, withdrawal, and anxiety in the child and family members because parents had a marked preoccupation with their sons and a diminished expression of enjoyment.[313] Predictably, the integrity, strength, and intragenerational and intergenerational function and coping styles of the child's family contribute a great deal to the way the family responds to the child's progressive deterioration. Extended periods of anxiety and depression should be treated vigorously with cognitive interventions, support groups, respite care, and, when appropriate, short-term anxiolytics and antidepressants. Repeated opportunities to discuss end-of-life care must be given to both the child and parents. Professionals, however, tend to underestimate the quality of life for patients with end-stage DMD; therefore patients and family members must be educated about long-term options for ventilatory support or palliative care well ahead of any respiratory emergency that might occur to ensure that the patient's desires are respected.[214,318]

Because of the extended life opportunities for DMD patients who may now live into their 20s, home care requirements, the impact of in-home care on family members, and the financial impact must be fully reviewed and support systems put in place before caregiving stress becomes overwhelming. Positive family functioning while caring for a dependent child or adult with DMD is correlated with caregiver health and hardiness and requires multiple levels of family support from family, friends, and professionals.[319] Increasingly, young men with DMD are attending college even though they may require 24-hour assistance with ADLs and monitoring of ventilation equipment. To date, parents are providing most of the care to their children with DMD by attending colleges or living in dorms or apartments with their child. With life extended with ventilation, parents and the young person with DMD should begin early to plan for a future with maximal decision making by the young adult with DMD. This mindset of a "future" requires considerable problem solving by all people involved in the care of the young adult. Parents of children with DMD should involve their child early in life to make appropriate decisions about care, learn about medical needs and practices, and deal with finances necessary to run a home or hire an attendant. These issues related to independence (even though physically dependent) and caregivers are now being discussed by patients with DMD and their caregivers.[320]

Parents and the child should be given the opportunity to discuss the impending death in an accepting environment with persons who are experienced in dealing with degenerative diseases. Because the child and family have long anticipated the child's death and have made transitions through many levels of grieving, the process of separation and mourning may have occurred before the child's death. Each child and family member should therefore be helped to deal with the process according to his or her own pace and in response to individual needs. The child's death is sometimes considered a welcome relief.[321] This feeling of relief, however, is often accompanied by survivor guilt and a tremendous sense of loss of life focus for the family members whose lives have been so intertwined with that of the child's. Ideally, arrangements should be made for the family to meet with the professionals with whom they feel most comfortable several weeks after the child's death and again several months later so that the family (and caregivers) can deal with their thoughts and feelings (Case Study 17-3).[322,323]

CASE STUDY 17-3 ■ JEREMY

Jeremy was 3 years old when he was diagnosed with DMD. He lived at home with his mother and a 5-year-old sister. There was no known family history of DMD, although family lore suggested that a cousin died quite young from pneumonia and a "wasting disease." Jeremy was referred for a medical evaluation when a playground supervisor at his preschool noted that he was clumsy when running and that he had difficulty on the playground climbing equipment and the slide. He also had difficulty rising from the ground and needed to hold on to a railing when stepping up a stair.

During a medical history, Jeremy's mother said that she had noticed that he was "slow to develop" but was not worried because she thought he was just a "late bloomer." A muscle biopsy was positive for a diagnosis of DMD. A physical therapy evaluation 3 months after diagnosis showed ROM to be within normal limits for all joints. Muscle weakness was evident on

CASE STUDY 17-3 ■ JEREMY—cont'd

MMT with G− (4−) hip abduction and extension and quadriceps strength bilaterally. Hip flexion, knee flexion, dorsiflexion, and toe extension were in the G (4) range. Plantar flexion was G+ (4+) with evident hypertrophy. Shoulder abduction and flexion was in the G (4) range, although the patient had difficulty sustaining abduction for more than 5 seconds.

Jeremy had a moderate head lag when moving from supine to sitting, because of G− (4−) anterior neck muscles. The therapist made an on-site school visit to help the teachers identify obstacles to Jeremy's full integration with his classmates. The school custodian built some ramps to help Jeremy use the playground equipment.

Jeremy ambulated independently until age 8 years. His gait pattern was typical of late-stage ambulation (marked equinus, knee hyperextension during stance, bilateral Trendelenburg on stance, marked lordosis with a protuberant abdomen with arms held posterior to hips). He had 40-degree hip flexion contractures with iliotibial band tightness, no knee contractures, and 25-degree plantar flexion contractures. MMT showed the expected decrease in strength, with pelvic and shoulder girdle muscles being weaker than more distal musculature, except that the anterior tibialis and the peroneals were F+ (3+). He was unable to rise independently from the floor and needed assistance with stairs. Because his gait pattern was slow and he needed to rest frequently when walking more than 20 feet at school, Jeremy had been using a manual wheelchair for long-distance mobility since the age of 7 years.

On the recommendation of orthopedist consultants, Jeremy underwent bilateral percutaneous hip flexor lengthening, iliotibial band fasciotomy, and heel cord release. Bilateral KAFOs had been fitted before surgery, and Jeremy was placed in the braces after surgery. No casting was done. Despite his complaints, he was gradually brought to the full weight-bearing standing position by late afternoon on the day after surgery. Adjustments were made in his pain medication schedule to allow him to tolerate the process more comfortably. By the third hospital day, Jeremy participated in two therapy sessions per day and was standing in the parallel bars, where he was taught lateral and anteroposterior weight shifting in preparation for ambulation. Active assisted and passive ROM exercises were performed without the KAFOs twice a day. On the fourth hospital day, Jeremy began to take short steps using the parallel bars for balance. His mother was also taught his exercises so that Jeremy could have more than two therapy sessions a day. On the fourth day, he practiced walking for 10 minutes six times a day with full physical therapy treatment twice a day.

Because Jeremy was from a rural area and daily physical therapy would not be available on discharge, he was kept in the hospital for 3 additional days for intensive rehabilitation. An OT worked with Jeremy to provide adaptive equipment for reaching, self-care, and eating (he was unable to raise his arms above 45 degrees and needed his left arm to assist the right when reaching). He was discharged home on the eighth day. An Elks traveling therapist arranged to visit the family once a week for the next month to continue ambulation training and to guide the mother in a home positioning and ROM program. The therapist also helped the mother adapt the home environment and his school to adjust expectations of Jeremy so he was less prone to falling and excessive fatigue.

The family was lost to follow-up, but by report Jeremy continued to ambulate in his KAFOs for approximately 9 months after surgery, when he chose to use his wheelchair full time. A motorized wheelchair was recommended; however, his mother believed that Jeremy was easier to handle in his manual chair. The Muscular Dystrophy Association loaned Jeremy a motorized wheelchair for school use. He had developed moderate scoliosis but did not report pain. He refused to wear a molded spinal corset, but the padded thoracic pads fitted to his chair increased his comfort. By age 15 years, Jeremy was dependent for all care except feeding. He was able to sit with support in a large living room chair and he enjoyed watching television and playing card games with a few friends who visited his home. He was disinterested in continuing school and missed more days than he attended. He was not cooperative with his home-based teacher.

During his fifteenth year, Jeremy had repeated episodes of chest congestion and difficulty handling stringy foods. The visiting therapist taught his mother some postural drainage and breathing exercises for Jeremy; however, the mother did not follow through with the recommendations. Because his mother had to work full time, a public agency provided in-home care during the days when Jeremy was not at school or after he returned from school. The mother refused in-home nursing care, preferring to continue with the attendant, who was not comfortable carrying out Jeremy's exercises or pulmonary care. The family refused counseling or support from parents of other children with disabilities. Jeremy died at home after a brief bout with pneumonia.

SUMMARY

In this chapter, discussion of three different diseases reveals the varied effects of neuromuscular pathology on a person's day-to-day function. ALS is an adult-onset degenerative disease of the upper and lower motor neurons; GBS is an inflammatory process affecting the PNS of children and adults; and DMD is an inherited degenerative disease manifesting in childhood that affects muscle tissue. In all three conditions the therapist must design a therapy program that will provide the patient with the impetus to become or remain as active as possible without causing possible muscle damage from excessive exercise demands or overwork.

Therapists must be aware of their own feelings and reactions to patients with severe neuromuscular diseases. Working with patients with GBS is usually a positive experience because most patients attain full recovery despite their often severe disability during the acute illness and long recovery period. Working with patients with degenerative terminal diseases, however, draws deeply on the therapist's emotional and spiritual strength. A typical response of health care professionals is to view these patients' conditions as hopeless and to assume that the patients must also perceive their existence as hopeless, depressing, and without value. Research does suggest an increased incidence of depression and demoralization in patients with degenerative, terminal diseases compared with nonaffected populations. Other research, however, has indicated that many patients perceive their own life satisfaction much more positively than professionals would believe.[318,324] Therapists must tap into patients' positive energy to design treatment programs that respect patients' goals and life plans within the context of their environment.

Limited evidence exists to document the effectiveness of rehabilitation for patients with progressive neurological diseases. Determining the most appropriate exercise and therapeutic intervention programs therefore requires diligent examination of the dysfunctions and needs of the individual patient and assessment of the effects of interventions appropriately adapted from use in other populations. Because few medical-clinical facilities see a large enough sample of patients with any of these three diagnoses, therapists must align with their professional organizations to institute nationwide, multisite research studies to provide clear evidence of effectiveness of therapy in these populations.

References

To enhance this text and add value for the reader, all references are included on the companion Evolve site that accompanies this textbook. This online service will, when available, provide a link for the reader to a Medline abstract for the article cited. There are 326 cited references and other general references for this chapter, with the majority of those articles being evidence-based citations.

CHAPTER 18

Beyond the Central Nervous System: Neurovascular Entrapment Syndromes

BRADLEY W. STOCKERT, PT, PhD, LAURA J. KENNY, PT, OCS, FAAOMPT, and PETER I. EDGELOW, PT, MS, DPT

OVERVIEW

The purpose of this chapter is twofold. The first purpose is to develop the concept that the entire nervous system forms a continuous tissue tract. This concept is central to the idea that movements of the trunk and/or limbs can have a profound biomechanical and physiological impact on the peripheral nervous system (PNS) and central nervous system (CNS). Mobility of the nervous system and some of the responses of the system to movement in normal and sensitized states are discussed.

The second purpose of this chapter is to develop in the reader an understanding of neurovascular entrapment syndrome. This is an underrecognized impairment present in some patients with a wide variety of diagnoses—for example, nonspecific arm pain, repetitive strain injury, carpal tunnel syndrome, and thoracic outlet syndrome. Standard medical care frequently fails with these patients. A theoretical model for the development and perpetuation of neurovascular entrapment syndrome is presented. Background information regarding the syndrome is provided, and the appropriate screening tools for assessment of the impairment are discussed. Treatment suggestions and a case study are presented at the end of the chapter.

PERIPHERAL NEUROANATOMY

The PNS is generally regarded as the portion of the nervous system that lies outside the CNS (i.e., the brain and spinal cord).[1,2] The major components of the PNS include motor, sensory, and autonomic neurons found in spinal, peripheral, and cranial nerves. Although this partitioning is valid from an anatomical perspective, it often leads to a lack of appreciation as to the truly continuous nature and integrative function of the nervous system as a whole. The concept that the entire nervous system is a continuous tissue tract reinforces the idea that limb and trunk movements can have a mechanical effect on the PNS and the CNS that is local and global.

The nervous system is composed of two functional tissue types. One type of tissue is concerned with impulse conduction. This functional category includes nerve cells and Schwann cells. The second functional tissue type provides support and protection of the conduction tissues—that is, the connective tissues.

Three levels in the organization of a peripheral nerve have been described[2,3] (Figure 18-1). At the innermost level the nerve fiber is the conducting component of a neuron (nerve cell). A connective tissue layer called the *endoneurium* surrounds each nerve fiber. The endoneurium surrounds the basement membrane of the neuron and plays an important role in maintaining fluid pressure within the endoneurial space. There are no lymphatic channels within the endoneurial space. The pressure within the endoneurial space increases with compression of the neuron.[4]

The second level of organization consists of a collection of many nerve fibers (a fascicle) surrounded by a layer of connective tissue called the *perineurium*.[2,3] The perineurium acts as a selective barrier to diffusion and as such exerts significant control over the local movement of fluid and ions. This connective tissue layer acts like a pressurized container—that is, extrusion of the contents occurs if the membrane is cut. The compartment enclosed by the perineurium does not contain lymphatic channels.[4] This may be a problem during inflammatory states when edema is present deep to the perineurium. The perineurium is the last connective tissue layer to rupture in tensile testing of peripheral nerves.[5] The outermost connective tissue layer of a peripheral nerve is called the *epineurium*. The epineurium surrounds, protects, and enhances gliding between the fascicles. Lymphatic channels are found within the epineurial compartment.

All three connective tissue layers are interconnected—they are not separate and distinct, but continuous tissue layers.[2,3] Each of the connective tissue layers contains free nerve endings from the nervi nervorum. As a result, all three connective tissue layers are a potential source of pain. In addition, all three layers are continuous with the homologous connective tissue layers of the CNS—for example, the dura mater and the epineurium.

The vascular supply for peripheral nerves is designed to provide uninterrupted blood flow regardless of the position of the trunk and limbs. Extrinsic vessels provide blood flow to segmental vessels that in turn supply an extensive intrinsic (intraneural) vasculature within the PNS. These segmental vessels branch off of the extrinsic vessels and enter peripheral nerves in areas of low nerve mobility relative to the surrounding tissue. The intrinsic vasculature supplies all three connective tissue layers within the PNS. Arterioles and venules are found in the epineurial and perineurial spaces, but only capillaries are found in the endoneurial compartment.

Peripheral nerves are regularly subjected to compression and elongation (stretching), which have been shown to increase intraneural pressure. An increase in intraneural pressure decreases the diameter of the intrinsic blood vessels and results in a reduction in blood flow within the nerve. Compressive forces of 20 to 30 mm Hg have been shown to adversely affect intraneural blood flow,[6] and compressive forces of 50 to 70 mm Hg have been shown to result in complete arrest of blood flow[7] and cause damage to myelin and axons.[6] A strain (elongation) of 6% to 8% has been shown

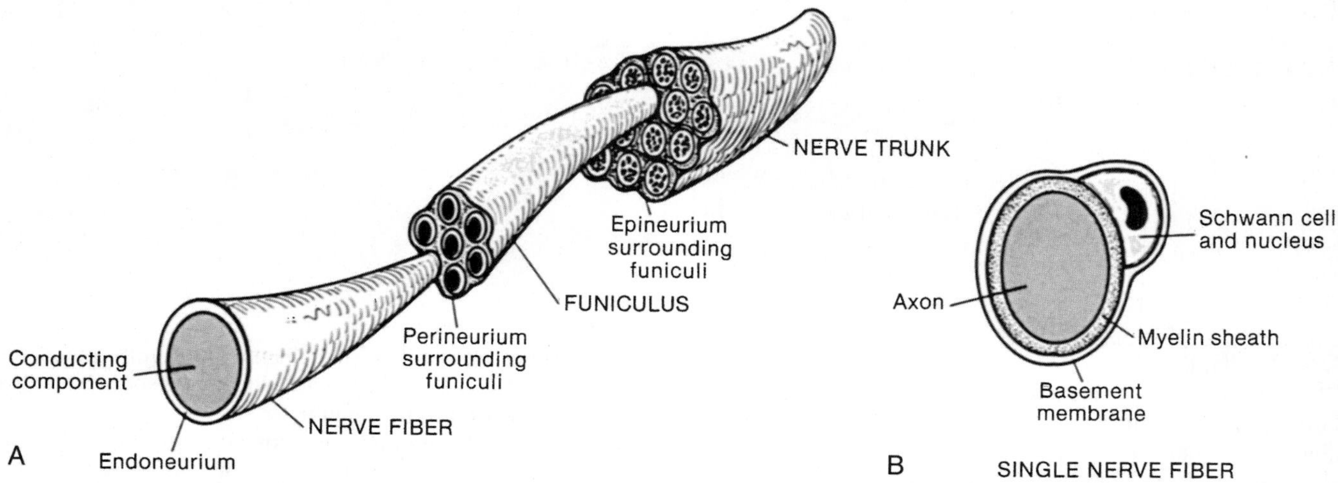

Figure 18-1 ■ Three levels of organization of a peripheral nerve or nerve trunk. **A**, Nerve trunk and components. **B**, Microscopic structure of nerve fiber.

to decrease intraneural blood flow by 50% to 70% in the sciatic nerve of rats.[4,8,9] A strain of 15% in the sciatic nerve of a rabbit has been shown to result in complete arrest of blood flow,[7] and the same strain produces an 80% reduction in blood flow in the rat sciatic nerve.[9] Strains of 11% or greater are produced by some of the positions used in neurodynamic tests of the upper limb.[6] Significant increases in intraneural pressure and concomitant decreases in intraneural blood flow have been shown to adversely affect neuronal conduction.[7,10,11]

The cytoplasm in cells moves and has thixotropic properties—that is, the viscosity of cytoplasm is lower when it is continuously moving.[4] In neurons the movement of the cytoplasm from the cell body through the axons (anterograde movement) occurs at two speeds. Fast axoplasmic flow occurs at a rate of about 100 to 400 mm/day and is used to carry ion channels and neurotransmitters (i.e., materials required for normal impulse conduction) to the nerve terminals. Slow axoplasmic flow occurs at a rate of about 6 mm/day and is used to transport cytoskeleton proteins, neurofilaments, and other materials used to maintain the physical health of the cell. A third flow occurs in the opposite direction (retrograde) at a rate of about 200 mm/day. Retrograde transport carries unused substances and exogenous materials taken up at the terminus—for example, neurotrophic factors. The material carried back to the cell body by retrograde transport has been shown to influence activity in the cell nucleus.[4]

Compression raises intraneural pressure, which has a negative impact on the flow of cytoplasm.[4] Anterograde and retrograde flow of axoplasm is impaired with 30 mm Hg compression on the nerve, hypoxia, or a strain of 11% or greater.[12-14] Prolonged or intense exposure to compression can result in conduction abnormalities, endoneurial edema, fibrin deposition, demyelination, and axonal sprouting. Each of these events increases the likelihood of developing adhesions and abnormal impulse-generating sites (AIGSs).[4] (The negative impact of AIGSs is discussed in the section on adaptive responses to pain.)

MOBILITY OF THE PERIPHERAL NERVOUS SYSTEM

Several types of tissues (e.g., bone, fascia, and muscle) surround peripheral nerves as they "travel" to target tissues. Peripheral nerves can be thought of as passing through a series of tissue tunnels composed of various biological materials. The composition of the tissue tunnel changes with the passage of the nerve from the vertebral column (an osseous tunnel) to the target tissue—for example, from an osseous tunnel to a soft tissue and/or fibro-osseous tunnel. A "mechanical interface" exists at the junction between the nerve and the material adjacent to the nerve that forms the tissue tunnel. Movement of the trunk and/or limbs can cause three types of movement to occur in the peripheral nerves: unfolding, sliding, and elongation.[15]

When there is little or no tension in a peripheral nerve, the axon typically contains undulations (folds). As tension is applied the axon will "unfold" so that the undulations disappear. "Sliding" can be defined as movement between the nerve and the surrounding tissues at the mechanical interface (extraneural movement). Sliding by itself does not cause significant elongation or tension to develop within the nerve, so intraneural pressure remains relatively unchanged. Ultrasound studies have shown that the median, ulnar, sciatic, and tibial nerves undergo extraneural movement (sliding) with movement of the upper and lower limbs, respectively.[16-19]

"Elongation" of the nerve occurs when tension is applied to a nerve and there is little or no unfolding and sliding at the mechanical interface. Elongation causes movement to occur between the neural elements and connective tissue layers (intraneural movement). Elongation decreases the diameter of the nerve, resulting in an increase in the intraneural tension and pressure.[15] An increase in intraneural pressure has been shown to decrease the flow of blood and axoplasm, resulting in altered neural function (see previous section). Elongation within the median and ulnar nerves has been shown to occur with movements of the upper limb.[6]

Both extraneural and intraneural movements may occur simultaneously within a nerve, but they may not be uniformly distributed. When a body moves, some parts of the PNS will undergo primarily extraneural movement (sliding) with little or no development of tension while other areas undergo intraneural movement (elongation) that results in an increase in intraneural tension and pressure. As a consequence, some areas within a nerve slide, developing little or no tension, whereas other areas of the same nerve elongate significantly, increasing the amount of intraneural tension.[6] In areas repeatedly exposed to high amounts of tension, for example, the median nerve at the wrist, the nerves are found to contain a higher-than-average amount of connective tissue.[15]

If one considers the entire nervous system as a continuous tissue tract, then the idea that movement and/or tension developed in one region of the nervous system can be distributed and dissipated throughout the entire nervous system becomes apparent.[20,21] The inability of a component within the nervous system to dissipate and/or distribute movement and tension can lead to abnormal force development and lesions elsewhere in the continuous tissue tract.[22]

PERIPHERAL NERVE ENTRAPMENT

Seddon's classification of nerve injury is based upon mechanical trauma.[23] Schaumberg[2] modified this paradigm into an anatomically based scheme containing three classes of injury (Table 18-1). Injuries in class II and III are caused by macrotrauma that results in some disruption to the integrity of the nerve fiber. The following discussion of entrapment is focused on microtrauma in which there is no breach in the anatomical integrity of the nerve fiber (class I). Mechanical microtrauma resulting in nerve entrapment can occur with excessive or abnormal friction, compression, and/or tension (elongation).[2]

Tissue tunnels, peripheral nerves, and the mechanical interfaces between them are all vulnerable to mechanical microtrauma—that is, abnormal friction, compression, and/or tension.[2,15] Some peripheral nerves are exposed to bony hard interfaces, for example, the lower cords of the brachial plexus at the first rib, which are potential sources of abnormal friction. Inflammation and swelling within a tissue tunnel can produce compression of a nerve, for example, the median nerve within the carpal tunnel. The point at which a nerve branches limits the amount of gliding (extraneural movement) available at that location and increases the amount of local intraneural tension developed with movement, for example, the tibial nerve in the popliteal fossa.[2,15]

Microtrauma can produce an intraneural lesion that causes a decrease in intraneural flow of blood and axoplasm, demyelination, and/or conduction defects.[2,15] If the lesion occurs in the connective tissues of the nerve, there may be pain, inflammation, proliferation of fibroblasts, and scar formation (fibrosis). Ultrasound studies have shown that the median nerve in patients with carpal tunnel syndrome is enlarged approximately 30%.[24] An intraneural scar decreases the compliance of the nerve and increases the amount of intraneural pressure and tension generated with elongation.[21] Intraneural lesions can impair or completely block the ability of the nerve to conduct action potentials.[2,15,25] Partial or complete conduction blocks can result in abnormal sensation, loss of motor function, autonomic dysfunction, and atrophy of target tissue, for example, muscle and/or skin.

Microtrauma can produce an extraneural lesion.[2,15,21,25] The damage in an extraneural lesion occurs in the tissue surrounding the nerve or at the mechanical interface. Swelling within the tissue tunnel can produce compression of the nerve. Fibrosis can produce adhesions at the mechanical interface leading to a decrease in sliding of the nerve. A decrease in the ability of a nerve to slide within a tissue tunnel will result in an abnormal increase in intraneural tension and pressure as movement is imposed on the nerve. The increase in local intraneural tension can produce abnormal changes in the conduction of action potentials, and the tension will be distributed in an aberrant pattern throughout the continuous tract of the nervous system. The resultant abnormal distribution of tension predisposes the nervous system to the development of lesions at other sites.[15]

Friction, compression, and tension can produce microtrauma that results in intraneural and extraneural pathology.[2,15] For example, fibrosis can produce a combined pathological state that results in a substantial reduction in the ability of a nerve to slide within the tissue tunnel and a substantial increase in intraneural tension during nerve elongation as the compliance of the nerve is decreased. Movement of the median nerve at the carpal tunnel has been shown to occur with movements of the upper limb.[16-19] Longitudinal and transverse movements of the median nerve at the carpal tunnel have been shown to be reduced in the presence of microtrauma, that is, carpal tunnel syndrome,[24,26] nonspecific arm pain,[27,28] and whiplash injury.[28]

Intraneural and extraneural lesions result in an abnormal distribution of sliding and tension throughout the nervous system with movement of the trunk and/or limbs. The abnormal distribution of tension within a nerve increases the probability of a second lesion or abnormality developing within the nerve. This situation led Upton and McComas[29] in 1973 to first use the term "double crush injury." (This term should be considered a misnomer because a "crush" does not necessarily occur.) For example, entrapment of the

TABLE 18-1 ■ CLASSIFICATION OF ACUTE TRAUMATIC PERIPHERAL NERVE INJURY

ANATOMICAL CLASSIFICATION	CLASS I	CLASS II	CLASS III
Previous nomenclature	Neuropraxia	Axonotmesis	Neurotmesis
Lesion	Reversible conduction block resulting from ischemia or demyelination	Axonal interruption but basal lamina remains intact	Nerve fiber and basal lamina interruption (complete nerve severance)

Modified from Schaumberg HH, Spencer PS, Thomas PK: *Disorders of peripheral nerves,* Philadelphia, 1983, FA Davis.

median nerve at the carpal tunnel can cause the development of abnormal tension in cervical spinal nerves, resulting in a lesion at that site. Upton and McComas[29] have shown that a lesion at the carpal tunnel increases the risk of having a second neural lesion in the cervical region.

PATHOGENESIS OF NEUROVASCULAR ENTRAPMENT

Neurovascular entrapment can occur at any point along the continuous tract of the nervous system. The carpal tunnel, a common site of entrapment, has been studied and provides a framework of information regarding the pathogenesis of neurovascular entrapments. Sunderland[30] has reasoned that a change in the normal pressure gradients within the carpal tunnel can lead to compression of the median nerve. In order to maintain homeostasis in the carpal tunnel and the median nerve, blood must flow into the tunnel, then into the nerve and back out of the tunnel. For normal blood flow to occur in the median nerve the blood pressure must be highest within the epineurial arterioles and becomes progressively lower in the capillaries and epineurial venules and lowest within the extraneural space of the carpal tunnel. Any increase in the pressure of a single compartment has the potential to disrupt the normal pressure gradients and impair the flow of blood within the compartments of the carpal tunnel and median nerve. Impaired intraneural blood flow can lead to localized hypoxia, edema, inflammation, and fibrosis.[30]

An increase in pressure within the carpal tunnel can occur for a variety of reasons, for example, synovial hyperplasia, thickening of tendons, venous congestion, inflammation, and/or edema. Venous blood flow within a nerve will be impaired and venous stasis will develop if pressure within the extraneural space of the carpal tunnel becomes greater than the pressure within the epineurial venules. Because blood pressure within venules is relatively low, partial occlusion of blood flow can begin to occur with pressures as low as 20 to 30 mm Hg.[15,31]

The pressure within the carpal tunnel is normally about 3 mm Hg with the wrist in a neutral position.[4] The pressure can rise to over 30 mm Hg when the wrist is placed in 90 degrees of extension[32] or with the functional task of using a computer mouse to drag or point at an object.[33] Studies have shown that the pressure within the carpal tunnel in someone with carpal tunnel syndrome can be 30 mm Hg, or more, with the wrist in neutral and can increase to about 100 mm Hg when the wrist is in 90 degrees of flexion[4,12,13] or extension.[12] Compressive forces of 20 to 30 mm Hg have been shown to adversely affect intraneural blood flow,[6] whereas compressive forces of 50 to 70 mm Hg have been shown to result in complete arrest of blood flow[7] and cause demonstrable damage to myelin and axons.[6] Motor and sensory abnormalities begin to manifest at about 40 mm Hg, and complete blockade of the median nerve has been shown to occur at 50 mm Hg.[34] The pressure found in the carpal tunnel of people with carpal tunnel syndrome is clearly adequate to disrupt the normal flow of blood, axoplasm, and action potentials within the median nerve, causing severe impairment to normal nerve functions.

Sunderland[30] proposed that venous congestion or stasis within the carpal tunnel will lead to localized hypoxia, edema, and fibrosis. Hypoxia causes capillary endothelial cells to deteriorate and local C fibers to secrete substance P and calcitonin gene–related peptide,[4] which in turn cause mast cells to release histamine and serotonin.[35,36] Together these chemical mediators augment the inflammatory state and cause the endothelial cells of capillaries to further deteriorate by becoming flatter, larger, and leakier, enhancing exudation and edema.

Deterioration of the capillary endothelium results in exudation and the formation of a protein-rich edema in the interstitial space. Protein-rich edema stimulates proliferation of fibroblasts, resulting in fibrosis, and intensifies the abnormal pressure gradients, resulting in more tissue hypoxia—that is, a positive feedback or self-perpetuating cycle of pathology is initiated. Intraneural fibrosis decreases compliance of the nerve, and extraneural fibrosis results in the formation of adhesions at the mechanical interface between the nerve and tissue tunnel. Fibrosis causes a nerve to become stiffer and less mobile, resulting in an abnormal increase in tension when movement is imposed on the nerve.

The set of circumstances described earlier may be referred to as a *neurovascular entrapment syndrome,* and it has the potential to cause the development of problems elsewhere in the system—that is, a double crush injury (see previous section). Upton and McComas[29] studied 115 subjects with carpal tunnel syndrome or ulnar impingement at the elbow. They found that 81 of the 115 subjects also had evidence of a neural lesion at the neck. Because all nerves essentially travel within tissue tunnels, the potential exists for this scenario to occur elsewhere in the continuous tissue tract of the nervous system, for example, the capsule of the dorsal root ganglion and the thoracic outlet.[5,15,37]

ADAPTIVE RESPONSES TO PAIN

A thorough discussion of the pain associated with neurovascular entrapment is beyond the scope and intent of this chapter. The topic of pain management is discussed in Chapter 32 of this book. However, we would like to describe the development of hyperexcitable states and AIGSs in neurons as well as their role in the development of pain associated with neurovascular entrapment.

"Normal" or physiological pain occurs when peripheral nociceptors are subjected to a stimulus that is at or above the threshold for firing. "Abnormal" or pathological pain can occur when there is a change in the sensitivity (threshold) of the somatosensory system.[38] Devor[39] wrote that "the crucial pathophysiological process triggered by nerve injury is an increase in neuronal excitability."

Neurons that become inflamed, hypoxic, and/or demyelinated can enter a hyperexcitable state.[2,39-47] A neuron in a hyperexcitable state can begin to discharge spontaneously and/or develop a sustained rhythmic discharge after stimulation. In addition, hyperexcitable neurons can develop mechanosensitivity,[41] chemosensitivity,[4] and/or thermal sensitivity,[45] all of which can result in the production of allodynia, a form of pathological pain.* These changes in the behavior of a nerve can occur in the absence of detectable degeneration.[40-42] The changes in impulse generation and neuronal sensitivity are characteristics of an AIGS.[4] A hyperexcitable state and an AIGS can develop with the mechanical microtrauma and inflammation often

*References 28, 39, 43, 45, 47, 48.

associated with peripheral nerve pathology, for example, compression, tension, and friction.[2,39,48,49] A variety of chemical mediators have been implicated in the development of a hyperexcitable state in a neuron—for example, neurotrophins,[50,51] histamine,[52] and other inflammatory mediators,[53] which are thought to act through changes in gene expression,[45,50,51] changes in voltage gated sodium channel expression,[45] and a reduction in anterograde axoplasmic transport.[44,52]

The dorsal root ganglion appears to play a significant role in the pain associated with peripheral nerve pathology.[38,41] Mechanical microtrauma to and inflammation of peripheral nerves can cause the dorsal root ganglion to become hyperexcitable (sensitized).[41] The change in sensitivity allows what were weak, subthreshold stimuli to evoke pain and suprathreshold stimuli to evoke exaggerated pain (hyperalgesia). In addition, the dorsal root ganglion can develop mechanosensitivity, chemosensitivity, and thermal sensitivity, resulting in allodynia.[45] This change in sensitivity reflects a change in the physiology of the nerve and may be a component in the development of enhanced central sensitivity to pain and development of a chronic pain state.[38]

As noted previously, the PNS and CNS represent a continuous tissue tract. The pain and symptoms associated with musculoskeletal injury and/or peripheral nerve pathology can include changes that are the result of an alteration in the autonomic nervous system, which is considered part of the continuous tissue tract of the nervous system.[2,54] For example, catecholamines do not normally elicit pain. However, if a nerve is injured or if there is local inflammation, the catecholamines can induce pain (chemosensitivity) and they can maintain or enhance pain in inflamed tissues.[4]

Some patients who are treated for musculoskeletal injuries have signs that may be related to autonomic dysreflexia.[37] Wyke[55] demonstrated that stimulation of nociceptors in spinal joints resulted in reflex changes in the cardiovascular, respiratory, and endocrine systems. Dysregulated breathing has been documented in patients with chronic pain.[56] Patients with nonspecific arm pain have a reduced sympathetic vasoconstrictor response in the hand of the affected limb.[57] Thermal asymmetry has been documented in the hands of patients with neurogenic thoracic outlet syndrome.[58] Feinstein[59,60] has shown that injecting saline solution into the thoracic paraspinal muscles caused pallor, diaphoresis, bradycardia, and a drop in the blood pressure. These cardiovascular and respiratory changes are often associated with an alteration in the output from the autonomic nervous system.[37,54,61]

In patients with cumulative trauma disorder (CTD), signs of abnormal autonomic nervous system output can include (1) vasomotor reflexes leading to cool, pale skin,[57] (2) changes in the pattern of sweating (hypohidrosis and/or hyperhidrosis), (3) trophic changes in the skin, (4) hyperactive flexor withdrawal reflexes, and/or (5) paradoxical breathing patterns.[37] Edgelow has described paradoxical breathing as the predominant use of the scalene muscles for ventilation during quiet breathing versus normal ventilation, which is predominantly a function of the diaphragm.[37] Edgelow found that paradoxical breathing is present in most patients with CTD of the upper extremity.[37] A better appreciation of the contribution of the autonomic nervous system to the pathology and symptoms present in some patients with neurovascular entrapment may enhance the effectiveness of their treatment.

CLINICAL EXAMINATION AND TREATMENT OF NEUROVASCULAR ENTRAPMENT

For an effective evaluation of a patient with a neurovascular entrapment problem, the whole person must be addressed and involved in the evaluation and treatment processes. This philosophy requires the therapist to become the evaluator, teacher, and guide for the patient. Wherever possible the testing procedures should be performed by the patient so that he or she can learn to self-assess his or her status before and after treatment procedures. This self-assessment gives the patient control, thus decreasing the fear of movement or reinjury. In some cases, if a therapist uses his or her hands it may be detrimental to the patient in a lifelong sense if it leads to dependence. The concept of the patient gaining control of the problem(s) is fundamental and must be integrated into the initial patient contact for development of an effective self-management approach. Without an effective self-management strategy, the patient is at risk for recurrent problems and development of a chronic condition.

The Edgelow protocol for examination and treatment of neurovascular entrapment challenges the traditional musculoskeletal paradigm by placing the primary emphasis on the response of the neurovascular and neuromotor systems to injury.[62-64] The standard musculoskeletal evaluation centered on a biomechanical model of the musculoskeletal and nervous systems is adequate for patients with straightforward symptoms that appear to be of biomechanical origin. However, a biomechanical approach is inappropriate for patients with severe or irritable signs and symptoms that may be neurological or vascular in origin. Patients with neurovascular entrapment often have severe, irritable symptoms. First a subjective evaluation is conducted in a patient with a potential neurovascular entrapment problem to determine how the objective examination should proceed. The history of the condition is discussed with the patient. Key components that should be discussed include history of trauma, repetitive activities, sustained static or tension postures, such as computer keyboard work, or physical activities performed with a high level of cognitive demand, as seen in a pianist. The history should include a discussion of general health, including any potentially relevant medical conditions (e.g., asthma, diabetes, hypothyroidism). Phase I of differential diagnosis (medical screening) should be completed to ensure that the patient is appropriate for evaluation and intervention. (See Chapter 7 on medical screening.)

A discussion of the patient's symptoms and complaints should include questions that determine whether the neural or vascular system is a potential source of the problem. Symptoms relevant to the potential problem of neurovascular entrapment include complaints of fullness in the upper extremity; a feeling of swelling, tingling, pain, coldness, or numbness; or dropping things. In addition, the progression of the symptoms or complaints and the level of irritability should be determined. If pain is a major factor, then a functional pain questionnaire should be completed (see Chapter 32 on pain management). Motor changes of relevance to the potential problem of neurovascular entrapment include complaints of dropping things, weakness, or an inability to perform motor tasks that were done previously without difficulty. The level of neural irritability and the presence of peripheral or central sensitization should be determined by asking the patient what activities aggravate and ease the symptoms. When an extended period of time is required for symptoms to ease after provocation, irritability may be a cause. Sensitization is indicated when minor mechanical or normally nonnoxious stimuli, such as clothing on the skin, provoke pain. Vascular complaints relevant to the potential problem of neurovascular entrapment include complaints of fullness, swelling, abnormal skin color, or cool skin temperatures. A change in the vascular symptoms with a change in limb position is particularly significant.

In a biomechanical evaluation model the therapist examines the quantity and quality of active movements and determines whether there is pain, spasm, or resistance at an end feel. In patients with neurovascular entrapment, this procedure may evoke a significant flare and worsening of symptoms. In patients with neurovascular entrapment the "feel" of involuntary muscle tension can be the first sign of abnormality in assessing movement. This tension is often subtle and may occur earlier in the range of motion than where traditional biomechanical symptoms or the end feel normally occurs.[65] Moving into the range of motion to the initial onset of tension minimizes the risk of provoking adverse neurological or vascular consequences. In patients with suspected neurovascular entrapment who have symptoms suggestive of neural irritability and sensitization, the biomechanical examination and treatment techniques should be modified or deferred until the sensitivity and irritability of the nervous system are improved. See Table 18-2

TABLE 18-2 ■ SUGGESTED MODIFICATIONS TO A STANDARD BIOMECHANICAL EVALUATION

OBSERVATION			
Cervical and thoracic:	WNL	Kyphosis	Flat
Scapula:	Equal	High R/L	Low L/R
Lumbar:	WNL	Lordosis	Flat
Hands and feet: swelling, discoloration, other			
ACTIVE RANGE OF MOTION (FOR A PATIENT WITH UPPER QUADRANT SYMPTOMS)			
Cervical			
Flexion:	__________degrees		causes/increases symptoms
Extension:	__________ degrees		causes/increases symptoms
Rotation: (R):	__________ degrees		causes/increases symptoms
Rotation: (L):	__________ degrees		causes/increases symptoms
Lateral flexion (R):	__________ degrees		causes/increases symptoms
Lateral flexion (L):	__________ degrees		causes/increases symptoms
Shoulder Flexion			
(R) (with elbow extension):	______ degrees		causes/increases symptoms
(L) (with elbow extension):	______ degrees		causes/increases symptoms
(R) (with elbow flexion):	______ degrees		causes/increases symptoms
(L) (with elbow flexion):	______ degrees		causes/increases symptoms
Shoulder Internal Rotation (Reaching behind Back) (Functional Tension Test with Radial Nerve Bias)			
(R) position:		causes/increases symptoms	
(L) position:		causes/increases symptoms	
NEURAL EXAMINATION			
Passive Neck Flexion			
no/yes	_________ degrees		causes/increases symptoms
Upper Limb Neural Dynamic Test[4]			
(R) position:	_________		causes/increases symptoms
(L) position:	_________		causes/increases symptoms
Straight Leg Raising Test or Lasegue Test[66]			
Right:	_________ degrees		causes/increases symptoms
Left:	_________ degrees		causes/increases symptoms
Tinel Sign[66]			
(Normal = 0; Mild = 1+; Moderate = 2+; Severe = 3+)			
Supraclavicular region:		Right	Left
Elbow:		Right	Left
Wrist:	Median	Right	Left
	Ulnar	Right	Left

TABLE 18-2 ■ SUGGESTED MODIFICATIONS TO A STANDARD BIOMECHANICAL EVALUATION—cont'd

KABAT TESTS[71]

Strength Tests[71]

Flexor carpi ulnaris:	(R)/5	(L)/5
Adductor pollicis:	(R)/5	(L)/5

Thinker Pose[71] (Isometric Contraction of Longus Colli) (Temporary Strengthening of the Flexor Carpi Ulnaris and Adductor Pollicis)

no/yes—Which muscles are affected and by what amount?

VASCULAR INTEGRITY

Temperature of Hands (Ambient Room Temperature)

Right: (index)	(digiti minimi)
Left: (index)	(digiti minimi)

Adson Test[66] (Change in Pulse Pressure)

Right after:	1 minute	2 minutes	3 minutes
Left after:	1 minute	2 minutes	3 minutes

Elevated Arm Stress Test (EAST)[66] (Change in Pulse Pressure)

Right after:	1 minute	2 minutes	3 minutes
Left after:	1 minute	2 minutes	3 minutes

SENSATION[66]

Localization

Stereognosis

Graphesthesia

BREATHING PATTERN (ABILITY TO RELAX THE SCALENE MUSCLES WITH QUIET BREATHING)

Normal or dysfunctional pattern

PALPATION FINDINGS

(Tenderness: Normal = 0; Mild = 1+; Moderate = 2+; Severe = 3+)

Scalene muscles:	Right:	Left:
Subclavius:	Right:	Left:
Pectoralis minor:	Right:	Left:

L, Left; R, right; WNL, within normal limits.

for suggested modifications to a standard biomechanical evaluation.

One component of the examination involves evaluating the integrity of the vascular system in the extremities. The hands or feet should be inspected for discoloration, and the skin temperature should be determined in each of the peripheral nerve territories present in the affected limb. Cool, cyanotic skin can be an indication of arterial insufficiency or sympathetic dysreflexia in the area, whereas swelling can be an indication of inflammation and venous or lymphatic insufficiency. An Adson test and the elevated arm stress test (EAST) can be used to evaluate vascular integrity by determining whether the pulse pressure decreases with a change in the position of the limb.[66] The Adson test and EAST should be performed on both upper extremities, and the pulse pressure evaluated at 1, 2, and 3 minutes. These tests may be modified or deferred depending on the level of neural irritability found.

Sensory changes may be subtle and are not always accompanied by obvious motor dysfunction. The most common complaint with neurovascular entrapment of the upper extremity is "I drop things," yet standard tests of strength, light touch, and two-point discrimination may have normal results. Therapists often think of this problem as motor until our standard tests fail to demonstrate motor dysfunction. Subtle changes in the somatosensory cortex can occur as a consequence of repetitive motions, particularly when performed under conditions of intense concentration or in the presence of pain.[67-69] Byl observed severe degradation in the representation of the hand in the somatosensory cortex of owl monkeys that were trained in a behavior of rapid, active opening and closing of the hand under conditions of high cognitive drive.[68] In addition, Byl[67] found a significant difference in response on some sensory integration and praxis tests in human subjects with diagnoses of tendinitis and focal dystonia. Byl has postulated that similar changes can be identified in humans with repetitive strain injuries with the use of Jean Ayers's tests of sensory localization, stereognosis, and graphesthesia.[69]

An assessment of the patient's breathing pattern at rest and palpation of the subclavius, pectoralis minor, and scalene muscles should be performed. The normal breathing pattern at rest is primarily diaphragmatic (Figure 18-2). However, patients with neurovascular entrapment often demonstrate a breathing pattern at rest that relies predominantly on the scalene muscles. The scalene breathing pattern mechanically narrows the thoracic outlet area, thus potentially perpetuating a neurovascular entrapment syndrome in the area. The scalene breathing pattern may be a sign of protective posturing. Palpation is used to determine whether tenderness or tightness is present. Palpation of the subclavius, pectoralis minor, and scalene muscles is significant because of the relationship these muscles have with the subclavian vein, brachial plexus components, and subclavian artery, respectively. The results of the palpation should be correlated to the neurological and vascular changes found elsewhere in the extremity.

Neurovascular Entrapment Examination

There are some common symptom patterns characteristic of neurovascular entrapment that alert the therapist to modify the physical examination. In addition to the symptoms mentioned previously, the following patterns help the therapist recognize a patient with a potentially sensitized nervous system.

Symptom Patterns Characteristic of Neurovascular Entrapment

1. Symptoms are severe and irritable.
2. Function is markedly reduced in the target task (injury-producing activity) and activities of daily living.
3. The patient reports feeling that his or her emotions are in a state of "being out of control."

In a modified examination scheme designed to evaluate for the presence of a neurovascular entrapment syndrome, patients typically have six signs. These signs, in addition to the more traditional musculoskeletal signs, are used as guides in determining the effectiveness of treatment.

Six Common Signs of Neurovascular Entrapment

1. Abnormal hand temperature within the following parameters:
   a. Cold hands defined as in the 70° F range at rest and during activity at the target task
   b. Asymmetry between the temperatures of the second digit and the fifth digit, with the fifth digit being colder.[70]
   c. Asymmetry between hands in which there is an abnormal temperature cooling response to diaphragmatic breathing, aerobic walking, and repeated use of the upper extremities in an activity such as bouncing a gymnastic ball.
2. Abnormal breathing pattern: accessory, chest, or paradoxical rather than diaphragmatic.
3. Abnormal mobility and sensitivity of the nervous system: specifically the dura, the brachial plexus, or the sciatic nerve or sacral plexus.
4. Cardiovascular deconditioning: patient has a low level of endurance and is easily fatigued.
5. Sensory dysfunction of the hand at the cortical level: abnormal tactile localization, graphesthesia, and stereognosis.
6. A positive Kabat[71] sign: weakness of the flexor pollicis brevis in the shortened range of adduction that is unilateral and reversed with a gentle 30-second isometric contraction of the longus colli obtained with the "thinker pose" (Figure 18-3).

This combination of symptoms and signs identifies neurovascular consequences of the injury. Improvements in these signs and symptoms serve as markers that identify treatment effectiveness—namely, decrease in pain, improvement in function, and a feeling of being more in control.

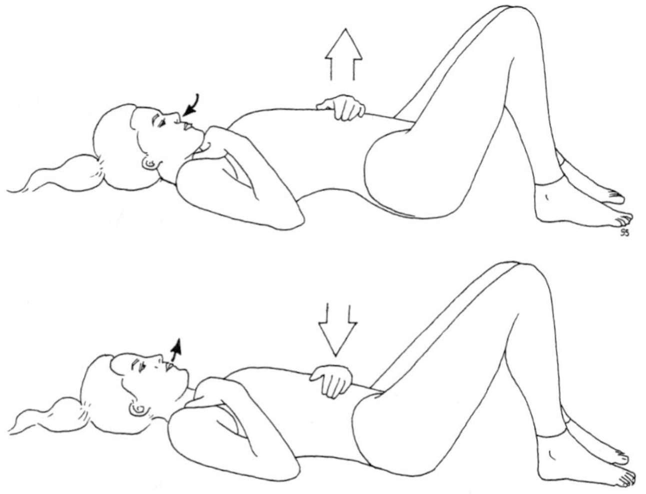

Figure 18-2 ■ Diaphragmatic breathing. As the client inhales, the stomach should rise and the lordosis in the low back should increase. During exhalation the stomach should fall and the back should flatten against the floor.

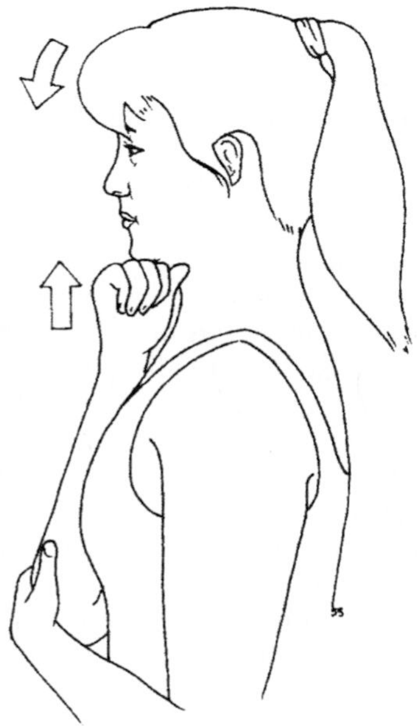

Figure 18-3 ■ The "thinker pose." Self-traction is applied by using gentle upward pressure from one upper extremity onto the chin.

Neurovascular Entrapment Examination Procedures

Neurodynamics of the upper extremity is assessed with the use of upper limb neural dynamic tests as described by Butler.[4] Passive neck flexion is examined to assess dural sensitivity, whereas the straight leg raise test is used to assess the sensitivity of the sciatic nerve and sacral plexus. In addition to these passive neural dynamic tests performed by the examining therapist, the patient is taught an "arm self-test" to use as a self-assessment technique.

The arm self-test is an adaptation of the brachial plexus tension test. This is an active test that the patient, the medical provider, and the physical therapist can use as an indicator of upper quarter neural sensitivity. The test provides immediate feedback regarding the patient's response to an exercise or other form of intervention. The test results can be used as an indicator of a change in patient status. The test is nonspecific, meaning that it does not indicate which structure is the source of the protective tension response. The test is an important tool that helps the patient recognize and manage symptom flares. The arm self-test is one of the self-assessment tools that encourage the patient to take control of his or her treatment.

The arm self-test is performed by guiding the standing patient through a series of positions using the upper extremity (Figure 18-4). The sequence goes from position zero to five, with zero being the position of least general tension on the brachial plexus and five being a position of maximum elongation and general tension on the brachial plexus. Care must be taken to educate the patient to stop at the first sensation of tension and not linger with the arm in any self-test position that provokes symptoms. The test sequence begins in the *zero position* with the patient's hand resting on the chest. In *position one* the patient's arm is straight at the side; in *position two* the patient abducts the arm to shoulder height with the palm pronated. In *position three* the patient maintains abduction to shoulder height while supinating the forearm and hand; *position four* is performed by maintaining position three while extending the wrist. If the patient does not experience tension or pain in the previous positions, he or she can progress to *position five* by adding cervical lateral flexion away from the side being tested. Coppieters,[72] in a cadaver study of nerve gliding, noted increased strain on the medial nerve in positions of wrist extension combined with elbow extension; thus position four of the arm self-test can be too provocative to use on the affected extremity in a patient with severe symptoms. (Please refer to the references at the end of this chapter for more information on neural dynamic tests.)

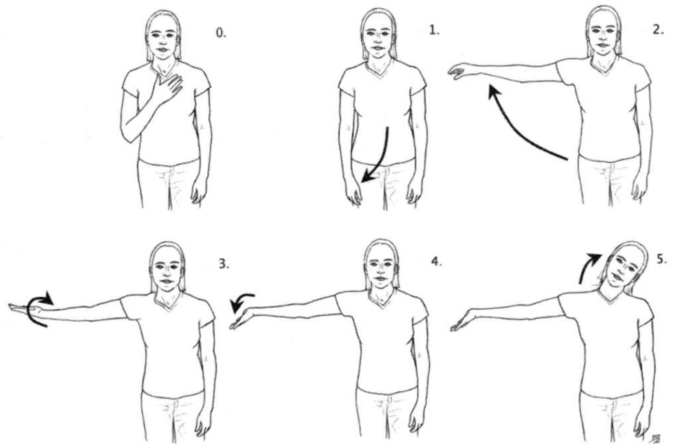

Figure 18-4 ■ Demonstration of arm self-test positions. The arm self-test is an active upper extremity neural dynamic test.

Hand temperature is assessed with an infrared hand-held thermometer. Measurements are made of the second digit (innervated by the upper roots of the brachial plexus) and fifth digit (innervated by the lower roots). Temperature is assessed during rest, diaphragmatic breathing, walking on a treadmill, and repeated movements of the upper extremities while a gymnastic ball is being bounced. A normal response is an increase in temperature in response to these activities. A cooling response is considered abnormal.

Breathing pattern is assessed by palpating the scalene muscles in the area between the inferior border of the sternocleidomastoid and superior to the clavicle. This procedure is best done while the patient performs relaxed inhalation. The scalene muscles are normally quiet during relaxed inhalation. Contraction of the scalene muscles and elevation of the sternum are considered to be abnormal during quiet inhalation. Patients are instructed to breathe with the "belly" only (diaphragmatic breathing). If they are unable to do this, breathing is considered to be paradoxical.

Cardiovascular fitness is assessed by treadmill walking. The patient is instructed to walk at a speed that does not cause an increase in symptoms for up to 20 minutes. Over time, patients are encouraged to increase their walking speed until they reach a level where they are aerobically fit on the basis of standard measures.

CNS sensory dysfunction of the hand (specifically tactile localization, graphesthesia, and stereognosis) is assessed by the methods of Byl.[69]

Hand strength is assessed by examining for the presence of a Kabat sign.[71] The patient is instructed to hold the arm at the side with the elbow flexed to 90 degrees and fully supinated. The wrist is positioned in neutral flexion-extension with the fingers fully extended and the thumb in the shortened range of adduction and flexion (thumb in the plane of the palm). The distal phalanx of the thumb is held in full extension. This starting position inhibits the median innervated muscles of the palm and finger flexors. A manual muscle test is done to test the strength of flexor pollicis brevis and adductor pollicis in the shortened range. If there is a "giving way" at the metacarpophalangeal joint, then this is quantified using a "thumbometer," an inexpensive device consisting of an eye drop bottle attached to a blood pressure cuff sphygmomanometer. Clinical experience demonstrates that after longus colli isometric contraction there is a strengthening of the affected muscles in the thumb. There will be a weakening effect on thumb strength if the patient has cervical instability during the performance of activities or exercises. This indicates the activity is too much for the patient at that time. If there is no effect on thumb strength then the patient is stable enough for the activity.

Neurovascular Entrapment Interventions

Treatment must follow the same principles that guide the examination. The patient is taught self-assessment techniques and strategies so that the patient has control of the progression of treatment and activities of daily living. The patient may use any of the following self-assessment techniques, as appropriate, to guide the course of treatment: a pain scale, a thermometer to test skin temperature, a neurodynamic test, or a Kabat strength test. Any treatment or activity that increases symptoms, protective posturing, or tension is modified or discontinued.

Treatment is begun using sensory motor integration with an emphasis on functional skills (e.g., breathing, balance, and hand function) in a manner that does not cause irritation of the patient's condition. The patient is guided through a series of breathing exercises designed to improve the circulation to the extremities, calm the nervous system, and retrain the scalene muscles, if appropriate. The breathing exercises are progressed through the use of foam rollers (Figure 18-5). These are used to increase the mobility of the spine and rib cage. The breathing exercises are combined with functional movements of the trunk and extremities in a manner that mobilizes the nervous system. Once the patient is able to manage the symptoms, the treatment can progress to stabilization exercises with a gym ball (Figure 18-6). If the patient has vestibular, balance, or sensory integration deficits, then specific techniques for vestibular, balance, or sensory retraining would be added.

Our intention is not to present every component of a total treatment program but rather highlight those core components that address the neurovascular consequences of the injury. Our experience is that modifying these neurovascular consequences is the first step and the foundation for recovery.

Core Components of Treatment

The reversible weakness of the thumb is addressed by strengthening the longus colli muscle. This is accomplished by a 30-second isometric contraction using the "thinker pose" (see Figure 18-3) and specific muscle reeducation for

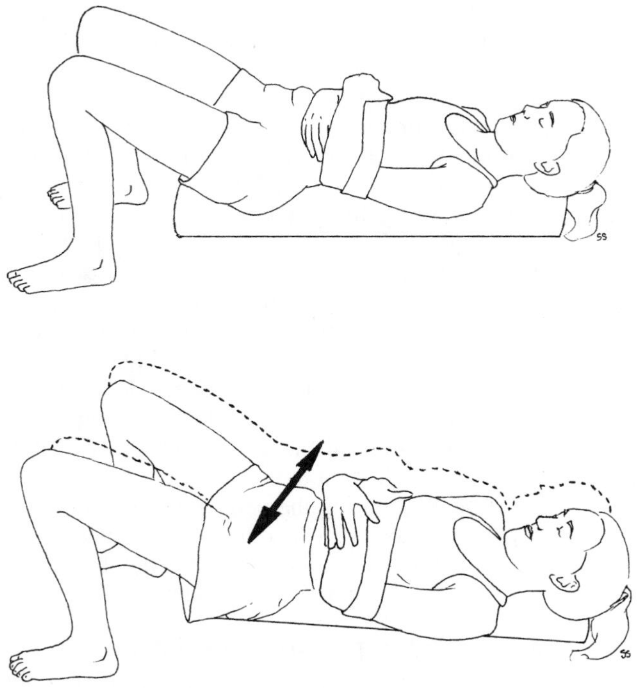

Figure 18-5 ■ Foam roller exercise for mobilization of the spine. The roller is placed underneath the spine with the client in the supine position. The client gently rolls from side to side to increase mobility of the spine.

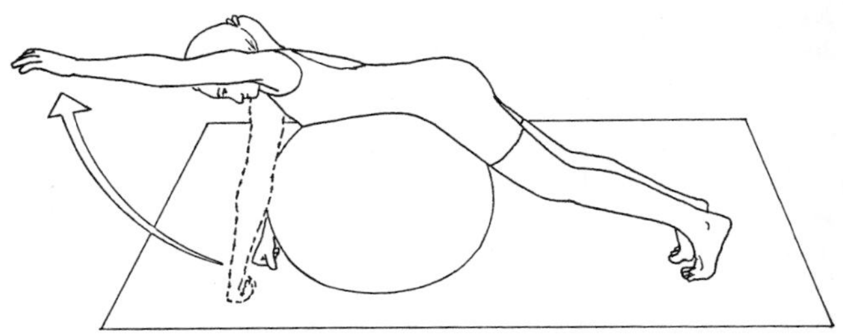

Figure 18-6 ■ Patient in a quadruped position on a therapy ball with the chin tucked and the neck straight. The patient can lift an upper or lower extremity to provide a challenge to the muscles that stabilize the spine.

the longus colli with Jull's protocol.[73] The expected effect of the thinker pose is to reverse the identified weakness of the thumb. The patient is taught to minimize mechanical stress to the cervical and thoracic spine through instruction in body mechanics. An important concept is to train the patient to identify the coactivation position for stability of the neck and to visualize that position before moving the body away from the center of gravity or moving the arm. This method has the patient assume the thinker pose to stimulate the deep neck flexors to contract before the movement is performed.

The temperature, neurodynamic, and breathing dysfunctions are addressed by training the patient to perform relaxed diaphragmatic breathing with spinal motion (see Figure 18-2). The expected outcomes are to normalize hand temperature and increase the range of motion while decreasing sensitivity to the neurodynamic tests. Low cardiovascular endurance is addressed by having the patient begin a progressive aerobic conditioning program of walking. Because the examination identifies six signs of dysfunction, the goals of treatment are to normalize these six signs. Clinical experience teaches that as these signs improve there is a reduction in pain and an increase in function.

Role of the Patient

Maximizing the treatment response requires a unique partnership between the physical therapist and the patient that facilitates the patient's feeling of being in control. The feeling of being in control is thought to have a positive impact on the response to treatment. Patients are taught methods for self-assessment of the immediate effect of the treatment. They are taught to assess their responses to the core program on the basis of signs of hand strength and hand temperature and mobility and sensitivity of the nervous system. The patients are provided with self-assessment tools and treatment devices. The details of the exercise program are provided in a patient booklet, audiotapes, and a videotape, which can be found at www.edgelow.com.

References

To enhance this text and add value for the reader, all references are included on the companion Evolve site that accompanies this textbook. This online service will, when available, provide a link for the reader to a Medline abstract for the article cited. There are 73 cited references and other general references for this chapter, with the majority of those articles being evidence-based citations.

CASE STUDY

The following case example describes brief components of this patient's physical therapy encounter. This presentation is not meant to describe a complete case but rather to illuminate key concepts in the clinical reasoning behind the physical therapy examination, assessment, and plan of care in a patient with signs and symptoms of neurovascular entrapment. Video clips of the patient using self-assessment techniques to evaluate his response to treatment are included.

PATIENT DESCRIPTION

The patient is a 27-year-old, right-handed caterer who 3 weeks ago, while lifting a box, felt a "pop" and strain in his right forearm. He was referred to physical therapy with a diagnosis of "forearm strain." He has avoided using his right arm for 3 weeks, but his symptoms have not significantly improved.

The patient drew a body chart indicating symptoms not only in his right forearm but also in his upper arm, his wrist, and the right side of his neck (Figure 18-7). On further questioning he stated that another component of his work was developing menus. He develops menus using a laptop computer perched on some shelves in a cramped office space with his right arm sustained overhead in an awkward position.

Clinical Reasoning

Diagnostic hypothesis is based on the subjective examination findings:

1. Potential soft tissue strain of forearm flexors based on the mechanism of injury
2. Potential altered neural dynamics with sensitization on the basis of:
   a. History of receptive use of the upper extremities in sustained awkward positions
   b. Pattern of symptoms that do not fit localized forearm strain or cervical radiculopathy
   c. Lack of response to 3 weeks of rest and self-care measures.

PHYSICAL EXAMINATION

Figure 18-8 is a photograph of the patient's sitting posture on initial examination. He demonstrated forward head posture and mildly protected posture of his right arm. Based on the patient's history, the nervous system was considered a potential source of dysfunction. (See Table 18-2 for suggested modifications to a biomechanically based musculoskeletal examination to use when the nervous system is considered a significant source of dysfunction.)

The patient was instructed to complete active movement testing just to the point of feeling tension or resistance to movement. This modification to the physical examination was meant to minimize the potential for a significant flare of symptoms from provocation testing of potentially irritable neurovascular structures while still providing a repeatable measure for reassessment.

The patient moved through full cervical range without complaints of tension or resistance. On palpation the scalene muscles were noted to be active during quiet breathing. The arm self-test indicated a restriction of mobility in his right brachial plexus as compared with his uninvolved left side. He indicated the onset of tension and the reproduction of his forearm symptom with the arm self-test.

Clinical Reasoning

Diagnostic hypothesis is based on physical examination findings:

1. Cervical postural dysfunction
2. Altered neural dynamics based on the presence of:
   a. Early onset of protective muscle tension and reproduction of symptoms with arm self-test (indicator of possible neurovascular entrapment)
   b. Scalene breathing pattern (indicator of possible adaptive response to pain)

INTERVENTION

The patient was taught a neural dynamic self-assessment technique to evaluate his response to activity. We called this his "arm self-test." If he had a negative response to an exercise or activities of daily living, as evidenced by an increase in symptoms or a decrease in the range of his arm self-test, he was instructed to modify or discontinue the activity and perform a self-treatment that restored his tension-free range.

Videos 18-1 through 18-3 demonstrate the patient performing his arm self-test, engaging in an exercise on a foam roller, and repeating his arm self-test immediately after engaging in the foam roller exercise. The intention of the foam roller exercise was to help him mobilize his thoracic spine to improve his ability to correct his cervical posture on his own. After the roller exercise he demonstrated a dramatic increase in tension-free range of his right arm self-test. The difference was readily apparent to the patient and helped him grasp the concept of sensitivity of the nerves as well as the concept of the nerves as a continuous tract in which cervical posture correction was a key component of his treatment.

After the foam roller exercise his right-sided neck discomfort was unchanged. A trial of cervical traction with the use of a towel (Figure 18-9) was found to relieve his neck discomfort without producing forearm symptoms or worsening his arm self-test. During the first treatment, the techniques that he found successful for restoring his neural mobility were foam roller exercises, diaphragmatic breathing (see Figure 18-2), and supine cervical traction (see Figure 18-9). Therefore those interventions were the focus of his home program instruction.

The patient was issued a foam roller and instructed in spine mobilization exercises (see Figure 18-5). He was instructed in the towel cervical traction technique for symptom management (see Figure 18-9). A cervical posture correction exercise termed the "thinker position" (see Figure 18-3) was added to his home exercise program as a form of dynamic cervical posture correction. In addition, he was instructed to walk daily to maintain his aerobic capacity. Figure 18-8 shows the patient's posture before the initial examination. Figure 18-10 shows the patient's posture immediately after the initial treatment that included foam roller exercise, towel cervical traction, instruction in the self-assessment of upper extremity neural dynamic test, and dynamic cervical posture correction via the thinker position.

At 4 weeks (visit 4) treatment progressed to light resistive exercises. At this stage the patient no longer demonstrated signs of neural irritability. The patient was placed prone on a therapy ball to perform exercises that promote scapular

Continued

CASE STUDY—cont'd

stabilization, postural strengthening, and functional grip (see Figure 18-6). At visit 5 he reported a flare of his symptoms and what he did to resolve the problem. The patient experienced a flare of symptoms after an attempt to progress his strengthening exercises. He discontinued the strengthening exercise and used his symptom relief techniques of breathing exercises and towel cervical traction. He subsequently used the arm self-test to determine which strengthening exercise he could tolerate without producing a protective tension response of his arm. The sixth and final treatment session focused on problem solving related to symptom management, upper-quarter stabilization during simulated work tasks, and progression to recreational activities. Emphasis was placed on continued self-assessment of the response of the nervous system to the progression of activity.

OUTCOME

The early success with self-guided treatment set the stage for teaching the patient to evaluate the effect of any activity, manage symptoms with one or two easing techniques, and ultimately progress his own activity level. This approach gave the patient control of his problem so that he was capable of managing a flare of his symptoms.

The patient received a total of six treatments. At the time of discharge his grip strength was equal bilaterally and his upper extremity neural dynamic test results were equal bilaterally. At this point he was working full-time, regular duty with ergonomic improvements at his workstation.

DISCUSSION

This case illustrates the importance of evaluating the role of the nervous system in patients with symptoms associated with repetitive use of the upper extremity. In this case example the patient's problem did not seem to be chronic, because he reported a specific recent injury. However, on further investigation he also reported symptoms that were chronic in nature, which could have delayed his recovery if not appropriately assessed on initial examination. There can be a wide spectrum of presentations of neurovascular entrapments ranging from subtle signs and symptoms of nervous system involvement to dramatic, life-altering, complex problems in patients who have undergone multiple medical and surgical interventions without obtaining symptom relief. The key to success in treating patients with neurovascular entrapments is recognizing the signs and symptoms of subtle nervous system involvement early. Neural sensitization[4] and possible processing changes in the CNS[67-69] necessitate evaluation of the nervous system as a potential source of symptoms in patients with symptoms of CTD. If the issues of nervous system irritability and sensitization are not addressed during evaluation and throughout treatment, then the risk for increasing the patient's symptoms and continuing the cycle of nervous system hypersensitivity is high.

The indicators that this patient may have had a nervous system dysfunction were his history of repetitive work in an awkward position, the pattern of his symptoms, and his lack of response to standard medical care and rest. The indicators of nervous system dysfunction on physical examination were the restricted upper limb neural dynamic test (arm self-test), altered breathing pattern, and lack of objective signs of a localized soft tissue strain. Other objective indicators not assessed initially that may have further guided the treatment would be Kabat testing,[71] measuring the temperature of the hands,[70] and sensory testing of localization, graphesthesia, and stereognosis.[69]

A key concept to keep in mind is the role of education in treating patients with a problem such as neurovascular entrapment. Patient-clinician communication is extremely important when dealing with all patients, but the clinician's communication skills are really challenged when dealing with a patient who has a neurovascular entrapment. Describing the dysfunction of a neurovascular entrapment to the patient in succinct, nonmedical terminology can be quite difficult, but it is a critical step in the patient encounter to help him or her develop an understanding of what is wrong so he or she can engage in self-treatment. Teaching the patient self-assessment tools restores the patient's control, allowing the patient to guide his or her own treatment and to be more responsible for his or her own well-being.

QUESTIONS

1. How would you describe a form of neural sensitization (mechanical allodynia) to a patient?

   Answer: I say to the patient: Have you ever touched a hot plate? When you touched that hot plate what did your hand do? It quickly pulled away. Your body has reflexes that protect you, like tightening the muscles in your arm so you can pull your hand away from the hot plate. What if you touched this smooth, cool sink, but your finger did not recognize the smooth, cool sink. Instead your finger sent a signal to your brain that it was touching a hot plate. That's what your body does when it has experienced pain for a period of time—it becomes sensitized, meaning it starts to sense things that are normally not painful as now being painful. The body then tenses or tries to withdraw and get away from what it senses as pain.

2. How would you instruct a patient to do an active self-test of the arm?

   Answer: I say to the patient: I am going to ask you to place your arm in a sequence of positions. The positions are numbered from 0-5. I want you to stop when you feel tightness anywhere in your arm or if you feel an increase or change in your pain. Remember the number where you stopped. We will redo the self-test after we have done some exercises. That way you can decide which exercise helps you the most.

   After the patient has completed one self-test and one form of treatment followed by a reassessment self-test, then I help the patient interpret the body's response. If your self-test result was worse (lower number, less arm range), it means that your body responded as though it were touching the hot plate—it tightened and tried to withdraw. This means that the exercise we tried is not a helpful exercise for you at this time. If your self-test result was better (higher number, greater range), then this exercise was helpful; your body responded in a way that indicated calming of the protective response. The self-test is something you can always use to help you evaluate whether an exercise or activity is going to be helpful or hurtful for your arms.

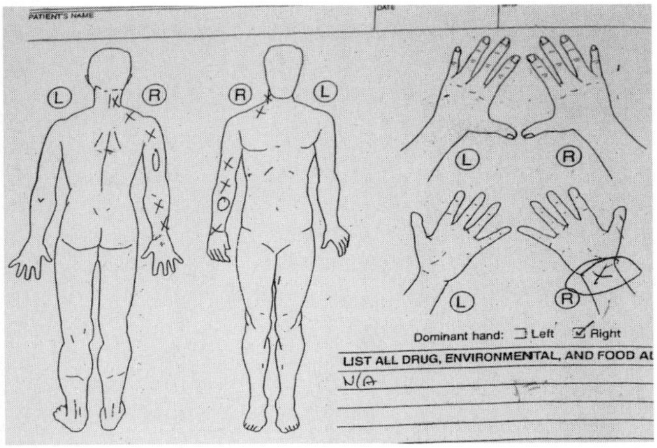

Figure 18-7 ■ Body chart with symptomatic areas marked by the patient.

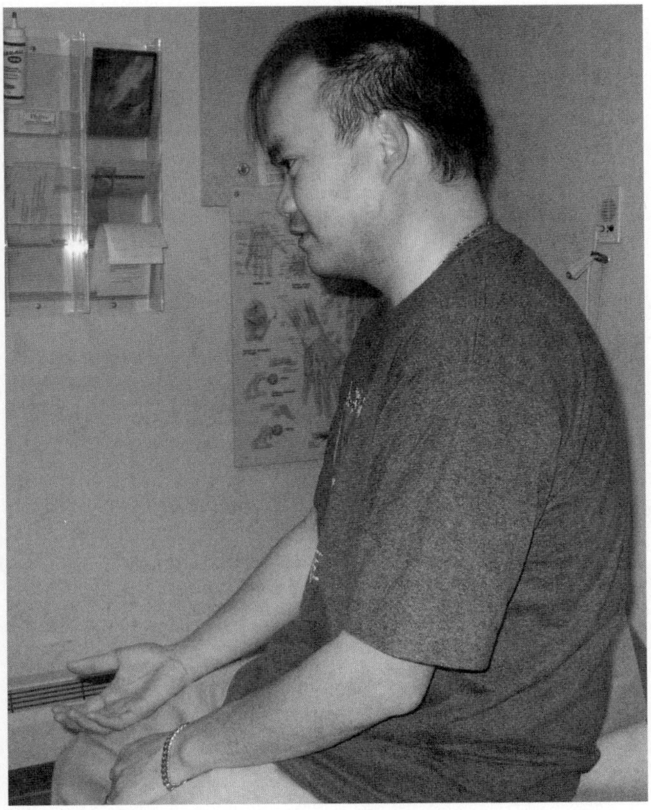

Figure 18-8 ■ The patient's posture before initial examination.

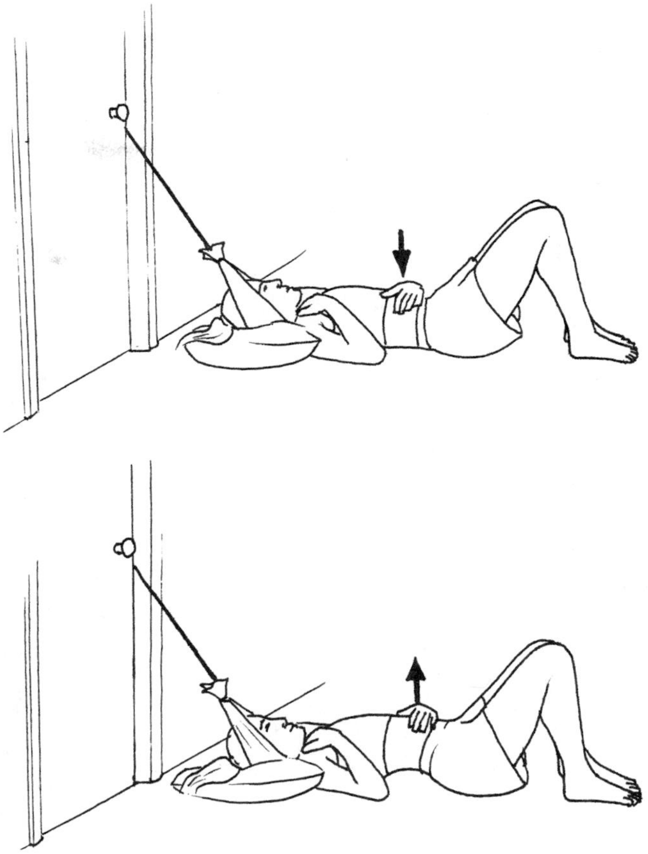

Figure 18-9 ■ Towel traction unit. Through arching of the low back, the amount of traction is increased slightly. Through flattening of the low back, the amount of traction is decreased slightly.

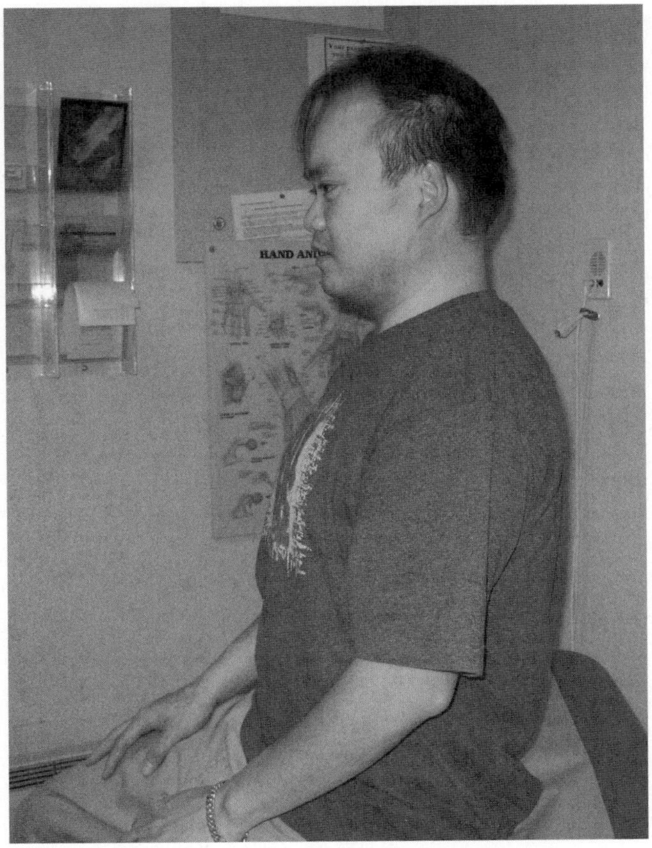

Figure 18-10 ■ The patient's posture immediately after the initial treatment.

CHAPTER 19 Multiple Sclerosis

GAIL L. WIDENER, PT, PhD

KEY TERMS

autoimmune disease
axonal damage
benign
demyelination
disease-modifying agents
exacerbation
immune system
lesion
neuroprotection
plaques
primary progressive
progressive relapsing
relapse
relapsing remitting
remission
secondary progressive

OBJECTIVES

After reading this chapter the student or therapist will be able to:

1. Describe the pathological processes, prevalence, and clinical presentation of people with multiple sclerosis.
2. Compare and contrast the types of multiple sclerosis and the common disease progression in each.
3. Discuss the medical management of the disease and the disease symptoms.
4. Describe how the International Classification of Functioning, Disability and Health provides a common language for describing the impact of disease on people with multiple sclerosis and how it provides a framework for rehabilitation management.
5. Describe the outcome measures that can be used to examine people with multiple sclerosis that cover body system problems (impairments), functional skill and activity limitations, and participation restrictions.
6. Develop a rehabilitation plan of care using evidence-based interventions to maximize patient function and quality of life.

OVERVIEW OF MULTIPLE SCLEROSIS

Pathophysiology

Multiple sclerosis (MS) is a chronic, inflammatory disease of the brain, optic nerve, and spinal cord mediated by the immune system.[1] It is characterized by lesions of disseminated focal demyelination accompanied by variable axon damage and destruction and reactive gliosis. Initially, MS was thought to be a disease of the white matter (WM); however, recent investigations have shown that the gray matter (GM) is significantly involved. Lesions found in the GM typically contain demyelination and loss of neurons without the immune system infiltrates and inflammation characteristic of lesions in the WM. Tissue damage has been found outside the focal lesions throughout the GM that is associated with brain and spinal cord atrophy. These areas of demyelination and axonal damage interfere with normal conduction of neural signals, leading to a disruption of function.

Early in the course of the disease, focal inflammatory WM lesions are composed of immune system components that produce demyelination, axonal injury, and loss of oligodendrocytes. Astrogliosis activated by the damaged neurons produces gliotic scarring (visualized as sclerosis in postmortem brain tissue) called *plaques*. Active disease is followed by periods of remission in which acute inflammation is reduced. Axonal remyelination occurs but is highly variable and is related to recovery of function during periods of remission. The degree of axonal loss is associated with the severity of the inflammation; however, axons are spared in the majority of WM lesions. Treatment in the initial stages of the disease is aimed at reducing inflammation and immune system infiltration with disease-modifying agents (DMAs).

Later in the course of the disease, inflammation becomes uncommon while demyelination and axonal loss continue, suggesting replacement by a neurodegenerative disease process. Disease progression becomes more constant with a lack of exacerbation. The motor, sensory, and cognitive disability that accumulates in the advanced stages of the disease appears to be associated with the cortical GM pathology.[2] Owing to the lack of inflammation, DMAs have not been shown to be beneficial in the later stages of the disease.

Incidence and Prevalence

MS is the primary cause of nontraumatic disability in young and middle-aged adults and the most common inflammatory condition of the central nervous system (CNS). It is reported that approximately 350,000 to 400,000 people in the United States and over 2.5 million people worldwide have the disease.[3,4] People are most commonly diagnosed at age 20 to 50 years, with an average age of 32. However, MS can be diagnosed in people of any age. Approximately 5% of all patients with MS are diagnosed before their sixteenth birthday.[5]

MS is found in people who reside above the northern or below the southern 40° latitude with greater frequency than those who live closer to the equator (Figure 19-1). Given the

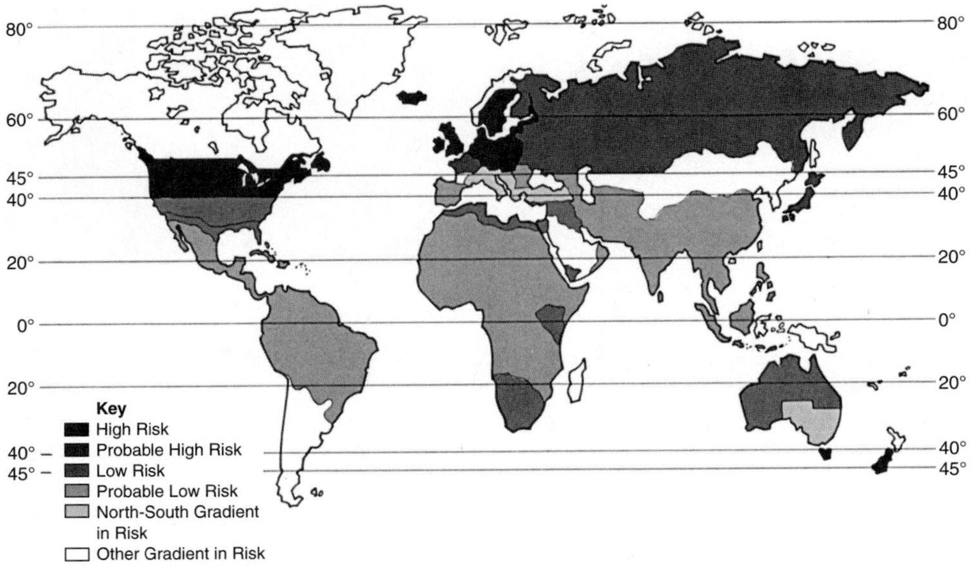

Figure 19-1 ■ World distribution of multiple sclerosis. (From Multiple Sclerosis Resource Center, www.msrc.co.uk.)

increased sun exposure of people living closer to the equator, lack of vitamin D is being investigated as a potential factor contributing to disease development.[6] Many researchers believe that exposure to an infectious agent may trigger the disease process: Epstein-Barr virus is currently considered a likely candidate.

Women are affected two to four times more frequently than men. Even so, men are more likely to have a more aggressive disease progression and a worse prognosis.[4,7] Caucasians with Northern European ancestry have the greatest incidence of MS, whereas people of Asian, African, or Hispanic ethnicity are at lower risk. African Americans have a lower incidence, but become disabled earlier than Caucasians, suggesting that tissue destruction occurs earlier and more rapidly.[8] Inuits, Yakutes, Hutterites, Hungarian Romani, Norwegian Lapps, Australian Aborigines, and New Zealand Maoris do not appear to develop MS.[9] Being diagnosed with MS may be related to age, gender, genetics, geography, or ethnic background. An identical twin with MS means that the other twin will have a 25% chance of diagnosis, suggesting something beyond genetics. Having a first-degree relative with MS will increase the risk of disease from 1/750 to 1/40.[3]

Types of Multiple Sclerosis and Clinical Characteristics

At least four types of MS have been identified (Figure 19-2). Although the course of the disease is highly variable even within a subtype of MS, there are characteristics common to each.

The initial neurological episode or attack is typically identified as *clinical isolated syndrome* (CIS). Symptoms must last for at least 24 hours and can be monofocal or multifocal. If there are lesions present on magnetic resonance imaging (MRI), there is a high risk of developing MS. In one group of people with CIS followed for 20 years, 63% were diagnosed with definite MS.[10]

Relapsing remitting MS (RRMS) represents about 85% of people with MS, characterized by exacerbations (attacks, flairs, relapses) that can last days to months and are typically followed by periods of improved function. During remissions, function can return to prerelapse levels, but most frequently it does not recover fully. Attacks normally occur with a frequency of one or two per year. Approximately 90% of people with RRMS transition to SPMS after 20 years or around 40 years of age.

In *secondary progressive* MS (SPMS), relapses decrease in frequency over time and convert to a slow steady progression of increasing disability or disease severity. Relapses may occur early in SPMS but gradually lessen over time. People with RRMS eventually convert to SPMS 10 to 20 years after diagnosis.[11]

It is thought that the clinical disability associated with SPMS results from the neurodegeneration that occurs as a result of tissue injury that accumulates from early in the disease process. In addition to less inflammation, there is a greater amount of brain atrophy in people with SPMS compared with RRMS. Figure 19-3 shows the natural history of RRMS and SPMS, comparing the change in brain volume with increasing clinical disability and disease burden.[2]

Primary progressive MS (PPMS) is less common, affecting only 10% to 15% of people with MS. From disease onset, progression results in a gradual worsening of symptoms without relapses. People tend to be older when diagnosed (late 30s or early 40s), have fewer abnormalities on brain MRI, and respond less favorably to standard MS therapies. Progressive myelopathy is commonly associated with PPMS.

Progressive relapsing MS (PRMS) is the least common form (5%). This form of MS typically begins with a progressive course with clear relapses or exacerbations.

Benign MS is identified when symptoms occur once and never recur. This happens in roughly 25% of cases.[12] Recently, Sayao and colleagues[13] reported that 52% of people with benign MS had not developed MS 20 years later. However, the remainder of people went on to develop MS, with at least 21% requiring the use of a cane.

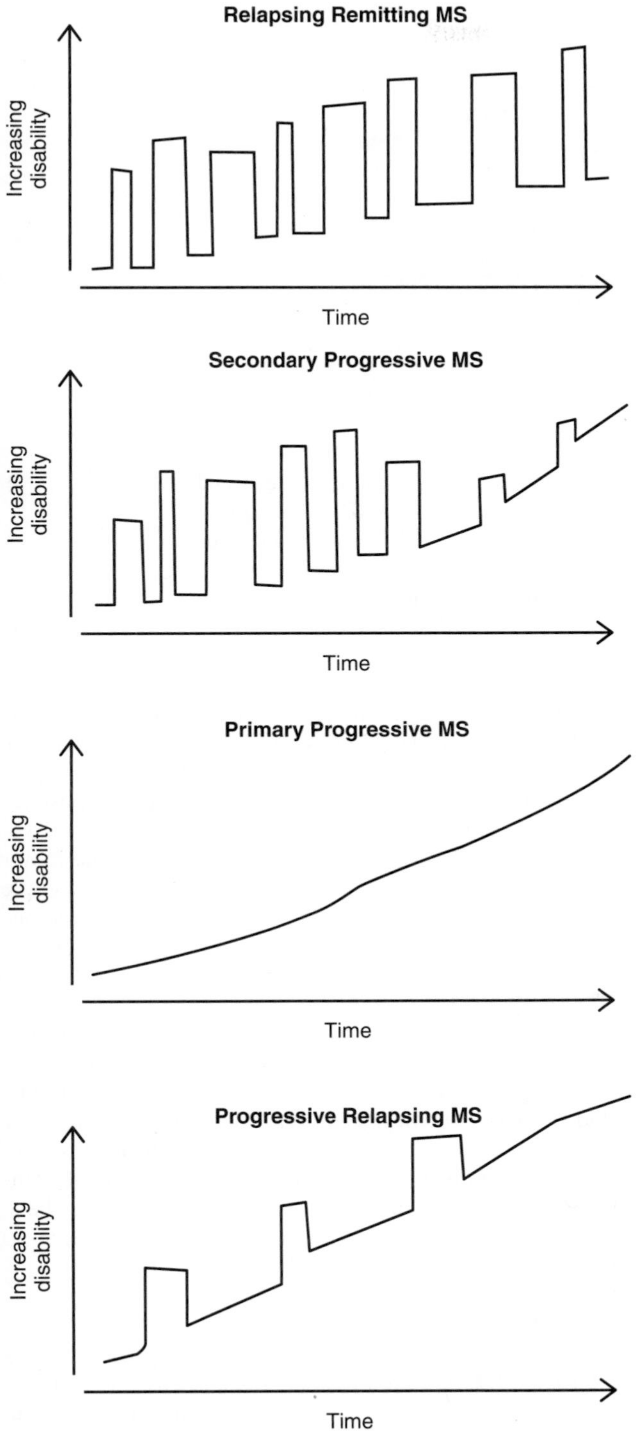

Figure 19-2 ■ Types of multiple sclerosis.

The authors could not identify any criteria associated with either developing MS or continuing to have the benign form.

The risk of a more rapid disease progression is correlated with older age at diagnosis; male sex; initial symptoms involving the motor, sphincter, or cerebellar systems; multifocal disease at onset; shorter time between first and second attacks; and frequent attacks in the first 5 years postdiagnosis.[7,14]

Clinical Manifestations

MS can affect the optic nerve and any tissue within the brain or spinal cord, so almost any neurological symptom can result. Individual assessments are required to identify the problems present. Even so, the following list constitutes the most common problems encountered by people with MS.

Fatigue

Of people with MS, 65% to 97% report fatigue during the course of the disease; as many as 40% of people with MS state that fatigue is their most disabling symptom.[15] There are two types of fatigue in people with MS: primary and secondary. Primary fatigue, often called *lassitude,* is caused by the effects of the demyelination and axonal destruction and its effect on nerve conduction. Restorative rehabilitation has little effect on primary fatigue from neurodegeneration. Secondary fatigue results from problems such as deconditioning, infections, sleep disturbances, poor nutrition, medication side effects, other medical conditions (such as thyroid disease), and heat intolerance. Clinicians should be extremely careful to separate the types of the fatigue in order to determine the most appropriate interventions.

Sensory Impairments

Sensory impairments are among the most common symptoms associated with MS and can affect the visual, somatosensory, and vestibular systems.[16] The most common problem of the visual system is optic neuritis, which can produce blurry or double vision and/or painful eye movements and nystagmus. Somatosensory or proprioception disturbances can include dysesthesias (tingling, buzzing, or vibrations) or anesthesias (complete loss of sensation in part of the body). People may experience paresthesia or anesthesia in half of the body—upper or lower or side to side—or below a certain spinal cord level. Dysesthesias may be limited to small body areas such as a patch of skin on the head or a single upper or lower extremity. Vestibular system involvement occurs in 20% of people with MS at some time during their disease course[17] and may manifest as dizziness and/or vertigo.

People with MS can have pain associated with the damage to neural tissue (neuropathic pain). This may manifest as neuralgias with burning, itching, or electric shocklike sensations. Lhermitte sign is an electric shock–like shooting sensation that can run into the upper extremities or down the back in response to flexion of the neck.

Motor Systems Impairments

Deficits in the motor system include weakness, spasticity, ataxia, and tremor. Paresis or muscular weakness is frequently seen in people with MS and is associated with several causes. Like fatigue, weakness can be caused by damage to the myelination and axons of motor and premotor neurons in the CNS that can manifest in many different patterns including monoparesis, paraparesis, hemiparesis, or quadriparesis. However, additional causes of muscle weakness can also be associated with disuse deconditioning and may also result in muscle atrophy. When muscle weakness or loss of motor control is seen in the muscles of speech, it results in dysarthria. Paralysis or total loss of muscle strength occurs with less frequency but can be devastating for patients. Several patterns of paralysis (or "-plegia") occur in people with MS including paraplegia, hemiplegia, and quadriplegia.

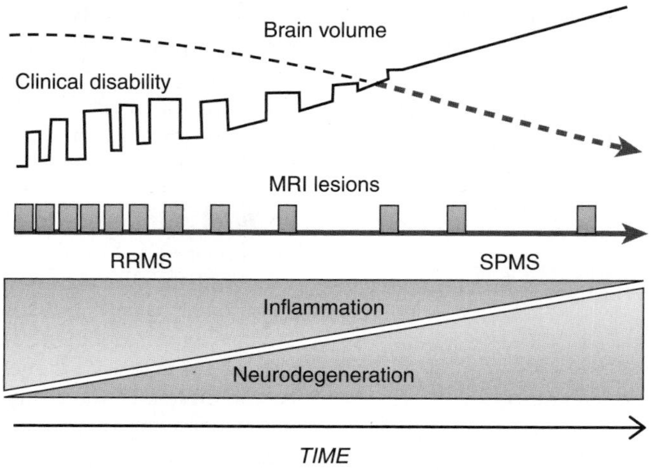

Figure 19-3 ■ Natural history of relapsing remitting multiple sclerosis (RRMS)—conversion to secondary progressive multiple sclerosis (SPMS). Figure shows the typical clinical course of RRMS with conversion to SPMS. Magnetic resonance imaging (MRI) activity *(gray line and boxes)* indicates the inflammatory lesions; they occur more frequently early in the disease and occur with greater frequency than in clinical disability *(solid black line)*. Brain volume indicated by the stippled line shows brain atrophy increasing as the inflammatory component of the disease slows and is replaced by neurodegeneration.

A broad clinical definition of spasticity is a velocity-sensitive resistance to muscle stretch or a muscle spasm during movement.[18] Some people report heaviness in the limbs, difficulty moving a joint, jumping of the extremities, or involuntary painful movements. Muscle spasms or cramping are frequently experienced by people with MS. Eighty four percent of people with MS report spasticity, with 34% indicating that their spasticity is moderate to severe.[19] Female sex or longer disease duration are both associated with higher prevalence of spasticity. Spasticity has been highly correlated with patient-reported disability and poorer quality of life (QOL).[19] Spasticity may change according to position and may result from increased effort during activity or from the presence of a noxious stimulus such as an infection, skin lesions, fractures, renal stones, distention of bladder or colon, or other physiological stressors such as certain medications (DMAs or serotonin reuptake inhibitors) or psychological distress. Environmental factors such as tight clothing, hunger, or elevated body or air temperature may also lead to increased spasticity. Spasticity can cause muscle contractures, skin breakdown, pain, and sleep disturbances, which often lead to secondary activity limitations and participation restrictions that limit performance of activities of daily living (ADLs) and mobility.

Ataxia occurs in up to 80% of people with MS at some point in their disease progression.[20] This motor deficit can occur from disturbances in the vestibular system or cerebellum or a loss of proprioception. Ataxia or a lack of coordination can manifest as difficulty with walking to difficulty with movements of the extremities such as overshooting or undershooting targets (dysmetria) or an inability to produce rapid alternating movements (dysdiadochokinesia). Occasionally, patients experience sustained body positioning (dystonia) of the extremities or head and neck. In different research studies, tremor is reported by 25% to 58% of people with MS, with the majority of people experiencing mild to moderate dysfunction.[21,22] Action tremor, both postural and intention, are found in people with MS, pointing to the cerebellum as a likely source (see Chapter 21). Tremors affect the head, neck, vocal cords, limbs, and torso, with the upper extremities having the greatest occurrence.[21,22]

MS affects many of the systems required for postural control and balance, including sensory input (visual, somatosensory, and vestibular), central processing, and motor output. Therefore it is not surprising that over 50% of people with MS report falling one or more times in the previous 6 months.[23-26]

Bowel and Bladder Dysfunction

The incidence of bowel problems (35% to 68%) and bladder problems (52% to 97%) make them common in people with MS, as reported by two research studies.[27,28] Symptoms include urinary urgency, nocturia, or retention of urine or feces.[29] Incontinence of either system can also occur. Neurogenic detrusor muscle overactivity is the most common urological impairment in people with MS; 20% have detrusor muscle underactivity, and only 10% report no symptoms.[28]

Sexual Dysfunction

Sexual dysfunction affects 40% to 85% of women with MS and 50% to 90% of men. It can manifest as erectile dysfunction, impotence, inability to achieve orgasm, and, in men, retrograde ejaculation.[28,30,31]

Cognitive Impairments

Cognitive dysfunction occurs in roughly 40% to 70% of people with MS, with 70% demonstrating mild to moderate impairment.[32,33] Although cognitive problems can occur at anytime, abilities affected early in the course of the disease are verbal fluency and verbal memory.[34] Other cognitive dysfunctions common in people with MS include impairments in memory, processing speed, executive functioning, attention, and visuospatial learning. There is a fair correlation between cognitive decline and ability to work and unemployment because of the impairments in short- and long-term memory, problems with concentration, forgetfulness, and slowed word recall.[35,36] This is a likely source of frustration for both patients and caregivers alike.

Depression

Depression is two to three times more common in people with chronic health conditions than in the general population and has a greater incidence than other neurological conditions.[37] From 26% to 50% of people with MS have been reported to experience depression during the course of the disease.[32,38] Several factors contribute to the high incidence of depression in people with MS. The fact that MS is a chronic, progressive, and unpredictable disease that affects people in their early to middle adult years, is often invisible, and limits participation in many life roles often leads to a perceived reduction in QOL.[39] Suicide is of great concern for people with depression, and rates are significantly higher in people with MS than in the general population.[40] Depression is associated with a lower QOL and other symptoms of MS including fatigue, disability, pain, and cognitive impairment.[41]

Heat Intolerance

Uhthoff phenomenon is a temporary worsening of MS-related problems associated with an increase in core body temperature. Such increases can occur with physical exertion such as exercise or with a change in the environment such as hot baths or showers, hot weather, and hot air temperature.

MEDICAL MANAGEMENT

Diagnosis

Historically, people with MS would wait for a diagnosis for a year or more. Although there are no definitive tests that diagnose MS, the addition of MRI has accelerated diagnosis. In 2001 the International Panel on the Diagnosis of Multiple Sclerosis updated criteria to include MRI, visual evoked potentials, and cerebrospinal fluid (CSF) analysis. The 2005 Revised McDonald Criteria for MS diagnosis were designed to make the diagnostic process even more efficient and easier.[42] The Poser criteria require the presence of two separate episodes over time, plus evidence of two or more lesions in separate brain or spinal cord regions identified by radiological imaging studies. Even with the improved technological measures used to facilitate diagnosis, an accurate clinical history is critical. Often patients will recall episodes of transient symptoms that did not last long enough to require attention by a primary care provider.

In addition to the clinical history, MRI studies have improved diagnosis of MS. Although T2-weighted MRI images show MS lesions as hyperintense and identify new or active lesions, MRI has been shown (Figure 19-4) to overestimate clinical relapses. Conventional MRI with T1 weighting identifies lesions as hypointense (black holes) and is able to identify brain atrophy. T1 imaging demonstrates a stronger correlation with clinical status and disease severity than the lesion load found with T2 weighting. Gadolinium-enhanced T1-weighted MRI images show active MS lesions as hyperintense (white).

Two additional medical tests can be used to aid in the diagnosis of MS and differentiate it from other diseases and conditions. The first is the analysis of CSF. This requires a lumbar puncture in which CSF is gathered and analyzed to identify oligoclonal bands representing the presence of immune system proteins indicating that the body is attacking itself. The majority of people with MS have oligoclonal bands; however, because people with other diseases or conditions also have oligoclonal bands, the test is not specific for MS. The lack of oligoclonal bands at diagnosis has been related to a slower progression of the disease and increased time to reach markers of disability such as walking with an assistive device or confinement to a wheelchair.

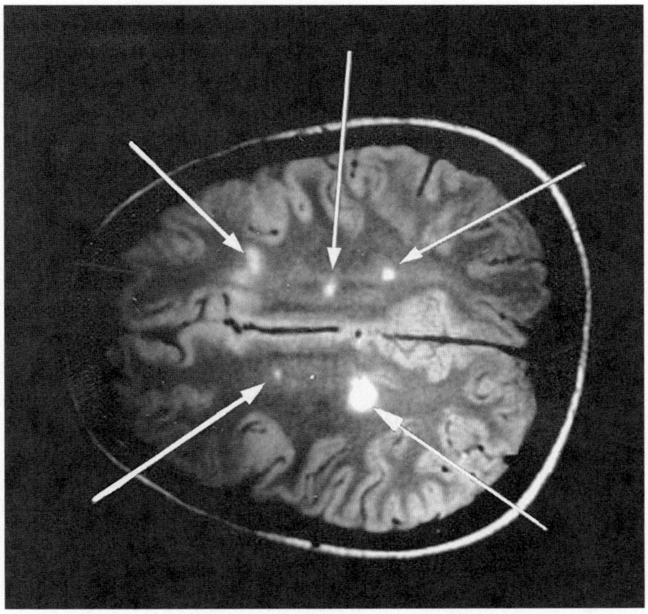

Figure 19-4 ■ T2-weighted magnetic resonance imaging (MRI) scan of plaques associated with multiple sclerosis. Plaques are indicated by arrows. (From Frey H, Lahtinen A, Heinonen T, Dastidar P: Clinical application of MRI image processing in neurology. *Int J Bioelectromagnet* 1(1), 1999.)

Evoked potentials record the nervous system's response to stimulation of a specific sensory pathway (visual, auditory, vestibular, or general somatosensory). Demyelination and axonal degeneration cause a slowing of signal transmission along neurons and therefore will increase the response time to an externally applied sensory stimulus. Damage to the optic system is a common first symptom in MS, and therefore visual evoked potentials are often most helpful in diagnosis.

Disease severity and progression are monitored by ongoing medical checkups, MRI imaging, and the use of several outcome measures. The Kurtzke disease severity scale was developed to allow primary care providers a way to measure clinical disability and chart disease progression. It has been replaced by the Expanded Disability Status Scale (EDSS) (Table 19-1).[43] The EDSS is a 10-point ordinal scale completed by a physician or physician extender, with 0 indicating no disability and 10 indicating death caused by MS. Using a cane relates to an EDSS score of 6.0. The National MS Society (NMSS) Task Force on Clinical Outcomes Assessment also recommends the Multiple Sclerosis Functional Composite (MSFC)[44] as a measure of disease severity and progression. This set of outcome measures is used to

TABLE 19-1 ■ ABBREVIATED EXPANDED DISABILITY STATUS SCALE

SCORE	FUNCTION
1.0	Normal neurological examination findings
2.0	Minimal disability
3.0	Moderate disability
4.0	Ambulates 12 hours without aid
5.0	Disability impairs activity (walks 1500 feet without assistance)
6.0	Intermittent or unilateral constant assistance
6.5	Bilateral support required (walker, crutches, two canes)
7.0	Unable to walk 15 feet without assistance
8.0	Basically constrained to bed
9. 0	Bedridden
10.0	Death from multiple sclerosis

chart change in physical and cognitive function and will be discussed later in this chapter. It includes three tests that measure upper-extremity function (Nine-Hole Peg Test [NHPT]), lower-extremity function and mobility (25-Foot Timed Walk [25FTW]), and cognitive function (Paced Auditory Serial Addition Test [PASAT]).

Medical management of MS has two major goals: long-term management of the disease and exacerbations and symptomatic management. Early after diagnosis with CIS, it is recommended that people take DMAs. Recent evidence suggests that as the disease progresses it becomes less inflammatory and more neurodegenerative. Therefore medications aimed at reducing inflammation will be less effective as the disease progresses. Fox[2] suggests that early treatment is needed to compensate for the later stages of the disease when inflammation is less prevalent.

Medications

Disease-Modifying Agents

DMAs are aimed at reducing immune system dysfunction, thereby reducing damage to neural tissue and long-term disability for people with RRMS. There are several different medications that act on various components of the immune system with the intention of modifying the course of the disease (Table 19-2). In general, these drugs are approved for use with RRMS and are used off-label for other forms of MS and have been shown to reduce the number of attacks experienced. The majority of the drugs require injections; however, in 2010 the U.S. Food and Drug Administration (FDA) approved the first oral DMA, fingolimod. Measurement of therapeutic effectiveness includes relapse rate, progression of disability (EDSS), and quantitative evidence of lesions on MRI. All DMAs have side effects (see Table 19-2), but rarely are they serious. These medications are costly, and some people do not respond well or tolerate the side effects. It is common that people will try more than one type before finding the DMA they tolerate the best.

Antiinflammatory Medications

High-dose corticosteroids (such as prednisone or methylprednisolone) are used to reduce inflammatory response during exacerbations for people with RRMS. Although no medications have demonstrated effectiveness in people with

TABLE 19-2 ■ DISEASE-MODIFYING AGENTS: INDICATIONS AND SIDE EFFECTS

FDA-APPROVED DISEASE-MODIFYING AGENTS	INDICATION	COMMON SIDE EFFECTS
IFN beta-1a (Avonex)	CIS	Flulike symptoms
IFN beta-1a (Rebif)	RRMS	Injection-site reactions
IFN beta-1b (Betaseron)	SPMS	Depression
IFN beta-1b (Extavia)		Elevated liver enzymes
Glatiramer (Copaxone)	CIS	Injection-site reactions
	RRMS	Systemic reactions, immediately postinjection
		Elevated liver enzymes
Natalizumab (Tysabri)	RRMS	Progressive multifocal leukoencephalopathy
		Infusion reactions
		Hepatotoxicity
Mitoxantrone (Novantrone)	RRMS	Cardiotoxicity
Intravenous infusion	SPMS	Treatment-related leukemia
	PRMS	Infection risk
		Alopecia
		Amenorrhea
Fingolimod (Gilenya)	RRMS	Flulike symptoms
		Increased liver enzymes
		Headache
		Diarrhea
		Back pain
		Cough

CIS, Clinical isolated syndrome; *FDA,* U.S. Food and Drug Administration; *IFN,* interferon; *RRMS,* relapsing remitting multiple sclerosis; *SPMS,* secondary progressive multiple sclerosis.

PPMS, anecdotal evidence suggests that intermittent pulses of intravenous methylprednisolone can help slow progression of clinical disability in some patients.[2]

A host of additional medications are used to manage the symptoms associated with MS. Each will be discussed as part of symptom management. Also refer to Chapter 36 for additional information.

Symptom Management

Fatigue

The fatigue experienced by people with MS is generally divided into primary and secondary causes. Fatigue from primary causes results from the disease itself or to heat intolerance and is defined by the term *MS lassitude.* Heat intolerance may result in a temporary worsening of symptoms. It is sometimes referred to as *pseudoexacerbation* and occurs when core body temperature rises with exposure to raised ambient temperature or metabolic activity such as exercise. However, in addition to MS lassitude, other causes can include side effects of medications used in the treatment of MS, deconditioning from reduced activity levels, poor nutrition, infections or other medical conditions, depression, or sleep disturbances. Several medications combined with rehabilitation strategies have been recommended for management of fatigue. Amantadine (Symmetrel) and modafinil (Provigil) are frequently prescribed.

Spasticity

Spasticity can interfere with physical function and hygiene. However, spasticity can also add support to weakened limbs, allowing more effective mobility. The goal of medical management of spasticity is to maintain full range of motion (ROM) of muscle and soft tissue structures to allow maximal physical function and proper hygiene. Haselkorn and colleagues[18] describe the clinical practice guidelines for managing spasticity in people with MS written by the Multiple Sclerosis Council. A complete assessment of the spasticity and how it affects the individual's life is required. Typically, successful management includes both pharmaceuticals and rehabilitation.

When spasticity is the result of CNS impairments, medical management often includes the use of oral pharmacotherapy including baclofen (Lioresal) or tizanidine (Zanaflex). Adjuvant therapies include diazepam (Valium) or clonazepam (Klonopin), dantrolene (Dantrium), gabapentin (Neurontin) or levetiracetam (Keppra), clonidine (Catapres), or muscle relaxants. Each of these drugs can have negative side effects that interfere with movement and therefore rehabilitation.

Management of focal spasticity may include local anesthetics such as lidocaine, bupivacaine, etidocaine, all of which are short acting with side effects of CNS and cardiovascular toxicity and hypersensitivity. Neurolysis treatment with phenol or alcohol is longer acting; however, these agents can have the side effects of pain, swelling, fibrosis, and dysesthesias. Focal spasticity affecting functional muscle groups can also be effectively treated with neuromuscular blocking agents including alcohol, phenol, or botulinum toxin. Botulinum toxin type A (Botox) has been shown to improve spasticity as measured by the Ashworth Scale and the hygiene score, but no changes were noted in spasm frequency score.[45] Blocks last 1 to 3 months with relatively few side effects. Similarly, botulinum toxin type B was shown to reduce hip adductor spasticity.[46] Clinical practice guidelines[18] recommend that neuromuscular blocks be performed by appropriate specialists in conjunction with a rehabilitation program.

Refractory spasticity is defined as unsuccessful treatment with oral medications and/or rehabilitation. In this situation two other options exist: surgery or placement of an intrathecal baclofen pump (ITB). Surgical procedures include tendon lengthening or tendon transfer and are performed to maintain adequate hygiene or prevent or correct contractures and therefore preserve function. Intrathecal pumps, inserted into the spinal cord, allow adjustable drug delivery. Baclofen, the drug of choice for the intrathecal pump, can be given in higher doses; use of the pump avoids the side effects often encountered when the drug is taken orally. Relapses are more commonly reported in people on oral medications than those using ITB. People using ITB also report higher levels of satisfaction, less spasticity, and fewer painful spasms compared with those on oral medications.[19]

Pain

Both nociceptive and neuropathic pain can be present in people with MS. Therefore it is important to discern the type of pain in order for the most appropriate treatment to be rendered. Nociceptive pain can often be treated with analgesics (acetaminophen, nonsteroidal antiinflammatory drugs [NSAIDs], or opioids) and is more amenable to physical therapy (discussed later under rehabilitation management). Neuropathic pain generally requires pharmacological intervention, although an interdisciplinary team approach may be valuable. First-line medications for neuropathic pain that occurs in the spinal cord are calcium channel blockers (gabapentinoids) or *N*-methyl-D-aspartate (NMDA) antagonists (ketamine). When pain is present in the head, the primary treatment is opioid drugs such as antidepressants (tricyclics) or anticonvulsants (gabapentin or pregabalin).[47] In the case of trigeminal neuralgia, the first choice is often carbamazepine. Refer to Chapter 32 on pain management for additional information.

Mobility

Physical rehabilitation is the primary intervention used to manage mobility dysfunctions. However, one medication has recently been FDA approved to improve gait. In clinical studies dalfampridine (Ampyra) demonstrated the ability to improve walking speed in people with MS.[48] However, changes in the quality of gait or movement were not measured.

Tremor

Tremor management using medications such as isoniazid, carbamazepine, ondansetron, or cannabis extract has been minimally effective.[49] Surgical interventions including stereotaxic thalamotomy and deep brain stimulation have been studied, but the evidence to support the effects on functional status and disability is lacking. The effectiveness of other options including physical therapy, tremor-reducing orthoses, and extremity cooling have yet to be proven beneficial in clinical trials.[49]

Bowel and Bladder Management

Behavioral modification and rehabilitation are used to help alleviate the symptoms of bladder incontinence or detrusor muscle overactivity. A few medications have been shown to be helpful: anticholinergic agents are used to manage detrusor overactivity or dyssynergia, and underactivity is treated with cholinomimetic agents.[2]

People with constipation are encouraged to combine adequate fluid intake with dietary fiber or bulk-forming medications.[2]

Depression and Cognitive Impairments

Depression is very common in people with MS, yet it is infrequently identified or treated.[50] Therapy can include supportive psychotherapy and medication given individually or in combination. To date two pharmacological therapies have shown the most promise in reducing cognitive deficits (L-amphetamine sulfate and donepezil), and neither has serious adverse effects.[51,52]

REHABILITATION MANAGEMENT

Overview

Chronic neurodegenerative conditions, such as MS, result in a loss of physical and cognitive function from the destruction of neurons and from a lack of activation of the affected systems. People with MS experience physical and cognitive impairments potentially leading to inactivity and resultant deconditioning (Figure 19-5). This often becomes a cycle that is difficult to break. One question that frames the rehabilitation strategy chosen is whether the focus should be compensation for or restoration of lost function. Compensation includes interventions such as wheelchairs or walkers to assist with mobility or braces for absent or inadequate muscle power. Restoration is aimed at increasing the capacity of the system—for example, maximizing cardiovascular endurance by increasing maximal oxygen uptake or restoring full ROM. Therefore, prescribing programs, activities, and exercises that provide an adequate stimulus to produce adaptation is critical to restore function or improve motor and cognitive performance. Although each patient case is unique, the most likely answer is that both strategies will be employed. The challenge for rehabilitation professionals is to sort out how much of a patient's dysfunction arises from neurodegeneration, which necessitates compensation, and how much occurs from inactivity and system deconditioning, in which case system capacity can be restored to some extent. Rehabilitation professionals must choose therapeutic interventions based on whether compensation or restoration is the goal.

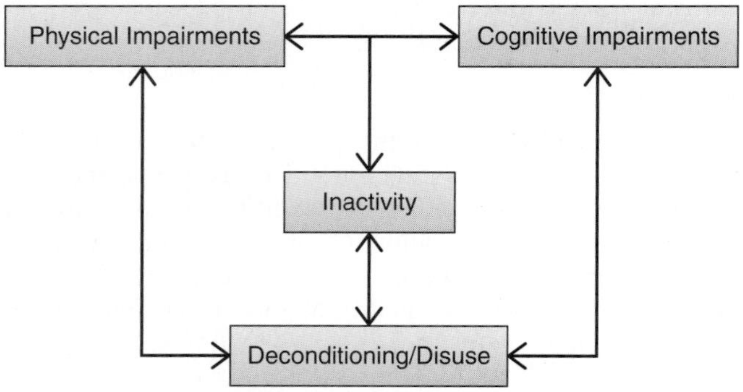

Figure 19-5 ■ Interaction among impairments, inactivity, and deconditioning. People with multiple sclerosis often experience physical and/or cognitive impairments that can lead to or be increased by inactivity. Deconditioning and disuse can reduce activity levels or be caused by inactivity. This can become a cycle that is self-perpetuating. (Modified from Multiple sclerosis treatment: impact on quality of life (Clinical monograph, p. 10): Proceedings from Clinical Medical Education/Clinical Education Symposium at the Consortium of Multiple Sclerosis Centers Annual Meeting. Washington, DC, June 2007.)

Rehabilitation for people with MS occurs in every setting: inpatient hospitals, outpatient clinics, skilled nursing facilities, home care settings, and the community. With the current climate of decreasing access to and reducing coverage for rehabilitation, therapists must be able to make evidence-based arguments to primary care providers and insurers, as well as patients, to support effective therapeutic interventions that will achieve the goals of optimal physical and cognitive functioning, safety, and QOL.

For rehabilitation professionals managing people with MS, the International Classification of Functioning, Disability and Health (ICF) model (refer to Chapter 1) provides an excellent framework for assessment and management regardless of the setting in which the patient or client is encountered.[53] Although guided by the opening interview and chart review, the initial assessment must include how the individual with MS is functioning in home, at work, and in recreation environments and which impairments of bodily structure or function might be contributing to the identified activity limitations and participation restrictions. Rehabilitation professionals must consider how personal and environmental factors may impede or facilitate achievement of rehabilitation goals. Personal factors in people with MS may include whether the patient is heat intolerant, experiences MS-related fatigue, or has the confidence or motivation to perform certain tasks. Environmental factors that may be of particular importance for the patient with MS may be living in a hot climate or having access to cooling equipment such as air conditioning or cooling garments. It is critical to understand how the disease affects the lives of both individual patients and their caregivers. Outcome measures designed to test impairments, activity, and participation, along with assessments of environmental and personal factors, will help health care professionals understand the deficits of their patients and determine the best place to focus rehabilitation efforts and monitor the patient's response to intervention.[54]

Because of the myriad CNS lesions and variable clinical presentations in people with MS, there is no one approach that is the gold standard for rehabilitation management. Whatever the approach, evidence is growing that rehabilitation is beneficial. Intensive inpatient therapy programs provide long-term improvement in a number of functional skills, participation, and QOL but may not change underlying impairments. Prospective studies have shown that intensive inpatient rehabilitation improves disability and QOL and that these benefits can be long lasting.[55-58] High-intensity programs in the outpatient clinic or home environment offer evidence of short-term symptomatic changes that have translated into improved participation and QOL.[56,59]

Assessment

The initial interview must include a quick screen or questioning about the body systems and areas that are commonly impaired in people with MS and the problems commonly encountered: motor strength, coordination, spasticity, sensory disruption (vestibular, visual, and somatosensory), bladder control, depression, and cognition. If impairments are present, there is a strong likelihood of negative impact on the patient's ability to perform ADLs or participate in activities related to work, home, and leisure. All patients with MS must be asked if they have fallen in the last 6 months because of the high rate of falling in people with MS.[23-25,26] Results of the interview and chart review will help develop hypotheses about which potential impairments might be contributing to the patient's or client's physical or cognitive dysfunctions. Therefore the examination needs to be designed to observe the problematic tasks and test the hypotheses developed.

During the assessment, examiners must determine if the problems identified by the patient (or those found by the assessor) fit within their scope of practice or whether the patient requires a referral to an appropriate health care professional. A good example is identifying people with depression using a quick two-question screen. According to Mohr and colleagues,[60] these questions are 98.5% sensitive for identifying major depressive disorder. The two questions are (1) "During the past 2 weeks, have you often been bothered by feeling down, depressed, or hopeless?" and (2) "During the past two weeks, have you often been bothered by having little interest or pleasure in doing things?"[61] An answer of yes to either question should trigger a referral to the patient's primary care provider for follow-up.

The physical examination might then start with testing the patient's ability to perform functional activities that the patient or his or her caregivers have identified as problematic. This might include performance of transfers, gait, ADLs, or cognitive tasks as well as the specific activities that the person states are compromised in his or her work, home, and recreational life. There are several measures of QOL that also cover participation issues relevant to people with MS.

Comprehensive lists of standardized tests and measures for impairment, activity limitations, and participation restrictions or QOL are provided in Chapter 8. The next section of this chapter will primarily focus on the tests and measures found to be valid and reliable in the examination of individuals with MS.

Assessing Body System Problems Contributing to Activity Limitations

In general, standardized methods of examining muscle strength and endurance, somatosensation, vision, coordination, cardiovascular status and endurance, posture, muscle tone, reflexes, ROM, pain, and cognition are useful in examining patients with MS. As with many neurological conditions, abnormal posturing or pain may necessitate using nonstandardized test positions or methods that must be noted in the patient documentation. If a patient is unable to attain the normal test position while performing a muscle strength test, the assessed strength is noted along with the position in which the muscle or muscle group was tested.

Spasticity. Spasticity can be measured using resistance to passive ROM and Ashworth[62] and Modified Ashworth Scales.[63] However, because these scales measure spasticity at rest, they may not reflect the degree to which spasticity may be interfering with function. Careful observation of the patient's movements may also inform the clinician about how spasticity is affecting the patient's ability to move.

Ataxia and Incoordination. Few standardized tests have been developed to specifically measure ataxia. One recent test is the Scale for the Assessment and Rating of Ataxia (SARA). Although this test has yet to be validated in people with MS, it has good reliability and validity in patients with cerebellar dysfunction, a common problem in people with MS.[64,65]

Tests of nonequilibrium coordination are designed to measure the presence of dysmetria or dysdiadochokinesia, both of which occur in patients with MS. However, these tests (including finger to nose, heel to shin) are somewhat subjective and are therefore difficult to use to demonstrate improvement after an intervention. However, using a stopwatch during these tests can be an important tool to record objective data. Count the number of repetitions of a given activity performed in a set amount of time (e.g., how many alternating forearm supinations and pronations can be performed in 30 seconds), or record the time it takes to complete a set number of repetitions of a given activity (e.g., how long it takes to complete five alternating supination-pronation movements). Refer to Chapter 21 for additional assessment tools.

Vestibular Dysfunction. The vestibular system is affected by MS both centrally (lesions in the vestibular nuclei or cerebellum) and at the entry site of cranial nerve VIII.[66] However, benign paroxysmal positional vertigo (BPPV) can also occur.[67] The techniques used to assess and treat the effects of vestibular disorder in an individual with MS are the same as those discussed in Chapter 22. When vestibular symptoms are present, Williams and colleagues[68] suggest evaluation using computerized platform posturography (CPP) in people with MS with minimal to mild disability. It is important to keep in mind that the patient with MS will often have additional problems that might require modification of the vestibular intervention—for example, heat intolerance or additional visual or somatosensory deficits.

Fatigue. Identifying if and when fatigue occurs in individuals with MS is important to assessment and the structuring of intervention. Questions should address the type of fatigue, whether mental or physical; when during the day it occurs; whether it is related to physical or mental exertion; and what the person with MS does, if anything, to relieve it. In addition, fatigue-related self-report scales can help the rehabilitation professional gain an understanding of the perceived impact that fatigue may be having on a patient with MS. Two of the commonly used scales are the Modified Fatigue Impact Scale[69] and the Fatigue Severity Scale.[70] These measures may also aid the therapist in determining if the intervention had any impact on the patient's perceived level of fatigue.

Cognition. The PASAT,[71] recommended by an expert panel of the National MS Society, is a test for cognitive impairments in people with MS. A more recent test, the Audio Recorded Cognitive Screen (ARCS),[72,73] appears to be a more comprehensive cognitive assessment developed for people with dementia but the psychometric properties have not yet been determined in people with MS. However, Lechner-Scott and co-workers[74] found that compared with the PASAT, the ARCS was similar in detecting impairments of cognition and more sensitive at identifying problems with memory or executive impairments.

Assessing Activity Performance and Participation

Outcome measures assess the ability of an individual to perform an activity or task as well as assess the perception of the person to use those tasks to fulfill life roles. Following are activity and participation measures commonly used in people with MS. An individual's perceived ability to participate may also be included in some QOL outcome measures that are included in the following sections.

Balance. Balance is foundational to upright movement and is produced by a complex interaction among sensory inputs, central processing, and motor responses. It can be discussed under both body structure and function or activity. In either case balance dysfunction has been identified in people with MS with minimal as well as more advanced disability.[75-79] Cameron and Lord[80] report the three most common problems with balance to be delayed response to postural perturbations, increased body sway while standing quietly, and an inability to move outside the base of support.

Whereas some balance tests focus on stationary or static tasks that allow observation of body sway in standing, including single-leg stance test, Romberg test with eyes open or eyes closed, tandem stance, and CPP, others add movement and challenge dynamic balance (Functional Reach Test,[81] Tinetti Performance-Oriented Mobility Assessment [POMA],[82] and Berg Balance Scale [BBS][83]). Other tests challenge anticipatory balance (reactions to perturbations related to self-generated movement) or reactive balance (perturbation tests, CPP). Frzovic and co-workers[84] found that single-leg stance, tandem stance, response to external perturbations, and the Functional Reach Test were able to distinguish people with MS from healthy controls.

Several authors have studied measures of balance in people with MS. Cattaneo and colleagues[85] determined that four tests measuring balance during standing and gait and self-perception of balance had good intrarater and interrater reliability. The two tests measuring balance during standing and movement were the BBS and the Dynamic Gait Index (DGI).

CPP provides an objective assessment of sensory contributions to balance dysfunction in people with MS.[86] In particular, the Sensory Organization Test is useful in identifying the relative sensory contributions (visual, vestibular, and proprioceptive) to stationary balance and response to perturbation. Understanding the sensory conditions under which the patient loses balance and falls assists the therapist in providing exercises that will challenge those conditions in a safe and controlled manner. For example, the patient who relies heavily on visual input to maintain balance (conditions with eyes closed in the Sensory Organization Test) would be provided exercises and activities that challenge the vestibular and proprioceptive systems, such as standing on foam while the eyes are closed.

Developed by Horak and colleagues,[87] the Balance Evaluation Systems Test (BESTest) is an instrument examining complex balance disorders that includes the six domains that underlie orientation and postural stability: biomechanical constraints, stability limits and verticality, transitions and anticipatory postural reactions, reactive postural responses, sensory orientation, and stability in gait. Both interrater reliability in people with parkinsonism and content validity are good, but testing in other populations has not yet been completed. There is an abbreviated version of the BESTest, the mini-BESTest,[88] that covers four of the six systems, focusing on dynamic balance. These promising tests may offer the clinician a better way of identifying which components of orientation and postural control are dysfunctional, which may allow more targeted interventions.

The Activities-specific Balance Scale (ABC)[89] is a questionnaire that rates people's self-perception of how confident they are to perform activities that challenge their balance. The Dizziness Handicap Inventory (DHI)[90] assesses three domains of disability related to dizziness: physical, emotional, and functional. The sum score or each subscale score can be reported. Higher scores mean greater levels of handicap and disability. Cattaneo and colleagues[91] found that both the ABC and DHI tools discriminated between fallers and nonfallers and were therefore good predictors of fall status in people with MS. Refer to Chapter 22 for additional information on balance.

Gait. Gait can be measured in myriad ways depending on the goal of the assessment. Speed, distance, and quality may all be important to the patient and therapist. Observational gait analysis is the gold standard for clinical measurement of gait quality. Although motion-analysis laboratories are able to provide detailed kinetic and kinematic assessment of joint angles and gait cycle, it is costly and typically not available in most clinical settings. Instrumented mats such as the GaitRit can provide clinicians with temporal and spatial gait parameters such as step length, step width, cadence, and single-leg support and double-leg support times. Although this is less costly than motion analysis, it may still be out of reach for many clinics. Gait speed and velocity can also be measured by having the patient walk a given distance while being timed. These walks can occur at a self-selected pace or as fast as the person can walk safely. Several short-distance timed tests exist, the 25FTW and the timed 10-meter gait test,[92] both of which have been shown to have good reliability and sensitivity to change.[93,94] The 6-minute walk test (6MWT) measures walking endurance and is recommended by the NMSS Task Force on Clinical Outcome Measures as a measure of walking ability that is sensitive to change. Gijbels and co-workers[95] report that the 6MWT was better at predicting habitual walking in people with mild to moderate MS than the 25FTW. However, the 25FTW may be more sensitive to change when compared with the EDSS.[96] The 6MWT distance was reduced in people with MS compared with healthy controls and was inversely related to disability.[97]

Two additional performance-based tests, the DGI and the Timed Up-and-Go Test (TUG), combine walking with other functional tasks. The DGI measures the ability of an individual to walk while adding various challenges such as slowing down or speeding up, head turning, stepping over or around obstacles, and stair climbing. It was developed to assess gait dysfunction associated with peripheral vestibular disease.[98] McConvey and Bennett[99] found the DGI to be a reliable and valid tool for use in people with MS. The TUG test combines walking with transfers and turning. It is frequently used in both clinical and research settings and has been shown to be reliable in measuring function in people with MS.[93]

The Multiple Sclerosis Walking Scale–12 (MSWS-12) is a 12-item patient-rated questionnaire that measures the perception of the impact of MS on walking ability. This scale has good reliability and validity and may be very useful to document patient perceived change in walking ability before and after intervention.[100,101]

Upper-Extremity Tests of Function. Movement impairments of the upper extremities can result in decreased ability to perform ADLs and other functional activities. Standardized tests such as the Box and Block Test (BBT)[102] or the NHPT[103] provide objective data about unilateral manual dexterity or the ability to manipulate objects. Both tests are inexpensive but do require some equipment and a stopwatch. The NHPT is part of the MSFC and therefore has been used extensively in evaluating people with MS.

Composite Tests. An expert panel of the NMSS recommended the use of the MSFC,[44,104] including the 25FTW, the NHPT, and the PASAT. The MSFC has been tested against lesion load as measured via MRI, EDSS scores, and QOL measures, showing that it has good validity and reliability and is sensitive to change.[104-106] Each component scale of the MSFC can also be used independently to monitor physical and cognitive function as written previously.

Assessing Quality of Life

QOL measures are patient-report tools that evaluate the value a person places on his or her abilities and limitations and how these affect the individual's social, emotional, and physical well-being. Many of these tools include questions that address an individual's perception of how well he or she is able to fulfill life roles and how the disease affects this participation. In a meta-analysis of exercise training on QOL in people with MS, Motl and Gosney[107] found that disease-specific measures of QOL detected larger changes than generic QOL measures. Several measures have been commonly used to evaluate people with MS: the Multiple Sclerosis Quality of Life–54 (MSQOL-54)[113] and the Multiple Sclerosis Quality of Life Inventory (MSQLI).[114] The multidimensional MSQOL-54 was based on the Health Status Questionnaire (SF-36), with 18 additional items specific to MS covering fatigue, and cognitive and sexual functioning. There are 12 subscales that cover physical function, role limitations—physical, role limitations—emotional, pain, emotional well-being, energy, health perceptions, social function, cognitive function, health distress, overall QOL and function, and change in health. The measure takes about 15 minutes to complete and requires 15 to 20 minutes to score. Reliability is good to excellent in people with MS.[113]

The MSQLI was developed by the Consortium of Multiple Sclerosis Centers Health Research Subcommittee in 1997. It is composed of 10 components covering issues important in MS. It includes the Health Status Questionnaire, Modified Fatigue Impact Scale, MOS Pain Effects Scale, Sexual Satisfaction Survey, Bladder Control Scale, Bowel Control Scale, Impact of Visual Impairment Scale, Perceived Deficits Questionnaire, Mental Health Inventory, and MOS Modified Social Support Survey. It takes about 45 minutes to administer the complete set of questionnaires and does not provide a sum score for all tests. There is good test-retest reliability for the MSQLI even in people with MS and cognitive dysfunction.[108] A shortened version of the tool exists, but the psychometric properties have not been thoroughly tested.

Disease Severity Measures

Disease severity is a measure of disablement. Interventions that change function (e.g., improve walking distances or decrease reliance on assistive devices to move) can reduce disability. There is also compelling evidence that exercise may actually modify disease progression in people with MS. Therefore disease progression may be used to assess the impact of an intervention on the patient's perceived level of disability. Although the EDSS[43] is the gold standard for assessing disease severity, it requires a trained primary care provider to administer. Disease Steps[111,112] and Guy's Neurological Disability Scale (GNDS)[109] are two additional disability scales that have demonstrated good correlation with the EDSS. Whereas Disease Steps must be administered by a professional, GNDS can be given to patients to complete on their own.[110]

Interventions

The goals of rehabilitation for persons with MS are to maximize and maintain function and prevent complications so that they can participate fully in all aspects of their lives. The variable presentation that people with MS can manifest requires rehabilitation professionals to be flexible and creative. The plan of care developed to manage a patient must be linked to the impairments, activity limitations and participation restrictions identified during the assessment. Research provides evidence for the most effective interventions and must be coupled with the desires and needs of the individual with MS. The rehabilitation program must be negotiated with the patient/client in consultation with caregivers when available or appropriate.

The National Clinical Advisory Board of the National MS Society recommends that rehabilitation occur whenever there is a sudden or gradual decline in function or an increase in impairment that has a negative impact on an individual's safety, independence, mobility, or QOL. In addition, it is recommended that rehabilitation be a part of a comprehensive health care plan at all stages of the disease.[115]

Regardless of the type of intervention chosen, evidence is growing that increased activity, whether cognitive or physical, may have a neuroprotective effect on the brains of people with neurological insults. In fact, Golzari and colleagues[116] demonstrated that an 8-week, 24-session, combined exercise program improved muscle strength and balance and reduced disability in people with MS. In this study, levels of proinflammatory immune system mediators were measured before and after the intervention. The authors demonstrated that this dosage of exercise reduced markers of inflammation in the blood. This is one of the first studies in people with MS showing that inflammation and therefore the disease process may be altered by the application of an exercise intervention, suggesting a role for rehabilitation in neuroprotection and not simply symptom management. This also implies that rehabilitation, specifically exercise, should occur early in the course of the disease and not only after clinical disability has occurred. However, the exact dosage, intensity, or type of exercise required to produce activity-dependent neuroplasticity is not yet known. At least one study in an animal model of MS, experimental allergic encephalomyelitis, has shown the beneficial effects of exercise.[117]

In prescribing a rehabilitation program for persons with MS, each individual's level of fitness and physical and cognitive resources including memory, judgment, strength, endurance, spasticity, balance, and coordination must be taken into consideration. In addition, therapists must investigate the person's level of fatigue and heat sensitivity. If present, these factors will require modification of the rehabilitation program, including where the activity is performed, in what environment, and the time of day in relation to fatigue level and the other tasks the individual must perform. In other words, to be successful, the rehabilitation program must fit into the framework of the person's life.

Rehabilitation can occur in a variety of locations: inpatient, outpatient, home, and the community. Figure 19-6 shows a physical therapy–led community-based exercise program for people with MS in which group activities addressing strength, balance, and endurance are modified for each individual. In addition, a number of health providers can be members of the rehabilitation team, including nurses, occupational therapists, physical therapists, speech-language pathologists, psychologists, neuropsychologists, and physicians.

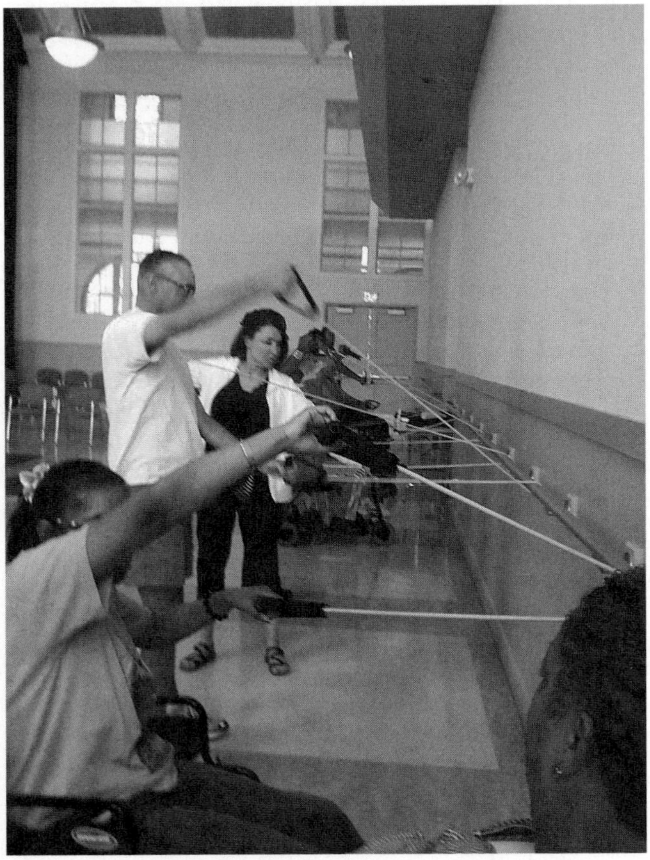

Figure 19-6 ■ Community exercise class for individuals with multiple sclerosis. A physical therapy–led community exercise class is shown. Participants perform group strengthening and balance activities that are modified for each individual.

Exercise

Historically, exercise was thought to worsen disability and bring on exacerbations. Medical advice warned patients that overexertion could hasten relapse and progression. There now exists clear evidence that this is not the case. Regular, appropriate exercise has been shown to increase strength, aerobic capacity, overall function, and QOL. In 1996 Petajan and colleagues published a seminal study in which a 60% $\dot{V}O_2$max aerobic ergometer exercise program was well tolerated in people with MS and did not provoke remission.[118] After 10 weeks, participants had improvements in $\dot{V}O_2$max, work capacity, isometric strength, and blood lipids and reduced depression, anger, and fatigue. In a 2009 systematic review of the literature,[119] exercise was shown to be an effective intervention for people with MS to improve muscle strength, endurance, mobility-related actions, and to a lesser extent mood compared with control conditions. This evidence did not suggest the superiority of one particular type of exercise program over others. It is very important to note that adverse effects were rarely seen in any of the exercise studies, and when they did occur they did not last for longer than 24 hours, indicating that exercise is safe for people with MS.

In a review of the exercise literature, White and Dressendorfer[120] recommend that endurance exercise programs for people with MS with mild to moderate disability use the following guideline: perform regularly, two or three sessions per week, at an intensity of 65% to 75% heart rate maximum, and last 20 to 30 minutes per session. Resistance exercise should include 15 to 18 repetitions for one to three sets initially with a goal of increasing to three to four sets. Training should last at least 12 weeks.[121] Owing to heat intolerance, exercise should incorporate intermittent rest periods that allow heat to dissipate.[120] Heesen and colleagues[122] developed a guideline for exercise prescription for people with MS for all levels of disability (Table 19-3).

Prescribed early in the course of the disease when mild to moderate disability is present, exercise can be used to restore function by reducing physical or cognitive decline from disuse or deconditioning. As clinical disability accrues in the later stages of the disease, exercise may then be used to compensate for missing function or prevent secondary complications—for example, stretching hip adductor muscles with decreased range of motion to allow adequate personal hygiene to occur.

Evidence-Based Interventions for Specific Problems

Fatigue

Fatigue is one of the most frequent and disabling symptoms associated with MS and is best managed with a multidisciplinary team composed of physicians, physical therapists, occupational therapists, and nurses. As described earlier, the causes of fatigue can be divided into two basic categories:

TABLE 19-3 ■ GENERAL EXERCISE GUIDELINES FOR LEVELS OF DISABILITY

LEVEL OF DISABILITY	EDSS LEVEL	TRAINING PROGRAM
None: no fatigue or thermosensitivity	0	Full exertion, aerobic and resistance exercise, no extreme sports
Minimal: limited fatigue and heat sensitivity; minor balance or gait problems	1-2	Monitored exercise program including strengthening and endurance using a variety of exercise types, precooling if heat-sensitive, avoid overtraining
Moderate: limited gait; may have spasticity, weakness, ataxia, balance problems	3-5	Deficit-driven exercise protocols including strengthening and endurance training using methods tolerated, walking, cycle ergometry, precooling if needed
Severe: cannot participate in all daily activities; short-distance, aided walking only	6-7	Movement preservation, stretching, targeted strengthening needed for task-specific training
Bedridden	8-9	Primarily passive movements to maintain motion, breathing exercises

Modified from Heesen C, Romberg A, Gold S, Schulz KH: Physical exercise in multiple sclerosis: supportive care of a putative disease-modifying treatment. *Expert Rev Neurother* 6:347–355, 2006.

EDSS, Expanded Disease Severity Scale.

primary and secondary. Primary fatigue related to demyelination and neurodegeneration may have fewer options for treatment. Secondary fatigue caused by deconditioning, comorbidities, depression, poor nutrition, heat intolerance, sleep disturbance, and medications may be more easily managed. Several strategies for fatigue management have been reported and show promise; however, few research studies have demonstrated effectiveness in randomized controlled trials or in comparisons among approaches. Interventions for fatigue management include cooling devices, energy conservation education training, exercise, and a multifaceted class aimed at teaching people with MS how to manage their fatigue.

One study found that the cooling suit was shown to improve all dimensions of fatigue on the Fatigue Impairment Scale (physical, cognitive, and psychosocial) in a small multiple-case study.[123] Although recommended in the clinical practice guidelines on fatigue and MS by expert opinion and anecdotal reports of people with MS, little additional evidence exists to support cooling as a therapeutic intervention. Two additional studies have shown that cooling garments can reduce symptoms of fatigue and improve ambulatory ability.[124,125]

Exercise shows promise as an intervention that can improve fatigue for people with MS that may improve muscle weakness caused by disuse and deconditioning. However, no one type of exercise, resistance or aerobic, or program has been proven most effective. One program included a 5-day-per-week, 30-minute bicycle aerobic training program for 4 weeks that improved fitness and showed a tendency for reduced fatigue. This study had an age, sex, and activity level control group.[126] Di Fabio[58] showed that a prolonged outpatient rehabilitation program in patients with progressive MS led to a decrease in MS-related symptoms, including fatigue. However, there was no control group. A randomized study comparing bicycle training with yoga found that fatigue improved in both groups, with neither group shown to be better than the other.[127]

Energy conservation is defined by the fatigue and MS guidelines of the Multiple Sclerosis Council for Clinical Practice Guidelines[128] as energy effectiveness and includes an analysis of individuals' home, work, and leisure activities and the environments in which they occur in order to develop activity modifications designed to reduce fatigue. This can include a variety of strategies such as reducing energy expenditure through activity and modification, workspace organization and improving efficiency of movements; balancing work and rest periods; delegating tasks; evaluating standards and prioritizing activities; and using assistive technologies that conserve energy usage.[129,130] In a randomized controlled trial, a 6-week community-based energy conservation class using the strategies listed previously was compared with a wait-list control group. Immediate post-course improvements in fatigue were noted[129] and were present after a 1-year follow-up period.[131]

The multidimensional fatigue management class "Fatigue: Take Control" was developed based on the recommendations of the Fatigue Management Guidelines of the NMSS from 1998.[132] The content of the 6-week class includes many of the aspects of fatigue management education and training that were described previously. The pilot study found that participants had less fatigue compared with a wait-list control group.[132] These classes are often offered by local chapters of the NMSS.

Patients may need to be prescribed assistive devices for ADLs. People with MS who have spasticity have a greater cost of walking.[133] Using wheeled mobility for longer-distance outings (to the shopping mall, an extended event, on vacation) can conserve energy and extend the time a person can participate in activities of importance to him or her. However, therapists should be aware that using assistive devices such as walkers or crutches actually increases energy expenditure for elderly people,[134] and therefore the need for improved support must be balanced with the increased energy burden an assistive device might add.

Spasticity

Several rehabilitation strategies to manage spasticity are available, including ROM, stretching, light pressure or stroking,[135] cold therapy, electrical stimulation, and education. Although none of these interventions is supported by strong research evidence, many are used routinely in clinical practice (ROM, stretching). Other approaches (cold therapy, light pressure or stroking) are recommended for use in conjunction with stretching or ROM programs. Regardless of the technique employed, educating individuals and caregivers about the importance of adhering to a spasticity management program is essential. The Multiple Sclerosis Council for Clinical Practice Guidelines[18] recommends, based on expert opinion, stretching a muscle with spasticity for 60 seconds or longer or using a prolonged stretch, lasting hours, with braces or splints.

Cold can be applied in a number of ways: baths, towels, or cooling garments. There are multiple quasi-experimental research studies that suggest an improvement in spasticity for a brief period after cooling[18]; however, the number of subjects and study methods make these results equivocal. Nilsagård and co-workers[136] found subjective reports of improved spasticity after a single session of cooling, although no statistically significant differences in spasticity measures were found.

Balance and Postural Control

Balance is foundational to the ability to stay upright and perform dynamic movements. It is a frequent problem in people with MS and results in a person limiting his or her participation in home, work, and leisure activities. Abnormalities of balance along with cane use and poor performance on tests of balance and ambulation can increase the risk of falling.[26] Other fall risk factors that have been identified include fear of falling, male sex, poor concentration or forgetfulness, and urinary incontinence.[25] Rehabilitation programs must be based on a thorough understanding of the impairments and personal and environmental factors that may be contributing to the balance dysfunction. Cattaneo and co-workers[137] compared the effects of three balance interventions on falling and other measures of balance. Three rehabilitation groups were included: one in which motor and sensory strategies were targeted, the second focusing on motor strategies alone, and the third group not receiving balance-specific training. The greatest reduction in falls and improvement on the BBS were associated with group one, and the least with group three. Hayes[138] compared 12 weeks of standard physical therapy with high-intensity resistance exercise (60% to 80% maximal contraction) added to standard therapy and found that standard therapy produced better balance outcomes. In addition, strength and the ability to ascend and descend stairs were all better in the standard therapy group. Importantly, people with MS tolerated the high intensity resistance exercise without problems. One pilot study found that a 12-week, biweekly aerobic exercise program did not improve balance as measured by the Functional Reach Test but did result in an improvement in walking distance.[139] For additional intervention strategies on balance, refer to Chapter 22.

Mobility

People with MS rate gait as one of the most important bodily functions[122]; gait is often adversely affected in people with MS. Gait disturbances have been observed in people with MS even before disability is measured on the EDSS scores.[140] Lesions in the brain and spinal cord produce a wide variety of potential impairments that can adversely affect gait. In a review article by Kelleher and colleagues,[141] imbalance, fatigue, spasticity, incoordination, muscle weakness, and sensory system impairments were all reported to negatively affect ambulation ability. Therefore addressing each of these impairments has the potential to improve gait. A recent literature review of therapeutic interventions for mobility problems suggests that a variety of different methods can be used to improve ambulation.[142] Snook and Motl[143] performed a meta-analysis of exercise studies aimed at improving walking mobility in people with MS and found that greater effects were associated with supervised exercise training, programs of less than 3 months' duration, in mixed samples of people with RRMS and progressive MS.

Task-specific gait training has been evaluated in people with MS. A randomized controlled trial compared two different treatment groups—facilitation and task-specific training—that each received 15 to 19 1-hour treatment sessions over 5 to 7 weeks and found that both improved 10-m gait speed, stride length, and balance; however, there was no control group.[144] Treadmill training has been investigated in several small, pilot or case studies with promising results of improved QOL, energy expenditure, and gait parameters.[145-147]

Several exercise studies have an association with improved gait. A combined resistance and aerobic home program lasting 23 weeks improved gait speed for short and longer distances in exercise compared with a control group.[148] Rampello and co-workers[149] compared a neurorehabilitation program with an aerobic training program of similar duration (three times per week for 8 weeks). The authors found that aerobic training improved walking distances and speeds and measures of aerobic capacity over the neurorehabilitation group. Both groups had QOL improvements in emotional well-being and health distress; the neurorehabilitation group demonstrated improved mental health.

An additional technique that shows promise for improving mobility in people with MS is an evaluation and intervention approach that uses small amounts of weight placed on the torso in response to identified balance dysfunction. Balance-Based Torso-Weighting (BBTW) is an intervention that uses directional loss of balance in both static and dynamic assessment to determine where small amounts of weight (generally less than 1% to 1.5% of body weight) are placed in a treatment orthotic called BalanceWear. The BalanceWear orthotic can be worn during the performance of activities in therapy or daily for home, work, or leisure activities. A recent randomized controlled trial in people with MS who reported gait abnormalities showed that when wearing the weighted BalanceWear orthotic participants increased their gait speed compared with no weight controls, and improved TUG scores compared with a standard weighted control.[150]

When people with MS do not respond to therapeutic interventions to restore function, mobility assistive devices such as canes, crutches, walkers, wheelchairs, and scooters are used to enhance mobility through compensation. Mobility-assisted technology (MAT) can improve function in people with moderate to severe impairments of ambulation and may reduce activity limitations and participation restrictions by reducing fatigue and enhancing energy conservation to allow greater involvement in work, family, social, vocational, and leisure activities. Other MAT technologies include functional electrical stimulation (FES), neuroprostheses, and orthotics. FES is applied to specific muscles or muscle groups to activate weak muscles. Some of these stimulators can be built into a neuroprosthesis that can be set up for use during exercising or walking.[151] Orthotics such as the ankle-foot orthosis (AFO) or hip flexion assist orthosis (HFAO)[152] can compensate for muscle weakness in the lower extremity, improve foot and knee positioning, and reduce energy expenditure. Therapists often work cooperatively with orthotists to ensure proper fit. Use of wheeled mobility devices such as a manual wheelchair, power wheelchair, or scooter requires a formal evaluation by an occupational or physical therapist with justification that it is required for mobility at home at least on a part-time basis. Therapists must take a long-term view of the projected needs of the patient when prescribing wheeled mobility, as most insurance companies will replace this equipment only every 5 years.

Pain and Dysesthesias

The occurrence of pain in people with MS is often underestimated. Pain can be acute, as in optic neuritis or Lhermitte syndrome, or chronic, as in dysesthesias in the limbs or joints or mechanical pain related to abnormal positions or repeated movements that cause abnormal wear and tear on the musculoskeletal system. Occupational and physical therapists can address poor body mechanics and weakness and poor movement patterns with retraining, and soft collars may help reduce Lhermitte syndrome. However, little evidence supports these interventions.[153] Transcutaneous electrical nerve stimulation has been suggested anecdotally by Kassirer[154] as beneficial for reducing pain. Cognitive-behavioral therapy has been researched for managing chronic pain[155]; however, little evidence exists for using it in people with MS.

Bladder Dysfunction

Urinary incontinence and retention are common and often embarrassing problems for people with MS. Patients may be advised to avoid bladder irritants including caffeine, alcohol, concentrated urine, and infection. Physical therapists may work with patients to assess the factors contributing to bladder dysfunction by retraining hyperactive or weak pelvic floor muscles using biofeedback techniques and exercise. Nurses may need to teach patients with urinary retention intermittent catheterization. Refer to Chapter 29 for additional information on pelvic floor dysfunction and its treatment.

Cognition

Strategies for managing cognitive impairments include compensation techniques such as memory notebooks, diaries, calendars, and computer-assisted programs for memory, attention, or other executive functions. Neuropsychologists, speech-language pathologists, and occupational therapists can all direct cognitive rehabilitation programs. Strategies for coping with cognitive impairments are often shared with the other members of the health care team for reinforcement with patients.

There is growing evidence to support psychological interventions for people with mild to severe MS-related cognitive deficits, aimed at alleviating depressive symptoms and helping people cope with and adjust to their impairments.[156,157] However, the evidence is not yet convincing for specific programs addressing attention and executive functioning. O'Brien[156] was able to recommend the use of a modified story technique to address learning and memory deficits in people with MS. In a systematic review Maitra[158] found that cognitive behavioral therapy programs performed by occupational therapists were positively correlated with improvement in Functional Independence Measure (FIM) scores. Refer to Chapter 27 for additional information regarding interventions with individuals with cognitive problems.

Dysphagia and Dysarthria

Dysphagia or difficulty with chewing and swallowing becomes more prevalent in people with MS as the disease progresses.[159] Therapists facilitate proper swallowing with exercises that will improve posture to prevent aspiration and strengthen muscles of mastication. Other interventions may include diet modifications and education for the patient and his or her family or caregivers. Dieticians may be consulted to facilitate proper food choices.

Dysarthria from the disruption of muscular control in the central and peripheral speech mechanisms leads to abnormalities of speed, range, timing, strength, sound, and accuracy of speech movements. Speech-language pathologists determine therapy programs that take into consideration the stage of the disease and speech quality. Typical programs may include exaggerating articulation, increasing voice volume, and increasing strength of oral musculature. Exercise programs designed to increase respiratory muscle strength have not been successful in improving voice quality or production.[160]

SUMMARY

This chapter has focused on the pathophysiology, clinical presentation, medical management, and rehabilitation of people with MS. Understanding the type of MS, clinical disability, and stage of the disease will help therapists determine the best assessment and intervention strategies for management of the rehabilitation program. Using the ICF framework will facilitate the assessment of the impairments, activity limitations and participation restrictions affecting patients and clients. In addition, including the environmental and personal factors present will help tailor the program to the patient's needs. Using QOL measures developed for people with MS should help the therapist understand the entire range of problems that patients may have.

Many websites are available to assist therapists and their patients with MS to understand the disease and find resources to help them manage the disease. The National MS Society (www.nationalmssociety.org) and the Multiple Sclerosis Foundation (www.msfocus.org) are both excellent resources.

References

To enhance this text and add value for the reader, all references are included on the companion Evolve site that accompanies this textbook. This online service will, when available, provide a link for the reader to a Medline abstract for the article cited. There are 160 cited references and other general references for this chapter, with the majority of those articles being evidence-based citations.

CASE STUDY 19-1

INITIAL INTERVIEW

Mrs. P. is a 54-year-old woman with a 28-year history of RRMS. She was first diagnosed after her third daughter was born and remembers having a lot of trouble walking. Mrs. P. is concerned about her trunk weakness, back pain, and difficulty with walking; she often stumbles, especially when she does not use her single-point cane. She reports having fallen twice in the past year when she lost her balance and was unable to catch herself. One fall was at home, and one in the backyard. Therefore she has been using the cane more, especially on days when she feels off balance. Mrs. P. is limited to 10 minutes of walking and standing secondary to trunk fatigue and difficulty balancing. She is overweight and reports some bladder incontinence and heat sensitivity. Mrs. P. is a homemaker with 4 children; the youngest is 11. Leisure activities include playing the piano, singing, doing the Wii balance exercise for 20 min/day, and doing 10 minutes of treadmill walking at 3.0 mph after using a cooling vest. After her treadmill walking, she feels fatigue for 3 to 4 hours. Recently she has noted having more difficulty with singing and at times feels out of breath. Mrs. P's goals are improved posture, better breath control, no back pain, the ability to walk without stumbling or using a cane, and the ability to keep up with her children and her busy life.

ASSESSMENT

Mrs. P.'s Disease Steps classification is 3 (she uses a cane intermittently and is able to walk for 100 feet without it), and her EDSS score is 6.0. Vital signs are within normal limits (WNL) at rest and for exercise. This patient is cognitively intact and reliable in her response to questions. Her active and passive ROM is WNL throughout her extremities, trunk, and neck. She has selective motor control with normal tone. Manual muscle tests of bilateral upper extremity (UE) were normal, with the lower extremity (LE) 4/5 except for right hip flexion 3+/5, hip extension-abduction and plantarflexion 3/5. Abdominals 2/5, back extensors 3/5 (able to lift trunk against gravity through full range with difficulty and unable to take resistance). Sensation to light touch (LT), pain, and proprioception are intact throughout except for bilateral (B) feet, noted to have diminished sensation to LT. In sitting her posture is extremely slumped (from 30 to 45 degrees when fatigued) with notable thoracic kyphosis. She requires standby assist from supine to prone secondary to trunk weakness and instability. She requires use of B UEs in weight bearing to move from sitting to standing. During observational gait analysis, she demonstrates an asymmetrical step length with the left longer than the right and a right heel strike that is notably loud or audible. Her TUG score is 8 seconds using B UEs to stand up. Tinetti balance (POMA) = 14/16 and gait = 6/12 for a total score of 20/24 (19 to 24 risk for falls). Single-limb stance on the right = 4 seconds and left = 6 seconds, tandem stance = 4 seconds. Perturbation tests reveal loss of stability with an anterior nudge (posterior loss of balance [LOB]), posterior nudge (anterior LOB), and lateral and upper and lower trunk (LOB to opposite side). Rotational resistance tests to the right upper and lower trunk result in a stepping response, and the patient is unable to maintain stability, resulting in a stepping response. Results of rotational resistance tests to left upper and lower trunk are normal.

PLAN OF CARE AND GOALS

Mrs. P. had weakness in B LEs, balance problems, and an unsteady gait with an increased risk of falling, interfering with her functional mobility and QOL. The physical therapy plan included balance and gait training, improved posture and time standing, and increased endurance and cardiovascular fitness. Goals included a decreased fall risk with an improved Tinetti score of 25/28, improved B LE and trunk strength (4/5 in all muscle groups), improved endurance to stand and walk to 30 to 45 minutes, decreased back pain to 0 to 1/10 on most days, and improved endurance and cardiovascular fitness to 45 minutes to 1 hour in 12 to 24 weeks.

INTERVENTION

BBTW placement of 1.5 pounds of weight to the torso to address the perturbation and rotational asymmetries (posterior right upper and lower trunk and anterior near navel) was effective in reducing her kyphotic posture and impaired reactive balance control. The rigid component of the BBTW resolved back pain immediately; she felt better breath control and trunk support, and her Tinetti balance 15/16 and gait 12/12 = 27/28 significantly improved. TUG score remained the same, but she no longer needed her UE to stand up. Her posture also improved to 50% less kyphosis. During gait while weighted, a softer (inaudible) right heel strike was noted, and her step length was even. Mrs. P. expressed that she felt much steadier and more balanced with the BBTW BalanceWear vest and was thrilled to have no back pain.

Mrs. P. was seen in a managed care setting and was able to make significant progress with her physical therapy program. She was seen in physical therapy (1×/week × 1 month, 2×/week × 2 months, 1×/month × 3 months) to improve her posture, strength, balance, and fitness. Breath-control exercises using her diaphragm were implemented to improve singing, monitoring progress with an inspiratory spirometer. Because this patient understood the principles of exercise, she was advised to perform the specific exercise until she experienced a decrease in the quality of movement or the muscles fatigued. A general stretching program was initiated, including specific stretches to improve her posture in sitting and standing. For strengthening exercise she started with one set of 8 to 15 reps; resistance was increased by 2% to -5% when 15 reps were efficient for major muscle groups including hip flexion-extension-abduction, heel raises for plantarflexion, rowing (shoulder retraction) with yellow Thera-Band in standing, curl-ups in hook-lying, and quadruped weight shifts, which were performed 2× to 3×/week. To address her deconditioning, an interval treadmill-training program was implemented on alternating days. Recommendation was to maintain the intensity of 3.0 mph at 65% to 75% of HRmax and do intervals of four blocks of 3 minutes with 1- to 2-minute rest breaks in between and to continue to use the cooling vest before exercise. She continued with the Wii balance program, increasing to 30 minutes on the days she was not doing the treadmill. On those days she also performed specific balance exercises in the corner, beginning with her eyes open (single-leg stance; tandem stance). Mrs. P. was advised to use the BBTW rigid vest for 2 hours during functional activities and walking and to perform her exercises with it every other day. If she became less steady, she was advised to wear the vest an additional 1 to 2 hours per day.

CHAPTER 20 Basal Ganglia Disorders

MARSHA E. MELNICK, PT, PhD

KEY TERMS

Basal ganglia
Dystonia
Huntington disease
Parkinson disease

OBJECTIVES

After reading this chapter the student or therapist will be able to:

1. Describe the circuitry of the basal ganglia.
2. Relate the anatomy and physiology of the basal ganglia to its roles in sensorimotor and cognitive processes.
3. Use the information on anatomy, physiology, and pharmacology to explain the signs and symptoms seen in classic disease states—for example, Parkinson disease, Huntington disease, and dystonia.
4. Develop an evaluation plan for patients with diseases of the basal ganglia.
5. Develop an intervention plan for patients, with the rationale for treatment methods.
6. Determine treatment effectiveness, especially in the case of degenerative disease.
7. Integrate the information in this chapter with the information provided in Section I of this book to develop treatment plans for patients with metabolic or toxic disorders.

This chapter considers the degenerative, metabolic, hereditary, and genetic disorders that typically have their onset in adulthood, including Parkinson disease, parkinsonian syndromes, Huntington chorea, Wilson disease, dystonias, heavy metal poisoning, and drug intoxication. Because of the wide variety of diseases with their wide variety of causes, the concentration is on understanding the clinical problems and commonalities that exist within this grouping. In general, the practice parameter of the diseases discussed in this chapter is the physical therapy diagnostic parameter 5E: Impaired motor and sensory integrity associated with progressive disorders of the central nervous system, from the *Guide to Physical Therapist Practice.*[1] Although the occupational therapy guide does not classify practice parameters in that manner, the concepts and clinical reasoning process can be used by both professionals. The predominant area of the brain affected by these disorders is the basal ganglia: this group of central nervous system (CNS) structures is therefore discussed in some detail.

THE BASAL GANGLIA

The most commonly seen disorders affecting the basal ganglia include Parkinson disease, Huntington chorea, and dystonias, including drug-induced dyskinesias. All of these medical diagnoses involve impairments in muscle tone, movement coordination and motor control, and postural stability and the presence of extraneous movement. Taken together, these disorders now affect approximately 1 million people in the United States.[2-4]

To understand how this area of the brain can account for such a wide variety of symptoms, the anatomy, physiology, and neurochemistry of the basal ganglia structures must be considered.

Anatomy

The dorsal or sensorimotor basal ganglia are composed of three nuclei located at the base of the cerebral cortex—hence their name. These nuclei are the caudate nucleus, the putamen, and the globus pallidus. Two brain stem nuclei, the substantia nigra and the subthalamic nucleus, are included as part of the basal ganglia because they have a close functional relation to the forebrain nuclei. In addition, connections between the basal ganglia and the pedunculopontine nucleus (PPN) are important in regulating underlying tone. Other parts of the basal ganglia, the ventral basal ganglia, are intimately related to the limbic system and are discussed in Chapter 5. The anatomical location of the various parts of the basal ganglia is shown in Figure 20-1.

The caudate nucleus and the putamen are similar structures embryologically, anatomically, and functionally and are often referred to together as the neostriatum—a term derived from the word *striate* and used to denote pathways from and to the caudate and putamen. An older term, *corpus striatum,* refers to the caudate, putamen, and globus pallidus. The various connections and interconnections of this system are discussed on the basis of these definitions.

Afferent Pathways

Functionally, the basal ganglia can be divided into an afferent portion and an efferent portion (Figure 20-2). The afferent structures are the caudate and putamen. They receive input from the entire cerebral cortex, the intralaminar thalamic nuclei, and the centromedian-parafascicular complex of the thalamus as well as from the substantia nigra and the dorsal raphe nucleus, both located within the brain stem. The projections from the cortex are systematically arranged so that the frontal cortex projects to the head of the caudate and putamen and the visual cortex projects to the tail. In addition,

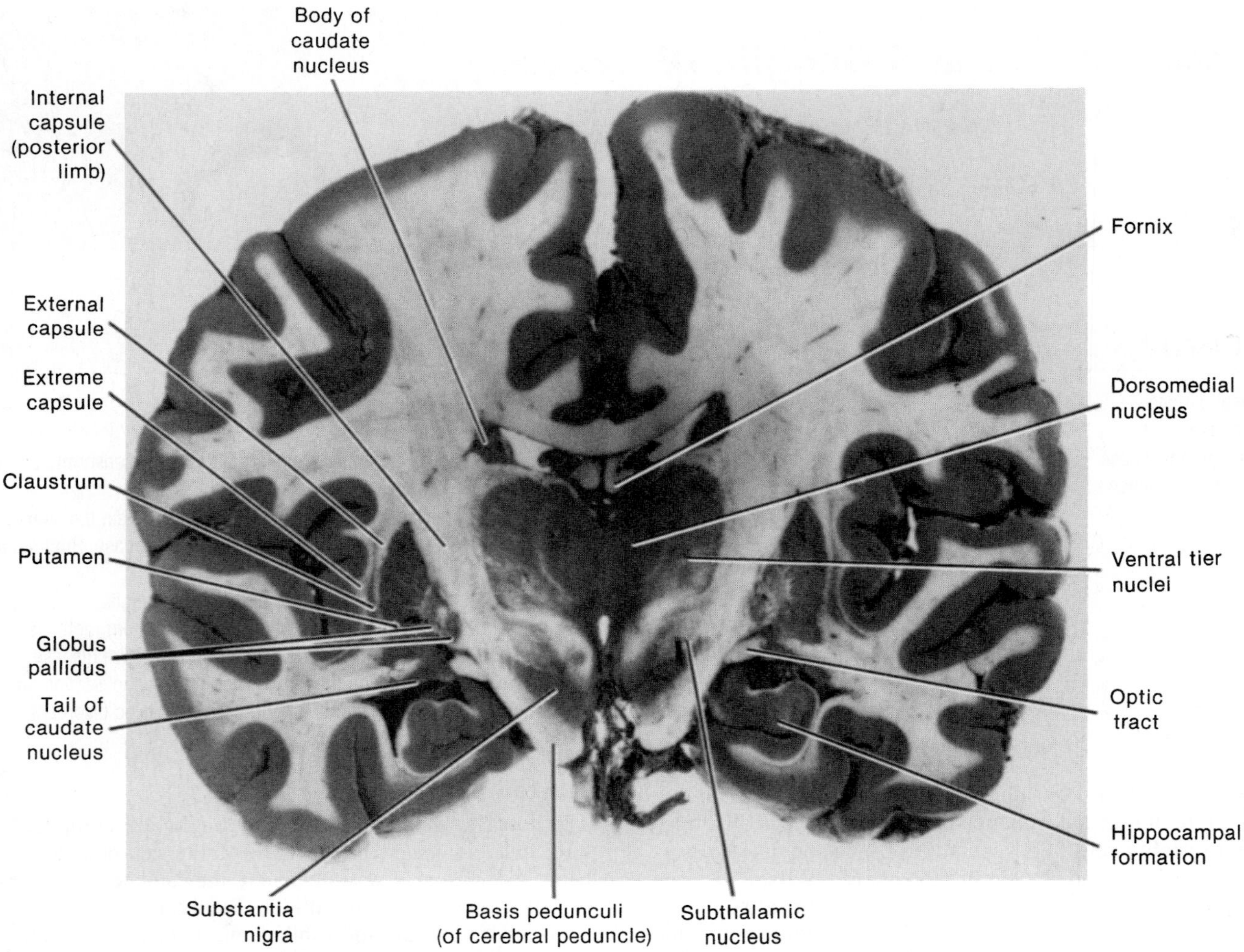

Figure 20-1 ■ A coronal section of the anatomical location of various parts of the basal ganglia. (Reprinted from Nolte J: *The human brain: an introduction to its anatomy,* St Louis, 1981, CV Mosby.)

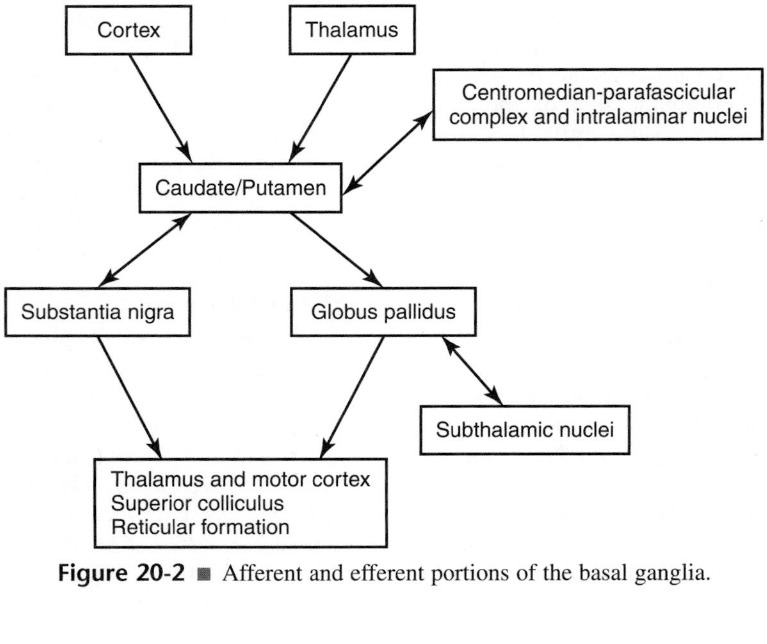

Figure 20-2 ■ Afferent and efferent portions of the basal ganglia.

the prefrontal cortex projects mainly to the caudate, whereas the sensorimotor cortex projects mainly to the putamen.[5-8] Projections from the cortical regions that represent the proximal musculature, and those from the premotor regions may be bilateral.[6,9-11] These close and profuse connections between the cortex and the basal ganglia suggest a close interfunctional relationship. The projections from the thalamus to the caudate-putamen are also somatotopically arranged. The heaviest projections are from the centromedian nucleus, and these nuclei also receive massive input from the motor cortex.[7-10]

The somatotopic arrangement of the cortico-striatal–thalamic-cortical pathways is maintained throughout the loop. This finding has led to an important functional hypothesis that the basal ganglia form parallel pathways subserving specific sensorimotor and associative functions.[5] The putamen is linked to the sensorimotor functions and the caudate to the associative, including cognitive functions.[9,12]

As knowledge of the circuitry of the basal ganglia has advanced, so has the knowledge regarding the microscopic structure. The caudate-putamen looks somewhat homogeneous because of the predominance of one cell type. Careful analysis using precise staining methods has demonstrated the appearance of patches within these nuclei. It is hypothesized that this organization is important for the ability of the basal ganglia to modulate ongoing sensory input and choose the appropriate motor response.[12] The intrinsic structure of the caudate-putamen also suggests that at least nigral input occurs in a way that could immediately modulate the input coming from the cortex.[13,14]

Efferent Pathways

The input that has been processed in the caudate-putamen is sent to the globus pallidus (pallidum) and substantia nigra (nigra), which constitute the efferent portion of the basal ganglia. The globus pallidus and substantia nigra are each divided into two regions. The globus pallidus has an external and an internal region; the substantia nigra consists of the dorsal pars compacta and the ventral pars reticulata. Embryologically and microscopically, the internal segment of the globus pallidus and the pars reticulata of the substantia nigra are similar. These two regions are the primary efferent structures for the basal ganglia. The projections from the caudate and putamen to the pallidum and nigra maintain a somatotopic arrangement.[10,15,16] From these structures the information is transmitted to the thalamus and then to the cortex, still maintaining somatotopy. The superior colliculus, the PPN, and other, less defined brain stem structures (perhaps the reticular formation) also receive pallidal and nigral output. All output of the basal ganglia has then been processed through the globus pallidus and/or the substantia nigra before proceeding to other areas of the brain (see Figure 20-2).

Pathways to the Motor System

Information processed in the basal ganglia can influence the motor system in several ways, but no direct pathway to the alpha or gamma motor neurons of the spinal cord exists. The first route is the projection to the ventroanterior and ventrolateral nuclei of the thalamus, which then project predominantly to the premotor cortex. Another pathway is through the superior colliculus and then to the tectospinal tract. Pathways exist from the globus pallidus and substantia nigra that terminate in areas of the reticular formation (e.g., the PPN) and thus may influence the motor system through the reticulospinal pathways. Anatomically the basal ganglia are therefore in good position to affect the motor system at many levels. Many of these connections are also areas that receive cerebellar input, and thus these two regions of the brain have ample opportunity to further integrate movement responses.[17]

The basic circuitry of the basal ganglia comprises two loops.[7] The loops for the sensorimotor system are shown in Figure 20-3. The direct loop is the loop that begins in the motor regions of the cortex and projects to the putamen and then directly to the globus pallidus, the internal segment, and on to the thalamus. The indirect pathway adds the subthalamic nucleus between the globus pallidus, external segment, and internal segment before sending the signal on to the thalamus. The subthalamic nucleus also receives direct

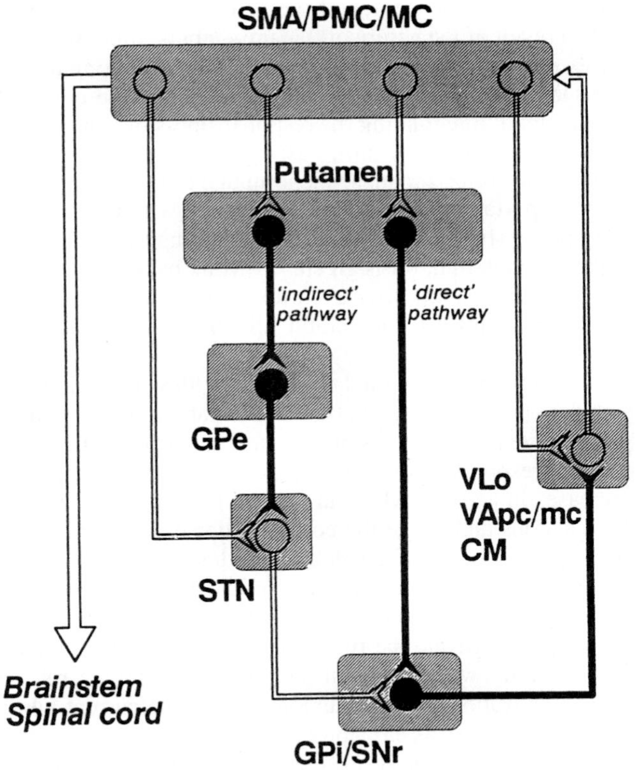

Figure 20-3 ■ Diagram of the sensory motor portion of the basal ganglia depicting the direct and indirect pathways. *Black circles* represent inhibitory neurons; *open circles* represent excitatory neurons. *CM,* Centromedian nucleus of the thalamus; *GPe,* globus pallidus external segment; *GPi,* globus pallidus internal segment; *MC,* motor cortex; *PMC,* premotor cortex; *SMA,* supplementary motor cortex; *SNr,* pars reticularis of the substantia nigra; *STN,* subthalamic nucleus; *VApc/mc,* ventral anterior pars parvocellularis and pars magnocellularis of the thalamus; *VLo,* ventral lateralis pars oralis nucleus of the thalamus. (Reprinted from Alexander GE, Crutcher MD: Functional architecture of basal ganglia circuits: neural substrates of parallel processing, *Trends Neurosci* 13:266-271, 1990.)

input from the premotor and motor cortex as well as from the pallidum.[18,19] The darkened neurons represent inhibitory connections, and the open neurons represent excitatory connections. In general, the direct pathway, by disinhibition, activates the thalamocortical pathway; the indirect pathway inhibits the thalamocortical system. The role of these loops in normal and diseased states is clarified in the discussion of the physiology and pharmacology of the basal ganglia.

In summary, input from the motor cortex, all other areas of the cortex, parts of the thalamus, and the substantia nigra enter the basal ganglia through the caudate and putamen. Here they are processed and sent on to the globus pallidus and substantia nigra. The appropriate "gain" of the system is adjusted, for example, how large a movement is necessary or how much postural stability is needed. The information is sent to the muscles by way of the thalamus and motor cortex, the superior colliculus, and/or the reticular formation.

Physiology

The caudate and putamen are composed of neurons that fire slowly; the globus pallidus neurons fire tonically at high rates. The low firing rates of the caudate-putamen are partially a result of the nature of thalamic inputs. Input from the cortex seems to have priority over input from the thalamus and substantia nigra. These data indicate that the cortex is instrumental in regulating the responsiveness of caudate and putamen neurons.[20] In turn, basal ganglia stimulation may prepare the cortex for subsequent inputs; this might be especially important when a response must be withheld until an appropriate stimulus occurs, such as keeping the foot on the brake until the light turns green.[20-23] Mink hypothesized that basal ganglia inputs to the cortex activate only the most necessary pathways and inhibit all unnecessary pathways (Figure 20-4).[24]

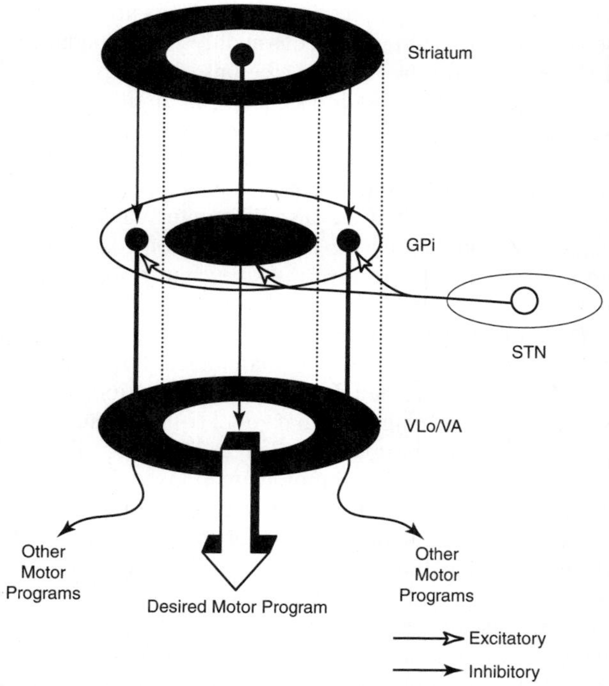

Figure 20-4 ■ The net effect of basal ganglia circuitry to produce an area of excitation (the desired program) surrounded by an area of inhibition (all other unnecessary programs). *GPi,* Globus pallidus internal segment; *STN,* subthalamic nucleus; *VLo/VA,* ventral lateralis oralis, ventral anterior. (Adapted from Mink JW: The basal ganglia: focused selection and inhibition of competing motor programs, *Prog Neurobiol* 50:381-425, 1996.)

The pattern of neuronal firing in the direct and indirect pathways also suggests that the basal ganglia modify input to the cortex. The neurons of the efferent portion of the basal ganglia respond with either phasic increases or phasic decreases in activity, which in turn will affect the activity in the thalamus and hence the cortex. A decrease in activity of the internal segment of the globus pallidus removes inhibition to the thalamus and thus enables cortical activation. Whether the two pathways are activated concurrently or whether different activities activate the two pathways separately is not yet known; either way, the basal ganglia would have a role in cortical activation and modulation. One of the current views in relationship to disease processes is that an underactive direct pathway and/or an overactive indirect pathway would lead to decreased activation of the cortex and hence bradykinesia and akinesia, whereas an overactive direct pathway and/or underactive indirect pathway would lead to the presence of extraneous movements (see Figure 20-3).[6,25]

How do these pathways relate to everyday function? Rigidity could be explained by too much muscle activity (through the pathways from the basal ganglia to the PPN and on to the spinal cord). Akinesia and bradykinesia typical of individuals with Parkinson disease are caused by insufficient excitation or too many conflicting patterns of movement. Increased extraneous movements are characteristic of basal ganglia diseases and can be attributed to the dysfunctions within these pathways. If the amount of muscle activity and the sequence and timing of activation are inappropriate, the individual will have difficulty in selecting the environmentally appropriate behavior.[24-27] Aldridge and colleagues found that the basal ganglia were modulated dependent on the purpose of the impending movement.[27]

Relationship of the Basal Ganglia to Movement and Posture

Lesion experiments; single and multiple unit recordings in awake, behaving animals; careful observations of the sequelae of human disease processes; and the results of functional magnetic stimulation studies in humans have provided some answers regarding the precise role of the basal ganglia in movement and posture.

Automatic Movement

The earliest view of the basal ganglia came from Willis in 1664. He hypothesized that the corpus striatum received "the notion of spontaneous localized movements in ascending tracts.... Conversely, from here tendencies are dispatched to enact notions without reflection [automatic movements] over descending pathways" (p. 7).[28] Willis possessed great insights in the discussion of the signs and symptoms of basal ganglia disease. Magendie in 1841 demonstrated that removal of the striatum bilaterally produced compulsive movements, whereas removal of only one striatum produced no visible effect.[29] Studies by Nothnagel[30] demonstrated that lesions of the nigra tended to produce immobility. With the advent of the use of electrical stimulation in the late nineteenth century, further information on the function of the basal ganglia was gathered. Stimulation of the caudate nucleus did not (and does not) produce movement of muscles or limbs as occurs with stimulation of the motor cortex. However, at higher levels of current, total body patterns and postures were usually evoked. The earliest stimulation of the caudate nucleus produced an increase of flexion of the head, trunk, and limbs and tonic contraction of the facial muscles.[31] These early studies are mentioned because of the insights they provide for the symptoms of the disorders of today.

Motor Problems in Animals

Contemporary experiments using lesion paradigms show a wide variety of motor problems in a variety of animals. Hypokinesia, a decrease or poverty of movements, a decreased amount of exploration of novel environments, and a tendency to assume a fixed posture are the most common problems after a lesion in the basal ganglia. These motoric dysfunctions are seen regardless of the method by which the lesion is made: pharmacologic, surgical, or by stimulation. In essence, movements are altered in scale (related to the gain), take longer for completion, and take place under altered conditions of antagonistic muscle interactions (e.g., contraction).[32-40]

Movement Initiation and Preparation

The hypothesis that the basal ganglia are involved in movement initiation and preparation is an area of some research disagreement. A "readiness potential," recorded from the scalp of human beings before movement and thought to reflect basal ganglia activity, is more apparent in complex than in simple movements, for example, before dorsiflexion with gait but not before dorsiflexion when sitting.[41-44]

Neuronal recordings from awake, behaving animals found that units in the basal ganglia alter their activity before changes in the electromyographic activity of the prime movers of the task.[45-51] Studies recording from multiple units in animals moving freely in their home environment suggest that neurons in the caudate-putamen and in the substantia nigra are activated in sequential, purposeful movements.[27]

Postural Adjustments

The basal ganglia have been implicated in the process of posture and postural adjustments. People with diseases of the basal ganglia assume flexed or other fixed postures as the disease progresses (Figure 20-5). In addition, these individuals have decreased postural stability and are therefore at risk for falls. Animal experiments indicate that a deficit exists in determining response based on one's own body position, or "egocentric localization."[52-54] This deficit decreases the ability of a person with basal ganglia disease to modify a postural response to the precise environmental demands.

Martin,[55] in his extensive studies of individuals with Parkinson disease, was the first to describe severe disturbances in posture, especially when vision was occluded. Melnick and colleagues[56] showed that a decrease in static postural adjustments in persons with Parkinson disease could be seen early in the disease process.[57] Bloem and colleagues[58-60] and Visser and colleagues[61,62] meticulously studied the reflexes involved in postural adjustments and

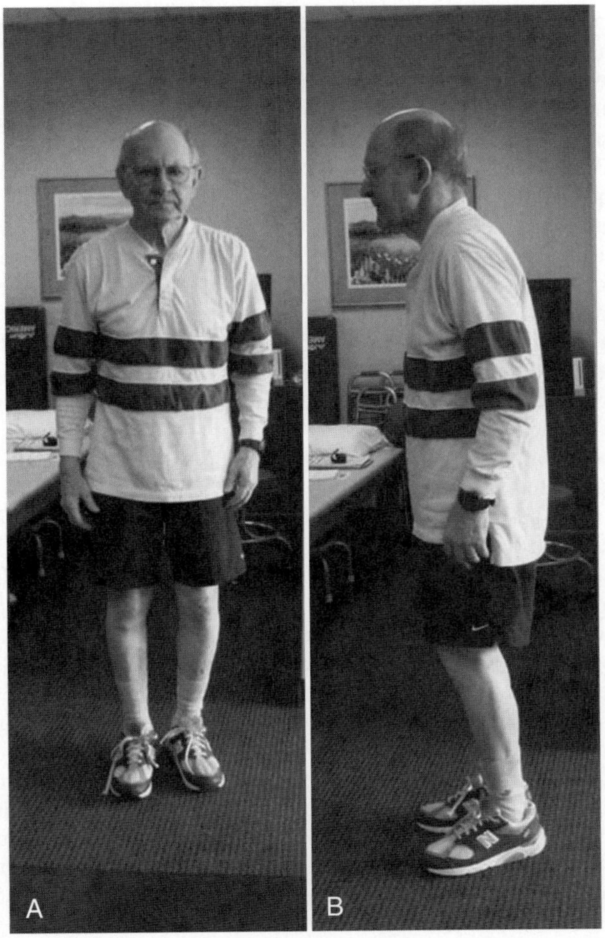

Figure 20-5 ■ Typical posture of a patient with Parkinson disease from the front and from the side. Note the flexed spine, mild flexion at the hips and knees, and excessive dorsiflexion with weight predominantly on the heels. Patient was at Hoehn and Yahr stage 2.5.

described deficits in the longer loop reflexes but not in the short latency reflex associated with the stretch reflex.

Others have investigated the interactions of the sensory systems involved in balance in those with Parkinson disease.[62-66] Bloem and colleagues[60] and Visser and colleagues[62] concluded that postural instability was caused by a decrease in proprioception. In a recent review of proprioception and postural stability and motor control, Nicola and colleagues also describe the kinesthetic and proprioceptive deficits in people with Parkinson disease. Nicola and colleagues concluded that there was a "failure" in the body map similar to the failure in egocentric localization described previously.[54] A decrease in the ability to use proprioceptive and kinesthetic information to properly scale the input and response also contributes to a loss of balance reactions.

Perceptual and Cognitive Functions

The basal ganglia are not solely motor systems. The previous paragraphs demonstrate the role of the basal ganglia in sensory integration. The basal ganglia are also involved in cognitive functions and responses associated with reward.[36,37,48,50,67-70] Researchers have found that learned movements are more affected by basal ganglia lesions than reflexes, that neurons in the basal ganglia are responsive to some sensory input, especially proprioceptive input, and that neurons in other parts of the basal ganglia are responsive to reward and anticipation of the reward.[26,71,72] Klockgether and Dichgans[73] as well as Jobst and colleagues[74] found that patients with Parkinson disease likewise had impairments in kinesthesia and that as a person moved a limb further from the body's center, kinesthetic sense decreased. Schneider and colleagues[75] found that animals that developed parkinsonian symptoms from a neurotoxin had deficits in operantly conditioned behavior. They suggested that the decrease in performance resulted from a "defect in the linkage" between a stimulus and the motor output centers. These sensory difficulties may be important factors in evaluation and treatment of basal ganglia diseases, especially those associated with dystonia.

The basal ganglia appear to be involved in the process of withholding a response until it is appropriate.[76] A deficit in alternation of response may be the result of a tendency toward perseveration of a previously reinforced cue.[77] Additional deficits exist in remembering or relearning tasks requiring a temporal sequence.[78] Graybiel[26] integrated the behavioral findings with information from her anatomical and chemical studies to suggest that the basal ganglia are important in providing behavioral flexibility. She hypothesizes that the basal ganglia are involved in procedural learning that leads to the development of habits. These habits become routine and are easily performed without conscious effort. Because these activities can proceed without thought, we are free to react to new events in our environment and to think. She and colleagues have performed electrophysiological experiments that explain this learning process, and these studies demonstrate great plasticity in basal ganglia networks.[79] This enables the individual to select the proper movements in the proper environmental context. An elegant study by Brown and colleagues[80] demonstrates a model of the basal ganglia that can reflect these cognitive and learning activities. Their model seems to integrate many of the functions of the basal ganglia with the physiology and pharmacology of the entire system. These cognitive dimensions are important to remember when developing a plan of care for a patient with basal ganglia dysfunction.

Humans with basal ganglia disease also show problems in perceptual abilities, including deficits in tasks that involve perception of interpersonal and intrapersonal space.[81] In pursuit-tracking tests individuals with Parkinson disease had particular difficulties in correcting errors[77]; if the motor system is inflexibly set, corrections can be made only by a complete reprogramming.

The ability to perform cognitive activities involves integrating sensory information and, on the basis of this information, making an appropriate response. The basal ganglia seem to have a sensory integrative function as evidenced by experiments that show a multisensory and heterotopic convergence of somatic, visual, auditory, and vestibular stimuli.[26,71,72] Segundo and Machne[82] hypothesized that the function of the basal ganglia was not subjective recognition of the stimuli but rather in the regulation of posture and movements of the body in space and in the production of complex motor acts. Nicola and colleagues had similar conclusions.[54]

For movements to be properly controlled and properly sequenced, the two sides of the body need to be well integrated. There is anatomical evidence that suggests some means of bilateral control for the basal ganglia. A lesion of one caudate nucleus or nigrostriatal pathway produces a change in the unit activity of the remaining caudate.[78,83] Studies of the dopaminergic pathway also indicate interactions between the two sides of the body.[83] For this reason one may find deficits in function even on the "uninvolved" side of an individual with disease of the basal ganglia. It is also possible that diseases of the basal ganglia may go unnoticed until damage is found bilaterally.

This summary of experimental results on the function of the basal ganglia illustrates several points. At least in some general way the basal ganglia are involved in the processes of movement related to preparing the organism for future motion and future reward. This may include preparing the cortex for approximate time activation, setting the postural reflexes or the gamma motor neuron system, organizing sensory input to produce a motor response in an appropriate environmental context, and inhibiting all unnecessary motor activity. Because of the multilevel involvement of the basal ganglia in movement, it is crucial that clinicians carefully observe all aspects of movement (simple and complex) with and without interference of sensory cues or performance of dual tasks as well as postural tone during examination and treatment and the responses to treatment (see Chapter 9).

Neurotransmitters

Before a detailed analysis of the diseases of the basal ganglia can be considered, a brief description of the neurotransmitters of this region is necessary. The most prevalent diseases discussed in this chapter indicate a deficit in specific neurotransmitters. The pharmacological treatment of Parkinson disease and, in the future, perhaps other "basal ganglia plus" diseases, is based on these neurochemical deficits. The basal ganglia possess high concentrations of many of the suspected neurotransmitters: dopamine (DA), acetylcholine (ACh), γ-aminobutyric acid (GABA), substance P, and the enkephalins and endorphins. This discussion, however, includes only the first three neurotransmitters. A diagram of the basal ganglia pathways, which includes the neurotransmitters, is shown in Figure 20-6.

DA is the major neurotransmitter of the nigrostriatal pathway. It is produced in the pars compacta of the substantia nigra. The axon terminals of these dopaminergic neurons are located in the caudate nucleus and putamen. DA appears to be excitatory to the neurons in the direct pathway (GABA and substance P neurons) and inhibitory to the neurons in the indirect pathway (GABA and enkephalin neurons).[2] This dual effect means that a loss of DA will lead to a loss of excitation in the direct pathway and an excess of excitation of the indirect pathway, leading to a powerful decrease in activation of the thalamocortical pathway.

Several DA receptors exist; however, their chemical interactions permit the continued use of D1 and D2 receptor classes.[7] The role of DA may modulate the effects of other neurotransmitters such as glutamate. Many new drugs (called the *dopamine agonists*) influence only one of these receptors. Recent experiments have been trying to determine which behaviors are mediated by which DA receptor in the

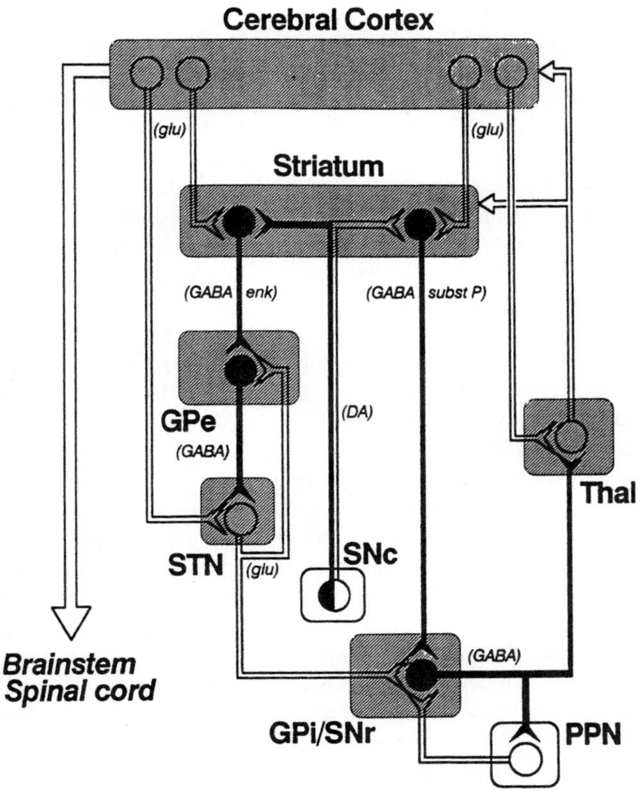

Figure 20-6 ■ The neurotransmitters of the direct and indirect pathways of the basal ganglia. *Black circles* represent inhibitory neurons; *open circles* represent excitatory neurons. *enk,* Enkephalin; *glu,* glutamate; *GPe,* globus pallidus external segment; *GPi,* globus pallidus internal segment; *SNr,* pars reticularis of the substantia nigra; *STN,* subthalamic nucleus; *subst P,* substance P; *Thal,* thalamus. (Reprinted from Alexander GE, Crutcher MD: Functional architecture of basal ganglia circuits: neural substrates of parallel processing, *Trends Neurosci* 13:266–271, 1990.)

hope that this research may lead to more effective drug treatment with fewer side effects.

Because various drugs and chemicals can act as agonists (similar to) and antagonists (blocking the action of) of DA, they are used in treating disease involving the basal ganglia. Agonists include amantadine, apomorphine, and a class of drugs called the *ergot alkaloids* (e.g., bromocriptine). Amphetamine, which prevents the reuptake of DA, can enhance the effect of any DA present in the system. Antagonists include haloperidol, clozapine, and antipsychotic drugs of the phenothiazine class. With time these drugs may deplete the basal ganglia of DA and thus cause Parkinson disease or tardive dyskinesia. Similar effects on the DA system are observed in a single dose of methamphetamine (see Chapter 36).[84]

ACh is believed to be the neurotransmitter of the small interneurons of the caudate and putamen. It is presumed to inhibit the action of DA in this region and classically must be "in balance" with DA (and GABA). Dopaminergic axon terminals are found on cholinergic neurons. Substances that increase dopaminergic activity decrease release of ACh and vice versa.[85] The antagonists of ACh, such as belladonna alkaloids and atropine-like drugs, were one of the first class of drugs used in the treatment of Parkinson disease. ACh antagonists are still used as adjuncts to treatment for patients with Parkinson disease. As some of the drugs to treat dementia are ACh agonists, care must be used when these are prescribed for the person with basal ganglia dysfunction, especially Parkinson disease.

GABA is an inhibitory neurotransmitter that is found throughout the brain. In the basal ganglia it is synthesized in the caudate nucleus and putamen and transmitted to the globus pallidus and substantia nigra.[86] GABA in the basal ganglia may permit movement to occur by allowing a distribution of neuronal firing. It also may provide a means of feedback inhibition in the efferent parts of the basal ganglia so that the program of activity is not repeated unless needed.[86] Individuals with Huntington disease have a deficiency of this chemical. Although agonists of GABA exist (e.g., muscimol and imidazole acetic acid), a successful drug for the treatment of Huntington disease has not yet been found. This may be a result of either the ubiquitous nature of GABA or the very complex circuitry and interrelationships that exist among GABA, ACh, and DA.

In addition to the transmitters discussed, co-transmitters may be found in the basal ganglia. Two such co-transmitters are cholecystokinin and neurotensin. The interactions of these co-transmitters may alter the sensitivity of DA receptors. Fuxe and colleagues[87] suggest that the interactions of co-transmitters may alter the "set point" of transmission in synapses. They may therefore be important in one of the side effects of DA therapy, supersensitivity.

Lastly, the neurotransmitter from the cortex to the caudate nucleus and putamen is glutamate. Studies are ongoing to investigate glutamate antagonists as a treatment for Parkinson disease. Glutamate receptors use calcium, and in the future, drugs affecting calcium channels may also have a therapeutic effect.

SPECIFIC CLINICAL PROBLEMS ARISING FROM BASAL GANGLIA DYSFUNCTION

Parkinson Disease

Parkinson disease, first described by Parkinson in 1807, is a disease characterized by rigidity, bradykinesia (slow movement), micrography, masked face, postural abnormalities, and a resting tremor. As might be suspected from the review of functional physiology of the basal ganglia, the postural abnormalities include an assumption of a flexed posture, a lack of equilibrium reactions, especially of the labyrinthine equilibrium reactions, and a decrease in trunk rotation. Parkinson disease is among the most prevalent of all CNS degenerative diseases. Presently there are an estimated 1 million people in the United States with this disease, with approximately 60,000 new cases each year; the incidence is 4.5 to 20.5 and the prevalence is 31 to 347 per 100,000. (Refer to the list of websites at the end of this chapter.) Incidence increases with advancing age, and it is estimated that one in three adults over the age of 85 will have this disease.[2] The personal and societal burden of Parkinson disease is great and includes the costs of actual treatment, the burden of caregiving, and the costs of lost earnings in patients under the age of 65.[88]

The pathology of Parkinson disease consists of a decrease in the DA stores of the substantia nigra with a consequent depigmentation of this structure and the presence of Lewy bodies (intracellular inclusions). It is DA that gives the substantia nigra its coloration (and hence its name); therefore the lighter the nigra, the greater the DA loss.

The cause of Parkinson disease remains unknown, and the consensus is that it is multifactorial.[89,90] A slow viral process or long-term effects of early infection were implicated in postencephalitic parkinsonism. Some evidence indicates involvement of environmental factors and that interaction of environment and aging lead to a critical decrease in DA. Several investigators have found a link between growing up in a rural area and Parkinson disease; the important factors include pesticide use, insecticide use, and elements in well water.[91-97] Accumulation of free radicals, cell death to excitatory neurons from toxins, and dysfunction of nigral mitochondria have all been implicated in the pathological process. The genetics of Parkinson disease is still debated. Although twin studies indicate that there may not be a single gene involved in Parkinson disease, as in Huntington disease, a family history may be an important risk factor.[93,98-101] Very recently a large-scale study found two genetic loci to be associated with Parkinson disease.[102] So the debate continues, with most neurologists agreeing that the multifactorial approach will yield the best opportunity to develop a cure.

In view of possible treatment effects for Parkinson disease, it is interesting that a study by Sasco and others[103] found an inverse relationship, albeit small, between participation in exercise or sports and later development of Parkinson disease. The loss of DA from the substantia nigra leads to alterations in both the direct and indirect pathways of the basal ganglia, resulting in a decrease in excitatory thalamic input to the cortex and perhaps a decrease in inhibitory surround that leads to the symptoms of Parkinson disease.

Symptoms

Bradykinesia and Akinesia. Bradykinesia (a decrease in motion) and akinesia (a lack of motion) are characterized by an inability to initiate and perform purposeful movements. They are also associated with a tendency to assume and maintain fixed postures. All aspects of movement are affected, including initiation, alteration in direction, and the ability to stop a movement once it is begun. Spontaneous or associated movements, such as swinging of the arms in gait or smiling at a funny story, are also affected. Bradykinesia is hypothesized to be the result of a decrease in activation of the supplementary motor cortex, premotor cortex, and motor cortex.[104] The resting level of activity in these areas of the cortex may be decreased so that a greater amount of excitatory input from other areas of the brain would be necessary before movement patterns could be activated. In the individual with Parkinson disease, an increase in cortically initiated movement even for such "subcortical" activities as walking supports this hypothesis. Automatic activities are cortically controlled, and each individual aspect seems to be separately programmed. Associated movements in the trunk and other extremities are not automatic. This means that great energy must be expended whenever movement is begun.[105]

Bradykinesia and akinesia affect performance of all types of movements; however, complex movements are more involved than simple movements, such as dorsiflexing the foot at toe-off in walking as opposed to dorsiflexing the foot in a seated position.[71,106-109] In addition, patients with parkinsonism have increased difficulty performing simultaneous or sequential tasks, over and above that seen with simple tasks. Parkinsonian patients must complete one movement before they can begin to perform the next, whereas control subjects are able to integrate two movements more smoothly in sequence. This deficit has been shown in a variety of tasks from performing an elbow movement and grip to tracing a moving line on a video screen. The patient with Parkinson disease behaves as if one motor program must be completely played out before the next one begins, and there is no advance planning for the next movement while the current movement is in progress.[106-108,110,111] Morris and colleagues demonstrated a similar phenomenon in walking. Patients with parkinsonism were unable to perform walking while carrying a tray with a glass of water and had even more difficulty when walking and reciting a numerical sequence.[112,113]

Sequential movements become more impaired as more movements are strung together; for example, a square is disproportionately slower to draw than a triangle; a pentagon, more difficult than a square.[5,106] These results indicate that patients with Parkinson disease have difficulty with transitions between movements. Transitional difficulties are more impaired in tasks requiring a series of different movements than tasks requiring a series of repetitive movements. For example, an individual will have less difficulty continually riding a stationary bike than movement requiring transitions such as coming from a chair to standing, walking, and turning a corner. Therefore treatment must include complex movements with directional changes to ensure that the patient is safe outside the treatment setting.

Bradykinesia is not caused by rigidity or an inability to relax. This was demonstrated in an electromyographic analysis of voluntary movements of persons with Parkinson disease.[114] Although the pattern of electromyographic agonist-antagonists burst is correct, these bursts are not large enough, resulting in an inability to generate muscle force rapidly enough. Even in slow, smooth movements, however, these individuals demonstrated alternating bursts in the flexor and extensor muscle groups. This type of pattern, expected in rapid movements that require the immediate activation of the antagonist to halt the motion, interferes with slow, smooth, continuous motion. Other researchers have found an alteration in the recruitment order of single motor units.[115,116] These alterations included a delay in recruitment, pauses in the motor unit once it was recruited, and an inability to increase firing rates. These persons therefore would have a delay in activation of muscles and an inability to properly sustain muscle contraction for movement, and a decreased ability to dissipate force rapidly.[24,115,117] Such changes may account for perceived decreases in strength that are seen in persons with Parkinson disease. They are also important to remember in both treatment planning and the efficacy of treatment efficiency.

Rigidity. The rigidity (increased resistance to passive movement) of Parkinson disease may be characterized as either "lead pipe" or "cogwheel." The cogwheel type of rigidity is a combination of lead-pipe rigidity with tremor. In rigidity there is an increased resistance to movement throughout the entire range in both directions without the classic clasp-knife reflex so characteristic of spasticity. Procaine injections can decrease the rigidity without affecting the decrease of spontaneous movements, confirming that rigidity is not the same phenomenon as bradykinesia.[118,119]

Rigidity is not caused by an increase in gamma motor neuron activity, a decrease in recurrent inhibition, or a generalized excitability in the motor system.[120] Long- and middle-latency reflexes are enhanced in parkinsonism, and the increase in long-latency reflexes approximates the observable increase in muscle tone. Short-latency reflexes (i.e., deep tendon reflexes), on the other hand, may be normal in persons with Parkinson disease.

Tatton and others[121] found differences in certain cortical long-loop reflexes in normal and drug-induced parkinsonian monkeys, which led them to speculate that the "reflex gain" of the CNS may lose its ability to adjust to changing environmental situations. For example, in normal persons the background level of motor neuron excitability is different for the task of writing than for the task of lifting a heavy object; in individuals with Parkinson disease motor neuron excitability would be set at the same level. Similarly, in the normal individual there would be a difference in excitability if the environmental demands were for excitation or inhibition of a muscle; for the individual with Parkinson disease, there would be similar motor neuron excitability regardless of task demands. Furthermore, this lack of modulation may mean that the person with parkinsonism perceives himself or herself to be moving farther than he or she is actually moving. It is also consistent with a decrease in system flexibility and an inability to adjust to equilibrium perturbations.[58,59,65]

An important aspect of rigidity is that it might increase energy expenditure.[122] This would increase the patient's perception of effort on movement and may be related to feelings of fatigue, especially postexercise fatigue.[123]

Tremor. The tremor observed in Parkinson disease is present at rest, usually disappears or decreases with movement, and has a regular rhythm of about 4 to 7 beats per second. Some people with Parkinson disease may have a postural tremor. The electromyographic tracing of a person with such a tremor shows rhythmical, alternating bursting of antagonistic muscles. Tremor can be produced as an isolated finding in experimental animals that have lesions in various parts of the brain stem or that have been treated with drugs, especially DA antagonists. DA depletion, however, is not the sole cause of tremor. It appears that efferent pathways, especially from the basal ganglia to the thalamus, must be intact because lesions of these fibers decrease or abolish the tremor.[124] Poirier and colleagues[124] proposed that tremor results from a combined lesion of the basal ganglia and cerebellar–red nucleus pathways. Because both the basal ganglia and the cerebellum project to the thalamus, a lesion of the thalamus can abolish the tremor regardless of the specific pathway(s). Although tremor may be cosmetically disabling, the tremor rarely interferes with activities of daily living (ADLs).

Postural Instability. Postural instability is a serious problem in parkinsonism that leads to increased episodes of falling and the sequelae of falls. More than two thirds of all patients with parkinsonism fall, and more than 10% fall more than once a week.[125] People with Parkinson disease have a ninefold risk of recurrent falls compared with age-matched control subjects.[60,126-130] Patients have an increased likelihood of falling as the duration of the disease increases. Drug treatment is not usually effective in reducing the incidence of falls. Deep brain stimulation and exercise, on the other hand, have been shown to be effective in increasing functional skills and/or motor performance; these improvements may decrease the number of falls.[131-134] Large randomized clinical trials have been performed to determine the efficacy of exercise.[135]

Although the causes of balance difficulties are not known, several hypotheses exist. One explanation for postural instability is ineffective sensory processing. Several investigators have found deficits in proprioceptive and kinesthetic processing.[55,74,117,136] For example, Martin[55] found that labyrinthine equilibrium reactions were delayed in patients with Parkinson disease. Studies of the vestibular system itself, however, have shown that this system functions normally. Pastor and colleagues[137] studied central vestibular processing in patients with Parkinson disease and found that the vestibular system responds normally and that patients can integrate vestibular input with the input from other sensory systems. This group hypothesized that the parkinsonian patients had an inability to adequately compensate for baseline instability. This theory is in partial agreement with studies by Beckley, Boehm, and others[58,59,65] demonstrating that patients with Parkinson disease were unable to adjust the size of long- and middle-latency reflex responses to the degree of perturbation. These patients are therefore unable to activate muscle force proportional to displacement. Melnick and colleagues[56] found that subjects with Parkinson disease were unable to maintain balance on a sway-referenced force plate. Glatt[138] found that patients with Parkinson disease did not demonstrate anticipatory postural reactions and, in fact, behaved exactly as a rigid body with joints. Horak and colleagues,[139,140] in a variety of studies, reported similar findings and found defects in strategy selection as well; patients with Parkinson disease chose neither a pure hip strategy nor a pure ankle strategy but mixed the two in an inappropriate and maladaptive response. Investigators have found that antiparkinsonian medications could improve background postural tone but did not improve automatic postural responses to external displacements.[58,59,65,139-141] Other studies have demonstrated deficits in proprioceptive perception—what has been termed an "impaired proprioceptive body map." Patients with Parkinson disease did not alter anticipatory postural adjustments in response to step width changes, unlike control subjects.[142] Increased step width requires increased lateral reactive forces to unload the stance leg. The lack of ability to prepare for these extra forces may indicate that narrow stance width, start hesitation, and freezing of gait are compensatory mechanisms to proprioceptive loss.[136] Likewise, when patients could not see their limbs, they had difficulty moving the foot to a predetermined location in response to perturbation. Control subjects had no difficulty.[143,144] Taken together, it appears that postural instability results from inflexibility in response repertoire; an inability to inhibit unwanted programs; the interaction of akinesia, bradykinesia, and rigidity; and some disturbance in central sensory processing.

Gait. The typical parkinsonian gait is characterized by decreased velocity and stride length.[145,146] As a consequence, foot clearance is decreased, which again places the individual at greater fall risk.[147] In many patients, especially as the disease progresses, speed and shortening of stride progressively worsen as if the individual is trying to catch up with his or her center of gravity; this is termed *festination.* Forward festination is called *propulsion;* backward festination is known as *retropulsion.* One hypothesis is that festinating gait is caused by the decreased equilibrium responses. If walking is a series of controlled falls and if normal responses to falling are delayed or not strong enough, then the individual will either fall completely or continue to take short, running-like steps. The abnormal motor unit firing seen with bradykinesia may also be the cause of ever-shortening steps. If the motor unit cannot build up a high enough frequency or if it pauses in the middle of the movement, then the full range of the movement would decrease; in walking this would lead to shorter steps. Festination may also be the result of other changes in the kinematics of gait.

The changes in gait kinematics include changes in excursion of the hip and ankle joints (Figure 20-7). Instead of a heel-toe, the patient may have a flat-footed or, with disease progression, a toe-heel sequence. The patient with Parkinson disease appears to have lost the adult gait pattern and is using a more primitive pattern. The flat-footed gait decreases the ability to step over obstacles or to walk on carpeted surfaces. The use of three-dimensional gait analysis has shown that there is a decrease in plantarflexion at terminal stance. Changes are also seen in hip flexion, which may alter ankle excursion. However, qualitative aspects of the timing of joint excursion appear intact. Figure 20-7 illustrates the joint angles in a 55-year-old patient with Parkinson disease compared with adults without basal ganglia dysfunction.[148]

Gait and postural difficulties are the two impairments that cause the greatest handicap to persons with parkinsonism. They have been found to be the major elements of disability at home and work for these patients.

Perception, Attention, and Cognitive Deficits. Especially in recent years, researchers have tried to address the cognitive and perceptual impairments of people with Parkinson disease.[136,149-152] Whereas the movement deficits are hypothesized to be caused by a decrease in putaminal excitation of the cortex, the learning and perceptual deficits are hypothesized to be caused by a decrease in cortical excitation from the caudate nucleus.[111] The deficits are of frontal lobe function and include an inability to shift attention, an inability to quickly access "working memory," and difficulty with visuospatial perception and discrimination. Research attention has focused on the specific deficits of parkinsonian patients compared with patients with Alzheimer disease, patients with frontal lobe damage, and those with temporal lobe damage.[149,152,153] The perceptual deficits of all groups appear to increase with progression of the disease process. In general, patients have difficulty in shifting attention to a previously irrelevant stimulus,[154] learning under conditions requiring selective attention,[154] or selecting the correct motor response on the basis of sensory stimuli.[155-157] There is also evidence that DA is involved in selection of responses that will be rewarding.[54] These impairments will affect treatment strategies.

Learning deficits also have been found in patients with parkinsonism; procedural learning has been particularly implicated, as would be indicated based on the physiology of the system. Procedural learning is learning that occurs

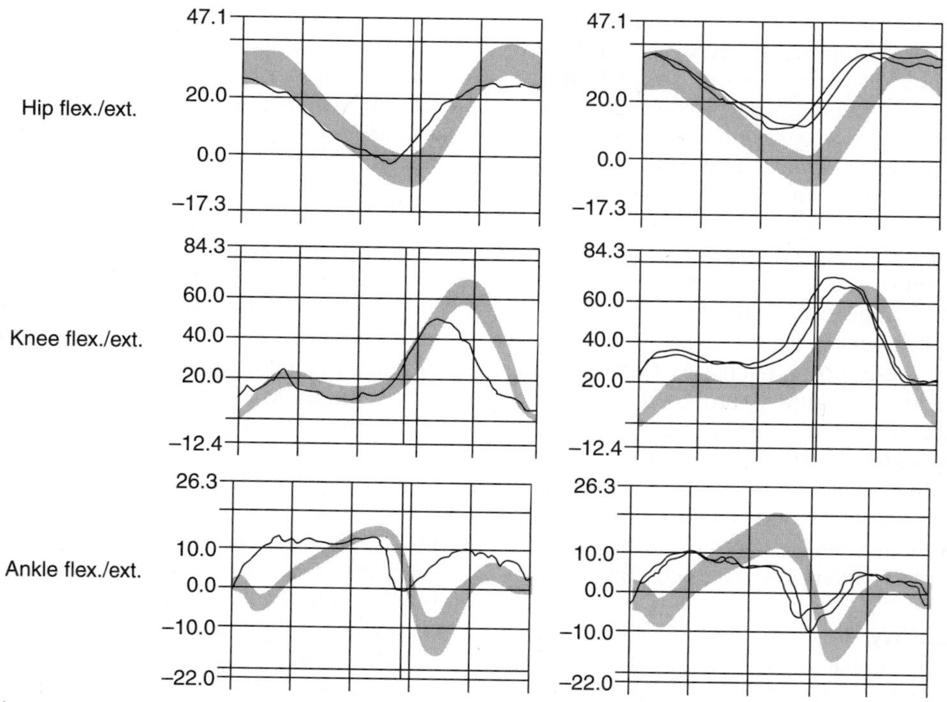

Figure 20-7 ■ Angles of excursion during gait in a patient with Parkinson disease. *Shaded areas* are mean ± standard deviations for adults *without* Parkinson disease; *black lines* represent a patient *with* Parkinson disease. Movement shown for right and left lower extremities. Note decreases, especially in left lower extremity for extension and bilateral decreased plantarflexion.

with practice or, as defined by Saint-Cyr and colleagues,[158] "the ability gradually to acquire a motor skill or even a cognitive routine through repeated exposure to a specific activity constrained by invariant rules." In their tests, patients with Parkinson disease did very poorly on tests of procedural learning, but their declarative learning was within normal limits. Pascual-Leone and colleagues[111] studied procedural learning in more detail. They found that patients with Parkinson disease could acquire procedural learning but needed more practice than control subjects did. They also found that the ability to translate procedural knowledge to declarative knowledge was more efficient if it occurred with visual input alone rather than the combination of visual input with motor task. This may be a rationale for more therapy, not less.

Nonmotor Symptoms. Nonmotor symptoms are consistently seen in patients with Parkinson disease and may be attributable to dopaminergic pathways outside the basal ganglia. Braak[159] hypothesized that Parkinson disease actually begins with DA deterioration in the medulla and progresses rostrally. Often the first signs are loss of sense of smell, constipation, vivid dreams (rapid-eye movement [REM] behavior disorder), and orthostatic hypotension.[160,161] Orthostatic hypotension may cause some dizziness and requires coordination of medications for other medical problems. L-Dopa and DA agonists may lower blood pressure; blood pressure medication may need to be altered once antiparkinsonian drugs have been prescribed. Although not all people with these problems have Parkinson disease, when they are combined they may indicate risk for this disorder. Because physical therapy may be most effective when started early, researchers are trying to learn more about these early symptoms.

Other nonmotor symptoms that decrease quality of life include incontinence in men and women, sexual dysfunction, excess saliva, weight changes, and skin problems. Nonmotor symptoms that can interfere with and complicate physical and occupational treatment include fatigue, fear, anxiety, and depression. Urinary incontinence is important because it increases the risk of hospitalization and mortality.[162]

Sleep disorders are widespread in Parkinson disease and include more than just REM sleep disorder.[163] The patient may experience daytime drowsiness and decreased sleep at night. There appears to be a lack of consolidation of sleep with decreased total sleep time as well as the presence of restless leg syndrome.[164] Daytime drowsiness may be a side effect of medication; however, it can also be exacerbated after therapeutic exercise, so a cool-down period is necessary before the patient sits down and relaxes.

Another side effect of medication is presence of hallucinations. Many patients report seeing very ugly creatures or monsters, and when such hallucinations occur in the therapeutic session they can be most uncomfortable for the therapist and the patient. These hallucinations also make it difficult for the patient to use adjunct treatments such as computer games and virtual reality activities.

Nonmotor symptoms often predominate as the disease progresses.[160] They contribute to severe disability, impaired quality of life, and shortened life expectancy. As the disease progresses, cognitive problems also become more frequent. Braak[159] hypothesized that this was an indication of rostral progression of dopaminergic involvement. Cognitive involvement can include memory loss, confused thinking, and dementia. Parkinson disease medications may worsen these cognitive impairments. The nonmotor symptoms of Parkinson disease have been addressed in a practice parameter recommendation by the American Academy of Neurology.[161]

Stages of Parkinson Disease

Parkinson disease is a progressive disorder.[165] The initial motor symptom is often a resting tremor or unilateral micrography (bradykinesia of the upper extremity). With time, rigidity and bradykinesia are seen bilaterally, and postural alterations and axial symptoms then begin to occur. This commonly starts with an increase in neck, trunk, and hip flexion that, accompanied by a decrease in righting and balance responses, leads to a decreased ability to maintain the center of gravity over the base of support.

While these postural changes are occurring, so does an increase in rigidity, which is most apparent in the trunk and proximal and axial musculature. Trunk rotation becomes severely decreased; there is no arm swing during gait and no spontaneous facial expression; and movement becomes more and more difficult to initiate. Movement is usually produced with great concentration and is perhaps cortically generated, therefore bypassing the damaged basal ganglia pathways. This great concentration then makes movement tiring, which heightens the debilitating effects of the disease.

Eventually the individual becomes wheelchair bound and dependent. In the late and severe stages of the disease, especially without therapeutic attention for movement dysfunctions, the client may become bedridden and may demonstrate a fixed trunk-flexion contracture regardless of the position in which the person is placed. This posture has been called the "phantom pillow" syndrome because, even when lying supine, the person's head is flexed as if on a pillow.

Throughout this progressive deterioration of movement, there is also a decrease in higher-level sensory processing. In addition, the patient can perform only one task at a time. Reports of dementia range from 30% to 93% in patients with Parkinson disease.[166] The presence of dementia in this population may indicate involvement of the ACh or noradrenergic mesolimbic system. In this case, treatment with anticholinergic drugs may increase a tendency toward dementia, especially in older patients. Sometimes cognitive deficits are inferred because of slowed responses, spatial problems, sensory processing problems, and a masked face (see Chapter 36).

The most serious complication of Parkinson disease is bronchopneumonia. Decreased activity in general and decreased chest expansion may be contributing factors. The mortality rate is greater than in the general population, and death is usually from pneumonia.

Staging of Parkinson disease uses the Hoehn and Yahr scale (Table 20-1).[165] Originally developed as a 5-point scale, in recent years 0, 1.5, and 2.5 measurements have been added. The 1.5 and 2.5 ratings have not been validated, but because their use is so common, the latest recommendation is to continue using them while the validity is studied.[167]

TABLE 20-1 ■ HOEHN AND YAHR STAGING SCALE FOR PARKINSON DISEASE

STAGE	PROGRESSION OF SYMPTOMS
0	No signs of disease.
1	Unilateral symptoms only.
1.5	Unilateral and axial involvement.
2	Bilateral symptoms. No impairment of balance.
2.5	Mild bilateral disease with recovery on pull test.
3	Balance impairment. Mild to moderate disease. Physically independent.
4	Severe disability, but still able to walk or stand unassisted.
5	Needing a wheelchair or bedridden unless assisted.

The Hoehn and Yahr scale is commonly used to describe how the symptoms of Parkinson disease progress. The original scale included stages 1 through 5.[165] Stage 0 has since been added, and stages 1.5 and 2.5 have been proposed to best indicate the relative level of disability in this population.[167]

Pharmacological Considerations and Medical Management

The knowledge that the symptoms of Parkinson disease are caused by a decrease in DA led to the pharmacological management of this disease. Because DA itself does not cross the blood-brain barrier, levo-dihydroxyphenylalanine (L-dopa), a precursor of DA that does, has been used to treat Parkinson disease since the late 1960s.[168-170] An inhibitor of aromatic amino acid decarboxylation (carbidopa) is usually given with L-dopa to prevent the conversion to DA before entering the brain. The decarboxylase inhibitor allows a reduction in dosage of L-dopa itself, which helps decrease the cardiac and gastrointestinal side effects of DA.

Amantadine is another drug that has been effective in the treatment of patients with Parkinson disease. Although the mechanism of action of this antiviral medication is unknown, it is thought to include a facilitation of release of catecholamines (of which DA is one) from stores in the neuron that are readily releasable. It is often administered in combination with L-dopa.

Treatment of Parkinson disease with L-dopa in these various combinations is extremely helpful in reducing bradykinesia and rigidity. It is less effective in reducing tremor and the postural instability. Because Parkinson disease involves the nigral neurons, the receptors and the neurons in the striatum (which are postsynaptic to dopaminergic neurons) remain intact and initially are somewhat responsive to DA.[171,172] With time, however, the receptors appear to lose their sensitivity, and the prolonged effectiveness (10 years or more) of L-dopa therapy is questionable.[173-175] A further complication of L-dopa therapy is the development of involuntary movements (dyskinesias) and the "on-off" phenomenon—a short-duration response resulting in sudden improvement of symptoms followed by a rapid decline in symptomatic relief and perhaps the appearance of dyskinesias and/or dystonias.[176,177] With time the "on" effect becomes of shorter and shorter duration.[173,176,178,179] Controlled-release or slow-release L-dopa may decrease these side effects. The effectiveness of L-dopa does not appear to be closely correlated with the stage of the disease.

The use of L-dopa alone or in combination with carbidopa has not provided a cure or even prevented the degeneration of Parkinson disease.[178,179] As more has become known about the DA receptor, specific agonists have been developed. Ropinirole, pramipexole, pergolide, and bromocriptine are examples of DA receptor D2 agonists that are used alone or with L-dopa. The agonists are thought to decrease the wearing-off effects as well as decrease the dyskinesias that occur with long-term L-dopa use, but L-dopa remains the most effective medication. It is quite likely that newer D2 and/or D2-D1 (DA receptor D1) agonists will be developed. Pharmacological interventions also include drugs that prevent the breakdown of DA (e.g., catechol-*O*-methyltransferase [COMT] inhibitors) and/or its reuptake. Entacapone is an example of a COMT inhibitor.[180]

Another approach to pharmacological treatment of individuals with Parkinson disease was developed from research on a designer drug that contained the neurotoxin 1-methyl-4-phenyl-1,2,3,6-tetrahydropyridine (MPTP). It was found that the conversion of MPTP to the active neurotoxin MPP+ could be prevented by monoamine oxidase inhibitors such as deprenyl and pargyline.[73,179] Deprenyl, rasagiline, and selegiline are now used before the initiation of, or in conjunction with, L-dopa and carbidopa.

Another treatment alternative is surgery performed in precise areas of the basal ganglia, known as *stereotaxic surgery.* Stereotaxic surgery is an old technique that has made a comeback based on the new knowledge of basal ganglia connectivity and improvements in the procedural instrumentation.* Initially, one of the structures of the basal ganglia was lesioned with freezing or high-frequency stimulation. Today the globus pallidus internal segment or the subthalamic nucleus is stimulated with implanted electrodes. This technique is known as *deep-brain stimulation (DBS).* DBS has now been approved by the U.S. Food and Drug Administration (FDA). An advantage of deep brain stimulation over permanent lesions is that DBS is reversible and is safer for bilateral surgeries. Stimulation of the globus pallidus internal segment or subthalamic nucleus has been shown to decrease all symptoms; subthalamic nucleus stimulation is also effective in reducing dyskinesias and may lessen the amount of medication taken.[183-185] Effects of stimulation are greater for symptoms manifested in the "off" state. Deep brain stimulation has been demonstrated to improve rigidity, bradykinesia, and akinesia, as well as gait[57,184,186-189] and balance.[56,190] It has also been demonstrated to improve movement velocity and speed of muscle recruitment for activity.[190,191] The proposed mechanism of action is interference with the abnormal neuronal firing.[192,193] In a randomized, controlled, clinical trial, DBS was more effective in reducing symptoms and increasing quality of life than medication.[194,195] This group also found that although some side effects were worse (e.g., brain hemorrhage), the total number of adverse reactions was greater in the medication group. Whether stimulation of the subthalamic nucleus is neuroprotective, that is, prevents further degeneration, is presently under investigation. Thalamic stimulation is used

*References 6, 7, 76, 173, 181, 182.

for decreasing tremor. Therapists may find that intense treatment immediately after these surgeries may be able to take advantage of neural plasticity.

Fetal transplantation of the substantia nigra to the caudate nucleus remains under investigation. A double-blind, placebo-controlled trial was completed with mixed results.[192,196-198] Studies continue, including those of dose, cell type, and placement of cells. Recently, however, there was a report of Lewy-body inclusions in grafted cells 14 years after the transplant.[199] The authors concluded that Parkinson disease was an ongoing process and that what caused the disease initially, also affected the grafted cells.

Examination of the Client with Parkinson Disease

The previous sections introduced the symptoms of Parkinson disease and hypothesized pathophysiological explanations for these symptoms. Examination of the client with Parkinson disease should include the degree of rigidity, bradykinesia, balance impairments, and gait abnormalities and how much these symptoms interfere with ADLs—that is, how the symptoms are influencing the client's participation in life. The outcome measures used in the examination of patients with Parkinson disease should be as objective as possible.

The Hoehn and Yahr Scale (see Table 20-1) is frequently used to describe the general severity of disease.[165] The Unified Parkinson's Disease Rating Scale (UPDRS) is the most widely used assessment tool to describe all facets of impairment: cognitive and emotional status, ADL ability, motor function, and side effects of medication.[200-202] The UPDRS is also frequently used to measure the efficacy of treatments. Another clinical scale is the Core Assessment Program for Intracerebral Transplantation (CAPIT), which includes timed tests.[203] This scale was designed to standardize assessments of patients with Parkinson disease who undergo surgical intervention. It is comprehensive and more time-consuming and therefore tends to be used more in research than in the clinic. Knowledge of these scales will help the physical therapist in communication and interactions with other health care professionals even though the scales may not be ideal for planning physical and occupational therapeutic interventions.

Assessment of functional activities will be most beneficial for treatment planning and reevaluation. In addition to assessing how the patient performs the activity, the time it takes to complete an activity must be measured. For example, gait is assessed by general pattern, speed, and distance, as well as the effects of interfering stimuli including walking while performing cognitive tasks. It is advantageous to evaluate forward and backward walking as well as braiding and the ability to alter gait speed in each of these conditions.[145,146] Available objective tests of gait and functional mobility include the Timed Up-and-Go Test, 10-meter walk test, the 5 or 10 Times Sit-to-Stand Test, the Dynamic Gait Index, or any of the objective standardized tests presented in Chapter 8. Careful observation of how the person performs a task would be useful for treatment planning. For example, when rising from a chair, does the patient move forward in the chair, place the feet underneath the knees, and lean forward before rising?

A careful analysis of balance is imperative for the patient with Parkinson disease. This must include assessment with and without vision and the differences between the two conditions (see the section on balance in Chapter 22). Assessing challenges to balance such as tandem walking or standing on a compliant surface is important, especially in the early stages of the disease. This may be the first sign of balance impairment. Posturography is the most sensitive measure of postural instability, especially in the early stages of the disease (Hoehn and Yahr stages 1 and 2).[58] A clinically useful tool to assess dynamic balance is the functional reach test, which has been shown to be an effective, predictive tool in people with Parkinson disease as it is in the elderly.[204] The Balance Evaluation Systems Test (BESTest) is also an appropriate comprehensive measure for those with Parkinson disease. Obtaining a falls history continues to be a reliable predictor of future falls and is easy to measure. (Refer to Chapters 8 and 22 for specifics on these tests.)

An assessment of chest expansion and vital capacity should also be included. This is important because of their contribution to the complication of pneumonia. For this reason, when rigidity is assessed, the muscles of respiration should be included, along with extremity and trunk assessment. Active and passive range of movement, general strength, chest expansion, and vital capacity should also be measured on regular intervals. At present a complete and easy-to-use form for evaluation does not exist for Parkinson disease.

General Prognosis, Treatment Goals, and Rationale

As with all treatment, the prognosis (functional goals and established time parameters) is based on the general goals related to the findings from the examination of each client and the client's expectations and functional requirements. Parkinson disease must be understood as a degenerative disease when establishing the prognosis and treatment plan. Nonpharmacological and surgical interventions, especially physical therapy treatment, are especially important in the beginning of the disease.[205] In general, goals include increasing movement and range of motion (ROM) in the entire trunk as well as the extremities, maintaining or improving chest expansion, improving balance reactions, and maintaining or restoring functional abilities. Increased movement may in fact modify the progression of the disease.[206,207] It may further help to retard dementia. Although L-dopa decreases the bradykinesia, it alone will not be effective in increasing movement or improving balance; therefore, aggressive intervention in the early stages is necessary. Increasing trunk rotation goes hand in hand with increasing range of movement and motion in general. The longer clients are kept mobile, the less likely they are to develop pneumonia and the longer they can maintain independence in ADLs. Ideally, rehabilitation interventions should begin at the first sign of the disease, but this is not always possible. Treatment initiated while the disease is still unilateral (Hoehn and Yahr stage 1) is more advantageous.[208,209]

Treatment Procedures

Overall, physical rehabilitation is effective in the treatment of people with Parkinson disease. The results are greater when treatment is started early in the disease process, but it has been shown to be effective in Hoehn and Yahr stages 1 to 3. The American Academy of Neurology recommends physical therapy in its practice parameters.[210] The bottom line is that treatment by movement specialists that incorporates complex, sequential movements with multiple sensory inputs creates demands for responses that are environmentally appropriate, challenges balance, uses large-amplitude movements, and is fun and effective. Many treatment regimens have been used, and almost all have been successful. Animal research indicates that exercise and forced functional movements may protect the dopaminergic neurons.[211] The following paragraphs will provide more precise information and more precise details.

Basic principles for treatment of the person with Parkinson disease will, of course, depend on the areas of impairment and handicap revealed in the evaluation. Certain principles, however, are true for all stages of the disease. First, the activities selected must engage the patient: the patient must find the activities interesting enough to do them regularly. Variety is important to facilitate shifts in movement as well as in thought. And movements must be *big!* (In fact, one treatment technique even uses that word in its name.) Activities that are designed to improve balance are valuable even in the early stages of the disease. To date, many rehabilitative techniques and exercises have demonstrated improvement in function for people with Parkinson disease, and there have now been a few randomized clinical trials with small numbers of patients to test efficacy of the varied techniques. Programs that emphasize sensory-motor integration, agility, and motor learning demonstrate decreased progression of disease and improved motor function.[212-227] Programs that involve the coordination of dual motor-cognitive tasks and complex sequences of movements and that force the participant to quickly change movements dependent on environmental conditions have resulted in improved performance on the Timed Up-and-Go Test, the UPDRS, the 10-meter walk test, and a variety of balance tests. Some of these programs include the Lee Silverman Voice Treatment (LSVT BIG) program, sensory attention focused exercise (PD SAFEx), ballroom dance, Zumba, tai chi, karate, computer game playing, and alpine hiking.

Most of the studies referenced previously have included people at Hoehn and Yahr stages 1 to 3. As the person progresses, practice of precise ADLs is advisable. These include rising from a chair, getting out of bed, turning in bed, adjusting covers, and being aware of posture. At the later stages of the disease, breathing exercises will need to be a more prominent aspect of treatment. Big movements still need to be stressed. At these later stages of the disease, use of assistive equipment may also need to be taught. What follows are ideas for treatment of more specific aspects of the disease. These are ideas and are not exhaustive. The words *big, fun,* and *novel* are good words to remember when planning treatment.

Decreasing Rigidity. Movement throughout a full ROM is crucial, especially early in the disease process, to prevent changes in the properties of muscle itself. In Parkinson disease the contractile elements of flexors become shortened and those of the extensor surface become lengthened, enhancing the development of the flexed posture that is traditionally present.[228] For most patients, treatment proceeds better if rigidity is decreased early in the treatment session. In fact, movement therapy interventions appear to have more lasting effects when the treatment is performed during the "on" phase of a medication cycle.

Many relaxation techniques appear to be effective in reducing rigidity, including gentle, slow rocking, rotation of the extremities and trunk, and the use of yoga (see Chapters 9 and 39). In the client with Parkinson disease, success in relaxation may be better achieved in the sitting or standing positions because rigidity may increase in the supine position.[91] Furthermore, because the proximal muscles are often more involved than the distal muscles, relaxation may be easier to achieve by following a distal-to-proximal progression. The inverted position may be used with care. Initially this position facilitates some relaxation (increase in parasympathetic tone) and then increases trunk extension, which is important for the parkinsonian client. Relaxation may also be effective in reducing the tremor of Parkinson disease. Once a decrease in rigidity has been achieved, movement must be initiated in order to use the newfound range in a functional way.

Therapeutic Programs. Exercise itself is important for the person with Parkinson disease. There is a relationship between longevity and physical activity.[229] Those who exercise have lower mortality rates.[229] Some evidence also indicates that exercise may alter the magnitude of free radicals and other compounds linked to aging and parkinsonism. Immunological function may also be improved with exercise. Sasco and colleagues[103] demonstrated a link between a lack of exercise and development of parkinsonism. Finally, the role of aerobic fitness itself may be a factor in reducing dysfunction.[103] Animal data indicate that functional exercise decreased DA loss after a variety of lesion models.[129,208,209,211,230] Some of the animal activities were similar to the complex, sensory-motor and agility programs now used in patient programs.[213,218,221,222] Aerobic exercise may improve pulmonary function in patients with Parkinson disease because these functions appear to suffer from deficiencies in rapid force generation of the respiratory muscles, similar to limb musculature.[231] Exercise is most beneficial when it is begun early in the disease process as is recommended in all books, pamphlets, and websites for the patient.[232] (Refer to the list of websites at the end of this chapter.) All research on the effects of exercise programs in parkinsonism indicates this point. When the use of forced functional activities is delayed too long, few beneficial effects of exercise on the DA system have been shown in animal studies.[208,209] Hurwitz[233] found that patients who were still independently mobile at home and in the community benefited the most from a home program. Schenkman and Butler[228] also indicate that patients in the earlier stages of the disease had the best potential for improvement. If patients practice regular physical exercise in conjunction with disease-specific exercises, the ill effects of inactivity will not potentiate the effects of the disease process itself. Although most patients with Parkinson disease can achieve an adequate exercise level, many clients have fitness levels that are poor or very poor before the medical diagnosis.[122] Exercise, even once a week, can be effective in improving gait and balance in clients with Parkinson disease when practiced over several months.[212,234]

So far almost all studies have found that exercise under the guidance of a therapist is effective.[213-227] Palmer and colleagues[235] used precise, quantitative measures to assess motor signs, grip strength, coordination, and speed as well as measurements of the long-latency stretch reflex after two exercise programs in patients with Parkinson disease. These two programs were the United Parkinson Foundation program and karate training. Their results indicated improvement over 12 weeks in gait, grip strength, and coordination of fine motor control tasks and no change in a decline in movements requiring speed. The patients all felt an increase in general well-being. A study by Comella and colleagues[236] as well as one by Patti and colleagues[237] also found decreases in parkinsonian symptoms with physical and occupational therapy. However, these studies found no long-term carryover once therapy had been discontinued. The authors never explain the exercise program precisely nor the instructions provided for a home program.

Rhythmical exercise has been shown to decrease rigidity and bradykinesia and improve gait over time.[212,238-254] Ballroom dancing is a form of rhythmical therapy for patients with Parkinson disease that incorporates rhythmical movement, rotation, balance, and coordination.[212] A program of tango versus waltz and foxtrot indicated that although both groups improved on the UPDRS motor scale, Berg Balance Scale, 6-minute walk distance, and backward stride length, the tango group had greater improvements.[214,217,225] The waltz and foxtrot, which are easier dances, may be beneficial for those at more advanced stages of the disease. The use of dance also facilitates changing direction. Our program using Latin dance (predominantly mambo and cha-cha) and other weight-bearing exercise demonstrated similar improvements in balance and especially initiation of gait.[212,234,247,255] Similar effects were seen in tai chi, which demands attention to movement and increases challenges to balance and control of movement. Tai chi has been shown to be effective in improving gait and balance parameters.[220]

Studies using a program emphasizing sensory awareness of the size of movement have shown improvement in both speed of movement and gait parameters.[224,226,227] PD SAFEx,[226] a program that focuses attention on sensory awareness, was shown to improve gait and function on the UPDRS in a randomized controlled study. A group that engaged in aerobic exercise alone improved gait but not symptoms. A group that continued usual activities did not demonstrate improvements on any outcome measure. These authors concluded that programs emphasizing increased sensory feedback and awareness were superior in reducing the symptoms and improving the function of patients with Parkinson disease.

Treadmill training has been used in Parkinson disease exercise programs. Use of the treadmill with body-weight support increases safety and allows the therapist to control speed of movement as well as perturbations. Some studies have used cued treadmill training with good results and carryover to the home.[256] Cognitive tasks and other dual tasks have also been added during treadmill training with good results.[257] These studies found collectively improved measures of balance and gait, as well as reduced fear of falling and number of falls.[213,221]

Physical activity and movement appear to increase quality of life by decreasing depression and improving mood and initiative.[248,258] Group classes can serve as an extra support system for patients with Parkinson disease and their spouses.* A carefully structured low-impact aerobics program appears to be beneficial to patients even with long-standing disease.[234]

*References 210, 226, 227, 238, 249, 258.

One program designed for those at Hoehn and Yahr stage 2.5 or 3 begins with seated activities for upper extremities (Figure 20-8, *A*) and combination movements for warmup (Figure 20-8, *B*). The participants then progress to standing and marching activities that incorporate coordinated movements of arms and legs as well as balance and trunk rotation (Figure 20-9). All movements are performed to music similar to that used in aerobics classes in any gym or health club (Figure 20-10). (The rationale for the use of external cues and the role of rhythm in gait training are discussed in subsequent paragraphs.) A cool-down period allows participants to practice fine motor coordination activities of the hands (Figure 20-11). Many Parkinson disease associations also have audiotapes for exercises (e.g., United Parkinson Foundation).

The use of computer games to improve symptoms is currently under investigation. These games force the participant to move in precise ways or to shift weight to score points. Many "off-the-shelf" games exist and have been used with older adults (the predominant patient population of those with Parkinson disease) to increase activity levels. For some with Parkinson disease, even in the early stages, these games

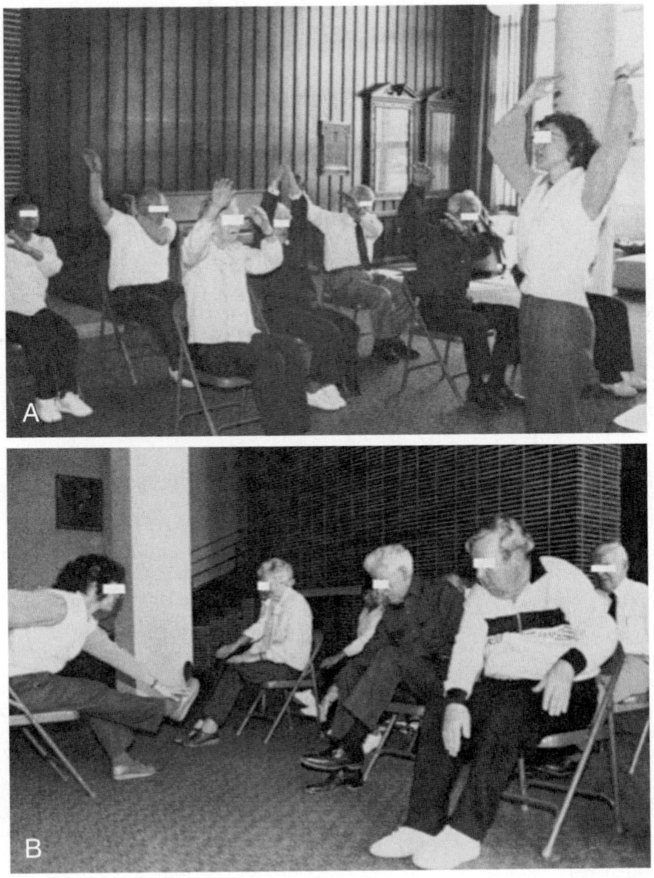

Figure 20-8 ■ Seated aerobics or warmup exercises. **A,** Clients are using bilateral upper-extremity patterns to facilitate trunk rotation. Instruction was to let the head follow the hands. **B,** This exercise encourages trunk rotation, large movements, and coordination of the upper and lower extremities. Clients are to reach with the arms and touch the opposite foot. This coordination is difficult for those with Parkinson disease, and many clients initially could not move the arms and legs at the same time.

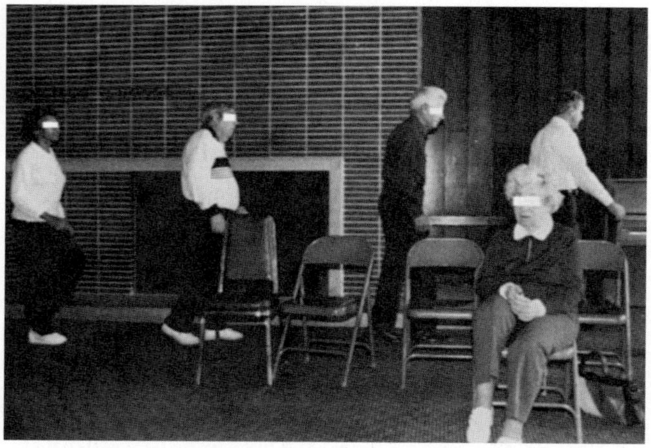

Figure 20-9 ■ Initial warmup in standing. Clients are to walk with the head up, with the back as straight as possible, and to take large steps. When the group began, walking was the major aerobic activity and was used to increase endurance and encourage movement. Nonambulatory patients march in place while seated.

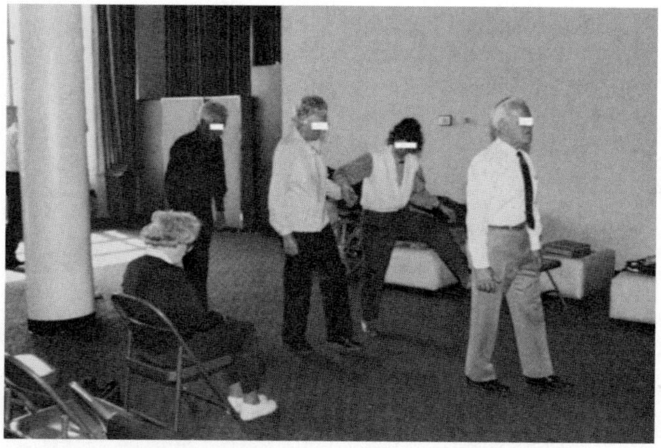

Figure 20-10 ■ Walking in a "waltz rhythm" (slow, quick, quick) emphasizes a big step for the slow step. Note lack of automatic arm swing. Also note flexed posture of seated patient during rest period.

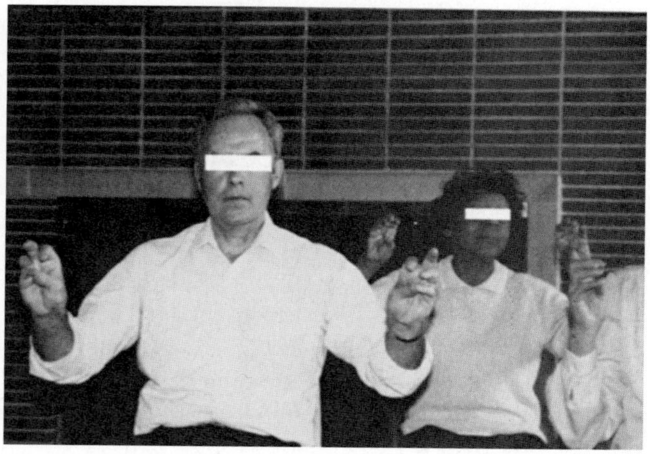

Figure 20-11 ■ Cool-down period allows time to work on fine finger movements. Thumb abduction with rounded fingers and various rhythms are used to increase coordination. Note "masked face" appearance.

are too fast or too confusing. A feasibility study showed that disease-specific games could be used, and enjoyed by those with Parkinson disease.[259]

The most successful exercise programs appear to be those that incorporate context-dependent responses and a varied environment. All of the previously listed examples of these activities are presented in Box 20-1. Aerobic exercises that are not as effective in requiring context-dependent responses are presented in Box 20-2. Research has shown the importance of adjusting the response to the specific task and has also demonstrated the importance of practice for the parkinsonian patient.[157,260] The principles of motor learning are of paramount importance in the treatment program of these patients. Random practice may enable the patient to learn the correct schema by which to regulate the extent, speed, and direction of the movement. Random practice also may be important in facilitating the ability of the patient to shift attention and to learn to access "working memory." The parkinsonian patient may benefit from visual instruction and mental rehearsal before performing the movement.[137,157] In addition, the instructions used need to be pertinent to the task at hand.

BOX 20-1 ■ EXERCISES THAT PROMOTE CONTEXT-DEPENDENT RESPONSES

The following exercises promote context-dependent responses and are recommended for people with movement disorders:

1. Walking outdoors
2. Karate and other martial arts
3. Dancing (all forms)
4. Ball sports (various types)
5. Cross-country and downhill skiing
6. Well-structured, low-impact aerobics classes
7. Treadmill training with guidance of a movement specialist

This list is a sample of activities; it should not be considered all inclusive.

BOX 20-2 ■ EXERCISES THAT PROMOTE FITNESS AND INCREASE RANGE OF MOTION BUT NOT CONTEXT-DEPENDENT RESPONSES

The following exercises promote fitness and increase range of motion but not context-dependent responses and are recommended for people with movement disorders.

1. Treadmill walking without guidance or supervision
2. Stationary bicycle riding
3. Using strengthening machines and free weights (with low weights or low resistance)
4. Using step exercises and stair climbers
5. Using rowing machines
6. Swimming laps

This list is a sample of activities; it should not be considered all inclusive.

Strengthening. Strengthening exercises have been promoted for the patient with Parkinson disease. With disuse comes decreased strength. Weakness occurs with initial contraction and also with prolonged contraction. Manual muscle testing may not reveal losses in strength; however, most of the successful exercise programs previously mentioned did include functional strength training as part of the program. High-resistance eccentric resistance can produce muscle hypertrophy and may effect improvements in mobility.[261] Another study used "sports activities" in a twice-per-week program.[158] The program included exercises on land designed to improve gait and balance and exercises in the water to increase strength. These investigators reported significant improvements in UPDRS scores, cognitive function, and mood in addition to ADL and motor scores during the 14-week program. Interestingly, they also found decreases in dyskinesia. The greatest changes in exercise appeared early and were maintained up to 6 weeks after cessation of the exercise program. According to the literature, functional strength training seems to be more effective than weightlifting if the goal is improvement in ADLs.[158] An important part of any strengthening program is the trunk musculature. Spinal extensors need to be exercised, and spinal flexibility likewise encouraged.[262]

Use of Cues for Improving Gait. As the disease progresses, intensive exercise programs may need to be revised or altered. By stage 2.5, gait disorders are the most common diagnosis for which the person with Parkinson disease will see a therapist. Many aspects of gait are amenable to treatment. The problems that cause the biggest ambulation limitation are freezing and small steps. Both auditory and visual stimuli have been used in treatment of parkinsonian gait disorders. Thaut and colleagues[263] demonstrated that use of a metronome or carefully synthesized music improves stride length and speed and that these improvements remain up to 5 weeks after the cessation of the auditory stimulus.[234] Melnick and colleagues[234] also demonstrated both immediate and longer-lasting improvements in gait with a rhythmical exercise program once a week in patients needing assistance to walk. A study by Nieuwboer and colleagues[256] used auditory, visual, or somatosensory cues in the patient's home. The patient chose the cue that was best for him or her. The cues were provided in a variety of tasks including walking with dual tasks and walking sideways and backward. Cues were effective in decreasing freezing, but there was only a small effect when the cues were stopped. There may be a difference in the use of cueing for those who freeze during gait and those who do not. The use of cues may be more effective for those who do not have frequent freezing episodes.[264]

People with Parkinson disease find climbing stairs easier than walking on a flat surface because of the visual stimulation provided by the stairs. Visual stimuli have been effective in freezing episodes. These include the use of lines on the floor and stair climbing. Martin[55] found that parallel lines were more facilitating than other lines and that the space between lines was also important; the lines cannot be too close together. The use of visual stimuli has scant evidence of carryover. One client used visual stimuli in special glasses that provided constant lines for the client to step over. At present these glasses are not commercially available. Dunne and colleagues[265] described a cane that could present a visual cue for the patient who has freezing episodes. Canes can be especially useful for patients who fall because of freezing. If a specialized cane is not available, the client can turn his or her own cane upside down. Other visual cues have been used to help initiate movement after freezing. For example, one patient tosses pennies ahead of him and steps over them. (He cautions that one should not bend to pick them up as this will again lead to freezing.) Another watches the movement of a person walking beside him; the movement of that person's feet encourages his feet to move. The U walker has a laser line that can be added to provide lines on the ground. Morris and colleagues[147] have tried to increase carryover of visual stimuli by incorporating them with a program of visualization. Their clients practiced walking with lines until the steps were near normal in size; the clients were then to visualize the lines on the floor as they walked. Their visualization program met with initial success. Increasing the magnitude of the step or the amplitude of the movement appears to be the most important component for improvement in gait and a decrease in freezing.[147] Tactile cueing has also been demonstrated to improve gait ability.[266]

Gait rehabilitation must include walking in crowds, through doorways, and on different surfaces. Practicing walking slowly and quickly is important, as is walking with differing stride lengths, because in the real world step length and speed must change with environmental demands. The principles of motor learning presented in Chapter 4 appear to be very helpful for facilitating carryover of the therapeutic effects in our preliminary studies. One word of caution, however; as previously mentioned, the person with Parkinson disease has difficulty performing two tasks at once, such as walking and performing math problems or walking with a glass of water on a tray.[113,130,155] The patient may have to concentrate only on walking as the disease progresses, to increase patient safety.

Balance. Another problem for which therapy is indicated is impaired balance, especially because drug and surgical treatments are ineffective in remediating this problem. This problem will eventually affect all persons with Parkinson disease.[267] If at all possible, the client should be instructed to practice balance exercises at the early stages of the disease. Equilibrium reactions in all planes of movement and under different controls should be encouraged. Techniques to increase dynamic balance control should be included, especially turning the body and turning the head. All three balance strategies need to be addressed and then practiced in a variety of environmental conditions. The newer computerized games that target balance have provided a fun and therapeutic method for keeping interest in balance exercises.[130,135,136,142,143] (See Chapter 22 for other procedures to improve balance.)

Dual Task Performance. Rarely will the client with Parkinson disease state that he or she has difficulty performing two tasks at once. Nonetheless, this is quite apparent in very simple activities, such as requiring the patient to count backward and walk at the same time.[146,268] One solution is to instruct the client to attend to only one task at a time. Another is to have the client practice doing two things at the same time and constantly alter activities in a random practice mode during treatment. The efficacy of these two approaches has yet to be studied.

Activities of Daily Living. Transitional movements pose great problems for the client, especially by Hoehn and Yahr stage 3. This is most likely because normal postural adjustments are no longer automatic and they become a sequential task. Practice with frequent review is helpful. Some researchers report improvement in moving from a seated to a standing position after practicing techniques designed to increase forward weight shift (e.g., leaning on a chair while standing up).[269,270] Visualization of this task has demonstrated carryover. If getting up from a chair becomes too difficult, chairs with seats that lift up have been used effectively.

Bed mobility is another important consideration for patients with Parkinson disease. Rolling in bed and rising from the supine position become difficult and need to be practiced, with increased emphasis on trunk rotation. A firm bed may make getting in and out of bed easier. Rolling and getting out of bed is a task that may be easy for the patient on the hard mat tables in the clinic but difficult on the softer bed at the client's home. Tempur-Pedic beds may make movement even more difficult than traditional beds by Hoehn and Yahr stage 3. Most patients report that satin sheets with silk or satin pajamas make moving in bed far easier. This is true in both the early and later stages of the disease. Teaching the client to roll onto the side and lower the legs off the bed facilitates getting out of bed; the client may not be using this method and so learning or relearning this movement is important. Beds with a head that can be raised electrically may be helpful as the disease progresses, but while sleeping the patient should lower the head as close to horizontal as possible.

Breathing exercises are crucial for the patient with Parkinson disease. As stated previously, the most common cause of death is pneumonia. Chest expansion may be included in upper-extremity activities such as swinging the arm. The clinician may also have the client shout—especially with some kind of rhythmical chant, even a simple "left, right" while walking. With disease progression, specific breathing exercises need to be incorporated. This is crucial for the patient who is no longer able to walk.

In addition to treatment in the therapy department, the parkinsonian client also should be given a home program. The home program should encourage moderate, consistent exercise as part of the normal day. Periodic checks may enhance compliance. Fatigue should be avoided and the exercise graded to the individual's capability. The therapist should keep in mind that learned skills such as various sports are sometimes less affected than automatic movements, perhaps because these skills may rely on cortical involvement.[16]

Fatigue is a frequent complaint of people with Parkinson disease. Although it has been correlated with disease progression, depression, and sleep disturbances, it also exists in up to 44% of those without depression or sleep difficulty.[271] This type of fatigue is over and above what is associated with the exertion of an exercise program and may be one reason people with Parkinson disease no longer exercise. The client with Parkinson disease frequently experiences postexercise fatigue. If a person is so tired after exercise that he or she cannot perform normal ADLs, exercise will not become a part of the client's daily routine. Postexercise fatigue is easily alleviated by a gradual and extended cool-down period.

Patients frequently ask about the timing of medication and exercise. For any form of exercise in parkinsonism to be effective, movement must be possible, especially movement through the full arc of the joint. It seems plausible, therefore, that exercise should be performed during the "on" period of the medication cycle. On the other hand, perhaps a more long-lasting effect would result if the patient with Parkinson disease tried to exercise without medication. The question of the effects of exercise on DA agonist absorption was investigated by Carter and colleagues.[272] These authors concluded that the effect was variable from patient to patient, but the response of each patient was consistent. However, none of the patients exercised vigorously, which may have skewed the results. Reuter and colleagues[273] interpreted a decrease in dyskinesia seen after an exercise program as indicative of more efficient DA absorption. Nevertheless, this study supports the concept that the patient needs to be "in tune" with his or her own response and adjust medications and exercise to a schedule accordingly. The therapist is also involved in the prescription of assistive devices. The use of ambulatory aids for patients with Parkinson disease is an area with no clear-cut guidelines. Because coordination of upper and lower extremities is often difficult, the ability to use a cane or walker is often limited. The patient may drag the cane or carry the walker. Walkers with wheels sometimes increase the festinating gait, and the patient may simply fall over the walker. Nonetheless, four-wheel walkers with pushdown brakes appear to work best for many clients. A walker that is in the brake condition at the start and requires the patient to push on handles to walk may also be safer. For patients with a tendency to fall backward, an assistive device may simply be something to carry backward with them. Therefore the reason for using the assistive device must be carefully assessed. Walkers, walking sticks, or canes can be helpful for the person who is able to walk with a heel-toe gait pattern but lacks postural stability. The height of walker or cane should be adjusted carefully to promote trunk extension and avoid an increase in trunk flexion. A walking stick, or the use of two sticks as in hiking, is less likely to promote flexion than a cane. A survey by Mutch and colleagues[250] in Ireland found that nearly half of the patients responding used some type of assistive device. These devices included devices for walking, reaching, rising from bed, and performing ADLs. Patients with Parkinson disease may also benefit from assistive devices for eating or writing.

As Parkinson disease progresses the patient may experience difficulty in swallowing and even chewing. Therapy for oral-motor control should be initiated, and a dietician consultation may be necessary to ensure adequate nutrition. A dietician may also be beneficial in guiding the patient's protein intake. A diet high in protein may reduce the responsiveness of the patient to DA replacement therapy.[146] Regulating the amount and timing of protein ingestion can improve the efficacy of drug treatment in some patients. Use of vitamins is a subject that appears on many websites for patients with Parkinson disease, and the patient should be reminded to consult with his or her physician when changing vitamins.

The resurgence of surgery as a treatment alternative in Parkinson disease, including stimulation of deep brain sites that may alter neuroplasticity, means that the therapist will face new and exciting challenges in treatment.[274] Intense physical therapy, especially incorporating complex motor skills, has been demonstrated to be effective in improving function after a subthalamic nucleus lesion in animal studies.[275] Therefore, intense physical therapy after surgery may be necessary to maximize benefits from all surgeries in Parkinson disease (as well as in Huntington disease and the dystonias).

Finally, therapeutic rehabilitation and exercise may modify but cannot halt or reverse the progression of this degenerative disease. The therapist can assist the client and family in coping with the constraints of this disease, enhancing the patient's quality of life throughout its course. As stated in one study of Parkinson disease, the total cost of treatment must also include the cost to the spouse or other family members.[2]

Differences between Parkinson Disease and Parkinson Plus Syndromes: Theoretical and Practical Considerations

Several other neurodegenerative diseases are grouped together as "Parkinson plus" syndromes. Clients with these syndromes usually do not respond to L-dopa intervention. The most common of these is progressive supranuclear palsy (PSP). Symptoms of this disease include bradykinesia, gait instability with frequent falls, rigidity, and a vertical gaze palsy. These clients can be evaluated and treated in a manner similar to clients with Parkinson disease. However, PSP usually involves more cognitive impairment and the progression is more rapid; within a decade the patient is typically immobile.

Multiple system atrophy (MSA) is a degenerative disease that affects various areas of the CNS, causing problems with movement, balance, and autonomic functions. The disease is characterized by bradykinesia and rigidity and a tendency to walk with a wide base of support. A person with MSA often has frontal lobe dysfunction as well. Unfortunately, L-dopa is not effective in treating this disorder.

Because these syndromes are more rare than Parkinson disease and far more variable, no studies have been undertaken regarding rehabilitation intervention efficacy. Because accurate differential diagnosis is important in patient planning, a thorough evaluation by a neurologist is highly recommended.

Huntington Disease

Huntington disease (formerly *Huntington's chorea*) is another degenerative disease of the basal ganglia.[276] It is the classic disorder representing hyperactivity in the basal ganglia circuitry.[277] This disease gets its name from the family of physicians who described its patterns of inheritance. Huntington disease is inherited as an autosomal dominant trait and affects approximately 6.5 per 100,000 people.[3] The defect is on the short arm of chromosome 4.[278] The defect alters DNA so that there is an increase in the cytosine-adenine-guanine (CAG) sequence; in normal individuals there are 10 to 28 CAG triple repeats, but in the individual with Huntington disease there are 36 to 120 repeats.[64] The longer the length of the CAG triple repeats, the earlier the onset of the disease. The CAG repeat is related to glutamine. The target protein affected by the polyglutamine expansion has been named *huntingtin.* Huntingtin combines with ubiquitin and induces intranuclear inclusions and interference with mitochondrial function. The defect is characterized by severe loss of the medium spiny neurons and preservation of the ACh aspiny neurons. There are decreases in choline acetyltransferase (CAT), ACh, the number of muscarinic ACh receptors, glutamic acid decarboxylase, and substance P. There is generally no decrease in DA, norepinephrine, or serotonin (5HT), although more recent studies with single-photon emission computed tomography (SPECT) indicate that DA does diminish significantly in the later stages of the disease.[279]

Huntington disease is usually manifested after the age of 30 years, although childhood forms appear rarely. Those younger than 20 years with the disease account for approximately 10% of all people with Huntington disease. Death from this disease occurs about 15 to 25 years after the onset of symptoms, although as in Parkinson disease the earliest symptom is not known.

A marker for the Huntington gene has been detected.[278] If the family pedigree is known and the chromosomes of the parents can be obtained, detection of which offspring have the faulty chromosome is possible presymptomatically. Of course, early detection of this disease involves ethical and practical issues. At present, although testing is available, it is not widely used. Furthermore, testing for Huntington disease is typically available only to those older than 18 years. Despite these problems, localization of the gene and the repeat is promising and offers hope for improved means of treatment.

Huntington disease affects neurons in the basal ganglia as well as the frontal cortex. The movement disorders are presumed to be related to degeneration of the striatal neurons, specifically the enkephalinergic neurons.[16] The cognitive and emotional symptoms are associated with cortical destruction.

Symptoms

Some of the signs and symptoms of Huntington disease are similar to those of Parkinson disease: abnormalities in postural reactions, trunk rotation, distribution of tone, and extraneous movements. Individuals with Huntington disease, however, are at the other end of the spectrum; rather than a paucity of movement, they exhibit too much movement, which is evident in the trunk and face in addition to the extremities. The gait takes on an ataxic, dancing appearance (in fact, *chorea* means to dance in Greek), and fine movements become clumsy and slowed.[280] As with the person with parkinsonism, there is a decrease in associated movements (e.g., arm swing). The extraneous movements are of the choreoathetoid type, that is, involuntary, irregular isolated movements that may be jerky and arrhythmical as in chorea, to rhythmical and wormlike as in athetosis. Usually, however, these occur in successive movements so that the entire picture is one of complex movement patterns. The "movement generator" aspects of the basal ganglia seem to be continuously active, as would fit the hypothesis of a disruption in the indirect pathway. As the disease progresses, the choreiform movements may give way to akinesia and rigidity.

Gait patterns of the person with Huntington disease are in some ways similar to those of Parkinson disease. Gait velocity and stride length are decreased. The decrease in velocity is correlated with disease progression. Unlike the person with Parkinson disease, however, the person with Huntington disease has a decreased cadence as well.[281] The base of support is increased (again unlike the pattern seen in Parkinson disease). In addition, lateral sway is increased along with great variability in distal movements.

Disruptions in movement for the person with Huntington disease reflect the role of the basal ganglia in movement. For example, the person with Huntington disease, like the person with Parkinson disease, has difficulty responding to internal cues; he or she also has difficulty with internal rhythms. Kinematic analysis of upper-extremity complex tasks demonstrates that the person with Huntington disease must rely on visual guidance in the termination of a movement. This has been interpreted to indicate impairment in the development and fine-tuning of an internal representation of the task.[282] These clients have increasing difficulty with more complex movements in the absence of advanced cues.[283,284] The lack of internal cuing in the person with Huntington disease has been linked to the increased variability of response seen in these clients.[285]

The face is also affected in Huntington disease. Speech, breathing, and swallowing lack normal control and coordination. Speech lacks rhythm, as might be expected with decreased internal timing, and is often soft. Swallowing and therefore eating may also be difficult, are common problems, and often are accompanied by weight loss. In fact, some suggest that a person with decreased body weight and a parental history of the disease is at greater risk.[286,287] Impaired voluntary eye movement is often the first sign of Huntington disease. The person with Huntington disease has difficulty with initiation and control of saccadic eye movements.

The exact mechanisms for the production of choreoathetoid movements are unknown. Because these extraneous movements are part of a person's normal repertoire of movement patterns, they may be "released" at inappropriate times and without any modulation. A postmortem examination showed a decrease in GABA that was greater in the globus pallidus external segment than the internal segment. This agrees with the previously described current model.[6] Recent use of positron emission tomography (PET) scans demonstrates loss of ACh and GABA neurons.[288] A pattern therefore may be executed before it is necessary, and inappropriate portions of a movement pattern cannot be inhibited. Petajan[289] found motor unit activity indicative of bradykinesia. Recordings of single motor units in the muscles indicates that persons with Huntington disease have a loss of control evidenced by an inability to recruit single motor units.[289] As the efforts at control increased, these individuals demonstrated an overflow of motor unit activity that resulted in full choreiform movements. Those in the earlier stages of the disease demonstrated what the experimenters termed "microchorea," or small ballistic activations of motor units.[289] As in Parkinson disease, difficulty occurs in modulating motor neuron excitability. Another finding in this experiment revealed motor unit activity indicative of bradykinesia. Yanagasawa[290] used surface EMG recordings to classify involuntary muscle contractions in Huntington disease patients with varying movement disorders from chorea to rigidity. He found brief, reciprocal, irregular contractions in those patients with classic chorea, and tonic nonreciprocal contractions in those patients with rigidity. Presence of athetosis or dystonia was associated with slow, reciprocal contractions. During sustained contractions, EMG activity demonstrated brief, irregular cessation of activity in the choreic patients. Thus patients with Huntington disease have interruption of normal motor function at rest and during sustained activity (e.g., stabilizing contractions).

The abnormal postural reactions of the person with Huntington disease may occur from a misinterpretation of sensory input, especially vestibular and proprioceptive (similar to the parkinsonian syndrome). However, the dementia of Huntington disease precludes further testing.

In addition to the involvement of the motor systems, the individual with Huntington disease also shows signs of dementia and emotional disorders that become worse as the disease progresses. Neuropsychological tests are therefore part of the Unified Huntington's Disease Rating Scale (UHDRS). The client may show lack of judgment and loss of memory, deterioration in speech and writing (i.e., severe decrease in ability to communicate), depression, hostility, and feelings of incompetence. IQ decreases, with performance measures decreasing more rapidly than verbal levels. Evidence of ideomotor apraxia is also present, especially as the disease progresses.[291] Suicide is fairly common.

Stages of Huntington Disease

Huntington disease is a progressive disorder. The initial symptoms are most often incoordination, clumsiness, or jerkiness. A classic test for eliciting choreiform movements in this early stage is a simple grip test. The client grips the examiner's hand and maintains that grip for a few seconds. The person with Huntington disease displays what is descriptively called the "milkmaid's sign"; alternate increases and decreases in the grip that are perhaps the equivalent of the electromyographic abnormalities seen during sustained contractions. Facial grimacing or the inability to perform complex facial movements also may be present very early.

In many cases the dementia and psychological symptoms of Huntington disease occur after the onset of the neurological signs. In cases in which very subtle personality changes occur first, the diagnosis may be more difficult. Such persons may appear forgetful or unable to manage appointments and financial affairs. They may be thought to have early senility, or they may show signs of severe depression or schizophrenia. Early diagnosis may be important, and SPECT is showing promise for early detection of the disease.[292]

With time, the combination of the psychological and neurological problems causes the individual to lose all ability to work and perform ADLs. This person eventually can be cared for only in an extended care facility. By this time the choreiform movements have given way to rigidity, and the patient is bedridden. Death is usually caused by infection, but suicide is also common. Figure 20-12 shows the stages of Huntington disease according to Shoulson and Fahn.[293]

Pharmacological Considerations and Medical Management

Advances in the pharmacological management of Parkinson disease have led to a great deal of research in an effort to find appropriate drugs for the management of Huntington

	Engagement in occupation		Capacity to handle financial affairs		Capacity to manage domestic responsibility		Capacity to perform activities of daily living		Care can be provided at	
		Score		Score		Score		Score		Score
Stage 1	Usual level	3	Full	3	Full	2	Full	3	Home	2
Stage 2	Lower level	2	Requires slight help	2	Full	2	Full	3	Home	2
Stage 3	Marginal	1	Requires major help	1	Impaired	1	Mildly impaired	2	Home	2
Stage 4	Unable	0	Unable	0	Unable	0	Moderately impaired	1	Home or extended care facility	1
Stage 5	Unable	0	Unable	0	Unable	0	Severely impaired	0	Total care facility only	0

Figure 20-12 ■ Functional stages of Huntington disease. (Reprinted from Shoulson I, Fahn S: Huntington's disease: clinical care and evaluation, *Neurology* 29:2, 1979.)

disease.[294-299] At present, however, no fully effective medication is available for this disease. Each symptom is treated with its own medication.

The symptoms of Huntington disease indicate an increase in dopaminergic effect. At autopsy a decreased number of intrinsic neurons of the striatum that contain the neurotransmitter GABA or ACh are found. Biochemical studies reveal a definite decrease in GABA concentration in addition to a decrease in ACh concentration in the basal ganglia. Therefore drug therapy depends on drugs that are cholinergic or GABA-containing agonists and those that act as DA antagonists. To date, the DA antagonists have been more effective in ameliorating neurological symptoms; however, these drugs have severe side effects including parkinsonism—for example, bradykinesia and rigidity—and tardive dyskinesia.[294] There is no evidence that improvement of the choreiform movements leads to improved function.

In general, pharmacological treatment is not started until the choreiform movements interfere with function because these drugs have side effects that may be worse than the chorea.[300] Perphenazine, haloperidol (Haldol), and reserpine are still the most commonly used medications. The first two block the DA receptors themselves; reserpine depletes DA stores in the brain. Side effects include depression, drowsiness, a parkinsonian type of syndrome, and sometimes dyskinesia. Drugs such as choline, which would increase ACh concentrations, have produced only transient improvement.[188] Many efforts have been undertaken to find a GABA agonist that would reduce the symptoms of Huntington disease, but these have been unsuccessful so far.[300,301] The problem with finding a medication to increase GABA is that such a drug will probably cause inhibition throughout the brain, not just in the basal ganglia. Thus the individual's level of alertness and ability to function might be reduced—something the person with Huntington disease can ill afford.[301] Riluzole, a drug that blocks glutaminergic neurotransmission, has been tried with initial success.[302] A 2009 Cochrane review concluded that no pharmacological intervention demonstrated disease-modifying or disease-progression effects.[303]

The dementia and personality problems interfere more with life tasks than do the presence of movement disorders. Medications are usually prescribed as combinations of drugs to treat the specific emotional and psychological symptoms. Cortical degeneration is most certainly involved, but disruption of the heavy corticostriate projections also may be a factor in the progression of this disease. Although alterations in DA have been implicated in psychotic problems such as schizophrenia, the role of the basal ganglia in thought processes is, at best, little understood. In the words of Woody Guthrie, "There's just not no hope. Nor not no treatment known to cure me of my dizzy called Chorea."[304]

At present the best hope for the person with Huntington disease lies in a better understanding of the genetic mechanisms causing destruction of the GABA-containing cells in the striatum and cortical destruction. In the meantime, correct and early diagnosis is important in providing the proper early intervention, which must include counseling.[305] In an effort to facilitate research into the causes as well as the treatment of the disease, the Commission for the Control of Huntington's Disease has set up several research centers, including a brain and tissue bank. Research has also begun on the use of tissue transplantation. As with Parkinson disease, the tissue does survive, but the results are even more preliminary than for parkinsonism.

Examination of the Client with Huntington Disease

The standard medical evaluation is the UHDRS.[306] This comprehensive evaluation examines cognitive function as well as motor function. The physical or occupational therapy evaluation of a person with Huntington disease must include an assessment of the degree of functional ability and how the chorea interferes with function. Which extremities, including the face, are involved? Does the client have any cortical control of the chorea or any means (i.e., tricks) of allaying these extraneous movements? What exacerbates the symptoms? What lessens them? A simple rating scale is the capacity to perform ADLs (see Figure 20-12). A standardized ADL assessment with space to write in how the client performs these activities or why she or he cannot perform them would be helpful.

Gait analysis can include a timed walk test and cadence assessment; stride length can then be calculated. A subjective assessment of variability and incoordination should also be made. In addition, posture and equilibrium reactions should be tested. What associated reactions, if any, are present? In assessing posture, care should be taken to observe the posture of the extremities in addition to the trunk, head, and neck. Dystonic posturing should be carefully noted, especially if the client is taking medication. Any changes should be reported to the physician.

A gross assessment of strength should be made, with particular attention paid to the ability to stabilize the trunk and proximal joints. To reduce the effects of rigidity, ROM measurements become important as the disease progresses.

In the assessment of the client with Huntington disease, the stage of psychological involvement and mental state must be reliably assessed during both evaluation and treatment. SPECT and other computer tomography scans may give some clues to the amount of cortical and basal ganglia degeneration, which can assist in determining possible cortical functioning. There does not seem to be a consensus in research or clinical practice for which measurements are most sensitive to change or best reflect function for the patient with Huntington disease.

General Treatment Goals and Rationale

Maintenance of the optimal quality of life is the most important goal for treatment of persons with Huntington disease and their families, including maintenance of functional skills and advice to the family on adaptive equipment. Techniques that reduce tone may also reduce choreiform movements. Increasing stability about the shoulders, trunk, neck, and hips helps maintain function. Respiratory function should be kept as high as possible. Again, the evaluation results dictate treatment procedures.

Treatment Procedures

The Commission for the Control of Huntington's Disease[307] stated that these individuals are underserved by physical and occupational therapy. Peacock[308] surveyed physical therapists in one state. Of the 585 therapists who responded, only 15.5% had worked with at least one patient with Huntington disease, and 6.2% had worked with more than one patient; this confirmed the underutilization of physical and occupational therapy today. Hayden[304] and Peacock[308] suggest that therapy can improve quality of life for this population. A 2008 article by Busse and colleagues[309] demonstrated that there is still underutilization of therapy services. They also found that there no routine outcome measurements for the stages of the disease, and they suggested that management of falls and decreased mobility dysfunction could be a treatment goal of physical therapy interventions. Although animal models of Huntington disease exist, there have been few studies investigating possible movement interventions. In one animal study even a little environmental enrichment improved the ability of Huntington mice on a rotarod test and slowed the progression of the disease.[310] The mice getting even more enrichment showed improvement on more behavioral tests as well as changes in the striatum. Recently a few articles have been published examining physical and occupational therapy treatment techniques for holistic therapy and for treating specific problems.[311-313] See Chapter 9 for other specific therapeutic interventions.

A study by Zinzi and colleagues[311] was a nonrandom pilot study that incorporated gait, balance, and transfer training. Strengthening of the extremities, trunk, and muscles of respiration as well as coordination and postural stability activities were included. The program was undertaken with occupational therapy to include cognitive, rehabilitation, and ADL training. Participants were engaged in the intensive inpatient program for 3 weeks for 8 hours per day, 5 days a week, 3 times a year. The data indicate that there was significant improvement in motor function and in ADL performance and that these subjects did not show deterioration over the 3 years of the study—a positive outcome for a degenerative disease.

Treatment of the person with Huntington disease has some parallels with the treatment of cerebral palsy athetosis. These techniques, however, must be adapted to the adult. Of critical importance are the techniques for improving coactivation and trunk stability. The use of the pivot-prone and withdrawal patterns of Rood are helpful, and their benefit may be increased with the use of Thera-Band. Neck cocontraction and trunk stability may improve, or at least oral functions may be maintained. In addition, the techniques of rhythmical stabilization in all positions as well as heavy work patterns of Rood should be helpful.[314] Yet movements practiced out of context may not carry over into functional activities; thus practicing coactivation in functional patterns during treatment if at all possible is recommended. Whereas in Parkinson disease the emphasis is on large-amplitude movements, movements for the person with Huntington disease need to be of smaller amplitude and controlled.

The gait disorder of Huntington disease has been shown to respond to rhythmical auditory stimuli in one study.[315] The ability to respond decreases in those most severely involved, indicating that treatment in the later stages of the disease may not be amenable to rhythmical stimuli. Another finding of this study was that cadence was a larger problem than stride length, especially at normal and fast speeds (compare this with the findings in Parkinson disease). Interestingly, people with Huntington disease were able to modulate gait to a metronome but had more difficulty with musical cues even when the tempos were identical. Subjects with Huntington disease demonstrated short-term carryover of metronome auditory stimuli to gait without auditory stimuli. Although the long-term carryover was not studied, using a metronome in gait training may be helpful in clients with Huntington disease. A more recent study using a metronome to cue gait during single and dual task gait activities found that participants with Huntington disease had difficulty synchronizing steps to a metronome in all conditions.[313]

Relaxation aids the reduction of extraneous movements. In the early stages of the disease methods that require active participation of the client, such as biofeedback and traditional relaxation exercises, may be included. As dementia becomes more apparent, more passive techniques such as slow rocking and neutral warmth must be used. These techniques are also helpful in reducing the choreiform movements of the mouth and tongue, which may prove useful for the dentist and those responsible for proper nutrition of the client. In most cases of Huntington disease, the individual is quite thin (almost emaciated) and begins to age rapidly as the disease progresses. The extraneous movements, especially as they become more severe, increase metabolic demands, and nutrition therefore becomes increasingly important. Attention therefore must be paid to head, neck, and oral-motor control. Increased pressure on the lips may aid in lip closure and facilitate swallowing. Special straws with a mouthpiece similar to a pacifier may be useful. A dietician should be consulted for assistance in teaching the family how to prepare balanced and appetizing meals and snacks that are still easy to swallow.

The degree of dementia influences treatment options. Conscious efforts to control extraneous movements will be more difficult as cognitive function decreases. New memories and new patterns of movements are more difficult to establish. The therapist therefore must use techniques that require subcortical control and must keep in mind that the client can sometimes remember old, normal patterns of movement. An encouraging treatment method may be the use of imagery. Yágüez and colleagues[312] found that patients with Huntington disease could use imagery to compensate for impairments in a graphomotor design task.

Peacock's study[308] suggests that group programs including strength, flexibility, balance, coordination, and breathing exercises may be very successful, especially in the early stages of the disease. This was confirmed in the study by Zinzi.[311] No amount of physical or occupational therapy, however, can prevent neuronal cell loss. Because Huntington disease is a progressive, degenerative disease, the client's condition will get worse, although the Zinzi study suggested that the progression might be slowed with integrated therapy.[311] Eventually, goals must be aimed at preventing total immobility and assisting caretakers in transfer techniques and advising them in the use of adaptive equipment. One aspect of treatment that cannot be measured but is important in my view is the degree of hope offered just by the fact that a health professional is providing ongoing care. This may lessen the client's degree of despair and depression and may help maintain quality of life.

Wilson Disease

Wilson disease, or hepatolenticular degeneration, is a disease caused by faulty copper metabolism. The toxic effects of copper lead to degeneration of the liver and the basal ganglia. Wilson disease, inherited as an autosomal recessive trait, affects a very small percentage of the population. If the disease is recognized and properly treated, the patient can expect function without restriction and a normal life span.

Wilson disease is characterized by an increase in the amount of copper absorbed from the intestinal tract, a subsequent elevation in the amount of copper in the blood serum, and an increase in the amount of copper deposited in tissue.[316] Ceruloplasmin is concomitantly reduced. The increase in tissue copper may interfere with various enzyme systems of particular cells. The connection of copper with DA metabolism may account for the basal ganglia involvement.

Neuronal degeneration is present in the globus pallidus and putamen and to a lesser extent in the caudate nucleus. Atrophy may be present in the gray matter of the cortex and the dentate nucleus of the cerebellum.

Symptoms

The deposition of the excess copper in the cornea results in the classic diagnostic sign of Wilson disease, the Kayser-Fleischer ring: a brownish-green or brownish-red ring found in the sclerocorneal junction.

Several forms of Wilson disease have been classified on the basis of the signs and symptoms. One type entails only liver involvement and no neurological signs. A dystonic form is most common in those with an onset of the disease after age 20 years. The individual shows the same abnormal positioning of the limbs and trunk that characterizes the dystonia, rigidity, and bradykinesia seen in Parkinson disease. Associated reactions and facial expressions are absent. Festinating gait and flexed posture are present. Tremor of the hand, head, and body may be present.

If the onset of the disease occurs before age 20, the appearance of choreoathetoid movements of the face and upper extremities is usually present. The gait resembles that of the individual with Huntington disease. This early-onset form is accompanied by a rapid deterioration.[317]

Common to all forms of Wilson disease that involve brain structures are difficulty in speaking and swallowing, incoordination, and personality changes. The personality changes are the first signs of the disease, especially emotional lability and impaired judgment. If the disease progresses, dementia and cirrhosis of the liver increase and motor function progressively decreases.

The postures and movement patterns seen in people with Wilson disease include dystonic movements involving twisting and rotation of limbs, with sustained contraction at the end of the movement.[16] As Wilson disease progresses, the classic abnormal posture of increased flexion occurs, along with rigidity that can progress to the inability to move if severe enough. Dystonia, like bradykinesia and choreoathetosis, belongs on a continuum of the extraneous movements present with basal ganglia involvement. Dysfunction of the cerebellum and intralaminar nuclei of the thalamus may also contribute to these impairments of posture and movement.[318] A peculiar aspect of dystonia is that it can be decreased with proprioceptive or tactile inputs.[16] As with other diseases of the basal ganglia, an imbalance or abnormal response in the neurotransmitters occurs in Wilson disease; however, the precise imbalance is not yet known.

Stages of the Disease

The first symptom of Wilson disease is usually a change in the individual's personality. Either when this becomes severe enough or when the movement disorder appears, a diagnosis can be made by the presence of the Kayser-Fleischer ring in the eye or by an analysis of copper metabolism. Because Wilson disease is now treatable by chemical means, the full progression of this disease is usually not seen. If left untreated, the dystonia becomes worse and the person becomes more rigid. In addition, muscle weakness can occur and progress, seizures may develop, and the dementia and personality disorder also become worse.

Medical Management

Wilson disease is usually one of the first diseases to be ruled out when a patient manifests movement disorders and behavioral problems, especially in the younger patient. Because the signs and symptoms of Wilson disease are caused by an increased absorption of copper, treatment consists of drugs that will inhibit this absorption. Concomitantly, copper intake in the diet is restricted; no nuts, chocolate, liver, shellfish, dried fruit, or mushrooms. Zinc salt, which blocks the absorption of copper in the stomach and has no side effects, is now the treatment of choice. Penicillamine and trientine increase urinary excretion of copper, but there are serious side effects to these drugs. If the copper imbalance is treated, the neurological signs do not progress.

Examination and Treatment Intervention

Because Wilson disease is fully managed medically and can be diagnosed early, it may not be of concern to the therapist. If the client is referred for therapy, treatment techniques should be wholly based on symptoms. Examination is similar to that of the person with Parkinson or Huntington disease. It consists of describing the type of extraneous movement present, when it is present, and factors that influence the degree of dystonia. Ease of movement should also be assessed and may be timed as for the patient with Parkinson disease. In addition, range of movement and strength should be evaluated, especially if the disease is progressing.

Treatment is then designed to alleviate the problems. Extraneous movements may be reduced by any technique that will reduce tone. Positioning is important. If bradykinesia is the major sign, then treatment would be similar to that used for people with Parkinson disease; if trunk stability is poor, the therapist proceeds as in Huntington disease. The client with Wilson disease has knowledge of what normal movement feels like and usually has good cognitive abilities at the time treatment is started. Because of the emotional lability, which is one of the first symptoms in this disease, the treatment session should be well planned and quite structured.

Tardive Dyskinesia

Tardive dyskinesia is usually a drug-induced disorder and thus will be used to indicate the problems that can arise from drug intoxication. In particular this section concentrates on the problems associated with drugs that affect DA metabolism and/or reuptake, including amphetamine, methamphetamine, haloperidol, and classes of drugs used in treatment of psychotic disorders: the phenothiazines, butyrophenones, and thioxanthenes. As the use and misuse of drugs becomes more common, these types of disorders may become more frequent. (Refer to Chapter 36 for additional information.)

The use of phenothiazines (one of the neuroleptics) has become a very effective and common treatment for schizophrenia. This treatment protocol has enabled many schizophrenics to leave the mental institution. These drugs are DA antagonists and thus decrease the amount of DA in the brain. The exact site of the brain involved in schizophrenia itself is not within the scope of this chapter, but the neurological signs that occur will be discussed. As might be expected, they involve structures within the basal ganglia. Tardive dyskinesia is a gradual disease that occurs after long-term drug treatment. The most typical involvement is of the mouth, tongue, and muscles of mastication; therefore tardive dyskinesia may be called *orofacial* or *buccolingual-masticatory* (BLM) dyskinesia.

Symptoms

Dyskinesia is defined as an inability to perform voluntary movement.[305] In practical terms, however, dyskinesia is usually a series of rhythmical extraneous movements. In tardive dyskinesia this typically begins with, or may be confined to, the region of the face. These extraneous movements may include choreoathetoid or dystonic movements. Because of abnormality in basal ganglia function, abnormalities in postural tone and postural adjustments are also present. Instead of the typical flexed posture of Parkinson disease, clients with tardive dyskinesia show extension of the trunk with increased lordosis and neck flexion.[319] This description of the disease is rather broad, but the problems of drug-induced movement disorders are varied. They may take the form of drug-induced Parkinson disease or dystonia. In tardive dyskinesia, akinesia and rigidity similar to that seen in parkinsonism may exist simultaneously with the choreoathetoid-like movements. The key factor in tardive dyskinesia is its slow onset after the ingestion of neuroleptic medications.

Etiology

Although many people take neuroleptic medication, only a small percentage acquires tardive dyskinesia. Many factors may predispose an individual to movement disorders. One of these is age.[320] This might be expected because of the influence of aging processes on the concentration of DA. Gender may also be a factor. Women, and older women in particular, are more at risk for tardive dyskinesia, perhaps because of decreased estrogen.[319] The absolute amount of neuroleptic ingested may also be a factor, but to date definitive studies have not been completed. So far the length of time the individual takes medication does not appear to be a strong predisposing factor. As the biological abnormalities of schizophrenia become better understood, further understanding of the causes of tardive dyskinesia also may be elucidated. The development of tardive dyskinesia is hypothesized to be caused by supersensitivity.[305,321] With the use of drugs that deplete the brain of DA, the brain becomes more sensitive to it. And, in fact, in humans the withdrawal of neuroleptics tends to heighten the disease; essentially, withdrawal of the DA antagonist means that far more DA is able to act on these already sensitive terminals.[305,321,322]

Because of the effectiveness of long-term treatment for schizophrenia provided by neuroleptics, research into the underlying cause and therefore treatment of the major side effect, the motor disorders, has greatly increased.[323] But as with Parkinson disease and Huntington disease, animal models are difficult to produce. However, experimental evidence indicates that the basal ganglia are involved in movements about the face, especially the mouth, and buccolingual dyskinesia is the most frequently encountered symptom in tardive dyskinesia.[69,70] The response of basal ganglia neurons to sensory input shows increasing localization of response with age; the region about the mouth becomes increasingly sensitive.[70] Further research along these lines, both in normal animals and in those with lesions, may answer the question of what is happening at a neuronal level. This would facilitate pharmacological and therapeutic interventions.

Pharmacological and Medical Management

The most important treatment for tardive dyskinesia is prevention. Today, DA receptor agonists are prescribed only when other, newer medications are not effective. Tardive dyskinesia is often irreversible. The withdrawal of medication, in fact, may increase the movement disorders. Or recovery may take even more time than that required for the onset of the disease. Strangely, sometimes the drug that caused the disease may be the drug that reduces the symptoms; that is, increasing the dose may lessen the movement disorder. This might be expected if supersensitivity to DA is involved. But again, with time the increased dose will also cause a reappearance of the symptoms. The Movement Disorder Society and WE MOVE recommend that the physician evaluate the schizophrenic patient at 3-month intervals to prevent the disease. (Refer to the list of websites at the end of this chapter.)

The use of other drugs in conjunction with the neuroleptics has been tried in various animal models of the disease. As might be expected, anticholinergic drugs (which would worsen an imbalance between DA and ACh) worsen the dyskinesia. Lithium has been successful in one animal model of dyskinesia.[305] Some neuroleptic drugs seem to have less effect on movement than others; however, the side effects of one such drug, chlorpromazine, are life-threatening. Reducing the buildup of phenylalanine is also indicated as a way to decrease occurrence of tardive dyskinesia. A medical food comprising branched-chain amino acids seems to reduce concentration of phenylalanine and was effective in reducing the movement disorder in one clinical trial. More research is needed into both the mechanisms of schizophrenia and the mechanisms for the production of the abnormal movements.

Evaluation and Treatment Interventions for Dyskinesia

The effectiveness of rehabilitation therapy intervention in drug-induced dyskinesia is, as yet, not completely known. However, because the neuroleptics do provide an effective long-term treatment of schizophrenia, and because amphetamines and methamphetamine are being abused, therapists need to become aware of the problem and offer some assistance. Early drug holidays (time without use of drugs) may be of value in treatment of tardive dyskinesia, and therefore early awareness of incipient changes in motor function may be of value. Assessment of patients receiving drug therapy could perhaps begin before treatment and then at prescribed intervals. The knowledge that postural adjustments are abnormal in most basal ganglia diseases means that analysis of posture statically and in motion might provide early clues of development of movement disorders. The same would be true for balance reactions and changes in tone with changes in position. Once movement disorders appear, an assessment of when and where the extraneous movements occur is important. (See Chapter 8 for general examination tools and Chapter 22 specifically for tests of balance.)

General treatment is similar to that used in Huntington disease; oral treatment corresponds to that for the athetotic child with cerebral palsy. If a hyperreactivity to sensory stimulus exists, then oral desensitization may be of value.

Ameliorating the oral grimacing, of course, would be helpful for the schizophrenic person who is trying to return to society. The effectiveness of physical and occupational therapy treatment cannot be assessed until therapists become involved with these clients and record the effectiveness of their interventions. In cases in which the parkinsonian-like symptoms are stronger than the dyskinetic movements, treatment would follow the plan for the individual with Parkinson disease. As yet, physical therapy for drug-induced dyskinesias is not mentioned on websites to the physician or the patient.

Other Considerations

Other drugs besides neuroleptics may also produce movement disorders. Amphetamine, for example, has been shown to cause long-term changes in brain function even with very small doses.[324-326] Adults who were hyperactive as children sometimes show a decrease in the readiness potential.[327] Further longitudinal research and research using PET scans and functional magnetic resonance imaging (fMRI) are underway to determine the role that medications used in treating hyperactive children, such as methylphenidate (Ritalin), might play in changing the architecture of the basal ganglia and causing movement disorders.[84] The problem of drug-induced movement disorders may become an ever-increasing one for the therapist.

In 1982 several young people were treated for rigidity and "catatonia" after the use of what they thought was heroin. Careful examination of these patients revealed that they had parkinsonian-like symptoms.[38,105] The chemical responsible for the symptomatology was MPTP, a meperidine analog that was an impurity in the designer heroin. This discovery has enabled research in animals and clinical studies in humans and may enable better understanding of the pathogenesis and, in turn, of the treatment of the disease. One hypothesized cause of Parkinson disease implicated environmental toxins (because some herbicides such as paraquat resemble the chemical structure of MPTP) and the involvement of superoxide free radicals.[92,328,329] More complete epidemiological studies are now underway to investigate Parkinson disease to determine the relationship to specific herbicides and pesticides.

Methamphetamine use also induces movement disorders. The MRI of even infrequent users shows damage to the basal ganglia.[330,331] A child born to a mother using methamphetamine may also have movement disorders and delayed achievement of developmental milestones. Another recreational drug, cocaine has long been known to produce parkinsonian movement disorders.[332]

Dystonia

General Information

Dystonia is a movement disorder characterized by sustained muscle contraction in the extreme end range of a movement, frequently with a rotational component. There are inherited dystonias that usually involve the entire body. These dystonias are most prevalent in those of European Jewish descent. Focal dystonias involve just one joint or a few neighboring joints, such as spasmodic torticollis or writing cramps. Full-body dystonia is a disease of the basal ganglia, and the current view is that focal dystonia also involves lesions of precise areas of the basal ganglia.

Generalized and focal dystonias manifest differently and have different pathophysiologies and therefore different treatments. They will therefore be separated in this part of the chapter. However, in all cases of dystonia, excessive coactivation of agonists and antagonists occurs that interferes with the timing, execution, and loss of independent joint motions. Rarely are any abnormalities of muscle tone present, per se—that is, no increase in deep tendon reflexes or rigidity occurs. Muscle strength and ROM are usually within normal limits unless disuse leads to weakness.

Generalized Dystonia

Symptoms. The person with generalized dystonia will begin a movement (such as walking) and then will experience a torsional contraction of the trunk; of the upper extremity, especially at the shoulder; and in the ankle, foot, and toes. These contractions may be so strong that further movement is impossible. Many patients experience pain as the muscles remain contracted for long periods of time.[333]

Etiology. The cause of generalized dystonia is predominantly genetic, involving the *DYT* gene.[334]

Pharmacological and Medical Management. There are few treatments for generalized dystonia. DA agonists and L-dopa are sometimes effective.

Evaluation and Treatment Intervention. Evaluation of the person with generalized dystonia will be similar to the evaluation of the person with tardive dyskinesia or Huntington disease. Several ADLs should be examined. And the way that dystonia interferes with these ADLs is of most importance for treatment. In addition to the full extent of the motoric abnormality, it is also important to test sensation, especially higher level sensory processing such as precise localization of touch, graphesthesia, and kinesthesia.

Movement therapy interventions are only now being developed for generalized dystonia. Overall, treatment similar to that in Huntington disease that emphasizes treating the symptoms may be beneficial. One successful program uses sensory integration and relearning techniques performed with attention.[335] Practice is a crucial element of treatment, and the client must be willing to practice the sensory tasks many, many times throughout the day for benefit.

Other Considerations. As with other extraneous movements associated with basal ganglia disorders, relaxation can reduce the muscle contraction. However, I have found that the time to incorporate the relaxation is before the full-blown development of the muscle contraction—a difficult task. Therefore clients should practice relaxation on a regular basis. There is frequently a psychological aspect to the focal dystonias that may necessitate intervention from a psychiatrist or psychologist.

Focal Dystonias

Spasmodic torticollis is the most common focal dystonia. The person with this disorder will have involuntary contractions of neck muscles that result in head turning and head extension and flexion movements that are often sustained for long periods of time. Other common sites of focal involvement are the vocal cords; the tongue and swallowing muscles; the facial muscles, especially about the eye; the hand; and the toes. Writer's cramp is a task-specific dystonia, unlike other focal dystonias. An interesting phenomenon of dystonia is the fact that many patients will develop a sensory or motor "trick" that will decrease the severity of the muscle contraction(s) and may even stop these movements.[333,336]

Symptoms. Symptoms of focal dystonia will depend on the site of involvement. For example, in the case of spasmodic torticollis, the symptom is pain and an inability to control a movement of the head to the side.

The signs and symptoms of focal hand dystonia are variable. The problem may initially manifest as an abnormality in the quality of sound produced by a musical instrument (e.g., a deterioration of vibration in a violinist),[337] increasing errors in task performance, unusual fatigue or sense of weakness, or involuntary or excessive movement of a single digit or multiple digits. Initially the symptoms are subtle and virtually indistinguishable from the normal variations that may be seen in the execution experienced by all musicians studying technically demanding music or software engineers who spend excessive hours at the computer. Frequently, a person engaged in a profession with high repetition of tasks who has minimal pain but vague motor control problems or somatosensory dysfunction is manifesting early signs of focal dystonia.[338] Although a co-contraction of flexors and extensors can be observed while an individual with hand dystonia performs the target task, at rest and during the performance of nontarget tasks the hand appears to function normally. Some patients demonstrate a variety of subtle abnormalities such as a reduced arm swing; loss of smooth, controlled grasping; a physiological tremor; hypermobility of the interphalangeal joints; decreased ROM in some upper limb joints (e.g., shoulder abduction, external rotation, finger abduction, forearm pronation); neurovascular entrapment; compression neuropathy; or poor posture.[339-344]

Etiology. The cause of focal dystonias is unknown and multifactorial. Frucht[344] observed that task-specific hand dystonia seemed to begin after motor skills had been acquired rather than during skill acquisition. Thus, focal hand dystonia in a musician is probably not a disorder of motor learning but a disruption of acquired, complex, motor programs. The data also suggested that peripheral environmental influences seem to play an important role in molding the dystonic phenotype. For example, the hand performing the more complex musical tasks (e.g., right hand in pianists and guitarists, left hand in violinists), seemed to be more predisposed to the development of dystonia. In addition, the dystonia usually began in one finger and spread to adjacent fingers, rarely skipping a finger. Furthermore, the ulnar side of the hand (fingers 4 and 5) was disproportionately affected, potentially because of the challenging ergonomics and technical stresses of the musical instrument required for this part of the hand in terms of gripping and activation of individual finger movements.[345]

Pharmacological and Medical Management. The most common medical treatment for the focal dystonias is botulinum toxin. This toxin binds with the ACh receptors on the muscle and prevents the muscle from contracting. The injections are made under electromyographic guidance so that only those motor units involved in the production of the extraneous movements are paralyzed. However, the treatment does not cause permanent change, so the patient must repeat these injections every 3 to 4 months. Some people develop antibodies to the toxin, rendering it then ineffective.[346,347] Therefore, medical management prevents the abnormal movement but is not a cure.

Evaluation and Treatment. Overall, treatment of focal dystonia will depend on the joint or joint involved. The duration of the dystonia, the trigger, and the person's trick, if any, to relieve the dystonia must be noted. Tricks are sensory in nature and help relieve the pain often associated with the extreme movement. The Toronto Western Spasmodic Torticollis Rating Scale (TWSTRS) is one evaluation for the person with spasmodic torticollis.[348]

Several ADLs should be examined. For example, in hand dystonia, the person should be evaluated using the instrument producing the dystonia (i.e., the pen in writer's cramp) as well as other tools (e.g., a fork). In addition, there seems to be position dependence, so writing while prone may not evoke the dystonia despite severe inability to hold the pen at a desk.[349]

In addition to the full extent of the motoric abnormality, sensation, especially higher-level sensations such as precise localization of touch, graphesthesia, and kinesthesia must be assessed. Byl and colleagues found changes in the sensory cortex after development of focal hand dystonia.[335,349-352] Recent evidence suggests that balance, particularly dynamic balance, should also be assessed in patients with torticollis.[353] These balance difficulties have not been relieved with botulinum toxin.

Movement therapy interventions are now being developed. One successful program uses sensory integration and relearning techniques performed with attention.[354] Practice is a crucial element of treatment and the client must be willing to practice the sensory tasks many times throughout the day for benefit. The client practices cognitively demanding sensory discrimination tasks throughout the day and tries to use only tension-free movements.[349]

Treatment for the person with torticollis must include a relearning of midline before the person can begin to practice normal movement away from midline. The client may find this relearning process easier after botulinum injection. See Chapter 9 for further treatment interventions appropriate for patients with focal dystonias.

Other Considerations. As with other extraneous movements associated with basal ganglia disorders, relaxation can reduce the muscle contraction. However, the time to incorporate relaxation is before the full-blown development of the muscle contraction—a difficult task. This task requires a shift in paradigm to a health and wellness model and prevention (see Chapter 2). Therefore clients should practice relaxation on a regular basis. A psychological aspect to the focal dystonias frequently necessitates intervention from a psychiatrist or psychologist.

METABOLIC DISEASES AFFECTING OTHER REGIONS OF THE BRAIN

All alterations of metabolism, if allowed to continue, will affect nervous system function. This includes alterations in sodium, water, sugar, and hormonal balance. Table 20-2 lists metabolic diseases that often have neurological sequelae. Proper treatment is usually medical management of the imbalance. Physical therapeutic intervention, if necessary, should address specific neurological symptoms.

Ingestion of or exposure to heavy metals may also lead to CNS disease. Table 20-3 describes the sequelae of these problems.

TABLE 20-2 ■ NEUROLOGICAL COMPLICATIONS OF METABOLIC DISORDERS

METABOLIC PROBLEM	TREATMENT	NEUROLOGICAL COMPLICATION
Decreased sodium (too much water)	Restriction of water intake	Muscle twitching, seizures, coma
Increased sodium	Slow rehydration	Cerebral edema, muscle rigidity, decerebrate rigidity
Decreased potassium (hypokalemia), often caused by aldosteronism	Restoration of potassium levels after assessing primary cause	Changes in resting potential of neuron; hyperpolarization; muscle weakness and fatigue with eventual total paralysis
Magnesium imbalance	Improved diet, intravenous magnesium	Mental confusion, muscle twitching, myoclonus, tachycardia, hyperreflexia, extraneous movements, seizures
Diabetes mellitus	Proper control of diabetes	Peripheral neuropathy, pseudotabes, possible seizures and coma
Hypoglycemia	Treatment of primary cause; diet adjustment	Anoxia of the brain, seizures, mental confusion
Hyperthyroidism	Thyroid-blocking agents; intravenous fluids, hydrocortisone, and propranolol if patient is in thyroid crisis	Hyperkinesia, irritability, nervousness, emotional lability, symmetrical peripheral neuropathy
Hypothyroidism	Thyroid supplement	Sluggishness, mental and motor retardation, muscle weakness, sometimes muscle pain
Hypercalcemia	Treatment of primary cause, which is often hyperparathyroidism, vitamin D malignancy (therefore surgical removal)	Headache, weakness, fatigue, proximal neuropathy, rigidity, tremor, disorientation
Hypocalcemia	Intravenous administration of calcium (possible medical emergency)	Hyperexcitability of the peripheral and central nervous systems, which can lead to tetany and convulsions

TABLE 20-3 ■ NEUROLOGICAL COMPLICATIONS OF HEAVY METAL POISONING

TYPE OF METAL	TREATMENT	NEUROLOGICAL COMPLICATION
LEAD		
Source: lead paint, industrial (fumes of molten lead)	Elimination of source, reduction of fluids, intravenous urea or mannitol, use of chelating agents	Interstitial edema and hemorrhage (especially in cerebellum) in acute poisoning; all levels of central nervous system affected in chronic long-term poisoning In children: seizures, mental retardation, behavior problems, hyperactivity In adults: spasticity, rigidity, dementia, personality changes Peripheral neuropathy may occur in adults and children
ARSENIC		
Source: paint and insecticides	Removal of source, gastric lavage, intravenous fluids, maintenance of electrolyte balance; penicillamine used in acute poisoning	Demyelinization of peripheral nerves in all extremities
MANGANESE		
Source: industrial if manganese dust is not removed; symptoms appear 2-25 yr after exposure	Levodopa	Neuronal loss in basal ganglia, substantia nigra, and cerebellum Initially psychiatric disturbances, including nervousness, irritability, and a tendency toward compulsive acts Later, muscular weakness and parkinsonian symptoms
MERCURY		
Rare, but may affect farmers and dental office workers	Penicillamine; function returns only with physical, occupational, and speech therapy	Loss of neurons, especially in cerebellum; also in cortex near calcarine fissure Alternating periods of confusion, drowsiness, and stupor with restlessness and excitability Ataxia, dysarthria, visual deterioration

SUMMARY

This chapter has focused on the pathophysiology, evaluation, and treatment of genetic, hereditary, and metabolic diseases affecting adults. In all of these diseases the therapist or movement specialist is an important (though sometimes underused) part of the rehabilitation team. Knowledge of the possible mechanisms involved in the production of the varying movement disorders may make the appropriate evaluation and subsequent treatment more meaningful. Even with degenerative, progressive disorders the therapist plays an important role in maintaining quality of life and assists the client and family in coping with the disease. The importance of documentation (see Chapter 10) and publication of cases and larger controlled studies cannot be overstressed. Both will assist in the development of improved therapeutic techniques and may help researchers in planning and interpreting appropriate experimental studies. Establishment of efficacy will be the first step toward evidence-based practice and a critical link in the evolution of professionals who have been identified as movement specialists.

With the advent of the Internet, many websites have been created to focus on diseases and conditions mentioned in this chapter. In addition, the organization WE MOVE (Worldwide Education and Awareness for Movement Disorders) has a website for both patients and care providers (www.wemove.org). These sites answer many questions for patients and provide information on making day-to-day life easier. Local and national support groups and foundations also provide information and support for the patient and caregiver. Most also have separate sections for health care providers.

Websites

National Institute of Neurological Disorders and Stroke, National Institutes of Health
A comprehensive index of neurological disorders.
www.ninds.nih.gov/disorders/disorder_index.htm

WE MOVE—Worldwide education and awareness for movement disorders
This organization is for professionals and patients and includes information regarding all movement disorders included in this chapter. Refer to Web booklet, *A Caregiver's Guide to Huntington's Disease.*
www.wemove.org

The Parkinson's Disease Foundation
This website includes an exercise program for people with Parkinson disease.
www.pdf.org

The National Parkinson Foundation
News, medical information, events calendar, and more for people with Parkinson disease, families, and caregivers.
www.parkinson.org

American Physical Therapy Association Podcast on Parkinson Disease

Schenkman M, Gill-Body K; Craik RL, moderator. Outcome measures for people with Parkinson disease. http://ptjournal.apta.org/content/suppl/2011/08/17/91.9.1339.DC2/ptj_201109_discussion_outcomes.mp3

Huntington's Disease Society of America

Information, research, and help for people with Huntington's disease, families, and caregivers.

www.hdsa.org

References

To enhance this text and add value for the reader, all references are included on the companion Evolve site that accompanies this textbook. This online service will, when available, provide a link for the reader to a Medline abstract for the article cited. There are 354 cited references and other general references for this chapter, with the majority of those articles being evidence-based citations.

CASE STUDY 20-1 ■ PATIENT WITH PARKINSON DISEASE, HOEHN AND YAHR STAGE 1

Ms. T. is a 55-year-old woman who was diagnosed with Parkinson disease 1 year ago. The disease began in her left arm and leg when she noticed increasing stiffness and difficulty moving. She complains of some instability in walking and recently has developed a slight resting tremor in the left hand. On initial evaluation she had full active and passive ROM in all extremities, neck, and trunk. There is a mild resting tremor present in the left hand. There is mild cogwheel rigidity in the left upper and lower extremities; there is some intermittent resistance to passive movement in the right upper extremity as well. Strength is grossly within normal limits throughout. Sensation is intact throughout. Equilibrium reactions are delayed, but the patient demonstrates an ankle strategy on a flat surface and a hip strategy when standing on the balance beam; there is no mixing of the synergies, and her balance responses are appropriate to the degree of displacement.

The patient is able to stand in the sharpened Romberg position for 30 seconds with the eyes open and 20 seconds with eyes closed. She can stand on the right leg for 30 seconds with eyes open and 15 seconds with eyes closed; she can stand on the left leg for 15 seconds with eyes open and 10 seconds with eyes closed. When walking, she has a heel-toe sequence, shortened stride length, and normal stride width. There is no arm swing on the left and a diminished arm swing on the right. There is no trunk rotation and very slight trunk flexion throughout the gait cycle. Speed is within normal limits for a 25-foot walk. The patient is able to turn freely. She has recently begun to experience a foot dystonia, which is worse with fatigue. It has interfered with her daily walking program and her tennis, an activity she enjoys with her husband twice a week. Her only medication is deprenyl.

This patient is in Hoehn and Yahr stage 1, with some beginning of bilateral symptoms and progression to stage 2. She is young, is employed full-time, and has been involved in regular exercise for the past 10 years. Her complaints are of stiffness, slowed movements, and foot dystonia. Because her symptoms are mild at present and she has good balance in standing and walking, this patient should be encouraged to continue exercising regularly. She should try to maintain her tennis, as this requires complex, sequential, context-dependent movements. Although tennis involves motor responses to external cues, it does necessitate rapid force generation and anticipatory movements. This should encourage continued motor learning. In addition, she should be encouraged to continue walking out of doors and practice alternating speed of walking. The dystonia is more difficult to resolve. It may be tied to medication, and differing medication schemes are now being tried. She is also on a program of stretching and strengthening of the ankle as well as a sensory stimulation program for the feet. Foam between the toes has helped to decrease dystonia early in the day.

Ms. T. has also been informed about the importance of maintaining chest expansion and monitoring her breathing. This will be important as the disease progresses. She attends a support group for young parkinsonian patients to increase her awareness of the disease, new treatments, and support. As the disease progresses, she will need a home program appropriate for her symptoms. The home program will be reassessed every 3 to 6 months.

CASE STUDY 20-2 ■ PATIENT WITH A SEVEN-YEAR HISTORY OF PARKINSON DISEASE, HOEHN AND YAHR STAGE 3

Mr. R. is a 68-year-old man with a 7-year history of Parkinson disease. He is currently in Hoehn and Yahr stage 3 of the disease progression. He falls two or three times a day, has difficulty eating, and has noticed weakness in his right hand. He would like to return to full activity including golf twice a week, swimming, and skiing. On evaluation he has moderate rigidity in all extremities; the right side is worse than the left. It is most marked in the right wrist, forearm, and hand. Shoulder flexion and abduction lack 15 degrees bilaterally. He has a 15-degree knee flexion contracture on the right; all other joints in the lower extremity have range within functional limits. Strength is grossly 4 to 4+/5 on manual muscle testing throughout including grip strength. Sensation is within normal limits throughout. Sitting balance is good during static and dynamic activities.

The patient sits with a posterior pelvic tilt, rounded shoulders, and flexed neck. On rising to a standing position, he does move forward in the chair, which positions his feet under his knees. He does not lean forward as he stands and momentarily loses his balance on rising from a chair. Static standing balance

Continued

CASE STUDY 20-2 ■ PATIENT WITH A SEVEN-YEAR HISTORY OF PARKINSON DISEASE, HOEHN AND YAHR STAGE 3—cont'd

is fair, and dynamic balance is fair. When pushed on the sternum, he takes one or two steps backward, even to a gentle push. When pushed from behind he takes several steps forward. He lost his balance and required assistance when trying to catch a large ball thrown to the side. His gait pattern is typical of a parkinsonian patient. There is a shortened step and a flat-footed foot contact. He complains of festination and of freezing, but neither are observed during the evaluation. He turns "en bloc," exhibiting no arm swing and no trunk rotation. He walks slowly and is unable to increase his speed measurably in a 25-foot walk. He is taking L-dopa–carbidopa and deprenyl. He tried taking another D2 agonist but experienced hallucinations. He was able to ski until last winter. At that time he found that he could not stand up once he fell down, and sometimes he fell without realizing that he was falling. He stated that he "did not think it was safe to ski." He also no longer swims because he has difficulty breathing in the pool and coordinating his breathing with the strokes. He does not play golf because it takes him so long.

This patient was encouraged to continue both to exercise and to socialize while exercising. He was encouraged to resume golf at times when his course is less crowded. In addition, he was given a home program consisting of activities to be performed in seated and standing positions that encourage trunk rotation and large movements and are coordinated with good breathing practices. He was given some balance exercises that challenge his equilibrium in a safe environment. His home program was monitored every 3 months because of the distance he must travel to come to the clinic. His wife was instructed to exercise with her husband and to exercise to music with him. He was referred to the speech pathologist for a swallowing evaluation and was given a therapeutic program for his speech and breathing. He is now able to play golf once a week; however he is not yet ready to resume swimming or skiing.

CHAPTER 21

Movement Dysfunction Associated with Cerebellar Damage

SUSANNE M. MORTON, PT, PhD, and AMY J. BASTIAN, PT, PhD

OVERVIEW

The cerebellum is a highly unique brain structure, easily recognizable by its location on the dorsal surface of the brain stem and the distinct, dense folia, or foldings, of its cortex. For centuries the cerebellum has been the object of intense investigation by scientists, in particular because of the extreme uniformity in the arrangement of neurons in the cerebellar cortex and the presence of very large Purkinje cells, which have an extensive fanlike dendritic arbor. The human cerebellum contains more neurons than any other brain region, suggesting that whatever its role in behavior, it requires the integration of vast amounts of information and may perform rather complex computations. Researchers agree that the cerebellum plays a critical role in coordinating and adapting movements, although how it does so is still not fully understood. It is now also clear that the cerebellum is connected to nonmotor regions of the brain, such as the prefrontal cortex, and therefore likely plays a role in cognitive and other nonmotor functions. Yet the most striking and debilitating effect of damage to the cerebellum is *ataxia,* which comes from the Greek and translates literally to "without order." We will focus on this hallmark feature of cerebellar damage, which is incoordination of movements without overt muscle weakness.

In this chapter we will review critical features of cerebellar anatomy and physiology that help reveal the role of the cerebellum in motor control, and we will describe the major movement deficits associated with damage to the human cerebellum. We will highlight the most valuable and unique components of the physical therapy examination for clients with suspected cerebellar dysfunction and review the evidence for and against specific rehabilitation interventions targeting recovery of body functions, activities, and participation. Emphasis is placed on the importance of the physical therapist's judgment in determining whether a recovery or a compensation approach should be implemented.

Types of Cerebellar Damage

Cerebellar ataxia can result from damage to the cerebellum itself or the pathways to or from it. Damage can occur from a number of different causes, such as stroke, tumor, degenerative disease, trauma, or malformation. The cause of cerebellar dysfunction is often an important consideration when determining a prognosis and developing a treatment plan. Other factors to consider include whether the cerebellar lesion is static versus progressive, whether it involves only the cerebellum or multiple neural structures, and whether it was present at birth or acquired.

Cerebellar strokes are rarer than cerebral strokes, but not entirely uncommon. They account for less than 5% of all strokes.[1] These strokes can involve any of the three arteries that supply the cerebellum: the superior cerebellar artery, anterior inferior cerebellar artery, and posterior inferior cerebellar artery. Depending on the territory supplied by the damaged vessel (Table 21-1), there are stereotyped patterns of cerebellar and extracerebellar motor dysfunction that result. However, there is certainly some variation in distribution from person to person. Stroke involving the superior cerebellar artery often leads to dysmetria of ipsilateral arm movements, unsteadiness in walking, dysarthric speech, and nystagmus.[1] Stroke involving the anterior inferior cerebellar artery often causes both cerebellar and extracerebellar signs (owing to involvement of the pons) including dysmetria, vestibular signs, and facial sensory loss.[1] Finally, stroke involving the posterior inferior cerebellar artery is usually, in the long run, the most benign, though initially it often manifests with vertigo, unsteadiness, walking ataxia, and nystagmus.[1] The best predictor of recovery from cerebellar stroke is whether the deep cerebellar nuclei are involved: recovery is best when they are not damaged.[2]

Tumors in the posterior fossa (i.e., in or near the cerebellum) do occur, though they are more common in children than adults. Depending on the type and location, tumors may be treatable with surgical resection, chemotherapy, radiation therapy, or some combination of these. Children with cerebellar tumors often have a good prognosis for recovery because many of the types of tumors most common in this population are benign and can be removed. Children also typically recover very well after cerebellar damage from tumor resection and show little signs of cerebellar ataxia. Tumors in adulthood often are caused by a more aggressive form of cancer and therefore may carry a poorer prognosis. Second to tumor type, damage of the deep cerebellar nuclei is an important factor that predicts recovery, even more so than age.[2]

Several neurodegenerative diseases can damage the cerebellum (Table 21-2). One of the more common types of degenerative diseases is a group of hereditary, autosomal dominant diseases referred to as the spinocerebellar ataxias (SCAs). Currently there are 30 known distinct SCAs, which are named by numbers (e.g., SCA1, SCA2). Depending on the genetic abnormality, they can cause either purely cerebellar damage or combined cerebellar and extracerebellar damage.[3,4] Most of the SCAs have onset in midlife and are slowly progressive, which means that children of an affected parent will likely not know if they are affected until adulthood. There are genetic tests for a subset of these diseases. Because onset of symptoms is delayed and there are no effective pharmacological treatments, genetic counseling is a must before families decide whether or not to have children undergo genetic testing. A related set of diseases

TABLE 21-1 ■ TERRITORIES OF THE CEREBELLAR ARTERIES

ARTERY	CEREBELLAR TERRITORY SUPPLIED
SCA	Superior or upper half (approximately) of the dorsal and upper third (approximately) of the ventral surface of the cerebellum except for the extreme lateral wing of the hemisphere Portions of the vermis and nodulus Substantial upper portions of the intermediate and lateral hemispheres Portions of the deep cerebellar nuclei Superior cerebellar peduncle
AICA	Middle 10%-30% of the ventral cerebellum, sometimes wrapping laterally to encompass a small portion of the most lateral aspects of the dorsal cerebellum Flocculus Small portions of the lateral hemisphere Middle and inferior cerebellar peduncles
PICA	Inferior or lower half (approximately) of the dorsal cerebellum and the inferior fourth to third of the ventral cerebellum Portions of the nodulus, vermis, intermediate and lateral hemispheres Portions of the deep cerebellar nuclei

Data from Amarenco P: The spectrum of cerebellar infarctions. *Neurology* 41:973–979, 1991; and Tatu L, Moulin T, Bogousslavsky J, Duvernoy H: Arterial territories of human brain: brainstem and cerebellum. *Neurology* 47:1125–1135, 1996.

AICA, Anterior inferior cerebellar artery; *PICA,* posterior inferior cerebellar artery; *SCA,* superior cerebellar artery.

Note: The cerebellar arteries also supply extracerebellar regions (i.e., portions of brain stem) not listed here.

TABLE 21-2 ■ SELECTED FORMS OF CEREBELLAR DAMAGE[102]

ACQUIRED	DEGENERATIVE NONHEREDITARY
1. Stroke (infarct, hemorrhage) 2. Tumor (primary brain tumor, metastatic disease) 3. Structural (Chiari malformation, agenesis, hypoplasia, etc.) 4. Toxicity (alcohol, heavy metals, drugs, solvents, etc.) 5. Immune-mediated (multiple sclerosis, gluten ataxia, etc.) 6. Trauma 7. Infection (cerebellitis, etc.) 8. Endocrine (hypothyroidism)	1. Multiple system atrophy (MSA) 2. Idiopathic late-onset cerebellar ataxia (ILOCA) HEREDITARY 1. Autosomal dominant disorders (episodic ataxias, spinocerebellar ataxias) 2. Autosomal recessive disorders (Friedreich ataxia, early onset cerebellar ataxia, etc.) 3. X-linked disorders (mitochondrial disease, fragile X-associated tremor, etc)

Data from Manto M, Marmolino D: Cerebellar ataxias. *Curr Opin Neurol* 22:419–429, 2009.

is the hereditary episodic ataxias,[5] which are rare autosomal dominant diseases. As the name implies, clients with episodic ataxia will have periods of ataxia lasting minutes to hours, brought on by exercise, stress, or excitement. Some of the episodic ataxias respond well to medications.[6]

Cerebellar damage can occur from other sources as well. In traumatic brain injury, damage of the cerebellum is almost always found in the presence of widespread brain damage and is seen as a predictor of poorer outcome.[7] The cerebellum is also particularly sensitive to toxins, including certain heavy metals and alcohol. Chronic alcoholism causes cerebellar atrophy preferentially involving the anterior superior vermis.[8,9] The inflammatory disorder multiple sclerosis also frequently produces lesions in the cerebellum. Finally, congenital brain abnormalities such as Chiari malformation damage the cerebellum by increased pressure and mechanical deformation. Recovery from cerebellar malformation is not understood; often these children have substantial damage to the brain stem or other neural structures, which may make therapy more challenging. A more comprehensive list of the variety of types of cerebellar damage is provided in Table 21-2.

Given the wide range of cerebellar disorders, it is useful for the clinician to categorize the damage as progressive or nonprogressive. Clients with progressive disorders, such as the SCAs, are likely to experience worsening ataxia and decreased mobility over time, and will need periodic therapy over the life span for optimal function. In contrast, the condition of patients with nonprogressive disorders would not be expected to worsen, and some may have the potential for substantial recovery. Note that when additional brain areas are involved, rehabilitation may be more challenging, theoretically because other, compensatory brain mechanisms may be impaired. This type of information is vital for making an appropriate prognosis and developing a long-term plan of care for clients with cerebellar dysfunction.

CEREBELLAR ANATOMY AND PHYSIOLOGY

A brief review of specific anatomical and physiological features is critical to understanding the mechanisms by which the cerebellum helps coordinate and adapt movement. Recall that most pathways between the cerebellum and spinal cord are uncrossed or double crossed, whereas pathways between the cerebellum and cerebrum are crossed. Hence a lesion to one side of the cerebellum produces ataxia and related cerebellar deficits involving the same side of the body as the lesion. Also note that the cerebellum has relatively few direct projections to the spinal cord. Instead, it exerts a strong influence on movement through its projections to cerebral and brain stem motor structures, as described later.

Anatomical Divisions

The cerebellum is part of the hindbrain and is positioned on the dorsal surface of the brain stem at approximately the level of the pons (Figure 21-1). It is connected to the brain stem by the superior, middle, and inferior cerebellar peduncles. The cerebellar peduncles contain all of the axons that transmit information to and from the cerebellum. The cerebellum can be anatomically divided into three lobes: the anterior, posterior, and flocculonodular lobes. The primary fissure divides the anterior and posterior lobes, and the posterolateral fissure divides the posterior and flocculonodular lobes (Figure 21-2).

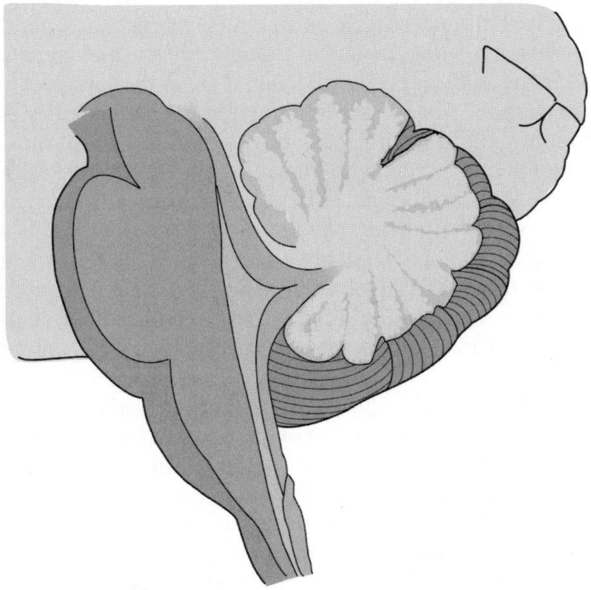

Figure 21-1 ■ The cerebellum, bisected through the midsagittal plane. (Redrawn from Kandel ER, Schwartz JH, Jessell TM: *Principles of neural science,* ed 4, New York, 2000, McGraw-Hill Medical.)

Looking at a sagittal slice through the cerebellum, distinct cellular regions can be visualized. The most superficial region is the cerebellar cortex, which, unlike the cerebral cortex, contains only three layers. The arrangement of cells within the cortex is strikingly uniform across all cerebellar lobes and plays a vital role in determining cerebellar function, which will be described later. Deep to the cerebellar cortex is the white matter layer, which contains the axons of Purkinje cells projecting out from the cerebellar cortex and the axons of mossy and climbing fibers entering the cortex from other brain and spinal regions (see Figure 21-1). The cerebellar nuclei are the output structures of the cerebellum, and they make up the deepest region. Groups of neuronal cell bodies receive information coming into the cerebellum from a variety of brain and spinal cord regions and also from the cerebellar cortex, via Purkinje cell axons. The deep nuclei are arranged in pairs, with one nucleus of each pair on each side of the cerebellum. Most medially are the fastigial nuclei, followed by the globose and emboliform nuclei and most laterally the broad dentate nuclei (see Figure 21-2). The medial and lateral vestibular nuclei also receive input directly from the cerebellar flocculonodular lobe and are therefore considered to play a role as an additional set of cerebellar output structures.

Functional Divisions and Their Afferent and Efferent Projections

Probably the most useful way of thinking about the anatomy of the cerebellum is to divide it into distinct functional longitudinal "zones."[10] Each cerebellar zone consists of a region of cerebellar cortex and its own pair of deep cerebellar nuclei. Each zone also has projections to and from distinct areas of the brain and spinal cord. Thus, despite the regular arrangement of cells over the entire cerebellum, each functional longitudinal zone is uniquely positioned to control certain types of movement but not others.[10-12] See Table 21-3 for a summary.

The medial zone consists of the midline structure, the vermis, and the fastigial nuclei. This region of the cerebellum predominantly receives afferent information from the brain stem vestibular and reticular nuclei and the dorsal and ventral spinocerebellar pathways,[13-18] which convey important information regarding the current sensorimotor state of the trunk and limbs.[19-21] In turn, its outputs, through the fastigial nuclei, are largely to reticular and vestibular nuclei that will form part of the medial descending system (reticulospinal and vestibulospinal tracts), with some additional projections to the cerebral cortex via the thalamus.[22-24] The medial cerebellar zone is involved in the control of posture and muscle tone, upright stance, locomotion, and in gaze and other eye movements.

The intermediate zone is made up of the intermediate hemispheres and the globose and emboliform nuclei. This region also receives inputs from the dorsal and ventral spinocerebellar pathways and brain stem reticular nuclei, as well as some projections from the cerebral cortex that arrive via the cerebropontocerebellar pathway.[11,13,14,25,26] Major projections from this cerebellar zone are to the cerebral cortex via the thalamus and to the red nucleus.[23,24,27] The intermediate zone is considered to be important in controlling coordination of agonist-antagonist muscle pairs during a variety of activities including walking and voluntary limb

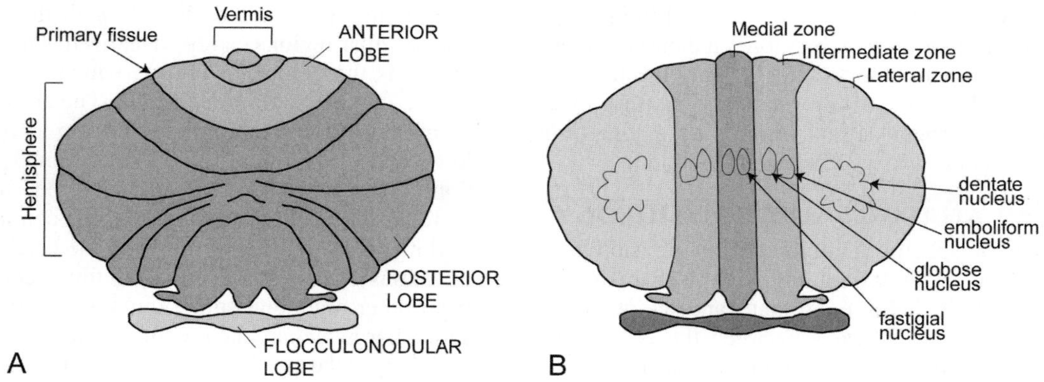

Figure 21-2 ■ The cerebellum, flattened, showing key structures. **A,** Different shading distinguishes the three lobes of the cerebellum. The cerebellar vermis and hemispheres are also identified. **B,** Functional longitudinal cerebellar zones, distinguished by different shading, and the locations of the deep cerebellar nuclei within each zone. (Redrawn from Kandel ER, Schwartz JH, Jessell TM: *Principles of neural science,* ed 4, New York, 2000, McGraw-Hill Medical.)

movements. The medial and intermediate zones of the cerebellum are collectively referred to as the *spinocerebellum,* because these are the only cerebellar regions that receive afferents from the spinal cord.

The largest region of the cerebellum is the lateral zone, which contains the two broad lateral hemispheres and their output structures, the dentate nuclei. Afferents to the lateral zone predominantly come from the cerebrum, from a wide variety of cortical areas including motor, premotor, and prefrontal cortices, parietal somatosensory and sensory association areas, and primary visual and auditory cortices.[25,26] Outputs from the dentate travel mostly back to large areas of the cerebrum (through the thalamus), to many of the same areas from which afferents arrived in the cerebellum. Again, these include vast regions of sensorimotor cortices.[27-33] Other efferent fibers project to the red nucleus in the brain stem. The lateral cerebellar zone plays a major role in control of complex, multijoint voluntary limb movements, particularly those involving visual guidance, and in the planning of complex movements and the assessment of movement errors. Because this region of the cerebellum interacts predominantly with the cerebrum, it is also commonly called the *cerebrocerebellum.* It is also sometimes referred to as the *neocerebellum* because it is considered to have arisen fairly recently in the phylogenetic tree, being much more expansive in primates than in lower animals.[34]

The flocculonodular lobe can be considered a fourth zone of the cerebellum. It receives afferent projections directly from the vestibular primary afferents (semicircular canals and otoliths) as well as from vestibular nuclei and visual brain regions.[11,13,14,16,18] Outputs from the flocculonodular lobe project directly to the medial and lateral vestibular nuclei of the brain stem, without a synapse in a deep cerebellar nucleus.[12,22,35] For this reason, these vestibular nuclei are sometimes considered an additional set of deep cerebellar nuclei. This cerebellar zone helps control eye movements and balance. The well known vestibuloocular reflex (VOR), which provides gaze stabilization during head turning or walking, relies on the cerebellum for proper functioning.[36,37] Because of its critical ties to the vestibular system, the flocculonodular lobe is also known as the *vestibulocerebellum* (see Figure 21-2).

Physiology of Cerebellar Neuronal Circuits

Within a longitudinal zone, thousands of microzones may exist,[11] each consisting of a highly organized group of connected cerebellar cortical neurons. A *microcomplex* is the name given to a neural circuit made up of a single microzone plus the other connected neurons with which it communicates directly. The following section provides a very brief overview of the circuits important for cerebellar function and reviews the flow of neuronal signals into and out of cerebellar microzones (Figure 21-3).

Most afferent information enters the cerebellum through one of two pathways: the mossy fiber pathway or the climbing fiber pathway. Both have important actions on cerebellar Purkinje cells. The mossy fiber pathway affects "beams" or rows of Purkinje cells oriented along the cerebellar folia. Dense mossy fiber inputs arise from a wide variety of regions, including the cerebral cortex, several subcortical areas, the brain stem, and the spinal cord. Mossy fibers enter the cerebellar cortex and synapse onto granule cells, whose axons ascend and branch into parallel fibers. Each parallel fiber extends long distances longitudinally and synapses onto many Purkinje cells, all located along the same beam.[38] Each parallel fiber has a relatively weak effect on single Purkinje cells, but the mass effect of many thousands of parallel fiber contacts with Purkinje cells drives the Purkinje cells to fire at high rates.[39] In contrast, each climbing fiber arises exclusively from the inferior olive, located in the brain stem, and contacts only a few (approximately 1 to 10) Purkinje cells.[12,40,41] Each Purkinje cell receives information from only one climbing fiber, yet the climbing fiber's effect on the Purkinje cell is powerful, causing large complex spikes.

The Purkinje cell provides the output for the cerebellar cortex; each Purkinje cell axon projects to one of the deep cerebellar nuclei. The mossy fiber and climbing fiber pathways affect Purkinje cells differently and are thought to transmit different types of information. Mossy fibers are active at very high rates (generating action potentials at approximately 100 Hz) and are highly modulated by various sensory stimuli and motor activity. They have been speculated to relay information related to the direction, velocity, duration, or magnitude of movements or sensory

TABLE 21-3 ■ FUNCTIONAL LONGITUDINAL CEREBELLAR ZONES

FUNCTIONAL ZONE	ALTERNATE NAME	MAJOR AFFERENTS	MAJOR EFFERENTS	ROLE IN MOVEMENT	CLINICAL SIGNS IF DAMAGED
Flocculonodular lobe Flocculo-nodular lobe; med & lat vestib nuclei	**Vestibulocere-bellum**	■ Vestib primary afferents ■ Vestib nuclei ■ Visual areas	■ Med & lat vestib nuclei	■ VOR ■ Gaze and eye movements ■ Posture and balance	■ Nystagmus ■ Impaired VOR ■ Imbalance
Medial zone Vermis; fastigial nuclei	Spinocerebellum	■ Vestib & retic nuclei ■ DSCT & VSCT	■ Vestib & retic nuclei ■ Cerebrum	■ Gaze and eye movements ■ Postural tone ■ Balance ■ Locomotion	■ Oculomotor deficits ■ Hypotonia ■ Imbalance ■ Falls ■ Gait ataxia
Intermediate zone Intermediate hemispheres; globose & emboliform nuclei	Spinocerebellum	■ DSCT & VSCT ■ Retic nuclei ■ Cerebrum	■ Cerebrum ■ Red nucleus	■ Limb movements ■ Coordinate agonist-antagonist muscle pairs	■ Imbalance ■ Gait ataxia ■ Tremor ■ Lack of check ■ Dysdiadocho-kinesia ■ Dysmetria
Lateral zone Lateral hemispheres; dentate nuclei	**Cerebro-cerebellum or Neocerebellum**	■ Cerebrum (wide range of areas: motor, premotor, prefrontal, somatosensory, sensory association, visual, auditory cortices)	■ Cerebrum (same areas as afferent projections) ■ Red nucleus	■ Complex, multijoint voluntary limb movements ■ Visually guided movements ■ Motor planning ■ Sensorimotor error assessment	■ Dysdiadocho-kinesia ■ Dysmetria ■ Dyssynergia ■ Decomposition

Med, medial; *Lat,* lateral; *Vestib,* vestibular; *Retic,* reticular; *DSCT,* dorsal spinocerebellar tract; *VSCT,* ventral spinocerebellar tract; *VOR,* vestibuloocular reflex.

stimuli.[42-45] Climbing fibers, however, are active at very low rates (approximately 1 to 4 Hz) and do not appear to be as strongly modulated by sensory stimuli or motor activity.[40,46,47] There is still some disagreement regarding what sort of information is encoded in the climbing fiber signals, but the frequency of discharge appears to be too low to transmit information pertaining to specific parameters of sensory or motor events. The role of the climbing fiber is clearly important, however, because its firing produces large complex spikes in the Purkinje cells and can also powerfully affect subsequent Purkinje cell firing.[41,48]

CEREBELLAR FUNCTION IN ADAPTING AND CONTROLLING MOVEMENT

The cytoarchitecture of the microzones is extremely stereotyped throughout the cerebellum, suggesting that it performs the same overall function regardless of whether it is acting on circuits controlling standing balance, eye movements, reaching and grasping, and so on. So what is the function of this cerebellar circuit? What aspect of motor control does it uniquely provide? Despite centuries of study, these questions have still not been answered completely. Although numerous theories of cerebellar function exist, here we limit the discussion to just a few that we view as particularly relevant.

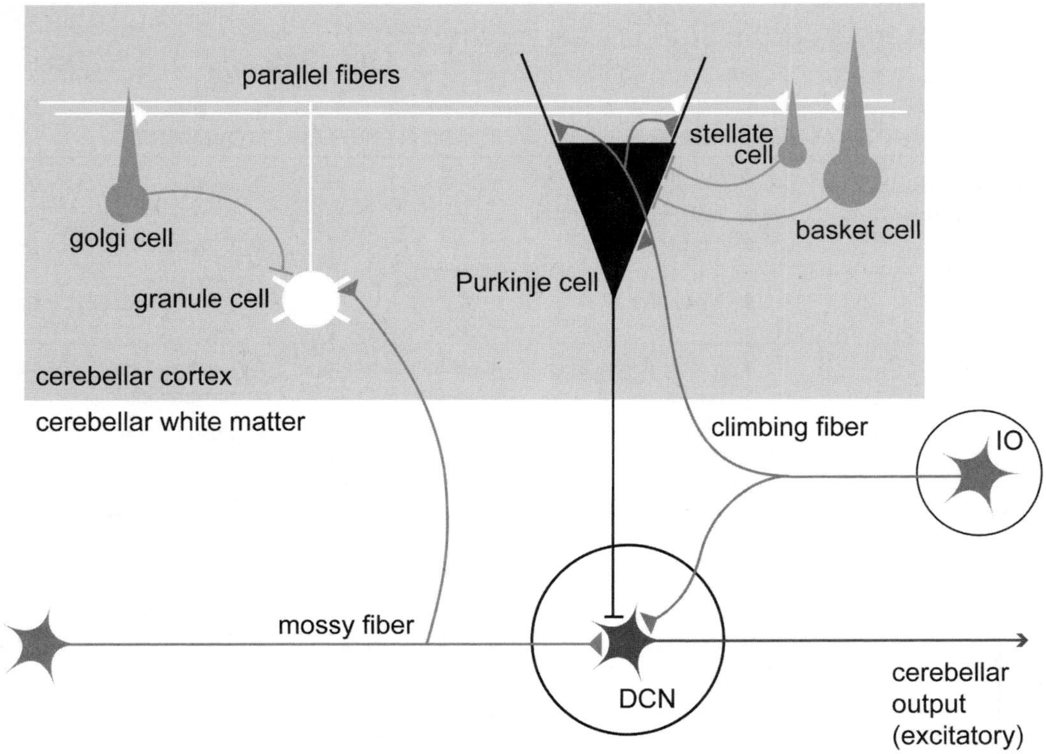

Figure 21-3 ■ Schematic of the major cell types and their connections within the cerebellum. Excitatory synapses are indicated with a triangle; inhibitory synapses with a bar. *DCN,* Deep cerebellar nucleus; *IO,* inferior olive. (Redrawn from Ito M: Cerebellar circuitry as a neuronal machine. *Prog Neurobiol* 78:272–303, 2006.)

Theories of Cerebellar Function

One general theory states that a primary function of the cerebellum is in coordinating multiple limb segments to generate smooth and fluid multijoint movements.[49-52] This "motor coordinator" theory has support from behavioral studies demonstrating that multijoint movements appear to be particularly impaired in clients with cerebellar lesions.[50] Multijoint movements are inherently more complex than single joint movements because they require control of mechanical interaction torques; those occurring at one segment but caused by movement of other linked segments.[53] This model suggests that the cerebellum predicts the mechanical interactions between segments based on a stored internal knowledge of limb dynamics, and helps generate the correct motor commands for appropriate multijoint movements.

A second popular theory is the timer hypothesis. This idea proposes that the cerebellum is the main site for the temporal representation of movements.[54,55] Supporters of this theory suggest that cerebellar output ultimately encodes the precise temporal sequence of muscle activation with such precision that a cerebellar lesion produces obvious deficits in the spatial domain (e.g., movement direction and magnitude) as well as the temporal domain.[56] Other studies have shown that individuals with cerebellar damage also have impairments in perceiving time intervals, suggesting that this could be a more general cerebellar function.[57,58]

A third idea is that the cerebellum acts as an internal model to allow predictive control of movement. Sensory feedback is inadequate for movements that need to be both fast and accurate: it is too slow, and as a result, motor corrections would be issued too late. Instead, the brain generates motor commands based on an internal prediction of how the command would move the body. This "feed-forward" control requires stored knowledge of the body's dynamics, the environment, and the object to be manipulated, and it is learned from previous exposure. The neural representation of this knowledge is referred to as an *internal model,*[59-62] as it provides the ability to reproduce the effects of motor actions in the brain. The internal model theory for cerebellar function states that the cerebellum serves as the site of an internal model for movement. Accordingly, the incoordination of movement associated with cerebellar damage is a consequence of an inaccurate internal model, which disrupts nearly all aspects of feed-forward motor control.[63] This idea is appealing, as it could help explain the wide variety of motor behaviors (e.g., reaching, standing balance, eye movements) and movement parameters (e.g., force, direction) that can be impaired after cerebellar damage. Likewise, human behavioral studies have recently pointed out that cerebellar damage is frequently associated with impaired feed-forward control but relatively intact feedback mechanisms.[64,65]

A related theory originates from the seminal works of Marr,[66] Albus,[67] and Ito,[68] in which the cerebellum was theorized to be a sort of "learning machine." This theory was based on careful examination of the anatomy and physiology within cerebellar microcircuits, and today it continues to provide the basis for many of the current theories of cerebellar function (i.e., those described earlier). Central to the idea of cerebellar involvement in learning was the discovery that Purkinje cell output can be radically altered by climbing fiber induction of long-term depression (LTD) of the parallel fiber–Purkinje cell synapse.[48] Hence, climbing fiber inputs onto Purkinje cells can be viewed as providing a unique type of teaching or error signal to the cerebellum. More recently, LTD, long-term potentiation (LTP), and nonsynaptic plasticity have all been shown to exist at numerous sites within the cerebellum, both in the cortex and in the deep cerebellar nuclei.[69-72] Thus there are multiple avenues for activity-dependent plasticity to occur within the cerebellum over relatively short time scales. It is presumed that the plastic changes in cerebellar output are responsible for changing motor behavior during the process of learning new skills.

To summarize, although the precise mechanisms are still under debate, a majority of researchers can agree on a few central themes of cerebellar function. First, the cerebellum is an integral structure for the coordination of movements. Second, precisely timed interactions between neurons produce activity-dependent plasticity at a number of different sites within the cerebellum. Presumably this plasticity plays a fundamental role in motor learning. Convergence of these two themes would seem to indicate that a major cerebellar function is to maintain optimal motor control through constant adaptive learning processes, so that movements are appropriately adjusted for varying environmental demands.

CLINICAL MANIFESTATIONS OF CEREBELLAR LESIONS

Ataxia is the primary sign of damage to the cerebellum or its input structures. *Ataxia* refers generally to uncoordinated or disordered movement, which, though most often associated with gait *(gait ataxia),* can also be used to describe uncoordinated arm or leg movements *(limb ataxia).* Ataxia is exacerbated by moving multiple joints together and by moving quickly. Because *ataxia* is a nonspecific term, it is important in both clinical and research settings to use more precise terminology to describe the specific aspects of motor performance that are impaired. Around the beginning of the twentieth century, Joseph Babinski and Gordon Holmes were two of the earliest investigators to describe many of these specific features we now discuss here.[73-75]

Dysmetria

Dysmetria specifically refers to an impaired ability to properly scale movement distance. Movements are described as either hypermetric or hypometric, referring to overshooting or undershooting of targets, respectively. Many clients with cerebellar lesions will show both forms of dysmetria even during successive movements (Figure 21-4).[49,50] Dysmetria can be seen in both proximal and distal joints and occurs during both single-joint and multijoint movements, though multijoint movements worsen dysmetria (Figure 21-5).[49,76-78] Slow movements tend to produce hypometria, whereas fast movements almost always bring about hypermetria.[49] For this reason, it has been speculated that hypometria represents more of a voluntary compensation for hypermetria than a primary impairment from cerebellar damage. Sometimes large end point errors can be reduced to some degree with visual feedback, but even the corrective movements themselves are still abnormal.[79]

One proposed mechanism for dysmetria is an impaired ability to predict and account for the dynamics of the limbs.

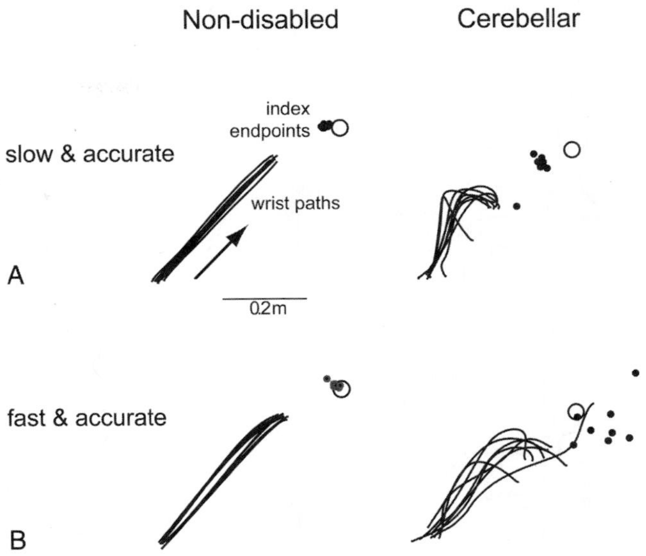

Figure 21-4 ■ Trajectories of the wrist *(solid lines)* and final end point positions of the tip of the index finger *(filled circles)* during **(A)** slow and accurate and **(B)** fast and accurate reaches from a typical nondisabled individual *(left)* and a subject with cerebellar damage *(right).* The subject with cerebellar damage shows dysmetria and an abnormally curved wrist path. Note also the tendency for hypometria during slow movements and hypermetria during fast movements (the same control and cerebellar subjects are shown in **A** and **B**). Several reaches are overlaid for each subject. *Arrow* indicates the reach direction. *Large open circles* indicate the target locations. (From Bastian AJ, Martin TA, Thach WT: Cerebellar ataxia: abnormal control of interaction torques across multiple joints. *J Neurophysiol* 76:492–509, 1996.)

In particular, clients with cerebellar lesions have been demonstrated to have a specific deficit in the ability to account for interaction torques,[49,50] the rotational forces that act on a limb segment when another linked limb segment is in motion.[68] When the cerebellum is intact, the central nervous system is able to predict the effects of interaction torques and appropriately counter or exploit them so as to produce a smooth, straight, and accurate reach in a feed-forward manner. When the cerebellum is damaged, an incorrect or absent accounting for interaction torques leads to an incorrect feed-forward motor plan and subsequently an uncoordinated, overly curved and hypermetric or hypometric reach that requires feedback corrections to reach the target location.

Dyssynergia

Originally, Babinski[80] coined the term *asynergia* to mean a deficit in the coordination of movements of one body region or in one limb segment with movements of another. Today, *dyssynergia* is used to describe impairment of multijoint movements, wherein movements of specific segments are not properly sequenced or of the proper range or direction, resulting in uncoordinated multijoint movement. As indicated earlier, it is nearly universally true that clients with significant cerebellar damage show greater impairments during multijoint movements than single-joint movements. However, it is not fully understood whether the reason for that is because the deficits of single-joint movements are

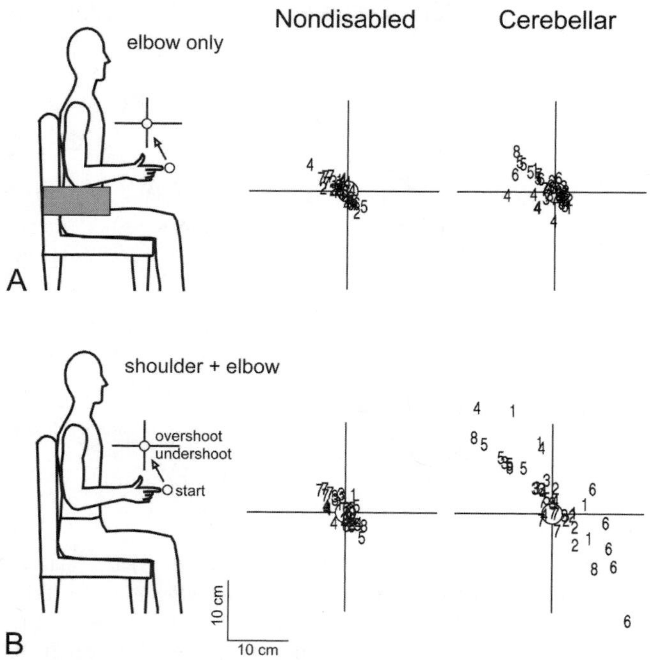

Figure 21-5 ■ Final end point positions of the tip of the index finger (numbers; each value corresponds to a different subject) during **(A)** single-joint (elbow only) and **(B)** multijoint (combined shoulder and elbow) reaches from nondisabled *(left)* and cerebellar *(right)* subjects. Cerebellar dysmetria (both hypometria and hypermetria) is greatly exacerbated during the multijoint reaching condition. Multiple reaches are shown for all subjects. *Arrow* indicates the reach direction. *Large open circles* indicate the target locations. (From Bastian AJ, Zackowski KM, Thach WT: Cerebellar ataxia: torque deficiency or torque mismatch between joints? *J Neurophysiol* 83:3019–3030, 2000.)

compounded during a multijoint movement or because the cerebellum plays a special and unique role in multijoint control. Dyssynergia appears to be related to dysmetria and therefore is probably also related to a deficit in predicting limb dynamics.[49]

Dysdiadochokinesia

Dysdiadochokinesia specifically refers to a deficit in the coordination between agonist-antagonist muscle pairs elicited during voluntary rapid alternating movements.[80] Such coordination is typically tested during performance of simple, fast alternating movements such as forearm supination-pronation or hand or foot tapping. Characteristic deficits are excessive slowness along with inconsistency in the rate and range of the alternating movements, which worsen as the movement continues.[74] Dysdiadochokinesia appears to be caused by poor regulation of the timing of cessation of agonist muscle activity and the initiation of antagonist muscle activity,[81,82] which could be related to a deficit in predicting limb dynamics. Indeed, rapid reversals in movement are dynamically difficult to control.

Decomposition

Movement decomposition refers to the breaking down of a movement sequence or a multijoint movement into a series of separate movements, each simpler than the combined movement.[75] An example of this is the well known finding that clients with cerebellar damage, when asked to reach to a target in front of and above the resting arm, will often flex the shoulder first and then, while holding the shoulder fixed, extend the elbow.[49] This approach is generally slower and will produce a more curved trajectory of the finger to the target compared with nondisabled individuals, who would typically perform the shoulder flexion and elbow extension at the same time to produce a nearly straight-line finger trajectory. Most likely, decomposition reflects more of a compensatory strategy for dealing with impaired multijoint movements than it does a primary sign of cerebellar damage.[49,83]

Lack of Check

Lack of check, sometimes also referred to as excessive "rebound," refers to the inability to rapidly and sufficiently halt movement of a body part after a strong isometric force, previously resisting movement of the body part, is suddenly released. Individuals without cerebellar damage can very quickly halt, or "check," this unintended movement. Individuals with cerebellar damage, on the other hand, are known to have considerable movement in the direction opposite the previous resistance, to the point that the unchecked movement risks loss of upright balance or self-injury. This phenomenon is presumed to be caused by delayed cessation of agonist and/or delayed activation of antagonist muscles.

Cerebellar Tremor

Despite being a very common neurological sign, tremor is poorly defined and not well understood. There are several different forms of tremor, many with different causes, only some of which are related to cerebellar dysfunction, so it is important to distinguish among them. Tremor associated with damage to the cerebellum is typically called *action tremor,* reflecting the fact that it is absent at rest and elicited during muscle activation and distinguishing it from the resting tremor associated with Parkinson disease. Action tremor can be classified as postural or kinetic tremor.[84] Postural tremor occurs in muscles maintaining a static position against gravity (e.g., holding arms out in front of the body or standing in place), whereas kinetic tremor occurs in muscles producing an active voluntary movement. Therefore the movement oscillations are most visible in the same plane as the voluntary movement. Kinetic tremor typically occurs at relatively low frequencies (approximately 2 to 5 Hz) and can be observed during simple nontarget-directed movements such as forearm pronation and supination or foot tapping, or during targeted movements such as pointing during the finger-to-nose test. Intention tremor is a specific form of kinetic tremor that occurs during the terminal portions of visually guided movements toward a target. It may actually represent the multiple corrective movements, driven by visual feedback, to reach the target. As such, intention tremor can be tested by repeating the test movement with eyes closed; if the tremor decreases substantially or disappears, it is an intention tremor.[79]

Classic cerebellar tremor is kinetic tremor with intention tremor at movement termination. In general, cerebellar tremor is thought to be caused by an insufficient ability to anticipate the effects of movement and excessive reliance on sensory feedback loops.[85] Cerebellar tremor is highly influenced by sensory conditions and has a strong mechanical component; it is significantly reduced during isometric conditions or when vision is removed. It also can be decreased in some clients by adding an inertial load to the limb,[86] though that strategy may also increase dysmetria.[87] There may also be a significant central component to cerebellar tremor, possibly related to influences from the thalamus or the inferior olive.[81,88]

Hypotonia

Hypotonia in clients with cerebellar damage was first described by Holmes.[75] It appears to arise from decreased excitatory drive to vestibulospinal and reticulospinal pathways, two major output pathways from the cerebellar vermis and flocculonodular lobe. The hypotonia usually manifests as a decrease in the extensor tone necessary for holding the body upright against gravity. In cats, lesions of either the vestibular or fastigial nuclei cause this sort of postural hypotonia.[51,89-91] More recent observations in humans indicate that hypotonia is typically most problematic in cases of severe cerebellar hypoplasias affecting the vermis, such as Joubert syndrome,[92] or in adults during the acute stage of cerebellar injury only. In cases of adult-onset acute injury, hypotonia usually resolves naturally over time and clients recover normal passive muscle tone and normal reflexes quickly. Thus hypotonia typically presents minimal to no problems for physical function.[81]

Imbalance

Another cardinal sign of cerebellar damage is postural instability in both static and dynamic conditions. Specifically, clients with cerebellar damage usually show increased postural sway; either excessive or diminished postural responses to perturbations; poor control of equilibrium during voluntary movements of the head, arms, or legs; and sometimes abnormal oscillations of the trunk, called *titubation.*

Classically, cerebellar imbalance during stance was considered to be of a similar magnitude whether or not the eyes are open; that is, little improvement noted with visual feedback[73,75] and a negative Romberg test result. However, more recently, investigators using posturography measures have been able to distinguish several different categories of cerebellar imbalance during quiet standing, some of which do show improvement with visual stabilization.[93,94] For instance, clients with cerebellar damage relatively isolated to the anterior lobe typically show increased postural sway, which is of a high velocity and low amplitude and occurs mainly in the anterior-posterior dimension. These individuals also tend to have associated postural tremor and increased intersegmental movements of the head, trunk, and legs and tend to improve when allowed visual information. On the other hand, localized damage to the vestibulocerebellum more often leads to increased postural sway that consists of low-frequency and high-amplitude movements without a preferred direction and without increased intersegmental movements. These individuals typically show no improvement with visual information. Clients with damage limited to the lateral cerebellum tend to have only slight or even no postural instability at all.[93-95]

Human cerebellar damage is also associated with hypermetric postural responses to surface displacements or during step initiation; that is, dynamic instability.[96,97] Specifically, clients tend to produce larger-than-normal surface-reactive torque responses and exaggerated and prolonged muscle activity, thereby overshooting the initial posture during the return phase of the recovery from a perturbation (Figure 21-6).

Gait Ataxia

Probably the greatest complaint and the most obvious sign of cerebellar damage is gait ataxia. This abnormal pattern of walking is often described as a "drunken" gait because clients often stagger and lose balance as if intoxicated. Early work of Holmes showed that patients with cerebellar lesions have severe difficulty maintaining balance during walking, which often leads to falls, typically directed backward and toward the side of the lesion. Holmes reported specifically that walking is slowed, with steps that are short, irregular in timing, and unequal in length. The legs sometimes lift overly high during the swing phase by excessive flexion at the hip and knee and then lower abruptly and with uncontrolled force. The trajectory of walking often veers erratically and patients have difficulty with stops or turns, especially if performed quickly.[75]

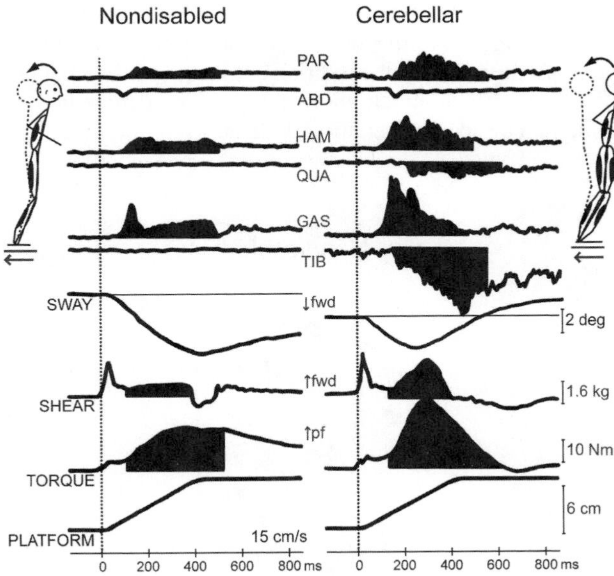

Figure 21-6 ■ Postural responses from nondisabled control and cerebellar groups (average of 10 trials from 10 subjects in each group) after backward platform translations of 15 cm/s for 6 cm. Traces show *(top to bottom)* electromyographic recordings from various postural muscle groups, postural sway, shear force, surface torque, and platform displacement. *Filled areas* indicate the first 400 ms of activation in the electromyographic traces and the active surface-reactive forces in the shear force and torque traces. Postural responses of the cerebellar subjects are increased, with excessive and prolonged muscle activity (note especially the abnormal activation of flexor muscle groups), larger sway, and greater torque production. *ABD,* Rectus abdominis; *fwd,* forward; *GAS,* gastrocnemius; *HAM,* biceps femoris; *PAR,* paraspinals; *pf,* plantarflexion; *QUA,* rectus femoris; *TIB,* tibialis anterior. (Adapted with permission from the American Physiological Society. From Horak FB, Diener HC: Cerebellar control of postural scaling and central set in stance. *J Neurophysiol* 72:479–493, 1994.)

Those initial reports have now been confirmed numerous times; clients with cerebellar damage walk without the consistency in timing, length, and direction of steps typical of healthy adults.[77,98] In some cases gait appears wide based. There is also increased variability in both the timing and movement excursion at the hip, knee, and ankle joints and irregularities in the resulting path of the foot during swing. Coordination between joints of one leg and between legs (intralimb and interlimb coordination, respectively) is also abnormal.[77,98,99] As an example, the timing of peak flexion at one joint with respect to other joints' positions may be altered or inconsistent. Often decomposition is also observed between hip and knee, knee and ankle, and/or hip and ankle joints.[99,100]

A critical component of locomotor control is the requirement for stability and dynamic balance while maintaining forward propulsion. Thus imbalance, described previously, is also a major contributor to many features of gait ataxia. In fact, it has been shown that clients with cerebellar damage and significant balance deficits also typically demonstrate nearly all the classic features of gait ataxia (i.e., reduced stride lengths, increased stride widths, reduced joint excursions, abnormal swing foot trajectories, increased variability in foot placement, and joint-joint decomposition). In contrast, clients with cerebellar damage and significant leg coordination deficits but minimal or no balance deficits typically have very few walking abnormalities (Figure 21-7).[101,102] Therefore during typical conditions of level walking, balance deficits contribute much more strongly to cerebellar gait ataxia than do leg coordination deficits.

Oculomotor Deficits

Eye movements are often dramatically impaired after cerebellar damage. Saccades are often slowed and dysmetric (can be hypermetric or hypometric).[103] Smooth pursuit may be "choppy," referred to as *saccadic pursuit,* wherein the smooth tracking of a target is degraded into a series of shorter saccadic movements following behind the target.[104] The ability to cancel, or suppress, the VOR may be impaired or absent.[105] Finally, abnormal nystagmus may also be present. The nystagmus may occur during central gaze, or there may also be alternating nystagmus or rebound nystagmus. The most common form of nystagmus in cerebellar dysfunction is gaze-evoked nystagmus, indicating nystagmus elicited toward the end ranges of lateral and/or vertical gaze.[106,107]

Clients with significant oculomotor abnormalities may be referred to vestibular specialists, but these deficits should never be ignored. Impaired eye movements may have a significant negative impact on physical function. For example, impaired saccades can prevent a client from reading, and saccadic pursuit can exacerbate already poor visually guided limb movements.[108] Perhaps most devastating, deficits related to impaired oculomotor control and vestibular reflexes often worsen dynamic balance and walking abilities.

Speech Impairments

Speech production may also be impaired when the cerebellum is damaged. Classically, the speech deficit associated with cerebellar damage is referred to as *scanning speech,* though it may be more generally referred to as *ataxic dysarthria.*

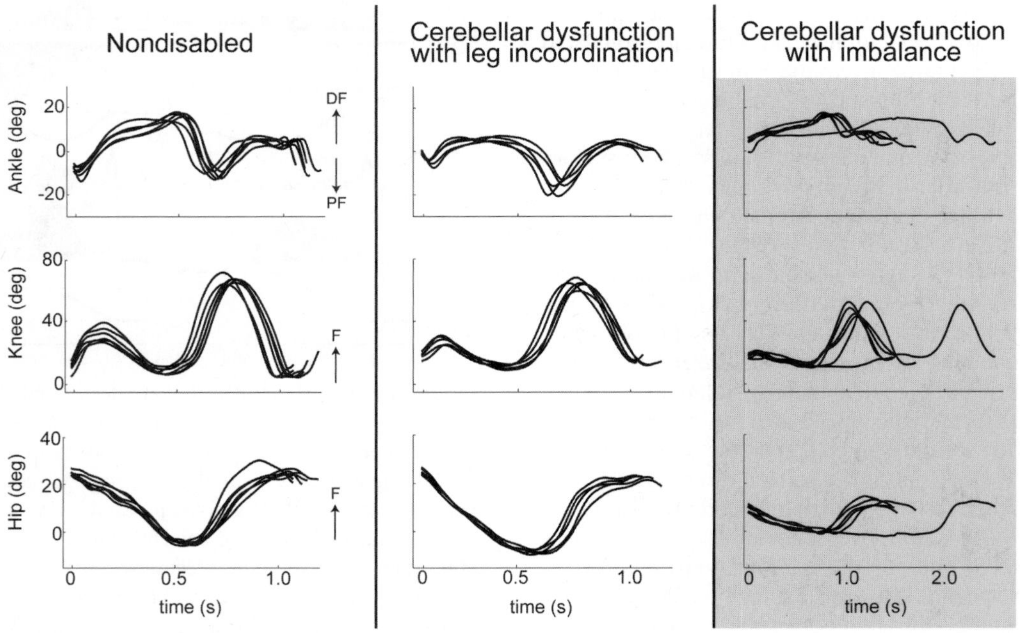

Figure 21-7 ■ Angular excursions at the ankle *(top row),* knee *(middle),* and hip *(bottom)* during fast walking from a typical nondisabled individual *(left column),* a subject with cerebellar dysfunction who has significant leg incoordination but minimal imbalance *(middle),* and a subject with cerebellar dysfunction who has significant imbalance but minimal leg incoordination *(right).* Several strides (from initial contact to next initial contact) are overlaid for each subject. The client with cerebellar imbalance *(shaded)* shows significant evidence of gait ataxia, including reduced joint excursions, excessive stride-to-stride variability, and abnormal timing between joints, whereas the client with cerebellar leg incoordination and no imbalance shows no evidence of gait ataxia. *DF,* Dorsiflexion; *F,* flexion; *PF,* plantarflexion. (Adapted with permission from the American Physiological Society. From Morton SM, Bastian AJ: Relative contributions of balance and voluntary leg-coordination deficits to cerebellar gait ataxia. *J Neurophysiol* 89:1844–1856, 2003.)

Similar to limb control deficits, the primary impairment of speech may be related to the planning and prediction of movements rather than the execution of speech components directly.[109] Also like limb movements, most speech impairments appear to be attributable to alterations in timing and coordination.[143a] The most consistent characteristics of ataxic dysarthria are impaired articulation (the correct pronouncement of speech sounds) and impaired prosody (the pattern of stress and intonation of certain syllables or words). Other common findings include slowed speech and either a lack of or excessive loudness variability.[109] Traditionally, speech impairments are treated primarily by speech and language pathologists.

Impaired Motor Learning

A critical problem associated with cerebellar damage is impaired motor learning. In humans the cerebellum has been linked to learning of a wide variety of motor behaviors, including recovering balance after a perturbation,[96,97] learning new walking patterns,[64,100,111] adjusting voluntary limb movements,[65,112,113] and making eye movements.[114,115] The type of learning that appears most reliant on the cerebellum is associative and procedural. Specifically, the cerebellum appears to be essential for learning to adjust a motor behavior through repeated practice of, or exposure to, the behavior and using error information from one trial to improve performance on subsequent trials. It is important to note that cerebellum-dependent motor learning is driven by errors directly occurring during the movement rather than by other types of feedback, such as knowledge of results after the fact (e.g., hit or miss). Studies have suggested that the type of error that drives cerebellum-dependent learning is not the target error (i.e., "How far am I from the desired target?"), but instead what has been referred to as a *sensory prediction error* (i.e., "How far am I from where I predicted I would be?").[113,116]

In the laboratory setting, cerebellar learning is most easily tested via motor adaptation, a form of motor learning that requires a modification of an already well learned motor behavior for new environmental or physical demands (in contrast to learning of a completely novel skill). Adaptation is an error-driven learning process that is acquired on a time scale of minutes or hours, as opposed to days or weeks.[117,118] It is an active process: movement adaptation takes trial-and-error practice of the task, in which errors during one trial change movement on the subsequent trial. Storage of the adapted movement is shown by the presence of aftereffects when the new demand is removed. Specifically, aftereffects are movement errors in the opposite direction to the original errors during adaptation and provide strong evidence that the central nervous system adjusts the predictive control for body movements with practice.[62,119] Thus when the new demand is removed, a process of active "unlearning" or deadaptation must occur to return the movement to its original form. An example of a locomotor adaptation is shown in Figure 21-8. In this case, a walking adaptation is induced by having subjects walk on a split-belt treadmill, where one belt is moving at twice the speed of the other, forcing the two legs to walk at different speeds. Control subjects are able to rapidly restore appropriate step length symmetry after only a few minutes walking on the split-belt treadmill. They also appear to store the newly learned set of (predictive) motor commands, demonstrated by large negative aftereffects (step length asymmetry in the reverse direction compared with early adaptation) when the treadmill belts are initially returned to a regular (nonsplit) pattern. In contrast, individuals with cerebellar damage typically show a slower rate of adaptation, a reduced magnitude of adaptation, or no adaptation at all, and small or no aftereffects (see Figure 21-8). All of these findings indicate a significant deficiency in the capability for motor adaptation in individuals with cerebellar damage. As indicated earlier, adaptation deficits have been demonstrated in this patient population with numerous behavioral tasks.*

Cerebellum-dependent adaptation is not the only form of motor learning, but it is an important one for rehabilitation for several reasons. First, adaptation is a highly automatic process to rapidly adjust movements for new, predictable demands (e.g., adjusting the walking pattern for snow or sand; adjusting eye movements for glasses). Individuals with impaired cerebellar adaptive learning must use other means to handle new task demands, such as conscious control strategies. This is obviously inefficient and difficult, as it means that the individuals must think much more about their movements and cannot tolerate distractions. Adaptation is also important because when it is repeated many times, it can result in more permanent storage of a movement pattern that can be called on immediately (i.e., no error-based period of adaptation required). A clear example of this is the use of new bifocal glasses. Initially, there is an adaptation process to adjust eye movements when switching between the top and bottom lenses because eye movements have to be bigger for magnified objects. Yet with repeated adaptation, the brain eventually stores two calibrations, one for making eye movements when viewing through the top lens and one for making eye movements when viewing through the bottom lens, that can be switched between instantly. Thus adaptation can lead to a more permanent, learned calibration that is used in specific situations. Clients with cerebellar damage will not be able to make these short-term adaptations normally, and theoretically one would expect that they will not be able to form the more permanent calibrations with repeated adaptation.

Other forms of motor learning may not depend on the cerebellum and thus may be particularly useful for rehabilitation for clients with cerebellar lesions, though this has never been formally tested. One example is use-dependent motor learning, in which a person strengthens a movement pattern with repeated practice of that same pattern.[120] It is not clear what mechanisms subserve this form of learning, though a Hebbian-like process in the cerebral cortex seems likely (i.e., repeated use strengthens the synapses in the brain that are engaged). Another form of motor learning is reward or reinforcement learning. This may involve basal ganglia circuits to strengthen movements that are rewarded.[121] Whether individuals with cerebellar damage can use either of these other forms of learning has not been experimentally tested. Yet if they can, these learning mechanisms might provide important compensatory strategies for the loss of error-dependent adaptations.

*References 56, 64, 65, 96, 97, 111-113.

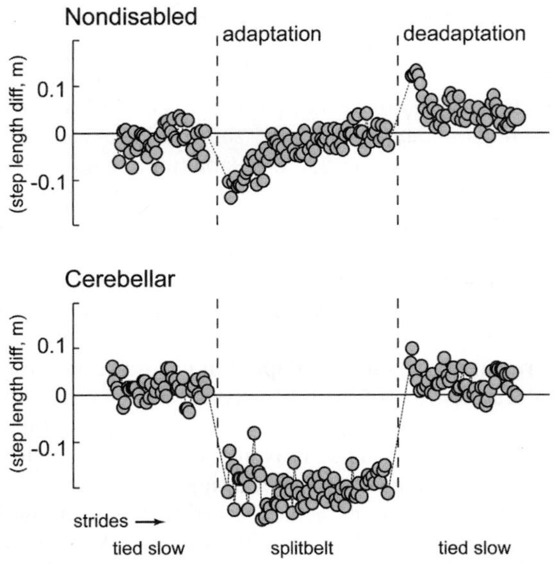

Figure 21-8 ■ Motor adaptation of step length symmetry during walking on a split-belt treadmill by a nondisabled individual *(top)* and a subject with cerebellar damage *(bottom).* Each data point represents the difference in step lengths between the legs (fast minus slow) for all strides during regular walking (belts tied, speed 0.5 m/s), split-belt adaptation walking (fast belt speed 1.0 m/s; slow belt speed 0.5 m/s), and deadaptation walking (belts tied, speed 0.5 m/s). Perfect symmetry between the legs is represented by a step length difference value of 0. Note that the split-belt condition perturbs step length symmetry initially in both subjects. The control subject rapidly adapts the walking pattern to restore appropriate step length symmetry while walking on split belts. The cerebellar subject does not adapt. Once the belts are returned to the tied condition, the control subject shows a large negative aftereffect; that is, perturbed step length symmetry in the reverse direction, which again is rapidly adjusted to restore near-symmetric step lengths. The cerebellar subject shows a reduced aftereffect and no deadaptation. (From Morton SM, Bastian AJ: Cerebellar contributions to locomotor adaptations during splitbelt treadmill walking. *J Neurosci* 26:9107–9116, 2006.)

Nonmotor Impairments

Within the last 25 years, researchers have exposed a possible role of the cerebellum in a number of nonmotor, cognitive behaviors. Much of the early evidence for cerebellar involvement in nonmotor tasks came from functional imaging studies showing increased activation within the cerebellum during performance of certain tasks with a predominant cognitive component, such as language processing.[122,123] Speculation has since arisen that the cerebellum may be involved in not only language, but also working memory,[124] learning nonmotor associations between objects,[125] and higher-order executive functions.[126] Loss of control over emotional behaviors[127] and certain neurodevelopmental and neuropsychiatric disorders have also been said to be linked to cerebellar damage.[128,129] However, interpretation of some investigations of the relationship between the cerebellum and cognition is limited in that it is sometimes difficult to separate the cognitive and motor components of a task, particularly in imaging studies in which subjects are instructed to perform some motor task to indicate a cognitive choice.[130,131] Nevertheless, anatomical studies have shown clearly that the cerebellum has connections to brain areas considered relatively purely cognitive in function, suggesting that a cognitive role for the cerebellum is likely.[132]

Clinical Signs by Functional Division

Because of the organizational structure of the cerebellum into functional longitudinal divisions, discrete areas are associated with specific signs and symptoms. Thus, depending on the location and volume of cerebellar damage, clients may have just a few or nearly all of the clinical manifestations described earlier. Clients with damage to the flocculonodular lobe or midline zone typically demonstrate some (though usually transient) loss of postural tone, impaired upright posture and balance, gait ataxia, and oculomotor deficits.[2,51] On the other hand, damage to the intermediate zone often results in action tremor, dysdiadochokinesia, and dysmetria of the limbs.[2,51] Finally, damage to the lateral zone commonly produces dyssynergia, dysmetria, and difficulty planning complex limb movements, especially those that are visually guided (see Table 21-3).[2,51]

Often, however, multiple longitudinal zones are affected at the same time. For instance, the arteries supplying the cerebellum each span more than one longitudinal zone, such that a stroke involving a single cerebellar artery would be likely to cause signs and symptoms associated with more than one zone (see Table 21-1). Degenerative disorders affecting the cerebellum also are typically pancerebellar, affecting large regions of the cerebellum. Hence these clients will also typically have a wide variety of signs and symptoms. A careful and thorough clinical examination is therefore a requirement before a diagnosis for physical therapy can be made in clients with cerebellar damage.

MEDICAL MANAGEMENT OF CEREBELLAR DAMAGE

The greatest limitation in caring for clients with cerebellar dysfunction is the lack of any curative treatment for most forms of cerebellar damage. Pharmacological agents have been used, but with limited success. Often, clients with ataxia and degenerative forms of cerebellar damage may be prescribed vitamin E, coenzyme Q10, and/or its synthetic analogs, but the effectiveness of these drugs in minimizing symptoms or otherwise slowing or halting the disease is largely unsubstantiated.[133,134] Other drugs that may be used include acetazolamide, amantadine, 4-aminopyridine, and buspirone chlorhydrate,[6,135-137] but these also have questionable effectiveness. Studies of the effectiveness of medications for cerebellar ataxia have been significantly limited by inadequate sample sizes, inappropriate outcome measures, and/or limited follow-up. Given the unsatisfactory results from pharmacological interventions thus far, most clients with cerebellar ataxias must rely primarily or solely on physical rehabilitation approaches to restore or reduce the symptoms of their disease.

PHYSICAL AND OCCUPATIONAL THERAPY MANAGEMENT OF CEREBELLAR MOVEMENT DYSFUNCTION

As is the case with all brain lesions, there is nearly always some level of natural, or spontaneous, recovery after damage to the cerebellum. The extent of recovery depends on complex interactions among numerous factors including the source of damage; the severity, location, and volume of damage; the presence or absence of damage to other brain regions; the presence or absence of other coexisting medical conditions; age; and other factors. Several studies have now indicated that motor recovery from a first-ever ischemic cerebellar stroke is generally excellent, with minimal to no residual deficits in up to 83% of patients.[138-140] On the other hand, individuals with degenerative cerebellar disorders tend to have progressively worsening clinical signs and symptoms.[141] One study has shown that people with damage to the deep nuclei do not recover as well as those with damage to only the cerebellar cortex and white matter.[2] Another consideration is the degree to which other brain regions are lesioned. Individuals with cerebellar stroke or tumor may also have damage of the brain stem. Clients with multiple sclerosis or head injury often also have cerebral and spinal cord lesions. Moreover, the majority of the spinocerebellar ataxias (SCAs) affect other neural structures well beyond the cerebellum; these are often the corticospinal tract, cerebral cortex, basal ganglia, and sometimes the peripheral nervous system. Generally speaking, the presence of multiple lesion locations is associated with a poorer outcome, possibly because circuits that could otherwise serve a compensatory role are also damaged.[142]

Physical/Occupational Therapy Evaluation

A majority of the components of the physical therapy examination for clients with cerebellar dysfunction are the same as would be performed with any client with a health condition that is primarily neurological in origin. Therefore we will discuss only the features that are unique or of critical importance for the client with cerebellar pathology. In the following sections we highlight just a few of these specific tests. Box 21-1 contains a more complete list. One important note is that many of the tests for cerebellar movement dysfunction are sensitive but not specific to cerebellar pathologies. That is, although they often will reveal abnormalities in a client with cerebellar damage, their results are frequently also observed to be abnormal in clients with other, noncerebellar disorders of a neuromuscular origin. Therefore they should not be used in isolation to rule in or rule out cerebellar pathologies.

Tests of Impairments of Body Functions or Structures

At the level of body functions or structures, physical/occupational therapists use a variety of simple tests and measures to detect the typical movement impairments associated with cerebellar dysfunction. Many of these fall into the category of limb movement coordination tests. Particularly useful in the upper extremity are the finger-to-nose test, the alternating forearm supination-pronation test, and the hand or finger tapping test. The heel-to-knee test and foot or toe tapping test provide similar information for the lower extremity. Each of these tests informs the therapist about the presence and severity of many components of ataxia, including dysmetria, dyssynergia, dysdiadochokinesia, decomposition, and kinetic and/or intention tremor. Some general rules should be applied when performing and interpreting the findings from these clinical tests. First, it is important to perform the test on and compare both sides. Each test should be repeated multiple times with the same limb, as subsequent movements may look strikingly different (e.g., hypometric on some trials, hypermetric on others). Comparing slow or preferred with "as fast as possible" speeds allows the clinician to determine the severity of the ataxia (generally worst with fastest movements) and how well the client is able to compensate when allowed full use of feedback mechanisms (the degree to which the movement is improved when performed slowly). It is also generally useful to compare the same movements with and without vision, to determine whether or not visual feedback improves movement quality. A final caution about the tests of voluntary movement coordination is that the examiner must carefully dissociate limb incoordination from deficits of balance and/or vision. For example, if the client has difficulty maintaining quiet unsupported sitting, he or she will most likely demonstrate several abnormal movement patterns that resemble classic limb ataxia when asked to move the limbs (e.g., dyssynergia, dysmetria) if tested in this unsupported position. In this situation the examiner cannot distinguish whether the deficits observed are caused by a true incoordination of voluntary limb movements or because of an inability to maintain the trunk in a stable and upright position that provides the limb a stable base from which to generate movement. Thus, to test coordination, the examiner must give the client the necessary head and trunk support required for the limb movement task (e.g., test sitting in a high-backed chair with manual support at the shoulders or perform in supine position) if the client is unable to provide this support by himself or herself. Similar confusion may arise if the client has significant visual or other oculomotor impairments such as diplopia. Here, the client would be likely to show apparent dysmetria during visually targeted movements, but it would not be possible to determine whether it was caused by real limb ataxia or a visual impairment preventing the client from accurately identifying the target location in space. This is not to say that it would not be beneficial to test limb coordination in positions or situations that also challenge balance and/or vision; only that during the initial examination of the client, one should be careful to ensure an accurate determination of the source of the movement impairment.

A major component of almost all physical therapy examinations of clients with cerebellar dysfunction is the posture and balance examination. Posture and balance should always be observed in both static and dynamic conditions and in both sitting and standing positions, as the client's capabilities allow. The examination is performed in the same manner as for clients with other neurological disorders and so is not described in detail here (see Box 21-1 for suggested components to emphasize with clients with cerebellar dysfunction). Important considerations specific for clients with cerebellar dysfunction include careful monitoring for symptoms of nausea or vertigo (common in acute cerebellar stroke, may resolve quickly), observation for postural tremor or titubation, and observation of the recovery from perturbations and the presence of lack of check. Although physical therapists most often deal with posture and balance, occupational therapists also need to identify and examine these components in order to analyze movement activity problems that are based upon a functional trunk such as dressing, feeding, and other daily living activities.

BOX 21-1 ■ TYPICAL CLINICAL TESTS AND MEASURES FOR THE PHYSICAL THERAPY EVALUATION OF CEREBELLAR DYSFUNCTION

TESTS OF IMPAIRMENTS OF BODY FUNCTION OR STRUCTURE

1. Muscle tone
   Hypotonia: Particularly involving postural extensor muscle groups. Can be assessed in supine, sitting, and/or standing position.
2. Voluntary movement coordination
   For all coordination tests, the following guidelines are recommended, when appropriate: (1) compare both sides; (2) repeat each test multiple times; (3) compare slow or preferred versus "as fast as possible" speeds; (4) compare with and without vision.
   Finger-to-nose test: Vary the target (fingertip) locations. Require near-full excursion at elbow and shoulder. Observe for speed, dysmetria, dyssynergia, decomposition, kinetic tremor, intention tremor.
   Alternating forearm supination-pronation: Do not allow bracing of upper arm against trunk. Require elbow flexion and extension along with forearm movements. Observe for speed, dysmetria, dyssynergia, decomposition, dysdiadochokinesia, kinetic tremor.
   Hand or finger tapping: Observe for speed, dysmetria, dysdiadochokinesia, kinetic tremor.
   Drawing or handwriting sample: Compare with and without permitting bracing upper arm against trunk and/or forearm on writing surface. Observe for speed, dysmetria, dyssynergia, decomposition, kinetic tremor, intention tremor.
   Holding static position, arms outstretched: Client holds position for several seconds. Observe for drift, postural tremor.
   Resisted movements: Compare different levels of resistance. Observe for lack of check (rebound). Note: Ensure client safety; rebound may be extreme, destabilizing, and/or injurious in severe cases.
   Heel-to-knee test: Client performs with shoes removed and in supine position to test full excursion at hip and to prevent bracing of thigh or hip on support surface. Client performs (1) repeated taps on knee with heel and (2) sliding the heel up and down the lower leg. Observe for speed, dysmetria, dyssynergia, decomposition, dysdiadochokinesia, kinetic tremor, intention tremor.
   Foot or toe tapping: Observe for speed, dysmetria, dysdiadochokinesia, kinetic tremor.
3. Static and dynamic balance
   Sitting balance: Client performs with and without upper and lower extremity support or with and without trunk support (as skill level permits), with and without vision. Test for recovery from self-imposed perturbations (upper extremity or head movements) or external perturbations (gentle pushes by examiner). Observe resting preferred posture, tremor, sway, ability and effort required to maintain position, recovery from perturbations or other loss of balance. Inquire about vertigo, nausea, and subjective perception of stability.
   Standing balance: Client performs with and without upper and lower extremity support, with and without vision, and with feet apart and together. Test for recovery from self-imposed perturbations (upper extremity or head movements) or external perturbations (gentle pushes by examiner). Advanced testing: assume and maintain tandem stance and single limb stance. Observe resting preferred posture, natural foot position (base of support), tremor, sway, ability and effort required to maintain position, recovery from perturbations or other loss of balance. Inquire about vertigo, nausea, and subjective perception of stability.
4. Oculomotor performance
   Smooth pursuit: Sitting, keeping the head still, client follows pen tip or similar small object with eyes. Test in all movement planes and directions and through full range of motion. Vary speed. Observe for saccadic (choppy) pursuit.
   Saccades: Sitting, keeping the head still and when verbally prompted, client alternately fixes gaze on one of two pen tips, or a pen tip and the examiner's nose, or other small objects. Vary the target (pen tip) locations, testing a variety of end point locations, directions of movement, and distances traveled, including full range of motion. Observe for dysmetria, particularly on initial trials.
   Gaze-evoked nystagmus: Sitting, keeping the head still, client maintains gaze in a variety of locations, including near end ranges of lateral gaze. Observe for nystagmus, particularly toward the direction of gaze.

TESTS OF ACTIVITY LIMITATIONS

1. Bed mobility
2. Transfers
3. Gait
   As skill level permits, client performs natural, narrow, and tandem gait. Compare preferred versus fastest speed and with and without vision. Test for recovery from self-imposed perturbations (upper extremity or head movements) or external perturbations (gentle pushes by examiner). Observe on inclines and declines, uneven surfaces, negotiating introduced obstacles. Observe walking while distracted (dual-task situation) and while holding an object with the upper extremity (e.g., hold a Styrofoam cup half-filled with water). Test turns and control through narrow areas such as a doorway. Observe for speed, irregularity of step height and distance, veering walking path, loss of balance, seeking out of upper extremity support surfaces or guarding, leg dyssynergia, decomposition (e.g., stiff knees, reduced ankle motion), widened base of support, truncal sway, kinetic tremor. Note distance tolerated and need for assistive devices and/or orthotics.
4. Stair climbing
5. Activities of daily living (ADLs): dressing, grooming, feeding, bathing, and so on

As described previously, because other areas of the nervous system are also frequently damaged along with the cerebellum, it may be appropriate to test for impairments of body functions or structures associated with pathology involving extracerebellar regions of the neuromuscular system. Most commonly this involves testing of muscle strength, somatosensation (including cutaneous sensation and proprioception), reflexes, passive muscle tone, and observation for signs of other motor abnormalities such as spasticity, dystonia, abnormal synergies, chorea, bradykinesia, or resting tremor.

It is also important to examine the client's initial level of endurance (fatigability), both in the cardiovascular and muscular systems. For the cardiovascular system, this can be approximated by recording the response to sustained aerobic exercise on one or more measurement scales (e.g., perceived exertion, heart rate, blood pressure, respiratory rate). See chapter 30 for additional information. For the muscular system, this can be approximated by recording the maximal number of repetitions of a specific set of muscle contractions or limb movements that can be tolerated before force output or range of motion is reduced. These types of measures can provide a gross gauge of the overall level of cardiovascular and musculoskeletal fitness of the client. Because cerebellar dysfunction often leads to movements being much more effortful and often exaggerated, it is extremely important that the client with cerebellar dysfunction obtain adequate endurance for safe participation in daily activities.

Tests of Activity Limitations

Tests of activity limitations should typically proceed similarly to the standard neurological examination. The observation of gait should be given particular attention, as gait ataxia is considered one of the most sensitive signs of cerebellar damage and the inability to walk safely is a major participation limitation for most clients with motor disorders.[143] Box 21-1 provides suggested components of the gait analysis for clients with cerebellar dysfunction. In addition, it may be necessary to evaluate the activity limitations related to speech, visual, and/or oculomotor deficits common to cerebellar dysfunction. With careful interviewing, the client may relay information about limitations in conversation and communication, reading, and so on that should be addressed in rehabilitation. The physical or occupational therapist may be the first health care professional to note these types of activity limitations and should refer the client to the proper professional for additional services.

Documentation of the body function or structure impairments and activity limitations should include not only the level of assistance, if any, required to perform the skill (or for the voluntary limb coordination tests, the degree of impairment, e.g., none, mild, moderate, or severe), but also a detailed description of the deficits observed during the attempted movement; that is, the movement quality. Specifically, the severity and frequency of the specific features of ataxia (e.g., decomposition, lack of check) should be reported when they accompany a given movement. Also useful is documentation of the time taken to perform certain tasks. For example, one might document performance of a functional reach and place task by a client with cerebellar dysfunction in the following way: "The client was able to perform five repetitions of a block-stacking task with the right upper extremity in 9.4 seconds without significant drops or placement errors. Decomposition was observed between shoulder and elbow joints and obvious intention tremor was present during terminal block placement. When asked to repeat at a faster pace, the client performed the same task in 6.0 seconds with one block dropped and two misplaced on the stack (dysmetria). Notable dyssynergia was also present."

Standardized Clinical Scales

There are two common standardized rating scales that quantify the severity of cerebellar ataxia. The more well known is the International Cooperative Ataxia Rating Scale (ICARS).[143a] This scale was first published in 1997 by the Ataxia Neuropharmacology Committee of the World Federation of Neurology in response to an established need for a universal scale to quantify ataxia in randomized clinical trials of pharmacological interventions for treating ataxia. The ICARS measures a client's ability to perform 19 specific activities or movements using an ordinal scale. The activities are grouped into categories based on whether they relate to cerebellar dysfunction affecting (1) posture and gait, (2) limb movements, (3) speech, or (4) oculomotor performance. A subscore is tallied for each category and a total score is obtained, ranging from 0 (no ataxia) to 100 (most severe ataxia). The ICARS has been found to be reliable in clients with cerebellar dysfunction and has established criterion-related and external validity.[144-147] More recently, it was shown that the ICARS is sensitive to increases in ataxia severity over one year in persons with chronic cerebellar degeneration.[141] The Scale for the Assessment and Rating of Ataxia (SARA) is a newer tool that was devised, at least in part, out of concern over the construct validity of the ICARS subscale structure.[148] The SARA is similar to the ICARS in that it quantifies performance of specific movements or activities on an ordinal scale (many of the test activities are the same or similar to those in the ICARS), but it does not categorize individual test items by body part. The SARA has fewer test items (only eight) and can therefore be administered faster in the clinical setting. The SARA has been shown to be reliable and valid for clients with SCAs.[148] Either the ICARS or SARA scale may be useful for longitudinal tracking of disease progression in cerebellar degeneration or for quantifying improvement of ataxia in clinical trials. The scales are detailed in Appendixes 21-A and 21-B.

Diagnosis, Prognosis, and Plan of Care

Clients with cerebellar dysfunction should be given a diagnosis by physical and occupational therapy that identifies the primary movement dysfunction and helps direct treatment interventions to return the client to his or her desired level of activity and participation, if possible. Typically, determination of a movement diagnosis is based largely on both the results of the therapist's examination and evaluation, as well as on knowledge of the cause of the disorder and the extent of the lesion. The prognosis for recovery likewise depends highly on the cause and extent of the lesion. It is important to make a determination whether the impairments in body function or structure and activity limitations are expected to improve or expected not to improve or potentially to worsen over time (e.g., with disease progression). For impairments and activity limitations that are expected to improve, emphasis should be placed on recovery of those skills; for those expected not to improve or to worsen, emphasis should be placed on instruction and practice of compensatory strategies and general conditioning to minimize degradation due to fatigue.

Physical/Occupational Therapy Interventions for Clients with Cerebellar Dysfunction

The literature on the effectiveness of rehabilitation interventions for individuals with primary cerebellar damage is extremely limited: there have been no randomized controlled trials published. Of the few studies on the effects of rehabilitation interventions in this patient population, all have been nonrandomized, noncontrolled small group[101,149,150] or case study[151-155] designs. The fact that there are so few studies available, each featuring different client populations (e.g., post-stroke versus post–surgical tumor resection versus cerebellar degeneration) and different outcome measures, makes determining the most effective interventions difficult. Therefore we provide here only a description of the major themes that have arisen from these studies to date.

Gait and Balance Interventions

Many of the intervention studies for cerebellar ataxia emphasize stability and balance, especially during gait.[101,149,153,155] This likely is a reflection of the tight link between gait and balance[102] and the fact that gait ataxia is one of the most common and debilitating signs of cerebellar damage.[100] Common interventions include combinations of exercises targeting gaze, static stance, dynamic stance, gait, and complex gait activities.[101,153] Some examples of exercises in each of these categories are detailed in Box 21-2. Dynamic balance activities performed while sitting, kneeling, and quadruped have also been advocated.[101] Other interventions specific to the client's individual impairments of body structure or function should be implemented as necessary, for example, stretching of short or tight ankle plantarflexors and exercises for the VOR.[101,153] Locomotor training over ground and on treadmills and with and without body weight support has also been used with some success in single case examples.[151,156] It is not clear how imbalance is corrected in the body weight support environment, however. With all gait and balance activities, it is critical that the exercise be sufficiently and increasingly challenging, so as to facilitate plasticity in the nervous system.[157,158] In a recent study in mice, it was suggested that trial-and-error practice is a requirement for regaining full motor recovery during cerebellar remyelination.[159]

Aerobic Exercise and Resistance Training

Integration of aerobic exercise and resistance training into the treatment plan is recommended for a majority of clients with cerebellar dysfunction, particularly if it is expected the client will not regain premorbid status. If full recovery is not attained, nearly all types of movements will be generally more effortful, requiring increased energy expenditure and demanding greater concentration. It is well known that repetitive fatiguing activity worsens postural control[160,161] and therefore may contribute to trips, falls, or other injuries.[162] Because imbalance is such a common outcome for clients with cerebellar dysfunction, incorporating both aerobic exercise to improve cardiovascular endurance and submaximal resistive exercise to improve muscle fatigue resistance appears appropriate. Aerobic exercise activities might include walking, dance, recumbent or stationary cycling, rowing, arm ergometry, swimming and aquatic exercise, as well as many other possibilities.

Consider More Intensive, Longer Duration Interventions

Because the cerebellum is thought to be a primary site of motor learning and individuals with cerebellar damage often have motor learning deficits, it is reasonable to consider whether these clients are capable of benefiting from any intervention that relies on trial-and-error motor practice.[101] It has been suggested that rehabilitation for clients with significant cerebellar dysfunction may take longer (more trials, more sessions) and might not ever be complete. The question remains unanswered thus far. Of course, cerebellum-dependent motor adaptation is only one of many motor learning mechanisms, so it is possible that other processes can be engaged during rehabilitation. In support of this idea, it now appears that at least partial "re-learning" of more normal movement patterns is possible with selected cerebellar patient populations.[101,150] Notably, in the literature, gains were reported under conditions of very frequent (10 hours/week) or very long (6 months) training schedules. This could be a necessity for clients with health conditions in which motor learning is impaired. Figure 21-9 shows improvements in SARA scores and self-selected walking speeds in a group of individuals with significant progressive ataxia, in response to an intensive rehabilitation program targeting balance and dynamic intersegmental control. Much more research is needed to determine the full range of improvements possible, the minimal dosage of intervention required, and whether the benefits can be retained over the long term in this difficult patient population.

Compensatory Strategies

Compensation is a common component of the plan of care for clients with cerebellar dysfunction. Many clients begin using compensations subconsciously, whereas others need to be taught these strategies and when to use them. If the client is not expected to recover premorbid movement patterns, compensation can enable the individual to regain a certain prior level of activity or societal participation despite an abnormal movement pattern. Instruction in compensation can also be valuable in situations when full recovery is expected but the client would benefit from the use of compensatory strategies for the short term, such as for safety purposes. One compensatory strategy that works well for clients with cerebellar dysfunction is the instruction to simply slow down movements. Recall that slower movements are less dyssynergic and less hypermetric.[49] Voluntarily reducing the number of segments moving at the same time (i.e., decomposition) also helps reduce dyssynergia and dysmetria.[49,83] In some cases, reminding clients to use visual cues can also be helpful, for instance, to use vertical markings of a doorway to maintain upright stability, although for certain types of cerebellar damage this is not effective.[93,94] For gait, deliberately widening stance can be helpful, both for maintaining balance and for preventing tripping over a

BOX 21-2 ■ COMMON GAIT AND BALANCE INTERVENTIONS FOR CLIENTS WITH CEREBELLAR DYSFUNCTION

1. Gaze and eye movements
   a. VOR: (i) visually fixate on stationary target, slow head movements; (ii) visually fixate on target moving in opposite direction, slow head movements; (iii) VOR cancellation, visually fixate on target moving in same direction, slow head movements. Progression: increase and vary speed, perform eyes closed, add complexity to background.
   b. Saccades: active eyes alone and combined eye and head movements between two stationary targets. Progression: increase and vary speed.
2. Static stance
   a. Feet together, arms across chest, eyes open and closed, with and without slow head movements. Progression: increase time with eyes closed, increase and vary speed of head movements.
   b. Stand on foam, feet apart, arms across chest, eyes closed briefly and intermittently. Progression: narrow base of support, increase time with eyes closed.
   c. Semitandem stance, arms across chest, eyes closed briefly and intermittently. Progression: narrow base to full tandem stance, increase time with eyes closed, perform semitandem stance on foam.
   d. Unilateral stance, arms across chest, eyes open. Progression: perform with intermittent then longer periods with eyes closed, perform on foam.
3. Dynamic stance
   a. March in place, arms across chest, eyes open and closed. Progression: increase time with eyes closed, add and incrementally increase pause time in unilateral stance, add head movements.
   b. Standing toe taps, forward, backward, to the side, alternating legs, arms across chest, eyes open and closed. Progression: increase step distance, increase time with eyes closed, add head movements.
   c. March in place on foam, arms across chest, eyes closed briefly and intermittently. Progression: increase time with eyes closed, add and incrementally increase pause time in unilateral stance.
   d. Standing 360-degree turn, rightward, leftward, arms across chest, eyes open and closed. Progression: tighten turns, increase speed.
   e. Standing reaches, feet apart and together, eyes open and closed. Progression: increase time with eyes closed, increase reach distance, vary directions, narrow base of support to feet together position.
   f. Standing bends and squats, feet apart and together, eyes open and closed. Progression: increase time with eyes closed, narrow base of support to feet together, reach to touch the floor.
   g. Transitions: standing to supine on floor and back up. Progression: transition into and out of all possible positions, with and without upper-extremity support, eyes open and closed, including kneel, half-kneel, quadruped, side sit, squat, and so on.
4. Gait
   a. Narrow base of support, arms at sides. Progression: increase gait speed.
   b. Normal base of support, arms at sides with periodic head movements. Progression: narrow base of support, increase and vary speed and frequency of head movements.
   c. Gait with wide turns, arms at sides. Progression: sharpen angle of the turn, increase gait speed, add head movements.
   d. Gait with eyes closed, arms at sides. Progression: add turns, add head movements, increase gait speed.
   e. Gait with perturbations: (i) self-imposed (e.g., large arm movements); (ii) external (e.g., pushes by therapist). Progression: increase speed and amplitude of perturbations, make external perturbations unexpected.
5. Complex gait
   a. Sideways and backward gait, eyes open, arms at sides. Progression: narrow base of support, add head movements, perform with eyes closed, increase gait speed.
   b. Incline and decline gait, eyes open, arms at sides. Progression: narrow base of support, add head movements.
   c. Gait on foam, padded or other compliant surface, eyes open, arms at sides. Progression: narrow base of support, add turns, add head movements, perform with eyes closed.
   d. Semitandem gait, eyes open, arms at sides. Progression: narrow base to tandem gait, add head movements, perform with eyes closed.
   e. Gait while negotiating obstacles, eyes open, arms at sides, avoid, step onto, step over. Progression: increase obstacle number and size, vary obstacle placement.
   f. Gait while distracted, eyes open, arms at sides. Add cognitive task as a distracter; start with responding to simple yes-no questions, progress to difficult tasks (e.g., counting, performing two- or three-digit addition, subtraction).

Adapted from Gill-Body KM, Popat RA, Parker SW, Krebs DE: Rehabilitation of balance in two patients with cerebellar dysfunction. *Phys Ther* 77:534–552, 1997; and Ilg W, Synofzik M, Brötz D, et al: Intensive coordinative training improves motor performance in degenerative cerebellar disease. *Neurology* 73:1823–1830, 2009.

VOR, Vestibuloocular reflex.

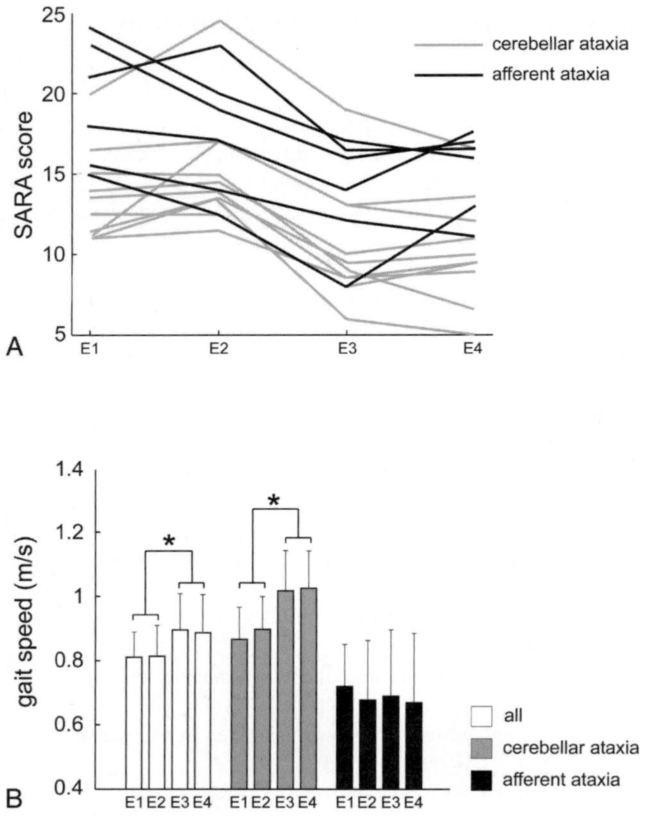

Figure 21-9 ■ Changes in **(A)** SARA scores and **(B)** self-selected walking speeds for 16 individuals with progressive ataxia who completed 4 weeks of intensive (1 hr/day, 3 days/wk supervised training plus 1 hr/day, 7 days/wk independent home exercise) rehabilitation emphasizing balance. Measures were recorded at four time periods (E1 to E4), corresponding to 8 weeks preintervention (E1), immediately preintervention (E2), immediately postintervention (E3), and 8 weeks postintervention (E4). Subjects were categorized as having either a predominant cerebellar ataxia (e.g., SCA2, SCA6, idiopathic cerebellar ataxia, or another autosomal dominant cerebellar ataxia) or a predominant afferent ataxia (e.g., Friedreich ataxia or other significant somatosensory neuropathy). The group overall showed significant improvements in both measures (reduced SARA scores and increased walking speeds) after the 4 weeks of exercise and retained these improvements over a further 8 weeks. When broken down by ataxia category, subjects with a predominant cerebellar ataxia, but not the subjects with a predominant sensory ataxia, showed a significant improvement in walking speed. (Asterisks [*] denote significant improvements immediately following the intervention, while no significant changes occurred during pre and post intervention periods.) *SARA,* Scale for the Assessment and Rating of Ataxia. (Adapted with permission from the American Academy of Neurology. From Ilg W, Synofzik M, Brötz D, et al: Intensive coordinative training improves motor performance in degenerative cerebellar disease. *Neurology* 73:1823–1830, 2009.)

foot. The use of assistive devices for gait should be considered on a case-by-case basis. For some clients, facilitating upper-extremity support and increasing the base of support improve balance during gait. However, for others, the level of skill required to coordinate controlling the device with the movements of arms and legs is too difficult, and using the device actually worsens the instability. Generally speaking, clients with significant imbalance and limb ataxia but who are ambulatory will often not be safe with any type of cane and instead require a wheeled walker and/or the physical assistance of a caretaker to walk. A final strategy is to remove or minimize distractions during effortful activities. Distraction, for example, dividing attention between a motor and a cognitive task, can worsen ataxia.[163]

The Controversy of Weighting

Rehabilitation textbooks have traditionally supported the use of weights for adults and particularly children with cerebellar dysfunction and ataxia. Either the trunk may be weighted by having the client wear a vest or pack that is weighted, increasing the load on the body axially,[164] or the limbs may be weighted individually[165,166] with simple wrist or ankle weights. Presumably this trend was based on the common finding, first noted by Holmes,[74] that clients with cerebellar dysfunction appear improved (move more smoothly and with reduced tremor) if they are asked to hold a heavy weight in the hand while moving the arm. Today it is known that cerebellar tremor is at least in part mechanical in nature, such that anything that adds inertia to the moving segment would reduce the amplitude of the tremor.[86] This most likely explains the improvement that has been reported. However, this apparent benefit would certainly not continue once the weight is removed, and a reduction in tremor does not indicate a normalization of any other parameters of movement. In fact, weighting of the extremities would seem a questionable choice, given the known difficulty of clients with cerebellar dysfunction to predict and account for limb dynamics or to account for interaction torques.[49,50] Addition of weights, particularly to the distal segments, would seem only to make this task more difficult. Evidence for this has been demonstrated in a study of patients with cerebellar ataxia in which it was shown that weighting the extremities worsens the amount of hypermetria during a simple single-joint wrist movement task.[87]

One unintended consequence of weighting is that it tends to slow movements down. As described earlier, slower movements are less hypermetric and less dyssynergic than preferred-speed or fast movements. In early studies of weighting, speed was not monitored or controlled for, so a simple reduction in movement speed could account for the immediate apparent improvement described in some reports.[165,166] Therefore weighting may indeed provide a benefit to some clients with ataxia but it is most likely an indirect one, related more to decreased movement speed. Accordingly, the significant potential for negative consequences of weighting (i.e., worsened hypermetria, increased interaction torques, and the annoyance and physical awkwardness of weights) makes this intervention option seem inferior to the simpler strategy of instructing the client in voluntarily moving more slowly.[167]

SUMMARY

The cerebellum is highly unique, in terms of its anatomy, its physiology, and the movement-related impairments individuals experience if it becomes damaged. Ataxia, or movement incoordination, is the major sign of cerebellar damage and can affect limb movements, eye movements, speech, balance, and walking. Depending on which cerebellar functional longitudinal zone is lesioned, one or more of these specific categories of movements will be impaired. Although the precise mechanisms are not yet fully understood, it is widely acknowledged that the cerebellum is integral to (1) coordination of movements, particularly fast, multijoint movements and (2) adaptation of movements to changes in body conditions or the environment and learning new movement patterns based on trial-and-error practice (motor learning). Unfortunately, evidence for the effectiveness of rehabilitation interventions for individuals with primary cerebellar damage is extremely limited and incomplete. One critical factor in the evaluative process is the determination of whether the body function or structure impairments and activity limitations are expected to improve or expected not to improve or even worsen, as is the case in progressive diseases. If expected to improve, emphasis should be placed on trial-and-error practice of increasingly challenging motor activities. Balance and gait skills may be highlighted. On the other hand, if recovery is not expected, instruction and practice of compensatory strategies and general conditioning may be effective in at least partially restoring prior participation levels.

Acknowledgments

The authors are supported by the following grants: NIH R01 HD040289 (AJB), R01 HD048741 (AJB), K01 HD050369 (SMM), and R21 NS067189 (SMM). Special thanks to Ms. Jennifer Keller for assistance with the videos and Ms. Tara Hackney for assistance with the illustrations.

References

To enhance this text and add value for the reader, all references are included on the companion Evolve site that accompanies this textbook. This online service will, when available, provide a link for the reader to a Medline abstract for the article cited. There are 167 cited references and other general references for this chapter, with the majority of those articles being evidence-based citations.

APPENDIX 21-A ■ International Cooperative Ataxia Rating Scale (ICARS)

I. POSTURE AND GAIT DISTURBANCES

1. **Walking capacities** (Observe walking 10 m, near a wall, including half-turn.)
   0 = Normal
   1 = Almost normal naturally but unable to walk with feet in tandem position
   2 = Walking without support but clearly abnormally and irregularly
   3 = Walking without support but with considerable staggering; difficulties in half-turn
   4 = Walking with autonomous support not possible; uses the episodic support of the wall
   5 = Walking possible only with one stick
   6 = Walking possible only with two special sticks or with a stroller
   7 = Walking only with accompanying person
   8 = Walking impossible, even with accompanying person (wheelchair)
   Score: _____
2. **Gait speed** (Observe only if subject scores <4 on preceding test; otherwise automatically score this test as 4.)
   0 = Normal
   1 = Slightly reduced
   2 = Markedly reduced
   3 = Extremely slow
   4 = Walking with autonomous support no longer possible
   Score: _____
3. **Standing capacities, eyes open** (Ask subject to stand on one foot; if impossible, ask to stand with feet in tandem; if impossible, ask to stand with feet together. For the natural position, ask subject to find a comfortable standing position.)
   0 = Normal; able to stand on one foot >10 s
   1 = Able to stand with feet together but no longer able to stand on one foot >10 s
   2 = Able to stand with feet together but no longer able to stand with feet in tandem position
   3 = No longer able to stand with feet together but able to stand in natural position without support, with no or moderate sway
   4 = Standing in natural position without support, with considerable sway and considerable corrections
   5 = Unable to stand in natural position without strong support of one arm
   6 = Unable to stand at all, even with strong support of two arms
   Score: _____
4. **Spread of feet in natural position without support, eyes open** (Ask subject to find a comfortable position, then measure the distance between medial malleoli.)
   0 = Normal (<10 cm)
   1 = Slightly enlarged (>10 cm)
   2 = Clearly enlarged (25-35 cm)
   3 = Severely enlarged (>35 cm)
   4 = Standing in natural position impossible
   Score: _____
5. **Body sway with feet together, eyes open**
   0 = Normal
   1 = Slight oscillations
   2 = Moderate oscillations (<10 cm at the level of head)
   3 = Severe oscillations (>10 cm at the level of head), threatening the upright position
   4 = Immediate falling
   Score: _____
6. **Body sway with feet together, eyes closed**
   0 = Normal
   1 = Slight oscillations
   2 = Moderate oscillations (<10 cm at the level of head)
   3 = Severe oscillations (>10 cm at the level of head), threatening the upright position
   4 = Immediate falling
   Score: _____
7. **Quality of sitting position** (on flat, hard surface, thighs together, arms folded)
   0 = Normal
   1 = With slight oscillations of the trunk
   2 = With moderate oscillations of the trunk and legs
   3 = With severe disequilibrium
   4 = Impossible
   Score: _____

Posture and Gait Subscore: _____/34

II. KINETIC FUNCTIONS

8. **Knee-tibia test: decomposition of movement and intention tremor** (Subject is supine with head tilted to allow visual control. Ask subject to raise one leg in the air (to a height of approximately 40 cm) and place heel on opposite knee and then slide the heel down the anterior tibial surface of the resting leg toward the ankle. On reaching the ankle joint, the leg is again raised, and the action repeated. Repeat for at least three trials on each side.)
   0 = Normal
   1 = Heel lowering in continuous axis, but movement is decomposed in several phases (without real jerks) or abnormally slow
   2 = Heel lowering jerkily in the axis
   3 = Heel lowering jerkily with lateral movements
   4 = Heel lowering jerkily with extremely strong lateral movements or test impossible
   Score right: _____ Score left: _____
9. **Action tremor in the heel-to-knee test** (Same test as preceding one; visual control required. Observe action tremor of the heel when asked to hold the heel on the knee for a few seconds before sliding down the leg.)
   0 = No trouble
   1 = Tremor stops immediately when the heel reaches the knee
   2 = Tremor stops in <10 s after reaching the knee
   3 = Tremor continues >10 s after reaching the knee
   4 = Uninterrupted tremor or test impossible
   Score right: _____ Score left: _____
10. **Finger-to-nose test: decomposition and dysmetria** (Subject sitting; visual control required. Start trials with hands resting on knees. Repeat for at least three trials on each side.)
   0 = No trouble
   1 = Oscillating movement without decomposition of the movement
   2 = Segmented movement in two phases and/or moderate dysmetria in reaching nose
   3 = Segmented movement in more than two phases and/or considerable dysmetria in reaching nose
   4 = Dysmetria preventing the subject from reaching nose
   Score right: _____ Score left: _____

APPENDIX 21-A ■ International Cooperative Ataxia Rating Scale (ICARS)—cont'd

11. **Finger-to-nose test: kinetic tremor of the finger** (Same test as preceding one; visual control required. Observe movement tremor occurring during the ballistic phase of the movement.)
 0 = No trouble
 1 = Simple swerve of the movement
 2 = Mild tremor, estimated amplitude <10 cm
 3 = Moderate tremor, estimated amplitude 10 to 40 cm
 4 = Severe tremor, estimated amplitude >40 cm
 Score right: _____ Score left: _____
12. **Finger-finger test: action tremor and/or instability** (Subject sitting. Ask subject to flex, abduct and internally rotate shoulders and then flex elbows so as to have both index fingers pointing at each other at midline. Subject is to maintain index finger positions for approximately 10 s, at distance of approximately 1 cm apart (not touching) and hands at the level of the thorax.)
 0 = Normal
 1 = Mild instability
 2 = Moderate oscillations of finger, estimated amplitude <10 cm
 3 = Considerable oscillations of finger, estimated amplitude 10 to 40 cm
 4 = Jerky movements, amplitude >40 cm
 Score right: _____ Score left: _____
13. **Pronation-supination alternating movements** (Subject sitting. Ask subject to raise the forearm vertically and alternate supinating and pronating the forearm on the lap, combining elbow flexion and extension with forearm supination and pronation.)
 0 = Normal
 1 = Slightly irregular and slowed
 2 = Clearly irregular and slowed, but without sway of the elbow
 3 = Extremely irregular and slowed movement, with sway of the elbow
 4 = Movement completely disorganized or impossible
 Score right: _____ Score left: _____
14. **Drawing of the Archimedes' spiral on a predrawn pattern** (Subject sitting at a table with a sheet of paper fixed in place. Ask subject to trace the spiral with a pen using the dominant hand; no timing requirements.)
 0 = Normal
 1 = Impairment and decomposition, the line quitting the pattern slightly, but without hypermetric swerve
 2 = Line completely out of the pattern, with recrossings and/or hypermetric swerves
 3 = Major disturbance caused by hypermetria and decomposition
 4 = Drawing completely disorganized or impossible
 Score: _____

Limb Kinetics Subscore: _____/52

III. SPEECH DISORDERS

15. **Dysarthria: fluency of speech** (Ask subject to repeat a standard phrase several times; for instance, "A mischievous spectacle in Czechoslovakia".)
 0 = Normal
 1 = Mild modification of fluency
 2 = Moderate modification of fluency
 3 = Considerably slow and dysarthric speech
 4 = No speech
 Score: _____
16. **Dysarthria: clarity of speech**
 0 = Normal
 1 = Suggestion of slurring
 2 = Definite slurring, most words understandable
 3 = Severe slurring, speech not understandable
 4 = No speech
 Score: _____

Dysarthria Subscore: _____ /8

IV. OCULOMOTOR DISORDERS

17. **Gaze-evoked nystagmus** (Ask subject to look laterally at examiner's finger. Observe for nystagmus, mainly horizontal, but could be oblique, rotary, or vertical.)
 0 = Normal
 1 = Transient
 2 = Persistent but moderate
 3 = Persistent and severe
 Score: _____
18. **Abnormalities of ocular pursuit** (Ask subject to follow the slow lateral movement of the examiner's finger.)
 0 = Normal
 1 = Slightly saccadic
 2 = Clearly saccadic
 Score: _____
19. **Dysmetria of the saccade** (Examiner's two fingers are placed, one in each temporal visual field of the subject, whose eyes are in the primary position. Ask subject to shift eyes to look laterally at the finger, first on the right and then on the left. Average overshoot or undershoot of the two sides is then estimated.)
 0 = Absent
 1 = Bilateral clear overshoot or undershoot of the saccade
 Score: _____

Oculomotor Subscore: _____/6

TOTAL ATAXIA SCORE (SUM OF FOUR SUBSCORES): _____/100

Modified with permission from Trouillas P, Takayanagi T, Hallett M, et al: International Cooperative Ataxia Rating Scale for pharmacological assessment of the cerebellar syndrome. The Ataxia Neuropharmacology Committee of the World Federation of Neurology. *Neurol Sci* 145:205–211, 1997.

APPENDIX 21-B ■ Scale for the Assessment and Rating of Ataxia (SARA)

1. **Gait** (Subject (a) walks at a safe distance parallel to a wall including a half-turn (turn around to face the opposite direction of gait) and (b) walks in tandem (heels to toes) without support.)
   0 = Normal, no difficulties in walking, turning, or walking tandem (up to one misstep allowed)
   1 = Slight difficulties but visible only when walking 10 consecutive steps in tandem
   2 = Clearly abnormal, tandem walking >10 steps not possible
   3 = Considerable staggering, difficulties in half-turn, but walks without support
   4 = Marked staggering, intermittent support of the wall required
   5 = Severe staggering, permanent support of one stick or light support by one arm required
   6 = Walking >10 m only with strong support (two special sticks or stroller or accompanying person)
   7 = Walking <10 m only with strong support (two special sticks or stroller or accompanying person)
   8 = Unable to walk, even supported
   Score: _____
2. **Stance** (Subject stands (a) in natural position, (b) with feet together in parallel (big toes touching each other), and (c) in tandem (both feet on one line, no space between heel and toe). Subject does not wear shoes, eyes are open. For each condition, three trials are allowed. Best trial is rated.)
   0 = Normal, able to stand in tandem for >10 s
   1 = Able to stand with feet together without sway but not in tandem for >10 s
   2 = Able to stand with feet together for >10 s but only with sway
   3 = Able to stand for >10 s without support in natural position but not with feet together
   4 = Able to stand for >10 s in natural position only with intermittent support
   5 = Able to stand >10 s in natural position only with constant support of one arm
   6 = Unable to stand for >10 s even with constant support of one arm
   Score: _____
3. **Sitting** (Subject sits on an examination table without support of feet, eyes open and arms outstretched to the front.)
   0 = Normal, no difficulties sitting >10 s
   1 = Slight difficulties, intermittent sway
   2 = Constant sway but able to sit >10 s without support
   3 = Able to sit for >10 s only with intermittent support
   4 = Unable to sit for >10 s without continuous support
   Score: _____
4. **Speech disturbance** (Speech is assessed during normal conversation.)
   0 = Normal
   1 = Suggestion of speech disturbance
   2 = Impaired speech but easy to understand
   3 = Occasional words difficult to understand
   4 = Many words difficult to understand
   5 = Only single words understandable
   6 = Speech unintelligible, anarthria
   Score: _____
5. **Finger chase** (Subject seated comfortably, feet and trunk supported if needed. Examiner sits in front of subject and performs five consecutive sudden and fast pointing movements in unpredictable directions in a frontal plane, at about 50% of subject's reach distance. Movements are approximately 30 cm in distance and occur at a rate of approximately one reach every 2 s. Ask subject to follow the movements, pointing with his or her index finger as fast and precisely as possible. Average performance of last three movements is rated. Rate separately for each side.)
   0 = No dysmetria
   1 = Dysmetria, undershooting or overshooting target <5 cm
   2 = Dysmetria, undershooting or overshooting target <15 cm
   3 = Dysmetria, undershooting or overshooting target >15 cm
   4 = Unable to perform five pointing movements
   Score right: _____ Score left: _____ Mean score ([R + L]/2): _____
6. **Nose-finger test** (Subject seated comfortably, feet and trunk supported if needed. Ask subject to point repeatedly with the index finger from his or her nose to examiner's finger, which is in front at about 90% of subject's reach distance. Movements are performed at moderate speed. Average performance of movements is rated according to the amplitude of the kinetic tremor. Rate separately for each side.)
   0 = No tremor
   1 = Tremor with an amplitude <2 cm
   2 = Tremor with an amplitude <5 cm
   3 = Tremor with an amplitude >5 cm
   4 = Unable to perform five pointing movements
   Score right: _____ Score left: _____ Mean score ([R + L]/2): _____
7. **Fast alternating hand movements** (Subject seated comfortably, feet and trunk supported if needed. Ask subject to perform 10 cycles of repetitive alternation of pronation and supination of the forearm on his or her thigh as fast and as precisely as possible. Demonstrate the movement at a speed of approximately 10 cycles in 7 s. Record times for movement execution. Rate separately for each side.)
   0 = Normal, no irregularities, performs in <10 s
   1 = Slightly irregular but performs in <10 s
   2 = Clearly irregular, single movements difficult to distinguish or relevant interruptions, but performs in <10 s
   3 = Very irregular, single movements difficult to distinguish or relevant interruptions, performs in >10 s
   4 = Unable to complete 10 cycles
   Score right: _____ Score left: _____ Mean score ([R + L]/2): _____
8. **Heel-shin slide** (Subject supine on examination bed without sight of his legs. Ask subject to lift one leg, point with the heel to the opposite knee, slide down along the shin to the ankle, and lay the leg back on the examination bed. The task is performed three times. The slide component of the movement should be performed within 1 s. If subject slides down without contact to shin in all three trials, rate as 4. Rate separately for each side.)
   0 = Normal
   1 = Slightly abnormal, contact to shin maintained
   2 = Clearly abnormal, goes off shin ≤3 times during 3 cycles
   3 = Severely abnormal, goes off shin ≥4 times during 3 cycles
   4 = Unable to perform the task
   Score right: _____ Score left: _____ Mean score ([R + L]/2): _____

Total Ataxia Score (Sum of Eight Test Scores): ____/40

Modified with permission from Schmitz-Hubsch T, du Montcel ST, Baliko L, et al: Scale for the Assessment and Rating of Ataxia: development of a new clinical scale. *Neurology* 66:1717–1720, 2006.

CHAPTER 22 Balance and Vestibular Dysfunction

LESLIE K. ALLISON, PT, PhD, and KENDA FULLER, PT, NCS

KEY TERMS

activity limitation
anticipatory postural adjustments
automatic postural responses
balance
base of support
body system problems
center of gravity
impairment
limit of stability
motor learning stages
participation
sensory conflict
sensory environment
strategies
systems model or systems approach
volitional postural movements

OBJECTIVES

After reading this chapter the student or therapist will be able to:

1. Describe both central and peripheral sensory and motor components of the postural control system.
2. List common postural control impairments found in clients with neurological problems.
3. List commonly used balance tests, and distinguish which are appropriate for clients at low, moderate, and high levels of function.
4. Differentiate how test results are used to identify body system impairments and activity limitations that limit participation.
5. Analyze the interaction of individual, task, and environmental factors that affect balance.
6. Describe how to plan and progress balance exercise programs to increase the use of, or compensation with, available sensory inputs.
7. Describe how to plan and progress balance exercise programs to facilitate anticipatory postural adjustments to prevent balance loss and provoke automatic postural responses to regain balance after unexpected disturbances.
8. Describe how to plan and progress balance exercise programs to increase the control of center of gravity in upright postures and during gait.
9. Describe how to increase the difficulty level of balance exercise programs in order to promote the automaticity of postural control during functional activities.
10. Identify and analyze the function of the vestibular system.
11. Describe how to facilitate adaptation and central nervous system reorganization to regain control of balance and decrease dizziness.
12. Identify patterns of recovery that influence choices of intervention.

Balance Function and Disorders

Leslie Allison, PT, PhD

No matter what the neurological diagnosis, a disease or injury that affects the nervous system is likely to compromise one or more of the postural control mechanisms. For example, clients with such diverse diagnoses as stroke, head trauma, spinal cord injury, peripheral neuropathy, multiple sclerosis (MS), Parkinson disease, cerebellar dysfunction, cerebral palsy, and Guillian-Barré syndrome all experience disequilibrium problems. One common thread among all these different medical diagnoses is the presence of balance impairments. Clients with different medical diagnoses may have the same balance impairments, and clients with the same medical diagnosis may have different balance impairments depending on which portions of the postural control system are involved.[1] To optimally understand and manage balance problems, a test of each balance component and the interactive nature of the components is important. The traditional medical "diagnostic" model does not provide this information and is not the most beneficial model for planning balance rehabilitation interventions. The medical diagnosis is relevant: knowing whether deficits are permanent or temporary, and whether recovery or progressive decline is expected, is critical. This medical prognostic information will assist physical and occupational therapists in goal setting and intervention planning.

The International Classification of Functioning, Disability and Health (ICF) model described in Chapter 1 and illustrated in Figure 1-1 describes the interactions of body function and structure problems (impairments) and activity limitations as seen in clients with balance disorders, and how these functional activity limitations restrict an individual's ability to participate in life situations, thus decreasing quality of life. Balance impairments negatively affect function, often reducing the individual's ability to participate fully in life.[2] These impairments often restrict activity levels, produce abnormal compensatory motor behavior, and may require devices for support or assistance from another person. Falls can result when imbalance is severe, leading to secondary injuries. To avoid these consequences and advance the functional status of clients, therapists should understand both the demands that various environments and functional tasks place on postural control systems and the impairments that may diminish the ability of those systems to respond adequately.

BALANCE

Definitions of Balance

Balance is a complex process involving the reception and integration of sensory inputs and the planning and execution of movement to achieve a goal requiring upright posture. It is the ability to control the center of gravity (COG) over the base of support in a given sensory environment.[3,4] The COG is an imaginary point in space, calculated biomechanically from measured forces and moments, where the sum total of all the forces equals zero. In a person standing quietly the COG is located just forward of the spine at approximately the S2 level. With movement of the body and its segments, the location of the COG in space constantly changes. The base of support is the body surface that experiences pressure as a result of body weight and gravity; in standing it is the feet, and in sitting it includes the thighs and buttocks. The size of the base of support will affect the difficulty level of the balancing task. A broad base of support makes the task easier; a narrow base makes it more challenging. The COG can travel farther while still remaining over the base if the base is large. The "shape" of the base of support will alter the distance that the COG can move in certain directions.

Any given base of support places a limit on the distance a body can move without either falling (as the COG exceeds the base of support) or establishing a new base of support by reaching or stepping (to relocate the base of support under the COG). This perimeter is frequently referred to as the *limit of stability* or *stability limit*.[3,5] It is the farthest distance in any direction a person can lean (away from midline) without altering the original base of support by stepping, reaching, or falling.

Environmental Context

This biomechanical task of keeping the COG over the base of support is always accomplished within an environmental context, which is detected by the sensory systems. The sensory environment is the set of conditions that exist, or are perceived to exist, in the external world that may affect balance. Peripheral sensory receptors gather information about the environment, body position and motion in relation to the environment, and body segment positions and motions in relation to the self. Central sensory structures process this information to perceive body orientation, position, and motion and to determine the opportunities and limitations present in the environment. Gravity is one environmental condition that must be dealt with to remain stable. It is a constant condition for everyone except astronauts in space. Surface and visual conditions, however, may vary significantly and may be stable or unstable. Unstable surface conditions might include the subway, a sandy beach, a gravel driveway, or an icy parking lot. Common unstable visual conditions are experienced on mass transit, in crowds, or on a boat. Rapid head movements may render even a stable visual environment unusable for postural cues, and darkness may preclude the use of vision. The more stable the environment, the lower the demand on the individual for balance control. Unstable environments place greater demands on the postural control systems.

Balance is also affected by an individual's intentions to achieve certain goals and the purposeful tasks that are undertaken. Volitional balance disturbances are self-initiated almost constantly, such as shifting from foot to foot, reaching for the telephone, or catching an object that is falling from a high shelf. Even reactions to involuntary balance disturbances, such as a slip or trip, are modified on the basis of the immediate task. A man carrying a bag of groceries who slips may drop the bag to reach with both hands and catch himself. If he is instead carrying his infant child, he may reach with only one hand or even take the fall if by doing so he can protect the infant from harm. Often in real life we perform several tasks at once, such as carrying a laundry basket while walking, or talking on a cellular phone while climbing a flight of stairs. When tasks are undertaken concurrently, attention must be divided between them, which may also affect balance abilities.

All these variables—the location of the COG, the base of support, the limit of stability, the surface conditions, the visual environment, the intentions and task choices—are inconstant, producing changing demands on the systems that control balance. The integrity and interaction of postural control mechanisms allow a wide range of movements and functions to be achieved without loss of balance.

HUMAN CONTROL OF BALANCE

Early studies of postural control mechanisms using selectively lesioned cats and primates focused on reflexive and reactive equilibrium responses that are relatively "hard-wired."[6] These valuable studies brought to light certain stereotypical motor responses to specific sensory stimuli, such as the crossed extension reflex or tonic neck reflexes. There is no doubt that these reflexive and reactive responses—for example, the vestibuloocular reflex (VOR) and the protective extension reactions—are foundational to normal postural control. However, the postural control system encompasses much more than these subcortically driven components. Balance abilities are heavily influenced by higher-level neural circuitry and other systems (e.g., cognitive, musculoskeletal), as well.[5] In addition, the nervous system is influenced by and responsive to the demands placed on it by the tasks being accomplished and the environments in which those tasks are performed.[7-9] All of these facets are included in a systems approach to dynamic equilibrium.[10-12] Examination and intervention methods based on this systems model have consequently evolved.[11,13]

The Systems Approach

The dynamic systems model for dynamic equilibrium recognizes that balance is a result of interactions among the individual, the task(s) the individual is performing, and the environment in which the task(s) must be performed. These interactions are represented in Figure 22-1. Within the individual, both sensory inputs and processing systems (left side of figure) and motor planning and execution systems (right side of figure) are critical. Both peripheral components (lower part of figure) and central components (upper part of figure) of the systems are involved in the cycle. The cycle is driven both by purposeful choices of the individual (tasks) and by demands placed on the individual by the environment. Successful function of the sensory systems allows recognition of body position and motion in relation to self and the world. The desired outcome from the motor systems is the generation of movement sufficient to maintain balance and perform the chosen, goal-directed task(s).

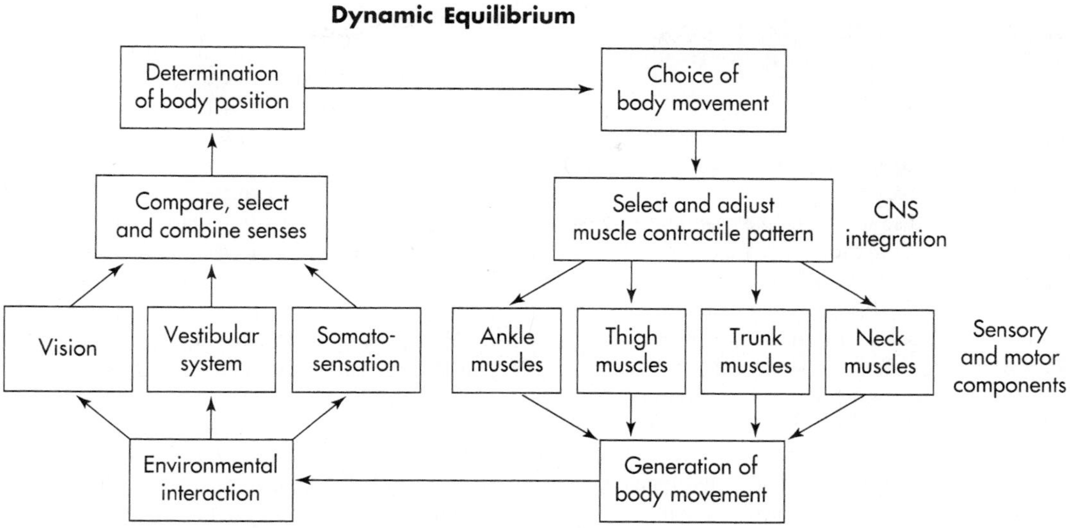

Figure 22-1 ■ The systems model of postural control illustrates the constant cycle that occurs simultaneously at many levels. (Reprinted with permission from NeuroCom International, Clackamas, Ore.)

Peripheral Sensory Reception

The three primary peripheral sensory inputs contributing to postural control are the bilateral receptors of the somatosensory, visual, and vestibular systems.[4,10] Somatosensory receptors located in the joints, ligaments, muscles, and skin provide information about muscle length, stretch, tension, and contraction; pain, temperature, and pressure; and joint position. The feet, ankles, knees, hips, back, neck, and eye muscles all furnish useful information for balance maintenance. Somatosensation is the dominant sense for upright postural control and is responsible for triggering automatic postural responses (APRs). Somatosensory loss significantly impairs balance. Loss of peripheral somatosensation occurs in clients with loss or disease of or injury to the peripheral sensory receptors or afferent sensory nerves. Examples include clients with diabetic neuropathy, peripheral vascular disease, spinal cord injury, and amputation.

Visual receptors in the eyes perform dual tasks. Central (or foveal) vision allows environmental orientation, contributing to the perception of verticality and object motion, as well as identification of the hazards and opportunities presented by the environment.[10] For example, a kayaker may see rocks in a stream as a hazard to be avoided, whereas a hiker who wants to cross the stream may see the same rocks as a welcome opportunity. Peripheral (or ambient) vision detects the motion of the self in relation to the environment, including head movements and postural sway. Peripheral vision is largely subconscious, whereas central visual inputs tend to receive more conscious recognition.[10] Both are normally used for postural control. Vision is critical for feed-forward, or anticipatory, postural control in changing environments. This includes planning for functional movements such as reaching and grasping, and especially for successful navigation during gait. Vision loss also impairs balance. Loss of peripheral visual inputs occurs in clients with disease of or injury to the eyes or afferent cranial nerves. Examples include clients with cataracts, macular degeneration, glaucoma, or diabetic retinopathy.

The vestibular system provides the central nervous system (CNS) with information about the position and motion of the head. The position of the head in relation to gravity is detected through the otolith system. Horizontal and vertical accelerations, as in riding in a car or an elevator, are also detected by the otoliths.[14] Movements of the head are detected through the semicircular canals. Head movement stimulates both sets of semicircular canals, so that the vestibular nerve on one side becomes inhibited while the other becomes excited. The vestibular system provides sensory redundancy in the information obtained from each separate vestibular apparatus. If the peripheral vestibular system is damaged on one side, the information can be captured by the intact canals on the opposite side. The vestibular system is critical for balance because it uniquely identifies self-motion as different from motion in the environment. Box 22-1 describes the sensory components of the vestibular system. Vestibular loss also impairs balance. Loss of peripheral vestibular inputs occurs in clients with disease of or injury to the peripheral sensory receptors or afferent cranial nerves. Examples include clients with head injury involving temporal bone damage, acoustic neuroma, benign positional vertigo (BPV), or Meniere disease. For a comprehensive review of the vestibular system and vestibular disorders, please see the vestibular section of this chapter beginning on page 689.

Orientation to the wider environment, primarily from vision, allows feed-forward, or anticipatory, postural adjustments. Prior experience and high attentional capacity improve anticipatory postural adjustments significantly. Detection of head movement by the vestibular and cervical somatosensory systems and of body sway by somatosensory and peripheral visual systems provides feedback for APRs. Note that the better anticipatory abilities become, the fewer balance errors occur. Fewer balance errors mean fewer losses of balance and a reduced need to produce APRs.

Disease of or damage to any of the peripheral sensory receptors or afferent pathways impairs or removes the detection capabilities of the system, rendering sensory information unavailable for use in postural control. Many patients with neurological diagnoses have peripheral sensory impairments.

BOX 22-1 ■ SENSORY COMPONENTS OF THE VESTIBULAR SYSTEM LABYRINTHS

SEMICIRCULAR CANALS

- Semicircular canals are ring-shaped, fluid-filled structures containing hair cells that respond to fluid movement when the head moves.
- The canals are arranged so that when the head moves, the direction and velocity in each canal are compared with a mutually perpendicular canal on the opposite side of the head.
- The brain uses the relative change in firing from each side to identify the direction of rotation. This provides for sensory redundancy; the brain interprets motion by comparing information from each side to calculate the velocity and direction of head turns.
- The orientation of the three semicircular canals on each side corresponds to the directions of neck motion, flexion and extension, right and left rotation, and right and left side-bending. This relation supports the integration of vestibular inputs with somatosensory information from the cervical spine.

OTOLITHS

- Located in the vestibule or central component of the labyrinth, the otoliths respond to gravity and linear acceleration through hair cell deflection.
- These compartments contain multiple hair cells attached to the walls and connected to the vestibular nerve. These hair cells are embedded in a gel-like substance called the *macula.*
- Sitting on top of the macula are crystals of calcium carbonate, known as *otoconia.* The purpose of the otoconia is to establish mass so that the hair cells can measure the effects of gravity as well as movement.
- The otoliths respond to movement of the head by the shearing effect of the otoconia pressing on the macula and displacing the hair cell in the opposite direction of the movement. These signals from the otoliths are used to compare this motion with the resting tone established by gravity.

Central Sensory Perception

The brain processes all the environmentally available sensory information gathered by the peripheral receptors in varying degrees. This processing is usually referred to as *multisensory integration* or *sensory organization.*[4,10] Central sensory structures function first to compare available inputs between two sides and among three sensory systems. The somatosensory system alone is unable to distinguish surface tilts from body tilts. Also, the visual system by itself cannot discriminate movement of the environment from movement of the body.[14] The vestibular system by itself cannot tell if head movement through space is produced by neck motion or trunk and hip motion. Therefore the brain needs information from all three senses to correctly distinguish self-motion from motion in the environment.

How are sensory inputs from separate senses combined to form perceptions of position and motion? For example, consider the movement of turning your head to one side to look over your shoulder. When the head turns to one side, firing will increase in one vestibular organ and decrease proportionately in the other. This is known as *push-pull function,* and the information from each side is considered to "match." With the same example, if the eyes are open while the head moves, the rate of the visual flow will be equal and the direction of the visual flow will be opposite to the rate and direction of information from the vestibular inputs. The muscles on one side of the neck will shorten and on the other side will stretch. The inputs from these three systems are congruent. If both sides and all three systems provide compatible inputs, the process of sensory organization is simplified.

When changes in the environment occur, the relative availability, accuracy, and usefulness of information from the three sensory systems may also change. Sensory organization also includes an adaptive process, called *multisensory reweighting,* that permits the CNS to prioritize the sources of sensory information when environmental conditions change.[15,16] Available, accurate, and useful information is "upweighted," whereas unavailable, inaccurate, or less-useful information is "downweighted." For example, in dark environments, vision would be downweighted and somatosensory and vestibular information would be upweighted. This adaptive process is imperfect, however, and balance is not as well controlled when any sense must be downweighted as it is when all three senses are available and accurate. Individuals with peripheral sensory loss or central sensory processing deficits may have difficulty reweighting quickly and fully. This impairs their ability to adapt to, and remain stable in, changing environments.[17]

Sensory conflict can arise when information between sides or between systems is not synchronous. Sensory organization processing then becomes more complex because the brain must then recognize any discrepancies and select the correct inputs on which to base motor responses. The vestibular system may be used as an internal reference to determine accuracy of the other two senses when they conflict. For example, a driver stopped at a red light suddenly hits the brake when an adjacent vehicle begins to roll. Movement of the other car detected by the peripheral visual system is momentarily misperceived as self-motion. In this situation, the vestibular and somatosensory systems do not detect motion, but the forward visual flow is interpreted as backward motion. Because the brain failed to suppress the (mismatched) visual inputs, the braking response was generated.

When the brain recognizes that the information coming from one sensory input is inaccurate or unavailable, as is the case when somatosensory information is diminished post-stroke, it must depend more on the remaining senses (in this case, vision and vestibular system) to determine position and motion in space. The brain then compares and uses information from senses it considers accurate for balance. An individual with the problem just described may compensate for the loss of somatosensory function by becoming visually dependent for balance during movement. If vision subsequently also becomes disrupted as this client ages, his ability to orient in space will be further compromised. This will impair balance and increase risk of falls.

Activities or environments that create sensory conflict or demand sensory resolution become more difficult to manage when the vestibular system is deficient or underused. These situations, such as going down stairs, riding escalators or elevators, walking on uneven ground, and making quick turns, are often avoided. When sensory conflicts cannot be resolved rapidly, dizziness or motion sickness occurs.

Intrinsic central sensory processing impairments also can produce sensory conflict. An adult hemiplegic patient with pusher syndrome illustrates an inability to integrate visual, vestibular, and somatosensory inputs for midline orientation. Within a single system, discrepancies between the sides are also problematic. Unequal firing from opposite sides of the vestibular system, as in unilateral vestibular hypofunction, produces a mismatch that is subsequently interpreted as head rotation when head movement does not occur. This spinning sensation is known as *vertigo.*[14] Vertigo is resolved if the brain is able to adapt to the mismatch. For further information on vertigo, refer to the section on the vestibular system.

Finally, the central processing mechanisms combine any available and accurate inputs to answer the questions "Where am I?" and "How am I moving?" This includes both an internal relation of the body segments to one another (e.g., head in relation to trunk, trunk in relation to feet) and an external relation of the body to the outside world (e.g., feet in relation to surface, arm in relation to handrail). CNS disease or trauma involving the parietal lobe may impair these processing mechanisms so that even available, accurate sensory inputs are not recognized or incorporated into determinations of position and movement.[18,19] Impairments of central sensory processing may occur after stroke, head trauma, tumors, or aneurysms; with disease processes such as MS; and with aging.

Central Motor Planning and Control

Whereas sensory processing allows the interaction of the individual and the environment, motor planning underlies the interaction of the individual and the task. Aside from reflexive activity such as breathing and blinking, most motor actions are voluntary and occur because some goal is to be achieved. That is not to say that reflexes occur separately from volitional movements; for example, the vestibuloocular reflex is active concurrently with visual tracking activity, but most actions occur because of some purposeful intent.[14] These task intentions precede motor actions.[10,20] Wrist and hand movements vary depending on what is to be grasped (a cup versus a doorknob); foot placement and trunk position vary depending on what is to be lifted (a heavy suitcase versus a laundry basket). The initiation of volitional motor actions depends on intention, attention, and motivation.[10,21]

Once an objective ("Where do I want to be?" "What do I want to do?") has been chosen, the next step in motor planning is to determine how to best accomplish the goal given the many options that are potentially available. For example, when the task demands fine skills or accuracy, the dominant hand is preferred; when the task involves lifting a large or heavy object, both hands are preferred. In addition to which limbs, joints, and muscles will be used, motor planning also adjusts the timing, sequencing, and force modulation. This can be demonstrated in various reaching tasks. Reaching to remove a hot item from the oven will occur slowly, whereas reaching to put an arm through a sleeve will occur more quickly. Optimal motor plans are developed with knowledge of self (abilities and limitations), knowledge of task (characteristics of successful performance), and knowledge of the environment (risks and opportunities).[21]

The motor plan must be transmitted to the peripheral motor system to be enacted. A copy of the intended movement plan is sent to the cerebellum during the transmission. When the movement begins, incoming sensory inputs (feedback) about the actual movements and performance outcome are compared with the intended movements and performance outcome. Movement errors (the difference between the intended and the actual movement) and performance errors (desired goal not achieved) are detected, and plans for correction are then formed and transmitted. This process of error detection and error correction is the foundation of motor learning.

Clients with CNS disorders often have central motor planning and control system problems. After a stroke, clients may have hypertonus and poor reciprocal inhibition; clients with head trauma may have difficulty initiating or ceasing movements; clients with Parkinson disease exhibit bradykinesia; and those with cerebellar ataxia display modulation problems.[22]

Peripheral Motor Execution

Movement is accomplished through the bilateral joints and muscles. Normal range of motion (ROM), strength, and endurance of the feet, ankles, knees, hips, back, neck, and eyes must be present for the execution of the full range of normal balance movements. Decreased ankle dorsiflexion ROM, for example, restricts the forward limits of stability. Strength deficits are a primary cause of movement abnormalities in both central and peripheral nervous system disorders. In addition, weakness may be the result of force modulation deficits or disuse.[11] Balance is directly affected by loss of strength. For example, weakness of the hip extensors and abductors will impede successful use of a hip strategy for upright trunk control. Initially adequate toe clearance may diminish with fatigue. Many clients with neurological issues also have stiffness and contractures as a result of persistent weakness or hypertonus. Restrictions in ROM also limit balance abilities.

The ability to achieve static postural alignment, although necessary for normal balance, is not sufficient to allow volitional functions. Adequate strength (to control body weight and any additional loads) through normal postural sway ranges is needed to permit dynamic balance activities such as reaching, leaning, and lifting. Postural control demands are increased during gait because the forces of momentum and the interaction between recruitment, timing, and velocity also must be regulated.[23] Traditionally considered orthopedic problems, deficits in strength, ROM, posture, and endurance have a great impact on balance abilities. Attention must be given to these musculoskeletal system problems in examination of and intervention for clients with neurological diagnoses.

Influence of Other Systems

Balance abilities are also influenced by other systems. Attention, cognition and judgment, and memory are critical for optimal balance function and are often impaired in hemiplegic and head-injured clients as well as those who have progressive neurological disorders. Attentional deficits reduce awareness of environmental hazards and opportunities, interfering with anticipatory postural control.[12] When balance is threatened, an inability to allocate attention to the necessary task of balance versus a secondary, less necessary task increases the risk of falls. Cognitive problems such as distractibility, poor judgment, and slowed processing also increase the risk of falls. Memory loss may preclude recall of safety measures. Depression, emotional lability, agitation, or denial of impairments also can increase the risks for loss of balance. In addition to having a direct impact on balance abilities themselves, these cognitive and behavioral problems impede motor learning processes, which are crucial for the relearning of balance skills.

Constant Cyclic Nature

The systems model of postural control previously presented illustrates the constant cycle that simultaneously occurs at many levels. Attention and intention allow feed-forward processing for active sensory search of the environment and motor planning, both of which are needed for anticipatory postural control. Movements are initiated and executed with resultant sensory experiences and error detection, or feedback. Successful movements are repeated and refined; unsuccessful ones are modified. The nature of this cycle presents the clinician with opportunities for intervention after the appropriate examination of sensory, motor, and cognitive functions. Through feedback and practice, balance abilities can improve.[24]

Motor Components of Balance

Reflexes

Many levels of neuromuscular control must be functioning to produce normal postural movements. At the most basic level, reflexes and righting reactions support postural orientation. The VOR and the vestibulospinal reflex (VSR) contribute to orientation of the eyes, head, and body to self and environment.[10]

When motion of the head is identified by the semicircular canals, it triggers a response within the oculomotor system called the *vestibuloocular reflex.* This causes the eyes to move in the opposite direction of the head but at the same speed. Stimulation of the otoliths drives the eyes to respond to linear head movement. Quick movements of the head will trigger the VOR.[25]

The VOR allows the coordination of eye and head movements. When the eyes are fixed on an object while the head is moving, the VOR supports gaze stabilization. Visuo-ocular responses often work concurrently with the VOR. They permit "smooth pursuit" when the head is fixed while the eyes move and visual tracking when both the eyes and the head move simultaneously.[10]

The VSR helps control movement and stabilize the body. Both the semicircular canals and the otoliths activate and modulate muscles of the neck, trunk, and extremities after head movement to maintain balance. The VSR permits stability of the body when the head moves and is important for the coordination of the trunk over the extremities in upright postures. Righting reactions support the orientation of the head in relation to the trunk and the head position relative to gravity and include labyrinthine head righting, optical head righting, and body-on-head righting.[10]

Automatic Postural Responses

At the next level, automatic postural responses operate to keep the COG over the base of support. They are a set of functionally organized, long-loop responses that act to keep the body in a state of equilibrium.[3,4] *Functionally organized* means that the responses, although stereotypical, are matched to the perturbing stimulus in direction and amplitude. If the stimulus is a push to the right, the response is a shift to the left, toward midline. The larger the stimulus, the greater the response. Automatic postural responses always occur in response to an unexpected stimulus and are typically triggered by somatosensory inputs. Because they occur rapidly, in less than 250 ms, they are not under immediate volitional control.

Four automatic postural responses have been described. Ankle strategy describes postural sway control from the ankles and feet. The head and hips travel in the same direction at the same time, with the body moving as a unit over the feet (Figure 22-2, *A*). Muscle contractile patterns are from distal to proximal (i.e., gastrocnemius, hamstrings, paraspinals). This strategy is used when sway is small, slow, and near midline. It occurs when the surface is broad and stable enough to allow pressure against it to produce forces that can counteract sway to stabilize the body. Ankle strategy is typically used to control anterior-posterior sway, because most of the degrees of freedom at the ankle are in this direction.

Hip strategy involves postural sway control from the pelvis and trunk. The head and hips travel in opposite directions, with body segment movements counteracting one another (Figure 22-2, *B*). Muscle contractile patterns are from proximal to distal (i.e., abdominals, quadriceps, tibialis anterior). This strategy is observed when sway is large, fast, and nearing the limit of stability or if the surface is too narrow or unstable to permit effective counterpressure of the feet against the surface. Hip strategy is used to control both anterior-posterior and medial-lateral sway. Hip strategy in the medial-lateral direction involves weight shifts from foot to foot; any client with difficulty weight-shifting quickly and accurately will have difficulty with medial-lateral hip strategy.

Suspensory strategy involves a lowering of the COG toward the base of support by bilateral lower-extremity flexion or a slight squatting motion (Figure 22-2, *C*). By shortening the distance between the COG and the base of support, the task of controlling the COG is made easier. This strategy is often used when a combination of stability and mobility is required, as in windsurfing.

Stepping and reaching strategies involve steps with the feet or reaches with the arms in an attempt to reestablish a new base of support with the active limb(s) when the COG

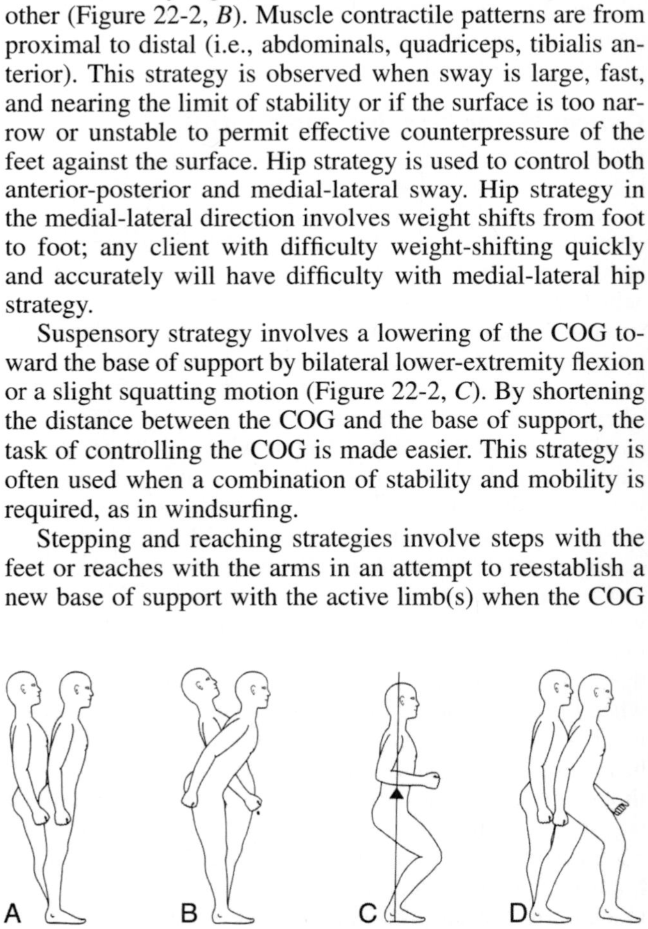

Figure 22-2 ■ Automatic postural responses. **A,** Ankle strategy. **B,** Hip strategy. **C,** Suspensory strategy. **D,** Stepping strategy. (From Hasson S: *Clinical exercise physiology,* St Louis, 1994, Mosby.)

has exceeded the original base of support (Figure 22-2, *D*). A successful stepping strategy is the best way to avoid a fall after a slip or trip.

Misconceptions about these APR strategies are common. First, these strategies do not function in daily life as separately as they are described in the early research literature. In quiet standing, for example, frequency analysis of unperturbed postural sway in healthy adults reveals that both ankle and hip strategies occur in combination, simultaneously.[26] In perturbation studies, mixed use of strategies is often seen unless the perturbation is clearly below or above certain-sized thresholds. Second, these strategies occur in response to disturbances from all directions, not just in pure anterior-posterior or medial-lateral directions.[27] Third, although these strategies are stereotypical in humans, great individual variation in strategy selection and performance comes from other influential factors. For example, many people use stepping strategy for most perturbations unless specifically instructed not to step or unless the conditions do not permit a step. An anxious person may reach or step much sooner than a relaxed person with similar physical deficits. Last, all these strategies do *not* occur in sequence with every balance disturbance.[28,29] In other words, individuals normally do not try ankle strategy and wait until it fails before trying hip strategy, then wait until it fails before trying stepping strategy (although early learning may involve such exploration). Because these responses must occur extremely rapidly to prevent balance loss, such a sequential approach would be inefficient and ineffective. Instead, the normal response is the emergence of the single strategy best suited to the particular perturbation, the limitations of the individual, and the conditions in the environment.

Abnormal use of automatic postural responses is often observed in individuals with neurological disorders. Clients with vestibular deficits typically rely on ankle strategy, which permits the head to remain aligned with the body and sustains congruence between vestibular and somatosensory inputs. Use of hip strategy may be modified or limited because when the head is moving in the opposite direction as the COG, vestibular and somatosensory inputs are not congruent. Activities that require use of hip strategy, such as standing in tandem or on one leg, can be a problem for clients with bilateral vestibular loss or an uncompensated vestibular lesion. However, some cases involve excessive use of hip strategy on a level surface (when an ankle strategy would suffice).[30] This may reflect abnormal integration of the somatosensory and vestibular information. If peripheral somatosensation is impaired, as in diabetic neuropathy, or central sensory weighting of somatosensory inputs is inadequate, hip strategy may dominate.

Clients with somatosensory loss, distal lower extremity weakness or hypertonus, restricted ankle ROM, and/or reduced limits of stability typically rely on hip strategy. This occurs because the client cannot feel the surface or the feet well enough to modulate foot pressure against the surface, because the person cannot generate sufficient force against the surface with the ankle muscles, or because restricted ankle ROM prevents COG sway. The use of hip strategy is normal when the COG is at or near the limits of stability and a step is either not possible or not desired.

When the hip or ankle strategy is not efficient enough to control the movement of the center of pressure, or if conditions and instructions permit a stepping response, stepping strategy may be preferred. Individuals who are fearful of falling often perceive even slight body sway as threatening instability. They may use stepping and reaching strategies exclusively whether or not these "rescue" strategies are actually necessary.

Anticipatory Postural Adjustments

Anticipatory postural adjustments are similar to automatic postural responses, but they occur before the actual disturbance.[20] If a balance disturbance is predicted, the body will respond in advance by developing a "postural set" to counteract the coming forces. For example, if an individual lifts an empty suitcase thinking it is full and heavy, the anticipatory forces generated before the lift (to counter the anticipated weight) will cause excessive movement and brief instability. Failure to produce these anticipatory adjustments increases the risk of sudden balance loss, creating the need to use rapid, reactive automatic postural responses to prevent a fall. For clients with deficits in reaction time or automatic postural responses, superior use of anticipatory postural control can help the client avoid the unexpected perturbations that make automatic postural responses necessary.

In balance laboratories, anticipatory postural adjustments are studied using electromyography so that muscle activity before observable movement can be measured. In the clinic, problems with anticipatory adjustments may be observed when the client fails to counteract a predicted disturbance, such as "don't let me push you backward," or fails to integrate postural control tasks during other activities, such as the inability to step smoothly over an anticipated obstacle during gait or inability to maintain sitting balance when both arms are intentionally lifted overhead.

Volitional Postural Movements

Volitional postural movements are under conscious control. Weight shifts to allow an individual to reach the telephone or put the dishes in the dishwasher, for example, are self-initiated disturbances of the COG to accomplish a goal. Volitional postural movements can range from simple weight shifts to complex balance skills of skaters and gymnasts. They can occur after a stimulus or be self-initiated. Volitional postural movements can occur quickly or slowly, depending on the goal at hand. The more complex or unfamiliar the task, the slower the response time. Use of a variety of movements that might successfully achieve a goal is possible. Volitional postural movements are strongly modified by prior experience and instruction. Automatic and anticipatory postural responses allow the continuous unconscious control of balance, whereas volitional postural movements permit conscious activity. This level of postural motor control is the most frequently tested and treated in clinical practice, but it is by no means sufficient by itself to produce normal balance.

CLINICAL ASSESSMENT OF BALANCE

Objectives of Testing

When present, activity limitations need to be identified and measured. Functional scales are typically used to determine the presence and severity of these limitations, not necessarily why those limitations exist. From these functional tests, decisions can be made about whether to treat and, if so, what tasks need to be practiced. If treatment is indicated, clinicians must make judgments about what to treat. Further testing to identify and measure impairments is then necessary to know what systems are involved. A comprehensive evaluation of balance includes both functional and impairment tests.[12]

No single quick-and-easy test of balance can adequately cover the many multidimensional aspects of balance, although many such tests have great value as screening tools. However, a comprehensive test battery, called the Balance Evaluation Systems Test (BESTest), based on the systems model has been developed that provides clinicians with a thorough examination at the impairment level (Figure 22-3).[31] The BESTest takes more time to administer than, for example, a single-leg stance test, but results from the BESTest give the clinician a far more complete and accurate picture of the client's balance impairments than any single-item test or screening test can. Armed with these results, the clinician can develop interventions specifically targeted to the impaired systems. For clients whose primary problems include imbalance, the clinician's investment of time to perform this comprehensive test battery yields a valuable outcome. A shorter version of this test, the mini-BESTest, has subsequently been published.[32] It takes less time to administer but likewise provides a less complete picture of the client's balance systems. Specifically, it does not include any items from the biomechanical constraints or stabilities limits categories. Even so, it is superior to single-item tests or screening tests that are not based on the systems model and do not identify balance system impairments that should be addressed in the intervention plan.

No single, simple test for balance is possible because balance is such a complex sensorimotor process.[33] Many relatively simple balance tests exist, but not all tests are appropriate for all clients. Different tests may be needed to answer specific questions. For example, several good tests have been developed to determine the risk of falls in elderly people. These would be insufficient to discern whether an injured dancer can resume practice or an injured roofer is ready to return to work. Clinicians should understand the advantages and limitations of different balance tests to be able to select appropriate evaluative tools.

In general, a balance test will not be useful unless it sufficiently challenges the postural control system being tested. Tests for stability ("static balance") are appropriate for clients who are having difficulty simply finding midline or holding still in sitting or standing. They are of much less value for clients with higher-level abilities. Conversely, single-leg stance tests or sensory tests with a foam surface may be far too difficult for clients with lower-level abilities to perform.

A word of caution about interpreting test results is indicated. Most clinical tests rely on observations of motor behavior to arrive at some conclusion about what systems have problems and how they affect movement. Abnormal motor behavior has many causes, and clinicians should be careful before concluding that an observed behavior is caused by problems in a certain system. For example, the Romberg test is commonly assumed to test the use of vestibular inputs. Yet during the test, both somatosensory and vestibular inputs are (normally) used for balance control. If balance control is deficient, is the vestibular system necessarily the culprit? Could somatosensory system deficits also result in a poor test result? Or, alternatively, because the Romberg test is performed with feet together, what effect would hip weakness have on the ability to stand with a narrowed base of support? When using a test whose results may be altered by problems in more than one system, any relevant system should be evaluated. If multiple system deficits exist, and they often do in clients with neurological conditions, then use caution in making "commonly assumed" conclusions on the basis of clinical test results.

Because so many balance tests are available, several questions must be asked to determine whether a test is appropriate for use.[33] For what purpose and population was the test designed? Can that test be used legitimately for a different purpose or with a different population? Is it valid? Is it repeatable by different examiners or by the same examiner multiple times? Are results reliable? In what populations are they reliable? What is the threshold for this test—that is, how large must performance changes be before this test can detect them? Are normative data available for comparison? These questions are being investigated but have not yet been answered for many of the clinical balance tests commonly used by therapists with the many different neurological populations they treat. Some of the evidence already reported may be frustrating to clinicians. For example, the Timed Up-and-Go test (TUG) predicts falls in community-dwelling older adults but not in acute-care hospital populations.[34,35] For several balance tests such as the Functional Reach Test, the Berg Balance Scale, and others, the cutoff scores used for accurate prediction of falls in clients with Parkinson disease are different from the cutoff scores used in older adults without Parkinson disease.[36] These examples make it clear that clinicians must understand their clients and the characteristics of the various balance tests in order to select the most appropriate tests and interpret test results for each client.

Types of Balance Tests

Balance tests can be grouped or classified by type. Different types of tests measure different facets of postural control (Table 22-1). Quiet standing (static) refers to tests in which the client is standing and the movement goal is to hold still. Disturbances to balance, called *perturbations,* may or may not be applied. Active standing (dynamic) tests also position the patient standing, but the movement goal involves voluntary weight shifting. Sensory manipulation tests use altered surface and visual conditions to determine how well the CNS is using and reweighting sensory inputs for postural control. Functional balance, mobility, and gait scales involve the performance of whole-body movement tasks, such as sitting to standing, walking, and stepping over objects. A few test batteries offer a combination of the preceding tests. The BESTest is the most comprehensive test battery to date. Dual-task tests have been developed to examine the effect of concurrent activities and divided attention on balance and mobility performance. A commonly accepted test for sitting balance in adults is not yet available, although clients with neurological problems often need sitting balance retraining in early stages. Clinicians typically modify standing tests or pediatric sitting tests to assess sitting balance in adult clients with neurological conditions. For example, the Functional Reach Test has been used to measure excursion in seated individuals with spinal cord injuries.[37]

I. Biomechanical Constraints	1. Base of support	2. CoM alignment	3. Ankle strength and ROM	4. Hip/trunk lateral strength	5. Sit on floor and stand up		
II. Stability Limits/Verticality	6. Sitting verticality (left and right) and lateral lean (left and right)	7. Functional reach forward	8. Functional reach lateral (left and right)				
III. Anticipatory Postural Adjustments	**9.** Sit to stand	**10.** Rise to toes	**11.** Stand on one leg (left and right)	12. Alternate stair touching	13. Standing arm raise		
IV. Postural Responses	14. In-place response, forward	15. In-place response, backward	**16.** Compensatory stepping correction, forward	**17.** Compensatory stepping correction, backward	**18.** Compensatory stepping correction, lateral (left and right)		
V. Sensory Orientation	**19.** Sensory integration on balance (modified CTSIB). **A:** Stance on firm surface EO, B: stance on firm surface EC, C: stance on foam EO, **D:** stance on foam EC			**20.** Incline, EC			
VI. Stability in Gait	21. Gait, level surface	**22.** Change in gait speed	**23.** Walk with head turns, horizontal	**24.** Walk with pivot turns	**25.** Step over obstacles	26. Timed "Get up & Go" Test	**27.** Timed "Get up & Go" Test with dual task

Figure 22-3 ■ Balance Evaluation Systems Test (BESTest) with modifications of both long and short forms. Short form identified by 14 components shown in BOLD. *CoM,* Center of mass; *CTSIB,* Clinical Test of Sensory Integration on Balance; *EC,* eyes closed; *EO,* eyes open; *ROM,* range of motion. (Data from Horak FB, et al: *Phys Ther* 89:484–498, 2009.)

TABLE 22-1 ■ TYPES OF BALANCE TESTS

TYPE	TESTS
Quiet standing (with or without perturbation)	Romberg Sharpened Romberg or tandem Romberg One-legged stance test (OLST) Timed stance battery Postural sway Nudge or push Postural Stress Test Motor Control Test
Active standing	Functional Reach Test Multi-Directional Reach Test Limits of stability
Sensory manipulation	Sensory Organization Test (SOT) Clinical Test of Sensory Interaction and Balance (CTSIB)
Vestibular	Vertiginous positions Hallpike-Dix maneuver Nystagmus Semicircular canal function Visual-vestibular interaction Visual acuity Oculomotor tests Fukuda Stepping Test Dizziness Handicap Inventory
Functional scales	Berg Balance Scale Timed Up-and-Go Test Tinetti Performance-Oriented Assessment of Balance Tinetti Performance-Oriented Assessment of Gait Gait Assessment Rating Scale (GARS) Dynamic Gait Index Functional Gait Assessment
Combination test batteries	Fregly-Graybiel Ataxia Test Battery Fugl-Meyer Sensorimotor Assessment of Balance Performance
Dual task	Stops walking when talking Multiple Tasks Test

Quiet Standing

The classic Romberg test was originally developed to "examine the effect of posterior column disease upon upright stance."[38] The client stands with feet parallel and together and then closes the eyes for 20 to 30 seconds. The examiner subjectively judges the amount of sway. Quantification of sway can be accomplished with a videotape, forceplate, or, more recently, accelerometer.[39,40] Excessive sway, loss of balance, or stepping during this test is abnormal. The sharpened Romberg,[38] also known as the *tandem Romberg,* requires the client to stand with feet in a heel-to-toe position and arms folded across the chest, eyes closed for 60 seconds. Often four trials of this test are timed with a stopwatch, for a maximum score of 240 seconds.

One-legged stance tests (OLSTs) are commonly used.[38,41] Both legs must be alternately tested, and differences between sides are noted. The client stands on both feet and places hands on the hips or crosses the arms over the chest, then picks up one leg and holds it with the hip in neutral and the knee flexed to 90 degrees. The lifted leg may *not* be pressed into the stance leg. This test is scored with a stopwatch. Five 30-second trials are performed for each leg (alternating legs), with a maximum possible score of 150 seconds per leg. Normal young subjects are able to stand for 30 seconds, but this may not be a reasonable expectation for frail older clients.[38]

In both the Romberg test and the OLST, problems in sensory organization processes can be observed. To determine how much of the stability is achieved through visual stabilization, each test can be repeated with eyes closed. The client with visual dependency for balance will often have an immediate loss of balance when the eyes are closed. (Remember, visual dependency may be a sign of somatosensory or vestibular loss, or both.) As noted earlier, the client with somatosensory or vestibular loss may have difficulty producing the hip strategy necessary to perform these tasks.

A battery of timed stance tests has been developed by Bohannon and Leary.[42] This set of tests varies the foot position (apart, together, tandem, and single leg) and the availability of visual information (eyes open and closed) to produce eight different combinations. Maintenance of balance in each condition is timed for a maximum of 30 seconds; the assigned score is the total number of seconds that balance could be maintained. The best possible score on this test is 240 seconds. This test is reliable, valid, and sensitive to change over time.[42]

A related test is the Balance Error Scoring System, or BESS test, which was developed for use with athletes to screen for concussion effects.[43,44] The original BESS test involved three stance positions (double-leg stance with feet together, single-leg stance, tandem stance) on two surfaces (firm and foam), thus providing six conditions. The eyes are closed in all conditions. Each trial is 20 seconds in duration. The examiner observes and counts the number of balance errors that are made in each condition. The six observed errors include hands lifted off waist; opening eyes; step, stumble, or balance loss; moving a hip past 30 degrees of abduction; lifting the forefoot or heel; and remaining out of the test position for more than 5 seconds. If more than one error occurs at the same time, for example, opening eyes and hands off waist, only one error is counted. When measured in high-level young adults, the reliability of this test improved with the removal of the double-leg stance condition, which produced few to no errors in this high-functioning population, and the addition of three trials in each of the remaining four conditions. The modified BESS test thus includes only four conditions.[45] This test has not been investigated for use in traditional neurological rehabilitation populations.

Objective postural sway measures can be obtained by computerized force plates (Figure 22-4) or wearable accelerometers (Figure 22-5).[40,46-48] The client is asked to adopt a standardized foot placement if possible (this varies by manufacturer) and to stand quietly with arms at the sides or hands on hips for 20 or 30 seconds. Sway with both eyes open and eyes closed is commonly measured. Graphic and numerical quantification is provided. Normative data may be provided. These more technical measures are able to detect more subtle problems and are more sensitive to change in performance after treatment than are rating scales or timed measures.

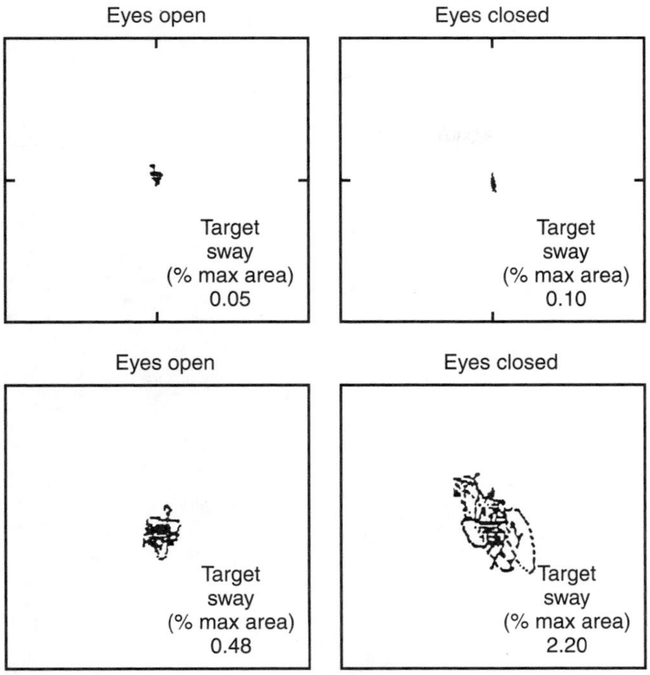

Figure 22-4 ■ Graphic and numerical postural sway measures using a computerized force plate system. *Top left,* Normal subject, eyes open. *Top right,* Healthy subject, eyes closed. *Bottom left,* Client with Parkinson disease, eyes open. *Bottom right,* Client with Parkinson disease, eyes closed. (Reprinted with permission from NeuroCom International, Clackamas, Ore.)

Automatic postural responses are assessed by the client's response to perturbations. It is imperative that clinicians include APR testing in their balance assessment because APRs are the motor responses necessary to prevent loss of balance and falls. The push-and-release test is a clinically useful method with a five-point ordinal rating scale.[31,49,50] Testing for ankle and hip strategies ("in-place" strategies) requires that the clinician (1) place his or her hands on the front or back of the patient's shoulders, (2) ask the patient to remain still and centered by resisting the pressure applied by the hands (producing isometric muscle activity), (3) watch for the toes or heels to begin to raise slightly (the clinician increases pressure until this occurs), then (4) suddenly release the push. Both forward and backward directions are tested; the clinician always stands where he or she can support the client in case of balance loss. Testing for stepping strategy follows the same concept but is performed differently. Instead of keeping the client's COG at midline, the client leans his or her weight into the clinician's hands, shifting the COG away from midline toward the outer limit of stability before the release. The correct client response is to step to reestablish a new base of support underneath the new position of the COG. Forward, backward, and both lateral directions are tested. When nudge or push tests are performed predictably (i.e., "don't let me push you backward"), this is assessment of anticipatory postural control. When the release happens unpredictably (no cues, unpredictable timing), automatic postural responses can be assessed. Perturbations of different strengths from multiple different directions should be given.

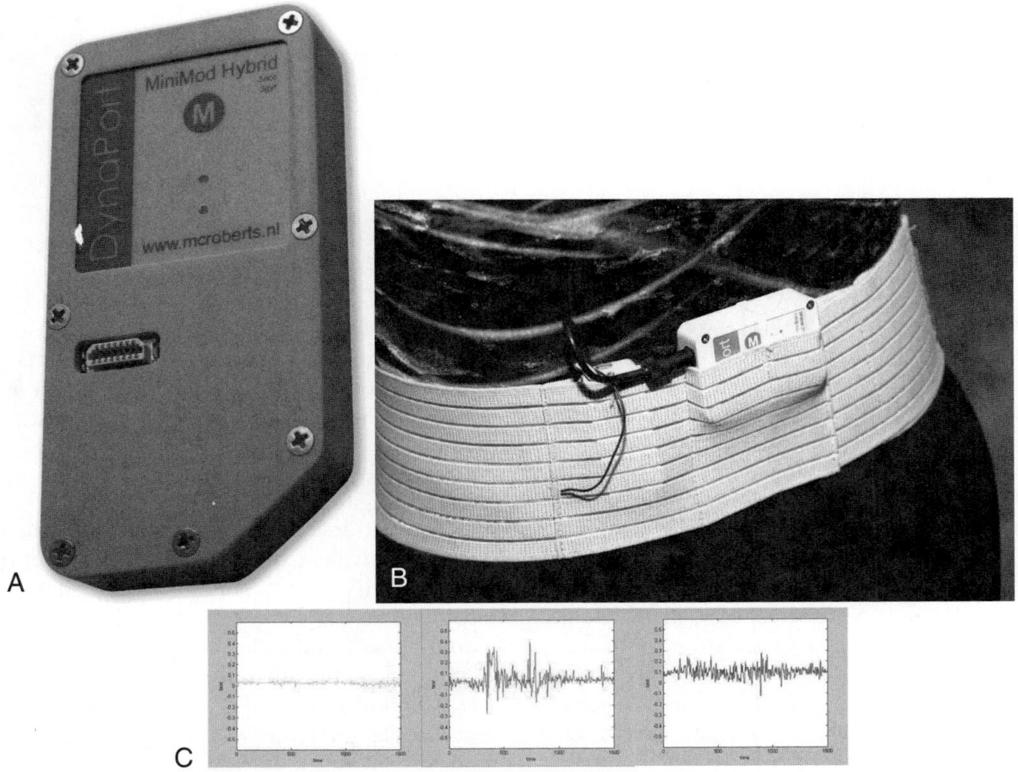

Figure 22-5 ■ **A,** A wearable accelerometer for motion detection that can be used to measure postural sway and other physical motions. **B,** The accelerometer worn in a belt at the L5-S1 level. **C,** Postural sway data recorded by the accelerometer. (Photographs courtesy McRoberts B, The Hague, The Netherlands.)

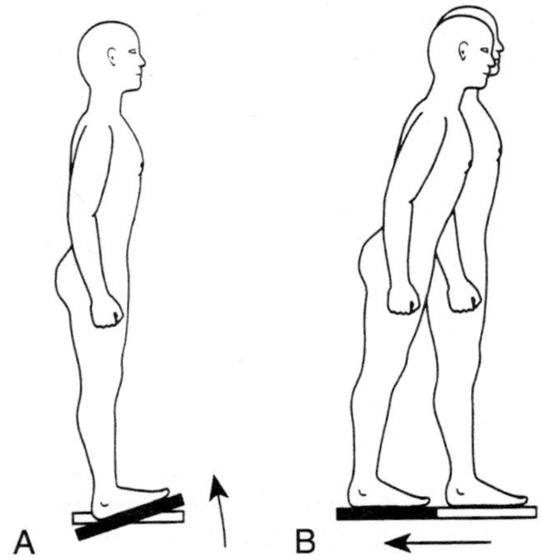

Figure 22-6 ■ Surface perturbations during **(A)** the adaptation test and **(B)** the motor control test using computerized dynamic posturography. Force plate measures include latency and amount of response and adaptation of the response to repeated perturbations. (From Hasson S: *Clinical exercise physiology,* St Louis, 1994, Mosby.)

The Motor Control Test (MCT) is a computerized test of automatic postural responses that perturbs the client through surface displacement (Figure 22-6, *B*).[3] The client stands on a dynamic (movable) forceplate with feet parallel and arms at sides. The support surface rapidly translates (slides) forward or backward. This surface displacement results in a rapid shift in the relation between the COG and the base of support. The expected responses are directionally specific (to the direction of the stimulus) forces generated against the surface to bring the COG back to the center. Response latencies, strength, and symmetry are measured. Normative data are available. This test can be used to look for abnormal stepping strategies when failure to select hip strategy occurs. The MCT is the most standardized and reliable test of automatic postural responses, but it is not widely used because it requires computerized equipment.

Active Standing

Volitional control of the COG is evaluated by asking the client to make voluntary movements that require weight shifting. The Functional Reach Test was developed for use with older adults to determine risk of falls.[51] The client stands near a wall with feet parallel. Attached to the wall at shoulder height is a yardstick. The client is asked to make a fist and raise the arm nearest the wall to 90 degrees of shoulder flexion. The examiner notes the position of the fist on the yardstick. The client is then asked to lean forward as far as possible, and the examiner notes the end position of the fist on the yardstick (Figure 22-7). Beginning position is subtracted from end position to obtain a change unit in inches. Three trials are performed. Normative data are available, and the test is reliable. However, the standard error of measurement for this test may be as high as 2 inches, meaning that a change in score of less than 2 inches cannot be attributed to clinical improvement because it may reflect only measurement error. Subsequent studies have not shown that this test is useful for fall prediction.[52-54]

One serious limitation of the Functional Reach Test is that it measures sway in only one direction (forward). An expansion of this test has been devised to measure sway in four directions.[55] The multidirectional reach test is conceptually equivalent but measures sway anteriorly, posteriorly, and laterally to both sides. This test should provide a more comprehensive picture of volitional COG control limitations. Validity and mean values have been established for community-dwelling older adults.[56]

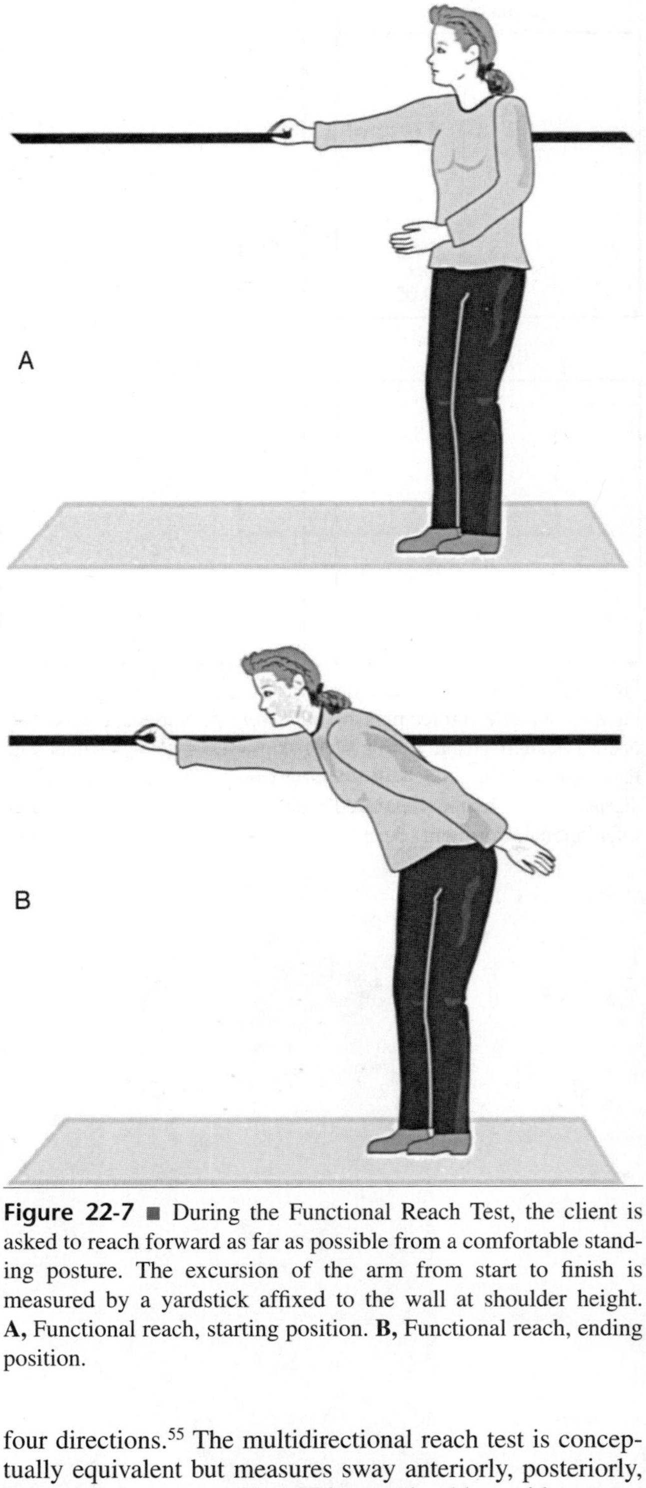

Figure 22-7 ■ During the Functional Reach Test, the client is asked to reach forward as far as possible from a comfortable standing posture. The excursion of the arm from start to finish is measured by a yardstick affixed to the wall at shoulder height. **A,** Functional reach, starting position. **B,** Functional reach, ending position.

The limits of stability test uses a computerized forceplate to measure postural sway away from midline in eight directions.[46,57] Clients assume a standardized foot position and control a cursor on the computer monitor by shifting their weight. They are asked to move the cursor from midline to eight targets on the screen (Figure 22-8). Measures include movement velocity, directional control (path sway), measures

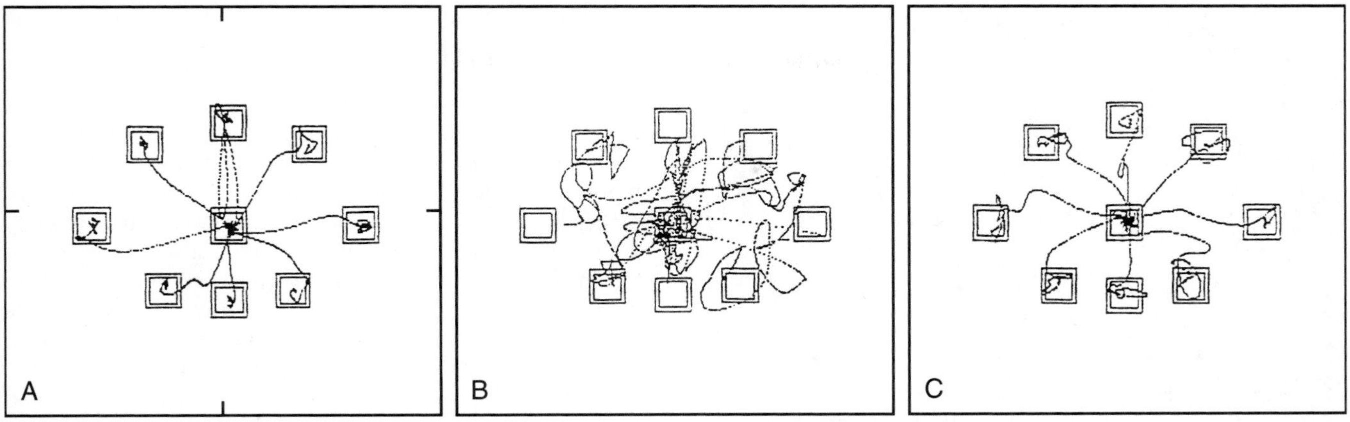

Figure 22-8 ■ Graphic postural sway measures from the limits of stability test using a computerized force plate system (numerical measures not shown). Clients are asked to move away from and return to midline. **A,** Subject with normal postural sway. **B,** Hemiplegic client on initial evaluation. **C,** Hemiplegic client on discharge evaluation. (Reprinted with permission from NeuroCom International, Clackamas, Ore.)

of excursion (length of the trajectory of the COG), and reaction time. This test should be performed once for familiarization, then a second time for scoring purposes. Second and subsequent tests are reliable. Normative data are available.

A very challenging test used primarily in athletic populations is the Star Excursion Balance Test (SEBT) (Figure 22-9).[58,59] The SEBT could be used, for example, in high-level traumatic brain injury (TBI) clients who require more demanding test conditions. However, although there is evidence for the validity and reliability of this test in orthopedic populations, as yet this test has not been investigated for use in neurological populations. The SEBT is in concept a lower-extremity functional reach test, requiring single-leg stance on one leg and a reach with the other leg. The original SEBT included eight directions; currently the SEBT is typically performed in three directions: center-forward, right-rear, and left-rear.[60] Three tape measures are taped to the floor, radiating out from the same center point. The two rear tape measures are at a 45-degree angle from the center line. The client stands on one foot with the great toe on the center point, then reaches the maximum distance away from the center with the lifted foot. The distance is recorded by the examiner. This is done in all three directions, with the lifted leg having to cross behind the stance leg to reach to the opposite-side rear tape. Six practice trials in each direction are given before recording scores to eliminate a learning effect, although recent evidence suggests four practice trials may be sufficient.[61] Three scored trials in each direction are performed. Both legs are tested.[61a]

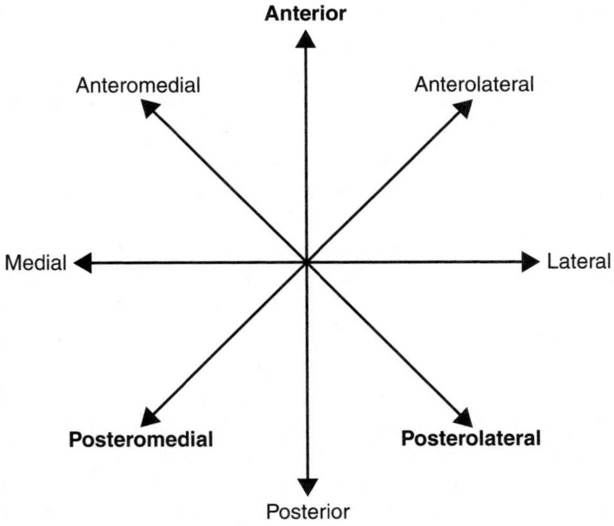

Figure 22-9 ■ The floor grid layout for the original Star Excursion Balance Test (SEBT) with eight directions. Bolded arrows in the anterior, posteromedial, and posterolateral directions indicate the three directions used in the modified SEBT. (From Brumitt J: Assessing athletic balance with the Star Excursion Balance Test. *NSCA Perform Train J* 7:6, 2008.)

Sensory Manipulation

Sensory inputs play a critical role in postural control, but few tests to measure their use to produce a balance performance outcome have been developed. The Sensory Organization Test (SOT) uses a computerized, movable forceplate and movable visual surround to alter the surface and visual environments systematically.[3,4] The client stands on the forceplate with feet parallel and arms at the sides and is asked to stand quietly. Three 20-second trials under each of six sensory conditions are performed (Figure 22-10). In conditions one, two, and three the support surface (forceplate) is fixed. During conditions four, five, and six the support surface is sway referenced to the sway of the client. In other words, the movement of the surface is matched to the movement of the client in a 1:1 ratio. This responsive surface movement maintains a near-constant ankle joint angle despite body sway, rendering the somatosensory information from the feet and ankles inaccurate for use in balance maintenance. Visual inputs are undisturbed in conditions one and four. Vision is absent (eyes closed) in conditions two and five. The movable visual surround is sway referenced in conditions three and six. This responsive visual surround movement maintains a near-constant distance between the eyes and the visual environment despite body sway, rendering visual inputs from

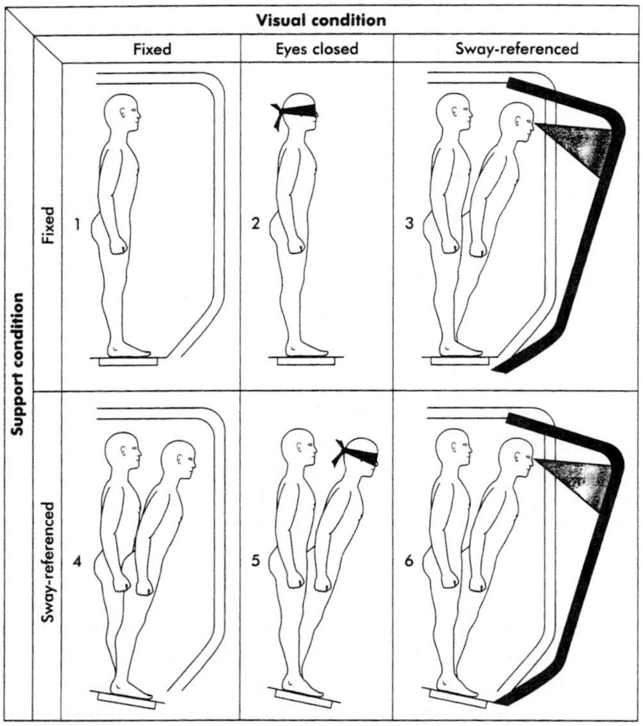

Figure 22-10 ■ The six Sensory Organization Test conditions. The Sensory Organization Test determines the relative reliance on visual, vestibular, and somatosensory inputs for postural control using computerized dynamic posturography. (From Hasson S: *Clinical exercise physiology,* St Louis, 1994, Mosby.)

the eyes inaccurate for balance maintenance in those two conditions.

Under condition one, all three senses (vision, vestibular sense, and somatosensory sense) are available and accurate. Body sway is measured by the forceplate; this initial measurement forms the baseline against which subsequent measures are compared (Figure 22-11). Under condition two the eyes are closed, so only somatosensory and vestibular cues remain. In an individual with normal movement function, the somatosensory inputs will dominate in this condition. By comparing sway during condition two with sway during condition one, detection of how well the client is using somatosensory inputs for balance control is possible. Clients with somatosensory loss from spinal cord injury, diabetes, or amputation have difficulty in condition two. Functional situations with inadequate lighting or unusable visual cues (e.g., busy carpeting) are similar to condition two.

Under condition four, the support surface is sway referenced (somatosensory cues are available but are inaccurate), so only visual and vestibular cues remain useful. In a normal client the visual inputs will dominate in this condition. Comparing sway during condition four with sway during condition one indicates how well the client is using visual inputs for balance control. Clients with visual loss caused by diabetes, cataracts, or field loss have difficulty in condition four. Functional situations that correlate with condition four include compliant surfaces (beach, soft ground, gravel driveway) and unstable surfaces (boat deck, slipping throw rug).

Under condition five, the eyes are closed (visual cues are absent) and the support surface is sway referenced (somatosensory cues are inaccurate), leaving the vestibular inputs as the only remaining sense that is both available and accurate. Comparison of sway during condition five with sway during condition one indicates how well the client is using vestibular inputs for balance control. Clients with vestibular loss caused by head injury, MS, or acoustic neuroma may have difficulty with condition five. Many elderly clients also may be unstable in this condition. Functional situations in which these clients may be at risk for falls would have both inadequate lighting and compliant or unsteady surfaces (e.g., walking on a gravel driveway or thick carpet in the dark).

Under both conditions three and six, the visual surround is sway referenced (visual cues are available but inaccurate). By comparing sway during these two conditions with sway in the absence of vision (conditions two and five, with eyes closed), determining how well the client can recognize and subsequently suppress inaccurate visual inputs when they conflict with somatosensory and vestibular cues is possible. Some clients with CNS lesions (e.g., head injury, stroke, tumor) may have difficulty with this condition. Clients who cannot recognize and ignore inaccurate visual cues cannot distinguish whether they are moving or the environment is moving. If they perceive that they are moving (away from midline) when they are not, they may often actively generate postural responses to "right" themselves. These responses, invoked to bring the COG to midline, then result in movement away from the midline. The inaccurate perception leads to a self-initiated loss of balance. Functional situations that correlate with this test condition include public transportation, grocery and library aisles, and moving walkways.

The SOT is valid and reliable in the absence of motoric problems, which increase sway for reasons unrelated to sensory reception and perception. Normative data are available.

The Clinical Test of Sensory Interaction on Balance (CTSIB) is a clinical version of the SOT that does not use computerized forceplate technology.[62] The concept of the six conditions remains intact (Figure 22-12). Instead of sway measures, the examiner uses a stopwatch and visual observation. A thick foam pad substitutes for the moving forceplate during conditions four, five, and six. In normal individuals and clients with peripheral vestibular lesions, measures with foam correlate to moving forceplate measures.[63] Originally, a modified Japanese lantern substituted for the moving visual surround in conditions three and six. Studies have not shown that measures using the Japanese lantern correlate with the moving visual surround measures. Most clinicians now perform the modified CTSIB with just four conditions, eyes open and closed on a firm surface and eyes open and closed on the foam surface. The client is asked to stand with feet parallel and arms at sides or hands on hips. At least three and up to five 30-second trials of each condition are performed.[18] The watch is stopped if the client steps, reaches, or falls during the 30 seconds. If the client is very steady for 30 seconds on the first trial of a condition, some clinicians choose not to test the remaining trials in that condition and will give the client a full score for that condition. A maximum score for five trials of each condition is 150 seconds. Individuals with normal movement abilities are able to stand without stepping, reaching, or exhibiting loss of balance for 30 seconds per trial per condition. It is

SENSORY ANALYSIS			
RATIO NAME	**TEST CONDITIONS**	**RATIO PAIR**	**SIGNIFICANCE**
SOM Somatosensory	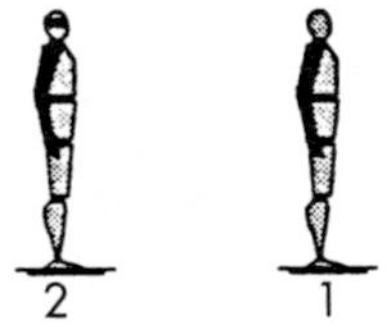 2 1	Condition 1 / Condition 2	Question: Does sway increase when visual cues are removed? Low scores: Patient makes poor use of somatosensory references.
VIS Visual	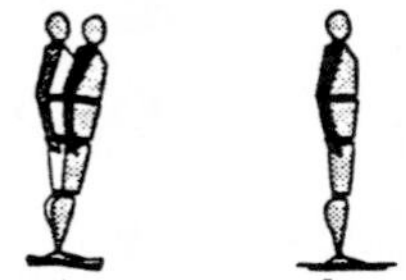 4 1	Condition 4 / Condition 1	Question: Does sway increase when somatosensory cues are inaccurate? Low scores: Patient makes poor use of visual references.
VEST Vestibular	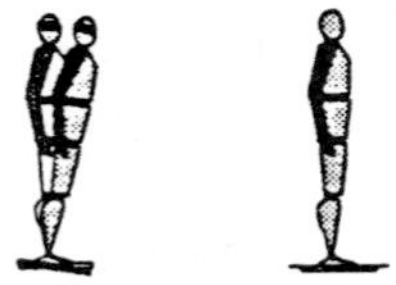 5 1	Condition 5 / Condition 1	Question: Does sway increase when visual cues are removed and somatosensory cues are inaccurate? Low scores: Patient makes poor use of vestibular cues, or vestibular cues unavailable.
PREF Visual Preference	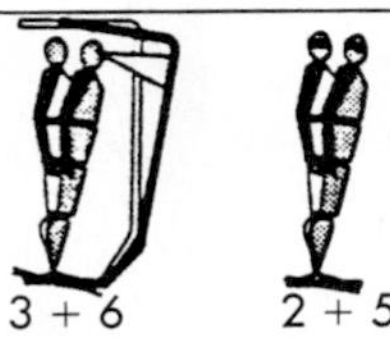 3 + 6 2 + 5	Condition 3 + 6 / Condition 2 + 5	Question: Do inaccurate visual cues result in increased sway compared to no visual cues? Low scores: Patient relies on visual cues even when they are inaccurate.

Figure 22-11 ■ Postural sway measures from each of the six Sensory Organization Test conditions are compared, and the ratios are used to identify impairments in the use of sensory inputs for postural control. (From Jacobson GP, Newman CW, Kartush JM: *Handbook of balance function testing,* St Louis, 1993, Mosby.)

normal for sway to increase slightly as the conditions increase in difficulty. The CTSIB may not be a reliable measure in clients with hemiplegia or other conditions that involve motor deficits in, or abnormal response time through, the lower extremities and trunk.[64] The clinician can use the information regarding client response in a variety of environmental conditions to determine intervention management strategies.[65]

Vestibular System Tests

Please refer to the vestibular section for a thorough presentation of vestibular disorders and their management.

Active Stepping

The ability to change the base of support without balance loss then to reestablish COG stability over the new base of support is a balance-dependent skill critical for functional activities. The four square step test is a timed stepping test in a standardized, structured format in forward, backward, and lateral directions (Figure 22-13).[66] A simple plus sign–shaped grid is laid out on the floor using four straight canes, dowel rods, or plastic piping. This creates four quadrants. The client begins standing in the rear-left quadrant, steps forward over the first bar to stand with both feet in the front-left quadrant, steps rightward over the second bar to stand with both feet in the right-front quadrant, steps backward over the third bar to stand with both feet in the right-rear quadrant, steps leftward over the fourth bar to stand with both feet in the left-rear quadrant (starting location), then reverses direction, going back through each quadrant in the same way until standing again with both feet in the rear-left quadrant. The outcome measure is the time it takes the client to perform this task correctly, clearing each bar completely with each foot. This test has been used with older adults, individuals with vestibular disorders, and clients poststroke.[67,68]

Functional Scales

A comprehensive balance evaluation must include both impairment-based tests of body systems and activity-based functional measures. Functional scales help address the activity limitations. By asking the client to perform functional tasks that demand balance skills, the clinician can determine the presence of activity limitations that will affect the individual's ability to participate in life, and identify the tasks that the client needs to practice. Three mobility scales and three gait scales focus on postural control; five of these were developed for the elderly population to determine risk of falls. Many clinicians are also using them to assess clients with neurological conditions, although their usefulness with neurological populations is less well-documented. Far fewer standardized tests for high-level balance skills have been developed; some clinicians adapt tests used by athletes, but

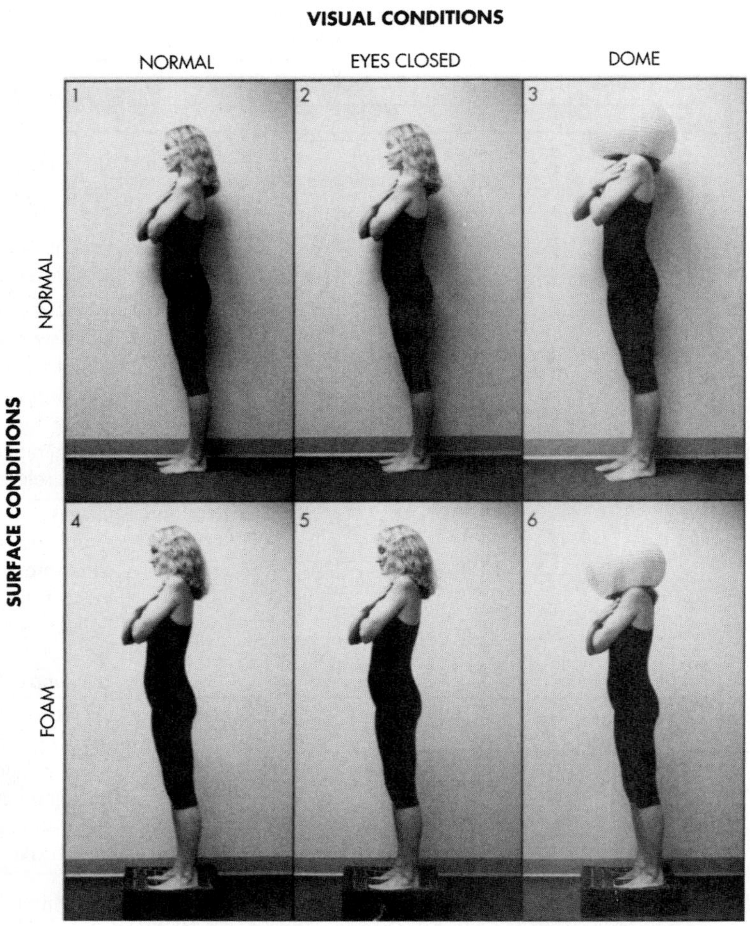

Figure 22-12 ■ The Clinical Test of Sensory Interactions on Balance uses foam and a Japanese lantern to replicate the six sensory conditions. A stopwatch is used to time trials.

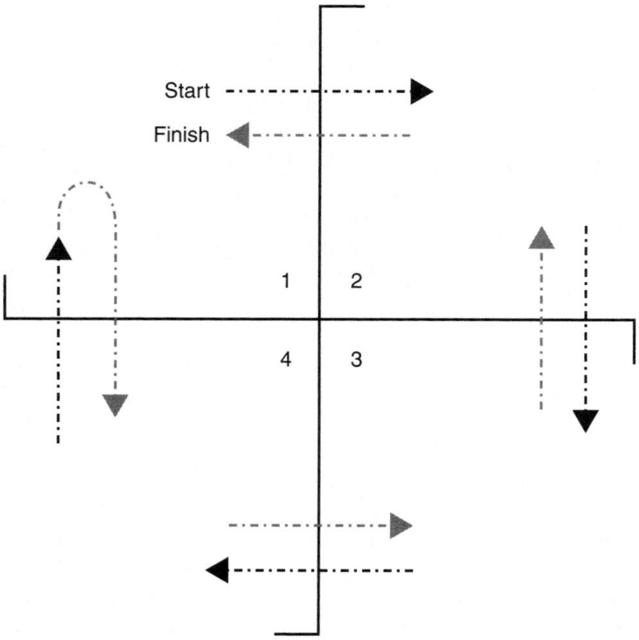

Figure 22-13 ■ The floor grid for the timed Four Square Step Test (FSST). *Arrows* indicate the direction of the steps. (From Dite W, Temple VA: A clinical test of stepping and change of direction to identify multiple falling older adults. *Arch Phys Med Rehabil* 83:1568, 2002.)

these are often too difficult for many neurologically involved clients.

The Berg Balance Scale consists of 14 tasks that the client is asked to perform.[69] The examiner rates the client on each task by using an ordinal rating scale of 0 to 4, in which 0 is unable to perform and 4 is able to perform without difficulty. This test is highly reliable. It was originally designed for assessing risk of falls in older adults, and cutoff scores for fall risk vary depending on which of several studies is consulted.[70,71] Use of higher cutoff scores may erroneously identify nonfallers as fallers; use of lower cutoff scores may erroneously identify fallers as nonfallers. The Berg Balance Scale has also been used with clients after stroke.[72-75]

The original Get-Up-and-Go Test is made up of seven items and subjectively scored on an ordinal rating scale of 1 to 5, in which 1 is normal and 5 is severely abnormal.[76] This test has been modified by making it a timed measure to increase its objectivity and reliability, which is now high. The TUG test eliminates the "standing steady" segment and uses a stopwatch to time the performance.[77] Clients are asked to rise from a chair with arms, walk 3 meters as fast as they safely can, turn, walk back to the chair, and sit down. This test may be performed with an assistive device; however, the use of a device will alter the speed at which the task can be accomplished, and any retesting must be done with the same device to produce comparable results. Originally designed to assess frailty in older adults, the test is now more commonly used to assess fall risk in this population. Young adults typically perform this task in 5 to 7 seconds, healthy older adults in 7 to 9 seconds (low risk), moderate-risk older adults in 10 to 12 seconds, and high-risk older adults in 13 seconds or more.[78,79] These cut-off scores are for older adults walking without assistive devices. Improvements in test performance that are not captured by the time score alone should also be documented, for example, if the client can now perform the test without the use of chair arms to stand up, or without an assistive device.

The Tinetti Performance-Oriented Mobility Assessment—Balance subscale (POMA-Balance) is a list of nine items scored on scales of either 0 to 1 or 0 to 2, with the higher numbers reflecting better (more normal) performance.[80] The score value is specific to the item. The best possible score is 16, with a score of 10 or lower indicating a high risk of falls.[81]

Most balance and mobility scales have been developed to assess risk of falls in older adults. Many share similar items. See Table 22-2 for a summary of scale items.

The Tinetti Performance-Oriented Mobility Assessment—Gait subscale (POMA-Gait) is a list of seven normal aspects of gait that are observed by the examiner as the client walks at a self-selected pace and then at a rapid but safe pace.[80] Scoring scales are again either 0 to 1 or 0 to 2, and higher numbers indicate better performance. Score values are specific to the item being observed (Table 22-3). The best possible score is a 12; scores of 8 or below indicate a high risk of falls. When combined, the Tinetti POMA balance and gait scales offer a best possible score of 28, with scores of 19 or less indicating a high fall risk.

The original Gait Assessment Rating Scale (GARS) is a list of 16 abnormal aspects of gait observed by the examiner as the client walks at a self-selected pace (see Table 22-3).[82] These abnormalities are commonly seen in older adults who fall, who are fearful of falling, or both. The items are scored on a scale of 0 to 3, with lower numbers reflecting better (less abnormal) performance. The best possible score is 0. This gait scale provides some relative numerical indication of the quality of gait. A shorter, modified version of this test, the Modified GARS, has been developed. The Modified GARS (GARS-M) includes nine of the original items plus a gait velocity measure. It provides equivalent sensitivity and takes less time to perform.[83] These two gait scales were developed to assess risk of falls in older adults.

The Dynamic Gait Index (DGI) is a gait test specifically designed to look at postural control during gait.[12] It includes eight items requiring changes in gait speed, walking with horizontal and vertical head turning, whole-body turns during gait, stepping over and around obstacles, and stair ascent and descent. Items on this test are scored on a 4-point ordinal scale of 0 to 3, with 3 being normal performance and 0 indicating severe impairment. The best possible score on this test is a 24, and scores of less than 19 points have been associated with impairment of gait and fall risk. The presence of head motion and whole-body turns in this test may help identify clients with potential vestibular dysfunction.

TABLE 22-2 ■ BALANCE AND MOBILITY SCALE ITEMS

ACTIVITY	BERG BALANCE SCALE	DYNAMIC GAIT INDEX	TIMED UP-AND-GO TEST	TINETTI BALANCE ASSESSMENT
1. Sitting unsupported	√			√
2. Sitting to standing	√		√	√
3. Standing to sitting	√		√	√
4. Transfers	√			
5. Standing unsupported	√		√	√
6. Standing with eyes closed	√			√
7. Standing with feet together	√			
8. Tandem standing	√			
9. Standing on one leg	√			
10. Rotating trunk while standing	√			
11. Retrieving object from floor	√			
12. Turning 360 degrees	√			√
13. Stool stepping	√			
14. Reaching forward while standing	√			
15. Sternal nudge				√
16. Walking		√	√	
17. Abrupt stop		√		
18. Walking then turning		√	√	
19. Stepping over obstacle		√		
20. Stairs		√		
21. Walking at preferred and varied speeds		√		
22. Walking with horizontal and vertical head turns			√	
23. Stepping around obstacles		√		

TABLE 22-3 ■ GAIT SCALE ITEMS

GAIT ACTIVITIES	TINETTI GAIT SCALE	GAIT ASSESSMENT RATING SCALE (GARS)
1. Initiation (hesitancy)	√	√†
2. Step length	√	√†
3. Step height	√	√
4. Step symmetry	√	√
5. Step continuity	√	√†
6. Path deviation	√	√
7. Trunk	√	√
8. Walking-heel distance	√	
9. Staggering		√†
10. Heel strike		√†
11. Hip ROM*		√†
12. Knee ROM*		√
13. Elbow extension*		√
14. Shoulder extension*		√†
15. Shoulder abduction*		√
16. Arm-heel strike synchrony		√†
17. Forward head*		√
18. Shoulders held elevated*		√
19. Forward flexed trunk*		
20. Gait speed		√†

ROM, Range of motion.
*During gait.
†Items that were retained for the Modified GARS.

The reliability of this test is high.[71,84,85] A modified and slightly more difficult version of this test, the Functional Gait Assessment (FGA), has been developed specifically for use with patients with vestibular disorders.[86] The best possible score on the FGA is 30 points, and a score of 22 points or below can be used to classify fall risk and predict unexplained falls in community-dwelling older adults.[87]

The three gait tests listed previously are distinct from traditional gait tests because they focus on elements of postural control during gait. One very important traditional gait measure that should be included in the assessment of balance and gait in older adults and clients with neurological disorders is gait speed. This measure has been termed "the sixth vital sign" for older adults because of its strong association with level of dependence in activities of daily living (ADLs) and instrumental ADLs (IADLs), probability of hospitalization, risk of falls, eventual discharge location, and ambulation category.[88]

Combination Test Batteries

Because no single test can give a complete picture of a client's balance abilities, individual test items are often combined to form a test battery. Several of the tests described earlier, such as the Berg Balance Scale and the Tinetti POMA, include a combination of multiple items and could be categorized as combination test batteries. Different items on a test may challenge different components of the postural control system to permit a more complete assessment of the client's balance abilities.

The BESTest is an excellent comprehensive test battery based on the systems model of postural control (see Figure 22-3).[31] It includes seven categories representing components of postural control: biomechanical constraints; stability limits; anticipatory postural adjustments; automatic postural responses; sensory orientation, and stability during gait. Within each category are individual test items and, in some cases, existing tests. For example, the sensory orientation category contains the individual item "Stand on incline with eyes closed" and the four-condition CTSIB discussed earlier. Although the BESTest takes approximately 30 minutes to administer, the information acquired helps to identify which underlying components of the postural control system are causing the observed balance problems. Armed with this critical information, the clinician can design a customized, individualized intervention program that targets the sources of imbalance in each client.

A shorter version of this test has been developed, the Mini-BESTest (see Figure 22-3).[32] It includes 14 of the original 36 items, has a compressed rating scale, and takes approximately 15 minutes to administer. It does not include any items from the biomechanical constraints category or the stability limits category. This does not mean that these components need not be measured. Biomechanical constraints such as hip and ankle weakness, and constricted limits of stability, seriously negatively affect balance and should be tested in addition to administration of the Mini-BESTest. The compressed rating scale may reduce the ability of this test to reflect a client's progress over time.

The Fregly-Graybiel Ataxia Test Battery is a more challenging test appropriate for clients with higher-level balance skills. It includes eight test items that the client must perform (Figure 22-14).[38] Standing trials in tandem stance both off and on a rail with eyes open and closed are timed. Timed single-leg stance trials also are performed for each leg. Walking 10 steps with eyes closed is included. Five trials of each task are given. Trials are stopped if the client uncrosses the arms, opens the eyes (during eyes-closed trials), steps (during standing trials), or falls. Trials are judged on a pass-fail basis. This test battery is valid for use with clients who have peripheral vestibular dysfunction. Normative data are available from a normative database composed primarily of findings in young men. As noted earlier, clients must be at a high level motorically to perform these tasks. This test is a good choice for clients with higher-level abilities because it does provide more demanding balance tasks. Interpretations regarding a client's use of sensory inputs when motor involvement is also present cannot be made with certainty.

The Fugl-Meyer Sensorimotor Assessment of Balance Performance is a subset of the Fugl-Meyer Physical Performance Battery, which was designed for use with hemiplegic clients (Figure 22-15).[18] Three sitting and four standing balance activities are listed. The items are scored on a 0 to 2 scale, with score values specific to each item. Higher scores indicate better performance; the maximum (best) score is 14. However, a client could achieve this score of 14 and still not have normal balance.

The Dizziness Handicap Inventory (DHI) was developed to identify specific functional, emotional, or physical problems associated with an individual's reaction to imbalance or

FREGLY TEST

Condition	Trials 1	2	3	4	5
1. Sharpened Romberg, EC (60 sec; feet in tandem)					
2. Walk on Rail, EO (5 steps; best 3/5 trials)					
3. Stand on Rail, EO (3 trials; 60 sec/trial)				x	x
4. Stand on Rail, EC (3 trials; 60 sec/trial)				x	x
5. Stand on Right Leg, on Floor, EC (5 trials; 30 sec/trial)					
6. Stand on Left Leg, on Floor, EC (5 trials; 30 sec/trial)					
7. Walk on Floor, EC (3 trials; 10 steps each)				x	x
8. Stand sideways on rail (characterize sway)*					

*Added by the author to observe the movement strategy used by the individual.
EO, eyes open; EC, eyes closed.

Figure 22-14 ■ A combination of tasks (Romberg test, one-legged stance test [OLST], walking) and environments (eyes open, eyes closed, rail) are included in the Fregly-Graybiel Ataxia Test Battery. (From Newton R: Review of tests of standing balance abilities. *Brain Inj* 3:335, 1989.)

FUGL-MEYER

Test	Scoring	Maximum Possible Score	Attained Score
1. Sit without support ________	0—Cannot maintain sitting without support 1—Can sit unsupported less than 5 minutes 2—Can sit longer than 5 minutes		
2. Parachute reaction, non-affected side ________	0—Does not abduct shoulder or extend elbow 1—Impaired reaction 2—Normal reaction		
3. Parachute reaction, affected side ________	Scoring is the same as for test 2		
4. Stand with support ________	0—Cannot stand 1—Stands with maximum support 2—Stands with minimum support for 1 minute		
5. Stand without support ________	0—Cannot stand without support 1—Stands less than 1 minute or sways 2—Stands with good balance more than 1 minute		
6. Stand on unaffected side ________	0—Cannot be maintained longer than 1–2 seconds 1—Stands balanced 4–9 seconds 2—Stands balanced more than 10 seconds		
7. Stand on affected side ________	Scoring is the same as for test 6		
		Maximum Balance Score	/14

Figure 22-15 ■ The Fugl-Meyer Sensorimotor Assessment of Balance Performance includes both low-level and high-level tasks. (From DiFabio RP, Badke MB: Relationship of sensory organization to balance function in patients with hemiplegia. *Phys Ther* 70:20, 1990.)

dizziness.[89,90] The DHI assesses the client's perception of the effects of the balance problem and the client's level of emotional adjustment. It also looks at perceived physical limitations as a consequence of the disorder. Twenty-five items are divided into three subscales in this self-assessment inventory. Included are a nine-item functional scale, a nine-item emotional scale, and a seven-item physical scale. Each item is assigned a value of four points for a "yes," two points for a "sometimes," and zero points for a "no." This inventory is reliable, is easy to administer, and can be used to evaluate treatment outcomes.[91] Changes in scores on the functionally based DHI correlate highly with changes in scores on the impairment-based SOT.[89]

The DHI can be given before the initial evaluation to help determine which physical tests should be performed. An astute clinician can see patterns of dysfunction within the reported symptom level. For example, visual motion sensitivity and visual dependency can be indicated from the answers about grocery stores, crowds, riding in a car, or difficulty at night. Imbalance usually is indicated when the client has difficulty walking down a sidewalk and using stairs. Patients with chronic mild head injury often will report many activities as most provoking because of their inability to integrate the sensory systems and poor motor control for balance.

Dual-Task Tests

In everyday life tasks, normal balance is largely unconscious and does not compete for attentional resources. In clients with balance disorders, however, the challenge of maintaining postural control during upright activities and gait is often sufficient to demand the use of attentional resources. The interaction of cognitive demands and postural control demands is examined in dual-task tests that add concurrent cognitive and motor tasks to gait tasks. At the simplest level are the walking while talking (WWT) and stops walking when talking (SWWT) tests.[92-95] In these tests the client is asked to walk and, while the client is walking, the clinician asks the client one or more questions and observes if the client must stop walking to answer the question(s). If so, the test result is positive—that is, the client must stop attending to the postural control demands of walking to reallocate attention to the cognitive task. These are gross measures, apt to identify only those with more severe attentional balance problems or to misidentify clients who prefer to chat and rest rather than keep walking. A more formalized dual-task test is the Multiple Tasks Test (MTT), which includes eight items involving gait plus other verbal cognitive and motor tasks such as carrying a tray and avoiding obstacles.[96,97] Two dual-task versions of the TUG have been developed. The TUG-Manual involves performing the TUG while carrying a cup nearly full of water. The TUG-Cognitive involves performing the TUG while subtracting backward from a randomly selected number or spelling words backward.[98] The Walking and Remembering Test (WART) requires the client to remember a set of numbers that the tester speaks aloud while the client walks as quickly as possible while trying not to step off of a narrow path.[99] Once the walk is completed, the client must repeat the numbers in sequence. For all dual-task tests, performance of each single task is measured separately first. Then the dual-task performance is recorded. The difference for each of the two scores (physical and cognitive performance) between undivided attention and divided attention conditions is calculated.

Balance Confidence Tests

Reduced participation in functional activities may occur not only because balance impairments impede participation, but also when clients are anxious about falling. Fear of falling may lead individuals to avoid activities that they remain quite capable of doing.[100] In turn, prolonged self-restriction of activity leads to the many negative consequences of being sedentary—decreased ROM, weakness, low endurance, and so on—and thus ironically further impairs balance and increases fall risk.[101,102] As this worsening balance and increased risk is perceived by the client, further activity restriction occurs, creating a self-perpetuating downward spiral leading to social isolation, anxiety, and depression.[103,104] It is just as important to address poor balance confidence as it is to address poor balance, for without sufficient balance confidence a client will not participate in activities even if balance abilities permit him or her to do so. The client will lose all the gains made in therapy if he or she does not remain active, and he or she will not be active if fearful of falling.

The two most commonly used measures of balance confidence are the Activities-specific Balance Confidence Scale (ABC Scale), and the Falls Efficacy Scale (FES).[105,106] Both are questionnaires that are easy to administer. The ABC Scale consists of 16 items that range in difficulty from "walk around the house" to "walk outside on icy sidewalks." Several of the items inquire about activities in public places, for example, parking lots and escalators. Clients are asked how confident they are that they could do each of the activities without losing their balance or becoming unsteady. Responses are given on a scale from 0 to 100 in increments of 10, with higher numbers indicating higher confidence. More recently a short version, the ABC-6, has been developed. It has six of the original 16 items and takes less time to administer, yet retains good reliability and correlation with balance and fall risk measures.[107] The FES consists of 10 activity items that are less difficult than the items on the ABC Scale. Items on the FES include getting in and out of a chair and answering the door or a phone. All of the items refer to activities done in the home. Clients are asked how confident they are that they could do each of the activities without falling. Responses are given on a scale from 1 to 10, with lower numbers indicating higher confidence. The Modified FES (MFES) has 14 activity items and includes two activities done outside the home and three activities done in public spaces. It also takes into account whether or not an assistive device is used.[108] Scoring is identical to that of the original FES.

A third measure of fear of falling is the Survey of Activities and Fear of Falling in the Elderly (SAFFE).[109] This measurement instrument is more involved than the ABC Scale or MFES; however, it provides additional information specific to activity restriction that is valuable to the clinician. The SAFFE has 11 activity items that are similar in nature to the items on the other two scales, including community activities. This questionnaire asks if the client actually does the activity or not. If he or she does the activity, the questionnaire asks how worried the client is that he or she might fall during the activity, on a scale from 1 to 4. Lower numbers indicate increased worry. If the client does not do the activity, the client is asked whether the reason he or she does not do the activity is fear of falling, with degree of fear scored on the scale from 1 to 4, or whether the client does not do the activity for reasons other than fear, and what those other reasons are. For each item, clients also indicate whether the frequency of doing the activity has increased, decreased, or remained the same. The SAFFE takes longer to administer than the ABC Scale or MFES but provides explicit results about activity restriction not obtained from the other two scales.

The Fear of Falling Avoidance Behavior Questionnaire (FFABQ) is a recently developed instrument with a focus on activity avoidance versus fear.[110] It lists 14 different activities, ranging in difficulty from walking and preparing meals to going up and down stairs to engaging in recreational activities such as sports or traveling. Clients rate whether or not they agree with a statement that they avoid a specified activity on a 5-point scale from 0 (completely disagree) to 4 (completely agree). This questionnaire is reliable, with scores that discriminate between previous fallers and nonfallers, and more versus less active individuals. The shift from an emphasis on fear or confidence as in the ABC and FES, to activity avoidance as in the SAFFE and FFABQ is an important and positive one for physical and occupational therapists. As the ICF health and disablement model describes, our goals are to increase activity and participation to achieve an improved quality of life for our clients.

Considerations in the Selection of Balance Tests

To determine the type and level of challenge of the tests to be used during the examination, a thorough subjective history is critical. In describing the symptoms and the situations that cause dizziness or imbalance, the client offers clues to possible deficits and thereby the measures that will help identify them.

Many of the functional scales previously reviewed were designed to determine whether balance is abnormal in elderly clients who have no medical diagnosis, in other words, as screening tools. Clinicians working with clearly diagnosed clients with neurological conditions often do not need such tools to establish that balance skills are abnormal because the deficits are patently obvious. These screening tools can be useful, however, to identify disabilities, establish a baseline, monitor progress, and document outcomes.

Many clinical facilities have their own therapy evaluation forms that include a section on balance. Items and scoring are usually defined by the facility. They are not standardized across sites, as are published scales, and are rarely tested for measurement qualities such as validity and reliability. As rehabilitation professions evolve toward evidence-based practice, nonstandardized tests with unknown measurement quality are no longer acceptable. Clinicians should use standardized, objective, quantifiable, valid tests with high reliability, sensitivity, and specificity whenever possible. Facilities insistent on using their own tests should conduct research to ensure that they are valid, reliable, and responsive to change over time. A functional balance rating scale is important in the evaluation of clients with neurological impairment. To be responsive enough to measure changes in clients who clearly are not (and may never be) clinically normal, scales should have at least five, and perhaps seven, possible relative scores.

In addition, additional tests are necessary to assess the systems that may affect postural control to help identify and measure impairments (e.g., ROM, strength, sensation and sensory organization, motor planning and control). These types of measures should be sensitive, objective, and quantifiable. Unfortunately, some body system components do not have objective, quantifiable clinical measures (e.g., motor planning, coordination). In these cases, clinicians must continue to use subjective rating scales.

Other factors to include when deciding what tests to use are the time required to perform the test, the number of staff members who must be present, and the space and equipment needed. Clinicians must weigh the potential benefits of technological tools (e.g., computerized forceplates, isokinetics, motion analysis, electromyography) against their cost and practicality (i.e., their cost-effectiveness). The test must be suitable for the client's level of functioning (physical and cognitive). Many head-injured clients, for example, cannot initially participate in traditional forms of testing because of cognitive limitations.

PROBLEM IDENTIFICATION, GOAL SETTING, AND TREATMENT PLANNING

Clinical Decision Making

Treatment of clients with neurological diagnoses is based on the particular set of impairments and activity limitations possessed by each individual. Remediation of balance deficits similarly must be specific to the involved body systems and functional activity losses in each client. Clinicians should generate an overall problem list for each client; if imbalance is a listed problem, then a sublist of balance problems also can be developed (Figure 22-16).

EXAMPLE OF BALANCE PROBLEM LIST

General Problem List	Balance Problem List
1. Decreased strength (L) side	
2. Decreased ROM (L) shoulder	
3. Decreased endurance	
4. Impaired sensation (L) side	
5. Decreased balance	a. Decreased weight bearing on left (L) LE b. Unable to maintain midline orientation c. Extraneous sway with eyes closed d. Unable to stand on (L) LE e. Decreased limits of stability to 40/100% f. Unable to shift to (L) side g. Unable to establish stable base of support h. Unable to stand on unstable surface i. Unable to perform hip strategy
6. Increased tone (L) side	
7. Synergistic movement (L) side	
8. Min. assist transfers	
9. Mod. assist ambulation	

Figure 22-16 ■ An example of a balance-specific problem list (as a subset of a general problem list), which should be developed to guide balance rehabilitation treatments.

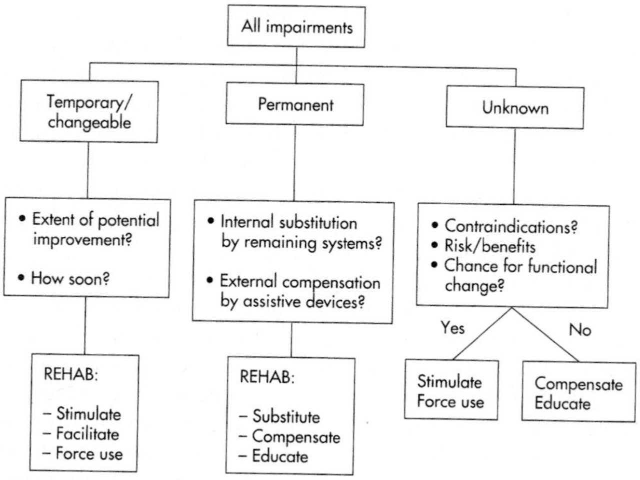

Figure 22-17 ■ A clinical decision-making tree to illustrate the treatment-planning process in balance rehabilitation.

To direct and establish priorities for treatment, clinicians must review the problem list and ask themselves the following questions (Figure 22-17): Which impairments are temporary and can be remediated? How much improvement can be expected? How soon will it occur? Which impairments are permanent or progressive and must be compensated for? What other body systems can be counted on to substitute? What external compensations may be needed?

For some clients with neurological impairments, knowing whether a problem is permanent or temporary is not possible, as in recovery from a stroke or head injury. In others with progressive diseases such as Parkinson disease or MS, the rate of decline is unknown and abilities may fluctuate. In these cases the clinician should consider the following issues: Would a consultation provide the required information? If so, referral is appropriate. Do any contraindications to treatment exist? What are the risks and benefits of providing versus withholding treatment? Is some amount of functional improvement possible? If no contraindications are present, the benefits outweigh the risks, and functional improvement is expected, then a trial of treatment may be given, even if knowing for certain whether the problem(s) will respond to the treatment is not possible. In these cases especially, a baseline must be established against which to measure any change. Change for the worse or no change after a reasonable trial period indicates that treatment should be altered or discontinued.

Using the Systems Model to Identify Postural Control Impairments

The systems approach is useful to develop a balance problem list because it can be applied to different diagnoses equally well and allows deficits in multiple systems to be recognized. Table 22-4 illustrates several examples of ways this framework is used to identify balance deficits in clients with different neurological diagnoses.

For each client, problems affecting postural control should be described in objective, measurable terms whenever possible. For example, the term "impaired vision" is too vague; "four-line drop on eye chart" is more specific. "Poor use of visual inputs for balance control" is an interpretation; the objective result could be stated "Loss of balance after less than 15 seconds on 5/5 trials of standing on

TABLE 22-4 ■ EXAMPLES OF MEDICAL DIAGNOSES AND RELATED IMPAIRMENTS AFFECTING BALANCE

IMPAIRMENTS FROM SYSTEMS MODEL	CLIENT WITH DIABETIC STROKE	CLIENT WITH PARKINSON DISEASE	CLIENT WITH INCOMPLETE PARAPLEGIA
PERIPHERAL SENSORY			
Vision	Retinopathy	Cataracts	
Vestibular		Hair cell loss	
Somatosensory	Peripheral neuropathy	Slowed transmission time	Complete loss
CENTRAL SENSORY			
Vision	Hemianopia	Vision dominant	Needs superior use to compensate
Vestibular	Failure to use inputs		Needs superior use to compensate
Somatosensory	Failure to use inputs	Failure to use inputs	
Strategy selection	Step dominant	Ankle dominant	Hip dominant
Perception of position in space	Midline shift with left neglect	Restricted limits of stability	
CENTRAL MOTOR			
Timing	Increased reaction time	Bradykinesia	
Sequencing	Disordered	Co-contraction	
Force modulation	Spasticity	Rigidity	
Error correction	Use right side only		
PERIPHERAL MOTOR			
Range of motion	Knee hyperextension	Bilateral ankle plantar flexor contractures	Hip flexion contractures
Strength	Decreased left side	Decreased bilateral extremities and trunk	Severe weakness bilateral lower extremities and trunk
Endurance	Severely impaired	Moderately impaired	Mildly impaired

foam, eyes open." Documenting problems in this manner makes goal writing (and subsequent treatment planning) much easier.

Writing Goals on the Basis of Body Structure and Function Impairments and Activity Limitations

Goals also should be stated in objective and measurable terms so that their achievement can be judged. "Improved balance" is open to any interpretation, whereas "able to stand on right leg for 30 seconds on 3/3 trials" and "walks tandem entire length of balance beam without misstep 7/10 times" are measurable goals. These types of goals may be helpful to the clinician who understands the link between impairments and function, but they may seem nonfunctional (and therefore unnecessary) to others who read them (e.g., case managers, third-party payers). From their standpoint, incorporating the functional task that will be positively affected by its achievement into the impairment goal is beneficial; for example, "able to stand on right leg for 10 seconds at a time so that stairs can be ascended and descended step-over-step without railing," or "walks tandem on balance beam to demonstrate ability to avoid falls using hip strategy." By describing the specific system problem (e.g., power, range, balance strategies) as it relates to function in the treatment objectives, clinicians force themselves to focus on functional outcomes and illustrate for others why these goals are meaningful. The need for and validity of the treatment are then more likely to be clearly perceived. At times, goal documentation requirements may specify that the goals be purely functional in nature. Writing goals without impairment components may meet the needs of the reviewer, but they will not help to direct clinical interventions to the specific components that need to be addressed in each individual client. Documentation must meet reviewer requirements, but for one's own benefit, writing a separate set of goals with the dual impairment-function component will assist the clinician with planning and prioritizing treatment.

If a problem cannot be alleviated and requires compensation, the goal(s) should reflect this as well. For example, a client with diabetes has progressive peripheral neuropathy with somatosensory loss and ineffective ankle strategy. If the client's visual and vestibular sensory systems and proximal strength are relatively intact, however, then the goals might mention improved use of visual cues and successful substitution of hip and stepping strategies. Educational and environmental modification goals for safety also are appropriate in these situations.

Developing a Treatment Plan

Once the goals have been listed and priorities established, the treatment plan is developed. The most effective and efficient treatments focus first on those problems with the greatest impact on function and address more than one problem at a time. Training balance on an unstable surface contributes to the use of visual and vestibular inputs as well as to the use of hip strategy, increased lower-extremity strength, and increased motor control (skill) on that type of surface. Training gait on an inclined treadmill with eyes closed or head movement increases the use of somatosensory and vestibular inputs, endurance, postural control, ROM, and lower-extremity strength. Creative clinicians develop comprehensive treatment plans with this type of multiple-problem approach to maximize the time available with clients.

The clinician must thoughtfully choose environments and tasks that together stimulate and challenge the appropriate postural control systems. To stimulate one sensory system, the other systems must be placed at a disadvantage to force reliance on the targeted system. The environment is then structured to put the other systems at a disadvantage (e.g., training with eyes closed or in the dark puts vision at a disadvantage and forces the use of somatosensory and vestibular inputs). If one side or limb is significantly more affected, such as in hemiplegia, then the other side must be disadvantaged to force reliance on the targeted side. Tasks are then selected to disadvantage the less affected side. For example, placing the less affected leg on a step or small ball makes it more difficult to use for balance and forces the transference of weight to the more affected leg. To achieve optimal function, however, all systems and all sides must be capable of working together, so training to improve balance impairments must be incorporated and interspersed with training functional tasks. For carryover of improvements into real-life situations, training tasks should be varied enough to promote motor problem solving on the part of the client.[111] For example, sitting balance and transfers should be taught using stable and unstable surfaces, with different heights and firmnesses, with and without armrests and back supports, and using both right and left sides. This technique may improve the client's abilities to perform safe sitting and transfers in new situations not previously practiced in therapy.[24]

Tables 22-5 through 22-7 illustrate the process of test choice, problem identification based on test results, goal setting based on impairments and disabilities, and treatment planning based on goals in three different types of clients. Note that only selected tests were performed for each client. Goals were directly related to the problems that were identified by the tests, and treatment plans followed directly from the goals.

BALANCE RETRAINING TECHNIQUES

Motor Learning Concepts

Although covering the principles of motor learning is not within the scope of this chapter (refer to Chapter 4), the discussion of balance retraining methods is not possible without some consideration of several motor learning concepts that must be incorporated into treatment. The clinician must remember that successful treatments address the interaction of the individual, the task, and the environment (Figure 22-18).[12,24]

Individual

Therapists should know their clients' impairments: sensory and motor, peripheral, and central. Whenever possible, therapists should know which impairments can be rehabilitated and which require compensation or substitution. Because of the nature of neurological insult, this includes an awareness of cognitive and perceptual impairments that may affect the ability to relearn old skills or develop new ones. Optimal learning of skilled movement requires that the client have (1) knowledge of self (abilities and limitations), (2) knowledge of the environment (opportunities and risks),

TABLE 22-5 ■ AN EXAMPLE OF TEST SELECTION, PROBLEM IDENTIFICATION, GOAL SETTING, AND TREATMENT PLANNING IN A CLIENT WITH PERIPHERAL VESTIBULAR DEFICIT

Patient profile: 50-year-old woman
Diagnosis: Uncompensated (R) unilateral peripheral vestibular deficit for 6-7 years
Course of examination and treatment: Otolaryngologist → psychologist → neuro-otologist → outpatient physical therapy

TEST	PROBLEMS IDENTIFIED	GOALS SET	TREATMENT PLAN
Visual acuity	Four-line drop on Snellen eye chart	Able to read chart with only one-line drop	Gaze stabilization exercises
Oculomotor	Positive nystagmus with Frenzel lenses		
Saccades			
Pursuit			
Nystagmus			
Gaze stabilization	Unable to perform test	Able to rotate head horizontally 2 min without problems	Gaze stabilization exercises
Visual-vestibular interaction	↓ Fixation with horizontal + vertical head movements after 5-10 s		
VOR cancellation		Able to perform visual-vestibular interaction test	
Hallpike			
SOT	Decreased use of somatosensory inputs 70/100	Somatosensory use 100/100	Sensory environment stimulation
	Decreased use of visual inputs 55/100	Vision use 90/100	
	Absent use of vestibular inputs 0/100	Vestibular use 70/100	
	Unable to resolve visual conflict 0/100	Visual conflict resolution 90/100	
Limits of stability	Restricted anteriorly and posteriorly to 35% limit of stability	Limits of stability expanded to 85% anterior and posterior at 5-s pacing	COG control training
	Slow movement time		
ROM and strength	None		
Gait			Gait training
Eyes open	Weaves side to side		
Eyes closed	Deviates to (R) with eyes closed	Walks in a straight line with eyes closed	
Head turning	Dizzy with horizontal head turns	Walks with only slight deviation with eyes closed and head turning	
Pivots	Loss of balance and dizzy with (R) pivot	Spins to (R), (L) with eyes closed	
Abrupt stops	Very unsteady with abrupt stop; feels "off"	Comes to abrupt stop steadily	

Reprinted with permission from NeuroCom International, Clackamas, Ore.
COG, Center of gravity; *(L),* left; *(R),* right; *ROM,* range of motion; *SOT,* Sensory Organization Test; *VOR,* vestibuloocular reflex.

(3) knowledge of the task (critical components), (4) the ability to use those knowledge sets to solve motor problems, and (5) the ability to modify and adapt movements as the task and environment change. To the extent that a client is missing these characteristics, the clinician should attempt to support his or her development or even supply them until they are present. Different types of clients vary with regard to which characteristics are likely to be missing. For example, a cognitively impaired, head-injured client may lack awareness of self and environment, even though his or her physical abilities make modifying and adapting movements possible. Conversely, a quadriplegic client may be aware of his or her limitations, the environment, and the task demands but may initially have limited experience to know how to solve a motor problem and limited physical ability to modify movements.

The clinician must also ask what motor learning stage the client is in for different tasks. Skill acquisition is the first stage. The objective is for the client to "get the idea of the movement" to begin to acquire the skill.[112] In this stage, errors are frequent and performance is inefficient and inconsistent. Within the nervous system only temporary changes are occurring. Skill refinement is the second stage. The goal is for the client to improve the performance, reduce the number and size of the errors, and increase the consistency and efficiency of the movements. Skill retention is the final stage. The ability to perform the movements and achieve the functional goal has been accomplished, and the new objective is to retain the skill over time and transfer the skill to different settings. Retention and transfer are the hallmarks of true learning, in which some relatively permanent changes have occurred within the nervous system. A client may have attained the skill retention phase for sitting balance tasks, be in the skill refinement stage for standing balance tasks, and be in the skill acquisition stage for locomotor balance tasks.

Therapists use practice and feedback to teach motor skills. Repetition is necessary to develop skill; feedback is necessary to detect and correct errors. During skill acquisition, frequent repetition of a movement or task and frequent feedback are beneficial to help the client begin to be able to

TABLE 22-6 ■ EXAMPLE OF HOW TREATMENT PLANNING FLOWS FROM TEST RESULTS IN AN ELDERLY CLIENT WITH FREQUENT FALLS

Patient profile: 72-year-old woman
Diagnosis: Disequilibrium of aging, frequent falls
Course of examination and treatment: Cardiologist → neurologist → outpatient physical therapy

TEST	PROBLEMS IDENTIFIED	GOALS SET	TREATMENT PLAN
Peripheral sensory Somatosensory Vision	Mildly decreased vibration sense bilateral lower extremity ↓ Acuity, cataracts ↓ Depth perception	Compensate for permanent sensory loss	Educate about safe surfaces and lighting Home safety evaluation
SOT	Absent use of vestibular inputs 0/100 Decreased use of somatosensory inputs 60/100 Dependent on vision	Increase use of vestibular inputs to 30/100 Increase use of somatosensory inputs to 75/100	Somatosensory and vestibular stimulation*
Static postural sway	Excessive sway—2 standard deviations outside normal range for age	Standing sway within normal limits for age	COG control training
Nudge or push test	No use of ankle or hip strategy Steps immediately	Survives 5/10 pushes with hip strategy	Hip strategy exercises*
LOS	No ankle strategy—uses hip strategy Sway to 45% LOS anterior, 35% LOS posterior Slow movement time	Uses ankle strategy to reach 40% LOS anterior and posterior Reaches 8/8 targets at 75% LOS using hip or ankle strategy within 4 s	COG control training
ROM	↓ Neck extension 0-10 degrees ↓ Lumbar extension 1-15 degrees ↓ Hip extension 0-5 degrees	↑ Spinal extension neck 0-20 degrees ↑ Lumbar extension 0-20 degrees ↑ Hip extension 0-10 degrees	ROM exercises*
Strength	Flexion 4/5 (B) Hip abduction 3+/5, extension 3/5 (B) Knee extension 4+/5, flexion 4/5 (R) Ankle dorsiflexion 3−/5 (L) Ankle dorsiflexion 2/5 (B) Ankle plantarflexion 3+/5	↑(B) Hip abduction and extension to greater than 4/5 ↑ (B) Ankle dorsiflexion and plantarflexion to 4−/5	Progressive resistive exercises, including bicycle*
Gait (GARS)	Score 35/48 Deviations Forward flexed trunk Double limb stance prolonged bilaterally Short step length	GARS scales 25/48 (I) Ambulation with walker in home, community	Gait training* 1—starts, stops, turns 2—treadmill 3—uneven surfaces, curbs, stairs, carpet, outdoors
Endurance	Fatigue after ambulating 60 ft	Ambulates more than 200 ft without stopping	Gait training as earlier
Tinetti balance scale	6/16 score	Tinetti balance score 10/16	Gait training as earlier
Tinetti gait scale	5/12 score Falls and catches self	Tinetti gait score 8/12	Gait training as earlier

Reprinted with permission from NeuroCom International, Clackamas, Ore.
LOS, Limit of stability; *(B),* bilateral; *COG,* center of gravity; *GARS,* Gait Assessment Rating Scale; *(I),* independent; *(L),* left; *(R),* right; *ROM,* range of motion; *SOT,* Sensory Organization Test.
*Also included in home exercise program.

perform the desired movements and tasks. As soon as the client progresses to the skill refinement stage (the clinician observes reduced errors and less variable performance), however, then practice should be varied and feedback briefly delayed. For example, the task of standing and reaching to one side to take an object from the therapist might initially be repeated to the same side and at the same height several times. Then the therapist should begin to vary the task demands gradually: reach farther or faster; take different objects of various weights, shapes, and sizes; and take the object from higher and lower heights and alternately reach to right and left sides. This variation introduces a problem-solving demand for the client: modifications in timing, force, and sequencing are now necessary.[111]

Feedback, which is especially helpful for those with sensory reception or perception problems, initially may contain information to assist the client in detecting errors about the goal achievement (knowledge of results, such as "you did

TABLE 22-7 ■ AN EXAMPLE OF HOW TREATMENT PLANNING FLOWS FROM TEST RESULTS IN A CLIENT WITH RIGHT HEMIPARESIS

Patient profile: 69-year-old woman
Diagnosis: Left cerebrovascular accident with right hemiparesis
Course of examination and treatment: Acute rehabilitation → home health → outpatient rehabilitation

TEST	PROBLEMS IDENTIFIED	GOALS SET	TREATMENT PLAN
Peripheral somatosensory		None	
SOT	Average overall stability 47/100 Absent use of vestibular inputs 0/100	Average stability 60/100 ↑ Use of vestibular inputs 15/100	Vestibular stimulation with forced use and head movements COG control training
Postural sway			
Functional reach	Forward lean restricted to 5 inches	Able to reach forward 8 inches	
Static balance	Weight shift asymmetry to left in static standing and medial or lateral sway, 25% LOS to left of midline	↑ Control of COG Stands midline	
Limit of stability	Forward weight shift restricted to 25% LOS	↑ Forward LOS to 50% ↑ Right LOS to 50%	
Rhythmic weight shift	Extraneous sway off desired path	↓ Extraneous sway scores by 50%	
OLST	Unable on right leg, 30 seconds on left leg	Stands on right leg, 10 seconds	COG control training
Nudge, push (motor strategy selection)	Switch from ankle to hip strategy noted but unable to withstand perturbation	Able to stand upright after mild perturbations 5/10 times Able to "catch" self by stepping or reaching 5/10 times	Hip and stepping strategy training
Range of motion	None		
Strength: right leg	4/5 Knee extension 3/5 Knee flexion 2/5 Ankle dorsiflexion 3/5 Ankle plantarflexion	↑ RLE strength 5/5 Knee 4/5 Ankle	Progressive resistive exercises
Endurance	Standing tolerance less than 10 minutes	Able to stand unaided for 15 minutes	Standing tolerance tasks
Gait	↓ Step length—RLE ↓ Step height—RLE ↓ Heel strike—RLE ↓ Toe-off—RLE	Symmetrical step height and length 5/10 times ↑ Heel strike RLE 5/10 times	Gait training on treadmill
Tinetti Gait Subscale	Unable to turn, reach, or bend without loss of balance Falls: Uneven surfaces Low lighting Head turning No community ambulation Requires cane Requires supervision for household ambulation	8/12 score No falls Gait independent without cane in household; with cane in community	Gait training on uneven surfaces, with head movements, with low lighting Safety education

COG, Center of gravity; *LOS,* limit of stability; *OLST,* one-legged stance test; *RLE,* right lower extremity; *SOT,* Sensory Organization Test.

not lean far enough to reach this last time") or about a movement error (knowledge of performance, "you did not straighten your knee enough last time").[113] Early feedback also may contain cues about what to do better next time, such as "straighten your knee before you shift weight onto that leg." If feedback is always provided by an external source, such as the therapist, a mirror, or a computer monitor, then the client is not given the opportunity to develop internal error detection and error correction mechanisms and will not be as likely to retain or transfer the skill. By delaying the feedback and asking the client to estimate or describe her or his own errors, and afterward providing the feedback, the therapist allows the client to compare her or his own developing internal frame of reference with the correct external frame of reference. By asking clients to suggest what might be done to correct the errors, the therapist shifts the error correction process from the external source to the clients, supporting motor problem-solving processes. As clients progress to the skill retention level, variations should increase (including task and environmental demands) and feedback delays should be longer. The clinician must develop a sense of how to use practice variation and feedback

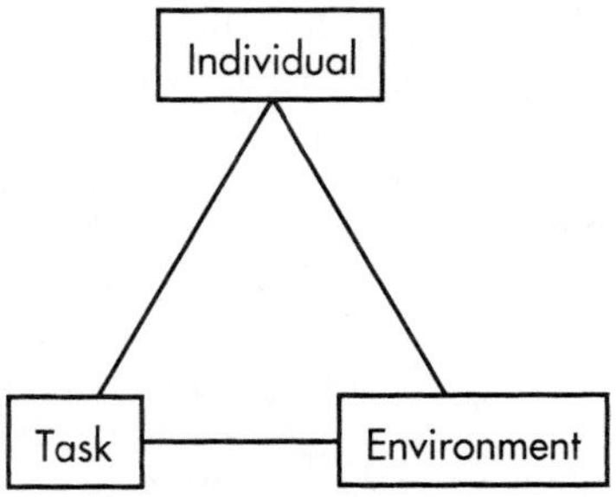

Figure 22-18 ■ Interactions of the individual, the environment, and the task are critical to postural control skills. Although they may be isolated in the mind of the clinician for assessment purposes, they are never isolated in the function of the client.

delay therapeutically to progress clients through the stages of motor learning. Too much variation and too little feedback early on impede skill acquisition; insufficient variation and excessive feedback later on hamper skill retention and transfer.

Task

Functional rating scales performed as a part of the evaluation yield information about what tasks, or functional activities, are limited by the postural control impairments. Bed mobility, sitting, sitting to standing, transfers, standing, walking, working, and sports participation may be affected. Repeating the problematic tasks over and over is one approach; however, analyzing the problematic tasks to determine what postural control demands are placed on the client when undertaking those tasks is far more productive for the clinician. Does a task demand predominantly stability? Mobility? Both? For example, standing to take a photograph demands the ability to hold still, standing to move laundry from the washer to the dryer requires weight shifting, and standing to don a pair of pantyhose calls for both steadiness and movement. All three are standing tasks, but each places different postural control demands on the client. By using task analysis, the therapist may consciously select or design tasks to place specific demands on the client such that the postural control systems that need improvement will be challenged to respond.

Analysis of mobility tasks includes attention to timing, force, and duration of movements. Consider the different timing demands for weight shifting and reaching to catch an item falling from a shelf, take a hot casserole out of the oven, or open a door. Compare the different amounts of force necessary to pick up a heavy suitcase, pick up a baby from a crib, or replace a ceiling light bulb. The duration of a balance demand may be brief, as in recovering from a trip, or extended, as in walking across an icy parking lot. Clinicians should choose tasks that vary these parameters to prepare clients for activities with various mobility demands. Activities that incorporate changing head positions will further challenge the individual with vestibular insufficiency.

Therapists also need to consider whether the elements of the task are predictable or unpredictable. In other words, will the postural control demand be a voluntary movement (e.g., sweeping the porch), an automatic postural response (e.g., missing the last step on a flight of stairs), or an anticipatory postural adjustment (e.g., preceding a lift)? Clients need to learn to respond in all three conditions, which are often combined. For instance, lifting is a voluntary movement. Predicting the load to be lifted leads to anticipatory postural preparation. Counteracting the destabilizing force of a greater-than-predicted load requires an automatic postural response. If, during therapy, the clinician says "don't let me push you" before nudging the client, the demand is for anticipatory postural adjustment. If the disturbance is provided without warning, the demand calls for APRs. If the clinician requests a lean to the right, that is a voluntary postural adjustment. Activities that demand all three types of balance control, either one at a time or in combination, should be included in balance retraining programs.

Environment

Just as tasks can be purposefully selected to promote postural control responses, environmental conditions also must be included in the design of the therapy plan to stimulate the necessary systems. Gravity cannot be manipulated by the clinician, but the client needs to learn to counteract it at different speeds and from different positions, among other things. Familiarity with how gravity can aid movement, as in walking, is also important. The therapist can vary the surface conditions. They may be stable, even, and predictable (hospital hallway, sidewalk), unstable (boat, subway, gravel driveway), uneven (grass, curbs, stairs), or compliant (beach, padded carpeting). Visual conditions also may be manipulated. Visual cues may be available and accurate (daylight, fluorescent lighting), unavailable (darkness or poor lighting, or lack of environmental cues such as a busy carpet pattern on a stairway), unstable (moving crowd, public transportation), used for purposes other than balance (fixation on a ball in tennis), or dependent on head movements. Clinicians should help prepare their clients to function in the real world by training them to maintain balance under different combinations of surface and visual conditions. This includes situations in which cues from the environment agree—that is, visual, somatosensory, and vestibular inputs are all sending the same message, so to speak—as well as in sensory conflict environments, where cues from one system may disagree with (not match) cues from the other sensory systems. Functional situations in which sensory conflicts may exist include elevators, escalators, people movers, airplanes, and subways. An emphasis on being able to adapt to changes in environmental conditions rapidly and effectively is important.

Intervention

Successful intervention for the individual with a balance disorder depends on the ability of the *clinician* to identify the components of the problem. The therapist must create a program that addresses several components at a time, not just for efficiency, but because these systems should be able to function together to perform functional activities in real-world environments. Treatment is oriented toward multiple impairments, with tasks and environments selected to best correct involved or facilitate compensatory systems.

The intervention must be matched to the level and combination of body system impairments. For example, tasks related to the different functions of the sensory systems should be identified and not treated as a single body system problem. The clinician should have a good idea of the level of stimulus during each exercise program so that the facilitation is as accurate as possible. Progression of the program follows the changes seen from one intervention to the next to promote carryover and retention of learning. The exercise progression integrates activities that reflect those changes. This usually involves more complex movement skills in a greater range of gradually more challenging environments.

Sensory Systems

In general, the less sensory information available, the more difficult the task of balancing. A treatment progression might therefore start with full sensory inputs (vision, somatosensory, and vestibular: 3/3) available in the environment and perhaps augmented feedback if intrinsic sensory channels are deficient, as with somatosensory loss or a vestibular disorder. Challenge is added by manipulating either visual or somatosensory inputs, so that equilibrium must be maintained by using only two of three senses (vision and vestibular or somatosensory and vestibular). If both vision and somatosensory inputs are manipulated, then only the vestibular inputs are a reliable source of sensory information and balance is accomplished with only one of three senses.[114]

Most patients with permanent or progressive vestibular or somatosensory losses naturally compensate and become visually dependent. In cases in which improving the use of somatosensory or vestibular inputs is necessary, the training of vision for stability can be counterproductive, teaching compensation versus improvement of normal function. On the other hand, visual retraining is entirely appropriate for the client with severely compromised somatosensation that cannot be changed, as is common in persons with diabetes.

To stimulate the use of visual inputs, environments are designed to disadvantage somatosensation while providing reliable visual cues (stable visual field with landmarks). Somatosensation cannot be removed as can vision, but it can be destabilized by having the client sit or stand on unstable surfaces (rocker board, biomechanical ankle platform system [BAPS] board, randomly moving platforms) or confused by having the client sit or stand on compliant surfaces that give way to pressure, such as foam, "space boots," or responsively moving platforms.

To stimulate the use of somatosensory inputs, environments are designed to disadvantage vision while providing reliable somatosensory inputs (stable surfaces, level or inclined). Having the client close the eyes or practice in low lighting or darkness removes or decreases visual inputs. For clients with an overreliance on visual input for balance, the somatosensory system needs to be facilitated while the visual system is disrupted. This can be accomplished by having the client sit or stand on a stable surface while performing quick head turns. For the client with self-limited head movement, the intervention may begin with head movement during quiet standing and progress to head movements during weight shifts and then walking. Eyes-closed standing and weight shifting also increase the use of somatosensation for balance. Optokinetic stimuli in the visual surround also stimulate use of somatosensory inputs.

To stimulate the use of vestibular inputs for adaptation of the CNS, environments are designed to disadvantage both vision and somatosensation while providing reliable vestibular cues (detectable head position). Practicing on unstable or compliant surfaces, with vision either absent (eyes closed), destabilized (eye movements or head movements), or confused (e.g., optokinetic stimulation) provides challenging combinations. Adding neck extension and rotation to place the vestibular organs at a disadvantaged angle can increase difficulty. Gaze stabilization with head turns while standing on an uneven surface or while walking creates a higher-level challenge. Quick movements of the head, head tilts, or forward bending trigger vestibular signals to add input to the system. Combining these types of activities can create progressively more complex challenges. Standing or weight shifting on foam with eyes closed, and head and eye movement while walking all require vestibular input for successful performance.

Additional vestibular challenge can be added by including activities that require quick changes of position in a superior or inferior direction, such as a lunge or going up and down stairs. Other exercises involving up-and-down body movements, such as sitting to standing, seated bouncing on a Swiss ball, and standing bouncing on a mini-trampoline, all with eyes closed to eliminate use of vision for stability, increase the demand on the vestibular system. To train the client who is overreliant on vision to improve the use of vestibular inputs versus vision, activities such as watching a ball being tossed from hand to hand while walking, walking backward, or walking with eye movements can be used. Reading while walking requires the use of vision for reading so that it cannot be used for postural orientation, forcing the other sensory sources to be used for orientation.

Multisensory and Motor Control Dysfunction

Older clients often have dysfunction in all three sensory systems—that is, a multisensory balance disorder. Disease-related disruptions of the somatosensory or visual system (e.g., a peripheral neuropathy or cataracts) are combined with age-related declines in the vestibular system. In some cases therapy aimed at increasing vestibular function can have a significant impact on postural stability. If sensory loss is permanent or progressive, safe function may require the use of an assistive device.[115] Choosing an assistive device for these clients can be a challenge. An individual with cerebellar or visual-perceptual problems may have more difficulty using an assistive device, and thus it may be contraindicated. For these clients, careful assessment of safety and gait both with and without the device is demanded. A single cane often does not allow for compensation for changes in direction of an impending fall, and a standard aluminum walker does not provide support when changing directions because it must be lifted. The ideal walker has four rotating wheels and thus the ability to change direction without being lifted. This device greatly increases stability, and the client usually describes a significant increase in confidence. Of course, the use of a walker also limits normal use of the upper extremities and trunk during gait and restricts the types of environments that can be negotiated. Making sure the client stands erect in walking versus leaning forward into a permanent flexed position is important in order to retain and/or improve existing postural function.

Many clients with neurological conditions have temporary difficulty with head control early in their recovery, and others have chronic head control problems. Their ability to orient the vestibular organs, eyes, and neck proprioceptors properly is impaired, which negatively affects the ability to perceive internal and environmental cues that could assist in balance maintenance. Thus, developing head control is very important. (Refer to Chapter 9 for examples of how to improve head control.) Clients with spasticity or contractures of the ankles and feet who cannot place their feet in full contact with the floor are at a biomechanical disadvantage and also have difficulty receiving somatosensory inputs that could support postural control processes. The more accurate and reliable sensory information available, the greater the chances that the sensoriperceptual processes that contribute to balance can fulfill their role. Treatment progressions should include attention to increasing the client's ability to receive and process sensory information pertinent to balance control through oculomotor, head, and peripheral limb positioning and movement.

Control of the Center of Gravity

Effective control of the COG depends on accurate awareness of body position and motion in space and the relation between body parts (perception) as well as biomechanical and musculoskeletal systems (execution). Trunk and head control abilities are primary. For clients with paralysis or degenerative disease that limits the ability of arms and legs to assist with postural stability, head and trunk control may be the dominant means of balance. Both the head and neck and the trunk need to be able to achieve and hold a midline position, rotate around this midline axis, and move away from and return to the midline without loss of balance. The term *midline* here refers not to a line between right and left sides but to a point at which the right and left and forward and backward components are centered in all planes—medial-lateral, anterior-posterior, rotary, and side bending (shortening and elongation on either side). Midline problems can certainly be caused by body system problems such as weakness, pain, or sensory deficits but can also be caused by perceptual problems that have nothing to do with balance deficits but do cause balance problems.

Sitting Balance. In sitting the pelvis and posterior thighs form the primary base of support, with additional stability provided by the feet in contact with the floor. The axis of anteroposterior movement rotates around the greater trochanter, and forward and backward leans are achieved through pelvic and trunk movement. Anterior pelvic tilt with upper trunk extension allows forward reaching and begins the sitting-to-standing transition. Lateral weight shifts with trunk elongation precede right and left reaching and scooting. Lateral weight shifts with trunk rotation permit cross-midline reaching and begin the sitting-to-supine progression. The use of arms to prop in sitting is an extension of the base of support.

Standing Balance. In standing, the feet form the base of support. The axis of anteroposterior movement rotates around the medial malleolus. Mediolateral movement occurs with weight shifts from foot to foot. Weight shifts move the COG through space for reaching and lifting tasks as well as in preparation for stepping. Ankle strategy is most effective for forward and backward movement of the COG through the limits of stability on a stable surface. As the COG nears the sway boundary, hip strategy works to restrict its travel. If this fails, stepping or reaching strategies are used to reestablish a new base of support.

Balance during Gait. During gait, the COG follows a sinusoidal path as forward progression of the body mass combines with alternating lateral weight shifts to the stance foot (Figure 22-19).[23] Each step creates a new base of support. Assistive devices such as canes, walkers, and crutches extend the base of support and thus reduce the demands on the intrinsic balance control system. In sitting, standing, and walking, control of the COG involves the ability to establish a stable base of support and transfer weight over it. Treatment progressions for COG control then involve training to establish, maintain, and reduce the base of support and to

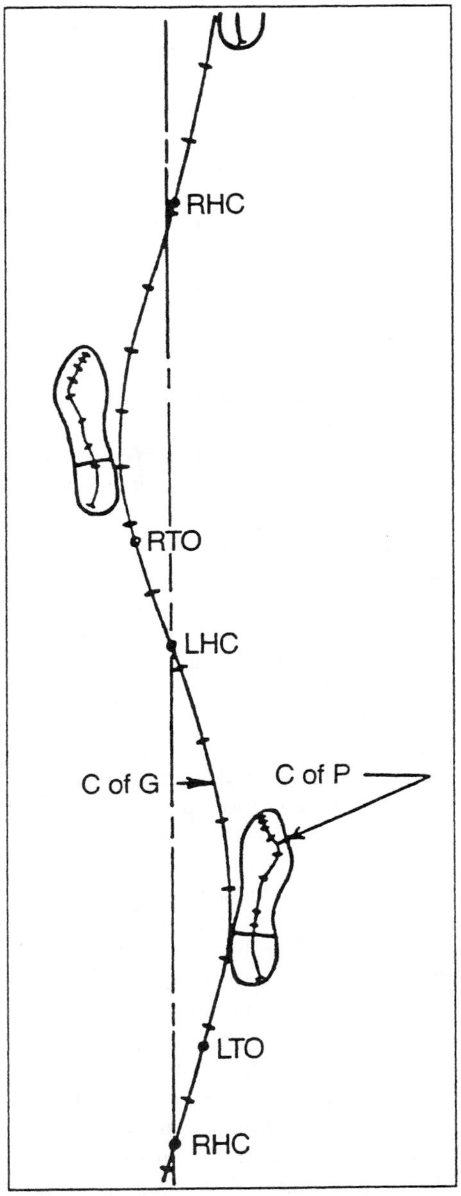

Figure 22-19 ■ The trajectory of the center of gravity *(C of G)* and the center of pressure *(C of P)* during a gait cycle. *LHC,* Left heel contact; *LTO,* left toe-off; *RHC,* right heel contact; *RTO,* right toe-off. (From Palia AE, Winter DA, Frank JS, et al: Identification of age-related changes in the balance control system. In Duncan P, editor: *Balance: proceedings of the APTA forum,* Alexandria, VA, 1990, American Physical Therapy Association.)

produce automatic, anticipatory, and voluntary postural responses to restrict or produce weight shifts.

Early treatment progression for COG control may include "neurodevelopmental sequence activities" (e.g., prone on elbows, all fours, kneeling, right or left side sitting, half-kneeling), not for the purpose of "reflex development" in the traditional sense but because the task demands are to balance with progressively less surface contact (i.e., shrinking the base of support). Additional benefits include greater control, coordination, and generation of power of the neck, trunk, and axial muscles. It also is useful for simultaneously addressing impairments such as lower-extremity extensor tone, trunk weakness and asymmetries, and head and neck extensor weakness. Functionally, bed mobility and floor-to-stand transfers are related to these progressive position exercises and should be practiced concurrently in low- and high-level clients, respectively.

Sitting balance can be progressed by (1) removing upper-extremity support (hands on firm surface to moveable surface [e.g., ball, bolster, rolling stool], one hand free and both hands free); (2) making the seating surface less stable (mat to bed to rocker board to Swiss ball); and (3) removing the use of one foot by crossing the leg or of both feet by raising the height of the seat so they do not touch the floor. Tasks might include multidirectional weight shifts with the hands in contact with a bolster or ball that is pushed or pulled to and fro, reaching or passing objects, performing upper body tasks (grooming, dressing), managing socks and shoes and wheelchair armrests and footrests, and so forth.

Sitting to Standing and Transfer Balance. Transitional movements such as sitting to standing and transfers involve large COG excursions over a stable base of support. For sitting to standing, the base of support must change from the seat to the feet. The feet begin to accept the weight first by downward pressure through the heels as the pelvis rolls anteriorly. The weight moves to the front of the feet as the trunk comes forward and the pelvis lifts from the surface, then backward toward midline as the trunk extends into standing. The COG stays near midline if both legs are participating equally, but it will often deviate to a preferred side during the transition in clients with hemiplegia. Training should include disadvantaging the preferred leg (perhaps by moving it a bit forward) to allow the more affected leg and foot to experience the weight transference. During transfers, a lateral weight shift is required in addition to the partial stand. The COG does not remain near midline; it instead moves forward to load the feet and then laterally toward the side of the transfer. Progression of balance skills in sitting to standing and transfer tasks may involve gradually lowering the height of the surface, removing armrests to preclude upper-extremity assistance, and transferring to surfaces of different heights and firmnesses. Remember that velocity is a normal part of sitting-to-standing movements because the momentum is used to assist the weight transfer from seat to feet, so the clinician must allow some speed during this task. If the client is unsteady on arising (cannot dampen or slow the speed in a controlled manner), working gradually from standing to sitting initially may be beneficial before progression to sitting to standing. Practice of sitting to standing with the eyes closed can be an effective way to train clients who are overdependent on vision for balance. Without the use of vision for stability, integration of vestibular and somatosensory systems can be facilitated.

Standing Balance. Standing balance tasks also can begin with finding midline and becoming stable there. Controlled mobility (volitional) should be encouraged as soon as possible, first on a stable surface with slow, small weight shifts. Challenge is added by increasing the distance traveled away from midline, moving toward restricted regions of the limits of stability, altering speed of sway, adding combined upper-extremity activities (e.g., dribbling a basketball, reaching), or adding resistance (manual, flexible bands). Narrowing the base of support (Romberg, tandem, single leg) makes control of the COG more demanding. Placing the feet in a diagonal stride position is more desirable for pregait weight shifting than is symmetrical double stance. Attention should be given to the stance (loading) leg with regard to pelvic protraction, hip and knee extension, and ankle dorsiflexion, with the tibia traveling forward over the foot. Focus on the swing (unloading) leg should include pelvic drop with knee flexion as the heel comes up and pressure through the ball of the foot and toes to load the opposite leg maximally. Standing balance exercises can be made more difficult by training on a less stable surface (carpet, foam, rocker board, BAPS board) and by adding combined head and eye movements or closing the eyes. The goals for dynamic sitting and standing balance exercises are to increase the size and symmetry of the limits of stability and improve the ability to transfer weight to different body segments with control at different speeds and with varied amounts of force. To facilitate somatosensory and vestibular integration, these activities can be performed with decreased or distorted visual cues. Closing the eyes, turning the head quickly, turning the lights down low, or wearing sunglasses may decrease the use of vision for stabilization.

Strategy Training. Training ankle, hip, and stepping strategies may begin in a voluntary manner but must progress to an automatic level of use to develop more normal balance and for real-life prevention of balance loss. Before strategy training, the clinician should be sure that the client has the ability to develop the desired strategies. The observed dominance of other strategies is appropriately compensatory, not dysfunctional, if a missing strategy cannot be effectively executed. Clients use these strategies to prevent loss of balance, so the clinician must take care not to reduce reliance on an effective strategy but to add additional strategies to the repertoire.

Ankle strategy should be practiced on a firm, broad surface. Clients can be asked to sway slowly in anterior-posterior, right-left, and diagonal directions, first to and from midline, progressing to passing midline, and finally progressing to sway toward the periphery without return to midline. Head and pelvis should be traveling in the same direction at the same time. Clients can practice standing near a wall with a table in front of them, swaying forward to touch the table with the stomach (leading with the pelvis) and backward to touch the wall with the back of the head. Cues are given not to "bow" to the table and not to touch the wall with the buttocks. As soon as the client is able to perform this protocol, functional meaning should be added with maneuvers such as forward or lateral reaching tasks, hands over head to take things off shelves, and leaning backward to rinse hair in the shower. To improve anticipatory and automatic ankle strategy use, add slight perturbations to the body or the surface when midline, progress to gentle perturbation when away from midline, and finally progress from predictable to unpredictable perturbations.

Hip strategy is practiced on either a narrow or an unstable surface, such as standing sideways on a balance beam, a two-by-four, a half-slice foam roller, foam, or a rocker board. The head and pelvis travel in opposite directions to counterbalance each other, in a forward bow–backward bending motion for anterior-posterior sway. Rapid sway is requested in forward-backward, right-left, and diagonal directions. By using the wall and table setting previously mentioned, clients can be cued to how to touch the nose toward the table while simultaneously touching the wall with the buttocks. Lateral hip strategy can be trained similarly, with the client standing sideways to the wall, touching the table with one hip and the wall with the opposite shoulder. Sway close to the edge of the client's limit of stability should produce a shift from ankle to hip strategy, so to enhance the use of hip strategy the client should practice sway control as far away from midline as possible without stepping. As soon as the client demonstrates the ability to perform this strategy, it should be incorporated into functional tasks such as low reaching (e.g., trunk of car, laundry dryer). To promote anticipatory and automatic use of hip strategy, the client is in midline and given moderate, rapid perturbations to the body or the surface such that ankle strategy will be insufficient to counteract the force. Then the size of the disturbance is increased, and the client is positioned away from midline when the perturbation is given so that righting to midline is appropriate. The shift should be made from predictable ("don't let me make you step or fall") to unpredictable perturbations.

Stepping strategy can be practiced first from atop a step, curb, or balance beam. Both legs should be included in training because real-life situations such as a slip or trip often preclude the use of one limb and demand the use of the other. It may be necessary to fix one foot in position to prevent stepping by the less affected leg in order to allow a stepping response on the more affected leg to emerge (a forced-use paradigm). Progress is made by stepping on a level surface and then to stepping up onto a step or curb or over progressively larger obstacles (appliance cord, shoe, phone book). All directions should be practiced, including lateral and diagonal perturbations, if safe recovery from real-life unexpected balance losses is to be learned. Large, rapid perturbations are given such that ankle and hip strategies will be inadequate and stepping or reaching is demanded. Again, progress should be made from predicted to unpredictable disturbances. For any automatic postural response—ankle, hip, stepping, protective reaching—to be effective in real life, successful demonstration of the response to *unexpected* perturbations is imperative.

Many clients, especially those who are fearful of falling, are dependent on the use of hands for stability. Therapeutic balance retraining activities should provide the maximal level of challenge that can be managed without the need for upper-extremity support. If the client physically needs to hold on, then the activity is at too high a level and should be modified. Otherwise, what is being taught is a "hand strategy" that will not be useful if the client experiences loss of balance when nothing firmly fixed is available to grasp for stability. Extremely anxious clients may initially benefit from training with an overheard harness system that will permit hands-free motion but provide tangible reassurance that a fall will be prevented if balance loss occurs. In this case, treatment progression would include weaning the client off the use of the harness. If the only harness available is on a body-weight support treadmill or gait system, move the balance retraining to that harness. The treadmill does not need to be moving.

Gait Training. The initial focus for controlling the COG during gait is a stable base of support that can be continually reestablished quickly and reliably through stepping. Unlike standing balance, in which the base is stable and the COG moves over it, during locomotion the base is moving and the COG moves to stay over the base. Achieving a symmetrical, smoothly oscillating COG movement is the objective, with the forces of gravity and momentum being exploited.

The training is begun first in the forward direction but also includes backward and sideways directions (sidestepping, braiding, or carioca) to increase postural control demands. Challenge can be added by narrowing the base of support (tandem) or reducing the foot-surface contact (walk on toes or heels). Training to integrate postural control with locomotor skills is best accomplished not through continuous, steady-pace walking, but by starting, stopping, turning, bending, varying the speed, and avoiding or stepping over obstacles. Difficulty is added by increasing the abruptness, frequency, and unpredictability of these types of tasks and by adding tasks such as carrying or reading while walking. Altered surface conditions (carpets, ramps, curbs, stairs, grass, gravel) or reduced lighting conditions also heighten the challenge. Head and eye movements while walking should be added as the client improves. Walking quickly while reading signs on the wall or room numbers, for example, or looking toward and away from the therapist while walking makes vision more difficult to use for stability. Walking in crowds or in busy, cluttered environments is also challenging. Locomotion training on the treadmill reduces some abnormal asymmetries and increases control of gait with increased extension of the trailing limb.[116] Again, gait training specifically for balance enhancement should occur without holding onto fixed surfaces with the hands, for example, parallel bars or the side rails of the treadmill. This is because the nervous system needs to learn to solve the balance problem using the legs and trunk, not the hands.

Clients with somatosensory loss in the feet should use a cane or walker. They may not need the device for biomechanical support, but they do need to obtain as much information about the surface as possible. Through use of a cane or walker, preserved somatosensation in the hands can detect surface information that is important for balance control, and biomechanical support is available if needed in case of balance loss.

Other Considerations

Treatment Tools

Therapists use both high-technological and low-technological equipment in the remediation of balance deficits; each has advantages and disadvantages. High-technological options include accelerometers with motion biofeedback, forceplate systems with postural sway biofeedback, electromyographic biofeedback, optokinetic visual stimulation (from visual surround or moving lights), videotaping, and treadmills with biofeedback. Options for the evaluation and treatment of balance and gait deficits are expanded with the addition of advanced technology such as forceplate measures of postural sway and pressure mat measures of gait, giving the therapist a more quantitative and sensitive measurement than visual observation or timed measures. Most high-technological systems provide computer-generated reports with charts and graphs quickly. For training, overhead harness systems allow safe, hands-free practice, and computerized sway feedback supports motor learning (Figures 22-20 through 22-23). Computerized systems allow advanced monitoring of progress and biofeedback, which supports motor learning.[117] Figure 22-20 is an example of technology in which forceplates measure pressure-generated signals (center of force [COF]). The systems shown use height and COF data to calculate the COG, which is used to measure postural sway. The COG icon may be displayed on the monitor screen for feedback to the individual if desired. Figure 22-21 is an example of how surface motion provides both biomechanical and somatosensory challenges. Balance measurement characteristics vary: some systems measure the motion of the surface (Figure 22-21, *A*), whereas others use motion sensors on the body placed at the level of the COG (Figure 22-21, *B*). Other systems provide the ability to generate visual motion. Figure 22-22, *A*, shows a system with a three-sided booth with unidirectional motion combined with a moveable forceplate with unidirectional motion. Both visual and somatosensory inputs can be manipulated for testing (e.g., SOT) and training. Omnidirectional visual motion (Figure 22-22, *B*) can be produced by rotating display systems that are used in a dark room.

The ability to challenge balance during gait training is improved if the client is secure in an overhead harness system as seen in Figure 22-23, *A* and *C*. These systems allow

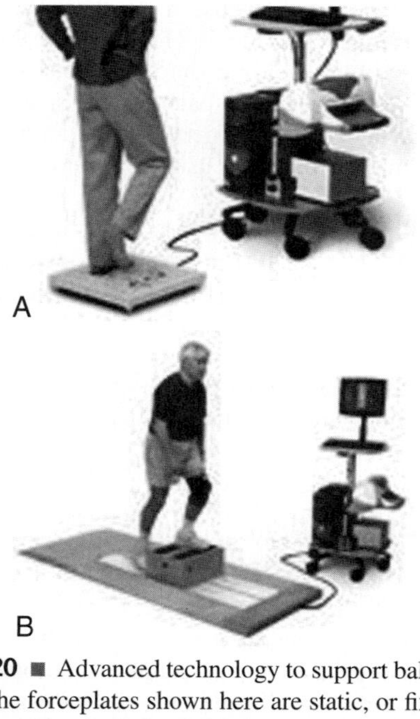

Figure 22-20 ■ Advanced technology to support balance and gait retraining. The forceplates shown here are static, or fixed. They are somewhat portable. **A,** Balance Master Basic. **B,** Balance Master. (Courtesy NeuroCom, a division of Natus, Clackamas, Ore.)

hands-free training as soon as possible, to increase reliance on the lower extremity and trunk reactions critical for balance recovery strategies. Rapid and recordable measurement of gait characteristics (e.g., velocity, step length, step width) is possible with instrumented systems. Some systems are made for overground walking (Figure 22-23, *B*) and are portable. Other systems are incorporated into treadmills and provide feedback during gait training. All motorized systems provide the ability to manipulate the environment easily and efficiently and to graduate tasks and environmental challenges safely. Drawbacks to high-technological equipment include cost, space requirements, and operator training requirements.

Low-technological options include mirrors, soft foam pads, hard foam rollers, rocker boards, BAPS boards, tilt boards, Swiss balls, mini-trampolines, balance beams, and wedges or incline boards. All these items are accessible (low cost, easy to obtain), portable, and easy to use. The main drawbacks for low technological equipment are that it does not provide novel feedback, objective scoring, or graphic recording, and clinicians must be skilled and creative in the use of such equipment in order to provide appropriate gradation of task difficulty and environmental conditions.

Safety Education and Environmental Modifications

Remediation of balance deficits is not always possible, but the clinician is always responsible for ensuring the safety of each client. When permanent deficits exist, the client and the family should be taught in what environments the client is at risk (e.g., a client with vestibular loss on a gravel driveway at night), what tasks are unsafe (e.g., ladder climbing, changing ceiling light bulbs), how the client can compensate (e.g., use a cane at night or in crowds), and what changes in the home or workplace are needed (e.g., night lights, stair stripes, raised toilet seats). Clinicians can ask the client (or family) to problem solve risky situations: "What would the client do?" Home evaluations should be followed by a list of recommended safety modifications. Falls are frightening and dangerous; clinicians should do their utmost to prevent them. If falls are likely, clients and families should be taught what to do if a fall occurs and, once the client is on the floor, how to perform floor-to-standing or floor-to-furniture transfers. Home monitoring services such as Lifeline may be indicated if the client lives alone and is prone to falling. Hip protectors will not prevent falls but do significantly reduce the risk of hip fracture.

Home Programs

Strengthening, stretching, posture, and endurance exercises can all be performed safely at home so that time in the clinic can be spent on balance-challenge exercises requiring supervision. Improvements in strength, ROM, posture, and endurance support improvements in balance. Many balance exercises can and should be performed at home if safety and adherence can be ensured; however, *unstable clients should always be supervised.* Standing balance tasks can be completed in a corner or near a countertop so that in case of balance loss the client can use the hands (reaching strategy) to prevent a fall if other automatic postural response strategies are inadequate. However, balance exercises should not be routinely done while holding onto countertops, furniture, or other surfaces. If the client needs to use her or his hands to perform the balance task, the task is too difficult and

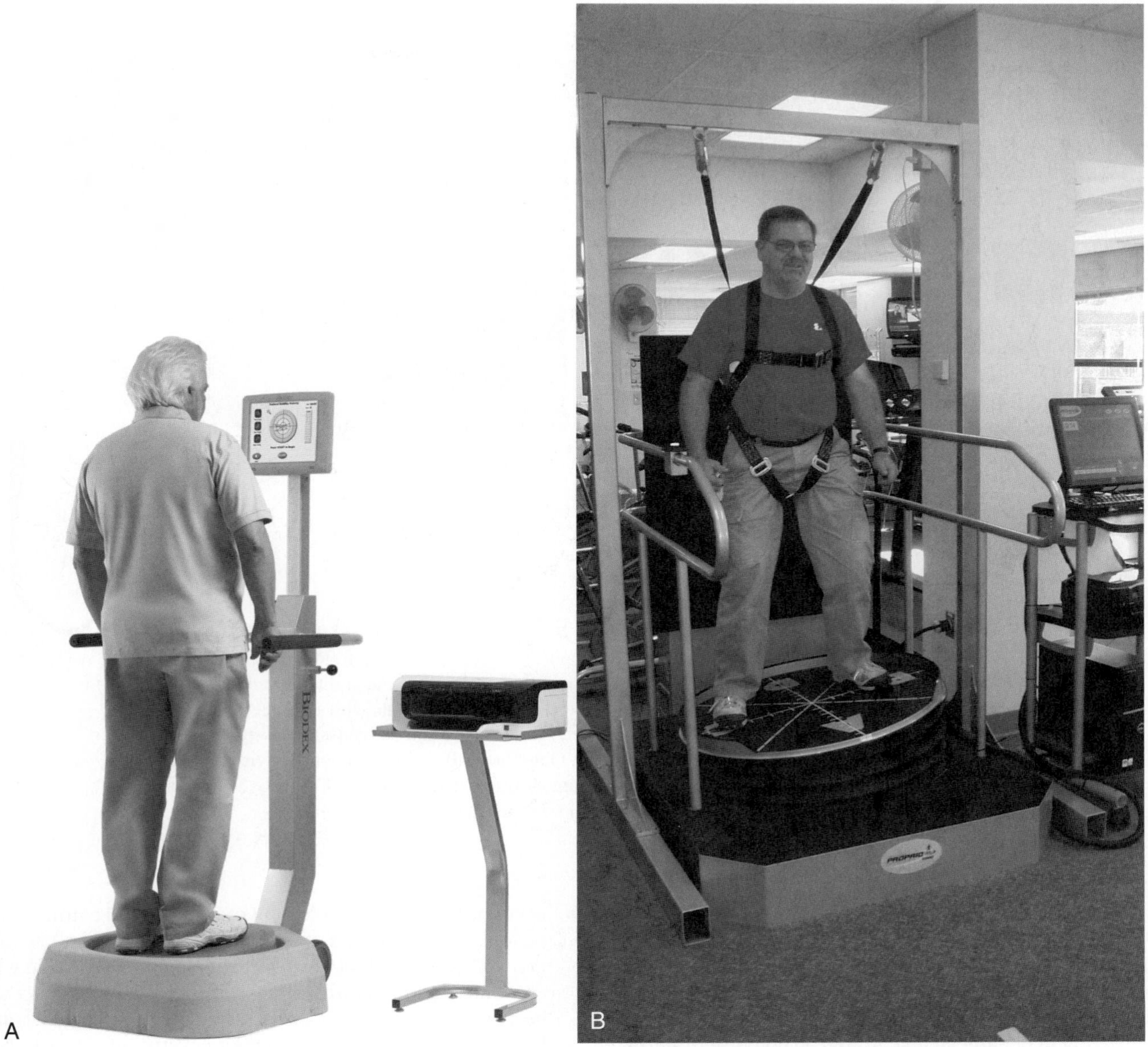

Figure 22-21 ■ Advanced technology to support balance and gait retraining. Other systems provide surfaces that can be made unstable **(A)** or made to move **(B).** The surface motion provides both biomechanical and somatosensory challenges. Amplitude and velocity capacity also vary from system to system. Both systems shown here provide omnidirectional motion. **A,** Biodex Balance System SD measures the motion on the surface, **B,** Proprio Reactive Balance System uses motion sensors on the body placed at the level of the COG (**A,** Courtesy Biodex Medical Systems, Shirley, NY; **B,** Courtesy Perry Dynamics, Decatur, Ill.)

should be modified so that it can be safely performed without needing to hang onto a stable object. The community setting is ideal for postural control gait training. Grocery or library aisles, public transportation, elevators, escalators, grass, sandboxes or beaches, ramps, trails, hills, and varied environmental conditions in general provide both challenge and functional relevance.

Concurrent Tasks

Normal balance is largely subconscious. One objective in balance retraining is to force the nervous system to solve postural control problems at the automatic, subconscious level. A great deal of practice and dual-task training are necessary to accomplish this; the conscious brain is focused on accomplishing some other goal(s) and thus balance control must be achieved at a less conscious level. Alternative tasks can be physical in nature, such as carrying a tray or dribbling a basketball, or cognitive, such as conversing or solving verbal or math problems, or a combination of physical and cognitive demands.

This objective is not universal. Clients with permanent or progressive deficits in automatic motor processing, particularly those with Parkinson disease, lose automaticity. They must learn to produce motor actions volitionally, with attention and intention, unless there are external sensory cues to drive the motor system.

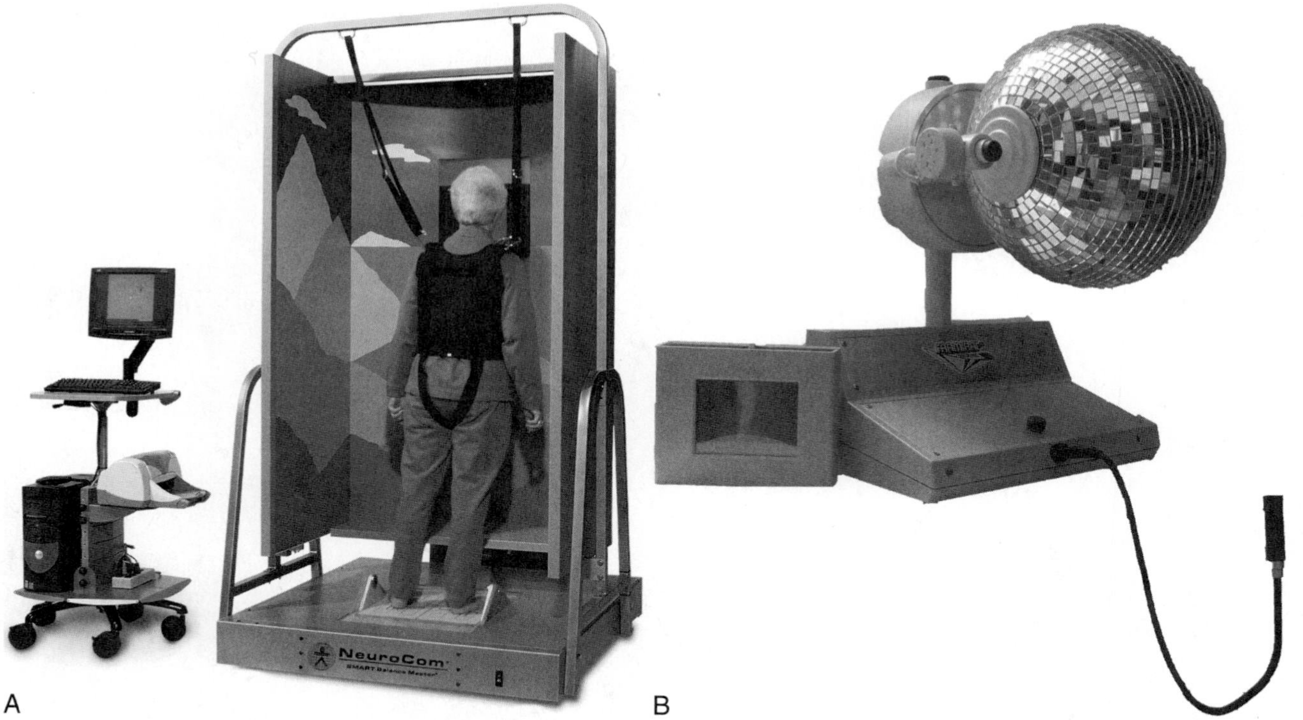

Figure 22-22 ■ Advanced technology to support balance and gait retraining. Visual motion may provoke instability for certain individuals. Some systems provide the ability to generate visual motion. **A,** SMART Balance Master is a system with a 3-sided booth with unidirection motion combined with a unidirectional movable forceplate. Both visual and somatosensory inputs can be manipulated for testing and training. **B,** Stimulopt Optokinetic Ball. Omnidirectional visual motion can be produced by rotating display systems that are used in a dark room. (**A,** Courtesy NeuroCom, a division of Natus, Clackamas, Ore; **B,** courtesy Framiral, Cannes, France.)

Fall Prevention

Client safety is always paramount; for any client with balance deficits the risk of falls is increased and must be addressed in every clinical management program. In older adults without documented neurological conditions, falls are prevalent and lead to severe injury (including head trauma) and death. Fall risk is even greater and is especially high in persons with stroke and Parkinson disease. Fall prevention is a critical primary objective for clinicians serving clients with neurological conditions who have impaired balance and gait.

Fall risk factors are categorized as intrinsic, relating to the individual, and extrinsic, relating to the environment. Intrinsic risk factors include but are not limited to medical conditions (e.g., stroke, Parkinson disease); medications; impaired balance and gait; somatosensory, visual, or vestibular sensory loss; central processing problems; slow reaction time and other central motor deficits; lower-extremity weakness and decreased ROM; cognitive deficits; depression; urinary urgency or incontinence; and footwear. Extrinsic risk factors are hazards in the environment, such as inadequate lighting or excessive glare, slippery or cluttered surfaces, lack of handrails or grab bars, attention distracters, and timing demands (e.g., hurrying to answer the phone). The more risk factors present, the greater the likelihood of falls. Most falls in community-dwelling older adults are trips and slips and occur because of a combination of intrinsic and extrinsic risk factors. For example, a client with hemiplegia who has limited ability to rapidly and maximally dorsiflex the ankle who encounters a trip hazard such as a rumpled doormat may not be able to clear the obstacle by lifting the hemiplegic leg and foot quickly. If the number and/or severity of intrinsic risk factors is great, falls may occur without any provoking extrinsic hazard.

Additional factors influence fall risk levels. The location of the client may have an effect on fall risk. While in an institutional setting, the physical environment may be safer and the level of supervision and assistance higher, thus lowering risk. Yet if the surroundings are unfamiliar or confusing to the client, the client does not remember to call for assistance before getting up, or the environment holds barriers such as bedrails, wheelchair footrests, and so on that must be dealt with when hurrying to the bathroom, then an institutional setting may pose increased risk. The amount of supervision or assistance the client receives may alter risk level. Confused or forgetful clients in facilities with high staff-to-client ratios or who have family or caregiver supervision most of the time will have lower risk than those in facilities or homes where supervision and assistance are sparse. Lastly, the relative dependence-independence level of the client, both physical and cognitive, affects risk level. Very dependent clients who cannot get up by themselves, and very independent clients with high-level balance and

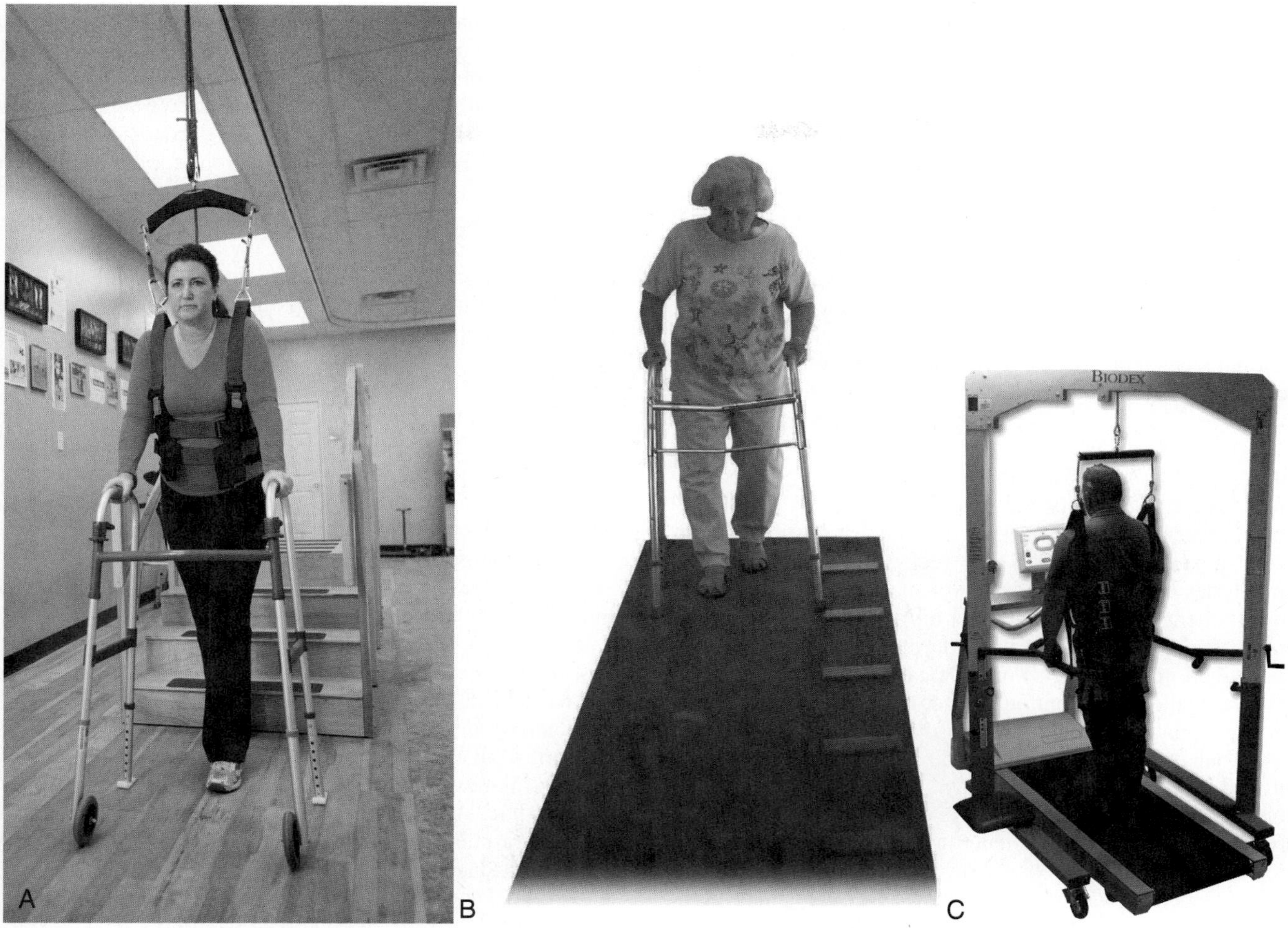

Figure 22-23 ■ Advanced technology to support balance and gait retraining. High technology used to challenge gait. The ability to challenge balance during gait training is improved if the client is secure in an overhead harness system. These systems allow hands-free training to increase reliance on the lower extremities and trunk reactions critical for balance recovery strategies. Rapid and recordable measurement of gait characteristics is possible with instrumented systems. **A,** Biodex FreeStep SAS uses overhead harness system to challenge balance during gait. **B,** GAITRite Portable Walkway System challenges gait during overground walking. **C,** Biodex Gait Trainer 3 with Unweighting System is another example of how to challenge balance during gait training. (**A** and **C,** Courtesy Biodex Medical Systems, Shirley, NY; **B,** courtesy CIR Systems, Havertown, Pa.)

gait skills, are both at lower risk than clients in the middle of that spectrum. Clients who have sufficient ability to get up out of the bed or chair, and perhaps to walk, but who have impaired balance and gait skills and poor judgment or memory are at a much higher risk level.

A separate but equally important risk to consider is the risk of injury from a fall. Injury risk also depends on both intrinsic and extrinsic factors. Clients with low bone mineral density, low body mass, and impaired protective responses (automatic postural responses, especially reaching or protective extension) are more likely to be injured. Falls that occur from a greater height onto a harder surface are more apt to result in injury. An overweight client with adequate bone mineral density (BMD) who, while in her yard gardening, stumbles and falls to the grassy ground from standing height with both arms out to break her fall would have a lower risk of injury. A thin client with osteoporosis who, while at the store shopping, stumbles off a curb and falls to the concrete parking lot without getting her arms out in time to protect her would have a higher risk of injury.

Clinicians should consider fall risk and injury risk factors as they carry out their assessments and evaluation. This would begin with the chart review or history taking; as problems are noted, the clinician should be "red-flagging" those that are risk factors for falls. For example, you might note that the client is on more than six prescription medications; polypharmacy is a risk factor for falls. You also note that one of the medications is a drug to remediate bone loss, and further inquiry reveals that the client does have a diagnosis of osteoporosis, a risk factor for injury. During your own therapy assessment, you find substantial lower-extremity weakness, balance impairments, and gait limitations requiring the use of an assistive device, all major risk factors for falls. One of the identified balance impairments includes deficient automatic postural responses, a risk factor for injury. Later, during a team meeting to discuss the new client, you learn from the occupational therapist that the home safety survey completed by the client's spouse indicates numerous safety hazards, extrinsic risk factors for falls and perhaps injury. For fall prevention and injury prevention purposes, a list of all fall and injury risk factors pertaining to that client should be generated for use in treatment planning.

The aim of intervention for fall prevention is to eliminate or minimize risk factors, with emphasis on four risk factors that appear to be more influential than others (in community-dwelling older adults). These four interventions are exercise, medication management, home safety modification, and vision management. The single best intervention for fall prevention is exercise—specifically, individualized exercises that target balance, gait with balance challenges, and leg strength. The challenge level of the balance and gait exercises should be high. The balance and gait training program must be of high intensity and frequency and of long duration. For a reduction in fall rates in community-dwelling older adults, a bare minimum of 5 to 6 weeks, with sessions two to three times a week, is required. For more neurologically involved clients, the overall amount of practice would need to be greater. Gains that are made during therapy will not be maintained unless exercise or physical activity that includes balance challenge is continued after therapy. Clients should be intentionally transitioned from therapy to a community-based balance exercise or physical activity program as an integral part of their discharge plan. Clinicians may consider doing their last treatment or two at the community-based program to support the client through the transition and increase the probability of follow-through. It is critical for clients to persist with physical activity to maintain or even further lower their fall risk level.

The second area of intervention is medication management. This requires a team approach and tactful, professional communication with the client's physician(s). The goal is to have the client take as few medications as possible, in the smallest doses possible, and to eliminate or when necessary replace certain drugs that are known to raise the risk of falls substantially (e.g., benzodiazepines). (Refer to Chapter 36 for a discussion of the impact of drug therapy on patients undergoing neurological rehabilitation.) Clinicians must understand that medication management for fall prevention is a difficult balancing act for the physician. For example, antidepressants and sleeping pills raise the risk of falls. Yet depression and sleep disorders are serious conditions with many negative effects, and depression, inattention, and fatigue are all risk factors for falls. Both the condition and its treatment increase risk! Clients on blood-thinning medication who are at risk for falls are also at risk for serious bleeding problems should a fall occur; the physician, client, and family or caregiver should all be alerted to this risk. Medication management guidance for fall prevention directed to physicians is available from the American Geriatrics Society.

Home safety modification is an effective intervention for those who are already at high risk for falls. Ideally an in-person home safety evaluation is performed by a trained professional, usually a physical or occupational therapist. If this is not possible, a home safety survey may be completed by a reliable source (client, family member, or caregiver). The clinician and client or their responsible decision makers should then have a frank discussion about recommended home safety modifications. The clinician should convey what is recommended and why, highlighting the benefits. However, factors such as time, expense, and personal preference also influence client and family decisions. Identification of barriers to safety modification implementation is helpful and may lead to solutions that permit initial resistance to be overcome.

Vision management is critical for any client with visual deficits. (Refer to Chapter 28 for a discussion of disorders of vision and visual-perceptual dysfunction.) These visual impairments might be at the peripheral level, such as macular degeneration, or the central level, such as homonymous hemianopsia. Occupational therapy is recommended for a visual-perceptual evaluation and potentially for low-vision rehabilitation if needed. Vision professionals (ophthalmologists, developmental optometrists), preferably those with specialization in neurological populations if indicated (e.g., TBI, cerebrovascular accident [CVA], MS), should also be involved. Objectives include maximizing vision for the client and including visual support within the home safety modification plan if needed.

Footwear assessment is important. Walking indoors barefoot or in socks is associated with increased fall risk. The footwear most highly associated with hip fractures is slippers. Shoes and slippers that do not provide adequate foot support, or that have slick soles, are unsafe and not recommended. Footwear lacking a secure back (flip-flops, mules, or sling-backs), high-heeled shoes, and platforms are poor choices for clients at risk for falls. Running shoes with very thick, cushioned soles and a heavy tread are also not ideal. The optimal shoes for fall risk reduction are well fitted with thin, hard soles. Shoes with a tread sole and a tread beveled heel are more stable on wet or slippery surfaces.[118] Just as with home safety modifications, factors such as expense, habit, and personal preference may create obstacles to client adoption of suggested footwear changes. These obstacles should be recognized, respected, and addressed directly with professional communication strategies designed to facilitate positive behavior change.

Clinicians should assume that clients at risk for falls will fall when they are discharged home. Though we work to ensure this will not happen, we also prepare for the possibility that it will. Clients who are able must be taught how to get up from the floor independently, with and without furniture if the latter is possible. If clients cannot get up from the floor by themselves, then family members or caregivers should be taught how to assist clients to get up from the floor. This may be as simple an act as bringing a chair close to the client so the client can use the chair to get up independently. Clients at risk for falls who will be home alone for extended periods of time would benefit from a wearable home alerting system. If such a system is cost-prohibitive, the client should develop the habit of carrying a cell phone at all times. For clients without cell phones, a landline phone should be left on the floor or a chair seat so that it is within reach from the floor should a fall occur. Older clients with osteoporosis should consider wearing hip protectors. Hip protectors do not reduce the risk of falls but when properly fitted and worn may reduce the risk of hip fracture. Adoption of and adherence to wearing hip protector apparel is typically low and requires commitment and effort.

The combined aim of balance retraining and fall prevention is to assist the client to become as active as is safely possible. With improved balance and gait skills, the client achieves higher levels of function and physical activity. With attention to and emphasis on fall prevention, safety is maintained, injury is prevented, and the opportunity for improved quality of life is preserved.

Vestibular System

Kenda Fuller, PT, NCS

OVERVIEW: THE ROLE OF THE VESTIBULAR SYSTEM

The CNS integrates the information from visual, somatosensory, and vestibular inputs to determine the most appropriate response to maintain stability and homeostasis.[119] These three senses play an important role in dynamic equilibrium (Figure 22-24). In fact, the somatosensory system is necessary to interpret vestibular information.[120] The activity of the vestibular system must be recognized in order to interpret balance testing. This chapter provides background information that has been incorporated into the earlier portion on balance.

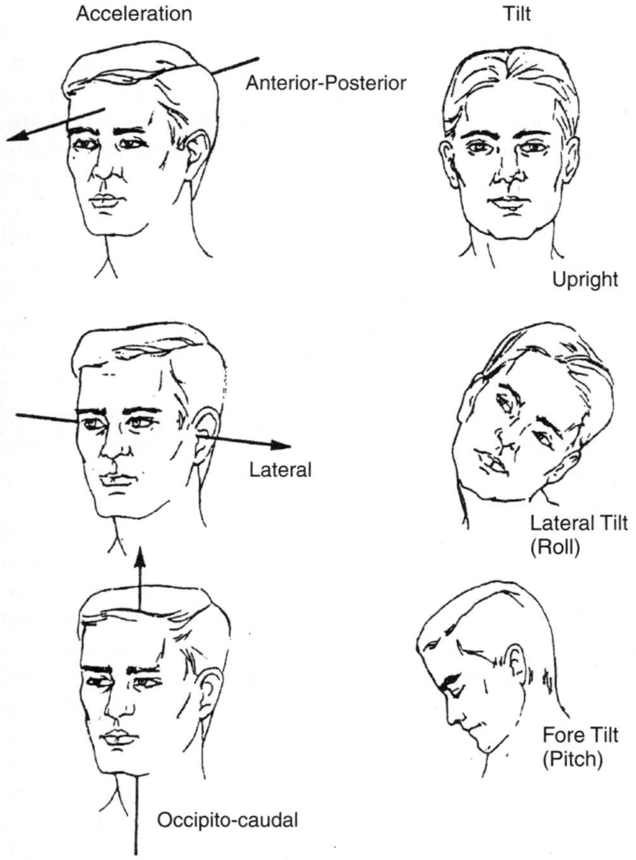

Figure 22-24 ■ The otoliths register linear acceleration and static tilt of the head. (From Hain TC, Ramaswany TS, Hillman MA: Anatomy and physiology of the normal vestibular system. In Herdman SJ, editor: *Vestibular rehabilitation,* ed 3, Philadelphia, 2007, FA Davis.)

The role of the vestibular system is to maintain clear vision during head motion as well as to orient head and trunk in space with respect to gravity when the visual and surface references are not sufficient. Horizontal and vertical accelerations, as in riding in a car or an elevator, are also detected by the vestibular otolith mechanism as seen in Figure 22-24.[121] The vestibular system is critical for postural control because it uniquely identifies self-motion as different from motion in the environment. Recognition of self-movement as it relates to visual movement can be disrupted momentarily in a normal individual experiencing unexpected movement in the peripheral visual environment. This is a common sensation noticed, for example, when the car next to you moves backward, and you press the brake, thinking that you are rolling forward. Unless the system fails, the vestibular system is noticed only when it is stimulated beyond the level at which it is typically activated, as in a fast spin or the drop of a roller coaster. The dizziness that occurs in the normal individual when the vestibular system is overstimulated is reflective of the dizziness that occurs when the brain encounters sudden changes or losses of input from the vestibular system.[122]

Disorders of the vestibular system can cause devastating lack of visual stability, loss of balance, and inaccurate sense of movement. There is an initial loss of trunk and gaze stability with vestibular dysfunction that improves as a result of CNS adaptation. The CNS adaptation is critical to recovery of function.[123] In the course of recovery, the visual or somatosensory systems may be chronically used in preference to the vestibular system, causing abnormal sensory dependence patterns.[123,125] Comorbid dysfunction can affect functional recovery, especially if it affects the visual or somatosensory inputs. Prior trauma, either physical or psychological, can cause maladaptation resulting in responses to intervention that are inconsistent with typical recovery patterns.[126-128]

Clinicians are exposed to patients at many different levels of adaptation, from the ones who show adequate adaptation with minimal intervention to those who have recovered only limited independence after disruption of vestibular system inputs. Successful intervention is achieved by accurately analyzing both the missing and the available components of the system, facilitating adaptation, avoiding excessive sensory substitution, and determining appropriate compensatory strategies.[129] If maladaptation is not understood and treated properly, it can lead to frustration for the patient and clinician, resulting in less than optimal outcomes.

VESTIBULAR SYSTEM DISORDERS

There are many types of common vestibular disorders. This chapter cannot provide a total discussion of all these disorders. They have been summarized in Appendix 22-A.

RECOVERY OF FUNCTION: NEUROSCIENCE OF THE VESTIBULAR SYSTEM

Recovery of function is related to the mechanism of injury and where the damage is located. In order to understand how the system recovers, we must first understand how it works. The end organ of the vestibular system is basically a mechanical, fluid-filled system activating afferent signals that travel through the vestibular nerve to the brain stem nuclei.[130,131] Figure 22-25 shows the relative relationship of the canals to the otoliths and the cochlea. This demonstrates

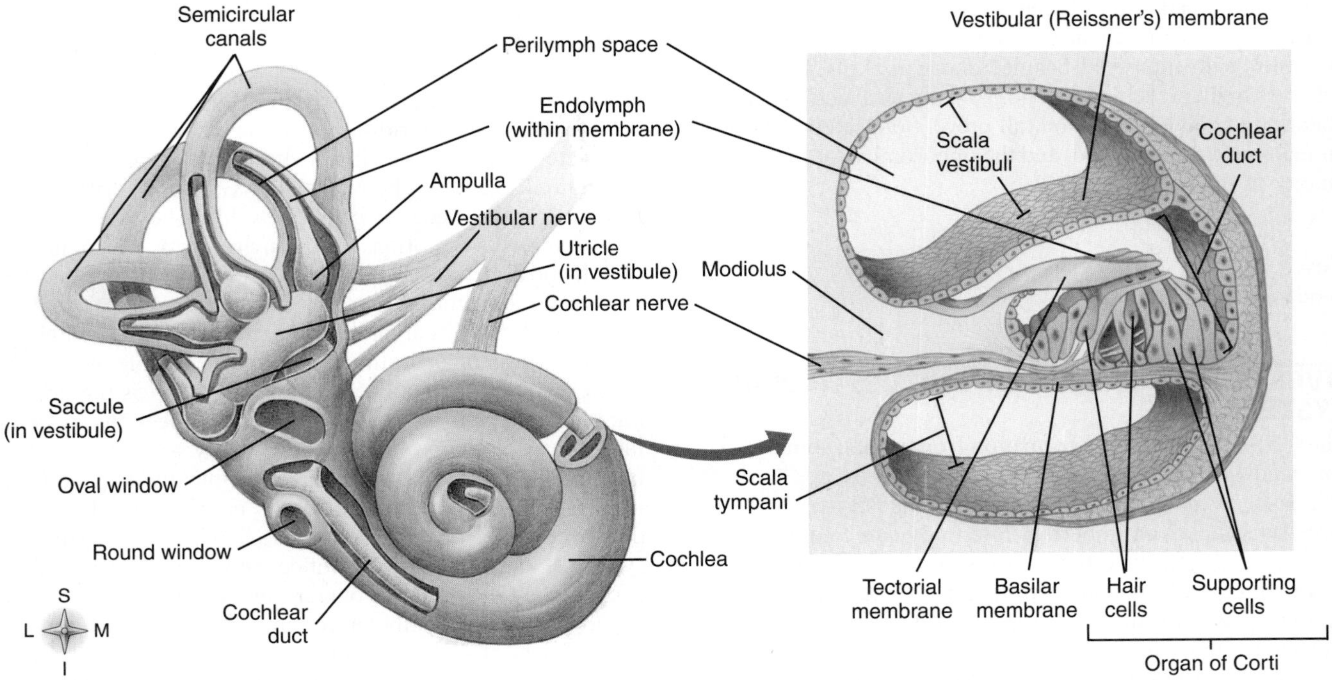

Figure 22-25 ■ Components of the vestibular system and cochlea with distribution of neural connections. (From Thibodeau GA: *Anatomy and physiology,* ed 6, St Louis, 2006, Mosby.)

why there is often a connection between loss of hearing and vestibular dysfunction, especially when the fluid mechanism is part of the impairment. Box 22-1 describes the sensory components of the vestibular system. At the level of the nuclei, the brain stem receives input from the other sensory systems related to orientation of the head and body. The combined input is further modulated by the cerebellum, providing further calibration. Purkinje cells in the cerebellum provide inhibitory control of the vestibular nuclei. The flocculonodular lobe and medial zone of the cerebellum affect postural control.[132] Input continues to the cortex via the vestibular projections (Box 22-2).

Recalibration at Rest

The tonic firing of the vestibular system when the head is in a neutral nonmoving state is symmetrical on both sides of the system at approximately 50 spikes per second. The brain is able to compare this symmetrical resting level tone to the information coming from the visual and somatosensory systems' feedback about the position and movement of the head.

BOX 22-2 ■ POTENTIAL LOCATION OF LESIONS THAT MAY AFFECT THE VESTIBULAR SYSTEM

- Vestibular end organ and vestibular nerve terminals
- Vestibular ganglia and nerve within the internal auditory canal
- Cerebellopontine angle
- Brain stem and cerebellum
- Vestibular projections to the cerebral cortex

From Goodman CC: *Pathology: implications for the physical therapist,* ed 3, Philadelphia, 2008, WB Saunders.

When there is disruption of signal from one side of the vestibular pathway, it will change the relative input into the CNS, resulting in a perception of the head rotating toward the intact side when the head is not actually moving (Figure 22-26). Initially, as well, there will be a phenomenon of spontaneous nystagmus, a reflex-driven movement of the eyes. In an acute asymmetrical vestibular system disruption, the eyes will move away from the perceived direction of head motion, and that movement of the eyes will cause a sensation of dizziness with the head still, eyes open. The brain quickly identifies this as an abnormal state and begins CNS recalibration so that the vestibular system input from each side becomes calibrated to match the visual and somatosensory system input. The system is able to determine that despite the uneven signals, the head is not really moving.[133] There is usually adequate central adaptation to stop the spontaneous nystagmus in a lighted environment within 3 days.[134] The spontaneous nystagmus may continue to be active in a dark room, and there may still be a sensation that the head is rotating when the eyes are closed for weeks after the insult. Increasing somatosensory input about stability can help in the central recalibration process. Input through the joint surfaces by establishing a stable joint reference can facilitate calibration. This appears to be most effective through mechanical pressure through the top of the head or with the use of weights on the shoulders to increase the vertical reference of the spine in a neutral position. Figure 22-27 shows how weights are placed on the shoulder to provide somatosensory input. The brain can then match or recalibrate the abnormal perception of head movement induced by the inaccurate vestibular system to the correct reference of the stable somatosensation. It is critical in the rehabilitation process to achieve accurate CNS recalibration with the head at rest before initiating intervention that requires movement of the head.

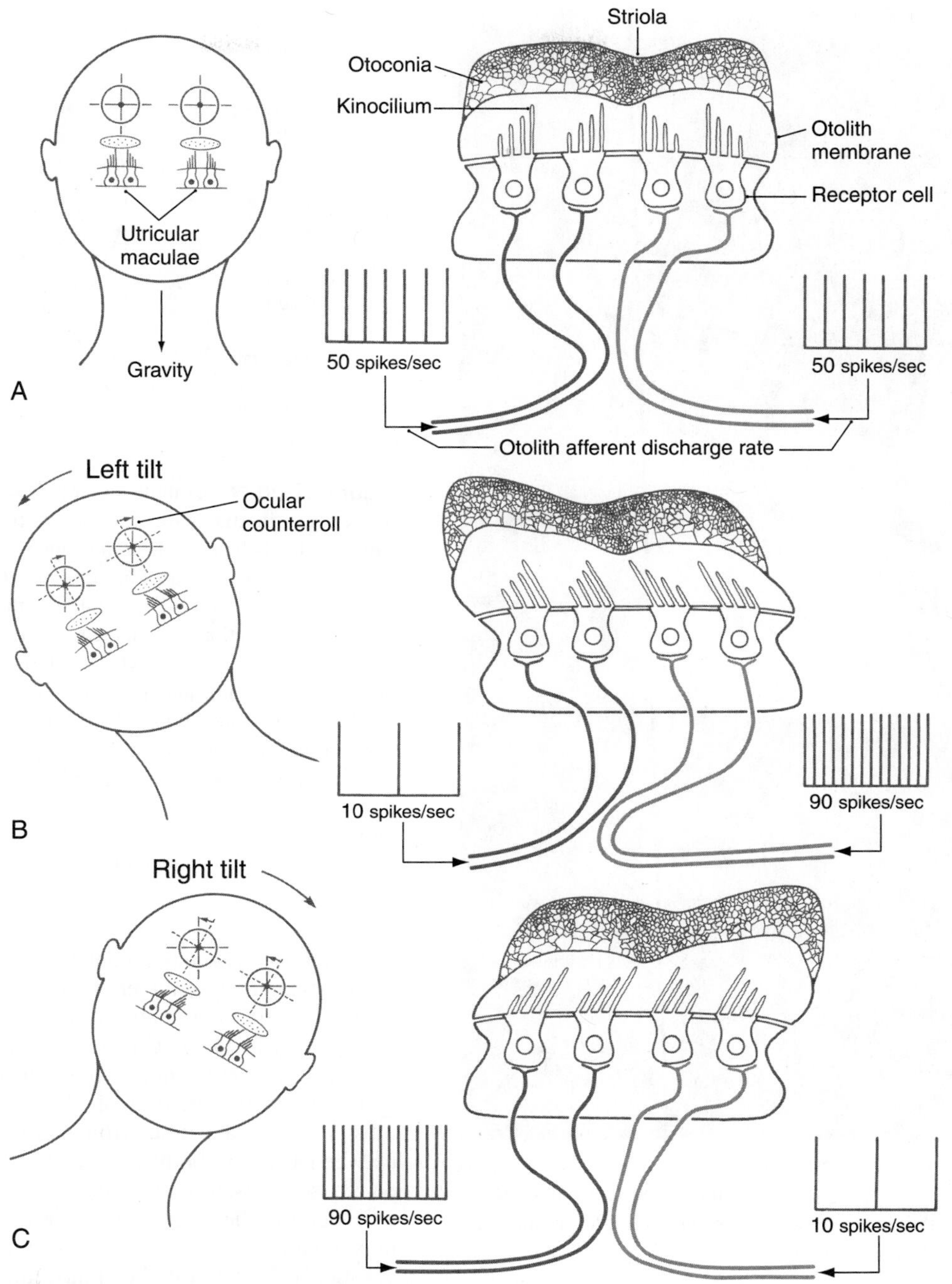

Figure 22-26 ■ Patterns of excitation and inhibition for the left utricle and saccule when the head is upright **(A),** tilted with the left ear 30 degrees down **(B),** and tilted with the right ear 30 degrees down **(C).** The utricle is seen from above and the saccule from the left side. (From Haines DE: *Fundamental neuroscience for basic and clinical applications,* ed 3, Philadelphia, 2006, Churchill Livingstone.)

Head Movement and Gaze Stability

As the head starts to move, the signal from each part of the vestibular system activates as a result of fluid movement against the cupula. The direction of movement is determined by the relative firing pattern of the vestibular system from each side of the head. The vestibular system on the side toward the movement increases in firing, and the side opposite decreases its firing rate. The resulting signal to the brain stem drives the VOR to move the eyes in opposition to the head movement, and the gain remains 1:1. Figure 22-28 shows the neural connections involved in activation of the VOR. If the vestibular system does not drive the eyes to the correct position for stable gaze, the result is vestibular-driven oscillopsia, and again, objects can appear to move as the head moves. This disorder has significant functional implications and works in conjunction with both smooth pursuits and saccades to interpret the relationship of the body to the environment (Figure 22-29).

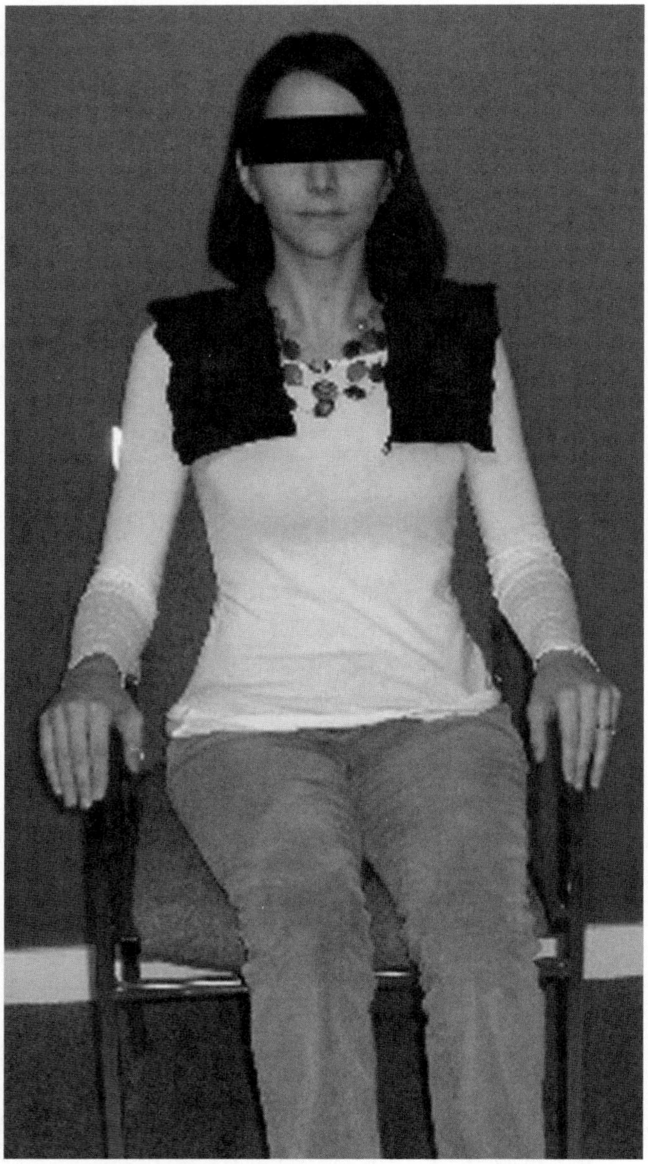

Figure 22-27 ■ Use of 5-pound weights on each shoulder to increase the somatosensory reference allows the vestibular system to recalibrate to the body reference. Eyes are closed to so that head position is not referenced by vision.

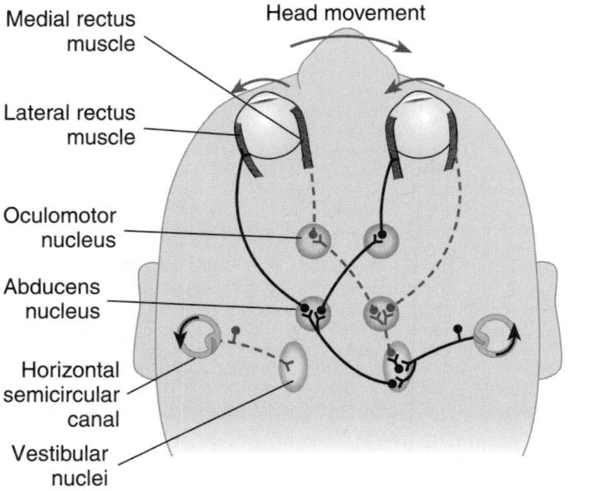

Figure 22-28 ■ Vestibuloocular reflex. When the head is turned to the right, inertia causes the fluid in the horizontal semicircular canals to lag behind the head movement. This bends the cupula in the right semicircular canal in a direction that increases firing in the right vestibular nerve. The cupula in the left semicircular canal bends in a direction that decreases the tonic activity in the left vestibular nerve. Neurons whose activity level increases with this movement are indicated in solid lines. Neurons whose activity level decreases are indicated in dotted lines. For simplicity, the connections of the left vestibular nuclei are not shown. Via connections between the vestibular nuclei and the nuclei of cranial nerves III and VI, both eyes move in the direction opposite to the head turn. (From Lundy-Ekman L: *Neuroscience: fundamentals for rehabilitation,* ed 3, Philadelphia, 2007, Saunders.)

The VOR is reported as abnormal only if there is loss of gaze stability, or blurring of target objects with head movement at 1 to 3 Hz. Rotation or pitch of the head during testing of the VOR may cause dizziness because of the differences in firing patterns from each ear that are not yet efficiently calibrated. This is especially noted when the head is moving in the direction of the abnormal ear. It is important to note that head motion–provoked dizziness can persist even when gaze stability has normalized.

The clinician must also be aware that the peripheral visual field will appear to move in the opposite direction as head movement during these testing procedures. This normal visual phenomenon can cause dizziness in the patient with visual dependence or visual motion sensitivity (described later). It is the vestibular system that provides the reference of head movement and position so that the perceived movement in the environment is properly identified.

The quality of somatosensation in the spine and muscles of the upper body can contribute to dizziness with head motion. The vestibular nuclei have the job of integrating somatosensory information on its way to the cortex. There must be adequate input from both systems to distinguish between head-on-body and body-on-head movement. Impaired somatosensation, pain, and guarding of movement will disrupt the accuracy of calibration related to head movement. The patient who has an abnormal VOR will be constantly decelerating head movement to less than 2 Hz in order to prevent blurred vision. That unconscious deceleration by the muscles in the neck can cause stiffness and decrease the sensitivity of the somatosensory mechanisms in the neck. Two simple tests will alert the therapist to abnormalities of head motion related to the quality of somatosensation. Holding the head upright and still, in gravity-neutral position, while the patient rotates in a chair (body on head) provides information about the somatosensory reference. The movement may elicit dizziness if the somatosensation is impaired. If the patient has been relying on somatosensation as a primary reference for head position, there may be resistance or guarding against allowing the body to move in a direction different from the direction of the head movement.

Rotating in a chair at 1 to 3 Hz and allowing the head to move at the same speed as the body will eliminate somatosensation reference through the neck receptors and isolate the vestibular system response to rotation of the head. This should

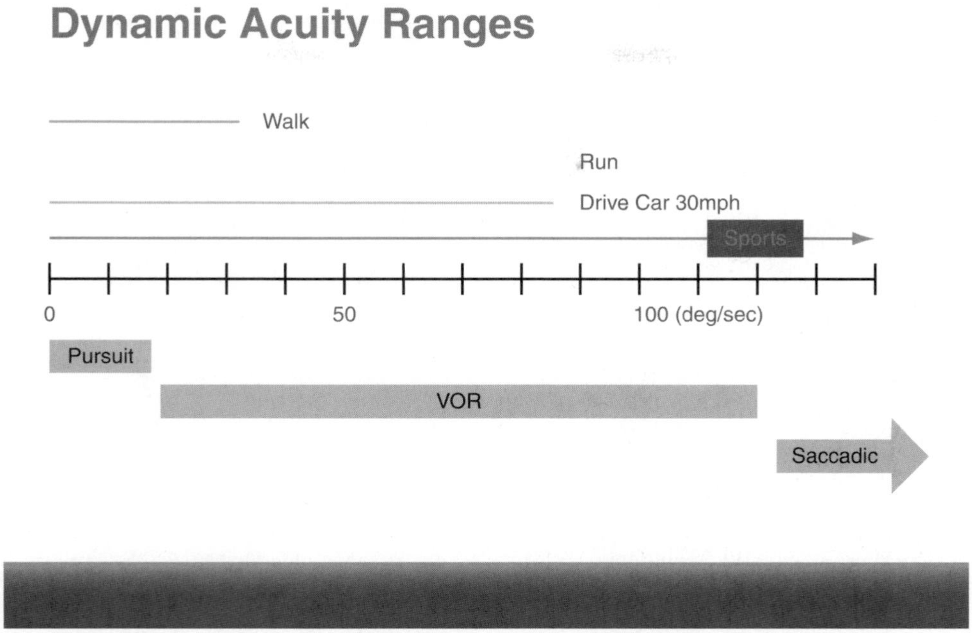

Figure 22-29 ■ Dynamic acuity ranges. (From NeuroCom beta-testing data and analysis (2004-2008), used by permission.)

be done with the eyes closed to eliminate the sense of visual motion. Movement at this speed will cause an increase in dizziness even in a normal system, but it should resolve in less than 10 seconds. If the dizziness persists for longer than 15 seconds, it is considered to indicate abnormal vestibular calibration.

Head Position Changes

Head position changes in reference to gravity can cause dizziness as a function of the vestibular system under certain circumstances. The most common form of head position dizziness in adults is BPV (see Appendix 22-A). In this condition, debris (otoconia) from the utricle moves into the semicircular canal, and there is suddenly mass in a system that is designed to calculate only fluid pressure changes in response to head movement. The added mass causes excessive deflection of the hair cells in the cupula when the head is moved into a gravity-dependent position. The otoconia move in the direction of gravity through the endolymph, causing a pull on the cupula and increased firing of the hair cells as if the head were moving quickly in that direction. Figure 22-30 shows the movement of the otoconia in relationship to head movement in a gravity-dependent state. The brain activates the VOR in response to the message that the head is moving quickly, and there is nystagmus based on the same mechanism as described previously. The nature of this nystagmus reflects the canal in which the debris is floating. As soon as the otoconia come to rest, the pressure on the hair cell is gone, and the nystagmus subsides. This takes about 20 seconds. There is no nystagmus until the head is moved into another gravity-dependent position causing the otoconia to roll through the canal.

Top-down Reference for Postural Control

The most important role of vestibular information for postural control relates to orientation of the head and trunk in space with respect to gravitational forces.[135-137] Orientation to gravity is most critical when balancing on unstable surfaces when vertical and horizontal visual reference is not adequate. The vestibular system provides a top-down reference for the head and trunk stability in line with gravity while the leg segment is coordinated to maintain surface reference. Vestibular inputs are critical to determine whether the body is swaying or the surface is perturbed.[138] The conscious perception of verticality used to orient to gravity when the support surface is perceived to be unstable is provided by the vestibular system. Vestibular inputs are used in order to recognize the changes in angle of the support surface.[139-141]

Surface perturbations or oscillations provide a method to examine the ability of the vestibular system to maintain the head and trunk in gravity-neutral position as the legs move in reference to the platform movements. When standing on a surface that tilts both anteriorly and posteriorly at 4 degrees per second, patients with bilateral vestibular loss will lose balance and fall.[120,140,141] A normal person should be able to position a hand-held rod in vertical while standing or sitting on an oscillating surface, irrespective of the angle of the surface, even with eyes closed. Individuals with loss of orientation to gravity will orient the hand-held rod with respect to the angle of the moving surface.[142]

It is important to remember that at the same time the vestibular system is activated in this moving surface condition, the somatosensory system is still providing feedback about the relationship of the head that is provided by vestibular inputs to the base of support.[2] Resulting patterns of muscle activation reflect vestibular and somatosensory integration to maintain continuous upright postural control. As a surface rotates to greater degrees, there is more weighting of the system away from the somatosensory reference toward the gravity reference.[138,143] Patients with noncompensated vestibular dysfunction will report lack of awareness of angle changes when standing on an oscillating support surface. Therefore, instead of changing the ankle angle to

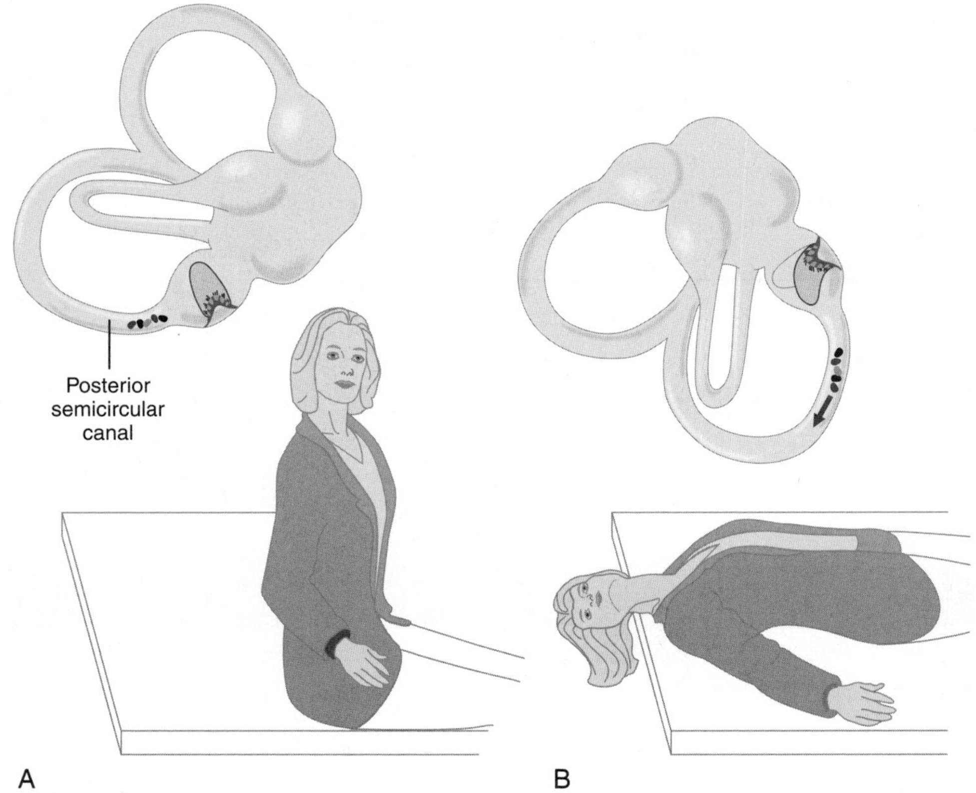

Figure 22-30 ■ The Hallpike-Dix maneuver. **A,** Starting position with head rotated toward the side to be tested. **B,** Lowering the patient's head backward and to the side allows debris in the posterior canal to fall to its lowest position, activating the canal and causing eye movements and vertigo. (From Lundy-Ekman L: *Neuroscience: fundamentals for rehabilitation,* ed 3, Philadelphia, 2007, Saunders.)

adjust to the tilt, the torque around the ankle remains locked, holding the leg, trunk, and head at 90 degrees to the surface. The head then follows the direction of the surface tilt as seen in Figure 22-31. As the surface tilt angle exceeds 8 degrees, the individual who cannot activate gravitational reference or adjust the ankle angle will be unable to maintain balance.[143] Lateral tilt can activate the system in the same way; with the head following the direction of the downward tilt, the weight is typically shifted to the downward-most leg. Patients report lack of awareness of the movement generated. Figure 22-32 shows the abnormal shift of weight as the patient attempts to orient to the surface rather than gravity.

Bottom-up Reference for Postural Control

The somatosensory system can determine the orientation of the head in reference to the surface through cutaneous, proprioceptive, pressure, and stretch receptors of the muscles and joints, primarily related to pressure through the balls of the feet. Although overreliance on this surface reference can be destabilizing in some conditions, it contributes to balance when the surface is stable or moving slowly (at less than 4 degrees per second). At the other end of the spectrum, in very fast oscillations the muscle spindles provide stabilizing information that can contribute to head and trunk stability.[144]

It is critical to remember that the vestibular spinal system also activates the neck muscles in response to head perturbations and modulates somatosensory-driven activity of muscles in the neck. When the vestibular system function is missing or inaccurate, there is abnormal muscle activation in the muscles of the neck.[120] One way this function can be tested is by observing head-righting response when a patient has vision blocked and is tilted while sitting on a tilt board so that the perturbation starts at the surface instead of the head. In the patient with vestibular dysfunction, when gravity vertical reference is lacking, lateral head righting back to center, or neutral is inadequate. This can be a result of co-contraction of the neck muscles to lock the head into position, with the trunk maintaining the same tilt as the trunk. The head stays in reference to the surface in much the same way as described earlier regarding locking of the ankle joints. This is evidenced in higher-level activities that require gravity reference such as tandem walking in visually stimulating environments or with vision occluded. As the patient tries to use somatosensation to determine head position instead of gravity reference, the head becomes locked onto the trunk through abnormal muscle activation. The narrow stance limits the contribution of surface reference in the lateral plane, and the patient must take a step out to control the excessive lateral tilt of the trunk and head. Figure 22-33 represents the abnormal and normal views of head righting in both sitting on a tilted surface and standing in tandem. It is the vestibular inputs that should drive the appropriate head righting and resulting postural strategies that are required in these conditions.

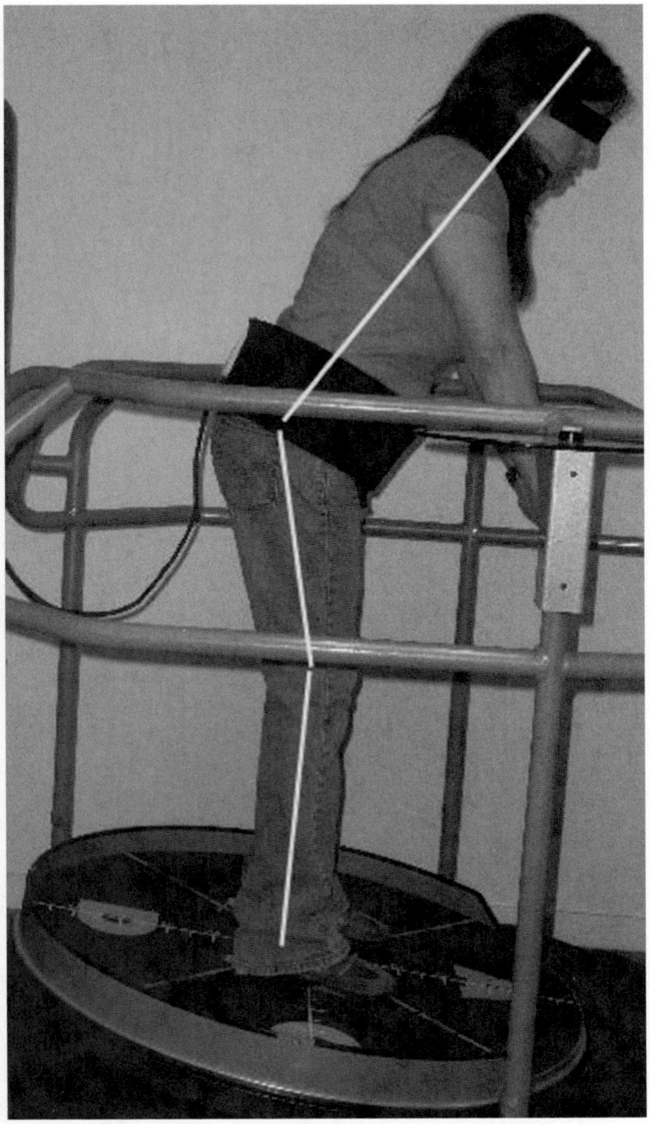

Figure 22-31 ■ In anterior tilt of the platform, the head and trunk follow the reference of the platform rather than maintaining a gravity-neutral position. This is reported as surface reference. (Courtesy Perry Dynamics, Decatur, Ill.)

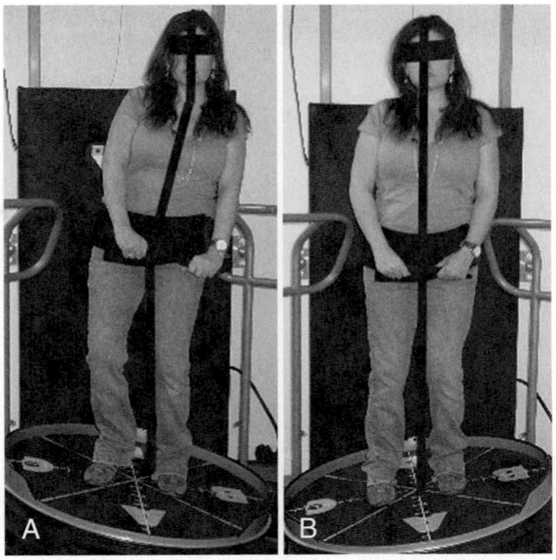

Figure 22-32 ■ **A,** The patient references her trunk to the platform, shifting weight downhill to the downhill leg. **B,** The patient has referenced her trunk and head to gravity, resulting in improved postural control. (Courtesy Perry Dynamics, Decatur, Ill.)

Having even the slightest touch reference so that the somatosensory system can orient the trunk through upper-extremity joint position sense is another way to substitute somatosensation for vestibular reference.[145] The position of the head and trunk can be determined by this touch even when the vestibular system function is missing and eyes are closed. Because the arm stabilizes the trunk more than the legs do, reaching for a stable surface is a common way to maintain balance when challenged. The therapist must recognize when the patient is using this touch reference to substitute for gravity. This is why allowing a patient to touch a stable surface during balance training should be quickly eliminated from intervention to avoid dependence on surface reference when attempting to activate the vestibular system.

When the brain is not able to use somatosensation to identify the relationship between appropriate body segments and the surface, the patient often will report feeling lightheaded or having the sense of floating. When somatosensory inputs from the neck are reduced, absent, or distorted, the result is poor spinal segment stabilization. Excessive muscle activity, including co-contraction of the sternocleidomastoid (SCM), levator scapulae, upper trapezius, and superficial neck extensors indicates poor stability, altered afferents, and recruitment patterns that are ineffective. Nociception from cervical segments can create "noise" in the postural control system contributing to dysmetric postural responses and nausea. Impaired cervical afferents will cause changes in cadence and length of stride when neck motion is introduced to gait. Diminished gait measures have been seen on the DGI in the presence of neck pain. When abnormal somatosensation is concurrent with CNS vestibular adaptation, the result is less than satisfactory. Because brain pattern learning is task specific and dependent on high repetition, it is not helpful to practice poor motor recruitment patterns during balance retraining.

Visual Reference for Postural Control

Orientation of the head in space is possible through predictive control of vision. A stable environment provides visual vertical and horizontal references for balance. Patients with vestibular loss are able to substitute vision for vestibular reference, even during surface perturbations.[146,147] Destabilization occurs when the peripheral visual references are moving slowly or are not in alignment with gravity. When eyes are tracking something moving in central gaze field, the background or peripheral visual field will appear to move in the opposite direction. In the patient with lack of gravity reference, when performing diagonal smooth pursuits, postural adjustment patterns are activated as if the room were tilting, because that is the dominant sensory reference being used. The patient is pulled off balance when aligning himself or herself with the apparent visual vertical. This is most pronounced and can be tested easily when a patient is standing

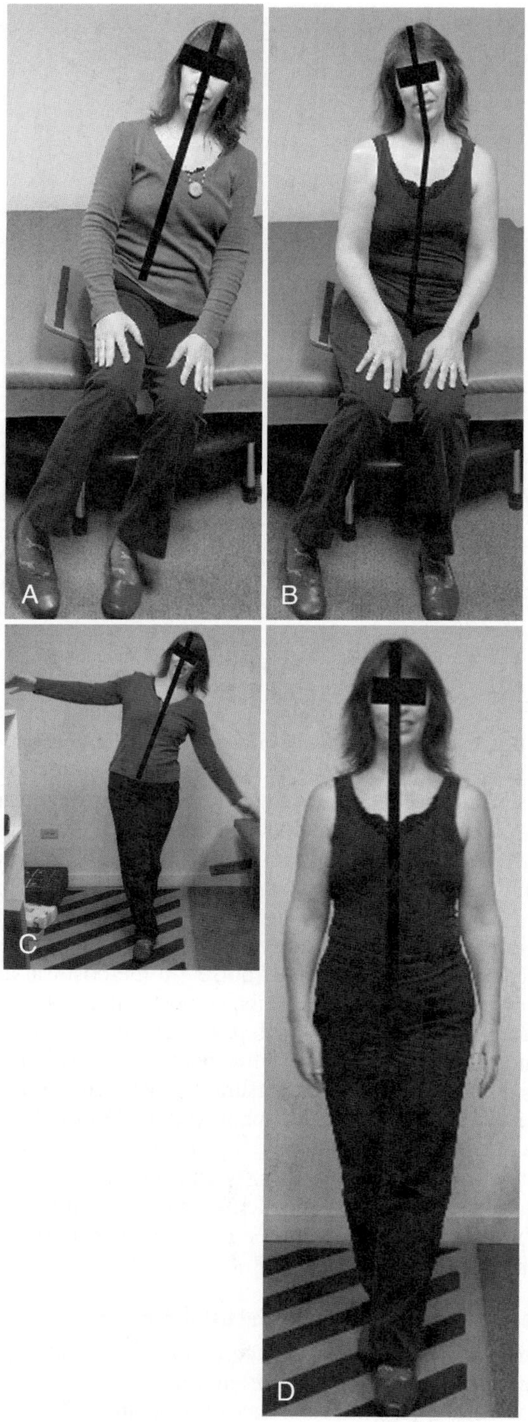

Figure 22-33 ■ **A,** When surface reference is used in preference to vestibular cue, the head remains in alignment with the surface. **B,** As the patient is able to regain vestibular function and gravity reference, the head remains in alignment with gravity, as a head-righting response. **C,** Lack of head-righting responses can cause excessive use of upper-extremity activity to try to reference to the surface, with bottom-up firing patterns; hip strategy is activated but inefficient. Abnormal reference patterns result in loss of balance in tandem stance with eyes closed. **D,** When the vestibular reference is restored, the head remains over the feet, so balance is restored. This is why it is important to observe the angle of the head during examination of tandem stance or gait. (Courtesy Ray Hedenberg, IRB Solutions, Silverthorne, Colo.)

on a compliant surface, tracking a target moving in a figure-of-eight configuration. Head and trunk sway match the apparent visual field movement instead of actual gravity vertical in the patient who is visually dependent. This test can be used in a clinical battery to determine the level of visual dependence or substitution related to lack of gravity reference. Figure 22-34 shows the effect of visual dependence on head position and the resulting balance responses.

Visual disorders can disrupt balance, cause sensation of dizziness, and lead to limitation of function. Accurate evaluation of the visual system is critical in differential diagnosis (see Chapter 28 on disorders of vision and visual perception). Disorders of convergence are common in the vestibular-deficient patient and can cause delay in the process of adaptation. Sensitivities to physiological diplopia develop, causing visual motion hypersensitivity during daily activity (Box 22-3). Remember, too, that abnormal responses in neck muscle activity associated with eye motion have implications for control of posture and movement. The smooth pursuit neck torsion test (SPNT) is used to delineate abnormal cervical afferent influences on oculomotor function from vestibular influences (Box 22-4).

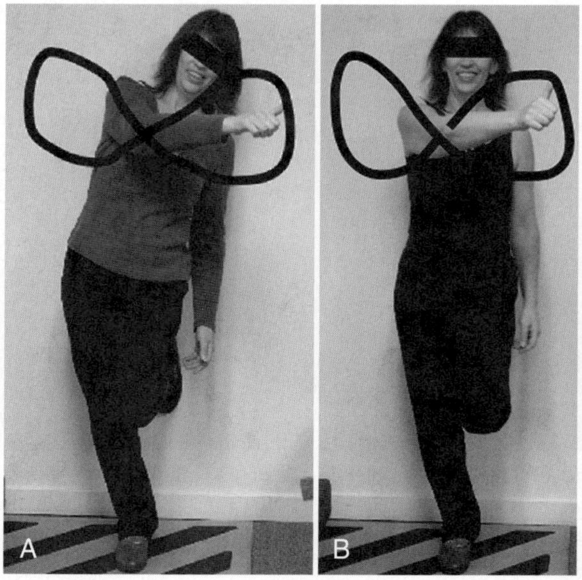

Figure 22-34 ■ When the visual reference is dominant for head position, the position of the head changes to match the tilted peripheral visual reference that results from the eye following the thumb in a figure-of-8. **A,** The head tilts off center as the perception of the visual field tilts. **B,** If the vestibular system is dominant, suppression of the apparent shift in the visual field allows the head to stay in alignment over the base of support. (Courtesy Ray Hedenberg, IRB Solutions, Silverthorne, Colo.)

BOX 22-3 ■ PHYSIOLOGICAL DOUBLE VISION

- Everything in front of and behind the central focal point is perceived as double.
- The closer the focal point, the more distance appears to be between the *perceived* double images.
- As the central focal point moves in space, the background image appears to move.

BOX 22-4 ■ SMOOTH PURSUIT NECK TORSION TEST (SPNT)

Test: Smooth pursuits tested in head neutral and then compared with head rotated right and left
Findings: Compare gain in three head positions
Considerations: Shows relationship to cervical pain, proprioception, and oculomotor control

Sensory Substitution for Postural Control

When, as noted several times earlier, critical information from one system is absent or inaccurate, the CNS will begin to rely more heavily on the other systems for necessary reference. Although this is used initially to provide stability during the recalibration process, it can limit adaptation over the course of recovery.[125] Visual or somatosensory dependency patterns develop when the patient persistently makes use of either or both of those systems in preference to vestibular references when the most efficient reference for the environmental condition would be the vestibular system. This phenomenon has been identified in individuals with unilateral vestibular loss, thought to be compensated for. On testing there was an average of only 50% use of vestibular system weighting (trunk in gravity neutral), resulting in trunk sway in reference to the surface tilt, when tested on a rotating (tilting) surface at 8 degrees. Individuals with normal functioning systems showed 100% reliance on gravity by the time the surface made the 8-degree rotation, with minimal head and trunk sway following the surface tilt.[120]

Dependency patterns are typically observed in an individual who does not recover satisfactory adaptation and integration of the sensory systems required for normal balance responses in a variety of environmental conditions. Clinically, these substitution patterns often manifest as hyperreliance on vision or somatosensory cues even when the vestibular system may have adequate potential for recovery. When given standard vestibular rehabilitation, these patients often do not recover a full return to activity and are left with functional limitations or symptoms that have a negative impact on their lives. They may experience discomfort every time they close their eyes or may find it impossible to walk down an incline in a visually challenging environment. Increased vestibular weighting can improve the ability to accomplish ADLs and improve balance confidence.[148] Interventions are now possible that provide both the therapist and the patient with feedback regarding trunk movement during surface perturbations.

Inadequate Use of Available Sensory Reference

Central maladaptation is a term used for what appears to be a condition that limits the use of any of the sensory systems so that each system seems to be inadequate for reference. The vestibular, visual, and somatosensory systems may test normal, but the individual is not able to use them adequately for functional activity. Patients report chronic subjective dizziness and have a tendency to develop hypersensitivities to stimuli in their environment.[149,150]

Hypersensitivity patterns result in a patient who is intolerant of typical environmental conditions that include apparent visual motion, ground vibrations, or conflict between sensory references. Avoiding provoking environments such as airports or malls, wearing dark glasses inside, limiting driving, and using bracing techniques for balance are common behaviors in this group of patients. Box 22-5 presents conditions that may drive hypersensitivities. These patients have typically lost their jobs and generally underperform in life roles. Routine vestibular rehabilitation is usually not successful. Unless sensitivities are identified at initial presentation, a patient in this category may become recognized only when several treatment regimens fail. Based on the status of normal test results for individual systems, the patient has often been told that there is nothing wrong and therefore the problem is "in his head." Indeed, this category of patient often has an overlapping psychological disorder that should be treated concomitantly. Anxiety, depression, posttraumatic stress disorder, and a history of physical or verbal abuse are common comorbidities that will affect intervention and successful outcomes. It is sometimes possible to identify the condition within the initial evaluation. These patients often report abnormal sensations with the head at rest with eyes closed, such as "flickers," "explosions," or "racing," that do not reflect vestibular or somatosensory deficits. These patients will often demonstrate fear of the testing process but perform better on the higher-level tests of balance, such as eyes closed on foam, especially when distracted by a concurrent mental task. Visual motion hypersensitivity during oculomotor testing is common, and excessive startle is often seen during tests of head righting.

BOX 22-5 ■ ENVIRONMENTAL CONDITIONS THAT MAY CAUSE VISUAL MOTION HYPERSENSITIVITIES

Grocery stores—cans and boxes appear to be moving backward when one walks down isle
Airports with moving sidewalks
Malls with open walkways and glass elevators
Disco lights
Escalators, if the "down" and "up" escalators are side by side
Department Stores, especially during holidays or when displays are moving
Large "box" stores where the ceiling is unusually high
Large-format TV and movies, especially IMAX or 3D
Walking outside when the wind blows the tree limbs
Driving in rain or snow with windshield wipers active

Vestibular Contributions to Movement

Vestibular system losses can result in motor responses that are larger than necessary for the task, which can predispose a patient to falling. This can be seen in the gait cycle when the body's center of mass moves faster and farther than the individual can control. This movement appears similar to that of the patient with cerebellar dysfunction (see Chapter 21), and indeed may represent the loss of vestibular input to the Purkinje cells in the cerebellum that would normally modulate vestibular pathways.[120,151] The earlier portion of Chapter 22, which discusses balance, describes automatic postural responses and describes balance testing in detail. It is important to understand the role of the vestibular system in movement disorders related to balance. Patients with vestibular deficits typically rely primarily on their ankle strategy, which permits the head to remain aligned with the body and sustains congruence between vestibular and somatosensory inputs, with the somatosensory system being the dominant reference. Use of hip strategy may be modified or limited in the vestibular-deficient patient because when the head is moving in the opposite direction as the COG, vestibular and somatosensory inputs are not congruent.[126]

Activities that require use of hip strategy, such as standing in tandem or on one leg, can be a problem for clients with bilateral vestibular loss or an uncompensated vestibular lesion.[152] However, some patients demonstrate excessive use of hip strategy on a level surface when an ankle strategy would suffice. This often is related to a maladaptation or somatoform dizziness.

The vestibulospinal system is responsible for initiation of muscle activity in the neck in response to perturbations of the head as stated earlier. Abnormal integration of the vestibular responses can be seen in excessive co-contraction of the muscles of the neck when attempting to stabilize on unsteady surfaces. Responses to postural perturbations that start at the surface instead of the head may be exaggerated and poorly timed in the patient with insufficient use of vestibular system input. Understanding the critical link between the sensory input and motor output of the structures in the neck in relation to VSR activity is critical. Comorbid dysfunction of the cervical spine can negatively affect the reactions driven through the vestibular and somatosensory systems.

EXAMINATION OF THE VESTIBULAR SYSTEM AND DEVELOPMENT OF SPECIFIC MOVEMENT DIAGNOSES

Assessment of eye movement control can help diagnose dysfunction of the peripheral and central vestibular pathways. In particular, tests for a specific type of abnormal eye movement called *nystagmus* should be performed in clients with dizziness and those with known neuropathology involving these pathways. Nystagmus is involuntary, rhythmic oscillation of the eyes, with movement in one direction clearly faster than movement in the other direction. The client with nystagmus will also usually report vertigo. There is more than one type of nystagmus; identification of the particular type can direct the clinician toward the area of dysfunction. Visually induced, optokinetic, and end-gaze nystagmus should not be confused with conditions having a vestibular cause.[134,153]

Spontaneous Nystagmus

Spontaneous nystagmus results from imbalance in the vestibular signals through their transmission to the oculomotor neurons. This imbalance produces a constant drift of the eyes in one direction interrupted by brief, fast movement in the opposite direction. Spontaneous nystagmus occurs after acute vestibular lesions and usually lasts approximately 24 hours. Peripheral versus central lesions may be distinguished by asking the patient to fix his or her gaze on a stable target. Nystagmus from peripheral vestibular lesions is easily inhibited with visual fixation. Nystagmus caused by central lesions of the brain stem or cerebellum is not easily inhibited with visual fixation.

Positional Nystagmus

Positional nystagmus is induced by a change in head position. Nystagmus caused by stimulation of the peripheral semicircular canals from movement of the otoconia or canaliths typically lasts up to 30 seconds and then dissipates. Static nystagmus occurs with lesions to the peripheral otolith system through connections in the vestibular nuclei and cerebellum. It is provoked with change of head position in relation to gravity and continues as long as the position is maintained, although it can fluctuate in frequency and amplitude. Nystagmus caused by central vestibular system damage lasts minutes or longer before abating.

Gaze-Evoked Nystagmus

Gaze-evoked nystagmus occurs when clients shift the eyes from a primary central position to a second location. It is caused by the inability to maintain stable gaze position, and the eye drifts back toward the center or primary position. Usually indicative of a CNS problem, it is common in MS, brain injury, and congenital lesions.

Video Nystagmography

Video nystagmography (VNG) captures eye movements related to vestibular dysfunction using video goggles or electrodes surrounding the orbit of the eye. Oculomotor testing is performed to determine the ability to move the eye at normal speeds. Abnormal responses can indicate central dysfunction. Another component of the VNG is the caloric test, in which warm and cold air are introduced into the external ear canal to manipulate the fluid in the horizontal canal to isolate the ear and indicate the relative function on one side compared with the other. Central disorders will produce nystagmus patterns that are different from those related to a peripheral lesion.

Vestibular-Evoked Myogenic Potential

Vestibular-evoked myogenic potential (VEMP) is based on the principle that the saccule is sensitive to sound and responds in a similar fashion to clicking sounds as it does to tilt. A click produced in the ear stimulates the saccule, which in turn inhibits the synchronous discharges of muscles in the SCM on the same side. The rate of firing or tone of the SCM is inhibited during the recorded sounds, and this change is captured using surface electromyography (sEMG). The response in one ear can be compared with the response on the other side in the same person. VEMP findings are considered to be abnormal when they are very asymmetrical such that one side is more than twice as large as the other, low in amplitude, or absent. It is thought that this inhibition allowed the head to turn reflexively to sound, as was critical for survival of early humans.[131] An abnormal VEMP can indicate ipsilateral lesion in the saccule, the inferior vestibular nerve, the lateral vestibular nucleus, or the medial vestibulospinal tract. Conversely, dysfunction of the motor neurons of the SCM will cause abnormal findings that are not related to vestibular disorder.

Subjective Visual Vertical

Subjective visual vertical (SVV) is used to test the degree of ocular torsion present in unilateral lesions. The SVV is tested in absolute darkness or an environment that prevents visual reference to vertical. The patient is asked to orient a rod to gravity, and the degree of off-axis tilt represents the torsion of the eye that is common in acute unilateral lesions.[154]

Gaze Stability and Vestibuloocular Reflex

The ability to hold the eyes fixed on a target while the head is moving is known as *gaze stabilization.* To test the accuracy of the vestibular system gain, the head is rotated or moved up and down at a rate of about 2 Hz. This is the rate at which the head moves during typical daily tasks, moving up to about 3 to 4 Hz with activities such as sports. When an individual is unable to achieve similar clarity of vision at rest and at 2 Hz, it would be expected that the VOR is not sufficiently calibrated.[155] If the image blurs, the gain of the system is abnormal, meaning that the vestibular system is unable to move the eyes at the exact speed in the opposite direction as the head movement. The ratio of eye velocity to head velocity is known as the *gain* of the VOR. The gain of an intact VOR is usually equal to one, which means movement of the eyes is equal to the movement of the head.[156] Testing of dynamic visual acuity assesses the acuity that can be obtained during a specific rate of rotation of the head. It can be tested with manual head turn using a Snellen eye chart (the same chart that is used to determine visual acuity, with normal vision recorded as 20/20) with the patient reading the smallest line that is comfortable, then having the head moving at 2 Hz in attempts to read the same line.[157] When acuity drops more than three lines, it is clear that the patient will be unable to maintain visual acuity during typical daily activity. Quantified dynamic visual acuity can be recorded as the logarithm of minimal angle of resolution or LogMAR. This can be tested and quantified by use of equipment such as inVision (NeuroCom International). Gaze stability can also be quantified using the same equipment, but the measure is one of function, reporting the head speed that can be obtained while maintaining gaze stability. This is a good way to clarify the amount of deceleration that is necessary in order for the patient to maintain proper vision. Figure 22-35 shows testing and treatment available using quantified dynamic visual acuity.

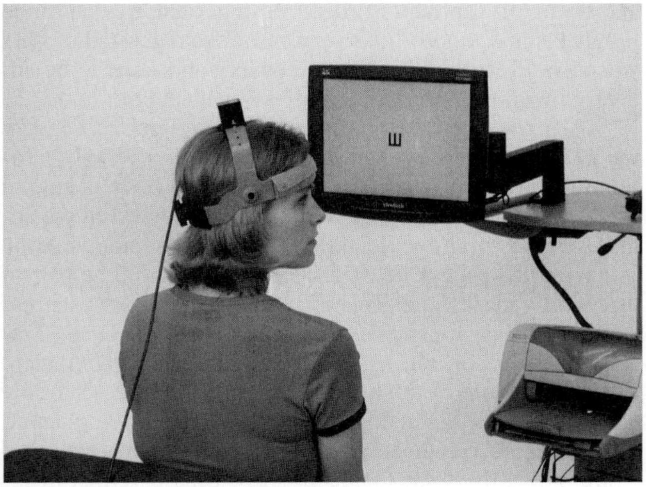

Figure 22-35 ■ Quantified dynamic visual acuity is possible with systems such as inVision. (Courtesy NeuroCom International, Clackamas, Ore.)

Vestibuloocular Reflex Cancellation

VOR cancellation reflects the ability to synchronize simultaneous eye and head movements in the same direction and is associated with the ability of the brain to suppress the VOR. This function allows an individual to track an object while moving the head at the same speed. Testing results are reported as normal if the eye can remain in the center of the orbit as the head and eyes track an object as it moves across the visual field. If the central integration capabilities are abnormal, the client will not be able to override the reflex activity and cannot keep the eye and head moving at the same rate in the same direction.

Gait

Vestibular control of position for the upper body and head appears to be separated from the lower body in gait in a similar pattern as noted during perturbed stance. Head and trunk stability remain constant throughout the phases of gait, and vestibular inputs appear to be most critical during initiation of gait, toe-off, and heel strike. Vestibular information contributes to the planned foot trajectory and placement of the foot to prevent disequilibrium. It is interesting to note that during steady-state gait, and even more so with running, vestibular contribution appears to diminish in importance. This may be because running is so highly automated and the trajectory remains fairly steady.[157]

The gait pattern reflected by vestibular dysfunction, or lack of integration, involves flat-foot gait with minimal heel strike, abnormal foot placement requiring larger-than-normal trunk adjustment. In order to control the position of the trunk, the base of support is widened. Speed of gait is another indication of vestibular function from the perspective that patients with bilateral vestibular loss demonstrate a slower self-selected speed. Typically, increased double-limb stance time and decreased stability at heel strike are present.[158] Walking with head turns becomes even more challenging as the vestibular system is activated and the somatosensory and visual systems are disadvantaged. Vestibular contributions to stability during transitions from sitting to standing, initiation of gait, and abnormal foot placement can be identified during standard tests such as the TUG, the Tinetti, and the DGI. Scores are adversely affected when vestibular system functions are diminished. The FGA was developed specifically for use with patients with vestibular disorders.[159] For a more complete description of tests of balance, see the earlier portion of Chapter 22.

Movement diagnoses related to vestibular examination are presented in Box 22-6.

BOX 22-6 ■ MOVEMENT DIAGNOSES RELATED TO VESTIBULAR EXAMINATION

- Spontaneous nystagmus inhibited by fixation
- Sensation of motion with body held still
- Instability or dizziness during head motion
- Loss of adequate head righting
- Head position dizziness
- Dependency patterns
- Inadequate use of available sensory reference

INTERVENTION

Positional Dizziness

The Hallpike-Dix maneuver is a positional test used to determine if otoconia are present in the posterior or anterior semicircular canal. Figure 22-30 demonstrates the position of the head and movement of the otoconia. A positive response is a delayed nystagmus of about 3 to 15 seconds, which determines potential diagnosis of BPV.

To test, the client is positioned in long sitting on a mat or plinth such that, when supine, the head and neck extend over the upper edge of the surface. The examiner holds the head of the sitting client between both hands and then rapidly moves the client backward and down with the head turned to the side and the neck extended 30 to 45 degrees below the horizontal position. The head is held in this position for 20 to 30 seconds. The examiner monitors for symptoms of vertigo and observes the eyes for nystagmus.[121]

When the Hallpike-Dix test position indicates BPV, specific, highly effective procedures can be performed in the clinical setting to remediate the disorder.[160]

Canalith repositioning is a series of passive movements designed to move loose debris (otoconia) through the canal and back into the otolith. The client is first brought down into the extended and rotated position that causes the nystagmus and vertigo (the positive Hallpike-Dix position). The head is held in that position until the symptoms fade completely or for 60 to 90 seconds. The head is maintained in extension and then slowly rotated toward the unaffected side and kept in that position for an additional 1 to 2 minutes to allow movement of the otoconia through the canal. The client then rolls so that she or he is side-lying and the head is turned to a 45-degree position relative to the ground. This position often produces more vertigo and nystagmus as the otoconia continue to move through the canal. In the next movement, the head is tipped toward the chest and the client is assisted into the sitting position. Figure 22-36 shows the sequence of the Epley maneuver. The client must then follow specific instructions for 24 hours.[161] These include avoiding forward, backward, or lateral head tilts or bending activities. Clients should also sleep with the head elevated to at least 30 degrees and avoid turning to the involved side.[162]

When the BPV is within the horizontal canal, dizziness or vertigo is reported when rolling, especially if the head is elevated on a pillow because that puts the canal in a position perpendicular to the ground. The symptoms are reported when the head is turned in either direction, but the side that triggers the worse symptoms is thought to be the side of the dysfunction.

Horizontal canal BPV is tested for in the supine position with the head held in 30 degrees of flexion to keep the lateral canal perpendicular to the ground or in the neutral position for ease of positioning. The head is then turned in each direction and the eyes observed for horizontal nystagmus. This must be distinguished from static positional nystagmus by the fact that the nystagmus will fatigue if it is caused by movement of the otoconia but otherwise persists.[163]

The repositioning intervention then begins with the client supine with the head turned toward the more affected ear. The head is then turned away from the affected ear and the client is slowly rolled 360 degrees (essentially staying in the same place) until the head is returned to the original position. The client sits back up with the head tucked. Side tilts of the head, as well as forward and backward movements of the head and trunk, are avoided for 24 hours.[164]

Position-provoked dizziness may alternatively be related to canal sensitivity or abnormal firing through the brain stem when BPV is not found to be the cause. In this case, exercises should be done to increase the client's tolerance to the provoking position(s). This involves having the client perform the provoking positions to give the CNS the opportunity to adjust to the sensation that the position triggers. Rolling on a bed or spinning in a chair can help adapt when stimulation to the horizontal mechanism is disrupted. In cases of maladaptation causing sensitivity of head position, moving gradually into the position of discomfort while minimizing input from the other sensory systems can be successful. In addition to exercise sessions, incorporating the provoking positions into daily activities is also important

Adaptation

Adaptation represents the highest level of recovery in the patient with a vestibular dysfunction, and therefore as much adaptation as possible should be facilitated for the final outcome.[129,133] As noted earlier, the patient may be at any level of adaptation when intervention is initiated, and it is critical to be able to recognize the symptoms and behaviors associated with lack of adaptation and those that represent sensory substitution. Overdependence on nonvestibular sensory reference must be extinguished. Isolating specific components of the symptoms reported and understanding how impairments can manifest across several different testing procedures will guide intervention. Activation of an error signal starts the recovery process, and the environment must be carefully manipulated to challenge the patient at the right level for the correct impairment. Substitution strategies must be eliminated during exercise even if they are still in use during activity. To stimulate the use of vestibular inputs for adaptation of the CNS, environments are designed to disadvantage both vision and somatosensation. Practice can be on unstable or compliant surfaces, with vision either absent or destabilized by eye and head movements, progressing to optokinetic stimulation.[140,165-168] Central dysfunction will negatively affect recovery rate, and knowledge of the degree and form of central disorders is important to determine prognosis and modify interventions. Psychogenic disorders will also affect the process of recovery and need to be addressed with the appropriate professional support.

When the integration of vestibular and somatosensory inputs is not congruent even at rest, there is a reported sensation of movement inside the head when the body is held at rest in supported sitting. In this instance, enhancing the somatosensory input by weighting through the spinal column or having the patient lie on a firm surface should be part of the initial intervention. This allows the vestibular system to calibrate using somatosensory input as a reference. This activity, known as *settling,* is a good way to allow the patient to manage symptoms when they have been exacerbated by activity. Use of distracting mental tasks pushes the adaptation to the subconscious level. Figure 22-27 shows the setup of weighting the spine to encourage settling of symptoms.

On the other hand, if the use of weights increases the sensation of movement, the clinician should suspect abnormal central sensory weighting of somatosensory inputs.

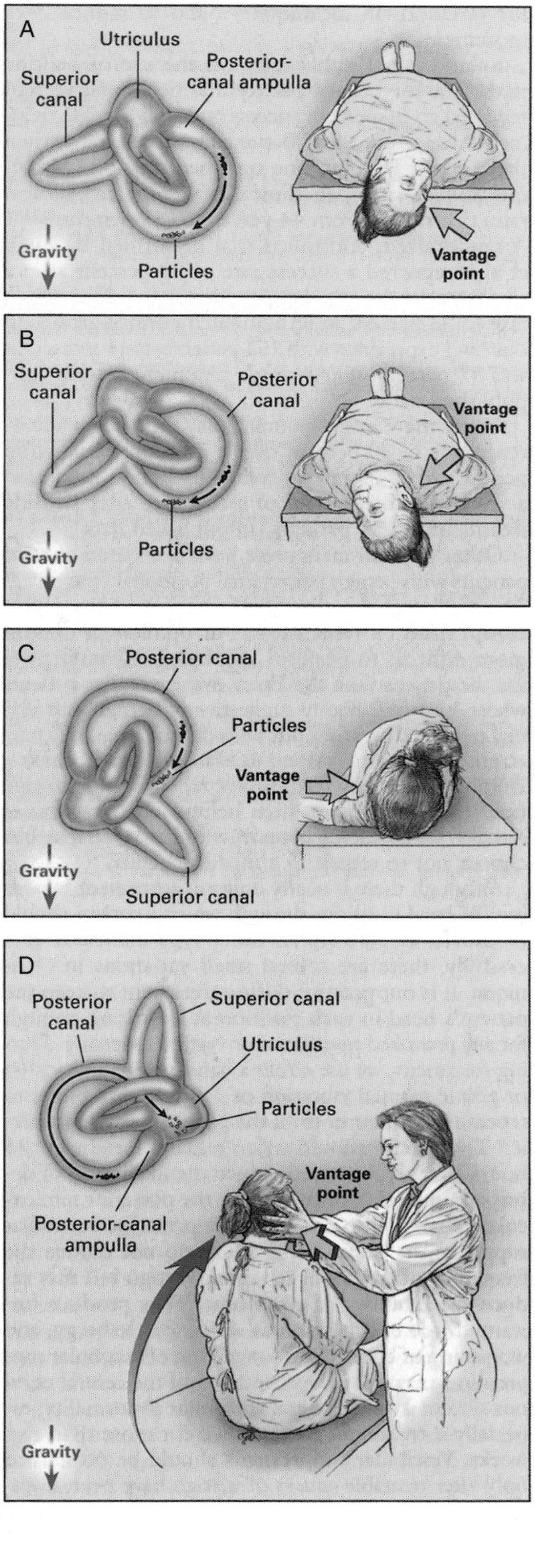

Figure 22-36 ■ Epley maneuver: Canalith repositioning maneuver for the patient with posterior canal benign positional vertigo (BPV). Figure represents procedure for right-side BPV. Movement of particles through the canal is shown in each position. (From Furman JM, Cass SP: Benign paroxysmal positional vertigo. *N Engl J Med* 341:1590–1596, 1999. Copyright 1999 Massachusetts Medical Society. All rights reserved.)

Slow progressive introduction of weights may be necessary to achieve decreased sensation of movement.

VOR adaptation requires movement of images on the retina, or retinal slip. Therefore intervention begins with head movement at the speed that allows stable vision.[156,169] Adaptation of the VOR is accomplished by having the patient move his or her head while trying to maintain gaze stabilization by keeping a stationary object in clear focus.[128] As the system adapts, speed of head movement increases, with the goal of achieving head movement at 2 Hz without the object blurring. Initially the client can focus on the thumb or a business card held at arm's length. The activity is progressed to a higher level of difficulty by adding a background visual stimulus such as a television set or a visually complex environment. Gaze stabilization with head turns while standing on an uneven surface or while walking creates a higher-level challenge. Many clients have avoided head movement, so simply turning the head may initially trigger dizziness. As stated previously, dizziness with head motion should not be confused with abnormal VOR; in VOR dysfunction the visual image blurs as the head moves.

As stated previously, the vestibular system provides a top-down point of reference that the somatosensory system uses to prevent the head and trunk from aligning with surface changes. Perturbations in the form of oscillating surfaces provide a mechanism to activate the gravity receptors, and feedback about the alignment of the trunk to gravity neutral can help to discourage surface dependence when it should not be the dominant reference.[140]

Ineffective head-righting responses observed during sharpened Romberg or standing on a narrow surface should be treated as such and activated for efficiency starting in a sitting tilt. Activities that require quick changes of position in a superior or inferior direction, such as a lunge or going up and down stairs, can be difficult when the otoliths are damaged. Good program components for otolith stimulation are activities involving up-and-down body movements. Examples include sitting to standing, seated bouncing on a Swiss ball, and standing bouncing on a mini-trampoline, all with eyes closed to eliminate use of vision for stability. Certain positions or movements of the head during upright activities can affect balance if just one part of the vestibular system has abnormal function. If the otoliths are damaged or hypersensitive, a voluntary lateral tilt of the head when standing with the eyes closed can cause destabilization.

A vestibular adaptation program should challenge the patient at the limit of his or her ability. Clients often choose to do the easiest exercise and avoid the more difficult exercises if they are not educated about the need to trigger the symptoms. Conversely, if the challenge is too far above the ability of the patient, the CNS will fail to adapt and symptoms will not decrease.

Elimination of Visual Dependence

When the use of vestibular inputs has been minimized through self-limitation of head and eye movements to control dizziness and imbalance, the visual system often becomes dominant for balance. Testing as identified in Figure 22-34 can be used for intervention. Another way to train the client to use vestibular input versus vision is watching a ball being tossed from hand to hand while standing on a compliant surface (Figure 22-37). This can also be done while walking. Clients with visual dependency often report excessive fatigue after activity because of the strain of using vision for postural stability. When these clients are in situations with excessive visual stimulation, reports of dizziness increase. The subtle eye movements associated with viewing a computer monitor cause more fatigue for the individual with vestibular disorder. These individuals also often avoid crowds as in a mall, grocery store, or airport. Attending church services, which are often characterized by low lighting, visual stimulation, and the need to stand with eyes closed or read a hymnal while singing challenges the vestibular system. Figure 22-38 shows the use of optokinetic stimulus to decrease visual dependence and to improve the ability to maintain gaze reference when there is movement in the visual background.

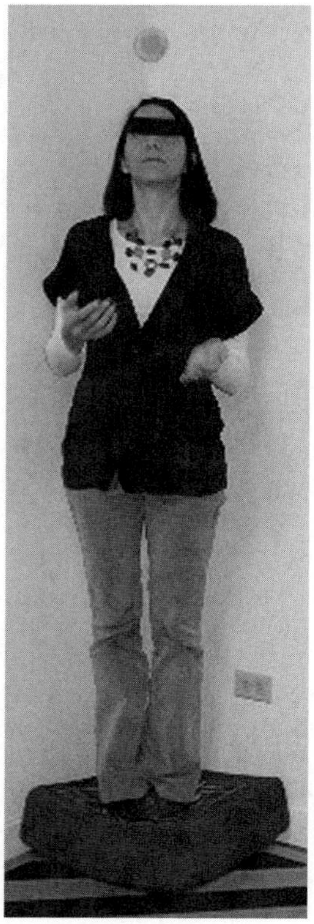

Figure 22-37 ■ Keeping the gaze directed at the moving ball while standing on a compliant surface eliminates the primary use of visual targets to stabilize the head and is an effective way to shift reference from visual to vestibular. (Courtesy Ray Hedenberg, IRB Solutions, Silverthorne, Colo.)

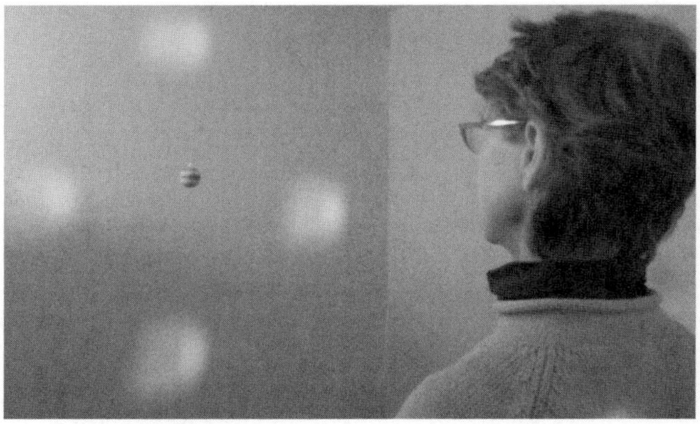

Figure 22-38 ■ Projecting peripheral movement activates the optokinetic response. Individuals with visual dependence for balance, or visual motion hypersensitivity are not able to adequately achieve gaze stability of the central object or will lose balance as they match head position to the peripheral reference. In the patient with maladapted responses, this stimulus can cause significant nausea and other abnormal autonomic nervous system (ANS) responses.

Gait

Gait with head motion is important for the individual with vestibular dysfunction. Because head movement causes visual disturbances and dizziness, the client with a vestibular disorder will significantly limit head movement while walking. When visual cues are used predominantly for balance, the client will try to keep the body in line with vertical and horizontal visual targets. This will decrease the small, natural movements typically made during the gait cycle. Patients with potentially recoverable vestibular function should be trained to walk with eye and head movements, trunk rotation, and arm swing. Figure 22-39 shows abnormal placement of the foot for stability when the individual is unable to use the head orientation to gravity as the primary reference.

When the vestibular system does not accurately inform the client about the speed and direction of head movement, visual cues are used to determine movement speed and direction in relation to nonmoving objects. However, in environments with a lot of motion, or when someone approaches in the opposite direction, determining speed and direction of self-movement becomes more difficult. Clients often report dizziness and imbalance in a crowd. Changing visual environments can trigger imbalance in the client with visual dependency. Walking into a darkened room, especially if the surface is uneven (as in a theater), can often trigger a fall or stumble. Clients with permanent vestibular loss should be educated about these potentially high-risk environments and taught compensatory strategies to ensure safe mobility. If improvement in vestibular function is anticipated, however, then progressive exposure to these busy environments is needed to prepare the client for real-world mobility.

To increase somatosensory input, clients with a vestibular disorder often put the whole foot down at once to get better input on the position of the body relative to the ground. The normal heel-toe weight progression over the ball of the foot

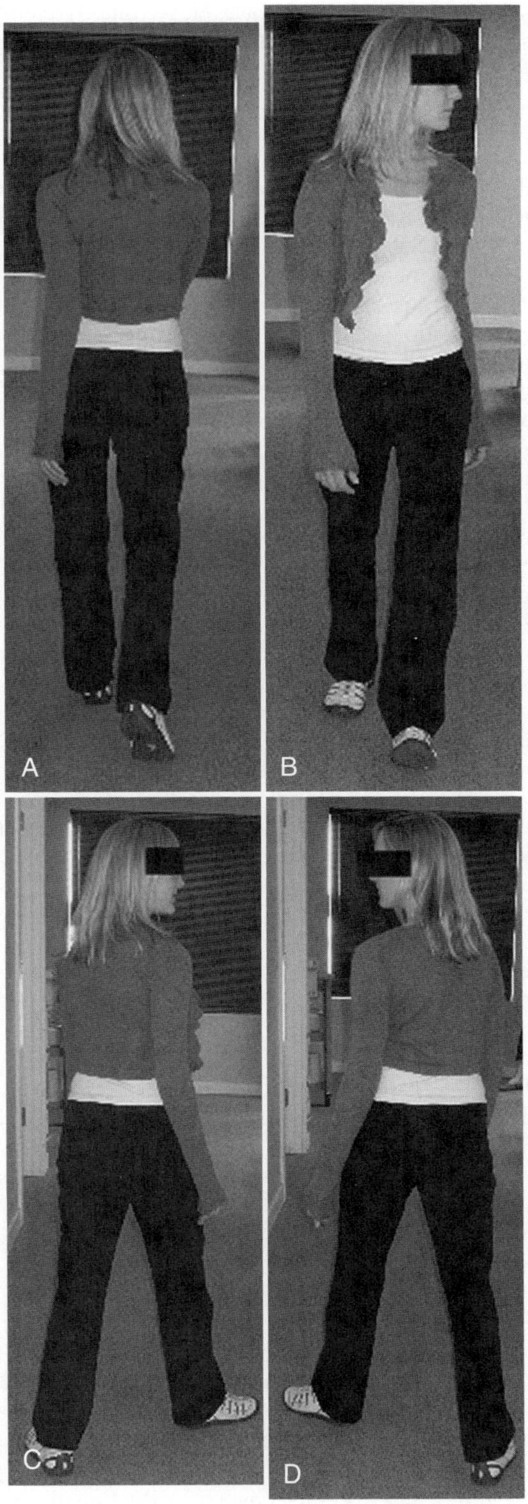

Figure 22-39 ■ **A** and **B,** When the vestibular, visual, and somatosensory systems are integrated properly, the movement of the head does not change the pattern of the step. **C** and **D,** When the vestibular system is not primary for reference, step outs occur during head rotations. This demonstrates the foot moving in the direction of head turn, causing a staggering gait pattern seen often with patients with lack of ability to activate primary dominance of the vestibular system. (Courtesy Ray Hedenberg, IRB Solutions, Silverthorne, Colo.)

is diminished. This is often seen in conjunction with increased step width while walking. This compensatory strategy is acceptable in clients with permanent loss but should be discouraged in clients who do not need to be overreliant on somatosensation for balance control during walking. Walking on uneven surfaces can be a challenge if the client is primarily reliant on somatosensory input and has poor visual-vestibular interaction. This is one reason why walking indoors is less of a problem than walking outdoors. Again, clients who are not expected to recover vestibular function should be educated about these potentially hazardous environments and encouraged to develop compensatory mechanisms to permit safe mobility. Gait training on progressively less stable surfaces is appropriate for clients who need to reduce dependence on somatosensory cues and improve visual-vestibular interaction.

Substitution

Permanent bilateral vestibular loss, however, requires substitution of somatosensation and vision to orient to the environment. Use of a cane or walking stick to increase use of somatosensation and allow more time to prepare for the next step can increase confidence in gait. Control of turns can be achieved by a quick stop while the head is turning, rapid saccade to stable target, and then completion of the turn with a fixed gaze. Figure 22-40 shows the sequence of the spot turn. This process can become second nature and can be performed on a regular basis to increase stability during daily tasks.[170] Driving can be trained in a safe manner in reference to head turns and visual references by doing a slow blink to decrease distracting visual flow.[171]

Maladaptation

Clinical interactions have an important influence on the course of maladapted responses. Explaining the psychosomatic connections in detail can be the first step in recovery. This is critical in order to engage the patient who demonstrates strong avoidance behaviors. Successful outcomes are possible; however, the process may take longer because the central modulation of sensory input is compromised, and therefore adaptation will occur in smaller increments. Proper referral to someone to assist with the management of the psychological or psychiatric condition should always be considered.

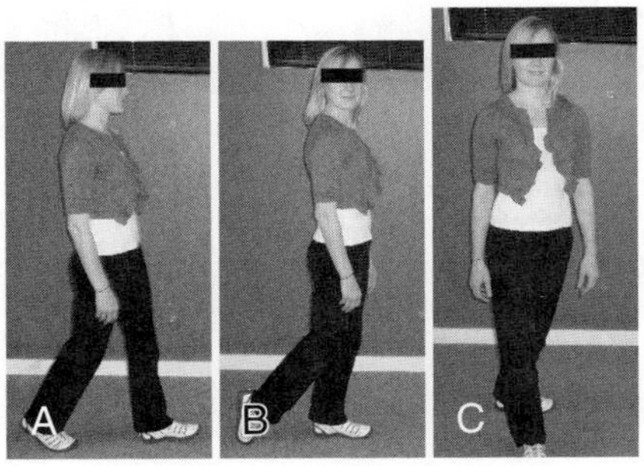

Figure 22-40 ■ The "spot turn" for the patient with bilateral vestibular loss. **A,** When the patient is ready to turn, the front foot is planted to provide somatosensory reference. **B,** Once the foot is planted, the head is turned. **C,** Visual reference on a nonmoving target is maintained while the body turns under a stable head. (Courtesy Ray Hedenberg, IRB Solutions, Silverthorne, Colo.)

FEEDBACK

Biofeedback can be used in a variety of ways. Feedback about correct postural responses remains the task of the therapist in the training paradigm. Visual feedback has been used to supplement center of pressure reference for control of weight shifting using vision to supplement vestibular integration to somatosensory inputs. Visual feedback about the head and trunk movement versus total movement on a perturbed surface is available on the Proprio 5000 (Figure 22-41).

Use of the Nintendo Wii Fit has been popular and provides information about results of weight shifting integrated into games that integrate a balance task into an activity that may represent another activity. Training is performed on a nonmoving surface, so somatosensory drive is activated. Patients with visual motion hypersensitivities may find the games overstimulating at the beginning of the session, but playing them may also be an appropriate method to increase adaptation so that more visual stimulus can be tolerated.

Audio feedback has long been used in the patient with vestibular system loss to provide information about sway when surface and visual reference is lacking. It can be used in many different ways for intervention.

Vibrotactile feedback using accelerometer or gyroscopic information has emerged in recent years. This has been successful on many levels, and the modes of input are becoming less intrusive to those who wear them. The input typically provides immediate positive changes in performance of a task, with behaviors that represent improved postural response to gravity reference; however, the rate of retention or carryover may still be related to available plasticity within each system.

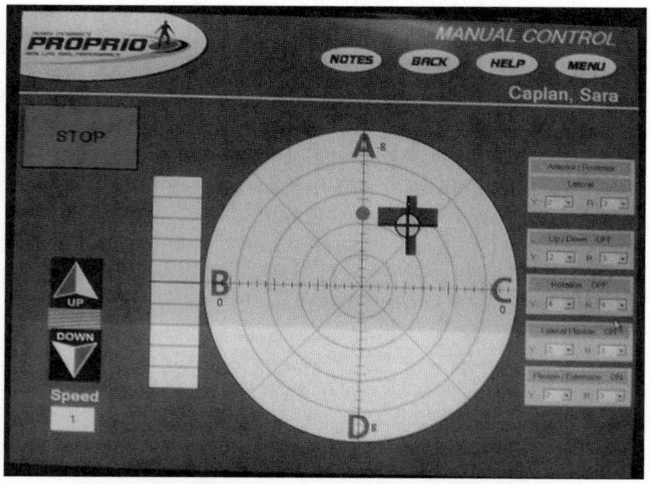

Figure 22-41 ■ Feedback about the position of the trunk in relation to the center of the platform, as well as feedback about the amount of trunk flexion and extension and rotation, can be provided to the patient during the perturbations. The patient can also receive summary feedback after sessions performed with the eyes closed. (Proprio 5000, Perry Dynamics, Decauter, Ill.)

CONCLUSION

This chapter has been divided into two sections owing to the specificity and amount of information specific to both areas. Balance was presented first because of the general nature of this topic and because it lays the foundation for discussion of vestibular problems. Although vestibular disorders have a direct effect on balance, not all balance dysfunction is caused by vestibular problems. With the amount of research available in both areas and the areas of specialization separating, the chapter was separated to aid the readers in focusing on specific problem areas. The references have been placed chronologically as appearing in the chapter, but the reader will see that the two portions have been clearly identified to assist in finding materials specific to the topic of interest. The complexity of these two topic areas has grown as new research and new technology have become available. Outcomes of treatment once thought unrealistic have become reality. Many patients who once thought their quality of life was permanently diminished and their ability to participate in meaningful activities had been taken away now show tremendous improvement in functional movement. The effectiveness of therapists working with these patients depends on understanding the specificity of the clinical problems and applying interventions that show measurable change. The importance of active patient participation cannot be overemphasized when discussing motor control and motor learning principles needed to optimize positive changes in balance and in specific vestibular disorders. These problems dramatically affect an individual's quality of life, and the role occupational and physical therapists play in providing appropriate interventions has established efficacy in practice.

Acknowledgment

Thanks to Janet Helminski, PT, PhD; Linda Horn, PT, NCS; Pat Huston, MS, PT; Leslie Allison, PT, PhD, NCS; and Kenda Fuller, PT, NCS, for their significant contributions to the development of this chapter. Gratitude is also extended to Darcy Umphred, PT, PhD, FAPTA, and our families for their patience and support.

References

To enhance this text and add value for the reader, all references are included on the companion Evolve site that accompanies this textbook. This online service will, when available, provide a link for the reader to a Medline abstract for the article cited. There are 182 cited references and other general references for this chapter, with the majority of those articles being evidence-based citations.

CASE STUDY 22-1 ■ ANDY

Andy is a 27-year-old man who sustained a severe closed-head injury in a skiing accident. He was hospitalized for 2 months and resided at a long-term care facility for 6 months before cranial surgery for removal of bilateral subdural hygromas and revision of a ventriculoperitoneal shunt. After surgery he demonstrated marked improvement and was transferred to a rehabilitation unit. His initial physical therapy assessment revealed the following impairments, which had a negative effect on postural control:

1. Oculomotor deficits (difficulty tracking to the right and upward)
2. Disorientation
3. Delayed and slow motor responses
4. Bilateral ankle plantarflexion contractures (1 to 10 degrees left, 1 to 15 degrees right); limited right shoulder flexion (0 to 100 degrees) and external rotation (0 to 20 degrees)
5. Hypotonic trunk (right, moderate; left, mild), hypertonic (extensor) lower extremities (right, moderate; left, mild), hypertonic right upper extremity (mild)
6. Fair head control
7. Poor trunk control with right scapular atrophy, shortened right side, strength 3−/5
8. Left upper and lower extremity movement isolated and coordinated but slow, strength 4/5 at shoulder, 4+/5 elbow, wrist, hand, 4/5 hip and knee, 3+/5 ankle, able to place and hold for weight bearing
9. Right upper extremity rests and moves in synergistic pattern but can move out of synergy with request or demonstration; strength 3−/5 at shoulder and 4−/5 distally; coordination is poor; can place and hold for weight bearing if cued but not spontaneously
10. Right lower extremity moves in flexor-extensor pattern, grossly 3+/5 in hip and knee flexion, 2+ hip extension, 3+/5 knee extension, no isolated ankle movement, cannot place or hold for weight bearing

Functional tests found the following activity limitations:

1. Minimum assist supine-to-sit
2. Sitting balance, poor
3. Moderate assist sit-to-stand
4. Standing balance, unable
5. Moderate assist transfers
6. Nonambulatory

Body system impairment goals were the following:

1. Increase ROM to within normal limits throughout
2. Increase trunk tone to normal and strength to 4+/5
3. Decrease right-sided tone to normal
4. Increase spontaneous use, isolated movement, and strength (4+/5) in right extremities
5. Able to place and bear weight on right lower extremity

Short-term functional goals were the following:

1. Independent in all bed mobility
2. Independent in wheelchair transfers
3. Good static and fair dynamic sitting balance
4. Contact guard sit-to-stand
5. Minimal assist static standing balance

Note: Ambulation goals were temporarily deferred because of the ankle contractures and balance deficits.

Early treatments included the following:

1. Standing frame activities for head control, visual tracking, trunk control, reduced lower-extremity extensor tone, and heel cord stretching with ultrasound
2. Neurodevelopmental sequence activities for head and trunk control; trunk strengthening; decreased lower-extremity extensor tone; balance on all fours, heel-sitting, kneeling
3. Supine to and from sitting, especially over the right arm
4. Sitting balance with upper-extremity functional tasks (e.g., putting glasses on and taking them off, taking shirt off and putting it on, wiping nose with tissue), with focus on right visual tracking, right trunk elongation, and incorporation of right lower-extremity ground pressure for stability
5. Transfer training with incorporation of right upper extremity to push up, reach and grasp, and right lower-extremity placing and weight bearing

As soon as Andy's ankle dorsiflexion ROM was near neutral on the right (was then 0 to 5 degrees on the left), neurodevelopmental activities were phased out and standing balance and pregait activities in the parallel bars were initiated with moderate assistance. He rapidly progressed to minimal-assistance gait in the parallel bars but with significant scissoring of the lower extremities. Gait outside the bars was begun with a quad cane on the left, but Andy was not able to organize the sequence for cane use and did not use the cane when loss of balance occurred, so use of the cane was discontinued. Gait without an assistive device required moderate assistance from the therapist for balance. A line drawn on the floor provided a visual cue to remind him to keep his feet apart; when walking without this cue, approximately 25% of his steps were close or crossed.

At discharge, 2 months after admission, Andy had good visual tracking; normal ROM with the exception of right lower-extremity dorsiflexion, which was limited to 0 to 5 degrees; normal tone in the left extremities; mildly increased tone in the right extremities with slight extensor patterning in the leg; good head and trunk control; and strength grossly 4+/5 throughout. Functionally, he was independent in bed mobility, wheelchair mobility, and sitting balance. He required supervision for safety in transfers and standing activities and minimal to moderate assistance for indoor ambulation without an assistive device depending on his fatigue level.

CASE STUDY 22-2 ■ DORIS

Doris is a 73-year-old woman with a long history of Parkinson disease who had fallen four times within the 6 months before referral to physical therapy. As a result of her most recent fall, during which she hit her head, Doris had ear pounding, lightheadedness, and headaches. After referral to an otolaryngologist, she was diagnosed with unspecified peripheral vestibular dysfunction and referred to outpatient therapy. Her therapist found that Doris reported increased lightheadedness and dizziness, with anterior-posterior head movements, rolling in bed, sit-to-stand, and the Hallpike-Dix maneuver (worse to the right). Multiple impairments that could be contributing to her instability and falls, as well as symptoms related to the vestibular disorder, were also noted. Doris had mildly decreased ROM in her left ankle, shoulders, and neck; mild left-sided weakness and lack of coordination; marked bilateral upper-extremity tremor; and moderately forward-flexed posture.

She could not perform an ankle strategy at all and continually used hip strategy; she also used stepping strategy frequently with the least shift or sway. Static postural sway tests indicated that Doris had excessive sway when attempting to stand still and that she kept her COG slightly posterior and to the right of midline. Sway increased tenfold with eyes closed, indicating poor use of somatosensory inputs for postural control. Doris could not perform repeated weight shifts in either anterior-posterior or medial-lateral directions. Her limits of stability were severely restricted to less than half of normal sway range anteriorly, and her movement time was slow.

Functional testing revealed that Doris had several disabilities. She had to use a walker or have manual assistance to ambulate and could negotiate level surfaces only. Without her walker or handhold assistance, Doris could stand for less than 30 seconds and take a maximum of 10 steps. For community ambulation, Doris needed minimum assistance with her walker and could go only short distances. She also required minimum assistance with bathing and household tasks.

Doris participated in therapy twice a week for 6 weeks and also performed a home exercise program daily. Her treatment plan included vestibular exercises for the dizziness and balance retraining exercises for instability and falls. The vestibular exercises she was given were designed to provoke her symptoms repeatedly and included head turning in supine and sitting (progressed to standing), rolling in bed, rocking in a rocking chair, and sit-to-stand practice. As her dizziness subsided, her home program was modified to increase the number and rate of head movements. To improve her use of somatosensory and vestibular inputs, Doris also practiced standing on a firm surface with eyes closed (with family supervision). In the clinic, Doris did stretching, strengthening, and postural extension exercises to address her musculoskeletal limitations. For increased use of somatosensory and vestibular inputs, she practiced standing and weight shifts with optokinetic stimulation. By using postural sway biofeedback, she practiced achieving the midline position, controlled anterior and left-sided weight shifts at progressively faster speeds, and ankle strategy. Gait training included starts, stops, turns, and obstacle avoidance and progressed to community ambulation tasks such as curbs and ramps. As her endurance improved, she also did gait training on the treadmill to increase the gait speed, stride length, hip strength, and use of vestibular inputs.

Despite her multiple problems, Doris was able to reduce the severity of her impairments and consequently improve her functional level. Her dizziness resolved completely. Although she still had excess sway during static standing, she was able to achieve and hold a midline position, and her sway with eyes closed reduced by more than half. Doris could shift her weight in both anterior-posterior and medial-lateral directions at moderate speeds by using ankle strategy without stepping. Her limits of stability were expanded from 35% to 80% of normal, and she was able to shift her weight much more quickly. Functionally, she could stand without the walker for 8 minutes and walk independently indoors on level surfaces without the walker for short distances. She was independent in community ambulation with the walker. At a 3-month follow-up visit, Doris reported that she had experienced no more falls.

APPENDIX 22-A ■ Common Vestibular Disorders

Benign Positional Vertigo (BPV)

The otoconia in the otolith can become loose, clump together, and form densities known as *canaliths,* which can move into a semicircular canal and become a cause of vertigo. In cases of BPV, the involved side is distinguished by which ear is toward the ground when the symptoms occur. The critical hallmark of BPV is that the vertigo usually starts after 5 to 10 seconds and resolves or fatigues within 20 to 40 seconds. A less common variant of BPV, cupulolithiasis reflects the adherence of the otoconia to the cupula. The vertigo associated with change of head position is caused by the direct pressure deflection of the cupula. The vertigo appears with less latency and is often more persistent, taking up to 60 seconds to resolve after change of head position.

Benign positional nystagmus or vertigo is a common sequela of head concussion, viral labyrinthitis, hydrops, and vascular occlusion in the distribution that feeds the inner ear. It can also develop without a known external cause and is the most common cause of vertigo.[172] Other conditions that can cause head position dizziness are described in Appendix Box 22-1.

BPV may involve any semicircular canal, although the posterior canal is most common because of its relationship to the otoliths when the person is in the recumbent position. The horizontal canal can also collect otoconia, and the result is horizontal nystagmus generated with head movement; dizziness often occurs as the head is going backward, when the horizontal canal moves into the gravity-responsive position. The dizziness is also triggered in the head rotated and flexed position.

Despite the use of the term *benign,* the symptoms related to positional vertigo are intense and can cause significant disability. There is often a strong sense of falling or spinning out of control, even when the individual is lying on a bed. Before the individual is aware of the mechanism, it seems to be something that is uncontrollable because it is associated with head movement. Spontaneous remissions are common and may reflect an underlying disorder such as hydrops or migraine-induced ischemia. Infections or inflammations may occur months or years before the onset of BPV. Adverse life events are reported to trigger an event, especially in individuals with an underlying disorder.

APPENDIX BOX 22-1 ■ ALTERNATIVE CAUSES OF HEAD POSITION DIZZINESS AND NATURE OF DIZZINESS

Unilateral vestibular dysfunction: Dizziness when changing head position while supine
Vestibular migraine: Episodic dizziness that can usually be related to specific triggers
Cerebellar nodulus: Nystagmus is downbeat without torsion without fatigue or habituation
Vertebral artery compression: Nystagmus with extreme rotation or extension of neck
Central vestibular pathways: Nystagmus without dizziness, usually unidirectional
Geriatric supine nystagmus: Vertical nystagmus when supine
Perilymph fistula: Episodic dizziness after trauma, increases with Valsalva or head hanging
Superior canal dehiscence: Dizziness with loud noises or change of head position
Hypermobile stapes: Unstable at oval window; allows fluid pressure changes that cause dizziness with head positions
Head extension: Otoliths outside of functional range, causing dizziness
Orthostatic intolerance: Dizziness when bending or quickly standing from sitting, never when lying

Infection

Acute unilateral vestibulopathy affects the vestibular nerve. Most often the infection is viral in nature and is known as *neuronitis* or *neuritis.* It can also be caused by bacterial infection from a variety of causes, either as a primary infection or secondary to bacterial meningitis or encephalitis. Vestibular neuritis can be partial, affecting the superior afferents from the horizontal and anterior semicircular canals primarily.

The infection often is preceded by a systemic illness or an upper respiratory tract infection, but it can be an isolated infection affecting the nerve or labyrinths. This causes an acute, severe dizziness often accompanied by nausea and vomiting. Initial impairment may include ocular tilt, skew deviation, or lateropulsion. Recovery reflects central adaptation to loss of input on one side of the vestibular system.

Endolymphatic Hydrops

Increased fluid pressure within the labyrinth, known broadly as *hydrops,* will cause vertigo. The fluid pressure may increase because the fluid cannot move out of the system through the endolymphatic sac, which normally absorbs excess fluid. As the fluid pressure increases, the brain receives abnormal signals from the cupula of the labyrinth on one side, and the result is the sensation of spinning. There is often concurrent low-frequency loss of hearing related to the fluid pressure in the cochlea. The episode can last from just a few minutes to a day but usually lasts 2 to 4 hours. The use of diuretics can control the fluid changes and decrease the number and intensity of symptoms. Meniere disease is a type of hydrops that occurs intermittently; the person has normal balance when not having an episode.

Over time there appears to be a gradual degradation of the vestibular system, resulting in symptoms associated with chronic unilateral vestibular loss. These patients often have a diffuse dizziness and report imbalance between episodes. Intervention is targeted at adaptation of the abnormal vestibular responses, and this can improve symptoms, although it cannot remedy the disease itself. Traumatic hydrops can be the result of a blow to the head during a fall or whiplash injury. The mechanism is not fully understood, but it may be related to damage to the endolymphatic sac during the trauma, resulting in inflammation or scarring that limits the regulation of fluid in the sac. Patients often appear drunk during an episode and therefore may limit social interactions or driving for fear of an attack. In some individuals an attack can include the "crisis of Tumarkin," resulting in feeling as if they have been thrown to the ground without a sensation of dizziness.

Perilymph Fistula

Fistula, or an abnormal communication of the inner and middle ear, can occur at the round or oval windows. This may have a congenital cause or may be related to trauma through the middle ear from surgery, blasts, head injury, or even sneezing. The Valsalva maneuver can trigger an intense sensation of dizziness owing to increased pressure in the system, and daily activity can produce an almost

Continued

APPENDIX 22-A ■ Common Vestibular Disorders—cont'd

persistent sense of dizziness that is relieved by recumbent positions with minimal head movement. Typical vestibular testing is nondiagnostic, but use of pressure in the ear may assist this diagnosis. Vestibular rehabilitation for adaptation fails because the system has a persistent fluctuating nature. Successful surgical repair of the fistula produces the stability needed to resume rehabilitation efforts.

Superior Semicircular Canal Dehiscence Syndrome

Dehiscence or thinning of the bone overlying the superior (anterior) semicircular canal creates a "third mobile window," and the effect of change in pressure of the canals appears to be similar to the fistula. Loud noise or pressure can cause disequilibrium. Surgical repair usually produces good results.

Vertiginous or Vestibular Migraine

The aura or even the primary symptom of migraine may be dizziness. Diagnosis is based on the episodic nature, recognition of triggers, history of migraine, and combination of dizziness with the other typical prodromes of migraine including photophobia, nausea, and vestibulocochlear symptoms of tinnitus and sensitivity to sound. The pathophysiology follows that of migraine headache, in which there are multiple levels of dysfunction from gene defects that drive familial autosomal disorders and an inherited migraine threshold, brain stem activity that can trigger vascular responses of dilation or restriction, serotonin platelet activity, and spreading neuronal depression. Medical management follows the criteria for migraine. Rehabilitation is indicated when avoidance of activity has changed the sensory integration, or when multiple episodes have influenced the system toward dependency or hypersensitivity patterns.[173]

Vascular Disorders

Ischemia in the areas of the vestibular system (brain stem, cerebellum, parietal-insular cortex) can cause dizziness and imbalance. Vertebral basilar artery insufficiency syndrome, for example, classically produces these problems. Ischemia is usually seen in individuals older than 50 years, but it can also be associated with bleeding disorders such as leukemia. Migraine headache can cause intermittent dizziness from compromise of blood flow in the areas of the vestibular system.

Neoplasia

Neoplasia can compromise vestibular function when it occurs near any part of the vestibular system. Vestibular schwannoma (commonly but mistakenly known as *acoustic neuroma*) can cause damage as it slowly grows on the sheath of the vestibular nerve. The schwannoma can grow into the pontocerebellar angle and cause symptoms typically associated with cerebellar lesions. Meningiomas (encapsulated tumors found most often deep in the brain) growing in the area of the temporal lobe can cause pressure on the vestibular mechanism. In some cases, damage to the vestibular nerve occurs as a result of surgical removal of the tumor.

Ototoxicity

Aminoglycosides, antibiotics used in cases of massive or systemic infection, can be ototoxic (causing damage to the vestibular hair cells). Although a small percentage of users experience this adverse effect, it can affect both sides of the bilateral vestibular apparatus and cause significant disability. Often the client does not begin to experience the symptoms until the medication has been used for more than a week.

Traumatic Brain Injury (TBI)

TBI can affect the vestibular system in several ways. It can cause direct damage to the vestibular end organ (in the temporal bone); BPV; and, in many cases, disruption of the integration of the vestibular nuclei (in the brain stem) and cerebellum. Sensorimotor disturbances are common with TBI involving the cerebellum or parietal lobe. Visual dysfunction results from damage to brain stem areas such as the pontine gaze centers or central damage in the medial longitudinal fasciculus. Frequently the third, fourth, or sixth cranial nerve is damaged, and this affects the ability to move the eyes for conjugate gaze. In some extensive TBI cases the brain loses its ability to use any of the three sensory systems accurately. Dizziness and imbalance are prevalent complaints from client with TBI because there are often situations in which they cannot acquire accurate sensory information.[174]

Each system should be evaluated individually for its function. In patients with TBI, the adaptation of the vestibular system occurs more slowly and with more effort than in other clients with vestibular deficits. The client with vestibular problems associated with TBI requires significantly more intervention initially, and the outcomes are less favorable than for other clients experiencing vestibular dysfunction.[175]

Allergies

Persons with allergies are often predisposed to episodes of dizziness. Foods, airborne allergens, and chemicals can trigger dizziness in these individuals.

Metabolic Disorders

Vertigo and dizziness are often reported with metabolic disorders such as diabetes. Autoimmune diseases such as rheumatoid arthritis, lupus, and human immunodeficiency virus infection can also cause symptoms when the disease process damages components of the vestibular system.

Autoimmune Ear Disease

Autoimmune responses may result in rapid decline of hearing with intermittent symptoms of vertigo, aural pressure, and tinnitus. It is caused by the deposition of antibody-antigen complex in the capillaries or basement membranes of inner ear structures. It can appear in the same manner as hydrops, with fluctuations of hearing loss and vestibular function. The Western Blot is one of the most widely used diagnostic tools.

Autonomic Related Vertigo

The autonomic and vestibular systems are physiologically connected, and significant activation of the vestibular system will cause nausea, pallor, sweating, and clamminess. Autonomic dysfunction can contribute to dizziness and is reported in conjunction with palpitations, chronic fatigue, sleeping disorders, cold extremities, headaches, gastrointestinal disorders, medication intolerance, and fainting.

Mitral valve prolapse can be found in patients with such signs and symptoms, and disorders of circulation should be considered. Orthostatic concerns should be considered, and often patients are found to have abnormal tilt-table test results. Often patients will have been diagnosed with Meniere disease but do not respond to diuretics and, when observed carefully, have signs as described previously, with lightheadedness a component of the dizziness, along with vertigo.[176]

APPENDIX 22-A ■ Common Vestibular Disorders—cont'd

Mal de Debarquement (Disembarkment Syndrome)

The symptoms of continued rocking or a sensation that one has just gotten off a boat is the hallmark of disembarkment syndrome. Indeed it comes often after a long boat or airplane ride, often when there is turbulence. The vestibular system seems to be activated to a high degree, then is unable to calibrate back to normal in reference to the somatosensory input available.[177]

The sensation is greater when the patient is at rest, and movement is actually preferable to standing or sitting. The system remains maladapted, and the condition can persist over months and years, causing significant disability and frustration. Rehabilitation is directed toward recalibration of the somatosensory and vestibular systems.

Somatoform Dizziness

Forty percent of dizzy patients have psychological disorders, and individuals with psychological disorders report more disability related to dizziness. There are connections between the locus coeruleus and lateral vestibular nucleus within the brain stem, and both nuclei are affected by serotonergic processes. Primary somatoform disorders, dissociative (conversion) disorders, and anxiety disorders produce dizziness without organic cause.[178] Secondary, reactive, or comorbid disorders can emerge as a consequence of identifiable organic dysfunction, but the recovery process is derailed owing to an underlying psychiatric disorder. Vestibular disorders have an influence on autonomic regulation, and symptoms such as heart palpitations, fainting spells, and chronic fatigue are reported to a higher degree when there is an additional psychogenic component. Vertiginous migraineurs have a higher frequency of comorbid anxiety disorders. The common neuroanatomic pathways provide focus for interventions. Antivertiginous medications are not effective, and challenging the vestibular pathways can often lead to increased avoidance behaviors, more dizziness, and actual decline in function.[179] Determination that there is a psychogenic or somatoform component of the disorder is often made late in the diagnosis when treatment from the ear, nose, and throat specialist, neurologist, or internist has failed.[180-182] Appendix Box 22-2 describes the relationship of the disorders.

APPENDIX BOX 22-2 ■ RELATIONSHIP BETWEEN OTOLOGICAL CONDITIONS AND ANXIETY

Otogenic: Primary otological conditions that can trigger secondary anxiety disorders

Psychogenic: Anxiety disorders as primary cause of dizziness

Interactive: Otological conditions that exacerbate preexisting anxiety

CHAPTER 23 Movement Dysfunction Associated with Hemiplegia

SUSAN D. RYERSON, PT, DSc

KEY TERMS

atypical movements
clinical hypertonicity
composite impairments
edema
evaluation of movement control
goal setting
hemiplegia
movement deficits
muscle activation deficits
orthoses
postural control
predictors of recovery
primary impairments
secondary impairments
shoulder pain
shoulder subluxation
significant impairments
standardized evaluations of function
trunk and arm linked movements
trunk control
trunk and leg linked movements
undesirable compensations

OBJECTIVES

After reading this chapter the student or therapist will be able to:

1. Identify the various types of neurovascular disease.
2. Identify the atypical patterns of movement in clients with residual hemiplegia.
3. Identify significant primary and secondary body system problems (impairments) that interfere with functional movement patterns and limit ability to participate.
4. Describe a reeducation intervention strategy for improving functional movement in clients who have had a stroke.

OVERVIEW

The treatment of hemiplegia from vascular insult is controversial. Various treatment methods have been devised and advocated. Recent scientific theories have changed the focus of treatment from one of inhibition of abnormal tone and facilitation of normal movement to reeducation of control and weakness, and functional retraining. In this chapter, pathological conditions, body system problems (impairment), functional limitations, and intervention strategies for clients with hemiplegia from stroke are reviewed. Although hemiplegia from neurovascular pathological conditions is the focus of the chapter, therapists can use this information and apply it to adults with hemiplegia caused by other central nervous system (CNS) pathological conditions, such as tumor (see Chapter 25), trauma (see Chapter 24), multiple sclerosis (see Chapter 19), and demyelinating diseases (see Chapter 17). Movement components and their relationship to functional performance are used as the basis for selection of therapy techniques and training.

Definition

Hemiplegia, a paralysis of one side of the body, is the classic sign of neurovascular disease of the brain. It is one of many manifestations of neurovascular disease, and it occurs with strokes involving the cerebral hemisphere or brain stem. A stroke, or cerebrovascular accident (CVA), results in a sudden, specific neurological deficit and occurs when a brain blood vessel is either occluded by a clot or bursts. It is the suddenness of this neurological deficit—occurring over seconds, minutes, hours, or a few days—that characterizes the disorder as vascular. Although the motor deficits of hemiplegia may be the most obvious sign of a CVA and a major concern of therapists, other symptoms are equally disabling, including sensory dysfunction, aphasia or dysarthria, visual field defects, and mental and intellectual impairment. The specific combination of these neurovascular deficits enables a physician to detect both the location and the size of the defect. CVAs can be classified according to pathological type—thrombosis, embolism, or hemorrhage—or according to temporal factors, such as completed stroke, stroke-in-evolution, or transient ischemic attacks (TIAs).

Epidemiology

In the United States, stroke is the third ranking cause of death—more than 137,000 people die each year—and is the leading cause of adult disability.[1] The National Stroke Association estimates that 795,000 new or recurrent strokes occur each year. The incidence of stroke rises rapidly with increasing age: two thirds of all strokes occur in people older than the age of 65 years; and after the age of 55 years, the risk of stroke doubles every 10 years. With the over-50-years age group growing rapidly, more people than ever are at risk. In the United States, the incidence of stroke is greater in men than in women, and it is twice as high in blacks as in whites. Cerebral infarction (thrombosis or embolism) is the most common form of stroke, accounting for 70% of all strokes. Hemorrhages account for another 20%, and 10% remain unspecified. Stroke is the largest single cause of neurological disability. Approximately 4 million Americans are dealing with impairments and disabilities from a stroke. Of these, 31% require assistance, 20% need help walking, 16% are in long-term care facilities, and 71% are vocationally impaired after 7 years.[1] One study reported that 12% of subjects have complete functional arm recovery and 38% have some dexterity 6 months after stroke. In addition, loss of leg movement in the first week after stroke and no arm movement at 4 weeks are associated with poor outcomes at 6 months.[2]

The three most commonly recognized risk factors for cerebrovascular disease are hypertension, diabetes mellitus, and heart disease. The most important of these factors is hypertension.[3] Because high blood pressure is the greatest risk factor for stroke, human characteristics and behaviors that increase blood pressure, including increased high serum cholesterol levels, obesity, diabetes mellitus, heavy alcohol consumption, cocaine use, and cigarette smoking, increase the risk of stroke.

Ostfeld[4] noted that mortality rates for stroke declined, slowly at first (from 1900 to 1950) and then more quickly (from 1950 to 1970), with a sharp drop noted around 1974. Experts have speculated that the greater use of hypertensive drugs in the 1960s and 1970s started this decline, and the creation of screening and treatment referral centers for high blood pressure may account for the marked decline in the late 1970s.

Outcome

The long-term follow-up on the Framingham Heart Study revealed that long-term stroke survivors, especially those with only one episode, have a good chance for full functional recovery.[5] For people left with severe neurological and functional deficits, studies have demonstrated that rehabilitation is effective and that it can improve functional ability.[6,7] It has been demonstrated that age is not a factor in determining the outcome of the rehabilitation process.[8] Currently it is thought that clients should be given an opportunity to participate in the rehabilitation process, regardless of age, unless it is medically contraindicated.

The prediction of ultimate functional outcome has been hampered by the inaccuracy of commonly used predictors (medical items, income level, intelligence, functional level). Computed tomography (CT), functional magnetic resonance imaging, and regional cerebral blood flow studies are used in diagnosis and increasingly as predictors of functional recovery after stroke. Positron emission tomography and single-photon emission CT are newer techniques that are used in research centers to define areas of dysfunctional but perhaps "salvageable" tissue.[2,9]

Pathoneurological and Pathophysiological Aspects

Classification

The pathological processes that result from a CVA can be divided into three groups—thrombotic changes, embolic changes, and hemorrhagic changes.

Thrombotic Infarction. Atherosclerotic plaques and hypertension interact to produce cerebrovascular infarcts. These plaques form at branchings and curves of the arteries. Plaques usually form in front of the first major branching of the cerebral arteries. These lesions can be present for 30 years or more and may never become symptomatic. Intermittent blockage may proceed to permanent damage. The process by which a thrombus occludes an artery requires several hours and explains the division between stroke-in-evolution and completed stroke.[10]

TIAs are an indication of the presence of thrombotic disease and are the result of transient ischemia. Although the cause of TIAs has not been definitively established, cerebral vasospasm and transient systemic arterial hypotension are thought to be responsible factors.

Embolic Infarction. The embolus that causes the stroke may come from the heart, from an internal carotid artery thrombosis, or from an atheromatous plaque of the carotid sinus. It is usually a sign of cardiac disease. The infarction may be of pale, hemorrhagic, or mixed type. The branches of the middle cerebral artery are infarcted most commonly as a result of its direct continuation from the internal carotid artery. Collateral blood supply is not established with embolic infarctions because of the speed of obstruction formation, so there is less survival of tissue distal to the area of embolic infarct than with thrombotic infarct.[2]

Hemorrhage. The most common intracranial hemorrhages causing stroke are those resulting from hypertension, ruptured saccular aneurysm, and arteriovenous (AV) malformation. Massive hemorrhage frequently results from hypertensive cardiac-renal disease; bleeding into the brain tissue produces an oval or round mass that displaces midline structures. The exact mechanism of hemorrhage is not known. This mass of extravasated blood decreases in size over 6 to 8 months.

Saccular, or berry, aneurysms are thought to be the result of defects in the media and elastica that develop over years. This muscular defect plus overstretching of the internal elastic membrane from blood pressure causes the aneurysm to develop. Saccular aneurysms are found at branchings of major cerebral arteries, especially the anterior portion of the circle of Willis. Averaging 8 to 10 mm in diameter and variable in form, these aneurysms rupture at their dome. Saccular aneurysms are rare in childhood.

AV malformations are developmental abnormalities that result in a spaghetti-like mass of dilated AV fistulas varying in size from a few millimeters in diameter to huge masses located within the brain tissue. Some of these blood vessels have extremely thin, abnormally structured walls. Although the abnormality is present from birth, symptoms usually develop at ages 10 to 35 years. The hemorrhage of an AV malformation presents a pathological picture similar to that for the saccular aneurysm. The larger AV malformations frequently occur in the posterior half of the cerebral hemisphere.[10]

Clinical Findings

The focal neurological deficit resulting from a stroke, whether embolic, thrombotic, or hemorrhagic, is a reflection of the size and location of the lesion and the amount of collateral blood flow. Unilateral neurological deficits result from interruption of the carotid vascular system, and bilateral neurological deficits result from interruption of the vascular supply to the basilar system. Clinical syndromes resulting from occlusion or hemorrhage in the cerebral circulation vary from partial to complete. Signs of hemorrhage may be more variable as a result of the effect of extension to surrounding brain tissue and the possible rise in intracranial pressure. Table 23-1 summarizes the clinical symptoms and the anatomical structures involved according to specific arterial involvement.

The frequencies of the three types of cerebrovascular disease—thrombosis, embolism, and hemorrhage—vary according to whether they were taken from a clinical study or from an autopsy study, but they rank in the order presented in this section. Ischemic strokes, thrombotic or embolic, account for 80% of strokes, and hemorrhagic strokes account for 20%.[11] The clinical symptoms and laboratory findings for each type are condensed in Table 23-2.

Medical Management and Pharmacological Considerations

Acute Medical Care

Thrombosis and Transient Ischemic Attacks. Although infarcted tissue cannot at present be restored, medical management of the acute stroke from thrombosis or TIA is geared toward improving the cerebral circulation as quickly as possible to prevent ischemic tissue from becoming infarcted tissue. Cells that have 80% to 100% ischemia will die in a few minutes because they cannot produce energy, specifically adenosine triphosphate. This energy failure results in an activation of calcium, which causes a chain reaction resulting in cell death.[1] Around this area of infarction is a transitional area where the blood flow is decreased 50% to 80%. Cells in the transitional area are not irreversibly damaged.[12,13]

One of the newer drugs available for immediate stroke treatment is tissue plasminogen activator (t-PA) (see Chapter 36). It is approved for use within 3 hours of symptom onset but is most effective if used within the first 90 to 180 minutes. Recent studies indicate that 42% of patients who have sustained a stroke wait 24 hours before getting care, with the average being 13 hours.[13] The importance of community-wide programs to increase awareness of symptoms and effectiveness of emergency medical responses is immense for this drug's usage. The American Heart Association and the National Stroke Association are creating community campaigns to increase awareness of the medical emergency nature of stroke symptoms. These campaigns encourage people to call 911 immediately when any of the following warning signs occur:

- Sudden numbness or weakness of the face, arm, or leg, especially on one side of the body
- Sudden confusion or trouble speaking or understanding
- Sudden trouble walking, dizziness, loss of balance or coordination
- Sudden severe headache with no known cause
- Sudden trouble seeing with one or both eyes

Anticoagulant drugs are used to prevent TIAs and may stop a stroke-in-evolution. Before anticoagulant drugs are used, an accurate differential diagnosis is necessary because of the danger of excessive bleeding if hemorrhage is present. Heparin is often used in the early stage of the stroke, and warfarin (Coumadin) or dabigatran (Pradaxa) is commonly used in the months after the stroke. Cerebral edema, if present, is managed pharmacologically during the first few days. Antiplatelet drugs such as aspirin, dipyridamole (Persantine), and sulfinpyrazone (Anturane) are used to prevent clotting by decreasing platelet "stickiness."[10]

Surgical treatment (thromboendarterectomy or grafting) is used when TIAs are the result of arterial plaques. Areas accessible to and suitable for surgery include the carotid sinus and the common carotid, innominate, and subclavian arteries. Although both surgery and anticoagulant therapy are used for TIAs, Adams and Victor[10] extensively reviewed the wide divergence of opinions. For clients who have had a stroke yet recovered quickly and well, medical care focuses on prevention. Prevention usually includes maintaining blood pressure and blood flow, monitoring hypotensive agents (if given), and avoiding oversedation, especially for sleep, to prevent cerebral ischemia.

Embolic Infarction. Management of embolic infarction is similar to that of thrombotic infarction. The primary emphasis is on prevention. Long-term anticoagulant therapy is effective in preventing embolic infarction in clients with cardiac problems such as atrial fibrillation, myocardial infarction, and valve prostheses. The diagnostic use of CT is important in anticoagulant therapy to rule out hemorrhage after the infarct.

Hypertensive Hemorrhage. Medical procedures for hypertensive hemorrhage parallel those for thrombosis and embolism. Surgical removal of the clot and lowering of the systemic blood pressure to decrease hemorrhage have generally not been helpful. Again, the preventive use of antihypertensive drugs in clients with essential hypertension is the soundest medical management available.[10]

Ruptured Aneurysm. Comatose clients are not good candidates for surgery. However, if the client survives the first few days and if the state of consciousness improves, surgical intervention, whether extracranial or intracranial, is the treatment of choice. Medical treatment consists of lowering arterial blood pressures. Bed rest for 4 to 6 weeks with all forms of exertion avoided is prescribed. Antiseizure medication may be used. Often a systemic antifibrinolysin is given to impede lysis of the clot at the site of rupture. Vasospasm, resulting in severe motor dysfunction, occurs with the use of drugs such as reserpine (Serpasil) and kanamycin (Kantrex) (see Chapter 36).

Regardless of the cause of the stroke, comatose clients are managed by (1) treatment of shock; (2) maintenance of clear airway and oxygen flow; (3) measurement of arterial blood gases, blood analysis, CT, and spinal tap; (4) control of seizures; and (5) gastric tube feeding (if coma is prolonged). Hypertensive hemorrhage is one of the most common vascular causes of coma.[14]

TABLE 23-1 ■ CLINICAL SYMPTOMS OF VASCULAR LESIONS

AFFECTED VESSEL	CLINICAL SYMPTOMS	STRUCTURES INVOLVED
Middle cerebral artery	Contralateral paralysis and sensory deficit	Somatic motor area
	Motor speech impairment	Broca area (dominant hemisphere)
	"Central" aphasia, anomia, jargon speech	Parieto-occipital cortex (dominant hemisphere)
	Unilateral neglect, apraxia, impaired ability to judge distance	Parietal lobe (nondominant hemisphere)
	Homonymous hemianopia	
	Loss of conjugate gaze to opposite side	Optic radiation deep to second temporal convolution
	Avoidance reaction of opposite limbs	Frontal controversive field
	Pure motor hemiplegia	Parietal lobe
	Limb—kinetic apraxia	Upper portion of posterior limb of internal capsule
		Premotor or parietal cortex
Anterior cerebral artery	Paralysis—lower extremity	Motor area—leg
	Paresis in opposite arm	Arm area of cortex
	Cortical sensory loss	
	Urinary incontinence	Posteromedial aspect of superior frontal gyrus
		Medial surface of posterior frontal lobe
	Contralateral grasp reflex, sucking reflex	Uncertain
	Lack of spontaneity, motor inaction, echolalia	Uncertain
	Perseveration and amnesia	
Posterior cerebral artery		
Peripheral area	Homonymous hemianopia	Calcarine cortex or optic radiation
	Bilateral homonymous hemianopia, cortical blindness, inability to perceive objects not centrally located, ocular apraxia	Bilateral occipital lobe
	Memory defect	Inferomedial portions of temporal lobe
	Topographical disorientation	Nondominant calcarine and lingual gyri
Central area	Thalamic syndrome	Posteroventral nucleus of thalamus
	Weber syndrome	Cranial nerve III and cerebral peduncle
	Contralateral hemiplegia	Cerebral peduncle
	Paresis of vertical eye movements, sluggish pupillary response to light	Supranuclear fibers to cranial nerve III
	Contralateral ataxia or postural tremor	
Internal carotid artery	Variable signs according to degree and site of occlusion—middle cerebral, anterior cerebral, posterior cerebral territory	Uncertain
Basilar artery	Ataxia	Middle and superior cerebellar peduncle
Superior cerebellar artery	Dizziness, nausea, vomiting, horizontal nystagmus	Vestibular nucleus
	Horner syndrome on opposite side, decreased pain and thermal sensation	Descending sympathetic fibers Spinal thalamic tract
	Decreased touch, vibration, position sense of lower extremity greater than that of upper extremity	Medial lemniscus
	Nystagmus, vertigo, nausea, vomiting	Vestibular nerve
Anterior inferior cerebellar artery	Facial paralysis on same side	Cranial nerve VII
	Tinnitus	Auditory nerve, lower cochlear nucleus
	Ataxia	Middle cerebral peduncle
	Impaired facial sensation on same side	Fifth cranial nerve nucleus
	Decreased pain and thermal sensation on opposite side	Spinal thalamic tract
Complete basilar syndrome	Bilateral long tract signs with cerebellar and cranial nerve abnormalities	
	Coma	
	Quadriplegia	

TABLE 23-1 ■ CLINICAL SYMPTOMS OF VASCULAR LESIONS—cont'd

AFFECTED VESSEL	CLINICAL SYMPTOMS	STRUCTURES INVOLVED
	Pseudobulbar palsy	
	Cranial nerve abnormalities	
Vertebral artery	Decreased pain and temperature on opposite side	Spinal thalamic tract
	Sensory loss from a tactile and proprioceptive	Medial lemniscus
	Hemiparesis of arm and leg	Pyramidal tract
	Facial pain and numbness on same side	Descending tract and fifth cranial nucleus
	Horner syndrome, ptosis, decreased sweating	Descending sympathetic tract
	Ataxia	Spinal cerebellar tract
	Paralysis of tongue	Cranial nerve XII
	Weakness of vocal cord, decreased gag	Cranial nerves IX and X
	Hiccups	Uncertain

Modified from Adams RD, Victor M: *Principles of neurology,* New York, 1981, McGraw-Hill.

TABLE 23-2 ■ CLINICAL SYMPTOMS AND LABORATORY FINDINGS FOR NEUROVASCULAR DISEASE—RUPTURED SACCULAR ANEURYSM

DISEASE TYPE	CLINICAL PICTURE	LABORATORY FINDINGS
THROMBOSIS	*Extremely variable* Preceded by a prodromal episode Uneven progression Onset develops within minutes or hours or over days ("thrombus in evolution") 60% occur during sleep—patient awakens unaware of problem, rises, and falls to floor Usually no headache, but may occur in mild form Hypertension, diabetes, or vascular disease elsewhere in body	Cerebrospinal fluid pressure is normal Cerebrospinal fluid is clear Electroencephalogram: limited differential diagnostic value Skull radiographs not helpful Arteriography is definitive procedure; demonstrates site of collateral flow CT scan helpful in chronic state when cavitation has occurred
TIA	Linked to atherosclerotic thrombosis Preceded or accompanied by stroke Occur by themselves Last 2-30 min A few attacks or hundreds are experienced Normal neurological examination findings between attacks If transient symptoms are present on awakening, may indicate future stroke	Usually none
EMBOLISM	*Extremely variable*	
Cardiac	Occurs extremely rapidly—seconds or minutes	Generally same as for thrombosis except for the following:
Noncardiac Atherosclerosis Pulmonary thrombosis Fat, tumor, air	There are no warnings Branches of middle cerebral artery are involved most frequently; large embolus will block internal carotid artery or stem of middle cerebral artery If embolus is in basilar system, deep coma and total paralysis may result Often a manifestation of heart disease, including atrial fibrillation and myocardial infarction Headache As embolus passes through artery, client may have neurological deficits that resolve as embolus breaks and passes into small artery supplying small or silent brain area	If embolism causes a large hemorrhagic infarct, cerebrospinal fluid will be bloody 30% of embolic strokes produce small hemorrhagic infarct without bloody cerebrospinal fluid

Continued

TABLE 23-2 ■ CLINICAL SYMPTOMS AND LABORATORY FINDINGS FOR NEUROVASCULAR DISEASE—RUPTURED SACCULAR ANEURYSM—cont'd

DISEASE TYPE	CLINICAL PICTURE	LABORATORY FINDINGS
HEMORRHAGE		
Hypertensive hemorrhage	Severe headache Vomiting at onset Blood pressure >170/90; usually from "essential" hypertension but can be from other types Abrupt onset, usually during day, not in sleep Gradually evolves over hours or days according to speed of bleeding No recurrence of bleeding Frequency in blacks with hypertensive hemorrhage is greater than frequency in whites Hemorrhaged blood absorbs slowly—rapid improvement of symptoms is not usual If massive hemorrhage occurs, client may survive a few hours or days as a result of brain stem compression	CT scan can detect hemorrhages larger than 1.5 cm in cerebral and cerebellar hemispheres; it is diagnostically superior to arteriography; it is especially helpful in diagnosing small hemorrhages that do not spill blood into cerebrospinal fluid; with massive hemorrhage and increased pressure, cerebrospinal fluid is grossly bloody; lumbar puncture is necessary when CT scan is not available Radiographs occasionally show midline shift (this is not true with infarction) Electroencephalogram shows no typical pattern, but high voltage and slow waves are most common with hemorrhage Urinary changes may reflect renal disease
Ruptured saccular aneurysm	Asymptomatic before rupture With rupture, blood spills under high pressure into subarachnoid space Excruciating headache with loss of consciousness Headache without loss of consciousness Sudden loss of consciousness Decerebrate rigidity with coma If severe—persistent deep coma with respiratory arrest, circulatory collapse leading to death; death can occur within 5 minutes If mild—consciousness regained within hours then confusion, amnesia, headache, stiff neck, drowsiness Hemiplegia, paresis, homonymous hemianopia, or aphasia usually absent	CT scan detects localized blood in hydrocephalus if present Cerebrospinal fluid is extremely bloody Radiographs are usually negative Carotid and vertebral arteriography is performed only when diagnosis is certain

Modified from Adams RD, Victor M: *Principles of neurology,* New York, 1981, McGraw-Hill.

CT, Computed tomography; *TIA,* transient ischemic attack.

Medical Management of Associated Problems

Spasticity. Spasticity and its treatment constitute a major medical problem after stroke because clients complain about it, it may fluctuate, and it does not respond to one fixed treatment. The relationship between spasticity and movement after stroke is an area of continued interest for researchers. Recent studies have refuted the earlier belief that spasticity was inversely related to voluntary movement.[15,16] Although therapists are more hesitant to treat spasticity now, physicians continue to treat it aggressively. Various pharmacological, surgical, and physical means are used to decrease spasticity. The pharmacological and surgical means are examined here, and therapy management is discussed later.

Two types of drugs are used to counter the effects of spasticity: centrally acting and peripherally acting agents. Centrally acting drugs, such as diazepam, have been used to depress the lateral reticular formation and thus its facilitatory action on the gamma motor neurons. This form of drug is used widely to treat spasticity, although the greatest disadvantage of centrally acting drugs is that they depress the entire CNS. Drowsiness and anxiety are common side effects.

Peripherally acting drugs are used to block a specific link in the gamma group. Procaine blocks selectively inhibit the small gamma motor fibers, resulting in a relaxation of intrafusal fibers. The effect of procaine blocks is transient. Intramuscular neurolysis with the injection of 5% to 7% phenol has been used to destroy the small intramuscular mixed nerve branches.[17] Phenol blocks relieve hypertonicity and improve function, especially when followed by an intensive course of therapy.[18] It can provide relief for 2 to 12 months, and the effects have been documented to last as long as 3 years.[17,18] Disadvantages of phenol use include its toxicity to tissue and the complications of pain that occasionally result.

Botulinum toxin type A (Botox) is also used to decrease the effects of hypertonicity on functional movement in hemiplegia.[19-21] Local injection of the toxin into spastic muscles produces selective weakness by interfering with the uptake of acetylcholine by the motor end plate. The effect of the toxin is temporary, depends on the amount injected, and is associated with minimal side effects. Repeat injections are recommended no sooner than 12 to 14 weeks to avoid antibody formation to the toxin. Researchers report positive functional results when botulinum toxin A injections are followed by intensive muscle reeducation and appropriate splinting.[22]

Dantrolene sodium is used to interrupt the excitation-contraction mechanism of skeletal muscles. Trials have shown that it has reduced spasticity in 60% to 80% of clients while improving function in 40% of these clients. The side effects—drowsiness, weakness, and fatigue—can be decreased through titration of dosage. Serious side effects, including hepatotoxicity, precipitation of seizures, and lymphocytic lymphoma, have been reported when the drug has been used in high doses over a long time.[17]

Baclofen, in pill form, is used as a skeletal muscle relaxant to decrease spasticity. It can now be delivered intrathecally into the spinal cord with a pump that is surgically inserted into the body. It relieves spasticity with a small amount of medication (10 mg/20 mL, 10 mg/5 mL). Intrathecal baclofen has had dramatic results in cases of severe spasticity because it acts directly on the affected muscles instead of circulating in the blood. It is used for extremity spasticity that interferes with the ability to assume functional positions in patients with severe stroke, multiple sclerosis, head injury, and cerebral palsy.[23]

The surgical treatment of spasticity through tenotomy or neurectomy is considered when all other treatments fail, and it is used to correct deformity, especially of a hand or foot. A peripheral nerve block is often used as a diagnostic tool to evaluate the effect of surgical treatment. If anatomical or functional gains are made through a temporary nerve block, consideration is given to surgical release. The surgical treatment of spasticity does not necessarily result in increased movement control and, with the increased understanding of the causes of spasticity, does not seem appropriate in stroke.

Seizures. The highest risk for seizure after a stroke is immediately afterward; 57% of seizures occur in the first week and 88% occur within the first year.[24] Seizures after thrombotic and embolic stroke are usually of early onset, whereas seizures after hemorrhagic stroke are of late onset. The management of seizures after stroke is usually with antiseizure medication. Commonly used drugs include phenytoin (Dilantin), carbamazepine (Tegretol), gabapentin (Neurontin), and divalproex (Depakote).[25] Side effects that interfere with movement therapy include drowsiness, ataxia, distractibility, and poor memory.

Respiratory Involvement. Fatigue is a major problem for the person with hemiplegia. This fatigability, which interferes with everyday life processes and active rehabilitation, is attributed to respiratory insufficiency resulting from paralysis of one side of the thorax. Haas and colleagues[26] studied respiratory function in hemiplegia and found decreased lung volume and mechanical performance of the thorax to be significant factors, in addition to abnormal pulmonary diffusing capacity. Clients with hemiplegia consume 50% more oxygen while walking slowly (regardless of the presence or absence of orthotic devices) than that used by subjects without hemiplegia.[26] The decreased respiratory output and the increased oxygen demand that result from atypical movement patterns are responsible for early fatigue in persons with hemiplegia. Treatment objectives and techniques must reflect the understanding of this respiratory problem. For clients who walk at velocities greater than 0.48 m/s, a gain in walking capacity is associated with an increased peak Vo_2. Research exploring the role of exercise after stroke indicated that gains in respiratory fitness were associated with increased walking capacity. In clinical practice, therapists should remember to include standard respiratory measures and functions to evaluate the efficacy of treatment techniques.[27]

Cardiovascular Health. In the chronic stage of recovery, clients may have significant cardiovascular deconditioning with half the fitness levels of age-matched controls. This decrease in fitness affects the performance of daily activities and adds to these clients' morbidity and mortality risk. This decreased fitness results in part from decreased mobility of the leg, muscular atrophy, altered muscle physiology, increased muscular fat, and altered peripheral blood flow.[28,29]

Fractures. If the hemiplegic client has severe extremity or trunk weakness and relies heavily on the nonparetic extremities for function, poor balance and falls are possible. After a stroke the risk of hip fracture is greatest in the first year of recovery. Eighty percent of hip fractures occur on the paretic side and are the result of bone loss or falls. In addition, other common fracture sites are the humerus and wrist.[30]

Therapy intervention for a hip fracture with a hemiplegia is complicated by increased difficulty sustaining a symmetrical trunk posture over the fractured hip, decreased strength in the leg, pain, and spasticity. In addition to the loss of balance and protective mechanisms, the development of osteoporosis from disuse is a limiting factor for functional recovery after a fracture.[31]

Thrombophlebitis. Thrombophlebitis may occur in the early stages of rehabilitation. Vascular changes are often premorbid. Deep vein thrombosis is caused by altered blood flow, damage to the vessel wall, and changes in blood coagulation times. The vascular changes are aggravated by the inactivity and dependent postures of the weak extremities. Deep vein thrombosis is many times more common in the weak leg.[32]

Complex Regional Pain Syndrome. Formerly known as reflex sympathetic dystrophy, *complex regional pain syndrome* is a chronic pain condition affecting the paretic arm or leg. The extremity pain is reported as intense and burning and may be accompanied by swelling and redness. It leads to changes in bone and skin and, if left untreated, becomes debilitating. Medical treatment includes the use of chemical sympathetic blocks and oral or intramuscular corticosteroids. The use of blocks and corticosteroids often stops the burning pain. The length of time of the relief varies from client to client. Adverse reactions from blocks and corticosteroids occur about 20% of the time[33,34] (see Chapter 32).

Pain. The pharmacological management of joint pain after stroke (usually shoulder pain) includes the local injection of corticosteroids. (For additional information regarding pain and its management, see Chapter 32.)

Sequential Stages of Recovery from Acute to Adaptive Phase

Evolution of Recovery Process

The evolution of the recovery process from onset to the return to community life can be divided into three stages—acute, active (rehabilitation), and adaptation to personal environment.

The acute state involves the stroke-in-evolution, the completed stroke, or the TIA and the decision whether to hospitalize.

The stroke-in-evolution develops gradually with distinct demarcation of the damaged area over 6 to 24 hours. Thrombosis, the most common cause of stroke, results first in ischemia and finally in infarction. Its gradual onset has led researchers to believe that a "cure" may be found for this type of stroke. If ischemic tissue can be treated and saved before infarction occurs, the neurological damage may be reversible. Small hemorrhages also may become a stroke-in-evolution by effusing blood along nerve pathways and by attracting fluid.[35] A completed stroke has a sudden onset and produces distinct, nonprogressive symptoms and damage within minutes or hours. In contrast, the TIA has a brief duration of neurological deficit and spontaneous resolution with no residual signs. TIAs vary in number and duration.

The physician decides the extent of hospitalization. The trend to hospitalize is more common today than years ago.[36] However, a mild stroke or TIA may produce minimal physical and mental symptoms, and the person may not even seek medical help. Cost-containment measures in hospitals and managed care have led to decreased lengths of stay and the development of critical pathway plans to deliver services more efficiently. Critical pathways are plans that describe the duration and extent of services after a stroke. The inpatient length of stay for acute stroke is currently 2 to 4 days. After the inpatient stay, the client follows one of four pathways: he or she returns home with or without home care services, goes to a rehabilitation hospital for a 2- to 4-week stay, goes to a subacute facility to become strong enough for the rehabilitation regimen, or goes to a long-term care facility for rehabilitation or maintenance care.

Once the stroke is completed, the clinical symptoms begin to decrease in severity. A person with a stroke caused by an embolic episode may have symptoms that reverse completely in a few days; more frequently, however, improvement takes place very slowly with a marked deficit. The fatality rate is high within the first day but decreases substantially in the following months of recovery.[36] Evidence from efficacy studies of rehabilitation programs that aim at improving functional performance is limited. Studies by Bamford and colleagues[37] indicate that early rehabilitation intervention reduces disability and improves compensatory strategies.

The Framingham Heart Study has revealed that long-term stroke survivors have a good chance of returning to independent living. The greatest deficit in persons with hemiplegia who have recovered basic motor skills and who have returned home is in the psychosocial and environmental areas.[5]

Recovery of Motor Function

Recovery of motor function after a stroke was thought historically to be complete 3 to 6 months after onset. More recent research has shown that functional recovery from a stroke can continue for months or years.[38,39] Measuring recovery is difficult because the definition of "successful" or "complete" recovery varies greatly. Duncan reports that if recovery is defined at the disability level (Barthel score greater than 90), 57% of stroke survivors have a complete recovery. However, if impairments are measured, less than 37% recover fully. And if recovery is related to prior physical functioning, less than 25% are considered completely recovered.[40]

The initial functional gains after the stroke are attributed to reduction of cerebral edema, absorption of damaged tissue, and improved local vascular flow. However, these factors do not play a role in long-term functional recovery. The brain damage that results from a stroke is thought to be circumvented rather than "repaired" during the process of functional recovery. The CNS reacts to injury with a variety of potentially reparative morphological processes. Two mechanisms underlying functional recovery after stroke are collateral sprouting and the unmasking of neuropathways: regeneration and reorganization.[38] Research continues to provide important insights into the fundamental capabilities of the brain to respond to damage. Methods of intervention that use the environment and help the client learn lead to long-term improved recovery.

The CNS has some predictable traits in response to injury. Twitchell, in his classic study, first documented the initial loss of voluntary function.[41] Although paralysis with flaccidity initially exists, there is seldom, if ever, total paralysis. He reported both an increase in deep tendon reflexes after 48 hours and the emergence of synergistic patterns of movement.[41] The synergistic movement patterns of the upper extremity and lower extremity have been described in detail by many.[42-44] Verbal description of a visual phenomenon often leads to differences in written and spoken communication, yet the visual array or behavioral patterns may be exactly the same.[45] Synergistic patterns may not be the same as movement combinations necessary for function. Although it is stated that the leg recovers more quickly or better than the arm, a leg that is bound by an extensor synergy and that is as "rigid as a pillar" during gait has not recovered more quickly and has no better function than an arm that is flexed and held across the chest and that can only grasp in a gross pattern with no ability to release.

Although studies are investigating the exact nature of the relationship between voluntary movement and spasticity, clinical evidence demonstrates that as voluntary function increases, the dependence on synergistic movement decreases.[16] With the knowledge that the CNS is capable of reacting to injury with a variety of morphological processes, we should no longer view the effect of a stroke as a fixed event. Because the brain immediately institutes neuromechanisms that reconstitute typical functions, therapy interventions should emphasize use of movement patterns on the affected side to maximize return and to help the client achieve the highest level of function.

Predictors of Recovery

Research in motor recovery shows that although motor recovery may continue after 6 months, the functional status usually remains constant, and that 86% of the variance in 6-month recovery is predictable at 1 month.[46]

In one study, although 58% of the patients regained independence in activities of daily living (ADLs) and 82% learned to walk, 30% to 60% of patients had no arm function.[47] Initial return of movement in the first 2 weeks is one indicator of the possibility of full arm recovery. But failure to recover grip strength before 24 days was correlated with no recovery of arm function at 3 months.[47] In another study that used the modified Rankin scale as the outcome measure, half of the patients recovered within 18 months with the greatest amount of recovery present at the 6-month mark. Predictors of recovery in this group included stroke severity, no previous ischemic stroke, peripheral artery disease, or diabetes.[48]

One problem inherent in prognostic research is the lack of a movement-based classification system. The clinical "predictors" in regression models are assumed to be static, whereas in fact they may change over time. Another problem is that there may be a lack of accuracy because of differences in researchers' objectives.[49]

As clinicians we can help minimize the problems in research methods by precisely formulating functional goals, stating movement components and significant impairments that interfere with functional performance, and following a model when making clinical decisions to postulate cause and effect during intervention.

Classification of Atypical Movement Patterns

Although the *Guide to Physical Therapist Practice* groups patients with neurological dysfunction according to pathological condition, therapy intervention rarely is directed by the diagnosis of stroke and resultant hemiplegia.[50] The World Health Organization (WHO) classification system, the International Classification of Function (ICF-2), provides a structure that allows us to evaluate by health condition, impairment, or activity or participation limitation.[51,52]

Impairment-related classification systems for stroke are just beginning to be researched.[53] Currently, atypical movement patterns in stroke are classified according to type of lesion (embolism, thrombosis, TIA) or side of weakness. The classification models make it easier for therapists to identify and define the focus of their intervention for the neurological patient. These models help us organize our interventions into two categories: (1) interventions that aim at improving relevant impairments that contribute to functional limitations and disability and (2) interventions that focus on the activity or participation limitations. The treatment interventions in this chapter try to relate limitations in activities to relevant underlying impairments.

Although the main focus of this chapter is the evaluation and treatment of activity limitations and impairments resulting from a loss of movement control, a stroke may result in damage to other systems that affects the client's ability to perform functional skills. There may be deficiencies in sensory processing (vision, somesthetic sensation, and vestibular systems) and disorders of cognitive integration (arousal and attention, awareness of disability, memory, problem solving, and learning), which all have a large impact on functional retraining. Depression and, most important, problems of language and communication also affect the client's ability to participate in a therapy program.

Impairments Contributing to Activity and Participation Limitations

Clients with hemiplegia from stroke have movement problems—impairments—that lead to activity and participation limitations. These movement problems manifest themselves as loss of movement in the trunk and extremities, atypical patterns of movement, and involuntary nonpurposeful movements of the affected side that lead to compensatory functional strategies. These impairments interfere with normal functional movements and may lead to loss of independence in daily life.

Impairments are the signs, symptoms, and physical findings that relate to a specific disease pathology. Schenkman and Butler were the first to apply a model of impairments to neurological physical therapy practice. Ryerson and Levit, using a similar format, specifically defined the impairment categories as primary, secondary, and composite[54,55] (Box 23-1).

Primary Impairments. Primary impairments are physical findings that are associated with the specific brain lesion. The primary impairments of stroke that relate to functional recovery of movement include changes in strength, changes in muscle tone, muscle activation or control changes (sequencing, firing, initiation), and changes in sensation. Cognitive and perceptual, emotional, and speech and language changes are also primary impairments that have an effect on function but are less of a focus of this chapter.

Secondary Impairments. Secondary impairments involve systems of the body other than the neurological system. They occur as a consequence of the stroke or because

BOX 23-1 ■ IMPAIRMENTS THAT INTERFERE WITH FUNCTIONAL MOVEMENT

PRIMARY IMPAIRMENTS

Changes in muscle strength
- Paralysis or weakness

Changes in muscle tone
- Hypotonicity
- Spasticity
- Clinical hypertonicity

Changes in muscle activation
- Inappropriate initiation
- Difficulty sequencing
- Inappropriate timing of firing

Changes in sensation
- Awareness
- Interpretation

SECONDARY IMPAIRMENTS

Changes in alignment and mobility
Changes in muscle and soft tissue length
Pain
Edema

COMPOSITE IMPAIRMENTS

Movement deficits
Atypical movements
Undesirable compensations

Modified from Ryerson S, Levit K: *Functional movement reeducation: a contemporary model for stroke rehabilitation,* New York, 1997, Churchill Livingstone.

of other medical and environmental influences, such as a fall, pneumonia, or phlebitis. As they develop, they influence one another and the primary impairments. Secondary impairments influence the client's level of disability by contributing additional physical problems. There are four major categories of secondary impairments: orthopedic changes in alignment and mobility, changes in muscle and soft tissue length, pain, and edema.

Composite Impairments. Composite impairments are the combined effects of the primary and secondary impairments, motor recovery, treatment, and behavioral factors. Movement deficits are the missing pieces of movement control that the client needs to move normally. Atypical movements are movements that deviate from normal coordinated movement. Undesirable compensations are alternative, severely one-sided strategies used to perform a functional activity because of loss of normal movement patterns.

Patterns of Recovery

In the 1970s, "neurophysiological" theories and approaches changed therapy treatment for adults with CNS lesions. The founders of these approaches described positions and patterns of trunk and extremity movement.[42-44] These patterns were described in terms of spastic synergies, reflexive patterns, and position. Extremity movements were described as patterns of flexor or extensor synergies, arm and leg patterns were changeable according to the influence of tonic reflexes, and trunk position was always short on the affected side with scapular and pelvic retraction. The intervention techniques followed the descriptions and understanding of the movement problems. As knowledge from orthopedics, manual therapy, and motor control grew, therapists looked more closely at movement patterns and body position in clients with hemiplegia and expanded the categories. As early as 1982, new descriptions emerged that combined synergistic patterns and biomechanical influences on the musculoskeletal systems.[56] Today, descriptions of position and patterns of movement follow the impairment categories. The composite impairment category used in this chapter has three generalized movement patterns that create one model of classification: (1) movement deficits, (2) atypical movements, and (3) undesirable compensatory patterns.[54]

Movement deficits result from severe weakness or paralysis with either gradual, balanced return or no significant return. Functional movement patterns and levels of independence are based on the distribution and amount of return: trunk control greater than extremity control, extremity control greater than trunk control, distal extremity return greater than proximal extremity return or vice versa, and arm control greater than leg control or vice versa. These clients do not have problems with spasticity but, when weakness is severe, have long-term problems with the secondary impairments of muscle shortening and loss of joint range.

In the acute stage, the arm hangs by the side, the humerus is internally rotated, the elbow is extended, and the forearm is pronated. Inferior shoulder subluxation is common. The trunk is weak, the ribs flare, and posture is impaired, with a convex lateral curve seen on the affected side. (Appearances of lateral trunk flexion with the concavity on the affected side exist with compensatory upper- and lower-trunk movements.) In standing, the client has problems recruiting strength on the affected leg. The pelvis lists downward, and the hip and knee flex. The hip and knee flexion combined with a tendency to place more weight on the stronger leg places the ankle in plantarflexion, and no weight is borne on the heel. As the client learns to walk, either the knee flexes because of weakness or the patient compensates and "locks" the knee in extension.

Over time, the heavy arm pulls the upper body into flexion, creating an appearance of a low shoulder. To stand and walk, a compensatory shift of the upper body onto a cane helps the client balance. This overshifting of the upper body also makes it easier for these clients to initiate stepping with the use of pelvic elevation (Figures 23-1 and 23-2).

Atypical movement patterns are found in clients with unbalanced muscle return and deficits in muscle activation. These clients have difficulty organizing and sequencing muscle return, quieting muscles after active firing, and grading strength of contractions. Clients with unbalanced return can be further divided into two subcategories: (1) those with greater weakness, that is, unbalanced return, with secondary

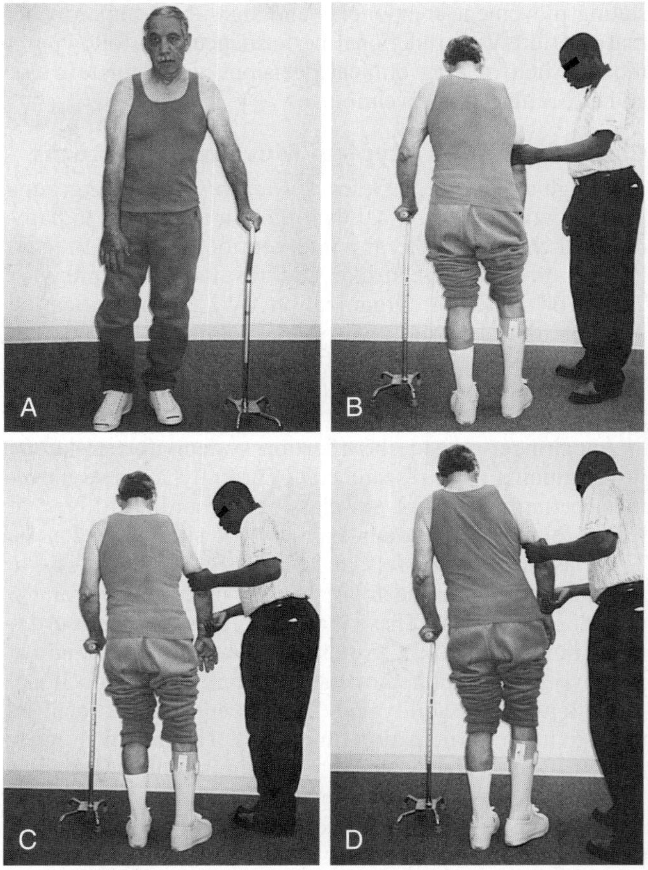

Figure 23-1 ■ **A,** Client with right hemiplegia. Movement deficit: paralysis; client was unable to move arm or leg in standing or sitting. **B,** Client uses cane and tries to shift to the right as he gets ready to step forward with the left leg. Note how the heavy weight of the right arm pulls the upper body into forward flexion and rotation left. **C,** Client prepares to step forward with the right leg. Note that his attendant has corrected his upper-body position. **D,** Client leans heavily onto cane (his upper body translates laterally to the left) to lessen weight on the right leg. He will accomplish the "step" by rotating his upper body to the left, a compensation for the loss of leg control in standing.

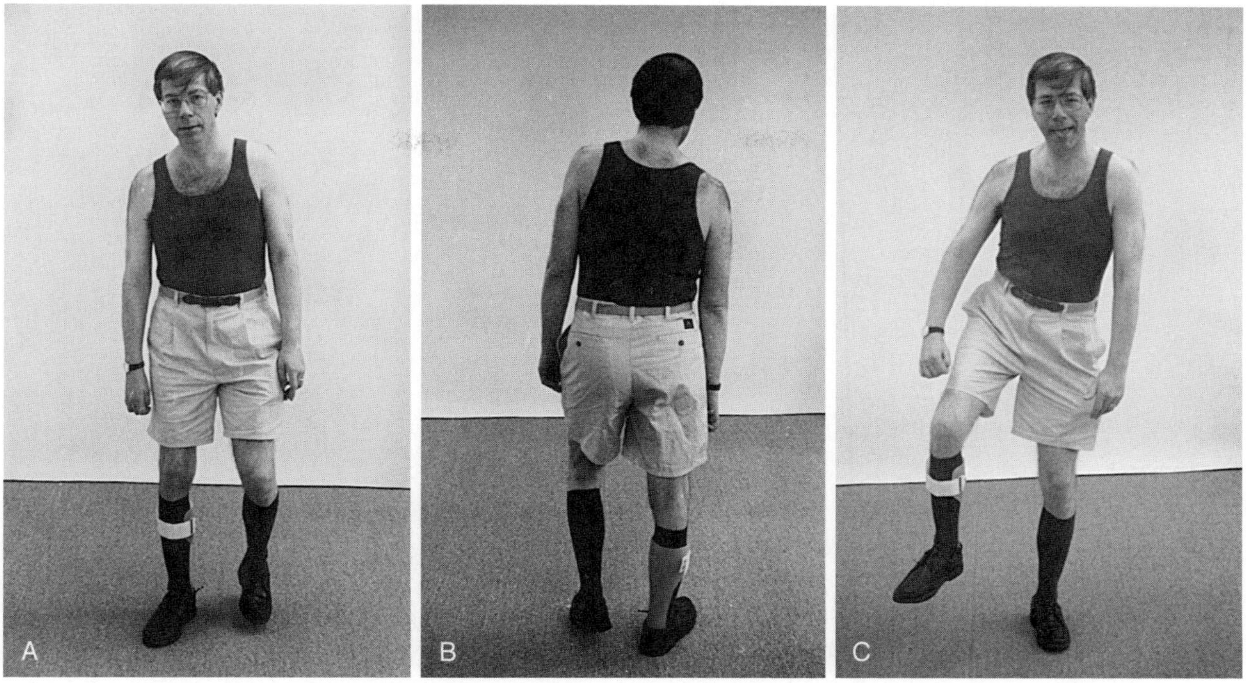

Figure 23-2 ■ **A,** Client with right hemiplegia. Movement deficit: weakness; client is able to walk with a brace and does not need a cane. **B,** During stance, his upper body moves laterally to the right and his right femur internally rotates as his knee hyperextends. **C,** He has enough trunk control to stand and balance and sufficient leg control to lift the leg with knee flexion.

problems of muscle shortening and poor alignment, and (2) those with greater return, with more problems of hypertonicity in the arm and leg.

These clients move and function with patterns that were formerly described as "spastic" or "synergistic." They have either anterior or superior shoulder subluxations, which determine the possibilities for fractionated movement in the arm. Common atypical leg movement patterns used for walking include *swing*—proximal initiation patterns of pelvic hiking or rotation toward the affected side, hip flexion with internal rotation and knee extension, or pelvic posterior tilting with hip abduction and knee flexion—and *stance*—contact with ground via toe strike or foot flat, loss of hip extension, and using excessive forward trunk flexion to initiate forward progression instead of moving the shank and lower leg over the foot.

Regardless of the proximal trunk and extremity patterns, the ankle-foot and wrist-hand patterns are predictable on the basis of the amount of distal return and the effects of proximal alignment. With weakness, the ankle plantarflexes and the wrist flexes. The foot or hand rotates on the ankle or wrist according to the pattern of and amount of return of proximal movements. Finger and toe patterns (curling or fisting, clawing) follow biomechanical rules of compensation or correlation (Figure 23-3).

Although the main movement problems of stroke occur because of weakness and atypical muscle activation patterns (e.g., sequencing, initiation), other movement disturbances, such as ataxia, may occur. In clients with ataxia, the main movement problem is one of wide swings of tone and muscle activation disturbances with fewer problems of weakness. These clients demonstrate trunk instability, excessive extremity movement, and overshooting of distal targets. Voluntary extremity movements are usually present but uncoordinated (see Chapter 21).

Undesirable compensatory patterns are patterns of function that may arise from either of the two previously described movement categories. Compensations are alternative movements or movement substitutions used to circumvent the challenge to the impaired side during daily activities. Although compensatory movements may be necessary and desirable to achieve the highest level of activity performance when there is no ability for recovery to occur, some may be more desirable than others. Undesirable compensatory patterns are noticeably one sided; they rely on movements of the uninvolved arm and leg and are accompanied by asymmetrical postural trunk movements. They lead to unsafe patterns, or to secondary impairments, or contribute to strategies that may have the potential to block or hinder future motor recovery. These undesirable compensatory patterns create "learned nonuse" of the affected arm and leg and foster asymmetrical postural patterns. Recent research findings indicate that limiting compensatory trunk movements may actually increase the performance of arm-reaching activities.

Patients who come into therapy with strongly established undesirable compensatory patterns do not respond quickly to any type of intervention. Although therapists may be tempted to train a one-sided pattern in early rehabilitation to quickly meet a stated goal, the long-term effects of learned nonuse of one side of the body include increased severity of secondary impairments and poor balance with an increased chance of falls (Figure 23-4).

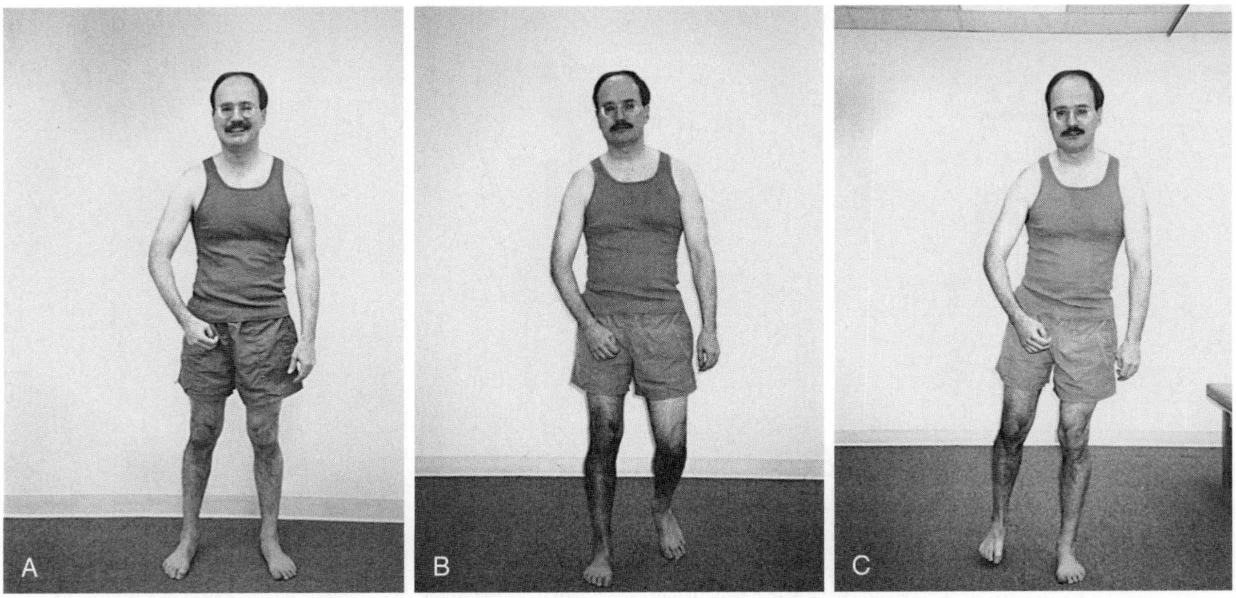

Figure 23-3 ■ **A,** Client with right hemiplegia. Movement deficit: loss of control of firing patterns, timing, and sequencing. **B** and **C,** Client walking.

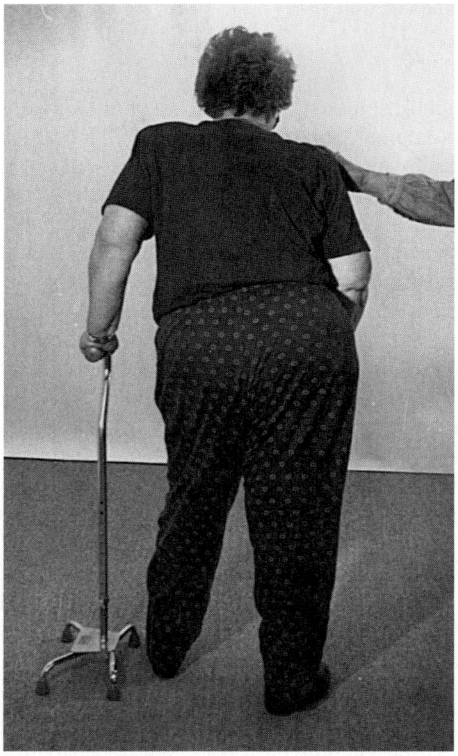

Figure 23-4 ■ Client with right hemiplegia. Severe compensatory patterns. She walks with a quad cane and standby assistance. Pelvis rotates to the right, upper body rotates to the left, hip flexes, and knee hyperextends. There is strong lateral translation of upper body to the left (to the stable cane).

EVALUATION PROCEDURES

Evaluation is a process of collecting information to establish a baseline level of performance to plan interventions and to document progress. This section reviews medical evaluations, standardized evaluations of functional performance (disability scales), evaluation of motor function and balance, and evaluation of secondary impairments that interfere with motor performance.

Medical Evaluation

After or during the evolution of a stroke, a thorough medical examination is conducted. All systems are surveyed, with emphasis placed on the level of consciousness; mental, affective, and emotional states; communication; cranial nerves; perceptual ability; sensation; and motor function. The National Institutes of Health (NIH) Stroke Scale is often used to evaluate the level of these common impairments poststroke.[57]

Levels of Consciousness

Scales of varying types are used to measure the client's level of consciousness, to assess the initial severity of brain damage, and to prognosticate recovery curves. The Glasgow Coma Scale, devised by Teasdale and Jennett in collaboration with Plum,[58] has been used for nontraumatic comas caused by stroke, head injury, and cardiac disease. This scale records motor responses to pain, verbal responses to auditory and visual clues, and eye opening. It assigns numerical values according to graded scales. Plum and Caronna[59] and Levy and colleagues[60] have also established criteria for correlating clinical signs of coma with prognosis.

The standard descriptions of level of consciousness—normal, semistupor, stupor, deep stupor, semicoma, coma, deep coma—are categorized by objective medical data but often leave a gap in the understanding of how the client functions in life.[58] This gap was closed by the creation of a scale, Levels of Cognitive Functioning, at Rancho Los Amigos Hospital. This behavioral rating scale is not a test of cognitive skill but an observational rating of the client's ability to process information[61] (see Chapter 24).

Mental, Emotional, and Affective States

The history portion of the neurological evaluation leads to an assessment of the mental, emotional, and affective states. The client's ability to describe the illness gives information on memory, orientation to time and place, the ability to express ideas, and judgment. If the examiner suspects a particular problem, a more thorough review is undertaken of the higher cortical function: serial subtraction, repetition of digits, and recall of objects or names. Clients with right hemiplegia may be cautious and disorganized in solving a given task, and clients with left hemiplegia tend to be fast and impulsive and seemingly unaware of the deficits present. These different response patterns stem from hemispheric involvement and prior hemispheric specialization.

Loss of emotional control often exists after a stroke. Crying is a common problem. Although excessive, inappropriate, or uncontrollable crying is usually a result of brain damage and a sign of emotional lability, crying can also be an expression of sadness as a result of depression. This difference is distinguishable by the ease with which the crying can be stopped. Other signs of emotional lability in persons with hemiplegia from stroke include inappropriate laughter or anger.

Communication

A general evaluation of communication disorders is noted while taking the history. Cerebral disorder resulting from infarct or hemorrhage can produce a loss of production or comprehension of the spoken word, the written word, or both. The therapist should be familiar with all types of communication disorders and with alternate modes of communication to establish a good client relationship.

Cranial Nerves and Reflexes

Thorough cranial nerve evaluation is necessary in hemiplegia because a deficit of a particular cranial nerve helps to determine the exact size and location of the infarct or hemorrhage. In hemiplegia, it is imperative to check for visual field deficits, pupil signs, ocular movements, facial sensation and weakness, labyrinthine and auditory function, and laryngeal and pharyngeal function.

Standard areas of reflex testing include the triceps, biceps, supinator, quadriceps, and gastrocnemius muscles. According to Adams,[10] there are four plantar reflex responses: (1) avoidance–quick, (2) spinal flexion–slow, (3) Babinski–toe grasp, and (4) positive support.

Perception

Perceptual deficits in clients with hemiplegia are complex and intimately linked to the sensorimotor deficit. Sensory integration theory has begun to establish normative values and objective data for testing and documenting perceptual deficits in children. Currently, norms and testing procedures for adults have not been standardized, but perceptual deficits have been identified in clients with hemiplegia. Common perceptual deficits found in left and right brain damage are listed in Box 23-2.

BOX 23-2 ■ PERCEPTUAL DEFICITS IN CENTRAL NERVOUS SYSTEM DYSFUNCTION

LEFT HEMIPARESIS: RIGHT HEMISPHERE—GENERAL SPATIAL-GLOBAL DEFICITS

Visual-perceptual deficits
- Hand-eye coordination
- Figure-ground discrimination
- Spatial relationships
- Position in space
- Form constancy

Behavioral and intellectual deficits
- Poor judgment, unrealistic behavior
- Denial of disability
- Inability to abstract
- Rigidity of thought
- Disturbances in body image and body scheme
- Impairment of ability to self-correct
- Difficulty retaining information
- Distortion of time concepts
- Tendency to see the whole and not individual steps
- Affect lability
- Feelings of persecution
- Irritability, confusion
- Distraction by verbalization
- Short attention span
- Appearance of lethargy
- Fluctuation in performance
- Disturbances in relative size and distance of objects

RIGHT HEMIPARESIS: LEFT HEMISPHERE—GENERAL LANGUAGE AND TEMPORAL ORDERING DEFICITS

Apraxia
- Motor
- Ideational

Behavioral and intellectual deficits
- Difficulty initiating tasks
- Sequencing deficits
- Processing delays
- Directionality deficits
- Low frustration levels
- Verbal and manual perseveration
- Rapid performance of movement or activity
- Compulsive behavior
- Extreme distractibility

Perceptual retraining without standardized norms for the deficit is at best difficult. The soundest course currently available appears to be one that relates perceptual and motor learning rather than retraining perception in isolation (see Chapters 4 and 14).

Sensation

Traditional sensory testing is used to assess sensory deficits in the adult with hemiplegia: light touch, deep pressure, kinesthesia, proprioception, pain, temperature, graphesthesia, two-point discrimination, appreciation of texture and size, and vibration. A comparison of the differences in the two sides of the body and qualitative and quantitative measurements are important features of sensory testing. Sensory testing is difficult because it relies on the client's interpretation of the sensation, the client's general awareness and suggestibility, and the client's ability to communicate a response to each test item.

The presence and quality of sensory loss must be considered during the process of reeducating motor control. Although Sherrington established the principle of interdependence of sensation and movement, current researchers have refined the concept and hypothesize that sensation modifies continuing movement by providing feed-forward information, feedback, and corollary discharge. They have provided evidence that sensation is not an absolute prerequisite for movement.[62]

Evaluation of motor function includes both standardized evaluation of functional performance and evaluation of movement control. Manual muscle testing, although used by physicians to determine a general level of strength, is not widely used by therapists to measure strength in individuals with CNS dysfunction because of the insensitivity of the test to loss of trunk and limb linked control. New measures of manual muscle testing for stroke are now beginning to be investigated.

Standardized Evaluations

Functional Performance

During the initial interview the therapist and the client together form a list of limitations and relate them to the client's goals and needs. The client can state his or her perceived functional limitations, or the therapist can ask the client to perform tasks. Commonly used standardized tests and scales for activity and participation limitations are listed here. Additional information can be found in Chapter 8.

Scales

The *Barthel Index* is one of the oldest measures of disability.[63] It has excellent validity and reliability and is simple to use, but it does not discriminate at higher levels of activity.

The *Motor Assessment Scale* (MAS) comes from the intervention theory of Carr and Shepherd.[64] Its reliability is high, it is simple to administer, and it takes only 15 minutes to perform. Although it mainly evaluates mobility skills, there is an arm and hand function section. The tests of arm function include movement patterns without tasks, and the hand function section uses object manipulation.

The *Functional Independence Measure* (FIM) is commonly used in rehabilitation centers, takes 45 minutes to perform, and measures ADLs, mobility, cognition, and communication.[65,66] It has good to excellent reliability.

The *Rivermead Mobility Index* measures common mobility functions, takes 5 minutes to perform, and has been tested for reliability and validity.[67]

The *Assessment of Motor and Process Skills* (AMPS) is a standardized test that measures task-performance abilities and efficiency during instrumental ADLs (IADLs).[68]

Tests of Motor Function and Balance

The *Fugl-Meyer Assessment* is a measure of extremity impairment severity. It is weighted, with more items measuring arm movement than leg movement. The test factors in reflexes and sensation and has good validity and reliability. It requires from 45 minutes to 1 hour to perform.[69]

The *Berg Balance Scale* is easy to administer, takes 5 to 10 minutes, and has norms specific to clients who have had a stroke.[70,71]

The *Balance Evaluation Systems Test* (BESTest and Mini-BESTest) is a balance evaluation that helps clinicians identify the impaired underlying system that is contributing to poor dynamic balance. The mini-BESTest is composed of 14 items and can be administered in 10 to 15 minutes.[72,73]

The *Postural Assessment Scale for Stroke* is a clinical balance measure that has been found to have better psychometric characteristics than the Berg Balance Scale or the balance subtest of the Fugl-Meyer test for people with severe stroke during the acute recovery phase. It has excellent reliability and validity and is easy to perform.[74,75]

The *Functional Reach Test* provides a measure of balance in standing. It measures control only during anterior (forward reach) weight shifts. Reliability is high, and the test is fast and easy to perform.[76]

The *Wolf Motor Function Test* is used to measure upper-extremity movements and functional tasks. It is a timed test, has been tested for reliability and validity, and is the assessment used in constraint-induced treatment studies.[77]

The *Trunk Impairment Scale* measures trunk movement patterns and dynamic and static sitting balance. It has high test-retest reliability and excellent concurrent validity.[78]

Gait

The evaluation of gait patterns includes the assessment of gait speed, a description of gait deviations, and, ideally, the assignment of a value representing the efficiency of ambulation.[79] Therapists are encouraged to measure gait speed throughout the rehabilitation process to quantitatively identify improvement in walking ability.[80,81]

The 5-meter walk test is responsive to changes in the acute phase of recovery especially the first 5 weeks poststroke. The 10-meter walk test has excellent reliability in the chronic recovery phase and is correlated with walking parameters and endurance.[82]

The 2-, 6-, and 10-minute walk tests are measures of walking endurance with high reliability and validity.[83]

The *Functional Ambulation Profile* is a system that attempts to relate the temporal aspects of gait to neuromuscular and cardiovascular functioning and converts this relationship to a single numerical score.[84]

The *Timed Up-and-Go Test* measures (in seconds) the ability to rise from a chair, walk 3 meters, turn, walk, and return to a seated position. It is frequently used in geriatric populations, but there is no validity testing for people poststroke.[85]

The temporal characteristics of gait—step time, cycle time, step length, and stride length—can be measured with a piece of chalk and a stopwatch or with more sophisticated equipment such as a gait analyzer. These parameters provide an objective measurement of performance and a baseline from which the efficacy of treatment procedures and client progress can be assessed.

Gait deviations in persons with hemiplegia have been described according to their biomechanical and kinesiological abnormalities and in terms of the loss of centrally programmed motor control mechanisms.[86,87]

Perry[87] described common problems of the hemiplegic person's gait as loss of controlled movement into plantarflexion at heel strike, loss of ankle movement from heel strike to midstance (resulting in loss of trunk balance and forward momentum for pushoff), and loss of the normal combination of movement patterns at the end of stance (hip extension, knee flexion, and ankle extension) and at the end of swing (hip flexion with knee extension and ankle flexion).

Knutsson and Richards[86] classified the motor control problems of the hemiplegic gait into three descriptive types. Type I is characterized by inappropriate activation of the calf muscles early in the gait cycle with corresponding low muscular activity in anterior compartment muscles. In the type I activation pattern, the calf musculature is activated before the center of gravity passes over the base of support. This thrusts the tibia backward instead of propelling the body forward in a pushoff as normally occurs. The client with hemiplegia compensates for the backward thrust of the tibia by anteriorly tilting the pelvis or flexing forward at the hip. Type II consists of an absence of or severe decrease in electromyographic activity in two or more muscle groups of the involved lower extremity. This pattern of markedly decreased muscular activity results in the adoption of compensatory mechanisms to gain stability. Type III activation patterns consist of abnormal coactivation of several limb muscles with normal or increased muscular activity levels in the muscle groups of the involved side. This type of pattern results in a disruption of the sequential flow of motor activity.

The Stroke Impact Scale (SIS) and the short version, the Stroke Impact Scale–16 (SIS-16) are measures with high reliability and validity for people poststroke. The long version assesses eight domains: strength, emotion, hand function, memory, physical function and mobility, communication, ADLs, and social participation. The SIS-16 includes most of the original items in the SIS physical function and mobility domain.[88,89]

Evaluation of Movement Control

After the standardized testing has been performed, the therapist continues to a subjective evaluation of movement components to gather information to answer the question "why" it is difficult for the client to perform specific movements or tasks.

Clients who have sustained a stroke have difficulty moving the trunk and the arm and leg on the affected side because of the presence of primary and secondary impairments. Objective standardized measures for the primary impairments are few; standard muscle testing has been questioned for CNS deficits because of the numerous degrees of freedom available and the discrepancy in functional strength on the basis of the increasing degrees of difficulty of controlling linked trunk and extremity patterns as the body moves from function in supine to function in sitting to function in standing.

Active Movement and Strength

When active movement patterns in the trunk and extremities are assessed, the therapist measures both strength and control. Paralysis, weakness, and imbalanced return are determinants of strength. Initiation pattern, sequencing, and control of firing patterns are indicators of control. Weakness and paralysis after stroke have been largely ignored because of a lingering focus on spasticity. Some recent studies have shown that muscle weakness is, in fact, present and interferes with the ability to generate enough force to achieve functional performance.[90-92] Motor weakness is present in 75% to 80% of clients after a stroke. There appears to be no difference in clients with left- or right-sided hemiplegia in terms of frequency or severity of weakness.[93] In contrast to these studies, Landau and Sahrmann[94] investigated the degree of functional impairment in strength that was a result of deficits in the contractile element of the affected muscles. Their findings from comparisons of maximal tetanic contraction of the anterior tibialis muscle suggest that maximal voluntary muscle strength was *not* impaired. Although recent research has moved weakness back into the impairment list, there is much more to be learned about the nature of weakness in CNS dysfunction.

The objective assessment of active movement in hemiplegia is commonly documented by therapists through the use of the Fugl-Meyer assessment scale, derived from synergistic stages as outlined by Brunnstrom,[43] and is similar to a version of Bobath's long evaluation form, which gradually builds series of selective or fractionated movement in the arm, trunk, and leg.[95]

When clinically assessing weakness and control of active movement patterns, the therapist analyzes and identifies the client's patterns of posture and movement in the trunk and extremities by position (supine, side lying, sitting, and standing) and in linked combinations. Active movement control is evaluated in individual muscles, movement components, and movement sequences.[54] Verbal directions or demonstrations may be necessary to help the client understand what is desired. In this phase of the evaluation, the therapist should not physically assist the client's movement but should be prepared to prevent loss of balance.

While evaluating force production or weakness in all these categories, the therapist gathers information about sequencing movements in increasingly complex patterns, timing of muscle firing, and speed of movement. Muscle activation deficits in these categories may explain why some clients with minimal weakness do not regain spontaneous functional use of the extremities.[54]

Assisted Movement

After the evaluation of active movement, therapists use their hands while retesting the movements to gain additional information about the relationships between impairments. Whereas the use of handling must be judicious, handling is used during an assessment for the following purposes:

1. To correct alignment to gather additional information about strength, control, and orthopedic impairments (Figure 23-5)
2. To limit degrees of freedom of one of the joints to assess relationships between intralimb segments
3. To assist the movement of a weak muscle
4. To block or stabilize a joint to assess the performance of a weaker muscle group or to limit the degrees of freedom of an intralimb segment[54] (Figure 23-6)

Example

Step 1. *Assessment of forward reach in sitting by client with left hemiplegia.* Active movement patterns on left: client initiates movement proximally; shoulder flexes to 60 degrees, with internal humeral rotation; abducted, downwardly rotated scapula elevates during the movement; elbow flexes, forearm supinates to 10 degrees; wrist remains in flexion and radial deviation. Client leans trunk

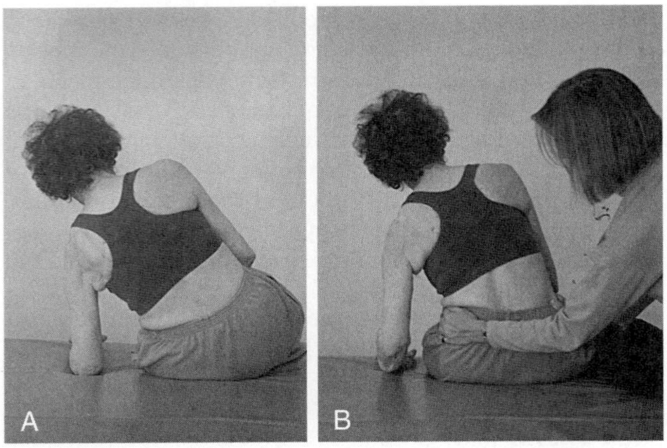

Figure 23-5 ■ **A,** Client with right hemiplegia trying to perform an upper-body–initiated lateral weight shift to the left. Note that the spine is straight and the right hip is off the surface. **B,** Therapist uses her hands to correct and stabilize the lower trunk as the client initiates the upper-body lateral movement to the left. The therapist gains information about trunk and hip control and secondary impairments of trunk muscle tightness. Note that the spine is beginning to curve as the client uses eccentric activity of the right lateral musculature to control the movement. Active stretching of the right quadratus lumborum and latissimus occurs if tight muscles are present.

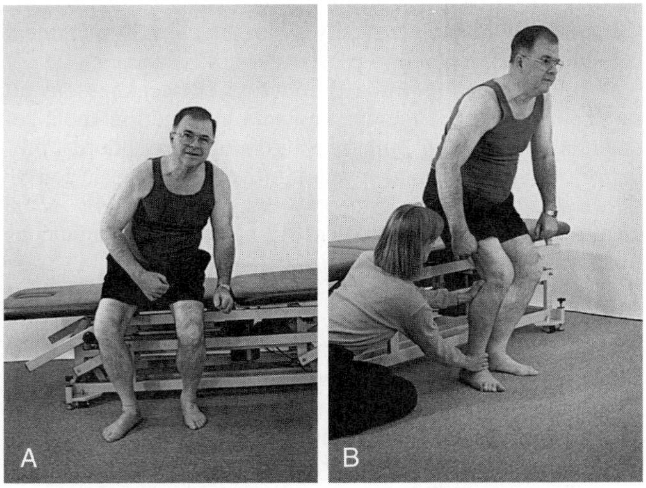

Figure 23-6 ■ **A,** Client with right hemiplegia moving from sitting to standing. Note the tendency to use the left leg more than the right, the left rotation of the upper body, and the position of the right arm. **B,** Therapist uses her hands to stabilize the lower leg and to assist lower-leg movements as the client initiates sit to stand. Note the change in upper-body position and the decrease in arm posturing.

forward to assist with task but cannot reach arm forward to place it on table.

Step 2. *Clinical judgment or hypothesis 1:* Weakness of scapula and humeral external rotators prevents antigravity use of elbow extensors during forward reach. Supination of forearm comes from strong proximal initiation and use of elbow flexors to lift arm. *Clinical judgment or hypothesis 2:* Forearm, wrist, and hand position prevents distal initiation and biases shoulder in internal rotation, thus blocking use of elbow extensors.

Step 3. *Test hypothesis 1:* Therapist uses her or his hands to externally rotate the humerus to neutral and asks client to reach again. *Result:* Client activates elbow extension halfway through range with shoulder forward flexion and places wrist and hand on table. *Clinical intervention implication:* Increased control of humeral external rotation and increased control of accompanying scapular pattern are important intervention goals to regain forward reach of arm. Retrain trunk, scapular, and humeral movement patterns, with emphasis on shoulder external rotation and scapular upward rotation. Assess secondary impairments of pectoral and rotator cuff tightness (rotator cuff is shortened if scapula is in an abducted position). *If result is unchanged, test hypothesis 2:* Therapist supports wrist and hand with wrist splint or with his or her hand and asks client to reach again. *Result:* Client activates elbow extension and places the wrist and hand on the table. *Clinical intervention implication:* Prevention or blocking of wrist flexion limits the degrees of freedom, changes the internal rotation moment on the distal portion of the lever arm, and allows use of existing elbow extensors. Use small wrist splint during independent practice or use object to assist or preset distal segment during practice.

Tone

The evaluation of extremity tone, sometimes referred to as *spasticity,* continues to be an integral part of poststroke movement research and is part of the physician's neurological examination. Over the years, leading physiologists have split into two camps over the definition of tone. During the beginning of the 20th century, tone was thought of as postural reflexes. In the 1950s the concept of tone was thought of as a state of light excitation or a state of preparedness.[96] Granit[97] later encouraged us to think of the relatedness of both these views. He believed that the same spinal organization is mobilized by the basal ganglia to produce both manifestations of tone: a state of preparedness and the postural reflexes.[97] In the 1980s, scientists challenged the concept that what led to a spastic movement pattern was hypertonicity resulting from an exaggerated stretch reflex.[98,99] A new construct emerged in the following years that acknowledged the contribution of both neural and nonneural elements to the phenomenon of "spasticity." This newer concept of spasticity explains why the stretch reflex or tendon tap response (performed in a passive condition—during rest) is an "epiphenomenon and is not the cause of the "spastic movement problem" that interferes with movement."[100] Although the Modified Ashworth Scale is an objective measure of spasticity caused by the stretch reflex,[101] it is not a measure of the functional problem that interferes with skilled movement. It is heartening to hear such discussions occurring among physiologists because therapists are also questioned about their notations of and changes in tone and they often have no objectively derived standard clinical system for measurement. The debate over tone continues, but clients with CNS dysfunction clinically display changes of muscle tone that result in longer rehabilitation stays and problematic secondary impairments.[102]

The response of a spastic muscle to stretch differs during passive and active movements, leading some to question the usefulness of the classic numerical test of spasticity, the Ashworth Scale. The Ashworth Scale rates the severity of tone from 1 to 5.[103]

The first noticeable change in tone is the change from the premorbid state. Clients in the acute phase of hemiplegia exhibit, for varying periods of time, a lower than normal tonal state. Clients with paralysis of the extremities exhibit low tone or hypotonicity. The extremities feel like "dead weight" as the therapist moves them. As neuromuscular return slowly begins, the extremities feel heavy, but some "following" of passive movement patterns is detected.

As the client becomes more active, he or she uses all available movement patterns. Ryerson and Levit have described three specific situations, which in reality have overlap, wherein tone increases (see page 23 for a detailed discussion).[54] This increased tone, or clinical hypertonicity, occurs in the arm and leg if the client's trunk control is less than the demand of the task, if altered joint alignment increases the tension of the muscle, or if the voluntary movement pattern of the extremity is unbalanced and disorganized.[54,104]

One clinical description of increased extremity tone put forth in the 1970s is still somewhat useful today: severe hypertonicity makes coordinated movements impossible; moderate hypertonicity allows movements that are characterized by great effort, slow velocity, and abnormal coordination; slight hypertonicity allows gross movement patterns to occur with smooth coordination, but combined, selective movement patterns are uncoordinated or impossible.[105]

Equilibrium and Protective Reactions

Equilibrium reactions help us to maintain or regain balance by keeping the center of gravity within the base of support. Equilibrium reactions are often referred to as the body's "first line of defense" against falling. They occur when the body has a chance of winning the battle against gravity. If equilibrium reactions cannot preserve balance, the second line of defense emerges: protective reactions. One of the best known protective responses in the arm is the "parachute reaction." Protective responses in the leg in standing positions include hopping and stepping.

When assessing equilibrium or balance reactions in clients with hemiplegia, the therapist remembers the distinction between equilibrium reactions and protective reactions. Equilibrium reactions should be assessed while slowly moving either the limb or trunk away from the base of support. The amount of control in the trunk and supporting limb, the size of the base of support, and the available range of motion as well as the evaluator's handling skills affect the response (see Chapter 22).

Descriptive Analysis of Functional Activities

When evaluating functional activities, the therapist assesses three phases of the movement pattern. The first phase is the *initiation* of the act, which includes the body segment initiating the movement, the direction of movement, and the establishment of antigravity control. *Transition,* the second phase, represents the point in the functional activity at which there is a switch in the muscle groups that provide antigravity control. The third phase is the *completion* of the activity, involving a final weight shift and the ability to maintain postural control.[54]

If assistive devices are used, the following questions should be asked: Is the device always used? If not, when is it used? How is the device used? Could the device be used another way that would foster trunk symmetry and allow activity of the affected extremities?

Evaluation of Secondary Impairments

Loss of Joint Range and Muscle Shortening

In hemiplegia, loss of joint range is caused by muscle shortening from poor alignment that is the result of weakness or muscle activation problems. Loss of alignment occurs early in recovery, whereas muscle shortening and loss of range occur over time. When measuring joint range of motion and muscle shortening, the therapist must remember to consider the functional consequences of two-joint (multijoint) muscle tightness.

Example 1. In sitting (knee bent), the client has ankle joint dorsiflexion range from 0 to 10 degrees; but in standing (knee and hip straight), ankle joint dorsiflexion range is −20 degrees. This functional loss of ankle range causes significant problems for standing and walking. Loss of ankle joint range in standing may be the result of gastrocnemius and soleus, tensor fasciae latae, or hamstring muscle tightness (Figure 23-7).

Range-of-motion measurements should be documented in terms of functional position. Extremity muscles that cross multiple joints are the most common groups to shorten and limit joint range in hemiplegia. Muscle shifting (changes in the resting position of muscle bellies and tendons) occurs with prolonged changes in alignment and loss of joint range.

Example 2. Long-standing wrist flexion may cause the ulnar wrist extensor to slip volarly and function as a wrist flexor. Similarly, a position of knee flexion with ankle plantarflexion and subtalar varus may lead to lateral shifting of the anterior tibial muscle belly. As the muscle shifts laterally, the tension increases distally and foot supination becomes more pronounced.

Pain

Two commonly used standardized pain measurement scales are the visual analog pain rating scale and the McGill Pain Questionnaire.[106,107] These scales focus primarily on the intensity of pain but provide an objective measure of intervention effectiveness. For an in-depth discussion of the topic of pain management, see Chapter 32.

The presence of pain in hemiplegia is devastating for the client and makes movement reeducation difficult. Shoulder pain is the most frequent pain complaint after stroke.[11,108] Pain must be evaluated specifically and should not be allowed to occur during intervention; the "no pain, no gain" message that is sometimes used in sports or orthopedic intervention should not be used in neurorehabilitation. Pain is an indicator that joint alignment or movements are incorrect. See Box 23-3 for general questions.

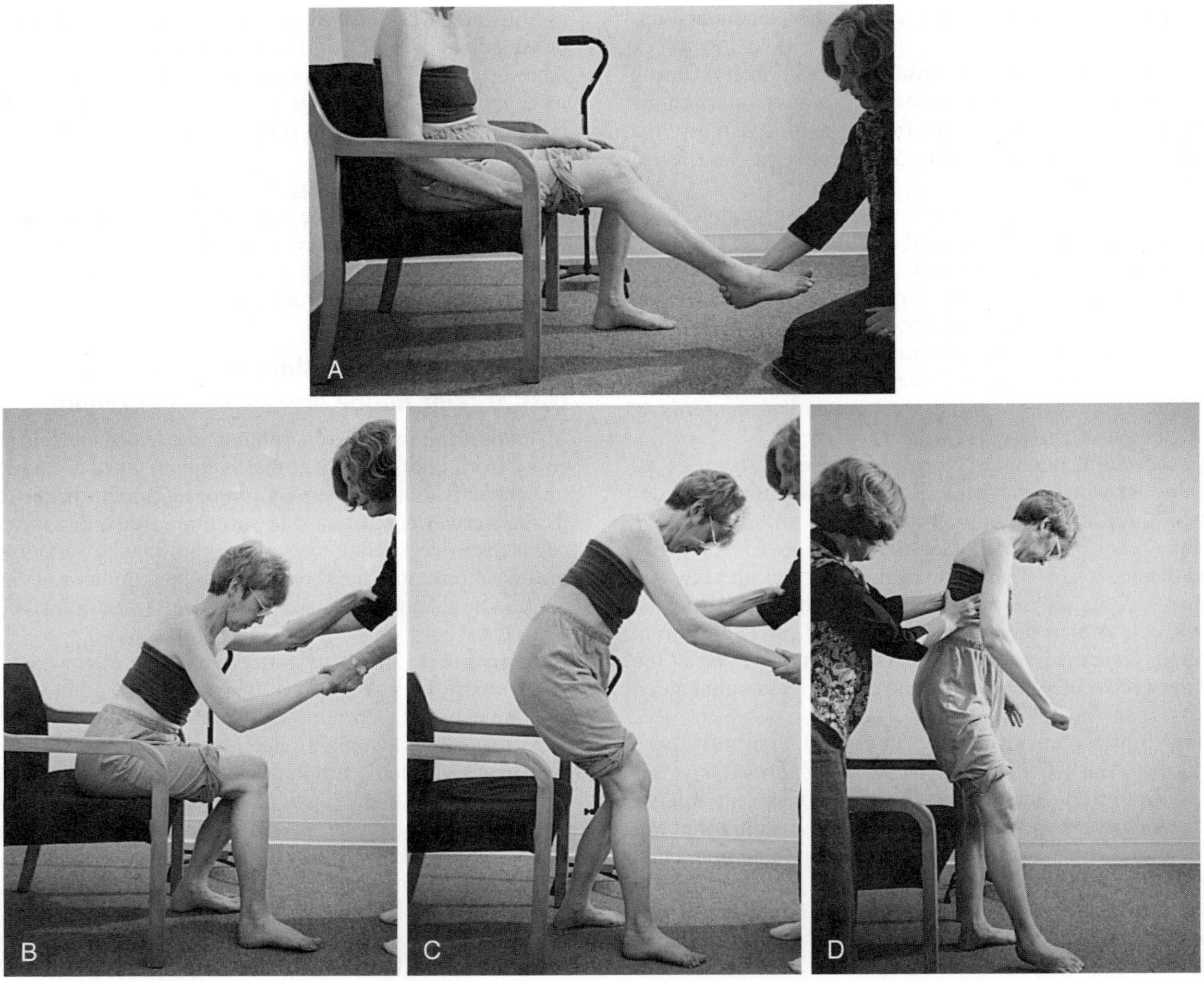

Figure 23-7 ■ **A,** Client with right hemiplegia with limited range in hamstring, tensor fasciae latae, and gastrocnemius and soleus muscles. **B,** Client has sufficient range at ankle to keep foot on the floor in sitting and as she initiates the rise to standing. **C,** As she stands and reaches the limit of range of these two muscle groups, her body compensates. The pelvis rotates right, and the tight medial hamstring adducts and internally rotates the femur and pulls the knee into extension as its medial insertion becomes more anterior to the joint. **D,** As the knee extends more, the calcaneus moves into equinus and varus. The foot supinates as a result of calcaneal varus and external tibial rotation from the tight tensor fasciae latae.

Motor Evaluation Forms

The foregoing information, once gathered, can be placed on an evaluation form in many ways. Every medical institution seems to have its own evaluation form and its own system of recording data. Active movement at the shoulder joint may be described in one institution in terms of percentages of synergistic stages, at another institution by a narrative of degrees and planes of movement, and at still another by functional outcomes of shoulder movement. At one hospital the documentation of pain may be descriptive, and at another it may be numerical. It is important to keep in mind the substance of the evaluative material, not the form in which it is described. A detailed motor evaluation form is necessary for the establishment of realistic goals and for subsequent treatment planning, but the specific form depends both on the needs of the specific clinical setting and on the clinician's choice.

BOX 23-3 ■ QUESTIONS FOR SUBJECTIVE EVALUATION OF PAIN

Location: Where is the pain? Pinpoint the location.

Type: What does it feel like?

- Pins and needles
- Sharp and stabbing
- Aching
- Dull
- Pulling

Occurrence: When does the pain occur?

- At rest
- During movement
    - Range-of-motion exercises
    - Weight-bearing exercises
    - A specific part of the movement

Recognizing Needs

The information obtained from the total evaluation provides the basis for answers to the following questions:

- What activities are possible?
- What activities are not possible?
- How do the movement impairments and secondary impairments relate to activity performance?

By understanding the impairments and their relationship to activity limitations, the therapist can answer the following question: What significant movement components are missing? The answer to this question becomes a hypothesis for intervention planning. How the possible is accomplished and why the impossible exists provide logical suggestions for selection of intervention techniques.

Therapy intervention occurs at either the level of activity limitation or the level of movement-related primary and secondary impairments. The process of establishing goals and selecting activities for intervention begins with clinical decision making or problem solving.

CLINICAL DECISION MAKING AND PROBLEM SOLVING

Problem solving is a process of gathering and analyzing evaluation information from movement analysis, organizing and reflecting on this information to develop hypotheses for causal relationships between activity limitations and significant impairments, and establishing and prioritizing goals for therapeutic intervention. The problem-solving process is also used to hypothesize how the movement problems of the trunk, arm, and leg are interrelated and how these problems relate to the ability to perform tasks. Movement control deficits, secondary impairments, and compensatory or atypical movement patterns should be identified in relation to each significant activity limitation.

Analyzing Evaluation Material

The relationship between activity performance and primary and secondary impairments in stroke has not been researched. Therefore, this relationship, which is the basis for therapy intervention, must be derived from clinical experience and judgment. Clinical reflection guides the evaluation process—what should be evaluated and how. As a result of the evaluation, the therapist has a list of functional skills that are difficult or impossible for the client to perform and a list of primary and secondary impairments that relate to the attempted performance of that task. The therapist analyzes this information with the goal of identifying common impairments in categories of tasks: Which primary impairments are major impediments in each task analyzed? Are there secondary impairments that interfere with the client's ability to perform specific critical movement components? What is the level of trunk-extremity control during task performance in each functional position evaluated? While analyzing the evaluation material, the therapist pays attention to all significant factors that limit performance of tasks, including environmental, cognitive, perceptual, and emotional barriers.

Example

A patient after an acute stroke with left hemiplegia cannot perform morning daily care activities at the sink while sitting in a wheelchair, cannot transfer from bed to chair, and cannot rise to stand. Common primary impairments include paralysis or weakness of the left arm and leg, a loss of muscle activation resulting in an inability to coordinate trunk and lower-body movements to allow forward weight shifts in sitting and/or to perform transfers from bed to chair and/or inability to sequence forward arm movements, and impaired proprioception in the extremities. Secondary impairments that begin to appear by the end of the acute recovery phase might include trunk asymmetries (lateral trunk flexion with a left spinal convexity; inferior shoulder subluxation; loss of ankle joint dorsiflexion range; muscle shortening in the pectoralis, wrist flexors, and gastrocnemius; and edema in the hand and foot.

In the rehabilitation phase of care, the primary impairments of weakness and loss of muscle activation pattern (motor control) begin to improve. As the client performs tasks that exceed his or her level of trunk strength and control, clinical hypertonicity in the arm and leg may increase as a strategy for maintaining balance or reinforcing trunk control. Secondary impairments of shoulder pain increase, along with increasing instances and degrees of muscle tightness and continued loss of trunk-extremity alignment.

Developing Hypotheses for Significant Impairments

The process of motor performance evaluation results in a list of activities and related impairments. However, not all these impairments directly relate to each activity limitation of the client. The therapist, using clinical judgment, hypothesizes a causal relationship between frequently occurring impairments and activity limitation. These impairments, called *significant impairments,* are the ones that must be changed for measurable changes in movement and function to occur.[54] The other impairments are not forgotten but are reevaluated later as improvement begins and new activity goals are chosen. The significant impairments are often used as the focus of short- and long-term goals because they are the underlying building blocks of the selected activity goal. Because functional movement depends on the linkage of trunk and extremity movements, the therapist develops hypotheses between impairments in the extremities and specific levels of trunk control to set goals that result in improved activity performance. If weakness and control deficits of the trunk, arm, and leg are treated separately, the client may see improvement in the impairments but not see a change in function (Box 23-4). (See Chapters 4 and 9 for further discussion.)

Goal Setting

Once the therapist reviews the desired functional goal and identifies the underlying significant impairments, the intervention plan is created and discussed with the client.

Functional Goals

Functional goals are based on the needs and desires of the client and on the functional impairments that were identified by the therapist during the initial assessment. Functional goals should represent a significant change in the patient's level of independence, be practical, and reflect improvement in a specific activity limitation. They state the desired function and the expected level of performance.[54]

BOX 23-4 ■ MOVEMENT COMPONENT CONTROL MODEL OF POSTURAL CONTROL

Postural tone and stability
Trunk control
- Level I: Basic movement components
  - Upper-body– and lower-body–initiated movement
    - Anterior
    - Posterior
    - Lateral
- Level II: Coordinated trunk and extremity patterns
- Level III: Power production

Equilibrium and protection

Example. Client will stand independently and safely while performing self-care activities at the bathroom sink.

Long-Term Goals

A long-term goal should reflect a major improvement in a primary or secondary impairment or an increase in level of performance of an existing skill. The accomplishment of a long-term goal brings the client closer to the functional goal. The time it takes to accomplish a long-term goal varies tremendously depending on the frequency of treatment and the length of time after stroke. The therapist may set many short-term goals to achieve one long-term goal. Long-term goals may be stated in functional terms, but they usually reflect a change in a primary impairment: an increase in strength, movement control, or balance.[54]

Examples

Functional Goal. Client will be able to perform meal preparation activities in the kitchen safely (while standing).

Long-Term Goals

1. Client will perform upper-body–initiated movement (lateral and rotational) while standing, supporting hips against a kitchen counter.
2. Client will safely stand near the kitchen counter and maintain balance during far-reach movements of the uninvolved arm.

Short-Term Goals

A realistic short-term goal should be achievable quickly and should be based on the result of the patient's response to handling during the evaluation of movement. Short-term goals should directly relate to the accomplishment of the long-term goal. There are multiple short-term goals that relate to one long-term goal. Short-term goals are compiled from the list of relevant secondary impairments or desired increases of strength or movement control. These goals are measurable but do not in and of themselves result in a functional change.[54]

When stated in terms of movement control rather than functional performance, these goals include the reestablishment of generalized movement patterns that link movement patterns of the trunk and extremities (Box 23-5).

Example. Decrease tight hamstring and gastrocnemius muscles in standing position to allow the foot to remain flat on the floor during assisted and independent upper-body movements while standing (e.g., forward reach beyond arm's length).

BOX 23-5 ■ COMPONENT GOALS IN FUNCTIONAL TRAINING

Component goal (power): Restore strength in trunk and extremity patterns (individual muscles, components, sequences)
Component goal (structure): Minimize or eliminate secondary impairments
Component goal (control): Reeducate patterns of control (sequencing and timing)

Choosing Intervention Techniques

Once the problem-solving process of goal setting is finished, therapists can select specific intervention techniques and activities. Therapists have many techniques to choose from to meet their goals. After a stroke, most clients will not fully regain normal movement patterns regardless of the type of intervention they receive.

Controversy exists as to the means of increasing functional mobility and performance in clients who have had a stroke. One school of thought teaches compensatory patterns or hopes for some use of the affected side through task-specific practice without direct intervention for the neurological impairments. The other prevalent practice pattern is to increase functional movement patterns on the affected side to help achieve an activity goal by increasing control and strength of movement sequences of the trunk and limb through specific levels of reeducation.[54,109-111]

A combination of these two practices may be useful: impairment-based intervention strategies to reeducate movement and training strategies to foster desirable compensations—a functional reeducation strategy. This type of intervention includes strengthening trunk and extremity linked patterns of movement, minimizing or eliminating secondary impairments that interfere with regaining control, teaching appropriate compensations, and training the client to practice functional movement patterns in the context of daily tasks[54,112] (Box 23-6). Research findings support a link between the trunk and upper extremity and the trunk and lower extremity during reaching activities.[113,114] One result of this research has been to design treatment interventions that restrain trunk movements during forward reach retraining to increase control of elbow extension movement in the paretic arm.[115,116]

For reeducation to be effective, therapists must allow the patient to initiate the active trunk and extremity pattern,

BOX 23-6 ■ REEDUCATION STRATEGY FOR INTERVENTION

Reeducating basic trunk movement components
Linking coordinated trunk and extremity patterns
- Weight bearing
- Movements in space

Preventing, minimizing, eliminating secondary impairments
Teaching appropriate compensations
Teaching independent practice routines

must move from assisted practice to independent practice with the assistance of appropriately selected objects or verbal cues, and must teach the patient appropriately staged practice patterns. Studies based on the "learned nonuse" phenomenon described by Taub have shown that when patients are encouraged to use the affected arm rather than receiving pessimistic messages about its potential, movement and functional use, even if limited, are possible.[117,118]

Regardless of intervention type used, task-performance practice or a reeducation strategy, there comes a time in the recovery process when therapists help the client select practical compensatory strategies. Compensatory strategies are taught when the client needs to function independently and cannot yet use the affected arm because of insufficient recovery or the severity of damage. To be appropriate, the strategy should incorporate the use of the involved extremities and use appropriate trunk movement patterns to maximize future return of movement. Undesirable compensations are patterns that are so asymmetrical that they fail to incorporate available movements of the affected trunk and extremities (Figure 23-8).

Although current literature generally applauds function-based techniques, therapists in clinical settings use hands-on approaches to increase muscle strength and control and to decrease impairments that block the emergence of new functional patterns.[54] As research in movement science and recovery of movement increases, therapists must critically analyze research findings and judiciously integrate them with their clinical experience and judgment.

COMMON IMPAIRMENTS AND INTERVENTION SUGGESTIONS

Weakness and Loss of Control

Diminished muscle strength, either paralysis or weakness, is an important category of impairment in hemiplegia. A paralyzed muscle is unable to contract to produce enough force for movement. A weak muscle contracts insufficiently for joint or body segment movement or to allow functional performance.[90-92] In a client who has sustained a severe, acute stroke, the paralysis or weakness affects the majority of muscles and results in a loss of functional movement in the face, trunk, arm, and leg. In clients who have had less severe strokes, some muscle groups are weak and produce movement, whereas other muscles are paralyzed and cannot be activated.[119]

Weakness from stroke differs from generalized weakness and orthopedic weakness: it involves one entire side of the body and includes the trunk and extremities. After a stroke, the trunk, perhaps because of its bilateral cortical innervation, does not display the degree of weakness found in the extremities. As a result of differences in testing methods,

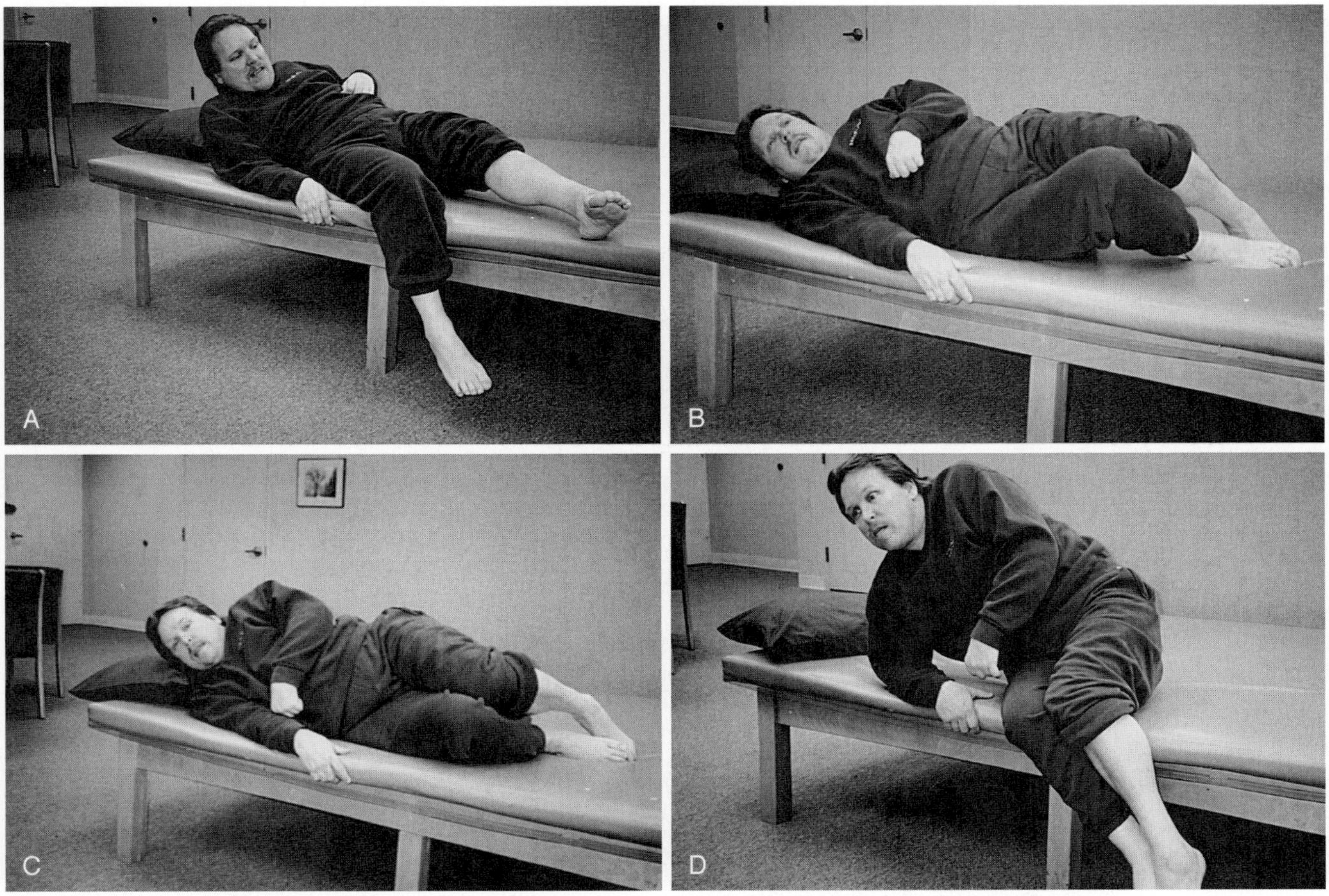

Figure 23-8 ■ **A,** Client with left hemiplegia using his right side to move to sitting and not incorporating movement of the left side—an undesirable compensation. **B** to **D,** Client moving to sitting while using as much control as possible on the left side to assist the movement to sitting.

position, and design, there is no consensus on the degree of trunk muscle weakness after a stroke: some research findings indicate a loss of lateral paretic-side trunk strength,[120] others report no significant difference in lateral trunk strength,[121,122] and others find slight weakness in the trunk extensors.[123,124] However, it is clear that weakness in the extremities interferes with functional use in either weight bearing or movement in space.[54,125]

Model of Postural Control

Trunk control allows the body to remain upright, to adjust to weight shift, to control movements against the constant pull of gravity, and to change and control body position for balance and function. Therapy based on neurophysiological models stressed facilitation of trunk rotation to gain trunk control. Newer clinical models of postural and trunk control began appearing around 1990.[104,126,127] Information from motor control science has resulted in revision of therapists' thoughts on trunk control.[128-130]

In a movement component model of postural control, trunk control has levels of increasing difficulty[131] (see Box 23-4). Trunk control not only helps us remain upright but also allows weight transfer to free an arm or leg for function. For some functional movements, such as sitting, trunk control keeps the upper and lower trunk stable during weight shifting and balance. For other tasks, such as reaching forward beyond the length of the arm, the upper trunk is stable and adjusts to the lower-body–initiated anterior weight shift.[54]

Additional postural control models, based on a developmental or systems model, are well documented.[105,132-134] Research in the field of postural control shows that the level of trunk control and trunk strength correlates with sitting balance, that extremity function correlates with trunk control, and that loss of trunk strength occurs in all planes.[135-137]

Postural Tone and Stability. Clients with hemiplegia frequently have alterations in both muscle tone and postural tone. *Postural tone* refers to the overall state of tension in the body musculature. Postural tone is tone that is "high" enough to keep the body from collapsing into gravity but "low" enough to allow the body to move against gravity. It is influenced by the input from the corticospinal tracts, the vestibular system, the alpha and gamma systems, and peripheral-tactile and proprioceptive receptors.[138] Normal postural tone allows a constant interplay among the various muscle groups in the body and imparts a constant readiness to move and to react to changes in the environment (internal and external). It provides an ability to adjust automatically and continuously to movements. These adjustments provide the proximal fixation necessary to hold a given posture against gravity while allowing voluntary and selective movements to be superimposed without conscious or excessive effort.

Trunk Control. Trunk control can be divided into levels of increasing complexity. The first level of trunk control is the ability to perform the basic movement components. Trunk strength and control at this level provide a base that allows extremity movement to be combined and used for function. Retraining strength and control of basic trunk movements in the three cardinal planes is a prerequisite for the coordination of trunk and extremity patterns for tasks.

Trunk movements in sitting are initiated from the upper trunk or the lower trunk according to the demands of the task. In standing, functional trunk movements are initiated from the upper trunk (if the head or arm is initiating a task) or the lower extremity. The two initiation patterns result in different spinal patterns, different types of muscular activity, and changes in the distribution of weight[54] (Tables 23-3 and 23-4). These basic movement patterns allow the body to be positioned for functional use.

The second level of trunk control, coordination of trunk and extremity patterns, may best be explained through the concept of anticipatory postural control. Anticipatory control allows the coordinated linkage of trunk and extremity patterns before the activation of extremity movements: it allows us to sit and reach beyond arm's length without falling forward or to step forward with one leg as walking is initiated. Researchers have identified altered anticipatory postural responses in people after stroke in both sitting and standing positions. The pattern of anticipatory responses poststroke appears to be preserved, but the timing of the response is slowed.[139,140]

TABLE 23-3 ■ UPPER-BODY–INITIATED WEIGHT SHIFT PATTERN: SITTING

WEIGHT SHIFT	SPINAL PATTERN	MUSCLE ACTIVITY
Anterior movement—reach down to floor	Flexes	Eccentric extensor activity
Posterior—to sit back up	Extends	Concentric extensor activity
Lateral—reach sideways and down to right	Laterally flexes with concavity on right	Eccentric lateral activity on left
Lateral—comes back up to middle	Spine moves back to neutral	Concentric lateral activity on left

TABLE 23-4 ■ LOWER-BODY–INITIATED WEIGHT SHIFT PATTERN: SITTING

WEIGHT SHIFT	SPINAL PATTERN	MUSCLE ACTIVITY
Posterior weight shift	Flexion	Concentric flexor activity
Anterior weight shift	Extension	Concentric extension activity
Lateral weight shift to right	Lateral flexion—convexity to right	Eccentric lateral activity on right Concentric lateral activity on left

This level of trunk control allows the trunk to remain stable yet adapt to movement of the arms and legs. There are two different ways this happens: trunk movements occur as postural adjustments to extremity movement around midline, or trunk movements can precede voluntary movements to help extend the reach of the extremities. These coordinated movements can occur in supine, sitting, or standing positions as demonstrated in the following three examples.

1. While sitting, the client reaches down or sideways to the floor to pick up an object. As the arm reaches down, the upper body initiates the anterior weight shift. To extend the reach of the arm, the lower body provides stability yet adjusts and adapts.
2. When the client lifts up a leg to tie a shoe, the lower body initiates a posterior weight shift. The upper body adjusts to the weight shift and to the demands of the arm and hand as they tie the shoe.
3. In standing, upper-trunk movements occur as postural adjustments as the legs initiate both the stance phase (forward weight shift) and swing phase (stepping) of walking.

The third level of trunk control allows strength and stability for power production from the arm or leg. The movement and control of the trunk are used to support power production in the extremities for propulsive activities such as stair climbing, jumping, running, throwing, hitting, and rowing.

The entire model is summarized in Box 23-4.

Extremity Weakness

Weakness in the arm and the leg results in ineffective and inefficient functional patterns in daily life. Intervention for weakness in the extremities includes reeducation of movements in space, reeducation of weight-bearing movements, and training of and appropriate initiation and sequencing of movement. Most clients with hemiplegia regain enough control in the leg to stand and walk, but those same patients may not be able to use the arm for any purpose. Today the concept of "learned nonuse" may help therapists understand why the discrepancy between arm and leg recovery exists. Wolf and colleagues[118] conclude from studies of hemiplegic patients that learned nonuse does exist in some patients who have had a stroke and suggest a program of "forced use" training. Although the research training model may not be directly transferable to the clinic, this study points out the benefits of incorporating the use of the affected side in intervention strategies.

Distal reeducation is an important component of early reeducation that has been neglected by therapists because of a previous belief that proximal return comes before distal. Distal reeducation trains the client to be able to initiate movements from the hand or foot, instead of the common proximal initiation patterns seen during attempted reach or stepping (Figure 23-9).

Weight bearing on either the forearm or the extended arm is used as a postural assist during transition activities such as side lying to sitting, or as a means of supporting the weight of the upper trunk in sitting or standing, and is used to stabilize objects during task performance. The activity of accepting weight through the arm is not passive but extremely active and dynamic. Forearm weight bearing in sitting or standing is used to activate trunk movements, to reestablish scapulohumeral rhythm, to maintain range of motion in the arm, or to strengthen movement sequences in the arm. It is not used to inhibit tone (Figure 23-10). The muscles of the arm are linked with trunk weight shifts during active weight bearing.[54] Table 23-5 presents the linked trunk and arm muscle activity during active weight bearing for one functional task.

The ability to support body weight on both legs for stability and movement control is important in sitting, standing, and walking retraining. Movements of the trunk in sitting and standing occur with constant changes of muscle activity in the legs as part of the base of support, to adjust to demands of weight shifts, and to increase activity levels of leg muscles to initiate standing weight shifts. Loss of control of weight bearing on both legs or on one leg has an immediate effect on balance. Problems of weight-bearing control of the leg may exist because of weakness; because of muscle shortening in the pelvis, hip, knee, or ankle; or because of posturing. When the leg cannot actively support body weight, undesirable asymmetrical compensations result. A significant and often overlooked prerequisite for active control of the leg in weight bearing is a stable, aligned upper body. The use of forearm or extended-arm weight bearing in standing provides external stability to the upper body while allowing the therapist to reeducate control of bilateral or unilateral weight-bearing movements in the leg.

Muscle Activation (Motor Control) Deficits

Common muscle activation deficits include improper initiation, the inability to grade timing and force production, and the inability to sequence muscles for task performance.

Improper Initiation

Improper initiation of movement occurs when the client attempts to move the arm or leg in space and substitutes the stronger proximal muscles for weaker distal muscles.[54]

Example 1. If we ask a client to lift a hemiplegic arm and reach forward for an object, she or he often initiates the movement proximally instead of distally with the hand and forearm, using the stronger elevators and abductors instead of the weaker hand and forearm muscles.

This is also seen during walking.

Example 2. The client initiates the swing phase of gait proximally instead of distally with the foot, using the stronger pelvic elevators or rotators instead of the weaker ankle and foot muscles.

Inappropriate Muscle Selection

Inappropriate muscle selection for the task occurs when the client substitutes a strong muscle group for a paralyzed muscle although it is inappropriate for the function.

Example. When the hamstrings are weak, the client may use the quadriceps to lift the leg up a step. This results in strong overshifting in the trunk and makes balance precarious.

Inappropriate Sequencing

Inappropriate sequencing includes improper initiation and excessive co-contraction. Excessive co-contraction occurs when the client activates too many muscles either at the same time or out of sequence for the task.

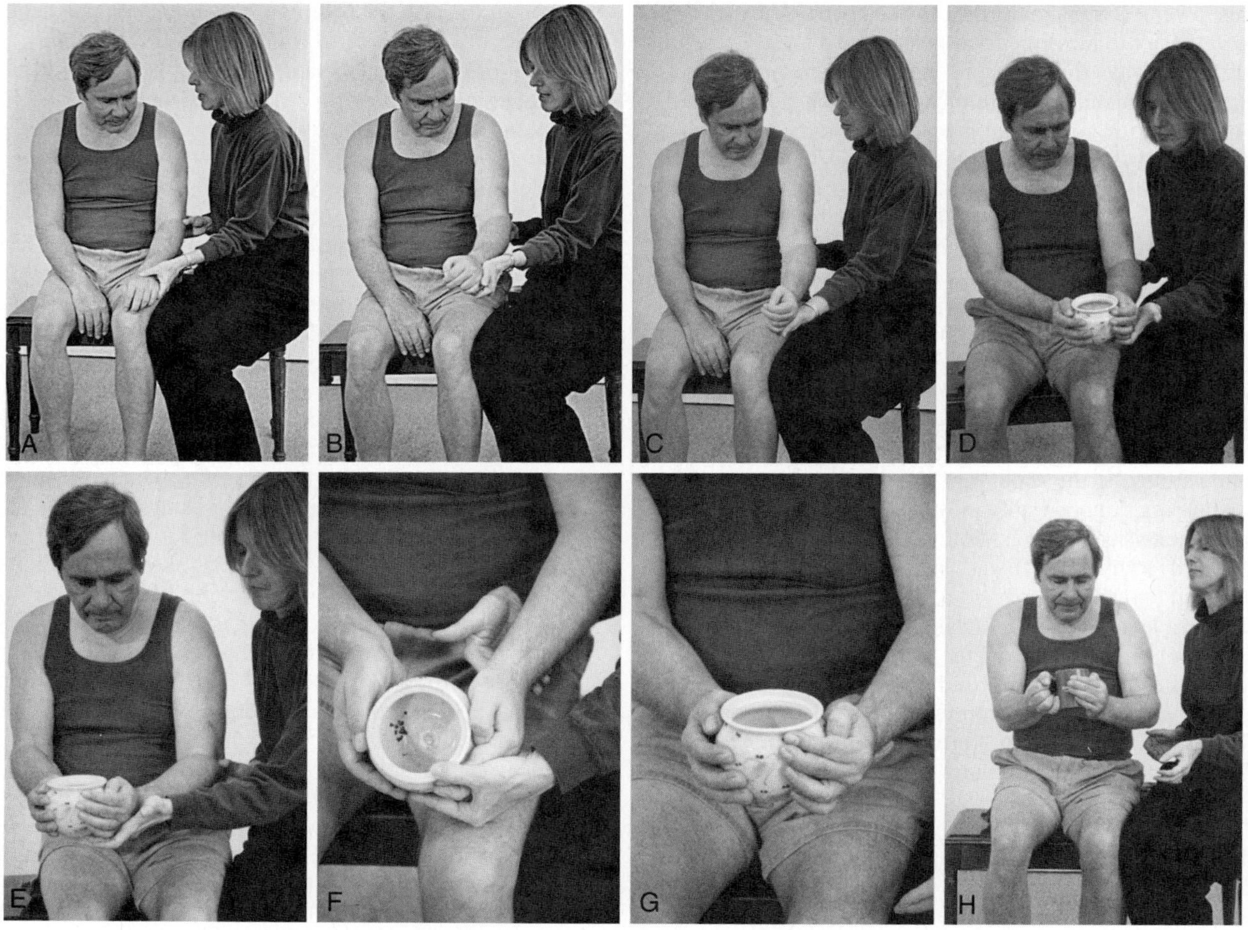

Figure 23-9 ■ **A** to **C,** Client with left hemiplegia. Therapist assists movements of forearm, wrist, and hand as client practices increasing distal arm control. **D** to **F,** Therapist introduces object and assists client as he learns to control the object and the movement. **G,** Independent practice. **H,** Client uses same movements with a similar object.

Excessive Force Production

Excessive force production occurs when the patient activates muscles with inappropriate effort during voluntary movement. When force is excessive, the movement pattern is slow and the extremity feels stiff. Frequently, these muscles easily fatigue and the extremity slowly falls back to the starting position. Therapists often label this movement a "spastic" pattern and intervene with inhibition techniques. However, if this pattern is not from spasticity but from a muscle activation pattern, the intervention should focus on reeducation of control, not inhibition.[54]

Hypotonicity

Hypotonic muscles offer no resistance to passive movement and are clinically associated with paralysis and weakness. Clients who have had a severe stroke may have no visible movement in the extremities; the extremities display no resistance to passive movement and feel heavy. As strength and control in the muscles of the trunk and extremities increase, the hypotonicity lessens. If weakness persists, the secondary impairments of poor joint alignment, muscle and soft tissue tightness, and eventually joint deformity or contracture will be more predominant than problems of spasticity.

Spasticity

There is considerable debate in the academic and clinical therapy community over the clinical relevance of spasticity and the need to address it in treatment.[90,141] Characteristics of a spastic muscle include increased velocity-dependent resistance to stretch, a clasp-knife phenomenon, and hyperactive tendon responses. It is important to remember that spasticity is the increased tension in a muscle when it is passively stretched. The type of high tone that occurs with active, voluntary movement is a different phenomenon: it is the result of both neural and nonneural changes in the muscle. As described earlier in this chapter, Dietz[100] recommended that we assign different names to these two different phenomena of increased tone: he suggested "spasticity" and "spastic movement disorder." Clinicians realize that although movement interventions may not change spasticity, if the "spastic movement disorder" is left untreated the task of muscle reeducation becomes more difficult. Additional, secondary problems such as joint dysfunction, pain, and undesirable compensatory movements may result. I suggest renaming Dietz's second category of spastic movement disorder to *clinical hypertonicity*.

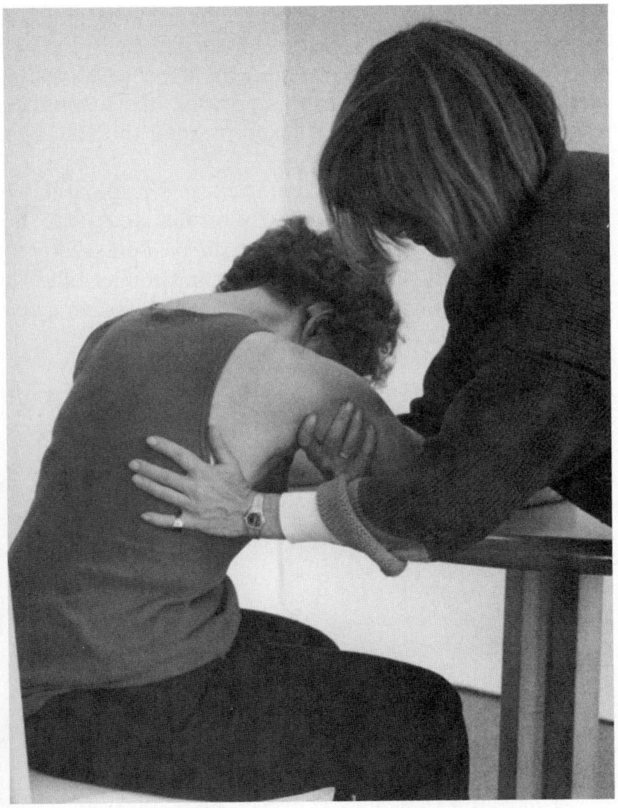

Figure 23-10 ■ Client performs lower-body–initiated posterior movement during forearm weight bearing at a table. The therapist uses her hands to stabilize the humerus, and as the patient moves back, the therapist's left hand slowly stretches or releases tight tissue in the rotator cuff.

TABLE 23-5 ■ TRUNK AND ARM–LINKED MOVEMENTS IN FOREARM WEIGHT BEARING

FUNCTIONAL TASK

Sit at a table with both forearms supported on the table. Keeping both arms on the table, move forward toward the table, and then move body back away from the table.

TRUNK AND ARM LINK	BODY MOVES FORWARD	BODY MOVES BACK
Spine	Extends	Flexes
Scapula	Adducts and depresses	Abducts and elevates
Glenohumeral joint	Less flexion	More flexion
Elbow	Flexes	Extends

Clinical Hypertonicity

Clinical hypertonicity can be separated from spasticity, in part, because clinical hypertonicity responds to movement interventions. Research findings have helped clinicians realize that spasticity is not the *major* problem in hemiplegia. However, for interventions to be successful, it is important to understand the situations in which hypertonicity occurs. At least three different situations result in an increase in clinical hypertonicity: (1) increased tone as a result of proximal instability, either insufficient trunk control for the task or instability of proximal limb musculature (e.g., hip weakness), (2) increased tension on a two-joint muscle caused by poor joint alignment and the resultant shortening or shifting of muscles, and (3) increased tone that is voluntarily produced during attempts at active movement, especially in the extremities.[54]

These situations are divided into three groups for ease of description, but, in reality, overlap occurs between groups. *Insufficient postural stability and control* in the trunk is the first explanation for arm and leg clinical hypertonicity. The extremity patterns of arm flexion or leg extension occur as an atypical balance strategy when the body is unstable.

Example 1. If a client has sufficient trunk control in sitting, the arm and leg display normal resting positions. However, during the rise to stand, the arm postures in flexion. The arm postures most obviously during the transition phase of the stand when the hips are off the surface and the center of gravity of the body is behind the feet, the new base of support.

Treatment of the increased tone, in this case, would not be directed at the arm. Rather, intervention would focus on increasing stability of the upper body during lower-trunk–initiated sit-to-stand patterns and on increasing strength and control of the leg in weight bearing. As the trunk and leg gain more control, the arm posturing decreases (see Figure 23-6).

A second situation in which clinical hypertonicity exists is when muscle tension increases in a two-joint muscle because of changes in alignment of one of the joints.

Example of Second Situation. In sitting, tightness in the gastrocnemius muscle across the knee may not affect the ability to keep the heel on the floor. However, as the client extends the knee, the limit of tightness in the gastrocnemius is reached and the distal end of the tendon shortens and the ankle plantarflexes. When gastrocnemius tightness pulls the calcaneus into equinus, it also moves the calcaneus into varus because of the position of its insertion on the sustentaculum tali. The resultant position, ankle plantarflexion and foot supination, has been labeled a "spastic foot position" (see Figure 23-7).

However, after lengthening of the gastrocnemius across the ankle and knee in standing and correction of the calcaneal position, the patient can stand and keep the foot on the floor.

Example 2 of Second Situation of Clinical Hypertonicity. In an anterior shoulder subluxation, the anterior movement of the humeral head increases tension on the biceps proximally, resulting in elbow flexion. As the tension increases, the forearm begins to supinate. As the humeral head and scapula are repositioned, the tension on the biceps is diminished. If the therapist holds this proximal correction, the elbow and forearm posturing activity stops; the forearm slowly pronates and then the elbow extends.

For the posturing to permanently stop, therapy intervention must help increase strength and control in linked trunk and scapulohumeral patterns to prevent the malalignment.

The third situation, *inappropriate voluntary muscle activation,* occurs when the client is trying to move the arm or leg. The client uses the muscles that have returning strength in the only way he or she knows how. Historically, these patterns were labeled "synergistic or spastic." This label resulted in intervention strategies of inhibition. If these patterns are thought of as unbalanced or inappropriately initiated, or inappropriately sequenced, therapy intervention is more appropriately directed. The abnormally extended or flexed leg movement changes when the patient learns new activation patterns or strengthens weaker muscle sequences. Often, these are "learned" patterns and are difficult to change. Early reeducation should include training in these skills of controlling sequencing, intensity, and duration of firing.

The underlying cause of each of these situations is weakness or loss of control. Therefore, for changes in clinical hypertonicity to last, treatment interventions must address the underlying causes. In each of these situations, the cause is weakness or loss of control of activation patterns.

In this model, generalized inhibition is inappropriate because it does not focus on the underlying cause. Intervention techniques that focus on global inhibition of extremity tone—maximal elongation, vibration, biofeedback, cold, or relaxation—rarely result in a permanent change in the tone. The temporary decrease of clinical hypertonicity that occurs with any of these methods does not by itself directly lead to an increase in function. If used, they must be immediately followed by therapeutic exercise to create a learning environment that improves motor performance.[142,143]

Toe Posturing

There are two patterns of toe posturing: toe clawing and toe curling. Toe clawing, metatarsal hyperextension with phalangeal flexion, is a result of loss of alignment; and toe curling, metatarsal and phalangeal flexion, is a response to instability of the trunk and leg during standing, that is, part of a balance response.[54]

Toe curling and toe clawing interfere with comfort during standing and walking. Problems of blistering on pads of the toes and on the top of the proximal interphalangeal joint and toe pain occur in the intermediate and long-term stage of hemiplegia as the result of the toes rubbing on the tops of the shoes and digging into shoe soles. Relief from pressure and pain on the toe pads (tips) comes with use of commercially available "hammertoe crest pads" available from distributors (e.g., AliMed) or from medical pharmacies.

Loss of Alignment

Muscle weakness or atypical anticipatory control in the trunk leads to atypical alignment patterns in the trunk and shoulder and pelvic girdle. This loss of alignment creates an atypical starting position for functional movement, interferes with muscle activation patterns, and limits weight transfer between extremities. Loss of alignment in the trunk in sitting and standing is analyzed and incorporated into intervention goals to reeducate functional trunk and limb coordinated movements. The commonly described pattern of trunk shortening (lateral flexion with the concavity) on the affected side is only one of the possible alignment problems. More routinely, weakness of the trunk on one side results in a flaring of the rib cage and lateral flexion of the spine with the *convexity on the affected side.* The "appearance" of shortening on the side comes from a number of compensatory adjustments to balance or as a result of the heavy weight of a weak arm. Often therapists confuse the lower contour of the shoulder on the hemiplegic side with shortening of the trunk and concavity of the spine. The heavy weight of the weak arm pulls the upper quadrant into *excessive forward flexion.* In this position, the scapula elevates and tips forward on a flexed, rotated thoracic spine (Figure 23-11).

Another compensatory pattern is excessive spinal flexion throughout the spine, the convexity on the weak side, and *spinal rotation toward the affected side.* Clients with this asymmetry usually shift weight onto the stronger hip. This pattern viewed from the front or rear gives the appearance of

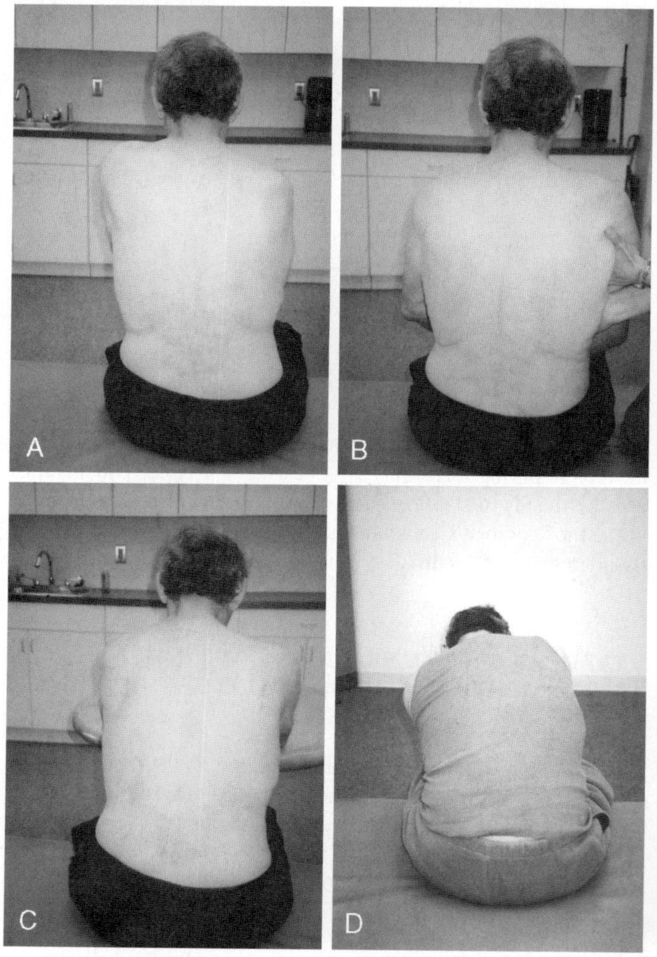

Figure 23-11 ■ **A,** Client with right hemiplegia. Contour of right shoulder appears lower and longer than on the left. Pelvis lists downward on the right. **B,** Therapist lifts the client's upper body up out of forward flexion and corrects the position of the glenohumeral joint. Note that the contour of the right shoulder is now higher and shorter than the left shoulder contour. The trunk is laterally flexed with the convexity on the right. These movement components, convexity of a lateral curve, high shoulder, and low pelvis, are compatible. **C,** Client's arms are supported symmetrically by a table. Note the convexity of the curve on the right and the low pelvis on the right. **D,** Same client moving forward and down with an upper-body anterior weight shift. This position allows the therapist to evaluate the position of the trunk. Note the tendency to avoid weight on the right hip. The trunk is laterally flexed with the convexity on the right, and the right shoulder is higher than the left shoulder.

a low shoulder. This pattern of rotation to the weak side does not occur acutely but develops over time in clients who sit more than they stand or walk.

Lateral translation of the thoracic spine from the hypermobile point of T10 occurs as a means of balancing when trunk weakness results in a lateral curve, with the convexity on the affected side. This asymmetry is common in sitting when the client is encouraged to stand by pushing up with the good arm without putting any weight on the affected leg. It occurs in standing when quad canes or hemiwalkers are used before standing control on both legs is reeducated. The stable external cane acts as a "third stable leg," and the "long, weak" side translates laterally as the unaffected arm pushes down into the cane for stability. This pattern creates a "skinfold" on the affected side that has been confused with shortening of the affected side (see Figures 23-1 and 23-4).

In standing, because the need for leg stability and movement control is much greater than in sitting, the trunk compensates to accommodate the demands of the leg. Often the upper-body and lower-body patterns are opposite one another (i.e., counterrotational). If the leg is in a position of ankle plantarflexion and knee extension, the hip flexes with pelvic rotation toward the affected side. The upper body then counterrotates to provide an equal and opposite balance pattern to allow the client to stand. The opposite may also occur: if the pelvis and hip rotate toward the unaffected side because of learned compensatory swing and/or stance patterns, the upper body rotates toward the affected side to provide a counterrotation for balance (see Figure 23-4).

The atypical alignment pattern in one client may be different in sitting and standing as a result of the pattern of loss of control in the leg. In sitting, the hip is in flexion and provides support, a base, for the upper and lower trunk. Weakness in the knee and lower leg is not as critical to sitting balance and function as it is to standing functions. In standing, the hip demand is one of neutral extension to support the trunk; and complex combinations of knee, ankle, and foot movements are necessary for functional activities.

Shoulder girdle asymmetries are described in the sections on shoulder subluxation, and pelvic girdle and leg asymmetries are described in the sections on standing and walking.

Alignment problems in the distal extremity segments are related to loss of movement control and proximal alignment changes. Patterns in the distal arm and distal leg are strikingly similar. When the midjoint, elbow or knee, is extended, the proximal rotational alignment asymmetry translates down the lower segment into the hand or foot. Shoulder internal rotation translates across an extended elbow, causing the forearm to pronate and the hand to fall into carpal pronation (often confused with ulnar deviation) (Figure 23-12, *A*). Similarly, with knee extension, hip internal rotation asymmetries translate across the knee and cause tibial internal rotation and midfoot pronation. However, as the midjoints gain flexion activity, the proximal pattern no longer dictates distal asymmetries. The distal weight-bearing pattern or active initiation pattern causes a distal rotation that may be opposite to the proximal rotational pattern. When this occurs, the midjoint may posture with a result of incompatible intralimb alignment.

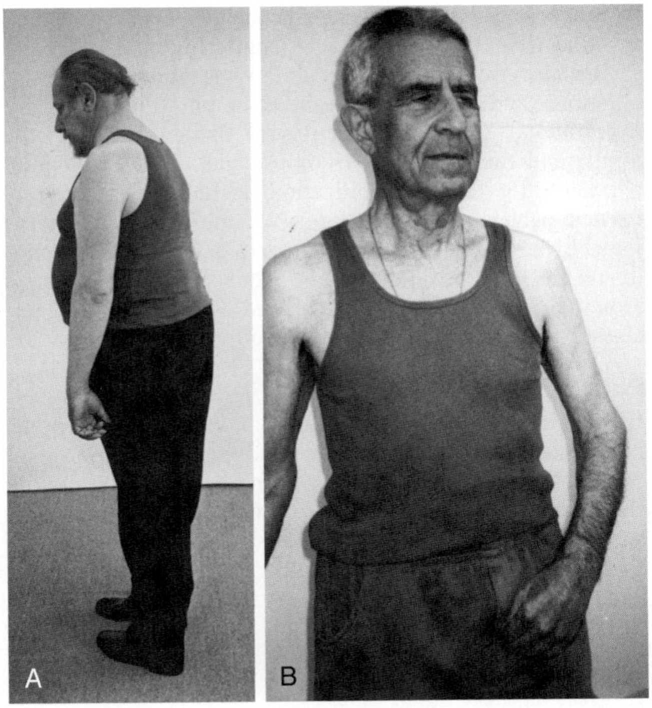

Figure 23-12 ■ **A,** Client with left hemiplegia and severe weakness. The left arm and hand are in shoulder internal rotation, elbow extension, and forearm pronation. The left wrist flexes, and the hand pronates and radially deviates on the wrist. **B,** Client with left hemiplegia with atypical movements. The left arm is positioned in shoulder internal rotation and elbow flexion. As the elbow flexes, the forearm begins to supinate on the internally rotated humerus. The wrist flexes and radially deviates with finger flexion.

Example

A client has a shoulder subluxation resulting in humeral internal rotation. This tendency for internal rotation places tension on the biceps tendon, resulting in beginning elbow flexion and forearm supination. With unbalanced return and weakness of arm muscles, the emerging biceps activity predominates and reinforces a posturing pattern of shoulder internal rotation, elbow flexion with forearm supination (Figure 23-12, *B*).

The weakness pattern of ankle plantarflexion and calcaneal equinovarus biases return in the anterior and posterior tibialis. During movements of the leg in space with hip and knee flexion, this distal supination pattern pulls the tibia into external rotation. To place the supinated foot on the ground, the client compensates proximally by rotating the pelvis and femur, as a unit, toward the unaffected side. This incompatible tibial external rotation and femoral internal rotation result in knee hyperextension.

Muscle and tissue tightness is a common result of alignment problems. Techniques of lengthening muscle and tissue tightness must be balanced with muscle reeducation. Isolated stretching does not result in a lasting improvement in range and may decrease functional ability if not combined with activities designed to increase control. In hemiplegia, slow stretching in functional positions through active weight shifting (i.e., functional stretching) is more effective than "orthopedic" stretching because it reeducates the weakness that underlies the loss of muscle length (Figure 23-13).

Because weakness is the underlying cause of loss of alignment and joint range, in the acute phase the *joints are hypermobile.* Over time the tissues tighten around some joints, and therapists often confuse that "feel" with joint hypomobility. Joint mobilization techniques are rarely needed because the weakness in hemiplegia renders the joints hypermobile. It is important to avoid excessive mobility in the intricate joints of the hand and foot. Tightness around a joint may indicate the need for lengthening exercises, but the joint almost never requires mobilization.

Pain

In the client with hemiplegia, arm pain can be caused by an imbalance of muscles, improper movement patterns, joint dysfunction, improper weight-bearing patterns, and muscle shortening, or it may be related to diminished sensation and sensory interpretation. Although evidence-based approaches should be used to manage shoulder pain after stroke, systematic reviews show that there are few rigorous studies that can be used to guide treatment.[144]

Joint Pain

Joint pain is caused by poor shoulder joint mechanics during movement. Two common alignment problems are loss of scapular and humeral rhythm and insufficient humeral external rotation.[108,145] With a shoulder subluxation, the humeral head is not seated in the fossa and passive movements of the shoulder will not occur with scapulohumeral rhythm. At 60 to 90 degrees of forward flexion, impingement of the capsule will occur and the client will report sharp pain on the superior aspect of the shoulder joint. The pain ceases when the arm is lowered. The subluxation and loss of scapulohumeral rhythm result from loss of trunk and arm movements or muscle tightness from either persistent arm posturing or weakness.

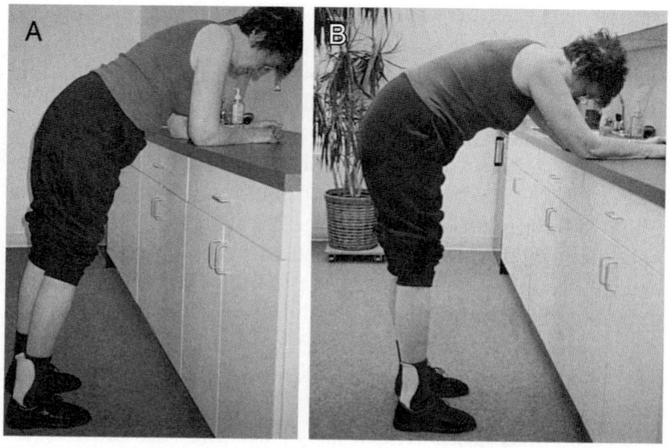

Figure 23-13 ■ **A,** Client with right hemiplegia practicing home program. During standing forearm weight bearing (providing upper-body stability), she initiates a lower-extremity forward-backward movement. As she moves her hips and lower leg forward, she thinks of keeping her knee straight and stretching her calf. **B,** As she moves her hips backward, she may feel a stretch in the back of her thigh, on the lateral aspect of her trunk, or under her axilla.

If the client reports joint pain, the therapist should lower the humerus immediately, reestablish the mobility of the scapula, reseat the humerus if necessary, and maintain appropriate humeral rotation while moving the arm up again. Trunk movements in forearm weight bearing are used to teach a self-ranging practice routine that ensures scapulohumeral rhythm.

Muscle and Tendon Pain

When a shortened or posturing muscle is stretched too quickly or beyond available length, a strong "pulling" type of pain is often reported in the region of the muscle belly being stretched. If the amount of stretch is decreased a few degrees, the reported pain subsides.

If the inappropriate stretching is not stopped, muscle pain progresses to tendon pain. Proximal biceps tendonitis, distal biceps tendonitis radiating into the forearm, and wrist flexor tendonitis are most common. The usual cause of tendonitis is improper weight bearing, with an inactive trunk and "hanging" on the arm with forced elbow extension and shoulder internal rotation. The treatment of tendonitis is rest and modalities (i.e., heat, ultrasound, or electrical stimulation) or injection of corticosteroids. When movement reeducation is restarted, it is important to avoid the "exercise" that caused the pain and to create a new intervention plan.

Complex Regional Pain Syndrome—Shoulder-Hand Syndrome

One type of complex regional pain occurs in the shoulder and hand. It begins with tenderness and swelling of the hand and diffuse aching pain from altered sensitivity in the shoulder and entire arm.[146] This pain interferes with the reeducation of movement patterns and causes a general desire on the part of the client to "protect" the arm by not moving it. Limited shoulder, wrist, and finger range of motion soon occurs.

The second stage includes further loss of shoulder and hand range of motion, severe edema, and loss of skin elasticity. This is followed by the third stage, which includes demineralization of bone, severe soft tissue deformity, and joint contracture.[146,147]

Not every edematous hemiplegic hand leads to shoulder-hand complex regional pain syndrome. Hand edema results from an upper extremity that remains dependent and that does not move for long periods of time. It is essential to teach the person with hemiplegia how to properly care for the hand and to give the responsibility for the care of the hand and arm to the client.

Ryerson and Levit[54] propose five steps for intervention for severe or chronic arm pain: (1) eliminate pain from intervention or the home program, (2) desensitize the arm and hand to touch, (3) eliminate hand edema, (4) introduce pain-free arm movements by reestablishing scapular mobility, and (5) beginning with guided arm movements below 60 degrees, gradually increase the variety and complexity of arm movements.

Edema

Edema in the hand and foot is another common secondary impairment that develops as a consequence of loss of movement control and hospitalization factors such as intravenous infiltrates and limb positioning. Edema limits joint range and tissue mobility. The edematous fluid places the skin on stretch and acts as an interstitial "glue" that bonds the skin, fascial tissue, muscle tissue, and tendons. Hand edema is associated with the development of shoulder-hand syndrome. Foot edema is as common as hand edema, limits ankle joint dorsiflexion range, and is often ignored during intervention programs. Edema begins on the volar surface of the hand and foot, progresses dorsally, and then continues proximally across the wrist or ankle.

Edema interferes with the retraining of functional movement patterns by preventing the smooth glide of tissues. It must be eliminated before active reeducation begins.

Edema has defined stages. When the involved tissue feels soft and fluid, the condition responds to retrograde massage and elevation. When the tissue is gelatinous and pitting, the edematous fluid cannot be physically expressed. At this stage, it begins to adhere to underlying tissues. The edema must be softened and liquefied through transtissue massage. The last stage of edema is characterized by hard, lumpy tissue that does not "pit" in response to manual pressure. This stage of edema requires gentle bilateral compression to break up the hard, solid areas into regions of softness. The soft regions then act as open spaces into which fluid released by massage of hard tissue is directed. The goal is to reverse the process of hardening—from hard, to pitting, to soft and fluid. In the pitting and hard stages, when the edematous tissue is not fluid, elevation, elastic gloves, bandaging, and retrograde massage are not effective. When edematous tissue is soft and fluid, active and active assistive extremity movement patterns produce muscular contractions that assist venous and lymphatic return of the fluid.[54]

Shoulder Subluxation

Shoulder subluxation occurs when any of the biomechanical factors contributing to glenohumeral joint stability are interrupted. In persons with hemiplegia, subluxation is related to a change in the angle of the glenoid fossa occurring because of muscle weakness. In the frontal plane the scapula is normally held at an angle of 40 degrees. When the slope of the glenoid fossa becomes less oblique (and more vertical), the humerus will "slide" down and out of the fossa.[148] Ryerson and Levit[149] first described three types of subluxation in clients with hemiplegia: inferior, anterior, and superior.

Inferior Subluxation

The most common type of subluxation is an inferior subluxation. It occurs in clients with severe weakness and it is present in the acute stage. Weakness and the weight of a heavy arm result in downward rotation of the scapula. Downward rotation orients the glenoid fossa vertically, the unlocking mechanism of the capsule is lost, and the humerus subluxates inferiorly with internal rotation. As the humerus internally rotates, the bicipital tuberosity rolls anteriorly; this anterior prominence is often confused with an anterior subluxation.[54] As subluxation occurs, the shoulder capsule is vulnerable to stretch, especially when the humerus is dependent and resting by the side of the body. In this position the capsule is taut superiorly, so any downward distraction of the humerus will place an immediate stretch on the upper part of the capsule. The coracohumeral ligament reinforces the superior portion of the capsule, which is crucial for shoulder stability. Jenson[150] has discussed the implications of rupture of this ligament as a result of forced abnormal passive motion as a cause of shoulder pain in subluxation.

Anterior Subluxation

Anterior subluxation occurs when the humeral head separates anteriorly from the glenoid fossa. Anterior shoulder subluxation occurs when the downwardly rotated scapula elevates and tilts forward on the rib cage and the humerus hyperextends with internal rotation. In an anterior subluxation, as tension increases on the proximal biceps tendon, the elbow flexes and the forearm supinates. This subluxation is found in clients with atypical patterns of return and trunk rotational asymmetries.[54]

Superior Subluxation

A superior subluxation occurs when the humeral head lodges under the coracoid process in a position of internal rotation and slight abduction. The humeral head is "locked" in this position so that every movement of the humerus is accompanied by scapular movement. The scapular position in this subluxation is one of abduction, elevation, and neutral rotation. The forearm adducts across the body as the humeral abduction and elbow flexion increase. A superior subluxation occurs in clients with inappropriate muscle firing and co-contraction.

Subluxation is not painful but results in changes in muscle length-tension relationships, muscle shortening, and permanent stretch of the joint capsule. If a subluxation exists, the therapist reduces the subluxation by correcting trunk, scapula, and humeral alignment patterns before attempting to reeducate arm movement patterns. A discussion of these subluxations, accompanying trunk movement patterns, and intervention suggestions can be found in therapy literature.[54] As the client learns to move the arm in patterns of functional coordination, subluxation and associated arm posturing decrease.

Prevention of subluxation requires (1) proper assessment of secondary alignment problems (rib cage, scapular, humeral position), (2) early reeducation of trunk and arm linked patterns in sitting and standing, and (3) prevention of shoulder capsule stretch, including support and positioning as the client sits, stands, and practices walking.

FUNCTIONAL ACTIVITIES

Functional mobility movement analysis, intervention techniques, unilateral compensatory strategies, and suggestions for task practice are documented in therapy literature.[151-153] In this section, representative mobility skills are selected in three functional positions: supine, sitting, and standing. For each task selected, the focus is on the basic trunk and extremity control patterns used, significant impairments in addition to weakness that make it difficult for the client to perform the task, and observations from the clinic that relate to intervention and practice. Detailed descriptions of each trunk pattern and trunk and extremity linked pattern can be found in the literature.[54]

Supine

Rolling

Basic trunk movement patterns for rolling include (1) upper-trunk flexion and rotation initiation, (2) lower-trunk extension and rotation initiation, and (3) symmetrical (log-rolling) lateral flexion initiation. These patterns link the trunk with either the arm or leg during the roll.

Trunk and Extremity Linked Patterns. The *upper-trunk flexion-rotation initiation pattern* links upper-trunk flexion-rotation with arm reach across the body. Active assistive patterns, with the client holding both hands together for a bilateral arm reach, are encouraged when strength is insufficient to lift the arm against gravity or, through therapist handling, when arm muscle weakness results in such a heavy feeling that the patient cannot control the extremity with the unaffected hand. If the therapist assists the arm, the goal of practice is for the client to initiate the active antigravity trunk pattern.

A *lower-trunk extension-rotation initiation pattern* is coordinated with either a leg-reach pattern or a flexed-leg "push" pattern. Active assistive patterns can be implemented through therapist handling to help train the sequencing or to grade the firing patterns of the leg when it is pushing into the bed. As the lower body moves from supine toward side lying, the upper body and arm follow the movement. The client is encouraged to practice independently with a focus on the sequence. During independent practice, the therapist may provide verbal cues to help the client time the movement of the upper body.

The *symmetrical lateral flexion initiation pattern* is known as "log rolling." In this pattern, the trunk does not rotate but is active in a coordinated fashion with the arm and leg on the same side; the arm and leg "reach or push" on the leading side. In rolling from supine to side lying, the trunk flexors initiate the antigravity movement, and when rolling from side lying to supine, the trunk flexors are the antigravity movement initiators.

Impairments that Interfere. Shoulder joint pain may occur when the client rolls onto the affected side. Pain occurs if the shoulder is trapped under the trunk as the client moves to side lying or when the humeral-scapular alignment causes the shoulder capsule to be impinged. If pain occurs during the roll, the therapist should teach the client to stop, roll back a few degrees, adjust the position of the arm away from the trunk, and then continue the roll. Therapists should teach their clients how to avoid shoulder pain during all activities, especially during rolling or when lying on the more affected side.

In rehabilitative or outpatient care, muscle tightness in the latissimus, quadratus lumborum, biceps, or tensor fasciae latae may limit trunk rotation or trunk and extremity linked movements.

Clinical Observations. Weakness in the extremities is a significant factor during rolling because the arm and the leg assist the trunk initiation patterns. Rotational patterns are difficult in the acute stage because they require an integration and sequencing of flexor and extensor muscle patterns. Symmetrical rolling may be an easier independent pattern to train. Therapists should incorporate active assistive strategies and extremity strengthening in the early recovery period. Clients have an easier time rolling to the affected side because they use the strength of the unaffected side to initiate the roll. But they may not want to stay on that side because of shoulder pain, instability of the hip, or decreased sensation and the fear that ensues. The client may prefer rolling to the unaffected side because it is easier to rest on, but initiating the movement is difficult because of loss of control on the affected, leading side.

The family is educated to understand the nature of the loss of movement and sensation and the effects of these losses on body awareness and early bed mobility. Family members are encouraged to sit with, visit, talk to, feed, and touch the person from the client's affected side. They are instructed in simple movements such as rolling to promote symmetry, midline control, and activation of trunk and extremity muscles.

Feeding and Swallowing

Although detailed facilitation and inhibition of oral and neck muscle movement for feeding and articulated language are a specialty of speech pathologists, the movement therapist activates upper-body control to prepare for more automatic chew and swallow.

Basic trunk patterns to be reeducated include (1) lower-body anterior and posterior movement control to move toward a table and back into a chair and (2) upper-body anterior and posterior and lateral movement control to provide control for head and arm movements.

Impairments that Interfere

Oral problems include the following:

- Forward head, poor lip closure, loss of saliva and food
- Facial asymmetry during function greater than at rest
- Inability to swallow
- Inability to chew
- Inability to lateralize foods
- Inability to take liquids from cup or spoon
- Muscle weakness

Central problems are as follows:

- Poor postural control
- Inability to feed self

Compensations include the following:

- Use of gravity—head and neck extension
- Chewing on one side only
- Using the hand to place food in the mouth
- Using the hand to pull food from the cheek
- Using thicker food than liquids

Clinical Observations

Excessive drooling occurs with loss of head control and a decreased ability to automatically close the mouth and swallow. If the client tries to lift the head from a flexed position and the cervical spine remains flexed, the head may jut forward into a position of axial extension. As a result of the biomechanics of the forward head position, the jaw opens, automatic swallowing becomes difficult, and saliva runs out of the open mouth.

Drooling from one side of the mouth is annoying and embarrassing. The client may not be able to maintain lip closure and, in addition, may not feel the saliva running out or may not identify a need to swallow. Drooling lessens as upper-body control increases.

In the majority of cases, swallowing problems are transient in persons with hemiplegia. After the initial insult, many clients exhibit a decreased gag reflex. In acute care settings, where liquid diets are often routinely given to persons with hemiplegia, education of hospital staff regarding the merits of using thicker foods should be considered. Thicker, chopped food is easier to swallow than soft food. Soft food is easier to swallow than liquids. Liquids with distinct taste or texture are easier to swallow than water. Specific feeding programs are noted in Chapters 9, 11, and 12.

Sitting

Function in sitting is based on the ability to maintain the trunk in an upright position, to automatically adjust the trunk when the arms or one leg moves around midline, and to follow movements of the arm and leg as they extend their reach. Control in sitting is also used to help change position, such as moving from sitting to standing, or lying down. The reestablishment of control in sitting for function is an important early goal in rehabilitation care.

Basic trunk movement patterns include the following:

1. Anterior, posterior, and lateral upper-body–initiated movements. Upper-body movements are easier to retrain than lower-body movements because the base of support (contact of the buttocks and thighs) remains on the surface.
2. Anterior and posterior lower-body–initiated movements. With lower-body–initiated movement, the upper body needs to be stable yet adjust to and follow the movement of the lower body. The reeducation of upper-body control allows the therapist to begin retraining lower-body control.
3. Lateral lower-body–initiated movements. These movements are more difficult to reeducated than upper-body movements because as the movement begins, the base of support narrows.
4. Rotational movements. In sitting, upper-body rotational movements are easier to perform than lower-body rotational patterns for the reason noted previously.

Trunk and Arm Linked Patterns (Representative Examples)

Postural adjustments to arm movements around midline require the trunk to be upright, to be active, and to perform small adjustments. When the hand functions in front of the body, the trunk adjusts with small posterior weight shifts and increased flexor control, whereas as the hand(s) move to function behind the body, the trunk adjusts with a small anterior weight shift.

The trunk moves with an arm to extend reach. If the reach is forward and down to the floor, as if to reach a shoe, the upper body initiates an anterior weight shift and the spine moves into flexion with control from eccentric contraction of the spinal extensors. If the reach is forward as if to grab an object on the far side of a table, the lower body initiates an anterior weight shift as the upper body remains stable and adjusts to the demands of the arm movement.

Trunk and Leg Linked Patterns (Representative Examples)

Small trunk adjustments occur with leg movements around midline. If the feet move back under the hips, the trunk adjusts with a small amount of anterior weight shift. When one foot is lifted up to slide into a slipper, the lower body adjusts with a small lateral weight shift. Upper-trunk stability allows lower-trunk–initiated patterns when rising to stand. As the legs extend and the buttocks lift off the chair, trunk adjustments accompany the changing leg pattern to control trunk position over the legs.

Impairments that Interfere

Changes in alignment of the arm resulting from weakness and muscle shortening affect the position of the thoracic spine and rib cage. The weight of an extremely weak arm pulls the upper trunk into forward flexion; an increase of flexor tone in the arm influences scapular and rib cage positions.

Shoulder subluxation results in muscle shortening (biceps, pectorals, latissimus, subscapularis), alters the line of muscle pull, and interferes with scapulohumeral rhythm. Muscle shortening contributes to loss of upper-body alignment and interferes with reestablishing arm and trunk control.

Loss of trunk alignment as a result of extremity weakness and loss of trunk control creates an atypical starting position for movement and can become an undesirable compensation.

Clinical Observations

Alignment changes in the arm influence strength and control of the upper body. Therefore intervention techniques to restore alignment and control of the arm in relation to the upper trunk must be included in the list of short-term goals to achieve the functional goal of safe, independent task performance in sitting.

Active control of the pelvis in a neutral position is necessary for the reeducation of lower-body lateral and rotational weight shifts. Pelvic position influences leg position. If the pelvis is held in a posterior tilt, the leg initially tends to abduct; and if it is held in an anterior tilt, the leg initially adducts.

Clients with poor hip control do not regain functional trunk patterns while sitting until they can activate and strengthen hip muscles for stability during weight shifts. Weakness of the hip joint results in a desire to shift weight to the stronger side, thus creating a spinal or pelvic asymmetry. Clients who push to the affected side in sitting need strength from the weak leg for stability as a prerequisite for midline control of the trunk.

Lower-body–initiated lateral weight shift patterns are difficult to train because they require a narrowing of the base of support. Forearm weight-bearing movement patterns are used to increase the base of support to allow practice of these patterns, which are needed for functional activities such as scooting, toileting, and lifting one leg off the surface. This movement is difficult to practice without upper-body stability (external or internal).

Transfers

Transfers in the half-stand, pivot pattern require upper-body control over the lower body and combined trunk and leg control patterns. The squat, pivot position is trained when leg strength and control are weak and the goal is to train the client to use the affected leg. Transfers involve interim patterns that are trained before safe standing is possible.

The client practices transfers to different objects (chair, bed, toilet) to either side. This promotes symmetry, encourages the use of the affected leg, and allows practice with varying environmental constraints. Transfers to the unaffected side have the advantage of being familiar to hospital staff because they are the "traditional" textbook way of transferring the person with hemiplegia. Nevertheless, transfers to the affected side need to be trained by therapists to allow function in either direction.

Sitting to Standing

Moving from sitting to standing is an important skill to retrain early after a stroke because it is used many times a day during functional activities. In a study investigating the relationship between sitting to standing and walking, Chou and colleagues[154] found that a critical component of sitting to standing was vertical force displacement, the amount of weight transferred down into the floor. Those who had a maximal vertical force difference of less than 30% body weight between both legs displayed faster walking speeds and more typical gait parameters.

Two initiation patterns are commonly used, with or without the use of momentum, to train sitting to standing. A *lower-body–initiated* anterior weight transfer occurs with a straight spine as the shoulders move forward. Therapists should emphasize the forward weight shift component of this pattern rather than the anterior pelvic tilt component; the requirement of sitting to standing is a forward shift of the upper body and shoulders. An anterior pelvic tilt usually results in a backward movement of the shoulders. The confusion over this movement occurs because clients often sit in a position of flexion with a posterior pelvic tilt. To come to upright, they must extend the spine and move the pelvis to neutral. Although individuals with a tendency for lumbar extension may have an anterior pelvic tilt as they shift forward, the anterior pelvic tilt is not as important a component as is a forward weight shift.

An *upper-body–initiated* anterior weight transfer during sitting to standing requires control in spinal flexion. This pattern keeps body weight over the feet, the new base of support, but does not link the extension of the legs with the lower trunk. The demand on the trunk from liftoff to standing is greater than in the previous pattern because of the need to move the spine from flexion to upright neutral. In the previous pattern the spine starts and remains in a neutral position through to standing. The upper-body–initiated pattern is used in rehabilitative and extended care centers because it allows caregivers to keep weight firmly over the feet, thus allowing a safe, maximal-assistance transfer.

During transfer and sitting-to-standing training, techniques of directing manual pressure from the top of the knee through the tibia into the foot help the client remember to keep weight on both feet and increase the dorsiflexion movement at the ankle. Full standing should not be attempted if loss of control in the leg results in nonuse. If the client cannot activate leg muscles in a weight-bearing position in attempts to stand, the standing position will be precarious with undesirable trunk compensatory patterns.

Standing

Standing Control

Control in standing is a difficult early goal to achieve because not only is there a need for trunk and leg coordinated movements, but there is also a prerequisite need for upper-body (trunk and arm) control over the lower body. Control of basic movement patterns in standing is divided into upper-body–initiated control patterns and lower-extremity–initiated control patterns.[134] Upper-body control in standing includes the ability to move the upper trunk and arm in all planes with appropriate leg responses and the ability to respond and adjust to weight transfer to each leg and to provide postural stability for movements of each leg in space. Lower-extremity control in standing has a weight-bearing component and a movement in space component. As a prerequisite for reeducation of these movements, the upper body must have enough strength and control to provide stability and postural adjustments for movements of the leg.

Basic trunk movements to be reeducated include the following:

1. Upper-body–initiated anterior, posterior, lateral, and rotational patterns with critical corresponding adjustments in the leg (either hip, knee, or ankle strategies).
2. Control of the upper body over the lower trunk during lower-extremity–initiated weight-bearing movements.
3. Linked trunk and leg patterns during movements of the leg in space. These are easiest when the leg moves around midline and increase in difficulty as movement in space increases in amplitude or speed.
4. Increased upper-body control to support power production of the arms for pushing, pulling, or lifting objects and increased lower-body control to support power production of the legs for jumping, running, and stair climbing.

Trunk and Arm Linked Patterns

Trunk and arm linked patterns include the following:

1. Upper-body–initiated flexion movements that occur with forward and downward arm-reach patterns
2. Upper-body–initiated extension that occurs when the arm reaches up or up and back
3. Upper-body–initiated lateral flexion when the arm reaches down and to one side
4. Upper-body flexion and rotation when the arm reaches down and to one side.
5. Upper-body extension and rotation when the arm reaches up and back to one side

Trunk and Leg Linked Patterns in Weight Bearing

Control of the upper and lower trunk during unilateral stance on either leg is one of the most difficult patterns to retrain. Control of the trunk in unilateral stance is linked with the need for abduction control on the stance leg. In clients with hemiplegia, the complicated control demands for leg and trunk control in standing combined with the presence of weakness and control problems result in loss of alignment in multiple joints and undesirable compensatory patterns.

Trunk and Leg Linked Patterns as the Leg Moves in Space

When the leg moves in space in small ranges, the movement of the upper trunk is small and occurs as a postural adjustment. The movement pattern of the femur and pelvis has a linked rhythm similar to that of scapulohumeral rhythm: the first 30 to 45 degrees of hip flexion occurs with no pelvic movements; from 45 to 90 degrees the pelvis flexes (posteriorly tilts) with the flexing hip; with continued hip flexion the upper trunk flexes. This pelvic-hip relationship occurs in the other planes of movement as well and is seen during the following functional movements:

1. Pelvic and lower trunk flexion occurs when the leg reaches forward and up; stepping up.
2. Pelvic and trunk extension occurs when the leg reaches back.
3. Pelvic elevation or depression with trunk lateral flexion occurs when the leg moves laterally.

Impairments that Interfere

In standing, loss of alignment in the upper body on the hemiplegic side may result in undesirable compensatory patterns that interfere with functional standing movements and balance. These patterns include (1) forward flexion of the upper trunk, (2) upper-body rotation toward the affected side, and (3) upper-body rotation away from the affected side.

Ankle range may decrease within a few days after stroke and needs to be minimized to allow early standing functions. Loss of ankle joint dorsiflexion range interferes with the ability of the body to recruit ankle strategies, and limited ankle joint dorsiflexion range is one cause of knee hyperextension in standing.

Loss of knee control during standing may result from leg weakness or loss of intralimb sequencing. Loss of knee control is also influenced by the position and movement control of the hip and ankle joints. Initially the knee flexes as more weight is shifted to the unaffected side, and the pelvis lists downward. If the pelvic position is not corrected (leveled) and the client actively straightens the knee, a compensatory pelvic rotation (toward the affected side) may occur. Because of the instability of a weak, flexing leg, the client may learn to "lock" the knee in hyperextension as a means of gaining stability (Figure 23-14).

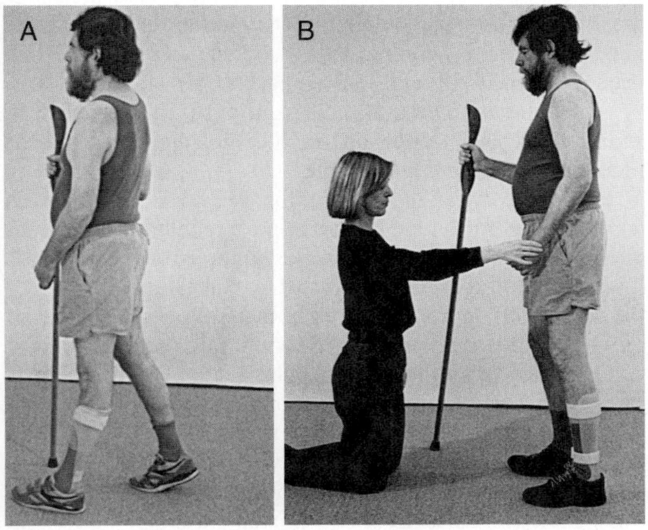

Figure 23-14 ■ **A,** Client with left hemiplegia with knee hyperextension wearing a lightweight prefabricated posterior leaf-spring brace that does not control his knee hyperextension. **B,** A solid ankle brace with foot control that decreases knee hyperextension by providing distal stability.

Clinical Observations

In the acute phase, therapists can help the client practice standing with the hips and shoulders back against a wall to provide support for the trunk and pelvis while creating a safe situation for practicing active self-initiated leg weight-bearing movements. The client can slide down the wall, activating eccentric control in the legs, and then slide back up, activating concentric control. By using the wall to assist the stand, the therapist frees his or her hands to help correct leg alignment problems and lets the client practice the initiation of movement early, independently, and safely.

The client can practice controlled lateral weight transfer with appropriate trunk activity in this position. Whereas one study concluded that there is no relationship between lateral weight shift and walking, therapists should not conclude that unilateral weight acceptance is inappropriate functional training.[155] What may be more important than the lateral weight transfer over the leg is learning to depress the foot into the floor, as it equalizes weight between the two legs.[156]

Upper-extremity forearm or extended-arm weight bearing provides upper-trunk stability for lower-extremity–initiated practice. This practice pattern also allows a means of self-ranging for the ankle, knee, hip, and pelvis. This position is used not to inhibit tone in the extremities but to activate and strengthen the trunk and legs in linked patterns.

Walking

Independent, functional, and safe walking is difficult to retrain in the early phases of intervention because it requires refined degrees of trunk and extremity control. It requires an advanced level of trunk control, linked trunk and leg movements, and enough strength and control in the leg to support body weight, to move the multiple joints of the leg in complex patterns, and to control speed, momentum, and balance. Walking patterns in clients who have experienced stroke are characterized by slow speed, uneven step and stride lengths, impaired balance with resulting arm and leg posturing, and reliance on adaptive equipment.

In the current health care environment with the emphasis on limited therapy visits, therapists are confronted with major intervention dilemmas: Should they force the client to walk without minimal prerequisites? Should they allow undesirable compensations although they predict future secondary problems? Should they use the benefits of the large health care systems to divide responsibility for continued gait training among therapy divisions (inpatient, rehabilitation, home care, outpatient)?

Prerequisites for functional, safe walking include the following:

- Upper-body control to support leg movements in unilateral stance and during swing
- Lower-trunk control to prevent atypical pelvic patterns
- Strength and control of the leg to initiate weight shifts
- Strength and control of the leg to move in space

Because gait is the most extensively studied, analyzed, and discussed in terms of intervention, this section describes the prerequisites for walking training and common impairments that interfere with walking.[157-159] Common impairments that interfere with walking are separated into three divisions of the walking cycle: (1) forward progression, (2) single- and double-limb support, and (3) swing.[160,161]

Impairments that interfere with functional walking are summarized in Box 23-7.

Research on and equipment for partial–body-weight supported treadmill walking training with or without robotic assistance have increased over the past 10 years.[162-166] In a 2004 review of randomized controlled studies, there was strong evidence for poststroke treadmill training with or without body-weight support[167] (Figure 23-15). Task specificity, speed, intensity, and symmetry of practice in this type of equipment were thought to contribute to improved overground walking performance.[162] However, the most recent Cochrane review reports no statistically significant effect of treadmill training with or without body-weight support.[168] A 2011 randomized controlled trial comparing body-weight–supported locomotor training with a therapist-supervised home progressive exercise and balance program reports improvements with both training methods.[169]

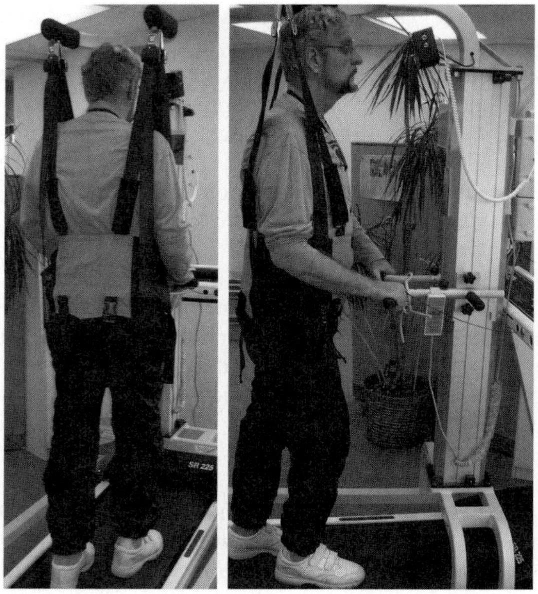

A B

Figure 23-15 ■ **A** and **B,** Client with right hemiplegia walking on a treadmill with partial body weight support.

BOX 23-7 ■ SUMMARY OF SIGNIFICANT FUNCTIONAL IMPAIRMENTS

FORWARD PROGRESSION—HEEL STRIKE TO MIDSTANCE

Poor trunk control
- Loss of alignment of upper trunk over lower trunk
- Loss of control of upper trunk as leg initiates weight shift forward

Lack of proper initiation pattern and direction
- Excessive forward trunk flexion
- Excessive lateral weight shift

Insufficient ankle joint dorsiflexion range
- Muscle tightness
- Loss of control
- Edema

Inappropriate foot contact
- Weakness of foot and ankle muscles
- Muscle tightness
- Foot posturing

SINGLE AND DOUBLE LIMB SUPPORT

Insufficient trunk control to maintain position over one leg
- Asymmetries during unilateral stance
- Loss of control of upper trunk over lower trunk

Poor lower-extremity control
- Hip instability
- Loss of knee control in unilateral stance
- Loss of ankle joint dorsiflexion range
- Toe clawing or curling

Loss of ability to transfer weight through foot
- Inability to maintain leg on floor behind body
- Muscle tightness
- Weakness or inappropriate activation of leg muscles

SWING—EARLY AND LATE

Atypical leg muscle firing patterns
- Lack of proper initiation
- Loss of ankle and foot dorsiflexion
- Inability to control trunk and lower-extremity initiation pattern
- Initiation pattern

Inability of the body to continue to move forward as leg swings

Foot posturing

Clinical Observations

If weakness in the foot and ankle creates difficulty clearing the foot during stepping, compensatory strategies of hip hiking, circumduction, or posterior pelvic tilting arise. If allowed to persist, these atypical initiation strategies become difficult to retrain. This points to a need to consider minimal ankle and foot support during early walking as a means of creating appropriate distal initiation patterns and limiting the need for proximal compensatory strategies (Figure 23-16). (See Chapter 34 for additional suggestions.)

After the identification of significant impairments in swing phase and stance phase, specific intervention techniques are chosen. See example.

Example. After the description set forth by Knutsson and Richards,[86] in a type I motor control problem with premature activation of the calf muscles, intervention may stress lower-extremity–initiated forward weight shift. Control of the ankle with appropriate knee activity allows the center of gravity to advance ahead of the foot before the activation of calf muscles pulls the lower leg backward. With a type II disturbance, training to improve control and power of the leg while standing or during sitting to standing under varied conditions may be indicated. In a type III problem, intervention is directed at achieving stability control of the upper trunk during lower-extremity–initiated patterns.

EQUIPMENT

Equipment for persons with CNS dysfunction can be thought of as supports or extra help to allow better alignment or stabilization so that the client can move and function more

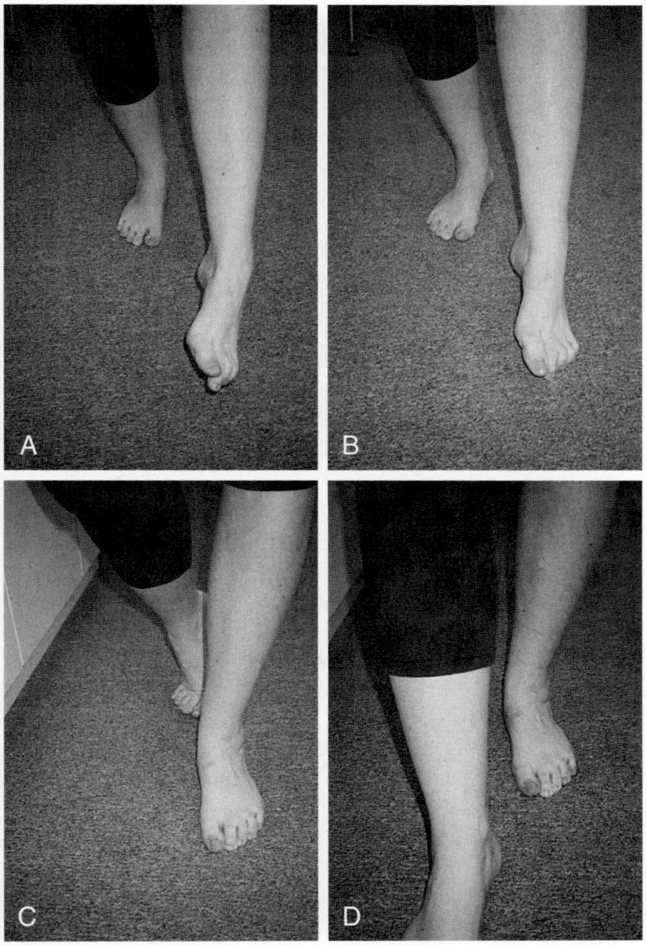

Figure 23-16 ■ **A** and **B,** Client with left hemiplegia. Supination of the foot during swing and during foot contact with ankle joint plantarflexion and calcaneal varus. **C** and **D,** Compensatory pronation of the midfoot to allow the foot to contact the ground during stance.

independently. Too much support or equipment may hinder the development of new movement control. Equipment should never be a substitute for treatment and should not be given without practice during treatment. One-handed equipment that is used as a compensation for trunk control is less successful than equipment that is used to compensate for loss of extremity function. Therapists should perform continuing assessments of the appropriateness of the equipment in relation to gains made in therapy.

Example

A "reacher" compensates for loss of trunk and limb linked control (reach beyond arm's length), but use of a reacher may prevent the development of this control; whereas an electric can opener designed for one-handed use substitutes for the ability to use the affected hand (when recovery is not possible).

Bedside Equipment

In acute and rehabilitation settings, pillows, blankets, or towels are used to position the client in bed. With the client in the supine position, the head pillow can be angled so that it slips under the shoulder and scapula to prevent loss of alignment: to prevent humeral hyperextension and internal rotation. A soft towel roll or pillow under the leg—greater trochanter or knee—maintains alignment of the leg in the first few days after a stroke. Once the client begins to move to both sides in bed, the use of pillows for support is not necessary.

Wheelchairs

Wheelchairs must have a solid surface and, when possible, a supportive backrest. The soft leather seats and backs of transport chairs act as slings and allow the pelvis to posteriorly tilt and the spine to flex. Solid seats and backs allow the pelvis, trunk, and extremities to be more normally aligned. Wheelchairs specifically for clients with hemiplegia who are not expected to become household ambulators have lower seat heights and one-armed drive (two hand rims on one wheel). These adaptations make it easier for clients to propel the chair with the unaffected hand and foot.

Support for the hemiplegic arm when the client is sitting in a wheelchair reduces the effect of the downward pull of gravity on the weak or paralyzed arm. Lapboards support both arms and provide symmetry for the upper body. However, in some health care settings, they are considered a form of restraint and cannot be used. The use of a pillow in the lap is another option for bilateral support of the arms. Half-lapboards or arm troughs are used to support the arm. If an arm support is used, the client should be taught how to protect the arm and hand while on the support.

Slings

Slings are used to support the glenohumeral joint to prevent capsular stretch, to temporarily maintain alignment that is gained in treatment, and to take some of the weight of the paralyzed arm off the upper trunk as the client begins to learn to stand and walk. Capsular stretch accompanies shoulder subluxation, and it is difficult to reverse an existing subluxation once the capsule is stretched. Because subluxation is not inherently painful, a sling is not used to prevent pain. However, use of a sling can help break the cycle of pain from shoulder-hand syndrome.

Various reviews and comparisons of slings are available.[170,171] Shoulder subluxation is the result of loss of strength and control in the shoulder girdle and trunk, especially scapular upward rotation. There is no sling available that corrects a subluxation because no existing sling provides scapular upward rotation control. Slings act as an assist to "hold" a scapulohumeral position that has been restored in treatment.

The ideal shoulder sling helps maintain the normal angular alignment of the glenoid fossa, decreases the tendency of the humerus to internally rotate, takes some of the weight of the arm off the upper trunk, and allows the upper extremity freedom of movement. Therapists should not prescribe slings that cradle the arm in front of the body, prevent any movement, and in effect teach learned nonuse. The orthopedic-type *envelope arm sling* was used in the 1950s and 1960s. In the 1970s, influenced by Bobath,[105] sling use was thought to be undesirable. As more information about tone and movement became available, new slings were designed to allow the arm to be supported while movement was reeducated. Slings have different suspensions, provide different means of control for the arm, give differing "messages" to the arm and trunk, and have individual uses. Table 23-6, adapted from the work of Levit,[172] lists available slings and their characteristics.

Clients who come into therapy with a sling but who do not require one are weaned from a supportive sling into a less controlling one. Clients state that the *clavicle support* provides support during household tasks that require upper-body flexion, such as bed making or vacuuming. Clients who complain of "aching" in the arm at the end of the day may relieve this ache by using a support for a few hours around midday.

If the arm dangles or bangs against the body during active periods, the *shoulder saddle sling* can be adjusted to protect the arm from bruising. This sling is also helpful to clients with severe shoulder-hand pain because it allows full support of the arm and can be adjusted by the client to allow the elbow to extend as the pain subsides. The *GivMohr sling* combines a humeral cuff with a hand support. *Humeral cuff slings* are the least practical from a functional standpoint because they do not affect scapula or trunk position.

Canes

Canes are given to clients with hemiplegia to provide extra balance, not as a means to support body weight. Canes should be used after upper-body control and lower-extremity–initiated movements have been practiced.

If quad canes or hemiwalkers are used before trunk and leg activity is minimally established, they encourage lateral translation of the spine or rotation of the spine and ribs. When clients shift off the weak leg onto the stable cane, the cane acts functionally as a third leg. This one-sided compensation encourages learned nonuse of the affected leg.

Single canes provide a balance assist. Often clients use the cane while walking outdoors or in crowded situations but not inside their homes. Reliance on a cane for walking eliminates the possibility of carrying objects and makes it difficult to perform one-handed tasks such as opening a door. Wrist loops allow the client to use the unaffected hand without having to put the cane aside. Weighted cane tips, such as the AbleTripod cane tip, are a bridge between quad canes and straight canes and allow a standard cane to remain upright.

Orthotics

Ankle-foot orthoses (AFOs) are used to allow foot clearance during walking, to ensure heel strike, to provide distal stability for early standing and walking in clients with severe weakness, to provide lateral lower-leg stability in clients who need an assist because of lateral hip weakness, and to control knee hyperextension caused by loss of ankle dorsiflexion control. Different design types provide different functions. Solid ankle bracing with plastic beyond the malleoli limits distal freedom but allows clients with severe weakness to practice gaining control of trunk and hip movements.

The use of polypropylene bracing to control foot posturing in adults began in the 1970s with information from pediatrics and podiatry. Foot control in a brace stops supination of the foot in swing and compensatory pronation of the foot in stance. This control is achieved through neutral rear foot positioning and long medial and lateral foot counters.

TABLE 23-6 ■ AVAILABLE SLINGS AND THEIR CHARACTERISTICS

BASIC TYPE	SUPPLIER	SUSPENSION	MESSAGE	COMMON USE
Clavicle support	DePuy (clavicle fracture sling with 1-inch soft foam axilla pad)	Figure-of-8 between scapulae Support under axilla	"Spine extend, scapula adduct"	Acute care Minimal support To wean out of other supports
Humeral cuff	Rolyan Hemi Arm Sling	Figure-of-8 between scapulae Velcro cuff support to humeral shaft	"Arm up"	Rehabilitative care
Unilateral shoulder orthosis	Bauerfeind Rolyan	Across body Elastic or spandex cuff support to humeral shaft	"Lift humerus up"	Rehabilitative care
Shoulder-saddle sling	Sammons	Saddle sits on top of shoulder Strap across body Forearm cuff—adjustable straps allow changes in elbow position	Maximal support of arm	To prevent "banging" of flaccid arm in active patients or during sports activities To provide support for painful arm
GivMohr sling	GivMohr	Figure-of-8 between scapulae Plastic cone in palm of hand	"Arm up"	To relieve weight of "heavy" flaccid arm

Techniques of Aquaplast fabrication have created new possibilities for inexpensive, immediate, remoldable bracing for the foot and ankle.[173]

Custom-made AFOs provide the best fit and control, but excellent prefabricated polypropylene braces are available through companies such as Friddle's Orthopedic Appliances, Orthomerica, or Wheaton Brace. These orthoses have long medial and lateral foot edges for control of foot posturing, come in multiple models and sizes, and can be ordered with regular or long foot plates or as blanks that can be self-trimmed (see Chapter 34).

Functional electrical stimulation foot-drop systems, the Bioness L300 and the WalkAide, are now available for clinical use. These systems use low-level electrical activity to stimulate the nerves that lift the foot and are timed with walking stance and swing patterns.

Clients should be encouraged to spend time standing or walking short distances without the brace so that dependence is not established. Clients like to be able to walk to the bathroom at night without a brace. Orthopedic ankle and foot supports provide alternatives to plastic bracing. The MalleoLoc ankle support controls rear foot equinus and varus while allowing ankle and forefoot movement (Bauerfeind USA/AliMed). Clients with moderate supination posturing report a reassuring feeling of security with this support while walking short distances and during sports participation. This support, a substitute for the Aircast and Ace support, is a good choice for sports activities such as golfing, bicycling, jumping, and running.

Functions and limitations of commonly used braces are found in Table 23-7 and orthotic manufacturers in Appendix 23-A.

Movable Surfaces

Movable surfaces such as gymnastic balls of varying sizes, large rolls, and adjustable stools with casters are used as assistive devices to help clients increase trunk and extremity strength and control. To encourage trunk and leg activity, the

TABLE 23-7 ■ ANKLE-FOOT ORTHOSES (AFOs) USED IN CLIENTS WITH HEMIPLEGIA FROM STROKE

ORTHOTIC DESIGN	FUNCTION	LIMITATIONS	PATIENT TYPES (CATEGORIES)
Solid ankle with foot control	Heel strike Distal stability Lateral hip stability Assists forward progression Assists knee control Stops foot posturing	No ankle mobility No toe break	Severe weakness in trunk and leg Need for distal stability
Modified solid ankle with foot control	Heel strike More distal mobility, less ankle control Stops foot posturing	Less knee control Reduced message of forward progression No control of knee	Increasing leg strength Increasing trunk and leg control
Posterior leaf spring	Toe clearance	No control of foot posturing	Good return of control in trunk and leg Need for minimal dorsiflexion assistance
Articulated ankle	Free dorsiflexion Heel strike if plantar stop used	Limited control of foot posturing Bulky at ankle	Normal ankle range—if range is limited, the movement of brace is translated into foot Functional needs; climb hills, stairs, move to and from ground
Supramalleolar foot orthoses in Aquaplast	Foot control Assist heel strike Used for weaning from AFOs Sports	No knee control Short shelf life of material	Increasing leg control Desire to begin increasing activity level
Foot orthoses	Balance small asymmetries of foot	No control of foot posturing No ankle or knee control	Persistent but minimal rear foot–forefoot asymmetries
Klenzak metal, double upright	Toe clearance Reminder of forward progression	No foot control Control of ankle and foot through shoe	Used before creation of polypropylene to provide heel strike and stop foot supination
ALTERNATIVE FUNCTIONAL ELECTRICAL STIMULATION FOOT DROP DEVICES			
Bioness L300	Foot control Knee control assist Operates via heel pressure switch	Expensive Requires cognitive ability to don and adjust settings	
WalkAide	Foot control Operates via tibial tilt	Requires cognitive ability to don and adjust settings	

See Chapter 34 for additional suggestions.

client sits on the ball and moves it in small ranges to the limits of perceived balance. This is an activity that increases trunk and leg control but does not lead directly to improvements in standing or walking. Gymnastic balls provide symmetrical support to the rib cage when used in the hands-and-knees position and are used to stretch specific tight tissues. Routines of lifting the ball with either the arms or legs strengthen extremity movements in space.

When spasticity was considered the major impairment in hemiplegia, therapists often placed clients prone over balls to "inhibit" tone. This is an inappropriate technique, considering advances in understanding of movement control and recovery.

Hand Splints

The practice of splinting the hemiplegic hand is controversial. Historically, the hand in clients with hemiplegia was splinted in a "resting" position. After the introduction of neurophysiological approaches, splinting became "inhibitory" in design.[174-176] Now, with the understanding that spasticity is not the major problem, splinting the wrist and hand has undergone another change. A splint designed in 1982 by Levit[177] as a neutral functional splint promotes functional retraining and hand use while minimizing secondary impairments. This splint, designed to hold the wrist and hand in a position of orthopedic neutral, decreases clinical hypertonicity that occurs either from poor alignment or unbalanced muscle return. The splint promotes support of the wrist and hand to avoid the secondary impairments of muscle tightness, muscle shifting, and overstretching of weak wrist and finger muscles. This type of splinting has been reported to decrease hand edema and pain.[178]

Therapists custom make the splints with the goals of supporting the wrist in neutral, preventing radial or ulnar deviation with long, high sides, and maintaining the palmar arches. The fingers are not incorporated into the splint but are left free, to allow movement reeducation and practice.

The increased tone in finger flexors, previously labeled "spasticity," comes in part from incomplete return or weakness of finger muscle activity on a poorly aligned wrist. A position of wrist flexion results in a drop of the proximal row of carpals and a flattening of the palmar arches. If the wrist is supported in neutral and the arches are preserved, returning muscle activity is reeducated in functional patterns. Finger support in a splint should be used only when there is a serious deformity with a need to serially, systematically, and slowly lengthen tight tissues.

This functional type of splint is worn mainly during the day when arm posturing is greater and when support of critical joints allows beginning hand use. Hand posturing is less of a problem when the patient lies down because of decreased demands on the trunk and legs. Clients are instructed not to wear the splint at night.

Design Considerations

If joint range is limited, the therapist makes the splint to support available range. The splint can be revised as range increases. Alignment is corrected in three steps: (1) keeping the wrist in flexion, the lateral deviation is corrected by aligning the third metacarpal with the middle of the radius; (2) the carpal position is corrected (usually by gently lifting up from a low position under the radius); and (3) the hand is moved to wrist neutral (see *Functional Movement Reeducation*[54] for a step-by-step analysis). The warmed, soft splinting plastic captures this corrected position as it cools. The length of palmar support is decided by the therapist after assessment of degree and distribution of muscle return and muscle tightness patterns. The thumb is supported at its base in a neutral position, not one of abduction. As beginning grip returns, the thumb hole is widened to allow function.

A variety of neutral functional splints have been designed. The neutral wrist and thumb hole splinting design makes the splint hard to keep on the hand of patients with severe weakness. They sometimes find ulnar or radial trough splints or wide opponens splints easier to keep on.

As wrist extension control against gravity emerges, the therapist can fabricate a wide opponens splint to maintain the palmar arches as the client begins practicing finger movements. The wide opponens splint supports the base of the hand and assists in maintaining carpal alignment. Patients can switch between the two splints as needed.

Clients with severe hand pain prefer a neutral wrist splint with a resting area for the thumb. This splint is fabricated with little or no correction initially but with gentle support for the wrist and palmar arches. As the pain decreases, this splint is modified to become the original neutral functional splint.

Although the move away from "inhibitory" splints and from night splinting to daytime functional splinting breaks many of the "rules" from the past, it is more compatible with concepts from research and clinical experts.

Recommended resources for practical solutions to one-handed functioning and devices that assist in independence are listed in Appendix 23-B at the end of this chapter.

PSYCHOSOCIAL ASPECTS AND ADJUSTMENTS

The suddenness of a stroke and the dramatic change in motor, sensory, visual, and perceptual performance and feedback may leave the person with hemiplegia confused, disoriented, angry, stressed, frustrated, and fearful.

Psychosocial issues may be more detrimental than any functional disability to long-term stroke survivors.[179] Decreased interest in social activity inside and outside the home and decreased interest in hobbies as a result of psychosocial disability hamper the hemiplegic person's return to a normal social life.[180] Feelings of rejection and embarrassment may interfere with the hemiplegic person's interaction with people outside the home environment. Individuals with long-standing hemiplegia often become clinically depressed with symptoms of loss of sleep and appetite, self-blame, and a hopeless outlook. The usual psychosocial adjustments to disability are compounded in persons with hemiplegia resulting from stroke by the issues associated with aging.

Family members and spouses may have difficulty assessing the capabilities of the hemiplegic person and may be overprotective. Overprotection among spouses may be a sign of affection and support or a sign of guilt.[181] Long-standing marriages do not tend to dissolve when one member has a stroke. However, previous marriage problems and personality traits may become exaggerated as a result of the presence of increased and changing demands and stresses that occur when the person returns home.

A comparison of occupational status of long-term stroke survivors in the United States and in Sweden reveals that 40% of the Swedes returned to a form of employment (including part-time work) but none of the U.S. group returned to work.[182] The scarcity of part-time work and a shorter treatment period dictated by third-party payers in the United States may account for this discrepancy.

Age is a general predictor for return to employment, and younger people are more attractive to employers. Barriers to return to work for the person with hemiplegia include speech, perceptual, and cognitive deficits along with a need for psychosocial support. Architectural barriers also can create severe problems for hemiplegic clients with regard to both work and recreational activities. Stroke clubs, usually organized through hospitals, the National Stroke Association, or the American Heart Association, provide educational, social, and recreational support for the hemiplegic person and her or his spouse.

The impact of psychosocial disability and the need for its long-term treatment is great. Programs need to be established and continued for years to allow clients and their families to deal with the many problems that result from the stroke. Refer to Appendix 23-C for resources.

Sexuality

Most persons with hemiplegia experience a decline in sexuality through a decrease in frequency of sexual intercourse without a change in the level of prestroke sexual desire.[183] On return home, the person with hemiplegia faces uncertainty about sexual skills and the risk of failure. Sexual dysfunction that results from a stroke depends on the amount of cerebral damage and includes a decreased ability to achieve erection and ejaculation in men and decreased lubrication in women.[184] The sensory, motor, visual, and emotional disturbances of hemiplegia may cause awkwardness, but these disturbances can be overcome through the education of the spouse in alternate positioning and ways to provide appropriate sensory experiences. The normal factors of aging also interfere with the sexual performance of persons with hemiplegia. A person's prestroke sexual activity is a good indicator of poststroke sexual activity. The closeness between partners achieved through a satisfactory sexual relationship can add to the quality of life after stroke (see Chapter 6).

SUMMARY

This chapter reviews the neuropathology of stroke, the evaluation of impairments that interfere with functional movement patterns, and intervention planning. Both evaluation of outcomes and evaluation of movement components are described. The chapter highlights significant impairments and provides clinical observations on critical areas of intervention. A detailed process of clinical problem solving helps the therapist organize and prioritize impairments to plan intervention programs that retrain movement components and train desirable compensatory patterns to help the client gain the highest level of functional performance and independence in daily life. An example of the synthesis of this chapter's concepts and ideas can be found in Case Study 23-1.

References

To enhance this text and add value for the reader, all references are included on the companion Evolve site that accompanies this textbook. This online service will, when available, provide a link for the reader to a Medline abstract for the article cited. There are 184 cited references and other general references for this chapter, with the majority of those articles being evidence-based citations.

CASE STUDY 23-1

A client with left hemiplegia was seen 4 days after stroke on admission to a rehabilitation center. The classification of movement disorder was composite movement category with severe movement deficits.

FUNCTIONAL LIMITATION 1: CLIENT IS UNABLE TO PERFORM MORNING SELF-CARE AT BEDSIDE OR SITTING IN WHEELCHAIR IN FRONT OF A SINK

Why?

Client cannot perform anterior and posterior or lateral trunk movements in sitting without loss of balance and falling to left. Client cannot feel left arm, and it hangs by side.

Evaluation

Primary Impairments

Weakness in left arm and leg
Impaired motor control: inability to coordinate trunk–limb movements
Decreased sense of touch in left arm, trunk, and leg
Loss of postural control

Secondary Impairments

Loss of trunk alignment in sitting
Left shoulder subluxation
Muscle tightness—pectorals, latissimus, wrist flexors, ankle dorsiflexors
Loss of alignment of lower trunk and pelvis in sitting—spine laterally flexed, convexity on left, left pelvis lists downward
Loss of 10 degrees of left ankle joint dorsiflexion range

FUNCTIONAL LIMITATION 2: CLIENT IS UNABLE TO TRANSFER FROM BED TO CHAIR INDEPENDENTLY

Why?

Client cannot control upper body while trying to activate bilateral leg activity when initiating transfers to either side. Left arm hangs by side with an inferior shoulder subluxation. Cannot lift left leg against gravity in sitting. Cannot depress left leg into surface. Tends to use right side exclusively during transfer with loss of balance. Client uses right arm to support self at edge of bed.

Primary Impairments

Weakness in upper trunk
Weakness in left leg and trunk–leg patterns
Inability to coordinate trunk–limb patterns in weight bearing
Inability to sequence movement patterns in left leg in weight bearing

Continued

CASE STUDY 23-1—cont'd

Secondary Impairments

Loss of upper-body alignment

Loss of left ankle joint dorsiflexion range

FUNCTIONAL LIMITATION 3: CLIENT IS UNABLE TO STAND UP FROM CHAIR INDEPENDENTLY

Why?

Client is unable to control upper body over lower trunk during lower-body–initiated transfers and sit to stand. Client is unable to use left leg for support and movement during the transition of sit to stand. Client is unable to keep weight (depress leg into floor) on left foot in standing.

Primary Impairments

Inability to control upper body over lower body, resulting in an inability to initiate lower trunk and leg movements

Weakness in left leg

Inability to coordinate trunk–leg patterns in weight bearing

Secondary Impairments

Loss of left ankle joint dorsiflexion range

Tightness in left gastrocnemius

SIGNIFICANT IMPAIRMENTS FOR FUNCTIONS EVALUATED

1. Loss of upper-body control during lower-body–initiated movements, especially anterior-posterior plane
2. Shoulder subluxation contributes to loss of upper-body control
3. Loss of control and weakness of left arm and leg
4. Loss of ankle joint dorsiflexion range

Treatment Goals

I. Functional Goals

A. Perform morning self-care activities in wheelchair in bathroom independently
B. Transfer from chair to bed and back with contact guarding
C. Rise to standing with assistance of one person

II. Long-Term Goals

A. Sit safely while performing tasks with right arm and leg around midline; that is, perform upper-body– and lower-body–initiated trunk movements in sitting independently
B. Increase upper-body control to prepare for independent, safe, lower-body–initiated movement patterns (extended-arm reach, sitting to standing, and standing balance)
C. Increase leg strength and establish trunk and leg coordinated patterns in weight bearing (to allow transfers, rising to stand, and standing with minimal assistance to the upper body)
D. Establish a home or bedside program that the client can perform independently

III. Short-Term Goals

A. Perform basic trunk movement patterns in sitting with contact guarding
B. Increase control in upper body and shoulder girdle to decrease shoulder subluxation
C. Protect shoulder joint from excessive capsular stretch
D. Strengthen left arm, be able to lift weak arm up onto sink with unaffected arm, maintain sitting balance during morning ADL activities
E. Increase ankle joint dorsiflexion range in standing
F. Increase strength in leg and in trunk and leg linked patterns during lower-body–initiated transfers, during sitting to standing, and in supported standing to allow lower-extremity–assisted practice

APPENDIX 23-A ■ Product Manufacturers

Wheaton Brace Company
391 S. Schmale Road
Carol Stream, IL 60188

Orthomerica
505 31st Street
Newport Beach, CA 92663

Friddle's Orthopedic Appliances
12306 B-HP Highway
Honea Path, SC 29654

AliMed
P.O. Box 9135
Dedham, MA 32703

DePuy Orthotech
700 Orthopedic Drive
Warsaw, IN 46581-0988

Patterson Medical/Sammons Preston
1000 Remington Boulevard, Suite 210
Bolingbrook, IL 60440

Bioness, Inc
25103 Rye Canyon Loop
Valencia, CA 91355

WalkAide System
www.walkaide.com

APPENDIX 23-B ■ Resources for One-Handed Adaptations

One-Handed in a Two-Handed World
Tommye K. Mayer
Prince Gallison Press
P.O. Box 23
Boston, MA 02113

Adaptive Resources: A Guide to Products and Services
National Stroke Association
8480 E. Orchard Road
Englewood, CO 80111

APPENDIX 23-C ■ Stroke Survivor Resources

Internet Links

National Stroke Association: www.stroke.org
American Stroke Association: www.strokeassociation.org
American Stroke Foundation: www.americanstroke.org
Stroke Survivor: www.strokesurvivor.com
Resource site: www.strokecenter.org
Stroke journal: http://stroke.ahajournal.org
Neurology stroke information: http://brainattacks.net
Useful stroke information: www.strokehelp.com

Audiovisual and Literary Resources

Films and Videotapes

Inner World of Aphasia, 35-minute film
American Journal of Nursing Film Library
267 W. 25th Street
New York, NY 10001

Candidate for Stroke, 35-minute film
American Heart Association

I Had a Stroke, 35-minute film
Filmmakers Library, Inc.
290 West End Avenue
New York, NY 10023

Living with Stroke
Rehabilitation Research and Training Center
The George Washington University
2300 I Street, NW, Suite 714
Washington, DC 20037

Evaluation of the Hemiplegic Patient (sensory and motor)
Audio-Visual Department
School of Allied Health
University of Maryland
32 Greene Street
Baltimore, MD 21201

Books

Children

First One Foot, Then the Other, by Tomie dePaola. This book explores the feelings and fears of children about a relative who has had a stroke.

Adult

How to Conquer the World with One Hand...and an Attitude, by Paul E. Berger. Merrifield, Virginia, 1999, Positive Power Publisher.

Stroke of Insight: A Brain Scientist's Personal Journey, by Jill Bolte. Taylor, 2008.

The Stroke Recovery Book: A Guide for Patients and Families, by Kip Burkman, MD, 2010.

CHAPTER 24 Traumatic Brain Injury

PATRICIA A. WINKLER, PT, DSc, NCS

KEY TERMS

anticipatory responses
knowledge of results
learning theory
motor control
motor learning
motor skill
neuroplasticity
systems theory
traumatic head injury

OBJECTIVES

After reading this chapter the student or therapist will be able to:

1. Describe the application of current concepts in motor control and motor learning theories for clients with traumatic brain injury.
2. Understand the meaning of *impairment, activity limitation,* and *participation limitation* and their interrelationships as they apply to clients with traumatic brain injury.
3. Prescribe methods of examining, evaluating, and developing interventions for clients with brain injuries on the basis of task, impairment, and activity limitation analysis.
4. Describe prognosis and outcomes for clients with traumatic brain injury.
5. Differentiate between development of basic movement patterns and motor skills.
6. Understand the role of synergy formation, synergy selection and modification, and anticipatory and feedback information as used in motor skills.
7. Describe the long-term effects of different types of feedback and practice on learning.

Traumatic brain injury (TBI) is defined as a blow or jolt to the head or a penetrating head injury that disrupts the function of the brain. Not all blows or jolts to the head result in a TBI. The severity of such an injury may range from mild—a brief change in mental status or consciousness—to severe—an extended period of unconsciousness or amnesia after the injury. A TBI can result in short- or long-term problems with independent function.[1]

OVERVIEW OF BRAIN INJURY

Epidemiology of Traumatic Brain Injury

One and three-quarter million people sustain a TBI every year.[1] Of these, 1.3 million are treated in emergency departments and 275,000 injuries are severe enough to require hospitalization.[2] Fifty-two thousand people die yearly of TBI, 80,000 injuries result in disabilities, and 5.3 million people are living with permanent disabilities from TBI. It is the leading killer and disabler of children and young adults. Motor vehicle crashes cause 20% of all TBIs, falls cause 28%, violence causes 11% (the majority from firearms), and sports and recreation account for 10%. Child abuse accounts for 64% of infant brain injuries.[1] Fifty-thousand children sustain bicycle-related brain injuries, and 400 of them die.[3] Two thirds of firearm-related TBIs are suicidal. Falls are the leading cause of TBI in people aged 65 years and older, with 11% proving fatal. The incidence of TBI is 506.4 per 100,000 population, with 43% of those hospitalized having long-term activity limitation.[4]

Population of Clients with Brain Injury

The incidence of brain injuries is higher for the male population than for the female population by more than 2:1. Most of those injured are 15 to 24 years old.[4] The greatest risk of injury is for those younger than 10 years old or older than 74. American Indians and African Americans have the highest rate of TBI. People in lower socioeconomic status also have a higher rate of injury.

Cost

The estimated lifetime cost for each individual with severe brain injury exceeds $4 million. Annual costs for all TBIs in the United States exceed $60 billion.

Mechanisms of Injury

There are four main types of injury, as follows:

1. Those from external forces hitting the head or the head hitting hard enough to cause brain movement. Injuries include those with skull fracture and those without skull fracture (closed head injuries). Direct blows to the head can cause coup injuries (at the site of impact) and contrecoup injuries (distant from the site of impact).
2. Severe acceleration and deceleration of the head can cause TBI without the head hitting an object. An example is shaken baby syndrome.
3. Blast injuries have become very common in the past 10 years, mainly affecting military personnel.
4. Penetrating objects cause direct cellular and vascular damage. Injuries to the face and neck can cause brain injury by damaging the blood supply to the brain.[5]

Pathophysiology of Injury

Acceleration, deceleration, rotational forces, and penetrating objects cause tissue laceration, compression, tension, shearing, or a combination, resulting in primary injury.

Primary Damage

Contusions—a bruise or bleeding on the brain—and lacerations can occur with or without skull fractures. Either an object hits the head, neck, or face, or the head hits an object. Damage can be to any area of the brain. Occipital blows are more likely to produce contusions than are frontal or lateral blows. Areas in which the cranial vault is irregular, such as on the anterior poles, undersurface of the temporal lobes, and undersurface of the frontal lobes, are commonly injured. Lacerations of blood vessels within the brain itself or of blood vessels that feed the brain from the neck or face reduce the flow of blood carrying oxygen to the brain. Contusions and lacerations can also injure the cranial nerves. The most commonly injured are the optic, vestibulocochlear, oculomotor, abducens, and facial nerves. Lacerations of the dura or in the arachnoid space may cause cerebrospinal fluid to discharge from the nose (cerebrospinal fluid rhinorrhea discharge increases with neck flexion, coughing, or straining).[6] An example of a computed tomography (CT) scan of a cerebral contusion can be found in Chapter 37, Figure 37-17, *B*.

Epidural hematomas or hemorrhages occur mostly in adults when tearing of meningeal vessels results in blood collecting between the skull and dura. Skull fracture is present in the majority of cases. This is accompanied by intervals of lucidness and can result in death unless treated early.

Subdural hematomas occur with acceleration-deceleration injuries when bridging veins to the superior sagittal sinus are torn. Blood accumulates in the subdural space. Symptoms include weakness and lethargy. Symptoms such as weakness and lethargy that come on acutely are life-threatening. Symptoms caused by slow bleeding may not be present for several weeks. A CT scan of this problem can be found in Chapter 37, online image Figure 37-17, *A*. Also, note on the same figure the midline shift of the brain.

Diffuse axonal injuries, or shearing injuries, are among the most common types of primary lesions in patients with brain trauma.[7,8] Brain tissues that differ in structure or weight experience unequal acceleration, deceleration, or rotation of tissues during rapid head movement or during impact, causing diffuse axonal injury and changes in chemical processing. Refer to Chapter 37, Figure 37-17, *D* for an illustration of what axons are most affected by this shearing motion. Severing of the axons may be severe enough to result in coma. In milder forms, more spotty lesions are seen, including deficits such as memory loss, concentration difficulties, decreased attention span, headaches, sleep disturbances, and seizures. Damage often involves the corpus callosum, basal ganglia, brain stem, and cerebellum.[6,8] For a complete image of how the axons diffuse throughout the entire CNS, refer to Figure 37-17, *C*.

Penetrating objects with high velocities, such as bullets or shrapnel from explosives, can cause additional damage remote from the areas of impact as a result of shock waves. Foreign objects such as sticks and sharp toys cause low-velocity injuries, directly damaging the tissues they contact.

Blast injuries occur when a solid or liquid explosive material explodes, turning into a gas. The expanding gases form a high-pressure wave (overpressure wave) that travels at supersonic speed. Pressure then drops, creating a relative vacuum (blast underpressure wave) that results in a reversal of air flow, which is in turn followed by a second overpressure wave. Blast-related injury can occur through several mechanisms. The primary blast wave generates extreme pressure changes that can cause stress and shear injuries. For example, rupture of the tympanic membranes is very common after blast injury, and lung and gastrointestinal injuries also occur. The exact mechanism of injury to the brain is unknown, with speculation about both axonal shearing and shearing of vasculature.[9,10]

Secondary Damage

Secondary injuries are mainly caused by a lack of oxygen in the highly oxygen-demanding brain. Secondary problems may result from the following:

- *Increased intracranial pressure* (ICP) (resulting from swelling or intracranial hematoma). Swelling of the brain causes distortion because the brain is held in the skull, a rigid, unyielding structure. The resultant increased ICP can lead to herniation of parts of the brain. The most often seen herniations include cingulate herniation under the falx cerebri, uncus herniation, central (or transtentorial) herniation, and herniation of the brain stem through the foramen magnum.[11] Acute hydrocephalus occurs when blood accumulates in the ventricular system, expanding the size of the ventricles and causing increased pressure on brain tissue being compressed between the skull and the fluid-filled ventricles. The increased pressure can then result in changes in PCO_2, which is also harmful to nervous tissue. Increased ICP has been correlated with poorer outcomes and higher mortality rates.[12]
- *Cerebral hypoxia or ischemia* (occurring when blood vessels are ruptured or compressed). Hypoxia can occur from a lack of blood to the brain or from lack of oxygen in the blood as a result of airway obstruction or chest injuries.
- *Intracranial hemorrhage* causes hypoxia to tissues fed by the hemorrhaging blood vessels and adds pressure and distortion to brain tissue. Metabolic products from damaged cells and blood bathe the brain. Cell death occurs within minutes after injury from ischemia, edema, necrosis, and the toxic effects of blood on neural tissues.
- *Electrolyte imbalance and acid-base imbalance.* Secondary cell death occurs either by swelling and then bursting of the cellular membrane (necrosis) or by destruction from within the cell through changes in the deoxyribonucleic acid (DNA) (apoptosis). Cell death can occur days, weeks, or months after injury.[13]
- *Infection from open wounds.* Infection in brain tissue may cause swelling and cell death.
- *Seizures from pressure or scarring.* Seizures are most common immediately after injury and 6 months to 2 years after injury. The seizures can cause additional brain damage owing to high oxygen and glucose requirements.

Physiological, Cognitive, and Behavioral Changes after Brain Injury

Autonomic Nervous System

Box 24-1[14] lists possible autonomic nervous system symptoms resulting from brain injury.

BOX 24-1 ■ AUTONOMIC NERVOUS SYSTEM SYMPTOMS RESULTING FROM BRAIN INJURY

- Changes in pulse and respiratory rates or regularity
- Temperature elevations
- Blood pressure changes
- Excessive sweating, salivation, tearing, and sebum secretion
- Dilated pupils
- Vomiting

Motor, Functional, Sensory, and Perceptual Changes

Motor abnormalities after severe head trauma are common. More severe head injuries tend to manifest more persistent physical problems.[6] In at least two studies[6,15] a fourth of the cases had no neurophysical sequelae. Changes in muscle tone may reflect the physiological effects of changes in the amount of tissue compression or irritation.[16] Box 24-2 lists motor changes and provides symptoms of sensory and perceptive involvement.

Cognitive, Personality, and Behavioral Changes

Cognitive and behavioral sequelae can result from generalized or focal brain injuries. Memory impairments are an aftermath of generalized lesions. Emotional changes may be seen with lesions in the orbitofrontal areas. Behavior may be excessive and disinhibited. Septal area lesions result in rage and overall irritability. Pseudobulbar injuries can result in emotional lability of involuntary laughing or crying not associated with feelings of emotions. Behavioral changes can be present even without cognitive and physical deficits. Although actual psychoses can be sequelae, they appear to be neither common nor definitively related to the brain injury.

The social consequences of inappropriate behavior can be disastrous and a stumbling block to achieving therapy goals. A correlation between preinjury personality and postinjury changes has not been established.[6] It does seem reasonable, however, that factors within an individual's psychological makeup may affect reaction to the injury. Brain trauma frequently happens to adolescents—an age group fraught with its own problems that may be aggravated by the injury. Outcomes at 1 year postinjury have shown the most common problems to be poor memory and problem solving, problems managing stress and emotional upsets, and an inability to control temper. Finally, managing money and paying bills were still a problem at the 1-year mark.[17] Box 24-3[18] lists both cognitive and behavioral changes resulting from brain injury.

Changes in Consciousness and Coma

Coma and changes in consciousness result from conditions in which there are diffusely extensive and bilateral cerebral hemispheric depression of function, direct depression or destruction of the brain stem–activating system that is responsible for consciousness or a combination of the two. In moderate or severe head injury, unconsciousness can be prolonged. Plum and Posner's definitions[16] of various stages of acutely altered consciousness are briefly presented, intermingled with some insights from the descriptions offered by

BOX 24-2 ■ MOTOR, FUNCTIONAL, SENSORY, AND PERCEPTUAL CHANGES RESULTING FROM BRAIN INJURY

Motor changes may include any or all of the following:

- Paralysis or paresis such as monoplegia or hemiplegia.
- Cranial nerve injury resulting in paralysis of eye muscles, facial paralysis, vestibular and vestibulooocular reflex abnormalities, slurred speech (dysarthria), swallowing abnormalities (dysphagia), and paralysis of the tongue muscles.
- Poor coordination of movement.
- Abnormal reflexes.
- Abnormal muscle tone: flaccidity, spasticity, or rigidity. (The terms *decorticate rigidity* and *decerebrate rigidity* are often used to denote abnormal posturing. *Decerebrate rigidity* denotes extension in all four limbs. *Decorticate posturing* includes flexion of the upper extremities and extension of the legs.)
- Combinations of asymmetrical cerebellar and pyramidal signs and of bilateral pyramidal and extrapyramidal signs have all been reported.[15]
- Loss of selective motor control.
- Poor balance.
- Loss of bowel or bladder control.

Sensory and perceptive involvement may include any or all of the following:

- Hypersensitivity to light or noise
- Loss of hearing or sight
- Visual field changes
- Numbness and tingling (peripheral nerves are often injured)
- Loss of somatosensory functions
- Dizziness or vertigo
- Visuospatial abnormalities
- Agnosia
- Apraxia

Gilroy and Meyer.[11] Plum and Posner[19] do not equate the presence or absence of motor responses with the depth of coma. These authors point out that the neural structures regulating consciousness differ from and are more anatomically distant from those regulating motor function.

Concussion. In mild concussion, the loss of consciousness may not occur or lasts a relatively short time (20 minutes or less) and there is little or no retrograde amnesia. A concussion can cause diffuse axonal injury and result in either temporary or permanent damage. The client may be irritable or distractible and have difficulty with reading and memory. There may be complaints of headache, fatigue, dizziness, and changes in personality and emotional disposition. This group of symptoms constitutes what is called *posttraumatic syndrome.* The effects of repeated concussions (second impact syndrome) are cumulative.[20]

Coma. *Coma* is defined as a complete paralysis of cerebral function; a state of unresponsiveness. The eyes are closed, and there is no response to painful stimuli. Within

BOX 24-3 ■ COGNITIVE, PERSONALITY, AND BEHAVIORAL CHANGES RESULTING FROM BRAIN INJURY

Cognitive changes might include any or all of the following:

- Temporary or permanent disorders of intellectual function
- Memory loss
- Shortened attention span
- Concentration problems
- Confusion
- Changes in motivation
- Difficulty sustaining attention
- Executive function loss (executive functions are those that affect how behavior is regulated); Lezak[18] outlined four functions:
  1. Choosing a goal
  2. Developing a plan
  3. Executing a plan
  4. Evaluating the execution of the plan
- Reduced problem-solving skills
- Lack of initiative
- Loss of reasoning
- Poor abstract thinking
- Shortened attention span

Behavioral changes could include the following:

- Lability
- Uncontrolled anger
- Irritability
- Euphoria
- Intolerance
- Inappropriate sexual behavior
- Perseveration (repetition of movements or sounds)
- Impulsiveness
- Hyperactivity

2 to 4 weeks, nearly all clients in coma begin to awaken. Oculomotor and pupillary signs are valuable in assisting with the diagnosis, localizing brain stem damage, and determining the depth of coma.[19] In coma, brain stem responses may include grimacing to pain, which is frequently associated with a flexor or localizing motor response, loss of hearing or balance, abnormal palate and tongue movements, and loss or distortion of taste.

Stupor. Stupor is a condition of general unresponsiveness. The client is usually mute but can be temporarily aroused by vigorous and repeated stimuli.

Obtundity. *Obtundity* describes the condition of a client who sleeps a great deal and who, when aroused, exhibits reduced alertness, disinterest in the environment, and slow responses to stimulation.

Delirium. Delirium is often observed in recovery from unconsciousness after severe brain injury. Disorientation, fear, and misinterpretation of sensory stimuli characterize this state. The client is frequently loud, agitated, and offensive.

Clouding of Consciousness. Clouding of consciousness is a state of quiet confusion, distractibility, faulty memory, and slowed responses to stimuli.

Persistent Vegetative State. Finally, no discussion of changes in consciousness would be complete without mention of those unfortunate enough to remain in a "persistent vegetative state." This state is characterized by a wakeful, reduced responsiveness with no evident cerebral cortical function. The vegetative state can result from diffuse cerebral hypoxia or from severe, diffuse white matter impact damage. The brain stem is usually relatively intact. Clients may track with their eyes and show minimal spontaneous motor activities that even appear purposeful, but they do not speak, nor do they respond to verbal stimulation.[21] Life expectancy can be weeks, months, or years.[22,23] Clients with brain injury who remain vegetative for 3 months rarely achieve an independent outcome. However, the term "persistent" should not be added to "vegetative state" until the injury has stabilized or the state has lasted for approximately 1 year.[24] Functional magnetic resonance imaging (fMRI) was recently used to test clients who were diagnosed as being in persistent vegetative states. Five of 54 clients diagnosed as in a persistent vegetative state demonstrated "willful, neuroanatomically specific blood-oxygenated–level–dependent responses when told to visualize one of two tasks."[25] The diagnosis of persistent vegetative state indicates lack of cortical function, and fMRI may be useful in this diagnosis in the future. Recovery of consciousness, if it occurs, includes a gradual return of orientation and recent memory.[19] The duration of each of these stages is variable and can be prolonged. Improvement can stop at any point.

Other Complications

A list of the complications that may accompany brain injury would be limitless. In addition to any concomitant injuries, some of the diagnostic, monitoring, and therapeutic procedures themselves carry hazards. So does prolonged bed rest. Catheters, nasogastric tubes, and tracheotomies can cause iatrogenic injuries. Infections, contractures, skin breakdown, thrombophlebitis, pulmonary problems, heterotopic ossification (HO), and surgical complications are but a few of the risks. Posttraumatic epilepsy is also a possible sequela. Depression occurs frequently after brain injury, and it can alter functional outcome. It appears that a combination of neuroanatomical, neurochemical, and psychosocial factors are responsible for the onset and maintenance of the depression.[26]

Locked-in Syndrome. Locked-in syndrome occurs rarely and can be confused with coma. The client cannot move any part of the body except the eyes but is able to think and is conscious.[27]

Communication Disorders. Communication disorders include expressive and receptive language aphasia and dysarthria.

Amnesia. Two types of amnesia are frequently associated with brain injury: retrograde and posttraumatic.[28] Cartlidge and Shaw[14] define *retrograde amnesia* as a "partial or total loss of the ability to recall events that have occurred during the period immediately preceding brain injury." The duration of the retrograde amnesia may progressively decrease. *Posttraumatic amnesia* (PTA) is defined "as the time lapse between the accident and the point at which the functions concerned with memory are judged to have been restored."[14] The duration of PTA is considered a clinical indicator of the severity of the injury.[14] An additional deficit can be the inability to form new memory, referred to as *anterograde memory.* The capacity for anterograde memory is frequently the last function to return after recovery from loss of consciousness.[29]

Memory. The client's inability to develop continuing short-term memory can be quite frustrating for the rehabilitation team as well as for the client because memory is an important component of learning.[30] There are two types of memory: *declarative* and *procedural.* Memory in which the client can recall facts and events of a previous experience is declarative memory. Explicit learning, a conscious verbal learning, is based on declarative memory. However, many clients who cannot reproduce memories through conscious recollection do have the ability to learn new motor skills. Implicit learning, a noncognitive type of learning in which clients can show changes in performance after prior experience, is based on procedural memory. Clients can show the ability to change motor, perceptual, or cognitive behaviors with practice or training but may lack declarative memory. That procedural memory may be present without declarative memory in clients with TBI has been demonstrated.[28]

Initial Care and Medical Interventions

On the client's admission to the hospital, a neurosurgeon usually assumes initial and primary responsibility for the client. The first priority in medical care is resuscitation, after which baseline assessments are made and a history is obtained. Immediate surgery may or may not be indicated. Surgery is indicated when blood and necrotic tissue are present in the cranial vault. Early concerns may include the management of respiratory dysfunction, cardiovascular monitoring, treatment of raised ICP by means of pharmacological, mechanical, or surgical procedures,[14] and general medical care. Examples of general medical care are familiar: maintenance of fluid and electrolyte balance, nutrition, eye and skin care, prevention of contractures, postural drainage, and safety considerations.[6] The need for this type of care gradually lessens as the client responds, or it may continue if unconsciousness persists. Initially, a determination of Glasgow Coma Scale[31] (GCS) score (Box 24-4) is performed to test the function of the brain stem and the cerebrum through eye, motor, and verbal responses. It provides a measure of the level of consciousness. Scores range from 3 to 15, with lower scores associated with lower levels of function. Scores from 13 to 15 indicate a mild brain injury, 9 to 12 a moderate brain injury, and 8 or less a severe injury.

Several scales define TBI as mild, moderate, or severe based on specific measurements (Table 24-1). Because the definition of mild brain injury has varied so widely, the CDC convened a panel of experts to further define it. The new definition of mild TBI is an injury to the head (arising from blunt trauma or acceleration or deceleration forces) that results in one or more of the following: any period of confusion, disorientation, or impaired consciousness; any dysfunction of memory around the time of injury; loss of consciousness lasting less than 30 minutes; or the onset of observed signs or symptoms of neurological or neuropsychological dysfunction.[2] According to the Brain Injury Association of America, with a moderate TBI the client experiences a loss of consciousness that lasts from a few minutes to a few hours; confusion that lasts from days to weeks; and physical, cognitive, or behavioral impairments that last for months or are permanent. A severe brain injury occurs when a prolonged unconscious state or coma lasts days, weeks, or months. With the possible exception of the diagnosis and hence prognosis of diffuse white matter impact damage,[32] one third of clients hospitalized with brain injuries have extracranial injuries,[6] which are explored with a physical examination and appropriate special tests. Additional testing depends on the client's particular dysfunctions. CT,[33] MRI, positron emission tomography (PET), radioisotope imaging, ventriculography, echoencephalography, electroencephalography, monitoring of ICP, measurement of cerebral blood flow and metabolism, monitoring of cardiorespiratory and cardiovascular function, and tests of cerebrospinal fluid and other biochemical studies all provide important information. Changes in electrocerebral potentials that occur in response to specific stimuli also are studied. Visual, auditory, and somatosensory evoked potential examinations are used with

BOX 24-4 ■ GLASGOW COMA SCALE

Eye Opening	**E**
Spontaneous	4
To speech	3
To pain	2
Nil	1
Best Motor Response	**M**
Obeys	6
Localizes	5
Withdraws	4
Abnormal flexion	3
Extensor response	2
Nil	1
Verbal Response	**V**
Oriented	5
Confused conversation	4
Inappropriate words	3
Incomprehensible sounds	2
Nil	1
Coma Score (E + M + V) =	**3 to 15**

From Jennett B, Teasdale G: *Management of head injuries,* Philadelphia, 1981, FA Davis.

TABLE 24-1 ■ SEVERITY OF TRAUMATIC BRAIN INJURY

MEASUREMENT	MILD	MODERATE	SEVERE
Glasgow Coma Scale	13-15	9-12	3-8
Loss of consciousness	<30 min	30 min-24 hr	>24 hr
Posttraumatic amnesia	0-1 day	>1 to ≤7 days	>7 days

clients with brain injury but are more effective when combined with other examinations.[34] These examinations make it possible to observe the presence, evolution, and resolution of a lesion.[6] Reflex motor responses in unconscious clients are tested by applying a noxious stimulus, such as pressure on a nail bed with a pencil or supraorbital pressure, and observing the response. Most responses generally fall into three categories: appropriate, inappropriate, or absent.[19] Testing for cognitive and behavioral functions is usually done via neuropsychological tests. In some circumstances the results of IQ tests, achievement tests, and Armed Forces tests may be available for comparison. Differentiating changes in cognitive and behavioral functions caused by brain injury from posttraumatic stress syndrome, conversion or hysterical reactions, malingering, depression, and anxiety is extremely important.

Surgical Interventions

Patients with epidural hematomas often undergo craniotomies with blood evacuation. Subdural injuries are frequently treated by removing the blood through bur holes.

Pharmacological Interventions

Medications are chosen according to symptoms to be treated. Many of these recommendations are from a meta-analysis of management of severe TBI published in 2007.[35-39]

Drugs that Decrease Intracranial Pressure. When ICP increases, changes in PCO_2 are seen. The maintenance of a PCO_2 at 30 to 40 mm Hg appears most appropriate. Osmotic agents such as mannitol are used to pull fluid from brain tissue back into the blood system, thus lowering ICP. Propofol, a barbiturate, is recommended for control of ICP if it cannot be controlled by other means.[35] Use of mannitol is recommended for clients who have profusion problems.[35] ICP has been lowered by intentional hyperventilation, which causes an increase in blood PCO_2, resulting in vasoconstriction of the central vessels and reduced cerebral blood flow. However, Muizelaar and colleagues[40] as well as information from the Traumatic Coma Data Bank[41] showed that dramatically reducing a client's PCO_2 in this manner resulted in a worse outcome than that in clients managed with medication. Therefore hyperventilation is currently used only for nonresponsive cases and for short durations. Glucocorticoids (dexamethasone [Decadron], methylprednisolone [Solu-Medrol]) have been used to treat cerebral edema, but most studies show no long-term changes in outcome, and methylprednisolone is contraindicated because it increases mortality.[39] See Chapter 36 for additional information.

Drugs that Control Blood Pressure. Blood pressure control is important in clients with brain injury. Cerebral perfusion pressure[42] or adequate blood pressure to maintain cerebral blood flow against increased ICP is calculated by subtracting the ICP from the mean arterial pressure. If fluid management cannot keep the blood pressures elevated, then vasopressor drugs such as phenylephrine (Neo-Synephrine) are used to constrict peripheral vessels but not the vessels of the brain.

Drugs that Affect the Motor, Behavioral, and Cognitive Functions (See Chapter 36). Medications also may be prescribed for motor abnormalities involving increases in tone. Baclofen is now used more frequently with clients with brain injury; however, it can produce lethargy, confusion,[43] and reduction in attention span[44] in some clients. These effects are greatly reduced with implantation of a pump to deliver the drug. Dantrolene sodium is another medication used to decrease spasticity and rigidity. This drug works directly at the muscle level and therefore is less likely to cause cognitive disturbances but more likely to cause generalized weakness.[45] Botulinum toxin type A (Botox) is widely used to inject into specific muscles, such as the finger flexors, biceps, or gastrocnemius, to decrease their tone. Diazepam (Valium) initially was the drug most commonly administered for spasticity or high tone. However, diazepam also promotes drowsiness and decreased responsiveness and can increase muscle weakness and ataxia.[43] These side effects actually hinder rather than assist in rehabilitation. Glenn and Wroblewski[44] conclude that "rarely, if ever, are the benefits of diazepam's antispasticity effect great enough to justify its use in the brain-injured population." Drugs to treat behavioral or cognitive dysfunction have not been particularly successful. Antidepressive drugs as well as carbamazepine (Tegretol) and propranolol (Inderal) have been used to treat aggression and agitation. Carbamazepine appears to reduce agitation or aggression in clients with brain injury.[46] Confusion and other neuropsychotic symptoms have been treated using neuroleptic medications. A recent review article suggests that these drugs may negatively affect motor outcomes.[47] Sedative drugs prescribed in an attempt to control delirium may add to the client's confusion and may also contribute to a decreased responsiveness. Later in the rehabilitative process, various antidepressants may be used to treat aggressive and disruptive behaviors. These, too, may have deleterious side effects. Antidepressants other than the tricyclics appear to be the most effective for treating depression.

Attention Deficits. Methylphenidate may increase information processing in some clients, but the evidence is still weak.[48] Traumatically acquired neuroendocrine dysfunctions, such as hyperphagia and thermal regulation, also may be treated with pharmacological agents.[49]

Pain. Severe, intractable pain may be present in clients who have had injury to the thalamus. In these cases, some of the antiseizure drugs appear to be more effective, including phenytoin (Dilantin) and gabapentin (Neurontin). Late seizure control is usually through valproic acid (Depakote or Depakene).

Prevention of Brain Cell Death. Hypothermia is frequently used in acute severe TBI. Although it does not appear to change the mortality rate, it is associated with improved functional outcome on the Glasgow Outcome Scale (GOS) (Box 24-5).[36]

For a variety of reasons, other pharmaceutical agents are prescribed as an adjunct to care. Antibiotics may be used with respiratory complications or with compound fractures and infections.

Prognostic Indicators

Numerous problems are encountered in trying to predict outcome. Included among these problems are the validity and reliability of the tests used, the uniform implementation and interpretation of predictive factors, the percentage of error in prediction, the possible effects of intervention strategies and

BOX 24-5 ■ GLASGOW OUTCOME SCALE

VEGETATIVE STATE

A persistent state characterized by reduced responsiveness associated with wakefulness. The client may exhibit eye opening, sucking, yawning, and localized motor responses.

SEVERE DISABILITY

An outcome characterized by consciousness, but the client has 24-hour dependence because of cognitive, behavioral, or physical disabilities, including dysarthria and dysphasia.

MODERATE DISABILITY

An outcome characterized by independence in activities of daily living and in home and community activities but with disability. Clients in this category may have memory or personality changes, hemiparesis, dysphagia, ataxia, acquired epilepsy, or major cranial nerve deficits.

GOOD RECOVERY

Client able to reintegrate into normal social life and able to return to work. There may be mild persisting sequelae.

Modified from Jennett B, Bond M: Assessment of outcome after severe brain damage: a practical scale. *Lancet* 1:480, 1975.

bias in treatment on the basis of predictions, and, finally, the definition of what constitutes a "successful" outcome. Understanding these problems is imperative because the therapist can provide persuasive suggestions regarding the type and intensity of rehabilitative care after injury. The differences in operational definitions, types and sizes of populations, and length of time after injury when the outcome assessment was made contribute to the lack of consistency in studies of predictive factors for clients with brain injury. For example, several authors have found that clients younger than age 20 years usually recover better[50-52]; however, this has not been uniformly confirmed. A reason for caution in using tests for prediction is the percentage of error in prediction. If prediction is 80% or even 90% accurate, there are still 10% to 20% of the clients with head trauma whose outcome may be predicted incorrectly.[53]

Lesion Size and Area

There is conflicting evidence regarding recovery outcomes on the basis of lesion size and area because the type of lesion and the rapidity with which lesions occur have an impact on both the deficits and the size. There is some evidence that lesion area rather than size is important. Van der Naalt and co-workers[54,55] looked at 67 patients with brain injuries in the mild to moderate injury categories and found that frontal and frontotemporal lesions were predictive of poorer outcomes than lesions in other areas. However, Kurth and colleagues[56] looked at number of acute hemorrhages, lesion volume, and location in TBI using neuropsychological outcome measures and found no relationship between the numbers of hemorrhages and the volume of injury. Brain MRI in 80 adult patients (6 to 8 weeks after injury) was predictive of nonrecovery from persistent vegetative states at 12 months when the client had corpus callosum and dorsolateral brain stem lesions.[57] Lesion location is not a significant predictor of GOS scores. Lesions in the brain stem do appear to cause poorer outcomes on the GOS than other lesions.[58,59]

Time Since Lesion

Better functional outcomes were found in monkeys when rehabilitation occurred earlier after the lesion. Black and colleagues[60] created lesions in the motor cortices of 27 adolescent rhesus monkeys and then trained them in motor tasks involving the arm. Active postoperative training of the weak hand led to recovery of 82% of the preoperative function in 6 months if the therapy was initiated immediately. Recovery was only 67% of preoperative control if training was delayed 4 months.

Age

Age is an important factor in recovery. Beginning at age 40 years, older patients have significantly longer PTA and worse functional outcome at any severity.[61]

Posttraumatic Amnesia

PTA duration is better related to outcome than either lesion area or size.[61] Postinjury amnesia had a predictable relationship to length of coma in patients with diffuse axonal injury. Duration of PTA was strongly correlated with the GOS score at 6 and 12 months after injury in patients with diffuse axonal injury but poorly correlated in patients with primarily focal brain injury. Van der Naalt and colleagues'[54] study of the GCS indicates that this scale, applied 12 months after injury, is a simple and consistent predictor of outcomes in clients with a score of 9 to 11 (mild to moderate brain injury). PTA is a strong predictor of outcome as measured by the Functional Independence Measure (FIM) (an activity level measurement tool)[62]; and when PTA is combined with age, sitting balance, and limb strength at admission, prediction of productive outcome is high.[63] Walker and colleagues[64] also found that when PTA lasted less than 4 weeks, a severe activity limitation was unlikely; and if longer than 8 weeks, a good recovery was unlikely when measured by GOS.

Sitting and Standing Balance

Age younger than 50 years had a significant association with normal sitting and standing balance. Measures of severity of TBI, including admission Glasgow Coma GCS score, length of PTA, length of coma, and acute care length of stay, were also each significantly related to impaired sitting and standing balance. Initial abnormalities in pupillary response, respiratory failure, pneumonia, soft tissue infections, and urinary tract infections had a significant relationship with impairment of sitting but not standing balance. Presence of intracranial hemorrhages did not have a significant relationship with either sitting or standing balance. Intracranial compression had a significant relationship with standing balance. Discriminant functional analysis showed no relationship between balance ratings and neurological or radiological findings, injury severity, or medical complications.[65]

Other Factors

Finally, several studies have reported that absence of previous TBI,[42] a higher level of educational achievement, and stable work history also are positive preinjury variables for a better prognosis.[66] The Wechsler Adult Intelligence Scale (WAIS)—Revised IQ test may correlate with prognosis according to other studies.[66]

Motor disturbances resulting from brain injury generally have a good prognosis.[14] Of the physical deficits encountered, dysfunctions in the cerebral hemispheres and of the cranial nerves are the most common disorders, and these may partially resolve. Losses of these functions can be more permanent,[11,14] especially without skilled rehabilitation interventions. Complete recovery is rare except with hearing, vestibular function, and smell. In one Glasgow study, some degree of hemiparesis was present 6 months after injury in 49% of the 150 clients who regained consciousness after severe brain injury.[6]

Psychosocial outcomes vary after severe brain injury.[67] Psychosocial variables that significantly increased life satisfaction for persons with TBI were total family satisfaction, being employed, being married, having memory, bowel independence, and not blaming oneself for the injury. Those who do not blame themselves show a greater number of functional activities as indicators for their self-satisfaction.[68]

See Box 24-6 for factors that can influence recovery and management.

CONCEPTUAL FRAMEWORK FOR THERAPEUTIC INTERVENTION

Motor Control Theory

Motor control and learning theories try to explain how the central nervous system (CNS) accomplishes the miracle of coordinated, meaningful movement. Motor control theory and factors affecting effectiveness and speed of motor learning are reviewed in this section and are discussed in detail in Chapter 4. This chapter's examination, evaluation, and intervention technique sections are based on that framework. A quick review of basic principles follows.

Synergistic Organization

Synergies, or motor patterns, were viewed by Bernstein[69] as the basis of movement. The need for the brain to use synergistic organization comes from the infinite number of movement combinations that are available. By use of motor patterns, which decrease the number of degrees of freedom, speed and efficiency are added while flexibility of response is maintained. Force (amplitude) of contraction, velocity, and timing can still be changed to meet task demands. Research suggests that motor patterns are shaped

BOX 24-6 ■ FACTORS THAT CAN INFLUENCE MANAGEMENT AND RECOVERY AFTER A TRAUMATIC BRAIN INJURY

PREINJURY CHARACTERISTICS

Cognitive Factors
1. Intelligence*
2. Memory
3. Level of education

Behavioral Factors
1. Personality*
2. Psychological status

Social Factors
1. Vocational skills
2. Avocational skills
3. Interpersonal skills
4. Family and friends support systems

Physical Factors
1. Age*
2. General health and physical fitness
3. Existing physical deficits
4. Morphology
5. Level of motor skill development and capacity for motor learning

POSTINJURY CHARACTERISTICS

Static Factors
1. Trauma factors (neurological)
   a. Location(s) and extent of injury
   b. Cause and type of injury*
   c. Immediacy of injury*
2. Cognitive factors
   a. Ultimate duration of retrograde amnesia*
   b. Ultimate duration of posttraumatic amnesia*
3. Physical factors: extracranial injuries

Dynamic Factors
1. Trauma factors (neurological)
   a. Depth and duration of coma*
   b. Secondary brain damage
   c. Brain stem reflexes
   d. Special investigations (radiological and laboratory tests)
2. Cognitive factors
   a. Rate of recovery of intellectual and memory functions*
   b. Quality of recovery of intellectual and memory functions*
   c. Communication disorders
3. Behavioral factors
   a. Primary personality changes*
   b. Secondary personality changes*
   c. Psychological status
4. Social factors
   a. Opportunity to reenter occupation or school
   b. Avocational reintegration abilities
   c. Reaction to family and friends
   d. Family adjustment and support capabilities*
5. Physical factors
   a. Pattern and quality of sensorimotor recovery*
   b. Rate of recovery of sensorimotor function*
   c. Range of motion and muscle flexibility
   d. Cranial nerve deficits
   e. Concomitant disabilities
6. Environmental factors
   a. Staff, facilities, equipment available
   b. Attitude of health care providers
   c. Expertise of health care providers
   d. Room or housing and treatment settings

*Discussed in the text.

through experience and that they develop before birth (innate) and after birth (learned). Early experiments on motor learning demonstrate how motor patterns may develop. Payton and Kelley[70] showed that with practice of a novel motor task, movements become more organized and skilled.

Characteristics of a Learned Skill (Motor Pattern). In learning a new skill, movement begins with a "gross approximation" of the movement that includes agonist-antagonist co-contraction. As movement is refined, reciprocal movement replaces co-contraction.[71] In electrophysiological studies of skill acquisition, less electrical activity is seen on electromyography (EMG) and less time to peak activation of the muscle is noted in motor tasks after they become skillful. In addition, fewer muscles are recruited for the same movement.[72] PET scans have confirmed these EMG findings, demonstrating decreasing areas of brain activity after skill acquisition. Neuronal changes brought about through long-term potentiation and long-term depression are a basis for learning new tasks and developing motor patterns and behavioral changes.[73] As neurons are repetitively fired at the same time, networks develop. These neuronetworks, or cell assemblies, are formed with increasing complexity and self-organization. The more they are used, the stronger and more permanent are the changes that occur. Finally, a specific stimulus now provokes a learned or skilled response as an organized synergy. The output of the networks is not a summation of individual functions but has "emergent properties" that are more than the sum of the output of individual neurons.

The best understood motor patterns are the balance and reaching patterns. Both appear to be basic innate synergies. Quiet standing in humans is maintained by somatosensory, visual, and vestibular inputs (see Chapter 22). It requires the coordination of many muscles, especially those of the hips, knees, and ankles, to maintain the body's center of gravity over its base of support. This complex coordination of muscle control is accomplished by sequences of stereotyped patterns mediated through the brain stem, cerebellum, and spinal cord. Somatosensory input during body sway stimulates the response in which posture is stabilized by small changes in the angle between the foot and the leg. For small and slower center of gravity movements, these synergies are sequenced in a distal to proximal manner. The direction of sway determines the particular synergy elicited to correct for the shift in the center of gravity. In forward losses of balance, the posterior extensor muscles of the legs and trunk respond at about 100 ms. In backward losses the anterior muscles respond, including the anterior tibialis, hip flexors, and abdominals. The timing between muscle contractions and the proximal-to-distal sequence are preset. The amplitude of contraction varies with the environmental demands and the amount and velocity of sway. In larger or more rapid sway, a different synergy is used; the person may bend at the hips and knees, or a hip strategy or a combination of hip and ankle strategies is used. If the balance loss is great enough, the person takes a step to maintain upright balance.[74] (For additional information, see Chapter 22A on balance and 22B on vestibular dysfunction). In gait, weight shifts from one leg to the other and stability after the weight shift are other aspects of dynamic balance performed through motor patterns. The movement pattern of the swing leg in gait is limited in the number of degrees of freedom at each joint and the sequence of movement by motor patterns. There is also a specific coordination and timing of swing leg movement in relation to the stance leg movement (interlimb timing and coordination) accomplished through motor patterns. In gait, the sequence of contraction of the leg muscle from ankle to hip, the time of onset of the contraction of each muscle, and a ratio of force for each muscle is preset in the motor control program of the brain or spinal cord. If an increase in speed is needed, step length, cadence, and force can be increased within the synergy, but the basic synergies, or motor patterns, are what give identity to a gait pattern. Whether the person is walking quickly or slowly, there is an individually recognizable pattern.

In the reaching and grasping pattern, three components have been identified: the reaching portion (transport), the grasping or prehension portion, and the maintenance of balance. Reaching and maintenance of balance are accomplished through motor patterns.[75,76] The target determines the reaching pattern. Characteristics of the reaching synergy include a distal-to-proximal sequence of firing, and movement is in a straight line with a bell-shaped velocity curve.[77] The prehension portion of reach and grasp is not a synergistic movement, and the motor-sensory cortex helps with force production and selection of muscles[78] during hand movement to meet task demands. This may be why more severe deficits are seen in the hand after cortical injury.

Anticipatory and Adaptive Responses

To meet the motor task (external) requirements, motor patterns are used and modified through a feed-forward and feedback system of control. The brain adapts motor patterns to environmental constraints, such as obstacles, by modifying the basic motor patterns' velocity, intensity, or duration of contractions before the movement even begins. Feed-forward or anticipatory responses (often from vision and past memory of successful movements) are provided by muscles that will stabilize before the prime mover of a motion begins to fire and thus are the first muscle contraction that occurs during a movement that might disrupt stability. For example, before a rapid forward reach, the gastrocnemius muscles fire to reduce the amount of forward sway that would occur secondary to the forward movement of the center of gravity.[79]

Adaptive responses use sensory feedback (visual or proprioceptive feedback is most commonly used) to improve the effectiveness of a response. After a movement, the brain checks to determine that the motor pattern matched the original "planned" pattern. Adaptive responses provide for modifications of movements, especially when the environment is changing. An example would be the ability to change the balance response when stepping from a firm surface onto a surface that is unexpectedly soft. A person will lose balance the first time but should be able to perform with good balance after several attempts. Sensory information helps fine-tune or adapt the subsequent movements within a synergistic movement. For gait, sensory impulses drive motor system adaptations to the environment. In the reaching-prehension pattern, tactile input from the fingertips (feedback) is used to make adjustments in grip force if the initial grip was not effective.[80] Once movement occurs, there is a final comparison of the original planned pattern with the executed pattern to see whether they match; if not, then more adaptations are made.

Dynamic Pattern Theory and New Patterns

Once called *motor control theory,* the dynamic pattern theory[81,82] addresses problems when motor behavior changes and also uses concepts of basic patterns of movement. This theory states that certain patterns are stable or unstable and that transition between patterns or to a new pattern depends on pattern stability. (See Giuliani[83] for a summary of this theory.) The challenge for therapists is to identify what makes these "stuck" behaviors become unstable and perhaps amenable to change. Patterns that are "set" are much more difficult to change than those that are more variable. In fact, phase transitions between old and new patterns are noted by periods of increased variability. The client appears to vacillate between the old and the new behaviors during transition phases and before new behavior establishment points. Transition phases are often frustrating for clients, as they feel unstable and may think that therapy is making them worse. Repetition is important to develop more consistent motor patterns and new establishment points; however, more important is preparing the client to expect this change.

Motor Learning

Three stages have been identified for motor learning: the cognitive stage, during which the performer begins to understand the task; the associative stage, in which performance is refined; and the autonomous stage, in which the task performance is skilled (a consistent motor pattern is formed).

Byl[84] noted that motor cortex (M1) changes occurred (motor learning) when (1) new or novel tasks were used, (2) movements were practiced together (spatial organization and temporal organization), (3) movements were frequently repeated, and (4) movements were important to the individual.

Interventions are designed to produce a task-oriented behavioral change that becomes permanent without continued therapist help or intervention. When this does not happen, the client performs well during therapy but does not seem to carry the improved performance outside the clinic. This difference between performance and learning is discussed by Schmidt.[85,86] Many things affect motor learning, among which are knowledge of results (KR) and type of practice. (See Chapter 4.)

Knowledge of Results

Information on how successful the movement was in meeting the task goal is basic to learning. Knowledge of results (KR) consists of extrinsic information over and above that provided by the task itself.[87] During the practice portion of most tasks, increasing any type of feedback appears to improve task performance.[88] But long-term learning may be improved when KR is provided less often. The relative frequency with which KR is provided in relation to the number of trials is important in learning. Bandwidth KR, in which information is given about trials falling outside a certain range, and a random schedule of feedback appear to be effective for many learning situations in therapy. Delaying KR also improves learning.[87]

Practice Type

The type of practice is important for clients who are learning new skills. A commonly used technique to simplify a task by practicing at a slower speed or practicing a part of a motor task is often not effective. For example, weight shifting is often practiced as a component of gait before walking is initiated. Winstein and colleagues[89] demonstrated that this part practice did not transfer to gait in a group of clients who had had a stroke. In a study by Man and colleagues,[90] a complex task was broken down into adaptive training methods (e.g., slower motions) and part-task training (on components of the task). Subjects who practiced the whole task had better performance than either of the other groups. A finding that practicing small components of a task does not make one better at the whole task is not too surprising. Many of us can jump, have good shoulder power, and can throw overhead but cannot, without practice, put this together to play basketball. A minimum basic amount of strength, range of motion (ROM), and interlimb sequencing is necessary to play basketball but is not adequate to play without the actual practice of the sport.

However, practicing other than the whole task may be possible. By use of the same task as that used by Man and colleagues,[90] Newell and colleagues[91] showed that part-task training was effective when it was conducted in natural subtasks of the whole. These subtasks are part of the whole task but are distinguished by changes in speed or direction. This area of skill acquisition has not been studied adequately to identify subtasks of most common movements. A recent meta-analysis reviews use of part practice and methods of part practice for the most effective motor learning.[92] Whole practice appears best for tasks low in complexity and high in organization as well as for discrete or serial tasks with high organization. An example might be a golf swing. Part practice appears effective for tasks high in complexity and low in organization, for example, dancing.

Finally, many therapy techniques that improve a client's immediate performance inhibit learning because they are based on the external controls and support provided by the therapist's manipulations, markedly changing the basic task. The types of feedback and the methods by which they are provided are critical to learning new motor skills. For example, when the hip stabilization component of walking is externally provided by the therapist during gait training, the client has no need to develop his or her own hip stabilization patterns, and feedback lacks a basic component of gait. Therefore the manual guidance may give the client a feeling of the movement pattern, but to continue to provide the hands-on control deprives the client of learning the balance and anticipatory components himself or herself.

To review, the conceptual framework for the evaluation and intervention of clients with TBI is based on distributed motor control theory, which states that movement is task or goal oriented and a result of combined systems working together to produce synergistic movement (motor pattern). Synergistic movement has an anticipatory component that is matched with sensory feedback and previous experience to contribute to task refinement through adaptation. Changes in motor behavior may be determined by how "set" the patterns are (dynamic pattern theory). They are influenced by the type of practice, knowledge of the effectiveness of the results, and how the motor skills are broken down for practice.

EXAMINATION, EVALUATION, PROGNOSIS, DIAGNOSIS, AND INTERVENTION

Terminology and Structure for Client Management

The World Health Organization (WHO), in the International Classification of Functioning, Disability and Health (ICF),[93] has developed a common terminology that is used in this chapter. Definitions are as follows (also see Chapter 1 and Figure 30-2):

- *Body functions* are physiological functions of body systems (including psychological functions).
- *Body structures* are anatomical parts of the body such as organs, limbs, and their components.
- *Impairments* are problems in body function or structure such as a significant deviation or loss.
- *Activity* is the execution of a task or action by an individual.
- *Participation* is involvement in a life situation.
- *Activity limitations* are difficulties an individual may have in executing activities.
- *Participation restrictions* are problems an individual may experience in involvement in life situations.
- *Environmental factors* make up the physical, social, and attitudinal environment in which people live and conduct their lives.

The American Physical Therapy Association has published levels of client management leading to optimal outcomes.[94] The Association's *Guide to Physical Therapist Practice,* which uses examination, evaluation, diagnosis, prognosis, intervention, and outcomes as its basis, will be followed in this chapter. Although this is the terminology used by physical therapists, its application and integration into the profession of occupational therapy should be simultaneously acknowledged. The method used in this chapter for gathering the guide information is based on the Hypothesis-Oriented Algorithm for Clinicians (HOAC II) model.[95] See Box 24-7 for an overview of this method, and see the text that follows for details of how to perform these items.

BOX 24-7 ■ DEVELOPMENT OF INTERVENTION APPROACHES LOOSELY BASED ON HOAC II MODEL[95]

Collect initial data.
Have client and family identify client problems with activity and participation limitations.
Develop an initial set of hypotheses based on a task analysis of identified activity limitations; choose and apply examinations to test those hypotheses.
Reassess hypotheses in light of examination findings and confirm or deny. Repeat first three steps if denied.
Develop list of non–client-identified problems, including anticipated problems (such as skin breakdown when sensation is impaired).
Choose and apply appropriate outcome measures to monitor progress that address the impairments or activity limitations.
Develop an evaluation and diagnosis identifying why the problems exist or are likely to occur in the future.
Establish a prognosis, and set goals with time frames for achievement.
Develop interventions that most effectively ameliorate the problems based on current literature or best practice.
Reexamine using outcome measures to determine progress.

Examination

Data are collected from referral information, from the medical record, via observation, and from the client or family interview. A history is taken and should include information regarding the mechanism, GCS score initially, extent and time since onset of injury, client's age, and duration of PTA. This information will be used to help establish a prognosis. Other information about education, family support, and living circumstances will also help with the prognosis as well as with discharge planning. Complications as well as coexisting diseases are reviewed with the client in order to discuss a thorough care plan as well as determine appropriate referrals. Finally, the therapist will develop a list of patient-identified problems (PIPs) and a list of potential problems that could develop secondary to the injury (non–patient-identified problems [NPIPs]).

Examination should lead to an understanding of the underlying causes of the activity or participation limitations and should be the basis of the intervention program. Clients usually present their problems as activity limitations, for example, "I can no longer walk very far."

Once activity limitations have been determined, a task analysis can be completed by having the client demonstrate the problem—in this case, walking. The therapist will develop a hypothesis as to why the observed deviation from typical performance is present. Tests and measures will be chosen on the basis of the therapist's knowledge of their importance in the task being performed to confirm the hypothesis. For example, in a client who drags his foot in initial swing, the client might lack 45 degrees of full passive knee flexion, but this is not critical in the task of walking. However, being able to dorsiflex the foot at initial swing is important. Therefore testing of both the ability to dorsiflex with the leg in the extended position and the speed at which the client can perform this task would be appropriate. The tests and measures should be chosen on the basis of the hypothesis that the therapist generates from the task analysis. For the components of examination, see Box 24-8.

Evaluation identifies the problems that can be managed by the therapist; serves to "tease" out those factors that influence or restrict the choice of therapeutic approaches; and states which components are most critical for the identified activity limitations. Evaluation provides a qualitative means of determining why a problem is present. It includes considerations of testing, motivation, and psychosocial areas. The evaluation thus determines intervention and goals. The purpose of the evaluation is to determine what prevents the client from performing in a functional, acceptable manner as identified by the client, the therapist, and society.

Diagnosis states the various causes of the problem to determine which are most critical. The therapist has a multilevel task that includes (1) identification of the components

BOX 24-8 ■ COMPONENTS OF EXAMINATION

I. History: injury, age, PTA, GCS score, job, home environment, educational level, previous injuries, and so on
II. Client and family data: client and family perception of the limitations, goals, personal factors, socioeconomic factors relating to participation limitations
III. Other health care team member evaluations
IV. Screens
  A. Systems review to emphasize precautions during intervention and to identify any "red flags" that will require referrals.
    1. Circulatory and respiratory
    2. Integumentary
    3. Musculoskeletal
    4. Autonomic nervous system—bowel, bladder
    5. Cognitive
    6. Language
    7. Emotional
V. Task analyses of client-identified problems
VI. Formation of hypotheses from the task analyses
VII. Choose specific tests and measures to confirm the hypotheses; these might include:
  A. Sensory
    1. Somatosensory
    2. Vestibular
    3. Visual
    4. Hearing
  B. Integrated, perceptual
  C. Motor
    1. Muscle strength
    2. Muscle flexibility
    3. Response speed
    4. Tone
    5. Movement speed
    6. Endurance and fatigue
    7. Complex impairments
      - Basic motor patterns available
      - Modification of motor patterns possible
      - Anticipatory and adaptive responses
      - Variability of performance
  D. Autonomic nervous system
  E. Cognitive
  F. Language
  G. Emotional

GCS, Glasgow Coma Scale; *PTA,* posttraumatic amnesia.

that compose a complex task or activity, and (2) evaluation of the degree to which a component's deficit contributes to loss of body function, activity limitation, or participation limitation. Prognosis is used to determine the optimal level of improvement that may be attained based on factors as discussed earlier. Prognosis includes short- and long-term goals that are specific to improved functions along with duration and frequency of intervention to achieve those goals. The interventions are provided by skilled professionals to treat the impairments and activity and participation limitations to achieve optimal outcomes.

Outcomes must be tested and usually are chosen to measure all levels of dysfunction from impairment through participation limitation to determine effectiveness of the intervention strategies and whether or not the client has met the goals. An example of the process is presented in Box 24-9.

Examination of the Client with Brain Injury

Cognitive, Behavioral, and Communication Deficits. Figure 24-1 depicts the close association of cognitive, behavioral, and physical functioning soon after injury. The three domains gradually become more distinguishable in later stages of recovery and can be assessed more independently; however, their interrelationships remain exceedingly complex. Cognition includes many aspects of function, including memory, learning, information processing, attention span, motivation, and initiation. Cognitive impairment was the primary contributor to activity limitation in most clients with TBI who scored at moderate to severe levels on the GOS.[96] Neuropsychologists, speech pathologists, and occupational therapists all perform testing of cognitive function. These tests may include word association, written word fluency, figural fluency, and card-sorting tests. Attention can be tested with the digit span and arithmetic tests on the WAIS[97] and by serial counting by 7. Information processing is reflected in reaction time tests and digit symbol tests. Choice reaction time is an indicator of information processing and commonly remains below normal in clients with brain injury.[98] Testing of intellectual functions is often done with the WAIS. However, formal testing of intellectual function can be hampered by inadequate perceptual, visual, and motor performance. Memory can also be tested with the WAIS and with the Galveston Orientation and Amnesia Test.[99] The Mini-Mental State Exam[100] is a memory screen often used by health care providers to determine whether further testing is indicated. Language and cognitive problems are frequently examined by speech pathologists and/or neuropsychologists using naming tests, aphasia examinations, and tests of auditory comprehension and speed of comprehension. A widely used system of cognitive function at the activities level is based on numerous observations of clients with brain injuries at Rancho Los Amigos Hospital. This has resulted in a descriptive categorization of various stages of "cognitive function," as shown in Appendix 24-A, with use of the Rancho Los Amigos Levels of Cognitive Functioning Scale.

Examination of Motor Functions

Although most of the following sections describe motor function, motor function is only a small part of the problem of the client with TBI. Social and family problems will likely be the most devastating in the long term. Motivation, attention skills, emotional instability, memory, learning, and social deficits are all cognitive processes that prevent or retard clients' progress in the therapy program as well as in home and work environments. Working with professionals who specialize in these areas will improve the client's chances to escape deficits that are permanently handicapping.

Task Analyses and Common Activity Level Impairments after Moderate to Severe Injury. Often the physical therapist begins the examination at the activity limitation level. This usually involves observing those functions

BOX 24-9 ■ CASE EXAMPLE OF EXAMINATION, EVALUATION, PROGNOSIS, INTERVENTION, AND OUTCOME MEASURES FOR A CLIENT WITH TRAUMATIC BRAIN INJURY

EXAMINATION

A client comes to your clinic reporting that he falls several times a week during walking and would like to improve his balance. He is 21 years old and suffered a moderate traumatic brain injury (TBI) 6 weeks ago. He had a Glasgow Coma Scale (GCS) score of 11 initially and 1.5 days of posttraumatic amnesia. He was at ABC Rehabilitation Center for 5 weeks and was discharged home last week. He lives with his parents in a single-story house. He is in his third year of college studying geology.

His systems review demonstrates slight decreased vital capacity of 3.8 L (4.6 L would be normal), but no abnormalities in the musculoskeletal systems or integumentary system. His cognitive functions are within normal limits according to neuropsychological testing, except for memory deficits.

TASK ANALYSIS

You observe this client during walking and note that he has decreased knee flexion in preswing and decreased dorsiflexion throughout swing phase, with the toe intermittently catching on the carpet when you have him speed up his walking. He also has decreased dorsiflexion at initial contact and in terminal stance.

HYPOTHESIS AND HYPOTHESIS TESTING

Because of the decreased dorsiflexion in terminal stance (which is passive), you hypothesize that the decreased dorsiflexion is secondary to gastrocnemius-soleus muscle tightness rather than anterior tibialis weakness. You test the range of motion (ROM) at the ankle, and it is within functional limits. You now develop a second hypothesis that there is increased tone in the gastrocnemius-soleus. On an Ashworth test, the client scores a level 3 for the gastrocnemius-soleus. Because the client does not get adequate plantarflexion at pre-wing (neutral versus 15 degrees for typical adults), you also hypothesize that the client is unable to generate plantarflexion fast enough in preswing to achieve the normal 15 degrees of plantarflexion. Testing by having the client plantar flex rapidly in standing shows that it takes a full 3 seconds to achieve 15 degrees of plantar flexion—much too long to be used in walking.

EVALUATION

The client is experiencing multiple weekly falls secondary to toe drag at initial swing when walking at speeds over 70 m/min. The toe drag comes from decreased dorsiflexion and decreased knee flexion at initial swing because of inadequate plantarflexion. Testing demonstrated both increased gastrocnemius-soleus tone (Ashworth level 3) and decreased ability to generate adequate plantarflexion to achieve the normal 40 degrees of knee flexion during preswing.

PROGNOSIS AND GOALS

The client has a good prognosis. He is early postinjury, is young, and has good family support and a high education level. There is no history of previous TBI. The client started rehabilitation immediately and in a center specialized for people with TBI. His posttraumatic amnesia was short.

Goals

1. The client will achieve 15 degrees of plantarflexion in preswing during walking at 90 m/min within 3 weeks and will be seen 3 × weekly × 3 weeks.
2. The client will not experience any toe drag during swing phase of gait while walking at 90 m/min or faster in 6 weeks. The client will receive 4 × weekly × 30 min body-weight–supported treadmill training (BWSTT) with functional electrical stimulation (FES) to the anterior tibialis muscle to accomplish this.

OUTCOME MEASURES

Gait speed, electromyography (EMG) for onset of contraction of the gastrocnemius-soleus, Rancho Los Amigos observational gait evaluation.[212]

INTERVENTIONS

BWSTT: Because there is only one study of BWSTT in subjects with acute TBI that did not measure changes in ankle motion or gait speed, the literature for cerebrovascular accident (CVA) was used. This literature shows improved gait speed overground and improved findings on EMG of ankle dorsiflexors in organization of contractions and timing.[186]

FES to gastrocnemius-soleus to improve timing and angle of plantarflexion during gait.

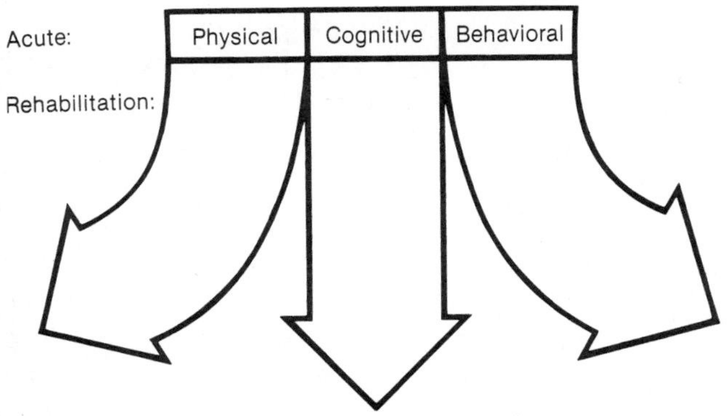

Figure 24-1 ■ Schema representing the close association of cognitive, behavioral, and physical functioning soon after injury. The three domains gradually become more distinguishable in the later stages of recovery.

that the client or family identifies as problems. Activity limitations in clients with TBI range over the entire spectrum of problems depending on the severity of injury. They may include loss of mobility in bed, coming to sit, sitting to standing; loss of household and community ambulation; loss of running, jumping, and kicking skills; poor reach and grasp; loss of throwing and batting skills; loss of activities of daily living (ADLs) such as dressing, toileting, and feeding; and loss of instrumental ADLs such as shopping and driving. The physical or occupational therapist performs a task analysis of the impaired function by comparing the client's performance of the task with typical task performance. For example, the therapist would observe the client performing the sitting-to-standing activity, observing that there is inadequate forward trunk momentum in the preextension phase.[101] A reasonable hypothesis may be that the client is fearful of falling forward.

If the problem is loss of balance in the extension phase, a hypothesis may be poor timing of the gastrocnemius firing. Both these hypotheses are based on the task analysis but also on the literature, which defines the importance of trunk momentum to initiate seat-off and timing of gastrocnemius firing during the end of the sitting-to-standing activity to maintain balance.

Examining activity limitations requires the understanding of the performance of the task in healthy individuals of about the same age as the client. Tasks that are described in the literature for typical performance include rolling, rolling to sit, sitting, sitting to standing, standing to sitting, standing balance, walking, hopping, jumping, kicking, running, reach and grasp, throwing, batting, and golfing. Task descriptions are part of therapists' basic educational programs. An example of a task analysis form developed at Regis University, School of Physical Therapy for sitting to standing is shown in Appendix 24-B.

Impairments

Once the task has been analyzed, the impairments leading to poor performance of the task are identified. Breaking motion down to its most basic components may be helpful, but two caveats are necessary. First, improvement in abnormal components may not lead to improvement in activity limitations.

Impairments can be identified and evaluated for their contribution to an activity or participation limitation. Some critical impairments will have more influences on an activity than will others. For example, in children with cerebral palsy who have gait disabilities, Olney and colleagues[102] demonstrated that poor force output by ankle plantarflexors during the late stance phases of gait was the most important factor in poor gait performance within this population. Another example comes from Perry and colleagues,[103] who showed that for normal walking velocity to be attained, although cadence and stride length are important, a strength level of 3+/5 is a critical component in the ankle muscles. Deficiencies of timing, strength, or sequencing can contribute to poor hand function, but sensory deficits at the hand level may be the critical impairment related to poor manipulation skills. In addition, impairments in the circulatory, respiratory, integumentary, and musculoskeletal systems can account for activity limitation in the client with TBI (Figure 24-2). Relative contributions of the impairments to the activity limitation or participation limitation are addressed by the therapist's task analyses, hypothesis, subsequent evaluation, and diagnosis,[104] which will determine the focus of the intervention program. Second, treating the individual impairments will not necessarily result in the client learning a skill. Skills result from an organization of many motor functions together and require whole task practice. Conversely, not having a critical component, such as arm strength, may be the one factor preventing a person from learning to perform a skill (e.g., enough force cannot be generated to throw a ball 5 feet in the air to hit a basket).

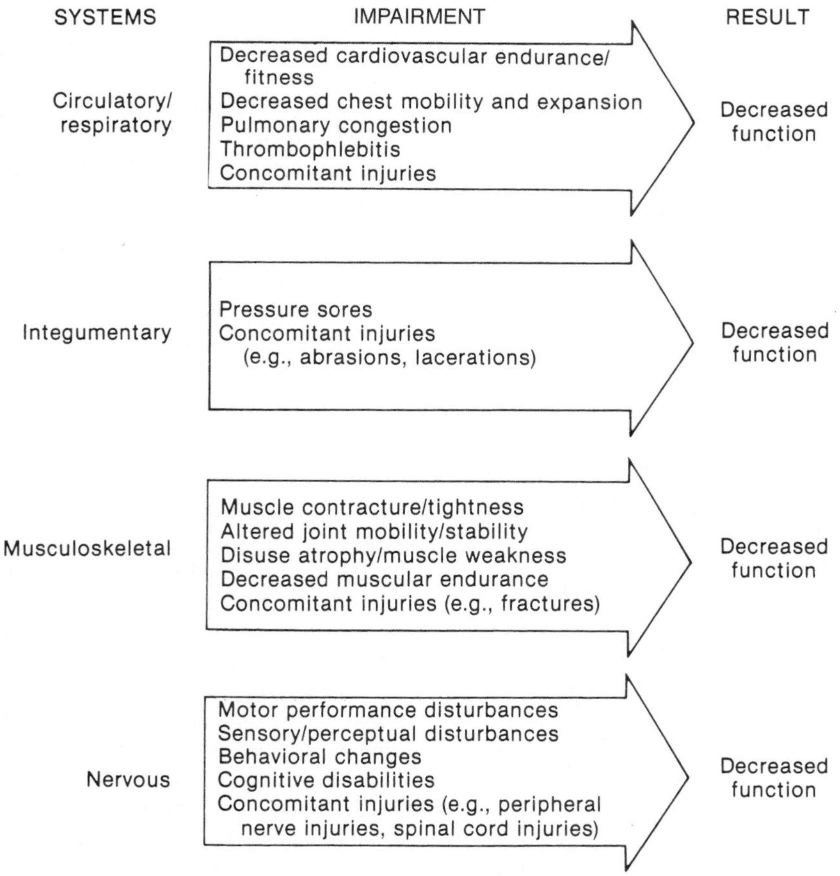

Figure 24-2 ■ Therapists develop intervention strategies to deal with functional deficits that may result from a variety of problems occurring primarily in one or more of the body systems depicted.

Many examinations address the impairment level. These include muscle strength tests, flexibility (ROM) tests, speed of motion, reaction time, sensation, vision, vestibular, tone, and proprioceptive examinations (see Chapter 7).

Impairments that Are Common after Traumatic Brain Injury and Measuring Impairments

Strength or Force Production

Evidence consistently shows that strength and force production are problems in both the upper extremities and lower extremities after TBI. In cases in which strength control or force gradations are significantly impaired at initial admission (about 25% of clients), these problems had generally resolved at a 2-year follow-up, with only 12% of problems remaining in the upper extremities and 7% in the lower extremities.[105]

In the case of upper motor neuron lesions, weakness can be a major problem. The number of motor neurons activated and the type of motor neurons and muscle fibers recruited affect force. Motor neurons in the motor cortex can be deficient, leading to disordered and reduced recruitment. Individuals with brain damage show early atrophy and loss of motor units, as well as motor units that fatigue easily.[106,107] Disuse, cast immobilization, joint dysfunction, improper nutrition, drugs, and aging can cause differential weakness with altered morphological, biochemical, and physiological characteristics within the muscle.[108] EMG studies by numerous investigators[109,110] suggest that reduced activity alters motor unit properties, discharge frequency, and recruitment patterns. Performance problems are reflected in the inability to generate force in different directions and against different loads as well as in problems sustaining force output.[11]

Changes in muscle length affect strength. In clients who have had a cerebrovascular accident (CVA), shortened muscles tend to be strong in short ranges and lengthened muscles are strongest in lengthened ranges but weak in shorter positions compared with the strength-length curves of normal muscles.[111]

Strength or force may be examined functionally—for example, by seeing if the client has enough strength to lift the arm overhead, out to the side, and up to the mouth or is able to go from sitting to standing. In some cases, such as those in which the client is unable to perform balance reactions or has been on extended bed rest, testing individual muscles may be important. Traditional manual muscle testing (MMT) with force transducers or strength testing with isokinetic testing[112] throughout the range provides good strength information. The level of testing chosen should be consistent with the deficit and the therapist's knowledge of its importance in contributing to the activity limitation.

Flexibility

Flexibility at the muscle and joint level is important. Muscle atrophy occurs rapidly[106] and changes in muscle fiber type and function can be seen as early as 3 days. Viscoelastic properties change with paralysis so that the muscle feels stiffer.[113,114]

Examinations should determine the contribution of both tone and tissue factors in limiting flexibility. Active and passive motion should be compared because stiffness (not contracture) often prevents good function. For example, active dorsiflexion is often limited in clients who have full passive ankle ROM because stiffness begins at neutral. The functional result is foot drop or toe catch in the early part of the swing phase of gait because the anterior tibialis muscle cannot generate adequate force production to overcome the stiffness in the gastrocnemius and soleus. This restriction also may limit forward movement of the tibia over the foot during the stance phase of gait, resulting in hip retraction or an apparent balance loss. Knee hyperextension also can result from lack of forward motion of the tibia.

Flexibility measurements are done with goniometers, motion analysis systems, tape measures, inclinometers, photographs, or electronic devices. Taking both passive and active measurements is critical in identifying intervention approaches.

Tone

In the motor learning theories of today, many of the behaviors and resulting motor patterns after brain injury are seen as attempts by the CNS to compensate for loss. For example, spasticity (increased tone) may be the result of an attempt to compensate for the client's inability to increase force. When the amplitude of a contraction cannot be increased because of the injury, the CNS may increase the length of time the muscle fires or may recruit muscles not normally used in a particular pattern of movement; both are characteristics seen in spasticity.

Whatever the cause of increased tone, the therapist can evaluate tone at two levels: is it interfering with function, and, if so, can it be changed? Spasticity is not a single problem.[107-110,113,115-119] Spasticity can have any or all of the following characteristics:

- Changes in response to stretch
- Decreased ability to produce appropriate force for a specific task
- Increased latency of activation
- Inability to rapidly turn off muscles
- Loss of reciprocal inhibition between spastic muscles and their antagonists
- Changes in the intrinsic properties of the muscle fibers
- Inability to generate enough antagonist power to overcome spastic muscles

Examination begins with identifying whether there is increased or decreased muscle tension at rest. If it is increased, is the tension at the muscle level (stiffness or sarcomere involvement) or the neurological level? Muscle stiffness resulting from tissue changes is common in the client with brain injury. If there is increased tone during movement, EMG may be beneficial to determine the nature of the tone. Is it a problem of co-contraction of agonist and antagonist at a joint? Is it a problem of prolonged contraction? Or is it poor sequencing, either temporally or spatially, of other muscles involved in the movement?

Spatial sequencing of movement involves the contraction of a preset group of muscles. Temporal sequencing involves muscles contracting in a fixed sequence. EMG and video analysis provide additional depth of information regarding the sequence and timing of movement patterns (Figure 24-3). For example, is the normal temporal sequencing in the distal-to-proximal manner present in the upper extremity during a reaching task? In a balance reaction, are the ankle, hip, and

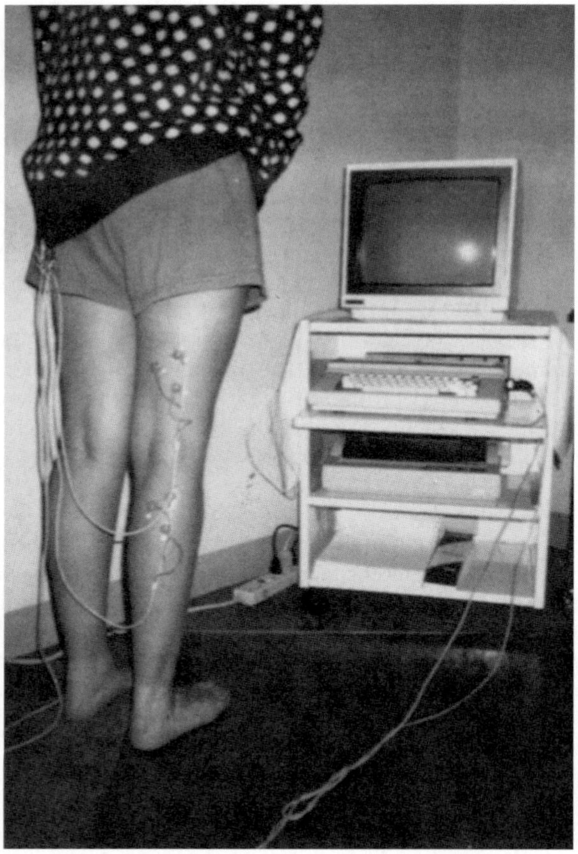

Figure 24-3 ■ Measurement of the sequence of contraction of gastrocnemius and hamstring in forward perturbation with dual-channel electromyographic surface electrodes.

back extensors (spatial sequencing) all contracting in response to a forward perturbation? The most commonly used tool in examination of tone is the Ashworth Scale or Modified Ashworth Scale[120] (Box 24-10). The Tardieu Scale[121] is similar, but testing is done at three different velocities and may provide a clearer picture of what is caused by tone versus muscle shortening. Testing of deep tendon reflexes identifies problems with stretch reflexes, and surface EMG (sEMG) can determine the presence of co-contraction, prolonged contraction, sequence and timing problems, and increased latencies.

BOX 24-10 ■ MODIFIED ASHWORTH SCALE

Grade	Description
0+	No increase in muscle tone
1+	Slight increase in muscle tone, manifested by a catch and release or by minimal resistance at the end of the range of motion (ROM) when the affected part(s) is moved in flexion or extension
1+	Slight increase in muscle tone, manifested by a catch, followed by minimal resistance throughout the remainder (less than half) of the ROM
2	More marked increase in muscle tone through most of the ROM, but affected part(s) easily moved
3	Considerable increase in muscle tone, passive movement difficult
4	Affected part(s) rigid in flexion or extension

Reprinted from Bohannon R, Smith M: Interrater reliability of a Modified Ashworth Scale of muscle spasticity. *Phys Ther* 67:207, 1987, with permission of the American Physical Therapy Association.

Speed of Motion

Research shows that seemingly different movements may actually be spatially the same (same muscles involved) but may appear different because of pauses within the movements, velocity, or speed.[122]

Measurements include how quickly a joint can be moved actively. Recording the number of repetitions of a movement in a specific time frame provides an easy clinical measurement. Isokinetic instruments can measure partial- and whole-extremity motion speed. Speed of movement at each joint in a synergistic movement (videotaped or movement analysis systems) can help with analysis of function. Is poor performance the result of speed of movement problems in just one part of the motor pattern or in all parts? Computerized motion analysis techniques can also help examine speed of motion relationships between and among limb segments, which is particularly useful in assessing upper-limb movements such as reaching and grasping activities.

Reaction Time

How fast can the client begin motion? This parameter can be measured by EMG or with other computerized equipment.

Simple reaction time examination gives insight into the time for neurological processing because it is the measurement of time from a stimulus to a response. Rapid reaction times may be critical for many patterns to be effective, but especially for automatic patterns such as balance responses. Simple reaction times appear impaired even long after TBI (moderate to severe),[123] although there is conflicting literature in this area.

Testing of reaction times is usually performed with computerized testing with a visual or auditory cue used as a stimulus, then the time to a motor response (usually at the hand or foot) is measured.

Endurance and Fatigue

Fatigue, which is separate from impaired endurance, may result from increased energy requirements resulting from less efficient motor patterns or from more CNS activity. Fatigue is a common complaint after TBI[124] and is associated with insomnia.[125] Testing for fatigue is difficult. There are a few paper and pencil tests, including the Chalder fatigue scale.[126]

Muscle endurance refers to the ability of a muscle to produce the same level of contraction over time. The subjective feeling of effort and weakness after fatiguing exercise may be related to the need to recruit more motor units and to increase the mean firing frequency of the motor units to maintain constant force output.[127] EMG with medium-frequency analysis can test this type of fatigue. Fatigue can also be assessed by measurement of maximal voluntary force, maximal voluntary shortening velocity, or power.[127] Decreased force production, prolonged time to relaxation of muscle fibers, and recruitment of additional muscles during an activity are characteristic of fatigue.[128] Although repeated muscle testing can pick up decreased strength in specific muscles, in most instances overwork fatigue is first noted by an altered pattern of movement of body segments during activity.

Cardiovascular endurance determines how effectively the body can use oxygen and how soon fatigue sets in. This type of endurance can be measured with several bicycle tests[129,130] and with a treadmill using the Bruce[131] protocol or a branching protocol for clients with less endurance. A simple test is heart rate before and after activity; the less change and the more rapid the return to resting rate, the better the client's fitness level. The 3- and 6-minute walk tests are also reliable and valid for endurance testing.[132]

Incoordination

Ataxia was one of the most common findings among military personnel who had sustained TBI,[105] with 32% of clients showing ataxia initially and 14% at the 2-year follow-up. There are many subcategories of ataxia, including dysmetria, rebound, diadochokinesia, and intention tremor. Many clinical tests are available. Common tests include having the client touch an index finger to the examiner's finger and back to the client's nose. Running the heel up and down the opposite shin is a test for ataxia in the lower extremity. For a list of coordination tests see Chapter 21.

Sensory Function

Various sensations can be impaired. Problems in the sensory system are often reflected in the motor system, creating distorted movement through faulty information in the feed-forward or feedback processes.

Two broad categories of sensations can be defined on the basis of the type of information: primary sensations and cortical (or integrative) sensations. This arbitrary division is useful functionally but it is not anatomically based. Primary sensations include exteroception and proprioception. The exteroceptors of smell, sight, and hearing are sometimes referred to as *teloreceptors*. Vision, hearing, olfaction, gustation, pain, touch, temperature, position sense, and kinesthesia are commonly checked primary sensations. Sensations cannot be clinically tested definitively without client participation. Further evaluations of sensation are provided in specific systems.

Proprioception, Light Touch, Two-Point Discrimination, and Stereognosis. After TBI, sensory deficits are common. Deficits associated with poor balance included a high number of subjects with discriminative touch deficits (20 of 27 subjects),[133] an impairment related to poor upper-extremity function.

Traditional examinations of proprioception include the ability to distinguish motion and motion direction at each joint. Some clients who cannot distinguish direction or movement still function well. They may have proprioceptive function at the unconscious level (e.g., cerebellar) while not perceiving the input at the parietal level (conscious level).

Testing is performed by having the client close his or her eyes; then the therapist places a joint in a specific position (e.g., flexed, extended) and asks the client to copy the position with the uninvolved limb. Asking the client to close the eyes and identify when the therapist passively presents small movements of a joint while the client indicates specific direction of movement can also test proprioception, especially for those with multilimb involvement. Very small joint movements of about 1 degree are within the discrimination level of typical individuals.

Light touch is tested with a brush for localization and quality of sensation. For more definitive light-touch discrimination, especially on the hands and feet to determine peripheral neuropathies, a monofilament test[134] can be used. Two-point discrimination can be tested with instruments specifically designed to measure how far apart two separate spots of contact need to be to identify them as distinct. For clients who are thought to be ignoring stimuli on one side, testing at the same time bilaterally is first performed, and then each limb is retested separately. Clients who extinguish stimuli will respond that they feel only one stimulus when both limbs are tested simultaneously but will perceive the stimulus just fine when each limb is tested separately. This is called the *bilateral extinction test.*

Stereognosis. Stereognosis, the ability to identify objects placed in the hand without visual assistance, may be critical to normal hand use. The therapist places multiple objects, such as pens, coins, and safety pins, in the hand and asks the client (eyes are closed) to identify the objects.

Vision and Visual Perception. Vision is critical in recovery of many motor functions because it is responsible for much of the feed-forward or anticipatory control of movement as well as the initial development of a movement pattern. For example, balance can be maintained through the visual system by modifying synergies before surface change occurs. Feedback through the peripheral field through the movement of the visual array on the retina can also trigger balance responses. Campbell[133] found problems with visual functions in most clients with mild to moderate TBI; these problems involved poor visual acuity (48%) and problems with vergence (85%), which can cause blurring and doubling of vision, and smooth pursuit (63%), which can cause a "jumping" of the visual image.

Some clients are able to use their hands for grasp and release, in spite of severe somatosensory deficits, when they are able to use vision to guide the motion; therefore many of the standard movement tests should be performed with and without vision.

General visual functions can be screened by the physical or occupational therapist as follows:

1. Tracking is assessed by use of an H pattern of movement of the object being tracked. The examiner observes any nystagmus or refixation saccades. Eye muscle paralysis can be observed during tracking if the client cannot move the eye(s) laterally, up, down, or medially.
2. Focus or accommodation can be checked by observing constriction and dilation of the pupil. Constriction occurs as an object is moved toward the nose, and dilation as the object is moved away from the nose.
3. Binocular vision is controlled through feedback from blurred or doubled vision. This reflex signals whether the eyes and fovea are focused on a single point or target, as the images in both eyes fall on the same retinal points. A "cover test" can screen for binocular vision. The client stares at an object at about 18 inches from the nose. The therapist covers one eye. If there is movement to adjust the remaining uncovered eye back to the object, both retinas may not be focusing on the same point. Observing whether light reflections fall on

exactly the same place on both pupils is useful in evaluating binocular eye focus. Vergence testing can also be an indicator of binocular visual functions.

4. Visual fields can be grossly tested by having the client look forward at a point (observer sits in front of the client to be sure the client remains focused straight ahead [Figure 24-4]). The client indicates when he or she first sees an object coming into the peripheral field from behind, or the "spotter" notes when the client looks toward the object.
5. Vergence is tested by having the client observe an object or pen tip as it is brought from about 20 inches away. The client is told to follow the object with his or her eyes. The object is moved at a moderate speed toward the bridge of the nose, and the client reports when the object becomes blurred or doubles. When typical convergence is present, there will be no blurring or doubling until the object is 2 inches away or closer, and when the object is moved back out, the client will report the object as single within 4 inches.
6. Visual interactions with the vestibular system are assessed through the vestibuloocular reflex (VOR). This reflex maintains a fixed gaze on a target as the head moves. The object should not appear to blur, move, or double during head motion at various speeds.
7. Perceptual tests that evaluate how visual information is used include visual memory tests, cancellation tests, and figure-ground tests.
8. Visual acuity is tested using a Snellen eye chart. Poor acuity can affect balance responses.

Neuro-optometrists and neuro-ophthalmologists are appropriate referrals for clients needing in-depth visual workups, especially when visual perception is involved.

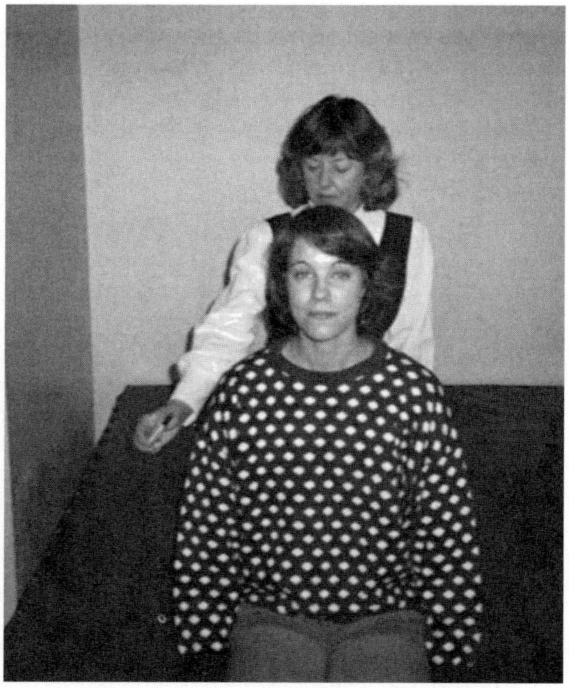

Figure 24-4 ■ Testing of peripheral visual fields from behind the client.

See Chapter 28 for additional information on vision and visual testing.

Vestibular System. The vestibular system monitors the position of the head in space and helps distinguish when the body is moving from when the visual surround is moving. It also provides a vertical reference to gravity to maintain the head upright. Vertigo, dizziness, eye-head incoordination, and postural and balance complications occur as a result of problems in the vestibular-cerebellar systems.

Clients with mild or moderate TBI have a high rate of complaints of dizziness.[135] In many cases the dizziness is a sign of vestibular dysfunction.[105] Campbell and Parry[133] found that 26 of 27 clients with TBI and poor balance also had abnormal VOR testing results. Impairments that can occur with vestibular injury after TBI include verticality and orientation dysfunctions.[79,116,117,133,136]

The VOR is indicative of vestibular system dysfunction. Vestibular tests can be performed at the screening level to note dizziness with body, head, or eye motions. A practical division includes testing head movement in lying, sitting, and standing positions. Vestibular system evaluation and training[137] is one such outcome test. Symptoms occurring only with specific head movements can be an indicator of problems in the semicircular canals. Benign paroxysmal positional vertigo (BPPV) is common after brain injury. Dizziness with head tilts might indicate problems in the otolithic system. In-depth evaluation tools may be used when clients are symptomatic, and clients can be referred for electronystagmography, the gold standard for diagnosing unilateral peripheral vestibular dysfunction. See Chapter 22 for additional information on balance and vestibular testing.

Anticipatory Reactions

Anticipatory reactions are dependent on learning. They require combining past information with present information to make motor responses appropriate to internal and external needs. Forces that stabilize limbs or the trunk during movements occur before the firing of the prime mover. The disruption of balance that would occur before moving must be anticipated and counterbalanced before the movement even begins. For example, does the gastrocnemius muscle contract before forward-reaching activities to prevent forward movement of the center of gravity? Does the client shape the hand for picking up objects? Almost all motor functions have an anticipatory component. Use of sEMG can help determine the presence of common anticipatory responses. Visual observation may provide some information about anticipatory responses also. For example, does the client walk smoothly over or around objects, or does he or she need to stop, slow down, or make corrective responses? When reaching or stepping during sitting or standing, does the client fall or lean in the direction the limb moves?

Adaptation

Feedback is used to modify and fine-tune responses. Observation is often used by providing the client with an unexpected perturbation after several expected perturbations. The initial response is usually poor, but as the same perturbation is repeated, the response improves. Other observations can include whether the activity is corrected to meet changing environmental conditions. When not successful at task performance, does the client use the information to modify or adapt subsequent responses? Is the adaptation appropriate, or does it result in poorer performance?

Activity Level Dysfunction and Testing

Although there are no data on frequency of problems with rolling and rolling to sit in the literature, a recent study of multiple centers that treat clients with acute TBI showed that sitting balance,[138] sitting to standing,[139] and losses of standing balance, gait, running, and reaching and grasping have high incidences of impairments at admission.

Sitting Balance

Brown and colleagues[138] found sitting balance to be impaired in 52% of the clients with TBI at initial examination in their review. Testing includes static sitting without arm support and dynamic sitting with the client reaching in multiple directions.

Standing Balance

Standing balance after TBI is usually affected in mild, moderate, and severe injuries, with 82% of clients showing standing balance problems. Problems include both motor strategy problems and appropriate use and integration of somatosensory, visual, and vestibular information. Newton[140] reported that clients with moderate and severe TBI showed significantly impaired reaction times to perturbation in standing. Although they could grade their responses to the perturbations appropriately, the responses were often asymmetrical.

Balance is tested with feet shoulder width apart, feet together (Romberg), and feet in tandem (sharpened Romberg) with eyes open and eyes closed. A Clinical Test of Sensory Interaction on Balance (CTSIB) test[141] is used to test sensory balance components. Perturbations to balance can be used to examine motor components of ankle, hip, and stepping strategies. See Chapter 22.

Gait

People with TBI walk with a significantly slower speed than matched healthy controls. There is a significant difference between groups for cadence, step length, stance time on the affected leg, double support phase, and width of base of support. The most frequently observed biomechanical abnormality is excessive knee flexion at initial foot contact. Other significant gait abnormalities are increased trunk anterior and posterior amplitude of movement, increased anterior pelvic tilt, increased peak pelvic obliquity, reduced peak knee flexion at toe-off, and increased lateral center of mass displacement. Walker[105] found that testing of clients using the tandem gait identified the most frequent physical impairment remaining at a 2-year follow-up in a group of people with TBI. He suggests using tandem gait as one part of the clinical examination for all clients with TBI.

The Barthel Index,[142] FIM,[143] Tinetti assessment,[144] Gait Assessment Rating Scale,[145] and Motor Assessment Scale[146] also examine different components of gait but more at the activity limitation level. Speed of walking for functional activities such as crossing a street at a stoplight and endurance can be measured by distance and a stopwatch.[147] Endurance can be measured with a 6-minute walk test.[132]

Reach and Grasp

Numerous problems occur during reaching and grasping. Tests such as the Nine-Hole Peg Test and the Purdue Pegboard Test provide a standardized means of measuring reach and grasp using a timed method. The Motor Assessment Scale has an upper-extremity component that is validated to use alone. The Frenchay Arm Test measures functional use of a dominant hand.

Grip Force. Problems with grip include inability to gradate force. Measurements can be done using hand-held dynamometers and asking clients to reproduce specific amounts of force.

Complex Task Level Problems

Although many of the movement problems observed in clients with TBI are at the impairment level, some are at a higher level. Complex task evaluation—evaluation of how movement works as a whole—requires extensive knowledge of abnormal and normal movement. This type of evaluation looks at larger movements involving many joints or even the entire body and may be considered from the point of view of motor control theory as described in the following sections.

Are Basic Motor Patterns Available, Accessible, and Used Appropriately?

Are the three basic components of movement all present? They are as follows[148]:

1. Reflex responses that are involuntary, such as the withdrawal reflex.
2. Rhythmic motor patterns, such as walking, that initiate and terminate a sequence of voluntary movements; the movements are relatively stereotypical and almost automatic.
3. Voluntary (volitional) movements that are purposeful, goal directed, complex, and learned. Playing the piano would be an example of this type of movement.

Starting at the reflex level, are reflexes such as swallowing, visual tracking, and smiling intact? Injury at this level may affect basic motor program production and sequencing. Are automatic movement patterns present (e.g., balance synergies, walking, and running)? Are volitional or voluntary movements present?

Are the Basic Motor Patterns Being Selected or Modified to Meet Specific Task Requirements?

Many of these functions are associated with cerebellar functions, which provide tone, timing, coordination, and amplitude of motions. The synergistic system smooths out the motor program and provides adaptability. One of the contributions of synergy use is the ability to limit the degrees of freedom in a movement. Is the client able to use the basic motor patterns in a functional manner? Is the client able to modify and then accomplish activities such as rolling over, coming from sitting to standing, standing, walking, reaching, picking up objects, and ball catching? Is there good interlimb coordination as demonstrated by coordinated two-handed activities, good timing between limbs in walking, and jumping? Does the client appear to have the ability to coordinate motions (decrease the degrees of freedom), or are they limited by too few degrees of freedom? Does the client respond correctly to environmental changes or stimuli such as stepping over or around objects or being able to walk on different terrain? When motor patterns are used, are they appropriate for the stimulus? For example, is the ankle strategy used for standing on a firm surface and when stopping walking?

Variability of Performance

The plastic nervous system can adapt and change its motor output to meet different requirements. VanSant[149] showed that children and adults vary in the way they stand from supine, even under the same environmental conditions. She states that the most striking observation in nondisabled individuals is this variability of performance. The lack of variability has been suggested as a sign of system damage.[86] When the client with brain injury is assessed, the therapist should look for variability of performance in basic motor acts. Can the client accomplish the same task in several ways? Can the client adapt to different task demands? As the complex task is being performed, keep in mind that the extent of deficit is important. To what extent is the observed motor behavior involved? Is the behavior totally absent, is it deficient, or are there signs of substitution of function or adaptation?

Following is an example of the examination process. The client complains of difficulty in walking and is experiencing several falls daily. Walking requires several complex elements including extensor strength, postural control, and balance.[150] First, a task analysis is performed, and in this case the therapist would look at the gait pattern, perhaps using the Rancho Los Amigos Observational Gait Analysis to analyze the kinematic aspects of the pattern. The therapist then hypothesizes about specific problems observed during the task (gait) analysis. For example, if the client is dragging his toe in swing and does not have adequate knee flexion in this phase, the therapist might hypothesize that the thigh is advancing too slowly (speed of motion impairment) to promote good knee flexion and that dorsiflexion is limited because of poor anterior tibialis activation (force production problem). Timing the speed of hip flexion and doing MMT might confirm or rule out these hypotheses.

If postural control appears to be the problem, the therapist observes the client in standing, noting that the client leans to the left. The therapist may hypothesize that head-righting reflexes are not intact. This might be tested by leaning the client to the side with eyes closed to determine head-on-body righting. Is the head righted to the body or to gravity (as is normal in adults)? Examination for verticality would include lying, sitting, or standing with the body vertical, both with eyes open where vision can control verticality and with eyes closed to examine somatosensory and vestibular control of posture and verticality. If the walking problem appears to be in the client's balance system, then use of sEMG on the leg muscles will determine whether the client is using balance synergies with a temporal sequence of distal to proximal contraction (ankle strategy) during small perturbations. Does the client use only the appropriate muscles in balance responses (spatial sequence)? Or is the client co-contracting, indicating a temporal or spatial sequencing problem that disrupts the normal motor patterns? Is there efficient movement in the swing leg? Does it move in a straight line, and is foot placement on the floor appropriate (coordinated movement)? Does closing the eyes change the character of the movement? If it does, the client may be controlling movement by vision without regard to vestibular and somatosensory input. The therapist may hypothesize that sensory influences on balance are impaired and choose to do the CTSIB to confirm this hypothesis. Does the client step over objects placed or rolled in front of him (anticipatory and adaptation)? If not, was it because the client misjudged the height of the object (visual anticipatory responses) or misjudged the distance to move the leg (modification of the locomotion synergy at the amplitude level)? Is movement too disorganized (uncoordinated) to clear the object? The therapist may hypothesize a problem in timing of the leg movements and confirm the hypothesis diagnosis with sEMG.

Prognosis for Improvement by Activity Limitation

In a review[63] of long-term problems after moderate or severe TBI, standing balance was most impaired initially (82%) and at 1-year follow-up (24%) compared with other systems. Sitting balance was impaired 52% of the time initially but only 5% at the 1-year follow-up. Strength was more often impaired (about 42% of clients) than coordination (40%) or tone (20%) but showed significant improvement, with less than 20% of clients being impaired in strength and less than 10% in coordination or tone at the 1-year follow-up. Dysphagia was present in 40% of the clients but in only 0.4% at 1 year.

INTERVENTION

Intervention Efficacy

The goals of intervention are to help a client work in the environment to produce movements that are efficient, successful, and to some extent socially acceptable, and to prevent secondary problems from developing. Bach-y-Rita[151] and others [152] stated that long-term rehabilitation is key to improved motor control and that recovery can continue to occur as long as the brain is challenged.

The concept that the external environment influences structural neural changes is basic to physical and occupational therapy interventions—that is, activities in which a client participates change brain structure and organization.

Evidence that mammalian brain anatomy and function are modifiable by environmental factors was first irrefutably demonstrated by Wiesel and Hubel,[153-155] who described the importance of environmental experience on functional development of brain cells in the visual cortex of kittens. These experiments showed that visual experiences determine the synaptic organization of neurons in the visual cortex. Devor and Wall[156] demonstrated this same type of plasticity in other sensory systems.

That intervention makes a difference in recovery after brain injury has been shown in many studies. In studies by Mitchell and colleagues,[157] kittens were deprived of sight by having one eye sutured shut. Recovery of vision occurred in the sutured eye only if the animal was forced to use that eye. Tower[158] demonstrated that when brain lesions caused limb dysfunction, monkeys did not use the involved limb, but if the remaining useful limb was restrained, the monkeys used the original "useless" limb for climbing and other activities. Similarly, Wolf and colleagues[159] and Taub and colleagues[160] showed that function in hemiplegic upper extremities is improved through use of constraint-induced therapy (CIT) by constraining the uninvolved arm, thus forcing use of the involved arm. Liepert[161] demonstrated neuroplastic changes in the motor cortex of clients who had sustained a stroke as the basis for improvement with CIT. Whether this is from learned disuse, as suggested by Taub and colleagues,[160] or by deactivation of silent synapses is unknown.

Jones and colleagues[162] looked at the effects of general versus complex exercise in rats after cortical injury on plasticity by use of a general exercise of walking through a tunnel versus a complex exercise (acrobatics). The researchers monitored recovery by looking at upper-limb coordination tasks and also by the number of new synapses per neuron and the number of multisynapses formed. The rats doing complex exercise showed significantly more multisynaptic formations and better limb coordination. Avoiding excessive use of the intact limb may also prevent impaired recovery of the involved limb, according to a study on rats by Jones and Schallert.[163]

Active participation is also important in motor learning, as Held's[164] experiments demonstrated. Activities that allow practice of the specific task have been proven effective. Walking on a treadmill with partial body-weight support (Figure 24-5) provides practice of the walking pattern and has been widely effective in improving overground gait parameters such as speed and improved pattern in a variety of neurological dysfunctions.[165,166] Whether treadmill walking is as effective as body-weight–supported treadmill training (BWSTT) for clients with TBI has not yet been determined, but there is evidence that this may be the case.[139]

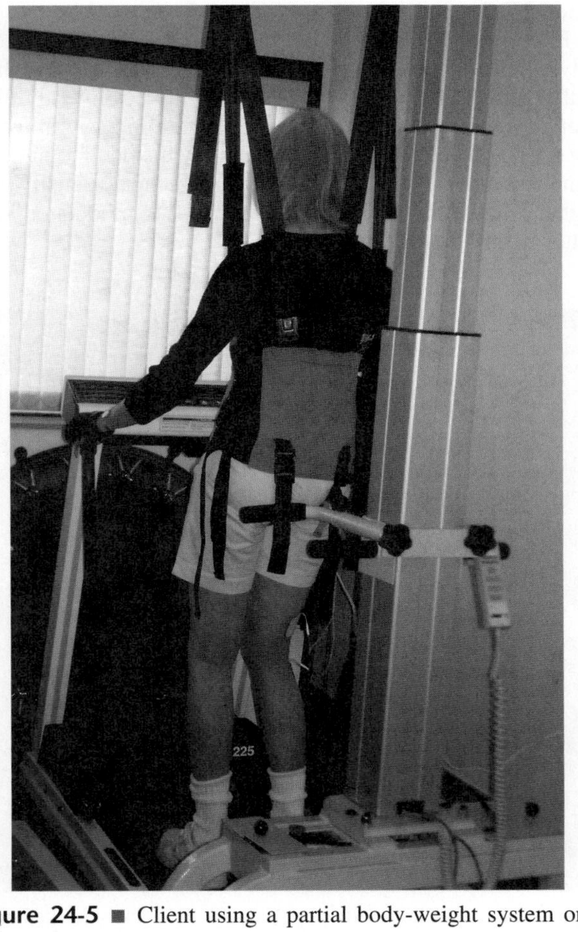

Figure 24-5 ■ Client using a partial body-weight system on a treadmill intervention with functional electrical stimulation on the right peroneal nerve to assist with dorsiflexion during the swing phase of gait.

Several authors have suggested that activation of the motor patterns by imagining movement[84] may be possible. In a study by Porro and colleagues,[167] motor imaging activated the same regions of the brain as motor performance; signal density was 30% as great as in real practice. Mental practice has been effective to improve multiple motor activities in clients with neurological disorders[168,169] but has not been reported on for clients with TBI.

The neurophysiological mechanisms thought responsible for CNS recovery[161,170,171] after injury are discussed in earlier chapters.

Because the therapist can identify a deficit during the examination does not mean the deficit can be fixed. The ability to "fix" impairments does not depend solely on the therapist's skills but includes inherent properties within the client such as the amount of physical damage, cognition, family support, and motivation. Just as critical are external constraints, for example, the availability of treatment devices such as EMG for biofeedback, stimulation devices, pools, and other equipment; travel to and from treatment; availability of qualified providers of care; and financial constraints on intervention.

Based on the evaluation, two levels of intervention are likely to be ongoing. At the impairment level, basic components of performance that are faulty and are contributing to lack of motor performance are addressed. Loss of complex movements, functional activities, and reestablishment of typical motor patterns for rolling, roll to sitting, sitting, sitting to standing, standing balance, gait, running, upper-extremity reach and grasp, and throwing and batting activities will also be part of the rehabilitation targets.

For those clients whose evaluations suggest that recovery of typical function at the body function, impairment level is not probable, substitutions for loss of function such as bracing, wheelchairs, functional electrical stimulation (FES), ambulation devices, environmental changes such as ramps, mobility devices, bath benches, padding for skin care, and reachers provide immediate change and improve the activity limitations almost immediately. The reader must remember that colleagues often use this model to clarify areas needing improvement to reach the goals established by the patients that allow them to participate in the highest quality of life.

With use of the ICF (WHO) model of impairment, activity limitation, and participation restrictions, the therapist determines whether improvement is possible at the level of impairment and then addresses these specific impairments. For example, for a client who is unable to roll over and is both weak and has contractures, strengthening, stretching, and casting may be done. For task-oriented practice, practice of rolling may be used. In the client with a permanent contracture or paralysis, a cloth loop may be provided to allow rolling over by pulling with the arm, a substitution technique at the activity limitation level. This adaptation to rolling allows the patient independence and participation in daily living activities that lead to a quality of life that may not be attained without environmental adaptation.

An example of the ICF intervention model for walking is presented in Box 24-11.

For skill in an activity to be developed, many, many repetitions must be performed. KR and feedback are also important in motor practice.[172] Attention span and motivation factors alone can impede skill acquisition.

Areas of Intervention

Multiple problems may occur after brain injury, most of which are amenable to interventions. A partial list of the most common problems is in Box 24-12.

Motivation, Cognition, and Memory

Multiple cognitive problems remain even after physical problems have resolved for the person with TBI. Fortunately, these problems do appear to improve with intervention. In a study of clients with TBI, Feeney and colleagues[173] demonstrated an 82% improvement in cognitive, memory, behavioral, and emotional problems in clients with severe problems in the home and community.

The motivational aspect of TBI may be one of the most difficult for the therapist to deal with. Clients' initiation and practice of movement are dependent on the internal control of the client and not easily dealt with from the external environment.

Working on client goals helps to establish motivation. Client goals that seem unrealistic should not be dismissed as inappropriate. The high school athlete who wants to play basketball next week and currently has no postural control can focus on how he will learn to sit, stand, walk, and run to play (Figure 24-6). Most clients who go through rehabilitation programs begin to assess their own potential more appropriately once they have worked through part of the program. Many clients and their families believe that the brain heals like any other part of their body and expect full recovery provided a client tries hard enough.[174] Sometimes giving clients time out of therapy to experience everyday life at home and work helps them to determine and readjust goals and skills and to set new priorities. The client who could not understand the point of "silly exercises" comes back asking to learn ADLs. In many cases it is the families who need help understanding their family member's social and behavioral changes.

The neuropsychological evaluation becomes crucial for treatment of clients who have a short attention span and confusion. Early on, techniques to increase attention span will probably include removing distracting stimuli from the client's environment, including auditory, tactile, and visual distractions. But slowly, distracting stimuli need to be reintroduced and attention maintained. (See Chapter 9 for additional information.)

Exercises requiring active involvement in the problem-solving process (e.g., crossword puzzles, study) may help with memory and perceived quality of life.[175] General fitness exercises may also affect cognitive functioning by influencing neurotransmitter functions that slow the decline in dopamine and muscarinic acetylcholinergic receptor density.[176] A higher total number of these receptors is associated with better mental function.

BOX 24-11 ■ ACTIVITY LIMITATION: NOT ABLE TO WALK

IMPAIRMENT: P+ LOWER-EXTREMITY HIP EXTENSOR AND QUADRICEPS STRENGTH

Can improve: Use weights, resistive exercises, antigravity work, stepping up and down steps, functional electrical stimulation (FES), and so on.

Cannot improve (significantly): Address at activity limitation level; use wheelchair, cane, walker, bracing, and so on.

IMPAIRMENT: DISRUPTED SEQUENCE OF MUSCLE CONTRACTION

Can improve: Use exercises to sequence muscles distally to proximally; use electromyographic feedback and so on.

Cannot improve: Use bracing, electrical stimulation for bracing, wheelchair.

BOX 24-12 ■ PROBLEMS AFTER TRAUMATIC BRAIN INJURY

- Impaired affect
- Impaired arousal and attention
- Impaired expressive or receptive communications
- Impaired motor function, including oculomotor and oral motor
- Altered muscle elastic properties
- Impaired respiratory function
- Impaired autonomic nervous system
- Impaired cognition
- Impaired learning
- Impaired sensory integrity and perception
- Impaired adaptive and anticipatory reactions

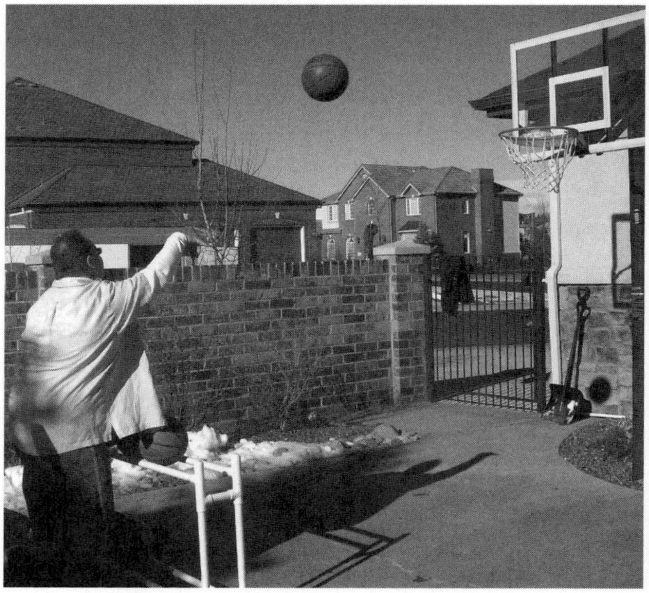

Figure 24-6 ■ Client with poor balance throwing a basketball to improve anticipatory and perturbation aspects of balance. Motivation for balance practice is high for this client, who loved to play basketball before his injury.

Interventions for Motor and Sensory Impairments

There are few randomized controlled trials to guide interventions for TBI for the physical and occupational therapist. A recent systematic review by Hellweg and Johannes[177] showed the following:

Level A (A to D with A highest, D lowest) evidence for:

- Functional training for sitting to standing, upper-extremity use, and gait (body-weight support or conventional gait training).
- Highly intensive rehabilitation programs leading to improved functional skills (activity level).
- Improving cardiovascular fitness with fitness or aerobic training (but no carryover to activity or participation level).
- Not using overnight splinting in functional positions. No clinical improvements were seen.

Level B evidence for:

- Serial casting to improve passive ROM.

Level C evidence for:

- Serial casting to reduce muscle tone.

Only a limited number of interventions were reviewed, leaving out many interventions such as use of sEMG, mental imaging, and FES.

Some interventions are effective for multiple impairments, for example, FES for improving force control and decreasing fiber type changes. At the impairment level are numerous and well known approaches to intervention. Following is a review of the current basis of some impairment interventions and more nontraditional approaches that may prove beneficial and have some evidence to support their use in clients with neurological diseases, although few studies include people with TBI.

Strength or Force Production. Muscle tension is increased and decreased by the number of motor units firing (spatial summation) and the rate at which they are fired (temporal summation). Literature for changing force production and strength after TBI is poor; however, there is strong evidence in other types of brain injury such as stroke.

FES for recruiting more nerve and motor fibers and changing type I back to type II[178,179] appears effective. FES applied to the peroneal nerve for improved dorsiflexion in gait also improves force production.[180] sEMG has also been shown effective in changing motor function after neurological injury.[181,182] It improves force control and is more effective than feedback of angles of movement and traditional treatment in gait retraining.[183]

Traditional strategies have also been effective. Movements that include resistance in eccentric and concentric contractions and movements through varying amplitudes effectively strengthen clients with neurological injury.[184] Using functional tasks for strengthening is often most effective. For example, practicing sitting to standing will help strengthen the hip and knee extensors.

Functionally oriented tasks such as stepping up and down small steps and progressing to larger steps with proximal body-weighting changes force production and require both eccentric and concentric contractions. Changing lever arm length also changes the need for force production; for example, lifting the arm in overhead prehension with the elbow bent, straight, and with weighting during the activity is effective. Picking up and releasing (concentric and eccentric contractions) objects with differing sizes and weight such as weighted silverware, brushes, or cooking utensils also can improve strength. Throwing weighted balls to different targets can improve force control if done at different speeds. Remember $F = ma$? These tasks also promote more interest and attention.

Improvements in strength are usually speed specific, so use of resistance at different speeds is critical. Body position in space may also be related to differences in force production. Current thought is that the brain uses different spatial maps for movement; therefore use of the extremities and trunk in multiple positions is important to address all different types of patterns of muscle activation. Consideration of how much work is asked of weak muscles is important. Weak muscles sometimes fail to respond well if overworked and can actually get weaker. Treatment in the pool or decreasing the number of repetitions and weight during strengthening may lead to more efficient strengthening and faster recovery.

Flexibility. Loss of sarcomeres and tissue shortening can occur rapidly in muscle and joints when clients are less active and in those with high levels of muscle tone. Flexibility can be addressed with traditional orthopedic techniques, including joint mobilization, stretching, and serial casting. Casting or ankle-foot orthoses may be used to prevent sarcomere loss and promote adaptive changes.[185] To prevent length-tension curves shifting left or right, early attention to maintaining middle length of muscles is probably important. In addition, electrical stimulation[179,181] is extremely effective in improving flexibility, especially in dorsiflexion, and can substitute for bracing in clients who need assistance for dorsiflexion during gait. For example, a small spot electrode placed over the peroneal nerve at the fibular head and a 2-inch-square electrode medial to the lateral hamstring 2 to 3 inches above the knee works well (Figure 24-7). Wrist flexor tightness has been treated with electrical stimulation with good results. However, electrical stimulation in the unconscious client with increased ICP or one who is agitated is usually contraindicated because noxious stimuli can increase these problems.

Speed of Movement. Speed of movement may be trained with isokinetic equipment, manually during resistive exercises, with proprioceptive neuromuscular facilitation, or with computerized equipment such as force platforms. Having clients vary speed is important with activities. Many gait studies show that activity limitation becomes most apparent when the speed of gait is increased. Walking at slow speeds, less than 50% of the normal gait velocity, also results in disruption in the walking rhythm.[147] BWSTT has shown good carryover in clients with stroke to improve overground walking,[186] especially when working at 1.8 to 2.0 mph.

Reaction Time. Reaction time training can be performed on force platforms with the client sitting or standing. In a pilot study by Winkler,[187] exercise performed while standing on foam pads (10 inches thick and of medium density; Figure 24-8) significantly improved reaction times during weight shifting to a visual stimulus in a group of eight clients with neurological deficits. Work on compliant surfaces may require that the client make faster corrections to avoid falling.

Endurance and Fatigue. Use of repetitions and increasing duration and intensity can improve endurance. BWSTT has been effective in improving cardiovascular

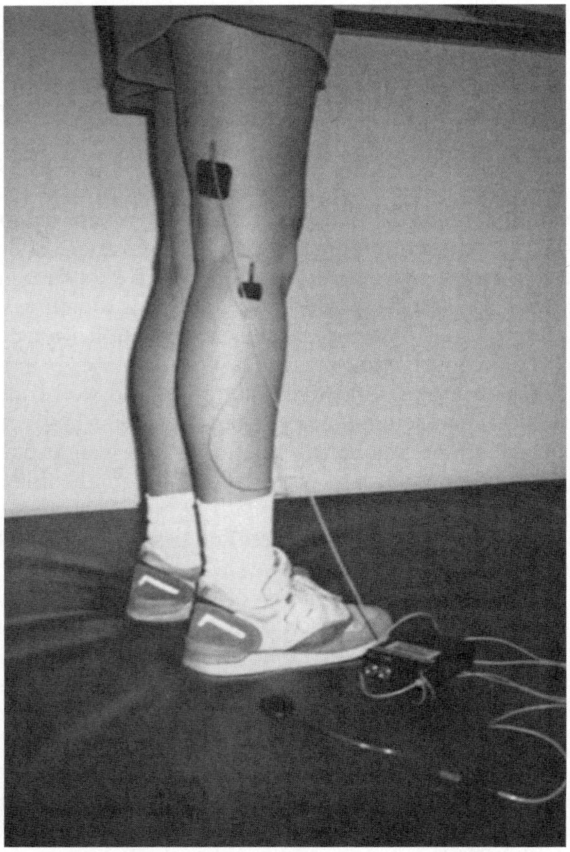

Figure 24-7 ■ Placement of electrical stimulation electrodes for peroneal nerve to attain dorsiflexion for stretching a tight gastrocnemius or for electrical bracing when used with a heel switch.

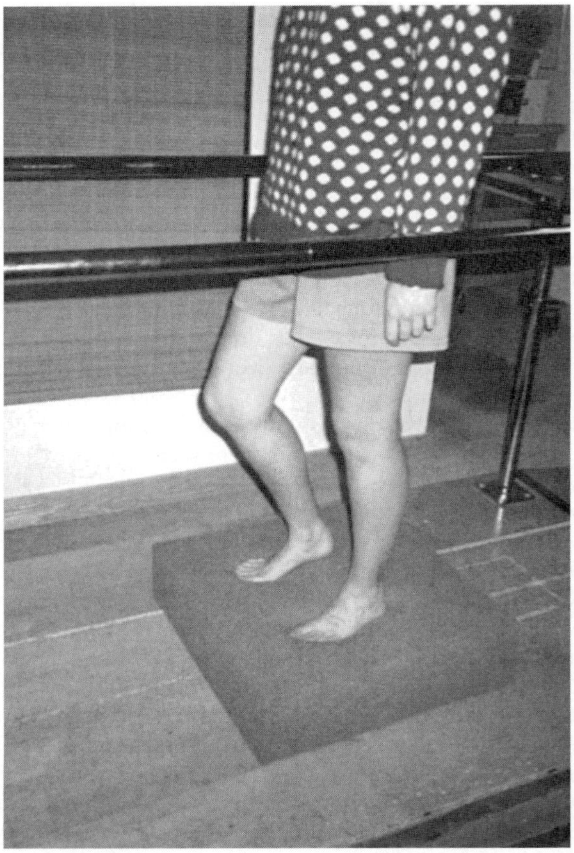

Figure 24-8 ■ Foam block to improve speed of motion and reaction time.

function in clients with TBI.[188] Upper-extremity ergometry can enhance cardiovascular conditioning in clients who are unable to walk or ride bicycles.

Tone. As previously discussed, problems with tone are caused by a variety of issues. Problems in spatial and temporal sequencing seem better addressed with multiple-channel sEMG (see Figure 24-3). The client can see both the level of muscle recruitment and the sequence in which the muscles function if dual channels are used. Co-contraction can be decreased during functional activities such as gait or reaching by using EMG biofeedback. Activation of muscles omitted in the gait or reaching patterns can be enhanced and the ability to "turn off" muscles with prolonged contractions are also effectively treated by sEMG (see Chapter 33). In clients unable to use EMG biofeedback information to make changes, FES may achieve some of the goals (see Figure 24-7). For example, gait training with use of an electrical stimulator on the dorsiflexor or plantarflexor nerves can achieve more normal activation patterns of the foot while providing some internal feedback information about sequencing and may decrease tone.[180] A heel switch and a unit with separate channel controls and ramp adjustment are necessary. Use of electrical stimulation on the gastrocnemius and hamstrings, with a slight delay of hamstring activation, has been effective in assistance with ankle strategy retraining. The goal is to slowly remove the "artificial" assistance over time. Strengthening exercises may also assist in improving central control of muscles and therefore improve tone control. Botulism toxin is very effective to reduce spasticity in specific muscles of the upper and lower extremities.

Somatosensory. Incorporating sensory function into movement is critical. Having the client actively involved by differentiating various textures and items is important to recovery.[189] Clients with poor tactile function can perform activities such as manipulation of objects, first in view and then out of view (nuts and bolts of different sizes are useful); using tactile discrimination to pick out objects from other objects (e.g., safety pins in a bowl of rice) is also challenging. The difficulty of the task can be increased by initiating treatment with visual and verbal cues and then removing all cues as the client progresses. Changing the surface of the objects that are manipulated from rough to increasingly smooth and slippery also increases difficulty. Activities can progress from one-handed to two-handed tasks for interlimb coordination. Proprioception at the shoulder and elbow can be enhanced by using a marking pen in the involved hand (a utility cuff may be required for securing) and then having the client practice writing, tracing, and drawing on paper or a blackboard while sitting or standing with eyes open and then closed. sEMG biofeedback can be used to help retrain the feeling of movement by having the client perform a movement based only on the EMG pattern and then reproduce the movement without vision. Lower-extremity sensory retraining can also use targets with and without vision and with shoes on and off. Clients can stand with eyes closed and practice leaning to a predetermined position while receiving feedback about their success (random or blocked). Tai chi has been shown to improve plantar sensation in clients with plantar sensory losses.[190]

Vestibular System. Basic research has resulted in a strong recommendation for vestibular rehabilitation, according to a 2007 Cochrane review.[191] Clients with sensory mismatches may require treatment that enhances input from the two normally functioning systems, somatosensation and vision, to adapt or retrain the faulty vestibular system. For example, the client who is dizzy when moving the head may need increased somatosensory input to provide information about the specific body motion that is occurring. The client can perform head motions while supine or sitting with the feet and arms well supported (proprioceptive and tactile input) and eyes open. Progression of treatment occurs by decreasing the additional somatosensory input as symptoms decrease until the client is finally standing and can increase the amount of movement without dizziness or imbalance occurring. Visual cues can be altered by adding movement in the visual surround. This causes the visual system to perceive body motion when there is none and forces the use of the somatosensory and vestibular systems to determine the real motion. Wearing bicycle glasses or taping the medial or lateral aspects of glasses can reduce peripheral visual input, enhancing vestibular and somatosensory input in clients with dizziness caused by visual movement or visual-vestibular conflicts. Provoking imbalance through unexpected perturbation especially of the standing surface helps promote reintegration of the vestibular system. Working on the motor aspect of balance by using soft or inclined surfaces and narrow beams to facilitate hip strategies (see Figures 24-8 and 24-9) and using small perturbations and quick stops to facilitate ankle strategies are important. Typical balance exercises using narrow bases of support in standing and walking can improve the balance problems related to vestibular dysfunction. For clients whose vestibular systems no longer function at all, enhancing visual and proprioceptive information is critical.

Many clients with brain injury who have vertigo have BPPV and will need a canalith repositioning maneuver for effective treatment (see Chapter 22 section on Vestibular Problems for more in-depth discussion of treatment).

Visual System. The visual system can have impairments in the oculomotor areas of tracking, convergence and divergence, the VOR, saccadic motion, and so on. These can be treated with oculomotor exercises, such as looking from a near object to a far object, tracking the movement of the thumb in figure-of-8 patterns, and fixing the eyes on a target during head movement (VOR). Occipital lobe injuries generally result in more perceptual problems—those of making sense of the visual environment. Professionals specializing in these types of problems, such as neuro-optometrists, and occupational therapists usually handle these deficits.

The visual system has separate pathways for movement, color, and form. Therapy can enhance visual input by increasing contrast between objects, such as light objects or print on dark backgrounds. Colors also can assist in easier object identification. Red is a strongly recognized color in deficient systems. Moving visual targets are easier to perceive than stationary ones. Finally, objects with sharp edges and vertical or horizontal lines are easier to perceive than objects with less distinct or curved lines. (See Chapter 28 for more information on visual problems and treatments.)

Anticipatory Responses. More complex activities such as postural stability require work at the anticipatory response level and at the stability level. Moving the extremities, adding weights to extremities during forward movement, and increasing motion speeds are effective techniques. Pulling and pushing activities require an anticipatory set. More dynamic movement may be practiced with ball activities. Using punching, catching, throwing, and kicking activities with weighted balls and regular balls will change the force and speed involved, requiring the client to adapt responses to the changing environmental demands. Treadmills help clients to adapt their motion to environmental changes and to make anticipatory responses. But remember, treadmills cause sensory conflicts because the somatosensory system and vestibular systems report movement but the visual system reports no forward movement of the head or body as would be normal in walking.

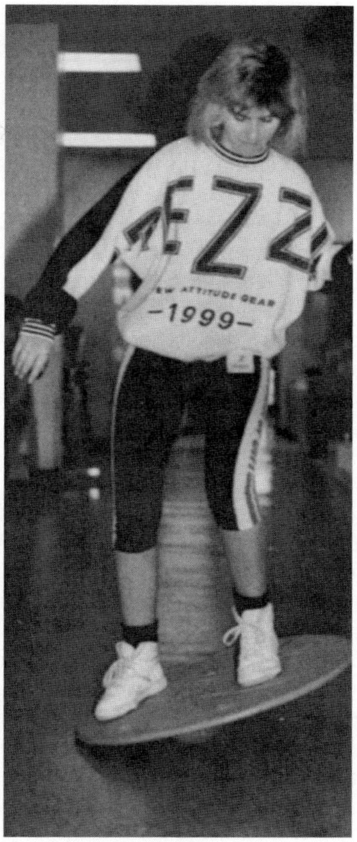

Figure 24-9 ■ Providing the appropriate sensory input is critical to stimulating the correct movement synergy or balance response. Although treatment of mechanoreceptive balance problems requires use of flat, firm surfaces, visual and vestibular balance problems are best treated on irregular, compliant, or moving surfaces, such as the multidimensional balance disk shown. The client should not be permitted to hold onto the therapist or to assistive devices because use of the arms changes the balance responses.

Activity Level Intervention

Activities. In clients in whom the basic body functions are available, basic synergy or skill acquisition should be based on whole-task and natural subtask work. As stated earlier, using subtasks of a whole task improves performance. Identifying natural subtasks is difficult. Winstein[172] suggests that "natural breaks in the resultant velocity profile of a multisegment movement may signify the end of one subunit and may identify natural subtasks of a movement."

Rolling impairments have been found to be amenable to intervention, showing significant improvements between initial admission and 6 weeks later in clients with severe TBI.[192]

The variability shown in the task performance by nondisabled subjects also may help elucidate subtasks. Assessment of a task, as done by VanSant[149] in her supine-to-standing studies, may provide a model to identify subtasks. In VanSant's studies, the upper-extremity patterns varied in six ways: push and reach to bilateral push, asymmetrical push, symmetrical push, symmetrical reach, asymmetrical push with thigh push, and push and reach to bilateral push with thigh push. The head and trunk movement patterns varied in five ways: full rotation abdomen down, full rotation abdomen up, partial rotation stomach down, partial rotation stomach up, and partial rotation. The lower-extremity patterns varied in five ways: kneel, jump to squat, half kneel, asymmetrical squat, and symmetrical squat.

A subtask exercise program to teach a client to get up from supine might work as follows: upper-extremity patterns of asymmetrical push with the trunk in partial rotation are practiced until successful; then lower-leg patterns are added; and finally, whole-task training is used. Natural subtask work probably will be more effective if it is performed in the environment in which the pattern is normally used.

When difficulty is encountered in moving from sit to stand, sliding the hips forward and coming to the point of hips-off appears to be a subtask unit and may be practiced. Dependent sit-to-stand is associated with institutionalization.[193] Sitting to standing practice is outlined in other chapters in detail. Intensive practice of sitting to standing resulted in significant improvements in a group of clients with TBI.[194] Having visual guidance may also help in practice with sitting-to-standing. The shoulder, if tracked visually, will make a reverse C pattern as the client stands up. Having that pattern drawn on a piece of paper and attached to the wall next to the client's shoulder often helps with achieving the movement more smoothly.

Working on improving balance usually occurs at the impairment level, including use of perturbations for reactive responses and quick arm reaching and leg kicking for anticipatory responses. Following a program of decreasing the base of support during each activity helps improve control of the center of gravity. Sensory components of balance require activities with eyes closed, head turning, or working on compliant surfaces.

Ambulation training requires working in the upright position. A common impairment is a slower swing phase in the more involved leg. This problem is often accompanied by decreases in total knee flexion ROM leading to problems of toe clearance and increased time on the stance leg. To work on this impairment, gait may be broken down into more natural subtasks, for example, working on half a gait cycle by stepping from the fully extended position (initial swing) to initial contact position. Practicing pulling the thigh forward rapidly and changing speeds of thigh flexion can also be helpful to increase knee flexion.

Whole-task practice of gait in clients with brain injury leads to the question of safety. How does the therapist allow a client who cannot walk without falling to practice walking, in light of research indicating that holding onto or using assistive devices changes the very skill the therapist is trying to teach? If the deficit is in balance, then walking without assistance may be critical to progress. The best the therapist may be able to do is to change the environment. Allowing a client to walk between parallel bars increases the likelihood that the client will catch himself or herself or that the therapist will catch the client during falls. Use of the body-weight support system with full weight bearing and a loosely worn harness provides safety within the clinic. Walking on mats may allow both for an environmental stimulus for soft, uneven surface work and for safer falling. Falling may be critical in relearning ambulation. Little research is available in this area, but in a study by Cintas,[195] children who performed more daring gait activities fell more often (more problem-solving experiences and stronger error signals?) but gained better gait skills. The therapist should work on techniques to reduce injuries from falling and getting up from the floor.

Goal-oriented tasks are mandatory in working with upper-extremity losses, just as with lower-extremity problems. Significant improvements were seen in a group of clients after CVA and TBI using a task-oriented intervention program for the upper extremity.[196] Many clients with minimal function can pick up and carry boxes. Often grip but not release is present. Again, EMG biofeedback is useful in helping develop release.[197] Functional release in clients with grip can be achieved by use of an electrical stimulator on the finger extensors with a hand switch.[198] Some clients respond to continuous low-level stimulation of the finger extensors and can learn to release by relaxing the grip. These activities are practiced while grasping and releasing objects. Feeding can be performed with this technique, as can other ADL tasks such as hair combing, turning on and off light switches, and opening doors. Games including those for the Wii and other interesting activities such as puzzle solving (Figure 24-10) may also be beneficial.

CIT has also proven effective with clients with TBI. They show improvements across a wide number of upper-extremity outcome measures.[199]

Reversing tasks for some clients allows them to develop increased control but requires modifying a task or synergy and working muscles both eccentrically and concentrically. For example, slowly lowering a spoon from the mouth may improve lifting the spoon to the mouth by improving motor control of the biceps during eccentric contractions. Wrist weights can be added to improve somatosensory feedback as long as the client does not have ataxia, in which case the wrist weight could increase the imbalance between agonist and antagonist.

Variability. VanSant[149] stated that variability of performance in her study had "something to do with body size, strength and ROM." Because force production (strength) and ROM may be critical components in variability, work in

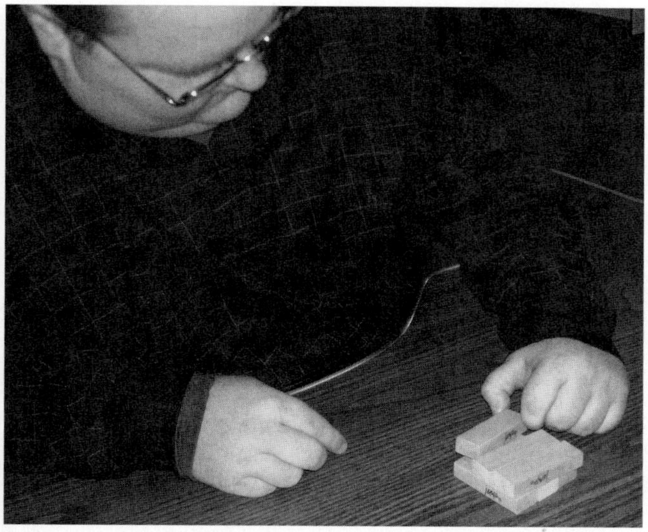

Figure 24-10 ■ Games that are challenging for both the mind and the hand provide interesting ways to work on upper-extremity function. This client lacks refined prehension skills in the left hand.

water or with weight to change force production and ROM may also enhance different responses. It is important to build environmental constraints so clients can perform functional movements in alternative ways. Adding environmental changes by having clients stop and start at different points in an activity or changing directions also develops improved responses as well as flexibility. The client is asked to stop without taking another step when he or she comes to a tape line, and to step over objects that are static or moving. The client may have to feed himself or herself while sitting with the involved extremity up against a wall. These techniques provide external influences on motor activities, helping to establish flexibility into responses. Adding objects to the environment to avoid or manipulate and exposing the client to changing environments also develop adaptations and modifications to motor patterns. Obstacle courses promote flexibility in responses. Activities such as tai chi and dancing require refinements in balance and speed of movement. Finally, for clients who are unable to produce movement, guided movement techniques may help with rolling and coming to sit or stand in clients who have lost basic motor patterns.[200]

Learning, Feedback, and Practice

Learning studies tell us that neuroplasticity underlies both recovery after injury and new learning. Neuroplasticity is facilitated when the activity is goal or task oriented. Novel tasks are better attended and therefore improve learning. Feedback type is critical.

Feedback is essential for learning to occur. According to Winstein,[172] KR research currently suggests a need to reexamine intervention approaches that advocate performance accuracy, strong guidance (manual, tactile, or verbal), frequent and continuous feedback, and avoidance of errors or "abnormal movements." Mistakes the person makes are a powerful type of feedback called *error signals.* For example, when a person drops a ball thrown to him or her, the brain notes the amount of grip, finger ROM, and so on and modifies them on the next attempt to improve the outcome. This is called *intrinsic feedback.*

Knowledge of Results

KR feedback is about the outcome of the task. The problem solving is done by the individual. An example of this feedback might be "You stepped into your walker five of 10 steps."

Knowledge of Performance

Knowledge of performance (KP) relates to the movement pattern used to achieve the goal, for example, "Your knee did not bend on five of the 10 steps."

KR appears more effective in general than KP.

Frequency of Feedback

Faded feedback (KP and KR) improves learning long term. The KR research findings are consistent with the motor control model that requires the client to be actively involved in problem solving through trial and error and adapting to new environmental situations. The higher-level client needs help to solve his or her own motor problems and thus needs less physical support but expanded environmental experiences. Conversely, the client with minimal motor function or the client who is in an early recovery state may require a great deal of external help with basic components of movement before learning how to access or develop basic motor patterns and skill. Assisting movement is appropriate for the level of this client's functioning. For example, in training upper-extremity reaching patterns, this client may need trunk support intermittently; then slowly decreasing the support will help develop the balance component necessary for successful reaching. Because feedback is so critical to learning and improving motor performance, especially at the higher levels of functioning, the method of treating highly functioning clients by assisting motion comes into question. Normal movement is unique in that it will change depending on the context in which it is performed and on the task constraints. The client being assisted in ambulation will not be making balance responses if the therapist is providing balance support. The same problems may be inherent in the use of assistive devices such as canes and walkers. For example, Horak and colleagues[79] showed that using a cane for balance disrupts the normal distal-to-proximal sequence in the lower extremities, and much of the balance responses are transferred to the arm, shoulders, and trunk. Canes also cause a shift in the center of gravity.[201] The same may be true of many externally guided motions. The therapist must provide the client with opportunities to practice all parts of the complex motor tasks, or the task requirements are not the same. Practice needs to be task specific, and changing environmental and task constraints can build in flexibility of response.

Types of Practice and Their Effects on Learning

Constant Practice. A person practices three different tasks, one at a time, before moving to the next task. This results in better performance during acquisition of the skill.

Random Practice. A person practices the tasks in random order and alternates the practice of tasks. This results in better learning in generalizing and transfer of the skill to other environments and conditions.

Massed Practice. Massed practice consists of sessions in which the amount of rest between trials is less than the length of the practice (Practice > Rest). Although fatigue may occur, learning continues. Do not mistake errors made during acquisition of a skill as the final product.

Distributed Practice. Distributed practice consists of sessions in which the amount of rest between trials is longer than the length of practice (Rest > Practice). It is used for clients with poor endurance and early in rehabilitation.

Substitution

Mobility and prehension are the two most frequent activity limitation losses after brain injury. For clients who will not be able to reestablish walking or prehension skills, functional devices are provided for substitution of the lost skills (e.g., use of a wheelchair for the client who will not be able to walk or use of a feeding cuff for a client who will not develop adequate motor function in the hand for feeding). At this level, the therapist also teaches functional tasks such as sitting transfers, cooking, and self-care with assistive devices and modified techniques.

Summary of Intervention Concepts

In choosing interventions for a client with TBI, both the client's and the family's goals are basic. Once the therapist has examined the activities that the client or family reports are impaired, the therapist determines what potential future problems may also occur. With the problem list established, the therapist begins the task analysis to determine the underlying causes of the activity limitations. Interventions are guided by the literature. There are some global principles that apply to all interventions. Evidence is strong that neuroplasticity underlies the majority of recovery. Interventions that promote neuroplasticity (see Chapter 4) include use of novel situations that are important to the client and also the need for many repetitions. The type of practice and feedback are critical for improvement. Intensity of practice is highly related to outcomes. In general, the more physically involved clients (those with losses of basic motor patterns and with multiple activity limitations or cognitive changes) need more hands-on help from the therapist while trying to develop basic motor programs. Interventions may need to focus at the impairment level, establishing strength, flexibility, timing, and sequencing of movements. Assistive devices such as braces, neck supports, and postural seating systems are often used to substitute for missing components of function. For clients who cannot manage multiple tasks, such as balance, coordination of trunk and limbs, and adaptive and anticipatory reactions, the therapist may choose to work in subtasks. Many less physically involved, functioning clients benefit from high-level functional activities. Square dancing, line dancing, karate, tai chi,[202] handball, running, and other sports often promote additional progress in balance, sequencing, and speed of movement. The clever therapist will tease out those components of the activities that best address the deficits in the client and structure enjoyable activities that provide specific training for the deficits in balance, gait, or upper-extremity use. No matter at what level the client is functioning, the teaching of functional skills is critical. More involved clients may learn to roll over and assist with eating and other ADLs by using assistive devices. Modern equipment can enhance all types of function. Computers communicate for those with severe dysarthria, and power wheelchairs with switches to run lights, television, and so on are available. These devices assist clients in their societal interactions and reduce participation restrictions. Remember, the main purposes of motion are exploration and getting the brain to a place where it can be used!

OUTCOME

Leahy,[203] in a discussion of brain-injured adults, suggested a general categorization of clients for prognosis by a combination of levels of cognitive and physical functioning. Cognition is rated as low, moderate, or high level and physical dysfunction as severely impaired, moderately impaired, or minimally impaired. The therapist may use the GOS and the Rancho Los Amigos Scale of Cognitive Function to determine the categories. This system provides a means of predicting return of functional skills and long-term activity limitation. As Leahy points out, clients with higher-level physical skills and moderate-level or low-level cognition skills often have the most difficult time reintegrating into the family and society. Therefore they may have the higher levels of participation restrictions remaining after rehabilitation because family and co-worker expectations are high on the basis of motor function, but it is the cognitive functions that make a person more successful in society.[98] These clients need aggressive help in the behavioral and cognitive areas early on. Neuropsychologists and counselors can suggest interventions that help with cognitive functions, especially techniques to deal with memory problems, attention span decreases, and inappropriate behavior. These programs can make a difference. Brotherton and colleagues[204] documented long-term social behavior improvement in four severely impaired clients with brain injury who had undergone traditional social skills training programs. Clients with low-level motor skills and higher-level cognitive skills do better because adaptive devices are available for these clients. These devices help substitute for the loss of motor functions. These include head-, mouth-, or hand-controlled electric wheelchairs; computerized communication systems; electric lifts for vans and hand controls for driving; books on tape; and numerous upper- and lower-extremity devices to help with hand control and ADLs. (See Chapter 16 on spinal cord injury for all types of substitution devices.)

Outcome Measures Appropriate for Use with Clients with Brain Injury

Wade[205] provides an in-depth presentation of examinations useful as outcome measures for the activity limitation level. Choosing tests and measures validated on clients with TBI is important, but equally important is ensuring that a test is reliable. The Barthel Index[142] is an example of a simple tool for gross measurement of overall activity limitation. It simply asks whether functional skills can be performed within a reasonable time limit. The FIM[143] is widely used in the United States and incorporates the concepts of the Barthel Index. It has six categories that evaluate independence. Twelve items relating to swallowing, community functions, and cognition (Functional Assessment Measure)[206] have been added to the FIM to make it useful for TBI clients. The Disability Rating Scale[13,207] is also widely used for clients with brain injuries. The High Level Mobility Assessment Tool (HIMAT) was specifically designed to test higher-level functions and has been shown to be reliable and valid in people with TBI.[208,209] It is very useful for clients who may be able to jump and run. Upper-extremity movement patterns and function can be examined with use of functional tests such as the Nine-Hole Peg Test,[210] the Frenchay Arm Test,[211] or the arm portion of the Motor Assessment Scale.[146]

These types of indexes should be chosen to address what abilities the client can accomplish. They are not intervention tools. Their purpose is to identify activity limitations and sometimes impairments and to monitor client progress. However, many are not effective in measuring changes in the client with higher-level functioning because they have a ceiling effect. Timed tests tend to have less floor and ceiling effects than other tests. So use of tools such as the Timed Up-and-Go Test (TUG), 3-minute sit-to-stand test, and timed walking tests can be particularly useful as outcome tools.

SUMMARY

The following concepts summarize the theory, research, and intervention concepts presented in this chapter.

1. Intervention is based on the nervous system's ability to learn through environmental influences.
2. The client's goals must be addressed to provide motivation and persistence in exercise and practice.
3. As a starting point, examination (task analysis) and evaluation are done at the activity limitation level.
4. Hypotheses are generated to explain the basic causes of the activity limitations by identifying the impairments that are major contributors.
5. Tests and measures are performed in the examination to confirm the hypotheses.
6. Interventions for prevention of secondary complications such as contractures, skin breakdown, and muscle contractures begin early to prevent loss of function.
7. Neuroplasticity is promoted when the task is novel, is important to the client so that it is well attended, and is repeated.
8. Changing speed of motion and varying the context and environment are necessary for thorough skill reacquisition.
9. Once components of movement are in place, motor pattern development—that is, skill learning—should be stressed through repetition of functional activities.
10. Interventions should be task oriented and performed with the goal of the movement incorporated into the intervention.
11. Practice is necessary in multiple environments and conditions.
12. The client should be allowed to problem solve.
13. Physical assistance by the therapist should be kept to a minimum but used when clients cannot produce movement at all.
14. Variability in performance is normal.
15. sEMG biofeedback, FES, isokinetic methods, and kinematic feedback should be used to modify responses that appear more resistant.
16. Environmental situations that cause changes in responses should be identified and used.
17. Feedback should be provided in well thought-out patterns; random and summary feedback promote learning better than continuous feedback.
18. Substitution devices, assistive devices, and environmental changes should be provided for clients who will not recover from their impairments.
19. Remember that the therapist's uniqueness lies in the ability to perform evaluation and effective intervention.

QUALITY OF LIFE

A life has been saved. The job of the rehabilitation team is to help improve the quality of that life. But what is quality of life? Family members knew the client before injury. The "rehabilitated" client may be dramatically different from their expectation. The rehabilitation team members, who can contrast the client's progress only since the injury, may be quite pleased. Is quality measured by past performance, past potential, present performance, or future potential? Clients themselves may or may not have insight into past, present, or future performance and potential. What is the standard by which quality of life is measured? Is it income, reduction of dependence, contribution to society, or social interaction? Each of these indicators has been used as a standard. Ultimately, the determination of successful rehabilitation relies on the answers to these questions. Jennett and Teasdale[6] suggest six aspects of living: ADLs, mobility and life organization, social relationships, work or leisure activities, present satisfaction, and future prospects. Most of these factors, although important, cannot be quantitatively measured, and they do not entirely answer the question of what is quality of life. However quality of life is estimated, those who have chosen to help rehabilitate clients with brain injury continue to pursue an ideal of quality for each life that has been saved and may, by doing so, enhance the quality of their own lives.

References

To enhance this text and add value for the reader, all references are included on the companion Evolve site that accompanies this textbook. This online service will, when available, provide a link for the reader to a Medline abstract for the article cited. There are 212 cited references and other general references for this chapter, with the majority of those articles being evidence-based citations.

CASE STUDY 24-1 ■ Mrs. E. K.

EXAMINATION

History

Mrs. E. K. is a 60-year-old woman who sustained a brain injury in a fall 1 year ago. Injury was to the cerebellum and brain stem, resulting in left-sided body involvement and incoordination. Currently she reports falling about two times monthly. She complains of feeling tired constantly and not having enough energy to even accomplish her housework. She lives with her husband and 29-year-old son in a two-story house 1.5 hours from a large western city. Her son is an alcoholic and unable to keep a job. Client goals included being able to sew again and to square dance with her club.

Task Analysis

Gait (with Use of the Observation Gait Analysis Based on the Rancho System)

Mrs. E. K. walks with a normal pattern on the right. She has significantly decreased trunk rotation during right leg swing and a right pelvic drop in left leg stance. On the left during swing phase, hip flexion is limited, and the leg circumducts. The left knee has limited flexion and the foot has excessive plantarflexion. In stance phase on the left, there is limited hip extension during midstance and late stance and flat foot contact at initial contact. The left arm is held tightly against her chest with the elbow in flexion and the forearm in full supination. When the client is asked to put her arm to her side during ambulation, the arm swings uncontrolled in large arcs, actually hitting her in the chest. Speed of walking is slow at 50 m/min. Cadence is 73 steps per minute with a 0.8-m stride length.

Hypothesis 1

Gait

Gait is impaired in kinematics and speed as a result of poor force production in the left hip flexor and dorsiflexors complicated by quadriceps and gastrocnemius hypertonia. Slowed gait is also present because of poor trunk rotation during arm-fixed gait and instability when the arm is not fixed to her chest. Flexibility of tissue in the quadriceps and gastrocnemius-soleus may also contribute to the poor movement patterns, and there may be a disruption of the normal temporal sequencing of muscle firing in stance on the left. Question whether proprioceptive problems may be present because of poor foot placement in stepping. Mrs. E. K. may have anticipatory problems because gait is not compensated during the arm movements.

Hypothesis Testing

Force production: Manual muscle strength (on MMT): 2+/5 left hip flexor and ankle dorsiflexors. Flexibility: ROM testing. Left rectus femoris tight at 100 degrees knee flexion test in prone. The gastrocnemius-soleus is tight at neutral. Tone: Modified Ashworth level 3 in left quadriceps and gastrocnemius-soleus.

Balance testing: no ankle strategy, only combined hip-ankle strategy to all perturbations. There is a proximal-to-distal balance response during small perturbations (EMG).

Proprioception is impaired when Mrs. E. K. is asked to note small changes in flexion and extension of the great toe and ankle within normal limits for knee and hip.

Motor patterns are poor in trunk. There is no trunk rotation during walking, and anticipatory responses are poor as measured by rapid forward reaching resulting in forward balance loss in standing and no sEMG activation of the gastrocnemius-soleus before deltoid firing.

Evaluation and Diagnosis

Poor walking ability and lack of automatic balance reactions as a result of decreased use of proprioceptive information, decreased strength in the hip flexors and ankle dorsiflexors, tone and limited flexibility in the quadriceps and gastrocnemius, and poor anticipatory responses disrupting balance when the upper extremities are moved rapidly or when the left arm flails.

Sewing (Large 4-Inch Needle with Yarn through 1-Inch Square Holes in Plastic Grid)

Mrs. E. K. hits the hole with the needle averaging one in three attempts. The left hand does not work in a distal-to-proximal manner. The scapula and shoulder initiate the motion and show excessive motion during the reaching phase of the movement. There is minimal braking of the motion as she approaches the target, resulting in overshooting or undershooting of the target. The hand remains excessively supinated throughout the task. Fine motion of the fingers appears within normal limits.

Hypothesis 2—Upper Extremity

Unable to perform sewing task because of poor timing and coordination of the scapula and shoulder muscles producing a sequentially uncoordinated movement pattern. The triphasic velocity pattern of movement is severely disrupted.

Impairments—Tests and Measures

Timing and coordination: sEMG—Poor sequencing and timing of movement of the scapular muscles with hand and wrist motion. Tremor of high frequency in the scapular stabilizers, especially in the external rotators at rest and with movement. There are lower-frequency tremors of larger amplitude in the wrist flexors and extensors during voluntary motion. Co-contraction of the biceps occurs with all shoulder and hand motions.

Adaptation: Modification of motor patterns is poor for upper-extremity reaching. Amplitudes of movement are far too large for tasks but are repeated with each trial without modification.

Evaluation and Diagnosis

Upper extremity is not being used functionally secondary to poor sequencing and timing of muscle firing during activities. Mrs. E. K. is unable to limit the degrees of freedom in the arm during upper-extremity activities. The arm is held in co-contraction during walking and other activities to decrease the instability in balance caused by large movements of the entire arm.

Participation Limitations

Mrs. E. K. has decreased social interaction with friends; she is unable to attend sewing circle and square dance clubs.

Outcome Measures

The TUG was chosen as it measures gait speed and sitting to standing, both problems for this client. Time was 30 seconds. A 15-m timed walk was used for gait speed. Step length was measured on paper using an inked heel during walking. She had 10 degrees hip flexion and lacked 10 degrees to neutral dorsiflexion. Measurements of hip flexion and dorsiflexion angles in midswing were done from videotape stop when the client was even with the camera.

CASE STUDY 24-1 ■ Mrs. E. K.—cont'd

INTERVENTIONS

Mrs. E. K. was referred to a psychologist, as there appeared to be no other reason for the fatigue on further examination. She was diagnosed with depression. Mrs. E. K.'s physician then prescribed an antidepressant medication.

Because Mrs. E. K. lived 70 miles from the treatment clinic, much of her treatment consisted of a home program. She was seen in the clinic once every 3 weeks for 3 months and then once a month for a year.

The initial home program focused on the basic impairments of reducing quadriceps and gastrocnemius-soleus tightness and increasing hip flexor and dorsiflexor strength in the lower extremity with functional activities such as wearing a 1-lb weight around the foot during walking practice and stepping exercises, tapping a target on the wall with her left knee as many times as possible in 1 min. Exercises included sitting-to-standing repetitions with the knees bent past 100 degrees, keeping the heels on the floor. Mrs. E. K. walked on a treadmill starting at 1.8 miles/hr at home to increase her speed of walking and endurance. She practiced a mental imaging exercise for 20 minutes a day, using sewing as the task. sEMG was used in the clinic to improve scapular-humeral rhythm during functional activities such as drinking from a cup and her sewing task. sEMG was also used to decrease the co-contraction of the biceps during functional use of the arm. At first the sEMG provided continuous feedback with the client observing the screen. After she was able to achieve a particular goal for the session, the visual sEMG was provided only randomly to the client. Practice of activities was for short periods interspersed with different activities. To reestablish some control of amplitude of motion in the left arm, gross movement activities of the hand were done with the elbow stabilized on the support surface and a wrist splint to limit the degrees of freedom—for example, drawing large circles with a pen and pulling long pieces of yarn through some large holes. She also used her left forearm to stabilize paper while writing, finally progressing to using the hand only for stabilization.

The remaining program focused on hand-guided movement activities such as sewing with yarn on a mat with large (1-inch) squares), combing hair, molding clay, playing the organ, and other functional tasks. These activities were first performed with the elbow stabilized and a wrist splint, then with the elbow not stabilized, and finally without the wrist splint.

Lower-extremity work included improving the use of proprioceptive function. Standing exercises with the eyes closed or occluded progressed to stepping activities and finally walking. Ankle strategies were promoted through rapid walking while the client's husband told her to stop abruptly and the client tried not to take a step after being told to stop. She also stood 6 inches from the wall and kept the upper body rigid while she swayed back and forth around the ankle joints. This was progressed to doing the same activity with eyes closed.

sEMG was used in standing to increase the force of contraction of the anterior tibialis.

As the amplitude of arm motion decreased with use, Mrs. E. K. was able to walk with her hands clasped behind her back and worked on trunk rotation coordinated with gait. When this was accomplished, she was able to allow her arm to hang freely at her side and had a natural trunk rotation in walking. Mrs. E. K. practiced line dancing with her husband, using an introduction videotape on line dancing. This activity promoted higher-level balance exercises and provided enjoyment.

OUTCOMES

At discharge, Mrs. E. K. had good motor patterns and improved patterns of motion in the left lower extremity. An articulated ankle-foot orthosis was used for long walks or when she was fatigued. She walked with 90 steps per minute with a 1.2-m stride length. The TUG result was 10 seconds. Tone was a level 2 Ashworth. She performed within normal limits on the CTSIB. Hip flexion improved to 20 degrees in midswing but dorsiflexion still lacked about 5 degrees to neutral.

Upper-extremity testing showed 100% accuracy in putting the needle through the 1-inch squares. She was able to sew and use the left arm for most activities, although a much smaller tremor persisted with volitional movement. She only occasionally (once every 3 months or so) went to the square dancing club. Medication had controlled her depression, and her fatigue was resolved.

CASE STUDY 24-2 ■ C. H.

EXAMINATION

History

C. H., a 21-year-old woman, was in an automobile accident and sustained a severe brain injury and fractures of the left scapula, left radius, right ankle (fused), and jaw. She developed heterotopic ossification (HO) in the right elbow. C. H. was in a coma for 1 month and a stupor for 2 more months. Her GCS score was 8/15 at 2 hours after the accident. She had 8 days of PTA. Her Rancho Los Amigos Scale of Cognitive Function score was a level V (confused, inappropriate) at 2.5 months. She is now at 5 months postinjury and her Rancho Cognitive Function level is a VII (automatic, appropriate).

Expressive language is minimal with severe expressive aphasia and dysarthria. C. H. appears to understand well, following directions and nodding appropriately to questions. Currently, she has dysarthria and is still very difficult to understand.

Behavior is immature. For example, C. H. continuously hugged and kissed her boyfriend when he was in the room. She was easily frustrated by difficult tasks. At these times she became extremely agitated and scratched herself to the point of bleeding.

Her memory was poor, as noted by her score of 19/30 on the Mini-Mental State Examination.

Continued

CASE STUDY 24-2 ■ C. H.—cont'd

Mobility is by manual wheelchair. C. H. is independent in transfers. She can roll and come to sitting independently, but she needs moderate assistance to come to standing, minimal assistance for standing with feet shoulder width apart, and maximal assistance to walk. She is unable to perform self-care such as personal grooming, hygiene, and dressing or to do household chores. Her chin rests on her chest; however, she lifts her head volitionally when asked to lift.

C. H. was a junior in college majoring in elementary school teaching. She worked part time in a clothing store, where she had to wait on customers, put out stock, and ring up purchases. She lives at home with her mother in a single-story house. Dancing and cooking were her hobbies.

C. H.'s goals include use of the left arm to put on makeup and dance with her boyfriend. Her mother, who is a psychologist, would like her daughter to hold her head upright and have better balance and walking.

Review of Systems

Musculoskeletal system: C. H. had HO in the right elbow; this was surgically removed 1 month ago. ROM is 25 to 110 degrees. Scapular and clavicle fractures are healed.

Left gastrocnemius is restricted in ROM to neutral dorsiflexion. Left shoulder has active flexion to 20 degrees but can hold at 90 degrees. Left elbow ROM is 20 to 135 degrees.

Strength screen demonstrates weakness in the left shoulder rotator, lower trapezius, and deltoid. Strength decreased on third repetition with resistance. There is stretch weakness in the gluteus maximus, which tests 4 in 30 degrees of hip flexion, but 2+ in neutral extension.

Cardiopulmonary system: She demonstrated poor endurance. Preexamination heart rate was 85 beats per minute (bpm) and 130 bpm after 5 minutes of standing balance and upper-extremity exercise. There was a 10-mm Hg increase in blood pressure of 115/65 to 125/72 after 5 minutes of examination. Vital capacity is documented as low normal (3 L).

Integumentary system: Unremarkable. No pressure sores since her injury. Incision healed over right elbow.

Cognitive and behavioral system: C. H. became easily frustrated and on each occasion she scratched her left forearm with her right hand. These episodes lasted 30 seconds or so. C. H. probably needs referral to a psychologist for suggestions for handling these episodes.

Task Analysis

Reach and grasp with left hand: C. H. is right handed. The task was picking up an eyeliner pencil, switching it to her right hand, and applying the eyeliner to the eyes, using the left hand to hold the eyelid taut. Her chin was resting on her chest. There was no anticipatory hand shaping before initiating the reach on the left. Reach component was with forward trunk lean, 20 degrees of left shoulder flexion, and elbow remaining at 90 degrees. She picks up the pencil with inferior lateral pinch and excessive grip force. She was able to switch the pencil to the right hand but able to get her left hand only to clavicle level and so was unable to hold the eyelid for applying the liner.

Complex movements: Motor patterns appear intact except in the cervical area, where the head is not held upright to maintain the eyes level, and the left arm, in which there is a proximal-to-distal pattern of movement.

C. H. is unable to modify the motor patterns in the left elbow, and intralimb joint coordination was poor.

Anticipatory responses were absent in reach and grasp; there was no hand shaping before the reach was initiated, and fingers were held wide open even as she approached the pencil.

Variability of performance: C. H. was able to reach and grasp and bend in many different ways with the right arm and was limited only by elbow ROM. The left arm was maintained in an adducted, internal rotation pattern with the elbow flexed at 90 degrees on the left. She also appeared limited in the degrees of freedom available at the forearm and hand.

Hypotheses: Upper-Extremity and Head Righting Dysfunction

Disuse weakness and limited ROM in the left deltoid and rotator cuff group from immobilization after scapular fracture and prolonged bed rest. Increased tone at the elbow and wrist on the left, causing immobility during reaching. Problems with force production and gradation of force are the result of poor somatosensory function in the left hand. Poor anticipatory control of reach and grasp.

Flexibility loss in the right elbow from postoperative swelling after HO removal.

C. H. is unable to maintain her head in upright on an automatic basis owing to visual and proprioceptive verticality impairment, lack of head-righting reflexes, and overstretch weakness of the neck extensor muscles.

Hypothesis Testing

Strength: MMT—neck extensors: 3−/5. Left arm—not able to actively abduct shoulder but able to actively hold if placed at 90 degrees. Shoulder flexion and external rotation, elbow flexion and extension—3/5 (but range was limited). Wrist extension—2+/5 (half range) and flexion 3+/5.

Force gradation was poor on use of a dynamometer. C. H. could not regulate her force output; she either gripped with full grip or used minimal force when asked to change her grip from minimal, 1 pound per square inch (psi) to 5 psi to 8 psi to 12 psi.

Flexibility: Passive ROM—Left shoulder limited to 100 degrees of flexion and abduction, 45 degrees of external rotation. Right elbow ROM—20 to 90 degrees in flexion and extension and 10 degrees in supination.

Tone: Modified Ashworth—Left arm, 3 in biceps, triceps, and wrist flexors, 2 in the finger flexors, otherwise 0 or 1 throughout. The tone was of a co-contraction nature at the elbow. There was poor spatial sequencing throughout the limb as tested during forward reach on sEMG.

Sensory and perception: Proprioception was impaired for the left hand; movement was perceived but direction was not consistent. Stereognosis—identified four of 10 objects placed in the left hand.

Visual-perceptual: C. H. complained of diplopia and identified a pen as vertical when in a left 10-degree tilt.

Task Analysis

Standing Balance

C. H. stood in quiet standing, feet shoulder width apart. There was hip flexion of 20 degrees with forward trunk lean. More weight was on the right leg than left. Shoulders were rotated 20 degrees to the left, and she had a 15-degree upper-trunk left

CASE STUDY 24-2 ■ C. H.—cont'd

lean. Her chin was resting on her chest. Standing is with increased sway in the fore-aft direction and no loss of balance in 30 seconds; sway increased moderately with eyes closed. Feet-together stance caused loss of balance in 15 seconds and in 10 seconds with eyes closed. When asked to reach rapidly forward, she fell forward and needed maximal assistance to recover her balance. Responses to small perturbations were with flexion at the hips and knees, and she continued to flex at the hips and knees with larger perturbations, again requiring assistance to recover her balance. When asked to take a step with the right foot in response to a perturbation, C. H. did not shift the weight to the left and required maximum assistance for balance recovery.

Hypotheses: Standing Balance

Forward lean is secondary to poor vertical perception (seen with lack of head righting with and without vision) from visual, proprioceptive, and vestibular dysfunction. There is overuse fatigue of hip extensors for maintaining continuous contraction whenever C. H. is upright. Trunk rotation secondary to increased left side tone in trunk, upper extremity (scapular retraction), and lower extremity. Balance losses were secondary to lack of anticipatory responses when reaching forward and for weight shift before right-foot stepping. The losses of balance with perturbation were secondary to a lack of stepping strategy and exclusive use of a mixed strategy for all standing conditions. Weakness of the gastrocnemius resulted in the early use of the hip strategy. Reaction times increased in response to perturbations, also contributing to imbalance.

Hypothesis Testing

Strength: MMT: 3/5 strength in left leg except 2+/5 in the left hip extensor and gastrocnemius.

Tone: Modified Ashworth 3 in the left quadriceps and gastrocnemius. The left lumbar extensors have above-normal tone and often elicited an extensor spasm during forward bending.

Muscle endurance: Poor in trunk and lower-extremity muscles; there was a reduction in amount of resistance tolerated after approximately five repetitions with isolated muscle testing of the quadriceps, hip extensors, back extensors, and cervical extensor muscles.

Sensory and perceptual systems: Proprioception was decreased (needs larger movement for accuracy) in the left ankle, knee, and hip.

Visual testing: C. H. had a left hemianopsia. No nystagmus was present. (Vision and vestibular systems are also addressed under the activity limitation.) Left tilt off vertical 15 degrees in standing with eyes open and with eyes closed.

Vestibular testing: C. H. complained of double vision and objects "jumping" with moderate and fast head motion with trying to maintain eye fixation on a pen tip. C. H. had increased sway during this test (in sitting). Unable to maintain balance for CTSIB testing.

Verticality: Unable to hold head up consistently; no head righting reflexes to tilts. Did not right lower body to floor in standing. No change with eyes closed.

Balance synergies to large and small perturbations: sEMG—appeared intact, in the right lower extremity, but ankle strategy is absent in the left. Small perturbations at the chest to balance are responded to with synergies showing a proximal-to-distal firing beginning in the trunk flexors and extensors. Amplitude of muscle contraction at the gastrocnemii was small even for large perturbations, less than 25% of her maximal contraction.

Gastrocnemius reaction times were 400 ms to perturbation on sEMG.

Anticipatory responses were generally absent in the left lower extremity and trunk during stepping. C. H. fell to the right each time she tried to raise her right leg. There was no anticipatory shift of weight to the left. sEMG showed no left gastrocnemius firing before rapid forward reaching.

Attention span was about 2 minutes during therapy.

EVALUATION AND DIAGNOSIS

Poor force control, timing and sequencing, lack of wrist and finger proprioception, co-contraction of the biceps and triceps, and poor anticipatory hand shaping during reach and grasp resulted in nonuse of the left hand. Contributing to the lack of use of the hand was poor strength in the scapular stabilizers after a scapular fracture that was immobilized and prolonged bed rest from decreased consciousness for 3 months. Lack of adequate elbow ROM from HO and postoperative swing in the right elbow prevented independent grooming, personal hygiene such as teeth brushing, and applying makeup when combined with deficits in the left hand.

C. H. appears unable to stand or walk without moderate to maximum assistance because of a lack of appropriate balance synergies in response to perturbations, lack of anticipatory responses to movements of her center of gravity, and impaired perception of vertical. Poor left gastrocnemius strength contributes to lack of an ankle strategy. Standing posture is with a forward lean owing to poor perception of vertical. The forward lean has in turn overstressed the back and hip extensors, and perhaps the gastrocnemius, which is consistent with disuse weakness from prolonged bed rest during the time when C. H. was in a coma and stupor and overuse weakness secondary to chronic forward lean position.

C. H. has problems perceiving the vertical position in sitting and standing because of visual, vestibular, and proprioceptive impairments.

Head righting is absent owing to loss of visual and proprioceptive head righting as well as overstretch weakness of the cervical extensors.

She has poor muscular endurance from prolonged bed rest.

Participation Limitations

Immature behavior and inappropriate anger and self-destructive responses resulting in loss of friends. Inability to balance and reach and grasp with the left hand restricts her from performing her job in a clothing store.

Outcome Measurement Tools

FIM score 79/126. Gait requires maximum assistance of 1. Romberg 15/30 seconds, Nine-Hole Peg Test 1 minute, Frenchay = 1/5.

Prognosis

Long-term goals: In 4 months, C. H. will be independent in all self-care activities and ADLs using the left hand as an assist. C. H. will be able to participate in activities with appropriate emotional responses (no episodes of scratching herself) and will have independent standing balance with and without perturbation using appropriate strategies.

Continued

CASE STUDY 24-2 ■ C. H.—cont'd

Short-term goals: Improved force production and timing of left gastrocnemius using FES daily for 15 minutes on a home exercise program and EMG biofeedback 3 × weekly for 2 weeks in clinic.

Improved force gradation for grasp so C. H. can grasp and release a paper cup filled with water and not deform the cup or spill the water in 2 weeks.

The prognosis for meeting the goals was good because C. H. is young, has a supportive family (sister and mother), and showed more focal lesions on MRI. The literature shows that problems of force production, flexibility, and ambulation modification in clients with brain injury have shown good modification. Decreasing the overall frustration level by working on achievable short-term goals and doing behavior modification should result in more appropriate emotional responses and improve her compliance.

INTERVENTIONS

Initial goals included addressing those impairments that did not allow higher levels of functioning. These were improvements in neck and hip strength and overstretch; gastrocnemius strength and flexibility; visual skills, particularly in tracking of objects into the left visual field; and awareness of vertical.

The head was the first focus. FES was applied to the posterior cervical muscles (5:1 duty cycle and frequency at 35 pps) for strengthening and upright head position. A sterno-occipital-mandibular immobilization support (SOMI) was worn intermittently to prevent further stretch weakness; later the SOMI was changed to a Philadelphia collar. Visual focus on a door frame was used to encourage visual control of head and body position for improved alignment. Complex neck activities to encourage basic synergy use and modification included seated activities in which C. H. wore a "hat" with a flat top from which she tried to prevent an object from falling off (first flat stable objects and later more rounded objects). This exercise was performed first on a firm, flat-seated surface and progressed to sitting on an exercise ball. The ball promoted automatic neck muscle motor patterns in which the body moves and the head is kept upright and still. To make the activity at the automatic level, C. H. did side-to-side leans while sitting on the ball, looking in a mirror to monitor head verticality and then doing the activity without the mirror.

Upper extremities: Traditional basic left upper-extremity strengthening exercises included the use of Thera-Band. Functional activities that required scapular use such as emptying the dishwasher with the left hand were assigned homework. Bilateral hand use was allowed early on. After C. H. could accomplish this, then only left hand use was allowed; a 1-lb wrist weight was added, which was gradually increased to 3 lb.

Electrical stimulation twice a day for 15 minutes to the right triceps and biceps gained 20 degrees of extension and 100 degrees of flexion. In the clinic, C. H. worked on picking up and manipulating objects of different sizes and shapes, throwing balls at targets, and doing two-handed carrying with a laundry basket and quick release of the basket. She sorted different-sized objects by retrieving them from a bucket which also contained marble-sized balls with her vision occluded to force the development of stereognosis.

C. H. enjoyed cooking, so tasks were given that used elbow extension, such as rolling out cookie dough. Exercises such as washing the dishes with hands in soapy water for proprioceptive feedback and practice of slip grip for enhancement of feedback through the fingertips were used. Setting the table with the left hand helped establish better functional use (plastic dishes).

Doing two-handed activities facilitated complex functions in manipulation with the left arm. C. H. hooked a small rug. When able, she began trying two-handed typing. Two of the most motivating activities were applying makeup and inserting contact lenses.

Visual treatment used exercises that required visual fixation at different points in space and at different distances using letters and objects, while moving the head left and right with the goal of seeing only one image. These exercises advanced to include moving objects and head moving with a fixed object and progressed to both the object and head moving while a single image was maintained. Finally, full body movement with eyes fixed on a moving object was accomplished. Vergence exercises were worked on, first using a ball with an "X" marked on it on a string, swinging the ball toward and away from her. She did five swings at a time and wrote down how many times the X stayed single. The ball was swung side to side, and C. H. had to point at it with her finger for left visual field loss.

Standing balance exercises focused on developing anticipatory responses. Exercises early on used a Gymnastik Ball, as well as wrist-weighted reaching exercises. Different weight balls were thrown and returned to C. H. She also worked on kicking a ball to a goal with the right foot. First the kick was very slow, and then the ball was made smaller and the kick faster. Kicking with the left leg was with eyes closed to promote increased proprioception. Exercises to promote ankle strategy such as swaying around the ankles were practiced to increase gastrocnemius control and timing.

After C. H. was able to stand and weight shift without support, small-angle, slow random tilts on a tilt board were used to promote both vertical upright and vestibular responses for balance. To promote vertical trunk control as well as anticipatory responses, C. H. practiced taking a full step forward on each foot. C. H. had a penlight attached by Velcro to a belt she wore on her waist. The goal was to keep the light, aimed at a wall target in front of her, from moving more than 2 inches side to side. This was also facilitated by moving the parallel bars extremely close together (about 1 inch from each hip) and asking C. H. not to touch the bars with either hip as she practiced stepping.

Tone was addressed with exercises to promote less co-contraction and distal-to-proximal sequencing in both the left leg and left arm. sEMG with a two-channel setup on the triceps and biceps and wrist flexors and wrist extensors was used with a faded schedule of feedback to teach decreased co-contraction during activities such as reaching and lifting.

C. H. used a NordicTrack machine for general cardiovascular fitness work. The gliding motion with toe loops allowed her to keep her feet near the ground when moving forward, and the arm work encouraged free movement of the trunk in rotation and hip extension without having to flex the hips through large ranges, that is, work her hip extensors in the shortened range to avoid overstretch positions.

CASE STUDY 24-2 ■ C. H.—cont'd

The goal C. H. had when first starting therapy was "to dance with my boyfriend." To encourage functional use of postural and balance motor patterns, dancing was used. She started first with slow dancing with her boyfriend. Gradually she was able to dance to faster music without being held, by using trunk and arm motion and a sidestepping motion. Finally, forward-backward movements and turning and bending were added. In addition, C. H. agreed to model in the brain injury association fashion show in 6 months, which provided motivation to walk independently.

Home exercises were not popular with C. H. A behavioral modification program was established so that she was given control to stop activities that were too stressful for her. She participated in a volunteer program on a farm feeding and watering animals two or three times a week on a fixed schedule to establish personal responsibility and provide a positive learning environment. A program of rewards and withholding of rewards was established to extinguish self-destructive behavior. Verbal feedback was provided when immature behavior was exhibited.

C. H. kept a diary of duties and accomplishments to help with memory and reinforce successes.

Motor learning was enhanced by using a program of blocked feedback to start, with only three trials before feedback was given. The number of trials increased to about 10, and then she progressed to random feedback, as C. H. was able to tolerate higher frustration levels. She began doing her own self-assessment of her performance after about 2 months of therapy for each of her activities.

OUTCOMES

C. H. reached the goals of independent standing both quiet and perturbed in about 6 weeks. She had vertical upright trunk and head posture but still needed the collar support intermittently for the neck. The left arm had good assistive and gross independent use. Tone in the left arm and left quadriceps was at a level 2 (Modified Ashworth Scale) at 6 weeks; however, the trunk tone was still interfering with standing posture and left side rotation remained, although at only about 50% of the initial rotation. C. H. was independent in all grooming and all but the most difficult of ADLs. The FIM score was 110/126, TUG 13 seconds, Frenchay 5/5, and Nine-Hole Peg Test 18 seconds. C. H. had no episodes of scratching herself and much higher tolerance for more difficult tasks. She continued to have some immature behaviors, but the work at the farm helped her to assess her own deficits better. She made friends, had a strong social life, and participated in the fashion show as a fundraiser activity for the Brain Injury Foundation.

APPENDIX 24-A ■ Patient Information

Family Guide to the Rancho Levels of Cognitive Functioning

Cognition refers to a person's thinking and memory skills. Cognitive skills include paying attention, being aware of one's surroundings, organizing, planning, following through on decisions, solving problems, using judgment, reasoning, and being aware of problems. Memory skills include the ability to remember things before and after the brain injury. Because of the damage caused by a brain injury, some or all of these skills will be changed.

The Rancho Levels of Cognitive Functioning is an evaluation tool used by the rehabilitation team. The eight levels describe the patterns or stages of recovery typically seen after a brain injury. This helps the team understand and focus on the person's abilities and design an appropriate treatment program. Each person will progress at his or her own rate, depending on the severity of the brain damage, the location of the injury in the brain, and the length of time since the brain injury. Some individuals will pass through each of the eight levels, whereas others may progress to a certain level and fail to change to the next higher level. It is important to remember that each person is an individual and there are many factors that need to be considered when assigning a level of cognition. There are a range of abilities within each of the levels, and your family member may exhibit some or all of the behaviors listed below.

Cognitive Level I
No Response

A person at this level will:

- not respond to sounds, sights, touch, or movement.

Cognitive Level II
Generalized Response

A person at this level will:

- begin to respond to sounds, sights, touch, or movement.
- respond slowly, inconsistently, or after a delay.
- responds in the same way to what he hears, sees, or feels. Responses may include chewing, sweating, breathing faster, moaning, moving, and/or developing increased blood pressure.

Cognitive Level III
Localized Response

A person at this level will:

- be awake on and off during the day.
- make more movements than before.
- react more specifically to what he or she sees, hears, or feels. For example, he or she may turn toward a sound, withdraw from pain, and attempt to watch a person move around the room.
- react slowly and inconsistently.
- begin to recognize family and friends.
- follow some simple directions such as "Look at me" or "Squeeze my hand."
- begin to respond inconsistently to simple questions with "yes" and "no" head nod or shakes.

What family and friends can do at Cognitive Levels I, II, and III:

- Explain to the individual what you are about to do. For example, "I'm going to move your leg."
- Talk in a normal tone of voice.
- Keep comments and questions short and simple. For example, instead of "Can you turn your head toward me?" say, "Look at me."

Continued

APPENDIX 24-A ■ Patient Information—cont'd

- Tell the person who you are, where he or she is, why he or she is in the hospital, and what day it is.
- Limit the number of visitors to two or three people at a time.
- Keep the room calm and quiet.
- Bring in favorite belongings and pictures of family members and close friends.
- Allow the person extra time to respond, but don't expect responses to be correct. Sometimes the person may not respond at all.
- Give the person rest periods. He or she will tire easily.
- Engage the person in familiar activities, such as listening to favorite music, talking about the family and friends, reading out loud to the individual, watching TV, combing his or her hair, putting on lotion.
- The person may understand parts of what you are saying. Therefore be careful what you say in front of the individual.

Cognitive Level IV

Confused and Agitated

A person at this level may:

- be very confused and frightened.
- not understand what he or she feels or what is happening around him or her.
- overreact to what is seen, heard, or felt by hitting, screaming, using abusive language, or thrashing about. This is because of the confusion.
- be restrained to prevent injury.
- be highly focused on basic needs—that is, eating, relieving pain, going back to bed, going to the bathroom, or going home.
- may not understand that people are trying to help.
- not pay attention or be able to concentrate for a few seconds.
- have difficulty following directions.
- recognize family and friends some of the time.
- with help, be able to do simple routine activities such as feeding himself or herself, dressing, or talking.

What family and friends can do at Cognitive Level IV:

- Tell the person where he or she is and reassure the person that he or she is safe.
- Bring in family pictures and personal items from home, to make the individual feel more comfortable.
- Allow the person as much movement as is safe.
- Take the person for rides in the wheelchair, with permission from nursing.
- Experiment to find familiar activities that are calming to him or her, such as listening to music or eating.
- Do not force the person to do things. Instead, listen to what he or she wants to do and follow this lead, within safety limits.
- Because the person often becomes distracted, restless, or agitated, you may need to give breaks and change activities frequently.
- Keep the room quiet and calm. For example, turn off the TV and radio, don't talk too much, and use a calm voice.
- Limit the number of visitors to two or three people at a time.

Cognitive Level V

Confused and Inappropriate

A person at this level may:

- be able to pay attention for only a few minutes.
- be confused and have difficulty making sense of things outside himself or herself.
- not know the date, where he or she is, or why he or she is in the hospital.
- not be able to start or complete everyday activities, such as brushing the teeth, even when physically able. Step-by-step instructions may be needed.
- become overloaded and restless when tired or when there are too many people around.
- have a very poor memory (the person will remember past events from before the accident better than the daily routine or information the individual has been told since the injury).
- try to fill in gaps in memory by making things up (confabulation).
- get stuck on an idea or activity (perseveration) and need help switching to the next part of the activity.
- focus on basic needs such as eating, relieving pain, going back to bed, going to the bathroom, or going home.

What family and friends can do at Cognitive Level V:

- Repeat things as needed. Don't assume that the person will remember what you say.
- Tell the individual the day, date, name and location of the hospital, and why he or she is in the hospital when you first arrive and before you leave.
- Keep comments and questions short and simple.
- Help the person organize and get started on an activity.
- Bring in family pictures and personal items from home.
- Limit the number of visitors to two or three at a time.
- Give frequent rest periods when he or she has problems paying attention.

Cognitive Level VI

Confused and Appropriate

A person at this level may:

- be somewhat confused because of memory and thinking problems; he or she will remember the main points from a conversation but forget and confuse the details. For example, the person may remember having had visitors in the morning but forget what they talked about.
- follow a schedule with some assistance but becomes confused by changes in the routine.
- know the month and year, unless there is a severe memory problem.
- pay attention for about 30 minutes but has trouble concentrating when it is noisy or when the activity involves many steps. For example, at an intersection, the person may be unable to step off the curb, watch for cars, watch the traffic light, walk, and talk at the same time.
- brush teeth, get dressed, feed himself or herself, and so on, with help.
- know when he or she needs to use the bathroom.
- do or say things too fast, without thinking first.
- know that he or she is hospitalized because of an injury but will not understand all of the problems he or she is having.
- be more aware of physical problems than thinking problems.
- associate his or her problems with being in the hospital and think that he or she will be fine once at home.

What family and friends can do at Cognitive Level VI:

- You will need to repeat things. Discuss things that have happened during the day to help the individual improve his or her memory.
- The person may need help starting and continuing activities.
- Encourage the individual to participate in all therapies. He or she will not fully understand the extent of the problems and the benefits of therapy.

APPENDIX 24-A ■ Patient Information—cont'd

Cognitive Level VII
Automatic and Appropriate
A person at this level may:

- follow a set schedule.
- be able to do routine self-care without help, if physically able. For example, he or she can dress or feed himself independently.
- have problems in new situations and may become frustrated or act without thinking first.
- have problems planning, starting, and following through with activities.
- have trouble paying attention in distracting or stressful situations—for example, family gatherings, work, school, church, or sports events.
- not realize how the thinking and memory problems may affect future plans and goals.
- Therefore the person may expect to return to the previous lifestyle or work.
- continue to need supervision because of decreased safety awareness and judgment. He or she still does not fully understand the impact of the physical or thinking problems.
- think more slowly in stressful situations.
- be inflexible or rigid and may seem stubborn. However, these behaviors are related to the brain injury.
- be able to talk about doing something but will have problems actually doing it.

Cognitive Level VIII
Purposeful and Appropriate
A person at this level may:

- realize that he or she has a problem in thinking and memory.
- begin to compensate for the problems.
- be more flexible and less rigid in thinking—for example, the person may be able to come up with several solutions to a problem.
- be ready for driving or job training evaluation.
- be able to learn new things at a slower rate.
- still become overloaded with difficult, stressful, or emergency situations.
- show poor judgment in new situations and may require assistance.
- need some guidance to make decisions.
- have thinking problems that may not be noticeable to people who did not know the person before the injury.

What family and friends can do at Cognitive Levels VII and VIII:

- Treat the person as an adult by providing guidance and assistance in decision making. His or her opinions should be respected.
- Talk with the individual as an adult. There is no need to try to use simple words or sentences.
- Be careful when joking or using slang, because the individual may misunderstand the meaning. Also, be careful about teasing.
- Help the individual in familiar activities so he or she can see some of the problems in thinking, problem solving, and memory. Talk to the person about these problems without criticizing. Reassure him or her that the problems are because of the brain injury.
- Strongly encourage the individual to continue with therapy to increase thinking, memory, and physical abilities. He or she may feel completely normal. However, he or she is still making progress and may possibly benefit from continued treatment.
- Be sure to check with the physician on the individual's restrictions concerning driving, working, and other activities. Do not just rely on the individual for information, because he or she may feel ready to go back to the previous lifestyle.
- Discourage the individual from drinking or using drugs, because of medical complications.
- Encourage the individual to use note taking as a way to help with the remaining memory problems.
- Encourage the person to carry out self-care as independently as possible.
- Discuss what kinds of situations make the person angry and what he or she can do in these situations.
- Talk with the person about his or her feelings.
- Learning to live with a brain injury can be difficult, and it may take a long time for the individual and family to adjust. The social worker and/or psychologist will provide the family and friends with information regarding counseling, resources, and/or support organizations.

Level IX—Purposeful, Appropriate: Stand-by Assistance on Request

- Independently shifts back and forth between tasks and completes them accurately for at least 2 consecutive hours.
- Uses assistive memory devices to recall daily schedule, make "to do" lists, and record critical information for later use with assistance when requested.
- Initiates and carries out steps to complete familiar personal, household, work, and leisure tasks independently and unfamiliar personal, household, work, and leisure tasks with assistance when requested.
- Is aware of and acknowledges impairments and disabilities when they interfere with task completion and takes appropriate corrective action but requires standby assistance to anticipate a problem before it occurs and take action to avoid it.
- Is able to think about consequences of decisions or actions with assistance when requested.
- Accurately estimates abilities but requires standby assistance to adjust to task demands.
- Acknowledges others' needs and feelings and responds appropriately with standby assistance.
- Depression may continue.
- May be easily irritable.
- May have low frustration tolerance.
- Able to self-monitor appropriateness of social interaction with standby assistance.

Level X—Purposeful, Appropriate: Modified Independent

- Able to handle multiple tasks simultaneously in all environments but may require periodic breaks.
- Able to independently procure, create, and maintain own assistive memory devices.
- Independently initiates and carries out steps to complete familiar and unfamiliar personal, household, community, work, and leisure tasks but may require more than usual amount of time and/or compensatory strategies to complete them.
- Anticipates impact of impairments and disabilities on ability to complete daily living tasks and takes action to avoid problems before they occur but may require more than usual amount of time and/or compensatory strategies.
- Able to independently think about consequences of decisions or actions but may require more than usual amount of time and/or

Continued

APPENDIX 24-A ■ Patient Information—cont'd

compensatory strategies to select the appropriate decision or action.

- Accurately estimates abilities and independently adjusts to task demands.
- Able to recognize the needs and feelings of others and automatically respond in appropriate manner.

- Periodic periods of depression may occur.
- Irritability and low frustration tolerance when sick, fatigued, and/or under emotional stress. Social interaction behavior is consistently appropriate.

APPENDIX 24-B ■ Sit-to-Stand Task Analysis

DESCRIBE START POSITION		CHECK BOX FOR PATTERN FOR EACH PHASE OF THE TRANSITIONAL MOVEMENT				SUMMARIZE MOVEMENT PATTERN AND HYPOTHESIZE BODY STRUCTURE IMPAIRMENTS TO EXPLAIN DEVIATIONS FROM EXPECTED PATTERN
DESCRIBE END POSITION		FLEXION MOMENTUM	MOMENTUM TRANSFER	EXTENSION	STABILIZATION	
Critical Events (circle if observed)		Feet 10 cm back Momentum generation	Continued LE flexion	LE and trunk extension	Ankle strategy	
UE	UEs push on chair UEs reach forward					
Trunk	Insufficient speed Insufficient flexion Insufficient extension					
LE	Insufficient ankle dorsiflexion Insufficient knee flexion Insufficient tibial translation Insufficient hip extension Insufficient knee extension Unstable					

LE, Lower extremity; *UE*, upper extremity.

CHAPTER 25 Brain Tumors

CORRIE J. STAYNER, PT, MS, RACHEL M. LOPEZ, PT, MPT, NCS, and KARLA M. TUZZOLINO, PT, NCS

KEY TERMS

astrocytoma
biopsy
chemotherapy
Gamma Knife
glioblastoma multiforme
hospice care
Karnofsky performance status scale
meningioma
metastatic
radiation therapy
ventriculostomy

OBJECTIVES

After reading this chapter the student or therapist will be able to:

1. Identify the categories of primary brain tumors.
2. Recognize and interpret signs and symptoms of primary brain tumors specific to tumor location.
3. Recognize current diagnostic tests used to detect brain tumors.
4. Identity the types of medical and surgical management for brain tumors and how that management will affect functional movement.
5. Describe the side effects associated with the treatment of brain tumors and recognize their impact on therapeutic intervention.
6. Discuss the multiple considerations necessary to plan and execute an intervention program for the client with a brain tumor.
7. Recognize the emotional and psychosocial impact of the disease process on the client, the client's support system, and the interdisciplinary team.

AN OVERVIEW OF BRAIN TUMORS

The rehabilitation clinician serves many different populations, including clients with brain tumors. Despite the prognosis for limited survival associated with primary brain tumors, these individuals have shown progress in the rehabilitation setting similar to that noted in clients with diagnoses of stroke or traumatic brain injury.[1-3] Advances in medical and surgical treatment for clients with cancer have resulted in improved survival rates and longer life expectancy. However, individuals are often faced with progressive impairments resulting from the disease process.[2] These impairments may be physical or cognitive, or both, and require an interdisciplinary team approach to best facilitate the individual's participation in a meaningful lifestyle. In addition, clinicians must recognize the psychological and emotional needs of the individual given this diagnosis and be sensitive and flexible in accommodating the patient's feelings. Improved quality of life, especially the opportunity to return home, remains the ultimate goal of the rehabilitation process.

The clinical presentation of clients with brain tumors mimics that of persons with other central nervous system (CNS) conditions. The location of the tumor or vascular accident determines the impairments the client will exhibit. However, in the brain tumor client the burdensome effects of standard medical intervention and the aggressive nature of the disease course itself provide obstacles to therapeutic intervention. The client's probability of eventual body structure and function deterioration provides a challenge to the clinician attempting to formulate realistic goals and plan for future needs. Therefore a thorough knowledge of the tumor's natural history, the complications and side effects of treatment, and the neurological impairment the client exhibits will assist the clinician in best developing a comprehensive, individualized plan of care.

Incidence and Etiology

The incidence of adult brain tumors is on the rise in the United States, with an estimated 62,930 new cases of primary benign or malignant brain and CNS tumors for 2010. The statistics for children include 4030 new cases for the same 12-month period, of which 2880 will occur in children younger than 15 years of age.[4,5]

The exact cause of the increase in incidence of brain tumors is not known. Studies suggest that the increase is the result of more tumors being diagnosed with improved tumor imaging, rather than an actual increase in the occurrence of malignant brain tumors.[6,7]

In the United States, brain tumors typically occur in two distinct categories of patients: (1) children aged 0 to 15 years and (2) adults in the fifth to seventh decades of life. In adults, white Americans have a higher incidence than black Americans, and in both pediatric and adult populations males are more frequently affected than females.[8,9] In children, a primary brain tumor is now the most common cause of solid tumor cancer death in the 0- to 15-year-old age group and the second overall cancer after leukemia.[5]

The frequently occurring meningioma, typically benign, accounts for 33.8% of all primary brain tumors. Glioblastoma multiforme, a malignant tumor, accounts for 17.1% of adult primary tumors (Figure 25-1).[5] The largest percentage of childhood tumors (17%) are located in the frontal, temporal, parietal, and occipital lobes of the brain, followed by 16% in the cerebellum and 11% in the brain stem.[5]

The etiology of brain tumors remains unclear. Theories suggest that heredity is a contributing factor, but studies

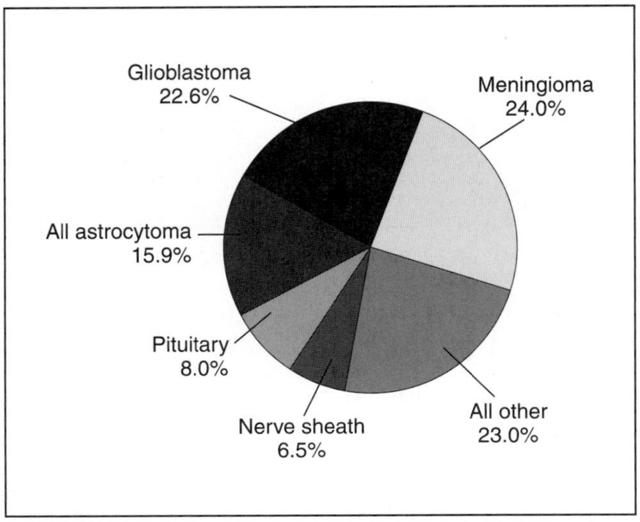

Figure 25-1 ■ Distribution of all primary brain and central nervous system tumors by histology. (From Central Brain Tumor Registry of the United States (CBTRUS): *2010 Statistical report: primary brain and central nervous system tumors diagnosed in the United States, 2004-2006,* Hinsdale, Ill, 2010, CBTRUS.)

show familial incidence can be explained by a common toxic or infectious exposure.[10,11] Research indicates an association, but not a causal relationship, linking brain tumors to certain chemicals and materials (petrochemicals, organic solvents, rubber). These materials are frequently found in specific occupations, such as farming and manufacturing. Electromagnetic field exposure is associated with an increased incidence of brain tumor.[12] Ionizing radiation, used therapeutically in high doses to treat tumors, was found to have a causal relationship to the development of a second brain tumor.[13]

Continued investigation into possible causal relationships with potential risk factors is essential if the incidence and mortality rate associated with brain tumors are to decrease.

Classification of Tumors

The World Health Organization (WHO) first published a universal classification system for CNS tumors in 1979. This system classifies tumors according to their microscopic characteristics and has been accepted as the universal method for the classification of brain tumors.[14,15]

Primary Brain Tumors

Primary tumors originate in the CNS, whereas metastatic or secondary tumors spread to the CNS from systemic cancer sites outside the brain. Characteristics of the most common brain tumors are discussed in the following paragraphs, with information provided regarding age at onset, location, medical treatment, and prognosis.

Gliomas are primary tumors that arise from supportive tissues of the brain and are frequently located in the cerebral hemispheres. These tumors may also occur in the brain stem, optic nerve, and spinal cord. In children, the cerebellum is a primary location for gliomas.[13,16] Gliomas have four primary categories and are classified by their predominant cellular components: astrocytomas and oligodendrogliomas originate from glial cells, ependymomas from ependymal cells, and medulloblastomas from primitive cells.[17]

Astrocytomas are derived from astrocytes, which are star-shaped glial cells, and are the most common primary brain tumor in adults and children.[18] Astrocytomas vary in morphology and biological behavior, from those that are diffuse and infiltrate surrounding brain structures, to those that are circumscribed with a decreased likelihood of progression. Astrocytomas are typically found in the cerebrum, originating in the frontal lobe in adults, and in the cerebellum in children. In adults the primary age at onset is typically in the third to fifth decades of life.[7,14]

Astrocytomas are further classified into four grades: pilocytic, well-differentiated, relatively benign low-grade tumors most common in childhood and young adults (grade I); diffuse, well differentiated, low-grade tumors (grade II); anaplastic, high-grade tumors (grade III); and glioblastoma multiforme, high-grade (grade IV). The higher the grade, the poorer the prognosis.[7]

Low-grade tumors (grade II) grow slowly and are typically subtotally resected through surgery when accessible, whereas grade I tumors occur primarily in children and are typically cured with complete surgical resection. As a result of incomplete resections, recurrence is common.[7] As these tumors recur, their form and structure often change to that of an anaplastic astrocytoma or glioblastoma.[17] Anaplastic, midgrade (grade III) tumors grow rapidly, typically carry malignant cell traits, and routinely progress toward glioblastoma multiforme tumors.[14]

Astrocytomas are typically treated with surgery, radiation therapy, and chemotherapy, depending on the grade, location of the tumor, age of the patient, and Karnofsky performance scale score (Table 25-1).[7,16,19] Pilocytic astrocytomas carry a 5-year survival rate of 94%; however, patients with grade III astrocytomas have a 5-year survival rate of only 27%.[5]

Glioblastoma multiforme is the distinct name given to the highly malignant grade IV astrocytoma. These tumors grow rapidly, invade nearby tissue, and contain highly malignant cells. Glioblastomas are predominantly located in the deep white matter of the cerebral hemispheres but may be found in the brain stem, cerebellum, or spinal cord. Fifty percent of these tumors are bilateral or occupy more than one lobe of a hemisphere.[7,14,16] Glioblastomas account for 17% of all primary brain tumors. They are most common in older adults and uncommon in children, with males having a 1.6:1 incidence rate over females.[5] The medical prognosis is poor for persons with glioblastoma: less than 33% survive more than 1 year and less than 5% survive 5 years.[5] The most important prognostic variables are age, tumor histology, and postoperative score on the Karnofsky performance status scale. These tumors are treated by surgical resection, radiation therapy, stereotactic radiosurgery, and chemotherapy.[7]

Oligodendrogliomas are slow-growing but progressive tumors that typically develop over a period of several years, with 50% involving multiple lobes. Fifty percent of these tumors occur in the frontal lobe, 42% in the temporal lobe, and 32% in the parietal lobe. Many clients have seizures as the only clinical manifestation of the tumor.[14,20,21] Oligodendrogliomas typically appear in the fourth to sixth decades of life, and the ratio of affected males to females is 2:1.[22] The prognosis with oligodendrogliomas varies considerably and

TABLE 25-1 ■ KARNOFSKY PERFORMANCE STATUS SCALE

CONDITION	PERFORMANCE STATUS (%)	COMMENTS
A. Able to carry on normal activity and to work; no special care is needed	100	Normal; no complaints; no evidence of disease
	90	Able to carry on normal activity; minor signs or symptoms of disease
	80	Normal activity with effort; some signs or symptoms of disease
B. Unable to work; able to live at home, care for most personal needs; a varying degree of assistance is needed	70	Care of self; unable to carry on normal activity or to do active work
	60	Requires occasional assistance but is able to care for most of personal needs
	50	Requires considerable assistance and frequent medical care
C. Unable to care for self; requires equivalent of institutional or hospital care; disease may be progressing rapidly	40	Disabled; requires special care and assistance
	30	Severely disabled; hospitalization is indicated, although death not imminent
	20	Very sick; hospitalization necessary; active supportive treatment necessary
	10	Moribund; fatal processes progressing rapidly
	0	Dead

Adapted from Karnofsky DA, Burchenal JH: The clinical evaluation of chemotherapeutic agents in cancer. In Macleod C, editor: *Evaluation of chemotherapeutic agents,* New York, 1949, Columbia University Press.

is dependent on age at diagnosis and tumor grade. Positive prognostic indicators have been age at onset of less than 40 years and a tumor grade of I or II. These patients have a 5-year survival rate of 79% and 10-year survival rate of 64%.[5] The 5-year survival rate decreases to 47% with anaplastic oligodendroglioma.[5] Treatment is dependent on symptoms and ranges from observation and seizure control with anticonvulsant drugs to surgical resection followed by radiation and chemotherapy.[7,17,20] Negative prognostic indicators include age at onset over 40 years, hemiparesis, and cognitive changes.[23]

Ependymomas and *ependymoblastomas* are tumors arising from ependymal cells, cells that line the ventricles of the brain and central canal of the spinal cord.[16,17] These cells have glial and epithelial characteristics. The tumors grow into the ventricle or adjacent brain tissue. The most common site is the fourth ventricle (70% originate here); they occur less frequently in lateral and third ventricles.[22] For supratentorial tumors, the age at onset is evenly distributed across the life span, whereas tumors originating in the fourth ventricle more frequently occur in childhood.[22] Ependymomas are primarily treated with surgical resection followed by radiation therapy, but chemotherapy is also used.[7,16,17,22] These tumors frequently recur, and prognosis is dependent on the success of resection, with a 5-year survival rate approaching 82%.[5]

Medulloblastomas are malignant embryonal tumors thought to arise from primitive neuroectodermal cells, specifically pluripotential stem cells that have been prevented from maturing to their normal growth-arrested state. The exact cell of origin, however, is still unknown.[22] These tumors are typically located in the posterior fossa, originating laterally in the cerebellar hemispheres in young adults and in the vermis in children.[14] Medulloblastomas typically grow into the fourth ventricle, blocking cerebrospinal fluid (CSF) flow, causing hydrocephalus and increased intracranial pressure (ICP).[7] These tumors primarily occur in children, accounting for 20% of childhood (0 to 19 years) brain tumors, with the most common age of onset being 4 to 8 years old; they are more prevalent in males than females.[22] An overall 5-year survival rate of 61% has been noted among adults and children; the most common treatment is surgery followed by radiation and chemotherapy.[5,14,22]

Meningiomas are slow-growing tumors that primarily originate from cells located in the dura mater or arachnoid membrane and account for 33% of reported brain tumors.[5,18,22] Frequently these tumors are found incidentally during imaging studies or at autopsy.[24] Approximately 25% of patients are symptomatic when diagnosed.[18,24,25] Meningiomas are classified by their cytoarchitecture and genetic origin into four categories: (1) meningothelial or syncytial, (2) fibroblastic, (3) angioblastic variants, and (4) malignant.[22] The incidence increases with age, and they occur in females at a 2:1 ratio over males.[3,5,26,27] Resectable tumors are primarily treated by surgery, and recurring tumors are treated with surgery, radiation therapy, or stereotactic radiosurgery.[17] Patients with nonmalignant meningiomas have a 5-year survival rate of 70% versus a 5-year survival rate of 55% with malignant meningiomas.[5,28]

Pituitary adenomas are benign epithelial tumors originating from the adenohypophysis of the pituitary gland and frequently encroach on the optic chiasm.[14,17,22] These tumors are characterized by hypersecretion or hyposecretion of hormones.[7,16] Age at onset spans all ages, but pituitary adenomas are rare before puberty.[7] The female-to-male ratio of incidence is 3:1.[5] These tumors are primarily treated by surgical resection and drug therapy.[7,16,17] Prognosis is related to size and tumor cell type, with a 5-year survival rate of 70%.[5]

Schwannomas are encapsulated tumors composed of neoplastic Schwann cells that can arise on any cranial or spinal nerve.[16,17] The eighth cranial nerve is the cranial nerve usually involved, and a schwannoma here is called an *acoustic neuroma*.[14] Acoustic neuromas produce otological, focal or generalized neurological impairments, depending on the location of the tumor. These tumors are typically located in the internal auditory canal but may extend into the cerebellopontine angle.[7,22] These tumors are frequently treated by surgical resection, but stereotactic radiosurgery is increasing in popularity as an alternative method of treatment.[16,29,30] The prognosis for patients with these tumors is good, yet complications can result from treatment, including facial paralysis, deafness, and equilibrium impairments. Resulting activity limitations after surgery vary depending on the size and location of the tumor. Currently these tumors rarely result in death, and with the increasing use of noninvasive procedures the eighth cranial nerve is more frequently being preserved.[30]

Primary CNS lymphoma represents only 1% of intracranial tumors, although the incidence has significantly increased in the last two decades. This increase may be a result of its frequency in individuals with acquired immunodeficiency syndrome (AIDS) and other immunosuppressed states. Surprisingly, there is an increased frequency in immunocompetent persons; however, no evidence-based explanation has been found. These lymphomas have a slightly higher incidence in men and peak in the fifth through seventh decades of life, or in the third and fourth decades in individuals with AIDS. The tumor cells are similar in histology to systemic non-Hodgkin lymphoma cells, but it is uncertain how this tumor arises, as the CNS lacks lymphatic tissue.[22,31] The tumor may be solitary or multifocal, forming a poorly defined mass that may be difficult to distinguish from an astrocytoma.[22] Although CSF cytology may be diagnostic, stereotactic brain biopsy is often needed for definitive diagnosis.[31] Primary brain lymphomas may arise in the cerebrum, cerebellum, or brain stem; however, 60% occur in the cerebral hemisphere. More frequently, presenting symptoms are behavioral and personality changes, confusion, dizziness, and focal cerebral signs rather than headache and other signs of increased ICP.[22] Surgical resection is typically ineffective because of the deep location of these tumors. Cranial irradiation and corticosteroids frequently yield a partial or complete response; however, the tumor recurs in 90% of these individuals.[22] A more recent favorable treatment includes the administration of intravenous methotrexate and leucovorin over 2- to 3-week intervals with corticosteroids to control neurologic symptoms.[22] CNS lymphoma carries a poor prognosis, with only 27% of patients surviving longer than 5 years.[5]

Secondary Brain Tumors: Metastatic Brain Tumors

Metastatic brain tumors originate from malignancies outside of the CNS and spread to the brain, typically through the arterial circulation.[7,22] Approximately 25% of individuals with systemic cancer develop metastatic brain tumors, approximately 80% in cerebral hemispheres and 20% in the posterior fossa.[22,31,32] One third of brain metastases originate in the lung, followed by the breast, skin, gastrointestinal tract, and kidneys in order of frequency. The frontal lobe is the most common site for metastatic disease from these systemic sources. Common clinical manifestations of metastatic brain tumors are similar to those of gliomas, including seizures, headache, focal weakness, mental and behavioral limitations, ataxia, aphasia, and signs of increased ICP.[22]

Treatment for these tumors is tailored to the individual and dependent on the management of the systemic disease, the accessibility of the lesion, and the number of lesions.[32,33] Current treatment regimens use combinations of corticosteroids, brain irradiation, surgical intervention, and chemotherapy.[22] The prognosis varies, with positive prognostic indicators including the Karnofsky performance scale score of 70 or greater, age 60 years or younger, remission or resolution of the primary cancer, and metastases located in the brain only.[32,33] The average survival with treatment is approximately 6 months but varies widely and is affected by the extent of other systemic metastases. With some radiosensitive tumors, survival increases to 15% to 30% for 1 year and 5% to 10% for 2 years.[22]

Signs and Symptoms

The clinical manifestation of a brain tumor can range from a decreased speed in comprehension or a minor personality change to progressive hemiparesis or seizure, depending on the type and site of the tumor. Patients with brain tumors typically have headaches, seizures, nonspecific cognitive or personality changes, or focal neurological signs.[22,34] The presenting sign in some may be a general sign, a specific neurological symptom, or a combination of both.

General Signs and Symptoms

General signs and symptoms of the presence of a brain tumor include headache, seizures, altered mental status, and papilledema. *Headache* is the presenting symptom in 30% of cases and develops during the course of the disease in 70% of cases. These headaches are generally dull, intermittent, and nonspecific and are usually on the same side as the tumor. They are often difficult to distinguish from migraine or cluster headaches. It is important to identify the specific nature of the headaches, because certain features often indicate the presence of a brain tumor. These features include the following:

1. The headache that interrupts sleep or is worse on waking and improves throughout the day
2. The headache that is elicited by postural changes, coughing, or exercise
3. The headache of recent onset that is more severe or of a different type than usual
4. The new onset of headache in a previously asymptomatic person
5. The headache associated with nausea and vomiting, papilledema, or focal neurological signs[1,7]

The mechanism of the headache is not clearly understood but may be related to local swelling, distortion of blood vessels, direct invasion of the meninges, and increased ICP. When the tumor has grown to a volume large enough to cause compression and displacement of the brain, the onset and severity of the headache seem to correlate with changes in ICP.[35] With increased ICP, a bifrontal or bioccipital headache is present regardless of the tumor location.[22,36]

Seizure activity is the presenting symptom in one third of cases and is present in 50% to 70% of cases at some stage of the disease.[13,34] Approximately 10% to 20% of adults with new-onset seizure activity have brain tumors. Seizures are usually focal but may become generalized and cause loss of consciousness.[37] Frontal lobe gliomas produce seizures in 59% of all cases. The percentages of patients exhibiting seizures from gliomas in other lobes are as follows: parietal, 42%; temporal, 35%; and occipital, 33%.[34]

Altered mental status is the initial symptom in 15% to 20% of individuals with brain tumors and is frequently present at the time of diagnosis. Mental status changes can range from subtle changes in concentration, memory, affect, personality, initiative, and abstract reasoning to severe cognitive problems and confusion.[34] Subtle changes may be incorrectly attributed to worry, anxiety, or depression.[22] Changes in mentation are common with frontal lobe tumors and in the presence of elevated ICP. Increased ICP causes drowsiness and decreased level of consciousness, which can progress to stupor or coma if treatment is not initiated.[34]

The incidence of *papilledema,* swelling of the optic nerve, is less frequent today because brain tumors are being diagnosed earlier with the use of sensitive imaging techniques. Papilledema is associated with symptoms of transient visual loss, especially with positional changes, and reflects evidence of increased intracranial hemorrhage transmitted through the optic nerve sheath. It is more common in children and with slow-growing tumors and posterior fossa tumors.[34] Other, less common symptoms are vomiting and frank positional vertigo, usually accompanying tumors found in the posterior fossa.[22]

Specific Signs and Symptoms

Certain clinical features are related to functional areas of the brain and thus have a specific localizing value in medically diagnosing a brain tumor.[34] Therefore it is essential that clinicians be familiar with the lobes of the brain and their distinct functions to effectively manage the impairments resulting from the tumor (Figure 25-2). These symptoms may vary among individuals and result in activity limitations that range from mild to severe.[35]

The *frontal lobe* is responsible for motor functioning, initiation of action, and interpretation of emotion, including motor speech, motor praxis, attention, cognition, emotions, intelligence, judgment, motivation, and memory.[38,39] Therefore frontal lobe tumors may result in movement disorders such as hemiparesis, seizures, aphasia, and gait difficulties. Initially the tumor may be clinically silent. As the tumor grows, however, there may be personality changes, including disinhibition, irritability, impaired judgment, and lack of initiation.[34] Bifrontal disease usually associated with infiltrative gliomas and primary CNS lymphomas may cause bilateral hemiplegia; spastic bulbar

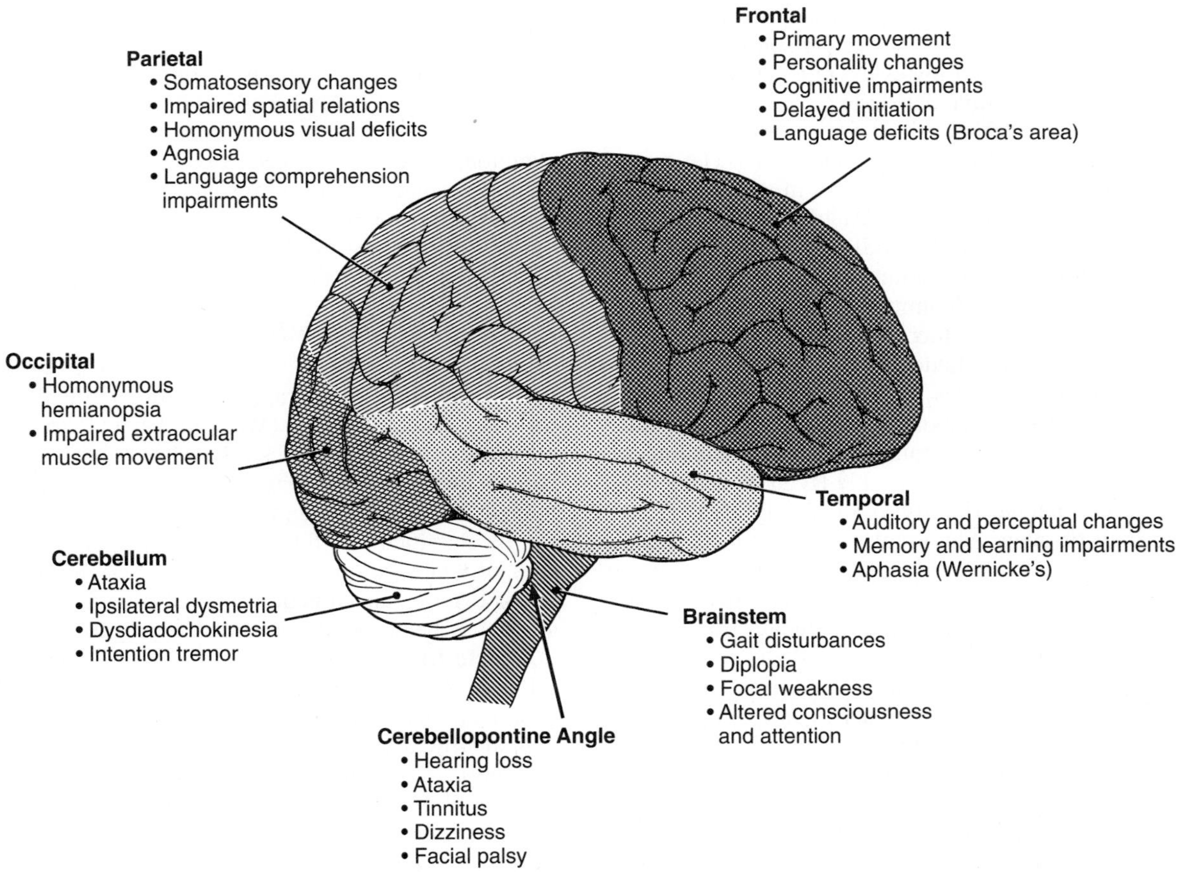

Figure 25-2 ■ Correlation between clinical symptoms and anatomical location of the tumor. (Used with permission from Barrow Neurological Institute.)

palsy; severe cognitive impairment; emotional lability; dementia; and prominent primitive grasp, suck, and snout reflexes.[35]

The *parietal lobe* processes complex sensory and perceptual information related to somesthetic sensation, spatial relations, body schema, and praxis. General symptoms of a parietal lobe tumor include contralateral sensory loss and hemiparesis, homonymous visual deficits or neglect, agnosias, apraxias, and visual-spatial disorders. If the dominant parietal lobe is involved, aphasia and seizures may be present. With nondominant parietal lobe involvement, contralateral neglect and decreased awareness of impairments can commonly be found.[26,34,36]

The *occipital lobe* is the primary processing area of visual information. Therefore lesions of the occipital lobe often result in dysfunction of eye movement and homonymous hemianopsia. If the parieto-occipital junction is involved, visual agnosia and agraphia are often present. Although less common, visual seizures may be present, characterized by lights, colors, and formed geometric patterns.[33,34,36] Bilateral occipital tumors may cause cortical blindness.[35]

The *temporal lobe* is responsible for auditory and limbic processing. Anterior temporal lobe lesions may be clinically silent until they have become quite large, resulting in seizures. If the lateral hemispheres are involved, auditory and perceptual changes may occur. When the medial aspects of the lobe are involved, changes in cognitive integration, long-term memory, learning, and emotions may be seen. When the dominant temporal lobe is involved, aphasia may be present. Anomia, agraphia, acalculia, and Wernicke aphasia, characterized by fluent, nonsensical speech, are specific to left temporal lobe lesions.[33,34,36] In comparison with bifrontal tumors, bitemporal tumor involvement is rare and causes memory deficits and possible dementia.[35]

The *cerebellum* is responsible for coordination and equilibrium.[26](Refer to Chapters 21 and 22A.) The most common symptoms of cerebellar tumors in adults include headache, nausea and vomiting in 40% of cases, and ataxia in 25% of cases. Lesions of the midline cause truncal and gait ataxia, and lesions of the hemispheres cause unilateral appendicular ataxia, most commonly seen in the upper extremities. Lesions of either hemisphere may cause ipsilateral dysmetria, dysdiadochokinesia, and intention tremor. If the tumor involves the cerebellopontine angle, hearing loss, headache, ataxia, dizziness, tinnitus, and facial palsy may occur. If the tumor invades the meninges at the foramen magnum or increased ICP causes cerebellar tonsil herniation, nuchal rigidity and head tilt away from the lesion may be seen. Abnormal posturing of the head is observed in children but not adults.[35] Because the cerebellum is located in an extremely confined space, even minimal increases in pressure can cause death from cerebellar tonsil herniation.[7,34,35,40]

The *brain stem,* which communicates information to and from the cerebral cortex via fiber tracts, controls basic life functions. The reticular formation specifically controls consciousness and attention. Even small changes in tumors invading or compressing the brain stem can lead to death or devastating signs and symptoms. Symptoms of a brain stem tumor have an insidious onset and may include gait disturbances, diplopia, focal weakness, headache, vomiting, facial numbness and weakness, and personality changes.[7] If the dorsal midbrain is involved, Parinaud syndrome, characterized by loss of upward gaze, pupillary areflexia to light, and loss of convergence, may be seen. If the reticular system of the pons and medulla is involved, symptoms of apnea, hypoventilation or hyperventilation, orthostatic hypotension, or syncope may occur.[7,40]

The *pituitary gland* is an endocrine gland that secretes hormones that regulate many bodily processes. Pituitary tumors are typically large and affect pituitary function by compressing its structure or hypersecreting hormones. An enlarging tumor causes a loss of pituitary function and decreases hormone secretion, resulting in pituitary disorders specific to the type of hormone involved (e.g., Cushing disease, hypothyroidism, Addison disease, diabetes). As the tumor enlarges it may invade or compress nearby structures. Lateral extension involving the third and fourth cranial nerves causes diplopia; fifth cranial nerve involvement causes ipsilateral facial numbness; and internal carotid artery occlusion causes cerebral infarction. Upward extension is more common and may compress the optic chiasm, hypothalamus, or third ventricle. Downward extension may compress the sphenoid sinus, typically without clinical signs.[7]

Medical Diagnosis of Disease or Pathology

Advances in research and imaging technology have greatly improved brain tumor medical diagnosis. When a physician suspects a brain tumor, many specialized tests may be used to gather clinical, radiological, pathological, and laboratory information to confirm the diagnosis.[31,34]

Clinical Diagnosis

A clinical diagnosis consists of information the physician gathers during a comprehensive evaluation. First, a thorough medical history, including the specific nature of signs and symptoms, must be obtained. A neurological examination is then performed to test reflexes and assess visual, cognitive, sensory, and motor function.[40] If the presence of a brain tumor is suspected after the neurological examination, the next diagnostic step, tumor imaging, is warranted.[22]

Radiological Diagnosis

The modern era of CNS imaging began with the introduction of computed tomography (CT) in 1973 and with magnetic resonance imaging (MRI) in 1979.[7] The availability of sensitive imaging allows for earlier tumor detection and has revolutionized the diagnosis and management of brain tumors.[34,41] Tumor imaging has continued to develop and can be classified into three categories: static, dynamic, and computer integration imaging. Each type of scan shows different features and function of the brain; therefore several scans may be needed for an accurate diagnosis.[16]

Static Imaging. Static neurological imaging includes CT and MRI, which are noninvasive techniques that provide accurate anatomical and functional analysis of intracranial structures.[34] CT uses ionizing radiation, thin bands of x-rays, to produce images of slices of brain tissue.[31] It was the first brain imaging technique to allow determination of tumor size. Contrast enhancement helps to identify isodense tumor from surrounding parenchyma, hypodense lesions in edematous areas, and optimal sites for tumor biopsy.[7,34] After surgical intervention, CT can be used to confirm the proper tissue biopsy site and determine the success of tumor resection. Although MRI has become the preferred method, CT scanning offers lower cost, a shorter scanning time, and a more sensitive method to detect calcification and bony involvement.[22]

Magnetic Resonance Imaging. MRI is the initial diagnostic imaging procedure of choice. MRI uses magnetic fields rather than ionizing radiation and is superior to CT scanning in detecting and localizing brain tumors, as well as evaluating edema, hydrocephalus, or hemorrhage.[22,34,35] CT scans can miss structural lesions, especially posterior fossa tumors and low-grade gliomas.[37] MRI is a more sensitive imaging modality than CT for identifying lesions and margin abnormalities by providing greater anatomical detail with thin slices and multiplanar images. With MRI, different signal intensities differentiate between normal brain and tumor. Contrast enhancement with gadolinium sharpens the definition of a lesion.[7,22,36] Under certain conditions, MRI enhanced with gadolinium can distinguish between tumor and edema. However, not all high-grade astrocytomas enhance with gadolinium, and MRI signals may imitate imaging abnormalities seen in low-grade astrocytomas or nonmalignant conditions. MRI also cannot accurately predict tumor type or grade of malignancy, for which surgical biopsy is necessary.[7,34]

Dynamic Imaging. Dynamic functional imaging includes positron emission tomography (PET), single-photon emission CT (SPECT), magnetic resonance spectroscopy (MRS), and functional MRI. PET is a noninvasive technique using a cyclotron and specific isotopes to obtain dynamic information about the metabolism and physiology of the brain tumor and the surrounding brain tissue. PET scans using radioactive markers to measure glucose metabolism can be useful in determining the grade of primary brain tumors and in differentiating tumor regrowth from radiation necrosis.[9,36,42] PET can also be helpful in studying the metabolic effects of chemotherapy, radiation therapy, and steroids on the tumor.[34] However, PET is expensive and less reliable in patients treated heavily with chemotherapy and radiation therapy.[7,22]

Single-Photon Emission Computed Tomography. SPECT is a functional imaging technique evolved from PET and uses isotopes without cyclotron to assess cerebral blood flow and determine tumor location.[7,22,34] SPECT is used to identify high- and low-grade tumors and to differentiate between tumor recurrence and radiation necrosis.[7,34] SPECT is used preoperatively with static imaging to localize the highest metabolic area within tumor for biopsy. Although SPECT is a less sensitive method of obtaining physiological information on brain tumors, it is more readily available and less expensive.[7]

Magnetic Resonance Spectroscopy. MRS is a noninvasive technique used in conjunction with static MRI to measure the metabolism of brain tumors.[7] MRS has been proved to differentiate successfully normal brain from malignant tumor and recurrent tumor from radiation necrosis. It also has been used to document early treatment response and provide information regarding histological grade of astrocytomas.[43,44] In the future, MRS targeting may enhance the diagnostic yield of brain biopsy and possibly be a noninvasive alternative to surgical biopsy.[43,45] Magnetic resonance angiography (MRA) generates images of blood vessels without dye or ionizing radiation to evaluate the blood flow and position of vessels leading to the brain tumor.[31]

Functional Magnetic Resonance Imaging. Functional MRI uses a conventional MRI scanner fitted with echo planar technology to map cerebral blood flow at the capillary level. Its intended purpose is to provide information regarding the diffusion of contrast into tumor, resulting in better resolution of tumor and edema.[7] Functional MRI can also be used to identify the motor, sensory, and language areas of the brain or the functional eloquent cortex.[16,46]

Modern computer technology allows for the two- and three-dimensional reconstruction of identical planes in cranial space by combining tumor images from different modalities, including CT, MRI, PET, and SPECT. *Computed integration imaging* involves the simultaneous display of images from different techniques in a single imaging system that is transposed to a reference stereotactic frame. This development has resulted in significant advances in stereotactic biopsy, interstitial radiotherapy, and laser-guided stereotactic resection.[7] By improving targeting and visualization of tissues, stereotaxis provides a safer, more accurate method of tissue acquisition and biopsy. A correct tissue diagnosis can be made in 95% of cases with this technique.[47] (Refer to Chapter 37 for additional discussion on all types of imaging and visual examples.)

Biopsy

Surgical biopsy is performed to obtain tumor tissue as part of tumor resection or as a separate diagnostic procedure.[13] Stereotactic biopsy is a computer-directed needle biopsy. When guided by advanced imaging tools, stereotactic biopsy yields the lowest surgical morbidity and highest degree of diagnostic information. This technique is frequently used with deep-seated tumors in functionally important or inaccessible areas of the brain in order to preserve function.[48]

Laboratory Diagnosis

Laboratory testing is often used to further assess focal deficits during the diagnosis and management of brain tumors. Perimetry is the measurement of visual fields used when evaluating tumors near the optic chiasm. Electroencephalography (EEG) is used to monitor brain activity and detect seizures but has limited value during screening because EEG findings are often normal in clients with brain tumors.[34] Lumbar puncture is used to analyze CSF, which is useful in the diagnosis and detection of dissemination of certain brain tumors. However, lumbar puncture is risky in patients with increased ICP and should be avoided in those cases.[22,34,36] Audiometry and vestibular testing are useful for diagnosing tumors in the cerebellopontine angle. Endocrine testing is used to examine endocrine abnormalities with tumors in the pituitary gland and hypothalamus.[34]

Medical and Surgical Management

After diagnosis of a brain tumor has been confirmed, specific treatment must be selected. The ultimate goals of tumor management are to improve quality of life and extend survival, by preserving or improving body function and structures.[49] These goals are accomplished by removing or decreasing the size of the tumor. Treatment techniques are determined by histological type, location, grade, and size of tumor; age at onset; and medical history of the patient.[7,17,49]

Four types of treatment are discussed: (1) traditional surgery, (2) chemotherapy, (3) radiation therapy, and (4) stereotactic radiosurgery.

Traditional Surgery

The primary goal of traditional surgery is maximal tumor resection with the least amount of damage to neural or supporting structures.[7] Gross total resection is associated with longer survival rates and decreased neurological impairment.[37] Benign tumors, if accessible, are resected completely, whereas malignant tumors are typically partially resected secondary to location or size of the tumor.[7,49] The *purposes* of surgery in the management of brain tumors include the following:

1. Biopsy to establish a diagnosis
2. Partial resection to decrease the tumor mass to be treated by other methods
3. Complete resection of the tumor
4. Provision of access for adjuvant treatment techniques[16]

Biopsies are performed through open, needle, and stereotactic needle techniques. Open biopsies involve exposure of the tumor followed by removal of a sample through surgical excision. Needle biopsies involve insertion of a needle into the tumor through a hole in the skull and the excision of the tissue sample drawn through the needle. Stereotactic needle biopsies use computers and MRI or CT scanning equipment to assist in directing the needle into the tumor. This type of biopsy is useful for deep-seated or multiple brain lesions.[7,16]

Partial and *complete resections* are accomplished through craniotomy. Craniotomy involves removal of a portion of the skull and separation of the dura mater to expose the tumor. Stereotactic craniotomy uses technology to create computed three-dimensional pictures of the brain to guide the neurosurgeon during the procedure. CT scanning and MRI scanners are used to provide an evaluation of the tumor resection during the procedure.[7,50] Awake craniotomy allows for intraoperative brain mapping that helps to identify and protect functional cortex and in recent years has become an alternative surgical treatment for most supratentorial tumors.[46]

Preoperative Management. Before surgery, clients are evaluated for general surgical risks and the possibility of tumors in additional locations. Unless medically contraindicated, steroids are administered before surgery if brain edema is present or if extensive manipulation will be occurring during surgery. Anticonvulsant medications are also administered preoperatively to prevent seizures during or after surgery.[7,49]

Intraoperative Management. During surgery, precautions are taken to prevent an increase in edema or ICP. Mannitol, a vasodiuretic to decrease ICP, is used to shrink the surrounding brain tissue, thus providing easier access to the tumor. Steroid use is continued and antibiotics are administered to prevent infection. Hyperventilation, with a CO_2 level of 25 mEq/L, is also used to reduce ICP.[7,49]

Postoperative Management. Patients are observed in an intensive care unit for at least 24 hours for possible intracranial bleeding or seizures. Blood pressure is monitored continuously. After surgery, patients are at risk for developing deep vein thrombosis or pulmonary embolism secondary to decreased muscle activity, but because these patients are at risk for intracranial bleeding, anticoagulants cannot be given.[51] Therefore compression stockings are used prophylactically in an attempt to prevent deep vein thrombosis. Steroids are tapered after surgery over 5 to 10 days. Anticonvulsant medications are continued after surgery, with the length of time dependent on the presence of seizure activity before and after surgery.[7,49] The primary limitations of traditional surgery include the following:

1. Medical complications such as hematoma, hydrocephalus, infection, and infarction from the surgical procedure
2. Complications resulting from general anesthesia
3. Increased cost of the hospital stay and surgical procedure[30,33,49]

Chemotherapy

Chemotherapy is another treatment frequently used to manage brain tumors. It can be used independently or as an adjuvant to surgery or radiation. Chemotherapeutic drugs are not effective on all types of tumors. Some tumors are known to be resistant to certain drugs, and therefore other treatments are more successful in treating these tumors. Drugs can be given in combination to target all cell types present within the tumor. Because different drugs have different modes of action and side effects, combined drug therapy often proves to be one of the most effective treatments.[52] Chemotherapy can be administered in a number of different ways. Most agents are given intravenously through a peripheral intravenous line or through a catheter such as a peripherally inserted central catheter (PICC) or Groshong catheter. Other drugs are placed directly into the tumor bed or are given intramuscularly, orally, or by means of an implanted device.

Chemotherapy drugs impede cellular replication of the tumor cells, interfering with their ability to copy deoxyribonucleic acid (DNA) and reproduce. Once the replicating capability of the tumor cell has been disrupted, the cell dies. In this way the tumor is prevented from growing and is destroyed at the cellular level.[52]

Methotrexate is a highly toxic drug and is usually paired with an antidote drug, leucovorin, to reverse the side effects on normal cells.[53] Typically methotrexate is used to treat cancer outside of the CNS; however, it is the major chemotherapy drug used to treat CNS lymphoma.[22] Methotrexate has been found to produce a high degree of neurotoxicity when used in combination with radiation therapy.[54]

Neurotoxic to surrounding tissue, methotrexate and ara-C are drugs able to be introduced directly into the CSF through an intraventricular Ommaya reservoir.[35] The reservoir, implanted under the scalp, is filled by use of a syringe, and the medication is then circulated through the ventricles to the brain.[52] The drugs are typically given in a clinic setting by a registered nurse certified in chemotherapy administration. A patient's chemotherapy schedule varies depending on the drug given. An on-off cycle is used to allow the patient to recover from the toxic effects of the drug.

One of the challenges in delivering cytotoxic drugs to the brain is the blood-brain barrier (BBB). The BBB is the brain's natural protective barrier against transmission of foreign substances from the blood into the brain.[52] One class of drugs that does penetrate the BBB is the *nitrosoureas.* These include BCNU (carmustine) and CCNU (lomustine), which are lipid soluble and cell cycle specific. These drugs are given in high doses and typically used to treat glioblastoma multiforme and anaplastic astrocytoma; however, often these high-grade tumors invade and destroy the BBB.

BCNU can also be administered in the form of wafers placed by the neurosurgeon directly into the brain tumor. An initial study for recurrent malignant gliomas found that patients' tumors responded to the treatment.[55] This report was followed by an up-front study for glioblastoma multiforme.[56] U.S. Food and Drug Administration (FDA) approval for these wafers (Gliadel) followed.

Temozolomide is an orally available chemotherapeutic agent introduced in the 1990s for the treatment of malignant gliomas.[57] Initial results in treating recurrent anaplastic astrocytoma[58] and glioblastoma[59] were so successful that the drug was approved for the treatment of recurrent brain tumors by the FDA. For recurrent tumors the drug is administered orally 5 days per month. Temozolomide was then tested for the up-front treatment of glioblastoma. This occurred in a multicenter study in which the drug was given daily as part of the initial treatment with radiation therapy, followed by five doses per month for maintenance treatment.[60] Survival increased substantially with this regimen, and as a result the FDA approved the use of temozolomide as part of first-line treatment of glioblastoma. Temozolomide is also used to treat anaplastic gliomas.

Another major breakthrough in chemotherapy of brain tumors was the finding that the antiangiogenesis monoclonal antibody Avastin (bevacizumab) improved the progression-free survival and the tumor images on MRIs of patients with glioblastoma.[61-63] The drug targets vascular endothelial growth factor (VEGF) and is administered intravenously. It has recently been approved by the FDA for the treatment of recurrent glioblastoma multiforme. It is usually administered with another chemotherapy agent, for example, irinotecan.

Radiation Therapy

Radiation therapy can be used alone or in conjunction with surgery or chemotherapy to treat malignant brain tumors. It is typically chosen as a treatment option for tumors that are too large or inaccessible for surgical resection and to eradicate residual neoplastic cells after a surgical debulking.

Radiotherapy consists of the delivery of high-powered photons, with energies in a much greater range than that of standard x-rays, as an external beam directly at the tumor site. The external beam is transmitted to the tumor through a linear accelerator or a cobalt machine that uses cobalt isotopes as the radiation source. External beam radiation is the most widely used form of radiation treatment.[7]

Conventional radiation therapy as described previously is fractionated into small doses delivered over a period of time.[16] Often, if a large fraction is to be delivered, the dose is divided and given more than once per day; this is called hyperfractionation. Hyperfractionated radiation therapy is believed to increase the efficacy and decrease the long-term side effects of radiation. More studies need to be completed to know its exact benefits.

Conformal radiation is the use of high-dose external beam radiation, produced by a linear accelerator, to precisely match or "conform" to the tumor shape. One such method of conformal radiation delivery is the Peacock system. This method attempts to deliver a uniform amount of radiation to the tumor and minimize irradiation of healthy brain tissue.[16]

Radiosurgery involves relatively high-dose hypofractionated radiation beams directed at small tumor areas through the use of computer imaging.[16] This type of treatment includes the Gamma Knife, linear accelerators, and the cyberknife, which are discussed later.

The radiation oncologist determines the dosage, frequency, and method of radiation delivery depending on tumor type, location, growth rate, and other medical issues for each client. A typical course of radiation therapy will last 6 weeks. Clients are irradiated for just 1 to 5 minutes, 5 days a week. The radiation is intended to kill the malignant cells and preserve healthy cells, but certain rapidly growing cells, those in skin tissue and mucosa, are killed as well. The side effects experienced by those undergoing treatment are a result of this destruction of healthy cells.

Radiation therapy has considerable limitations and disadvantages. There is an accepted maximum lifetime dosage of radiation that the brain and body can tolerate. As doses come close to this limit, the risk of radiation necrosis increases. Because the brains of young children are particularly vulnerable to radiation, other therapies, such as chemotherapy, are used until the developing brain is more tolerant of radiation. Metastatic lesions have invaded multiple organs or body systems, and a more systemic treatment such as chemotherapy is most effective for this type of brain cancer.[16]

Stereotactic Radiosurgery

Stereotactic radiosurgery is defined as delivery of a high dose of ionizing radiation, in a single fraction, to a small, precisely defined volume of tissue.[7,33,49,64] The high-energy accelerators involved with stereotactic radiosurgery improve the physical effect of radiation by allowing energy to travel more precisely in a straight line and penetrate deeper before dissipating.[64] The goal of stereotactic radiosurgery is to arrest tumor growth.[65] This technique has been shown to be most beneficial for treating centrally located lesions less than 3 cm in size and for patients with increased surgical risk factors.[33,64] Advantages of stereotactic radiosurgery are as follows:

1. Is a noninvasive procedure using local anesthesia and sedation to place the stereotactic frame
2. Avoids risks of general anesthesia and immediate postoperative risks such as bleeding, CSF leak, and infection
3. Lowers treatment cost and shortens hospital stays[7,30,64,66]

Stereotactic radiosurgery is used to treat benign and malignant tumors, vascular malformations, and functional disorders.[49,64] The primary modes of administration for stereotactic radiosurgery include the Gamma Knife, linear accelerators, and the cyberknife.[7,17,49]

The *Gamma Knife* was first introduced in Sweden in 1968 and is now used worldwide at 65 sites (Figure 25-3). The Gamma Knife uses 201 discrete sources of cobalt 60, which are focused precisely to one point in three-dimensional space within the cranium.[33,49,64,67] The Gamma Knife is typically used for deeply embedded small tumors that require precise delivery of radiation.[33]

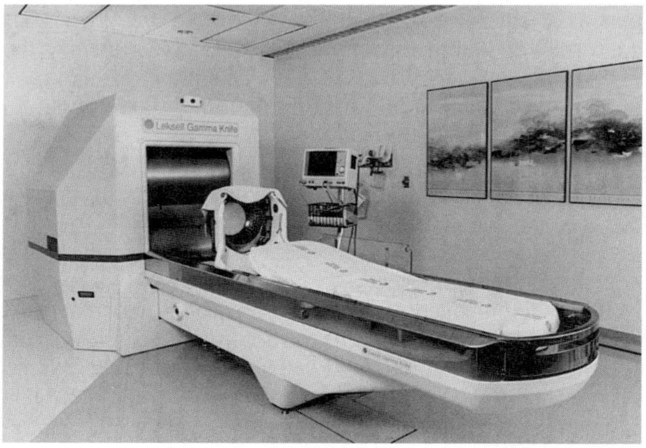

Figure 25-3 ■ The Leksell Gamma Knife.

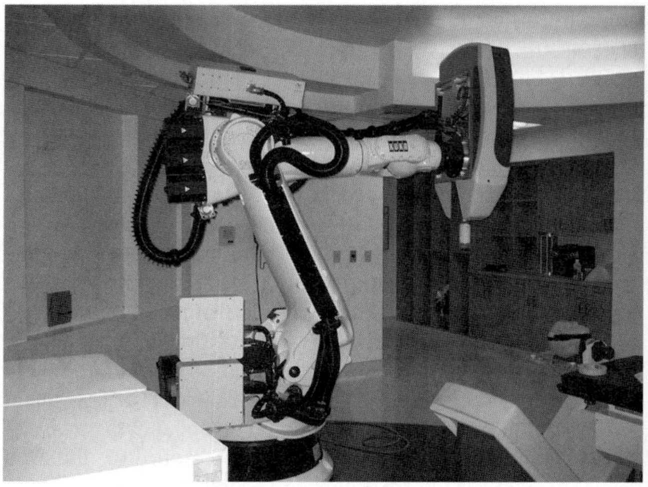

Figure 25-4 ■ The cyberknife.

MRI, CT scanning, or angiography is used to identify the exact location of the lesion to be treated after the stereotactic frame is placed on the client's head. The stereotactic frame is then fixed to the machine and attached to a collimator helmet containing 201 holes for the radiation to pass through. The patient is then locked into position. The prescribed dose is given over 20 minutes to 2 hours. After treatment the frame is removed; the client is observed and is frequently discharged after 24 hours. Return to previous activity typically occurs within a few days.[30,33,49,67]

With the Gamma Knife, the full dose of radiation is received only at the point where the 201 beams intersect, thereby giving only a minimal dose to uninvolved tissue when targeted accurately. Side effects are rare, but headache and nausea may occur.[7] The primary limitations of the Gamma Knife are the limited brain volume that can be treated with one dose and the cost of the Gamma Knife machine.[7,49]

Linear accelerators used for conventional radiation can be modified for stereotactic radiosurgery. The brain lesion to be targeted is stereotactically placed in the center of the arc of rotation of the machine. A single, highly focused beam of radiation is delivered over multiple sweeps around the brain lesion. Linear accelerators can be used to treat larger tumors with precise shape while maintaining uniform dose. Because linear accelerators are used for conventional radiation, a quality check for beam accuracy is imperative before the machine is used for stereotactic radiosurgery.[7,49]

The *cyberknife* uses a compact linear accelerator mounted on a robotic arm, with the robotic arm moving around the linear accelerator to multiple precalculated positions (Figure 25-4). At each position the accelerator fires a beam of radiation at the tumor or lesion. A high cumulative dose of radiation is achieved at the tumor or lesion because of the convergence of the beams. This dose is typically strong enough to destroy the abnormal cells while minimizing the damaging effects of radiation to healthy surrounding tissue. The cyberknife differs from other stereotactic radiosurgery because a linear accelerator is combined with an image guidance system. The robotic arm allows the cyberknife to target difficult-to-reach areas of the body, as well as adjust quickly for changes in target location during treatment.

Several research studies have reported on the use of stereotactic radiosurgery, including the Gamma Knife and linear accelerators, and compared this modality with microsurgery; however, studies involving the cyberknife are limited. In patients with brain metastases, the Gamma Knife is typically indicated for small lesions that are centrally located. Surgical resection is indicated for superficial lesions greater than 3 cm in diameter, when a significant mass effect of the tumor exists, or if edema is present in the cranium.[33] The Gamma Knife has been shown to achieve tumor control rates as high as those for surgery and whole-body radiation therapy combined and to halt or reverse neurological progression in 78% of patients treated.[68,69]

Microsurgical resection has shown a 90% cure rate for acoustic neuromas less than 3 cm in size. Stereotactic radiosurgery avoids the risk of an open procedure, but the tumor is controlled rather than removed. Thus far, a 92% tumor control rate has been noted, but the patients in this study have not had a 10-year follow-up.[29,30]

Research exists for both low- and high-grade gliomas, but large, controlled studies are few. With low-grade tumors, small studies have shown increased survival after stereotactic radiosurgery, but these studies are uncontrolled and limited by the small number of participants.[66] For high-grade tumors, recent studies have found median survival rates ranging from 9.5 to 17 months with use of stereotactic radiosurgery.[39,70-72] For recurrent malignant gliomas, survival after fractionated and nonfractionated stereotactic radiosurgery has been shown to be 8 to 11 months.[51,73-75] The addition of radiosurgery to surgery and radiation therapy produced only modest improvement when compared with surgery and radiation therapy alone.[66]

The preferred treatment for *meningiomas* is surgical resection, if complete resection is possible. When surgery is not an option and the tumor is less than 3 cm in size or 5 mm away from the optic nerve, stereotactic radiosurgery is indicated.[27,76,77] Four-year survival rates of 91% in benign meningiomas and 21.5% in malignant meningiomas have been demonstrated after use of the Gamma Knife.[27,76] In a survey taken 5 to 10 years after radiosurgery, 96% of patients believed radiosurgery had provided a satisfactory outcome.[76]

REHABILITATION

Overview

Rehabilitation is a key component in the management of the client with a brain tumor. With advances in technology and treatment intervention, survival rates of people with cancer have improved. Consequently, people are living longer with physical impairments resulting from the disease or its treatment, necessitating interdisciplinary therapeutic intervention.[2] Rehabilitating the body function and structural impairments complicates the medical and psychological issues typically associated with cancer diagnosis.[19] By preventing complications, maximizing function, and providing support, rehabilitation specialists ultimately improve the client's quality of life.[19] Research has shown that the functional outcomes and discharge to home for individuals with brain tumors are comparable to those of individuals with stroke or traumatic brain injury.[78] The most effective rehabilitation plan is flexible, to allow for increasing impairment, and sensitive, to accommodate the highly emotional impact that accompanies the diagnosis of a primary brain tumor. The tumor's invasion is marked by complaints of pain and growing activity limitations. These functional consequences of the disease process are the target of the rehabilitation team. In addition to the side effects of therapeutic intervention, functional progress may be affected by cerebral edema, hydrocephalus, tumor regrowth, infection, and radiation necrosis. Compared with clients with other diagnoses, clients with brain tumors have a higher rate of unplanned transfers back to acute care, primarily because of infection.[79]

The management of a client with a brain tumor is different from that of other CNS disorders, despite a similar clinical presentation. To establish an appropriate plan of care, the clinician must understand the nature of the specific tumor, consider the client's fluctuating neurological status, and prepare for the likelihood of progressive decline. The preferred approach is holistic, addressing quality of life issues such as physical, psychosocial, and emotional needs, incorporated into the systems model of motor control. Factors defining quality of life are unique to each individual, and therefore clinicians should identify and use these factors to construct a meaningful treatment program.[80] Individuals with advanced cancer who participated in exercise therapy have reported increased physical functioning, improved quality of life, and decreased fatigue.[78]

Evaluation, clinical analysis, intervention, discharge planning, and psychosocial issues specific to the management of the client with a brain tumor are discussed in the following sections.

Evaluation

The evaluation process must include a comprehensive examination and assessment of all systems in order to establish an appropriate impairment diagnosis, problem list, prognosis, and plan of care. Before a neurological assessment is performed, a thorough review of the client's medical history and an understanding of the medical diagnosis are necessary. The client's occupation, support system, personal goals, and role in the family are important psychosocial factors that should be identified in the evaluation. These factors, along with a thorough functional and neurological examination, assist the clinician through the diagnostic process. This process includes identification of clinical problems, establishment of realistic and appropriate goals, selection of the most effective intervention, and discharge planning.

Although the neurological examination yields important information regarding strength, reflexes, sensation, vision, and cognition, it is important not to rely solely on its findings to determine an appropriate intervention. Because multiple systems interact to produce normal movement, it is difficult to examine isolated systems and apply the findings accurately to movement patterns. Therefore clinicians are encouraged to examine all systems through functional tasks to understand how the impaired neurological, musculoskeletal, and cognitive systems are affecting the client's movement. During the evaluation process the clinician notes systems that are functioning normally, identifies abnormal components of movement, and determines appropriate interventions to optimize motor recovery.[38] The progressive nature of the disease necessitates ongoing evaluation followed by accommodating intervention.

Goal Setting

The functional impairments and objective neurological findings provide the clinician with valuable information to assess prognosis, establish goals, and determine a treatment plan. Despite the progressive nature of the disease, treatment goals should maximize the potential for function, introduce effective, task-oriented movement strategies, and offer multiple movement options.[38]

To set realistic and client-oriented goals, it is important for the clinician to envision where the patient will be at discharge based on present level of function, prognosis, and disease course, while considering client and caregiver personal goals. Appropriate goals range from comprehensive caregiver training to independent mobility with transition back to a work environment. Goals need to challenge the client to attain an optimal level of function but must also allow for fluctuations in potential resulting from the disease process. Clients who have the potential to return to work may require additional intervention from neuropsychology, vocational rehabilitation, or a multidisciplinary day program, depending on the nature of the job and the deficits.

Because the rehabilitation potential for clients with brain tumors varies greatly, it is imperative that the client, family members, rehabilitation team, and third-party payers understand and agree with the purpose of the client's rehabilitation program. Pathways can be extremely instrumental in clarifying rehabilitation goals and identifying the caregiver's role on discharge (Table 25-2). If a client has a poor prognosis, the rehabilitation team can successfully train family members and order equipment within 1 week if the family understands the goals and the need to be present during treatment sessions. The pathway serves as a guideline assisting the rehabilitation team in achieving the client's goals in an effective and efficient manner.

Functional Assessment

Historically persons with primary malignant brain tumors have not been considered rehabilitation candidates because of the progressive nature of their disease. Physicians, health care providers, and third-party payers have questioned the efficacy of rehabilitation in this population because of poor

TABLE 25-2 ■ BRAIN TUMOR CLINICAL PATHWAY: 1-WEEK STAY

	DAY 1	DAY 2	DAY 3	DAYS 4-5	DAYS 6-7
Nursing	Medical and functional assessment Establish LOS with MD Initiate care plan with caregivers	Provide education regarding sequelae of diagnosis and treatment Facilitate team meeting Collaborate with CM	Provide nutritional and dietary education prn Train caregiver with tube feedings prn	Skin care B&B training Home safety Address medical questions	Provide info regarding medications (i.e., pain and antiepileptics) Review side effects of radiation and chemotherapy Refer to palliative care or hospice prn
Physicians	Provide education and handouts to patient and family regarding diagnosis, prognosis, and treatment plan	Prescribe medications to minimize side effects (e.g., seizure, pain) and maximize rehabilitation potential	Maintain open communication between oncologist and rehabilitation physician		Recommend follow-up appointments and treatment
Physical Therapy	Functional evaluation Assess family support Schedule home evaluation prn	Provide education and handouts for caregiver body mechanics, physical therapy positioning, and mobility techniques Determine and order equipment	Continue mobility training—different types and surfaces Educate regarding safety precautions and energy conservation	Caregivers return demonstrate competency with mobility techniques Home evaluation completed	Patient discharged if caregivers competent in all necessary mobility techniques and equipment obtained
Occupational Therapy	Functional evaluation Discuss home environment Schedule home evaluation prn	Provide education and handouts for caregiver body mechanics, extremity management, and ADLs techniques Determine adaptive equipment needs and place order	Continue training Train caregivers in visual-perceptual needs	Caregivers return demonstrate competency with ADL techniques Home evaluation completed	Patient discharged if caregivers competent in all necessary ADL and mobility techniques and equipment obtained
Speech and Language Therapy	Bedside swallow evaluation performed Diet recommended MBS and FEES scheduled prn	MBS and FEES completed prn Provide education and handouts regarding precautions and strategies for safe swallowing, appropriate diet Signs of aspiration	Initiate cog/com evaluation Monitor diet Continue caregiver training for swallowing	Complete cog/com evaluation Provide family with ideas to modify environment to improve cog/com function Educate caregiver regarding signs of functional decline	Continue to monitor diet Continue caregiver education regarding swallowing, safety and judgment, and cog/com function
Therapeutic Recreation	Evaluate patient's leisure interests		Leisure skill building with holistic approach	Review community resources	Discharge
Neuropsychology	If indicated				
Case Management and Social Services	Initiate assessment	Complete assessment Inform physical therapy and caregiver of team recommendations and LOS	Order DME	Arrange for continued therapies prn	Review discharge plans and recommendations with patient and caregivers

Adapted with permission from Barrow Rehabilitation.

ADLs, Activities of daily living; *B&B,* bowel & bladder; *CM,* case manager; *cog/com,* cognition and communication; *DME,* durable medical equipment; *FEES,* fiberoptic endoscopic evaluation of swallowing, *LOS,* length of stay; *MBS,* modified barium swallow; *MD,* medical doctor; *prn,* when necessary.

prognoses and limited survival rates. However, advances in medical diagnosis and intervention are resulting in longer survival of people with multiple limitations that require rehabilitation. Functional assessment scales provide objective evidence that rehabilitation is effective and worthwhile for these clients.[3,78,81]

The functional assessment is a critical component in the development of the treatment intervention. It provides a method of analyzing deficits, compiling a problem list, developing a treatment plan, and measuring functional outcomes. The Functional Independence Measure (FIM) is a functional assessment tool used to measure degree of disability, regardless of underlying pathology, and burden of care to demonstrate functional outcomes of rehabilitation and assist clinicians with discharge planning.[51]

Functional outcome scales such as the FIM provide a means of documenting the client's response to therapy intervention for clinicians, physicians, and third-party payers in the rehabilitation setting. Research using FIM data demonstrates efficacy for inpatient rehabilitation of brain tumor clients similar to that noted in those with traumatic brain injury or stroke when matched by age, sex, and functional status on admission.[1,3,29,81]

Physicians use specific functional evaluation scales to measure the success of treatment. The Karnofsky performance scale, which rates patients' functional performance, is the tool most widely used in clinical research and treatment decisions (see Table 25-1).[19] The client receives a score from 0 to 100 based on independence or level of assistance required for normal activity. The scale is used in research to evaluate an individual's physical response to treatment.[19,51,82,83]

Side Effects and Considerations

Through advances in chemotherapy and radiation therapy, the ability to reduce tumor mass has greatly improved. Unfortunately, despite the often favorable long-term results of these treatments, the immediate effects create physical and psychological challenges for the client and clinician. Clients who are being treated aggressively during the rehabilitation phase will probably experience a decline in neurological or hematological status. These declines often limit the individual's tolerance for treatment intervention and increase client and caregiver feelings of depression and hopelessness. Clinicians have the opportunity to provide more than physical restorative services and should offer psychosocial support when possible to enhance successful rehabilitation.[84]

The side effects and special considerations that arise with this population range from physical to cognitive to psychosocial and emotional. The following paragraphs relate the spectrum of complications and side effects the client may experience when undergoing medical treatment, and the impact these may have on therapeutic intervention.

Not everyone undergoing chemotherapy or radiation treatment will experience physical side effects; however, the possibilities include hair loss, fatigue, nausea, skin burns or irritation, difficulty eating or digesting food, anorexia, and dry, sore mouth.[53,85] The side effects are caused by the toxic effects the drugs have on healthy, rapidly dividing cells, including bone marrow cells, cells lining the mucosa, and hair cells.[52,85]

The toxic effect chemotherapy has on bone marrow impairs the client's ability to produce red and white blood cells and platelets.[5,52] The client may develop anemia, infection, or hemorrhage as a result of depressed hematological values.

The lining of the mouth, esophagus, and intestines may become inflamed and irritated and interfere with the ability to eat or digest food. The client may experience nausea, vomiting, diarrhea, or constipation, any of which will impair mobility and energy for daily activities.[17]

Hair loss is a common side effect of brain radiation and chemotherapy. This requires an especially difficult adjustment for most people because it causes a drastic change in appearance.[16,52]

Clinicians involved in the management of clients who are currently receiving radiation therapy or chemotherapy need to be mindful of these side effects when developing a plan of intervention. Fatigue, low blood count, and gastrointestinal complaints may limit a client's ability to fully participate in the planned therapy session or may call for a modification in activity or environment. Moreover, the clinician must use these factors to determine if the client's health or safety would be jeopardized by therapeutic intervention at any particular time. In addition, the clinician must be flexible to determine the optimal time when intervention is most effective and does not interfere with medications or meals.

Together with the physical side effects mentioned previously, many clients with brain tumors have changes in cognition or personality as a result of the tumor's location. A patient with a frontal lobe tumor who was previously quiet and withdrawn may, over time, become loud and disinhibited as a result of tumor growth. Tumors that invade the speech-language area cause communication and comprehension difficulties that create challenges for the client and clinician. The client who has a left parietal tumor may be aphasic and not respond to verbal commands. In this case, the clinician must engage in alternate means of communication or provide therapeutic facilitation with tactile cues. An observant, critical analysis of the client's physical deficits and impaired communication, comprehension, and feedback mechanisms is essential to select an effective, client-specific intervention plan.

Because of the emotionally charged nature of the disease process, psychosocial and emotional issues frequently arise. Clinicians should be sensitive to fluctuations in temperament and mood that the diagnosis itself and subsequent treatment strategies create. Clinicians can offer psychosocial support and direct the client and family to resources that may give direction and guidance during difficult transitions.

Intervention

The ultimate goal of rehabilitation is to achieve maximum restoration of function, within the limits imposed by the disease, in the client's preferred environment. The clinician must recognize that the physical, cognitive, and emotional status of these individuals is inconsistent and changing as a result of the disease process or medical intervention. Treatment plans must be flexible to effectively manage fluctuations in the client's presentation. A comprehensive rehabilitation plan is individualized to accommodate progressive changes in functional mobility and provides problem-solving experiences to prepare the client and caregiver for these situations. The rehabilitation process typically begins in the intensive care unit and continues in the inpatient, outpatient, and home health settings.

In the intensive care unit, communication with nursing staff regarding the client's present medical status and an understanding of ICP, hemodynamic values, and monitoring devices are crucial to determining tolerance for therapy intervention (Figure 25-5). For a ventriculostomy, a catheter is placed in the third ventricle to drain CSF and to monitor ICP. Mobilizing a patient with a ventriculostomy is possible, but nursing staff must close the drain before any positional change and should inform the clinician of appropriate treatment measures. A client's dependence on these monitoring devices does not prevent therapeutic intervention, but the critical status of these individuals must be considered. The monitoring equipment provides constant feedback that assists the clinician in assessing the client's tolerance to activity and his or her ability to proceed with treatment.

As the client becomes more medically stable, the clinician upgrades mobility and prepares the client for the next stage of rehabilitation. Despite clients' decreased medical acuity in the rehabilitation setting, clinicians must continually reassess functional and neurological status and alert physicians to any changes. Clinicians spend many hours with clients during their rehabilitation stay. This daily interaction gives the clinician the opportunity to connect with the client on a personal level and observe her or him in many settings. Intuitive therapists are often the first to notice physical, cognitive, and emotional changes. Communication to the physician of significant changes is imperative for appropriate follow-up procedures and referrals to provide optimal care.

In the inpatient rehabilitation setting, treatment focuses on optimizing functional capabilities to prepare the client and family for discharge. Integrating the client's personal goals and interests into therapeutic intervention invests the client and family in the rehabilitation process. The incorporation of these quality-of-life issues encourages the pursuit of a meaningful lifestyle on discharge. If clinicians believe the client's goals are unrealistic, gentle redirection is helpful to channel energy toward achievable goals. Goals for inpatient rehabilitation range from returning the client to an independent lifestyle to training family members to be caregivers in the home environment.

The restoration of previous functional movement patterns is desired. The literature reports increasing evidence that the CNS has dynamic properties, including neural regeneration and collateral sprouting, which supports the concept of plasticity. Plasticity allows intact neural centers to recognize and assume functions of areas of the brain impaired or destroyed by the lesion or its medical management.[86] The treatment focus may need to turn to compensatory strategies if the potential for motor recovery and learning is lacking. Once compensatory patterns are established, it is not clearly known whether recovery of normal movement will be achieved.[86] Compensatory techniques may be beneficial in increasing safety and efficiency with mobility and activities of daily living, or in providing more independence for the client.[51] Increasing independence can assist in improving quality of life for the client and may permit return to work or participation in previous recreational activity.[51] For example, an avid golfer with right-sided hemiparesis and impaired standing balance can modify his clubs and return to the game at the wheelchair level.

The rehabilitation program should prepare the client and caregivers for an efficient transition from the structured care setting to the home. Using motor learning principles (refer to Chapter 4) to teach functional mobility will best produce transfer of learning from a constant environment to an unpredictable home environment. Repetitious practice of specific parts of a skill in fixed surroundings, with physical and verbal guidance throughout the movement and frequent feedback during and after completion of the task, are beneficial in teaching acquisition of a specific movement or activity.[87-89] Practicing the whole activity in a variable context, with irregular feedback and decreased physical and verbal guidance, expedites learning.[89-91]

Learning results in the ability to execute a task in any setting. Community outings and home passes naturally provide an environment that facilitates learning. The clinician can measure retention and transfer of learning by the client's performance in the community or at home. This information should be used to adjust the treatment plan and make

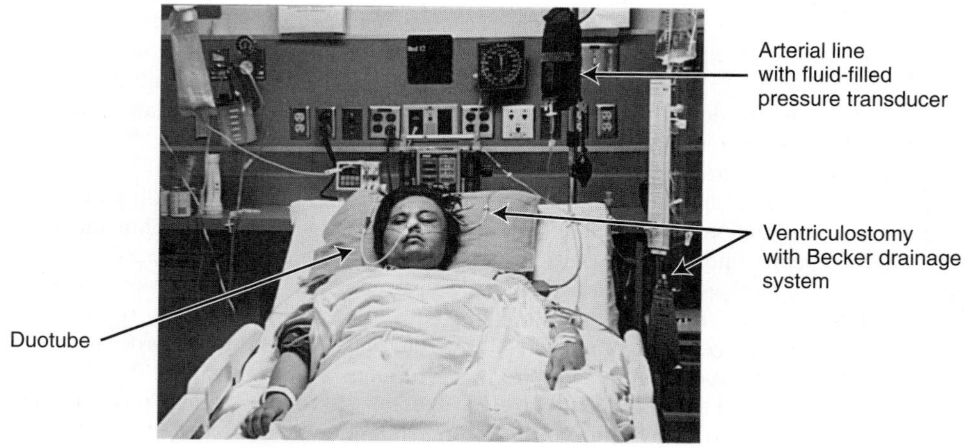

Figure 25-5 ■ A patient after a partial tumor resection. Labels indicate the equipment commonly seen in the neurological intensive care unit.

recommendations for environmental modifications that minimize physical and cognitive demands on the client. A client whose individual treatment focus is transfers gains confidence when able to transfer from a wheelchair to a table chair in a crowded restaurant.

An interdisciplinary team approach is used for community reentry to provide a meaningful experience for the client. Recreational therapists play an integral part in identifying the individual's interests, reintegrating the client into the community, and modifying leisure activities to meet physical abilities. Activities addressed in daily therapy sessions are practiced in the community, and feedback is provided to the appropriate clinician as well as the client. Initial reentry into the community can be intimidating to the client and may cause changes in the client's behavior that will affect mobility performance. Therefore it is necessary for the clinician to be sensitive and recognize the issues the client may be experiencing.

For caregiver training and education to be successful, a good rapport must be established among clinician, client, and the family members or caregivers. Caregiver training includes mobility training and education regarding the effect the tumor may have on the client's present and future mobility. Instruction should be given based on present level of function, but the probability of progressive decline should not be overlooked. An intuitive clinician should offer effective techniques and problem-solving to address potential obstacles created by the disease process. For example, when performing transfer training, the clinician may demonstrate a stand-pivot transfer but may also suggest a squat-pivot transfer if physical or cognitive changes mandate increased assistance by the caregiver.

Discharge Planning

Discharge planning is initiated early, continues throughout the rehabilitation process, and must allow for changes in the client's functional status. On discharge from the rehabilitation setting, the client will make the transition to one of the following settings: home, skilled nursing facility, or hospice. The transition to home is typically preferred by the client, caregiver, and interdisciplinary rehabilitation team. If the client cannot be physically or medically managed at home, then placement in a skilled nursing facility may be necessary. The client may choose hospice care when medical treatment is no longer providing control of the tumor and the physical demands of the client are not manageable by the caregivers. The case manager contacts insurance providers to determine coverage and, after conferring with the interdisciplinary team, gives the client and family information regarding discharge options.

Client and caregiver training and education constitute an integral part of discharge planning. Before discharge, the client and caregiver should be instructed in functional mobility and activities of daily living, informed of equipment needs and vendor resources, and provided with community resources for support and education. During individual training, the clinician is able to provide feedback to the caregiver and client to facilitate an easier transition to home. Documentation of caregiver education and training should be included in the progress and discharge notes. A sample form for interdisciplinary documentation of education is provided in Figure 25-6.

Equipment necessary to assist the client and family with mobility and activities of daily living is recommended by the appropriate clinician. When equipment is ordered, fluctuations in the client's present status, as well as the probable progressive decline in function, are considered. If the client is functioning without equipment at discharge, resources such as equipment vendors or local charitable organizations for future equipment needs should be provided.

Information about local community and national resources specific to brain tumors also should be provided before discharge. These resources can be found on the Internet, in the local phone book, or through communication with previous patients or other health care professionals familiar with these organizations. Support groups provide the caregiver and the client with an opportunity to share experiences and information, prevent isolation, foster hope, allow the client and caregiver to discover coping skills, and offer emotional support.[92] A study conducted to describe experiences and needs of clients with brain tumors found that "attendance and participation in a support group empowers people to seek the most out of life following a brain tumor diagnosis."[92] (Refer to Chapter 6 for additional information regarding support groups.) National organizations can provide educational information and support to clients (Box 25-1). These organizations can help the client find local resources unfamiliar to the clinician.

Hospice Care

A time may come when traditional tumor treatment is ineffective and local control is no longer expected. Patient and family must make a decision regarding the living environment and type of care desired. One option available is hospice care. In the United States, the hospice movement in health care has evolved to include specific standards, licensure requirements, and certification. Providing physical, emotional, and psychosocial support to patients and their families in their final days is the intent of hospice care.[93] Hospice recognizes the impact terminal illness has on a patient's family system, and the demands, both physical and emotional, it places on the caregiver.[94] The use of hospice implies a holistic approach that allows families the opportunity to be directly involved in the patient's care and encourages the expression of grief, love, support, and acceptance.

Inpatient hospice facilities provide continuous nursing care in a structured, supervised environment. Hospice services in these facilities offer ongoing pastoral counseling and emotional support to patient and family. However, if patient and family prefer, hospice care can be provided in the patient's home, with home health aides and nursing staff giving limited physical care or providing respite care.

Typically, mobility and caregiver training for the hospice patient are addressed by a therapist earlier in the patient's disease process. However, positioning, range of motion, and pain relief are important to the patient's continued comfort throughout the course of the disease and in any setting.

PSYCHOSOCIAL CARE

With many clients living extended lives with brain tumors, it is important to measure the efficacy of treatment not only in terms of functional outcome, but also in terms of its effect

St. Joseph's Hospital and Medical Center
Mercy Healthcare Arizona

NEURO REHABILITATION UNIT

BRAIN TUMOR TEACHING GOALS

ADULT BRAIN TUMOR

* Please note: For the brain tumor patient who is able to completely or partially use his or her extremities and cognitive abilities, the emphasis on rehab is to maximize the patient's own ability to be independent. It is also to educate and teach the family or care giver appropriate care and safe assistance with the patient and his or her equipment. Efforts will be directed to facilitate the patient's return to home and to resume work (if able) in his or her community in the most efficient and practical manner possible for the patient and the family.

Initials = Full Name & Title

=	=	=
=	=	=
=	=	=

KEY

I = Instructed	RD = Return Demonstration	NI = Not available for instruction
D = Demonstrated	VD = Verbally directs care	NA = Not Applicable
C = Comprehended	DC = Discharge review	

PATIENT NAME: ______________________ DATE __________

NURSING

	PATIENT								CARE GIVER						
	I	D	C	RD	VD	DC	NI	NA	I	D	C	RD	DC	NI	NA
1. Anatomy and physiology of brain tumor															
2. Application of braces-splints															
3. Bowel elimination															
4. Circulation															
5. Depression / grieving															
6. Family adjustment															
7. Hydrocephalus															
8. Medications															
9. Nutrition															
10. Safety															
11. Seizures															
12. Sensory stimulation															
13. Skin integrity															
14. Sexuality															
15. Stress management															
16. Tube feedings															
17. Treatments															
18. Urinary elimination															
19. Other ______________															
20. Other ______________															

RESPIRATORY

	PATIENT								CARE GIVER						
	I	D	C	RD	VD	DC	NI	NA	I	D	C	RD	DC	NI	NA
1. CPR training															
2. List emergency numbers															
3. Suction (in hospital) - (in community)															
4. Trach care															
5. Other ______________															

A

Figure 25-6 ■ Interdisciplinary education inventory for brain tumor teaching. (From Barrow Neurological Institute, St Joseph's Hospital and Medical Center, Phoenix, Arizona.)

OCCUPATIONAL THERAPY (OT)

UPPER EXTREMITY

		PATIENT								CARE GIVER						
		I	D	C	RD	VD	DC	NI	NA	I	D	C	RD	DC	NI	NA
1. R.O.M. - exercise	1.															
2. Positioning	2.															
3. Splinting	3.															

SELF CARE

		PATIENT								CARE GIVER						
		I	D	C	RD	VD	DC	NI	NA	I	D	C	RD	DC	NI	NA
1. Swallowing	1.															
2. Self-feeding	2.															
3. Hygiene	3.															

PATIENT NAME: ______________________ DATE __________

OCCUPATIONAL THERAPY (OT)

		PATIENT								CARE GIVER						
		I	D	C	RD	VD	DC	NI	NA	I	D	C	RD	DC	NI	NA
4. Bathing	4.															
5. Dressing	5.															
6. Adaptive equipment - vendors	6.															
7. Home management	7.															
8. Cooking	8.															

TRANSFERS

		PATIENT								CARE GIVER						
		I	D	C	RD	VD	DC	NI	NA	I	D	C	RD	DC	NI	NA
1. Toilet - Commode	1.															
2. Tub - Shower	2.															

PHYSICAL THERAPY (PT)

		PATIENT								CARE GIVER						
		I	D	C	RD	VD	DC	NI	NA	I	D	C	RD	DC	NI	NA
1. Range of motion exercise	1.															
2. Bed mobility	2.															
3. Bed transfers	3.															
4. Car transfers	4.															
5. Wheelchair mobility and management	5.															
6. Ambulation	6.															
7. Safety precautions	7.															
8. Equipment vendor resources	8.															
9. Other ______________________	9.															

SPEECH LANGUAGE PATHOLOGY

		PATIENT								CARE GIVER						
		I	D	C	RD	VD	DC	NI	NA	I	D	C	RD	DC	NI	NA
1. Aphasia	1.															
2. Dysarthria	2.															
3. Dysphagia	3.															
4. Cognitive deficits due to tumor-surgical area	4.															
5. Cognitive deficits (generalized)	5.															
6. Other ______________________	6.															

THERAPEUTIC RECREATION

		PATIENT								CARE GIVER						
		I	D	C	RD	VD	DC	NI	NA	I	D	C	RD	DC	NI	NA
1. Community re-entry skills ______________________	1.															
2. Community leisure referrals ______________________	2.															
3. Adapted recreation resources and or referrals ______________________	3.															
4. Community mobility skills ______________________	4.															

PATIENT NAME: ______________________ DATE __________

SOCIAL SERVICES-CASE MANAGEMENT

Referrals to community resources:

		PATIENT								CARE GIVER						
		I	D	C	RD	VD	DC	NI	NA	I	D	C	RD	DC	NI	NA
1. ______________________	1.															
2. ______________________	2.															
3. ______________________	3.															
4. ______________________	4.															
5. ______________________	5.															

B

Figure 25-6—cont'd

BOX 25-1 ■ NATIONAL ORGANIZATIONS

NATIONAL BRAIN TUMOR SOCIETY
East Coast Office
124 Watertown St., Suite 2-D
Watertown, MA 02472
West Coast Office
22 Battery St., Suite 612
San Francisco, CA 94111
(800) 770-8287
www.braintumor.org
e-mail: info@braintumor.org

AMERICAN BRAIN TUMOR ASSOCIATION
2720 River Rd.
Des Plaines, IL 60018
(800) 886-2282
www.abta.org
e-mail: info@abta.org

on quality of life. Quality of life is the individual's subjective sense of well-being as a whole and has been studied closely in the treatment of clients with brain tumor.[83] *Health-related quality of life* (HRQOL) refers to an individual's overall quality of life—physical, emotional, spiritual, and intellectual functioning. HRQOL has become an important secondary end point for treatment and clinical studies of individuals with gliomas and metastatic brain tumors. Recently, several self-reporting instruments to measure HRQOL specific for individuals with brain tumors have been developed.[95] Some additional tools used clinically include the Functional Living Index, the Karnofsky performance scale, the Index of Independence in Activity of Daily Living, the State-Trait Anxiety Inventory, and the Self-Rating Depression Scale.[96] The World Health Organization (WHO) has developed two additional scales to measure quality of life used in all types of medical as well as movement diagnoses that might lead to a decrease in perceived quality of life.[97,98] For further discussion and general information refer to the WHO website.[99]

The development of a strong supportive relationship with client and caregivers is key to successful rehabilitation. This process begins with respecting the client's unique experience and involves continually evaluating and addressing his or her changing psychosocial needs.[86] Many individuals with brain tumors experience higher levels of anxiety and depression as well as feelings of a loss of independence, loss of self, and loss of relationships.[100] The clinician must feel invested, demonstrate good communication skills, and exhibit self-confidence in discussing sensitive issues for a caring relationship to develop. By active listening, the clinician can identify the client's true concerns and feelings and assist the client and family in coping with cancer. The clinician's consistent interaction with the client can foster a supportive and safe environment in which emotional and spiritual feelings can be shared. Once a trusting relationship has been established, the clinician's empathy can help decrease common feelings of isolation and helplessness and support the client through the different stages of the disease.[86]

Hope is a key psychosocial need of the individual with cancer. It is an important coping strategy that can help clients with brain tumors face an uncertain and often fearful future. Hope gives the client something to look forward to each day. Clinicians can create a hopeful environment by encouraging clients to share their expectations, identify realistic short-term goals, and acknowledge hopes, even if they are unrealistic. It is important to recognize that hope must be balanced with reality and honest disclosure regarding diagnosis and prognosis.[86,101]

Psychological and social problems are not identified in 80% of physically ill persons, possibly owing to clinicians' personal behaviors or beliefs. Clinicians may find it easier to focus on the physical aspect of care to avoid becoming emotional or experiencing the client's distress. Persons with cancer often experience feelings of powerlessness and isolation, which may be increased by distancing behaviors demonstrated by clinicians. Before offering support to clients, clinicians need to examine their own thoughts, feelings, and past experiences with death and dying. This awareness may prevent the clinician from internalizing the client's grief, from protecting the client and family members from the pain of grieving, and from allowing personal values to adversely influence their psychosocial support.[101] By recognizing that psychosocial care involves holistic healing, clinicians will be able to develop the best environment for interventions to improve multiple aspects of the client's quality of life.[101]

SUMMARY

It is important for the clinician involved in the treatment of a client with a brain tumor to anticipate the activity limitations that will develop as a result of the medical intervention or the tumor itself. These limitations provide the foundation for treatment planning and goal setting. Improved quality of life is the goal of the rehabilitation process. This means restoring the client to maximal functional capacity with the least amount of assistance from others. Regardless of the client's life expectancy, the rehabilitation process should enable the client to pursue a productive and meaningful life. Case Study 25-1 is an example of the complexity of the problems faced by an individual with a CNS tumor. These problems include both the medical condition and the functional activity limitations caused by the tumor and/or the medical management.

References

To enhance this text and add value for the reader, all references are included on the companion Evolve site that accompanies this textbook. This online service will, when available, provide a link for the reader to a Medline abstract for the article cited. There are 101 cited references and other general references for this chapter, with the majority of those articles being evidence-based citations.

CASE STUDY 25-1 ■ MEDICAL DIAGNOSIS: LOW-GRADE ASTROCYTOMA

Mrs. S. is a 46-year-old woman diagnosed 9 years ago with a low-grade astrocytoma in the right posterior frontal lobe. Before this diagnosis, she had a 4-year history of seizures. She underwent a partial resection of a microcystic pilocytic astrocytoma. Postoperative medical management focused on controlling seizure activity. Radiation therapy and chemotherapy were not provided. Physically, she had resultant left foot weakness and minor seizures characterized by tingling numbness and tremors in the left foot. She was able to continue to work, but a career change was necessary owing to cognitive changes, including the inability to perform fast calculations, impaired memory, and decreased recall.

Three years later, imaging studies revealed tumor enlargement and Mrs. S. underwent Peacock radiation therapy. She remained independent for an additional 2 years. Mrs. S. then developed left facial weakness, progressive left hemiparesis, and hyperreflexia on the left side; 2 weeks later, MRI scans revealed a lesion in the right midcerebral hemisphere below the original tumor site. A stereotactic biopsy confirmed a diagnosis of glioblastoma multiforme. She then underwent a gross total tumor resection, received Gamma Knife radiosurgery, and was subsequently treated with chemotherapy.

Mrs. S. was admitted to the neurological rehabilitation unit for comprehensive rehabilitation. During the examination, it was noted that her speech was fluent and she tended to be hyperverbal, distractible, and perseverative. Manual muscle testing revealed functional strength in the right hemibody and $0/5$ strength in the left hemibody except for hip flexion of $2^{-}/5$. Decreased sensation to light touch and proprioception in the left hemibody were noted. Because of the location of the lesion, Mrs. S. experienced left seventh cranial nerve involvement, left homonymous hemianopsia, severe left-sided neglect, and right gaze preference. These visual-perceptual deficits greatly impaired her mobility. She was able to attend to the left side with maximal cues, but carryover was not observed.

Functionally, Mrs. S. required moderate assistance to assume sitting on the edge of the bed, where she demonstrated fair sitting balance. Owing to poor standing balance, she required maximal assistance to stand and pivot to her wheelchair. In standing, her head was rotated to the right and flexed, her pelvis was rotated to the right, her hips were flexed, her left knee was buckled, and her left foot was inverted. She was able to ambulate 15 feet in the parallel bars with maximal assistance to address these postural impairments and to advance the left leg. She was able to propel her wheelchair with her right arm and leg with much assistance and encouragement.

Mrs. S. refuses to use a wheelchair at home because her goal is to walk. She is married with three children and lives in a single-story house. Her husband works full-time, necessitating independent and safe mobility to return home. Mrs. S. and her family demonstrate poor understanding of her prognosis and express unrealistic goals. They frequently refer to her previous return to independence after her first resection and expect a similar outcome this time.

The clinician, in consideration of the client's goal to walk, incorporated standing, pregait, and gait training into treatment sessions. However, Mrs. S was encouraged to propel her wheelchair as a means of independent mobility on the rehab unit. A knee-ankle-foot orthosis (KAFO) was fabricated to provide stability in the left leg and assist in her goal of walking again.

Two weeks into her rehabilitation program, Mrs. S. began to demonstrate increased lethargy, decreased ability to participate in treatments, and increased weakness. She required more assistance with mobility. The clinician modified the treatment intervention to an appropriate yet challenging level. Sitting balance and transfers became the focus rather than standing balance and gait. The therapy team notified the physician of these changes and the client was transferred to acute care. She underwent additional surgery to drain a cyst and remove necrotic tissue within the tumor.

On her return to rehabilitation Mrs. S. became more alert and able to participate in therapy sessions. She and her family expressed hope that this surgery would cure the tumor. The clinician expressed encouragement but gently reminded the client and family members that although the drainage of the cyst may have allowed for functional improvements, the tumor was still present. The client's strength continued to improve and functional gains were observed. In gait, her left leg became able to stabilize during the stance phase; however, an Ace bandage was necessary to control foot drop. The client was able to ambulate household distances with minimal assistance.

The interdisciplinary team provided the client and family with the appropriate resources to choose a facility where Mrs. S. could continue her therapy and the family could easily visit. They also were provided with referrals regarding support groups and hospice care if needed in the future. At the time of discharge, Mrs. S. was delighted with her ability to walk but was disappointed that her left arm remained flaccid and that she was not returning home. The client and family continued to search for hope daily, but left with a better understanding of the poor prognosis.

CHAPTER 26 Inflammatory and Infectious Disorders of the Brain

JUDITH A. DEWANE, PT, DSc, NCS

KEY TERMS

brain abscess
encephalitis
functional activities
hypertonicity
hypotonicity
intervention goals
meningitis
postural control

OBJECTIVES

After reading this chapter the student or therapist will be able to:

1. Identify and comprehend the terminology for classifying different types of inflammatory and infectious disorders within the brain.
2. Discuss the range of neurological sequelae that occur.
3. Discuss the components of the comprehensive evaluation process and their interrelationships.
4. Structure the examination process to gather the information required to generate an appropriate plan of care.
5. Discuss the general goals of the intervention process.
6. Plan the interventions to meet the needs of the client.

The diversity of neurological sequelae that may occur after an inflammatory disorder in the brain (brain abscess, encephalitis, or meningitis) provides a range of challenges to the rehabilitation team. The therapist must identify the problems underlying the individual's movement dysfunctions without the template of the cluster of "typical" problems available with some other neurological diagnoses. Each client presents a combination of problems that is unique to that client and that requires the creative design of an intervention program. The following discussion of the therapeutic management of individuals recovering from an inflammatory disorder in the brain focuses on the process of designing an intervention plan to address the specific dysfunctions of the individual client. Because the management of the clinical problems is built on an understanding of the underlying pathological condition and because therapists may not be as familiar with these disease processes, an overview of the inflammatory disorders of the brain is presented.

OVERVIEW OF INFLAMMATORY DISORDERS IN THE BRAIN

Categorization of Inflammatory Disorders

Inflammatory disorders of the brain can be categorized based on the anatomical location of the inflammatory process and the cause of the infection, as follows:

A. Brain abscess
B. Meningitis (leptomeningitis)
  1. Bacterial meningitis
  2. Aseptic meningitis (viral)
C. Encephalitis
  1. Acute viral
  2. Parainfectious encephalomyelitis
  3. Acute toxic encephalopathy
  4. Progressive viral encephalitis
  5. "Slow virus" encephalitis

In most individuals, the defense mechanisms of the central nervous system (CNS) provide protection from infecting organisms. Compromises of the protective barriers can result in CNS infections as complications of common infections. The response of the CNS to the infection depends on several factors, including the type of organism, its route of entry, the CNS location of the infection, and the immunological competence of the individual. CNS infections occur with greater frequency and severity in individuals who are very young or elderly, immunodeficient, or antibody deficient.

The inflammatory process may be a localized, circumscribed collection of pus; may involve primarily the leptomeninges; may involve the brain substance; or may involve both the meninges and the brain substance. The infecting agents may be bacteria, viruses, prions, fungi, protozoa, or parasites. The most common agents producing meningitis are bacterial; the most common agents producing encephalitis are viral. However, bacterial encephalitis and viral meningitis also are disease entities. The following overview of the inflammatory processes within the brain is organized based on the anatomical location of the infection. More comprehensive discussions based on specific infecting organisms can be found in the references at the end of the chapter.[1] The site of the infection will determine the signs and symptoms of the CNS infections, whereas the infecting organism determines the prognosis, including the time course and severity of the problems.[2]

Brain Abscess

Brain abscesses occur when microorganisms reach brain tissue from a penetrating wound to the brain, by extension of local infection such as sinusitis or otitis, or by hematogenous spread from a distant site of infection. The route of infection influences the CNS region involved. The extension of a local infection tends to produce a solitary brain abscess in an adjacent lobe. Multiple abscesses may originate from the spread of microorganisms through the blood. The introduction of microorganisms by a penetrating trauma may result in an abscess soon after the trauma or several years later. As with the disorders presented in the subsequent discussions, circumstances that result in a compromised immune system (chronic corticosteroid or other immunosuppressive drug administration, administration of cytotoxic chemotherapeutic agents, or human immunodeficiency virus [HIV] infection) may predispose the individual to develop opportunistic infections.

The site and size of the abscess influence the initial symptoms. Evidence of increased intracranial pressure, a focal neurological deficit, and fever are described as the classic presenting triad.[3] However, the classic triad occurs in less than 50% of patients.[4] Most individuals experience an alteration of consciousness. In 47% of the cases, the frontal, parietal, or temporal lobe is involved.[4,5] Medical management of the abscess typically consists of antibiotic therapy (depending on the infecting agent and size and site of the abscess) and, often, surgical aspiration or excision. Bharucha and colleagues[3] describe neurological sequelae in 25% to 50% of the survivors, with 30% to 50% having persistent seizures, 15% to 30% having hemiparesis, and 10% to 20% having disorders of speech or language.

Meningitis

Meningitis (synonymous with leptomeningitis) denotes an infection spread through the cerebrospinal fluid (CSF) with the inflammatory process involving the pia and arachnoid maters, the subarachnoid space, and the adjacent superficial tissues of the brain and spinal cord. Pachymeningitis denotes an inflammatory process involving the dura mater. Meningitis can be caused by a wide variety of organisms, some of which cross the blood-brain barrier and the blood-CSF barrier. The CSF also can become contaminated by a wound that penetrates the meninges as a result of trauma or a medical procedure, such as implantation of a ventriculoperitoneal (VP) shunt. Once the organism compromises the blood-brain and blood-CSF barriers, the CSF provides an ideal medium for growth. All the body's typical major defense systems are essentially absent in the normal CSF. The blood-brain barrier may impede the clearance of infecting organisms by leukocytes and interfere with the entry of pharmacological agents from the blood. The infecting organism is disseminated throughout the subarachnoid space as the contaminated CSF bathes the brain. Entry into the ventricles occurs either from the choroid plexuses or by reflux through the exit foramen of the fourth ventricle. The spread of the organism through the CSF circulation accounts for the differences in the variety and extent of the neurological sequelae that can result from meningitis.

Bacterial Meningitis

Clinical Problems. The diagnostic categorization of meningitis depends on the infecting agent (e.g., *Haemophilus influenzae* meningitis, *Streptococcus pneumoniae* meningitis, and viral meningitis) and on the acute or chronic nature of the meningitis (acute, subacute, or chronic meningitis). The term *acute bacterial meningitis* denotes infections caused by aerobic bacteria (both gram-positive and gram-negative).[5,6] The most common infecting organism producing acute bacterial meningitis varies according to the age of the population. During the neonatal period and in the older adult, infections by gram-negative enterobacilli, especially *Escherichia coli,* and group B streptococci occur most frequently. Typical causative agents in children include *H. influenzae, Neisseria meningitidis,* and *S. pneumoniae.*[7] *S. pneumoniae, N. meningitidis,* and *H. influenzae* are the most common causes of community-acquired meningitis.[5,7,8] Individuals with a condition such as sickle cell anemia, alcoholism, or diabetes mellitus and individuals who are immunosuppressed are at increased risk.[1,9] Meningococci have been implicated in meningitis that strikes young children most often but can also infect adolescents and young adults. Freshman who live in dormitories are almost four times more likely to get meningitis than other college students.

An example of an organism that uses a typical systemic route of bacterial infection is the *H. influenzae* organism—a member of the normal flora of the nose and throat. During an upper respiratory tract infection, the organism may gain entry to the blood. The route of transmission of the organism from the blood to the CSF is not well established.

The circulation of CSF spreads the infecting organism through the ventricular system and the subarachnoid spaces (Figure 26-1). The pia and arachnoid maters become acutely inflamed, and as part of the inflammatory response, a purulent exudate forms in the subarachnoid space. The exudate may undergo organization, resulting in an obstruction of the foramen of Monro, the aqueduct of Sylvius, or the exit foramen of the fourth ventricle. The supracortical subarachnoid spaces proximal to the arachnoid villi may be obliterated, resulting in a noncommunicating or obstructive hydrocephalus caused by the accumulation of CSF. As the CSF accumulates, the intracranial pressure rises. The increased intracranial pressure produces venous obstruction, precipitating a further increase in the intracranial pressure. The rise in the CSF pressure compromises the cerebral blood flow, which activates reflex mechanisms to counteract the decreased cerebral blood flow by raising the systemic blood pressure. An increased systemic blood pressure accompanies increased CSF pressure.

The mechanism producing the headaches that accompany increased intracranial pressure may be the stretching of the meninges and pain fibers associated with blood vessels. Vomiting may occur as a result of stimulation of the medullary emetic centers. Papilledema may occur as intracranial pressure increases.

Other routes of bacterial infection may involve a local spread as the result of an infection of the middle ear or mastoid air cells. Meningitis may occur as a complication of a skull fracture, which exposes CNS tissue to the external environment or to the nasal cavity. Fractures of the cribriform plate of the ethmoid bone producing CSF rhinorrhea provide another route for infection. Meningitis may be a further complication to the clinical problems of a traumatic head injury.

Clinical features of acute bacterial meningitis include fever, severe headache, altered consciousness, convulsions (particularly in children), and nuchal rigidity. Nuchal rigidity is indicative of an irritative lesion of the subarachnoid space. Signs of meningeal irritation are painful cervical flexion, the Kernig sign, the Brudzinski sign, and the jolt sign.[10] Cervical flexion is painful because it stretches the inflamed meninges, nerve roots, and spinal cord. The pain triggers a

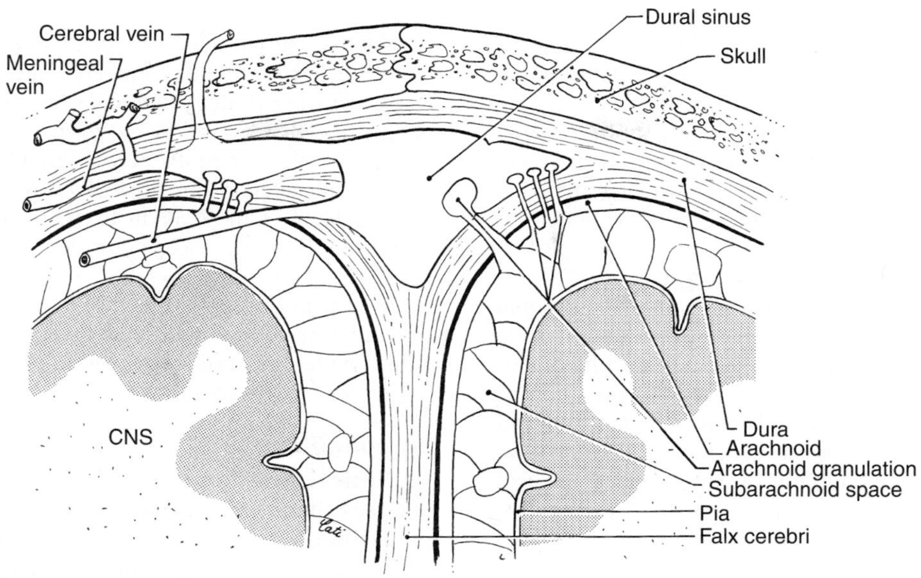

Figure 26-1 ■ The meninges, showing the layers of the dura, arachnoid, and pia mater and their relationship to the subarachnoid space and brain tissue.

reflex spasm of the neck extensors to splint the area against further cervical flexion; however, cervical rotation and extension movements remain relatively free.

The *Kernig sign* refers to a test performed with the client supine in which the thigh is flexed on the abdomen and the knee extended (Figure 26-2, *A*). Complaints of lumbar or posterior thigh pain indicate a positive test result.[10] This movement pulls on the sciatic nerve, which pulls on the covering of the spinal cord, causing pain in the presence of meningeal irritation. The same results are achieved with passive hip flexion with the knee remaining in extension. This is the same procedure described by Hoppenfeld[11] as the straight leg raising test for determining pathology of the sciatic nerve or tightness of the hamstrings. Passive hip flexion with knee extension can be painful because of meningeal irritation, spinal root impingement, sciatic nerve irritation, or hamstring tightness. The *Brudzinski sign* refers to the flexion of the hips and knees elicited when cervical flexion is performed[10] (see Figure 26-2, *B*). These signs will not be present in the deeply comatose client who has decreased muscle tone and absence of muscle reflexes. The signs may also be absent in the infant or elderly patient. Finally, the jolt test, which has the patient turn his or her head from side to side quickly (two to three rotations per second), has a positive result if the maneuver worsens the patient's headache.[10]

The diagnosis of bacterial meningitis can be established based on blood cultures and a sample of CSF obtained by a lumbar puncture. CSF pressure is consistently elevated. The CSF sample in bacterial meningitis typically reveals an increased protein count and a decreased glucose level.

The type and severity of the sequelae of acute bacterial meningitis relate directly to the area affected, the extent of CNS infection, the age and general health of the individual, the level of consciousness at the initiation of pharmacological therapy, and the pathological agent involved. Some of the common CNS complications include subdural effusions, altered levels of consciousness, seizures, involvement of the cranial nerves, and increased intracranial pressure.

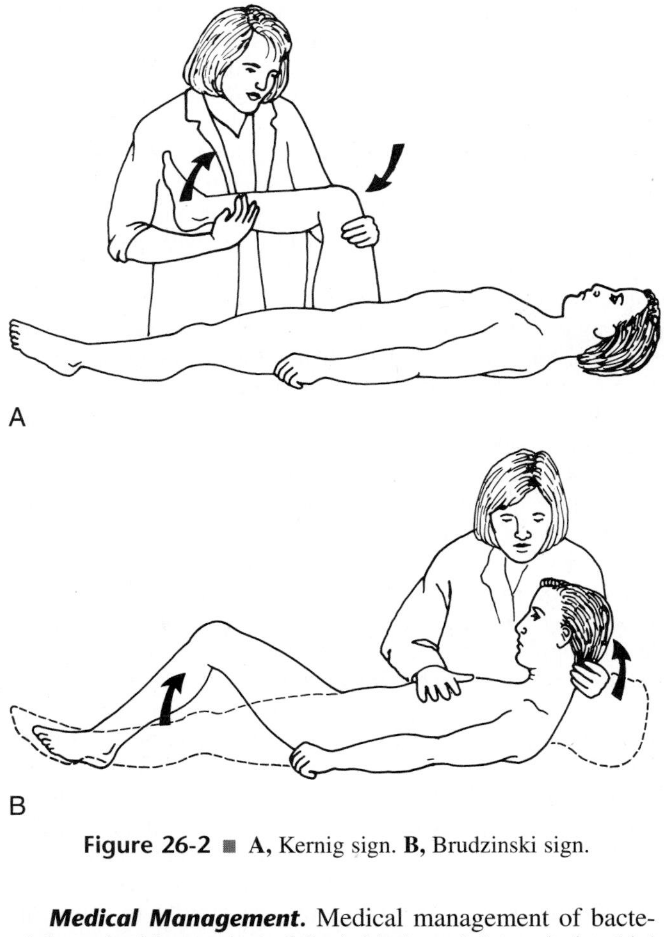

Figure 26-2 ■ **A,** Kernig sign. **B,** Brudzinski sign.

Medical Management. Medical management of bacterial meningitis consists of the initiation of the antimicrobial regimen appropriate to the infecting organism and procedures to manage the signs and symptoms of meningitis that have been described in the preceding paragraphs. Medical intervention strategies in both these areas change with the development of new pharmacological agents. Thus, medical management can change within short periods. The reader is encouraged to always review recent literature for additional information on current aspects of the medical management of the client with meningitis.

Prevention. Vaccination has significantly decreased the incidence of meningitis from *H. influenzae* type B in young children and infants. College freshmen who live in dormitories are four times more likely than other college students to develop meningococcus meningitis, and there is now a vaccine that has shown promise in reducing the outbreak rate.

Potential Neurological Sequelae. Even with optimal antimicrobial therapy, bacterial meningitis continues to have a finite mortality rate, which varies with the infecting organism, age of the individual, and time lapse to initiation of treatment, and has the potential for marked neurological morbidity. Neurological sequelae occur in 20% to 50% of the cases.[1,9] Bacterial meningitis is considered a medical emergency; delays in initiation of antibacterial therapy increase the risk of complications and permanent neurological dysfunction.[1,9]

Reports of the long-term outcome of individuals with bacterial meningitis indicate that up to 20% have long-term neurological sequelae.[1,5] The sequelae may be the result of the acute infectious pathological condition or subacute or chronic pathological changes. The acute infectious pathological condition could result in sequelae such as inflammatory or vascular involvement of the cranial nerves or thrombosis of the meningeal veins. Cranial nerve palsies, especially sensorineural hearing loss, are common complications. The risk of an acute ischemic stroke is greatest during the first 5 days.[9] Weeks to months after treatment, subacute or chronic pathological changes may develop, such as communicating hydrocephalus, which manifests as difficulties with gait, mental status changes, and incontinence.[10,12] Approximately 5% of the survivors will have weakness and spasticity.[6] Focal cerebral signs that may occur either early or late in the course of bacterial meningitis include hemiparesis, ataxia, seizures, cranial nerve palsies, and gaze preference.[1,13] Cognitive slowness has been found in 27% of clients after pneumococcal meningitis, even with good recovery as documented by a Glasgow Outcome Scale score of 5.[14]

Damage to the cerebral cortex can result in numerous expressions of dysfunction. Motor system dysfunction may be the observable expression of the damage within the CNS, but the location of the damage may include sensory and processing areas, as well as those areas typically categorized as belonging to the motor system. Perceptual deficits or regression in cognitive skills may present residual problems. Cranial nerve involvement is most frequently expressed as dysfunction of the eighth cranial nerve complex and produces auditory and vestibular deficits.

Aseptic Meningitis. Aseptic meningitis refers to a nonpurulent inflammatory process confined to the meninges and choroid plexus, usually caused by contamination of the CSF with a viral agent, although other agents can trigger the reactions. The symptoms are similar to those of acute bacterial meningitis but typically are less severe. The individual may be irritable and lethargic and complain of a headache, but cerebral function remains normal unless unusual complications occur.[5,15] Aseptic meningitis of a viral origin usually causes a benign and relatively short course of illness.[16,17]

A variety of neurotropic viruses can produce aseptic (viral) meningitis. The enteroviruses (echoviruses and the Coxsackie viruses), herpesviruses, and HIV are the most common causes.[5,7,18] The primary nonviral causes of aseptic meningitis are Lyme *Borrelia* and *Leptospira*.[19] The diagnosis of this type of aseptic meningitis may be established by isolation of the infecting agent within the CSF or by other techniques. The glucose level of the CSF in bacterial meningitis is usually depressed; however, the glucose level in viral meningitis is normal.[2]

Treatment of aseptic meningitis consists of management of symptoms. The condition does not typically produce residual neurological sequelae, and full recovery is anticipated within a few days to a few weeks.

Encephalitis

Clinical Problems. *Encephalitis* refers to a group of diseases characterized by inflammation of the parenchyma of the brain and its surrounding meninges. Although a variety of agents can produce encephalitis, the term usually denotes a viral invasion of the cells of the brain and spinal cord.

Different cell populations within the CNS vary in their susceptibility to infection by a specific virus. (For example, the viruses responsible for poliomyelitis have a selective affinity for the motor neurons of the brain stem and spinal cord. Viruses such as Coxsackie viruses and echoviruses typically infect meningeal cells to cause the benign viral meningitis discussed in the previous section.) In acute encephalitis, neurons that are vulnerable to the specific virus are invaded and undergo lysis. Viral encephalitis causes a syndrome of elevated temperature, headache, nuchal rigidity, vomiting, and general malaise (symptoms of aseptic or viral meningitis), with the addition of evidence of more extensive cerebral damage such as coma, cranial nerve palsy, hemiplegia, involuntary movements, or ataxia. The difficulty in differentiating between acute viral meningitis and acute viral encephalitis is reflected in the use of the term *meningoencephalitis* in some cases.

The pathological condition includes destruction or damage to neurons and glial cells resulting from invasion of the cells by the virus, the presence of intranuclear inclusion bodies, edema, and inflammation of the brain and spinal cord. Perivascular cuffing by polymorphonuclear leukocytes and lymphocytes may occur, as well as angiitis of small blood vessels. Widespread destruction of the white matter by the inflammatory process and by thrombosis of the perforating vessels can occur. Increased intracranial pressure, which can result from the cerebral edema and vascular damage, presents the potential for a transtentorial herniation. The likelihood of residual impairment of neurological functions depends on the infecting viral agent. Patients with mumps meningoencephalitis have an excellent prognosis, whereas 55% of the individuals with herpes simplex encephalitis treated with acyclovir have some neurological sequelae.[6] Because of the slow recovery of injured brain tissue, even in patients who recover completely, return to normal function may take months.[20]

Plum and Posner[21] discuss viral encephalitis in terms of five pathological syndromes. Acute viral encephalitis is a primary or exclusively CNS infection. An example would be herpes simplex encephalitis, in which the virus shows a partiality for the gray matter of the temporal lobe, insula, cingulate gyrus, and inferior frontal lobe. Other examples are the mosquito-borne viruses, such as the St. Louis encephalitis, California virus encephalitis, and most recently the West Nile virus (WNV). From 1999 to 2005 in the United States, the incidence of infection from the WNV has increased from 62 cases to 3000 cases.[22] Currently all states have some level of WNV activity, and only four states are without human cases (Figure 26-3). The majority (80%) of people infected by the WNV will be asymptomatic; of the remaining people infected, less than 1% will develop severe illness.[23] Risk of neuroinvasive disease from WNV is 40%; neuroinvasive disease involves meningitis, encephalitis, or poliomyelitis, with wide variety in clinical presentation (Figure 26-4).[24] Parainfectious encephalomyelitis is associated with viral infections such as measles, mumps, or varicella. Acute toxic encephalopathy denotes encephalitis that

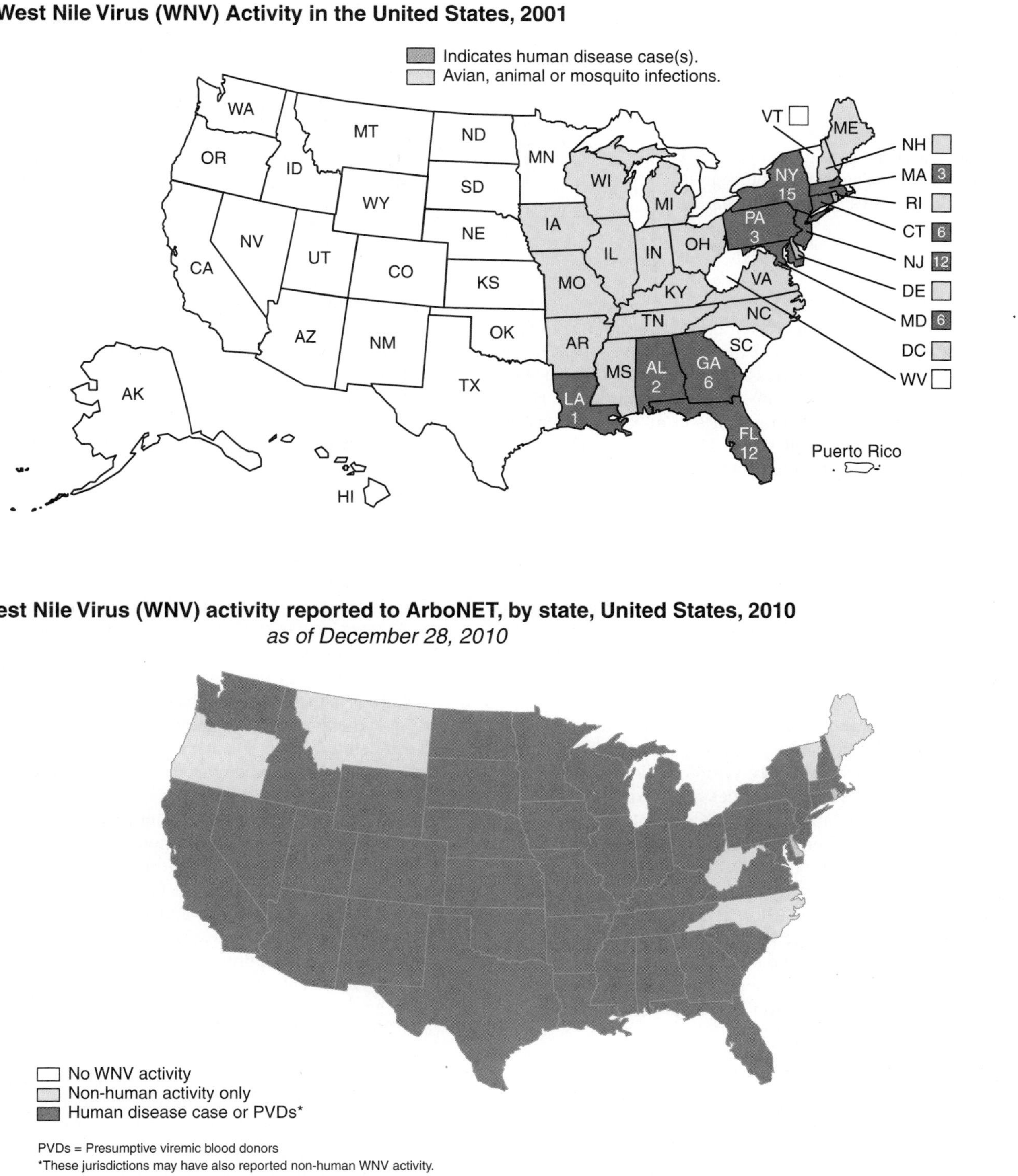

Figure 26-3 ■ West Nile virus (WNV) activity in the United States. (From www.cdc.gov/ncidod/dvbid/westnile/Mapsactivity/surv&control10MapsAnybyState.htm.)

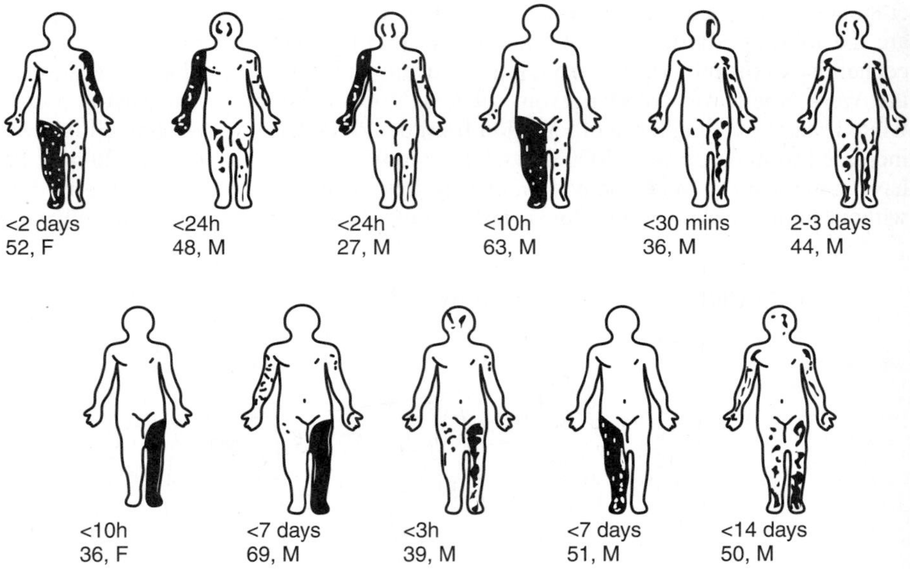

Figure 26-4 ■ Clinical presentation of West Nile virus. Weak limbs at the peak of paralysis are darkened. Degree of darkness corresponds to the severity of weakness. Duration of weakness and characteristics (age [years] and sex [*F,* female; *M,* male] are listed below each patient). (From Cao NJ, Ranganathan C, Kupsky WJ, Li J: Recovery and prognosticators of paralysis in West Nile virus infection. *J Neurol Sci* 236:73–80, 2005.)

occurs during the course of a systemic infection with a common virus. The clinical symptoms are produced by the cerebral edema in acute toxic encephalopathy, which results in increased intracranial pressure and the risk of transtentorial herniation. Reye syndrome is an example. Global neurological signs, such as hemiplegia and aphasia, are usually present, rather than focal signs. The clinical symptoms of the previous three syndromes may be similar. Specific diagnosis may be established only by biopsy or autopsy.

Progressive viral infections occur from common viruses invading susceptible individuals, such as those who are immunosuppressed or during the perinatal to early childhood period. Slow, progressive destruction of the CNS occurs, as in subacute sclerosing panencephalitis. The final category of encephalitis syndromes consists of "slow virus" infections by unconventional agents (the prion diseases) that produce progressive dementing diseases such as Creutzfeldt-Jakob disease and kuru.[25]

Medical Management. The medical management of virally induced encephalitis has been, and with many infecting agents remains, primarily symptomatic. In some cases, intensive, aggressive care is necessary to sustain life. Pharmacological interventions are available to treat some viral infections, such as herpes encephalitis. The probability of neurological sequelae differs according to the infecting agent. Aggressive management of increased intracranial pressure is required because persistently elevated intracranial pressure is associated with poor outcome.[1,26] Further information concerning the clinical features, medical management, and potential for neurological sequelae of a specific type of encephalitis should be sought in the literature based on the infecting agent.

Clinical Picture of the Individual with Inflammatory Disorders of the Brain

An individual within the acute phase of meningitis or encephalitis or with residual neurologic dysfunction from these disorders may demonstrate signs and symptoms similar to those of generalized brain trauma, tumor disorder, or other identified abnormal neurological state. The variability in the clinical picture is reflected in the inclusion of the category "infectious diseases that affect the central nervous system" in the *Guide to Physical Therapist Practice.*[27] Practice patterns for physical therapists that apply to this population include the following:

- 5C: Impaired Motor Function and Sensory Integrity Associated with Nonprogressive Disorders of the Central Nervous System—Congenital Origin or Acquired in Infancy or Childhood
- 5D: Impaired Motor Function and Sensory Integrity Associated with Nonprogressive Disorders of the Central Nervous System—Acquired in Adolescence or Adulthood
- 5I: Impaired Arousal, Range of Motion, and Motor Control Associated with Coma, Near Coma, or Vegetative State
- 5A: Primary Prevention/Risk Reduction for Loss of Balance and Falling

Although these patterns have been identified within the physical therapy practice patterns, the concepts and selection of evaluation and intervention procedures are just as applicable for occupational therapists and other individuals working on movement dysfunction. In the acute phase the inflammatory process may result in impairments in arousal and attention that range from nonresponsiveness to agitation. The degree of agitation may range from mild to severe, depending on both the client's unique CNS characteristics and the degree of inflammation. The agitated state may be the result of alterations in the processing of sensory input, with the consequence of inappropriate or augmented responses to sensory input. The client may respond to a normal level of sound as though it were an unbearably loud noise. Low levels of artificial light may be perceived as extremely bright.

Perceptual and cognitive impairments may be present, resulting in a variety of functional limitations and disabilities. Clients may have distortions in their perception of events as well as memory problems. As their memory returns, accuracy of time and events may be distorted, leading to frustration and anxiety for both the client and those family members and friends who are interacting within the environment.

In addition to alterations in mentation, the individual may demonstrate impaired affect, such as a hypersensitivity or exaggerated emotional responses to seemingly normal interactions. For example, when upset about dropping a spoon on the floor, a client may throw the tray across the table. When another individual was told his girlfriend would be a little late for her afternoon visit, the client became extremely upset and stated his intent to kill himself because his girlfriend did not love him anymore.

Because of the variety of pathological problems after acute inflammation, the client may have residual problems manifested as generalized or focal brain damage. The specifics of these impairments cannot be described as a typical clinical picture because they are extremely dependent on the individual client. These variations require the therapist to conduct a thorough examination and evaluation process to develop an appropriate individualized intervention program. Although content from the *Guide to Physical Therapist Practice* has been incorporated into the discussion of the examination, evaluation, and intervention processes, the model presented provides a structure that can accommodate the specific disciplinary expertise of both occupational and physical therapists.

EXAMINATION AND EVALUATION PROCESS

Just as the medical intervention with clients who have an inflammatory disorder of the CNS is, to a large extent, symptomatic, so is the intervention by therapists. Designing an individualized intervention program based on the client's problems requires a comprehensive initial and ongoing evaluation to define the impairments, functional limitations, and disabilities and to note changes in them. Although the discussion of examination procedures is separated from the discussion of intervention strategies, it must be recognized that the separation is artificial and does not reflect the image of practice. The evaluation process should be considered in relationship to both the long-term assessment of the individual's changes and the short-term within-session and between-session variations. For example, documentation of the level of consciousness of a client on day one of intervention will provide a starting point for calculation of the distance spanned at the time of discharge. Perhaps more critical to the final outcome is determination of the level of consciousness before, during, and after a particular intervention technique to determine its impact on the individual's level of arousal and ability to interact with the environment. The evaluation process is a constant activity intertwined with intervention. The observations and data from the process are periodically recorded to establish the course of the disease process and the success of the therapeutic management of the client.

Observation of Current Functional Status

The examination process should be conceptualized as a decision-making tree that requires the therapist to determine actively which components are to be included in a detailed examination and which can be eliminated or deferred. The first step in this process is the observation of the client's current functional status. If the client is comatose and nonmobile, the focus of the initial session might be an assessment of the stability of physiological functions, level of consciousness, responses to sensory input, and joint mobility. If the client is an outpatient with motor control deficits, the initial session might focus on defining motor abilities and components contributing to movement dysfunctions with a more superficial assessment of physiological functions and level of consciousness. The therapist must be alert to indications of the need for a more detailed evaluation of perceptual and cognitive function (e.g., the client cannot follow two-step commands, indicating the need to assess cognitive skills).

Some of the components discussed in this process may be examination skills that are more typically possessed by other professions (e.g., assessment of emotional or psychological status). The inclusion of these items is not meant to suggest that the therapist must complete the formal testing. The items are included to indicate factors that will affect goal setting for the client and that will have an impact on the intervention strategy. Although the therapist may not be the health care team member who has primary responsibility for evaluation of these areas, he or she should recognize these areas as potential contributors to movement dysfunctions.

Observation of the current functional status of the client provides the therapist with an initial overview of his assets and deficits. This provides the framework into which the pieces of information from the evaluation of specific aspects of function can be fit. The therapist must not allow assumptions made during the initial observation to bias later observations. The therapist might note that the client is able to roll from the supine to the side-lying position to interact with visitors in the room. When the same activity is not repeated on the mat table in the treatment area, the therapist, knowing the client has the motor skill to roll, might conclude that he is uncooperative or apraxic or has perceptual deficits. The therapist may have failed to consider that the difference between the two situations is the type of support surface or the presence or absence of side rails, which may have enabled the client to roll in bed by pulling over to the side-lying position. It is characteristic of human observation skills that we tend to "see" what we expect to see. The therapist must attempt to observe behaviors and note potential explanations for deviations from normal without biasing the results of the subsequent observations.

The following discussion of the specific considerations within the examination process does not necessarily represent the temporal sequence to be used during the data collection process. As different items are discussed, suggestions for potential combinations of items will be made. The sequence of the process is best determined by the interaction of therapist and client. Figure 26-5 outlines the components that should be considered during the evaluation process and provides a synopsis of the following discussion.

The general philosophy in the evaluation of the client with neurological deficits as a result of brain inflammation is a whole-part-whole approach. General observations of the client's performance provide an overall description of the client's abilities while indicating deficits in his or her performance. The cause(s) of the deficits (impairments) are explored to provide the pieces of data defining her or his performance. These pieces of data then are arranged within the framework provided by the general observation to define the whole of the client's assets and deficits. As the whole picture is established (with the realization that it will be constantly adjusted), the process of goal setting is initiated.

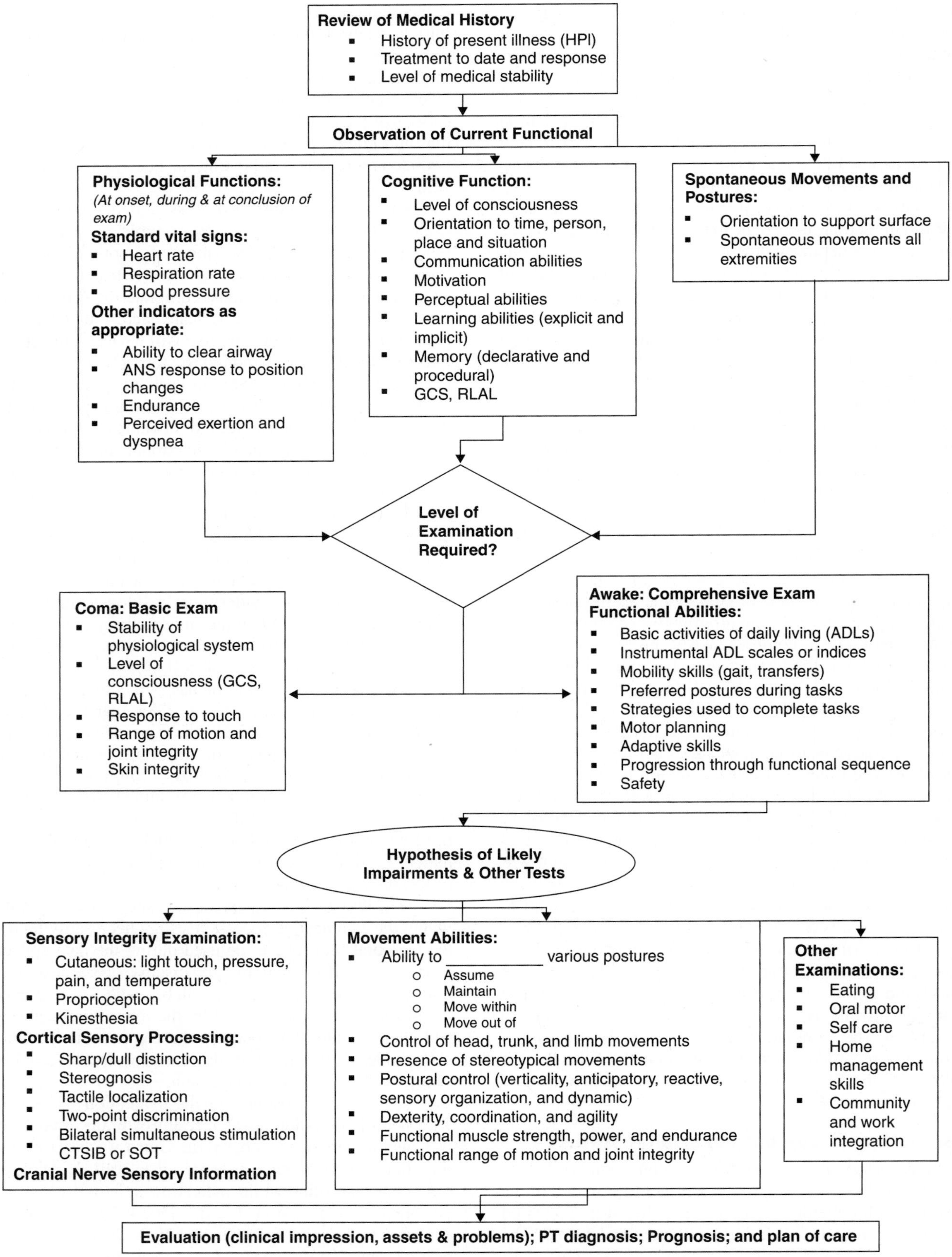

Figure 26-5 ■ Flow chart of the evaluation process.

These goals need to consider the patient's and family's desires. The process presented for refining evaluation data into an intervention plan is applicable whether the client's neurological dysfunction is the result of a bacterial or viral infection, cerebrovascular accident, trauma, or other factors.

Evaluation of Physiological Responses to Therapeutic Activities

It is assumed that the therapist enters the initial interaction with a client after reviewing the available background information. This may provide the therapist with information on the baseline status of the client's vital physiological functions. Any control problems in these areas should be particularly noted. Until the therapist determines that the vital functions, such as rate of respiration, heart rate, and blood pressure, vary appropriately with the demands of the intervention process, these factors should be monitored. The monitoring process should include consideration of the baseline rate, rate during exercise, and time to return to baseline. The pattern of respiration and changes in that pattern also should be noted.

Other tests and measures of the status of ventilation, respiration, and circulation may be indicated in specific individuals. Individuals with limited mobility or motor control of the trunk or those with cranial nerve dysfunctions may demonstrate difficulty with functions such as moving secretions out of the airways. Inactivity during a prolonged recovery period may result in cardiovascular adaptations that compromise endurance and contribute to increases in the perceived exertion during activities.

Autonomic nervous system dysfunctions may be expressed as inappropriate accommodations to positional changes, such as orthostatic hypotension. Clients with depressed levels of consciousness may display temperature regulation dysfunctions. One mechanism for assessing the client's ability to maintain a homeostatic temperature is to review the nursing notes. The events surrounding any periods of diaphoresis should be examined. If no causative factors have been identified, then interventions that involve thermal agents as discussed elsewhere in this text should be used judiciously.

Evaluation of Cognitive Status

Because the evaluation process encompasses the stages of recovery from the critical acute phase through discharge from therapy, a range of aspects are included under the evaluation of cognitive status. As indicated previously, the observation of current functional status will direct the therapist toward the appropriate component tests and measures.

Acute bacterial meningitis and various forms of viral encephalitis may result in changes in the client's level of consciousness. *Consciousness* is a state of awareness of one's self and one's environment.[21] *Coma* can be defined as a state in which one does not open the eyes, obey commands, or utter recognizable words.[28] The individual does not respond to external stimuli or to internal needs. The term *vegetative state* is sometimes used to indicate the status of individuals who open their eyes and display a sleep-wake cycle but who do not obey commands or utter recognizable words. DeMeyer[29] presents a succinct description of the neuroanatomy of consciousness and the neurological examination of the unconscious patient. Plum and Posner[21] also provide extensive information in this area.

Several scales have been developed to provide objective guidelines to assess alterations in the state of consciousness. The Glasgow Coma Scale[28] assesses three independent items: eye opening, motor performance, and verbal performance. The scale yields a figure from 3 (lowest) to 15 (highest) that can be used to indicate changes in the individual's state of consciousness. The evaluation format is simple, and the scale demonstrates both interrater and intrarater reliability. Refer to Box 24-4 for the specific scale. The Rancho Los Amigos scale assesses level of consciousness and behavior.[28] The therapist can use assessment tools such as the Glasgow Coma Scale and the companion Glasgow Outcome Scale to determine if the intervention program has resulted in any recordable changes in the client's level of consciousness. Ideally, the client with decreased levels of consciousness will be monitored at consistent intervals to determine changes in status. Any carryover or delayed effects of the intervention could then be noted. The record of the client's level of consciousness might also display a pattern of peak awareness at a particular point in the day. Scheduling an intervention session during the client's peak awareness time may maximize the benefit of the therapy.

Performed in conjunction with the assessment of the client's state of consciousness is the determination of the individual's orientation to person, time, place, and situation. Because the individual's level of orientation (documented as oriented times 4) is frequently recorded by multiple members of the rehabilitation team, the information in the medical chart may provide insights into fluctuations over the course of a day or a week.

Gross assessment of the individual's ability to communicate, both the expressive and receptive aspects of the process, is an important component of the examination. If a dysfunction is present in the client's ability to communicate, the client should be evaluated by an individual with expertise in this area so that strategies for dealing with the communication deficit can be developed. Evaluation of the movement abilities of the client with communication deficits requires creative planning on the part of the therapist but usually can be accomplished if generalized movement tasks are used. With the client who cannot comprehend a verbal command to roll, the therapist should use an alternate form of communication, such as manual cueing or guidance. The therapist could structure the situation to elicit the desired behavior by activities such as placing the client in an uncomfortable position or positioning a desired object so that it can be reached only by rolling.

As the therapist progresses through the examination and intervention process, ongoing data collection should be occurring on factors that influence the motivation of the individual. Individuals with damage to certain areas within the frontal lobe will have difficulty with committing to long-term projects and may not be motivated to work during a therapy session by an explanation detailing the relationship of the current activity to the larger goal of returning home. In these situations, the therapist must create appropriate immediate rewards, such as a 2-minute rest break after completion of a specific movement task.

Deficits in cognition may be evident as problems in the area of explicit (declarative) or implicit (procedural) learning. Explicit learning is used in the acquisition of knowledge that is consciously recalled. This is information that can be verbalized in declarative sentences, such as the sequential listing of the steps in a movement sequence. Implicit or procedural learning is used in the process of acquiring movement sequences that are performed automatically without conscious attention to the performance. Procedural learning occurs through repetitions of the movement task (refer to Chapter 4). Because explicit and implicit learning use different neuroanatomical circuits, implicit learning can occur in individuals with deficits in the components underlying explicit learning (awareness, attention, higher-order cognitive processes) (refer to Chapter 5 for additional information regarding implicit and explicit learning).

The emotional and psychological aspects of the client and the higher-order cognitive and retention skills of the client should be evaluated informally by the therapist, with referral to appropriate professionals if dysfunction in these areas is suspected. A coordinated team approach is necessary for clients with emotional and psychological, cognitive, perceptual, or communication problems or a combination of these problems. A consistent strategy used by all team members eliminates the necessity on the part of the client of trying to cope with different approaches by different people in an area in which she or he already has a deficit. The impact of cognitive deficits on the process of learning motor skills is further discussed in the next section on movement assessment. The assessment of the impact of perceptual dysfunctions is incorporated within the evaluation of sensory channels.

Examination of Functional Abilities

As indicated in the introduction to the evaluation of clients with inflammatory and infectious disorders of the brain, the examination process is not compartmentalized. As the therapist is examining the movement abilities of the individual through the format described in the previous section, he or she is also collecting information on the functional abilities of the individual. The components underlying the movement abilities of the client can be examined within the framework of the basic or instrumental activities of daily living (ADLs), depending on the functional level of the person. The treatment setting and documentation requirements within that setting will determine whether the data on basic ADL and instrumental ADL skills are recorded with use of a formal scale or index or are gathered through an individualized process.

The introduction of specific tasks provides the therapist with the opportunity to observe the preferred posture used to accomplish the different tasks. The therapist should construct situations that require the individual to respond to unexpected occurrences to provide some insight into the person's ability to adapt to the unexpected. Throughout the process of examining a patient's movement abilities and functional abilities, the therapist is assessing the individual's awareness of safety considerations and judgment in attempting tasks.

The presence of motor planning dysfunctions can be noted as the client attempts a movement sequence or a functional task. The therapist may have to cue the client physically to initiate the sequence, which then flows smoothly. The therapist may observe that the client has the correct components to a movement sequence, but that the sequence of the components is incorrect. Or the client may demonstrate the ability to produce a movement sequence under one set of conditions but not another. Indications of these types of motor planning problems can be observed during the initial interactions with the client. Similarly, the therapist also should be aware of indications of problems with dexterity, coordination, and agility, as well as with signs of cerebellar dysfunctions.

Another aspect of the evaluation process that can be integrated in the observations of movement abilities is identification of perceptual deficits. Aspects of the client's motor performance can provide indications for detailed perceptual testing to classify the deficits. This testing should be conducted by the health care team member qualified in the area of perceptual testing. During the general evaluation procedures, the therapist can screen the client for signs of perceptual deficits. Clients' abilities to cross their midlines with their upper extremities can be demonstrated in movement sequences, such as moving from the supine to the side-sitting to the sitting position (Figure 26-6). The quality of the integration of information from the two sides of the body can be indicated by the symmetry or asymmetry of posture in positions that should be symmetrical. The therapist may suspect that the client has a deficit in body awareness or body image by the poor quality of movement patterns that are within the motor capability of the individual. Spontaneous comments by the client as to how he or she feels when moving ("my leg feels so heavy") also add to the therapist's assessment of the client's body image. Problems with verticality can be seen with the client who lists to one side when in an upright posture. When the therapist corrects the list to a vertical posture, clients may express that they now feel that they are leaning to one side. Individuals who cannot appropriately relate their positions to the position of objects in their environments may have a figure-ground deficit or a problem with the concept of their position in space. When approaching stairs, these clients may fail to step up or may attempt to step up too soon. These examples should provide an indication of the observations that can indicate the need for detailed perceptual testing.

The preceding aspects of evaluation of movement abilities focused on facets of motor performance. Within this process the therapist should intertwine an appraisal of the individual's ability to learn motor tasks (or elements of the task). The therapist attempts to determine whether the client can maintain a change in the ability to perform a movement throughout a therapy session and into the next session. The client's ability to capture and integrate changes into the movement repertoire is fundamental to the success of the intervention program. The program can focus on the learning of movement sequences and the generalization of these sequences to movements within other contexts. Individuals with lowered levels of consciousness (typically Rancho Los Amigos Levels I to III) will be unable to learn or have difficulty learning and generalizing new motor skills. Therapy sessions may be more successful if the focus remains on the performance of motor tasks that were previously "overlearned" and automatic. Although the therapist may be able to manually guide the individual in coming to sit on the edge of the bed, until the individual demonstrates a higher level of processing, it may be unrealistic to expect that he or she will consistently reposition the legs without cueing before

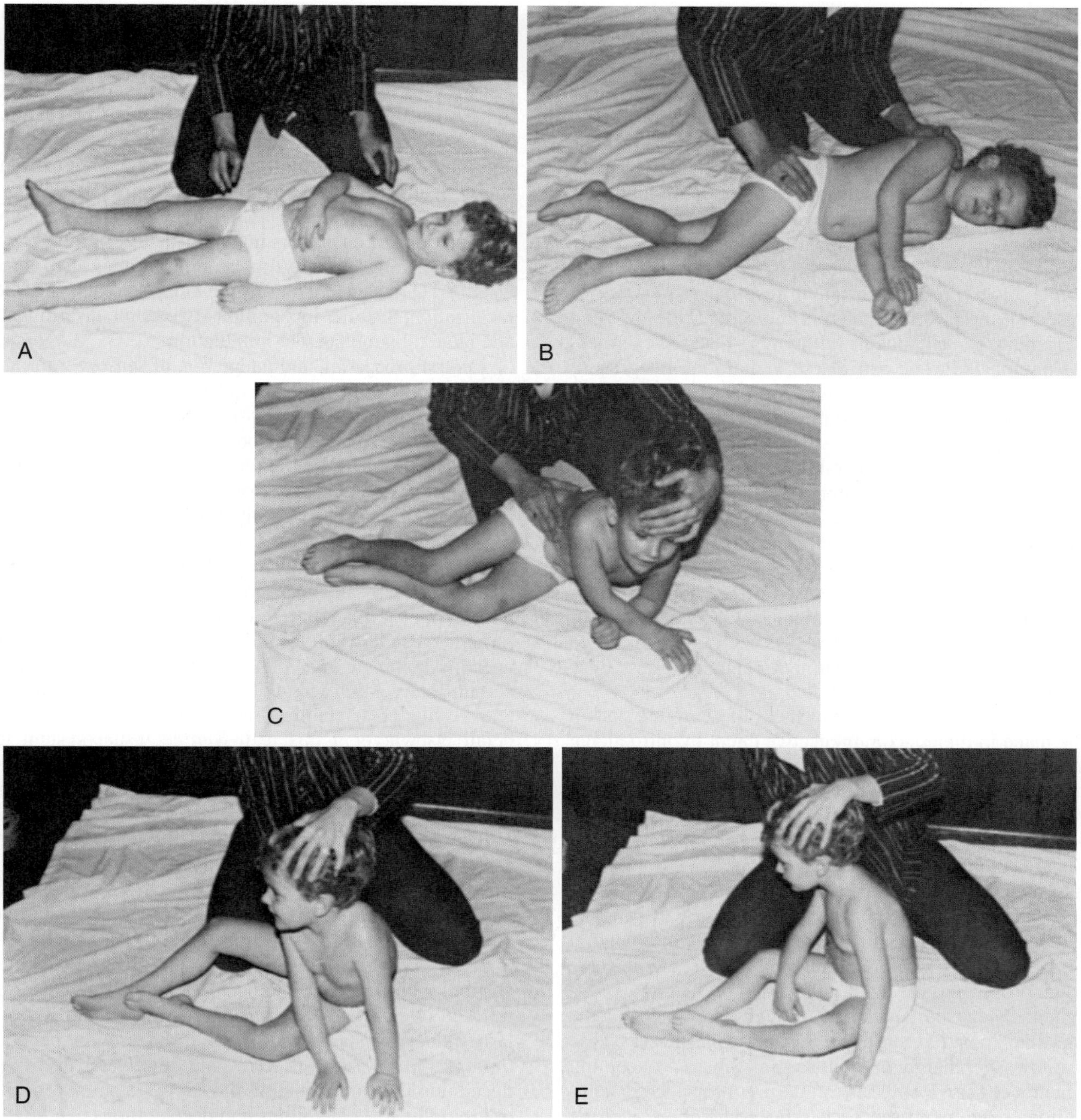

Figure 26-6 ■ Movement sequence from the supine to side-sitting to sitting positions. **A,** Supine position. **B,** Handling to side lying. **C,** Handling toward side sitting; arm positions are important. **D,** Side sitting; note propping patterns with arms. **E,** Handling to symmetrical sitting.

attempting the movement sequence. From looking at the "whole" of function, the therapist needs to determine the impairments that require further examination.

Evaluation of Sensory Channel Integrity and Processing

The examination process must include an assessment of the channels for sensory input. Knowledge gained in the assessment of the sensory systems will be used in the program-planning process to select the intervention strategies that have the highest probability of success. Although movements can be performed (and in some cases even learned) in the absence of typical sensory feedback, the presence of altered sensory function creates more challenges for both the client/learner and the therapist/teacher. The therapist assesses both the client's ability to perceive the sensory stimulus and the appropriateness of the response to the stimulus. Therefore it is important to determine if the sensory modality is intact, impaired, or absent, and if it is impaired, whether it hyperresponsive, hyporesponsive, or inconsistent. In addition, variations in the interpretation of sensory input may occur in some clients. Gentle tactile contact may be perceived by the person as a noxious input. Some individuals will have difficulty processing and discriminating information with high levels of one type of sensory input (e.g., the noisy clinic area) or with multiple simultaneous inputs (e.g., talking to the therapist while walking down a hallway with people moving toward the individual).

The therapist should develop a systematic approach to the initial cursory screen of the sensory systems. Deficits identified in the initial examination will provide structure for scheduling more comprehensive evaluation of deficits in specific systems. The therapist must also monitor changes in the status of physiological vital functions during sensory input, especially if the client has a history of instability of heart rate, blood pressure, or rate of respiration.

Based on the information from the screen, the therapist will organize the components of the more detailed examination. Components to be considered include the integrity of the peripheral sensory circuits, the cortical level processing of the sensory information, the integrity of the cranial nerve sensory circuits, and the processing of multichannel input.

Cutaneous input has several aspects that must be assessed. Some of the inflammatory diseases of the brain may result in cutaneous distributions in which sensation is absent or diminished. These areas should be routinely evaluated for changes in distribution of level of sensation. Tests of light touch, pressure, and pain can be used if the client can communicate reliably. In most cases, inclusion of assessment of differentiation of hot and cold will not add appreciably to the information needed for treatment planning unless thermal modalities are a consideration.

A gross assessment of the intactness of the touch system can be made in the noncommunicative client by introducing a mildly aversive (not painful) stimulus, such as a light scratch, while monitoring the client for changes in facial expression, posture, or tonus. The possibility of a spinal-level reflex response should be kept in mind when interpreting the results of such a gross assessment.

Assessment of the client's response to proprioceptive input is incorporated within the assessment of the client's movement abilities and is intertwined with the intervention process because a variety of intervention techniques are based on proprioceptive input. Evaluation of the proprioceptive channels can be conducted through assessment of the client's static position sense and dynamic kinesthesis. These tests allow the therapist to make inferences concerning the client's cognitive abilities to interpret proprioceptive information. Inherent in the successful completion of these tests is the necessity for the client to be able to understand directions and to be able to communicate data to the therapist. Because information input, processing, and output are involved in these tests, failure to comply with the test instructions cannot be definitively attributed to dysfunction of the proprioceptive system. The therapist also should consider information obtained from watching the client move before drawing a conclusion concerning the intactness of the proprioceptive channels. Some of the factors to consider include disregard of an extremity and variations in quality of performance between visually directed and non–visually directed movements. Although tests of position sense and kinesthetics provide one aspect of the evaluation of the proprioceptive system, the therapist also must be involved constantly in assessing the client's response to the intervention techniques that are part of the treatment plan. This again illustrates the intermingling of assessment and intervention. Intervention places a demand for movement on the client. As the movement occurs, the therapist assesses the quality of the movement. If the quality is not appropriate, the therapist initiates intervention to improve the quality. If the technique does not produce the desired result, a second technique can be tried and the cyclical process continues.

In addition to determining the integrity of the peripheral sensory pathways and recognition of the input, it is important to assess the individual's ability to process more complex presentations of cutaneous input. Difficulties in the cortical-level processing of cutaneous stimuli are identified through tests of sharp and dull discrimination, stereognosis, tactile localization, texture recognition, two-point discrimination, and bilateral simultaneous stimulation.

Central processing and integration of sensory information as it affects postural control can be examined using the Clinical Test of Sensory Integration and Balance (CTSIB)[30] or with computerized dynamic posturography using the Sensory Organization Test (SOT). With both tests, the effectiveness of using vision or somatosensory or vestibular sensation at the appropriate time (sensory weighting) and changing from one sensory system to the other is examined.

Assessment of the integrity of the cranial nerve sensory channels is typically incorporated within the standard cranial nerve examination. Review of the physician's notes may provide sufficient information; however, the therapist may need to complete more specific tests before considering certain intervention techniques. Of specific note are vision and vestibular screening, both of which are discussed in detail elsewhere in this text. Simple visual system tests, such as identification of field deficits, assessment of tracking abilities, and a gross evaluation of visual acuity, can be performed quickly.

The complex functions of the vestibular system can be assessed through a variety of avenues such as the Ayres Post-Rotatory Nystagmus Test,[31,32] the SOT, and tests of the vestibular ocular reflex (head-thrust test, head-shaking test, and test of dynamic visual acuity [DVA]), and are discussed in detail elsewhere in this text. It is important to examine the vestibular influence in both postural control and gaze stability. The integrity of the connections underlying a vestibularly induced nystagmus response is assessed by physicians through the caloric test (warm and cold water or air introduced into the ear channel to induce nystagmus). The effect of rapid linear accelerations and decelerations can be evaluated as potential activating mechanisms increasing the level of consciousness or level of muscle activity. An example is the Dynamic Gait Index, a functional test that incorporates changes in speed and head movements during walking.[33] Slow, rhythmical reversals of linear movements may have a calming effect on the client's behavior or level of muscle activation. Linear movements in all planes and diagonals should be explored.

During the evaluation of the client as well as during intervention with the client, the therapist must be aware of the potential to bombard him or her with sensory input and overload his or her ability to respond discriminatively to it. If the therapist detects that the client has difficulty in responding appropriately to sensory input, as with a client in a lowered state of consciousness or an agitated state, or demonstrating tactile defensiveness, sensory input should be used selectively during the initial examination or intervention sessions. If multiple sensory inputs are used, the positive or negative effects cannot be attributed to a specific input or necessarily to the series of inputs. Evaluation as well as intervention with sensory inputs should proceed in a controlled fashion. Inclusion of additional sensory modalities in the intervention plan should occur systematically.

The individual's response to multichannel sensory conflict input is typically assessed as a component of higher-level balance assessment and locomotor abilities. A more thorough discussion of sensory assessment is discussed elsewhere in the text. The therapist should apply these concepts during the evaluation of all motor tasks. Consider the following example: a client who relies on visual input to supplement vestibular and somatosensory information is performing the task of sitting on the edge of the mat table. She remains relatively steady until someone walks directly toward her from across the clinic. This change in the environmental context of the performance requires her to assess whether she is moving toward the individual or the individual is moving toward her. Without reliable vestibular and somatosensory check points, the client may activate a postural response to the incorrect assessment. As this example demonstrates, the evaluation of the sensory channels is intertwined with the evaluation of the person's movement abilities.

Examination of Movement Abilities

The initial assessment of the individual's movement abilities is conducted by observing as she or he moves through a sequence of functional postures. The therapist determines the functional postures to be examined for a specific client, ranging from bed mobility activities (assessment of movement in prone and supine positions) through upright ambulation. The medical status of the individual, the extent of involvement, the intervention setting, and the age of the individual are considerations in determining the appropriate functional postures to be examined. The therapist gathers information on the movement abilities of the client as he or she moves into, within, and out of the position.

The assessment focuses on both the quantity and quality of motor performance. The quantitative aspect of the movement assessment involves the number of different functional postures the individual can use. The quality of the movement abilities is assessed within the posture as well as in the process of moving between postures. For example, the therapist should assess the quality of the head, trunk, and extremity control demonstrated throughout the movement sequences. The use of stereotypical movement patterns should be noted because their presence may limit the adaptability of movements required to accomplish functional tasks. Other items relating to the client's movement abilities are assessed during this process.

Indications of abnormal ranges of movement of all joints can be obtained. The range may show a limitation of movement or an indication of joint instability. Once the gross deviations are identified, these joints can be examined to determine the source of the problem: joint capsular, ligamentous, bony, skin, or muscular and fascial dysfunction. Conducting the gross assessment of range while the client is moving eliminates the time spent in performing a joint-by-joint goniometric evaluation of articulations with normal excursions.

As the individual is moving (either independently or with the therapist assisting), an assessment of the distribution and fluctuations in muscle activity can be made and will provide information on functional muscle strength, power, and endurance. The timing, accuracy, and sequencing of muscle activation within the movement should be noted. The therapist can identify the postures that will be the most conducive to optimal motor performances and those that should be avoided. As the client is moving through various postures, the function of specific musculature can be examined. Muscle groups should be examined with regard to their ability to function in both stability (distal segment fixed) and mobility (distal segment free) situations. Because numerous demands are being placed on each muscle group, therapists can assess the ability to perform isometric and isotonic (concentric and eccentric) contractions. Each different posture introduces a new set of variables; therefore the performance of a muscle group must be reexamined as each new movement pattern is performed.

The therapist can identify postural control in a variety of functional positions. Within each posture, the therapist must examine the control the client displays over the posture. Because the assessment takes place as part of a dynamic sequence, the therapist can assess the client's ability to assume the posture. If the posture cannot be achieved independently, the therapist assesses the factors interfering with achieving the position, the type of assistance necessary to facilitate assumption of the posture, and the effect of the various intervention techniques used to assist the client in achieving the position. Once the client is in the posture, her or his ability to maintain the posture is examined. Factors that interfere with the performance are noted. The client's ability to move within the posture is identified. Movement demands placed on the client should include aspects of both static and dynamic equilibrium. Static balance in the sitting position (such as on the side of the bed) could be demonstrated by the individual matching the strength of a force attempting to displace him backward and maintaining the position when the force is suddenly released.

The presence of dynamic balance of the upper torso in the sitting position could be demonstrated by the individual reacting to a quick sideways displacement force administered to the shoulder by activating the trunk lateral flexors to compensate for the displacement. Equally important is the individual's ability to demonstrate appropriate equilibrium responses to self-imposed perturbations. The absence of anticipatory control in standing could be demonstrated by having the client do the rapid arm raise test with a 5-lb weight and noticing reactive stepping instead of doing a posterior weight shift in anticipation of the destabilizing force.

The final stage in examining the individual's movement abilities explores the individual's ability to move out of the posture. The client should have the ability to move out of the posture to a lower-level posture and to a higher-level posture before mastery of the posture is considered to have been achieved.

Many aspects of the client's performance are analyzed simultaneously. When the therapist assists the client in moving to a new posture, an analysis of the influence of facilitation and inhibition techniques is being conducted. The individual's response to these handling techniques cues the therapist in projecting the client's response to an intervention program. The therapist is constantly monitoring the client for changes in physiological functions or changes in the level of consciousness. Anything that results in expressions of pain by the client should be noted. Intervention programs should be a learning experience for clients. If they are attending to pain, they cannot attend to learning. The factor(s) producing the pain should be identified and measures instituted to eliminate the factor(s). If the factors producing the pain cannot be resolved, the intervention program should be designed to avoid triggering the pain.

In addition to looking at postural control in a variety of postures, it is also important to determine the type of postural control dysfunction, such as vertical orientation to the surface or to gravity as the situation dictates, anticipatory postural control, reactive postural control, sensory organization for postural control, and dynamic balance for gait.

PROGNOSING AND GOAL SETTING

Ideally, the process of establishing the prognosis and setting the goals for a client is a coordinated effort that involves all members of the health care team, including the client (if feasible) and family. If the therapist is not functioning in a setting where involvement of many disciplines is viable, the therapist can progress through the goal-setting process in the context of his or her role in the client's care.

Having collected data from the examination process, the first steps are to establish two lists: one dealing with specific problems (impairments, functional limitations, and disabilities) the client is encountering and the second dealing with her or his assets. Formulating an asset list focuses on the positive data elicited from the evaluation process and is critical for prognosing outcomes. Items on the asset list could be observations, such as the client being able to assume the position of sitting on the side of the bed with setup assistance only, improved head control in this posture being facilitated by approximation, and controlled weight shifting being elicited by alternated tapping. The asset list provides a reference defining the postures and intervention techniques that are effective. This reference is used to develop the intervention goals and plan. Formulating and recording a problem list and an asset list can be completed relatively quickly as one gains familiarity with the process. Whereas novice therapists will benefit from generating a written asset list, experienced clinicians may formulate a mental asset list while completing the written evaluation format required by the facility. Just as the evaluation process is ongoing, so are the steps involved in goal setting. The asset and problem lists are redefined as the client's status changes.

After assets and problems have been identified, the next step is to establish the expected outcomes from this episode of care. This is considered the prognosis. These outcome statements represent the general objectives toward which the intervention process is oriented. They identify the end point of the intervention process and are the exit criteria for terminating the episode of care.

The *Guide to Physical Therapist Practice* views outcomes in relationship to "minimization of functional limitations, optimization of health status, prevention of disability, and optimization of patient/client satisfaction," whereas goals "relate to the remediation (to the extent possible) of impairments."[27] The breadth of acceptance of these definitions with the neurorehabilitation professions remains to be determined. These definitions at least give professionals a place to start communicating with consistency. The International Classification of Functioning, Disability and Health (ICF) model of the World Health Organization provides similar definitions, with the focus being client centered.

Measurable, interim objectives should be established in relation to the outcome statements. To determine if the objective has been achieved, the objective should be measurable—either in terms of producing a numerical indicator of performance, such as time span, number of repetitions, distance covered, or accuracy of performance, or in terms of a precise description of the target motor behavior. The appropriate objective indicator must be carefully selected. Performing a movement more quickly may indicate that the individual is performing it with more normal control and therefore greater ease of movement, or it may indicate that the individual has become more skilled in using an abnormal pattern based on inappropriate muscle activation. If it is not appropriate to formulate the objective in terms of a numerical indicator, the objective can be formulated in terms of an observable behavior. The therapist can precisely describe body segment movements based on the component method of movement analysis presented by VanSant.[34] For example, the task of coming to standing from supine can be described in terms of the upper-extremity component, axial component, and lower-extremity component.[35] Formulation of an appropriate short-term objective could specify use of the upper extremities in a push-and-reach pattern during the task of coming to standing from supine. The interim objectives should be constructed so that observing the client's behavior will allow the therapist to state whether the criteria of the short-term objective were achieved. Table 26-1 gives an example of some components of short-term objectives leading to mastery of functional activities in sitting.

The outcome statements define the client's destination. The interim objectives define the mileposts. The therapist then uses the asset list to design the intervention program, which is the vehicle to get the client to his or her destination. From the asset list, the therapist knows the intervention techniques that have the highest probability of success. Adopting this process simplifies the task of outlining the strategy for intervention.

As the therapist considers the appropriate outcomes and goals for the client, a decision must be made as to whether the format of the intervention will focus on a "training" approach or a "motor learning" approach. During the assessment process, if the therapist concludes that the individual's level of cognitive function precludes the development of insight into movement errors (both the detection and correction of an incorrect performance) or the ability to retain the insight over time, then the therapist should delineate the outcomes and intervention plan to accommodate this limitation. The "training" approach requires more structure and repetition of activities within that structure. If it is more appropriate to design the intervention plan according to motor learning considerations, the therapist must consider the appropriate schedule and environmental context for the practice, the type and schedule for the feedback provided,

TABLE 26-1 ■ EXAMPLES OF SHORT-TERM OBJECTIVES RELATING TO MASTERY OF FUNCTIONAL ACTIVITIES IN SITTING*

	CONDITION VARIABLES†	ACTIVITY	CRITERIA
1. When sitting on a mat	a. Using the upper extremities for support	The client will maintain the posture	For ________ seconds
2. When sitting on the edge of a mat table	b. Using one upper extremity for support		
	c. Without using the upper extremities for support		
3. When sitting in a chair	d. With the therapist displacing the position of the: pelvis, shoulders, head, lower extremities	The client will make postural adjustments of the head and trunk	Appropriate to the degree of displacement
	e. Leaning forward and returning to erect sitting	The client will bring the right foot to the left knee (as if to put on a shoe)	

*Outcome: The client will master functional activities in sitting. Short-term objective: Select one phrase from each column.

†Therapist needs to consider all aspects of each variable (i.e., 1—a, b, c, d, e; 2—a, b, c, d, e; 3—a, b, c, d, e).

and techniques to promote the generalization of the learning beyond the specific practice session.

General Goals for the Intervention Process

Whereas the goal-setting process described earlier results in specification of the outcomes, goals, and objectives for a specific client, the general goals for the intervention process can be delineated to guide the process. As described in the overview of inflammatory disorders at the beginning of this chapter, the extent of the neurological sequelae may range from a single discrete problem to a devastating clinical picture composed of compromised functions in multiple areas. The goals for the intervention process address the problem areas that (1) jeopardize the efficiency and effectiveness of functional activities and (2) are the primary or secondary results of compromised neurological function. The listing of goals does not directly include consideration of secondary problems (such as decreases in joint range of motion [ROM], cardiovascular fitness, and endurance). The therapist should integrate these considerations in the overall assessment of the components of the movement problems.

The following goals are written as outcomes of the intervention process and not as goals for a specific client. Because of the broad nature of the goals, other professions also will contribute to the attainment of the goals. The goals of the therapeutic intervention program for clients with inflammatory CNS disorders are as follows:

Goal 1: Postural control is optimized as demonstrated by the ability to maintain a position against gravity and the ability to automatically adjust before and continuously during movement.

Goal 2: Selective, voluntary movement patterns within functional activities are optimized.

Goal 3: Performance of functional activities is enhanced.

Goal 4: Integration of sensory information is fostered.

Goal 5: Cognitive status and psychosocial responses are optimized.

Each of these goals is discussed in conjunction with the general therapeutic intervention procedures that can be used to achieve the goal.

GENERAL THERAPEUTIC INTERVENTION PROCEDURES IN RELATION TO INTERVENTION GOALS

■ *Postural control is optimized as demonstrated by the ability to maintain a position against gravity and the ability to adjust automatically before and continuously during movement.*

Because it is assumed that functional abilities are built on the base of the ability to control postures, the intervention goal of promoting optimal postural control underlies the ability to make selective, voluntary movement patterns (goal 2) and the performance of functional activities (goal 3). Optimization of a postural set includes the concepts of decreasing muscle activity that is too high to allow performance of movement sequences, augmenting activation that is too low to support the accomplishment of a movement sequence, and fostering proper timing of the postural responses. Intervention techniques to achieve this goal demand that the therapist constantly monitor the client's performance so that appropriate interventions are added when needed and continued only as long as they are needed.

Optimal postural control is defined by two elements. The client should have the ability to maintain a vertical orientation with regard to gravity and should be able to maintain balance in the presence of both internal and external perturbations. Automatic adjustments in the postural set should occur in anticipation of and continuously during movements (internal perturbations). Both elements should be performed with minimal physical or cognitive effort on the part of the client. Horak describes five components of normal postural control, including vertical orientation; anticipatory, reactive, sensory organization; and dynamic postural control for gait.[36] By looking at the subsets of postural control, interventions can be designed to specifically match the impairment (Table 26-2).

Verticality, or maintaining an upright posture, first requires the client to recognize the desired alignment. Augmenting internal feedback mechanisms with the use of mirrors, force plates, or scales or even using a flashlight attached to the client that shines on a target when he or she is vertical

TABLE 26-2 ■ INTERVENTIONS FOR POSTURAL CONTROL PROBLEMS

POSTURAL CONTROL PROBLEM	POSSIBLE INTERVENTIONS
Malalignment and verticality problems	Augment sensory feedback: ■ Mirror ■ Static force plate ■ Flashlight on target ■ Videotape ■ Align without vision and check (knowledge of results) ■ Stepping with eyes closed
Limits of stability perception problems	Computerized feedback of actual versus possible Weight shifting exercise with feedback and targets (somatosensory, visual, both) Surface orientation exercises (static, ankle sway, hip strategies)
Anticipatory control problems	Hold on and slow down (lessen the need for anticipatory control—substitution) Mental rehearsal (weight shift, then move) Practice limb movements where balance must be controlled (start slow and get faster) ■ Interactions with the environment with a static base of support, such as reaching up in a cupboard, opening a door, opening a drawer, lifting a suitcase, lifting a bag of groceries, wearing a backpack ■ Interactions with the environment with a dynamic base of support (stepping up a step, kicking a ball, stepping over an object, stepping around an object, changing the pitch of the surface—inclines) Practice rapid limb movements where balance must be controlled (opening a door, opening a drawer, lifting a briefcase, lifting a bag of groceries, lifting a suitcase, wearing a backpack). Practice order: ■ Practice the anticipatory postural adjustment ■ Practice the focal action while supported ■ Combine the anticipatory postural adjustment with the focal action unsupported (slow to fast) ■ Practice varying similar tasks (predictable to unpredictable) Example: After the patient is doing better on a lifting task involving one object, he or she can work to be successful with several objects of different weights; first cognitively solve what must change for achievement of success in lifting one object versus another; then much repetition of alternating one object versus another; and eventually, work with a variety of objects in a varied pattern.
Reactive postural control problems	Work to regain balance strategies (ankle, hip, and stepping) Remediate any biomechanical issues that affect use of balance strategies Begin with self-perturbation and progress to reacting to external perturbations Need to learn to match the magnitude and direction of perturbation Physioballs, T-stools, tilt boards, reaching, weight shifting
Sensory integration problems	If client is overreliant on vision, be sure to help patient with another strategy before you take vision away Surface orientation exercises (tuning into somatosensory feedback) ■ Textured surface ■ Textured surface + visual tracking ■ Textured surface with vision occluded Enhancing use of vestibular system: ■ Compliant surface with stationary visual target ■ Compliant surface + visual tracking ■ Compliant surface with moving visual background ■ Changing surface + head turns ■ Changing surface + head turns + moving visual background ■ Obstacle course with varying sensory demands
Dynamic balance problems in gait	Alter the sensory contexts (e.g., resisted walking) Walking and reading signs right and left Carrying objects and looking at items carried Walking with quick stops (predictable distances and reactive) Practice falling without injury and getting up; practice slips and trips Walking and negotiating obstacles (around and over) ■ Practice both around and over obstacles ■ Larger steps, standing on one foot, changing directions ■ Practice stopping quickly with feet in target ■ Practice shorter steps, on a slippery surface; braiding Gesturing while walking

can be effective. Manual skills such as positioning the client and using approximation to reinforce the position can be added to the treatment. Progression of intervention strategies can be done by having the client maintain the posture and then begin to manipulate objects with the extremities. Research suggests that the CNS is organized around tasks and not movement patterns. So, as the client is learning to maintain vertical and move in and out of the position, designing a task will likely give a better outcome. For example, Paul developed encephalitis, which left him with residual deficits in verticality. The simple task of keeping a book balanced on his head while sitting or walking gave him the type of feedback he needed without constant cues to "stand up straight" being the focus. Further progression involves teaching the client to move to his limits of stability and find vertical again.

Anticipatory postural control involves the postural preset, which positions the trunk to allow skilled use of the extremities without loss of balance. It requires the client to recognize the situation and the likely destabilizing force that will result, and posturally preset so destabilizing will not occur. The process requires memory and the ability to recognize the critical environmental and task cues. Interventions focus on practicing both the postural adjustment and the focal action before the two components are combined. Table 26-2 also has suggested interventions for reactive, sensory integrative, and dynamic balance in gait problems. Postural control is affected as well by biomechanical constraints, such as tonal abnormalities.

The client's ability to demonstrate optimal postural control may be restricted by the presence of hypertonicity or hypotonicity in various muscle groups. These states may be relatively static or may fluctuate with the demands of a particular situation. Inappropriately high levels of muscle activity may be present in a stereotypical muscle distribution in the extremities, whereas the activity of the trunk musculature may be too low to support an antigravity posture. The therapist must design the interventions creatively to meet the shifting responses of the demands of a particular activity.

Being cognizant that spasticity is a reaction to initial peripheral instability, the therapist must select treatment that deals with the fact that as spasticity is modified, weakness or hypotonicity may be present. Inappropriately high levels of activity in a muscle group or groups may limit the client's ability to demonstrate optimal postural control (and optimal selective movements as addressed in the second goal). The therapist can select intervention techniques that are mediated through any of the sensory channels functional for that client. The choice of which channel or combination of channels to use for the input is based on the therapist's initial and continuing evaluation of the client's response to specific types of sensory input.

The therapist must address the hypertonicity influencing postural control as a generalized problem before demanding selective voluntary activation of specific muscle groups. Vestibular input that is slow and rhythmical may promote a generalized relaxation of skeletal muscle activity. In some clients, the trunk remains "stiff" in movement sequences in which a segmental response between the upper and lower trunk should occur. Repetitions of rhythmical movements in side lying in which the therapist gently and progressively stretches the client's pelvis in one direction around the body axis while moving the shoulder girdle in the opposite direction and then reverses the movement may effectively alter the biomechanical and neurological contributions to the stiffness (Figure 26-7).

For some clients, changing the dynamics of a spastic extremity may permit the emergence of more optimal levels of postural control. The appropriately designed ankle-foot orthosis (AFO) may alter the individual's need to rigidly control the position of the pelvis to remain upright. Use of a soft webbing thumb loop to alter the resting position of the first metacarpal may change the overactivity of musculature throughout the upper extremity and allow appropriate adjustment of the shoulder girdle as part of postural responses.

If the client is sufficiently alert that attending to and understanding directions is a possibility, the therapist should direct the person to focus on the effects of the movement responses rather than focusing attention on the movement of the body.[37] As the person begins to appreciate the consequences of what is transpiring, he or she should be asked to assist in maintaining the changes that promote the more skillful movement response. Unless otherwise indicated by the client's status, interventions must actively involve the individual in the process of planning, initiating, completing, and evaluating the movement. Although the therapist may manipulate the environment (internal and external) in which the response is made, the client must be an active participant for learning to occur.

Although some clients will demonstrate a pattern of generalized overactivity of the postural muscles of the trunk, many will have difficulty generating sufficient activity in the appropriate groups to sustain a posture or to permit movement in the posture. With generalized hypotonia, temporary improvement in postural responses may occur by providing vestibular input that is characterized by rapid and irregular changes. The labyrinths should be stimulated by quick stops and starts with changes in direction. The program should include the introduction of movements in all planes. Approximation can be effective in developing appropriate postural activity from a state of either hypertonicity or hypotonicity. Empirically, it seems that more force is applied to increase than to decrease the postural response. Approximation appears to elicit a response in all the muscles surrounding a joint in preparation for responding to the demands on the erect posture or the demands of weight bearing. Approximation lends itself to combination with other proprioceptive techniques, such as quick stretch or tapping. Although the changes

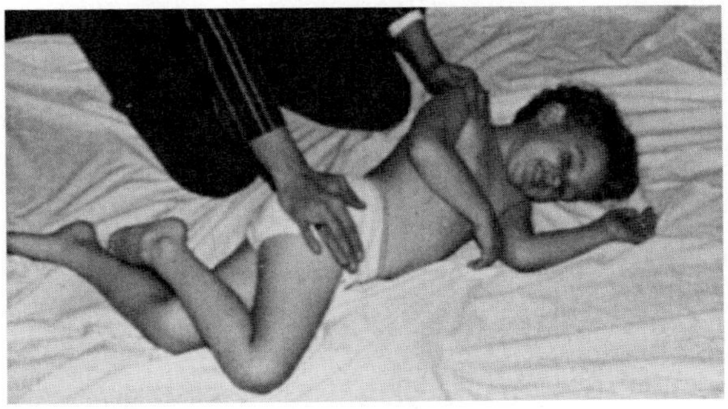

Figure 26-7 ■ Counterrotation of shoulder girdle backward (retraction) and the pelvis forward. Hand placement of therapist is important so that shoulder and hip movements can occur freely.

evoked by these techniques may be of short duration, the alterations can evoke movement components that would not otherwise occur and thereby provide the opportunity for the individual to learn from the movement. As the therapist applies various techniques in an attempt to elicit a specific response, the therapist must evaluate the desired response in relationship to the environmental context. If the client is sitting on the edge of a mat table, the activity of the trunk musculature will vary depending on whether the feet are flat on the floor, the client is engaged in an activity, the client is leaning on one arm for support, or the client is resting between activities. The client who slouches in sitting when fatigued, bored, or overwhelmed by the sensory input may present a different clinical picture when the appropriate factors are altered.

- *Selective, voluntary movement patterns within functional activities are optimized.*

The concept of the influence of the environment on the quality of a movement response, discussed in relation to the first goal of the intervention process, is also incorporated in the second goal. High-quality, selective, voluntary movement patterns are sought within the framework of functional activities, rather than as isolated and abstract movements. Optimization of the selective movement patterns may require a decrease in the stereotypical linkages of certain muscle groups, an increase in the ability to selectively activate certain muscle groups, the development of the ability to execute the movement in different postures, or a number of other variations.

Performance of functional activities requires that the individual have the capability of performing both mobility and stability patterns with the extremities. Mobility patterns are open kinetic chain movements in which the distal segment is free. These patterns are necessary for placing the extremities (e.g., swing phase of gait or reaching for a doorknob).

Clients who exhibit stereotypical posturing of the upper extremity with a restricted repertoire of available movement patterns require intervention to change the initial position of the extremity before movements are attempted. The influence of the spasticity that interferes with the repositioning of the extremity can be reduced by applying approximation through the long axis of the extremity. Preferably, the therapist's manual contacts for the application of the approximation force are on the weight-bearing surfaces of the hand. If the flexed position of the wrist prohibits application of the force to the heel of the palm, the approximation can be applied gradually through the fisted hand. As the resistance to passive movement diminishes, the wrist can be moved toward the neutral position so that the therapist can apply the approximation through the heel of the palm (Figure 26-8).

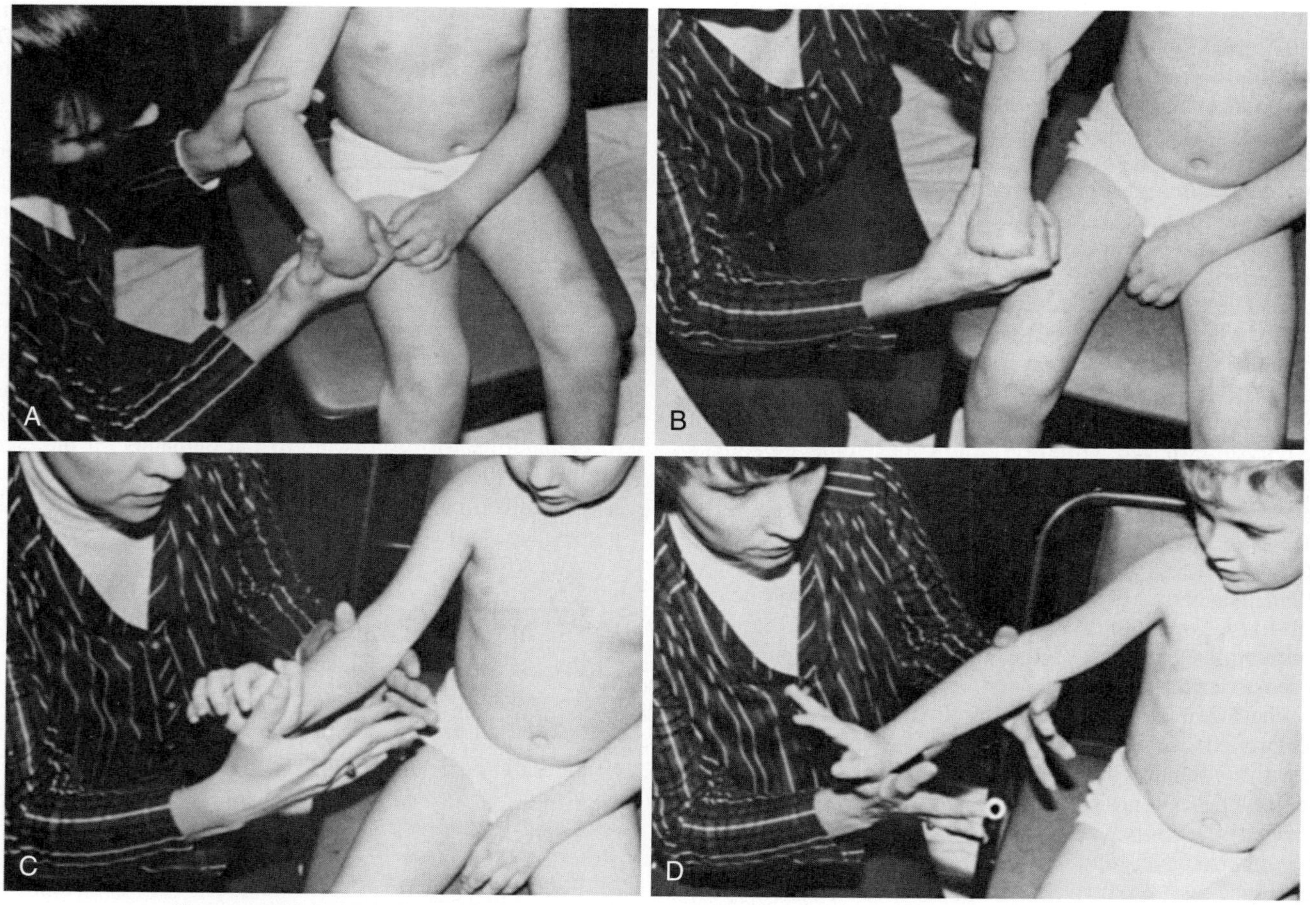

Figure 26-8 ■ Facilitating opening of the hand. **A,** Fisted hand; stretch to the extensors and approximation through hand, wrist, and elbow is applied. **B,** Approximation is continued; some resistance to the extensors may be applied. **C,** Approximation is applied to thenar eminence to further facilitate extensor tone. **D,** Full extension is achieved; approximation is maintained.

The therapist is moving the extremity toward an alternative resting position so that a new movement sequence can be attempted. It is important to use an intervention technique, such as approximation, to reduce the level of spasticity before passive movement is attempted so that a more appropriate position can be assumed without inappropriately stretching the spastic muscles.

The client is asked to assist the therapist with the movement, with the person being cued to do so with a minimum of effort. Too often, clients attempt to make a selective movement through a massive effort and overactivation of the muscle groups, which compounds the underlying spasticity. Clients should be encouraged to make easy, effortless movements—those they are instructed to perform with reduced effort so that they can relearn selective activation of motor units rather than mass firing patterns. Working "harder" often creates additional impairments versus increasing normal functional movement responses. It is critical that the movements requested relate to a functional activity or skill. Research suggests that skilled movements require attention and therefore motivation. Shaping the activity to both interest the client and afford some level of success is important.[33]

Electrical stimulation can be used as an adjunct to facilitate performance of a particular component of a mobility pattern. The wrist extension component of the proprioceptive neuromuscular facilitation (PNF) pattern of flexion, abduction, and external rotation can be reinforced by using a portable electrical stimulation unit with adjustable surge duration. The electrical stimulation elicits the correct movement so that the client could learn from the feel of the correct pattern. Adjusting the practice schedule so that the pattern is performed with and without the electrical stimulation support of the movement avoids the potential problem of reliance on the device to produce the movement. Electromyographic biofeedback can be a useful adjunct to achieve activation of specific muscle groups or to guide the client's attempts to reduce the level of activity of a muscle group.

Mobility patterns in the upper extremity have as their foundation the freedom of the scapula to adjust appropriately to the position of the humerus. The mobility of the scapula can be addressed through techniques that result in a general decrease in muscle activity and diagonal movement patterns of the scapula. The scapular stabilizers, such as the rhomboids, trapezius, and serratus anterior, must be capable of allowing appropriate adjustment of the scapula, as well as providing the fixation base on which humeral elevation can occur.

In stability patterns, the distal segment of the extremity is fixed (closed kinetic chain). These patterns are used in the weight-bearing components of the functional activities, such as the stance phase of gait or creeping. The components of the stability patterns are enhanced by proprioceptive input, such as approximation. During the performance of both stability and mobility patterns, the therapist should control the situation so that the client learns the appropriate movement patterns and not those imposed on top of inappropriate muscle activation.

Performance of movement patterns should progress toward an ability to easily reverse the direction of the movement. This can be promoted by incorporating rhythmical movements within a posture or between postures as early as possible in the intervention sequence. The end point at which the reversal is required should vary. In preparation for mastering the movements required to move from supine to sitting on the edge of the mat table, the client might be asked to move from the supine position to side sitting and back to supine; then the client could move from the supine position to side lying propped on one elbow (the halfway point in the overall movement), then reverse to supine. Incorporating reversal of movement patterns within the intervention program prepares the client to deal with situations that mandate unexpected adjustments in the movement sequence.

Clients who demonstrate problems with the sequencing of movements, such as those with motor dyspraxia, frequently perform better if the movement is performed at a speed that is close to normal. Clients who had normal movement sequences before the brain infection seem to be able to trigger better movement responses at normal speeds than at slower speeds. The slower movement speeds appear to disrupt the typical flow of the movement. In working with clients with sequencing problems, all team members should provide the same, consistent sensory cues to elicit a movement pattern. For example, the therapist may establish a coupling of the verbal cue "roll" with a quick stretch to the ankle dorsiflexors to elicit a rolling pattern. These same cues can be used by other team members to assist the client in changing positions in bed or in performing dressing activities. The consistency of cues may elicit a consistent response from the client. Once the pattern is well established, the intervention program can be designed to reduce the cues progressing toward the ability of the client to perform the activity in response to the demands of the situation rather than to externally imposed cues.

The flow of a movement pattern may be disrupted by problems categorized as incoordination. The origin of the coordination problems could be dysfunction of the visual-perceptual system (see Chapter 28) or vestibular system (see Chapter 22), dyspraxia (see Chapter 14), or dysfunction caused by cerebellar damage (see Chapter 21). If possible, the factors involved in producing a lack of coordination should be identified.

■ *Performance of functional activities is enhanced.*

As the client develops more appropriate postural control and the ability to perform selective movement patterns within functional activities, she or he is developing the basis to perform increasingly challenging functional activities. The movement patterns (and the postural control that underlies them) provide the building blocks for mastering an expanding variety of activities.

As the therapist designs the expansion of activities within the intervention program, the demands of each new functional activity and posture must be scrutinized. The client's ability to meet these demands was examined in the evaluation process. The intervention strategy must focus on the quality of the client's ability to assume a posture, maintain the posture, move within the posture (static and dynamic equilibrium responses to both self-generated and external perturbations), and move out of the posture. The therapist will change the sequence of this progression of activities to meet the needs of the client. The client may achieve independence in maintaining a posture while still requiring assistance in assuming the posture.

This progression should be grounded within the context of functionally relevant activities. Unless the individual has difficulty tolerating change, activities should be practiced within different environments to enhance generalization of learning. The creative therapist can design a variety of functionally relevant activities that require similar movement components.

With infants, the therapist may choose to use the developmental sequence as a general model for the functional activities progression. Progression through the developmental sequence should be viewed as a dynamic process so that the intervention incorporates movement both within and between postures. For individuals through the remainder of the life span, the focus should be on the age-appropriate functional activities essential to the individual's daily life, such as bed mobility, sitting to standing, standing to sitting, ambulation, reaching, and manipulation.

Examples of handling techniques that can be adapted to enhance the individual's progression through the sequence of functional activities can be found in the works of Bobath,[38] Carr and Shepherd,[39,40] Duncan and Badke,[41] Levitt,[42] Ryerson and Levit,[43] Sullivan and Markos,[44] and Voss and colleagues,[45] as well as throughout this book. These authors can provide the therapist with ideas for ways to enhance the client's performance within a specific activity.

■ *Integration of sensory information is fostered.*

At the same time that the therapist addresses the previous intervention goals, the goal of fostering integration of sensory input must be considered. Unless the therapist has advanced knowledge of sensory integration theories, this goal may be secondary rather than primary; nevertheless, it cannot be ignored.

The potential for an exaggerated and inappropriate response to sensory input was discussed as part of the clinical picture. Before the therapist expects the client to exhibit adaptive behavior to the potential bombardment of input from combinations of cutaneous, proprioceptive, auditory, and visual input, the therapist must assess the client's ability to respond to multisensory inputs. The ability to respond adaptively progresses from a response to a single sensory system input, to a response to the input in the presence of multiple system input, and then to an adaptive response based on inputs from two or more sources. The therapist must be sure that adding more sensory inputs augments an adaptive response rather than detracting from it. The client may respond to handling techniques that provide proprioceptive and cutaneous cues but may demonstrate a deterioration of performance when auditory input is added. When verbal cues are added, the therapist should follow the philosophy that verbal commands should be concise, sparse, and appropriately timed.[45]

All sensory inputs should evoke the correct response on the part of the client, rather than cause her or him to sift through the jumble of inputs to recognize the appropriate inputs to which a response should be made. At the highest level the client will demonstrate cross-modal learning in which input from one sensory system will evoke a response based on input previously obtained through a different system. Recognition of a comb by touch is based on the precept of "combness" usually obtained initially by visual input. If the therapist recognizes the hierarchy in the process of integrating sensory input, intervention situations that require too high a level of performance from the client can be avoided. The client who can respond adaptively to input from only one source would not be expected to perform in a crowded treatment area that presents extraneous visual and auditory input. The therapist will also recognize the need to include in the intervention plan situations that involve the controlled introduction of sensory inputs so that the client progresses toward the ability to deal with multiple inputs. Carr and Shepherd[40] discuss some general principles that can be used during the training of motor tasks in the presence of somatosensory and perceptual-cognitive impairments.

Dysfunctions in perceptual integration are addressed as the client moves through functional sequence activities. Although these movement activities would not provide the total program for an individual with a specific perceptual integration dysfunction, goals in this area can be addressed if the therapist is aware of indications of dysfunctions. The therapist must critically observe the performance of a movement sequence to identify substitute actions to compensate for problems such as inability to cross the midline. The therapist must then attempt to redesign the demands of the situation to elicit the desired behavior. The client who moves from the supine to the side sitting to the long sitting positions without the upper extremities crossing the midline could be required to side sit to the left and transfer objects with the right hand from the left side of the body to the right side (Figure 26-9).

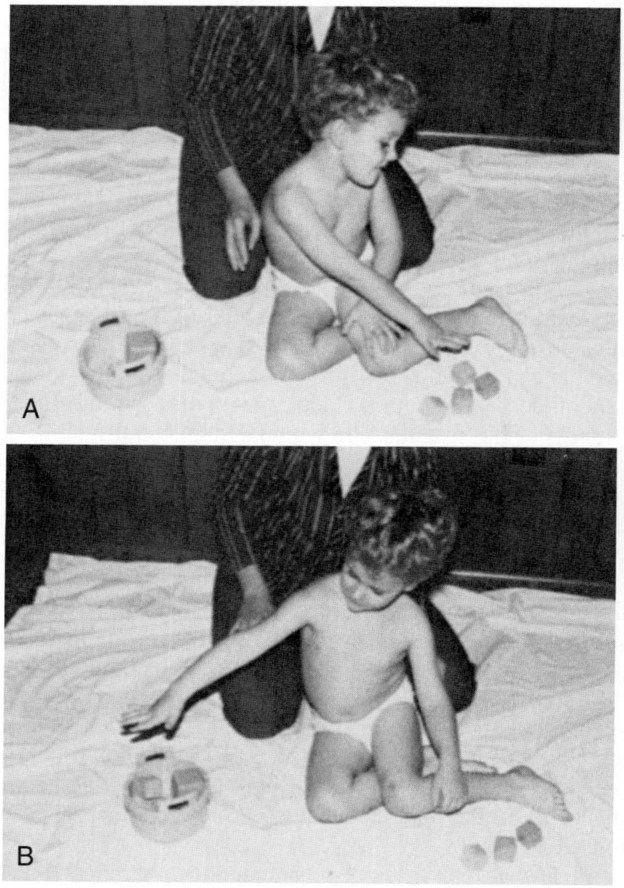

Figure 26-9 ■ Child crossing midline of body when transferring objects from left to right. **A,** Beginning act on contralateral side. **B,** Ending sequence by crossing midline and placing objects on ipsilateral side.

The therapist must determine whether the client is truly crossing the midline or rotating the midline of the body to continue to avoid crossing it.

Therapists may be most aware of disturbances in the client's ability to integrate sensory information into an appropriate response when this dysfunction disrupts balance. The ability to maintain and move in upright postures requires successful processing of information from the sensory triad of postural control: the visual, vestibular, and somatosensory systems. When one component is missing, unreliable, or discrepant with the other two, the person is at risk for loss of balance. During the ongoing evaluation process, the therapist gathers information on the integrity of each system and any evidence of central processing difficulties. Incorporated within the practice of activities to develop postural control, to promote selective movements with functional activities, and to develop mastery of increasingly difficult functional activities is the simultaneous practice of integrating sensory information so that a successful response can be generated.

Clients who are performing at higher levels can be challenged to maintain balance when one element of the sensory triad is missing (e.g., vision occluded) or altered (e.g., sitting, standing, or walking on a soft, compliant surface). Successful maintenance of balance outside the protective environment of the therapy clinic requires the ability to switch the primary information source to any one of the three systems. Walking in the dark requires the person to rely on vestibular and somatosensory input. Standing on a moving bus looking out a window requires resolution of the conflict between visual input (the external world is moving), vestibular input (you are moving), and somatosensory input (you are stationary). Movement experiences within the therapy program should foster practice of this sensory integration process (see Table 26-2).

■ *Cognitive status and psychosocial responses are optimized.*

In addition to attending to the factors directly related to motor performance, the therapist also must attend to the client's psychosocial and cognitive responses. Although the therapist does not have primary responsibility in this area, a goal of the intervention process should be to enhance the individual's psychosocial and cognitive responses.

Particularly in the agitated state that may be a component of the response to the inflammatory process, the client may demonstrate exaggerated and inappropriate emotional responses to events. Dealing with these emotional fluctuations can become a major determinant in goal attainment in the other areas. Maintaining a positive, nonthreatening interaction allows the client to use the therapist as a reference for judging the appropriateness of emotional responses.

If the client's state of agitation is interfering with the intervention program, the therapist may alter the program to include techniques that have a calming effect. For example, the individual can be wrapped in a cotton sheet blanket and rocked in a slow, rhythmical, repetitive manner to decrease agitation. Auditory and visual input should be controlled to avoid overloading sensory processing mechanisms.

Earlier in this text the psychosocial adjustment that occurs in the process of recovering from a neurological disability was discussed. The therapist must be aware of how the client's regression in affective and cognitive domains affects the intervention process. The therapist should seek assistance from the health care team members responsible for intervention in these areas to deal with the client constructively. The therapist must remember that both the family members and the client are in the process of adjusting to the client's changed and, it is hoped, changing status. Family members may be an asset or a liability to the client's recovery process. During the therapist's interactions with the family members in activities such as instructions in the client's home program, the therapist should be prepared to deal with expressions of the individual's difficulty in adjusting to the situation. The therapist also should be prepared to assist family members in identifying appropriate sources to help them deal with their problems.

Changes in mentation, perception of events, and memory losses present challenges to both the client and the therapist. Repetition in the recounting of past events may help reorder past knowledge. Use of brief verbal or visual cues may assist the client in recalling safety instructions or the components of the exercise program. The therapist should try to generate a nonstressful environment when working on these deficits so that attention and recall are not overshadowed by emotional pressure. As the therapist works with the client on an intervention program, situations arise that require problem solving to determine a way to accomplish a task. If the task is to accomplish an independent transfer from a wheelchair into a bathtub, decisions must be made concerning the sequence of movements. Therapists can approach this situation in two ways. They can instruct clients step by step in what to do, or they can involve clients to the extent possible in the process of deciding what to do. If the therapist instructs the client step by step, the client may master the task but may not be able to perform it under different conditions. If the therapist involves the client in the decision-making process, the client may be learning not only how to accomplish the specific task, but also how to accomplish the task under varied conditions. The intervention process should lead to the ability to respond to the demands of a situation, and involvement of clients in the problem-solving process helps prepare them for independence. The therapist must structure the client's role in decision making to the level of the client's ability to participate so that the experience is not frustrating. Although the client's participation may initially increase the time required to complete a task, it promotes skills that may lead more quickly to independence of function.

INTERACTION WITH OTHER PROFESSIONALS

The therapist needs to design an intervention program that is articulated with that of other members of the health care team. The recovery process of the client should be facilitated by a care plan in which each team member reinforces the goals of the other team members. The care of the person must be a collaborative effort. Each client deserves an intervention process that considers him or her as a whole person, not as a set of fragmented problems.

SUMMARY

This chapter has presented a brief discussion of the pathology and medical management of various inflammatory processes that affect the brain. The process of assessment, the role of assessment in designing an intervention program, the goals of the intervention process, and the means to meet those goals were presented to assist the reader in more effective management of clients with these diagnoses.

Although the problem-solving process presented in this chapter for assessment, prognosis, goal identification, and treatment planning is not limited to clients with inflammatory supraspinal disorders, its application in the presence of typical neurological sequelae has been described. When dealing with inflammatory disorders of the brain, the variability of neurological sequelae is examined based on the anatomical location of the inflammatory process and the cause of the infection.

Although the neurological disorders discussed in this chapter are life-threatening, many clients recover and return to their previous lifestyles. Clients will vary within the spectrum of minimal to severe involvement and from specific to generalized CNS dysfunction and will demonstrate little to full recovery after the acute distress. Prognosis for recovery depends on the type of infecting organism and the extent of involvement. The therapist must remain flexible and willing to adjust every aspect of therapeutic intervention to meet the specific needs of each client. Yet the therapist must also remember that learning requires active participation on the part of the client.

CASE STUDY 26-1

A 74-year-old client with cryptococcal *(Cryptococcus gattii)* meningitis was seen in the outpatient setting 1½ years after onset with residual complaints of constant dizziness, imbalance, and need for assistance with mobility tasks.

HISTORY OF PRESENT ILLNESS

Client manifested dementia and overt meningitis 1½ years prior. He was treated with liposomal amphotericin B + 5FC for 3 weeks and then put on fluconazole. He was transferred to a skilled nursing facility with dementia and need for significant assistance for all ADLs. His cognition and functional status continued to diminish over the next 3 months, when it was determined he had hydrocephalus, and a VP shunt was placed. This resulted in significant improvement in mentation and function, and he was discharged home with home care 3 months later.

PAST MEDICAL HISTORY

The past medical history included profound bilateral sensorineural hearing loss postmeningitis, chronic obstructive pulmonary disease (COPD), and possible Parkinson-like symptoms.

SUMMARY OF KEY FINDINGS

The client was alert and oriented to person, place, time, and reason for referral. He had some short-term memory loss. He lived with his wife in a single-story home. He was walking with a two-wheeled walker with standby assistance as his primary mode of mobility. He had difficulty with steadiness during transfers and when turning. He complained of constant dizziness, which he described as a sense of movement and at times spins. All movements worsened the symptoms, and being still decreased the symptoms.

Vision screen was normal, but he complained of increased dizziness with eye movement. Vestibular ocular testing findings were abnormal; client had a positive head-thrust test result bilaterally, and abnormal DVA with head movements at 2 Hz. Light touch and proprioception were intact for both legs. The accompanying table presents a summary of objective findings.

	FTSST	Strength	Berg	SOT	Ambulation	DVA (2 Hz)
Initial	18.73 s	LE 5/5 except hip extensor 4/5 and PF 2/5 bilaterally	38/56	28% (fell 9/18 trials—all sway referenced support)	Two-wheeled walker with SBA	20/200
1 month	15.12 s	Not tested	55/56	Not tested	Two-wheeled walker independent	20/125
2 months	Not tested	LE 5/5 except PF 4/5	Not tested	39% (fell 6/18 trials—conditions 5 and 6) Use of vision significantly improved from 0% to 55%	Single-point cane	20/80 horz
3 months	15 s	Not tested	55/56	Not tested	Single-point cane	20/63−2* at 2 Hz (horz); 20/80 (vert)
4 months	12.1	LE 5/5 with PF 4/5	Not tested	56% (fell 4/18 trials – first 2 attempts conditions 5 and 6)	No device on level surfaces, cane on uneven surfaces	20/50
5 months	51 s	Hip abductor 4/5 and ankle PF 2+/5	34/56	Fell conditions 3 and 4 of M-CTSIB in <5 s	Two-wheeled walker	20/100
10 months	16.9 s	LE 5/5 except PF only 2+/5	52/56	Only falls condition 4 of M-CTSIB	Single-point cane all surfaces	20/125

* The patient read the line with two errors.

DVA, Dynamic visual acuity test; *FTSST,* five-times-sit-to-stand test; *LE,* lower extremity; *horz,* horizontal; *M-CTSIB,* Modified Clinical Test of Sensory Interaction and Balance; *PF,* plantarflexors; *SBA,* standby assist; *SOT,* Sensory Organization Test; *vert,* vertical.

CASE STUDY 26-1—cont'd

PHYSICAL THERAPY MOVEMENT DIAGNOSIS

The client had an increased risk of falls, with significant balance impairment and gaze instability consistent with mixed peripheral (bilateral hypofunction) and central vestibular dysfunction postmeningitis (Physical Therapy Practice Patterns 5D and 5A). He also had lower extremity weakness and reduced vertical orientation. His strengths included supportive family and excellent motivation.

GOALS

1. Client will be able to ambulate independently in his home without assistive device (4 months).
2. Client will improve gaze stability to 20/80 with head movements at 2 Hz in either direction (4 months).
3. Client will be independent and safe to negotiate a flight of stairs with rail (2 months).
4. Client will be able to maintain standing with eyes open on foam surface >30 seconds (2 months).

INTERVENTIONS

The client lived 2 hours from the clinic, so many of the interventions were through progressive home exercises. Client was seen one or two times each month, and the program consisted of balance retraining, gaze stability exercises (vestibuloocular reflex [VOR] retraining beginning in sitting, plain background), lower-extremity strengthening, endurance activities, and gait training. Given the patient's hearing loss and memory deficits, teaching included demonstration, written instructions, and instruction of the client's wife. The client progressed steadily the first 4 months, then he began not feeling well. He complained of increased nausea and trouble eating and had a slow decline in mentation. At the 5-month visit, the client's condition had declined significantly, and after discussion with the client's physician, he underwent a series of tests which concluded that the patient was having intermittent shunt malfunction. After the shunt revision, the client did improve as noted at the 10-month follow-up visit.

KEY TAKE HOME POINTS

1. It is not unusual to have both cranial nerve and CNS involvement with meningitis.
2. Remember to monitor for signs of shunt malfunction, and the importance of educating the client and family members.
3. Use standardized objective measures in case management.

Acknowledgment

I would like to thanks Dr. Rebecca Porter, PhD, PT, for her contributions to the first four editions of this book. She not only has made a significant contribution through her publications and this chapter in the book but also is an inspiration to many of us within the profession of Physical Therapy.

Reference

To enhance this text and add value for the reader, all references are included on the companion Evolve site that accompanies this textbook. This online service will, when available, provide a link for the reader to a Medline abstract for the article cited. There are 45 cited references and other general references for this chapter, with the majority of those articles being evidence-based citations.

CHAPTER 27 Aging, Dementia, and Disorders of Cognition

OSA JACKSON SCHULTE, PT, PhD, GCFP/AT,
JAMES STEPHENS, PT, PhD, CFP, and JOYCE ANN, OTR/L, GCFP

KEY TERMS

aging
Alzheimer disease
caregiver training and support
dementia and delirium
function
physical and occupational therapy examination and intervention
problem solving
rehabilitation
therapeutic environment

OBJECTIVES

After reading this chapter the student or therapist will be able to:

1. Define the basic terminology and discuss the prevalence of cognitive disturbances seen in older persons.
2. Describe normative changes in brain function with normal aging and their relevance to the diagnoses of delirium and dementias.
3. Discuss how symptoms are altered with normal aging (specifically related to the Arndt-Schultz principle, law of initial values, and habitual biorhythms) for an individual.
4. Describe normal sensory changes with aging and how they alter a person's overall ability to adapt to stress.
5. Describe how, and for what type of patient, to use the Mini-Mental State Examination as a part of the physical or occupational therapy examination.
6. Describe common sensory changes with dementia and implications for adapting physical or occupational therapy evaluation and intervention.
7. Discuss common changes in learning styles with aging and implications for adapting physical or occupational therapy intervention to enhance patients' ability to perform at their highest functional level.
8. Describe how environmental design and ergonomics can enhance patient performance in activities of daily living and instrumental activities of daily living.
9. Describe a strategy to evaluate a patient's emotional capacity to participate in a learning task and its clinical relevance to both occupational and physical therapy outcomes.
10. Describe criteria for delirium and reversible dementia and sample strategies for modifying evaluation and treatment procedures.
11. Discuss symptoms and disease progression in irreversible dementia.
12. Discuss the therapist's role on the treatment team in educating key caregivers and support personnel and sample training strategies.
13. Discuss treatment skills that are helpful in working with persons who have irreversible dementia.
14. Describe research activities and new findings that affect physical evaluation and treatment of the patient with dementia or delirium.

THE STARTING POINT WITH OLDER PERSONS IN PHYSICAL OR OCCUPATIONAL THERAPY

Older persons can adapt to new physical problems. It is critical to use the processes of habilitation and rehabilitation to train caregivers (family, friends, or staff) to bring out the best functional performance in the older person. The health care staff, caregivers, family, and friends relating to the older person in a time of crisis need to prioritize creating a sense of safety, acceptance, and support based on the patients' preferences and habits. The specifics in this process include the following:

1. Evaluate, document, and make available to the hands-on caregivers what the patient "likes"—his or her preferences and habits for all activities of daily living (ADLs) and instrumental activities of daily living (IADLs).
2. Train caregivers to create a care plan for daily living and nursing that builds in the patients' preferences to support his or her personal identity and self-image.
3. Create specific physical therapy or occupational therapy functional goals that build on and reinforce patient preferences with regard to mobility, eating, bathing, grooming, dressing, socialization, and so on. (Note: If caregivers change, training needs to be added and new goals may need to be developed because not all caregivers have the same capacity to relate to the patient.)
4. Train caregivers with the older person to use specific neurofacilitation strategies to: (a) enhance breathing, (b) increase bed mobility, (c) improve balance in sitting

and standing, (d) perform active range of motion (AROM) and active assisted range of motion (AAROM) for ADLs and IADLs, (e) achieve skeletal weight shift for ADLs and IADLs, (f) encourage head, neck, and spine to upright postural response during ADLs and IADLs, and (g) encourage walking and stair climbing safely and as able.
5. Screen for signs of reversible cognitive losses.
6. Provide adaptations and training for performance of ADLs when chronic cognitive problems exist.
7. Train caregivers and the older person in ways to adapt the ADLs and IADLs to maximize ability.

PARADIGM FOR AGING, THE BRAIN, AND LEARNING

Life involves ongoing learning. The brain and human nervous system have at least 3×10^{10} parts. As Feldenkrais stated, "This is large enough for its balanced functions to obey the law of large systems. The health of such a system can be measured by the shock (stimuli) it can take without compromising the continuation of its processes."[1] Adaptability and health can be measured by the number of stimuli or amount of shock people can tolerate without their usual way of life being compromised. Aging is a process that requires ongoing adaptation to and compensation for the losses that are imposed on human beings from the *outside* world and the internal physiological changes that occur with the passage of time, physical activities, emotional state, fatigue, digestive and elimination processes, and habitual rest-activity cycle. If a person's health is altered by illness or trauma, then he or she goes through an adaptive process. If too many changes happen too quickly, the brain is not able to create a functional adaptive response, and the individual must alter or simplify her or his life processes or face negative mental or physiological reactions. The literature demonstrates that regression periods and illness seem to be linked.[2-5] As human beings explore coping with unfamiliar experiences, they require more nurturing, rest, and physical contact that is perceived as empowering.

Human beings progress to adulthood through the millions of perceptions and choices that are recorded and responded to through the developmental years. Human beings are not born with the brain and nervous system having the skills of an adult. In infancy the brain begins to learn during interactions with the environment. The kinesthetic and sensory connections provide data about the internal and external environments. Through this interactive learning process each human being (with a nondifferentiated nervous system) discovers new differentiations and thus new strategies for relating to the world. With advancing age there is a gradual decrease in the acuity of the kinesthetic and sensory information received. These changes can affect interactive learning for the older adult.[6-8] Active participation has a positive impact on recall and learning,[9] predictable events support recall,[10] and ordered events are easier to recall. Differentiation for human beings does not happen uniformly.[11,12] As a person grows, the result of this lack of uniformity is that some adults prefer to relate to the world visually, others aurally, and still others by touch or kinesthetically. In other words, people specialize with their sensory processing and at the same time become more vulnerable to issues of sensory adaptation and selection.[13]

The adult phase of brain and central nervous system development will, for most people, involve a gradual narrowing of the focus in the development of new skills as well as increased repetition of certain activities. The tendency is to have activity narrow more and more to the activities in which a person excels or feels comfortable. Intuitive or practical people continue to pursue self-knowledge and explore ways to maximize their talents. By accident or through mentoring, these people discover that lifelong learning is the gift of life itself. Ongoing and ever-increasing self-awareness allows for enhanced adaptability at any age.

What if rehabilitation after illness or trauma invited a guided examination of self-awareness and habitual strategies as the basis for inventing new functional adaptive strategies? The Feldenkrais Method is one model for neurological facilitation and enhancement of human learning and adaptability that is built on the concept of starting from the current habits of action of the person.[1,14,15] The Feldenkrais Method also uses several other basic learning strategies that make this approach helpful for the older patient: going slowly, simplifying the movement or stimuli, proceeding from the perception of the patient, learning to detect and respond to the smallest possible input, and increasing the awareness and use of the skeleton and the support it gives. Feldenkrais noted what a person automatically did during a crisis, such as a fall. He noted the automatic human response and then built in a self-defense response that took advantage of the innate reflex.[16] The result is that exploratory learning is easy for the patient because it builds on the automatic response with which the person is already familiar. The goal is to invent physical therapy interventions that encourage patient participation and that feel safe and useful to the patient.

In this chapter the paradigm for aging and lifelong learning presumes the following:

1. The brain and central nervous system are viewed as the master system and the controller of the other human systems (e.g., digestive, cardiovascular, muscular, hormonal).
2. Capacity exists for ongoing learning (self-awareness), self-regulation, and adaptability through the life span.
3. The whole (human being) is greater than the sum of its parts.
4. Language shapes reality and the experience and perceptions of life.
5. Enjoying a comfortable and easy pace for new learning is beneficial. Being able to learn new skills is important for adaptability and for lifelong well-being.
6. The mind and body are not separate.
7. Personal variations in learning style and preferences for relating can be used to maximize adaptation throughout life.
8. The activation of the limbic system for "fight or flight" is normal, and the ability to release the limbic activation and find the resting state when the crisis (real or imagined) is over becomes a critical skill for adapting as people grow older.[17]
9. Creation of environments that encourage safe exploration of new ideas and ways of self-expression can generate lifelong human growth and development.

FRAMEWORK FOR CLINICAL PROBLEM SOLVING

Therapists working with patients with cognitive impairments need to have received adequate advanced training in assessment of communication skills and neurological functioning as well as gerontology so they can work with maximal efficacy and enjoy the clinical interactions with each patient. In 37 BC the Roman poet Virgil wrote, "Age carries all things, even the mind, away."[18] Nearly 400 years ago, Shakespeare described the last stage of human life as "second childishness and mere oblivion, sans teeth, sans eyes, sans taste, sans everything."[19] This pessimistic view of the fate of the elderly persists among health care workers today despite the fact that significant cognitive deficits affect only 6.1% to 12.3% of the elderly (people older than age 65 years) in the United States.[20,21]

The clinician should not assume that an older person has impaired cognitive functioning. Perhaps the most crucial concept for clinical problem solving is that the clinician must not assume that the current abilities reflect the true capacity of the person. When a patient is observed to have altered brain function, description of the extent and type of the distortion of intellectual capacity and determination of the time of onset (sudden or gradual) are necessary to enable a diagnosis and the provision of appropriate and effective treatment and care. The capacity to learn is a possibility, although the process of learning may be altered or different from that of unaffected older adults.[22-25] When age, illness, or medications create a temporary or permanent change in cognitive abilities, all functional training requires alteration to meet the unique cognitive abilities of the patient at the moment. For example, the son of a patient who needed physical and occupational therapy showed staff how to communicate with his mother so she did not get scared. The therapist walked slowly into the room and greeted the patient by touching her softly on the cheek with the back of her hand. The patient looked up and smiled. The therapist smiled back and stroked the patient softly on the top of her head. The patient smiled again. The therapist kneeled down so that she was eye to eye with the patient sitting in the wheelchair. She took the patient's hand in her own hand and with her other hand slowly stroked the back of the patient's hand. The patient smiled again. The therapy session had begun. For this patient, words were actually confusing so they were avoided.[26] The need for tactile nurturing input stays and persists as people age.[27] Nurturing tactile input done at a pace that is pleasant for the patient can actually support a positive clinical outcome.[28]

Definition of Terms

Intellectual impairment falls into three categories: mental retardation, delirium, and dementia. A definition of terms is necessary to ensure that all personnel use the same framework for clinical problem solving.

1. *Mental retardation:* A person with mental retardation (also called *developmental disability*) has had some degree of intellectual impairment all her or his life. A person with mental retardation also can develop delirium or dementia. Delirium or dementia differs from mental retardation in that a change from the baseline level of functioning has occurred in that person.
2. *Delirium:* A person with delirium usually shows a change both in intellectual function and in level of consciousness.[29,30] The patient may be perplexed, disoriented, fearful, forgetful, or all of these. The patient is often less alert than normal and may be sleepy or obtunded; however, many patients with delirium are hypervigilant and may be extremely agitated and suspicious. Delirium frequently occurs in the presence of a concurrent dementia. Early identification of the symptoms and formal medical assessment and treatment are critical to ensure the return of a normal level of alertness and intellectual function and to prevent the development of secondary functional impairments and possible dementia.[31]
3. *Dementia:* Dementia is the impairment of some or all aspects of intellectual functioning in a person who is fully alert. Some diseases that can cause dementia are treatable, and if treated early and aggressively, the patient's deterioration of intellectual function may be either reversed or halted. Dementia usually involves cognitive impairment affecting memory and orientation and at least one of the following[32,33]:
   - Abstract thinking. This is a common loss and involves an altered ability to relate to anything other than tangible reality. In dementia or Alzheimer disease (AD), this skill is predictably missing in most cases. This is exacerbated by fear and anxiety.
   - Judgment and problem solving. This capacity decreases in the first stage of AD and is missing by the second stage.[34-36]
   - Language. Use of language for communication becomes altered in the second stage of AD, and by the third stage little verbal or no verbal communication is possible.[37]
   - Personality. A complex of all the attributes—behavioral, temperamental, emotional, and mental—that characterize a unique individual. A person makes choices that, whether remembered or not, make up his or her personality. Human beings live through these choices, which become filters for all future life experiences, and they believe that they are the truth. Caregivers and therapists must be aware of how the world is perceived by the patient. The staff must respect patients and their beliefs and work to minimize confrontation and agitation despite a person's beliefs, prejudices, and biases.
4. *Alzheimer disease:* This is not synonymous with dementia but rather is one of the many causes of dementia. The term should be used only as a diagnosis when a complete clinical evaluation has been performed, a diagnosis of dementia has been made, and all other possible causes of the dementia have been ruled out. Definitive diagnosis of this disease is not possible until an autopsy or brain biopsy has been performed. Although multiple putative causes of the disease have been proposed, the cause and pathogenesis are unknown. No curative treatment for AD is currently available. Some drugs appear to slow the process of cognitive deterioration in some patients, and patients and their families can be helped through rehabilitation to cope better with the vicissitudes of the disease (see Chapters 6 and 36).

Psychiatric problems may be present before old age or may develop as a result of dementia and need to be assessed and treated along with the dementia. Depression, for example, can mimic dementia.

Epidemiology

Currently 5.3 million Americans are estimated to have AD. One in eight people over the age of 65 has AD.[33] Researchers estimate that by 2050 13.2 million Americans will have AD if current trends continue and no cures are found.[38] Half the people aged 85 years and older will have some form of dementia (9.5 million in 2050).[39] Disorders causing cognitive deficits are expected to continue to be a growing public health problem for at least the next 50 years. The projected statistics, assuming no cures or effective means of preventing the common causes of dementia are discovered, are that by 2040 five times more individuals with dementia will be in society as today (7.4 million Americans). This increase is partially the result of the increased life expectancy of Americans.[40] The most rapid population growth in this country is in the oldest age group, hence the increase in the prevalence of severe dementia. The prevalence of dementia rises from approximately 3% at ages 65 to 74 years to 18.7% at ages 75 to 84 years and to 47% of those older than 85 years.[39] The increasing number of persons older than age 85 years will be paralleled by an increase in the incidence of dementia.

More than 70 conditions are known to cause dementia.[33] Secondary behavioral problems in the patient with dementia can be interpreted as a response to somatic, psychological, or existential stress. Because memory impairments, impairments of abstract thinking or judgment, or global cognitive impairments in an elderly person may be symptoms of acute physical illness, the patient's physical, emotional, social, and cognitive status and physical, social, and caregiver environment need to be systematically evaluated.[33]

Gradual or sudden changes in intellectual capacity or memory function are not a normal part of the aging process. Any change, whether it develops slowly over time or happens suddenly, should be diagnosed, and when possible the underlying cause(s) of the delirium or dementia should be treated. Even if the cause of the dementia is untreatable, teaching the patient and significant others strategies to make the patient's ADLs and IADLs easier to manage is always possible (see sample home program).

Physical and occupational therapists are an important part of the comprehensive evaluation, treatment, and caregiver training for patients with delirium or dementia. All treatment planning should occur as a part of a team effort in which the patient, the family or significant others, the physician, nurses, social worker, physical therapist, and occupational therapist collaborate so that a consistent treatment plan and orientation are followed. Inclusion of the day-to-day caregivers is crucial for all training because they most need to know and use the adaptations for the patient's personal style of communication and how to facilitate functional movement for ADLs and IADLs.

PHYSIOLOGY OF AGING: RELEVANCE FOR SYMPTOMATOLOGY AND DIAGNOSIS OF DELIRIUM AND DEMENTIAS

The Normal Brain

The brain of a normal person at age 80 years shows several significant anatomical, physiological, and neurochemical changes when compared with the brain of a younger person. Brain weight decreases with advancing age.[41] For example, the mean brain weight for women aged 21 to 40 years is 1260 g, whereas for women older than 80 years it is 1061 g.[42] Dickstein and colleagues[43] and Cabeza and colleagues[44] have noted that although the brain loses thousands of cells daily, the areas of the brain involved in language, memory, and cognition are relatively spared from significant loss of neurons. Normal age-related changes vary from person to person in degree and severity and can include the following:

- Disturbance in ability to register, retain, and recall certain recent experiences
- Slowed rate of learning new material[24]
- Slowed motor performance on tasks that require speed[24,45]
- Difficulties with fine motor coordination and balance[46-52]

A motivated, upbeat elderly person who is not undergoing emotional stress will show few negative changes in intellectual capacity and may actually demonstrate an increase in intellectual functioning over time.[19,53-55]

Because many of the variables that need to be considered as part of the clinical evaluation of the rehabilitation potential of the person with dementia are affected by both aging and disease, therapists working with the aged patient should be aware of these variables. The therapist explores ways to compensate for these changes; as a result, the patient will have a greater possibility of achieving her or his potential for self-care and contentment.

A slowing of the natural pace of movement is commonly noted in people older than 80 years. This slowdown is manifested in the brain as a slowing of resting electroencephalogram (EEG) rhythms. At age 60 years, the mean frequency of the occipital rhythm is 10.3 Hz; at age 80 years, the mean frequency is 8.7 Hz. The average change in EEG frequency is approximately 1 cps per decade during these years.[56] The speed of nerve conduction in the elderly can be 10% to 15% slower than in younger persons.[57-59] Because of these physiological changes, if the process and structure of evaluation and care of the healthy older person emphasize speed of execution or timed activities, older adults will appear less capable than they really are. The therapist may need more time when working with persons older than 70 years than is generally required with the younger adult.

For a person's brain to function effectively, it requires a delicate synchronization of a large number of variables. To maximize intellectual function, the brain must have the following:

- No genetic defects
- A constant supply of nutrients, neurotransmitters, and other neurochemicals from a personally suitable diet
- Functional daily elimination
- An unfailing supply of oxygen (implying appropriate blood count, collateral circulation, normal respiratory exchange and ruling out sleep apnea)
- Adequate cardiac output
- Fluid, rhythmic breathing that adapts to needed changes in posture and exertion of the activity
- Normal blood biochemistry, especially fluid and electrolytes; adequate fluid intake is critical, and dehydration can contribute to altered brain function
- Normal hepatic and renal function
- Freedom from noxious stimuli such as trauma, infection (including periodontal and gum disease), or toxins (including medications)

- Optimal levels of sensory stimulation and emotional stimulation balance
- Optimal levels of intellectual stimulation
- Adequate rest and sleep

The brain is the most physiologically active organ in the body. The brain represents only 2% of the total body weight, yet it consumes up to 20% of the oxygen and 65% of the glucose available in the circulation in the entire body.[18] The minimal cardiovascular output required to deliver this is 0.75 L/min, which is equal to 20% of the total circulation (also dependent on body size). Because of the high level of nutrient use by the brain, it is one of the organs of the body most likely to be affected by any acute change in homeostasis. The homeostasis of the elderly brain is more vulnerable to disruption because of the normal age-related changes already discussed, as well as the increased permeability of the blood-brain barrier and increased sensitivity of neurons to the effects of outside agents such as drugs,[60] junk food, allergies, and food sensitivities.

Arndt-Schultz Principle

The Arndt-Schultz principle summarizes the differences between the abilities of the younger brain and the aged brain to discriminate or respond to stimuli[61]:

1. The elderly require a higher level or a longer period of stimulation before the threshold for initial physiological response is reached. A related safety issue is that heat takes longer to be perceived, so the elderly are more likely to get a severe burn.
2. The physiological response in the aged is rarely as large, as visible, or as consistent as noted in younger people. In response to a heat pack, for example, the elderly skin may not turn bright red in response—the skin may turn white instead. When fever is present, they may not feel warm to the touch but instead may be very tired or clumsy.
3. The only similarity between the responses of the young and the elderly to stimuli is that once the threshold has been reached, then more stimuli result in an increase in response.
4. On average, the range of safe therapeutic stimulation is narrower for the elderly than for the young.

The implication of the Arndt-Schultz principle for clinical problem solving is that the level of a stimulus (e.g., heat, cold, sound, light, or emotional input) needs to be adjusted to compensate for the altered physiology of the aging patient. Optimal balance of the levels of sensory stimulation and emotional stimulation that is therapeutic for a young person may not be therapeutic for the older person. The stimulus may be too low so it does not reach the threshold for generating a physiological response, or it may go beyond the safe therapeutic range for the older adult and become harmful. Therefore when an elderly patient does not respond to treatment or presents an unusual physical response, the clinician needs to ascertain whether the strength of the stimulus is too strong or too weak and if modification of the stimulus is necessary because of factors associated with the aging process or the patient's cognitive deficits (he or she may be unable to accurately report the response because of a cognitive deficit). The older person with mild or moderate confusion needs small, slow clinical input and precise monitoring of the general response (heart rate, blood pressure, respiration) as well as local response. *(Clinical consideration—Use pulse oxygen meter to monitor exercise response on evaluation.)* This is especially true for persons who are hearing impaired. Because the patient may not hear what is being spoken, the therapist may assume that the patient does not have the capability to comprehend what is being said. Never assume that a person does not comprehend when she or he may simply be unable to hear what is being spoken.

Law of Initial Values

The law of initial values is both a physiological and a psychological principle stating that with a given intensity of stimulation, the degree of change produced tends to be greater when the initial value of that variable is low at the onset of stimulation. In other words, the higher the initial level of functioning, the smaller the change that can be produced.[62,63] The law of initial values, when defined and applied to younger persons, presumes that homeostasis is a stable and consistent process. When the law is used to describe physiological and psychological responses in older persons, it cannot be presumed that homeostasis for any variable is predictable or consistent from one person to the next, or even within a 24-hour period for the same individual. For example, an older person with mild dementia may eat only sweets if left without companionship at a meal. As a result, after the meal the individual may feel unsteady and afraid to walk back to the room. *(Clinical consideration—Check blood sugar for all diabetics on evaluation before exertion.)* In the young, defining the average times of peak activity for most physiological processes as well as for intellectual capacity is possible. In the clinical assessment of the older persons, defining the peak times of day for awareness and intellectual capacity for each individual is necessary. For example, some patients are best able to participate in learning a new skill in the early morning, and some only in the late afternoon.

Biorhythms

The brain has a biological clock that controls all physiological functions in a precise temporal course, whether daily (e.g., secretion of some hormones), monthly (e.g., menstruation), or during a certain period of the life cycle (e.g., ability to become pregnant).[2,64,65] Before evaluating a geriatric patient with dementia or disturbance of intellectual functioning, assessment of the patient's premorbid biorhythm is helpful. What was her or his daily schedule of activities before the medical crisis? The assessment or time study can map such things as rest periods, activities and level of exertion, sleep or rest periods, mental stimulation, emotional stimulation, eating, and elimination cycles across a 24-hour period. The patient assessment must allow for and assess the current and past variability of individual biorhythms. These biorhythms should be clearly documented and their stability evaluated and maintained as much as possible (critical if the patient will be going back to the family). For example, if a woman has worked for 40 years as a night nurse, being primarily active from 11 PM to 7 AM, she will most likely be alert and best able to participate in a rehabilitation program during those hours. In most cases the patient should be allowed to choose the best time for treatment. For patients whose dementia is too severe for them to make this determination, the staff, by monitoring the patient's behavior, can choose a time for treatment when the person is most alert. For the elderly, and particularly for those who have dementia, the time of assessment and treatment must be documented to maximize the person's rehabilitation potential.[66,67]

Sensory Changes with Aging

Aging can also be defined in terms of adaptation. Aging is the progressive and usually irreversible diminution, with the passage of time, of the ability of a person or body part to perform efficiently or adapt to changes in the environment. The consequence of the process is manifested as decreased capacity for function and for withstanding stresses.[68] Because the rehabilitation evaluation identifies functional problems, therapists should examine the possibility that sensory losses or disturbances (e.g., vision, hearing, touch, taste, smell, proprioception, temperature, and kinesthesia) are contributing to the functional impairments.[61] A partial or total loss of one or more of the normal sensory inputs can result in disturbance of an individual's mental status.

The more sudden the loss of a sense, the more difficult is the adaptation to the sensory disability. This is especially true for elderly persons because several mild sensory changes related to normal aging are already taxing their capacity to adapt. Adaptation to a sensory loss in one modality is typically accomplished through increased use of the other senses. For example, a young blind patient can adapt by using hearing and kinesthesia and usually learns to function well in spite of the loss of visual input. The older the patient is when blinded, however, the more difficulty she or he will have in making this adaptive crossover to other senses. At some time in any person's life, adaptive crossover from one sense to another becomes exceedingly difficult, if not impossible. Thus psychopathological or behavioral changes may occur if a sensory impairment develops.[69] This situation becomes more likely if the disruption is caused by a central nervous system deficit with multiple and abrupt simultaneous sensory input loss, such as might occur from a stroke.

The poliomyelitis epidemics of the early 1950s demonstrated the relationship between sensory input and abnormal behavior. Patients with poliomyelitis who were placed in tank-type respirators developed intermittent disruptions in mental state, including hallucinations, delusions, and dreamlike experiences while awake. The patients were deprived of normative input to the senses (kinesthesia and proprioception) and had severely restricted vision and hearing because of the nature of the construction of and the noise that emanated from the respirator. Solomon and Shackson[70] and Solomon[71] called this problem "sensory deprivation psychosis," but this clinical situation may include cognitive changes in addition to psychotic symptoms. This type of problem often occurs today after a hip fracture when, to control the pain, a patient is given a medication that has the side effect of disrupting orientation to time and place. Until other medication can be tried to control the pain, the patient is described as "out of his or her mind," especially at night. The patient may try to remove all clothing or call out to people for help, often a mother or father. The psychosis stops when the medication is removed. Recovery is also enhanced when consistent nurturing is provided. Note: Other common triggers can be the requirement to stay in one position (e.g., sleep on the back after surgery) or the need to have a spacer between the knees after surgery.

Sensory changes associated with normal aging can lead to the same degree of loss or distortion of significant sensory input as previously described.[72-74] A bilateral loss of vision may lead to agitation and disorientation. Elderly people with hearing impairments often have grave difficulty relating to the world. Elderly persons who become deaf commonly experience some episodes of paranoid behavior.[69] The problems for hearing-impaired elderly persons are often exacerbated by health care professionals who do not know how to place a hearing aid in a patient's ear, replace a battery, adjust the volume on the aid, remove excess ear wax from the aid, identify the need to trim ear hair, or consider the possibility of a malfunctioning aid. Finally, sensory impairments may become exacerbated by surgical or medical interventions.

Certain medications, as well as some diseases, can also distort kinesthesia or retard the activity and movement of the patient.[60] Movement is significant in the maintenance of an efficient nervous system. Anything that denies a person the ability to perform physical movement (e.g., drugs, restraints, traction, passive motion machine, positional props, or architectural designs not adapted to the elderly) hastens and increases the difficulty of adapting to functional limitations. The patient loses her or his freedom to move and may feel trapped and helpless. This can trigger memories of other trauma or violent experiences that involved feeling helpless or victimized. Movement is necessary for accurate sensation.[14,75] It has been demonstrated that if movement of the eyes does not occur properly, vision becomes ineffective. The same is true to a lesser degree for hearing. If movement does not occur in the course of the hearing process, hearing can become distorted and misrepresented at the central level.

New research on brain function in the elderly points to the following ideas for clinical consideration and possible modifications to enhance functional performance:

1. Evaluate the capacity to demonstrate the visual search response. This eye response is a tool to verify that the patient is relaxed and ready for new learning. A clinical example would be to have the person rest supine (with props for comfort as needed under the head, wrists, knees, ankles) and then begin a very slow passive rolling of the head 1 to 4 degrees per second to one direction and observe the eye response. The eyes of a relaxed person will naturally follow objects in the visual field in a functional tracking response as the head is rolled. The skill of visual search is altered (i.e., eyes dart around in a rapid visual search process or rest passively and do not move actively in the direction of the rolling of the head) when limbic activation or actual brain damage is present (90% discrimination).[13,76,77] When the visual search is compromised, the Feldenkrais Method or other neurofacilitation techniques can be used to normalize the resting pattern of the neck and chest and invite the enhanced functional response for eye-head righting. Therapeutic exercise and neurofacilitation to encourage eye participation and other eye-body coordination training strategies have resulted in good functional improvements for persons with AD.[78]
2. Evaluate the capacity to use symbols. Assess the capacity to use signage in the building; does the patient comprehend and demonstrate comprehension by performance?

For example, when an arrow points left, does the patient turn left?
3. Evaluate the capacity to perform complex motor skills (e.g., consistent step-by-step sequence). Even if the skill is not mastered, does the patient show improvement in the speed of a repetition task or increased emotional ease and willingness to participate even if verbal or physical cuing is still needed? Even if the patient cannot perform one motor skill, she or he may still show normal capacity to learn another motor skill.
4. If anxiety is present, try to alleviate it because anxiety interferes with integration of sensory learning (e.g., try a hot pack to the belly area for 5 to 10 minutes to promote relaxation).

Cognitive Changes in Normal Aging

The idea that cognitive decline is a necessary part of aging is a myth. This belief has been debunked by research on crystallized and fluid intelligence.[79,80] Crystallized and fluid intelligence are components of general intelligence. Crystallized intelligence involves the ability to perceive relationships, engage in formal reasoning, and understand intellectual and cultural heritage. Crystallized intelligence can be affected by the environment and the attitude of the individual.[81] Crystallized intelligence can increase with self-directed learning and education as long as a person is alive. The measurement of crystallized intelligence is usually in the form of culture-specific items such as number facility, verbal comprehension, and general information.

Fluid intelligence, what has been called "native mental ability," is the product of the brain's information processing system. It includes attention and memory capacity and the speed of information processing used in thinking and acting.[82] It is not closely associated with acculturation. It is generally considered to be independent of instruction or environment and depends more on the genetic endowment of the individual.[9] The items used to test fluid intelligence include memory span, inductive reasoning, and figural relationships, all of which are presumed to be unresponsive to training. Because fluid intelligence involves those intellectual functions most affected by changes in neurophysiological status, it has been generally assumed to decline with age. Several studies have shown this to be untrue; one study noted that during middle age, scores on tests for fluid intelligence are similar to scores in midadolescence.[53,83] These changes, however, are primarily associated with processing speed and working memory and executive function.[12,84]

Recent studies that have looked at the effects of cognitive changes in activities have shown that older people perform activities at a slower rate and use different areas of the brain in the process compared with younger people. Those additional areas of the brain used have mostly to do with monitoring and processing the ongoing activity.[13,85] Activities are therefore performed more in a feedback rather than a feed-forward manner, which also requires more time. So, if older adults are given time to complete tasks, they usually do well.

Botwinick[35] described the classic pattern of changes in intelligence with aging. In the adult portion of the life span, verbal abilities decline little, if at all, whereas psychomotor abilities decline earlier and to a greater extent (greater decline if the individual is not engaged in regular physical activity). The period between ages 55 and 70 years is a transition time, and some decreases in performance are noted on many cognitive tests. A substantial decline on laboratory tests of cognitive function is generally limited to those older than 75 years.[40] In these latter years, however, the decline in fluid intelligence is offset by the growth in crystallized intelligence for most people unless dementia is present. Although changes may be demonstrated in the laboratory, they may not be significant in the "real world," and the elderly may be as capable as the young of participating in rehabilitation training. For elderly people to benefit maximally, however, they must control the pace of training because the tasks that are the most difficult for older adults are those that are fast paced, unusual, and complex.[86] All physical and occupational therapy treatments with older patients need to be structured to encourage the patient to set his or her own pace. The goal is to have a pace that allows ease of breathing and a comfortable, functional upright posture so that the person can enjoy the experience. Interventions should be predictable and progress by adding one new concept at a time.

"Terminal drop" is another type of cognitive change that differs from those that occur in normal aging and in those with dementia. This involves a decline in IQ scores in persons within the year before their death. This change in intellectual function is thought to result from some predeath changes in brain physiology. Research studies that show drastic decreases in intellectual function with advanced age may have a large percentage of subjects who were near death as a part of the sample.[87] Subjects who did not experience this terminal drop would then appear similar to those in studies on normal elderly persons.

Stress and Intellectual Capacity

Selye[55] defined stress as the nonspecific response of the body to any demand made on it. All human beings require a certain amount of stress to live and function effectively. When a stressor (stimulus) is applied, the body predictably goes through the three stages of response called the *general adaptation syndrome* (GAS). The first response is a general alarm reaction, a "fight-or-flight" response that mobilizes all senses in an effort to make a judgment about the response needed. The older person is at a disadvantage because collecting and processing accurate sensory data are decreased with normal aging owing to short-term memory loss. This will manifest in a patient asking the same question repeatedly during a crisis. The sensory memory in an older person lasts less than 1 second.[24] The next stage involves judgment and the selective adaptation to the stressor. A decision is made regarding which action is needed, and all other bodily activities return to homeostasis. The older person is slower to search and retrieve the information from storage. If the stimulus continues and goes beyond the therapeutic or functional level, then the body system or part will gradually experience physiological exhaustion. A person in physiological exhaustion is likely to manifest abnormal responses to any new stimulus. Paradoxical reactions are unusual physiological or psychological responses to stimuli (e.g., an erythematous response when an ice pack is applied or a patient becoming more agitated after receiving a sedative).

When a person is under perceived stress (whether real or imagined), a predictable set of cognitive changes can occur. These cognitive functional changes can include preoccupation; forgetfulness; disorientation; confusion; low tolerance to ambiguity; errors in judgment in relation to work, distance, grammar, or mathematics; misidentification of people; inability to concentrate, solve problems, or plan; inattention to details or instructions; reduced creativity, fantasy, and perceptual field size; decreased initiative; decreased interest in usual activities, the future, or people; and irritability, impatience, anger, withdrawal, suspicion, depression, and crying. Differentiating whether the patient is having a stress reaction or has dementia is critical. If the changes occur with a sudden onset, they are probably related to a medical or pharmaceutical problem and may be reversible.

With aging, the brain undergoes physiological changes that make the older person less physiologically efficient in her or his response to stressors. The general alarm reaction is poorly mobilized and takes longer to become activated (Arndt-Schultz principle). The stage of resistance should yield a series of responses that allows the body to economize in its response to stress. In persons of all ages who receive too many different stimuli and in the elderly who experience normal levels of stimuli, the body becomes less efficient at turning off the general alarm response and replacing it with more appropriate and limited responses. When a person is overwhelmed by this type or level of stress, the individual may demonstrate mild global or specific cognitive impairments, especially mild short-term memory loss.[88]

The historical clinical data become the only means of establishing a diagnosis because no tests are currently available to distinguish acute dementia from emotional exhaustion. In cases of domestic violence that have been kept secret for years, this can be a difficult problem. For example, a 90-year-old man had beaten his wife a few times early in their marriage. They later came to an agreement and their marriage had continued with only verbal abuse and no physical abuse. As he approached 85 years of age, however, he again began to get violent and would shove her during arguments. At one point she fell, broke her hip, and ended up in a nursing home for 8 weeks. Another time he was bringing her to therapy and on the way he became angry and let go of the wheelchair, and it ran into a wall. The wife chose to do nothing and say nothing. The only sign was that she always cried in physical therapy when she started to relax. The client eventually confided to the physical therapist and was referred to a crisis counselor to determine how to proceed. She saw the counselor weekly for more than 4 years. Another incident happened in which the wife was hurt and protective services were called. The patient refused to press charges and returned to the home, stopped all counseling, withdrew in embarrassment, and within several weeks became confused. The husband placed her in a nursing home and she was given the diagnosis of dementia and placed on haloperidol (Haldol). No other therapeutic services were offered. Access to one-on-one counseling and family therapy is critical. What if support had been offered? Could this situation have turned out differently? If the person had been 36 years old, a psychiatric evaluation would likely have been made and treatment could have reversed the confusion that masked the severe depression.

The assessment of an elderly person, with or without dementia, must include a determination of the type, number, and severity of the patient's current stressors. Positive life events (e.g., marriage or the birth of a grandchild) are also stressful life events. Scores that rate stressful life events can identify patients who are at greatest risk of physiological and emotional exhaustion.[89] Developed in the 1970s, the Holmes-Rahe Social Readjustment Rating Scale is still a commonly used life stress evaluation tool (see www.stresstips.com).[90] Elderly patients, with their numerous psychosocial problems and chronic and acute illnesses, are likely candidates for physiological and emotional exhaustion and the development of psychopathology. Thus the environment and process of rehabilitation care need to be modified to counteract the effect of stress on the intellectual capacity of the older patient. Any action that modifies stress so that a deterioration of intellectual function is stopped or reversed is an efficient and cost-effective part of the total rehabilitation effort.

STRATEGIES FOR ASSESSING, PREVENTING, AND MINIMIZING DISTORTIONS IN INFORMATION PROCESSING

Each person acts on the available data perceived at a specific moment. This stimulus-response cycle has four major steps; each step contains a possibility for distortion or error. When a person is presented with a stimulus, the brain processes all the data (physiological, psychological, sociological, and environmental) collected and then integrates it with data from past experience. Based on this process, a response is elicited, which is then followed by the behavior appropriate for this response.

At the outset of the process of patient assessment, *it is important to identify whether the patient communicates best with verbal, written, or a combination of both strategies.* With an overview of the patient's cognitive capacity, the rehabilitation staff may be able to modify the process of evaluation to maximize the patient's performance (e.g., several 15-minute interactions spread over the 8-hour workday instead of an hour without rest; performing the assessment in the presence of a regular caregiver the patient trusts). A basic assessment of the patient's functional abilities (ADLs and IADLs) at a given moment to allow a comparison of cognitive capacity at other times in the 24-hour cycle provides the clinician a specific description of what aspects of intellectual function appear to be impaired and pinpoints those aspects of intellectual functioning that are still intact. Based on this approach, the rehabilitation evaluation can proceed in a language (perhaps the native language of childhood) and at a pace that are comfortable for the patient and at the time of day when the patient is most alert.

Mini-Mental State Examination and Other Cognitive Scales

The Mini-Mental State Examination (MMSE) was developed as a result of a study noting that 80% of cognitive disorders among elderly people were not detected by the general practitioner.[20,91] It appears to be the most predictable test but is only helpful if all caregivers can monitor the cognitive state of the older patient. All caregivers must be part of the team effort to get a real 24-hour picture of the cognitive capacities of the patient. Although training is improving in this area, most professionals on the rehabilitation team (physicians, nurses,[92,93] physical therapists[94] and social workers[95]) are likely to have had only minimal specialty training in gerontology and the unique symptoms and needs of the elderly.

The MMSE provides a screening test for identifying unrecognized cognitive disorders in the elderly (Figure 27-1).[21,96,97] The MMSE assesses only cognition and does not examine other aspects of the traditional mental status examination such as mood, delusions, or hallucinations. The test can identify whether the patient is oriented; remembers (short term); and can read, write, calculate, and see and reproduce in drawing the relation of one object or figure to another. The examination is used to screen for cognitive dysfunctions, much as a measurement of blood pressure or blood sugar is used to screen for significant medical disorders. The MMSE also may be used in a serial fashion to quantify changes in a patient's cognitive status over time. This examination can be used as a springboard for planning how to carry out the traditional rehabilitation evaluation of a patient who has some intellectual dysfunction.[98,99]

The MMSE has been standardized for elderly persons living in the community. The scores on this test correlate significantly with the Wechsler Adult Intelligence Scale and the Wechsler Memory Test. The MMSE is reported to have a high test-retest reliability for both normal and psychiatric sample populations with $r = 0.89$ or greater. It has been found that when a cutoff score of 24 is used for the detection of dementia, the MMSE had a sensitivity of 87.6% and a specificity of 81.6%.[96] Several studies have noted that interviews with informants are highly consistent with elderly persons' scores on the MMSE.[100]

The examination takes only a few minutes to administer, is scored immediately, and can be administered by any member of the rehabilitation team. The entire examination grades cognitive performance on a scale from 0 to 30. A score of 24 or less usually indicates some degree of cognitive dysfunction,

MINI-MENTAL STATE EXAMINATION

Maximum score	*Score*	
		ORIENTATION
5	( )	What is the (year) (season) (date) (day) (month)?
5	( )	Where are we: (state) (county) (town) (hospital) (floor)?
3	( )	REGISTRATION
		Name 3 objects: 1 second to say each. Then ask the client all 3 after you have said them. Give 1 point for each correct answer. Then repeat them until the client learns all 3. Count trials and record.
		TRIALS
5	( )	*Attention and calculation*
		Serial 7's. 1 point for each correct. Stop after 5 answers. Alternatively spell "world" backwards.
3	( )	*Recall*
		Ask for 3 objects repeated above. Give 1 point for each correct.
9	( )	*Language*
		Name a pencil and watch. (2 points)
		Repeat the following "No ifs, ands, or buts." (1 point)
		Follow a *3-stage command:* "Take a paper in your right hand, fold it in half, and put it on the floor." (3 points)
		Read and obey the following: "Close your eyes." (1 point)
		Write a sentence. (1 point)
		Copy design. (1 point)
30	( )	TOTAL SCORE

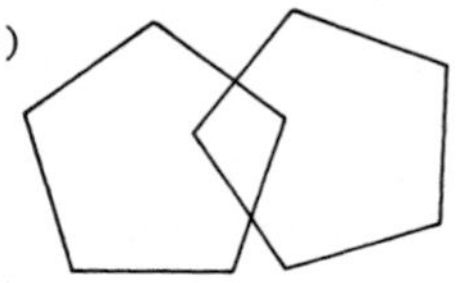

Assess level of consciousness along a continuum.

Alert — Drowsy — Stupor — Coma

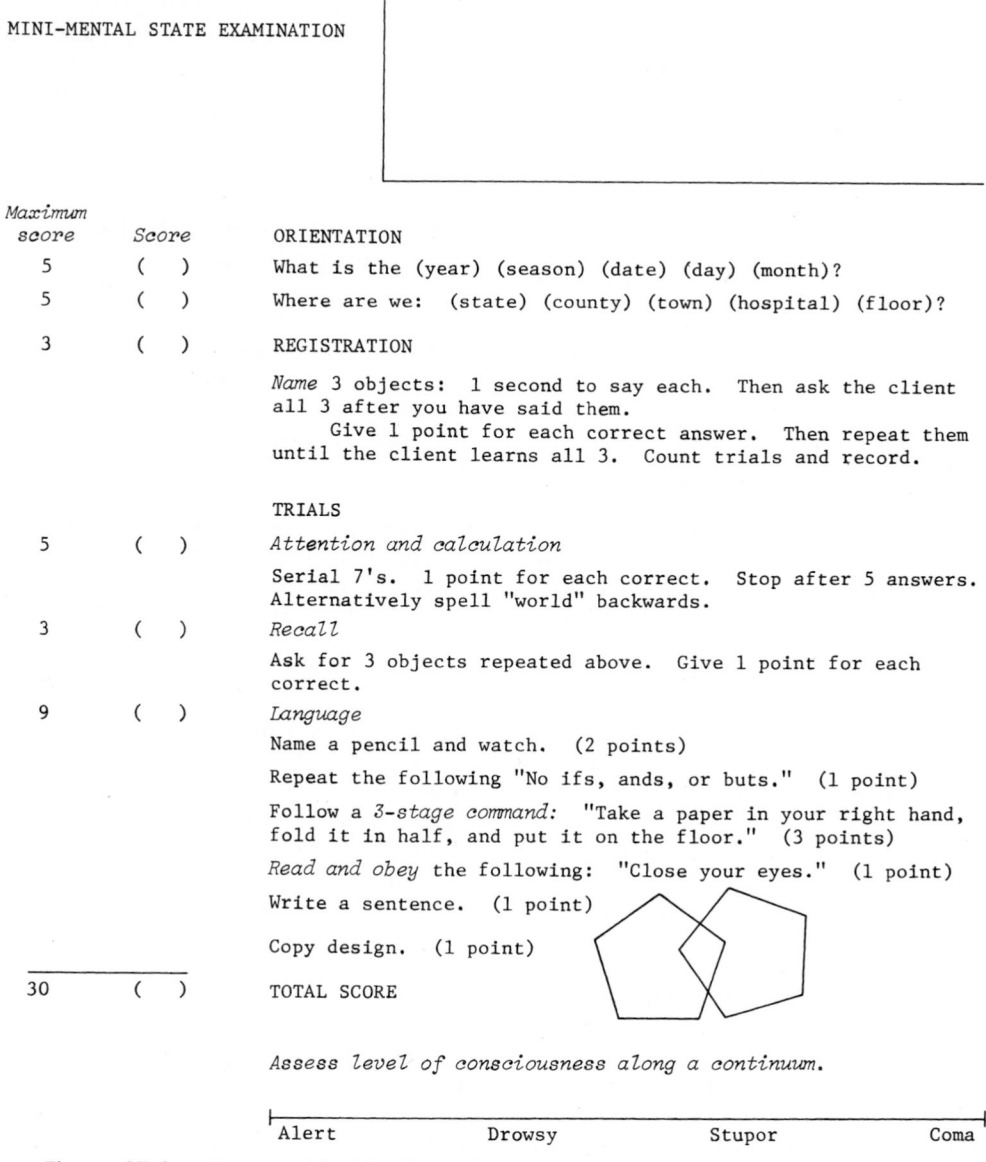

Figure 27-1 ■ Form used for Mini-Mental State Examination (MMSE) to assess cognition.

but some patients with dementia may score above 24 and some with depression or delirium may score significantly below 24. A low score on this examination can mean that the patient probably has dementia, delirium, mental retardation, amnestic syndrome, or aphasia. A low score on the MMSE can indicate the areas of specific cognitive impairment and gives the rehabilitation team data about how to best communicate with the patient. MMSE scores are also correlated with educational level, with scores dropping 10% to 20% for people with an eighth-grade education or less if older than 70 years.[101] A shortened version of the MMSE has been developed that uses only 12 of the 20 original variables. Although the original study suggested that the shortened version of the MMSE is equally as effective as the full MMSE in identifying elderly patients with cognitive deficits, more recent studies have questioned these findings. Another test recently developed to screen for cognitive deficits is the Mini-Cog. It is reported to have higher sensitivity and accuracy of classification because it is not biased by language or educational level.[102]

Older persons may show changes in mental abilities immediately after surgery, after hypoxia (low oxygenation), with delayed care after a fall, or after hitting the head during a fall or other trauma. The Glasgow Coma Scale and the Rancho Los Amigos Cognitive Scale can be used in many ways to assess the cognitive status of an individual, especially if brain injury results from an impact to the head or severe whiplash, for example. First, the extra testing helps staff choose which patients can live safely and compatibly in the same unit. The Rancho Los Amigos Scale can help identify the need to segregate the patients who are prone to screaming incomprehensible words over and over. The coma state may be temporary as a result of medication, anxiety, or anesthesia. Test scores may be used to create a patient group that allows calm and functional use of the shared living space. Another purpose in using these additional tests is to create small groups where patients at level 4 (confused, agitated, alert, active, aggressive or bizarre behaviors, nonpurposeful motor movement, short attention span, inappropriate verbalization) are segregated from those at level 5 (agitated by too much stimulation, require continual redirection) to allow level 5 clients to live and function to their full capacity and allow level 4 patients to have room to move and express. A level 4 patient may become upset and cry on a unit that has mostly level 5 and a few level 3 (inconsistent response to commands, turns toward or away from sound) patients. The biggest factor is to use the test scores to target activities and recreation to a specific cognitive level so that satisfaction and social comfort are possible.

Sensory and Perceptual Changes with Dementia

Patients with dementia may have specific problems that inhibit the integration of sensory input. Aphasias and disruption of association pathways may inhibit the patient's ability to integrate accurately perceived sensory information in a meaningful way. Bassi and colleagues[103] and Fozard[104] have demonstrated that patients with AD, multiinfarct dementia,[105] and alcoholic dementia may demonstrate disturbances in visual acuity, depth perception, color differentiation, and differentiation of figure from ground when compared with normal age-matched control subjects and normal younger subjects.

An assessment of specific sensory systems is necessary when a person demonstrates cognitive losses. The challenge in rehabilitation is to design a process and environment of care so that compensation and modification maximize the ability of the elderly patient with sensory deficits to adapt to most life situations. The example of visual deficits is a case in point. One of every two blind persons in the United States is older than 65 years (see www.afb.org/ and click on AFB senior site).[106] Techniques of environmental adaptation and special measures to organize care to help elderly blind people have allowed many of them to live independently in the community.[107] However, many elderly people with visual impairments are not blind. Some of the structural changes that result in mild to moderate deficits of vision include yellowing; uneven growth, striation, and thickening of the lens; increasing weakness of the muscles controlling the eye; alteration in the perception of color (especially fine distinctions in tone and brightness); and slower adaptation to light.[104] Modifications of the environment can include adequate effective lighting (including adequate intensity and controlling of reflection), dark and clear large-print, low-vision aids (e.g., magnifying glass), verbal orientation and escort by persons accompanying patients in a new environment, consistent furniture placement, explanation when changes occur, clear hallways, a systematic storage system for clothes and toilet articles, and the use of consistent contrasting colors to identify doors, windows, baseboards, and corners.[77,92,104,108]

Older Adult Learning Styles and Communication

Learning occurs throughout life.[86] In physical and occupational therapy, habilitation occurs when the client learns new skills, and rehabilitation occurs when the person relearns old adaptive skills. As with intelligence, the learning process does not change abruptly when an individual reaches old age, but differences in performance have been reported. One challenge for rehabilitation therapy is to find ways to improve the efficiency of learning by the older person.

Botwinick[35] has noted that learning and performance are not the same. Poor performance on a learning task may mean that insufficient learning has occurred, that learning has not transferred to a new environment or task, or that the performance does not accurately reflect the extent of learning achieved.[9] The key variables that affect a person's ability to participate in a learning task can include intelligence, learning skills acquired over the years, and flexibility of learning style. Noncognitive factors also can have a strong bearing on an individual's performance. The noncognitive factors include visual and auditory acuity, health status, motivation to learn, level of anxiety, the speed at which stimuli and learning are paced, and the meaningfulness to the individual of the items or tasks to be learned. Research has shown that learning styles change over the life span and that people learn better when instructional approaches are matched to their learning style.[25] Therefore a rehabilitation assessment needs to include a review of the preferred learning style of the patient. This is particularly important before discharging a patient from a rehabilitation program. The rationale is that a lack of progress may not reflect the patient's lack of capacity for rehabilitation, but rather may reflect a dissonance between the patient's learning style and skills with the presentation of materials in the treatment program (e.g., verbal input has not been adapted to match the level or pace of comprehension of a person who may have a strong preference for visual learning and slower pace).

Interference

Interference can make the learning process less efficient in two major ways.[109] First, interference can result from a conflict between present knowledge and the new knowledge to be learned. Second, if the task to be learned has two or more components, secondary components may interfere with the learning of the primary components. This is particularly true if secondary components overlap in time or use the same sensory modality.[82] The elderly have special difficulties if they must concentrate on intake, attention, and retrieval processes at the same time. Therefore the process and therapeutic environment of rehabilitation for the elderly patient must not be disturbed by background noise, other stimuli in the environment, or anxiety. When learning a new task, the elderly patient may require a quiet room with no stimuli other than that offered by the therapist. The need to rid the environment of distractions is particularly important when working with an elderly patient with dementia because this patient will have greater difficulty filtering out irrelevant sensory inputs compared with elderly patients without dementia.

Pacing

The pacing of therapeutic intervention is a significant variable in helping an elderly person learn. Elderly persons (with or without dementia) perform best if they are given as much time as they need and when learning is self-paced.[35] The major drawback of a fast pace (as perceived by the patient) is that the elderly person generally chooses not to participate rather than risk making a mistake. A lack of response by the patient is often interpreted as apathy, poor motivation, or "confusion."[110] Patient participation is increased when extra time to complete a rehabilitation task is offered. After the individual assessment, group work (where concepts can be presented, reviewed, and examined at leisure) also can be used to reduce the psychological pressure of faster paced one-on-one learning. The details of therapy must be planned carefully, including how questions are asked (this involves asking clear and precise questions in nonmedical language) and, most important, setting aside enough treatment time so the patient can respond at a manageable pace.

Organization

If data are organized in the brain as part of the learning process, the retrieval of these data becomes easier. Older persons are less likely than members of other age groups to organize data spontaneously to facilitate learning and later retrieval (memory) of that learning.[37] Elderly people who are highly verbal show fewer weaknesses in the ability to organize stimuli. Elderly persons with poor verbal skills show significant improvement in data retrieval when strategies for organization of data are provided by others (e.g., the therapist). Older learners have difficulty following content because they cannot anticipate what will be taught and do not see the "whole picture" of what is being presented.[111] This is an example of how organization may influence the learning process.

Organizing therapy by beginning with an overview in outline form of the entire lesson is helpful. This presents the patient with a conceptual map of the upcoming experience. The use of purposeful organizing also can help bridge the gap between what the older person knows and the new information or task to be learned. The use of neurolinguistic programming (NLP) is especially effective with elderly patients and patients with cognitive deficits because it builds consciously—through language, kinesthesia, and visual input—a picture of a new concept from a known and familiar frame of reference.[111]

Inefficient learning, and at times an inability to learn, occurs in the older adult if material is presented in one way and the older person is expected to apply it in some other way. Instructions need to be provided in the format and context in which they are to be used. If possible, one piece of new data should be presented at a time. A conscious transition needs to be made by the therapist from the patient's current frame of reference to the understanding of the new data, and the pace needs to be set by the patient.

Several other strategies exist for maximizing the efficiency of older adult learners based on awareness of normal age-related changes. Some of the more frequently used techniques are summarized in Box 27-1.

Communication

Therapists can begin by inquiring into what the reality of the patient looks like. The first goal should be to communicate with words, gestures, positioning, and so on so that stimuli

BOX 27-1 ■ TECHNIQUES FOR MAXIMIZING THE EFFICIENCY OF OLDER ADULT LEARNERS

1. Use mediators; the association of word, story, mnemonics, or visual inputs can help the person remember.
2. Choose learning activities that are meaningful for the client.
3. Use concrete examples to make learning easier.
4. Provide a supportive learning environment to prevent stress, which can interfere with efficient learning.
5. Use supportive or neutral feedback and avoid feedback that is presented in a challenging tone.
6. Reward all responses but reward correct responses more than incorrect responses. This can encourage elderly persons to decrease the number of errors by omission, which are often interpreted as apathy or lack of cooperation.
7. Use combinations of auditory and visual input to facilitate the learning process. This is effective only if the data presented are similar because variation between the two kinds of messages can result in interference and a decrease in the efficiency of learning.
8. Active learning is more effective. A patient who moves the involved body part while receiving verbal and visual input is likely to better master the new skill.
9. Design the learning situation so that successful completion of the task is likely. Older people are more likely to focus on errors, which increases anxiety and lowers self-esteem. Worst of all, with all the energy focused on the error, there is a strong chance of repeating the error.

bring out functional responses in the patient. All people have an ongoing internal dialogue. As a healthy adult, the therapist chooses to notice his or her own dialogue, hear the content, and then pursue the goals and commitments that enhance interaction with the patient.

The interaction with the patient needs to be grounded in the present moment. The power for action lies in the present moment. The patient will bring his or her authentic self to the conversation or the interaction. The therapist needs to be sensitive to the entire communication—what is said and what is withheld. The patient with cognitive problems may not understand the content, but many patients still have the ability to sense and respond to the therapist's affective state at the moment. When beginning communication, be clear of all previous concerns and bring no extra or extraneous emotions into the interaction. Caregivers and therapists bring into the conversation the power of intention to create a therapeutic interaction and the choice to stay on task. Patients bring their own sets of concerns at any particular moment. Knowing something about the patient's concerns helps the process.

Therapists and caregivers need to be self-aware. What is the therapist's favorite strategy for communication? What is the therapist's favorite sentence structure? Our habitual forms of presentation need to be assessed with regard to whether they are effective, because the patient needs to be the focus of attention. Honoring the communication habits of the patient is necessary if effective communication is to occur with a person with cognitive deficits. If the therapist chooses to speak to the patient as if there were no cognitive deficits, consistent results will not occur and the patient may be upset or agitated. The patient could be approached as if he or she were a person from another culture that has its unique customs, norms, and ways of communication. The patient-therapist interaction becomes an inquiry in which success is measured by the achievement of functional outcomes that are needed and wanted (e.g., the patient transferring into bed and feeling safe).

Now the question becomes what is the specific process of interaction with which the patient appears to be most comfortable and feels safe? Every patient is different, and it may depend on the time of day or whether the patient is tired or feeling threatened. Persons commonly respond best to one particular style of communication and are predictably upset or agitated by another style. If a patient wants to joke around and be playful, this should be a cue to staff that this is a workable style of communication. Another patient smiles whenever the tone of the conversation is soft, nurturing, and tender, and if staff is willing, this is where ease of relating can occur. Other patients relate best to rules and need predictable structures and boundaries. They love to know what is coming next. Still another category is people who can relate and communicate when definite admiration and respect are built into the conversation or when patient and therapist can agree to disagree. Each patient with cognitive problems needs to have caregivers develop a chart of what works to create a sense of relatedness and ease in communication. A challenge here for caregivers is that the patient's abilities can change; guidelines for communication when new caregivers are introduced to the patient can also be helpful. Someone who is familiar and enjoys interacting with the patient should introduce new staff to the patient.

For persons with cognitive disturbances, familiarity and rituals are keys to ease of adaptability. The basis for rituals is well-organized documentation to which all caregivers have access and contribute on an ongoing basis. This information needs to be filtered and organized so that each shift can see what is working for the patient today. Even a nonverbal patient can relate effectively to bathing if a ritual exists regarding dressing and undressing (e.g., the socks always come off first). Mace and Rabins[99] spelled out the details of the importance of caregivers being aware of the power of familiarity and rituals. Mintzer and colleagues[112] reinforced the same idea in their research on the effectiveness of alternative care environments for agitated patients with dementia. Another detail that requires staff or caregiver attention, evaluation, and adaptation in daily care is *ideational apraxia.* LeClerc and Wells[113] described this as "a condition in which an individual is unable to plan movement related to an object because he or she has lost the perception of the object's purpose." This is especially important in relation to feeding, dressing, toileting, and bathing. The authors described a tool that can help caregivers assess ideational apraxia and problem-solving compensations to prevent unnecessary agitation or disability and take actions to preserve existing abilities. Savelkoul and colleagues[114] emphasized the importance of effective communication between staff and patients and the importance of routines for patient care to maximize functional behaviors for institutionalized elderly living in residential homes. Another key point noted was that staff corrected and tested residents too often, which can create agitation and anxiety. This appeared to be related to lack of training and information on the part of the staff about the dementia and cognitive status of patients as well as a lack of support from other staff.

As a patient goes through gradual deterioration of cognitive status, as is common in AD, staff, family, and caregivers must be trained in nonverbal, positional, and manual cues and emotional communication techniques. Many patients come to a place in their lives with dementia when words are a source of confusion. Other strategies to communicate should then be used. Sign language is initially a possible tool until the associative functions begin to disappear. Accurate assessment needs to create adaptations in communication. It may be necessary to use hand-guided communication, in which the patient is led through a task or parts of a task to get his or her cooperation. At this stage of communication, ease and trust are the most important goals. It may take 5 minutes of tenderly holding a patient's hand before the patient is ready to walk to the dining room or bathroom. This requires much patience on the part of caregivers. Positional communication can be used as well as simple touch. As patients begin to feel safe with their state of being, they will relax and choose to participate. At times patients have unique needs, such as only wanting to be cared for by a female caregiver or a male caregiver. Honoring patient needs is critical because the cognitively impaired may not be able to learn or adapt to the demands of the staff member because of previous trauma (assault or incest, real or imagined).

As a way to summarize the considerations about communication with a person with cognitive impairment, therapists may find it useful to examine their own intentions from moment to moment. "What is my goal in this interaction?"

"Who am I being at this moment?" The task may be important and the "doing" of it may be critical. For the patient with cognitive disturbance, therapists must provide life-enhancing stimuli on the basis of the patient's perceptions. If in the zeal to "do," the patient is accidentally scared, intimidated, or bullied, the damage may not be able to be undone. The cognitively impaired patient presents a unique challenge if a threat has been created, because reestablishing their trust is often difficult. Often the patient may be afraid of the therapist and simply needs the therapist to leave the room for some time. The saving grace for many patients is that their short-term memory is poor so they may not remember the incident tomorrow. The problem with agitation occurs when other cognitively impaired clients in the area also get upset.

The solution to the crisis moment, when a breakdown in communication has occurred, is to redirect communication and the focus of the present moment effectively. For example, a staff member could purposely bump into a chair and knock it over, drop a cup of water or a book, start to sing, whistle loudly, or clap his or her hands. At that moment a distraction is created. If the distraction works, then the patient's attention is pulled away from his or her old thought and focused to a new topic. At that moment the staff needs to be intentional. The new focus needs to offer comfort or nurturing or a predictable sense of well-being (e.g., helping to clean up, eating some food, looking at a picture of a favorite thing, holding a favorite item, touching a favorite comfort object, hugging).

The research findings and techniques previously discussed describe many of the aspects of the Feldenkrais approach to learning.[1,14] The Feldenkrais Method has been applied to the needs of elderly persons with good results. The principle that learning needs to be pleasurable is especially applicable to elderly clients (with or without dementia) because they are often under more stress and have fewer supportive resources to cope with a crisis. Despite changes in learning style, the older person (with or without dementia) can be helped to learn more efficiently through well-planned instruction. The use of techniques to increase learning efficiency in the elderly has been demonstrated to decrease the stress that at times may result in emotional or cognitive overload and abnormal cognitive reactions.

Ann[115] notes that because habits and procedural memory (behaviors learned by doing) are two of the last areas of the brain affected by AD and dementia, individuals with these diseases can often walk around after they are no longer able to be aware of their surroundings, consistently communicate, or reason. The Feldenkrais Method taps into an individual's habits, producing positive and lasting results through the capacity of the individual to still use procedural learning (even though she or he is not able to describe verbally or be consciously aware of the learning that is achieved). One example of how the Feldenkrais Method taps into procedural memory follows. Lee, a man of age 92 years with advanced dementia, was able to achieve changes in his behaviors, even though he was worked with while he was sleeping, which changed his behavior while he was awake. Because of Lee's constant walking and potentially combative behavior, working with him initially was difficult. When he was asked to sit or lie down, he complained loudly and told the therapist to get away. Instead, the therapist worked with him during his frequent naps. He walked bent over with his feet and legs turned out and a wide stance. He held both arms close to his sides, with his elbows bent and no arm swing. He was unable to move isolated areas of his torso; he therefore did not turn his head to look at something next to him. Instead, he turned his whole body. Lee would decide to sit down without looking to see if a chair was behind him, partially because he did not have safety awareness and partially because he did not have the capability to rotate his body. Immediately after waking up or finishing a meal, he would start to walk. As a result of these limitations and actions, Lee was constantly falling. Lee needed to learn how to differentiate the movement pattern of turning his head separate from his trunk. Lee had a pattern that was "un"differentiated in which he moved his head and trunk as a single unit; he had no choice to do anything else. Through gentle movements while Lee was lying on his back or side, the first several sessions involved exploring passive movement of his pelvis and spine. The focus was to explore with Lee his capacity to move in diagonal patterns and to create a kinesthetic relationship between his right shoulder and his left hip and vice versa, the sensation of elongating his spine and learning to twist his torso. He began to demonstrate the capacity to breathe by allowing his chest to expand in the lower rib area. The passive movement explorations involved exploring upper torso rotation, including head turning, shoulder blade differentiation, and the ability to move the shoulder blades independently of his ribs, and connecting movements of the ribs and chest to flow with the movements of the upper spine. After the third session, Lee stopped falling while walking. Although he still exhibited rigid movements and difficulty moving his arms away from his body, he shifted weight a little more easily and demonstrated minimal trunk rotation for walking in both directions. Lee did not fall for several months until he stopped walking because of a sore on the ball of one foot. Lee gradually discovered how to allow the therapist to work with him and the protest stopped. This ability to learn to allow the therapist to sit next to him and touch him is an example of learning through use of emotional memory, another type of memory that seems to work in conjunction with procedural learning. Both procedural and emotional memory are preserved long after other memories are lost. Even without cognitive recognition, emotional memory capabilities in persons with AD allow them to communicate and establish trust with another human being and learn new functional ways to balance in gravity.

Another example is Dina, an 83-year-old with advanced AD, Parkinson disease, depression, and cataracts. The Feldenkrais sessions with her demonstrated the power of focusing the communication and interaction on keeping the activities pleasant and working within the comfort zone of the patient. The chief problem was that the patient had swollen knees and had not been able to straighten her knees past 90 degrees for the previous 2 years. Dina had received traditional physical therapy in which the intervention included attempting to straighten the knees by placing a weight on top of them. Dina cried during this treatment and reported pain. She could not propel her own wheelchair, and it took two staff members to transfer her to and from her wheelchair. Her reaction to their attempt to transfer her was to lift her legs off the floor and give them her entire weight. She did not rest her feet on the floor, even in sitting. Dina had difficulty lying in all positions. When on her back, her lower body twisted to the side. She stayed where she was placed and in the position she was placed in. Dina was unable to specifically point to a body part and say it hurt her. The focus of the first session was to explore how to help her rest more comfortably. The first efforts were to try to enhance mobility in her ribs and spine. After the first session, she was able to rest more fully on one side. After the second session she was able to rest more fully on both shoulder blades and on her pelvis evenly. After the fourth session, Dina began wheeling herself in the wheelchair with her feet, and staff reported that later in the day they saw her stand up from the wheelchair for about 1 minute by herself. None of the sessions had involved direct work with her legs, and the progress in her ability to participate in her life points to the fact that movement deficits are not always the root of problems. The capacity to feel safe and allow touch and other physical and social communication can create improvements in the ability to live in gravity and assist caregivers with the chores of life. The Feldenkrais Method is an example of effective, functional communication, manual therapy, and neurological rehabilitation that enhances daily living skills in people with AD and other dementias.[1,14,115]

ENVIRONMENTAL CONSIDERATIONS

Hypothermia

The temperature of the living environment must be carefully controlled because aged clients may not perceive that the environment is cold and may not experience shivering. Accidental hypothermia can develop in an older person even at temperatures of 60° F (15.5° C) to 65° F (18.3° C). Accidental hypothermia is a drop in the core body temperature to less than 95° F (35° C). Patients at risk for hypothermia are presented in Box 27-2.

The symptoms of hypothermia may include a bloated face, pale and waxy or pinkish skin color, trembling on one side of the body without shivering, irregular and slowed heartbeat, slurred speech, shallow and slow breathing, low blood pressure, drowsiness, and symptoms of delirium. The two principles of treatment of hypothermia are that the person will stay chilled unless the body temperature is slowly increased and that he or she should be evaluated by a physician, regardless of the apparent severity of the hypothermia.[9,116]

If a person continues to be at risk for hypothermia, specific measures can be taken to prevent subsequent distortions of cognitive status. First, the room temperature should be set to at least 70° F (21° C). Second, the person should wear adequate clothing; this may include long underwear and an undershirt. Adequate nutrition also may be a factor in preventing hypothermia.

Patients and their caregivers may attempt to save money by lowering room temperatures and thus inadvertently cause hypothermia. To prevent accidental hypothermia in institutions with central air conditioning, special accommodations for the elderly, such as a special wing of the building or individual temperature controls in the rooms, are required.[116]

BOX 27-2 ■ PATIENTS AT HIGH RISK FOR HYPOTHERMIA

- Persons older than 65 years
- Persons showing no signs of shivering or pale skin in response to cold
- Persons taking medications containing a phenothiazine (to treat psychosis or nausea)
- Persons with disorders of the hormone system, especially hypothyroidism
- Persons with head injuries, strokes, Alzheimer disease or other dementia, Parkinson disease, or other neurological conditions
- Persons with severe arthritis
- Persons with arteriosclerotic peripheral vascular disease, chronic ulceration, or amputation

Transplantation Shock

Some elderly persons seem to function well in a familiar environment but become severely disoriented and unable to perform ADLs if taken out of their own homes. As a general rule, these persons have mild symptoms of dementia that are not readily apparent when they remain in a structured, familiar, stable environment and maintain a consistent daily routine. When faced with the need to adapt to a new environment and bombarded with multiple unfamiliar sensory stimuli, however, their limited brain capacity is unable to make sense out of the large volume of new stimuli. If a patient was oriented before admission to an institution and then becomes disoriented, the patient's cognitive functioning will likely return to its baseline level of functioning on return to the familiar environment. Therefore all moves by a patient from one hospital room to another or from one institution to another, and all changes in a treatment regimen, need to be carefully planned. If a change is anticipated, the patient should be involved in the decision making. If the change is a permanent move, the patient needs to have a chance for one or two trial visits before the actual move. The patient needs to be informed of all changes well in advance, and this information needs to be given repeatedly to the patient with dementia. The precautions mentioned can help the patient relocate without creating transplantation shock and the negative cognitive and emotional changes.

EMOTIONAL CAPACITY TO PARTICIPATE IN A LEARNING TASK

Many elderly persons who come for physical therapy are in a state of emotional overload, as evidenced by disorientation, depression, anger, or a withdrawn and apparently uncooperative attitude. A person who is at or near the point of emotional overload needs to be evaluated regarding his or her ability to be involved in learning tasks that require active participation. If the patient is in emotional overload, forms of therapeutic intervention that temporarily allow the patient to be a passive recipient of therapeutic intervention can be used. Various types of therapeutic interventions, including massage, connective tissue massage, heat, breathing exercises, relaxation exercises, and *Feldenkrais Functional Integration,* can promote a relaxation response, lower the anxiety level, reinforce self-pacing of activity, and thereby prepare the patient to participate in more physically active types of therapeutic exercise.[117] If asked directly, most patients will state whether they feel able to participate actively.[1,14,115]

If for any reason the patient is not able or willing to state his or her feelings, evaluating the patient's ability to participate is still possible. If the therapist can get a patient's cooperation, the following movements can be attempted and then evaluated. (These active movements should be used only if active diseases involving the eyes are not present and no pain occurs during the movements.) The therapist asks the patient to do the following:

1. Close your eyes.
2. Close your eyes and keep them closed for 30 seconds, then for 1 minute.
3. Close your eyes; move only the eyes to the right and left slowly (slow movements with control is the goal).
4. Close your eyes; move your eyes diagonally: right and up, left and down, left and up, right and down.

If a patient is unable to perform these movements, feels they require too much effort, or experiences discomfort, a high level of tension is usually present. Another option is to create a screening of ease of movement and capacity for following increasingly complex directions using the mouth and tongue or movements involving the hands and face. When the patient is extremely tense, treatment should begin by using passive therapeutic procedures. If a person can comfortably execute the movements, she or he (i.e., the central nervous system and the body) is likely to be able to receive and integrate new data and act with ease. When the specific therapeutic intervention requires active participation by the patient, psychomotor readiness to participate can be explored using these kinds of screening activities.

Distortions in intellectual and emotional capacity to receive input, integrate input, and then act on the input affect a person's ability to participate in a learning task. This section has described the most common sources of distortion in information processing that are external to the patient and therefore under the direct control of the rehabilitation team. The rehabilitation team may choose to acknowledge the common age-related changes and common sources of stress response in the elderly and then design a learning process and environment of care that maximize the elderly patient's potential.

DELIRIUM AND REVERSIBLE DEMENTIA: EVALUATION AND TREATMENT

This section focuses on the patient's internal environment (physiological, psychological, spiritual, and pathological) and presumes that all unnecessary external environmental stressors have been removed. Delirium and dementia have been previously defined. Delirium can manifest suddenly or over a period of hours or days. Delirium may occasionally be chronic, but this is relatively infrequent. Dementia, whether reversible or irreversible, usually has a much longer time of onset, although an acute onset can occur.

The establishment of the diagnosis of the underlying cause of dementia or delirium is the key to effective care. Although the diagnostic process is primarily at the level of pathology, the therapist can obtain information, as part of a team evaluation, that will help establish the underlying diagnosis. Historical information needs to be obtained regarding the following:

- The amount of time that has elapsed since the onset of symptoms
- The progression or lack of progression of symptoms
- Associated functional impairments and associated medical signs and symptoms
- Use of prescription drugs, over-the-counter medications, home remedies, illegal drugs, alcohol, caffeine, and nicotine
- Exposure to toxins at work or during recreation

Even in a patient with cognitive disturbances, this information can frequently be obtained and corroborated by obtaining a history from significant others.

The causes of delirium and reversible dementia are many. In the elderly person, however, certain causes are more common than others (Box 27-3). Alcohol and drugs (prescribed, over-the-counter, or illegal medications and home remedies) are prime offenders (see Chapter 36). The delirium may be the result of intoxication, side effects, or withdrawal syndromes.[70] Benzodiazepines are among the most commonly prescribed offenders; even a low dose (2 mg) may cause demonstrable cognitive changes.[54] Other common drugs that cause delirium or reversible dementia are alcohol, oral narcotics, psychotropic medications, steroids, antineoplastic drugs, digoxin, anesthetic agents, antiparkinsonian drugs, and antihistamines. However, all drugs have the potential to cause significant cognitive problems in the elderly.[118] These symptoms often resolve with discontinuation of the offending agent or treatment of the withdrawal syndrome. For some patients a medication holiday of longer than 24 hours may be needed before a positive change in cognition can be noted.[67]

At times, the symptoms may be clearly correlated with the pharmacokinetic profiles of the medications taken by the client. The dose or frequency of administration of medications can be a contributing factor to a delirious state.[119] Every member of the rehabilitation team needs to document the patient's ability to participate in learning tasks and the time of the assessment because timing of medication administration can affect functional performance. The rehabilitation team needs the input of a clinical pharmacologist who can help the team focus on concepts such as biological half-life, clearance, bioavailability of drugs, and the time course of drug concentration in plasma as a function of dose and frequency.

Several medical diseases are likely to cause symptoms of delirium or reversible dementia, which will also reverse with treatment of the underlying disease. Urinary tract infections, more common in women, are the cause of delirium in 28%[120] of elderly patients. Fecal impaction is another common cause of acute cognitive change in elderly persons. Others are distended bladder caused by prostate enlargement or drug-induced urinary retention, dehydration, malnutrition, cardiovascular disorders,[116] metabolic disturbances (particularly undiagnosed diabetes mellitus),[18] endocrine diseases, renal diseases, hematological diseases, pneumonia or bronchitis,[116] and vitamin B_{12} deficiency.

Transient (and usually mild) cognitive deficits may be the result of a cerebrovascular accident (CVA). The cognitive deficits after a CVA are often reversible, although they may last for several months after the stroke. The rehabilitation

BOX 27-3 ■ COMMON CAUSES OF DELIRIUM AND REVERSIBLE DEMENTIA

ALCOHOL OR DRUG ABUSE OR DEPENDENCE
Intoxication
Toxicity
Side effects
Withdrawal

CARDIOVASCULAR OR PULMONARY CONDITIONS
Congestive heart failure
Cardiac arrhythmia
Hypertensive crisis
Hypoxia
Chronic obstructive pulmonary disease

METABOLIC OR ENDOCRINE CONDITIONS
Electrolyte disturbance (especially hyponatremia)
Hypercalcemia
Dehydration
Overhydration
Renal failure
Hypoglycemia
Diabetic ketoacidosis
Hypothyroidism
Hyperthyroidism
Malnutrition
Vitamin B_{12} or folate deficiency
Hepatic failure
Wernicke-Korsakoff syndrome
Cushing syndrome

INFECTION
Urinary tract infection
Pneumonia or acute bronchitis
Tuberculosis
Other acute infections

NEUROLOGICAL CONDITIONS
Stroke
Head trauma
Mass lesion (e.g., tumor, hematoma)
Seizure

PHARMACOLOGICAL CAUSES
Benzodiazepines
Barbiturates and other sedative-hypnotics
Antidepressants
Neuroleptics
Antihistamines
Anticholinergics
Cardiac glycosides
Steroids
Antineoplastic drugs
Narcotics
Antiarrhythmics
Antihypertensives

MISCELLANEOUS CAUSES
Sensory deprivation
Sensory overstimulation
Acute or chronic pain
Constipation or fecal impaction
Urinary retention

team needs to evaluate and regularly reevaluate the patient's cognitive capacity and build a program of care around current abilities. A program of therapeutic intervention that allows the older person to work in a self-paced program for 1 to 3 months can yield good therapeutic results and also prevent unnecessary secondary deconditioning until part or all of the patient's cognitive capacity returns.[121]

Depression is commonly misdiagnosed as dementia in the elderly.[116,122] For many years depression was thought to be a form of "pseudodementia" or false dementia.[123] Depression can result in mild and subtle cognitive changes affecting immediate recall, attention, and the ability to perform basic ADLs. Some reports noted that as many as 31% of those thought to have dementia have depression instead.[124] However, recent research has clarified the close relationship between structural changes in the elderly brain and the onset of depression, thus bringing the concept of pseudodementia, or depression as a reversible dementia, into disrepute.[125,126] Depression is a treatable disorder, and many patients with cognitive impairments show some improvement in their cognitive functioning if the depression is treated; however, the underlying cognitive problem does not resolve with treatment of the depression.[127]

Because the presence of depression can interfere with the progress of rehabilitation through cognitive deficits or its effects on motivation, this disorder needs to be diagnosed early and accurately. The Geriatric Depression Scale, a 30-item yes-no questionnaire, screens for this disorder.[128] No arbitrary cutoff score signifies depression in this test, and most individuals with a score of 15 or higher have this disorder. The higher the score, the more likely that the patient has depression and the severity of the depression is greater.

Depression after a stroke can produce a reversible decline in cognitive performance.[129] Depression after a stroke is more likely to occur in patients with left hemisphere lesions and as the site of the lesion moves toward the frontal pole.[9] The relation between site of lesion and depression also has been noted on neuropsychological testing.[87]

The treatment of major depression generally involves pharmacotherapy, psychotherapy, and environmental manipulation, which can require support from the entire rehabilitation team.[130] In the treatment of a patient with depression, therapeutic techniques can promote a relaxation response, enhance upright posture, decrease anxiety level (massage, heat, or Feldenkrais Functional Integration), and help bring the patient to the point at which aerobic training is possible, which is known to have a beneficial effect. All aerobic training for the elderly needs to begin with a stress test, modified as necessary to determine the patient's exercise target heart rate. The modification most commonly required is use of the upper extremities to achieve the training effect, because lower-extremity function may be limited, or use of major ADLs involving the upper extremities as the stress test or training program.

The causes of delirium and reversible dementia are usually treatable, and if diagnosis and care are provided in a timely fashion, the patient can likely regain full command of his or her cognitive processes. When this does not happen, the patient probably had mild, irreversible dementia that remained hidden until the onset of an acute problem that uncovered the poor cognitive functioning. The length of time in an institution (hospital or nursing home) needs to be kept as short as possible to avoid learned dependency and learned helplessness,[130] which make a return to full cognitive functioning and independent living difficult.[122]

Therapy for elderly persons with delirium or reversible dementia consists of treating the underlying causes of the cognitive changes. A close working relationship among all members of the rehabilitation team, including a geriatric psychiatric consultant, is necessary. Even before the cause of the disorder is elucidated, the patient should receive the same emotional and physical support as any patient with an irreversible dementia. The therapist must adapt all activities to the extent and types of cognitive losses that are present. The patient needs to feel secure, live in an environment that has as few changes as possible, and have a consistent and stable schedule for activities.

IRREVERSIBLE DEMENTIA

The course of irreversible dementia is unique for each patient. The variation in clinical course occurs based on the cause of the underlying disease and superimposed biological and psychosocial factors, including medications, concurrent illness (including delirium), the nature of the social support system, and the patient's premorbid personality structure. The causes of irreversible dementia are summarized in Box 27-4.

Regardless of the cause of the dementia, the clinical course of these disorders has several commonalities.[83] Most of these diseases are progressive. Symptoms may be subtle early in the course of the illness, and the onset of disease is usually noted by the person with the disorder, family members, friends, or colleagues at work rather than by a physician. The signs of impairment of mental ability are typically memory loss, poor judgment, or incompetence at work. The patient can often succeed at hiding his or her symptoms for a while. The social consequences of the cognitive impairment usually bring the patient to the attention of health care professionals. In addition, the patient with dementia can manifest a variety of psychiatric symptoms, including mood disturbance, agitation, violent behavior, socially inappropriate behavior, delusions, hallucinations, catastrophic reactions, and perseveration.[99,131] The pattern of onset and the types of psychiatric symptoms are often directly related to the underlying pathological condition.

When a physician is finally consulted, the diagnostic process can begin. When a complete diagnostic evaluation—including history, physical examination, neurological examination, neuropsychological testing, and laboratory testing (Box 27-5)—is performed, an accurate diagnosis can be made in approximately 90% of patients, although experienced geriatric psychiatrists can make an accurate diagnosis in more than 95% of patients.[132]

BOX 27-4 ■ COMMON CAUSES OF IRREVERSIBLE DEMENTIA

DEGENERATIVE CAUSES
Alzheimer disease
Parkinson disease
Huntington disease
Pick disease
Fahr disease
Multiple sclerosis

INFECTIOUS CAUSES
Neurosyphilis (general paresis)
Tuberculosis
Acquired immunodeficiency syndrome (AIDS)
Creutzfeldt-Jakob disease

VASCULAR CAUSES
Multiinfarct dementia
Stroke
Binswanger dementia
Anoxia
Arteriovenous malformation

OTHER CAUSES
Normal-pressure hydrocephalus
Mixed dementia
Alcoholic dementia
Toxins
Head trauma
Mass lesions

BOX 27-5 ■ LABORATORY EVALUATION FOR DELIRIUM AND DEMENTIA

Complete blood count
Thyroid function tests
Vitamin B_{12} or folate levels
Urinalysis
Blood levels of drugs patient is taking
Urine drug screen
Electrocardiogram
Magnetic resonance imaging scan of head (computed tomographic scan if magnetic resonance imaging is contraindicated)
Automated chemistries (including electrolytes, glucose, renal function, hepatic function, protein and albumin, cholesterol, and triglycerides)
Blood alcohol level
Human immunodeficiency virus (HIV) titer
Chest radiograph

Once the diagnostic process is completed, treatment can be started. Medications can assist in reversing underlying causes in only a small percentage of cases; patients in whom drug therapy is successful usually have potentially reversible dementia that has gone untreated and now have permanent sequelae of the disorder. Medications may be able only to slow the process of an irreversible disorder (e.g., tacrine for AD) or prevent further deterioration (e.g., aspirin for multiinfarct dementia). Psychotropic drugs may reverse depression or the behavioral symptoms associated with dementia.[124,130,133] Medical management also involves the prevention and treatment of other medical conditions and side effects of the new interventions as they are added.

Medical management of irreversible dementia focuses on maximizing the patient's remaining functions and roles, rehabilitating some lost functions, and providing family education and support.[99] Training caregivers to adapt to the patient (e.g., modifications for getting the patient out of bed, bathing), simplifying the individual's living space, and referring relatives to family support services are some of the issues to be addressed.[134]

Alzheimer Disease

The treatment of irreversible dementia is a long-term process. Recent studies have found that the average duration of illness from first onset of symptoms to death is 8.1 years for AD, 6.7 years for multiinfarct dementia,[135] and 5.6 years for Pick disease.[124] Medical and nursing care can extend the life expectancy of patients with dementia for up to 20 years or more.

In 1907, Alois Alzheimer[34] described the case and the neuropathology of a 54-year-old woman who developed morbid jealousy, which was followed by loss of memory, inability to read and understand, and death 4.5 years after onset of the illness. Since then, it has been noted that 50% of patients with dementia have AD.[101] In making the diagnosis of AD, all other causes of cognitive dysfunction must be ruled out. The disease can occur at any age, but the onset of the disease is almost always after age 65 years. The prevalence of the disease gradually increases to a rate of 20% in persons older than 85 years.[33]

AD can be clinically staged. The use of staging enables the family and health care team to plan ahead for the individual's needs. Staging helps the family prepare longitudinally for the process of interacting with the patient. It allows the treatment team to plan for appropriate levels of services as the individual's abilities decline. Finally, it allows the health care team to quantify change in functional and cognitive abilities over time, which helps assess the effectiveness of the patient's treatment plan and establish evidence-based practice. The use of staging requires an accurate description of the patient's behavior (without the use of jargon) as well as an assessment of the patient's mental state.

Traditionally the symptoms of AD have been thought to progress in three stages.

Stage 1 lasts from 2 to 4 years and involves loss of functional skills or orientation, memory loss, and lack of spontaneity. The patient is often aware of the losses and is, in many cases, able to cover up the cognitive losses by talking around the issues. During this stage the patient and family may need to deal with the issue of giving up a job, hobbies, or other types of meaningful activity because of the patient's inability to carry them out safely and independently. The patient begins to lose the ability to handle money and a personal budget, drive a car safely, and tell time. The family or significant others may have to come to terms with the question of whether the patient can live alone. Depression is common during this stage of the disorder.[130]

Stage 2 is characterized by progressive memory loss and the presence of a variety of neurological symptoms. Aphasias, apraxias, wandering, repetitive movements and stereotypical behavior, increased or decreased appetite, constant movement, and a peculiar wide-based gait can manifest. Psychotic symptoms (especially paranoid delusions and hallucinations), agitation, violent behaviors, and uncontrollable screaming are common symptoms during this stage of the disorder.

In stage 3 the patient develops vegetative symptoms. The patient may become mute, stop eating, and become incontinent of bowel and bladder. Muscle twitches or jerks, spasms of the diaphragm, and an inability to walk generally occur. The patient may develop seizures, and emotional responsiveness, if present, is at a primitive level. Eventually the patient dies from the disease.

The MMSE also may be used as a staging tool. Scores of 26 or more are generally associated with minimal, if any, dementia; scores of 21 to 25 are associated with mild dementia, scores of 15 to 20 with moderate dementia, scores of 10 to 14 with severe dementia, and scores of 9 or less with profound dementia. The severity of most other symptoms correlates well with the MMSE score.

There is wide agreement now on a seven-stage scale to describe the progression of Alzheimer's (see www.alz.org/alzheimers_disease_stages_of_alzheimers.asp). This scale is probably the most accurate staging system for AD and correlates more closely with the progression of different sets of symptoms through the course of the disease.

The Barthel Index

The Barthel Index (Table 27-1) is a profile scale that rates 10 self-care, continence, and mobility criteria.[136] The specific rating guidelines used in scoring are presented in Appendix 27-A. The advantage of the Barthel Index is its simplicity and usefulness in evaluating patients before, during, and after treatment. It is functionally oriented and may be best used when accompanied by a clinical evaluation.[87] The scale allows documentation of functional changes over time. It is useful when discussing with families the need for help for the patient who cannot manage self-care (ADLs and/or IADLs). Work continues to develop more effective and reliable scales for assessing function and status in people with AD.[137]

STRATEGIES FOR TREATMENT AND CARE

Most elderly people with decreased cognitive abilities live with family or friends and not in institutions. Because of this, the rehabilitation team needs to include the caregivers and the patient as much as possible in treatment planning. The goal of rehabilitation is to ensure that the patient remains safe, independent, and able to perform ADLs and IADLs for as long as is reasonable. The planning to reach these goals is best done within the context of the patient's social support system.

The rehabilitation process begins while the diagnostic workup is still in progress. At this stage of treatment, the rehabilitation plan includes basic training for the patient in performing and adapting the ADLs. It also includes caregiver training and support for significant others so they can make needed environmental modifications to ensure the safety of the patient with dementia.

Once the diagnosis is established, treatment planning for long-term care at home or in an institution must be carefully made. No matter where the patient will be living, involvement of the caregivers and significant others is essential to maximizing functional outcomes. The emotional, physical, and

TABLE 27-1 ■ BARTHEL INDEX

	WITH HELP	INDEPENDENT
1. Feeding (score as "with help" if food needs to be cut)	5	10
2. Moving from wheelchair to bed and return (including sitting up in bed)	5-10*	15
3. Personal toilet (wash face, comb hair, shave, clean teeth)	0*	5
4. Getting on and off toilet (handling clothes, wipe, flush)	5	10
5. Bathing self	0*	5
6. Walking on level surface (or if unable to walk, propel wheelchair)	10	15
7. Ascending and descending stairs	5	10
8. Dressing (includes tying shoes, fastening fasteners)	5	10
9. Controlling bowels	5	10
10. Controlling bladder	5	10

Modified from Mahoney FI, Barthel DW: Functional evaluation: the Barthel index, *Md State Med J* 14:61, 1965.

A patient scoring 100 is continent, feeds himself or herself, dresses, gets up and out of bed and chairs, bathes himself or herself, walks at least a block, and can ascend and descend stairs. This does not mean that he or she is able to live alone. The patient may not be able to cook, keep house, and meet the public but is able to get along without attendant care.

*A score of 0 is given in the activity when the patient cannot meet the criteria as defined (see Appendix 27-A).

financial resources of the patient and family or significant others who will be the caretakers must be ascertained. A review of the caretakers' willingness to perform basic tasks or make visits, their willingness to learn and teach the necessary skills, and the realistic need for respites must be determined.[138] Family training and orientation manuals that deal with all the details of caring for a person with dementia are available (see www.alz.org/living_with_alzheimers.asp).[99] The same detailed orientation is needed for institutional staff who care for elderly patients with dementia. The structure and process of care can help patients be maximally active in their self-care and prevent unnecessary anxiety and catastrophic reactions.

Supporting Families and Caregivers with Their Own Sense of Loss, Frustration, and Helplessness

Family, significant others, and caregivers go through their own coping and adaptive process as the patient experiences gradual or sudden cognitive disturbances.[139] These people have a history with the patient and have expectations about what the relationship and communication should be. As cognitive disturbance occurs, they experience a series of losses because the patient is no longer able to respond and interact as he or she has in the past. With progressive cognitive decline, family and friends experience ongoing losses because the patient is continually changing and less able to relate. For many patients with cognitive disturbances, at the final stage all communication disappears and the family is left with only nonverbal communication or no communication at all. Staff who work with a patient over a period of time also face their own personal reactions of loss, unfulfilled expectations, and a continual need to reassess how to relate effectively to the patient. The responsibility for creating a positive relationship falls on the people who are interacting with the patient. The family and caregivers themselves need training and ongoing support in learning how to nurture and maintain an ongoing relationship with the patient. This requires that caregivers and family members be aware that they are in a healing process as they relate to the loss of the relationship that previously existed.

Epstein: Stages of Healing for Caregivers

Epstein[140] provides a workable description of the stages of healing that occur when major trauma or loss occurs. Epstein defines *healing* as "putting right our wrong relation to our body, to other people and . . . to our own complicated minds, with their emotions and instincts at war with one another and not properly understood and accepted by what we call 'I' or 'me.' The process is one of reorganization, reintegration of things which have come apart."[140] When a patient experiences cognitive changes, the first stage of response by those who care for or love this person is suffering. Chaos exists during this traumatic time. For example, the patient suddenly cannot understand simple directions on how to operate the new electric cart and insists on getting the old one back. The family is upset and arguments ensue. The family and patient together eventually get a medical workup and they are told that "Mom has some type of degenerative cognitive problem." They all experience a profound sense that "something is wrong." The response to helplessness for most human beings is to resist. The lesson of this stage is acceptance. When acceptance is present, then detachment from the emotions is possible. With acceptance present, adaptation and compensation for losses are possible. In the example noted, this would mean that the family would return the new electric cart and have the old (familiar) model refurbished. The family would get training from the therapist in exactly what skills of interaction Mom does not have so that they can work to avoid creating situations in which she feels "stupid and helpless." When a cognitive loss is truly present, training in skills only creates frustration in the patient that may lead to anger and rage. The staff and family need to be trained to understand the exact nature of the losses and provide appropriate compensations in their oral communication and how they relate to the patient.

Stage 2 has been alluded to as a part of stage 1. Therapists, the family, and caregivers search for second opinions, see other types of physicians, and try alternative treatments to gain power over the sense of helplessness. The polarities and rhythms of this process define this stage. All persons involved, even the patient, eventually begin to note that the emotions of the interactions may actually be making things worse. Acceptance that no magic solution is available begins. Everyone involved looks with interest at the proposition, "What can I do to make *this* life—*this* person—cope more effectively and have a reasonable quality of life (regardless of my opinion about what cognitive loss means to me personally)?" The lesson at this stage is another level of acceptance.

The third stage invites an examination of the ways in which people are "stuck in a perspective." When overwhelming stimuli occur, people commonly resort to their favorite strategy from childhood. For some people the favorite strategy is to withdraw, for others it may be to eat to create a distraction, and for others it may be anger. The emotional and mental options created to adapt to a difficult situation are as varied as the human race itself. Human beings dwell in the desire to know why or how to fix something. The lesson of this stage is, again, another level of acceptance and insight about how involved individuals contribute to the problem by reactions at the moment.

Stage 4 begins the process of "reclaiming power." This is the stage at which people realize that the "script" (their internal dialogue) from the last three stages is not workable or even desirable. The anger is recognized and it brings an awareness that this reaction is not helping. Recognition begins that resisting is also not working because the condition of the patient is not affected in a positive way by the emotional reaction on the part of the caregiver(s). The truth of the matter is that the first four stages of healing often cause family and caregivers to be part of the problem and not part of the solution. The problem is how to support the patient to heal and adapt to the cognitive changes, whether temporary or permanent. Family and caregivers need to bring their healing process to their own support system, which needs to be separate from the patient. When caregivers attempt to share their frustration, suffering, sadness, or anger with the patient, the patient is usually upset because she or he cannot comprehend what the details of the issue really are. The patient knows only that people are upset. This will cause the patient to be further upset and agitated. The stages of healing in staff and family must be recognized and services created or referral to support groups made so the patient can interact with people who are able to adapt to his or her needs and not cause further upset.

Stage 5 is called "merging with the illusion" and represents the first step in being able to "relate to the facts in a powerful way" rather than resisting or trying to manipulate them. It is the step at which family and caregivers begin to integrate the facts into their view of the world. The adult son may say, "I hate the fact that my mom cannot live alone; it makes me feel so helpless [or frustrated or angry or upset or inadequate]." Many health care providers get upset when cognitive losses occur in their loved ones. The cognitive loss seems to be a failure that they take personally.

Stage 6 begins with active steps to prepare for the resolution of the emotions connected with the process. Many people describe this stage as the time when they really admit that their parents are never going to be able to give them advice again, babysit, or travel alone. The healing comes in allowing people to notice the emotions that come with accepting these big changes in reality.

Stage 7 brings the actual physical or emotional discharge. The process can be expressed as laughter, crying, fever, the urge to be physically active, sneezing, coughing, and so on. Resolution is marked by a deep sense of peace and inner strength. The person will have gone through the six stages, and the release of emotions or movement results in a deep shift away from resistance. *Family and caregivers need to create their own healing experiences separate from or away from the patient with cognitive losses.* When therapists work with the patient with cognitive losses, they must create for the patient a world that works and is safe and respectful of his or her unique abilities. In most cases the profound emotional and physical release that comes with resolution tends only to upset the patient.

At stage 8 affected individuals are emptied and the board has been wiped clean. In the space of nothingness is an opportunity for new possibilities for relating to the patient. *The relationship should not be based on the past but on moment-to-moment information that comes from the patient.* Therapists can now enjoy being with the patient and begin to feel gratitude. Family and caregivers begin to look for ways to make things work more easily.

Stage 9 is a time when the caregivers and family relate to the energy of the universe and begin to see the connections to all life around them. At this stage, involved individuals begin to see that they are also a part of the great flow of time and energy and that an opportunity for joy exists. The process of illness and dying becomes the focus of awe and a reason to connect with other people and appreciate other people because they are a part of the whole process of life.

Stage 10 is the time to connect with the creative force of the universe. The spiritual process is brought to the issue at hand. A sense of great wisdom and oneness with all creation is felt. *When working from this state of being, the caregiver has the unique capacity to speak or act to bring out the best in others.* In health care, some caregivers have the special gift of allowing themselves to step into the mental world of the other person and thereby create communication that will be heard and that can be acted on even by those with limited mental capacities. The most interesting thing is that the patients can often tell if a caregiver is in this unique state because they will come and sit next to the caregiver or want to hold hands. This state of ease and connection can be learned. A possible resource for exploring these skills is an organization called Landmark Education ([415] 981-8850; www.landmarkeducation.com), which provides programs and courses that examine how people listen, what bias they bring to the communication process, and specific speech strategies to bring out the best in others.

Epstein's stage 11 is when people live day to day without being attached to the situation. Epstein notes that in this stage, "we communicate with ourselves and others through our wounds instead of from them." As healing progresses, caregivers become part of the solution in the care of the patient with cognitive losses. They know they can make a positive difference and take action to create what needs to be done. *They are able to sort out the facts of a situation from the first impression, which is often loaded with judgments and wishful thinking. As caregivers relate to the verifiable facts, they speak to the issues at hand with power and create positive outcomes in which "win-win" becomes the norm.*

In the last stage, caregivers bring their unique individuality to the service of the community. They become aware that the limits to what they can bring to the community are connected to the limits to their sense of wholeness. This insight sends them back to their earlier stages of healing to create further self-awareness and healing on other issues.

In-service training can offer a basic introduction to strategies for lifelong learning, healing, and self-awareness. "What works for me?" "What is the easiest way to learn new skills?" "What strategies enhance adaptability?" This type of learning is nonlinear and is the model a scientist uses to conduct an inquiry. Recently more attention has been paid to managing stress and the role of spirituality in processing grief and loss among caregivers and family.[141-143]

Nonlinear Learning

Nonlinear learning begins with the posing of a question. Then data and information are collected, and additional questions are generated that are related to the first question. At some point an "Aha!" moment or insight occurs. A new relationship is suddenly made possible that was not possible before. Nonlinear learning is not about small gradual steps of progress but occurs as learning balance occurs when riding a bicycle—one minute balance is impossible, and the next is the breakthrough moment. Nonlinear training offers precise strategies that can enhance communication with someone who has cognitive deficits. Nonlinear learning is built on scientific communication that operates on the basis of verifiable facts at the present moment. Nonlinear learning invites each person to examine all strategies for communication to be sure that problems are not occurring as a result of misinterpretation of the facts. Communication can occur without verbal language, and fear does not need to be present. When a patient has cognitive deficits, the art and science of human interaction need to be precise so that caregivers do not speak in words that are not understandable to the patient. Which caregiver prejudgments are brought to the interaction with the patient needs to be understood: experiencing the stage of awe, sharing joy in the moment, or suffering because the person is "difficult"? The care and therapy provided to a person with cognitive disturbances need to be created based on the facts of the moment and carried out in a state of gratitude, vulnerability, and nurturing for the staff and the patient.

Role of the Physical Therapist: Development of Interventions and Caregiver Training

All persons with cognitive losses should have access to caregivers who are trained to manage emotional responses in order to provide precise strategies for communication with those with dementia. A gracious and secure existence is possible even when cognition is diminished if the caregivers are committed to adapting the environment and its demands to match the capacity of the patient. The challenge for health care is designing training programs that truly prepare families and caregivers to be effective, empowering communicators. All caregivers need training to create this experience for a person with cognitive deficits.

As a part of the rehabilitation program, caregiver training for this group of patients needs to emphasize reassurance, hands-on interventions, and communication to allow treatment to proceed at a pace perceived as reasonable by the patient.[67] In the early and middle stages of all dementias, physical therapy intervention usually can prolong the ability to move with ease in ADLs and IADLs and maintain the ability to participate in some social activities. This is extremely important for caregivers because deficits in the patient's ability to perform ADLs and IADLs often relate to the inability to physically perform these activities under supervision.[47] The ability to walk is lost late in most dementias, but gait and coordination disturbances are common and can benefit from physical therapy.[144-146] Therapeutic intervention to assist the patient and train the caregivers involves facilitation of ease of movement and motor planning and developing or refining environmental and cognitive cues to assist in carrying out complex tasks. Ultimately, caregivers require training in how to move, lift, and otherwise assist the patient.

Although not able to reverse the progressive cognitive decline, the exercise intervention that the physical therapist can develop may improve the level of function, confidence, vitality, and safety of the patient and ease the burden of care for the caregivers. Research is beginning to establish an important role for exercise in maintaining physical activity[147,148]; contributing to general health and slowing of cognitive decline[149-152]; as well as maintaining strength and aerobic conditioning.[153] Guidelines for exercise prescription include aerobic, strength, balance, coordination, and flexibility activities determined by direct assessment, and suggestions for motivational and problem-solving strategies. The Seattle Protocols are an important contribution in this area.[154,155] Research shows that exercise not only increases strength, coordination, and aerobic capacity but also creates beneficial changes in brain plasticity.[156-158] Further studies need to be done to work out more clearly what types of exercise are beneficial in what ways for what populations.[159]

Cognitive impairment is a key limiting factor in the performance of ADLs and IADLs as well as a limiting factor for participating in rehabilitation. Accurate assessment and training by the therapist helps the caregiver provide only the help that is absolutely needed, with patients continuing to perform for themselves as many ADLs as possible. For example, when brushing the teeth, the patient needs to be able to remember the command to brush, must recognize the toothbrush, and must perform a complex but repetitive motor action. The patient may only need the help of someone placing the toothbrush in his or her hand and slowly guiding it to the mouth to be able to safely brush the teeth.

The accurate assessment of IADLs and ADLs is more reliable than medical diagnosis for predicting the amount of assistance and interaction a person will need in a nursing home (see Table 27-1 and Appendix 27-A).[136] The first goal of rehabilitation for patients with dementia is to create a supportive emotional and physical environment. In other words, the environment must actively work to compensate for the patient's cognitive and functional losses as they occur. The ultimate goal is to help patients feel they are capable so that they will continue to try to do those things for themselves that they can do safely, whether they remain in their home or live in an institution. Orientation and training of significant others is also important so they feel comfortable allowing the patient to participate safely in activities and basic self-care tasks modified to their cognitive level.

The Alzheimer's Association ([800] 272-3900; www.alz.org) is a resource for professionals and caregivers of people with dementia. The goals of the association are the following:

- To support research related to the diagnosis, therapy, cause, and cure of AD and related disorders
- To aid in organizing family support groups; to educate and assist affected families
- To sponsor educational programs for professionals and laypersons on the topic of AD

- To advise government agencies of the needs of the affected families and to promote federal, state, and private support of research
- To offer help in any manner to patients and their caregivers to promote the well-being of all involved

The Alzheimer's Association promotes the provision of humane care to the patient with dementia or related disorders throughout the course of the illness. Other support groups have been tried in communities in which spouses have worked to develop ongoing respite care.[160]

As a member of the rehabilitation team, the physical or occupational therapist can conduct an inventory of services as a part of the annual review of the quality of care that is provided for a patient with dementia. Surveys of persons caring for patients with dementia listed the following services in their perceived order of importance[83,161]:

1. A paid companion who can come to the home a few hours each week to give caregivers a rest (respite)
2. Assistance in locating people or organizations to provide patient care
3. Assistance in applying for government programs, such as Medicaid, disability insurance, and income support programs
4. A paid companion who can come to the home for overnight care so caregivers can go away for one or more days (respite)
5. Personal home care for the person with dementia to help with activities such as bathing, dressing, or feeding in the home
6. Support groups composed of others who are caring for persons with dementia and other cognitive deficits
7. Special nursing home care programs only for persons with dementia and other cognitive deficits while the caregiver is away
8. Adult day care providing supervision and activities away from the home
9. Visiting nurse services for care at home

In the home care category, information about the availability of services and government programs and various forms of respite care were also ranked high in the survey. Overall, caregivers (family and friends) of the patient are often able and willing to provide care for the patient throughout the illness if appropriate professional consultation can help them cope with problematic situations and if adequate respite time is provided to the caregiver(s).

Not mentioned in this chapter was the need for psychological support for caregivers. The stress on caregivers is extreme, and symptoms of anxiety and depression are common. Because of the relative lack of counseling services for caregivers, however, the use of (and probable abuse of and dependence on) psychotropic medications by caregivers is high.[60,162] Because these medications may impair the cognitive functioning of caregivers, the risk of harm to the patient with dementia is also high.

DEMENTIA AND DELIRIUM: NEW FRONTIERS

Most current research in delirium and dementia is focused on AD. The Alzheimer's Association is the largest private foundation funding research on dementia, supporting on average about 100 projects totaling almost $15 million annually. Research is underway to explore possible causes of dementia, including work that examines the roles of neurotransmitters, structural brain changes, nutrition, viruses, drugs, immunological deficits, and heredity in the etiology of AD. Studies to increase the diagnostic accuracy of different forms of dementia, including making a distinction between cortical and subcortical dementia[161] or using *Diagnostic and Statistical Manual of Mental Disorders,* Fourth Edition, Text Revision (DSM-IV-TR) criteria[163] or neuropsychological criteria, are also underway. Newer diagnostic models of dementia, including that caused by stage II or III human immunodeficiency virus infection, are also being studied.[164,165] New research that may shed light on the mechanisms of the early stages of AD relates to other neurodegenerative diseases. Persons with dementia who also have parkinsonian symptoms, delusions, and hallucinations have been reported to experience faster decline that those who do not.[166] This research team found a relation between the presence of Lewy bodies (abnormal structures in the brain that contain a protein called *synuclein*) and parkinsonian symptoms; affected individuals had lower survival rates than those with either symptom present by itself.

The most exciting area of research is pharmacology (see Chapter 36). The advent of tacrine, a drug that slows down the progression of AD in some patients, has produced an explosion of research on drugs aimed at stabilizing or reversing the symptoms of this disease. Although no cures are available, some drugs, such as physostigmine, ondansetron, and nerve growth factor, have shown some promise. These studies have spawned a search for new drugs to treat both AD and the symptoms of other dementias.[167-169]

Research is also being funded that is investigating the best ways to provide care and support in the home and at long-term residential settings.[33]

SUMMARY

Why some people stay lively and creative in their older years is not known; Michelangelo designed St Peter's when he was nearly 90; Picasso painted at 90; and Arthur Rubenstein, Pablo Casals, and Martha Graham all worked creatively in their older years. What is clear is that lonely, isolated older people are much more likely to be confused and disoriented than their peers who remain actively involved with family and friends. Perhaps what is needed is to invite the world to explore rules of conduct in which older persons are honored and included.

In working with an older person with dementia or delirium, the therapist can do much to make the quality of life better for the patient, family, and caregivers.[99] A thorough listing of the details needed to develop an environment and process of care for elderly persons with cognitive deficits can be found in other texts (see www.alz.org/living_with_alzheimers.asp).[99,131]

Specific examples of modifications of physical and occupational therapy examination and treatment may include working in collaboration with the family, close friends, and other members of the rehabilitation team and developing a consultative relationship with key caregivers (professional and nonprofessional and all shifts of institutional staff) to encourage problem solving and patient participation in self-care. Another important modification includes the evaluation of each patient's communication abilities before the therapy assessment to adapt the assessment in such a way as to promote patient participation. Case Study examples are presented later in this chapter (refer to Case Studies 27-1 and 27-2) to provide clinical scenarios and corresponding physical and occupational therapy examination and treatment strategies.

CASE STUDY 27-1 ■ THE COMPLEXITY OF AGING

The patient was a 78-year-old woman who had the following deficits on the MMSE: was not aware of where she lived, the date, or the year; had poor short-term memory; could not spell the word "world" backward; could not copy two overlapping pentagons. The patient was generally happy and enjoyed having someone sit with her. The patient had fractured her femur and because of the location of the fracture site, a surgical procedure was performed to allow total weight bearing. The surgeon and the psychiatrist decided that partial weight bearing would not be a concept that the patient could understand. The physical therapist and assistant worked together with the family and caregivers in the nursing home to develop a plan of care. At the initial care conference, the main question was whether the patient should receive physical therapy. The family was fearful that the patient would fall again if she were taught how to walk. The focus of the conference was to educate the family and other staff regarding the importance of physical therapy so the patient could learn how to participate in and eventually perform transfers from wheelchair to toilet as well as to bed. The decision was made to begin physical therapy, with the initial goal being to achieve all functional ADL transfers with standby physical assistance.

The patient was not interested in walking and was fearful of falling. The key change in physical therapy intervention was in the style of communication used to teach basic bed mobility and the components of transfer skills. Through use of trial and error it was determined that the patient responded best to a smile, verbal encouragement, hand signals, and gentle manual pressure to indicate the desired task to be performed. If the task was broken down and components were identified, the patient became frustrated and refused to participate. If the patient was invited by manual cues and verbal reassurance to stand up and sit on the bed, the patient would hesitate for up to 1 minute and then she would attempt to perform the task. It became obvious that the patient needed at least 30 to 60 seconds of waiting time between when a verbal request was made and when she was ready to act on the request. If additional time was not given, the patient appeared to get frustrated and would refuse to cooperate. A sign was placed over her bed with instructions for communication: smile, reassure, use your hands to guide her to perform the desired action, and wait 60 seconds; let her feel there is plenty of time.

A sliding board was introduced in therapy, and the patient enjoyed the idea. The board allowed transfers for all ADLs to involve no lifting for the staff. The patient would lean her head on the shoulder of the staff member while sitting and then she would assist in sliding across on the board. All transfers for ADLs using the sliding board were possible within five visits of physical therapy. A bed was located that was 17 inches high to facilitate bed-to-wheelchair transfers. The bed could be raised to assist the nursing aide in cleaning activities. The decision was made to leave the bed at 17 inches unless the nursing staff needed to perform special in-bed procedures with the patient. The wheelchair footrests were modified so that they formed a solid flat surface to allow the patient to rest in a natural position. The patient was only 5 feet 2 inches tall, and the standard wheelchair allowed her only to comfortably put both feet on one foot pedal and sit with her weight mostly on one buttock. A smaller wheelchair and the adapted footrest gave the patient an equal pressure on both sitting bones, and the patient began to sit at rest in a natural upright posture. The other goal of physical therapy was to teach the patient wheelchair mobility by using her hands to push the chair. Once the patient was given gloves for her hands (she did not like germs), she was willing to try to push the wheelchair. The patient was instructed in the physical therapy department during two visits. The patient was next seen by the therapist on the unit to allow the nurse's aide to be a part of the physical therapy instruction. The rationale was that the nurse's aide would need to help reinforce the skills and encourage practice of wheelchair mobility skills as a part of daily activities. During the last visits the physical therapist watched daytime, afternoon, and evening staff practice with the patient and addressed new situations that arose. All caregivers on three shifts were trained to ensure consistency of verbal and manual cuing for the patient.

Before discharge to restorative nursing, the patient's current level of functional abilities was documented by using an ADL chart that specified time of day when tasks were easiest, task(s), equipment needs, special positioning, clothing and other assistive devices, verbal cuing, and other communication requirements for each critical task that had been mastered in physical therapy. The cataloging of functional skills reminded the nurse's aide of the ingredients involved for the patient to successfully perform ADLs. The other advantage of the detailed discharge summary to the nursing staff was that new staff could use the document and, as needed, contact physical therapy for clarifications if the patient suddenly were not able to perform the tasks (a signal of possible medical or psychosocial problems).

KEY POINTS

1. Common goals were identified and agreed on among all team members and the patient's significant others.
2. Education was provided as needed to allow for consistency of verbal and manual cuing to the patient.
3. Physical therapy treatment began in a quiet, undisturbed area where the patient could concentrate. As mastery of a skill was achieved, the skill was practiced with supervision, and instruction of other staff was provided as needed.
4. Equipment and furniture were adjusted to help the patient perform tasks with minimal assistance.
5. Discharge from therapy involved providing nursing staff with a detailed description of functional abilities and the conditions required to help maximize patient participation, sense of safety, and control (as had already been reviewed with all aides working with the patient).
6. The physical therapist was designated as a resource person for nursing staff for simplifying functional tasks in patient care, problem solving, communication, and movement-related issues.

CASE STUDY 27-2 ■ A CLIENT IN THE EARLY STAGE OF ALZHEIMER DISEASE

The patient was a 64-year-old man who until 1 month ago was working. He was forced to retire because he kept forgetting the natural sequences of the work tasks. For example, his partner would see him direct someone to wait for him in the waiting room and then he would forget the person was in the waiting room. On the MMSE, he had difficulty with date and year and would try to redirect the question in an apparent attempt to cover up for loss of short-term memory. He could not or would not spell the word "world" backward, and he poorly copied the overlapping hexagons (looked more like squares). He was a runner but now he apparently could not remember how to get home, and he would pretend to be hurt and get someone to drive him home. The man reported feeling restless.

The patient, his wife, and two sons were seen by the team at a psychiatric clinic. The wife was very upset and the family was asking for help. The role of therapy at this early stage of AD involved the following:

1. Functional assessment of basic ADLs and IADLs and home assessment.
2. Orientation of spouse and significant caregivers regarding the functional changes that could occur in the near future and how to compensate for current functional losses (e.g., patient had difficulty dressing in the morning and would get frustrated).
3. Orientation to the role of therapy in hands-on treatment related to techniques to help the patient relax. After initial evaluation, the team decided to teach caregivers massage techniques identified by the therapist as soothing and relaxing for the patient. (Note: The emphasis in hands-on intervention is to create slow, predictable, and nurturing contact that is perceived by the patient as soothing and relaxing.)
4. Orientation of caregivers to the use of manual contact and hand signals to communicate and reinforce the intention. Kinesthetic contact and the ability to follow kinesthetic cues can help the patient with ADL tasks at home. At this time the kinesthetic cuing may not be critical for the patient, but the caregivers need to get in the habit of cuing the patient as a compensatory tool for future cognitive losses.
5. Orientation of caregivers to the benefits of a ritualized schedule of daily events for the patient and assistance in developing the daily schedule. The predictability of the ritual would help the patient feel safe and in control. The ritualizing would be especially helpful to address the frustrations with dressing in the morning.
6. Written information about local support groups, day treatment centers, and the availability of the rehabilitation team, including therapy for problem solving.
7. Participation in evaluation of patient and family need for placement in a day treatment center or use of a home health aide. Supervision was needed for cooking (he would leave burners on), working in the woodshop (he would leave power tools running), and in self-care to ensure his safety. Supervision in the home was decided, with family members sharing the load. The idea of going to a new place was not positively received by the patient. (Note: The patient may function better in the environment where he or she has lived for a long time because of the familiarity with the details of the surroundings.)
8. The therapist participated in development of the home care plan and provided for home visits to accomplish tasks described in items 1 through 7. The next contact that the family made with therapy was 1 month later to address the patient's inability to settle down and be able to go to sleep at night. A home visit was made to evaluate the bedtime ritual, the relaxation strategies being used, and communication with the physician about current medications taken. The patient disliked bathing and undressing for bed. After discussion with caregivers the patient was allowed to go to bed in his clothes without bathing and undressing (bathing and undressing would be carried out in the morning when he was less tired). Relaxation massage was modified to involve the face, neck, hands, and feet, and the caregivers were instructed and practiced during two visits under the supervision of the therapist. A satisfactory bedtime ritual was developed, and home health care was workable for the patient and the caregivers.

The next request for therapy consultation came 4 months later when the wife and the daughter-in-law (who had been taking turns being the primary caregiver) both felt the need to hire and train an attendant-companion for the patient for 8 hours a day. At this time the patient preferred to be in the home, walk in the yard, or take long walks in the local park. The therapist, in cooperation with other team members, trained the patient and aide in how to sequence for ease in ADL tasks; use of kinesthetic cuing; how to facilitate ADLs, bathing, and dressing with a slow pace and ritualized format; and how to sequence the tasks and relaxation techniques to help the patient settle down and go to sleep. Foot massage was the only technique that the patient now allowed and appeared to enjoy. After three physical therapy visits over a 2-week period, the attendant was able to carry out home health care effectively for the patient.

The last request for help occurred when the family was concerned because the patient was trying to run away. The therapist made a home visit and found that the patient sat most of the day. The MMSE showed that he could not give his own first or last name and had no short-term memory. Based on the evaluation, the therapist proposed that the family or attendant go with the patient for a walk when the patient showed an interest in leaving the house. This strategy worked for a few months, but then the patient began to sit down on the sidewalk when he was tired. Another visit was made after a wheelchair was ordered to train the caregivers in use of the wheelchair and to orient the patient to the desired procedures and to reassure the patient. After this visit the patient showed gradually less interest in leaving the home over the next few months until he eventually stayed in the house constantly. At this time the patient also became incontinent of bowel and bladder. The patient refused to use the toilet and the decision was made to seek nursing home placement.

CASE STUDY 27-2 ■ A CLIENT IN THE EARLY STAGE OF ALZHEIMER DISEASE—cont'd

KEY POINTS

1. Physical (or occupational) therapy is a part of the team providing guidance and care for the patient and the family of the patient with AD and other dementias.
2. Evaluation of functional skills, communication related to functional skills, and home modifications to enhance patient participation in self-care can be continued as long as the caregivers request support and help problem solving.
3. Problem solving with caregivers and educating caregivers are the primary roles once the therapist has identified the intervention of choice to solve the key functional problems.
4. All therapy intervention needs to be coordinated with actions of others providing care for the patient (family, neighbors, and friends as well as other health care providers).

Modifications of treatment include the use of gentle, nonverbal neurological rehabilitation techniques (e.g., the Feldenkrais Method). The key is to acknowledge the now well-established research finding that nondeclarative learning and memory (procedural) are available long after declarative learning and memory (ability to consciously learn and remember facts and events) are lost for a person with AD. Motor ability is one of the last areas to be affected by AD.[170] Assisting a person with AD to edit procedural memory and increase walking safety is therefore possible. The functional outcomes of this learning can include a decrease in abnormal muscle tone, enhanced sensory awareness and organization for the position of the eyes and head in space, an increase in the ease of movement, an increase in the ease of breathing, enhanced endurance, minimized anxiety, minimized resting muscle rigidity in the chest, and increased patient coordination. The therapist needs to modify the process of neurological facilitation by decreasing patient effort and adding extra cuing and more frequent breaks for integration of learning. Tasks may need to be simplified so that the patient can perform them, and the caregiver is trained to perform only those tasks that the patient cannot perform.

Each month the therapist, treatment team, patient, and caregiver(s) need to identify safe physical activities that the patient can be encouraged to perform for recreation, relaxation, and overall fitness. The goal is to enhance the performance of simple ADL and IADL tasks (e.g., washing socks, setting the table), which can enhance patient self-esteem. In addition, the physical therapist, along with other members of the rehabilitation team and caregivers, needs to monitor the patient for new signs and symptoms of concurrent delirium or reversible dementia so that treatment can be initiated early and further deterioration can be prevented.

A hospital and nursing home patients' "Bill of Rights" defines the minimal quality of care required for any patient. The concepts presented apply to the care of patients with cognitive deficits no matter what the setting. The provision of considerate and respectful care for the patient with dementia or other cognitive deficits is possible and necessary. Well-planned and gentle care prevents unnecessary distortions in cognitive function brought on by feelings of fear or being rushed and thereby maximizes all remaining cognitive function. To use his or her remaining emotional and cognitive resources, the patient with cognitive deficits needs to live in an environment and experience a process of care that is modified to meet the special needs created by delirium or dementia.

Major efforts are underway in research to discover a cure for AD. In 1997 a consensus conference on the diagnosis and treatment of AD and related disorders was organized by the American Association for Geriatric Psychiatry, the Alzheimer's Association, and the American Geriatrics Society. The conclusions of the conference included the following statement:

"AD is the most common disorder causing cognitive decline in old age and exacts a substantial toll on society. Although the diagnosis of AD is often missed or delayed, it is primarily one of inclusion, not exclusion, and usually can be made using standardized clinical criteria. Most cases can be diagnosed and managed in primary care settings, yet some patients with atypical presentations, severe impairment, or complex co-morbidity benefit from specialist referral. AD is progressive and irreversible, but pharmacologic therapies for cognitive impairment and non-pharmacologic and pharmacologic treatments for behavioral problems associated with dementia can enhance quality of life. Psychotherapeutic intervention with family members is often indicated, as nearly half of all caregivers become depressed. Health care delivery to these patients is fragmented and inadequate."[36]

Physical and occupational therapy are key resources for the creation of a therapeutic environment and for the effective and timely assessment and treatment of the patient with cognitive deficits (presuming that the therapy can take into account the need to affect procedural learning directly—i.e., the Feldenkrais Method). The goal of therapy is to create a process of care in which the patient feels safe and the caregivers are given training and support in problem solving to guide the patient to participate in self-care, ambulation, and recreation as long as it is safe and functionally possible.

Caregiver agreements can enhance the capacity of older persons with dementia to participate in daily life—exploring the possibility of living a life with safety, dignity, and love. Following is a brief list of basic environmental supports for encouraging procedural memory to be activated:

1. I will ask my patient if he or she would like to pray or worship today, and I will make arrangements to meet those needs.
2. I will speak or communicate in a way that is functional and workable for the patient.
3. I will repeat what I hear and perceive back to the patient to ensure that I capture her or his perspective.
4. I will encourage natural participation by creating a pace that is pleasant for the patient.
5. I will close doors quietly.
6. I will not raise my voice and shout except in a real emergency.

7. I will talk to someone on staff when I get upset or take something personally so I can have peace with co-workers, creating a positive atmosphere for the patients to live in.
8. I will offer to warm up the patient's tea or coffee and make sure it is not so hot that it could cause a burn.
9. I will create only one choice at a time so the patient can understand and then choose yes or no.
10. I will know what "my" patient has eaten on my shift.
11. I will know my patients' timing for toileting so I can support their continence and dignity.
12. I will tell the patient I am going to touch him or her before I do so, to avoid surprises.
13. I will walk (rolling or ambulating) with every one of my patients outdoors as often as possible or at least every 3 days to encourage good sleep and mental and physical stimulation.
14. I will sit and visit with each of my patients for 10 minutes (every shift).
15. I promise to listen with an open heart to the patients' perception of life at the moment.
16. I promise to close the blinds in every room at night (unless the patient requests otherwise) and open blinds every morning to reinforce day-night orientation.
17. I will discover and use the "personal" get ready for bed routine for all patients so they sleep well.
18. I promise to talk and walk at a pace that encourages a sense of safety for my patients.
19. I promise to be self-nurturing and come to work well rested and ready to share myself.
20. I promise to avoid confrontational actions and body language except in an emergency.
21. I promise to respect the unique ergonomics of each patient and adapt as needed.
22. I promise to offer to add support to explore ways to increase comfort.
23. I promise to notice how my patients relate so no one agitates or bothers another.
24. I promise to be kind to myself, other staff, and my patients.
25. I promise to be of service and adapt to meet my patients' needs.
26. I promise to report problems (equipment, environment, relationships) to the person who can do something about them.
27. I promise not to gossip (talk about others so that it leaves a negative impression and no resolution of the problem).
28. I promise to leave my workspace clean and restocked after I have taken care of the patient (or at least to leave a note to alert the next shift about what has not been done).

DEDICATION

A personal note: This chapter was written for my grandmother. She had depression and related cognitive disturbances after World War II. She gradually got worse and worse in her ability to remember new information, but she could hold my hand and show me how to feed the ducks. We were great friends. I helped her remember to turn off the stove, and I remembered where she put her glasses. She could make sandwiches, and I could always find her comb. We empowered each other. Over 15 years she gradually grew more and more helpless in the adult skills of life. Even then she could give great hugs and loved to sit and drink tea with me. I remember her as a very frail woman. I watched the nurse's aide tuck her in, kiss her on the cheek, and hold her hand while they said prayers. The aide hummed a familiar song as she left the room. It was like those familiar songs that come from our childhood, and they wrap us in a sense of warmth and love and safety—we declare that all is well with the world and we go to sleep and dream of peaceful things.

References

To enhance this text and add value for the reader, all references are included on the companion Evolve site that accompanies this textbook. This online service will, when available, provide a link for the reader to a Medline abstract for the article cited. There are 170 cited references and other general references for this chapter, with the majority of those articles being evidence-based citations.

APPENDIX 27-A ■ Rating Guidelines for Barthel Index*

1. Feeding
   10 = Independent. The patient can feed himself or herself a meal when someone puts the food within reach. Patient must put on an assistive device if needed to cut up the food alone. The patient must accomplish this in a reasonable time.
   5 = Some help is necessary (with cutting up food, and so on, as listed above).
2. Moving from wheelchair to bed and return
   15 = Independent in all phases of this activity. Patient can safely approach the bed in the wheelchair, lock brakes, lift footrests, move safely to bed, lie down, come to a sitting position in the wheelchair if necessary to transfer back into it safely, and return to the wheelchair.
   10 = Either some minimal help is needed in some step of this activity or the patient needs to be reminded or supervised for safety in one or more parts of this activity.
   5 = Patient can come to a sitting position without the help of a second person but needs to be lifted out of bed, or he or she transfers only with a great deal of help.
3. Doing personal toileting
   5 = Patient can wash hands and face, comb hair, clean teeth, and shave. He may use any kind of razor but must put in blade or plug in razor without help as well as get it from drawer or cabinet. Female patients must put on own makeup.
4. Getting on and off toilet
   10 = Patient is able to get on and off toilet, fasten and unfasten clothes, prevent soiling of clothes, and use toilet paper without help. If a bedpan is necessary instead of a toilet, patient must be able to place it on a chair, empty it, and clean it.
   5 = Patient needs help because of imbalance or with handling clothes or using toilet paper.
5. Bathing self
   5 = Patient may use a bathtub or a shower or take a complete sponge bath. Patient must be able to do all the steps involved in whichever method is used without another person being present.
6. Walking on a level surface
   15 = Patient can walk at least 50 yards without help or supervision. Patient may wear braces or prostheses and use crutches, canes, or a walker (but not a rolling walker). Patient must be able to lock and unlock braces, if used; assume the standing position and sit down; get the necessary mechanical aids into position for use; and dispose of them when sitting. (Putting on and taking off braces is scored under dressing.)
   10 = Patient needs help or supervision in any of the above but can walk at least 50 yards with a little help.

6a. Propelling a wheelchair
   5 = Patient cannot ambulate but can propel a wheelchair independently. Must be able to go around corners, turn around, and maneuver the chair to a table, bed, toilet, and so on. Must be able to push a chair at least 50 yards. (Do not score this item if the patient gets a score for walking.)

7. Ascending and descending stairs
   10 = Patient is able to go up and down a flight of stairs safely without help or supervision. Patient may and should use handrails, canes, or crutches when needed. Must be able to carry canes or crutches when ascending or descending stairs.
   5 = Patient needs help with or supervision during any one of the above items.
8. Dressing and undressing
   10 = Patient is able to put on, remove, and fasten all clothing as well as tie shoelaces (unless adaptations are necessary). The activity includes putting on, removing, and fastening corset or braces when these are prescribed.
   5 = Patient needs help putting on and removing or fastening any clothing. Patient must do at least half the work. Patient must accomplish this in a reasonable time. Women need not be scored on use of a brassiere or girdle unless these are prescribed garments.
9. Continence of bowels
   10 = Patient is able to control bowels and have no accidents. Can use a suppository or take an enema when necessary.
   5 = Patient needs help in using a suppository or taking an enema or has occasional accidents.
10. Controlling bladder
   10 = Patient is able to control his or her bladder day and night. Patients who wear an external device and leg bag must put them on independently, clean and empty bag, and stay dry day and night.
   5 = Patient has occasional accidents or cannot wait for the bedpan or get to the toilet in time or needs help with an external device.

Modified from Mahoney FI, Barthel DW: Functional evaluation: the Barthel index, *Md State Med J* 14:63, 1965.

*A patient scoring 100 is continent, feeds, dresses, gets up and out of bed and chairs, bathes himself or herself, walks at least a block, and can ascend and descend stairs. This does not mean that he or she is able to live alone. The patient may not be able to cook, keep house, and meet the public but is able to get along without attendant care. A score of 0 is given in the activity when the patient cannot meet the criteria as defined.

SECTION III

Neurological Disorders and Applications Issues

CHAPTER 28 Disorders of Vision and Visual-Perceptual Dysfunction

LAURIE RUTH CHAIKIN, MS, OTR/L, OD, FCOVD

KEY TERMS

anatomy of the eye
eye diseases
functional visual skills
refractive error
strabismus
treatment
visual-perceptual dysfunction
visual rehab
visual screening

OBJECTIVES

After reading this chapter the student or therapist will be able to:

1. Identify and analyze visual anatomy and physiology as they pertain to visual function.
2. Analyze the functional visual skills and how visual dysfunction may affect functional performance.
3. Identify the symptoms of visual dysfunction.
4. Develop the skill necessary to take a visual case history by use of behaviors and clinical observations.
5. Identify the difference between phoria and strabismus.
6. Identify and evaluate the difference between visual field loss and unilateral neglect.
7. Identify and differentiate various pediatric and age-related disease conditions that may affect vision.
8. Clearly differentiate nonoptical and optical assessment and intervention adaptations for patients with low vision.
9. Differentiate basic tools for vision screening.
10. Identify when and why to refer and the tools necessary to document that decision.

Vision is an integral part of development of perception. Some aspects of vision, such as pupillary function, are innate, but many other aspects are stimulated to develop by experience and interaction with the environment. Visual acuity itself has been demonstrated to rely on the presence of a clear image focused on the retina. If this does not occur, a "lazy eye," or amblyopia, will result. Depth perception develops as a result of precise eye alignment. This ability will be delayed, less precise, or absent if correction of eye misalignment is not done within the first 7 years of life. Research has demonstrated that, in fact, most visual skills such as acuity, binocular coordination, accommodation, ocular motilities, and depth perception are largely intact by age 6 months to 1 year.[1] Visual skill development parallels postural reflex integration and provides a foundation for perception.

Early in infancy visual input is associated with olfactory, tactile, vestibular, and proprioceptive sensations. The infant is driven to touch, taste, smell, and manipulate what he or she sees. Primitive postural reflexes such as the asymmetrical tonic neck reflex help to provide visual regard and attention.

At some point the young child is able to look at an object and determine both the texture and the shape without having to touch or taste it. In adults, vision has moved to the top of the sensory hierarchy, providing full multisensory associations from sight alone. Even the visualized image of eating an apple can recreate the smell, sound of crunching, taste, and feel of the experience.

Early visual impairment and later acquired impairment can affect the quality of the image presented to the brain and thus affect the learning process. In addition, damage to association centers involved with spatial perception, figure-ground, and directionality can interfere with learning and performance. Altered function may be the result of congenital and developmental disorders, birth trauma, physical trauma, or neurological or systemic diseases. It is important, therefore, to isolate the primary visual processes of seeing from the secondary or associational processes of perceiving in the evaluation of perceptual disorders. The identification of a vision problem becomes part of the differential diagnosis of a perceptual deficit. Visual screening must be done before perceptual evaluation so that visual problems do not bias or contaminate the perceptual testing. It is just as important to eliminate vision as a contributing factor to a perceptual problem as it is to find a possible vision problem.

Our understanding of the ability to improve vision or recover visual function frequently needs to be updated as we apply new research and understanding of neuroplasticity. Principles of visual rehabilitation involve understanding how to provide visual feedback to the system in an optimal learning environment for the patient. The boundaries of improvement are slowly expanding as we refine this understanding.

ANATOMY OF THE EYE

An operational analogy of the eye as a camera may be useful up to a point in understanding the physical function of the structures. Once an image hits the retina and image enhancement begins, however, metaphors must change to match our ever-changing comprehension of brain function. Using computer analogies such as microprocessing of feature detectors comes closer. Many aspects of how we see remain a mystery inside the "black box" of our brain.

Eye Chamber and Lens

Structures and function are discussed from anterior to posterior (Figure 28-1). The first structure that light hits after it is reflected from an image is the cornea. (Technically, light first hits the tear layer, which has its own structure and rests on the corneal surface.) Corneal tissue is completely transparent. Light is refracted, or bent, to the greatest degree by the cornea because the light rays must pass through different media, which change in density, as in going from air to water.[2] The refraction of light can be observed by noting how a stick placed into water appears bent where it enters the water (Figure 28-2).

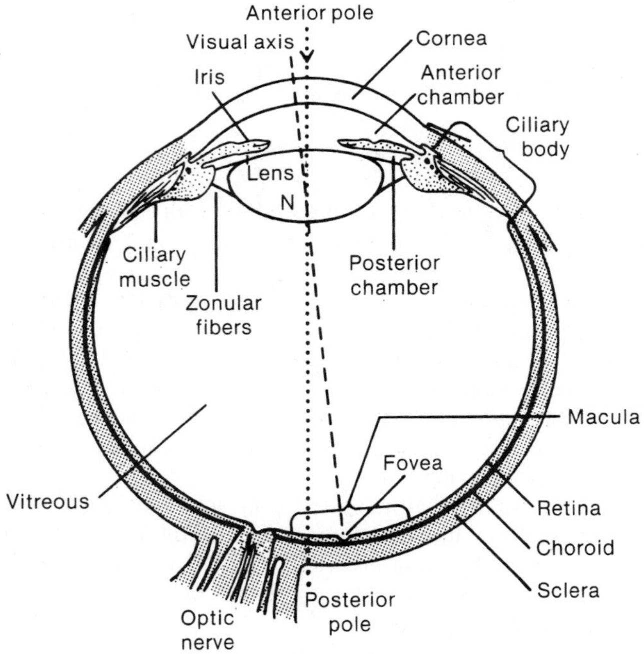

Figure 28-1 ■ Horizontal section of the eye. (Modified from Wolff E: *Anatomy of the eye and orbit,* ed 7, London, 1976, HK Lewis.)

Damage to the cornea from abrasions, burns, or congenital or disease-related processes can alter the spherical shape of the cornea and disturb the quality of the image that falls on the retina. Radial keratotomy, a surgical procedure done in the 1980s to reduce nearsightedness by placing spokelike cuts in the cornea, sometimes had the side effect of scarring the cornea and causing distorted vision. This surgery is no longer done. The newer surgeries such as laser-assisted in situ keratomileusis (LASIK) are far superior and more predictable in their reduction of refractive error (nearsightedness, farsightedness, or astigmatism) and induce virtually no scarring or distortion. In keratoconus the cornea slowly becomes steeper and more cone shaped, distorting the image and causing reduced vision.[3]

Iris

Behind the cornea is the iris, or colored portion, which consists of fibers that control the opening of the pupil, the dark circular opening in the center of the eye. The constriction and dilation of the pupil control the amount of light entering the eye in a similar fashion to the way the f-stop on a camera changes the size of the aperture to control the amount of light and the depth of field.[4] Under bright light conditions the opening constricts, and under dim light conditions it dilates, allowing light in to stimulate the photoreceptor cells of the retina. This constriction and dilation are under autonomic nervous system (ANS) control, with both sympathetic and parasympathetic components.[5] Under conditions of sympathetic stimulation (fight or flight) the pupils dilate, perhaps giving rise to the expression "eyes wide with fear." Under parasympathetic stimulation the pupils constrict. The effect of drugs that stimulate the ANS can be observed.[6] For example, someone who has taken heroin will have pinpoint pupils.

Exercise 28-1: Observation of Pupillary Constriction and Dilation

Observe pupillary dilation and constriction on a willing subject (or on yourself in a mirror) by flashing a penlight at her or his pupil. Observe the decreased size of the pupil. Remove the light and watch the pupil dilate.

Lens

Behind the iris is the lens. The lens is involved in focusing, or accommodation. It is a biconvex, circular, semirigid, crystalline structure that fine-tunes the image on the retina. In a camera the lens is represented by the external optical lens system. The ability to change the focus on the camera is achieved by turning the lens to change the distance of the lens from the film, which effectively increases or decreases the power of the lens, allowing near or distance objects to be seen more clearly. The same effect, a change in the

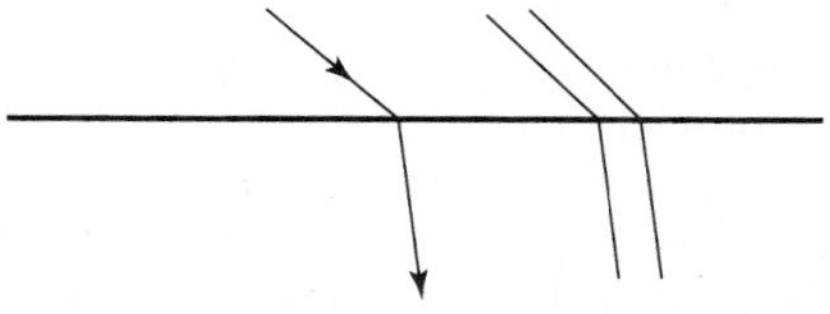

Figure 28-2 ■ Refraction: bending of light at air-water interface.

power of the lens, is achieved in the eye by the action of tiny ciliary muscles, which act on suspensory ligaments, thereby changing the thickness and curvature of the lens. A thicker lens with a greater curvature produces higher power and the ability to see clearly at near distances. A thinner lens and flatter curvature produces less optical power, which is what is needed to allow distant objects to be clear (Figure 28-3). The process of lens thickening and thinning is accommodation.[4,5]

Ideally the lens will bring an image into perfect focus so that it lands right on the fovea, the area of central vision. If the focused image falls in front of the retina, however, then a blurred circle will fall on the fovea (Figure 28-4). In this case the lens is too thick, having too high an optical power. One simple remedy is to place a negative (concave) lens externally in front of the eye in glasses (or contact lenses) to reduce the power of the internal lens and allow the image to fall directly on the fovea. In presbyopia (old eyes), the flexibility of the lens fibers decreases and the lens becomes more rigid.[7] Accommodation gets weaker until the image can no longer be focused on the retina. Normal-sighted individuals first begin to notice these changes in their early forties. When this occurs, a plus (positive) lens (or bifocals, progressive lenses, bifocal or monovision contact lenses) may be worn to aid in reading.[4]

Other solutions to the problems of aging can be implemented during the time of cataract surgery, where a bifocal

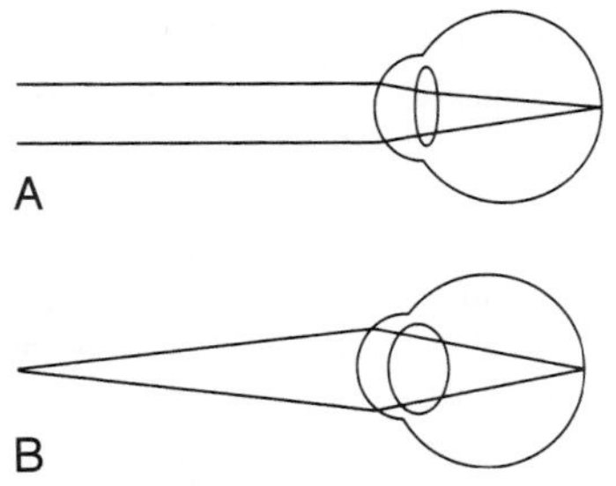

Figure 28-3 ■ Accommodation. **A,** Looking far away. **B,** Looking up close.

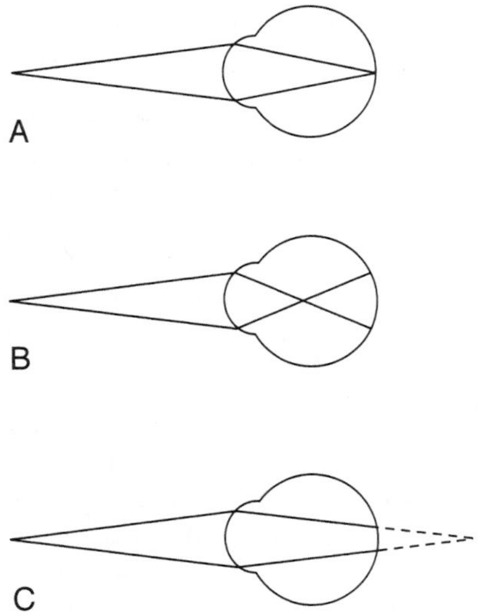

Figure 28-4 ■ Refractive error. **A,** Image focused on retina; no refractive error. **B,** A nearsighted or myopic eye. **C,** A farsighted or hyperopic eye.

implant may be inserted, or monovision implant correction performed in each eye.

The lens can be affected by the age-related process of cataract development, in which the general clarity of vision is impaired from a loss of transparency of the crystalline lens. Incoming light tends to scatter inside the eye, causing glare problems. When vision is impaired to such a degree that it affects function, the lens may be removed surgically and replaced with a silicone implant placed just posterior to the iris.

Vitreous Chamber

The space behind the lens, which is filled with a gel-like substance, is called the *vitreous chamber.* As we age, the gel tends to liquefy, and some of the remnants of embryological development that were trapped are released to float freely. This can cause the very common perception of "floaters," the shadows cast by these particles onto the macular region. They can be disturbing but generally float out of view over time.[5]

Retina

The retina at the back of the eye is the photosensitive layer, like the film in a camera, receiving the pattern of light reflected from objects. The topography of the retina (Figure 28-5) includes the optic disc, which is where the optic nerve exits and arteries and veins emerge and exit. This is also the blind spot because there are no photoreceptor cells on the disc. The macula is temporal to the optic disc and contains the fovea, providing central vision. The surrounding retina provides peripheral vision and defines a 180-degree half-sphere.[5]

Exercise 28-2: Blind Spot

Your blind spot may be observed by doing the following: draw two dots 3 inches (7.5 cm) apart on a piece of paper. The dots can be ¼ inch (0.5 cm). Cover your left eye and look at the dot on the left. Starting at about 16 inches (40 cm), slowly bring the paper closer. Make sure you can see the two dots—one you are looking at directly and the other peripherally. At approximately 10 inches (25 cm) the dot on the right will disappear. This is your blind spot! Why can this exercise only be done monocularly (with one eye)?

Visual Pathway

The visual pathway begins with the photoreceptor cells, which begin a three-neuron chain exiting through the optic nerve. This chain consists of the rods and cones, which synapse with bipolar cells that synapse with ganglion cells (Figure 28-6).[5,8]

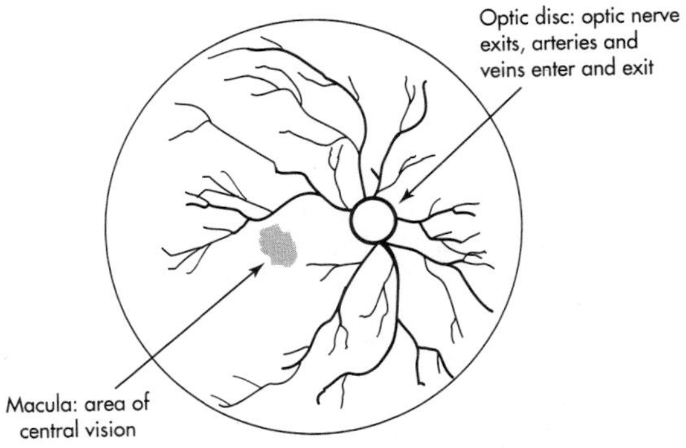

Figure 28-5 ■ Retinal topography.

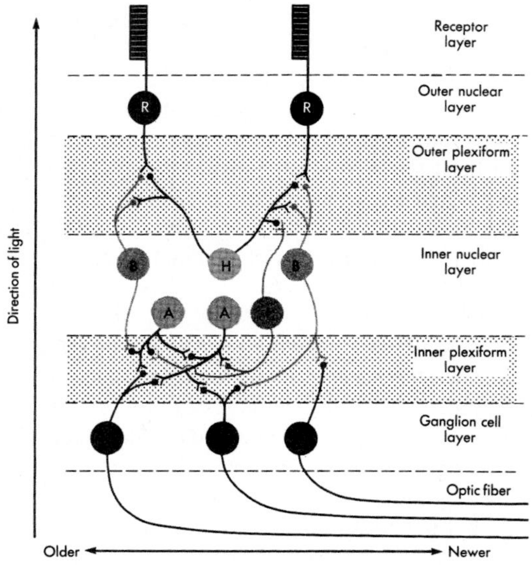

Figure 28-6 ■ The connections among retinal neurons and the significance of prominent layers. The neurons shown are photoreceptors *(R),* horizontal cells *(H),* bipolar cells *(B),* interplexiform cells *(I),* amacrine cells *(A),* and ganglion cells *(G).* It has been suggested that ganglion cells dominated by bipolar cell inputs represent newer circuitry. The arrow indicates the direction of light as it passes through the retina to reach the photoreceptors. (From Beme RM, Levy MN, editors: *Physiology,* St Louis, 1988, CV Mosby.)

There are two types of photoreceptor cells: rods and cones. The cone or rod shape is the dendrite of the cell. Variation in shape and slight variation in pigment give each one different sensitivities. The rod cell has greater sensitivity to dim light but less sensitivity to color, whereas the cone cell has greater sensitivity to color and high-intensity light and less to reduced light conditions. The highest concentration of cone cells is in the fovea and macula, with decreasing concentration of cone cells and increasing concentration of rod cells moving concentrically away from the macula. The high degree of low-light sensitivity can be most appreciated in survival mode conditions such as being lost in the woods on a moonless night. By swinging the eyes side to side one can maximize the image and keep the macula from interfering.

The phenomenon responsible for the high degree of neural representation of the foveal region and that accounts for the tremendous conscious awareness of the central view is called convergence.[5] At the periphery of the retina the degree of convergence is great; many photoreceptor cells synapse on one ganglion cell, which accounts for poor acuity but high light sensitivity. The closer to the macula, the less the degree of convergence, until, finally, at the fovea there is no convergence. This means that one photoreceptor cell synapses with one bipolar cell and one ganglion cell.

The awareness of what is seen is directly related to the amount of convergence, which reflects the extent of neural representation. The 1:1 correspondence between photoreceptor and ganglion cell at the fovea means that there is a high degree of neural representation of the foveal image in the brain. It is even greater than the neural representation of the lips, tongue, or hands.[9] This accounts for the primary awareness of what is in the foveal field and secondary awareness of the peripheral field. Conscious awareness of the environment is whatever is in the foveal field at the moment. But continuous information about the environment is flowing over the peripheral retina, usually subconsciously. Attention quickly shifts from foveal to nonfoveal stimulation when changes in light intensity or rapid movement are registered. This type of stimulus arouses attention immediately because it could have specific survival value. For example, a person is driving down the street and senses rapid motion off to the right. The foveas swing around immediately to identify a small red ball bouncing into the street. This information goes to the association areas, in which "small ball" is associated with "small child soon to follow." Frontal cortical centers are aroused and a decision is made to initiate motor areas to take the foot off the accelerator and put it onto the brake, while simultaneously moving the wheel away from the ball and scanning for the object of concern, that is, the child.

Exercise 28-3: Peripheral Central Awareness

We have a unique ability to change our awareness by consciously shifting attention from our foveal or central awareness to our peripheral awareness. For example, as you read these words, become aware of the background surrounding the paper; note colors, forms, and shapes; continue to expand your awareness to include your clothes, the floor, walls, and ceiling if possible. You are consciously stimulating your primitive, phylogenetically older visual system. The ability to do this has considerable therapeutic value because a typical pattern of visual stress is associated with foveal concentration to the exclusion of peripheral information. The ability to expand the peripheral awareness at will is a skill that can help you to relax while you drive, can improve reading skills, and can be used in visual training techniques.

The moment light hits the retina, the photographic film model must be abandoned for the image processing or computerized image enhancement model. The primary visual pathway at the retinal level is a three-neuron chain. From back to front the first neuron is the photoreceptor cell, rods or cones. They synapse with a bipolar cell, which in turn synapses with a ganglion cell. The axon of the ganglion cell exits by means of the optic nerve. Image enhancement occurs at the two junctions of the three–nerve-cell pathway. Lateral cells at the neural junctions have an inhibitory action on the primary three-neuron pathway, and through the inhibition of an impulse the image is modulated. For example, at the first junction between photoreceptor cell and bipolar cell, there are horizontal cells. These cells enhance the contrast between light and dark by inhibiting the firing of bipolar cells at the edge of an image. This makes the edge of the image appear darker than the central area, which increases the contrast and thereby increases attention-getting value. After all, it is by perceiving edges that we are able to maneuver around objects. In a similar manner, amacrine cells act at the second neural junction between bipolar and ganglion cells to enhance movement detection.[10]

This image enhancement process continues throughout the visual pathway. The process has been likened to the way in which a computer enhances a distorted picture of outer space received from a satellite. The image goes through a series of processing stations in the inner workings of the computer. The computer-generated, enhanced image shown on the screen is like the end product in the brain: the perceived image.

The visual pathway continues through the brain (Figure 28-7). The ganglion cell axons exit the eyeball by

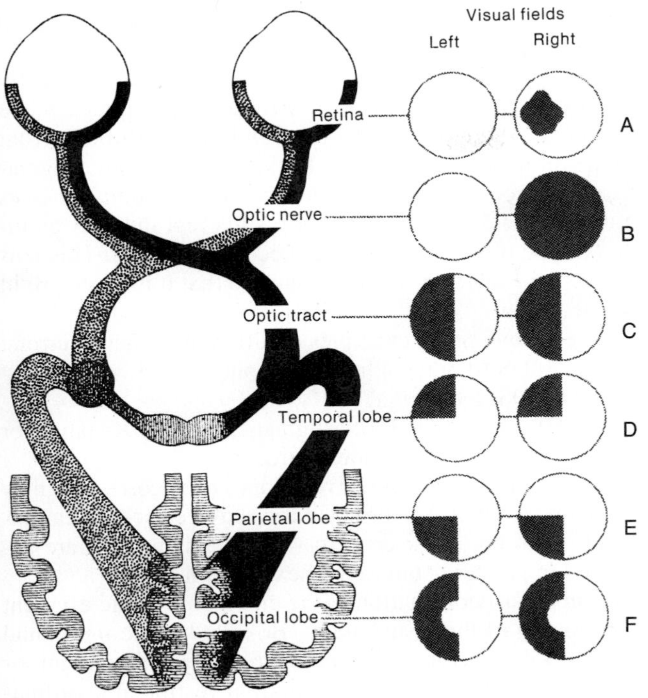

Figure 28-7 ■ Visual field disturbances at various points along the optic pathway. **A,** Retinal lesion: blind spot in the affected eye. **B,** Optic nerve lesion: partial or complete blindness in that eye. **C,** Optic tract or lateral geniculate lesion: blindness in the opposite half of both visual fields. **D,** Temporal lobe lesion: blindness in the upper quadrants of both visual fields on the side opposite the lesion. **E,** Parietal lobe lesion: contralateral blindness in the corresponding lower quadrants of both eyes. **F,** Occipital lobe lesion: contralateral blindness in the corresponding half of each visual field but with macular sparing. (Courtesy Smith, Kline & French Laboratories, Philadelphia, Pennsylvania.)

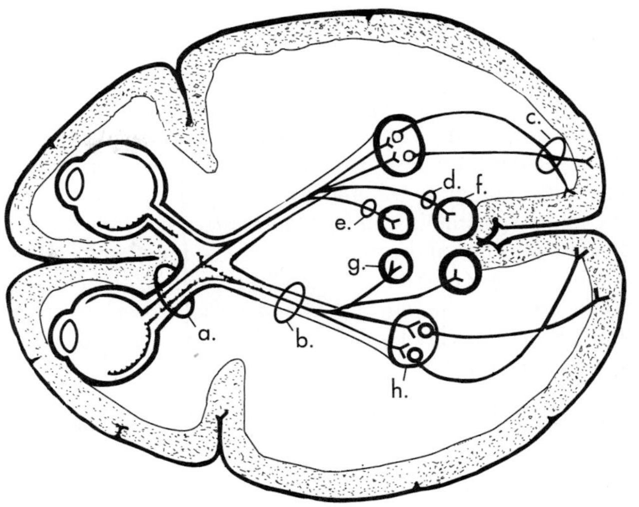

Figure 28-8 ■ Visual tract system: *a,* optic nerve; *b,* optic tract; *c,* geniculate-occipital radiators; *d,* retinocollicular radiation; *e,* retinopretecto tracts; *f,* superior colliculus (midbrain); *g,* pretectal area (tegmentum); *h,* lateral geniculate.

means of the optic nerve, carrying the complete retinal picture in coded electrochemical patterns. From there the patterns project to different sites within the central nervous system (Figure 28-8). Projections to the pretectum are important in pupillary reflexes; projections to the pretectal nuclei, the accessory optic nuclei, and the superior colliculus are all involved in eye movement functions.[5] The largest bundle, called the *optic tract,* projects to the lateral geniculate body in the hypothalamus, where additional image enhancement and processing occurs. The next group of axons continues to the primary visual cortex and from there to visual association areas.

At what point does the retinal image become a perception, and with what part of the brain does one see? Current theory regarding visual perception is the result of Nobel prize–winning research by Hubel and Wiesel in the 1960s called the *receptive field theory.*[11] This theory states that different neurons are feature detectors, defining objects in terms of movement, direction, orientation, color, depth, and acuity. Research in 1990 by Hubel and Livingstone[12] was able to locate a segregation of function at the level of the lateral geniculate body. They identified two types of cells, one type being larger and faster magno cells, which are apparently phylogenetically older and color blind but which have a high contrast sensitivity and are able to detect differences in contrast of 1% to 2%. They also have low spatial resolution (low acuity). They seem to operate globally and are responsible for perception of movement, depth perception from motion, perspective, parallax, stereopsis, shading, contour, and interocular rivalry. Through linking properties (objects having common movement or depth) emerges figure-ground perception. Much of this perception occurs in the middle temporal lobe.

The other type of cell, called the *parvo cell,* is smaller, slower, and color sensitive and has a smaller receptive field. These cells are less global and are primarily responsible for high-resolution form perception. Higher-level visual association occurs in the temporal-occipital region, where learning to identify objects by their appearance occurs. It appears that these two types of cells are functionally and structurally related to the two visual systems represented in retinal topography—the foveal (central) and peripheral visual systems.

Eye Movement System

The eye movement system consists of six pairs of eye muscles: the medial recti, lateral recti, superior and inferior recti, and superior and inferior obliques (see Figure 28-8). Together they are controlled by cranial nerves III (oculomotor), IV (trochlear), and VI (abducens). The eye movement system has both reflex and voluntary components. Reflexive movements are coordinated through vestibular interconnections at a midbrain level. The vestibuloocular reflex (VOR) functions primarily to keep the image stabilized on the retina. Through connections between pairs of eye muscles and the semicircular canals, movement is analyzed as being either external movement of an object or movement of the head or body. From this information the VOR is able to direct the appropriate head or eye movement.[5]

Two types of eye movements are the result. Smooth, coordinated eye movements are called *pursuits,* and rapid localizations are called *saccades.* Voluntary control of both these motions indicates cortical control. Pursuits are used for continuously following moving targets, and they are stimulated by a foveal image. Saccades are stimulated by images from the peripheral system, where a detection of motion or change in light intensity results in a rapid saccadic eye movement to bring the object into the foveal field. Either difficulties in the eye movement system or altered functioning of the vestibular system can affect the coordinated, efficient functioning of eye movement skills.

A third type of eye movement is specifically related to eye aiming ability. This is the coordinated movement of both eyes inward toward the nose, as in crossing the eyes, or outward along the midline, as when looking away in the distance. The inward movement is called *convergence,* and the outward movement is called *divergence.* The most important result of efficient vergence abilities is depth perception, or stereopsis. Small errors in aiming can dramatically affect stereopsis. Problems such as double vision, wandering eyes, and strabismus are discussed in greater depth in a later section.

Exercise 28-4: Pursuits, Saccades, Convergence

Pursuits. Follow a moving target such as a pencil point as you move it across your field of gaze, while keeping your head still. Continue to move it in different directions, vertically, horizontally, diagonally, and circularly to stimulate all pairs of eye muscles. For a more challenging demonstration, find a fly and follow its flight path around the room. If you lose sight of it, note that the detection of the movement of the fly will signal your eye movement directly toward it.

Saccades. Hold two pencils about head width apart. Shift your eyes from pencil to pencil without moving your head. Note that your awareness is of the two pencils, not of the background between them. Generally, perception occurs the moment the eyes are still, rather than while moving during saccades. For a more challenging exercise, move the pencil you are not looking at, then shift quickly to it; move the other pencil while looking at the one you just moved. In other words, you will pick up the location of the other pencil peripherally and direct your eyes to the foveal region. The size and degree of blur of the peripheral image will tell the brain where the image is and how far to move the eyes. This ability again is a result of the function of neural convergence, which is related to neural representation.

Convergence. Hold a pencil at arm's length along your midline. Slowly bring the pencil closer in toward you along your midline. Feel your eyes moving in (crossing). Try to bring the pencil to your nose, keeping the pencil visually single. (It is okay if you cannot.) Move the pencil away now, and your eyes are diverging.

FUNCTIONAL VISUAL SKILLS

Refractive Error

Before discussing binocular coordination and the individual visual skills, it is important to describe refractive errors and how they can affect binocular coordination. Three common types of refractive errors are myopia or nearsightedness, hyperopia or farsightedness, and astigmatism.[5,10]

The myopic eye is too long, or the cornea is too steep, so the focused image falls in front of the retina. It is easily corrected with a negative or minus lens, which optically moves the image back onto the retina.

The hyperopic eye is too short, or the cornea is too flat, such that the focused image falls behind the retina. A positive or plus lens optically moves the image onto the retina. A young hyperopic person will be able to use accommodation to bring the image focus back onto the retina, but because accommodation is finite, this can cause reading difficulties earlier than normal or can affect binocular coordination at near distances.

An eye will have astigmatism if it is not perfectly spherical. An aspherical eye will cause the image to be distorted, where part of the focused image will be in front of the retina and part on or in back. A person with astigmatism may see vertical lines clearly and horizontal lines as blurry, depending on the specific aspherical shape. A cylindrical type of lens is used to correct astigmatism. This lens corrects the distortion of the image so that it is placed right on the retina.

The following are examples of different refractive errors:

−5.50 DS (diopter sphere): myopia

+4.00 DS: hyperopia

+1.50 $\bar{c}$ − 1.50 × 180: astigmatism (Note: × stands for the axis of the cylinder correction.)

When significant refractive errors are uncorrected, they can reduce vision. Uncorrected refractive error also can interfere with binocular coordination. The symptoms are described in greater detail in the next section.

Binocular coordination is the end result of the efficient functioning of the visual skills (Box 28-1). The individual visual skills include accommodation, eye alignment or vergence, eye movements with normal vestibular coordination, stereopsis (depth perception), and peripheral and central coordination. During normal activities, all the skills are inseparable.

Accommodation

Accommodation is the ability to bring near objects into clear focus automatically and without strain. Relaxation of accommodation allows distant objects to come into focus. The primary action is that of the ciliary muscles acting on the lens, and the primary system of control is the ANS, with sympathetic and parasympathetic components.[5]

Both accommodation and pupil size changes are reflexes that work in concert: as accommodation relaxes the pupil dilates and as accommodation increases the pupil constricts.[4] As a person focuses on a near object, the lenses thicken, allowing the near object to come into focus. At the same time the pupils constrict to increase depth of focus (just as in a camera). As a person looks into the distance, the lens gets flatter, relaxing accommodation, and the pupil dilates, decreasing the depth of field.

Accommodative ability is age dependent. A young child can focus on small objects just a few inches in front of the eyes. At about the age of 9 years, the accommodative ability slowly begins to decrease. By the mid 40s the reserve focusing power diminishes to the point that near objects begin to blur. At this stage, reading material is pushed farther away

BOX 28-1 ■ BINOCULAR COORDINATION

- Corrected refractive error
- Accommodation
- Eye alignment
- Stereopsis
- Central and peripheral coordination
- Efficient eye movement skills

until the arms are not long enough, and then reading glasses are needed. This is called *presbyopia* (old eyes).

Problems in accommodation may contribute to myopia, hyperopia, and presbyopia. Symptoms include blurriness at either near or far distance, depending on the age and the problem.

Accommodation is important mainly for up-close activities: reading, hygiene, dressing (specifically, closing fasteners), use of tools, typing, tabletop activities, and games.

Exercise 28-5: Accommodation

Accommodation cannot be directly observed, but it can be implied indirectly through observation of pupillary constriction while doing an accommodative task. Cover one eye. Hold a finger in front at about 10 inches (25 cm). Focus on the finger, making sure that the fingerprint is clear. Shift focus to a distant object. Continue shifting far to near and near to far while a partner observes the pupil. The partner should be able to observe pupillary constriction with near focus and dilation with far focus.

Vergence

Vergence includes convergence and divergence. It is the ability to smoothly and automatically bring the eyes together along the midline to singly observe objects that are near (convergence) or conversely to move the eyes outward for single vision of distant objects (divergence). Specific brain centers control convergence and divergence.

With regard to reflexes, vergence is associated with accommodation: convergence with accommodation, and divergence with relaxation of accommodation. The function of this reflex is to allow objects to be both single and clear, at either near or far positions. Vergence has both automatic and voluntary components. Most of the time it is not necessary to think about moving the eyes inward while looking at a close object; yet if asked to cross the eyes, most people can do this at will.

Problems can occur in vergence ability when the eye movement system is out of sync with accommodation or from damage to cranial nerves III, IV, or VI. Problems can be slight, in which there is merely a tendency for the eyes to converge in or out too far, or the eyes can be grossly out of convergence. Tendencies to underconverge or overconverge are called phorias and are not visible except by special testing in which they are elicited. An individual may be asymptomatic, but symptoms may occur under conditions of increased stress or fatigue such as excessive reading or working at a computer terminal or from drug side effects (prescription and recreational).

Some phorias may worsen to the extent that binocularity breaks down, at which point the individual becomes strabismic. There are two main types of strabismus: esotropia and exotropia. An esotropia is an inward turning of the eye, and an exotropia is an outward turning. A third, less common type of strabismus is hypertropia, in which one eye aims upward relative to the other eye. Strabismus and dysfunctional phorias are discussed in greater detail in the next section.

Vergence ability is needed for singular binocular vision; thus it is basic to all activities. At near positions the patient may have difficulty finding objects; eye-hand coordination may be decreased, affecting self-care and hygiene tasks; and reading may be difficult. Distance tasks that may be affected include driving, sports, movies, communication, and, frequently, ambulation. Individuals with impaired vergence ability may also have difficulty focusing and may have decreased or no depth perception. Interpreting space can be quite difficult and confusing. If decreased vergence is a result of traumatic head injury or stroke, it may contribute to the patient's confusion, and he or she may not be able to identify or communicate the problem.

Exercise 28-6: Vergence

Hold a pencil in front of you at eye level at about 12 inches (30 cm). Look at the pencil. Look away into the distance. Looking at the pencil is convergence, and looking into the distance is divergence. As you converge and diverge slowly back and forth, note any changes you may feel: changes in how relaxed you feel, how focused or spaced out you feel, feelings of dreaminess, or nothing at all. Observe a partner's eyes as he or she shifts back and forth as well.

Pursuits and Saccades

Eye movement skills consist of pursuits and saccades. Pursuits are the smooth, coordinated movements of all eye muscles together, allowing accurate tracking of objects through space. Perception is continuous during pursuit movements. Saccades are rapid shifts of the eyes from object to object, allowing quick localization of movements observed in the periphery. The systems involved in eye movement skills are the oculomotor system with the VOR, in conjunction with coordination of the central and peripheral visual systems. The peripheral visual system is finely tuned for detecting changes in light levels and small movements.

Problems in pursuits or saccades can be the result of a dysfunction of any individual muscles, the VOR, or areas of the brain controlling pursuits or saccades.[13-15] Because the VOR helps to stabilize the image on the retina and to differentiate image movement from eye movement, simple tracking can be more difficult. In addition, visual field loss, either central or peripheral, can dramatically affect localization ability. People with blind half- or quarter-fields can be observed to do searching eye movements rather than directly jumping to the object.

Activities affected include searching for objects; visually directed movement for fine motor tasks, gross movement, and ambulation tasks; eye-hand coordination; self-care; driving; and reading.

Memory also may be affected by an eye movement dysfunction. Research by Adler-Grinberg and Stark[16] and Noton and Stark[17] examined patterns of eye movements as subjects looked at a picture. Distinct eye movement patterns, called scan paths, became apparent. When the subject was asked to recall the picture, the same eye movement pattern was elicited as when the subject originally saw the picture. It would appear that a type of oculomotor praxis is involved in recall. Applying this idea to the clinical setting, if a patient has inaccurate eye movement with poor pursuits or excessive saccades, then perhaps the stored memory is less efficiently stored and consequently more difficult to reconstruct from memory. Additionally, if a patient has a type of brain damage with generalized dyspraxia, the eye movement system could quite likely be affected and might be involved in the patient's perceptual dysfunction.

Another more recent example of the relationship between eye movements and memory is the use of eye movement desensitization and reprocessing (EMDR) therapy to help individuals with posttraumatic stress disorder reintegrate traumatic experiences.[18] Although the exact mechanism is at this time unknown, the prevailing hypothesis is that the lateral eye movements elicit an orienting response, scanning the environment for further danger, and that this is an investigatory reflex associated with a relaxed physical state.[19]

SYMPTOMS OF VISUAL DYSFUNCTION

History

The identification of a visual problem begins with case history. It is important to get some idea of the client's prior visual status or any history of eye injury, surgery, or diseases. Information can be elicited by direct questioning of the client or family members or by clinical observation. Sample questions include the following:

- Are you having difficulty with seeing, or with your eyes?
- Do you wear glasses? Contact lenses? For distance, near, bifocals, or monovision (one eye near, other distance)?
- Does your correction (glasses, contact lenses) work as well now as before the (stroke, accident, and so on)?
- Have you noticed any blurriness? Near or far?
- Do you ever see double? See two? See overlapping or shadow images?
- Do you ever find that when you reach for an object that you knock it over or your hand misses?
- Do letters jump around on the page after reading for a while?
- Are you experiencing any eye strain or headaches? Where and when?
- Do you ever lose your place when reading?
- Are portions of a page or any objects missing?
- Do people or things suddenly appear from one side that you did not see approaching?
- Do you have difficulty concentrating on tasks?

Clinical observations of the client performing various activities are a valuable source of problem identification. Therapists in general are in an ideal position to observe clients in a variety of functional tasks that require near vision, far vision, spatial estimations, depth judgments, and oculomotor tasks. This situation varies considerably from the physician's observations in the more contrived environment of the examination room. In addition, the therapist's initial observations can be used in documenting difficulties within the therapy realm that may be amenable to visual remediation in terms that can be applied to reimbursement of therapy.

Clinical observations include the following:

- Head turn or tilt during near tasks, or postural adjustments to task
- Avoidance of near tasks
- One eye appears to go in, out, up, or down
- Vision shifts from eye to eye
- Seems to look past observer
- Closes or covers one eye
- Squints
- Eyes appear red, puffy, or irritated or have a discharge (Notify nurses or physician of these observations.)
- Rubs eyes a lot
- Has difficulty maintaining eye contact
- Spaces out, drifts off, daydreams
- During activity, neglects one side of body or space
- During movement, bumps into walls or objects (either walking or in a wheelchair)
- Appears to misjudge distance
- Underreaches or overreaches for objects
- Has difficulty finding things

Near Point Blur

Blurred vision up close is not a symptom that by itself is indicative of a problem in any one area. It could indicate farsightedness (hyperopia), astigmatism, or reduced accommodative ability (insufficiency). The client may move objects or the head farther or closer, may complain of eye strain or headaches, may squint, or may even avoid near activities as much as possible. The therapist might observe excessive blinking, and the patient may complain of glasses not working well.

Distance Blur

Distance blur could also have a number of different causes, including nearsightedness (myopia), a pathological problem (such as beginning cataracts or macular degeneration), or accommodative spasm. Most people have some experience with accommodative spasm. After spending long periods of time either studying or reading a novel and then glancing up at the wall across the room, it may be blurry and then clear up slowly. For some individuals, this spasm eventually develops into nearsightedness if the reading habits continue for a long time.

Clients with distance blur may make forward head movements and frequently squint in an attempt to see. They may not respond or orient quickly to auditory or visual stimuli beyond a certain radius. The therapist may also note excessive blinking and a withdrawn attitude because the patient cannot see well enough to interact with the environment.

Visual hygiene can be recommended to assist in the development of good visual habits. This should include attention to good lighting and posture, taking frequent breaks, and monitoring the state of clarity of an environmental cue such as a clock across the room.

Phoria and Strabismus

The next area of eye alignment problems can be divided into two types of problems: phoria and strabismus. A *phoria* can be defined as a natural positioning of the eyes in which there is a tendency to aim in front of or behind the point of focus. It may or may not be associated with symptoms. Fusion is intact, and depth perception may also be intact to some degree.

Everyone has a phoria, just as everyone has a posture. It may be within normal range, or, just as someone may have scoliosis, a high phoria may cause problems. The following phorias may cause problems:

- Esophoria: The eyes are postured in front of the point of focus.
- Exophoria: The eyes are postured in back of the point of focus.

Phoria is measured in units of prism diopters, which indicate the size of the prism needed to measure the eye position in or out from the straight-ahead position.[4]

Phorias tend to produce subtle symptoms. These include having difficulty concentrating, frontal or temporal headaches, sleepiness after reading, and stinging of the eyes after reading.

A strabismus, or tropia, is a visible turn of one eye, which may be constant, intermittent, or alternating between one eye and the other. The person may have double vision, or if the strabismus is long term, the person may suppress or "turn off" the vision in the wandering eye. Suppression is a neurological function that is an adaptation to the confusing situation of double images. In the developing brain the individual must choose (unconsciously) which eye is dominant, and the image is confirmed by motor and tactile inputs as being the "real" image. The other fovea's image is then neurologically suppressed. The peripheral vision in the suppressing eye is still normal, and the eye still contributes to other aspects of vision such as orientation and locomotion.

The essential concept in understanding the difference between phoria and strabismus is that in strabismus fusion and depth perception are not present. Definitions of different types of strabismus are presented in Box 28-2. It is not a conclusive list; many other types and permutations are beyond the scope of this discussion. The intent here is to expose the therapist to different terms that may be used by the physician in diagnosing the type of strabismus.

In strabismus, one eye appears to go in, out, up, or down, and there is frequently an obvious inability to judge distances, especially if the strabismus is of recent onset (acquired). The client may underreach or overreach for objects, cover or close one eye, complain of double vision, or exhibit a head tilt or turn during specific activities. He or she may appear to favor one eye, have difficulty reading, appear spaced out, or avoid near activities. In addition, especially if the patient sees double but is unable or unwilling to talk about it, she or he may be confused or disoriented.

Certain postures may facilitate fusion for some clients. The eye doctor will be able to determine which head position may be best. Frequently, many clients will automatically move around to the best position. At other times, however, head position will be used to avoid using one eye. Head and body position, therefore, are important aspects to consider.

Many convergence problems are amenable to vision therapy,[20-22] but some are not.[23] Whether a particular problem can be helped by vision therapy can be determined by an eye doctor, who can prescribe specific exercises.

BOX 28-2 ■ TYPES OF STRABISMUS

Esotropia: One eye turns in.

Exotropia: One eye turns out.

Hypertropia: One eye turns up relative to the other eye.

Intermittent: The person is strabismic at times and phoric (fusing) at times. Fatigue or stress may bring out the strabismic state.

Alternating: The person switches from using the right eye to using the left eye. The person also switches the suppressing eye. If using the right eye, the person suppresses the left, and while using the left eye, the person suppresses the right; otherwise the person would see double.

Constant strabismus: One eye is always in or out (up or down), always the same eye.

Comitant and noncomitant strabismus: The amount of eye turn is the same regardless of whether the person is looking up, down, right, left, or straight ahead. People who have had the condition for a long time usually have comitant strabismus. People with new or acquired strabismus (i.e., from stroke or head injury) usually have noncomitant strabismus, in which the amount of eye turn changes depending on the direction in which the eyes are looking.

Oculomotor Dysfunction

Oculomotor dysfunction is a very common sequela of neurological deficits, with an incidence as high as 90% according to Ciufredda and colleagues.[24,25] Commonly the smooth pursuit system will be affected, such that the smooth movement is interrupted by a series of fixation stops and the movements appear jerky. Damage anywhere along the visual motor pathway may cause a variety of eye movement disorders. This includes injury to the pontine and mesencephalic reticular formation, oculomotor nucleus in the brain stem, caudate nucleus and substantia nigra, cerebellum, and vestibular nuclei.[24]

Patients with oculomotor disorders frequently also experience dizziness, nausea, and balance difficulties. Many times an eye movement will elicit dizziness and disorientation. It is thought that these symptoms are in part caused by a loss of integration of information coming from the two aspects of the visual system that process central vision (parvocellular pathway) and peripheral vision (magnocellular pathway).

As mentioned previously, detection of peripheral targets serves to direct an eye movement with a specific velocity and direction to bring the foveas in line for purposes of identification. Therapy for rehabilitation of eye movement disorders should be directed at using peripheral awareness with slow controlled eye movement toward the target. Once these movements are tolerated, head movement can be added, then slowly body movement.[26,27]

While doing any sort of tracking activity, the client is encouraged to maintain peripheral awareness. This technique will help the client keep her or his place. The oculomotor system is guided by the peripheral location of an object.

Visual Field Defects—Hemianopsia and Quadrantanopsia

Visual field loss may indicate damage that is prechiasmic, at the optic chiasm, postchiasmic, in the visual radiations of the thalamus, or in the visual cortex. The resultant visual field loss is characteristic (even diagnostic) in each case. The visual field loss pattern will generally reflect the location of the lesion. It could be bitemporal (outer half of each field), half-field loss (hemianopsia) with or without macular involvement, or quarter-field loss (see Figure 28-7). Some symptoms of field loss are an inability to read or starting to read in the middle of the page, ignoring food on one half of the plate, and difficulty orienting to stimuli in a specific area of space.

Hemianopsia is a loss of half of the visual field in each eye, and quadrantanopsia is loss of a quarter of the visual field in each eye. *Homonymous hemianopsia* refers to the inner or nasal half and the outer or temporal half of each eye being affected. The retina itself is intact, but a neurological lesion has interrupted the ability of the visual cortex to receive recognition of the image. Vision processing may be occurring at lower centers, such as the lateral geniculate body, but if signals are not being received by the cortex, then they are not recognized as "seen." In 1979, Zihl and von Cramon[28] published their findings that damaged visual fields could be trained by use of a light stimulus presented repeatedly at the border of the visual field defect. Balliet and co-workers[29] (when attempting to repeat the experiment, adding controls for oculomotor fixations) proposed that subjects were actually learning to make small compensatory eye movements rather than experiencing true improvements in the visual fields. In the 1980s and 1990s a group of German researchers developed a computer-based field training system for researching the question of visual field training. They found in their research that visual fields did expand on average by 5 degrees, with functional improvements noted by more than 80% of their patients (Figure 28-9).[30-34] A company called NovaVision introduced the computer-based visual field restitution training program in the United States with good results (see Appendix 28-A). This author has also noted documentable and functional improvements in visual fields even when trained with less sophisticated methods.

Compensation training may also be required to allow the client to resume activities such as reading. Compensation techniques include use of margin markers and reading with a card with a slit in it (typoscope) to isolate one line or a couple of lines at a time. Holding reading material vertically also can help.

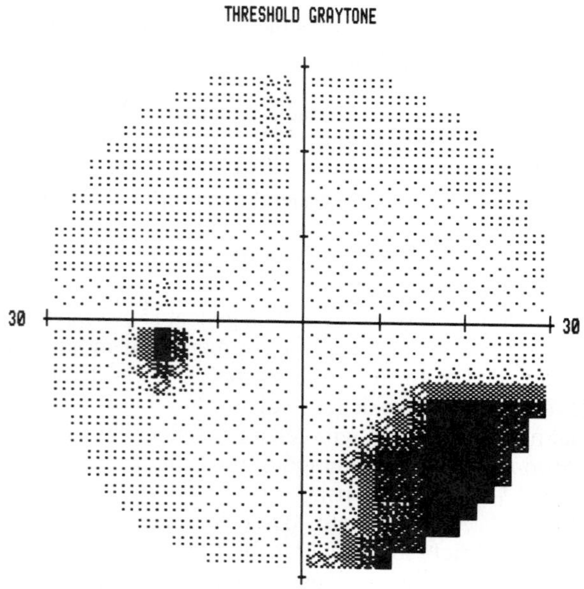

Figure 28-9 ■ Visual field defect (inferior temporal) as measured on Humphrey visual field tester.

SUMMARY OF DISORDERS OF VISION

Table 28-1 summarizes primary visual deficits. Once a therapist or other specialist has eliminated the possibility of primary visual deficits, the clinician must assess whether the identified problem is resulting from central associative processing that is causing visual-perceptual dysfunction.

EYE DISEASES

Areas addressed in this section are common ocular and systemic diseases of the pediatric and geriatric populations, an introduction to low vision, and recommendations for adaptations of the treatment plan. If reduced vision (low vision) is a result of eye disease, the client may be assisted by magnification aids. Also, the therapy treatment program may need to be altered to accommodate any special visual needs of the client (lighting, working distance, inclusion of magnifiers, use of filters, contrast-enhancing devices).

Pediatric Conditions

Retinopathy of Prematurity

The incidence of retinopathy of prematurity is increasing because of the improved survival of premature infants as a result of improved ventilation.[35] Immature retinal vessels are sensitive to high oxygen tension. The effect on the vessels is vasoconstriction, eventually leading to obliteration of the vessels. This creates a state of ischemia, which stimulates the growth of new blood vessels. These small, fragile vessels bleed easily, leading to fibrosis and traction on the retina. As a result of the traction, the macula gets stretched, interfering with the function of central vision.

The temporal vessels are most affected because they develop last. The degree of damage may be mild or severe, depending on the amount of prematurity.[7]

Retinoblastoma

Retinoblastoma is the most common malignant tumor in children.[1] The current incidence is 1 in 20,000 live births, a rate that has been increasing over the past 30 years, apparently owing to inheritance of a mutated gene.

The young child may have a strabismus resulting from impaired vision in the eye with the tumor. As the tumor grows, the pupil may appear milky white. If not detected early, the tumor will lead to loss of the eye; and if the tumor invades the brain, death will occur. Clearly, early detection is critical.

Mental Retardation

There are a higher number of visual problems in the mentally retarded populations.[1] These individuals have a higher incidence of refractive error (myopia, hyperopia, astigmatism), strabismus, nystagmus, and optic atrophy than do children with normal intelligence.

Cerebral Palsy

Therapists who work with children with cerebral palsy may have noticed a high incidence of vision problems. Many studies confirm these observations. A study by Scheinman[36] examining the incidence of visual problems in children with cerebral palsy and normal intelligence found the following incidences: strabismus in 69%, high

TABLE 28-1 ■ PRIMARY VISUAL DEFICITS ASSOCIATED WITH CENTRAL LESIONS, FUNCTIONAL SYMPTOMS, MANAGEMENT, AND TREATMENT

VISUAL DEFICIT	FUNCTIONAL DEFICIT	MANAGEMENT	TREATMENT
Decreased visual acuity (distance or near)	Decreased acuity for distance or near tasks (reading)	Provide best lens correction for distance and near vision	May not be correctable May be appropriate for low vision
Inconsistent accommodation	Inconsistent blurred near vision	Ensure appropriate lenses are worn for appropriate activities Determine whether bifocal is usable; if not, provide separate lenses for distance and near vision Enlarge target, control density, use contrast and task lighting	Accommodation training may be appropriate
Cortical blindness	Marked decrease in visual acuity Severe blurring uncorrectable by lenses	Evaluated by vision specialist to determine areas and quality of residual vision Present targets of appropriate size and contrast in best area of visual field	Use headlamp to improve visual localization (i.e., functional use of residual vision) Multisensory input
Visual field deficits include homonymous hemianopsia, quadrantanopsia, scotoma, visual field constrictions	Blindness or decreased sensitivity in affected area of visual field	Be aware of normal field position in all meridians of gaze Ask patient to outline working area before beginning task Partial press-on Fresnel prism to facilitate compensation	Scanning training to facilitate compensation Training in use of prism NovaVision VF training
Pupillary reactions	Slow or absent pupillary responses	Sunglasses to control excessive brightness	
Loss of vertical gaze (external ophthalmoplegia)	Inability to move eyes up or down	Raise target or working area to foveal level Teach patient head movement to compensate	Prism glasses to allow objects below to be seen as directly in front
Conjugate gaze deviation	Inability to move or difficulty in moving eyes from fixed gaze position		
Lack of convergence	Diplopia or blurred vision for near tasks Decreased depth perception for near tasks	Convergence exercises prescribed by vision specialist	
Oculomotor nerve lesion (strabismus)	Intermittent or consistent diplopia in some or all meridians of gaze Loss of depth perception	Fresnel prism to fuse image in select cases Occlude deviant eye	Oculomotor and binocular exercises with prism use prescribed by vision specialist
Pathological (motor) nystagmus	Movement or blur of image during reading, near activities, decreased activities	Enlarge print or target to decrease blur Contact lens provides feedback, reduces movement, and increases acuity	Rigid gas-permeable contact lens prescribed by vision specialist
Poor fixations, saccades, or pursuits	Erratic scanning Unsteady fixation	Decrease density of material Isolate targets during evaluation and treatment Sensory integration activities Scanning training Use of kinesthetic and tactile systems to lead visual system (eye movements)	Oculomotor exercises prescribed by vision specialist

phorias in 4%, accommodative dysfunction in 30%, and refractive errors in 63%.

Hydrocephalus

Various studies have found that the most common visual problem in children with hydrocephalus is strabismus, with an incidence of 30% to 55%. The strabismus may develop either from the hydrocephalus itself or from the shunting procedure.

Fetal Alcohol Syndrome

Children affected by fetal alcohol syndrome have several characteristic features and visual problems. They have a higher incidence of strabismus, myopia, astigmatism, and ptosis. These children frequently have some degree of mental retardation as well and are of small stature.

Age-Related Conditions

Cataracts. The most common malady affecting vision in elderly persons is cataracts. General clarity of vision is impaired from a loss of transparency of the crystalline lens of the eye.

In the senile cataract the lens slowly loses its ability to prevent oxidation from occurring, and liquefaction of the outer layers begins. The normally soluble proteins adhere together, causing light scatter.[3] Vision slowly declines as opacification and light scatter increase, until the lens must be removed.

Age-Related Macular Degeneration. Age-related macular degeneration (AMD) is the leading cause of blindness in the Western world and is the most important retinal disease of the aged (affecting 28% of the 75- to 85-year-old age group).[7]

Loss of central vision results from fluid that leaks up from the deeper layers of the retina, pushing the retina up and detaching it from the nourishing layer. New vessel growth and hemorrhage and atrophy further destroy central vision. There is much research going on regarding treatments for AMD. The most promising at this time is the use of bevacizumab (Avastin) or ranibizumab (Lucentis), which is injected into the eye; then the eye is treated with a laser. The drug targets the neovascular network of blood vessels, and the laser treatment obliterates the vessel network, sparing the photoreceptors.[37]

This condition has significant implications for independent functioning. Mobility tends to be less impaired because the peripheral visual system is still intact. All activities involving fine detail such as reading, computer use, sewing, and cooking are affected. Safety also can be affected.

Arteriosclerosis. In arteriosclerosis, vision may or may not be affected. There is a hardening of the retinal arteries, which may eventually lead to ischemia, with the areas of retina deprived of sufficient oxygen eventually dying.

Hypertension. Hypertension is usually accompanied by arteriosclerosis. There may be retinal bleeding and edema, which can affect central vision if the macula is involved.

Diabetes. Diabetes can affect the lens. In the diabetic "sugar cataract," sorbitol collects within the lens, causing an osmotic gradient of fluid into the lens, which leads to disruption of the lens matrix and loss of transparency. As the fluid increases and decreases within the lens, the patient's vision also can fluctuate, depending directly on the sugar level. This makes prescribing glasses during this time quite difficult. The cataract will need to be removed if vision is worse than 20/40.

The retinal effects include microvascular damage and the development of microaneurysms. Central vision may be reduced as a result of retinal ischemia. The ischemia leads to new blood vessel growth (neovascularization). These new vessels are weak, frequently leaking and causing hemorrhage. The hemorrhage leads to fibrosis, which puts traction on the retina, pulling it off and leading to retinal detachment and blindness. Laser treatment of the bleeding retinal vessels will stop the bleeding but also burns photoreceptors, creating blind spots. This result is far preferable to total retinal detachment and blindness.

Glaucoma. Glaucoma occurs in 7.2% of the 75- to 85-year-old age group.[7] It is generally caused by an increase in the intraocular pressure. This pressure interferes with the inflow and outflow of blood and nutrients at the optic disc. As it progresses, glaucoma can cause tunnel vision and, in some, complete blindness. Because of the type of vision loss affecting the periphery, mobility and safety are significantly impaired. Try walking around holding a paper towel tube to your eye while closing the other eye, and see what happens to your ability to maneuver around obstacles or find your destination.

A less common type of glaucoma is low-tension glaucoma, in which the internal eye pressures are essentially normal. The mechanism is not understood, and the disease is treated with eye drops to lower internal pressure, just like the other types of glaucoma.

In one type of glaucoma, called *open-angle glaucoma,* the outflow of aqueous humor is reduced, leading to increased intraocular pressure. There are no overt symptoms. In another type, closed-angle glaucoma, the outflow is blocked by the iris. Symptoms are a painful, red eye, which may be confused with conjunctivitis.

Corticosteroids used to treat many conditions in the elderly for long periods of time may have side effects in some people, such as glaucoma and cataracts.

Eye Muscle Dysfunctions. Eye muscle dysfunctions causing double vision may result from several disease conditions including thyroid disease (Graves disease and others), multiple sclerosis, myasthenia gravis, and tumors. The underlying condition must be diagnosed and treated.

Visual Field Loss. Visual field loss may be either central (macular degeneration, glaucoma, or retinal disease) or peripheral field loss from glaucoma, retinal damage, or stroke at any point in the visual pathway. This is potentially the most functionally disabling form of visual impairment (see Figure 28-7).

Implications for Functional Performance

Lighting

Lighting conditions are important and vary depending on the nature of the condition. The person with presbyopia requires more light because the aging pupil gets smaller. The smaller pupil has the advantage of increasing the depth of focus, allowing the presbyope to see clearly over a wider range, but it has the disadvantage of eliminating more light from the eye. Thus, providing a good source of direct lighting, especially on fine print, is helpful. Lighting for the low-vision client is critical. Direct sources of low-glare light such as halogen seem to work best. This is, however, quite individual, in that some clients actually see better in lower-light conditions.

Glare

People who have problems with glare, such as those developing cataracts or other disease conditions, can be helped by several approaches. Incandescent or halogen lighting is preferred over fluorescent lighting. The use of a visor or wide-brimmed hat will reduce one source of glare, improving overall comfort. For some individuals who have trouble reading because of the glare coming off the white page, a black matte piece of cardboard with a horizontal slit in it (called a *typoscope*) can be used to reduce the surrounding glare and enhance reading. Various colored filters can be quite helpful; frequently a light amber color reduces glare while enhancing contrast. Other colors such as light green, plum, or yellow can be tried. The improvement noted is quite individual to the client. Special photochromic, tinted antiglare lenses developed by Corning are available by prescription through the ophthalmologist or optometrist. An antireflective coating may also help.

Low-Vision Aids

Many types of low-vision optical and nonoptical aids are available, usually by prescription by a low-vision specialist. Clients with damage to their central vision as in AMD or diabetic maculopathy and who still have some reduced central vision may be able to use various types of magnification aids.

Hand and Stand Magnifiers. One type is a stand magnifier, which is placed directly on the reading material and is useful for patients who have a tremor. Hand magnifiers are held in the hand and moved away from the page to the focal point of the lens, which may range from half an inch to 5 inches, depending on the amount of magnification. Some are equipped with their own internal illumination, some with halogen lighting systems.

Telescopes. Telescopes can be used for a number of different functions. To increase independence in orientation and mobility, a "spotting" telescope is held in the hand and looked through to identify approaching bus numbers, public transportation signs, stop or walk signs, or aisle signs. There are also telescopes that are worn on the head for hands-free usage or for viewing the computer screen. A telescope system can be attached to the patient's glasses frames. Special driving telescopes called *bioptic telescopes* are ground into the patient's glasses, angled in such a way as to allow viewing straight ahead and, with a tip of the head, viewing through the scope to read a sign. The best corrected visual acuity needs to be at least 20/100, but regulations vary from state to state. The greatest disadvantages of scopes are the small visual field and the additional training required to learn how to effectively use them.

The implantable telescope is an exciting new option available for patients with end-stage AMD. After careful evaluation the patient may be considered to be a good candidate for implantation. The tiny telescope is surgically implanted near the lens inside the eye. It has the benefits of having magnification immediately available for use for distance targets and reading; however, the peripheral vision in the implanted eye is significantly reduced. Similar to someone adjusting to monovision contact lenses, the patient with the implanted telescope learns to look through either the telescopic eye or the other eye (Figure 28-10).[38-40]

Microscopes. Microscopes are high-powered reading glasses in which the magnification is created in the glasses rather than in the hand. The disadvantage of these is the close viewing distance, depending on the power. The viewing distance could be as close as 1.5 inches, creating discomfort in reading for many.

Electronic Digital Magnifiers. The best systems for severely impaired clients are the electronic digital magnifiers such as closed-circuit television (CCTV). The CCTV system consists of a camera housed in a device that can be directed at the object to be viewed. The scope of magnification is significantly larger, ranging from low power to 50×. Additional benefits include no distortion like that caused by optical magnifiers and a field of view limited only by the size of the screen. The housing for the camera may be in a stand, with a screen above, or portable, held in the hand or strapped to the head. Examples are the Merlin, Jordy, and MaxPort by Enhanced Vision Systems and the portable digital magnifiers such as Compact mini by Optelec.[41]

Nonoptical Aids. Nonoptical aids include large-print materials, available at many libraries, typoscopes, mentioned earlier, and reading stands. Talking books are available for those for whom reading is an important hobby. New developments include text-to-speech synthesizers, large-print computers, and image intensifiers. Other simple aids are available such as lined paper with dark slightly raised lines, felt-tipped pens for writing, talking clocks, needle threaders, and many cooking and measuring aids.

Visual Field Expansion. For clients with field losses, specially designed prism or mirror systems may be used. These frequently require training to get used to and are not useful for everyone. Compensation training also can be helpful, particularly in the use of eccentric viewing, or learning how to use a portion of the intact field by aiming the eye off center. Use of margin markers or reading slits and holding the book sideways so that the print is vertical are other helpful techniques.

Current Research. Areas of research have included mounting a video camera onto spectacles and then transducing the visual information to electrodes implanted in visual

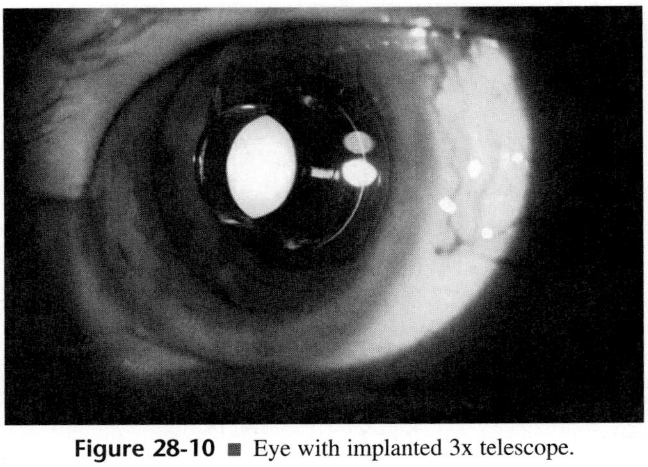

Figure 28-10 ■ Eye with implanted 3x telescope.

cortical centers. In one study this system allowed a low-vision patient to see the large E (20/400) and detect large contours.[42-44] Recently a company called Second Sight Medical Products developed the Argus II, which includes implantation of a 60-electrode grid on the retina, which is used in conjunction with a video camera mounted on eyeglasses. A wireless microprocessor with battery pack is worn on the waist. Altogether the system enables rudimentary perception of shapes and forms, allowing improved mobility in patients whose vision has been impaired by retinal diseases such as retinitis pigmentosa.[45]

VISUAL SCREENING

Primary visual dysfunction must be differentiated from a visual-perceptual disorder so that appropriate treatment can be addressed for each problem. Gianutsos and colleagues[46] found that more than half the individuals in their study admitted for general head injury rehabilitation who were eligible for cognitive services had visual sensory impairments sufficient to warrant further evaluation. Visual screening can identify the need for referral for a complete eye examination. The results of the examination become part of the differential diagnosis regarding a perceptual dysfunction. Box 28-3 presents key elements in vision screening.

This section describes vision screening tools and adaptations for various populations. The following principles should be kept in mind:

- Acuities: Acuities should always be tested first because decreased acuities will bias other tests except for ocular motilities and the peripheral field test.
- Positioning: The body and head should be in good alignment or straightened with positioning devices, with the head in midline.
- Glasses: If the client normally wears glasses, for either distance or near vision, the patient should be wearing glasses for tests for which spectacle correction is required. When in doubt, try it both ways, record the best response, and note whether glasses were worn.

Observations during Testing

The client's response during the test can provide important qualitative information about his or her visual system, including postural changes (head forward or back, body forward or back, head tilts or rotation [turning to either side]), squinting, closing one eye, excessive blinking, rubbing, signs of strain or fatigue, and holding the breath. Clients should be encouraged to relax, breathe normally, and not squint.

BOX 28-3 ■ KEY ELEMENTS IN VISION SCREENING

1. Distance and near visual acuities
2. Oculomotilities (pursuits, saccades, near point of convergence)
3. Measure of eye alignment to detect strabismus or high phoria
4. Measure of depth perception (stereopsis)
5. Measure of the visual fields

Distance Acuities

Equipment

Needed to measure distance acuity are a distance acuity chart, an occluder, a 20-foot measure, and the patient's corrective lenses if worn for distance.

Setup

A distance chart is taped on a well-lighted wall at the patient's eye level, and a distance of 20 feet is measured from the chart.

Procedure

One of the patient's eyes is covered and the patient is asked to read the smallest letters that he or she can see. Exposing one letter or line at a time can help if tracking or attention is a problem. The examiner should encourage the patient to guess and instruct the patient not to squint. The number of letters that were missed on the smallest line that the patient is able to see is noted. The procedure is repeated by covering the patient's other eye, and then both eyes are tested unoccluded.

Record

The smallest line the patient was able to read is recorded. If the client missed any letters on that line then the number of letters missed is subtracted. For example, if the client read four letters correctly on the 20/30 line but missed the other two, then it is recorded as 20/30−2. The scores for the client's right eye, left eye, and both eyes together are recorded.

If the patient is unable to see the top line at 20 feet, the patient is asked to move forward until able to identify the top letters. Then the distance and letter size (top line) are recorded. For example, if the patient had to move up to 4 feet to see the top line, then 4/100 is recorded. To calculate 20-foot equivalence, an equation is used where x equals the size of the letter (e.g., $4/100 = 20/x$); thus, $4x = 2000$ and $2000/4 = 500$. The client's vision is 20/500 (Box 28-4).

For clients whose attention is poor, the testing distance may need to be as close as 2 feet. Other testing stimuli can be used for children, such as the Broken Wheel Test* or the Lighthouse cards.* Acuity in low-functioning clients or infants can be evaluated by use of preferential looking methods. Targets are usually high-contrast grating patterns of decreasing size. One such type is the Teller cards.†

Implications

A patient who fails this test may require glasses or a change in the current prescription.

Near Acuities

Equipment

A near-point test card, an occluder, and the client's corrective lenses if normally worn for near vision are needed.

Procedure

The procedure is the same as for distance acuity. The standard test distance is usually 16 inches (40 cm).

---

*Bernell/USO, 4016 North Home Street, Mishiwaka, IN 46545; (800) 348-2225.

†Vistech Consultants, 4162 Little York Road, Dayton, OH 45414-2566.

BOX 28-4 ■ INTERPRETATION OR REFERRAL

20/20 is considered normal.
20/40 is required by the Department of Motor Vehicles (DMV) in most states for full-time day and night driver's license, although requirements vary in different states.
20/80 is required by the DMV for daytime driver's license.
20/40 or worse indicates referral to an eye doctor.
20/200 corrected (with spectacle prescription) is considered legally blind.
A difference of two lines or more between the two eyes indicates referral to an eye doctor (e.g., right eye is 20/20, left eye is 20/30).

Record

The smallest line read is recorded.

Interpretation and Referral

A test result of 20/20 is considered normal, 20/40 is required for reading newspaper-sized print, and 20/100 is needed for large print. Referral to an optometrist or ophthalmologist should be made if vision is 20/40 or worse or if a difference of two lines exists between the two eyes. Neurological damage can affect the accommodative system. Sometimes it corrects itself spontaneously, but not always.

Visual retraining of the focusing system may be appropriate, depending on the patient's age. This can be determined by an optometrist familiar with vision therapy.

Pursuits

Equipment

Any target that holds the patient's attention can be used, such as a pencil or small toy.

Setup

The patient is seated facing the screener.

Procedure

One pencil is held 16 to 20 inches in front of the client, and the client is asked to look directly at one part, such as the eraser, and to keep the head still, holding it if necessary. The pencil is moved around in the pattern shown in Figure 28-11, which is designed to incorporate all directions of gaze. The examiner should observe for smooth following, noticing and recording jerks and jumps, where they occur, or if the eyes stop at a certain point. If one or both eyes stop tracking, the client is encouraged to look at the pencil. If the patient is unable to do this, then the movement pattern is repeated with each eye separately and where the movement stops is recorded. Clients who have had a cerebrovascular accident (CVA) or head injury should be tested first monocularly (each eye separately).

Record

Results are rated as follows:

- Poor = Difficulty following target with any accuracy, jerky or jumpy, nystagmoid movements, incomplete range of motion

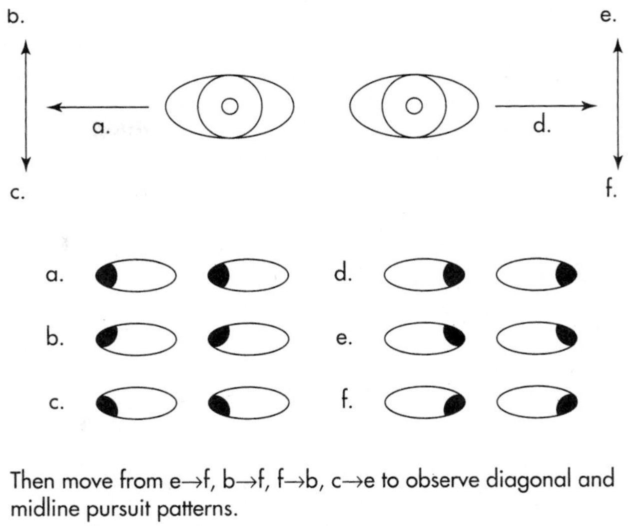

Figure 28-11 ■ Pursuit patterns.

- Fair = Generally able to follow target but goes off target occasionally (one to two times), with slight jerkiness
- Good = Eye movements smooth with no jerkiness

If one eye stops tracking at a certain point or if the client reports double vision (diplopia) in certain directions, the examiner should record which eye or in which direction the problem is noticed (e.g., the right eye does not pass midline when moving from left to right, or diplopia is reported on upward right gaze). This specific information can be helpful to the ophthalmologist or optometrist.

Saccades

Equipment

Tracking pencils can be used, although a few saccadic tests are available. One is the King Devick Saccadic Test; the other is the Developmental Eye Movement Test.* These both require form perception (number reading) and may be difficult, depending on the client's cognitive level.

Setup

The patient is seated facing the screener.

Procedure

A pencil is held in each hand about 17 to 20 inches from the client, and the client is told that he or she is going to be asked to look at one pencil while the other pencil is moved but not to look at it until told to do so. The client is to move the eyes only, keeping the head still. While the client looks at the first pencil, the other pencil is moved as the screener says "shift" or "look at this pencil." The screener then moves the other pencil, says "shift," then moves the pencil, says "shift," then moves the pencil, and so on, until a pattern of movement can be discerned.

*Bernell/USO, 4016 North Home Street, Mishiwaka, IN 46545; (800) 348-2225. Complete Visual Screening Kit: Laurie R. Chaikin, OD, OTR/L, 420 F Cola Ballena, Alameda, CA 94501; Laurie.chaikin@gmail.com.

This call-shift is repeated about 10 times, moving into different fields of gaze. The screener continues until the client is seen to respond. The screener observes for overshooting or undershooting the target, for the ability to isolate the eyes from the head (hold head still), for controlled eye movement, and for ability to wait until the verbal command to look. It is important to observe for the client's ability to shift to all fields of gaze. A lower level of testing would be to ask the client to move the eyes from one target to the other as quickly as possible (Figure 28-12).

Record

Results are rated as follows:

- Poor = Inability to control eyes with verbal command, consistent undershooting or overshooting, inability to isolate eyes from head
- Fair = Ability to maintain eyes on target with verbal command 50% of the time, with slight undershooting or overshooting, and ability to isolate eyes from head with verbal reminders
- Good = Ability to follow verbal commands 90% of the time, with no undershooting or overshooting, and complete eye from head isolation

Near Point of Convergence

Procedure

A pencil is introduced about 20 inches away from the client's midline. The client is asked whether the pencil looks single. If it is not, it is moved farther away. The client is told that the pencil will be moved toward her or him and that it will be getting blurry but to keep watching it as far in as possible. When the pencil appears single, it is moved toward the nose at a moderately slow rate (but not too slow). The screener should watch the client's eyes. As long as the client's eyes are tracking the pencil, the pencil is kept moving toward the nose. At the point where one eye moves out, both eyes move out, or the eyes simply stop tracking, the distance of the pencil to the nose is measured. If the client is wearing bifocals, it is important to make sure the patient is looking through the reading segment.

Record

The break point is the distance at which the eyes were observed to stop tracking the pencil. If the client was able to track the pencil all the way to the nose, then record this fact.

Interpretation and Referral

A score of poor or fair on saccades or pursuits suggests the need for training. A near point of convergence with a break point of 5 inches or more is suggestive of convergence problems, and recommendations for referral should be made.

Implications

Difficulties with smooth pursuit, accurate saccades, or convergence can all present tracking difficulties for the patient. These difficulties can cause loss of place in reading, rereading of words or lines, skipping lines, and lower comprehension and concentration. Inaccurate eye movements also may affect visual memory.

An eye movement problem may be the result of direct damage to the eye muscles themselves (Figure 28-13) or to the nerves controlling them, as in the case of a head injury. Damage to the vestibular center also may involve visual components. Neurons from cranial nerves III, IV, and VI synapse in the vestibular nuclei. Reflex control of eye movements occurs through the VOR and the optokinetic system.

Cover Tests

Purpose

There are two cover tests. The cover-uncover test is used to determine whether strabismus is present. The alternate cover test determines what type of phoria is present. The magnitude of the phoria generally determines the extent of the client's symptoms.

Equipment

An occluder and a tracking pencil or a small, distinct target is needed.

Setup

The client is seated facing the screener, who is also seated.

3		7	5			9			8
2	5			7		4			6
1			4		7		6		3
7		9		3		9			2
4	5				2			1	7
5			3		7		4		8
7	4		6	5					2
9		2			3		6		4
6	3	2		9					1
7				4		6	5		2
5		3	7			4			8
4			5		2			1	7
7	9	3			9				2
1			4			7		6	3
2		5		7			4		6
3	7		5			9			8

Figure 28-12 ■ Developmental eye movement test.

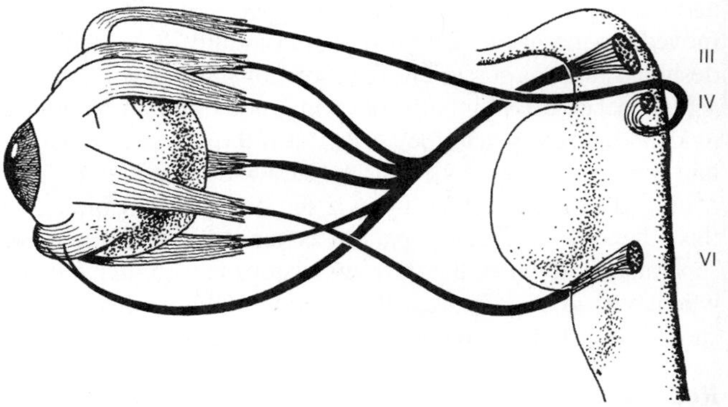

Figure 28-13 ■ Cranial nerves III, IV, and VI. Oculomotor, trochlear, and abducens nerves and their innervation of the extraocular muscles. (Courtesy Smith, Kline & French Laboratories, Philadelphia, Pennsylvania.)

Procedure

A pencil is held approximately 16 inches in front of the client, and the client is asked to look directly at the target and to keep it in focus.

Near Cover Tests

Cover-Uncover Test. The movement of the uncovered eye is observed. The client's right eye is covered, and the left eye is observed for movement in, out, upward, or downward. This is repeated a few times, allowing the eyes to be uncovered for about 2 seconds between trials. Then the left eye is covered to observe for movement in the right eye.

Alternate Cover Test. Eye movement is observed as the eye is uncovered. An occluder is held over the right eye for a few seconds while the client looks at a near target. The occluder is moved from the right eye to the left eye while the right eye is observed for movement in, out, up, or down. After a few seconds, the occluder is moved back to the right eye, observing the left eye for movement. This is repeated back and forth several times until the screener is sure of what is seen.

Far Cover Tests

The preceding procedure is repeated with the patient looking at a distant target.

Interpretation and Referral. Any visible eye movement seen during the cover-uncover test with good maintenance of fixation on the target indicates a strabismus. If there is no previous history of strabismus, referral is indicated. A large eye movement seen with the alternate cover test, along with the presence of symptoms such as eye strain, headaches, or apparent difficulty in making spatial judgments, also indicates referral. In the clinic the therapist may notice that the client has difficulty finding objects in a drawer, or that the client appears cross-eyed or seems to be looking past the target. He or she may have difficulty with spatial judgments in reaching for objects or in mobility, especially with stairs or curbs.

A visible eye movement may be part of a post-CVA client's premorbid pattern. This should be determined by asking the client or the family members before making a referral. Or the condition may be the result of neurological damage to cranial nerve III, IV, or VI from CVA, head injury, or cerebral palsy. Eye muscles are striated muscles, under voluntary control. Like other striated muscles that can be affected by neurological damage, they may recover spontaneously, they may not recover at all, or they may benefit from visual retraining. Many learning-disabled children with vestibular dysfunction have poor binocular skills. An ophthalmologist or optometrist specially trained in visual remediation can determine a patient's potential for vision therapy. Some published research has demonstrated the success of vision therapy for post-CVA patients.[47]

Stereopsis (Depth Perception)

Equipment

Any test that uses either Polaroid or red-green filters can test for stereopsis ability. Examples are the Titmus stereo fly, reindeer, and butterfly.*

*Bernell/USO, 4016 North Home Street, Mishiwaka, IN 46545; (800) 348-2225. Complete Visual Screening Kit: Laurie R. Chaikin, OD, OTR/L, 420 F Cola Ballena, Alameda, CA 94501; Laurie.chaikin@gmail.com.

Procedure

The client is asked to point to or say which test object appears closer. If the client is able to grasp for the object in space, some stereo ability is present.

Record

The client's response should be immediate. Long delays could indicate borderline ability.

Interpretation and Referral

If the client fails this test, a referral to an ophthalmologist or optometrist is recommended. The patient must have best-corrected acuities for this test; otherwise, the results are invalid.

Implications

A deficit in depth perception can interfere with all activities involving spatial judgments, in particular fine motor and eye-hand type activities in which judgments of relative depth are required (e.g., threading a needle, placing toothpaste on a toothbrush, hammering). Although ambulation itself may not be affected, ambulation involving curbs or stairs will be affected.

Vision therapy training can be helpful for clients with problems in binocular coordination. Proper diagnosis and therapy prescription are essential.

Visual Field Screening

Equipment

An occluder or eyepatch is required, and a black dowel with a white pin on the end or just a wiggling finger can be used as a peripheral target.

Setup

The client is seated facing the examiner.

Procedure

The client holds the occluder over the left eye. The examiner explains that he or she is going to wiggle a finger out to the side and that the patient is to say "now" when he or she first detects the movement of the wiggling finger. The client should look at the screener's nose the entire time and ignore any arm movement. The test is begun with the examiner's hand slightly behind the client about 16 inches away from the client's head. The hand is brought forward slowly while a finger is wiggled. Different sections of the visual field are randomly tested in 45-degree intervals around the visual field. The left eye is then tested after the client's right eye is occluded. Alternatively, if a dowel is used, it is slowly brought in from the side until the client reports seeing the small pin at the end of the dowel.

These confrontation field tests are considered gross tests compared with a visual field perimeter test. Many clients cannot do the perimeter test because it requires a higher cognitive level. Confrontation fields will reveal a hemianopsia and a quadrantanopsia (quarter-field cut). For lower-functioning clients the examiner can observe eye movements in the direction of the target to get a general idea of peripheral function once clients have seen it.

Record

The portion of field missing for each eye is noted.

Interpretation and Referral

If any hemianopsia or quadrantanopsia is noted, the patient is referred to an optometrist or an ophthalmologist.

Implications

A visual deficit has significant implication for the safe performance of many functional activities, including driving and mobility. Visually guided movement through space becomes impaired, as are efficient eye movements; if central field loss is present, reading and any other near activities are affected. The reader is referred to the discussion of assessment of unilateral inattention for differentiation between neglect and hemianopsia.

REFERRAL CONSIDERATIONS

The final outcome of the visual screening is referral to an optometrist or ophthalmologist, ideally to someone with an orientation toward visual rehabilitation. It is important not to make diagnostic statements but rather to indicate whether the client passed or failed the vision screening. By law, only optometrists or ophthalmologists can diagnose visual conditions.

It is not always clear when to refer a client or to whom. Many doctors do not test all areas of visual function. Generally, behavioral or developmental optometrists have a functionally oriented philosophy quite similar to occupational therapy models of functional performance.*

Recommended referral guidelines are shown in Box 28-5.

BOX 28-5 ■ REFERRAL GUIDELINES

1. Failure of either the distance or near acuity test (with glasses on). This could indicate an uncorrected refractive error, a disease process, or a neurological problem.
2. Failure of the oculomotility section only does not indicate referral because treatment of oculomotor dysfunction is currently within the scope of practice for rehabilitation. *Exception:* Failure of the pursuit test as a result of a reduced ocular range of motion in any direction of gaze, which indicates cranial nerve involvement.
3. Failure of the cover-uncover test indicates strabismus and is an indication for referral unless there is a history of an eye turn.
4. A large eye movement seen on the alternate cover test, along with apparent difficulties in stereopsis, such as spatial judgments, or symptoms, such as headaches, eyestrain, or difficulty with comprehension, constitutes an indication for referral.
5. Failure of the stereopsis test alone is an indication for referral if there is no history of an eye turn and if there is movement on either cover test.
6. Patients with quarter-field loss and half-field loss (hemianopsia) should be referred.

Rehabilitation Optometric Evaluation

Once the client has been referred for evaluation, the eye doctor will evaluate any changes in the refractive error and the need for new correction to achieve the best possible vision. The eye alignment will be quantified, and determination will be made regarding whether there is an eye muscle paresis, which cranial nerve is involved, whether strabismus or phoria is present, and whether the eye deviation is better or worse in particular directions of gaze.

Oculomotilities will be evaluated grossly, and more specific tests may be done. One test is the Developmental Eye Movement Test (see Figure 28-12). Another test is the Visagraph (Figure 28-14). This instrument records eye movements while the client is reading text. It will measure total reading rate, number of fixations and regressions per 100 words, span of recognition, and reading comprehension. The tool is excellent for in-depth evaluation and monitoring the progress of treatment over time.

Ocular health testing will include glaucoma testing, examination for cataracts, and retinal health evaluation. For visual field testing, either a screening field or a threshold visual field will be done on some type of automated perimeter such as the Humphrey Visual Field Analyzer or the Octopus. Threshold testing is done to determine the extent and depth of a defect, and it can help to determine whether there is potential for visual field retraining. In Figure 28-9 the black portions of the visual field are areas of absolute damage. The areas of white with small dots are intact visual fields. At the border of the damage area is a gray zone, which theoretically is amenable to training.[30-33]

The optometrist or ophthalmologist will deliver a report of the findings with recommendations for the treatment plan.

Visual Intervention

Early intervention is recommended when possible to identify ways in which a vision problem may be interfering with other therapies.[47-50] Some treatments may be applied early

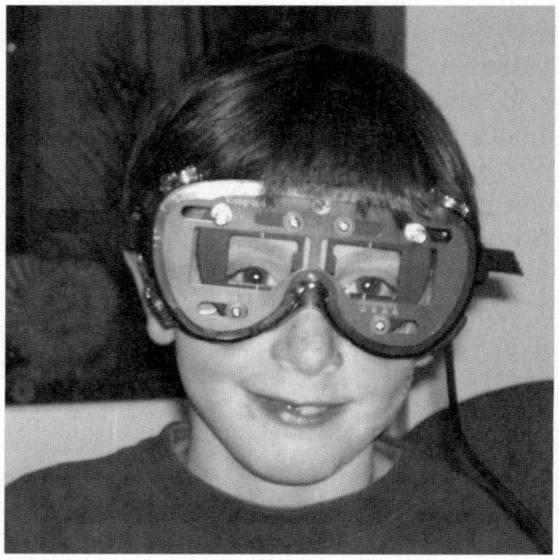

Figure 28-14 ■ The Visagraph (boy with goggles) measures eye movement while the subject is reading.

*College of Optometrists for Vision Development has a list of behavioral doctors: 234 North Lindberg Boulevard, Suite 310, St Louis, MO 63141; or Optometric Extension Program, 1921 East Carnegie Avenue, Suite 3L, Santa Ana, CA 92705-5510. Neuro-Optometer Rehabilitation Association, www.nora.cc/index.html.

on, as well. For example, if the client has an eye muscle paresis, range of motion exercises to the involved muscle can prevent the development of a contracture of the unopposed muscle.

In cases in which the client has double vision, a patching regimen can be instituted. One regimen is to alternate patching the eyes daily, allowing some time to experience diplopia, so that the eyes may attempt to make a fusion response. The stimulus to fusion is double vision. If one eye is always patched, spontaneous recovery may be slowed. Another patching regimen is binasal taping, and another is to use partially opaque materials to allow peripheral vision in the occluded eye. The patching regimen should be prescribed by an optometrist or ophthalmologist.

In some cases of double vision, a temporary plastic (Fresnel) prism can be applied to the client's glasses to reduce or eliminate the diplopia. This may significantly enhance the client's functioning in other therapies, particularly when spatial judgments are being made (e.g., in fine motor tasks or ambulation).

Documentation

Vision problems should be documented in functional performance terms—that is, how the vision problem affects activities of daily living. Improvement can then be monitored according to function. This will also help in reimbursement. For example, a client with an eye muscle dysfunction will have difficulty with spatial judgments such as placing toothpaste on a toothbrush, spearing objects, reaching for a cup handle, doing pegboard tasks, and using vision for balance.

THERAPEUTIC CONSIDERATIONS

Once a referral has been made, the client has been seen, and the examination report has been received, what else can be done? How the dysfunction affects therapy can be considered, and some visual training, prescribed by the optometrist, can be initiated.

Accommodative Dysfunction

If the client has an accommodative dysfunction, the treatment may be the prescription of glasses for reading or tabletop tasks or possibly near-far focusing exercises,[4] depending on the age of the client. "Flipper bars" are special lenses that exercise the focusing system.[51]

If the client needs glasses for near but cannot get them for some reason, the therapist can try moving the task farther away and increasing the lighting on the task.

Eye Alignment Dysfunction

If the client has a problem in the eye alignment system, several factors should be considered. If the client is able to fuse some of the time but loses fusion, seeing double when stressed or tired, then the most difficult tasks should be attempted when the client is least fatigued. Otherwise, if the client has constant double vision or the client is seeing double at the time the therapist is working with her or him, patching may be prescribed by the ophthalmologist or optometrist. This will reduce the client's confusion and increase attention to the task. For clients with acquired double vision, however, it is important to provide time without a patch so that the eyes will attempt to regain fusion. Wearing the patch constantly will discourage any attempts by the brain to overcome the double vision.

Visual Dysfunction and Balance Disorders

It is important to recognize the close interplay between the visual and the balance systems, including vestibular, proprioceptive and tactile receptors, in maintaining balance. Altered visual input can affect perception of space, even with something as simple as getting a new pair of glasses. The nonneurologically impaired individual will eventually adapt and reset the coordination of information. Neurologically impaired patients can have much greater difficulty in resetting the coordination of sensory information from multiple systems, resulting in a feeling of sensory overload or being overwhelmed. Conversely, damage to areas of the brain that process vestibular or somatosensory information can create altered maps of space, also affecting balance as the individual attempts to interact with the environment.

Therapy may be directed at both areas: improving balance by enhancing balance and proprioceptive mechanisms and/or by enhancing visual input through visual rehabilitation techniques. There has been recent research involving the strategic placement of small weights on the torso, which has had immediate and sometimes dramatic effects on balance.[52,53] Interestingly, these types of inputs to the torso can also affect visual processing (observations by BalanceWear vest developer Cindy Gibson-Horn, RPT, and me). It is hypothesized that the mechanism for this change may be mediated by cerebellar-visual pathways.[54]

VISUAL-PERCEPTUAL DYSFUNCTION

This discussion of visual-perceptual disorders is divided into a number of categories: unilateral spatial inattention; cortical blindness, defective color perception, and visual agnosia; visual-spatial disorders; visual-constructive disorders; and visual analysis and synthesis disorders. Cortical blindness is a disorder of primary visual input; however, because its variations may influence perceptual interpretation, it is discussed here. All other disorders listed involve direct problems with the interpretation of visual stimuli. Although each of these terms represents symptoms recognized by many authors, the reader is reminded that there are no clear boundaries between one deficit and another or one system and another. Apraxia and body image disorders are not discussed under separate categories because they are not considered "visual"-perceptual disorders per se, although their presence may influence and complicate an already dysfunctional visual-perceptual system.

Problems of Unilateral Spatial Inattention

Identification of Clinical Problems

General Category. In its purest form, unilateral spatial inattention is defined as a condition in which an individual with normal sensory and motor systems fails to orient toward, respond to, or report stimuli on the side contralateral to the cerebral lesion. Although this condition is not often seen in its pure form, inattention has been documented in persons who demonstrate no accompanying visual field defect (homonymous hemianopsia) or limb sensory or motor loss.[55] In most cases, however, unilateral spatial inattention is not seen alone but is associated with (although not caused by) accompanying sensory and motor defects such as homonymous hemianopsia and decreased tactile, proprioceptive, and stereognostic perception along with paresis or paralysis of the upper limb.[56]

It is easy to become confused by the numerous terms used in the literature, for example, *unilateral spatial agnosia, unilateral visual neglect, fixed hemianopsia, hemi-inattention,* and *hemi-imperception.* All terms describe the same deficit. Unilateral spatial inattention is used in this chapter because (1) in severe cases the syndrome most likely involves tactile and auditory as well as visual unawareness (i.e., a total spatial unawareness) and (2) the syndrome results in an involuntary lack of attention to stimuli contralateral to the lesion, whereas the term *neglect* implies a voluntary choice not to respond.

Unilateral spatial inattention occurs most frequently in individuals with a diagnosis of stroke (CVA), traumatic brain injury, or tumor. Most authors agree that unilateral spatial inattention occurs more often with right hemisphere than with left hemisphere lesions.[57-61] This frequency supports theories that the right hemisphere is dominant for visual-spatial organization. It is clear, however, that inattention may be present in individuals with left hemisphere lesions, but that the inattention tends to resolve more quickly.[62] The clinician should remember that, although the chances are statistically lower, the client with right hemiplegia may exhibit inattention to right stimuli.

Unilateral spatial inattention has been associated with lesions in both cortical and subcortical structures. It is most commonly seen in inferior parietal lobe lesions[60] but has also been observed in lesions in the inferior frontal cortex, the dorsolateral frontal lobe, the superior temporal gyrus, and the cingulate gyrus[63] and with basal ganglia, thalamic,[64] and putaminal hemorrhage.[65-67] Finally, lesions in the brain stem reticular formation have induced inattention in cats[66] and monkeys.[64]

Although a number of theories have been postulated regarding the mechanism underlying unilateral spatial inattention, no mechanism has been validly documented in human subjects. The one fact that is clear from all theoretical postulates is that inattention is a hemispheric deficit. LeDoux and Smylie[68] demonstrated this point effectively in an interesting case study of a right-sided lesion. During full visual exposure (bilateral hemispheric) of visual-perceptual slides, the affected individual made visual-spatial errors in left space. However, when the same slides were directed only to the right visual field (left hemisphere), performance improved substantially. It is as if the deficient hemisphere fails to receive or orient toward incoming information while the intact receiving hemisphere remains oblivious and goes about its own business. Treatment for inattention is problematic mainly because the mechanisms underlying unilateral spatial inattention are not clearly understood.

Theories on mechanisms underlying unilateral spatial inattention have attempted to explain it as an integrative associative defect as opposed to simply a problem of decreased sensory input. Theories include a unilateral attentional hypothesis, suggesting that inattention results from a disruption in the orienting response—that is, the corticolimbic hemisphere is underaroused during bilateral input, and therefore stimuli presented to that hemisphere are neglected.[60,63] Another theory is the oculomotor imbalance hypothesis, which suggests that individuals with inattention have a visual-spatial disorder worsened by oculomotor imbalance. The hypothesis suggests that the lesion disconnects the frontal eye fields in the damaged hemisphere from their sensory afferent nerves, resulting in an oculomotor imbalance deviating the gaze toward the lesion. This imbalance can be compensated for only momentarily by a voluntary effort to gaze toward the opposite hemispace (i.e., neglected space).[69]

Unilateral Spatial Inattention with Homonymous Hemianopsia. Inattention occurs more commonly with visual field defects and is generally better when the macular projections are not involved. Individuals with pure hemianopsia are aware of their visual loss and spontaneously learn to compensate by moving their eyes (foveae) toward the lost visual field to expand their visual space and thereby gather information right and left of midline. On visual examination other individuals may demonstrate no visual field defect on unilateral stimulation; however, during bilateral stimulation they extinguish the target contralateral to the lesion. Other persons may perceive both targets simultaneously, yet when engaged in activity they may not respond to visual stimuli in one half of the visual space contralateral to the lesion. These individuals are unaware of their inattention. Careful observation of their activity reveals few eye movements into the neglected space. The fovea does not appear to be directed to gather information in this space.

Unilateral Visual, Auditory, and Tactile Inattention. Inattention has been described as a multimodal sensory associative disorder involving not only visual but also tactile and auditory unawareness. Clinicians are well aware of the client with left inattention who continues to direct the head and eyes toward the right throughout an entire conversation although the therapist is standing on the client's left side. When one conceptualizes unilateral spatial inattention as a dynamic decrease or loss of sensory information within one half of the sensory-perceptual sphere (irrespective of hypothetical mechanism), the peculiar behaviors exhibited by these clients are more easily understood.

Unilateral Spatial Inattention and Body Image. Body image is often disturbed in individuals with inattention. The defect in these persons is unusual because it affects only that half of the body that is contralateral to the lesion, for example, the left side of the body in right-sided lesions. There appears to be a lack of spatial orientation and attention for one half of intrapersonal space. Those with severe inattention fail to recognize that their affected extremities are their own and function as though they are absent. They may fail to dress one half of the body or attempt to navigate through a door oblivious to the fact that the affected arm may be caught on the doorknob or door frame. In severe cases, individuals may deny their hemiparesis, or they may deny that the extremity belongs to them. This phenomenon is called *anosognosia.*

Behavioral Manifestations of Unilateral Spatial Inattention. Persons with inattention orient all their activities toward their "attended" space. The head, eyes, and trunk are rotated toward the side of the lesion for much of the time, including during gait. Careful observation of eye movements (scanning saccades) during activities indicates that all or almost all scanning occurs on only one side of the midline within the attended space; the individual never spontaneously brings the eyes or head past midline into contralateral "unattended" space. Oculomotor examination always shows full extraocular movements and no apraxia for eye movements.

Inattention, like all other perceptual disorders, may occur on a scale from mild to severe. Mild cases of inattention may go unrecognized unless behavior is carefully observed. Scanning is symmetrical except during tasks requiring increasingly complex perceptual and cognitive demands. Leicester and colleagues[70] believe that inattention occurs mainly when the individual has a general perceptual problem with the material, that is, some other problem with processing the task. This performance difficulty or stress brings on the additional inattention behavior; for example, neglect in matching auditory letter samples is more common in those with aphasia than in those with right hemisphere involvement without aphasia.

Independence in activities of daily living is often impossible because of inattention to both the intrapersonal and the extrapersonal environment. The individual may eat only half the food on the plate, dress only half the body, shave or apply makeup to only half the face, brush teeth in only half the mouth, read only half a page, fill out only half a form, miss kitchen utensils, carpentry tools, or items in the store if they are located in the unattended space, collide with obstacles or miss doorways on the unattended side, and, when walking or driving a wheelchair, veer toward the attended space rather than navigating in a straight line.

Assessment

Because most tests used to measure cognitive, language, perceptual, and motor skills require symmetrical visual, auditory, and tactile awareness, it is most important to rule out inattention early in the evaluation process of any client with a central lesion. The two most common methods used to distinguish inattention from primary sensory deficits are double simultaneous stimulation testing and assessment of optokinetic nystagmus reflexes. Double simultaneous stimuli should be applied in three modalities: auditory, tactile, and visual. Initially, stimuli should be presented to the abnormal side. If primary sensation is impaired (e.g., a visual field loss), this evaluation cannot proceed because double simultaneous stimulation testing is invalid in that modality. If responsiveness is normal, however, bilateral simultaneous stimuli should be applied. Unilateral stimuli should be interspersed with bilateral stimuli to ensure valid responses. Lack of awareness (extinction) of stimuli contralateral to the lesion during bilateral stimulation should be noted. Clients with extinction in only one sensory system often do not demonstrate inattention behaviors; however, those with extinction in more than one modality (e.g., tactile and visual) often demonstrate these behaviors. If critical diagnosis of inattention is necessary, the client may be referred for optokinetic nystagmus testing.

One of the best evaluation tools is a keen sense of observation. The position of the client's head, eyes, and trunk should be observed at rest and during activity. Persistent deviation toward the lesion may indicate unilateral inattention. The individual should be asked to track a visual target from space ipsilateral to the lesion into contralateral space and maintain fixation there for 5 seconds. The therapist may ask the client to quickly fixate on visual targets both right and left of midline on command. Problems with searching for targets in contralateral space should be noted. Some erratic oculomotor searching is normal when making saccades into a hemianoptic field because saccades are centrally preprogrammed by peripheral input. Slow searching or failure to search should be considered indicative of inattention.

Asymmetries in performance should be noted during spatial tasks. Specific spatial tasks have been designed for detection of inattention, including the following:

- Cancellation tasks. The client may be given a sheet of paper with horizontal lines of numbers or letters and asked to cross out all the 8s or As.
- Crossing-out tasks. In this standardized test the client is asked to cross out diagonal lines drawn at random on an unlined sheet of paper.
- Line-bisection tasks. The client is asked to bisect a 4- to 8-inch line on a piece of paper placed at the midline.
- Drawing and copying tasks. The client may be asked to draw or copy a house, clock, or flower or to fill in the numbers of a clock drawn by the examiner. For copying tasks, it is important that the copy be placed in the client's attended space.

Clients with inattention demonstrate one or more of the following behaviors: failing to cancel figures or cross out lines in the unattended space; bisecting the line unequally, placing their mark toward the side of the midline ipsilateral to their lesion; placing their drawing toward the edge of the paper ipsilateral to their lesion rather than in the middle of the page; drawing only the right or left half of the house, flower, or clock; crowding all the numbers of the clock into the right or left half of the clock; or completing numbers on only one half of the clock (Figure 28-15), and demonstrating differences in reaction time.[71] When interpreting performance, the examiner is looking specifically for asymmetries in performance. Clients with inattention often have other visual-perceptual deficits that result in faulty performance on these tasks; however, these deficits are always symmetrical, that is, evident in any space to which the individual attends.

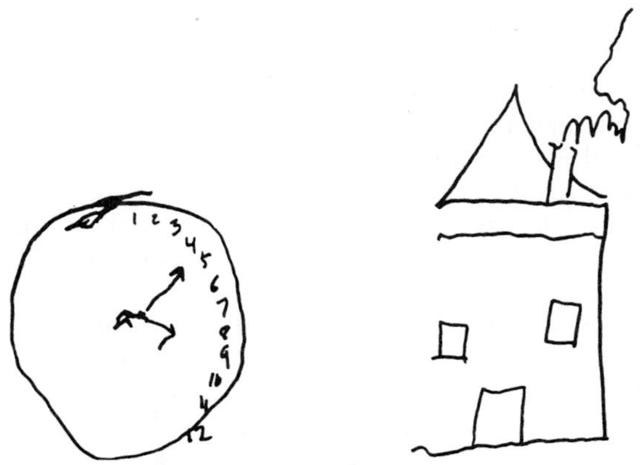

Figure 28-15 ■ Drawings of a clock and house by a client with a right hemisphere parietal lobe tumor. Note the left unilateral spatial inattention in the drawings.

Asymmetries in performance should be carefully observed during functional activities such as eating, filling out a form, reading, dressing, and maneuvering through the environment. The therapist may note unawareness of doorways and hallways in the unattended space; turns may be made only toward one direction. As a result, these clients lose their way in the hospital or even in the therapy clinic. This behavior should be distinguished from a topographical perceptual deficit in which the individual cannot integrate or remember spatial concepts well enough to find his or her way without getting lost. The Behavioral Inattention Test has recently been published as a standardized measure of functional inattention.[72]

Finally, various studies have shown that inattention may occur during testing that requires visual processing and therefore may invalidate test results.[57,73,74] Unresponsiveness to figures on one side of the page during visual, perceptual, cognitive, or language assessments may be subtle but must be documented to rule out the influence of inattention on raw score; that is, if the patient did not see the entire test display for an item, that test item is invalid. Responses to figures on the right half and left half of the test page should be counted. If the frequency of answers is noticeably less on one half of the page than would normally be expected, inattention may have occurred during testing. This may be used as additional evidence of inattention; but more important, this factor should be accounted for when computing the test score. Only those test items in which the correct answer was located in the attended space should be scored; that is, only those items in which the correct answer was right of midline in a client with left inattention should be scored.

Interventions

As previously stated, the mechanisms underlying unilateral spatial inattention are not well understood; however, recent research has uncovered a strong correlation between nonspatial aspects of attention called *tonic* and *phasic attention* and spatial aspects of neglect. Tonic attention is intrinsic arousal that fluctuates on the order of hours to minutes and contributes to sustained attention and preparation for more complex cognitive tasks. Phasic attention is a rapid change in attention in response to a sudden and brief event and is related to orienting responses and selective attention.[75] This research has postulated that nonspatial attention mechanisms affect spatial and nonspatial behavior. Some highly successful training protocols using these attentional mechanisms have been developed, and the researchers have been able to demonstrate improved responses with carryover in the environment (see Appendix 28-A). They also demonstrated that this remediation approach was more effective than just scanning strategies. A number of studies have investigated the remediation of unilateral spatial inattention. They have attempted to (1) define effective remediation techniques and (2) measure changes in trained tasks and generalization to untrained tasks, that is, determine whether inattention training in one task carries over to other unrelated tasks such as activities of daily living. Treatment techniques used in all these studies resulted in less inattention during trained tasks.[58,76,77] An overview of these studies suggests that training may decrease inattention, although extent of change and generalization to other tasks may vary widely. Discrepancies in these results may be related to neurological variables in the various client samples, severity of inattention, sample size, or tasks measured. A discussion of general principles of remediation follows.

Efforts should be made to increase the client's cognitive awareness of the inattention. The individual should be made keenly aware of what a peripheral visual field loss is and how it is affecting her or his view of the world. The person with normal visual fields but with visual extinction should be treated the same as the individual with an actual visual field loss because the visual experience is similar. Pictures of the visual field deficit may be drawn for illustration. Actual performance examples in the environment should be pointed out to the client to demonstrate the biased field of view.

Visual scanning should be emphasized. Initially, the client should be made aware of how eye and eye-head movements may be used to compensate for the deficit. The individual should be trained to make progressively larger and quicker pursuits and saccades and longer fixations into the unattended space. Training may be accomplished with interesting targets held by the therapist, for example, targets secured to the tips of pencils, such as changeable letters, colored lights, or bright small objects. Pursuit or tracking movements of the target leading the eye from attended into unattended space should be stressed first, followed by saccades into the unattended space. Initially the client may be allowed to move the head during scanning exercises; however, eye movements without head movements should be the major goal. Individuals with inattention often move the head into the unattended space while the eye remains fixed on a target in the attended space (i.e., the visual field remains the same). The client should be taught to independently carry out a daily right-left scanning program with targets appropriately positioned by the therapist. Eventually these targets can be moved farther into the unattended space.

Increased awareness and scanning abilities should be incorporated in increasingly complex visual-perceptual and visual-motor tasks. Because inattention often increases as task complexity increases, the therapist must select and structure tasks carefully. Examples of simple yet specific scanning tasks might include surveying a room repetitively, rolling toward and touching objects right and left of midline, assembling objects from pieces strewn on a table or the floor, completing an obstacle course, or selecting letters from a page of large print.

Scanning should be stressed during functional activities, for example, dressing, shaving, or moving through the environment. The client may be taught to constantly monitor the influence of inattention on functional performance, for example, "When something doesn't make sense, look into the unattended space and it usually will."

Diller[78] has designed a number of specific training techniques to decrease inattention during reading and paper and pencil tasks. With a little creativity, these techniques may be applied to other activities. For example, when the client is reading, a visual marker is placed on the extreme edge of the page in unattended space. The individual is instructed not to begin reading until he or she sees the visual marker. The marker is used to "anchor" the client's vision. As inattention decreases, the anchor is faded. Each line may also be numbered and the numbers used to anchor scanning horizontally and vertically. To control impulsiveness, which often accompanies inattention, clients are taught to slow down or pace their performance by incorporating techniques such as reciting the words aloud. Underlining and looping letters or words can also be used as a method to slow down impulsive scanning (Figure 28-16). Finally, the density of stimuli is reduced; decreased density appears to decrease inattention in these tasks.

To stimulate tactile awareness in clients with tactile extinction, Anderson and Choy[79] suggest stimulating the affected arm as the individual watches. A rough cloth, vibrator, or the therapist's or client's hand may be used. Eventually, this activity may be done before activities that require spontaneous symmetrical scanning, such as dressing or walking through an obstacle course.

During the early phases of treatment, when inattention is still moderate to severe, the client should be approached from the attended space during treatment for inattention or other deficits such as apraxia, balance, or speech. This ensures that the individual comprehends and views all demonstrations and treatment instructions. Subsequently, as orientation and scanning improve, activities should be moved progressively into the unattended space and the therapist should be positioned in the unattended space during treatment. In the final stages of treatment, the client should be able to symmetrically scan regardless of the therapist's position (i.e., the therapist should vary position).

To enhance the integration of scanning behavior during functional tasks such as gait and dressing, the client should be reminded of scanning principles and carried through a series of scanning exercises before initiation of the activity. If inattention reappears during the activity, the therapist should stop and assist the client in becoming reoriented before the activity is resumed. Inattention results in confusion, and confusion increases inattention. As will be pointed out repeatedly in the following pages, the therapist must control the perceptual environment continuously so that the client is able to sequence bits of information together meaningfully to learn or relearn.

Problems of Cortical Blindness, Color Imperception, and Visual Agnosia

Identification of Clinical Problems

Cortical Blindness. Cortical blindness is considered a primary sensory disorder as opposed to a secondary associative disorder. It is discussed here, however, because of the many variations of this lesion that may result in problems with interpretation of visual stimuli. Cortical blindness, also known as *central blindness,* is a total or almost total loss of vision resulting from bilateral cerebral destruction of the visual projection cortex (area 17). Similar destruction limited to one hemisphere results in hemianopsia.[55] The lesion may be ischemic, neoplastic, degenerative, or traumatic. The client may perceive the defect as a "blurring" of vision or as a marked decrease in visual acuity or may be unaware of the complete nature of the disability and even deny it, blaming the problem on eyeglasses that are too weak or a room that is too dark.

Color Imperception. Color perception may be impaired in the client with brain damage. This symptom is usually associated with right hemisphere or bilateral lesions.[80] This deficit is different from color agnosia, in which there is a problem with naming colors correctly. Clients with defective color perception may see colors as "muddy" or "impure" in hue, or the color of a small target may fade into the background, decreasing the ability to differentiate it from the background.[61,81] Total loss of color monochromatism is rare, but it can occur.

Visual Agnosia. A lesion circumscribed to the visual associative areas (areas 18 and 19) results in a number of unique visual disorders that are categorized as some form of visual agnosia. Lesions are usually bilateral with combined parietooccipital, occipitotemporal, and callosal lesions. Visual agnosia is defined as a failure to recognize visual stimuli (e.g., objects, faces, letters) although visual-sensory processing, language, and general intellectual functions are preserved at sufficiently high levels.[82] It also has been described as perception without meaning; perception apparently occurs, but the percept seems "disconnected" from previously associated meaning. In this pure form, visual

							0	1	2	4	5	6	7	8	9	10					
1.	1	2	3	5	4	9	7	8	0	6	3	2	10	1	2	3	5	4	9	7	1
2.	3	4	9	6	7	10	8	1	2	5	0	6	4	9	6	7	10	8	2	8	2
3.	8	0	6	2	1	3	5	4	7	9	10	1	8	0	6	2	1	3	5	7	3
4.	5	7	3	9	6	1	2	8	4	10	0	3	5	5	7	3	6	1	2	5	4
5.	6	5	1	4	2	3	8	10	9	7	9	0	6	5	1	4	2	3	8	9	5
6.	4	8	10	0	7	6	9	1	3	2	5	6	3	4	8	10	0	7	6	9	6
7.	9	6	5	3	8	4	2	0	10	1	7	2	4	9	6	5	3	8	2	4	7

Figure 28-16 ■ Underlining during visual discrimination tasks helps control eye movements (scanning).

agnosia is a relatively rare syndrome, and there is controversy as to whether it is simply an extension of primary visual sensory deficits (variations of cortical blindness) or whether it should be considered as a separate neuropsychological entity.

Three types of agnosia have been recognized: visual, tactile, and auditory. Agnosia is most often modality specific; that is, the individual who cannot recognize the object visually will usually give an immediate and accurate response when touching or hearing the object in use. In visual agnosia, then, poor recognition is limited to the visual sphere.

Visual agnosia is divided into a number of types: visual object agnosia, simultanagnosia, facial agnosia, and color agnosia. These deficits may be seen in isolation or in various combinations, depending on the size and location of the lesion.

Visual Object Agnosia. During evaluation for the presence of visual object agnosia, the individual is presented with a number of common objects (e.g., key, comb, brush) and asked to name them. The evaluator may assume that the object is recognized if the client (1) names, describes, or demonstrates the use of the object or (2) selects it from among a group of objects as it is named by the examiner. If the person recognizes (describes or demonstrates) but is unable to name the object, failure is most likely a result of an anomia rather than an agnosic defect. Individuals with real visual agnosia have no concept of what the object is.[82]

Simultanagnosia. Along the same vein are visual disorders that constrict or "narrow" the visual field during active perceptual analysis (i.e., when perceptions are tested separately, the visual field is within normal limits). Simultanagnosia is a disorder in which the person actually perceives only one element of an object or picture at a time and is unable to absorb the whole. As the individual concentrates on the visual environment, there is an extreme reduction of visual span. The problem is functionally similar to tubular vision. The narrowing of the functional perceptual field decreases the ability to simultaneously deal with two or more stimuli. It appears as if the person has bilateral visual inattention with macular sparing, although perimetric testing reveals full visual fields. A typical example is the individual whose visual attention is focused on the tip of a cigarette held between the lips and fails to perceive a match flame offered several inches away.[83]

Facial Agnosia. Another special type of agnosia that has been documented is failure to recognize familiar faces. The disorder is also known as *prosopagnosia.* The individual is able to recognize a face as a face but is unable to connect the face and differences in faces with people he or she knows. This person is unable to recognize family members, friends, and hospital staff by face. One must be careful not to confuse this with generalized dementia. There may be categorical recognition problems with items involving special visual experience, for example, recognition of cars, types of trees, or emblems. Facial agnosia is usually seen in combination with a number of other deficits, including spatial disorientation, defective color perception, loss of topographical memory, constructional apraxia, and a left upper quadrant visual field loss. These other symptoms are most likely not causative but rather a result of the similar neurological location of these functions.[84]

Color Agnosia. Finally, the individual may have difficulty recognizing names of colors, that is, an inability to name colors that are shown or to point to the color named by the examiner.[85] This defect is considered agnosic (as opposed to a defect in color perception) because the client is able to recognize all colors in the Ishihara Color Plates[86] and is also able to sort colors by hue. The determining factor here appears to be a problem with visual-verbal association. Color agnosia is most common in clients with left hemisphere lesions and is often accompanied by the syndrome of alexia without agraphia.[82]

Assessment

Cortical blindness and variations of it should be thoroughly assessed by the vision specialist. Assessment for agnosia must be preceded by a thorough assessment for visual acuity problems, visual field deficits, and unilateral visual inattention because these primary visual sensory and scanning deficits are often mistaken for agnosic performance. Next, basic color perception should be measured by use of the Ishihara Color Plates[86] and color-sorting or color-matching tasks. Individuals with defective color perception will have difficulty with some visual-perceptual tasks because contextual cues related to color and shading are unavailable to them. Agnosia is a valid diagnosis only if (1) the aforementioned primary visual skills are intact and (2) language skills are intact (i.e., there should be no word-finding difficulty in spontaneous speech).

Although there are no standardized tests for agnosia, commonly used assessment methods have been included. The presence of simultanagnosia is determined by keen observation of performance that indicates perception limited to single elements within objects, for example, describing only the wheel of a bicycle or, within the environment, describing only one part of a room or an activity.

Object agnosia is tested for by placing common real objects (e.g., comb, key, penny, spoon) in front of the client and asking the client to name or point to the item chosen by the examiner. In pointing and naming tasks, the therapist must be sure that the client is fixating on the appropriate target. The response is considered normal if the object is named correctly or described or its functional use demonstrated. Abnormal responses will be confabulatory or perseverative, with the individual often giving the name of a previous or similar object. Responses may also be completely bizarre and unrelated. The examiner may also present objects at an unusual angle. Abnormal responses will show lack of recognition or rotation of the head or body to try to view the object in the "straight on" position. The diagnosis of visual object agnosia is further confirmed if the individual can identify the object by touch or by hearing it in use, both of which should be attempted with vision occluded.

Color agnosia is evaluated by having the client name a color and point to colors named by the examiner. Facial agnosia is evaluated by presenting the individual with photographs of famous world figures, actors, politicians, and family members.[61]

Interventions

There are no reliable studies regarding treatment of cortical blindness, color imperception, or visual agnosia. Treatment principles presented here are based on the experience of

Bouska and Biddle[73] and Bouska and Kwatny.[57] If cortical blindness or simultanagnosia is suspected, the therapist must first attempt to increase the client's knowledge of foveal versus peripheral vision, that is, where the client is fixating. A small headlamp attached to the client's forehead may be used under conditions of subdued lighting. The headlamp should not be used in a completely darkened room because the client needs to use normal spatial cues from the environment. The movement of the projected light in the environment and kinesthetic input from the neck receptors augment knowledge of where the eye is fixed. To carry out this task, the client must learn to position the eyes in midline of the head. The individual is asked to move the light (i.e., head and eyes) to locate and discriminate fairly large, bright stimuli placed on a plain background (e.g., yellow block on a brown table). As acuity and localization skills improve, stimuli and background should be made smaller and more complex (e.g., paper clip on a printed background or letters printed at different locations on a large page). The client should be encouraged to accurately point to or manipulate targets once located with the light or to keep the light on a target as he or she slowly moves the target with one hand. Thus the kinesthetic input from the limb can augment visual localization abilities.[76] In patients with color imperception, treatment should initially involve materials and tasks with sharp color contrasts with minimal detail and should progress to less contrast (more hues) with more detail.

If the assessment has revealed a narrowing of the perceptual field, treatment should be aimed at progressively increasing the perception of large, bright, peripheral targets. For example, the client may be asked to fixate on a centrally placed target while another bright target is brought in slowly from or uncovered in the periphery.[87,88] The individual is encouraged to maintain fixation on the central target while remaining alert for the presence of another target somewhere in the periphery. As the client improves, targets should be smaller, multiple, and exposed for briefer periods. Peripheral targets should always have bright surfaces that reflect light because the peripheral receptors in the retina are mainly rods (light as opposed to color receptors). Another powerful variation of this technique is to involve hand use in peripheral location of objects. For example, the patient senses the presence of a peripheral object then reaches with the hand to pinpoint location, then shifts the eyes to identify it. This can further help to differentiate between central and peripheral vision.

The treatment of clients with object agnosia should progress according to the abilities that return first in spontaneous recovery from agnosia. Common real objects should be used before line drawings in treatment. Presentations should be given "straight on" rather than at an angle or rotated. The client should be asked to point to objects named by the examiner before being asked to name them. Manipulation of the object with simultaneous visual input should be attempted. This may help recognition, or it may simply confuse the client; each case is unique. In general, tactile input with or without simultaneous visual input should be encouraged as a compensation method, although it may not be helpful during treatment sessions.

Color and facial agnosia may be approached by simply drilling the individual with regard to two or three names of colors or names of faces of people important to her or him. The client may be helped to pick out or memorize cues for associating names with faces.[61]

Problems of Visual-Spatial Disorders

Identification of Clinical Problems

Individuals with brain lesions, particularly in the right posterior parietal and occipital areas, may have difficulties with tasks that require a normal concept of space.[55] Disorders of this nature have been termed *visual-spatial disorders, spatial disorientation, visual-spatial agnosia, spatial relations syndrome,* and numerous other names. Visual-spatial abilities are complexly interwoven within the performance of many perceptual and cognitive activities such as dressing, building a design, reading, calculating, walking through an aisle, and playing tennis. An attempt is made here, however, to discuss spatial disorders in their purest form—that is, basic disorders—before dealing with visual-constructive disorders and disorders of analysis and synthesis. Constructional tasks require spatial planning, a type of planning that involves the building up and breaking down of objects in two and three dimensions. Constructional apraxia is viewed as a particular type of spatial-perceptual disorder and therefore is discussed separately under visual-constructive disorders and disorders of analysis and synthesis. Similarly, although perceptual skills such as figure-ground, form constancy, complex visual discrimination, and figure closure involve spatial concepts, tasks involving these skills often require the intellectual operations of synthesis and deduction. They, too, are discussed in the section dealing with analysis and synthesis.

All visual-spatial disabilities involve some problem with the apprehension of the spatial relationships between or within objects. Benton[89] has categorized them as the following disabilities:

1. Inability to localize objects in space, to estimate their size, and to judge their distance from the observer. The client may be unable to accurately touch an object in space or indicate the position of the object (e.g., above, below, in front of, or behind). Relative localization may be impaired so that the individual may be unable to tell which object is closest. There may be difficulty determining which of two objects is larger or which line is longer. Holmes[90] reported cases of gross disorder in spatial orientation revealed through walking; affected individuals, even after seeing objects correctly, ran into them. In another example a man intending to go toward his bed would invariably set out in the wrong direction. Difficulty in estimating distances may also extend to judgments of distances of perceived sounds and lead to overly slow and cautious gait or fear of venturing into public areas.
2. Impaired memory for the location of objects or places. An example is not being able to recall the position of a target previously viewed or the arrangement of furniture in a room. Individuals with this difficulty often lose things because they have no spatial memory to rely on for recall.
3. Inability to trace a path or follow a route from one place to another. Persons without this ability, known as *topographical orientation,* have difficulty understanding and remembering relationships of places to

one another, so they may have difficulty finding their way in a space, as in locating the therapy clinic in a hospital or locating the housewares department in a store previously familiar to them. Normally functioning individuals often have mild signs of topographical disorientation. Everyone is familiar with the disoriented feeling of not knowing how to get out of a large department store or losing a sense of direction in a familiar city. Many of the topographical errors made by clients result from unilateral spatial inattention. For example, someone with left inattention may make only right turns. Topographical disorientation, however, may be seen in a person with no signs of unilateral inattention. This individual will demonstrate route-finding difficulties at certain points and will apparently randomly choose a direction.

4. Problems with reading and counting. These high-level tasks require directional control of eye movements and organized scanning abilities. Eye movements (saccades) during reading bring a new region of the text on the fovea, the part of the retina where visual acuity is the greatest and clear detail can be obtained from the stimulus. During reading, the line of print that falls on the retina may be divided into three regions: the foveal region, the parafoveal region, and the peripheral region. The foveal region subtends about 1 to 2 degrees of visual angle around the reader's fixation point, the parafoveal region subtends about 10 degrees of visual angle around the reader's fixation point, and the peripheral region includes everything on the page beyond the parafoveal region. Parafoveal and peripheral vision contribute spatial information that is used to guide the reader's eye.[91] Visual-spatial disorders appear to interfere to varying degrees with the spatial schema of a page of type or numbers and the dynamic organizational scanning that must take place to gather information appropriately. Clients with unilateral spatial inattention will miss words or numbers located on one half of the page. Other spatial problems unrelated to unilateral inattention include skipping individual words within a line or part of a line, skipping lines, repeating lines, "blocking" or having the inability to change direction of fixation, particularly at the end of a line, and generally losing the place on the total page. Performance usually deteriorates progressively as the individual continues to read. Eventually such persons cannot make sense of what they read, or if counting they complain of being lost or confused. This type of reading or counting disorder has nothing to do with recognition or interpretation of letters or numbers or their spatial configuration; rather, it represents a problem with dynamic sequential visual-spatial exploration during cognitive processing.

Other visual-spatial problems may include loss of depth perception, problems with body schema, and defective judgment of line orientation. There may also be difficulties with discrimination of right and left. Although unilateral spatial inattention is considered a visual-spatial disorder by many, it has been discussed separately in this chapter to increase clarity. Problems with judging line orientation (slant) or unilateral spatial inattention often interfere with a client's spatial ability to tell time with a standard watch or clock. Perception of the vertical may also be considered a visual-spatial skill. Verticality perception is the interpretation of internal and external cues to maintain body balance. This maintenance is a complex neuromuscular process involving visual, proprioceptive, and vestibular systems. Clients with right lesions, particularly in the parieto-occipital region, have more difficulty perceiving verticality than those with left lesions. This may affect posture and ambulation.[92]

Assessment

The client should be asked to accurately touch a number of targets in all parts of the visual field while fixating on a central point. Mislocalization should be noted as well as the part of the visual field in which it occurred. Mislocalization within the central field is infrequent; however, defective localization of stimuli on one or both extramacular fields is more frequently seen.[55] The client should be asked to determine which of a number of small cube blocks (placed perpendicularly in front of the client) is closest, which is farthest, and which is in the middle. Differences in binocular (stereoscopic) and monocular viewing should be measured in this and other tasks. Impairment in both of these types of depth perception and subsequent inaccuracy in judging distances have been described in individuals with brain injury.[89]

With regard to memory for the location of objects or places, clients should be asked to describe the position of objects in their room from memory. They may also be asked to duplicate from memory the position of two or more targets (on a table or piece of paper) that have been presented for a 5-second period. As the number of targets increases, individuals with short-term memory for spatial localization will begin to make errors in spatial placement. Visual memory per se should be ruled out as a conflicting variable.

Topographical sense is assessed by asking clients to describe a floor plan of the arrangement of rooms in their house or to describe familiar geographical constellations, such as routes, arrangement of streets, or public buildings. After therapy these persons may also be asked to find their way back to their rooms after being shown the route several times. Failure suggests a topographical orientation problem. Finally, such a client may be asked to locate states or cities on a large map of the United States. In all of these procedures, the examiner must be sure to separate unilateral spatial inattention errors from topographical errors.

The influence of spatial dysfunction on reading and counting written material may be measured simply by asking the client to read a page of regular newsprint. The examiner should observe performance carefully and document type and frequency of errors. If errors occur, eye movements should be observed to gather additional information. Pages of scanning material (letters or numbers) often give additional information on spatial planning during reading. These are pages of print in which the size and density of the print are controlled. Scanning behavior may be demonstrated by asking the client to circle specific letters. Switching direction in the middle of a line, skipping letters or lines, perseveration, or any other abnormal performance behavior should be noted. Benton's Judgment of Line Orientation

Test[93] may be used to document problems with directional orientation of lines. If there is no indication of apraxia, the client may simply be given a ruler and asked to match it to the directional orientation of the examiner's ruler.

Interventions

Treatment for visual-spatial deficits should follow basic developmental considerations, progressing from simple to more complex tasks. As with children, if the evaluation suggests disorders in body scheme, tactile or vestibular input, or right-left discrimination, these should be dealt with first.

Clients who do not know where they are in space need to internalize a spatial understanding before they can make judgments regarding the space around them. In gross motor spatial training, clients can be asked to roll and reach toward various targets. Supine, prone, sitting, and standing, with vision occluded, clients should try to localize tactile stimuli (various body locations touched by the therapist) and auditory stimuli (e.g., snapping fingers or ringing a bell) presented above, below, behind, in front of, and to the right and left of their bodies. The individual should state where the stimulus is and then point, roll, crawl, or walk toward it; this verbal, kinesthetic, and vestibular input augments spatial learning. In the occupational therapy kitchen, the client, once oriented to the room, may be asked to retrieve one type of object (e.g., cup) from "the top cupboard above your head," from "the bottom cupboard below your waist," from "the table behind you," or from "the drawer on your right [or left]." These clients may also place objects in various positions within a room. They should then stand in the middle of the room, close their eyes, and from memory visualize, verbalize, and point to where the objects are in relation to themselves. Having localized them, the clients should then walk through the space and retrieve the objects in sequence. Functional carryover should always be emphasized, such as having individuals remember through visualization where they put their glasses in the living room before they begin searching. Visualization is defined as the internal "seeing" of something that is not present at that moment: a vision without a visual input or internal visual imagery.[94] Visualization (spatial and other) is part of all perceptual tasks and may be used effectively as a treatment strategy. As previously discussed, a small feedback light placed in the middle of the client's forehead can help teach spatial localization through eye-hand movements.

More complex spatial skills may be taught by asking clients to "partition" space and then localize within it. An excellent activity is one in which clients use a yardstick to divide a blackboard into four or more equal parts and then number each section.

Objects may be presented to clients, who must select the largest, the farthest away, or the one placed at an angle; they may be asked to place various objects in certain relationships to one another. As shape, size, and angle begin to "make sense" to these individuals, form boards, simple puzzles, and parquetry blocks may be added to training.

Topographical abilities should improve as clients begin to better conceptualize space; however, they may be trained directly. The therapist may help such clients organize a basic floor plan of the hospital room and the furniture within it while looking at the room. They may then be asked to do this from memory. Activities can progress to drawing plans or larger areas with a number of rooms. These clients should first "navigate" tactually through the area with a finger. Eventually, they should walk or wheel through the route themselves, visualizing and repeating the route until spatial concepts are learned. Imaginary routes also may be taken through maps of cities, states, or countries.

Organized visual-spatial exploration (eye movements) during reading or other scanning and cancellation tasks may be taught. Number and letter scanning sheets may be used for such training. Initially the size of numbers and the spaces between numbers should be large; this places less stress on visual acuity while training scanning. Before beginning, clients should orient themselves to the page spatially by numbering the right and left edges of each line. These numbers are used as additional spatial localization cues if needed during the scanning task.[45] Clients should then be asked to circle a specific number (or numbers) whenever it occurs. To control erratic or impulsive eye movements, they should be instructed to use a pencil to underline each line and then loop the selected letter as it comes into view (see Figure 28-16). They may also be asked to read each letter. Underlining allows the kinesthetic and tactile receptors of the arm to control eye movements; verbalization allows the language and auditory systems to influence eye movements. Visual-spatial exploration exercises should progress to large-print magazines, books, or newspapers. The *New York Times* and *Reader's Digest* are both available in large print. In all training activities it is most important that before the activity begins the clients fully comprehend the total space in which they will work. It is equally important that they reorient themselves at any point where errors occur. Those who lose their place during reading will eventually lose it again if the therapist simply points to where they should be. Chances are better that they will not lose their place again if they reorient themselves to the page spatially when an error occurs.

Problems of Visual-Constructive Disorders

Identification of Clinical Problems

Clients with lesions in either the right or left hemisphere may have problems when trying to "construct." Lesions in the parietal, temporal, occipital, and frontal lobes have been documented in individuals with visual-constructive disorders.[55,95] The normal ability to construct, also known as *visual-constructive ability* and *constructional praxis,* involves any type of performance in which parts are put together to form a single entity. Examples include assembling blocks to form a design, assembling a puzzle, making a dress, setting a table, and simply drawing four lines to form a square (graphic skills). The skill implies a high level of dynamic, organized, visual-perceptual processing in which the spatial relations are perceived and sequenced well enough among and within the component parts to direct higher-level processing to sequence the perceptual-motor actions so that eventually parts are synthesized into a desired whole. Visual-constructive ability may be compromised if any part of this process is disturbed.

Typical tasks used to measure this ability include building in a vertical direction, building in a horizontal direction, three-dimensional block construction from a model or a picture of a model, and copying line drawings such as of houses, flowers, and geometric designs.[84]

Clients with visual-constructive deficits, especially those with right lesions, often also have visual-spatial deficits. These individuals may rotate the position of a part erroneously, place it in the wrong position, space it too far from another part, be oblivious to perspective or a third dimension, or simply be unable to complete more than two or three steps before becoming entirely confused. This is usually evidence of breakdown because of faulty or inadequate spatial information.

Other clients, usually those with left lesions, have an "executional" or apraxic problem; they seem to have difficulty initiating and conducting the planned sequence of movements necessary to construct the whole. The problem seems to be in planning, arranging, building, or drawing rather than in spatial concepts. This deficit in its purest form is known as *constructional apraxia.* Constructional apraxia lies clinically outside the category of most other varieties of apraxia and is considered a special kind of "perceptual" apraxia. It occurs frequently in aphasic individuals; therefore the underlying mechanisms of aphasia and constructional apraxia may be related.[96]

Assessment

Constructional abilities are generally measured through tasks that require (1) copying line drawings of, for example, a house, clock face, flower, or geometric design (drawing may also be done without copying); (2) copying two-dimensional matchstick designs; (3) building block designs by copying or from a model; or (4) assembling puzzles. Table 28-2 lists common tests. The more complex the picture or design to be copied, the more complex are the constructional tasks. The following are examples of drawing and block construction deficits:

1. Clients may crowd the drawing or design on one side of the page or in one corner of the page or available space on the working surface, usually a result of the influence of unilateral spatial inattention.
2. Lines in drawings may be wavy or broken, too long or too short.
3. One line may not meet another accurately, or lines may transect one another; in block designs, parts may not be neatly placed but rather may have small gaps.
4. There may be "overdrawing" of angles or parts of the figure because of graphic perseveration (scribble), spatial indecision, or problems with executive planning.
5. Clients may superimpose their copy on the model or superimpose one of their drawings on top of another. In block design construction, they may become confused between the model and their reproduction and use part of the model to complete their design. This has been termed the "closing-in" phenomenon, a failure to distinguish between model and reproduction.[55]
6. Parts of the drawing or design may be reversed. Horizontal reversals are more common than vertical reversals.

A note might be appropriate here regarding dressing apraxia. This problem occurs most frequently with right hemisphere damage. It is considered a "perceptual" apraxia rather than a motor apraxia because the inability to dress is believed to result from body scheme, spatial, and visual-constructive deficits rather than difficulty in motor execution. Persons with dressing apraxia cannot correctly orient their clothes to their body. They often put clothes on backward or inside out. Failure to dress one side of the body is also often noted and is directly related to unilateral spatial inattention.

Interventions

It must be remembered that both visual-constructive and visual analysis synthesis skills are often used almost simultaneously during task performance. Thus, treatment should not separate the two types of skills but rather should be a precise interrelationship of activities that require finer and finer levels of each facility. For example, arranging an office filing system is both an analytical-synthesis and a visual-constructive task. The individual must first analyze overall needs and translate them into an imagined visual-spatial plan (preliminary synthesis of the whole) that will help organization. Then the organizer begins to use the hands to categorize (segment visual space). This building is a visual-constructive task. Intermittently during building, new ideas of the whole surface, and visual-constructive tasks change in response to a "better idea" (final synthesis of the whole). Task performance, except for tasks that are rote, usually follows similar perceptual processes. Treatment therefore must be integral. Visual-constructive skills, however, may be emphasized more than visual analysis and synthesis skills or vice versa.

As previously mentioned, visual-constructive disorders are thought to result from different underlying problems in different individuals (e.g., visual-spatial disorders in persons with right hemisphere lesions and executive, planning, or synthetic disorders in those with left hemisphere lesions).

TABLE 28-2 ■ COMMON TESTS USED TO ASSESS VISUOCONSTRUCTIVE SKILLS

TEST	STANDARDIZATION
Drawing pictures or shapes with or without an example to copy	Not standardized
Reproducing matchstick designs	Not standardized
Assembling puzzles	Not standardized
Bender Visual Motor Gestalt Test	Standardized for children only
Kohs Blocks Test	Standardized for adults
WAIS Block Design Test	Standardized for adults
Benton's Three-Dimensional Constructional Praxis Test	Standardized for adults

There are few reliable studies on treatment strategies for visual-constructive disorders. One possible treatment strategy is known as *saturational cuing*.[97] This method involves presenting controlled verbal instruction on task analysis and sequence and presenting cues on spatial boundaries (cuing is also response related).

If there are problems with planning and sequencing of steps necessary to accomplish a visual-constructive task, the therapist should begin with simple tasks that require only three or four steps, such as positioning one place setting at a table. The client should discuss the plan and sequence of steps before initiating the activity, while looking at the parts to be used, such as silverware, plate, and glass. These steps may even be written down for additional input. The client should be helped to reorient the plan at any point during task breakdown. Eventually, tasks should increase in complexity (e.g., setting a table for five), and the client should be encouraged to function more independently. Another technique often used by clinicians is known as backward chaining. This involves presenting a partially completed task and asking the client to complete the final steps, for example, placing the knife and glass on a partially completed place setting. The perceptual cues of the task already begun appear to stimulate constructional abilities. As the client progresses, he or she should complete more steps.

Intervention for problems with spatial planning during visual-constructive tasks should begin with the simple spatial exercises discussed previously. If problems still exist, the individual may be asked to draw around shapes (blocks) one by one. These shapes should first have been placed in a simple two-dimensional design. The client is then asked to rebuild the design with the shapes alone. Therapy should progress from horizontal to vertical to oblique designs, from two-dimensional to three-dimensional designs, and from tasks with common objects to tasks involving abstract designs. For example, spatial problems with drawing, such as placing windows in a house or numbers on a clock face, are usually a result of an underlying spatial disorder. The client should use a ruler or protractor to segment the space and plan placement before drawing. Dot-to-dot tasks may be designed that actually lead and sequence the drawing into a spatial whole. Simple puzzles also may be used to increase visual-spatial abilities during visual-constructive tasks. Finally, if task breakdown results from impulsive visual or motor behavior, these symptoms should be dealt with before further visual-constructive treatment continues.

Examples of visual-constructive tasks that may be designed for therapeutic use include the following:

- Setting a table for one to five people
- Wrapping a gift
- Assembling a piece of woodwork, a toy, a tool, a motor
- Changing a tire on a car
- Organizing a shelf in a library or a kitchen
- Organizing a filing system or cabinet
- Putting pieces of a sewing pattern together
- Addressing an envelope
- Rearranging furniture according to a preset plan
- Assembling a craft according to a preset plan
- Drawing from memory or copy
- Copying two-dimensional block designs
- Copying three-dimensional designs with oblique components

The key to effective visual-constructive learning, however, is not the task itself but rather how carefully the therapist organizes it and monitors performance. Clients with visual-constructive disorders are often visually or motorically impulsive; they often move or draw parts before analysis has taken place. Once a part is placed inappropriately, it begins to confuse the whole visual-perceptual process. This confusion increases anxiety and contributes to further breakdown in analysis and synthesis. Treatment should be directed at the underlying causes of task breakdown if these can be determined.

Problems of Visual Analysis and Synthesis Disorders

Identification of Clinical Problems

This separate discussion of visual analysis and synthesis is arbitrary. There is never any clear demarcation among the processes of visual-spatial orientation, visual construction, and visual analysis and synthesis. Analysis of likes and differences, relationships of parts to one another, and reasoning and deduction occur simultaneously with more basic spatial and constructive percepts. The final visual concept of a task (e.g., what a place setting on a table should look like) is necessary before the task is begun. Similarly, synthesis of one part of a task may be necessary before synthesis of the entire task can occur. For example, the person who is setting a table for four people must be able to conceptualize one place setting before conceptualizing the table with four place settings. Those points during perceptual processing when there is a colligation or blending of discrete impressions into a single perception are known as *synthesis*. This final stage of coordination and interpretation of sensory data is thought to be deficient in many individuals with perceptual problems. Deficits may be present with either left or right hemisphere damage but are more common and more severe with right lesions.[61,98]

Visual-perceptual skills considered to be analytical and synthetic in nature include making fine visual discriminations, particularly in complex configurations; separating figure from background in complex configurations (figure-ground); achieving recognition on the basis of incomplete information (figure closure); and synthesizing disparate elements into a meaningful entity, as, for example, conceptualizing parts of a task into a whole.[5]

Assessment

Many tests have been designed to measure the capacity for analysis and synthesis. Test items include complex figures in which small parts of a figure differ from another figure. The client is asked to select the one that is different. Studies have shown that basic discrimination of single attributes of a stimulus such as length, contour, or brightness is intact in many clients.[99-101] The problem appears when these individuals are asked to discriminate between more complex configurations with subtle differences. Tests also measure figure-ground ability; the client must select the embedded figure from the background. Functional examples of this problem are the inability of a client to find her or his glasses if they are lying on a figured background, to find a white shirt on a white bedspread, and to find his or her wheelchair locks. Figure closure is measured by asking the client to complete an incomplete figure, such as part of the outline of a common shape. Finally, synthesis of parts into a whole, also known as *visual organization,* is measured by asking the client to conceptualize and organize the whole picture by, for example, looking at separate segments of the picture (e.g., cup or key) that have been divided and placed in unusual positions. This type of synthesis is necessary for high-level constructional tasks. Table 28-3 outlines examples of tests used to evaluate visual analysis and synthesis.

Interventions

Intervention for deficits in visual analysis and synthesis should follow developmental considerations described in the children's section. Visual discrimination tasks should begin with simple figures and obvious differences in complex figures. Color, size, texture, lighting, and verbal direction may help the client "cue in" on subtle differences among objects or figures. The therapist should determine the threshold at which the client is capable of discriminating differences and vary the dimension, contrast, and functional activity at this level. For example, if the individual cannot select a can of vegetables from a kitchen shelf stocked with cans of similar size, the therapist may simply change the task to fit that person's level of visual discrimination by removing some of the cans (decreasing the density of the display), replacing some of the cans with boxes of food (increasing the spatial contrast), moving the can to be selected forward or to one edge of the display (decreasing figure-ground difficulty), removing the label from the can (increasing the light and color contrast), or giving cues regarding what to search for (verbal direction). This example is described not as a method of compensation but rather as an approach to be used therapeutically in slowly building the client's visual discrimination abilities. Eventually, high-level visual discrimination skills should be incorporated within tasks requiring three or more steps, such as selecting a can of vegetables, opening the can (which involves selecting the can opener from the utensil drawer), and emptying the vegetables into a specific bowl (which involves selecting the bowl from among other bowls). Visual discrimination and figure-ground skills may appear normal until the client is required to do multiple-step activities, is given time constraints, or becomes anxious or confused. Tabletop games that require high levels of visual discrimination along with cognitive strategies may be therapeutic and motivating. Examples include Monopoly and card games such as solitaire. Matching and sorting tasks also may be helpful in enhancing visual discrimination. Examples include matching picture cards and sorting laundry, tools, silverware, or files.

Drawings of figures with subtle differences also may be used for therapy. The client should be encouraged to point to, verbalize, or outline the subtle differences in two or more pictures; this enhances visual attention to detail. If the individual cannot select the discrepant detail(s) among three or more figures, the problem most likely results from an inability to select one feature and compare it with elements in the other figures. This is a fairly high-level skill that requires selective attention and analysis with internal visualization while the individual is still viewing the complete figures. This type of client should practice feature detection and then begin systematic comparisons of similarities and differences between two figures, eventually progressing to three or more figures. The therapist may number or outline similar areas of each figure to help the client (1) direct attention to similar areas of all figures and (2) sequence comparisons appropriately. The client should verbalize, draw, or write details concerning similarities and differences in individual aspects of the figures. This enhances visual analysis and also informs the therapist about how the individual is selecting and comparing features. Eventually, speed should be stressed, the highest level being presentation of tachistoscopic designs.

Visual organization may be emphasized by presenting the client with activities that have multiple parts that must be sequenced together into a whole. Activities involving this type of synthesis are discussed in the preceding section on treatment of visual-constructive disorders. Figure closure may be emphasized by presenting parts of figures or objects (e.g., half a plate covered by a towel) and asking the client for identification. Figure-closure task difficulty may be increased by placing many objects on a table, some of which partially occlude others. Identification of objects in such a task requires figure closure simultaneous with figure-ground abilities.

Visual analysis and synthesis deficits reflect a disruption in cognitive function with specific regard to visual-perceptual features. The affected client may function normally when analytical tasks require another system, for example, language. In others with generalized brain damage (e.g., traumatic head injury and senile dementia), general cognitive analysis and synthesis may be at fault rather than visual analysis. Because most cognitive performance requires visual processing, however, increased ability to analyze and synthesize visual-perceptual material often generalizes to an increase in cognitive function.

TABLE 28-3 ■ COMMON TESTS USED TO ASSESS VISUAL ANALYSIS AND SYNTHESIS

TEST	USE
Hooper Visual Organization Test	Standardized for adults
Motor-Free Visual Perception Test	Standardized for adults
Raven's Progressive Matrices	Standardized for adults
Embedded Figure Test	Standardized for adults
Southern California Figure-Ground Test	Standardized for children only

PERCEPTUAL RETRAINING WITH COMPUTERS

During the past 15 years, numerous computer programs have been developed for rehabilitation of brain damage symptoms, including those affecting cognition (e.g., attention, sequencing, or memory) and perception. Because the computer is so highly visual, it becomes an obvious tool for treatment of visual-perceptual dysfunction. Treatment with computers has been named *computer-assisted therapy.* There is a growing interest in development of and research into programs for rehabilitation, for Alzheimer's prevention, and in normal healthy aging adults. The largest treatment study of 487 subjects was able to demonstrate statistically significant improvements in memory and attention by using a plasticity-based adaptive training program.[102] A number of other studies are in progress. Advantages of computer-assisted therapy include control and flexibility of perceptual variables during treatment (e.g., number, size, speed), immediate feedback regarding performance, automatic control for learning (e.g., items are repeated if incorrect to facilitate learning), and being motivational. Visual-perceptual training with computers, if used, should be viewed as one part of a patient's treatment program. One should always remember that the computer, monitor, and keyboard are just that: they do not require the many perceptual, vestibular, and motor responses typical of daily performance (e.g., scanning requirements may be bilateral, but they are not global and associated with head movement). A patient's total program may include computer-assisted therapy as an additional tool; however, it should never be substituted for more significant training within the multidimensional environment. Some computer programs for visual-perceptual training are listed in Box 28-6.

BOX 28-6 ■ COMPUTER PROGRAMS FOR VISUAL-PERCEPTUAL TRAINING

HTS Home Therapy Systems
www.homevisiontherapy.com

Visual Perceptual Diagnostic Testing and Training Programs
H. Greenberg and C. Chamoff
Educational Electronic Techniques
1886 Wantagh Avenue
Wantagh, NY 11793

Captain's Log Cognitive Training System
J. Sandford and R. Browne
Computability Corporation
www.braintrain.com/professionals/captains_log/captainslog_pro.htm
101 Route 46 East
Pine Brook, NJ 07058

Psychological Software Services Programs
Odie Bracey
www.psychological-software.com/psscogrehab.html
Psychological Software Services
P.O. Box 29205
Indianapolis, IN 46229

Life Science Associates Programs
R. Gianutsos
http://lifesciassoc.home.pipeline.com

Life Science Associates
1 Fenemore Road
Bayport, NY 11705 (Diagnosis and Training)

Posit Science
www.positscience.com
1 Montgomery Street, Suite 700
San Francisco, CA 94104
(866) 599-6463

On-Line Brain Training
www.lumosity.com

SUMMARY OF VISUAL-PERCEPTUAL DYSFUNCTION

Careful organized evaluation should delineate deficits well enough to result in a visual-perceptual function profile for each client, including both primary and associative visual skills. Clients rarely come with isolated visual-perceptual deficits; more often they exhibit a combination of visual-perceptual deficits usually interrelated with motor, language, and cognitive dysfunctions. For example, a visual-perceptual function profile may reveal strabismus, left unilateral visual inattention, visual-spatial deficits, visual-constructive deficits, and problems with visual analysis and synthesis, all affecting daily function. Treatment should be organized to progressively build skills, emphasizing one component more than another. The goal of treatment is eventual generalization of improvements in individual skills to spontaneous high-level function.

The presentation of information in this chapter is an attempt to use isolated and mechanistic terms to define a system that is extremely subtle, integrated, and complex. The reader is reminded that much of the normal and abnormal perceptual system has not been well defined. Preliminary studies cited throughout this chapter, however, suggest that disorders may be responsive to management and treatment. Research is needed to standardize evaluation procedures well enough to further define deficits and to investigate the effectiveness of various treatment approaches with various client populations.

References

To enhance this text and add value for the reader, all references are included on the companion Evolve site that accompanies this textbook. This online service will, when available, provide a link for the reader to a Medline abstract for the article cited. There are 102 cited references and other general references for this chapter, with the majority of those articles being evidence-based citations.

APPENDIX 28-A ■ Resources

Bernell/USO, 4016 North Home Street, Mishiwaka, IN 46545; (800) 348-2225

CCTVs: Enhanced Vision Systems, 5882 Machine Drive, Huntington Beach, , CA 92649, Tel: 888-811-3161, www.enhancedvision.com

Complete Visual Screening Kit: Laurie R. Chaikin, OD, OTR/L, FCOVD; 420 F Cola Ballena, Alameda, CA 94501; Laurie.chaikin@gmail.com

Teller Cards: Vistech Consultants, 4162 Little York Road, Dayton, OH 45414-2566

Helpful Websites

American Optometric Association, Position Statement on Optometric Vision Therapy (includes excellent reference list): http://www.aoa.org/x5411.xml

Annotated reference list: www.vtod.org/references.html

College of Optometrists in Vision Development: www.covd.org

Computerized home vision therapy system: www.homevisiontherapy.com

Enhanced Vision systems for closed circuit TVs: www.enhancedvision.com

Neuro-Optometric Rehabilitation Association: www.nora.cc

Optometric Extension Program Foundation: www.oepf.org

Parents Active for Vision Education: www.pave-eye.com/~vision

Vision Therapy Information and Referrals

NovaVision: www.novavision.com/Home.html
Information on the Visual Field Restitution Training System.

Optometrists Network: www.optometrists.org

Optometrists Network: All About 3D: www.vision3D.com

The Vision Help Network: www.visionhelp.com
Full Circle Cognitive Rehabilitation has unilateral inattention training programs via computer and the internet. Please see http://mytrainedbrain.com/. The developer Tom Van Vleet can be reached through his website email address at tomvanvleet@gmail.com or by phone at (925) 580-2806.
Motion Therapeutics: www.motiontherapeutics.com. For information on the Balance-Based Torso-Weighting vest, email Cindy Gibson-Horn, RPT at cindy@motiontherapeutics.com.

VisionCare Ophthalmic Technologies: www.visioncareinc.net
Information on the implantable telescope for macular degeneration.

CHAPTER 29 Pelvic Floor Treatment of Incontinence and Other Urinary Dysfunctions in Men and Women

BEATE CARRIÈRE, PT, CAPP, CIFK

KEY TERMS

functional training exercises
incontinence
pelvic floor dysfunction
recoordination of the functions of the abdominal compartment

OBJECTIVES

After reading this chapter the student or therapist will be able to:

1. Discuss factors that lead to incontinence.
2. Understand the neurophysiology involved in pelvic floor dysfunctions.
3. Describe the different layers of the pelvic floor and their functional connections.
4. Understand the importance of coordinating diaphragmatic breathing with pelvic floor activity.
5. Correct faulty breathing patterns to facilitate normal pelvic floor activity.
6. Apply motor learning and motor control principles when teaching exercises.
7. Select the most appropriate intervention to improve pelvic floor function.

OVERVIEW OF THE CLINICAL PROBLEM

History of Pelvic Floor Exercises

A different focus on how to view the pelvic floor and the problem of incontinence has evolved from new knowledge about neurophysiology, neuroplasticity, motor learning, motor control, and functional brain imaging.[1,2] Kegel[3-5] is considered the great American pioneer who, in the late 1940s, recognized the importance of exercises to help women with urinary incontinence (UI). Dr. Kegel, a Los Angeles physician, found that many women did not have any awareness of the function of the pelvic floor and that they were not always successful with the exercise he prescribed, which is drawing in the perineum. He therefore developed a pneumatic apparatus, the perineometer, which measured each muscle contraction in a manner visible to the patient. He instructed his patients to perform the exercise for 20 minutes three times daily, or a total of 300 contractions, and suggested weekly visits for instruction.[3,4] Kegel also recognized that evidence of bladder weakness was present in some women before childbearing and emphasized the importance of training the pubococcygeus muscle to achieve continence.[4,5] Considered visionary at that time, his approach to exercises demonstrates visual feedback combined with declarative learning. However, the treatment has not changed much since.[6-9] Kegel exercises are stereotypical and highly repetitive (300 repetitions until improvement, then 80 per day for life) with little functional value. More recent studies have investigated the effectiveness of Kegel's exercises.

Our current understanding of pelvic floor function shows the complex relationship of the pelvic floor with many systems and subsystems of the body, such as the nervous system (central, peripheral, autonomic, sensory, and limbic), musculoskeletal system, cardiopulmonary system, lymphatic system, and integumentary system, as well as with different organs in the abdominal cavity. The environment also has a profound influence on its function.

Given the complexity of the role of the pelvic floor muscles, procedural learning, sensory awareness, and functional retraining are now part of intervention strategies for an individual with pelvic floor dysfunction. Interventions may include breathing exercises, manual lymph treatment, visceral mobilization, manual therapy, connective tissue mobilization, and treatment of scars.

Prevalence of Urinary Incontinence

The prevalence of UI in men and women is high and costly. Mardon and colleagues,[10] who conducted a study of managed care beneficiaries, found the overall incidence of UI to be consistent with previous estimates. Fantl and colleagues[11] reported in 1996 that 10% to 35%, or 13 million adult Americans, have UI. In 2000 Hu and co-workers[12] estimated that 17 million community-dwelling persons had daily UI and 34 million had overactive bladder (OAB) syndrome, with 2.9 million of those reported to have had incontinence episodes.

In 1996 more than half of the 1.5 million nursing home residents in the United States were estimated to be incontinent. This condition is reported to be the most common reason for placing a family member in a home.[11-13] The number of adults in institutional care had risen to 1.89 million in 2000, and 945,000 of those were estimated to have UI.[12] Women older than 60 years have twice the prevalence of incontinence as men of that age.[11] The majority of patients with incontinence are parous women and older persons.[13] Goode and colleagues[14] report that UI is a common geriatric syndrome affecting at least one in three older women. "UI is not a normal result of aging, it is a medical problem that is often curable and should be treated."[15] Britton and co-workers[16] conducted a study of urinary symptoms in 578 men older than 60 years. Thirty percent of the men reported increased daytime frequency, and 27% reported urgency and a variety of other urinary symptoms, defined as OAB if nocturia (getting up at least once in the night to urinate) is included. Incontinence can also be found in the younger population. Nygaard and colleagues[17] investigated UI in nulliparous elite athletes and found that individuals who participate in gymnastics and sports that include jumping, high-impact landings, and running appear to score higher in the prevalence of UI than those who swim or play golf. Because exercises and activities during field training of soldiers can be strenuous, one third of 450 female soldiers experienced UI according to Sherman and Davis.[18] Baumann and Tauber[19] reported that 17% of boys aged 5 to 14 years are incontinent. Adedokun and Wilson[20] and Diokno and colleagues[21] provided thorough epidemiological overviews, collecting data from various sources all over the world.

Risk factors for incontinence include the following:

Obesity: This is a risk factor and can contribute to incontinence and make the treatment more difficult.[22,23]

Cigarette smoking: Smoking augments incontinence for three reasons: (1) it has been shown to interfere with collagen synthesis, (2) neuromuscular and anatomical changes likely occur from smoking that result in decreased functionality of the bladder, and (3) it causes coughing, which increases the strain on the weak pelvic floor muscles.[24] Moreover, cigarette smoking has been linked to erectile dysfunction and has an effect on sperm quality in men. In women, it is related to increased incidence of miscarriage and cervical cancer and reduced chance of conception.[25] It has been reported that smoking cessation, weight reduction, and regulation of bowel movements may reduce the risk of UI.[26]

Diabetes: Hunter and Moore[27] state that an estimated 13% of seniors have diabetes. Of these individuals, 32% to 45% have associated bladder dysfunction. The presence of UI in diabetics can be attributed to decreased bladder sensation, increased bladder capacity, and impaired detrusor contractility. Lee and colleagues[28] studied voiding patterns in women with type 2 diabetes and stated that peripheral neuropathy was an important factor associated with diabetic voiding dysfunction. They found that patients with diabetes had predominantly nocturia and a weak urinary stream, abnormal nocturnal urine production, and decreased voiding volumes and functional bladder capacity. In the same study, researchers noted impaired detrusor contractility, with 13.9% of 194 female patients having high postvoiding residual (PVR) urine of over 100 mL. The researchers suspected that the dysfunction in detrusor contractility was secondary to diabetes. Moreover, 14.4% of the women in the study had less than 70% efficiency of emptying the bladder.

Neurologic diseases associated with UI include the following:

Brain injuries: Leary[29] investigated incontinence after brain injury and reported that 50% of the patients had impaired bladder and bladder subscores on admission. Even though 90% of those patients were set goals for self-care and mobility, only 3.5% of the patients were set multidisciplinary goals addressing bladder and bowel function. The Agency for Health Care Policy and Research[30] reported that UI is most prevalent in persons with spinal cord injuries (SCIs) and people with multiple sclerosis (MS). Eighty percent of patients with SCI will have had at least one urinary tract infection (UTI) by their sixteenth year postinjury.

MS: Seventy percent to 90% of individuals diagnosed with MS develop bladder dysfunction, which places them at high risk for UTIs (Agency for Health Care Policy and Research). McClurg and colleagues[31] state that in patients with MS, bladder storage problems often coexist with inadequate emptying of the bladder because of detrusor sphincter dyssynergy. In their research with 30 patients with MS, they showed that a combined treatment of pelvic floor training and advice combined with electromyography biofeedback and neuromuscular electrical stimulation may reduce urinary symptoms in these patients. Schulte-Baukloh and colleagues[32] injected 11 women and five men with MS and drug-resistant OAB symptoms with botulinum toxin type A and found significant improvement for 4 weeks to 3 months (but not at 6 months), with reduction in frequency, nocturia, and pad use; however, buildup of residual urine remained a problem.

Spina bifida: Patients affected by spina bifida also can have various neurogenic urinary tract dysfunctions. Depending on the severity of the dysfunction, they may become socially dry with conservative therapy.[33]

Alzheimer disease: In patients with Alzheimer disease cognitive and central regulating mechanisms contribute to incontinence.[34] According to Holstege,[1] research has shown that "lesions in the pathway from prefrontal cortex and limbic system, to the PAG (periaqueductal gray) probably cause urge incontinence in the elderly."

Cerebrovascular accident (CVA): Brittain and colleagues[35] state that UI after a stroke is associated with poor outcome and depression in stroke survival and care. The overall prevalence of UI is high (32% to 79%) in older patients with stroke admitted to the hospital. At discharge the incidence of UI is 25% to 28%, and 12% to 19% continue to experience UI for months after the stroke. The inability to communicate, transfer, or walk and the use of drugs complicate matters. UI in stroke patients is similar to UI in patients without stroke and probably results from muscle weakness on the affected side. The patients may demonstrate stress UI (SUI), but urgency UI (UUI) and mixed incontinence are also common. Studies published from 1985 to 1997 suggest that 31% to 40% of hospitalized stroke patients have fecal incontinence on admission and 18% at discharge, and 7% to 9% still experience fecal incontinence 6 months after the stroke.[36] Unfortunately, treatment for these problems is rarely prescribed, even though it is very effective.[37]

Parkinson disease: In individuals with Parkinson disease, the prevalence of lower urinary tract symptoms (LUTSs) is 27% to 39%, most frequently nocturia (86%); 71% of patients have reported frequency, and 68% have reported urgency. According to a study by Winge and colleagues,[38] the patients were bothered most by the urgency symptoms. The authors inferred that the reason could be a progression of gait difficulties, decreased ability to separate and integrate sensory input, or both at a later stage of the disease. Zein and colleagues[39] agreed with increased incidence of voiding dysfunction with the progression of the disease. They also describe incomplete emptying (40%) and hesitation (37.3%) as problems in their prospective study of 110 patients with Parkinson disease. Fowler and Griffiths[2] suggest that the pathways from the PAG to the thalamus and insula do not conduct signals properly in Parkinson disease. Deep brain stimulation can restore the conduction.

Parkinsonian syndrome: Multiple system atrophy (MSA) is described in detail by Yamamoto and colleagues[39a] and Wenning and colleagues,[39b] who state that the clients have autonomic, cerebellar, and extrapyramidal symptoms. The syndrome presents as a more severe form of Parkinson disease and includes MSA, idiopathic Parkinson's, vascular parkinsonism, and supranuclear palsy. Clients with MSA can have severe blood pressure variations and sudden orthostatic hypotension secondary to autonomic system problems in addition to more severe bladder dysfunctions such as higher incidence for urinary urgency, retardation in initiating urination and incomplete emptying of the bladder that may require catheterization. Prolongation of urination and constipation are also more common in MSA clients than those with Parkinson disease. The physical treatment has to address more symptoms and it is more complex and more difficult to improve the client's quality of life.

Guillain-Barré syndrome (GBS): The prevalence and mechanism of bladder dysfunction were evaluated by Sakakibara and colleagues.[40] In their study of 65 consecutive patients urinary dysfunction was observed in 27.7%. Of those patients, 9.2% experienced retention, 24.6% had voiding difficulties, and 7.7% complained of urgencies. Overactive and underactive detrusor activity were the major urodynamic findings. The underlying mechanism, according to the authors, appeared to involve hypoactive and hyperactive lumbosacral nerves.

Cost of Incontinence

Wilson and colleagues[41] state that the cost for women over 65 years of age with UI is twice that for women younger than 65 years. Affecting 17% to 55% of community dwellers and up to 50% of nursing home residents, UI is one of the most prevalent chronic diseases. Only one-quarter to one-half of affected individuals seek medical attention. Within a 10-year period the direct cost increased considerably, more than could be accounted for by medical inflation. Hu and colleagues[12] adjusted and reported the cost of UI and OAB syndrome in 2000: $19.5 billion and $12.6 billion, respectively. Thirty-four million individuals had OAB syndrome, and 17 million had UI. Because individuals with OAB have fewer incontinence episodes, the per-person cost is higher in patients with UI—35% of patients with UI have SUI, which can involve expensive surgeries. However, the days spent in the hospital have declined since 1995.[12] The cost of UI escalated from $8.2 billion in 1984 to $16.4 billion in 1993 and to $26.3 billion, or $3565 per individual with UI, in 1995. Wagner and Hu[42] attributed this increase to the following three major changes in the previous 10 years:

- Introduction of more continence-related products to the marketplace
- Change in the age composition of the U.S. population
- Change in prevalence of UI

The authors stated that the cost for people younger than 65 years was not included in the study and that the true cost may be much higher because UI is underreported.

Definition of Incontinence

UI is defined as involuntary loss of urine.[43] Incontinence can have one or more causes, and in more than 90% of cases it can be improved or cured.[13] Treatment should be instituted only after a careful, thorough history and physical examination.[13]

SUI is defined as involuntary loss of urine on effort or physical exertion, for example, sporting activities or sneezing or coughing.[43]

UUI is considered to be involuntary loss of urine associated with urgency.[43]

Mixed UI is the complaint of involuntary loss of urine associated with urgency and also with effort or physical exertion, sneezing, or coughing.[43]

Symptoms associated with bladder storage disorders include the following:

Increased daytime urinary frequency: Micturition (emptying of the bladder) occurs more frequently during waking hours than previously deemed normal by the patient.[43]

Nocturia: Patient wakes up from sleep one or more times because of the need to micturate. Each void is preceded and followed by sleep.[43]

Urgency: A sudden, compelling desire to pass urine that is difficult to defer.[43]

OAB syndrome: Cluster of symptoms of urinary urgency, usually accompanied by frequency and nocturia in the absence of UTI.[43]

Symptoms associated with voiding disorders include the following:

Hesitancy: Delay in initiating micturition[43]

Straining to void: A need to make an intensive effort to either maintain or improve the urinary stream[43]

Feeling of incomplete bladder emptying: Report that the bladder does not feel empty after micturition[43]

Urinary retention: Inability to pass urine despite persistent effort[43]

In patients with nonneurological conditions, the most common forms of incontinence are SUI, OAB syndrome, UUI, and mixed incontinence. Weak pelvic floor muscles usually cause SUI. SUI occurs when the abdominal pressure is greater than the urethral pressure, resulting in a loss of urine with coughing, laughing, sneezing, lifting, and so forth. OAB syndrome, or detrusor overactivity, is associated with involuntary bladder muscle contraction during the filling phase, causing frequent urination; nocturia; and strong, sudden, and sometimes unpredictable urges to urinate but not always resulting in incontinence.[44]

UUI can be caused by detrusor instability, an involuntary contraction of the muscle of the bladder before it is full. It is associated with a sudden urgent need to void. The urgency can be so irresistible that it results in loss of urine before the individual reaches the bathroom.

ETIOLOGY

The causes of SUI and UUI in individuals with nonneurological conditions are as follows (Figure 29-1):

1. Functional causes include the inability to undress in a timely fashion and not being able to reach the bathroom in a timely fashion because of obstacles (e.g., no light, cannot enter the bathroom with the walker without maneuvering).
2. Weakening of the pelvic floor structures can result from childbirth (overstretching of muscles, injuries to the pudendal nerve, or ligaments), hysterectomy, prolapse (rectocele, cystocele, vaginal prolapse), straining with constipation, poor biomechanics when lifting, falls on the buttocks with shift of the pelvis affecting muscle length or stretching the nerves, and poor coordination of the pulmonary diaphragm with the pelvic floor, back, and abdominal muscles.[45,46] Scars in the perineal and pelvic area, aging (loss of muscle mass), obesity, smoking, poor posture, and pain in the pelvic area also can contribute to muscle weakness.
3. OAB syndrome and UUI can be caused by UTIs and other conditions that irritate the bladder: neoplasia, post–bladder or post–bowel surgery status, bladder outlet obstruction, anxiety, nervousness, and poor toileting habits. The condition can also be idiopathic. Some clients also have urgency to eliminate the bowels.
4. Over-the-counter medications with anticholinergic agents can cause retention (an inability to empty the bladder completely), overflow (leakage of urine when the bladder is overextended), and frequency; antipsychotic medications can cause sedation, rigidity, and immobility; and diuretics can worsen impaired continence. Medication for treatment of hypertension can also contribute to incontinence.[11,13,27,47,48]
5. Retention in nonneurological clients can occur in men with prostate problems; the enlarged prostate makes the passage of urine difficult.[16,49] Other causes in men and women are the hyperactive pelvic floor syndrome (HPFS),[50] an inability to relax the pelvic floor muscles. This can be caused by pelvic pain syndromes, by painful bladder syndrome (formerly *interstitial cystitis*), or by habits: trying to void in a hurry, squeezing rather than relaxing the muscles, and being unable to void because of stressful situations.
6. An overdistended bladder can cause overflow incontinence. It can manifest as constant or intermittent dribbling, sometimes combined with urgency or symptoms of stress incontinence. Patients often have high residual urine levels and feel that their bladder does not empty properly; sometimes secondary to sensory problems, the patients are unaware of the filling of the bladder.
7. Inadequate fluid intake (either too much or too little) and fluids that may be stimulants to the bladder can cause urgency incontinence or frequent trips to the bathroom. Smoking, obesity, and postmenopausal estrogen deficiency contribute to the problem.[11,22,24,47,48]

Neurogenic causes of bladder dysfunctions are as follows:

1. Lesions in the higher cortical areas and suprapontine lesions can be found in patients with MS, stroke, Alzheimer disease, Parkinson disease, traumatic brain injury, tumors, and dementia. Lateral prefrontal cortex activation probably regulates the desire to void and to remain continent.[2] Lesions in the pathways from the prefrontal cortex and limbic system to the PAG probably cause urgency incontinence in the elderly.[1] The emotional motor system (EMS) uses the cell group of the pontine micturition center (PMC), close to the locus coeruleus, which sends long descending fibers to the parasympathetic motoneurons to the sacral cord. Through inhibitory interneurons, fibers reach the nucleus of Onuf. Stimulation of the PMC therefore results in complete micturition.[1] Neurological diseases can cause many other symptoms such as retention and an inability to control the micturition reflex. Detrusor hyperreflexia (overactive detrusor during the filling phase) with coordinated urethral relaxation interferes with normal tonic inhibition of the parasympathetic pathways and the balance between facilitatory and inhibitory mechanisms in the PMC.[44,47,48,51]
2. Lesions in the upper motor neurons (UMNs) affect the spinal cord. Common problems resulting in urinary dysfunction are SCI, MS, cauda equina syndrome, tumors, inflammatory diseases such as transverse myelitis, infectious diseases such as syphilis (tabes dorsalis), injuries to the spinal column, prolapse of a disc, or stenosis of the spinal canal. A typical bladder problem is detrusor hyperreflexia without coordinated urethral relaxation (detrusor-sphincter dyssynergy).[47,48,51,52]
3. Lesions of the peripheral or lower motor neurons (LMNs) such as injuries from childbirth, traumatic injuries, diabetes, radiculitis (e.g., from herpes zoster), or tabes dorsalis can cause retention and detrusor areflexia. The inability to feel when the bladder is full can lead to an overflow bladder with symptoms of dribbling and incomplete or strained voiding. Patients may need to learn clean intermittent catheterization.[11,13,48,51,53]
4. Lesions stemming from injuries to the autonomic nervous system can be caused by surgery in the pelvic area, such as hysterectomy, rectum resection, and radical prostatectomy; injury; or inflammations such as chronic cystopathy in diabetic patients. Autonomic lesions can contribute to diffuse pain,[54] swelling, and altered sensory awareness. Patients with urinary problems can describe the feeling of having cold feet.[55,56] Patients with diabetic cystopathy (DC)—in addition to their symptoms of weak stream, hesitancy in starting urination, dribbling, and overflow from high residual urine levels (caused by decreased bladder sensation and increased bladder capacity, and impaired contractility)—may also have other symptoms of autonomic dysfunction. These can include orthostatic hypotension, nocturnal fall of blood pressure, and changes in heart rate.[7,27] Altered central nervous system (CNS) monoamines (serotonin and noradrenaline) can cause both depression and OAB.

Overview of bladder dysfunctions

Non-neurological

Stress urinary incontinence: *Weakness* of the pelvic floor muscles.
Reasons: Injury from childbirth; decreased function because improper use when coughing, lifting, breathing; straining with constipation or fecal impaction, estrogen deficiency, genetic make-up (possible collagen deficiency)

Bladder dysfunction

Urgency: *Detrusor instability*
Sudden urge to go to the bathroom, with or without loss of urine.
Possible reasons: Infection, prolapse of vagina, cystocele, weakness of the pelvic floor

Overactive bladder syndrome (OAB)
Urgency, frequency, and nocturia.
Possible reasons: Bladder spasm, bladder instability, neurological disease

Nocturia: Waking up from sleep one or more times to void.
Possible reasons: decreased bladder capacity, increased fluid intake or neurologic diseases (e.g., Parkinson)

Retention: *Inadequate emptying* of the bladder; can be associated with pressure/pain in the lower abdomen

Overflow: *Overdistention* of the bladder; it empties by constant dribbling of urine when the capacity is exceeded

Neurological

1. Lesions in higher cortical areas and suprapontine:
Possible causes: Multiple sclerosis (MS), stroke, Parkinson disease, traumatic brain injury (TBI), tumors, dementia, alcoholism, Alzheimer disease, Huntington disease

Possible symptoms: Retention, inability to control the micturition reflex resulting in detrusor hyperreflexia

2. Lesions in the upper motor neuron (spinal cord):
Possible causes: Spinal cord injury (SCI), MS, tumors, back injuries and prolapse of a disc, stenosis of the spinal canal, inflammatory and vascular diseases (e.g., transverse myelitis), infections (e.g., syphilis–tabes dorsalis), diabetes mellitus, cauda equina syndrome, herpes zoster

Possible symptoms: Detrusor sphincter dyssynergy with danger of urethrovesical reflux, decreased sensory awareness

3. Lesions in the lower motor neuron, peripheral nervous system, and in the autonomic nervous system:
Possible causes: Injuries to the spinal cord, radiculitis (e.g., herpes zoster), tabes dorsalis, radiation, radical abdominal/perineal surgeries, diabetes mellitus, autonomous neuropathy, Guillain-Barré syndrome

Possible symptoms: Areflexia of the detrusor muscle, decreased sensation, incontinence, void by straining.
Autonomic nervous system symptoms can include diffuse pain

Other causes

4. Psychogenic:
Nonneurogenic neurogenic bladder (Hinman syndrome), hysteria, schizophrenia, depression
5. Endocrine: e.g., diabetes, hypothyroidism
6. Hormonal deficiencies: e.g., lack of estrogen
7. Inflammatory: e.g., cystitis, vulvovaginitis, prostatitis, and painful bladder syndrome
8. Obstructive: e.g., tumor, prolapse
9. Pharmacological: e.g., some over-the-counter medications, medication for treatment of hypertension, depression

Possible symptoms: Retention, frequency, urgency, and stress incontinence, decreased sensory awareness

Figure 29-1 ■ Overview of reasons for incontinence of nonneurological and neurological causes.

Correction of some neurologic disorders can eliminate both depression and urgency incontinence.[57]

5. Psychogenic causes of urinary dysfunction include schizophrenia and depression. Patients can experience incontinence, hesitation, retention, and pain.
6. A nonneurogenic neurogenic bladder is called *Hinman syndrome.*[47]
7. Endocrine causes are hypothyroidism and diabetes, which may lead to a flaccid or areflexic bladder and require clean intermittent self-catheterization.[47,53] Diabetes can also increase the frequency of urination.

ANATOMY AND PHYSIOLOGY OF THE PELVIC FLOOR

The pelvic floor consists of all the muscles that close the pelvic cavity. It is part of the abdominal compartment that can be defined by the pulmonary diaphragm cranially, the pelvic diaphragm and perineal membrane caudally, the muscles of the abdominal wall ventrally, and the muscles of the back dorsally. This compartment houses the internal organs and the viscera.[13,45-47,58-61] All muscles of the abdominal compartment interact and support one another, providing postural stability and the ability to breathe, talk, and eliminate. The pelvic floor is essentially composed of three layers: the endopelvic fascia, the pelvic diaphragm, and the perineal membrane.

Endopelvic Fascia

The endopelvic fascia suspends and supports the organs within the pelvis. It is a mesh of connective tissue composed of collagen, elastin, blood and lymph vessels, and nerves. A thick, fibrous part of the endopelvic fascia, the pubocervical fascia, attaches to the cervix in a slinglike fashion and assists in supporting the urethra and the bladder. Laterally it connects to the fascia white line, the tendinous arch of the levator ani muscle. Injuries to this important fascial support can contribute to weakness of the pelvic floor, prolapse, and leakage with increased abdominal pressure.[13,48,61] One study[62] has shown that fascia may be able to contract in a smooth muscle-like manner and therefore may have the ability to influence musculoskeletal dynamics. This underlines the importance to not neglect the fascial structures surrounding the abdomen when treating pelvic floor dysfunctions. They are not purely passive structures.

Pelvic Diaphragm

The pelvic diaphragm consists mostly of the paired levator ani muscle (Figure 29-2). The levator ani is shaped like a hammock and has several parts. In the sagittal plane the muscle originates at the pubic bone and attaches to the coccyx, hence the name *pubococcygeus muscle.* The medial part of the pubococcygeus joins behind the rectum and therefore is named the *puborectalis muscle.* This part of the levator muscle provides continence of bowel by increasing the anorectal angle. Inability to relax the puborectalis therefore contributes to constipation in patients with HPFS. Other fibers of the levator ani form a sling around the vagina or prostate (pubovaginalis and levator prostate muscles). Each side of the muscle meets in the midline with the other half and attaches to the perineal and anococcygeal bodies. The compressor urethrae muscle is part of the external urethral complex. It originates from the rami of the ischium and pubis and runs fanwise forward and medially to arch over the anterior part of the urethral surface. The sphincter urethrovaginalis is part of the puborectalis.[63]

The posterior part of the levator ani has two paired sections. The coccygeus (or ischiococcygeus) muscle covers the sacrospinous ligament. The muscle arises at the spine of the ischium and extends to the lowest part of the sacrum and the coccyx. The iliococcygeus lies between the coccygeus and the puborectalis and passes in a diagonal direction between the coccyx to the spine of the ischium and the tendinous arch of the levator ani. This fibrous band of the arcus tendineus is suspended between the pubic bone and ischial spine.[13,47,48,61,63-65] The levator ani is a skeletal muscle with a high resting tone; it consists of approximately 70% slow-twitch fibers and 30% fast-twitch fibers.[48,61,66-68] Wall and colleagues[48] and Bump and colleagues[66] consider the high resting tone critical for pelvic support and for keeping the hiatus of the levator closed. Because the levator ani muscle is under voluntary control, it can be actively contracted and provide closure during an increase in abdominal pressure, such as when coughing or sneezing.[48,67-69] According to Retzky and Rogers,[13] the innervation of the levator ani muscles is under dual control: on the pelvic surface by motor efferents of the sacral nerve from S2 to S4, and on the perineal surface by the pudendal nerve.

Perineal Membrane

The perineal membrane (formerly *urogenital diaphragm*) is the outer layer of the pelvic floor. It is a thick, fibrous, and muscular layer of triangular shape immediately below the levator ani. In women the perineal membrane attaches the edges of the vagina to the ischiopubic ramus; in men it forms an uninterrupted sheet of tissue. The fibers of the deep and superficial transverse perineal muscles run primarily in a frontal plane and contain many fibrous tissues,[70] the ischiocavernosus muscle in a diagonal direction, and the bulbospongiosus muscle in a sagittal plane. The external sphincter muscle of the anus is part of the perineal membrane and is connected to the transverse perineal and bulbospongiosus muscle by the perineal body, which contains fibrous tissue. The dorsal attachment of the perineal membrane is achieved through the anococcygeal raphe, which connects the external anal sphincter (EAS) to the coccyx.[48,64,67,70]

The muscles of the perineal membrane include both smooth and striated muscles. The muscles become tight when the levator ani tone remains relaxed.[48] The anterior portion of the perineal membrane is closely connected to the urethral musculature. According to Wall and colleagues,[48] the perineal membrane does not substantially contribute to pelvic support; it is mostly the levator ani, which has much greater strength and bulk and can exert upward traction when contracting to maintain outlet support. The ischiocavernosus, bulbospongiosus, and superficial transverse perineal muscles function mainly in sexual responsiveness, serving to enhance and maintain penile erection in males and maintaining erection of the clitoris in females.[48,61] Trigger points in these muscles can cause a degree of impotence and pain with intercourse. According to Claes and colleagues,[71] Van Kampen and colleagues,[72] and Dorey,[73] strengthening exercises of the muscles of the perineal membrane can significantly improve impotence. In women the perineal membrane is often torn or injured during childbirth,

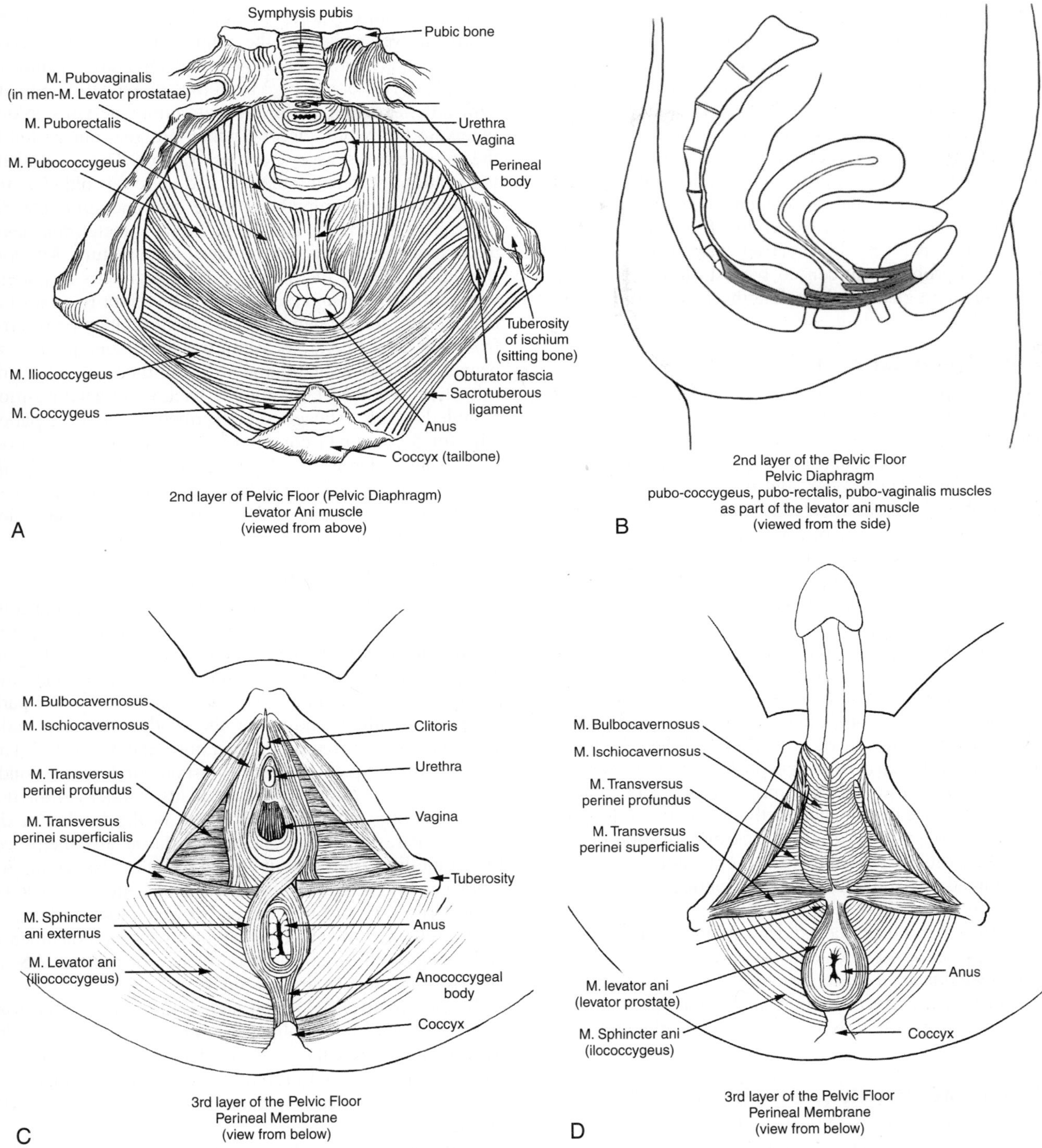

Figure 29-2 ■ Anatomy of the pelvic floor. **A,** Second layer of the pelvic floor, pelvic diaphragm viewed from above. **B,** Second layer of the pelvic floor, pelvic diaphragm viewed from the side. **C,** Third layer of the pelvic floor, perineal membrane viewed from below (female). **D,** Third layer of the pelvic floor, perineal membrane viewed from below (male).

and, if not properly repaired, injuries can cause sexual dysfunction, pelvic pain, and low self-esteem.

The complicated autonomic innervation of the pelvic area and its clinical relevance, including the perineal area, has been well described by Wesselmann and colleagues[54] as well as Fritsch and Umphred.[70] The pudendal nerve diverges from the sacral plexus, intermingles with the autonomic nerves, and then branches into several directions, innervating the EAS and the anterior perineal muscles.

Mucosal Coaptation of the Urethra

In addition to the three pelvic floor layers, an important contributor to continence is the mucosal coaptation, which is the arteriovenous complex between the epithelial lining and the smooth muscle coat of the female urethra. It is sensitive to estrogen, and with deficiency of this hormone the resting pressure of the urethra can decrease and cause leakage.[13] Wall and colleagues[48] compared it with an "inflatable cushion" helping to fill the urethral wall and sealing the 3- to 4-cm–long urethra in women. Because of possible serious side effects of estrogen treatment, it is now prescribed and applied to the vaginal area in low dosage and with caution. It can help some menopausal women increase the resting tone of the urethra and improve closure. The male urethra is not estrogen dependent. Its mucosal coaptation is highly vascular and probably influenced by testosterone. In addition, the prostate gland and the length of the male urethra may contribute to a sealing effect.

Internal Sphincter of the Urethra

The internal sphincter muscle at the junction of the bladder and urethra (urethrovesical junction) is an involuntary smooth muscle under autonomic control in both males and females. Its shape is circular and formed by the trigone, a smooth muscle in the bladder, and two U-shaped loops of muscles that derive from the bladder muscle. In females the urethra rests on a hammock of connective tissue (pubocervical fascia) and is held in a position that prevents descent into the vagina. The external sphincter muscle is able to close the middle portion of the female urethra.[13]

Incontinence usually happens when several factors come together. For example, men frequently leak after radical prostatectomy because the smooth internal sphincter urethra may have been damaged by the surgery and the pelvic floor muscles have to learn to substitute and provide closure of the urethra. A patient with dementia may not feel the need to go to the bathroom because of lesions in the limbic system or the cortex.[1,2] Parkinson disease may cause bladder outlet obstruction because of a noncontractile detrusor, resulting in large volumes of residual urine or lack of activation of the PMC.[2,74] In addition, the inability to quickly undress complicates an already existing problem of incontinence in such a client.

In healthy individuals the external sphincter and levator ani muscles serve as a backup system for continence. However, weakness of these structures leads to decreased bladder neck and urethral support and can lead to incontinence, especially with activities that increase the abdominal pressure.

VOIDING MECHANISM OF THE BLADDER

Many of the neurophysiological connections involved in functioning of the bladder and the surrounding muscles are not fully understood. A complicated coordination of many systems is involved in a properly functioning bladder and other pelvic organs. Elaboration on all the neural interactions, which take place at all levels, is not possible in this chapter. Wesselmann and colleagues[54] and Burnett and Wesselmann[75] provide comprehensive information about the neurobiology of the pelvis.

Sympathetic Innervation

The sympathetic innervation to the bladder, rectum, and sexual organs originates from the thoracolumbar segment of the spinal cord (T10 to L1-L2) as well as from the hypogastric plexus (the sympathetic hypogastric nerve), which descends from the aortic plexus (Figure 29-3). The hypogastric nerve feeds into the inferior hypogastric (pelvic) plexus, which is the major neuronal integrative center for multiple pelvic organs.[54,75] Both the sympathetic and parasympathetic divisions of the autonomic nervous system innervate the pelvic viscera, which are also innervated by the somatic and sensory nervous systems. The sympathetic innervation inhibits the bladder and increases bladder storage ability (it is sympathetic to be dry) and stimulates the muscles of the trigone and the internal sphincter muscles of the bladder as well as the muscles of the rectum. Attention should be paid to the T10 to L1-L2 segments in patients with tailbone pain and pain in the pelvic floor (e.g., testicular, buttock, scrotal pain) because the pain may be referred from that area. I recall a case in which tailbone pain disappeared instantly after treatment of the thoracolumbar area in a client who had fallen on the back in a flexed position. Doubleday and colleagues[76] described a case of a patient who for 5 years had complained of testicular and buttock pain along with posterior leg paresthesias. Treatment of the T10 to L1-L2 area (central disk protrusion at T12-L1) with direct and guided physical therapy resulted in complete symptom resolution.

Parasympathetic Innervation

The parasympathetic innervation exits the spinal canal at the level of S2 to S4. The nerves join the splanchnic nerve before entering the inferior hypogastric plexus (see Figure 29-3, *A*). The parasympathetic fibers stimulate the bladder and other pelvic organs, including the sexual organs.[54,75,77] The parasympathetic fibers ending in the bladder are especially sensitive to overstretching, infection, and fibrosis.[47] This explains the frequent urgency to urinate under such conditions. The parasympathetic nerve helps bladder contraction by stimulating muscarinic receptors in the fundus of the bladder. Parasympathetic nerve activation also helps colonic mobility. Therefore in an SCI when LMNs are injured (parasympathetic cell bodies in the cauda equina and conus medullaris), the result can be slowed stool propulsion with areflexic bowel. LMN injury causes constipation and increases the risk of incontinence from lax EAS, as described by Benevento and Sipski.[52]

In contrast an UMN lesion such as those from MS causes hyperreflexia with no voluntary control over the EAS. The patient cannot relax the EAS to defecate even though reflex coordination and stool propulsion are present. Urinary and fecal retention and constipation are common in such UMN injuries.[52]

Detrusor sphincter dyssynergia (DSD), caused by impaired coordination between bladder contraction and the external sphincter urethra, can be attributable to hyperreflexia or uncontrolled muscle spasm of the detrusor. This condition is common in patients with SCI[52] as well as MS but not in clients with cerebral vascular accident (CVA).

Somatic Innervation

The somatic innervation of the pelvic floor comes from the sacral plexus of S2 to S4 (see Figure 29-3, *A*). The pudendal nerve leaves the spinal cord at S2 to S4 and branches to innervate the striated muscles of the levator ani, the external sphincter muscles of both the urethra and rectum, the labia and clitoris, and the muscles of the perineal membrane. The

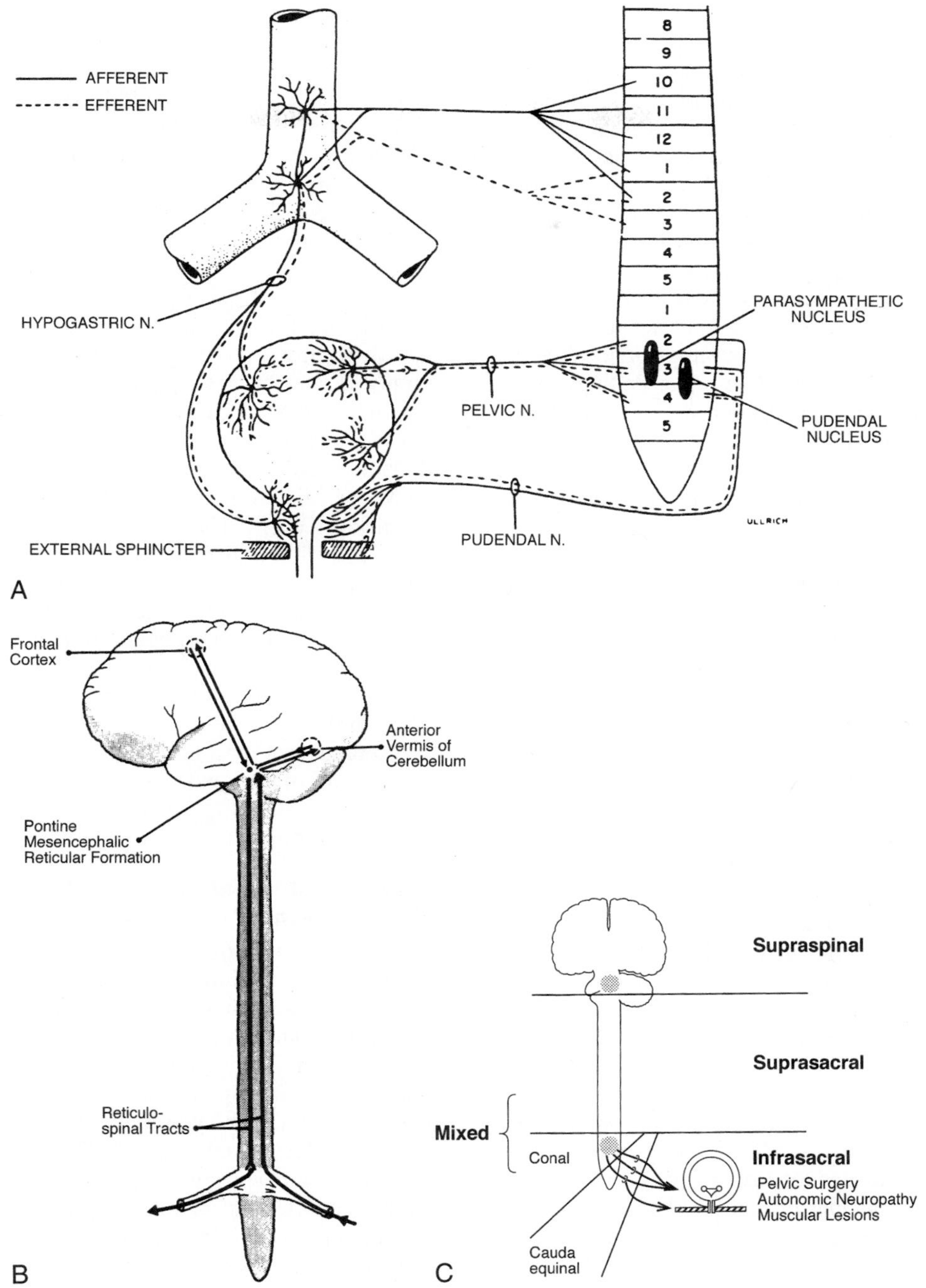

Figure 29-3 ■ Neurophysiology of the pelvic floor. (**A** from Blaivas JG: Management of bladder dysfunction in multiple sclerosis, *Neurology* 30:12, 1980; **B** from Bradley WE, Brantley SF: Physiology of the urinary bladder. In Harrison JH, Gittes RE, Perlmutter AD, et al, editors: *Campbell's urology,* Philadelphia, 1978, WB Saunders; **C** from Braddom RL: *Physical medicine rehabilitation,* ed 2, Philadelphia, 2000, WB Saunders.)

sacral plexus provides both efferent and afferent innervation; some of the fibers of the pudendal nerve intermingle with the autonomic pelvic nerves.[47,54,77] The somatic nerves can modulate the autonomic system. The complexity of the innervation of the pelvis and the influence of neurotransmitters in the bladder wall, as well as the control of higher CNS regulation (see Figure 29-3, *B* and *C*), can be appreciated in observing the filling and emptying phases of the bladder. Because of its topographical position the pudendal nerve is susceptible to nerve injury from stretching or compression (Alcock canal) from a fall on the buttocks or from slamming on the brake pedal during a motor vehicle accident (may alter pelvic alignment). Patients with pudendal nerve injury often have no problems when supine or standing but pain when sitting. Childbirth, especially during delivery of large babies, also can cause pudendal nerve injury.[13]

Sensory Innervation

The sensory innervation in the pelvic region is important to evaluate and restore in clients with motor control problems because sensation drives motor responses. The pudendal nerve carries both sensory and motor fibers. Absence of feeling in the perineal area can be caused by stress and memory of pain (e.g., abuse). For example, a client with symptoms of incontinence and pain with sexual intercourse and a history of considerable continuous stresses stated after few treatments, "I thought my pelvic region was dead; I had no clue how little I could feel before sensory awareness training. Feeling the pelvic floor, I can now contract and relax the muscles much better." Sensory innervation of the bladder comes primarily from proprioceptive nerve endings in the bladder and urethra. The afferent neuronal visceral system probably enters the spinal cord by way of the sacral and lumbar segments. These afferent nerve tracts may regulate pain, the absence of pain, and the feeling of having a full bladder.[47,77]

Filling and Storage Phase

The bladder is a smooth involuntary muscle with voluntary control. It stores the urine until it is emptied voluntarily. The normal bladder is a low-pressure system that accepts urine without a concomitant rise of internal pressure.[13,48] This is produced by sympathetic stimulation of the β-adrenergic receptors in the bladder wall. The sympathetic nervous system inhibits the parasympathetic activity while sympathetic stimulation of the α-adrenergic receptors in the internal sphincter muscle causes constriction and a rise in urethral pressure.[13,48] During the filling phase the bladder is inactive until it holds approximately 350 to 500 mL of urine, even though a first sensation of filling may occur with 150 to 250 mL of urine in the bladder.[77] When the bladder is full the receptors send a signal to the cortical centers of the brain, and as a result a voluntary micturition reflex is initiated to empty the bladder (see Figure 29-3, *B*).[13,48,77]

Involuntary contractions of the detrusor during the filling phase cause frequency and urgency (OAB syndrome). In neurological patients this is called *hyperreflexia;* if idiopathic, it is considered bladder instability.[47,48] Individuals with a hypersensitive bladder or painful bladder syndrome (interstitial cystitis) empty their bladders frequently to avoid pain, which results in a functionally small bladder. When the sensation of bladder filling is decreased or absent, the bladder will overfill and urine can back up into the kidneys, causing dysfunction. Symptoms of overflow from the overstretched bladder frequently cause dribbling. All these problems require thorough medical investigation of possible causes.

Preconditions for a normal storage phase as described by Henscher[78] include good distensibility of the bladder, stable bladder without premature detrusor contractions (adequate bladder sensation, i.e., intact CNS and peripheral nervous system), no obstruction between kidney and bladder, and positive urethral closure at rest and under load.

Emptying Phase

Micturition, or voiding, depends on the coordinated activity of the urethra and the detrusor muscle. The pelvic floor (levator ani and external sphincter muscles) has to relax when the detrusor muscle contracts. This occurs with activation of the parasympathetic cholinergic receptors in the bladder muscle. An afferent stimulus from the pelvic nerve (see Figure 29-3, *A*) reaches the PMC by way of the spinal cord. Efferent tracts inhibit the activity of the pudendal nerve, which results in relaxation of the external sphincter and levator ani. At the same time, sympathetic activity at the bladder neck is inhibited and postganglionic parasympathetic neurotransmitters are stimulated. This results in detrusor contraction.[13,19,47,77]

From the PMC, signals are also sent to the cerebral cortex, which allows voluntary control. An individual therefore can override the signal to empty the bladder and wait to empty it later or can empty the bladder when there is no signal that it is full. Suprapontine control of bladder function is a result of the modulating control of the brain stem, hypothalamus, and cerebral cortex.[1,77]

Many reflexes are involved in urine storage and voiding at various levels. The sacral reflex, for example, can be elicited by light stroking at the lateral aspect of the anus and should result in a symmetrical contraction of the anal sphincter ("anal wink"). Absence of the anal wink can be an indication of a neurological problem at S2 to S4, resulting in weakness or paralysis of the pudendal nerve.[13] The micturition reflex, on the other hand, depends on an intact PMC in the brain stem.[77]

Prerequisites for a normal emptying phase include intact neural control, adequate functioning of the detrusor, no increase in resistance to voiding by obstruction, and adequate pelvic floor relaxation.[78]

Pharmacological Treatment of Pelvic Floor Dysfunction

The great number of receptors in the bladder wall, as well as the ability to influence skeletal muscles with muscle relaxants, is the basis for pharmacological treatment of the symptoms found in patients with incontinence. Other treatments for urinary dysfunction address hormonal deficiency. Estrogen, for example, was prescribed for many postmenopausal women with symptoms of leakage and a feeling of dryness in the vaginal area.[13,47,48,51] However, treatment with oral estrogen is controversial, and reports of its efficacy for treatment of UI are mixed.[26] Topical vaginal application of Premarin and other drugs may be beneficial in the treatment of UI because estrogen deficiency decreases the turgor of the submucosa around the urethra.

Individuals with enuresis (bedwetting at night) or urge incontinence are frequently prescribed oxybutynin (Ditropan). Another prescribed drug is imipramine, an antidepressant. Patients with instability of the detrusor often receive anticholinergic agents or antispasmodic medications.

α-Adrenergic agents such as phenylpropanolamine or ephedrine increase striated muscle tone and are therefore used with SUI. α-Adrenergic antagonists, such as drugs for treatment of hypertension, can worsen incontinence. Caffeine, alcohol, and diuretics can increase urinary frequency, urgency, and SUI.[11,13,47,79] Antipsychotic agents are also α-adrenergic antagonists and reduce urethral pressure and can be used for treatment of urinary retention.[13] The problem with pharmaceutical treatment is the side effects, some of which may affect the pelvic floor adversely (e.g., constipation). Other clients describe severe dryness in the mouth and the need to drink or suck on candy constantly. Many other side effects have been described by the people taking these drugs, including dizziness, blurred vision, somnolence, confusion, hypertension or hypotension, and dryness of the mucosal membranes of the mouth, vagina, and eyes.[27]

New drugs have entered the market promising fewer side effects and help for patients with OAB syndrome and urinary frequency. Duloxetine, for example, works at the level of the spinal cord, inhibiting serotonin and regulating noradrenaline and thereby increasing the time between voids.

Solifenacin succinate is an antimuscarinic agent that blocks muscarinic receptors on bladder smooth muscles, relaxing them. It is therefore indicated for relief of urinary frequency, urgency, and UI associated with OAB syndrome. Other commonly prescribed antagonists of muscarinic acetylcholine receptors include darifenacin, fesoterodine, oxybutynin, propiverine, tolterodine, and trospium.[80]

These muscarinic receptor antagonists work on the OAB by relaxing the smooth muscle tissue in the bladder.

For clients with MS, anticholinergic medication is recommended for the treatment of neurogenic overactivity of the bladder. Intravesical treatments with vanilloids and botulinum toxin have been proposed, as well as sublingual cannabinoids. DasGupta and Fowler[81] also state that sildenafil citrate has been shown to be efficacious as a proerectile agent. Sildenafil (Viagra) has been shown to be efficacious in men with SCI; it also may improve arousal in women with SCI and is being evaluated for female patients with sexual arousal disorder.[82,83]

Intravesical resiniferatoxin (an analog of capsaicin with more than 1000 times its potency in desensitizing C-fiber bladder afferent neurons) is a new therapy for detrusor hyperreflexia for SCI, MS, and other neurologically impaired patients.[84]

The motivation to achieve a functioning pelvic floor without full dependence on drugs is high. Physical therapy may be the main contributor to reaching that goal. The combination of drug therapy and physical therapy can be helpful, and the therapist should know which medications the client is taking as well as their side effects.

EXAMINATION, EVALUATION, AND INTERVENTION

Medical Evaluation

Before a referral to physical therapy, a physician, preferably a urologist or gynecologist, should evaluate a patient with any urinary dysfunction. The patient's history will lead the physician to select appropriate diagnostic tests, including a urodynamic test, which helps explore the extent of the lesion, rule out causes that require other treatments, and determine if physical therapy may help.[13,47,48] Adams and Frahm[79] provide an excellent overview of the causes and the examination and intervention possibilities. Part of the evaluation process should be a bladder diary or voiding log completed over a several-day period (if possible including a weekend day) so that a clear picture emerges about fluid input and output as well as when frequency and incontinence episodes occur and to what extent. Patients can also weigh their pads or liners for 24 hours and that way get a clear picture of the loss of urine in 24 hours. Both "tests" can be repeated after a series of treatments to measure progress. If the physician has not done these tests, they should be included in the physical therapy evaluation.

Physicians should also include a muscle strength test of the levator ani when seeing a client with symptoms of UI to determine how much the muscle weakness contributes to the problem.[48,67,79]

Physical Therapy Examination

It is important to take a history of the client's problem in a quiet and pleasant setting. The ideal situation is a private room because it may be very uncomfortable for the client to discuss very private matters between curtains. Handouts and pictures of anatomy should be available in order to explain anatomy and physiological processes to the client. During the first visit a bladder diary and other evaluation tools or outcome measures such as the female NIH symptom index (NIH-CPSI), the Incontinence Impact Questionnaire—Short Form (IIQ-7), or other available questionnaires should be used. This enables the therapist to understand the extent of the problem. The same questionnaires should be used for reevaluation to verify progress and outcome. Only if the therapist listens carefully and attentively will the client provide necessary information. The therapist should always ask herself or himself what system of the body may be involved and require treatment. For example, a client who complains of feeling bloated or congested in the abdomen may have "trapped" fluid in the abdominal cavity and may benefit from manual lymph drainage (MLD). Lack of leakage of urine and difficulty initiating a urinary stream may be caused by hyperactive pelvic floor muscle, in which case strengthening exercises would be of no value. Urgency and frequency symptoms may necessitate bladder training, "Cold feet" or difficulty sleeping can indicate an autonomic system dysfunction. A frustrated and depressed state could be a result of limbic system dysfunction and could alter posture and pelvic floor muscle tone.

Careful observation of the client and good listening skills will help establish the client's level of functioning. At the same time, it validates the client's feelings, observations, and concerns, making the client feel taken seriously. This promotes client-therapist interaction and effective treatment. It is very important for the therapist to make sure the client understands why he or she has the problem and to empower the client to be part of the solution. The focus will be regaining the client's health. The first session also needs to be educational, with pictures or models of the pelvic floor, so that the patient understands how this invisible structure of the body works. The therapist should be able to explain to a 78-year-old patient with difficulty voiding after UTI that the advice of her doctor 20 years ago "to void each time she sees a bathroom" had decreased the volume of the bladder severely (maximum voiding was ⅔ cup, whereas the bladder can normally hold 2 cups) and this probably had decreased her ability to empty her bladder completely.

Usually, physical therapists trained in women's health assess the muscle strength of the pelvic floor of their clients by digital internal palpation. This may not necessarily take place on the first visit, and the patient must consent to such an evaluation. Because of the danger of re-traumatization, internal examination and use of instruments in the vagina (such as biofeedback probes) should not be applied to clients who have been abused.[85,86] Therapists should be reminded that such patients may say yes when they mean no because of their past experiences. It is possible to perform external palpations with the consent of the client and use other tests for evaluation of the extent of leakage and weakness with stress incontinence as described earlier, or the pad test, which can be performed by physicians or therapists.[47,48,79,87]

Conceptual Framework for Treatment

Therapy begins with a patient interview and appropriate tests and measures, which are necessary to determine which structures and systems are involved and what kind of impairment or activity limitations can be identified.[8,88,89] The information gathered leads to the development of a diagnosis and prognosis and selection of the intervention and, hopefully, the most efficacious treatment outcome.

Therapists working with female clients with incontinence have to ask about childbirth and related trauma or surgery, prolapses, and procedures such as cesarean delivery, hysterectomy, episiotomy, or sling suspension. Different questions need to be asked when a male patient is evaluated because the reason for his pelvic floor dysfunction will likely be quite different.

Evaluation of Female Clients with Incontinence

An example of an examination-evaluation process that might be used for female clients with incontinence is shown in Figure 29-4.

Question 1

This information gives the therapist a general idea of why the client was sent, how long the problem has existed, whether other illnesses may have contributed to the problem, and which body systems may be involved. Does the problem contribute to the inability to be socially active, travel, see friends, or pursue hobbies?

Question 2

The therapist learns from this information whether damage to the muscles or nerves supplying the pelvic floor muscles may be present as well as whether the surgery coincided with worsening, improvement, or the onset of symptoms. Because surgery produces scars, the possibility of scars being part of the problem should be considered. The therapist may also inquire if, for example, lifting the baby out of the crib increases the symptoms.

Even in older patients the questions about childbirth are important because, for example, a difficult delivery may cause problems much later in life. In some patients questions about the onset of menstruation or menopause may be indicated if, for example, hormone imbalance may be a contributing factor to vaginal dryness and pain with intercourse. It could also be that only later in life does fecal incontinence become a problem, although it originally stemmed from an injury sustained during delivery.

Thought Process. If the heaviest child weighed 9 pounds at birth, pudendal nerve damage could be contributing to the pelvic floor problem. The question of diabetes is important in the medical history because diabetic mothers are known to sometimes have big babies. The scars must be examined, especially if the client reports pain or constipation. With a hysterectomy, the bladder is not "stabilized" by the vagina, which normally leans against the bladder.

Question 3

Scars, especially in the pelvic and abdominal region, can cause pain, which can radiate to the hips or pelvic region. They can also contribute to constipation. Scarring may also necessitate more extensive examination of the thoracolumbar junction and mobility of both hips. The quality and intensity of pain may hint to autonomic or musculoskeletal dysfunction.

Thought Process. Any surgery can cause scar tissue or muscle weakness in the area surrounding the pelvic floor. Observation and palpation of the abdominal cavity may be necessary. If the surgery was recent, vigorous exercises should be avoided, and a review of body mechanics and lifting may be indicated.

Question 4

Diabetes and heart conditions can lead to increased fluid input and output. Diabetes also often causes a decreased sensory awareness of the bladder and decreased bladder contractility. Cancer can cause bony involvement, swelling, pain, and so on. Back pain can be caused by injuries to the back or injuries to the pelvic area, including the viscera. Pulmonary conditions may cause frequent coughing and leakage, which may prevent the patient/client from leaving the house for social activities.

Thought Process. Urine output can be increased in a patient with diabetes. A patient with frequent bladder infections may not drink enough water. The type of drink may stimulate the bladder, and the influence of medications on the medical condition may affect the muscle tone of the pelvic floor. Exercises need to be altered in clients with back pain or metastasis. Emphasis on tightening the pelvic floor before coughing needs to be addressed first in clients with pulmonary conditions. Weakness of the pelvic floor muscles can also contribute to low back pain and highlights the importance to look at the entire abdominal compartment. In addition to the pelvic floor muscles the patient may need to strengthen the transverse abdominis muscle to stabilize the back. Diaphragmatic breathing has to be addressed as well.

Question 5

Remember that antihypertension drugs, diuretics, antidepressants, and cough medicines can affect continence.

Thought Process. Is the client aware of what drugs may affect the incontinence problem? Coffee and alcohol are also considered drugs and can increase frequency of urination. For example, patients who have undergone prostatectomy and who already do well staying dry usually report problems of incontinence when drinking alcohol.

Question 6

This section obtains information about the extent of the problem of the pelvic floor dysfunction and what other areas may need to be addressed.

EVALUATION FORM

1. Medical diagnosis:

Onset:

2. Childbirth information:
How many gestations? births?
weight of heaviest child?
Cesarean, Y/N episiotomy
Vaginal/abdominal surgeries:
bladder suspension, hysterectomy,
other?

3. General surgical history:
Abdominal surgeries (please circle): hernia, appendix, gallbladder, kidney, laparoscopy, hemorrhoids, other?

4. Medical history:
Diabetes: Y/N heart problems Y/N
hypertension Y/N cancer Y/N
kidney/bladder infections Y/N
back pain Y/N neck pain Y/N asthma Y/N
bronchitis Y/N
other (e.g., neurological conditions)

5. Medications:

6. Current symptoms:
Do you have (please circle if yes) any leakage: with coughing, sneezing, straining?
While running and going up- or downstairs?
When resting? Are any other activities causing leakage?
Do you have: hesitancy, urgencies, do you push or strain?
(Please circle when applicable)
Does your problem cause you to have sexual dysfunction?
Do you have any pain? If yes, please describe:

7. Urination pattern:
How often do you have to urinate?
day night
How often do you leak?
daily times a week infrequent
Do you use one of the following during the day (d) or night (n)?
(Please circle and indicate how many):
liners d n pads d n
adult protection d n

8. Daily fluid intake (cups, glasses):
How much do you drink?
water coffee tea soda
alcohol citrus
other:

9. Bowel habits:
Regular Y/N, incontinent of bowel Y/N, gas Y/N, constipation Y/N. Do you use stool softenersY/N, fiber rich-dietY/N?

10. History of treatment:
Have you ever been treated for this condition before? Y/N Did you do Kegel exercises? Y/N
Other treatments? Y/N
Please describe:

11. Psychosocial history:
Current/previous employment: does it involve lifting?
Hobbies, sports:

12. Treatment goal of client:

13. Objective:
(Evaluate posture, ability to do diaphragmatic breathing, pelvic tilt, ability to "feel" the activity of pelvic floor muscles; evaluate muscle tone and strength of the pelvic floor muscles and of the surrounding muscle if indicated; evaluate scar tissue when applicable; check for contraindications.)

14. Evaluation/Goal:

15. Intervention:

Figure 29-4 ■ Evaluation form.

Thought Process. Which impairment needs to be addressed first, and does the medical diagnosis match the symptoms? Are any physical or emotional reasons causing sexual dysfunction and pain? Inability to have orgasm, pelvic pain, and dyspareunia (pain during intercourse) may be caused by hyperactive pelvic floor muscles and necessitate relaxation exercises for the pelvic floor muscles. Retention and hesitancy may also indicate tightness of the pelvic floor muscles. Urgency and frequency may benefit from bladder training to enable the patient to be socially active and participate in traveling, going to the theater, and so on.

Question 7

The pattern must be seen in light of the history and daily fluid intake. The information of the voiding diary should match the urinary pattern. Normal urination is six to eight times per day at a volume of at least 250 mL (9 oz), with a maximum of 500 mL. Many adults normally get up once a night to urinate; elderly people may need to get up twice each night.[47]

Question 8

Women normally drink and void 1500 to 2500 mL/day (50 to 80 oz). Aside from water, drinks that are carbonated, coffee, tea, citrus drinks, alcohol, and spicy foods are bladder irritants and can cause urgency or frequency.

Thought Process. A client who drinks below-average amounts of fluid may develop urinary frequency because the bladder is no longer used to store normal volumes. This prevents a patient from going to concerts and other events and being socially active. A person who drinks soda or alcohol before going to bed needs to evaluate if a change in drinking habits affects the incontinence or urgency. This can improve nocturia and help the patient to have a restful night.

Question 9

Many reasons exist for constipation; it can be related to difficulty going to the bathroom at work, being always in a hurry, or not relaxing the pelvic floor because of improper leg support when sitting on the toilet.[90] HPFS, eating hastily, and consuming constipating foods can contribute as well. Gastrointestinal problems, especially when combined with chronic pelvic pain or low back pain, can be the result of sexual abuse.[91] Fecal incontinence can result from weakness of the anal sphincter muscle, occult injuries or tears from difficult deliveries, hemorrhoids, insufficient fiber intake, poor bowel habits, and so on.

Thought Process. Eating habits may have to be reviewed as well as behavior during defecation. Pressing down, holding the breath, and straining during defecation as a result of constipation weaken the pelvic floor muscles and do not help clients who have prolapse. The abdomen needs to be evaluated and possibly treated (e.g., teach client colon massage, postural correction when sitting on the toilet, and diaphragmatic breathing). Should sexual abuse be suspected for any reason? Does the client appear to have low self-esteem? Are signs of fear or nervousness present during the evaluation, or a cluster of symptoms that could indicate sexual abuse?

Question 10

The therapist must find out if the patient has been treated for this condition before and whether the treatment was successful.

Thought Process. To motivate a patient, do not begin a treatment with exercises or modalities that have been used unsuccessfully in the past. The selection and explanation of the treatment intended are critical to success. Teach exercises the patient can do easily during the day, possibly combined with functions of daily life (lifting the baby), getting up from a chair, or favorite exercises. Custom tailor the exercises to activities the patient wants to do again (e.g., at home, practice delaying micturition while doing activities in house or garden to increase the time span between voids).

Question 11

Information about employment gives the therapist input about how work may contribute to the problem. How much does posture affect the pelvic floor dysfunction? How can exercises be integrated with activities at work? Hobbies and sports can be important motivational factors, but how the exercises or hobbies are done must be reviewed.

Thought Process. If poor postural alignment is part of the problem, stretching and strengthening exercises may have to be practiced for a neutral posture to be achieved. A client who can train the pelvic floor while doing his or her favorite exercises will be highly motivated. If the exercises can be performed while lifting at work, for example, the training effect will be greater.

Question 12

Client and therapist goals should ideally match, and goals should be directed toward activities the patient was able to do before he or she had the problem, such as travel without fear of leakage or embarrassment, and so on.

Thought Process. If a great discrepancy is present, more explanations or other questions may be required in the objective evaluation. Try to set a goal with the client that is achievable within a reasonable time frame. Then set new goals. Initially the goals can be having fewer episodes of wetness, sleeping through the night, having to wear a reduced number of pads, or urinating less frequently.

Question 13

Summarize the findings and consider the general cognitive status of the client and her or his mood. The therapist's goal should reflect the prognosis and the extent of the impairment or disability. The treatment intervention should be geared to an achievable goal that allows for more activity and participation and reduces social isolation.

Thought Process. A client who is cognitively impaired may require a different treatment approach. Individuals with good body awareness usually learn exercises and correct breathing patterns much faster and may require fewer treatments before seeing changes.

Question 14

Many treatment possibilities are available to choose from. Often various concepts lead to the same goal. The selection also depends greatly on the therapist's experience and preference for a certain type of treatment. The summary of the evaluation should be based on the International Classification of Functioning, Disability and Health (ICF).

Thought Process. The therapist should determine the patient's/client's level of functioning and consider the influence of the environment: Are there stairs that are obstacles within the home or that prevent access to the garden? Is help available from family or friends? The therapist also needs to think about which treatments or interventions can maximize the client's functioning and measure the outcome.

Body function and structures have to be evaluated to determine the extent of the impairment. The activity limitations and participation restrictions have to be considered in order to work to improve the activity level and achieve participation in various life situations. This has to be considered in connection with environmental factors that can help the patient to live a fulfilled life.

CASE STUDIES

Case Studies 29-1 and 29-2 give insight into how physical therapy can help clients with incontinence. Before presenting another case study, the conventional treatment approach to incontinence is discussed briefly, and then the Heller and Tanzberger concepts[92-98] are described in more detail.

CASE STUDY 29-1 ■ FEMALE CLIENT WITH INCONTINENCE

A 56-year-old woman was sent to therapy for biofeedback training and proper instruction in Kegel exercises. This alert librarian had a long history of mixed incontinence. Its onset had been approximately 19 years previously, but the condition had improved for 3 to 4 years after a hysterectomy and bladder suspension surgery in 1989. The client had had two vaginal deliveries and one episiotomy, and her heaviest child had weighed 8½ pounds. The client had urgencies more than once an hour and used one or two pads a day; wetting occurred one to three times a week. The client drank one cup of coffee in the morning and approximately two sodas per day. Her diet was regular, but she had constipation and took stool softeners.

The client liked to do brisk walking but had problems pursuing this activity because of the leakage. The client had received instructions for Kegel exercises elsewhere, but they did not help her. She had a history of chronic back and sciatic pain. The objective evaluation revealed good sitting and standing posture. Because the client exhibited a sensory awareness of the pelvic floor muscles, an internal strength test at that time was deferred. Her general strength appeared to be good, and the muscle tone of the abdomen was within functional limits.

IMPAIRMENT

The client had a poor awareness of a pelvic tilt motion and was a chest breather. There was incoordination of breathing with activity of the abdominal and back muscles and the pelvic floor muscles.

Activities

The client was unable to exercise without leakage and was required to wear one or two pads during the day. The assessment revealed a client who appeared motivated to achieve goals.

Participation

The patient no longer went to the theater, because of her urgencies.

GOALS

Goals included the ability to cough and sneeze without leakage, elimination of the need to wear pads during the day, ability to resume walking, ability to perform home exercises independently, and ability to participate in social activities without fear of leakage of urine.

INTERVENTION

She received a total of 10 treatments within 3 months based on the Klein-Vogelbach and Heller and Tanzberger concepts.[92-98,116-118] Treatment included breathing exercises, coordination of diaphragmatic breathing with pelvic floor contraction, and instruction in Swiss ball exercises for strengthening the pelvic floor muscles in all planes and during bouncing.[97,119,120] Colon massage,[121] treatment of scar tissue,[122] and biofeedback and electrical stimulation were considered as options if no improvement with the previous exercises had occurred after three to five treatments.

The client returned 6 days after the initial visit and reported decreased leakage with laughing. She received a colon massage and gentle scar tissue massage as well as more challenging exercises with the Swiss ball and elastic bands. Instruction in proper lifting with contraction of the pelvic floor was part of the treatment. A return visit was scheduled 3 weeks later for an additional treatment for the abdomen and exercises. The client reported feeling better, with improvement of the back pain, which she had had for 2 years. The abdomen had felt much looser after the treatment, and leakage with coughing and sneezing was further reduced. The plan was to review the exercises in 4 to 6 weeks. The client called 3 months later to report that she did not need further treatments.

TREATMENT OUTCOME

The client was able to hold urine for 2 to 3 hours without wearing pads. She had no more wetting episodes, and for safety she wore pads only when doing brisk walking for 45 minutes. Only occasionally did the client need to get up at night to urinate. She was able to travel and participate in all social activities she desired.

CASE STUDY 29-2 ■ MALE CLIENT WITH INCONTINENCE

Adjustments are required when taking the history of a man with pelvic floor problems (Figure 29-5). The client's answers are written in script typeface. A summary of treatment for one case follows.

The patient reported urgency, weakness of pelvic floor muscles (lost urine with straining and lifting the legs), and nocturia. He was educated about bladder training to improve the urgency by increasing his sensory awareness of the voiding pattern. He was instructed to count during urination and to keep a record of when he had gone to the bathroom last, what he had been drinking, and how much in order to evaluate whether the signal to void was correct. The patient knew that a high count during urination meant that the bladder was holding a greater volume than when the number was low. He therefore became more aware of when the urgency did not meet the need and learned to become his own "master" over the bladder. He also was instructed to do deep breathing to control the urge and to do quick flicks while standing without moving for one minute until the urgency disappeared.

In addition, the patient was instructed in fast fiber training and coordination with breathing. Before coughing or sneezing the client was instructed to do a quick contraction of the pelvic floor muscles. Slow muscle fiber contractions were taught as well, with submaximal contractions held for 6 to 10 seconds, increasing the repetitions until he could hold 10 times for 10 seconds with relaxation and breathing exercises between repetitions.

By the first return visit 4 weeks after the initial examination, the client was able to hold urine for longer periods and only needed to get up once during the night. The client also

Continued

CASE STUDY 29-2 ■ MALE CLIENT WITH INCONTINENCE—cont'd

reported being able to attend water aerobics classes without loss of urine. He was exercising for approximately 20 to 30 minutes each day. The exercises, based on the Heller,[94,95] Klein-Vogelbach, and Tanzberger concepts,[92,93,96-98,116-120] were reviewed with the client and new exercises were added. The client purchased a Swiss ball, and a return visit was scheduled approximately 3 weeks later. Before the next scheduled visit the client called to report that he was doing fine.

IMPAIRMENT

Impairments included weakness of the pelvic floor muscles, discoordination of breathing and pelvic floor contractions, and absence of tightening of the pelvic floor muscles before coughing, sneezing, or lifting his legs. The patient also had symptoms of OAB, including urgency and nocturia.

Activity

The patient had stopped doing water aerobics for fear of leakage and was worried about his urgency when teaching school at night.

Participation

Because of fear of leakage the patient's sexual life and intimacy were more stressful than he desired.

OUTCOME

The client no longer had leakage, and did not need to wear pads at night. He resumed all activities without problems, and intimacy and sexuality no longer caused stress and anxiety. He was able to exercise at home independently and did not require further treatment. His next attempt was to maintain his condition without the bladder medication tolterodine (Detrol).

CONVENTIONAL TREATMENT OPTIONS FOR STRESS URINARY INCONTINENCE, URGENCY URINARY INCONTINENCE, MIXED INCONTINENCE, AND OVERACTIVE BLADDER

Most therapists treating patients with incontinence are familiar with biofeedback, electrical stimulation, and vaginal cones, which are often used in combination with Kegel exercises. Kegel exercises have provided only limited success. Henalla and colleagues[99] found that 65% to 69% of patients in two hospitals became dry or significantly improved with exercises only. Wall and Davidson[68] stated that exercise programs have a place in the treatment of genuine SUI. Miller and colleagues[69] demonstrated how tightening the pelvic floor muscles before a cough significantly diminished leakage from the bladder. Bø and colleagues[100,101] found that intensive exercises taught by physical therapists over a long period provided better results, which was in agreement with a Danish study by Tilbæks.[102] Meaglia and colleagues[103] stated that motivation, close supervision, and encouragement are important for successful treatment. Holley and colleagues[104] found that a great number of patients stopped exercising because of lack of motivation. Bø and colleagues[105] found that intensive pelvic floor muscle training seen short-term was not maintained 15 years later. Bump and colleagues[66] found that brief verbal instructions in Kegel pelvic floor muscle exercises were not sufficient. Byl and colleagues[106] investigated the effect of repetitive movements (three to 400 trials per day) in skeletal muscle in primates compared with variable repetitive movements and found that the repetitive movements caused interference with motor control. Repetitive movements are also a problem in patients with focal dystonia. Stereotypical and nearly simultaneous movement causes problems in the brain.[107,108] Variable trials preserved motor control. The question must be asked: Is performing Kegel exercises 300 times a day beneficial? The question is appropriate because these exercises train the muscle in isolation and not as part of a functional activity. Do individuals believe that Kegel exercises do not help and therefore discontinue them? Similarly, a therapist would not ask a client to perform isometric exercises of a skeletal muscle 300 times a day and continue 80 times a day for the rest of the client's life once improvement became noticeable. This action does not seem any more appropriate if done with the pelvic floor muscles.

In a 1999 study by Salamey and Nof,[109] approximately 72% of the questioned therapists stated that they felt prepared to instruct patients in pelvic floor (Kegel) exercises. Only 18% of therapists were prepared to discuss UI with their patients, and the majority were not prepared to perform electrical stimulation, biofeedback, or other conservative treatments. For many years Kegel exercises were what the majority of therapists learned in the United States as treatment for incontinence.

Biofeedback and electrical stimulation, as well as vaginal cones, are recognized treatments for SUI. They are used either in combination with exercises or alone.[101,110-112] The effect of electrical stimulation alone on stress and urgency incontinence has been conflicting.[101,113] Bø[113] recommended its use only when a person is not able to contract the pelvic floor muscles and proposed continuing with the exercises when the individual is able to contract the pelvic floor muscles. Another study by Bø and colleagues[101] found pelvic floor exercises to be superior to electrical stimulation, vaginal cones, and no treatment.

The OAB syndrome was first defined by the International Continence Society (ICS) in 2002. Abrams describes this bladder storage problem as a combination of urgency with or without loss of urine, frequency, and nocturia.[114] Its prevalence is high, and it affects men and women. Twenty-four percent of men and 31% of women in a study by Temml and colleagues[115] reported a negative impact of OAB on sexuality. Even though it is common to treat the patients with antagonists of muscarinic acetylcholine receptors, physical therapy is very beneficial, and treatment has to address all three symptoms and include bladder training.

Exercises based on the Klein-Vogelbach and the Tanzberger and Heller concepts, the most common form of exercises for incontinence and pelvic floor dysfunction taught in Germany,[92-98,116-118] have been introduced and taught in a modified version in the United States by Carrière.[119,120]

Evaluation of Male Clients with Incontinence including Treatment Example

Name: **DOB:** *1926, 72 years old*

Tel #

MD: **Therapist:**

Diagnosis: *Status post prostate surgery 10 years ago*

Onset: *1989*

Surgical history: Abdominal surgeries (please circle): hernia, appendix, gallbladder, kidneys, laparoscopy, prostate, hemorrhoids, other? *Hernia, appendix, radical prostatectomy 10 years ago; hip and knee surgery 3 years ago*

Medical history: DM: Y/N heart problems Y/N CA Y/N pulmonary disease Y/N bladder or kidney infections Y/N history of bed-wetting? Y/N other:

Medication: *Detrol for the urgency, Prilosec for heartburn, medication for depression; sleep medication causes urinary accident*

Current symptoms and examination process:

Do you have difficulty urinating because of strictures (scar tissues in urinary tract, enlargement of prostate)? Y/N If yes, does your doctor know? Was any procedure done? *Strictures from the surgery were treated several times*

Do you have (please circle if yes) any leakage; with coughing, sneezing, straining? while running and going up or downstairs? *With straining and lifting the legs* when resting? Are any other activities causing leakage? *No*

Do you have: hesitancy, dribbling, urgencies? do you push or strain? (Please circle if applicable) *urgencies*

Do you have erectile dysfunction? *No*

How often do you have to urinate during the day? *Within normal limits* **night?** *Two times*

Do you have any pain? (If yes, please describe):

Daily fluid intake: (cups, glasses) **How much do you drink?** *6-8 glasses*

Water *at night* coffee tea *herb* soda alcohol *1 martini* citrus other:

Do you urinate: sitting down? *At night* Or standing? (please circle)

Do you use one of the following during the day or night? (Please circle and indicate how many):

Liners: d n **pads:** d n **adult protection:** d n *at night only*

Bowel habits:
Regular: Y/N incontinent of bowel Y/N gas Y/N constipation Y/N Do you use stool softeners? Y/N fiber-rich diet Y/N

History of treatment:

Have you ever been treated for this condition before? Y/N **Did you do Kegel exercises?** *Yes, the exercises did not help.*

Other treatment? Y/N **describe:**

Psychosocial history:

Current/previous employment: does it involve lifting? *Teaching night classes*

Hobbies, sports: *Water aerobics*

EVALUATION PROCESS

What is your treatment goal? *To be able to lift legs and do water aerobics without leaking, not to have to wear "Healthdry" at night.*

Objective: (evaluate posture, ability to do diaphragmatic breathing, pelvic tilt, ability to "feel" the activity of pelvic floor muscles; evaluate muscle tone and strength of the pelvic floor or surrounding muscles when applicable; evaluate scar-tissue when applicable)

Patient with a good posture and good mobility of the pelvis. Because the patient became aware of his pelvic floor during the evaluation, muscle testing of the pelvic floor was deferred. The patient was also a chest-breather and was instructed in diaphragmatic breathing.

Impairment: *poor awareness of the pelvic floor muscles, dyscoordination of diaphragmatic breathing with the pelvic floor while lifting legs, coughing, etc.*

Functional Limitation: *unable to lift legs or do water aerobics without leakage of urine. Leakage at night, urgencies at night*

Assessment: *very motivated client who stated during the evaluation that he now understood the function of the pelvic floor.*

Intervention: *teaching of diaphragmatic breathing and coordination of breathing with the muscles of the entire abdominal compartment.*

Goal: *having to get up at night no more than once. No Healthdry at night; ability to lift legs, do water aerobics without leakage of urine.*

Plan: *teaching correct breathing and functional exercises based on the Tanzberger concept[71] to restore pelvic floor function in 6-8 treatments over 3 months or until patient feels independent with the home exercise program.*

SIGNATURE: ______________________ **Date:** __________

Figure 29-5 ■ Evaluation of male clients with incontinence, including treatment example.

The goal of the exercises is to integrate the function of the entire abdominal compartment as a procedural program.[119] The exercises should teach patients fast and slow muscle fiber training, isometric, concentric and eccentric strengthening exercises, and relaxation of the pelvic floor muscles. Correct use of the pelvic floor muscles also requires restoration of diaphragmatic breathing, as does coordination with all muscles of the abdominal compartment. Hodges[59] and Massery[45,46,58] highlight the importance of integration of posture and breathing and treatment of all muscles of the abdominal compartment in order to restore the health of the pelvic floor. The Swiss ball allows for skill and coordination exercises and provides position to decrease the load of the pelvic floor muscles.

Client Education

A client needs to know where the pelvic floor muscles are, what their function is, and how they work with other systems of the body. The therapist should provide a clear picture of these muscles so that the client can visualize them and understand their function. Educational material and handouts are recommended.

Restoration of Proper Diaphragmatic Breathing

Every breath changes abdominal pressure. Forced exhalation increases the pressure; so do coughing and sneezing. Leaning forward or backward also changes abdominal pressure. Clients should learn to coordinate the contraction of the pelvic floor with changes of pressure. In addition, these activities cannot be done without the cooperation of the abdominal and back muscles. All abdominal muscles are important for posture and breathing.[58,59] Exercises designed to restore pelvic floor function must therefore include coordination of all muscles involved. A great number of individuals with incontinence are chest breathers, possibly because of the poor habit of constantly pulling the stomach in to appear more slender. Restoration of diaphragmatic breathing is therefore the first priority for clients with incontinence.[119,120]

Better breathing patterns may also help provide more oxygen to the pelvic region. Knowing how to control breathing may help a client relax when nervous or anxious (Figure 29-6).

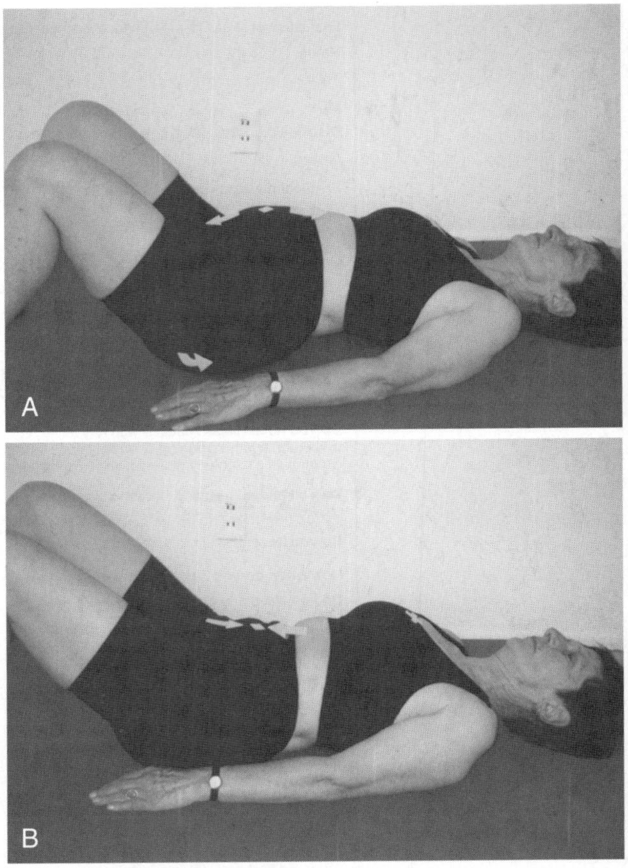

Figure 29-6 ■ Diaphragmatic breathing. **A,** Inhalation; **B,** exhalation.

Sensory Awareness of the Pelvic Floor

The pelvic floor muscles are in the shape of a hammock. Their resting tone is high, and relaxing the pelvic floor is required during urination and defecation as well as during delivery and sexual activity.[67,70] Thus sensory awareness is an important aspect of retraining the pelvic floor muscles. For all individuals, activities such as coughing, sneezing, lifting, and sexual activity require contraction and relaxation of pelvic floor muscles. The ability to relax and contract these muscles is a problem for clients with incontinence. For individuals to regain this control and sensitivity within the pelvic floor, certain treatment protocols must be established.

First, a client can feel landmarks such as the coccyx, the pubic bones, and ischium. Sitting on a firm surface, the client can first contract the gluteal muscles, then relax them, then try to feel the contraction of the anal sphincter and the muscles around the vagina by imagining holding a small object with those muscles without activation of the gluteal muscles. Imagery of voluntary movements of fingers, toes, and tongue has been shown to activate the appropriate sections in the contralateral primary motor cortex.[123] It is therefore probable that imagery of striated pelvic floor muscles would also activate sections in the primary motor cortex assigned to this body part.

In the side-lying position, the client can place a hand over the gluteal muscles while touching the anal sphincter with a fingertip (Figure 29-7). The client can then try to pucker the anal sphincter, similar to puckering the mouth.

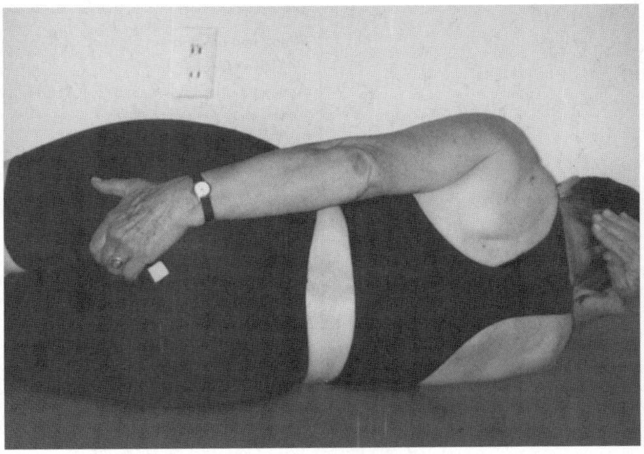

Figure 29-7 ■ Feeling the pelvic floor.

The contraction can be faint but is correct if the gluteal muscles remain relaxed. Tightening of the levator ani can be palpated at the perineum, between anus and vagina, or at the side of the tip of the coccyx. It can also be palpated deep in the groin and often can be distinguished from a contraction of the transverse abdominis. Clients learn that contraction of these muscles must precede any contraction of the surrounding pelvic floor muscles, such as the gluteal, adductor, and abdominal and back muscles. In the same position the client can also feel how a cough moves the pelvic floor muscles in a caudal direction. During proper breathing a gentle, rhythmical downward movement occurs during inhalation (eccentric for the pelvic floor and concentric for the pulmonary diaphragm). The client then tries to tighten the pelvic floor muscles before coughing and feels less caudal movement of the pelvic floor muscles.[119,120] Sensory awareness of relaxation of the pelvic floor muscles may require education, visualization, and tactile feedback. It may be very difficult to learn to relax muscles that have been tight for a long time.

Coordination of Breathing with Pelvic Floor Muscle Activity

The client learns to contract the pelvic floor muscles while exhaling (eccentric activity for the pulmonary diaphragm, concentric activity for the pelvic floor muscles) and relax those muscles while inhaling. This can be done in different positions, such as supine, side lying, on all fours, sitting, or standing. When coughing, sneezing, lifting, and changing positions, such as from supine to side lying, the pelvic floor contraction must precede the activity (Figure 29-8). In contracting the pelvic floor before saying an explosive word such as a forceful "kick," then relaxing the pelvic floor by slowly saying "aaaaand," before tightening once more before saying "kick" again, the sequence of contraction and relaxation is learned.[119,120]

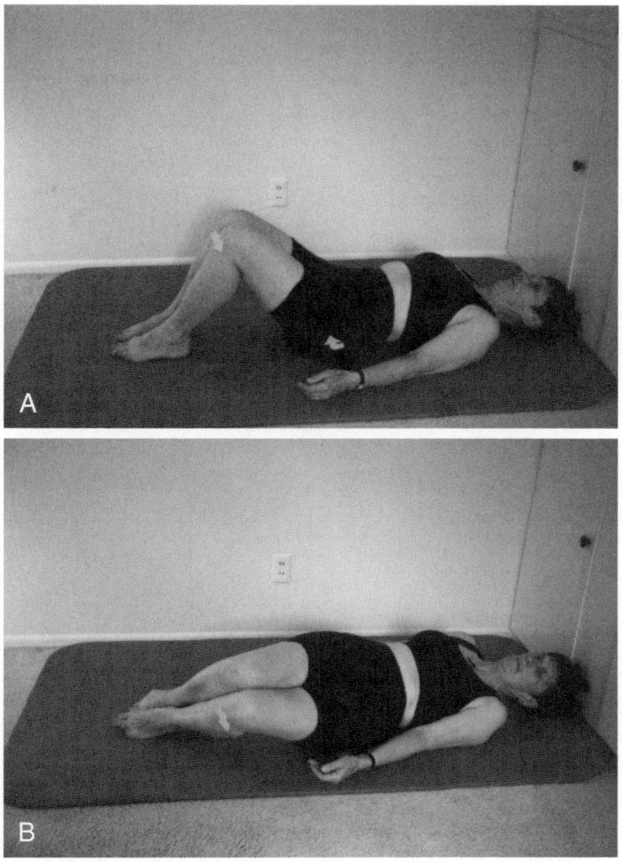

Figure 29-8 ■ Turning from lying on the back **(A)** to turning to the side while tightening the pelvic floor **(B).**

Strengthening Exercises

Strengthening exercises of the pelvic floor muscles must include fast-twitch muscle fiber training with quick fast-twitch muscle contraction, which can be done by bouncing on the ball as demonstrated in Figure 29-9.

Slow-twitch muscle fiber training requires holding the contraction at the end for 5 to 10 seconds. This is demonstrated in Figure 29-10; the client tightens the pelvic floor, gives herself resistance in a diagonal direction, and holds the contraction of the pelvic floor muscles for 5 to 10 seconds. The right ischial tuberosity initiates the movement toward the left knee, which should not move in space, as indicated by the *X.* The chest also is a "fixed" point marked by an *X.* All movement comes from the pelvis.

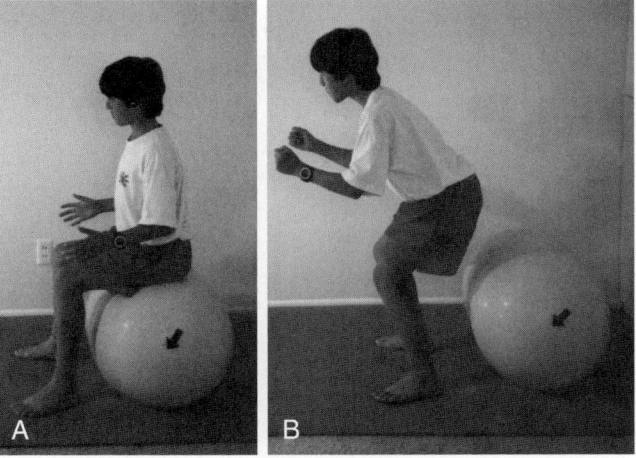

Figure 29-9 ■ **A,** Training fast fibers by bouncing on a double ball. **B,** Tightening the pelvic floor while lifting up.

Because the pelvic floor muscle fibers run in a sagittal and frontal plane as well as in a diagonal direction, movements in different directions should be included to maximize the benefit of strengthening exercises. The Swiss ball allows movement in all directions as a functional activity. When two persons sit back to back on a ball (Figure 29-11), one person can pull the ischium in the direction of the knees, which do not move, while the other person tries to slow down the movement. This requires eccentric activity of the pelvic floor muscles. Isometric muscle activity occurs when both pull at the same time with the same force. In Figure 29-12, two 12-year-old children tighten their pelvic floor muscles during exhalation while pulling the ball with the feet. Many exercises with or without the ball can be adapted with the Heller and Tanzberger concepts.[92,95,97,119,120] Muscle strengthening is not done in isolation but is trained during functional movement activities such as lifting a grocery bag or hitting a tennis ball.

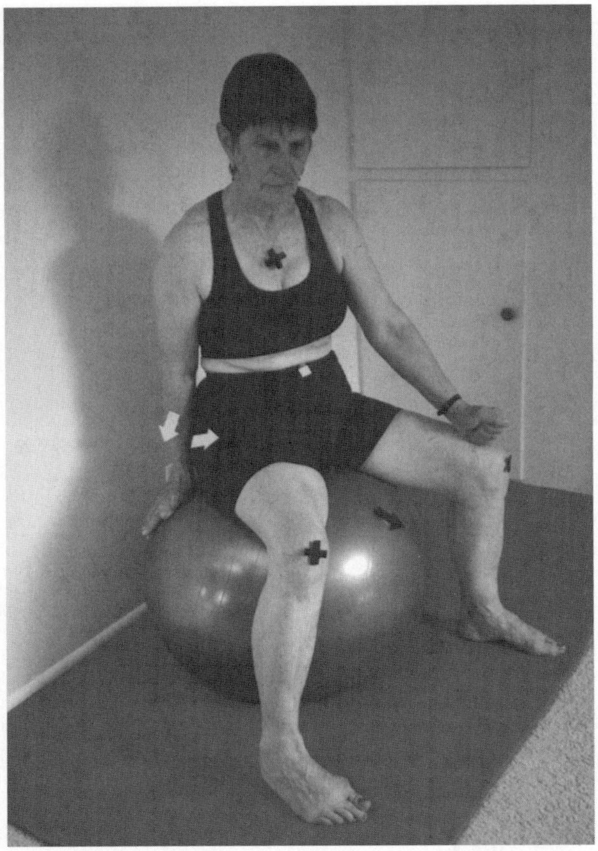

Figure 29-10 ■ Training of the slow muscle fibers by holding the contraction for 5 to 10 seconds at the end of the movement.

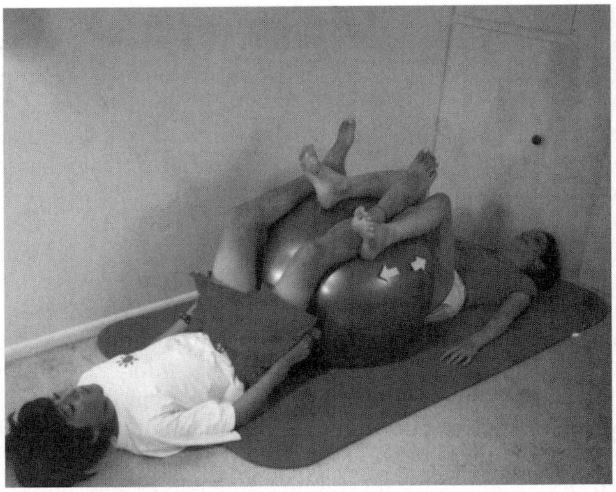

Figure 29-12 ■ Two children work on strengthening the pelvic floor during exhalation.

Teaching relaxation of the pelvic floor muscles is as important as strengthening exercises, especially in all clients with HPFS 60.

Programming of Functional Activities

Pelvic floor muscle activities must be tied to a function, such as getting up from a chair and tightening the pelvic floor muscles during exhalation (Figure 29-13). The exercises must be repeated many times in different combinations until they become automatic. The process of acquiring these skills is part of procedural learning.[7,8,124-128] The client must be empowered to make changes in lifestyle activity and be motivated to achieve the changes. Only then will the client be willing to exercise for months until the

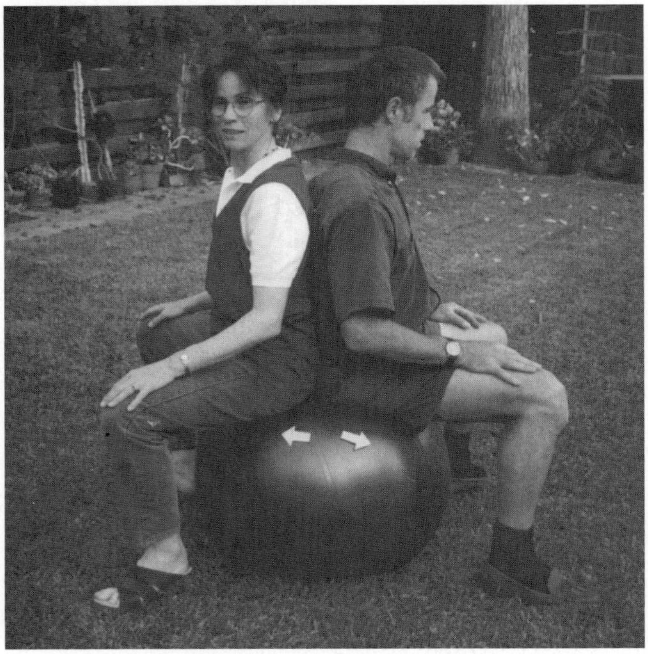

Figure 29-11 ■ Two adults sitting back to back on a ball doing eccentric and concentric pelvic floor contractions.

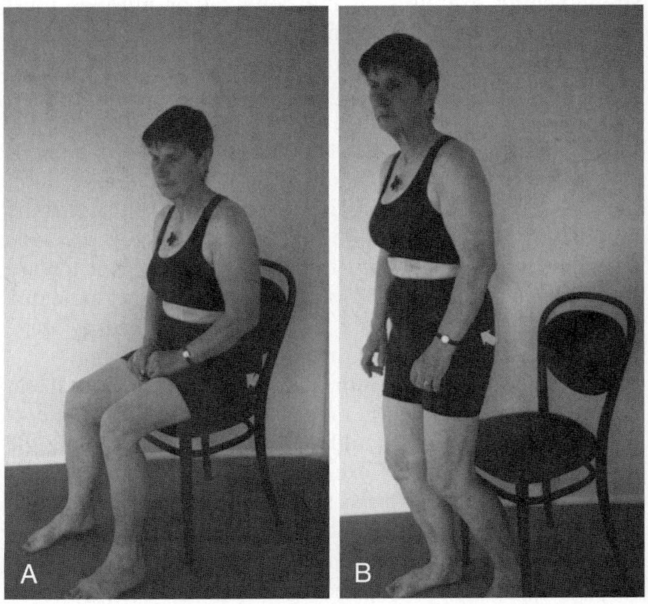

Figure 29-13 ■ **A** and **B,** Sit to stand can be done with integration of pelvic floor activity.

task becomes automatic.[8,9,124-128] To improve motor control of a task, the exercises selected must be meaningful and varied as well as challenging. Mental practice, visualization, part-to-whole task practice, prepractice instructions, appropriate feedback, and guidance are all part of motor learning and are incorporated in the Heller and Tanzberger approaches.[124-128]

Precautions

For clients who do not feel safe on a ball, a double ball, a ball base, or a flat ball that fits onto a chair (Figures 29-14 and 29-15) can be used. All are commercially available. Exercises also can be performed between two chairs or in a corner so that the ball cannot roll away. When learning the exercise, a belt can be used at first to hold onto a client. The ball should not be used if a severe cognitive deficit in the client makes the activity unsafe. Any medical condition that endangers a client on a ball makes these exercises contraindicated and requires a change of exercise and equipment.[119,120,129] Many possibilities for functional exercises exist that are based on motor learning and motor control principles as described by Umphred.[108] The client can walk or perform favorite gym exercises by incorporating pelvic floor strengthening and breathing coordination after learning how to do the exercises correctly. Functional training can also be achieved by incorporating the pelvic floor activity into certain movements that are done every day, such as lifting a child or grocery bag, getting up from a chair or out of a car, or turning in bed.

In addition, therapists must be aware of the involvement of other systems, such as the autonomic system or the limbic system. The patient may be nervous or fearful,

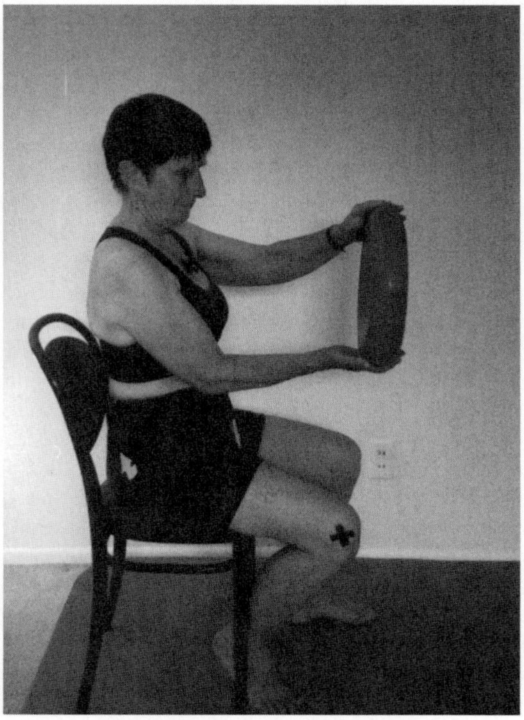

Figure 29-14 ■ Flat ball (sit fit).

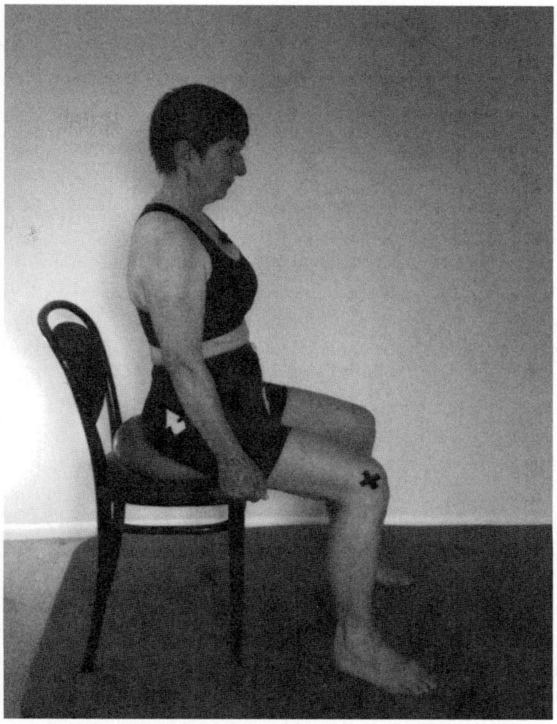

Figure 29-15 ■ Exercise for the pelvic floor; sitting on a flat ball.

depressed, and sleep deprived or may have pain in addition to the incontinence problem.[108,130] Some clients may have been abused, which may be manifested in multisystem involvement.[91] An environment of trust, understanding, and sensitivity toward the client's problems must be created.

Clinical Application of the Heller and Tanzberger Concepts

After a therapist has defined the aspects of pelvic floor dysfunction that require retraining, a specific exercise program can be custom tailored to the patient.

Case Studies

None of the four clients discussed in this chapter underwent biofeedback or electrical stimulation for treatment, and most of the clients had performed Kegel exercises without success. In clients who are unable to learn to feel their pelvic floor muscles, electrical stimulation or biofeedback may be helpful. Functional activities, including proper breathing, should be performed during biofeedback. Isolated contractions of the pelvic floor muscles by using a device without incorporating functional activities does not seem to restore the many different functions of the pelvic floor. Therefore the use of cones without proper pelvic floor muscle training remains questionable. All the clients mentioned in the case studies were extremely motivated, which is not uncommon in patients who have pelvic dysfunctions. They are more than willing to follow their regimen. Problems arise when the client is cognitively impaired or when an illness affects motivation (Case Studies 29-3 and 29-4).

CASE STUDY 29-3 ■ FEMALE CLIENT USING A WHEELCHAIR

A 25-year-old female client who used a wheelchair as a result of myelomeningocele was referred to therapy for upper-extremity strengthening exercises. The diagnosis was left biceps tendonitis, left wrist strain, and lumbar discogenic pain. During treatment the young woman was questioned about her bladder and bowel condition.

The patient had a history of bladder surgery as a child; placement of a suprapubic catheter and bowel reconstruction surgery were done at age 15. She reported that 50% of the time she leaked loose stool and she frequently did not make it to the bathroom in time. She was wearing up to two pads per day.

The client was shown a model of the pelvic floor muscle to illustrate visually how to contract her pelvic floor muscles. Although her sensory awareness of the perineal area appeared to be reduced, she stated that she could feel a faint contraction when trying to pucker the anal sphincter. The client was a chest breather and was instructed in abdominal breathing techniques. She then was instructed to try to coordinate the puckering of her anus with exhalation and work on relaxation of the pelvic floor, especially during defecation. She was told to place a stool in front of the toilet so she could rest her short legs when sitting on the toilet.

The highly motivated client returned 3 weeks later and stated, "I am very happy, I do not leak anymore and did not have to use any pads the last few weeks. I also feel my sphincter muscle now." The client had a total of six treatments. Four treatments were devoted to her arm and trunk problems (which resolved) and the last two treatments to the pelvic problem. Treatment then was discontinued because all goals had been met.

IMPAIRMENT

Impairments included anal incontinence, urgency, weakness of the anal sphincter, decreased sensory awareness of muscle contraction, and breathing dysfunction and discoordination.

Activity

The client needed to carry heavy pads to school; she worried about leaking stool and smelling bad.

Participation

The client felt social embarrassment with fear of leaking stool and smelling bad, and did not want to date. Because she was wheelchair dependent, it was difficult for her to find toilets where she could change her pads.

OUTCOME

The client, who was 25 years old, had never been given pelvic floor muscle training and had no clue that she could contract and strengthen her external sphincter anus. She was delighted to find out that she could exercise her pelvic floor muscles. Her student life became much better when she no longer was required to carry a bag of pads around. She no longer felt socially inept and was looking forward to socializing.

CASE STUDY 29-4 ■ CLIENT WITH VAGINAL PROLAPSE, ANAL SPHINCTER WEAKNESS, AND MIXED INCONTINENCE

A 38-year-old woman was referred to therapy because of anal sphincter weakness and incontinence of flatus for 5 to 6 years. She stated that she also had a prolapse. The client reported having SUI when laughing and running and during sexual intercourse, which affected her self-esteem (as she explained during a later visit). She had urgency, which made her run to the bathroom every hour during the day and get up twice each night. The bladder was painful when full. She also had pain in the lower abdomen. The client had constipation and had to strain during defecation. The surgical history was remarkable for difficult labor and delivery, one with forceps and two others with episiotomies. The patient also had had gallbladder surgery and hysterectomy over 10 years previously. The possibility of surgery for treatment of the prolapse and reconstruction of the vaginal area was discussed with the client and her physician. She had been instructed to perform Kegel exercises but they did not help. The client worked in an electrical assembly plant. The client's goals were to rid herself of the flatus and avoid surgery.

Objectively, she had decreased muscle tonus in the abdominal area and weakness of the abdominal and gluteal muscles. In addition, the client had incoordination between breathing and pelvic floor function. She developed some awareness of the pelvic muscles during the first evaluation. The impairment and the disabilities were considerable and the prognosis more guarded, but the goal was still to achieve anal continence, prevent surgery, and decrease urgency. The client was motivated.

The client was seen in therapy for 15 visits over a 7-month period, at first weekly, then every 2 weeks, and then for periodic reexaminations 3 to 4 weeks apart. Treatment began with teaching diaphragmatic breathing exercises and sensory awareness of the sphincter muscle. The client was able to distinguish between the activities of the anal sphincter and gluteal muscles and was also able to feel a faint contraction in the vaginal area. At first she had difficulty coordinating breathing with contraction and relaxation of the pelvic floor muscles, even when she practiced at home. At the second visit the client received a colon massage and gentle mobilization of the abdominal scars with connective tissue massage.[56,121,122] Home exercises for breathing and pelvic floor contraction and relaxation were reviewed with the client. At the third visit, the client reported that the flatus problem had improved and that the abdominal treatment lessened the constipation. New exercises were taught with the Swiss ball in supine and sitting positions. At the fourth visit, the client said, "I have less flatus, and I am able to control the sphincter. The pelvic floor is still a problem because of the prolapse; I have no more back pain after the visceral treatments." The client was also instructed regarding how to perform exercises with decreased load on the pelvic floor (supine, supine with the feet on the ball, side-lying, on all fours, and so on). The client was also instructed in how to self-massage the abdomen. At the fifth visit, the client said, "I am now taking medicine to help control the urgency and can hold urine for

CASE STUDY 29-4 ■ CLIENT WITH VAGINAL PROLAPSE, ANAL SPHINCTER WEAKNESS, AND MIXED INCONTINENCE—cont'd

3 hours. My husband massages my abdomen, which decreases the constipation. The bowel movements are now every 1 to 2 days instead of once a week."

The client reported only occasional pain with a full bladder, a reduction in the number of times she had to get up at night, and her ability to hold urine for 3 hours without pressure from the prolapse. The grateful client stated that her self-image had improved because she was no longer leaking urine during intercourse. According to the client's wishes, surgery was deferred. As the strength of the pelvic floor improved, the client stopped taking medication for the urgency and was still able to hold urine for 3 hours and sleep through the night. The client continued occasional follow-up sessions to monitor her progress and provide her with more challenging exercises.

IMPAIRMENT

Impairments included prolapse secondary to weakness of the pelvic floor muscles and difficult labor and delivery; urgency, nocturia and EAS weakness; constipation; and breathing dysfunction.

Activity

The patient had to go to the bathroom every hour. She could not laugh, cough, or run without leaking urine; she leaked urine during sexual intercourse, which caused embarrassment.

Participation

She avoided going out with friends, participating in sports, and having sexual intercourse.

OUTCOME

After treatment as described, the client could hold urine for 3 hours instead of 1 hour and could sleep through the night. Her bowel movements improved to one to two per day instead of one per week. The client could control flatus and was enjoying intimacy and sexual intercourse without fear of leakage of urine. Her self-esteem was restored, and at the time of discharge she no longer considered surgery. The client resumed her social activities.

TREATMENT OPTIONS FOR PELVIC FLOOR DYSFUNCTION

Cognitively Impaired Clients

Adjustments must be made and functional barriers decreased to help cognitively impaired clients maintain or achieve continence (Table 29-1). Prompted voiding, timed voiding,[16,131-133] and medicine can be used when a client has cognitive problems and cannot go to the bathroom independently. In prompted voiding, clients (e.g., with Alzheimer disease) are asked at regular intervals whether they have to go to the bathroom. In timed voiding, a client is placed on a commode or toilet at regular intervals. Many clients who are cognitively impaired probably would not be incontinent if they could reach a bathroom and if help were available to unbutton or unzip clothes, open a door, or assist in other aspects of toileting. Timely assistance could prevent falls (and therefore fractures) and incontinence episodes.[134]

Clients with a Cerebrovascular Accident, Multiple Sclerosis, or Parkinson Disease

Clients who have neurological deficits are usually not asked whether they have a urinary dysfunction. Not all clients with such diseases are incontinent; some had incontinence before the onset of the neurological disease. OAB syndrome and UUI are common in CVA,[35] MS, and other neurological diseases, whereas detrusor-sphincter dyssynergy is common in MS and SCI.[30,33] Patients with Parkinson disease can also have nocturia and retention. No matter what the cause, improvement can often be achieved by identifying the dysfunction, explaining the anatomy and physiology to the client, and then offering treatment options. Coordination of diaphragmatic breathing with pelvic floor muscle activity can improve self-control to relax the pelvic floor and improve oxygen supply to the pelvic region. Improving the posture and sensory awareness training can also be integrated to varying degrees. The therapist can help the client improve afferent sensory input and use visualization to learn to contract and relax the muscles properly. A client with retention can learn to emphasize relaxation of the pelvic floor muscles during urination through breathing, proper seating on the toilet, and self-relaxation. Double voiding technique encourages the patient with an overextended bladder to time voiding to every 2 to 4 hours during the day. The patient then attempts to empty the bladder by staying on the toilet longer and trying to void more than once with each trip to the toilet, with supportive cues and timed voiding when the patient has cognitive impairment.[34,131,133] Often, functional barriers can be eliminated or help can be provided. With clients who also need strengthening exercises for the pelvic floor and have difficulty sitting on a ball, a flat ball can be used in a chair, or exercises can be adapted to the client's ability without any devices.

Overdistended Bladder

Whether or not the overdistended bladder is neurogenic, the client must learn to time herself or himself to void at regular intervals. In other cases the client may learn to do clean intermittent catheterization and carefully monitor the output of urine. The residual urine in the bladder should be low, approximately 50 mL; measurements consistently higher require further evaluation by a urologist.[47] Proper relaxation of the pelvic floor is important; men often can relax the pelvic floor better when urinating in a seated position. Abdominal breathing and coordination with pelvic floor muscle activity are important for these clients and should be restored if a problem is present.

Areflexia

Education is always the most important part of intervention and is done at the beginning. Many clients may need to learn clean intermittent catheterization and timed intervals. In

TABLE 29-1 ■ POSSIBLE COMBINATIONS OF TREATMENT OPTIONS FOR BLADDER AND ANAL DYSFUNCTIONS

	FUNCTIONAL EXERCISES AND BREATHING	BIOFEEDBACK	ELECTRICAL STIMULATION	CONES	PROMPTED VOIDING	TIMED VOIDING	ABDOMINAL TREATMENT, SCAR TREATMENT	SELF-CATHETERIZATION	RELAXATION OF PELVIC FLOOR MUSCLES
Stress urinary incontinence	X	(x)	(x)	(x)			(x)		X
Urgency incontinence	X	(x)					(x)		X
Mixed urinary incontinence	X	(x)	(x)				(x)		X
Overactive bladder	X	X	(x)						X
Anal incontinence	X	(x)	(x)				(x)		
Constipation	X	(x)	(x)				X		X
Retention of urine	X					X	(x)	(x)	XX
Overdistention of bladder	X	(x)			(x)	X	(x)	X	XX
Areflexia of bladder, anus	(x)	(x)	X		(x)	X	(x)	X	(x)

X means recommended therapeutic intervention; (x) means additional treatment option. These options may be beneficial interventions, but evidence is mixed and outcomes may be patient specific.

some clients electrical stimulation or biofeedback may help restore some function of the pelvic floor activity; exercise may improve the strength of the pelvic floor muscles once some function returns. Obviously, all therapeutic interventions depend on the extent of the lesion, but as described in Case Study 29-3, discussion with the client regarding the exploration of treatment options is important. This client probably could have been spared wearing diapers for the previous 10 years. She also could have been condemned to wearing diapers for the rest of her life without intervention. All that was needed in her case was to ask about the problem and instruct her in achieving continence.

Anal Incontinence

The inability to hold gas or leaking stool can occur in neurogenic and nonneurogenic disorders. Clients who have had resections of the colon may have anal urgency incontinence. They must learn to evaluate what they ate, when the urgency is appropriate, and when a signal is false. They often cannot distinguish gas, liquid stool, and solid stool. A client, after instruction and explanation of the defecation process, stated, "I got it; it is mind over matter." He was also instructed to use deep abdominal breathing and quick flicks (activation of the fast fibers) and distraction to control the urgency. This helped him to stop and to control the need or motor program that could be identified as running to the bathroom every 30 minutes. He was asked to throw that program out consciously and replace it with breathing and reevaluation of each urgency, which enabled him in a short time to regain control, sleep through the night, and increase the intervals during the day. As with all clients with pelvic floor dysfunction, careful evaluation and education must be completed before beginning the treatment. In the presence of constipation, a careful abdominal evaluation and possible treatment of the viscera,[135] such as with colon massage,[121] may be indicated because constipation can also be present in clients who leak stool. The client needs to be educated about eating properly. Individuals who eat too much fiber need to drink large volumes of fluid to keep the stool soft. A client with a brain stem injury, for example, had bowel movements only every 5 days. When the family changed the breakfast to fruit and only minimal fiber, the client had daily regular bowel movements.

Electrical stimulation or biofeedback can in some cases be an adjunct or precede treatment of functional exercises of the abdominal compartment. It can be used to retrain when to contract the pelvic floor muscles and also to improve sensory awareness.

SUMMARY

Every client with UI, whether male or female, requires a thorough examination. To give the best possible chance for recovery, exercises must be custom tailored and modalities used with discretion. Electrical stimulation and biofeedback cannot replace functional exercises. Modalities may be helpful at the beginning of the treatment if the client has no sensory awareness of the pelvic floor but should be used in combination with exercises. Treatment of the viscera by a knowledgeable therapist should be considered in some clients to achieve full rehabilitation of the pelvic floor dysfunction.[135]

References

To enhance this text and add value for the reader, all references are included on the companion Evolve site that accompanies this textbook. This online service will, when available, provide a link for the reader to a Medline abstract for the article cited. There are 135 cited references and other general references for this chapter, with the majority of those articles being evidence-based citations.

CHAPTER 30 Cardiovascular and Pulmonary System Health in Populations with Neurological Disorders

MARILYN MACKAY-LYONS, PT, PhD

KEY TERMS

aerobic training
cardiovascular fitness
deconditioning
exercise tolerance
rating of perceived exertion

OBJECTIVES

After reading this chapter, the student or therapist will be able to:

1. Explain the physiological principles related to cardiovascular responses to exercise testing.
2. Discuss the evidence behind cardiovascular fitness and describe the factors that contribute to the deconditioned state in adults with neurological disorders.
3. Explain the adaptive responses to aerobic training in populations with neurological disorders and the factors underlying these responses.
4. Discuss general guidelines for designing exercise programs to improve cardiovascular health and fitness.

The cardiopulmonary health of individuals with residual movement dysfunction after a neurological insult is now regarded as a topic of interest in neurorehabilitation. In traditional practice, the state of the neuromuscular system preoccupied the attention of clinicians in the quest to optimize neurological recovery. Most interventions were based on strategies to improve the capacity of that system—an approach that has met with limited success in terms of restoring functional independence. It is now clear that recovery cannot be explained solely on the basis of improved neuromuscular function. For example, Roth and colleagues[1] determined that less than one third of the variance in functional limitations after a stroke can be explained by the extent of neurological impairment. Nevertheless, the current approach to neurorehabilitation is somewhat puzzling. Evidence has accumulated indicating that many people with neurological disabilities are woefully deconditioned. There has been widespread acknowledgement of the central role that aerobic exercise plays in improving cardiopulmonary health and fitness. Furthermore, application of the principles of exercise physiology in cardiac rehabilitation has been widely endorsed. Yet neurorehabilitation clinicians have been observed to practice without full knowledge of their patients' cardiac status or without monitoring heart rate (HR) and blood pressure (BP).[2] Moreover, there is evidence to suggest that patients with neurological insults have not been challenged enough in therapy to induce the metabolic stress needed to enhance their cardiopulmonary fitness.[3,4] A troubling explanation offered for these observations is that clinicians lack either an understanding or an appreciation of the basic physiological principles of exercise.[5,6]

Fortunately, attention has turned to the introduction of interventions that encompass the neuromuscular, cardiovascular, and pulmonary systems and promote a more holistic approach to neurorehabilitation. The challenge of improving cardiopulmonary health and fitness in these populations is not trivial. For individuals with chronic conditions, fitness is affected by a host of interacting influences such as the location and extent of the lesion, the presence of comorbidities (particularly cardiovascular disease), and the premorbid activity level. To complicate matters further, testing and training protocols for individuals with compromised motor and postural control need to be tailored to ensure safety and effectiveness.

This chapter begins with an overview of physiological principles related to cardiovascular responses to exercise testing. A summary of the evidence of cardiopulmonary fitness levels in adults and children with neurological disabilities is followed by a description of factors that contribute to the deconditioned state. Possible mechanisms responsible for reduced exercise capacity are then reviewed. Adaptive responses to aerobic training in patients with neurological conditions are examined, as are factors underlying these responses. The chapter closes with a summary of guidelines for the design of exercise programs that can be used to improve cardiopulmonary health and fitness. Appendix 30-A at the end of this chapter clearly identifies the meanings of the abbreviations used throughout the chapter.

PHYSIOLOGICAL RESPONSES TO EXERCISE

At rest the human body consumes roughly 3.5 mL of oxygen (O_2) per kilogram per minute, or 1 metabolic equivalent (MET).[7] In the resting state, skeletal muscle activity accounts for less than 20% of the body's total energy expenditure; the brain, making up only 2% of body weight, also consumes 20% of the available O_2.[8] Activities at rest such as breathing and contracting of the heart can be sustained indefinitely because the power demands of these activities are met by the rate of energy turnover. In other words, these activities occur well below the *critical power* of the muscles, defined as the maximal rate of work that can be endured indefinitely.[9] Any physical activity beyond the resting state requires more O_2; the increase is dependent on the intensity of the effort involved. The rise in metabolism relies on O_2 transport by the pulmonary and circulatory systems and O_2 usage by the active skeletal, cardiac, and respiratory muscles to convert chemical potential energy to mechanical energy.[10] The components of the O_2 transport system are outlined in Figure 30-1.

Selective distribution of the increased blood flow to regions with heightened metabolic demands—the working muscles—is largely a result of local vasodilation mediated mainly by metabolites acting on the vascular smooth muscle (e.g., carbon dioxide [CO_2], hydrogen ions [H^+], nitric oxide, potassium ions, adenosine) and vasoconstriction in tissues with low metabolic demands.[11] Blood flow to other vascular beds (e.g., renal and splanchnic bed) either is unchanged or decreases through active vasoconstriction resulting primarily from increased sympathetic discharge. Cerebral autoregulation maintains regional and total cerebral blood flow and normal tissue oxygenation over a wide range of BPs[12]; thus, cerebral blood flow and O_2 delivery during exercise either remain stable[13,14] or increase slightly.[15,16] As exercise intensity increases, systolic BP (SBP) increases markedly, whereas diastolic BP (DBP) either remains unchanged or lowers slightly, resulting in a moderate increase in mean arterial pressure.[17]

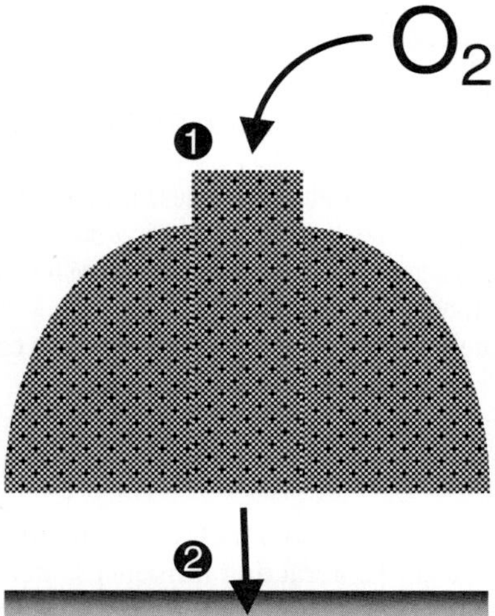

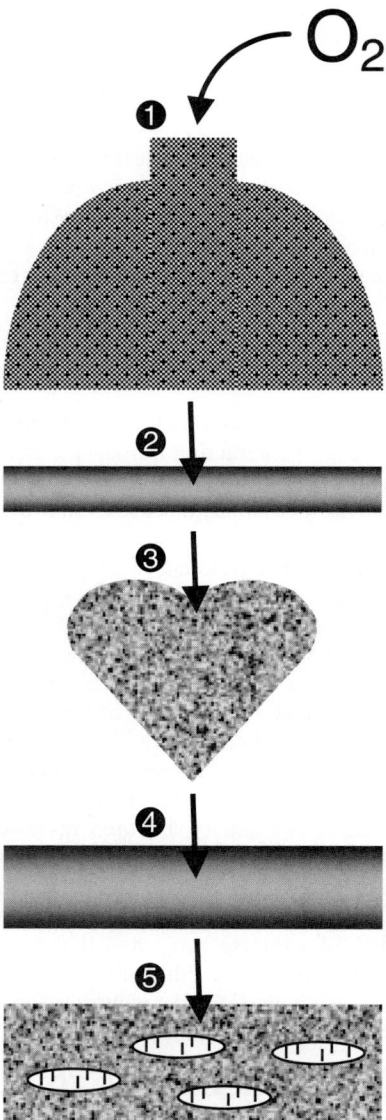

Figure 30-1 ■ Diagrammatic representations of the components of the O_2 transport system. *(1)* ⊇ During inspiration O_2 from the air is delivered to the alveolar gas space by the process of respiration. *(2)* ⊄ O_2 diffuses across the blood-gas barrier into the pulmonary capillary blood, where almost all of the O_2 is bound to hemoglobin. *(3)* ⊂ The heart acts as a pump and *(4)* ⊆ the vascular system acts as the plumbing to transport O_2 to the various tissues, including the exercising muscle *(5)* ∈ where it diffuses from the red blood cells into the mitochondria within the myocytes. Reduced conductance of any component impairs O_2 transport, whereas improved conductance of any component augments O_2 transport.

Extraction of O_2 from the muscle capillary blood to mitochondria is dependent on an adequate O_2 diffusion gradient. During a progressive increase in workload, the arterial hemoglobin saturation and arterial O_2 content remain relatively constant, whereas the venous O_2 content decreases substantially as a result of increased O_2 extraction in the active muscles.[18] As the metabolic rate rises, the minute ventilation (i.e., respiratory rate multiplied by the tidal volume) increases to remove CO_2 and to regulate pH balance of the active muscles. At low-intensity exercise, ventilation (mainly tidal volume) increases in a linear manner relative to the volume of O_2 use (Vo_2) and CO_2 production (Vco_2). Above the critical power, the energy demand of the muscle exceeds the capacity of the aerobic process to supply energy for muscle contraction; the additional energy is supplied by the anaerobic glycolytic system.

During more intense exercise, ventilation is extremely variable among individuals; the respiratory rate usually increases without a substantial change in tidal volume.[17] The point at which the rate of glycolysis exceeds that of oxidative phosphorylation is called the *anaerobic threshold* (which approximates the ventilatory threshold or lactate threshold).[17] Pyruvic acid is converted to lactic acid, which completely dissociates to lactate and H^+, resulting in a rise in blood lactate levels and a fall in intramuscular pH. Exercise-induced muscular fatigue is caused by the exponential accumulation of lactate and a drop in intramuscular pH, with negative effects on the actin-myosin turnover rate, enzyme activities, and excitation-contraction coupling.

Maximal oxygen consumption (Vo_2max) is defined as the highest O_2 intake an individual can attain during physical work.[17] The Fick equation describes the relationship between cardiovascular function and Vo_2max:

$$Vo_2max = Qmax \times a\text{-}vO_2diffmax$$

where Qmax is the maximal cardiac output and $a\text{-}vO_2diffmax$ is the maximal arteriovenous O_2 difference. Given that Qmax equals the product of maximal heart rate (HRmax) and maximal stroke volume, (SVmax),

$$Vo_2max = HRmax \times SVmax \times a\text{-}vO_2diffmax$$

Thus Vo_2max reflects both O_2 transport to the tissues and O_2 usage by the tissues. Increases in Vo_2 during exercise are caused by increases in both cardiac output and $a\text{-}vO_2diff$, with HR and stroke volume (SV) increasing progressively over the lower third of the workload range. Thereafter, HR continues to increase while SV remains essentially constant,[19,20] resulting, at maximal effort, in a cardiac output three to six times greater than baseline levels. An increase in SV (50% over resting volume) is caused by enhanced myocardial contractility and increased venous return resulting from compression of the veins by contracting muscles and reduced intrathoracic pressure.[21] At low-intensity exercise the increase in HR is mainly a result of decreased vagal tone, but as exercise intensifies, sympathetic stimulation and circulating catecholamines play a greater role, yielding, at maximal workloads, a rise in HR 200% to 300% above the resting level.[22]

MEASUREMENT OF CARDIOPULMONARY FITNESS

Exercise (aerobic) capacity is the principal determinant of the ability to sustain the power requirements of repetitive physical activity. Vo_2max is generally accepted as the definitive index of exercise capacity and cardiopulmonary fitness.[23] Vo_2max is a relatively stable measurement; variability of repeated measures of Vo_2max has been reported to be 2% to 4%[24] or 0.2 L/min.[25] Accurate determination of Vo_2max requires (1) adequate duration and work intensity by at least 50% of total muscle mass, (2) independence from motivation or skill of the subject, and (3) controlled environmental conditions.[26] Also, because test performance is sensitive to time of day, the time of repeat testing should be consistent.

Before any fitness test, a 3- to 5-minute warmup of slow treadmill walking on a level grade or unloaded pedaling that raises the metabolic rate twofold above resting should be performed.[27] A proper warmup prevents excessive local muscle fatigue from occurring before Vo_2max has been attained.[28] Furthermore, a 3- to 5-minute cool-down should follow test completion to aid in venous return to prevent blood pooling in the peripheral vasculature and a subsequent drop in DBP. The intensity of exercise can be increased in a continuous progressive manner (i.e., step or ramp protocol) or, less commonly, in a discontinuous progressive manner (i.e., subject rests between stages). Throughout testing, continuous monitoring of the electrocardiogram and periodic monitoring of BP are essential. The optimal duration of a graded exercise test is 8 to 12 minutes, with testing terminated when the subject can no longer generate the required power, is limited by symptoms, or is unable to continue safely.[29] Variables of interest during exercise testing include Vo_2max expressed in absolute terms (liters of O_2 per minute) or relative to body mass (milliliters of O_2 per kilogram of body weight per minute), MET level, percent of predicted HRmax, respiratory exchange ratio (RER; ratio of Vo_2 to CO_2), peak power, minute ventilation, tidal volume, respiratory rate, and rating of perceived exertion (RPE) according to the Borg scale.[30] Because there is considerable variability in HRmax among healthy individuals, the percent of predicted HRmax attained is not a robust indicator of exercise capacity.[31] Similarly, because both total exercise time and peak exercise intensity (or power attained, i.e., peak treadmill speed and grade or peak power on bike) are dependent on the test protocol, neither is a reliable measure of exercise capacity.[32,33] In addition, noninvasive estimation of the anaerobic threshold by identifying the point of nonlinear increases in minute ventilation and Vco_2 can be highly subjective and thus unreliable.[34]

The principal marker of exercise capacity is attainment of a plateau in Vo_2 beyond which there is a change of less than 100 mL/min, with further increases in workload dependent solely on anaerobic metabolism.[29] In cases in which a Vo_2 plateau is not observed (typically in deconditioned or elderly individuals or in patients with heart disease), the preferred term for the value obtained is *peak Vo_2* (Vo_2peak).[35] Criteria for attainment of Vo_2peak include achieving the age-predicted HRmax, RER in excess of 1.15, minute ventilation greater than the predicted maximal voluntary ventilation, tidal volume greater than 90% of the inspiratory capacity, and obvious patient exhaustion.[28]

Testing Modality

The modality of testing (e.g., treadmill walking, cycling, stepping, arm cranking) can affect Vo_2max values. The treadmill has the greatest potential to recruit sufficient muscle mass to elicit a maximal metabolic response, particularly in deconditioned individuals.[26] Bike ergometry yields 85% to 90%, and arm ergometry 70%, of the Vo_2max achieved with a treadmill.[26] Ideally the mode of exercise should be consistent with the patient's typical activity. Thus the treadmill is often preferred because the pattern of muscle activation during treadmill walking is similar to that for most mobility tasks. In patients with neuromuscular conditions, however, impaired balance and motor control often preclude the use of standard treadmill testing protocols. To resolve this limitation, we devised and validated an exercise protocol using a body-weight support system to permit safe and valid testing of Vo_2max early after stroke.[36] For subjects with paraplegia, tests with wheelchair treadmills are more functionally relevant than those using arm ergometry.

PREDICTING MAXIMAL OXYGEN CONSUMPTION WITH USE OF SUBMAXIMAL EXERCISE TESTS

Although submaximal tests do not measure the systemic response, they are inexpensive to administer and have a low risk of adverse events. The essentially linear relationship between Vo_2 and HR permits the estimation of Vo_2max from HR measurements taken during submaximal exercise. For example, for healthy people the HR increases approximately 50 beats per uptake of 1 L of O_2, independent of sex and body size.[37] For unfit individuals and patients with cardiac impairment, the increases in HR are greater per liter, except for patients taking β-blockers, who demonstrate blunting of the HR response throughout exercise. The Åstrand-Ryhming nomogram is often used to predict Vo_2max from submaximal HR.[38] The HR-Vo_2 relationship is independent of the exercise protocol. However, HR, unlike Vo_2max, is markedly affected by many stresses (e.g., dehydration, changes in body temperature, acute starvation), resulting in substantial error and inaccurate Vo_2max estimations.[26] In fact, discrepancies between estimated and measured Vo_2max in individuals with low exercise capacity can be as high as 25%.[39]

FITNESS LEVELS IN POPULATIONS WITH NEUROLOGICAL DISORDERS

Documentation of exercise capacity in populations with neurological disorders has been hindered by the lack of testing protocols that can safely and effectively accommodate the motor and balance disturbances common to these populations. Not surprisingly, the limited evidence to date suggests that most individuals with neurological disabilities are significantly deconditioned. A summary of Vo_2peak data from studies of common neurological conditions is presented in Table 30-1. Variability in the results from a multitude of factors, including differences in testing protocols, as discussed in the previous section, and differences in subject characteristics; these points are discussed in the following section.

Impact of Low Fitness Levels on Health of People with Neurological Disorders

People with high fitness levels use only a small fraction of the *physiological fitness reserve*[40] of the cardiovascular, respiratory, and neuromuscular systems to respond to the

TABLE 30-1 ■ EXERCISE CAPACITY IN COMMON NEUROLOGICAL CONDITIONS

DIAGNOSIS	TIME SINCE DIAGNOSIS	NO.	SEX (% MEN)	AGE (YR)	TEST MODALITY	VO_2PEAK (ML/KG/MIN)	VO_2PEAK % NORMAL
Cerebral palsy	N/A[296]	7	29	16 ± 1	Arm ergometer	18 ± 4	NR
	N/A[297]	11	64	10-16	Treadmill	34 ± 9	NR
	N/A[298]	12	100	21+	Arm ergometer	25.6 ± 3	87
Down syndrome	N/A[299]	16	100	21 ± 3	Treadmill	32 ± 5	NR
	N/A[300]	14	79	18 ± 3	Treadmill	27 ± 7	NR
Guillain-Barré syndrome	3 years[301]	1	100	57	Leg-arm ergometer	27	NR
	NR[221]	20	30	49	Cycle training	26 ± 8	NR
Multiple sclerosis	NR[229]	28	32	39 ± 10	Cycle ergometer	31.0 ± 7	NR
	12 ± 8 years[286]	26	81	45 ± 8	Cycle ergometer	22.5	70
	3 ± 5 years[302]	10	40	39 ± 6	Arm-leg ergometer	39.0 ± 8	87
	7 ± 1 years[199]	46	33	40 ± 2	Arm-leg ergometer	25.2 ± 1	79
	8 ± 5 years[303]	19	26	41 ± 8	Arm-leg ergometer	17.0 ± 7	58
Parkinson disease	6 ± 3 years[137]	16	81	54 ± 5	Cycle ergometer	28 ± 5	93
	8 years[304]	8	NR	60 ± 8	Cycle ergometer	17.7	NR
	9 ± 4 years[138]	20	65	64 ± 7	Cycle ergometer	22 ± 7	100
Postpoliomyelitis syndrome	11 ± 8 years[305]	68	34	53 ± 11	Cycle ergometer (n = 37) Arm ergometer (n = 31)	23 ± 5 15 ± 5	63 65
	11-45 years[306]	20	50	43 ± 6	Cycle ergometer	18 ± 6	73
	46 ± 3 years[307]	32	50	50 ± 10	Cycle ergometer	21 ± 7	74
Spina bifida	N/A[83]	37	51	16 ± 2	Arm ergometer	17 ± 6	64
	N/A[308]	23	54	10 ± 3	Treadmill	33 ± 2	NR
Spinal cord injury paraplegia	102 ± 62 days[180]	80	75	41 ± 15	Wheelchair ergometer	14.7 ± 5	NR
	6 months[309]	39	100	30 ± 1	Arm ergometer	1 ± 1	69
	>3 years[310]	46	100	33 ± 9	Wheelchair ergometer	24 ± 5	NR
	5 ± 4 years[83]	19		16 ± 3	Arm ergometer	17 ± 6	NR
	>0.5 year[311]	13	NR	29 ± 4	Arm ergometer	29 ± 10	NR
	21 ± 8 years[251]	9	100	30 ± 7	Arm ergometer	30.5 ± 8	71
	N/A[83]	19	53	16 ± 3	Arm ergometer	17 ± 6	64
Spinal cord injury tetraplegia	108 ± 67 days[180]	22	74	39 ± 13	Wheelchair ergometer	12 ± 4	NR
	7 ± 6 years[255]	8	100	24 ± 4	Arm ergometer	12 ± 1	NR
Stroke, subacute	15 ± 17 days[312]	36	61	65 ± 3	Semirecumbent ergometer	11.4 ± 1	NR
	15 ± 7 days[50]	12	100	59 ± 10	Cycle ergometer	8.3 ± 2	NR
	18 ± 2 days[313]	35	46	66 ± 3	Semirecumbent ergometer	11 ± 2	NR
	26 ± 9 days[314]	29	76	65 ± 14	Treadmill	14.4 ± 5	61
	29 ± 10 days[315]	17	76	61 ± 16	Semirecumbent ergometer	14.7 ± 4	51
	76 ± 3 days[204]	100	56	70 ± 10	Cycle ergometer	11.4 ± 3	NR
	120 ± 90 days[316]	8	100	52 ± 10	Cycle ergometer	16.1 ± 4	NR

TABLE 30-1 ■ EXERCISE CAPACITY IN COMMON NEUROLOGICAL CONDITIONS—cont'd

DIAGNOSIS	TIME SINCE DIAGNOSIS	NO.	SEX (% MEN)	AGE (YR)	TEST MODALITY	VO_2PEAK (ML/KG/MIN)	VO_2PEAK % NORMAL
Stroke, chronic (>6 months)	>6 months[185]	42	55	56 ± 12	Cycle ergometer	15.8 ± 5	NR
	>6 months[102]	26	85	66 ± 9	Treadmill	15.6 ± 4	NR
	3.0 years[317]	53	83	64 ± 8	Treadmill	14.7 ± 4	NR
	5 ± 5 years[318]	48	58	63 ± 9	Cycle ergometer	14.4 ± 3	NR
	10 months[319]	30	100	54	Cycle ergometer	17.7 ± 4	NR
	>12 months[320]	63	59	6 ± 9	Cycle ergometer	22.0 ± 5	NR
	13 ± 8 months[321]	20	70	50 ± 15	Treadmill (with harness)	16 ± 4.5	NR
Traumatic brain injury	17 ± 17 months[322]	36	78	32 ± 10	Cycle ergometer	22 ± 9	65
	2 ± 4 years[323]	13	NR	32 ± 8	Treadmill	27 ± 5	76
	2 ± 4 years[324]	40	73	33 ± 11	Treadmill	24 ± 7	NR
	NR[206]	14	93	29 ± 2	Treadmill	31.3 ± 2	67
	Pt. 1: 3 months[325] Pt. 2: 1 year	2	50	Pt. 1: 25 Pt. 2: 18	Treadmill (BWSTT)	Pt. 1: 17.1 Pt. 2: 14.6	NR NR

BWSTT, Body-weight–supported treadmill training; *NR,* not reported; *Vo_2peak % normal,* peak oxygen consumption expressed as a percentage of normative values.

metabolic challenge of activities of daily living (ADLs).[41,42] Thus, small declines in exercise capacity may not be noticeable in carrying out daily activities. In contrast, relatively minor reductions in capacity can substantially influence performance of ADLs by deconditioned individuals. Light instrumental ADLs require approximately 10.5 mL of oxygen per kilogram per minute (3 METs), whereas more strenuous activities have metabolic costs of about 17.5 mL/kg/min (5 METs).[43] Cress and Meyer[44] reported that the Vo_2peak of 20 mL/kg/min is needed for older adults to meet the physiological demands of independent living. From the data presented in Table 30-1, it is evident that many people living with neurological disabilities (particularly stroke, tetraplegia, and postpoliomyelitis syndrome) do not have the level of fitness required for the more strenuous ADLs and independent living. Moreover, relative exercise capacities (expressed as a percentage of normative values) associated with the disabilities in Table 30-1, with the exception of Parkinson disease, are of concern, given that Vo_2peak values less than 84% of normal are considered pathological.[45]

For individuals with neurological disabilities, the minimum Vo_2 requirements for ADLs are actually greater than the previously mentioned levels because of the increased energy requirements resulting from gross motor inefficiencies and other related factors.[46-48] In other words, the percentage of Vo_2peak required for activity at a fixed submaximal workload (termed *fractional utilization*) is increased. When the anaerobic threshold is exceeded prematurely and lactate accumulation is accelerated, accomplishment of low-intensity ADLs is unsustainable for extended periods and achievement of mid- to upper-intensity ADLs is virtually impossible. Moreover, the combination of poor exercise capacity and elevated energy demands results in diminished reserves to support other activities. For example, in the case of people with postpoliomyelitis syndrome, the energy costs of walking are about 40% higher than for healthy peers and are highly correlated with lower-extremity muscle strength.[49] Thus in the calculation of fractional utilization for walking, the numerator (Vo_2 during walking) is increased and the denominator (Vo_2peak) is decreased; hence, fractional utilization is substantially increased.

Of the neurological populations, people poststroke are the largest consumer group in need of rehabilitation services. This group also has received the most attention in the literature with regard to functional capacity. Exercise capacities documented in this population are consistently low—from 8.3 mL/kg/min in the subacute period[50] to 22.4 mL/kg/min in the chronic period.[51] As much as 75% to 88% of Vo_2peak (almost twice that of the healthy control subjects) is required to perform household chores[52] and one-and-a-half to three times the Vo_2 levels of healthy controls are needed to walk on level ground.[46,53,54] Not surprisingly, up to 70% of patients complain of fatigue after stroke[55] and rate poor energy levels ahead of mobility limitations, pain, emotional reactions, sleep disturbances, and social isolation as the area of greatest personal concern.[56]

In addition to contributing to reduced ADL performance and increased fatigability, low fitness levels are associated with higher mortality. Exercise capacity has been reported to be an independent predictor of mortality in persons with coronary artery disease (CAD), a comorbidity prevalent in some populations of people with neurological conditions.[57,58] Those with a Vo_2peak <21 mL/kg/min are classified as the high-mortality group and with greater than 35 mL/kg/min as the excellent-survival group.[59] Thus, determining an individual's Vo_2peak is of clinical value. Individuals who are being encouraged or are internally motivated to perform beyond their capacity and beyond the capabilities of the interaction of multiple systems are in a high-risk category. Conversely, individuals who are undermotivated or depressed and are performing below their capacity can be trained to self-monitor, which empowers them to reach goals that are safe and have the potential to improve the quality of their lives.

Factors Affecting Fitness Levels in People with Neurological Disorders

To identify appropriate measures to improve fitness levels in people with neurological disorders, the myriad factors at play that contribute to the deconditioned state must be considered. A useful conceptual framework to discuss the interaction of these factors is the International Classification of Functioning, Disability and Health (ICF)[60] (see Chapter 1). The ICF uses a biopsychosocial approach to organize factors related to the health conditions into two components: (1) personal and environmental contextual factors and (2) functioning and disability, which are further subdivided into components of body functions and structures, activity, and participation (Figure 30-2). Through application of the ICF framework, the complexity of interacting influences on cardiovascular and pulmonary health and fitness becomes more understandable.

Personal and Environmental Contextual Factors

For both able-bodied and disabled people, personal contextual factors contributing to individual differences in exercise capacity include age, sex, race, and lifestyle habits.

Age

A decline in Vo_2max of approximately 1% per year (0.4 to 0.5 mL/kg/min/year) occurs from 25 to 75 years of age.[61] In accordance with the Fick equation, a reduction in Vo_2max is caused by reductions in both O_2 transporting (i.e., Qmax) and O_2 utilization capacity (i.e., a-vO_2diffmax) associated with cardiac, respiratory, and muscular changes. Decreased Qmax is the result of increasing myocardial stiffness and decreased left ventricular contractility, manifested by reductions in both ejection fraction and HRmax—hallmarks of cardiovascular aging.[62] In fact, the reduction in HRmax, which decreases 6 to 10 beats per minute (bpm) per decade, is responsible for much of the age-associated decline in Qmax.[63] Evidence also suggests that older adults have a smaller SVmax[63] and that BP and systemic vascular resistance are higher during maximal exercise in older versus young adults.[64]

With advancing age, reduced elastic recoil of the lung and calcification and stiffening of the cartilaginous articulations of the ribs restrict compliance of the lungs, thus limiting increases in minute ventilation during exercise.[65] Age-related decline in oxidative capacity of the working muscles and hence decreased a-vO_2diff during peak exercise[66] have been attributed to alterations in mitochondrial structure and distribution, oxidative enzyme activity,[67] and skeletal muscle microcirculation, as well as sarcopenia resulting from a reduced number and size of fibers, particularly type II fibers.[68] Nevertheless, despite loss of aerobic capacity with aging, people without chronic health conditions retain adequate reserves for daily activities. However, for aging individuals with a neurological impairment, the decrease in aerobic capacity with age can further reduce their reserves and thus threaten living an independent lifestyle. In fact, in a population-based study, age was found to be a significant independent predictor of recurrent stroke.[69] Particularly disadvantaged are people with cerebral palsy (CP) or other developmental disabilities as a result of an incomplete development of their musculoskeletal and cardiorespiratory systems at the time of the neurological event, which accelerates the aging process.[70] In the case of people with Down syndrome, however, Baynard and colleagues[71] found that age-related changes in exercise capacity did not follow the typical pattern of decline after the age of 16 years. People with spinal cord injury (SCI) are at an increased risk for cardiac and respiratory complications with age.[72]

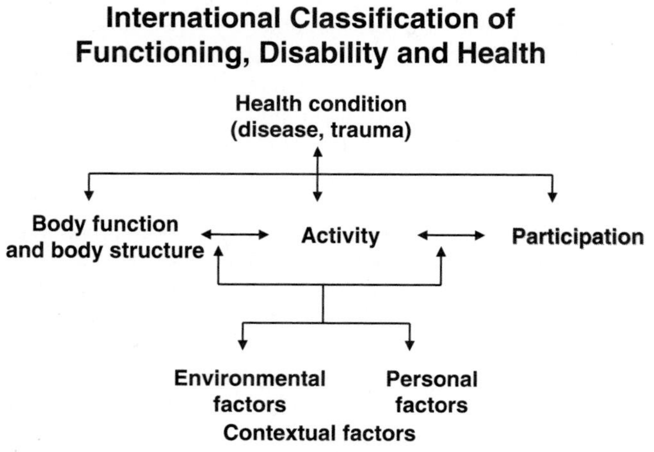

Figure 30-2 ■ Interaction of the various components of the International Classification of Functioning, Disability and Health (ICF). The ICF is a conceptual framework that uses a biopsychosocial approach to organize factors related to health condition into two components: (1) personal and environmental contextual factors and (2) functioning and disability, which are further subdivided into components of body functions and structures, activity, and participation.

Sex

The absolute and relative Vo_2max of women is about 77% of that of men, after adjustment for body weight and activity level.[73] For nondisabled older adults, Kohrt and colleagues[74] reported no significant gender difference in the percentage of improvement in Vo_2max; women had an increase in Vo_2max of 26% ± 12% (range 4% to 58%), and men demonstrated a 23% ± 12% (range 0% to 51%) increase. Although older men and women generally exhibit similar responses to maximal exercise, older women tend to have lower SBP during maximal exercise.[64]

Race

Little attention has been paid to the differences in exercise capacity among racial groups; however, in one study no differences were found between 66 black and 52 white stroke survivors in the level of physical deconditioning poststroke.[75]

Lifestyle Factors

Smoking is one factor that has been shown to impair exercise capacity in the general population.[76] Smoking causes increases in HR, myocardial contractility, and myocardial oxygen demand, which can lead to atherosclerosis and acute cardiovascular events.[77] In the stroke population, smoking doubles the risk of death (equivalent of a 7-year reduction in life span) when compared with the risk in nonsmokers and ex-smokers.[78]

Currently the relationship between cardiovascular disease and diet is receiving international attention.[79] Indeed, obesity increases the risk of cardiovascular risk factors such as impaired glucose tolerance and type 2 diabetes, hypertension, and dyslipidemia.[80] Specifically, abdominal obesity not only increases the risk of atherosclerotic disease but also the risk of primary ischemic stroke.[81,82] In addition, when compared with corresponding normal-weight populations, overweight youth with SCI and spina bifida have lower cardiovascular fitness.[83] Yet the lifestyle factor that has received the most attention in the literature is habitual activity. There is now irrefutable evidence of the link between physical activity and cardiopulmonary health and fitness.[76,84-86] In fact, in the stroke population, prestroke physical activity has been found to decrease stroke severity as well as to result in better long-term rehabilitation outcomes.[87] Cardiovascular alterations resulting from physical inactivity (i.e., reduced Vo_2max and Qmax) parallel, in many ways, the changes that occur with aging; in fact, sedentary lifestyles explain a significant proportion of these age-related declines. If physical activity levels and body composition remain constant over time, the expected rate of loss in aerobic power associated with senescence is reduced by almost 50%.[68] Nonetheless, people with chronic health conditions often rate poorly in terms of daily physical activity, in part because of underlying physical impairments (e.g., paralysis, pain). For example, people with SCI spend as little as 2% of their walking time participating in leisure physical activity,[88] making them the most sedentary members of society.[89] Some people with multiple sclerosis (MS) avoid physical activity to prevent elevated body temperature and minimize symptoms of fatigue.[90] Inactivity can lead to increased cardiovascular risk factors such as hypertension and dyslipidemia as seen in youth with chronic disabilities (including CP and SCI).[91] Bernhardt and colleagues[92] found that after a stroke, patients spend more than 50% of their time resting in bed. Short periods of bed rest cause rapid decreases in aerobic capacity—a 15% reduction in healthy, middle-aged men after 10 days of recumbency[93] and a 28% reduction in healthy young subjects after 3 weeks.[94] Inactivity-induced reductions in Vo_2peak have been attributed to both central changes (decreased SV from impaired myocardial function and increased venous pooling) and peripheral changes characteristic of aerobically inefficient muscle fibers (decreases in oxidative enzyme concentrations, mitochondria, and capillary density).[22]

Environmental Factors

Significant associations have been found between physical activity and physical environmental factors such as accessibility, esthetic attributes, and opportunities for activity within the general public.[95] However, the influence of such factors on cardiovascular and pulmonary fitness of people with neurological disabilities has received little attention in the literature.

Health Condition

Exercise capacity reflects both systemic capacity and the health of the component systems. Thus differences in Vo_2peak among individuals with neurological disabilities are a result of not only the contextual factors discussed previously but also pathological conditions involving the neuromuscular, cardiovascular, and pulmonary systems.

Neuromuscular System

For most individuals with neurological conditions, the existence of neuromuscular impairments confounds interpretation of Vo_2peak testing. When people with an intact nervous system are tested, normal biomechanical efficiency is assumed; an impaired nervous system increases the complexity of physiological responses. Both primary effects of upper motor neuron damage (e.g., paralysis, incoordination, spasticity, sensory-perceptual disorders, balance disturbances) and secondary "peripheral" changes in skeletal muscle (e.g., gross muscular atrophy[96] and changes in muscle fiber composition[97]) affect the response to exercise. As a result, people with neurological disabilities manifest not only metabolic but also biomechanical defficiencies, both of which contribute to reduction in functional capacity. Consequently, the decline in exercise capacity is greater than expected (e.g., in people with postpoliomyelitis syndrome, deterioration in Vo_2peak over a 3- to 5-year period was 12% greater than the predicted decline[98]).

Paresis reduces the pool of motor units available for recruitment during physical work,[99] thereby reducing the metabolically active tissue and lowering the oxidative potential.[100] In the case of stroke, an estimated 50% of the normal number of motor units are functioning,[101] and a strong relationship between bilateral thigh muscle mass and Vo_2peak has been reported.[102] In addition, along with altered joint kinematics and decreased postural reactions,[103] children with CP exhibit high levels of co-contraction (simultaneous contraction of agonist and antagonist muscle groups), which may prematurely induce skeletal muscle fatigue, further increasing the energy expenditure of walking and decreasing Vo_2peak.[104,105] Thus, when compared with able-bodied individuals, children with CP experience greater levels of fatigue at slower walking speeds.[104,105] For people with postpoliomyelitis syndrome, muscle weakness of the lower extremities is strongly associated with energy expenditure of walking.[49] In fact, when compared with healthy age- and sex-matched subjects, energy cost of walking is found to be significantly higher (40%) for people with postpoliomyelitis syndrome.[49]

Altered fiber composition and recruitment patterns of paretic muscle may also contribute to poor fitness.[97,106] Skeletal muscles are composed of fibers that express different myosin heavy chain (MHC) isoforms. Slow (type I) MHC isoform fibers have higher oxidative function, are more fatigue resistant, and are more sensitive to insulin-mediated glucose uptake; fast (type II) MHC fibers are recruited for more powerful movements, are more reliant on anaerobic or glycolytic means of energy production, fatigue rapidly, and are less sensitive to the action of insulin.[107] Although relatively equal proportions of slow and fast MHC isoforms are found in the vastus lateralis of healthy individuals,[100] elevated proportions of the fast, more fatigable fibers that are less glucose sensitive have been found in the paretic leg of people after a stroke.[97] Hence it is likely that reduced insulin sensitivity and increased use of the anaerobic processes during dynamic exercise at the level of the muscle contribute to reductions in Vo_2peak. Furthermore, alterations in the structure of mitochondria[100] and reduced activity of oxidative enzymes (e.g., succinate dehydrogenase)[108] may contribute to the reduced oxidative capacity of paretic muscles.

Cardiovascular System

Cardiovascular comorbidities, prevalent in populations with neurological disorders, contribute to metabolic inefficiency. In fact, cardiovascular complications are the leading cause of death in persons with stroke,[109] MS,[110] and SCI.[111] About 75% of patients who have had a stroke are hypertensive,[112] and the same proportion of patients have underlying cardiovascular dysfunction.[113] In fact, most persons who have had a stroke have atherosclerotic lesions throughout their vascular system,[114] and a high correlation has been reported between the number and degree of stenotic lesions in the coronary and carotid arteries.[115,116] The high prevalence of CAD in this population should not be surprising because stroke and cardiac disease share similar predisposing factors (e.g., older age, hypertension, diabetes mellitus, cigarette smoking, sedentary lifestyle, and hyperlipidemia) and pathogenic mechanisms (e.g., atherosclerosis).[117] Metabolic syndrome is a usual construct in identifying patients at high risk for future vascular events (e.g., a second stroke, myocardial infarction).[118] *Metabolic syndrome* refers to a constellation of markers of metabolic abnormalities (i.e., hypertension, abdominal obsesity, abnormal lipid profile) that interact to accelerate the progression of atherosclerosis and increase the risk of development of cardiovascular or cerebrovascular disease.[119] The prevalence of metabolic syndrome in neurological populations is high. A retrospective study reported that about 61% of 200 patients in stroke rehabilitation met the criteria for the syndrome.[120]

Factors that elevate HR for a given Vo_2, such as CAD, result in attainment of a peak HR (HRpeak) at a Vo_2peak below that predicted for that individual. Cardiac dysfunction contributes to a lower aerobic capacity through two principal mechanisms: ischemia-induced reductions in ejection fraction and SV with exercise[121] and chronotropic incompetence—the inability to increase HR in proportion to the metabolic demands of exercise.[21] For persons who can attain HRmax within 15 bpm of the predicted maximum, limitations in exercise capacity probably do not have cardiovascular causes.

Impaired peripheral blood flow also contributes to reduced cardiovascular fitness. Inadequate blood flow to the periphery impairs O_2 transport and limits energy production in the working muscles, thereby compromising the ability to sustain physical activity. Both resting blood flow and post-ischemic reactive hyperemic blood flow have been found to be lower (approximately 36% less) in the paretic leg of people poststroke.[122,123] In addition, despite near-normal (above 0.90) mean ankle brachial index values, arterial diameter has been found to be reduced poststroke.[122] Potential mechanisms responsible for reduced blood flow on the hemiparetic side include altered autonomic function,[124] enhanced sensitivity to endogenous vasoconstrictor agents,[125] and altered histochemical and morphological features of the vascular network itself.[126] However, the relative contribution of each of these factors is unknown. In addition, local metabolic mediators associated with changes in muscle fiber composition in the paretic limb (previously discussed) may contribute to impaired limb blood flow.[100]

Trauma to the spinal cord may disrupt the autonomic reflexes and sympathetic vasomotor outflow required for normal cardiovascular responses to exercise.[127] As a result, reduced venous return and cardiac output (referred to as *circulatory hypokinesis*) impair delivery of O_2 and nutrients to and removal of metabolites from working muscles, intensifying muscle fatigue.[128] For people with paraplegia, an exaggerated HR response may occur during exercise in order to compensate for reduced SV. However, adrenergic dysfunction associated with lesions above the T1 sympathetic outflow prevent this compensatory mechanism,[129] thereby increasing the risk of cardiovascular disease.

Pulmonary System

Typically in able-bodied individuals the pulmonary system does not limit cardiopulmonary fitness, because the lungs of people without chronic health conditions have a large reserve.[130] Nevertheless, at maximal workloads as much as 10% of Vo_2max is needed to support the mechanical work of the diaphragm, accessory inspiratory muscles, and abdominal muscles.[121] In contrast, people with neurological impairments may have limited O_2 availability for exercise as a result of pathological conditions involving the pulmonary system, either as a direct complication of a neuromuscular condition (e.g., muscle weakness, impaired breathing mechanics) or as a result of cardiovascular dysfunction, comorbidities (e.g., chronic obstructive pulmonary disease), or lifestyle factors (e.g., physical inactivity, smoking habits).[131,132] These impairments can reduce the *ventilatory reserve,* defined as the difference between the maximal available ventilation and the ventilation measured at the end of exercise.[133]

As previously mentioned, minute ventilation is closely associated with Vco_2 during exercise. At peak exercise, a ratio of minute ventilation to Vco_2 above between 35[134] and 40[135] indicates an abnormal ventilatory response. Neu and colleagues[136] reported an 87% incidence of obstructive pulmonary dysfunction in patients with Parkinson disease, despite the finding that Vo_2peak levels in this patient group tend to be in the normal range.[137,138] For children with CP, reduced exercise capacity may be partly caused by respiratory muscle spasticity resulting in reduced breathing efficiency.[105] In the case of stroke, pulmonary function is usually affected to only a modest extent, notwithstanding acute respiratory complications (e.g., pulmonary embolism, aspiration pneumonia).[131] Impaired respiration may be attributed to cardiovascular dysfunction or lifestyle factors (e.g., physical inactivity, high incidence of smoking)[139] or a direct result of the stroke, particularly brain stem stroke. The overwhelming fatigue felt by some persons after a stroke may be partly caused by respiratory insufficiency as manifested by low pulmonary diffusing capacity, decreased lung volumes, and ventilation-perfusion mismatching.[140] Impaired breathing mechanics with restricted and paradoxical chest wall excursion and depressed diaphragmatic excursion have been also reported.[131,141] Expiratory dysfunction appears to be related to the extent of motor impairment (e.g., hemiabdominal muscle weakness), whereas inspiratory limitations appear to be related to the gradual development of rib cage contracture.[142]

To summarize, a host of interacting factors are associated with abnormally low cardiopulmonary fitness in people with neurological disorders. Neuromuscular and respiratory dysfunctions are often superimposed on an already-compromised state as a result of comorbid cardiovascular disease and premorbid health- and lifestyle-related declines. Paresis and the subsequent reduction in lean muscle mass, changes in the muscle fiber phenotype, and increased reliance on anaerobic processes for energy production result in high metabolic costs of moving paretic limbs. As a consequence, cardiac reserves available for meaningful activity-level functions are limited, which in turn has a negative impact on participation-level functions. Collectively, impairments in the neuromuscular, cardiovascular, and pulmonary systems converge to promote a sedentary lifestyle and reduced health-related quality of life, which in turn leads to further inactivity and further reductions in cardiopulmonary fitness. The contribution of skeletal system impairments to this downward spiral has received little attention. Pang and colleagues[143] studied the relationship between bone health and physical fitness in patients who had had a stroke and found a significant correlation between paretic femur bone mineral density and Vo_2max. They concluded that further study is needed to determine the clinical implications of this finding.

ADAPTIVE RESPONSES TO AEROBIC TRAINING IN POPULATIONS WITH NEUROLOGICAL DISORDERS

It is now apparent that healthy young and old individuals who begin participating in regular activity even after years of inactivity can enjoy greater health and fitness than those who remain sedentary.[144] Training studies involving people with neurological disability, although limited in number and sample size and often lacking a control group, provide preliminary evidence of cardiopulmonary adaptations to physical work (Table 30-2). For example, for adolescents with chronic disabilities (including CP, SpinaBefida [SB], and SCI)[91] and children with CP,[145-148] cardiovascular fitness training is found to produce positive results on aerobic capacity and fitness. There is also growing evidence supporting the benefits of aerobic training in people with stroke of mild to moderate severity.[149] Exercise training has also been found to improve the physical capacity of people with

TABLE 30-2 ■ CARDIOPULMONARY ADAPTATIONS TO AEROBIC TRAINING PROGRAMS IN INDIVIDUALS WITH COMMON NEUROLOGICAL DISABILITIES

DIAGNOSIS	TRAINING MODE	NO.	PROGRAM WEEKS	FREQUENCY (TIMES PER WEEK)	DURATION (MIN)	INTENSITY	% VO_2PEAK CHANGE
Cerebral palsy	Uphill walking[296]	E: 7	12	3	20-22	65%-75% HRmax	E: +19
		C: 6					C: +0.6
Guillain-Barré syndrome	Arm-leg ergometer[301]	E: 1	16	3	20	75%-85% HRmax	E: +9
	Cycle training[221]	E: 20	12	3	NR	NR	E: +16
Multiple sclerosis	Arm-leg ergometry[199]	E: 21	15	3	30	60% Vo_2peak	E: +22
		C: 25					C: +1
	Leg cycle ergometer[303]	E*: 11	8	3	60	60%-80% maximum work rate	Aerobic: +17 Usual care: +0.6*
Postpoliomyelitis syndrome	Cycle ergometer[167]	E: 16	16	3	15-30	70% HRmax	E: +15*
		C: 21					C: +4
	Arm ergometer[306]	E: 10	16	3	20	70%-75%	E: +19
		C: 10				HRR or 50-60 rpm or RPE_{6-20} = 13	C: −1
	E1: Aerobic exercise, hospital[231]	E1: 15	8	3	30	50%-70% of Vo_2peak	E1: +23
	E2: Aerobic exercise, home	E2: 13					E2: +7
Spinal cord injury—C_7-T_{12}	FES-assisted rowing[166]	E: 6	6	3	30	75%-80% Vo_2peak	E: +11
	Circuit training[262]	E: 7	16	3	40-45	50%-60% 1 RM	E: +10
Spinal cord injury—tetraplegia	FES-assisted ergometry[164]	E: 18	12-16	3	30	0-31 W	E: +23
	Arm ergometer[255]	E: 8	8	3	30	50%-60% of HRR or 60 rpm	E: +94

Continued

TABLE 30-2 ■ CARDIOPULMONARY ADAPTATIONS TO AEROBIC TRAINING PROGRAMS IN INDIVIDUALS WITH COMMON NEUROLOGICAL DISABILITIES—cont'd

DIAGNOSIS	TRAINING MODE	NO.	PROGRAM WEEKS	FREQUENCY (TIMES PER WEEK)	DURATION (MIN)	INTENSITY	% VO_2PEAK CHANGE
Stroke—subacute	Stationary bicycle[204]	E: 44	12	3	20-30	40 rpm	E: +9
		C: 48					C: +0.5
	Treadmill[50]	E: 6	26	5	20	NR	E: +35
		C: 6					C: +1
	Cycle ergometer[312]	E: 23	3.3-4.1	3	30	50%-75% of Vo_2peak	E: +13
		C: 22					C: +8
Stroke—chronic	Cycle ergometer[207]	E: 37	26	3	10-20	40%-50% HRR	E: +18
		C: 24					C: −3[NS]
	Cycle ergometer[203]	E: 24	8	2	20	50%-60% HRR	E: +13
		C: 24					C: 0[NS]
	Treadmill with harness support[197]	E: 26	26	3	40	60%-70% HRR	E: +15
		C: 20					C: −3[NS]
	E1: Moderate intensity[326]	E1: 18	14	3	30-60	E1: 50%-69% HRR	E1: +4[NS]
	E2: Low intensity[326]	E2: 19				E2: <50% HRR	E2: +6[NS]
		C: 18					C: −3[NS]
	Treadmill[327] (plus strength training)	E: 14	12	5	90	E: 80% HRmax	E: +19
	Treadmill[321]	E: 20*	4	2-5	NR	80%-85% HRmax or RPE of 17	Immediate: +6 Delayed: +6
	Stationary bicycle[185]	E: 19	10	3	30	50-70 rpm	E: +13
		C: 23					C: +1
	Aerobic exercise[155]	E: 29	12	3	30	HR = (HR at RER = 1) -15	E: +8
	Treadmill[40]	E: 23	26	3	20	<60% HRR	E: +10
	Aerobic exercise[328]	E: 32	19	3	60	<80% HRR	E: +9
		C: 31					C: +1
	Water based[163]	E: 7	8	3	30	<80% HRR	E: +23
		C: 5					C: +3
Traumatic brain injury	Low-intensity aerobic exercises[324]	E: 40	16	3	15-20	"Low"	E: +3
	Circuit training[206]	E: 14	16	3	45	70% of Vo_2peak	E: +15
	Treadmill, walking, jogging[249]	E: 32	12	3	60	"Moderate intensity"	E and C: +14
		C: 30					
	BWSTT[325]	E: 2	Pt. 1: 11	2-3	17-32	Pt. 1: 60%-85% HRmax	Pt. 1: +24
			Pt. 2: 15			Pt. 2: <50% HRmax	Pt. 2: +16

*Crossover design.

BWSTT, Body-weight–supported treadmill training; *C,* control; *E,* experimental; *FES,* functional electrical stimulation; *HR,* heart rate; *HRR,* heart rate reserve; *NR,* not reported; *NS,* not significant; *RER,* respiratory exchange ratio; *RPE,* rating of perceived exertion; *rpm,* revolutions per minute; *RM,* repetition maximum.

SCI.[150,151] In the case of people with TBI, evidence regarding the effects of exercise training has been inconclusive.[152] However, in people with neurological disorders, cardiovascular adaptations in response to aerobic training enhance metabolic efficiency, and neuromuscular adaptations in response to strength and gait training improve mechanical efficiency. The result is improved functional capacity with lowered energy costs of ADLs, enhanced fatigue resistance, and increased exercise tolerance (Figure 30-3).

The magnitude of change in Vo_2peak in the training studies in Table 30-2 (mean gain of 20%) is comparable to the improvements of 10% to 30%[153,154] reported for healthy, sedentary adults and 13% to 15% for participants in cardiac rehabilitation.[155,156] The increases in Vo_2peak for clinically stable individuals with CAD have been reported to be 12% to 46%.[157-159] Substantial intersubject variability in results is attributable to many factors, including differences in neurological condition, severity, and time after insult, as well as variations in intensity of training, mode of exercise, and level of compliance with the exercise regimen. Within studies, considerable interindividual differences have been noted, of which only a small portion (about 11%) have been attributed to recognized covariates such as initial fitness status and an even smaller percentage (about 5%) to measurement error.[157-159] The most rapid improvements in exercise capacity are seen in previously sedentary people,[160] and similarly the highest overall gains occur in individuals with the lowest initial values of Vo_2peak.[161] Age and sex have not been shown to have a substantial effect on exercise trainability.[162]

The dramatic increases in exercise capacity reported in some of the studies (e.g., improvements of 23%[163,164] to 94%[50]) may not be possible for most people with neurological disabilities. Yet the subtle gains realized in other studies (e.g., 8%,[165] 11%,[166] 15%[167]) may yield meaningful dividends by extending the time in which muscle contraction can be sustained through oxidative processes, thus elevating the lactate threshold. Enhanced functional capacity could spell the difference between being dependent and independent. In other words, interventions that result in even small

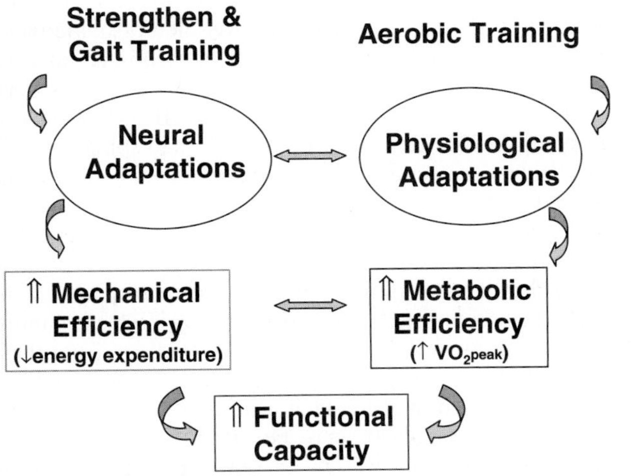

Figure 30-3 ■ Interaction of influences that enhance functional capacity. Neurorehabilitation interventions result in neural and physiological adaptations that in turn increase mechanical and metabolic efficiencies and ultimately improve functional capacity.

changes in aerobic capacity may be of practical significance for people with neurological disorders.

Mechanism of Improved Exercise Capacity in Neurological Disorders

It remains unclear whether training-induced increases in Vo_2peak in people with neurological disorders result from central mechanisms or peripheral mechanisms. In healthy individuals both peripheral and central adaptations occur; and in those with CAD and an intact nervous system, central[168,169] and peripheral[157,169,170] adaptations have been variably reported. In accordance with the Fick equation, central adaptations rely on improved SV because HRmax remains unchanged with training. Enhanced myocardial contractility, together with decreased vasoconstriction in the nonworking muscles and improved venous return, account for the higher Qmax[171,172] without a concomitant increase in mean arterial pressure.[171,172] The effect of training on ejection fraction remains unclear,[51] and lack of effect on blood hemoglobin content and coronary blood flow has been documented.[171,172]

Peripheral adaptations in the exercising muscle tissue include increases in capillary density,[173,174] size and number of mitochondria,[175] myoglobin levels, Krebs cycle enzymes (e.g., succinate dehydrogenase), and respiratory chain enzymes (e.g., cytochrome oxidase).[22] As a consequence of these skeletal muscle adaptations, a-vO_2diff and hence Vo_2peak increase.[61]

The possibility of "spontaneous" increases in exercise capacity during neurological recovery should not be overlooked. There have been several reports of non–exercise-induced adaptations after myocardial infarction.[176-178] In our lab we documented a significant increase (13%) in Vo_2peak over the course of a stroke rehabilitation program that lacked an aerobic training component.[179] Haisma and colleagues[180] reported that patients with tetraplegia and paraplegia demonstrated improvements in Vo_2peak of 17% and 23%, respectively, over the course of inpatient SCI rehabilitation; however, the extent and mode of aerobic training was not indicated. The authors speculated that the improved capacity could be, in part, a result of natural recovery and recuperation from trauma and complications. Dressendorfer and colleagues[181] hypothesized that the metabolic demands of unregulated daily activities after myocardial infarction may have an insidious training effect. In support of this prospect, a review of the threshold exercise intensity to improve cardiorespiratory fitness indicated that for deconditioned participants an effective training intensity is lower than previously reported.[182]

Additional Benefits of Aerobic Training

In addition to increased exercise capacity, other benefits of endurance training realized by healthy people appear to be attainable for individuals with neuromuscular disabilities. However, direct evidence of the impact on ICF-related domains remains limited.

Cardiopulmonary Function

Decreases in HR at a fixed submaximal workload after training have been attributed to increases in total blood volume[183] and vagal activity and to concomitant reductions in sympathetic-adrenergic drive and resting heart rate (HRrest).[184] However, according to Wilmore and colleagues[183] the decrease in HRrest is of minimal physiological significance. Potempa and colleagues[185] reported reduction in SBP at submaximal workloads after a 10-week training program for people after stroke. Related to this finding, training can also reduce the rate-pressure product (product of HR and SBP) at submaximal loads,[63] which reflects improvement in cardiac efficiency.[186] After a 4-week single-limb exercise training program with the hemiparetic limb, Billinger and colleagues[122] reported significant improvements in femoral artery blood flow and diameter compared with the nonhemiparetic limb poststroke. The authors reasoned that in order to maintain homeostasis, the diameter increased to adjust for the coupling of increases in metabolic demand and improved blood flow.

In patients with CAD, training has resulted in decreased ST segment depression (a marker of myocardial ischemia) during submaximal exercise performed at the same baseline rate pressure product,[168] thus raising the anginal threshold and extending the time that submaximal tasks can be performed without triggering myocardial ischemia. Cardiovascular and muscle adaptations also lower minute ventilation at a given submaximal workload, intimating improved ventilatory efficiency.[187] After training, Vo_2 at a given submaximal workload is either unchanged[19] or modestly reduced[188] because the increased a-vO_2diff in trained muscles is offset by reduced blood flow to the working muscles and a less pronounced decrease in blood flow to the nonexercising muscles resulting from depressed sympathetic reflex activity.[171] As a result of improved pulmonary function resulting from targeted expiratory[189] and inspiratory[190] muscle training in people with MS, it may be possible for members of this population to increase exercise tolerance.

Cardiovascular Risk Factor Reduction

Although limited physical activity is an independent predictor of risk of stroke,[191-193] the capacity of exercise to confer similar protective benefits against stroke recurrence is unknown. It is clear that endurance exercise training lowers resting BP in both young and older hypertensive adults.[194] Training is also associated with lower fasting and glucose-stimulated plasma insulin levels and with improved glucose tolerance (if initially impaired), insulin sensitivity,[195] and glycemic control in patients with type 2 diabetes.[196] A 6-month treadmill exercise training program reduced insulin resistance in stroke survivors.[197] Evidence suggests that populations with neurological disorders achieve similar training-induced improvements in lipid profile as previously documented for participants in cardiac rehabilitation.[198] Patients with MS showed reductions in triglyceride and very-low–density lipoprotein levels after a 15-week training program.[199] Similarly, an 8-week training program for individuals early after SCI led to improved lipid profiles, with more pronounced changes in response to high-intensity training.[200] However, these changes may be a result of training-induced reductions in body fat stores.[201] The potential for training to reduce intraabdominal fat is particularly significant because it is the body fat depot that increases the most with age and is associated with other cardiovascular disease risk factors.[202] Because of the positive effects on glucose homeostasis, lipid lipoprotein profiles, and cardiovascular fitness, exercise training has been found to be effective in reducing the risk of cardiovascular disease and comorbidities (e.g., type 2 diabetes, hypertension, obesity) in people with SCI.[151] Stroke survivors participating in a 10-week cardiac rehabilitation program obtained greater improvements in cardiac risk score when compared with stroke patients in usual care.[203]

Impairments in Body Structure and Function

The benefits of training to impairments in body structure and function of people with neurological disabilities, other than improved endurance and exercise tolerance, have not been well documented. In patients who have had a stroke, training studies have noted enhanced balance[204] and paretic lower-extremity muscle strength.[164] A 15-week aerobic training program for patients with MS resulted not only in improvement in exercise capacity but also in upper- and lower-extremity strength.[199] Children with CP have shown improved gross motor function after participating in an 8-month circuit-training program.[205]

An exercise training program designed to improve ambulatory efficiency of patients with traumatic brain injury failed to reduce energy costs of walking despite a 15% improvement in Vo_2peak.[206] In contrast, two studies reported mean reductions in energy costs of walking of 30%[53] and 23% after stroke rehabilitation,[54] and a pilot study reported a 32% reduction in the energy cost of walking in individuals with incomplete spinal cord lesions after a 12-week program of body-weight–supported treadmill training (BWSTT).[193] Macko and colleagues[40] interpreted gains observed in ambulatory workload capacity as a reflection of both improved exercise capacity and greater gross motor efficiency. The investigators postulated that central neural motor plasticity, mediated by the repetitive, stereotypic training, underlay these adaptations. In addition, Luft and colleagues[207] suggest that training-induced gains in walking ability[208,209] may be caused by neuroplastic mechanisms involving cerebellum-midbrain circuits.[207]

In recent years the possible role that dynamic exercise may play in enhancing cognitive function has come under investigation. In fact, in older adult populations without known cognitive impairment and in cardiac populations, there is evidence supporting the benefit of exercise training on improving cognition.[210-212] Neeper and colleagues[213] observed up-regulation of brain-derived neurotrophic factor (BDNF) in the cerebral cortex of rats housed in an environment with free access to a running wheel. Since then, several researchers have demonstrated increased BDNF production and synaptic plasticity in the brains[214,215] and spinal cords[216] of rodent models engaged in voluntary running. Tong and colleagues[217] reported that these responses appear to be dose dependent. Van Praag and colleagues[218] contributed to this line of inquiry by providing in vitro evidence of neurogenesis in the dentate gyrus of adult mice in response to an enriched environment that included voluntary wheel running. Gordon and co-workers[219] drew on the findings from these animal studies by suggesting that the improved cognitive function observed in individuals with traumatic brain injury who exercised regularly may be attributable to exercise-induced increases in BDNF or other growth factors. In another animal study, positive effects of aerobic training on neural functioning through the modulation of synaptic plasticity underlying neuroprotective and neuroadaptive processes were found.[220] In terms of fatigue, after an 8-week hospital-based training program, patients with postpoliomyelitis were found to have reduced levels of fatigue. However, limited evidence exists regarding the effect of exercise on fatigue in patients with Guillain-Barré syndrome[221] and MS.[222]

Emotional Well-Being

Increased exercise capacity has been shown to improve mental well-being (reductions in anxiety and depression) in cardiac patients.[223,224] There is moderate evidence regarding the effect of exercise training on improving mood in patients with MS.[222] Very limited evidence exists to support the relationship between aerobic exercise and emotional well-being poststroke. Yet 18% to 68% of stroke survivors are depressed,[191] making this population at an increased risk for depression.[225] High levels of physical disability, cognitive impairment, and severity of stroke have been found to be predictors of poststroke depression.[226] Stuart and colleagues[227] reported that stroke survivors participating in an exercise group improved their average score on the Hamilton Rating Scale for Depression, which for the control group remained constant. In addition, Lennon and colleagues[203] found that greater improvements in depressive symptoms were found in poststroke patients who participated in a 10-week cardiac rehabilitation program than in the usual care group.

Activity, Participation, and Quality of Life

Few investigators have studied training-induced changes in activity, participation, and quality of life for people with neurological disabilities. Evidence has been found regarding the positive impact of exercise training on quality of life for people with MS,[199,228,229] CP,[205,230] and postpoliomyelitis.[231] Turner and colleagues[228] reported better physical and mental health, as well as social functioning, in veterans with MS who exercised. However, only 26% of the 2996 veterans surveyed reported engaging in physical activity.[228] Dieruf and colleagues[230] found that after a 2-week intensive BWSTT program, children with CP reported improvements on a health-related quality-of-life measure. This finding may indicate that with a physically and psychologically challenging intervention program, along with encouragement from their parents and practitioners, children with CP may gain a better perception of their level of control and health and ultimately improve their quality of life.[230] In stroke survivors gains in walking capacity have been reported in terms of both gait speed[164,204] and walking tolerance.[204] However, there is insufficient evidence to support whether cardiovascular exercise improves quality of life after stroke.[225,232] Small improvements in Vo_2peak can have a substantial impact on the ability to perform daily activities, particularly in individuals with limited cardiac or ventilatory reserves, but there is a lack of documentation of these benefits in people with neurological disorders.

Aerobic Exercise Prescription to Optimize Fitness of People with Neurological Disabilities

Safety and Screening

In general terms, the risks imposed by lack of exercise are far greater than those imposed by exercise. Nevertheless, it is of paramount importance to recognize that symptomatic and asymptomatic cardiovascular disease, and related comorbidities such as diabetes, are much more prevalent in patients with many neurological conditions than in the general population. Because there is limited evidence regarding safety of aerobic exercise for people with neurological disorders, best clinical judgment should be used in aerobic exercise prescription. Thorough review of the health records of potential participants is critical to identify problems that may preclude safe participation in aerobic training programs. Cardiac screening, including a physician-monitored exercise stress test with continuous electrocardiographic and periodic BP monitoring, is essential for those with known or suspected cardiac comorbidities. Table 30-3 provides a compilation of contraindications to testing and training.[27,233] Before an exercise program is implemented without preliminary exercise testing, the following should be considered: (1) careful screening for possible contraindications must be conducted, (2) training must be done under the close surveillance of trained personnel, (3) a period of continuous electrocardiography and telemetry at the initiation of training is recommended, and (4) monitoring of BP, HR, and signs of exercise intolerance is essential. Furthermore, for subjects with pulmonary comorbidities such as chronic obstructive pulmonary disease, O_2 saturation levels should be monitored, with saturation levels less than 85% as the criterion to terminate exercise.[234]

In the past, clinicians were apprehensive about the possibility that the overload necessary to achieve an aerobic training effect could aggravate spasticity in patients with neurological disorders; however, such concerns have not been substantiated.[235-238] On observing that the muscles of most patients (81%) in the subacute stroke period were nonspastic, Sommerfeld and colleagues[237] postulated that focusing on spasticity may be out of step with its clinical importance. Furthermore, there is evidence from studies of cats[239] and humans after SCI[240] that treadmill training may, in fact, reduce spasticity by improving stretch reflex modulation.

Another concern raised regarding the implementation of aerobic training in neurological disorders is the potential for eliciting excessive fatigue. For people with MS, increased fatigue levels have been reported after high-intensity exercise[241]; however, exercising at an appropriate intensity has been shown to yield benefits without aggravating fatigue.[242] A preliminary study involving people with MS reported that although fatigue was a significant problem for most subjects, a single bout of low- to moderate-intensity exercise had no deleterious effects on fatigue levels immediately after, and at 24 hours after, the exercise session.[243] Dawes and colleagues[244] found that for most of their subjects early after traumatic brain injury, increasing the workload during cycling exercises did not elicit a disproportionate increase in Vo_2.

Initiation of Training

Most of the training studies on populations with neurological disorders have involved patients with chronic neurological impairments; however, the optimal time to introduce training is unknown. Macko and colleagues[245] expressed caution about training in the early poststroke period, speculating that abnormal cardiovascular responses to exercise (e.g., hypotension, arrhythmia) may impede perfusion of ischemic brain tissue during the period when cerebral autoregulation is most often impaired. Nevertheless, in one

TABLE 30-3 ■ CONTRAINDICATIONS TO EXERCISE TESTING AND AEROBIC TRAINING

ABSOLUTE CONTRAINDICATIONS	
Acute systemic illness or fever	
Shortness of breath at rest	
Suspected or known dissecting aneurysm	
Suspected or known active myocarditis or pericarditis	
Thrombophlebitis or intracardiac thrombi	
RELATIVE CONTRAINDICATIONS	
Myocardial infarction	Recent or complicated myocardial infarction
Heart surgery	Recent (within 3 months)
Angina	Unstable angina (within past 6 months), uncontrolled with medication, exertional angina at exercise intensities <3 metabolic equivalents (METs)
Ventricular arrhythmia	Uncontrolled with medication
Atrial arrhythmia	Uncontrolled atrial arrhythmia that compromises cardiac function
Resting ST segment displacement	>2 mm displacement
Atrioventricular block	Third-degree block without a pacemaker
Sinus tachycardia	HRrest >120 bpm
Pacemaker	Fixed rate pacemaker
Ventricular ectopy	Frequent or complex premature ventricular contractions at rest or during exercise
Congestive heart failure	Acute or uncompensated failure
Aortic stenosis	Moderate to severe aortic stenosis (peak systolic pressure gradient <50 mm Hg with aortic valve orifice <0.75 cm^2 in an average-sized adult)
Carotid stenosis	Severe stenosis
Large vessel intracranial stenosis	Severe stenosis
Systemic or pulmonary embolus	Recent embolus
Emotional distress or psychosis	Significant emotional distress
Hypertension	Resting SBP >200 or resting DBP >110 mm Hg
Valvular disease	Moderate or severe valvular disease
Electrolyte abnormalities	Hypokalemia or hyperkalemia or hypomagnesemia
Metabolic diseases	Uncontrolled diabetes with resting blood sugar >400 mg/dL, thyroiditis, myxedema
Orthostatic hypotension	>20 mm Hg drop with symptoms
Sudden weight gain	>2 kg increase in previous 1-3 days
Cardiac class	New York Heart Association functional class IV
Dizziness	Significant motion-induced dizziness or vertigo
Orthopedic conditions	Severe pain on weight bearing

study, training was initiated 8 to 21 days after stroke without complications.[50] In addition, an exercise rehabilitation trial, also involving patients in the hyperacute stage poststroke, began early mobilization within 24 hours of stroke onset.[246] The intervention group receiving early mobilization training reported fewer nonserious adverse events, and there were no differences in the total number of serious adverse events and fall rate when compared with the group receiving usual care.[246] Furthermore, because there is increased plasticity (e.g., axonal sprouting and neurogenesis) of the periinfarct cortex during the first month after an ischemic stroke, early training may accelerate functional recovery.[247]

Training Environment

High-risk individuals, such as patients in the early stages of neurological recovery or with cardiac comorbidities, should be trained in a setting with quick access to emergency medical equipment and trained personnel. An adverse event protocol should be posted and rehearsed. Lower-risk individuals, after appropriate screening to ensure an appropriate response to exercise, can be trained in supervised community[248] or home-based[204] aerobic exercise programs. One study involving postpolio patients reported reductions in fatigue and improvements in quality of life but found no changes in exercise capacity when patients were trained in either a hospital or home setting.[231] However, Hassett and colleagues[249] reported similar gains in cardiovascular endurance in poststroke patients training in either an unsupervised home-based or a supervised facility-based exercise program. Regardless of the setting, certain safeguards are required. Because thermal dysregulation is common in patients with neurological disability, particularly MS[250] and spinal cord injuries,[251] the ambient temperature should be carefully controlled and fans, spray bottles, towels, and a water cooler are recommended. Hydration before and during exercise and rehydration after exercise should be monitored by use of a water bottle with volumetric indicators. The exercise area should be wheelchair accessible, free of obstacles and blunt objects, and sufficiently large to permit safe transfer to and from exercise equipment.

Preparation of Participants

Participants should be advised to avoid eating 2 hours before training and to empty bowel and bladder before training, when possible, especially for patients with SCI above T6 at risk of autonomic dysreflexia. Comfortable clothing and supportive footwear, appropriate for dynamic exercise, prepare the participant both physically and psychologically for training.

Scheduling of Sessions

Many patients with neurological involvement report a decline in energy levels in the afternoon. If fatigability is a concern, training should be scheduled for morning hours, when circadian body temperature is at its lowest. For certain patient groups, including people with Parkinson disease, training should be coordinated with the timing of medication to optimize performance.

Duration of Program

A meaningful increase in aerobic capacity (i.e., greater than 10% improvement) of individuals without neurological impairment is unlikely to occur in less than 4 weeks.[252] The minimal exposure required for people with neurological disabilities has not been fully investigated. However, da Cunha and colleagues[50] reported a mean improvement of 35% in Vo_2peak after 2 to 3 weeks of treadmill ergometry in six people who had had a stroke less than 1 month previously. Regardless of the minimum, participation in training must be sustained indefinitely to prevent return to the deconditioned state measured at the beginning of the program. Therefore a maintenance program should be followed after termination of formal training sessions.

Frequency and Duration of Sessions

To optimize aerobic training, three to five sessions per week are required, although fitness can improve with twice-weekly sessions.[27] Although a minimum of 20 minutes of exercise within the target zone for training per session is required to elicit a training effect,[27] we documented that patients engaged in 1-hour sessions of stroke rehabilitation spent, on average, less than 3 minutes per session within the training zone.[4] For those with low fitness levels or who are very deconditioned (which would include the majority of patients with neurological involvement) training may be initiated with 5-minute exercise "bouts" with rest periods between bouts. Two additional 5-minute periods are required for warmup and cool down; hence the minimal time required to complete a training session is 30 minutes. Incrementally increasing the duration to a target of 40 to 60 minutes of aerobic training is recommended. However, the greater the intensity of exercise, the shorter the duration needed to achieve improvement in cardiopulmonary fitness; conversely, low-intensity exercise can be compensated for by longer duration.[253] As well, accumulation of 10- to 15-minute periods of activity throughout the day can yield similar physiological improvements, provided that the total volume of training is comparable.[254]

Mode of Training

To induce central adaptations, training must incorporate large muscle mass activities that require elevated levels of Vo_2. Treadmill or overground walking is a preferred mode because of its direct functional nature; however, a variety of disabilities may preclude this approach. Suitable alternatives include the cycle ergometer with toe clips and heel straps, recumbent ergometer, arm-leg ergometer, wheelchair ergometer, and stepping machine and swimming. Indeed, water-based exercise poststroke has shown positive effects on cardiovascular fitness and coping with life after stroke.[163] In addition, body-weight–supported treadmill training can also be used during early aerobic training poststroke.[50] Although arm ergometry activates a smaller portion of total muscle mass, its effectiveness in the aerobic training of patients with quadriplegia has been demonstrated.[255] Innovative approaches have been introduced to overcome limitations to exercise training imposed by upper motor neuron damage. For example, a combination of electric stimulation of lower-extremity muscles and voluntary upper-extremity rowing has been applied to augment the muscle activation of patients after SCI.[166] Grealy and colleagues[256] piloted use of a virtual reality recumbent ergometer with patients after traumatic brain injury, postulating that the interaction between the training apparatus and the participant might enhance attention to the task of exercising and increase the potential of structural changes in the brain.

A continuous, interval, or circuit training regimen may be used. Typically, training studies involving patients with neurological disabilities have used short bouts of exercise with a gradual transition to continuous training. However, it has been recommended for some time that if continuous training results in either a lack of improvement or a plateau in response, interval training should be instituted.[153,257]

Muscle Strengthening

Traditionally, aerobic training programs emphasized dynamic exercise. However, the addition of resistance training improves outcome.[238,258] Moreover, strength training decreases the cardiac demands of daily tasks such as lifting objects or carrying groceries while simultaneously increasing the endurance capacity to sustain these submaximal activities.[259] Muscle strengthening exercises should also be carried out 2 or 3 days per week. Key muscle groups (e.g., triceps, biceps, abdominals, hip and knee flexors and extensors, hip abductors, ankle dorsiflexors, and plantarflexors) should be strengthened with one set of 10 to 15 repetitions starting at a low weight and avoiding a Valsalva maneuver.[27] Including strength training with aerobic training may produce greater gains in functional and health outcomes. For example, engaging in a combined strength and aerobic training program has been shown to be more effective in improving Vo_2peak, walking endurance, and lipid profile in people with type 2 diabetes.[260] Improved fitness outcomes have also been reported in people who have had a stroke,[238] despite controversy about whether the benefits of strength training of the paretic upper limb poststroke outweigh the potential risk of increased tone and pain, particularly in the shoulder region. However, the meta-analysis by Harris and Eng[261] found no reported adverse affects after upper-limb strength training and concluded that upper-limb strength training improves upper-limb strength and function in people poststroke. In people with SCI, increases in fitness level and reduction in shoulder pain have been observed after circuit training involving resistance exercises and arm cranking.[262]

Intensity of Training

Determining an appropriate intensity is the most challenging aspect of exercise prescription. The cardiovascular system responds to overload; hence, the metabolic load must be sufficient to provoke central and peripheral adaptations.

TABLE 30-4 ■ FORMULAE USED TO DETERMINE THRESHOLD INTENSITY FOR EXERCISE TRAINING

FORMULA	COMMENTS
Karvonen method: HRrest + x% of heart rate reserve unfit (HRR), where HHR = predicted HRmax* − HRrest	Training intensities of 40%-85% HHR are recommended,[27] but for patients intensities of 30% HHR can be effective.[182]
x% of predicted HRmax = 220 − Age, where predicted HRmax = 220 − Age OR = 206.9 − (0.67 × age)[329]; if on β-blockers, predicted HRmax = 164 − 0.7 × Age[269]	Deconditioned individuals can benefit from intensities as low as 55%-64% of predicted HRmax.[27]
HRrest + x beats	The recommended intensity after myocardial infarction is HRrest + 20 beats and after cardiac surgery is HRrest + 30 beats.[27]
x% of Vo_2peak	Deconditioned individuals can benefit from intensities as low as 40%-50% of Vo_2peak.[27]

* *HRmax,* Maximal heart rate.

However, excessive stress imposed on the heart and contracting skeletal muscles can evoke abnormal clinical signs or symptoms. The initial exercise intensity and progression must be individualized using the participant's HR or Vo_2peak data (Table 30-4). The RPE can serve as a valid proxy to more physiological measures[30]; ratings of 11 ("fairly light") to 13 ("somewhat hard") on the RPE scale of 6 to 20 are recommended for initiation of training.[27] The RPE range associated with physiological adaptation to exercise is 12 to 16 on the Borg (6 to 20) category scale or 4 to 6 on the Borg (0 to 10) scale.[27] Despite considerable interindividual variation in RPE,[263] the ratings have been shown to correlate well with exercise intensity, even in patients taking β-blockers.[264] When exercise intensity is being established, other variables (e.g., anginal symptoms, arrhythmias) should also be considered. Continuous monitoring of HR and periodic monitoring of BP and RPE will ensure that an appropriate intensity is sustained during training.

In addition to the RPE, another proxy measure of intensity is the talk test, in which the participant's intensity is regulated by whether he or she can sing (in which case intensity should be increased) or whether he or she is unable to talk (in which case intensity should be decreased). At an appropriate intensity the participant should be able to talk while exercising, as the point of "hearing your breath" while exercising occurs at or near the ventilatory threshold.[265] This relationship was confirmed by Foster and colleagues,[266] who reported that the exercise intensity at the ventilatory threshold corresponds to the greatest intensity with which a participant can comfortably speak. Recently, the counting talk test (CTT) was introduced as another proxy measure; it measures how high the participant can count aloud without taking a second breath (e.g., "one, one thousand; two, one thousand…").[267] The percentage of resting CTT has been reported to be strongly correlated with the percentage of HR reserve, Vo_2 reserve, and RPE, with moderate intensity coinciding with 50% of CTT.[267] It should be noted, however, that the validity of the proxy measures of intensity has yet to be validated in neurological populations. For example, in the SCI population, no association was found between RPE and both HR and Vo_2.[129]

The American College of Sports Medicine guidelines recommend light- to moderate-intensity physical activities to optimize *cardiopulmonary health.*[254] In fact, a meta-analysis revealed that for very unfit patients (which would include many people with chronic neurological conditions), the initial intensity can be much lower than previously recommended.[182] However, the only consistent beneficial cardiovascular response to low levels of training is reduction in BP in older hypertensive adults. To reduce cardiovascular risk factors and increase *cardiopulmonary fitness,* moderate- or high-intensity exercise appears to be necessary.[202] In agreement, Fisher and colleagues[268] reported greater consistent improvements in gait parameters (self-selected gait speed, stride length, and step length), hip and ankle joint excursion, and sit-to-stand measures and lengthening of cortical silent period durations measured through transcranial magnetic stimulation in people with Parkinson disease participating in high-intensity BWSTT when compared with low-intensity or zero-intensity exercise programs. Nevertheless, light-intensity to moderate-intensity physical activity programs may prove adequate to reduce the rate of age-associated deterioration in a variety of physiological functions and in the long run may improve both quantity and quality of life.[202]

For many people with neurological involvement, determination of an appropriate intensity of exercise is confounded not only by cardiac status but also by the extent of neurological impairment. We have derived guidelines for determining the initial intensity of treadmill training for people after stroke, based on baseline cardiac signs, prescription of β-adrenergic blockade therapy,[269] fitness level, and motor control of the involved lower extremity (i.e., Chedoke-McMaster stage of recovery of the leg)[270] (Table 30-5).

Music to Pace Exercise

Music, if properly selected, can be helpful in pacing the repetitive, alternating movements characteristic of aerobic exercise such as walking or cycling. Rossignol and Jones[271] found that with close matching of the cadence of music and alternating movements, music can potentiate muscle activation. Similarly, McIntosh and colleagues[272] reported that music facilitated the gait pattern of people with Parkinson disease. (Refer to Chapters 4, 20, and 39 for additional information.)

Progression of Training Program

Exercise progression must be individualized because people with neurological disabilities have a wide range of functional capacities. Progression usually occurs over a 3- to 6-month

TABLE 30-5 ■ GUIDELINES FOR DETERMINING THE INITIAL INTENSITY OF TRAINING OF PEOPLE POSTSTROKE

	LOW INTENSITY	MODERATE INTENSITY	HIGH INTENSITY
Intensity	Minimum target HR = HRrest + 40% HRR	Minimum target HR = HRrest + 50% HRR	Minimum target HR = HRrest + 60% HRR
Cardiac signs	Mild-moderate abnormalities on ECG ± BP ± HR responses	Borderline abnormalities on ECG ± BP ± HR responses	Normal ECG ± BP ± HR responses
Fitness level	Vo_2peak <40% predicted	Vo_2peak 40%-60% predicted	Vo_2peak >60% predicted
Motor control	Chedoke-McMaster stage of leg: 1 or 2	Chedoke-McMaster stage of leg: 3 or 4	Chedoke-McMaster stage of leg: >4

BP, Blood pressure; *ECG,* electrocardiogram; *HR,* heart rate; *HRR,* heart rate reserve.

period from an initial conditioning phase to a training phase and then to a maintenance phase. Generally the first goal of training is to reach a target frequency (i.e., a minimum of 3 days per week), then duration (minimum of 20 minutes), and finally an appropriate intensity (40% to 60% of HR reserve, or 11 to 13 on the Borg scale). Subsequently, exercise duration should be increased as tolerated, every 1 to 3 weeks, with a goal of achieving 20 to 30 minutes of continuous exercise before increasing the intensity.[27] Patients with higher baseline fitness levels can be progressed more rapidly than those with lower initial capacities.

Laboratory Outcome Measures

Laboratory tests are useful not only to identify limitations in exercise capacity and establish exercise training protocols but also to evaluate the effectiveness of a training program. The principal indicator of a training effect is attainment of a higher Vo_2peak than was achieved in the pretrained state. The greatest increments occur in individuals with the lowest initial Vo_2peak.[161] Ideally, Vo_2peak should be measured directly because indirect methods of predicting exercise capacity are more variable and prone to error. However, because Vo_2peak testing requires special equipment and trained personnel, clinicians often resort to clinical measures of functional capacity.

Clinical Outcome Measures

Six-Minute Walk Test. The distance walked in 6 minutes is sometimes used as a clinical surrogate for Vo_2peak testing. However, the systemic response to the six-minute walk test (6MWT) is less than that of an incremental test using a treadmill cycle[273] or cycle ergometer.[274,275] Subjects tend to walk at a constant speed, achieve a Vo_2 steady-state condition after the first few minutes of exercise, and, with practice, walk at a pace approaching critical power.[275,276] Pang and colleagues[277] found a low correlation (r = 0.402) between 6MWT distance and Vo_2 in patients after stroke, concluding that the 6MWT alone should not be used as an indication of cardiopulmonary fitness after stroke. The same laboratory recommended that, to enhance the usefulness of the 6MWT, BP and HR should be recorded at initiation and termination of the test.[278] Reference equations for the 6MWT can be used to compute the percent of predicted total distance walked in the 6MWT: for men, Distance (m) = (7.57 × Height [cm]) − (5.02 × Age [yr]) − (1.76 × Weight [kg]) − 309; for women, Distance (m) = (2.11 × Height [cm]) − (5.78 × Age [yr]) − (2.29 × Weight [kg]) + 667.[279]

Shuttle Walk Test. The shuttle walk test is a standardized incremental test during which walking is initiated at an audio-guided set pace for a prescribed length of time.[280] Walking speed is increased at each stage until the subject can no longer maintain the required pace. Peak systemic responses have been reported to be consistent with those achieved during a progressive cycle test.[275] A variation of this test, the endurance shuttle walk test, involves walking as far as possible at a constant speed determined in a previously performed progressive walk test.[281]

Adherence to Program

The benefits of training are lost unless some form of training stimulus is maintained; therefore, sustained behavioral change must be an important goal in any exercise program. A decrease in mobility or inactivity can lead to rapid loss of cardiovascular and pulmonary fitness. For example, a 25% reduction in maximum oxygen uptake has been observed in nondisabled young adults after 3 weeks of bed rest.[94] In secondary prevention of stroke, behavioral modifications may be as beneficial as antihypertensive and cholesterol-lowering agents.[78] Yet establishing and maintaining a regular fitness regimen in patients with neurological impairments pose challenges. In one study, 39% of 691 patients did not engage in the exercise program created by their physical therapist.[282] In addition, 75% of people poststroke reported that they were not ready to incorporate exercise into their lifestyle.[203,283]

Some individuals are reluctant to engage in exercise owing to the fear of increasing their symptoms. Indeed, people with Parkinson disease avoid exercise out of fear they will increase their already high levels of fatigue.[284] Similarly, people with MS avoid exercising to avert increases in their level of fatigue and body temperature.[90] Furthermore, the frequency of MS-related symptoms has been found to be significantly and inversely related to physical activity.[285] It has been shown that less than 30% of 2995 people with MS reported engaging in any form of exercise,[228] with one study revealing an overall adherence rate of 65%.[286] Morris and Williams[287] reported that many individual factors (e.g., sex, level of disability), social factors, and environmental factors (e.g., access to facilities, travel) influence the level of engagement in exercise and physical activity in people with mixed disabilities. In addition, numerous psychological, cognitive, and emotional factors have been identified as potential mediators of engagement in physical activity (e.g., self-efficacy, attitude, competence, intention, knowledge of health and exercise benefits, motivation, readiness to change, and the value of exercise benefits).[288] One study involving people poststroke reported self-efficacy as an important psychological factor predicting engagement in exercise.[289] Snook and colleagues[285] reported that self-efficacy was significantly and moderately correlated with physical activity in people with MS.

A better understanding of theoretical frameworks of behavior change [see recent overview[290]] would be helpful for neurorehabilitation clinicians to increase participant engagement. Garner and Page[283] exposed community-based, chronic stroke survivors to a theoretically based intervention using the transtheoretical model with five stages of change (i.e., precontemplation, contemplation, preparation, action, and maintenance). Change is mediated at each stage by self-efficacy, decisional balance, and processes of change.[291] In a study by Gillham and Endacott,[292] a stroke-specific score based on the transtheoretical model was used to assess readiness to change behavior in patients undergoing enhanced secondary stroke prevention. The authors found that the prevention program, which consisted of conventional rehabilitation plus additional advice, motivational interviewing, and telephone support, improved exercise frequency and increased consumption of fruits and vegetables when compared with the control group receiving conventional rehabilitation.[292] They also reported a nonsignificant trend of more patients in the enhanced group progressing from contemplation to action stages of change.[292] Several other behavioral theories (i.e., social cognitive theory, theory of reasoned action, theory of planned behavior, health belief model, protection motivation theory, and self-determination theory) may also be useful in facilitating long-term engagement.[293] The American College of Sports Medicine (ACSM)[27] acknowledged that assessing the participants' self-motivation and readiness for change can provide important information toward adapting the exercise program to meet the specific needs of the participants.

In the cardiac rehabilitation literature, Piepoli and colleagues[294] recommended that in order for an individual to pursue and engage in an exercise program, both physiological and psychosocial changes are needed. Progression from promotion of physical activity within the patient's current domestic, occupational, and leisure settings to participating in vigorous and structured exercise programs is recommended.[294] In a systematic review also involving people with cardiac conditions, evidence supported the use of educational sessions, spousal and family involvement, flexible and convenient scheduling of sessions, ongoing positive reinforcement and enjoyment (e.g., motivational letters, pamphlets, conversations), and self-management aids (e.g., self-report diets, activity logs, individualized goal setting).[295] Other strategies to enhance long-term exercise adherence include gradually progressing the exercise intensity, establishing regularity of training sessions, minimizing the risk of muscular soreness, and exercising in groups. Training sessions should be scheduled at a convenient time and in an accessible location, and if feasible, assistance with transportation and childcare should be offered. With the established emphasis on patient-centered care, it is consistent to have the patient identify individual goals and time frames to achieve these goals. Incorporating physical activity within everyday life will help to promote cardiovascular and pulmonary fitness as a life activity and not solely an exercise program conducted within a medical environment or rehabilitation setting.

Lifestyle Modifications

Aerobic training alone is not sufficient to optimize the health and fitness of people with neurological disabilities. Education and counseling regarding daily physical activity, nutrition, energy conservation techniques, smoking cessation, and coping strategies are essential.

CONCLUSION

Several conclusions can be made based on available evidence. Neuromuscular, cardiovascular, and pulmonary impairments associated with most neurological conditions interact with contextual factors and the health condition itself to adversely affect exercise capacity and cardiovascular fitness. Aerobic training is now unequivocally regarded as an effective intervention to reduce the functional decline associated with the deconditioned state. Research, albeit limited, suggests that although patients with neurological impairments generally manifest poor cardiopulmonary fitness, they have the capacity to respond to exercise training in essentially the same manner as individuals without impairments. Trainability is evidenced by their ability to increase exercise capacity or Vo_2peak in response to the metabolic stress imposed by aerobic exercise. Although not abundant, research findings also suggest that involvement in aerobic exercise can also improve walking capacity and reduce risk factors for secondary complications. On the basis of the positive results of training studies, more aggressive training programs are now being introduced into neurorehabilitation, with the goals of interrupting the cycle of debilitation and enhancing neurological recovery. There is an obvious need for further, properly controlled research to examine the impact of aerobic training on all domains of function and quality of life, especially in a population in which chronic impairments might be diminished and quality of future life improved. Patients with neurological insults clearly have compounding system variables that interact when they are trying to perform any movement. A clinician who is assisting individuals to regain functional control over movement to improve their quality of life cannot afford to ignore the cardiovascular and pulmonary system regardless of the medical diagnosis.

References

To enhance this text and add value for the reader, all references are included on the companion Evolve site that accompanies this textbook. This online service will, when available, provide a link for the reader to a Medline abstract for the article cited. There are 329 cited references and other general references for this chapter, with the majority of those articles being evidence-based citations.

APPENDIX 30-A ■ Abbreviations Commonly Used When Discussing Cardiovascular and Pulmonary Problems and Their Effect on Function

6MWT: 6-Minute walk test
ADL: Activities of daily living
a-vO_2diff: Arteriovenous oxygen difference
a-vO_2diffmax: Maximal arteriovenous oxygen difference
BP: Blood pressure
CAD: Coronary artery disease
CO_2: Carbon dioxide
DBP: Diastolic blood pressure
ECG: Electrocardiogram
H^+: Hydrogen ion
HR: Heart rate
HRmax: Maximal heart rate
HRpeak: Peak heart rate
HRR: Heart rate reserve
HRrest: Resting heart rate
ICF: International Classification of Functioning, Disability and Health
MET: Metabolic equivalent
O_2: Oxygen
Q: Cardiac output
Qmax: Maximal cardiac output
RER: Respiratory exchange ratio
RERpeak: Peak respiratory exchange ratio
RPE: Rate of perceived exertion
SPB: Systolic blood pressure
SV: Stroke volume
SVmax: Maximal stroke volume
$V\text{CO}_2$: Carbon dioxide production per minute
$V\text{O}_2$: Oxygen consumption per minute
$V\text{O}_2$max: Maximal oxygen consumption per minute
$V\text{O}_2$peak: Peak oxygen consumption per minute

CHAPTER 31 Human Immunodeficiency Virus Infection: Living with a Chronic Illness

KERRI SOWERS, PT, DPT, MARY LOU GALANTINO, PT, PhD, MSCE, and DAVID M. KIETRYS, PT, PhD, OCS

KEY TERMS

AIDS
human immunodeficiency virus (HIV)
psychoneuroimmunology

OBJECTIVES

After reading this chapter the student or therapist will be able to:

1. Appreciate the role of the immune system in chronic HIV disease.
2. Discuss the neuropathological features of HIV infection and understand potential neurocognitive and neuropsychological alterations that may occur.
3. Understand the various systems (integumentary, musculoskeletal, cardiopulmonary, and neurological) that affect function in HIV-infected adult and pediatric patients.
4. Appreciate the role of psychoneuroimmunology in HIV rehabilitation management.
5. Establish safe exercise parameters in the HIV-positive population.

IDENTIFICATION OF THE CLINICAL PROBLEM

Initially recognized in 1982, acquired immunodeficiency syndrome (AIDS) has been one of the leading causes of death among young adults in the United States since that time. Even with significant advancements in the medical management of the disease, there continues to be a devastating impact in the developing world.[1,2] The course of human immunodeficiency virus (HIV) disease in industrialized nations, including the United States, has changed dramatically as a result of advancements in medications used to treat the disease, as well as increased public awareness and the expansion of programs in poverty-stricken areas. Although the disease was once considered a death sentence, the long-term prognosis for those diagnosed with HIV/AIDS has drastically changed in most industrialized countries. In the United States, HIV is no longer found in the top 10 causes of death for the entire adult population. Yet, HIV is the seventh leading cause of death in young adults (age 20 to 24 years); for both older teens (ages 15 to 19 years) and young teens (ages 10 to 14 years), HIV is ranked fourteenth; for children (ages 5 to 9 years), HIV drops to nineteenth on the list.[3] Although still alarming, this is actually an improvement compared with the 1990s. Most epidemiologists and clinicians attribute improved life expectancy to the impact of new, highly active antiretroviral therapies (HAART). Implementation of these medications has resulted in a decline in AIDS deaths nationally.[4,5] However, the incidence of HIV disease, which demonstrated some decrease in the 1990s, demonstrated an increase from 1999 to 2006. HAART regimens have fostered longevity for many, resulting in the evolution of HIV infection into a chronic disease. Individuals previously disabled by the disease now have the potential to return to work and functional activities and often can expect to live a normal life expectancy. Despite these gains, HIV disease, related comorbidities, and the side effects of medications used to treat the disease have a great impact on rehabilitative medicine because of the multisystem involvement, which often progresses slowly throughout the life span. The advancements in medications that have led to increased life expectancies and improved functional capabilities have also led to a greater demand for rehabilitative services.

HAART has slowed and prevented the progression from HIV infection to AIDS and from AIDS to death.[6] In communities with access to antiretroviral medications, the incidence of perinatally acquired AIDS has declined significantly as a result of administration of HAART during pregnancy.[7] Unfortunately, perinatal transmission of the virus in developing nations continues to be a crisis.

The clinical and pathological information about this disease is constantly increasing. Certainly, our understanding of the disease process and advances in drug regimens will change between the writing and the publication of this book. Changes in terminology reflect this evolution of clinical knowledge. The definitions used throughout this chapter reflect current usage.

The virus thought to be responsible for the transmission of AIDS was first identified in 1984; it was named *human immunodeficiency virus* in 1986 at the International Conference on AIDS in Paris. A second virus, HIV-2, was soon after identified in western Africa, and the original strain was renamed HIV-1. Infection caused by HIV-2, less widely distributed, has since been established in Europe and in South, Central, and North America. Both HIV-1 and HIV-2 have resulted in AIDS, but evidence suggests that HIV-2 may be less virulent than HIV-1. In addition to these subtypes, several strains or mutated forms of HIV-1 have been identified. Different strains reflect variations in cellular affinities and resistance to medications. The context of discussion for the purpose of this chapter will be HIV-1, herein discussed as *HIV.* HIV infection is identified via a positive HIV antibody screening test (enzyme immunoassay [EIA]) and confirmation with a supplemental HIV antibody test (Western Blot) or a positive result from an HIV virological test (nucleic acid detection test, p24 antigen test, or viral culture).

In 2008 the Centers for Disease Control and Prevention (CDC) revised its definition of AIDS and its classification system of HIV disease. To reflect current scientific knowledge, the new system elucidates the importance of $CD4^+$ T-lymphocyte cell counts as indicators for pharmacological disease management. Based on laboratory criteria and clinical presentation, the disease is classified into four stages. Stage 1 has no AIDS-defining condition and either a $CD4^+$ T-lymphocyte count greater than or equal to 500 cells/mcL or a ratio of $CD4^+$ T-lymphocytes to total lymphocytes greater than or equal to 29%. Stage 2 also has no AIDS-defining condition and either a $CD4^+$ T-lymphocyte count of 200 to 499 cells/mcL or a ratio of $CD4^+$ T-lymphocytes to total lymphocytes of 14% to 28%. Stage 3 is classified by the CDC as AIDS; it is defined as a $CD4^+$ T-lymphocyte count less than 200 cells/mcL or a ratio of $CD4^+$ T-lymphocytes to total lymphocytes less than 14% or documentation of an AIDS-defining condition (Box 31-1). A fourth stage was also identified as HIV Infection, Stage Unknown (for cases in which no information is obtained regarding the $CD4^+$ T-lymphocyte counts or ratios or regarding any AIDS-defining conditions); the primary use of this stage is for surveillance purposes.[8] The entire spectrum of illness from initial diagnosis to AIDS can be covered by the term *HIV disease.* In addition, the terms *acute HIV infection, asymptomatic HIV disease, symptomatic HIV disease,* and *advanced HIV disease (AIDS)* are used throughout this chapter. In general, asymptomatic HIV disease corresponds with Stage 1, symptomatic HIV disease with Stage 2, and advanced HIV disease (AIDS) with Stage 3. Table 31-1 presents the various modifiers of quality of life throughout the various stages of HIV disease.

Epidemiology

It is currently estimated that over 30 million people are infected with HIV globally. In the United States, the CDC estimated that 1.1 million adults and adolescents were HIV positive at the end of 2006. Because of complex social and economic factors, African Americans are disproportionally affected, with approximately half of the cases in the United States involving this minority group. Alarmingly, it is estimated that approximately 25% of individuals in the United States infected with HIV are unaware of the infection.[9]

In the most recent publication of the World Health Report from the World Health Organization (WHO), HIV/AIDS is the sixth leading cause of death worldwide, with an estimated 2.04 million deaths per year.[10] Worldwide, of the 33 million people (all ages) living with HIV, 30.8 million are adults, 15.5 million are women, and 2.0 million are children (under the age of 15 years). New HIV infections in 2007 totaled 2.7 million, with 2.3 million in adults and 370,000 in children under 15 years old. Global AIDS deaths totaled nearly 2.0 million; adult deaths were 1.8 million, whereas children under age 15 years totaled 270,000.[11] It was estimated that in 2006 the United States had approximately 14,561 deaths from AIDS-related illnesses.[9]

Tuberculosis (TB) is a former leading microbial killer; it is caused by infectious bacteria that spread through the air in microscopic droplets. WHO estimates that there were 9.27 million new TB cases in 2007; of those, 1.37 million cases (14.8%) were in HIV-positive individuals. Approximately 456,000 deaths caused by TB occurred in HIV-infected individuals (23% of the estimated 2 million HIV deaths were caused by TB).[12]

BOX 31-1 ■ AIDS-DEFINING CONDITIONS

Bacterial infections, multiple or recurrent*
Candidiasis of bronchi, trachea, or lungs
Candidiasis of esophagus†
Cervical cancer, invasive‡
Coccidioidomycosis, disseminated or extrapulmonary
Cryptococcosis, extrapulmonary
Cryptosporidiosis, chronic intestinal (>1 month's duration)
Cytomegalovirus disease (other than liver, spleen, or nodes), onset at age >1 month
Cytomegalovirus retinitis (with loss of vision)†
Encephalopathy, HIV related
Herpes simplex: chronic ulcers (>1 month's duration) or bronchitis, pneumonitis, or esophagitis (onset at age >1 month)
Histoplasmosis, disseminated or extrapulmonary
Isosporiasis, chronic intestinal (>1 month's duration)
Kaposi sarcoma†
Lymphoid interstitial pneumonia or pulmonary lymphoid hyperplasia complex*†
Lymphoma, Burkitt (or equivalent term)
Lymphoma, immunoblastic (or equivalent term)
Lymphoma, primary, of brain
Mycobacterium avium complex or *Mycobacterium kansasii,* disseminated or extrapulmonary†
Mycobacterium tuberculosis of any site, pulmonary,†‡ disseminated,† or extrapulmonary†
Mycobacterium, other species or unidentified species, disseminated† or extrapulmonary†
Pneumocystis jiroveci pneumonia†
Pneumonia, recurrent†
Progressive multifocal leukoencephalopathy
Salmonella septicemia, recurrent
Toxoplasmosis of brain, onset at age >1 month†
Wasting syndrome attributed to HIV

*Only in children aged younger than 13 years.
†Condition that might be diagnosed presumptively.
‡Only in adults and adolescents aged 13 years or older.

Normal Immunity

The immune system is complex and dynamic, comprising a multitude of components and subsystems, all of which interact continuously. The normal immune system has two main components, or lines of defense, against illness (Figure 31-1). The first is the innate, or inborn, component, which includes the skin, the cilia and mucosal linings of the respiratory and digestive systems, the gastric fluids and enzymes of the stomach, and the phagocyte cells. This innate component of the immune system keeps pathogens out of the body by creating barriers against them, by ejecting them, or by enveloping them and eliminating them. The second, the acquired component of the immune system develops defenses against specific pathogens, starts in utero, and continues throughout life. It is acquired (or antibody) immunity that is most pertinent to understanding HIV infection and its progression.

TABLE 31-1 ■ QUALITY-OF-LIFE ISSUES FOR HIV DISEASE STAGES

STAGE	$CD4^+$ COUNT	PHYSICAL INDICATORS	MODERATORS OF QUALITY OF LIFE	GENERAL QUALITY-OF-LIFE ISSUES
Stage 1: Asymptomatic Disease, HIV infection	>500 cells/mcL	May have persistent generalized lymphadenopathy	Appraisals: Anticipatory grieving, catastrophizing, and other cognitive distortions; changed expectations of future; identity and self-esteem issues Coping: Dealing with present and future uncertainties; at risk for denial, disengagement, substance abuse, risky sex, suicide; issues of eliciting social support	Emotional functioning: Anxiety, anger, often increasing at diagnosis and diminishing and recycling as individual confronts realities of living with HIV disease Role functioning: Often able to work; possible decrements in job mobility and career opportunities; job loss Social functioning: Fear, isolation, issues of trust in relationships; stigmatization; changes in social support networks because of deaths; relationship and sexual changes; isolation, withdrawal Physical functioning: Normal but may be altered because of depression or anxiety; may have hypervigilance regarding all physical symptoms Spiritual functioning: Opportunity to direct attention inward, thus yielding to contemplation of life's meaning, reassessment of spiritual and existential issues
Stage 2: Symptomatic Disease, HIV infection	201-499 cells/mcL	Emergence of symptoms such as thrush, night sweats, low-grade fevers, oral hairy leukoplakia, peripheral neuropathy; commonly taking antiretroviral drugs and/or *Pneumocystis jiroveci* prophylaxis	Appraisals: Anticipatory grieving, catastrophizing, and other cognitive distortions; changed expectations of future; identity and self-esteem issues related to threats to occupational and functional abilities Coping: Dealing with present and future uncertainties; at risk for denial, disengagement, substance abuse, and risky sex	Emotional functioning: Anxiety, anger, often increasing on emergence of symptoms and then fluctuating with challenges and threats to present and future functioning Role functioning: Often able to work; may take on new roles as part of HIV support–related network Social functioning: Changes in social support networks resulting from deaths, isolation, withdrawal, relationship and sexual changes, and stigmatization Physical functioning: May have reduced energy levels; moderate symptomatology; possible cognitive deficits; pain; wasting Spiritual functioning: Anticipatory grieving, sense of relatedness to something greater than the self, unavoidable confrontation with one's own mortality

Continued

TABLE 31-1 ■ QUALITY-OF-LIFE ISSUES FOR HIV DISEASE STAGES—cont'd

STAGE	CD4+ COUNT	PHYSICAL INDICATORS	MODERATORS OF QUALITY OF LIFE	GENERAL QUALITY-OF-LIFE ISSUES
Stage 3: AIDS Disease	<200 cells/mcL	Opportunistic infections such as extensive candidiasis, cryptococcal meningitis; Kaposi sarcoma; tuberculosis; *P. jiroveci* pneumonia; lymphomas; commonly taking antiretroviral drugs, chemotherapy, antibiotics, and so on	Appraisals: Facing chronic illness and death; grieving about current and anticipated losses; catastrophizing and other cognitive distortions; reassessment of spiritual and existential issues Coping: Coping strategies may be overwhelmed in dealing with current difficulties such as financial losses, medical costs, treatment and side effects, housing; may lose some traditional coping strategies such as recreational outlets	Emotional functioning: Anxiety, anger may cycle according to fluctuations in disease status and appraisals; relief from uncertainty Role functioning: Diminished capacity for work; role changes—often need care instead of being a caretaker Social functioning: May have diminished social networks because of lack of mobility, illness, and deaths among friends Physical functioning: Self-care difficulties; fatigue; wasting; much time spent in medical care; debilitation from infection and treatments; possible cognitive deficits Spiritual functioning: Essential worth is to provide a framework from which to pose and seek responses to metaphysical questions generated by presence of life-threatening disease; integration and transcending of biological and psychosocial nature, which gives access to nonphysical realms as prophecy, love, artistic inspiration, completion, and healing actions

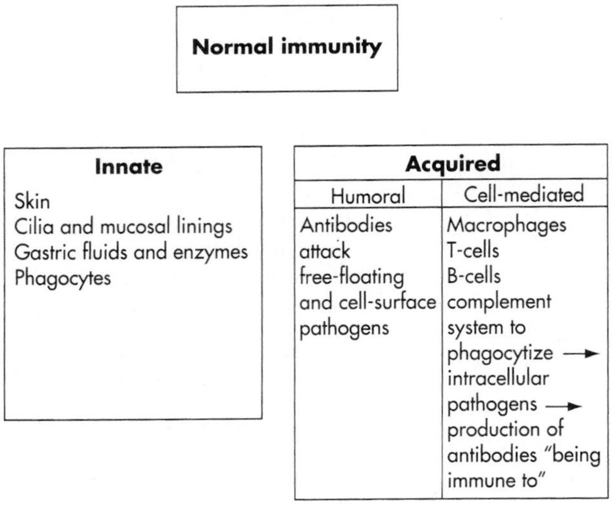

Normal immunity
Innate
Skin
Cilia and mucosal linings
Gastric fluids and enzymes
Phagocytes
Acquired
Humoral
Cell-mediated
Antibodies attack free-floating and cell-surface pathogens
Macrophages
T-cells
B-cells
complement system to phagocytize intracellular pathogens production of antibodies "being immune to"

Figure 31-1 ■ Main components of immunity.

Acquired Immunity

Acquired immunity is divided into humoral and cell-mediated responses. Humoral immunity depends on the production of antibodies. This response is effective for disposing of free-floating or cell-surface pathogens. The cell-mediated response is required to destroy infected cells, those with intracellular pathogens. Cell-mediated immunity is essential for destroying pathogens responsible for the opportunistic infections and neoplasms that are associated with AIDS.[13,14]

For the study of HIV pathology, it is important to consider three types of immune system cells: macrophages, T lymphocytes (T cells), and B lymphocytes (B cells). Macrophages originate in the bone marrow and then migrate to the organs in the lymphatic system. Macrophages recognize and then phagocytize antigens—substances deemed foreign to the body. All but a fragment of the antigen is digested by the macrophage. This remaining fragment protrudes from the cellular surface, where it is then recognized by T and B cells, allowing those cells to develop an appropriate immune response.[15]

Both of the lymphocytes (T and B cells) originate in the bone marrow. Their differentiation into T and B cells depends on where they develop immunocompetence. Immunocompetence is the ability of the immune system to mobilize in response to an antigen; it can be weakened secondary to age-related changes, radiation therapy, chemotherapy, or viral infections. T cells migrate to the thymus to develop this ability. B cells develop it before leaving the bone marrow. T cells travel to lymph nodes, the spleen, and connective tissues, where they wait to phagocytize the antigens in the manner previously described. B cells function in the same way against free-floating blood-borne pathogens.[15]

There are at least eight types of T cells with various functions. Two relevant types are helper T cells (CD4) and suppressor T cells (CD8). The helper T cells enhance the immune response, whereas suppressor T cells regulate the immune response. HIV primarily attacks these two types of T cells, impairing the body's immune response. On recognition of an antigen, CD4 cells chemically stimulate production and activation of other lymphocytes to destroy the foreign material. When the action of the T and B cells is a sufficient immune response, the CD8 cells will halt the action, thus preventing the destruction of normal (uninfected) cells. The HIV virus causes the destruction of the CD4 cells. Declining CD4 cell counts occur in untreated disease; in healthy (uninfected) individuals, CD4 counts should be 500 to 1600 cells/mcL. However, because T-cell counts fluctuate somewhat under normal circumstances, the ratio of CD4 to CD8 cells is considered a valuable laboratory value in tracking the progression of the disease.

In the process of identifying and destroying antigens, the acquired immune system retains a memory of the antigen. This allows the immune system to respond more rapidly and effectively to the pathogen if it is reintroduced into the body. Herein lies the pertinence of vaccination and the phenomenon of being immune to an illness.[15]

PATHOGENESIS OF HIV DISEASE

HIV belongs to a class of viruses known as *retroviruses,* which carry their genetic material in the form of ribonucleic acid (RNA) rather than deoxyribonucleic acid (DNA). HIV primarily infects the mononuclear cells, especially CD4 and macrophages, but B cells are also infected.[16] HIV binds to the receptor sites on the surface of the CD4 lymphocytes, eventually fusing with and then entering the cells. Reverse transcriptase released from the HIV allows a DNA copy of the virus to be made within the host cell, which then becomes integrated into the host cell genome. Other enzymes, such as integrase and protease, turn the lymphocyte into a "virus factory," and replicated virions bud out of the cell to infect others.

Within days of acute HIV infection, lymph nodes become sites of rampant viral replication, and viral loads in the blood are high. During the stage of acute HIV infection, the individual may remain asymptomatic or may experience nonspecific and self-limited flulike symptoms—fever, diarrhea, myalgias, and fatigue—for a period of 2 to 12 weeks. In the weeks after an acute infection, the body gradually produces an antibody response. The point at which antibodies can be detected with a blood test is known as *seroconversion.* Typically, seroconversion occurs within 3 months of the time of infection, but it can take as long as 12 months. Thus there is a period of time after HIV infection when the result of an HIV antibody test (the most commonly used test to determine HIV status) will be negative.

In asymptomatic HIV disease or Stage 1, individuals will have a positive antibody test result. This stage may last from 1 to 20 years. Although generally asymptomatic, individuals in this stage may express periods of generalized lymphadenopathy. Laboratory tests may reveal slowly declining immune dysfunction, as evidenced by an abnormally low CD4 cell count and an abnormal CD4/CD8 ratio. The viral load is typically at a "set point" during most of the asymptomatic stage of HIV disease. This set point is typically much lower than the viral load occurring during the period of acute infection. The viral load will inevitably escalate as the disease progresses.

As CD4 cell counts decline and viral load escalates, the individual will eventually enter Stage 2, or symptomatic HIV disease. With the continuing advancements in medications, this stage may last several years. Improved effectiveness of medications, increasing access to health care services, and medical comorbidities all have a large influence on the length of time a patient is considered to be in Stage 2. CD4 cell counts are declining and viral loads are increasing. Concurrently with these laboratory value abnormalities, the individual begins to have one or more of an array of symptoms such as weight loss, fatigue, night sweats, fever, thrush, yeast infections, prolonged recovery from other illnesses, or neurological complications.

When the CD4 cell count drops below 200 cells/mcL, the individual is diagnosed with an opportunistic infection or other AIDS-defining illness, or the individual demonstrates wasting syndrome or HIV-related dementia, he or she is reclassified as being in Stage 3—advanced HIV disease or AIDS. It is possible for patients in this stage to demonstrate remarkable recovery in terms of both laboratory values and function with HAART. Individuals who do not have access to HAART, or individuals in whom HAART has failed, will eventually die as a result of the effects of opportunistic infections that inevitably occur. Quality-of-life issues throughout the stages of HIV disease are described in Table 31-1.

Medical Management

Cell Counts and Prophylaxis

Pharmacological interventions to combat the opportunistic infections associated with HIV infection are beyond the scope of this chapter, but a simplified summary of clinical information is pertinent. Medical management of HIV infection is most often guided by the CD4 cell count and viral load.

For the healthy HIV-negative adult, the average CD4 cell count is approximately 1000 cells/mcL. However, counts fluctuate over time and may range from 500 to 1600 cells/mcL.[17] A CD4 cell count of 200 cells/mcL marks a critical point in the course of HIV infection, often indicating that the stage of advanced HIV infection or AIDS has been reached. Serious opportunistic infections are likely to occur once this level of immune depletion has been attained.[18-20]

Exercise, stress, seasons of the year, serum cortisol level, and the presence of acute or chronic illness and infection have all been reported to affect CD4 cell counts. Thus the initial CD4 lymphocyte numbers should be confirmed by repeat testing. Caution should be exercised to avoid overinterpreting small changes in CD4 lymphocyte test results. The overall trend of CD4 counts is more important than any single value. Testing is typically done at a frequency of four times annually. In addition to CD4 cell counts, CD4/CD8 ratios are used to evaluate the status of the immune system. CD4 counts above 500 cells/mcL indicate no need for antiretroviral therapy because individuals are generally asymptomatic. It is currently recommended that HAART be initiated when CD4 levels are below 350 cells/mcL, with individual parameters influencing the decision.[21] CD4 cell counts below 200 cells/mcL are an indication for prophylactic

Pneumocystis jirovechi (previously referred to in the literature as *Pneumocystis carinii;* this text will refer to the current terminology) pneumonia (PCP) and toxoplasmosis measures. Persons with counts below 100 cells/mcL may also receive prophylactic agents against cytomegalovirus (CMV) infection, infection with *Mycobacterium avium* complex (MAC), and fungal infections such as cryptococcosis and candidiasis.[13] In addition, it is recommended that HIV-positive pregnant women, those with HIV-associated nephropathy, and those co-infected with the hepatitis B virus be started on a HAART regimen immediately.[22] Table 31-2 is a summary of common pharmacological agents prescribed to combat opportunistic infections and, most pertinent to rehabilitation, their potential side effects.

TABLE 31-2 ■ HIV DRUGS BY CLASS

BRAND NAME	GENERIC NAME	DOSE	SIDE EFFECTS	FDA APPROVAL	COMMENTS
NUCLEOSIDE REVERSE TRANSCRIPTASE INHIBITORS (NRTIs)					
Combivir	Zidovudine and lamivudine	One tablet twice a day Contains two NRTIs in one tablet	Similar side effects to Retrovir (zidovudine) and Epivir (lamivudine). Please note Retrovir's and Epivir's Black Box warnings.	September 27, 2007	Take with or without food.
Emtriva	Emtricitabine	One 200-mg capsule once a day	Black Box warning: Buildup of acid in the blood; fatty liver; should be used carefully by people with hepatitis B. Otherwise, minimal side effects.	July 2, 2003	Take with or without food.
Epivir	Lamivudine	One 300-mg tablet once a day or one 150-mg tablet twice a day	Black Box warning: Buildup of acid in the blood; fatty liver; should be used carefully by people with hepatitis B. Otherwise, minimal side effects.	November 17, 1995	Take with or without food. Approved for treatment of hepatitis B virus infection at a lower dose. Individuals with both viruses should use the higher dose.
Epzicom (Kivexa in some countries)	Abacavir and lamivudine	One tablet once a day Contains two NRTIs in one tablet	Similar side effects to Epivir (lamivudine) and Ziagen (abacavir). Please note Epivir's and Ziagen's Black Box warnings.	August 2, 2004	Take with or without food. Need to be tested for the HLA-B*5701 gene to reduce the risk of a severe allergic reaction.
Retrovir	Zidovudine	One 300-mg tablet twice a day	Black Box warning: Anemia and decrease in white blood cells; damage to muscle; buildup of acid in the blood; fatty liver. Nausea, stomach discomfort, headache, insomnia, and weakness.	March 19, 1987	Take with food to minimize stomach discomfort. Do not take with Zerit.
Trizivir	Abacavir, zidovudine, and lamivudine	One tablet twice a day Contains three NRTIs in one tablet	Similar side effects to Retrovir (zidovudine), Epivir (lamivudine), and Ziagen (abacavir). Please note Retrovir's, Epivir's, and Ziagen's Black Box warnings.	November 14, 2000	Take with or without food. Need to be tested for the HLA-B*5701 gene to reduce the risk of a severe allergic reaction.

TABLE 31-2 ■ HIV DRUGS BY CLASS—cont'd

BRAND NAME	GENERIC NAME	DOSE	SIDE EFFECTS	FDA APPROVAL	COMMENTS
Truvada	Tenofovir and emtricitabine	One tablet twice a day Contains two NRTIs in one tablet	Similar side effects to Viread (tenofovir) and Emtriva (emtricitabine). Please note Viread's and Emtriva's Black Box warnings.	August 2, 2004	Take with or without food.
Videx EC (generic is now available in the United States)	Didanosine	One 400-mg capsule once a day or one 250-mg capsule once a day if <132 lb	Black Box warning: Damage to the pancreas (pancreatitis); buildup of acid in the blood; fatty liver. Numbness, tingling, or pain in the hands or feet (peripheral neuropathy); nausea; diarrhea.	October 31, 2000	Take on an empty stomach. Can be taken at the same time as other HIV medications except for the protease inhibitors (PIs) Aptivus, Prezista, and Reyataz. Avoid alcohol.
Viread	Tenofovir	One 300-mg tablet once a day	Black Box warning: Buildup of acid in the blood; fatty liver; should be used carefully by people with hepatitis B. Weakness, headache, nausea, vomiting, diarrhea, flatulence (intestinal gas), and kidney problems.	October 26, 2001	Take with or without food. Approved for treatment of the hepatitis B virus. Can raise Videx EC level in the blood and increase side effects.
Zerit	Stavudine	One 40-mg capsule twice a day or one 30-mg capsule if <132 lb	Black Box warning: Buildup of acid in the blood (has been fatal in pregnant women when combined with Videx/Videx EC); fatty liver; damage to the pancreas (when combined with Videx/Videx EC). Numbness, tingling, or pain in the hands or feet (peripheral neuropathy); lipodystrophy; muscular weakness (rare); increased cholesterol and increased triglycerides.	June 24, 1994	Take with or without food. Do not take with Retrovir or Combivir.
Ziagen	Abacavir	One or two 300-mg tablets once a day	Black Box warning: Severe allergic reactions (symptoms include fever; rash; severe nausea, diarrhea, abdominal pain; sore throat; cough; and shortness of breath); buildup of acid in the blood; fatty liver.	December 17, 1998	Take with or without food. Need to be tested for the HLA-B*5701 gene to reduce the risk of a severe allergic reaction.

Continued

TABLE 31-2 ■ HIV DRUGS BY CLASS—cont'd

BRAND NAME	GENERIC NAME	DOSE	SIDE EFFECTS	FDA APPROVAL	COMMENTS
NONNUCLEOSIDE REVERSE TRANSCRIPTASE INHIBITORS (NNRTIs)					
Rescriptor	Delavirdine	Two 200-mg tablets twice a day	Rash, increased liver enzymes, and headaches.	April 4, 1997	Take with or without food. May need to reduce the dose of any PIs being taken at the same time.
Sustiva (also known as Stocrin)	Efavirenz	One 600-mg tablet once a day.	Rash; central nervous system symptoms, such as drowsiness, insomnia, confusion, inability to concentrate, dizziness, and vivid dreams; increased liver enzymes; false-positive drug testing (marijuana); and birth defects if taken during pregnancy.	September 17, 1998	Take on an empty stomach at bedtime to reduce side effects. The dosage of some PIs may need to be increased or boosted with Norvir.
Intelence	Etravirine	Two 100-mg tablets twice a day.	Rash, nausea.	June 18, 2008	Take with food. May not be combined with certain Norvir boosted PIs, but other PIs must be boosted with Norvir; Do not use with other NNRTIs.
Viramune	Nevirapine	One 200-mg tablet once a day for 14 days, then one 200-mg tablet twice a day.	Black Box warning: Severe, life-threatening liver problems, notably among women with T-cell counts >250; severe skin reactions; careful dosing and monitoring needed at start of treatment.	June 21, 1996	Take with or without food. Dosage of certain PIs may need to be increased or boosted with Norvir. Do not use with Reyataz.
Atripla	Efavirenz, tenofovir, and emtricitabine	One tablet once a day. Contains two nucleoside reverse transcriptase inhibitors (NRTIs) and one NNRTI in one tablet.	Similar side effects to Sustiva (efavirenz), Viread (tenofovir), and Emtriva (emtricitabine). Please note Viread's and Emtriva's Black Box warnings.	August 2, 2004	Can be used with or without other HIV medications. Take on an empty stomach at bedtime to reduce side effects.
PROTEASE INHIBITORS (PIs)					
Aptivus	Tipranavir	Two 250-mg capsules plus two 100-mg Norvir capsules twice a day.	Black Box warning: Bleeding in the brain; hepatitis (extra care needed for HIV-positive people with hepatitis B or C). Rash, increased cholesterol, increased triglycerides, lipodystrophy, increased bleeding in patients with hemophilia.	June 22, 2005	Take with food. Approved only for treatment-experienced patients. Do not take with other PIs except for Norvir.

TABLE 31-2 ■ HIV DRUGS BY CLASS—cont'd

BRAND NAME	GENERIC NAME	DOSE	SIDE EFFECTS	FDA APPROVAL	COMMENTS
Crixivan	Indinavir	Two 400-mg capsules twice a day; preferred regimen is two 400-mg capsules twice a day plus one or two 100-mg Norvir capsules twice a day.	Kidney stones, nausea, vomiting, diarrhea, increased cholesterol, increased triglycerides, increased glucose (sugar), lipodystrophy, increased bilirubin (not harmful), increased bleeding in patients with hemophilia. Others: headache, weakness, blurred vision, dizziness, rash, metallic taste, low platelets, hair loss, anemia.	March 13, 1996	Take on an empty stomach or with a light, low-fat snack. If taking the preferred dose, take with or without food. Drink six glasses of water each day to prevent kidney stones.
Invirase	Saquinavir	Two 500-mg capsules plus one 100-mg Norvir capsule twice a day.	Nausea, diarrhea, stomach discomfort, headache, increased cholesterol, increased triglycerides, lipodystrophy, increased glucose (sugar), increased liver enzyme levels, and increased bleeding in patients with hemophilia.	December 6, 1995	Must be used with Norvir. Take with food.
Kaletra (also known as Aluvia)	Lopinavir and ritonavir	Two tablets twice a day or four tablets once a day. Contains two PIs in one tablet.	Nausea, diarrhea, stomach discomfort, headache, increased cholesterol, increased triglycerides, lipodystrophy, increased glucose (sugar), increased liver enzyme levels, and increased bleeding in patients with hemophilia.	September 15, 2000	Take with or without food. Must be taken twice a day and dose may need to be increased if taken with certain other medications.
Lexiva (also known as Telzir)	Fosamprenavir	Two 700-mg tablets twice a day or two 700-mg tablets plus one 100-mg Norvir capsule once or twice a day.	Skin rash, nausea, diarrhea, stomach discomfort, headache, increased cholesterol, increased triglycerides, lipodystrophy, increased glucose (sugar), increased liver enzyme levels, and increased bleeding in patients with hemophilia.	October 20, 2003	Take with or without food. If other PIs have been taken in the past, only take the twice-a-day, Norvir boosted combination.

Continued

TABLE 31-2 ■ HIV DRUGS BY CLASS—cont'd

BRAND NAME	GENERIC NAME	DOSE	SIDE EFFECTS	FDA APPROVAL	COMMENTS
Norvir	Ritonavir	Six 100-mg capsules twice a day.	Nausea, vomiting, diarrhea, appetite loss, numbness or tingling around the mouth, increased cholesterol, increased triglycerides, lipodystrophy, and diabetes.	March 1, 1996	The full dose is rarely used. It is most often used to boost the levels of other PIs in the blood. Needs refrigeration in hot weather.
Prezista	Darunavir	Two 400-mg tablets plus one 100-mg Norvir capsule once a day (for those starting HIV medication) or one 600-mg tablet plus one 100-mg Norvir capsule twice a day.	Nausea, diarrhea, stomach discomfort, headache, increased cholesterol levels, increased triglycerides, lipodystrophy, increased glucose (sugar), increased liver enzyme levels, inflammation of the nose and throat, and increased bleeding in patients with hemophilia.	June 23, 2006	Take with food. Must be used with Norvir.
Reyataz	Atazanavir	Two 200-mg capsules once a day or one 300-mg capsule plus one 100-mg Norvir capsule once a day.	Increased bilirubin (not harmful), abnormal electrocardiogram results, increased glucose (sugar), lipodystrophy, and increased bleeding in patients with hemophilia.	June 20, 2003	Take with food. Do not combine with Viramune. Regimen may vary depending on other medications being taken.
Viracept	Nelfinavir	Two 625-mg tablets twice a day or five 250-mg tablets twice a day or three 250-mg tablets three times a day.	Diarrhea, increased cholesterol, increased triglycerides, lipodystrophy, increased glucose (sugar), increased liver enzyme levels, increased bleeding in patients with hemophilia, increased liver enzymes.	March 14, 1997	Take with food. Can be dissolved in water (if trouble swallowing pill form).
Agenerase	Amprenavir	Twenty-four 50-mg capsules twice a day (to be combined with other HIV medications).	Nausea, vomiting, diarrhea or loose stools, taste disorders, tingling feeling (especially around the mouth), depression and mood problems, changes in body fat, high blood sugar or diabetes, diabetes complications, increased cholesterol, or increased triglycerides, severe or life-threatening rash.	April 15, 1999	Take with or without food. High fat meals will decrease the absorption of the medication. Do not take additional vitamin E. May need to adjust the dosage when taken with other HIV medications.

TABLE 31-2 ■ HIV DRUGS BY CLASS—cont'd

BRAND NAME	GENERIC NAME	DOSE	SIDE EFFECTS	FDA APPROVAL	COMMENTS
INTEGRASE INHIBITORS (INIs)					
Isentress	Raltegravir	One 400-mg tablet twice a day.	Diarrhea, nausea, and headache. In clinical trials, blood tests showed abnormally elevated levels of a muscle enzyme—creatine kinase—in some patients receiving Isentress. Isentress should be used with caution by patients who are at increased risk for muscle problems such as myopathy and rhabdomyolysis, which includes patients using other medications known to cause these conditions.	October 12, 2007	Take with or without food.
FUSION					
Fuzeon	Enfuvirtide	One 90-mg injection twice a day.	Skin reactions where Fuzeon is injected can include itching, swelling, redness, pain or tenderness, hardened skin, or bumps; increased risk of bacterial pneumonia; serious allergic reaction (rare).	March 13, 2003	Comes as a powder that must be mixed with sterile water in a vial before use.
RECPTOR SITE/ENTRY INHIBITOR					
Selzentry (also known as Celsentri)	Maraviroc	One 150-mg tablet or one 300-mg tablet or two 300-mg tablets twice a day. Reacts with many other HIV medications, which will affect the regimen.	Cough, fever, colds, rash, muscle and joint pain, stomach pain, and dizziness. Less common side effects include cardiovascular problems and liver toxicity. Because Selzentry blocks the CCR5 co-receptor located on some immune system cells, there is a theoretical risk of developing infections and cancers.	August 6, 2007	Take with or without food. Effective only against CCR5-tropic HIV.

FDA, U.S. Food and Drug Administration.

Viral Load Measurement

Testing for the amount of HIV in plasma by measuring viral RNA has become a standard component of the management of HIV-infected patients.[23] There are important prognostic implications for the amount of viral load in persons with HIV disease.[24] In patients with higher viral loads, disease progression is more rapid, both immunologically, in terms of the rate of CD4 cell count decline, and clinically, in terms of development of AIDS-defining illness. In addition, the plasma levels in HIV-positive pregnant women directly correlate with the risk of perinatal transmission.[25] Viral load is an important useful marker for judging the effectiveness of various antiretroviral drug interventions.[26,27]

There are several assays available for testing HIV for resistance to antiretroviral agents. Genotype or phenotype testing is used to determine whether the virus has mutated.

The results of genotype or phenotype testing provide important information about resistance to specific antiretroviral drugs. If a mutant form is resistant to a particular antiretroviral drug, the HAART regimen may be altered so that the potential for viral suppression is maximized. Changes in the drug combinations used for HAART to respond to viral resistance are referred to as *salvage therapy*. Like genotypic testing, phenotypic testing may not detect small subpopulations of resistant HIV.[28]

Researchers continue to work on developing effective HAART components and vaccines. The primary goal of antiretroviral therapy is to achieve prolonged suppression of HIV replication.[23,29] At this time, there are six classes of HIV medications. Two classes of drugs, receptor site inhibitors and fusion inhibitors (FIs), work to prevent HIV from successfully entering the cell. CCR5 inhibitors (CIs) include maraviroc (Selzentry), a CCR5 co-receptor antagonist (receptor site inhibitor). Receptor site inhibitors are the most recently approved class of drugs. FIs such as enfuvirtide (Fuzeon) or T-20 act outside the T cells by blocking the entry of HIV into the cell. T-20 is often used as part of salvage therapy; it is a twice-daily injectable drug with a cost of more than $25,000 per year.

The four other classes of drugs work within the cell by interfering with one of three enzymes that are involved with the replication process: reverse transcriptase, integrase, and protease. These classes include nucleoside reverse transcriptase inhibitors (NRTIs), nonnucleoside reverse transcriptase inhibitors (NNRTIs), integrase inhibitors (INIs), and protease inhibitors (PIs). In 1987, zidovudine (AZT), an NRTI, was first approved by the U.S. Food and Drug Administration. Since that time, several more NRTI drugs have been approved.[30] Other drugs, such as nevirapine and efavirenz, also inhibit the reverse transcriptase enzyme, but they are not nucleoside analogs. These NNRTIs bind to the enzymatic binding pocket of the reverse transcriptase gene and block binding by the nucleosides.[31] Like reverse transcriptase, integrase is an enzyme that is active in the early stages of the replication process, and INIs can be used to interrupt its function by preventing the integration of the virus in the host cell's DNA.[32] INIs, such as elvitegravir or raltegravir (Isentress), are one of the most recently approved classes of drugs. Another drug target for anti-HIV agents is the protease enzyme. The PI drugs are structurally different from other drugs and include agents such as ritonavir, indinavir, nelfinavir, and saquinavir.[33]

HAART may be NNRTI or PI based (i.e., NNRTI and PI drugs are used in combination with an NRTI such as AZT). There has been a gradual evolution of pharmacology that has allowed for multiple drugs to be combined into one pill. Thus the number of pills required per day as well as the administration schedule have become increasingly more manageable over recent years. However, drugs from different classes (NRTI, NNRTI, and PI) are typically included in HAART. The current recommendation from the Department of Health and Human Services for a treatment-naïve patient is either one NNRTI and two NRTIs or a PI (boosted with ritonavir) and two NRTIs.[22] Because of the rapidly evolving nature of HAART, the reader is advised to consult with the CDC for the most current clinical practice guidelines.

Side effects and toxicities are common with drugs used to treat HIV disease. Purported side effects of NRTIs include peripheral neuropathy, myopathy, anemia, gastrointestinal (GI) disturbances, hepatomegaly, and pancreatitis. NNRTIs may cause rash, liver dysfunction, cognitive problems, and lactic acidosis. PIs may cause lipodystrophy, peripheral neuropathy, GI intolerance, hyperlipidemia, hyperglycemia, and liver toxicity. Injection site reactions are common with T-20. This list of side effects is cursory, and the full impact of these and other HIV drugs on the various systems of the body is a continually emerging area. Occasionally an individual's HAART regimen is modified to mitigate the side effects that may occur with specific drugs.

Current medication regimens can significantly reduce the HIV level not only in the peripheral blood but also in the lymphoid tissue and the central nervous system (CNS).[34] The goal of HAART is to reduce HIV viral load to undetectable levels in serum. The greatest challenge with HAART is resistance to one drug in a class of agents, which may induce partial or complete resistance with other agents, depending on the specific mutations involved.[28,35] In a field that is rapidly changing, specific recommendations for antiretroviral therapy are best made by an infectious disease specialist with experience in the management of patients with HIV disease. The major therapeutic decisions include (1) when to initiate therapy, (2) what drugs to prescribe, (3) when to change therapy, and (4) which drugs to change to. When PIs were introduced as a complement to already existing NRTI and NNRTI drugs, the mortality rate of HIV-infected patients and the incidence of opportunistic infections decreased, most likely as a result of the increased use of combination HAART.[36] The role of drugs with immunomodulating activity in combination with HAART is also undergoing extensive research.[37,38] Drug regimens for HIV disease are dynamic, and clinical practice guidelines are consistently updated; many changes in the approach to drug interventions can be expected as HIV infection continues to be a chronic disease.[39]

Vaccines

HIV-positive individuals respond less well than do uninfected persons to most vaccines. The degree of immunodeficiency present at the time of vaccination has an impact on the response to hepatitis A or B, pneumococcal, and influenza A and B vaccines.[40] Patients with a CD4 count of more than 200 cells/mcL have a more successful response to the vaccine. Patients should be informed that the extent and duration of the protective efficacy of these vaccines are still uncertain.

Vaccination for HIV has the potential to prevent or control disease progression. The development of an effective preventative vaccine for HIV is an area of continuing research. The first human immunizations with the potential AIDS vaccine took place in 1986 in healthy seropositive volunteers in France and Zaire. Low levels of both humoral and cell-mediated immune responses resulted. One conclusion of this study is that booster vaccinations could be effective.[41] Several vaccine candidates have been developed and tested in human phase 1 or 2 trials. To date, at least 13 vaccine candidates have been created with use of different forms of recombinant proteins that target the HIV envelope. Research has found that the vaccine candidates introduced antibodies that rarely neutralized HIV progression, as evidenced by assessment of patient blood counts (i.e., CD4 counts). Furthermore, these recombinant proteins rarely produced a cellular response that would target and destroy cells already infected with HIV.[42] Currently there is no evidence of a vaccine that produces extended, high-titer neutralization across a variety of HIV strains.[42] The most recent clinic trial, the Thai Phase III HIV vaccine trial (also known as *RV 144*), was completed in September 2009. The study incorporated two vaccines, a prime vaccine (ALVAC-HIV) and a booster vaccine (AIDSVAX B/E), which were based on strains found in Thailand, where the clinical trial was conducted. The clinical trial involved over 16,000 volunteers who received either the vaccine combination or a placebo. The clinical trial found that the vaccine regimen was safe and modestly effective, demonstrating that the vaccine combination lowered the HIV infection rate by 31.2% compared with the placebo. The study also found that the vaccine had no effect on the viral load of those volunteers who became infected during the clinical trial.[43]

Genetic mutation of the virus further complicates attempts to disable it. Genetically similar but distinguishable strains of HIV can exist in one individual. Furthermore, drug-resistant strains of HIV have been identified.[44] Yet another difficulty with vaccination development is a lack of animal models. Chimpanzees replicate simian immunodeficiency virus, a similar but not identical disease. In addition, an average of 12 years and $231 million is required for a new drug to gain Food and Drug Administration approval. Many major pharmaceutical companies seem wary of the immense research expenses and potential liability risks linked to vaccine development. The result is that smaller biotechnology companies with fewer resources are assailing the complicated problems of HIV infection.[13] Recent advancements and plans for future clinical trials are largely supported by military or government programs. Researchers are optimistic that the vaccine will induce both humoral and cellular immune responses and have no toxic effects. It will protect against initial infection and retard disease onset in infected individuals.

In summary, as of July 2011 no HIV vaccines have been approved for use; there are clinical trials in process and research in this area is ongoing.

Nutrition

Involuntary loss of more than 10% of baseline body weight in a 12-month period or a 5% loss in baseline body weight in a 6-month period with chronic diarrhea or unexplained weakness and fever constitute HIV wasting syndrome.[45] Retrospective demographic research in the United States found that 17.8% of individuals with AIDS had wasting syndrome.[46,47] The ensuing malnutrition contributes to further immunosuppression.[48] Nutritional consultation is critical for those patients experiencing wasting syndrome and as a preventative measure for those who are HIV positive. Studies have been done investigating the effects of nutritional counseling and other measures such as medications, hormone supplementation, and exercise on lean body mass in patients with HIV wasting syndrome. It has been shown that nutritional counseling, medications to inhibit tumor necrosis factor, androgen supplementation, growth hormone administration, and resistance strength training have all been effective in improving lean body mass. Increased caloric intake alone increases lean body mass, but primarily through fat stores. Resistance strength training may prove to be the most beneficial in increasing lean body mass with minimal side effects and minimal cost.[49]

Weight loss or reduction in lean body mass is also a problem for patients using HAART. Comprehensive nutritional intervention is advocated during the early stages of HIV infection to maintain nutritional status. HAART compromises nutrition in HIV patients because of complicated drug and nutrient interactions, adverse side effects including diarrhea and nausea, and in some cases excessive pill loads that must be consumed. Furthermore, HAART has been linked to a condition identified as *HIV-associated lipodystrophy*. This syndrome is marked by various combinations of insulin resistance, hyperlipidemia, visceral adiposity, loss of peripheral fat stores, and dorsocervical fat accrual.[50] Lipodystrophy is a syndrome that makes the nutritional management of HIV more difficult and may necessitate exercise, pharmacological intervention, and diet modifications.[51]

Systemic Manifestations

Integumentary System and Neoplasms

Cutaneous disorders develop in 64% to 90% of all individuals infected with HIV. Most HIV-induced skin findings develop only when the CD4 count falls below 500 cells/mcL. As the CD4 cell count decreases further, multiple cutaneous disorders may develop.[52] There are three AIDS-defining malignancies: Kaposi sarcoma (KS), non-Hodgkin lymphoma (NHL), and cervical cancer. KS was the first neoplastic condition to be related to HIV infection and it remains the most common. However, over the past decade the incidence of KS has diminished as a result of the use of more powerful antiretroviral therapy and maintenance of immune status.[52] KS can involve almost every part of the body, but the most common site of initial KS presentations is the skin or mucous membranes.[53] The disorder manifests as cutaneous purple nodular lesions or as rife visceral lesions. AIDS-KS has been intimately associated with the lymphatic system, specifically, deficient lymphatic transport, nodal dysfunction, and tumors, which contribute to lymphedema.[54]

In KS there is a broad therapeutic spectrum from cryotherapy to systemic chemotherapy.[55] In NHL, early therapeutic intervention is necessary because of the fast progression of the tumor.[56] The cervical cancer in HIV-positive women seems to be more aggressive than in HIV-negative women and requires early therapeutic intervention.[57] The cancer incidence in patients with HIV is reported to be higher among non-black patients.[58]

Several other tumors occur in people with HIV infection: anorectal cancer, lung cancer, malignant testicular tumor, Hodgkin lymphoma, basal cell carcinoma, and malignant melanoma.[56,59] It is beyond the scope of this chapter to detail all aspects of cancer and dermatological concerns; however, the therapist needs to be aware of the importance of differential diagnosis because the skin is the first line of defense of the immune system and further workup may be warranted. See Table 31-3 for integumentary conditions associated with HIV.

TABLE 31-3 ■ HIV AND INTEGUMENTARY CONDITIONS*

VIRAL INFECTIONS	FUNGAL INFECTIONS	BACTERIAL INFECTIONS	ARTHROPOD INFECTIONS	INFLAMMATORY CONDITIONS	MALIGNANCIES	OTHER CONDITIONS
Acute morbilliform rash Herpes simplex Varicella zoster Molluscum contagiosum Human papillomavirus Oral hairy leukoplakia	Tinea Blastomycosis Candidiasis Cryptococcosis Histoplasmosis Pityrosorum folliculitis Pityriasis versicolor Systemic mycoses Pneumocystosis	Cellulitis Ecthyma Impetigo Folliculitis Bacillary angiomatosis	Insect bites Scabies Demodicosis	Seborrheic dermatitis Psoriasis Eczema Pruritic popular eruption of HIV	Kaposi sarcoma Cutaneous B-cell lymphoma Cutaneous T-cell lymphoma Skin cancer (melanoma, squamous cell carcinoma, basal cell carcinoma, and anal carcinoma)	Lipodystrophy Ichthyosis Eosinophilic folliculitis HAART medication side effects

HAART, Highly active antiretroviral therapies.

*Some skin conditions listed in this table are seen in the general population but may be more severe or more difficult to treat in HIV-infected patients.

Musculoskeletal System

Musculoskeletal manifestations of HIV infection are not as common as manifestations seen in other body systems, including the CNS, pulmonary system, and GI tract. Musculoskeletal disorders tend to occur in advanced HIV disease. Knowledge of the different abnormalities that may occur in the musculoskeletal system is crucial to patient management and affects morbidity and mortality. Primary abnormalities are seen as osseous and soft tissue infections, polymyositis, myopathy, and arthritis. Spinal infections such as pyogenic discitis, osteomyelitis, spinal TB, and epidural abscesses are more likely to occur in HIV-positive individuals than in those who are HIV negative. Discitis and osteomyelitis are more common in patients with CD4 counts >200 cells/mcL, whereas spinal TB and epidural abscesses are more common in patients with CD4 counts <200 cells/mcL.[60] Secondary musculoskeletal complications are often a result of the various compensatory patterns of gait as a result of HIV-related peripheral neuropathy syndrome or the change in biomechanics of the foot and ankle from KS and NHL.[61] These lead to potential spinal changes and back pain.

HIV-positive patients with acute myopathy typically have proximal muscle weakness and elevated creatine phosphokinase levels.[62] Patients may have initial symptoms of difficulty with basic activities of daily living (ADLs), such as rising from a chair or climbing stairs. If myopathy is in an acute inflammatory stage, resisted exercise is contraindicated.

Arthritis in HIV-positive individuals has a wide spectrum of presentations ranging from mild arthralgias to severe joint disability.[63] Arthritides seen in patients with AIDS have been classified into five groups on the basis of clinical presentation: (1) painful articular syndrome, (2) acute symmetrical polyarthritis, (3) spondyloarthropathic arthritis (Reiter syndrome, psoriatic arthritis), (4) HIV-associated arthritis, and (5) septic arthritis.[64] Standardized diagnostic tests and treatments are the same for HIV-positive individuals with musculoskeletal impairments. A key difference to consider is the effect of HAART medications. Side effects of HAART may evoke symptoms that may complicate the differential diagnosis. The HAART drugs taken by HIV-positive patients may limit pharmaceutical treatment options for musculoskeletal conditions, namely immunosuppressant medications. See Table 31-4 for musculoskeletal conditions associated with HIV.

Cardiopulmonary System

Pulmonary diseases continue to be important causes of illness and death in patients with HIV infection, but changes in therapy and demographics of HIV-infected populations are changing their manifestations. The risk for development of specific disorders is related to the degree of immunosuppression, HIV risk group, area of residence, and use of prophylactic therapies.[65] Sinusitis and bronchitis occur frequently in the HIV-positive population, more so than in the general public. The increasing population of HIV-positive drug users is reflected in the increasing incidence of TB and bacterial pneumonia.

Anti-*Pneumocystis* prophylaxis has reduced the incidence of and mortality from PCP. The PCP-causing organism is usually acquired in childhood, and 65% to 85% of healthy adults possess PCP antibodies. Reactivation of latent infection is responsible for the recurrent fever, dyspnea, and hypoxia that characterize PCP.[66,67] Adjunctive corticosteroid therapy has improved the outlook for respiratory failure.[65] Multiple studies have shown that the use of corticosteroids in HIV-positive patients in acute respiratory failure has not increased the risk for the development of opportunistic infections.[68]

Mycobacterial infections in HIV-infected individuals usually manifest as either MAC infection or TB.[5] Steadily increasing incidence of infection by *Mycobacterium tuberculosis* is likely the result of two factors: better medical management of HIV as a whole and the development of multidrug-resistant strains of mycobacteria. MAC infection

TABLE 31-4 ■ HIV AND MUSCULOSKELETAL CONDITIONS

CONDITION	SYMPTOMS AND COMMENTS	TREATMENTS
Reactive arthritis, septic arthritis, bursitis	Asymmetrical oligoarthritis or monoarticular arthritis, dactylitis, enthesopathy, joint effusion Most common in the foot and ankle May range from mild to severe Inflammation of synovial fluid, often gram negative	Surgical debridement Aspiration of fluid from the joint, antibiotics ROM activities
Idiopathic polymyositis	Bilateral proximal muscle weakness, elevated serum CK levels Often occurs early in infection Exact mechanism is still undetermined	Discontinue medication that causes inflammation or irritation of the muscle Antiinflammatory medications Corticosteroid medications
Zidovudine-associated myopathy	Causes mitochondrial toxicity Gradual myalgias, muscle tenderness, proximal muscle weakness, elevated CK levels	Discontinue AZT therapy CK levels return to normal within 4 weeks (of discontinuing AZT), weakness resolves in 8 weeks
Pyomyositis	Solitary or multiple muscle abscesses that are not formed by local extension from superficial subcutaneous tissue Acute, severe muscle pain with or without erythema, fever, edema Elevated ESR and CK levels Pathogen is most often *Staphylococcus aureus* Differential diagnosis includes muscle strain, contusion, hematoma, cellulitis, deep venous thrombosis, osteomyelitis, septic arthritis, and neoplasm	If not treated, septic shock and death can result in 3 weeks Open drainage or debridement of the site Antibiotic therapy
Psoriatic arthritis	Cutaneous manifestations (macropapules on the knees, elbows, scalp and trunk), nail changes, arthritic changes or deformities, soft tissue swelling, juxtaarticular erosions, osteopenia, osteolysis Five types: asymmetrical oligoarthritis, symmetrical polyarthritis, dominant desquamative interstitial pneumonia, arthritis mutilans, and sacroiliitis or spondylitis without peripheral involvement Synovial fluid usually contains 7000 to 15,000 white blood cells/mcL	NSAIDs Second-line agents (gold, methotrexate, and azathioprine) Intraarticular steroid injection (every 4 to 6 months) ROM activities
Reiter syndrome	Urethritis, conjunctivitis, and arthritis, nail involvement with subungual hyperkeratosis, circinate balanitis, keratoderma hemorrhagica, oral ulcers, uveitis, AIDS foot, weight loss, malaise, lymphadenopathy, and diarrhea Severe course of persistent and erosive polyarthritis, fevers, and enthesopathies, which responds poorly to treatment or has a mild and self-limited course Common enthesopathies include Achilles tendinitis, lateral or medial epicondylitis, rotator cuff tendinitis, and de Quervain tenosynovitis; axial skeleton involvement is rare Broad-based gait and stiff ankles with weight bearing through the lateral margins of the feet because of the painful heel; patients may become severely disabled and wheelchair bound	NSAIDs Second-line agents (gold, methotrexate, and azathioprine) Patients usually obtain relief after 5 to 7 days of therapy Intraarticular steroid injection (every 4 to 6 months) Methotrexate, other immunosuppressive agents, and phototherapy should be used only with extreme caution Early physical therapy and splinting of affected joints as needed to prevent atrophy and contractures
Diffuse infiltrative lymphocytosis syndrome (DLS)	Massive parotid enlargement, xerostomia, and lymphocytic hepatitis caused by CD8 lymphocytic infiltration of the liver Xerophthalmia (dry eyes), xerostomia (dry mouth), salivary gland enlargement, and arthralgias Extraglandular features may be pulmonary, neurological, gastrointestinal, renal, or musculoskeletal	Symptomatic treatment with artificial saliva and tears Antibiotics to address recurrent sinus, middle ear, and oral cavity infections Immunosuppressive therapy should be used only when patients are in life-threatening situations such as pulmonary insufficiency or renal disease Corticosteroids can be used for extraglandular features Radiotherapy to reduce the enlarged parotid gland

Continued

TABLE 31-4 ■ HIV AND MUSCULOSKELETAL CONDITIONS—cont'd

CONDITION	SYMPTOMS AND COMMENTS	TREATMENTS
Avascular necrosis or osteonecrosis	Results from direct or indirect damage to the vascular supply of the affected bone, leading to in situ death of subchondral bone Most common sites are the femoral head followed by the humeral head; may occur in other locations including the wrist (scaphoid [Preiser disease] or lunate [Kienböck disease]), knee, and ankle Deep, throbbing, intermittent pain that may be insidious or sudden in presentation and, in later stages, a loss of motion	Early osteonecrosis may be treated by minimizing the forces across the joint, either through avoiding weight-bearing activity (lower extremity) or through greatly limiting activity such as lifting and carrying (upper extremity) Advanced stages require surgical intervention in an attempt to restore vascularity, provide stabilization, or replace the joint ROM activities
Hypertrophic osteoarthropathy	Systemic disorder affecting bones, joints, and soft tissues, often develops in patients with PCP Severe pain in the lower extremity, digital clubbing, arthralgias, nonpitting edema, periarticular soft tissue involvement of the ankle, knees, and elbows; skin over the affected areas is glistening, edematous, and warm; chronic erythema, paresthesias, and hyperhidrosis may be noted in the hands and feet Radiography reveals extensive periosteal reaction and subperiosteal proliferative changes in the long bones of the lower extremity; bone scan demonstrates increased uptake along the cortical surfaces	Treatment of PCP usually alleviates this condition Surgical or chemical vagotomy or radiation therapy may be necessary in refractory cases
Acute symmetrical polyarthritis	Acute symmetrical polyarthritis exclusive to HIV-infected patients; resembles rheumatoid arthritis, develops in the small joints of the hand Characterized by ulnar deviation of the digits and swan neck deformities Acute onset and negative rheumatoid factor test result help differentiate it from rheumatoid arthritis Radiographic results also mimic those of rheumatoid arthritis, with periarticular osteopenia, joint-space narrowing, and marginal erosions	Gold therapy is effective treatment ROM activities
HIV-associated arthralgia	Asymmetrical, oligoarticular arthritis exclusive to HIV-infected persons; usually occurs in the late stages, but may occur in any stage Characterized by an acute onset of severe pain and disability, predominantly in the large joints such as the knees or ankles Self-limiting; may be mild to moderate severity; usually lasts a few weeks to 6 months Synovial fluid commonly contains only 50 to 2600 white blood cells/mcL Radiography may show diffuse osteopenia but without erosive changes; serum is negative for HLA-B27 and rheumatoid factor Synovial biopsy reveals a chronic mononuclear cell infiltrate	Symptomatic relief with NSAIDs Intraarticular corticosteroid injections ROM activities

AZT, Zidovudine; *CK,* creatine kinase; *ESR,* erythrocyte sedimentation rate; *NSAIDs,* nonsteroidal antiinflammatory drugs; *PCP, Pneumocystis jiroveci* pneumonia; *ROM,* range of motion.

tends to appear late in the course of HIV infection. Initial infection involves the GI and pulmonary tracts and eventually disseminates throughout the body. This disorder probably is caused not by latent reactivation of the organism but rather by primary infection by ingestion or inhalation.[69] Signs and symptoms of MAC infection include pneumonia, fever, weight loss, malaise, sweats, anorexia, abdominal pain, and diarrhea.

As in many other infections, initial signs and symptoms of TB include fever, weight loss, malaise, cough, lymph node tenderness, and night sweats. Pulmonary involvement accounts for 75% to 100% of cases of TB infection in

HIV-positive patients, but extrapulmonary infection, especially in lymph nodes and bone marrow, occurs in up to 60% of these individuals as well.[66,69-71] Less common areas of infection include the CNS, cardiac, and mucosal tissues. TB is communicable, preventable, and treatable. Tuberculin skin testing with follow-up chest radiographs when appropriate should be available and routinely offered to individuals at HIV testing sites. Individuals at highest risk for concomitant HIV and TB infections include the homeless, intravenous drug users, and prison inmates.[66,71] The risk of infection in health care personnel and in the general public is a concern. Isolation rooms that provide negative-pressure, nonrecirculated ventilation, specific air filters, and higher air exchange rates offer the best protection to health care providers exposed to TB-infected individuals. Properly fitted face masks that filter droplet nuclei should be worn. Monitoring of personnel who work with these populations will identify the need for necessary preventive therapy.[66] The majority of health care facilities require personnel to have yearly screenings and have established guidelines to prevent the spread of TB in their patient population and within their workforce.

CMV can affect the GI and respiratory tracts but primarily targets optic structures and the CNS; 40% to 100% of healthy adults possess CMV antibodies.[72] However, an individual who is immunosuppressed becomes more vulnerable to symptoms of infection with CMV. Predominant consequences of HIV-CMV co-infection are unilateral or bilateral deficits in visual acuity, visual field cuts, and blindness.

Although most other organ system involvement has been extensively described in studies and reviews, cardiac complications related to HIV infection have remained less characterized. Most studies have described cardiac problems as postmortem findings, although some clinical series have been reported. It is now clear that cardiac involvement in people living with HIV infection is quite common. Pericardial effusion and myocarditis are among the most commonly reported cardiac abnormalities. Cardiomyopathy, endocarditis, and coronary vasculopathy have also been reported. It is now apparent that HIV infection itself, the medical management of HIV disease, and secondary opportunistic infections can all affect the myocardium, pericardium, endocardium, and blood vessels.[72,73] Cardiovascular risk in HIV-positive patients depends on several factors: direct and indirect vascular effects of chronic exposure to the virus, metabolic effects from prolonged HAART, the normal aging process (important to consider given the increased life expectancy of HIV-positive patients), and other cardiovascular risk factors (such as diet and genetics).[74]

Body fat changes and lipid abnormalities have been reported in individuals with HIV disease.[75] Known as *lipodystrophy* or *fat redistribution syndrome,* these body fat and metabolic changes have been connected to PI use.[76] It is estimated that 50% of HIV-positive individuals taking HAART develop these metabolic conditions.[77] These body fat changes may have strong implications for patients undergoing rehabilitation interventions. Signs and symptoms of the syndrome vary, and not all need to be present in any particular patient. However, in both men and women, three main components of the syndrome have emerged. These include changes in body shape, hyperlipidemia, and insulin resistance. Clinically, distinct body shape changes are apparent. The most prevalent include increased abdominal growth, dorsocervical fat pad, benign symmetrical lipomatosis, lipodystrophy, and breast hypertrophy in women.[78,79] The increased abdominal growth is characterized by a redistribution and accumulation of fat in the central visceral areas of the body.[79,80] Corresponding symptoms include GI discomfort, bloating, distention, and fullness.[80]

In addition to visible signs and symptoms, adverse changes in lipid, glucose, and insulin levels have been reported.[81] A number of studies have revealed hyperlipidemia to be present in HIV-positive patients, many of whom, but not all, were undergoing PI therapy.[82]

To date, the exact cause of lipodystrophy has not been determined, but two main theories have been hypothesized. Each is still in the process of being studied.[75,83] As individuals live longer with HIV disease, they are at greater risk for development of cardiac disease. Therapists need to be apprised of various changes in laboratory results and signs and symptoms of cardiac disease when designing an exercise program and facilitating the return to functional activities. Screening guidelines (from the Infectious Diseases Society of America HIV Medicine Association [IDSA HIVMA]) include the following:

- Monitor fasting lipid levels before beginning HAART and during the first 4 to 6 weeks of treatment
- Monitor fasting glucose levels before and during HAART
- Monitor body weight and body shape changes on a routine basis

See Table 31-5 for effects of HIV treatment on cardiovascular factors and Table 31-6 for cardiovascular risk factors associated with HIV.

Neurological System

The neurological manifestations of HIV disease are numerous and involve the autonomic nervous system (ANS), CNS, and peripheral nervous system (PNS).[84] Over the course of the disease, up to 70% of patients have some form of neurological symptom.[85] Significant progress in understanding and treating the neurologically involved HIV patient has been made over the past decade.[86] However, HIV continues to affect every division of the human nervous system (Box 31-2). HIV-positive infants show early, catastrophic encephalopathy, loss of brain growth, motor deficits, and cognitive dysfunction.[87] Unfortunately, neurobehavioral dysfunction in early pediatric AIDS remains unchanged after therapy. Dementia develops in some adult patients in spite of the multidrug therapies, and other patients have subtle neurobehavioral changes that diminish the quality of their prolonged lives. Thus HIV infection of the CNS remains an important clinical concern. A variety of host and viral factors are associated with an increased risk of developing HIV-associated neurocognitive disorders (HANDs). Studies are demonstrating similarities between factors that predispose HIV-positive patients to HANDs and the risk factors of Alzheimer dementia, suggesting the potential for a common pathological mechanism.[88] Evidence has shown that HIV-infected monocytes are carried across the blood-brain barrier and infect the macrophages and microglia in the CNS.[89,90] HIV enters the CNS early, yet HANDs often do not occur until advanced stages when the patient is

TABLE 31-5 ■ EFFECTS OF HIV TREATMENT ON CARDIOVASCULAR FACTORS

CARDIOVASCULAR FACTOR	INCIDENCE WHEN TREATED AND UNTREATED	EFFECTS
Lipid metabolism (HDL-C)	Decreases in early infection. With viral suppression it will increase modestly, but not to premorbid levels.	Greater increases seen with NNRTI medications. Increased visceral adipose tissue and upper trunk fat associated with low HDL-C.
Lipid metabolism (LDL-C)	Decreases later in infection. With viral suppression it will increase modestly.	No evidence of direct medication effects on LDL-C.
Lipid metabolism (triglycerides)	Increases in late infection with viral suppression; decreased in early studies of AZT use.	No decrease or increase (primarily with PIs) with HAART medications. Increased visceral adipose tissue and upper trunk fat associated with elevated triglyceride levels.
Glucose metabolism (insulin sensitivity)	Current studies show a decrease if untreated. With viral suppression there is a trend toward decreased insulin sensitivity regardless of the medications; some insulin resistance shows a return to good health.	Some PIs and NRTIs may decrease insulin sensitivity. Increased visceral adipose tissue and upper trunk fat associated with insulin resistance.
Glucose metabolism (insulin secretion)	No evidence of effect if untreated. With viral suppression no evidence of effect.	Some PIs may decrease insulin secretion.
Glucose metabolism (fasting glucose)	No evidence of any effect if untreated. With viral suppression no evidence of effect.	Some PIs may increase glucose production.
Glucose metabolism (glucose tolerance)	No evidence of any effect if untreated. With viral suppression no evidence of effect.	With HAART there may be higher rates of impaired glucose tolerance.
Glucose metabolism (diabetes)	No evidence of differences in prevalence or incidence rates if untreated. With viral suppression there may be a higher prevalence of diabetes.	Higher prevalence of type 2 diabetes associated with certain PIs and NRTIs.
Body composition (lean body mass)	Decreases disproportionately with severe wasting if untreated. Increases modestly with the initiation of effective HAART.	No consistent evidence of direct medication effects.
Body composition (peripheral fat)	Decreases proportionately with wasting if untreated. Will initially increase with the start of effective HAART.	Subsequent depletion of subcutaneous fat in the face, arms, legs, and buttocks is associated with some NRTIs.
Body composition (visceral fat)	Decreased minimally when untreated; increases with effective HAART.	Preserved or increased visceral fat in some patients on HAART.
Renal function (renal disease)	HIV-associated nephropathy, proteinuria, microalbuminuria and elevated cystatin C if untreated. Decreased HIV-associated nephropathy but still have microalbuminuria and elevated cystatin C with viral suppression.	Some HAART may cause impaired renal function.

AZT, Zidovudine; *HAART,* highly active antiretroviral therapies; *HDL-C,* high-density lipoprotein cholesterol; *LDL-C,* low-density lipoprotein cholesterol; *NNRTI,* nonnucleoside reverse transcriptase inhibitor; *NRTI,* nucleoside reverse transcriptase inhibitor; *PI,* protease inhibitor.

categorized as having AIDS. Hypotheses for the development of HANDs in the advanced stages include the loss of immune control with disease progression, heightened immune activation, increased transfer of infected monocytes into the CNS, and variations or mutations in the virus. Because current HAART medications have poor CNS penetration, HANDs continues to pose significant challenges for advanced HIV/AIDS patients.[91] See Table 31-7 for neurological conditions associated with HIV.

Autonomic Nervous System. Dysfunction of the ANS has been associated with HIV infection. This has implications for overall function and the design of a rehabilitation program for people living with HIV disease. In one study, individuals with the greatest ANS involvement had dementia, myelopathy, and sensory peripheral neuropathy. Variations in heart rate, including resting tachycardia, were common. Abnormal blood pressure readings were identified in response to isometric exercise and positional changes (sit to stand and tilting).[92]

Central Nervous System. HIV enters the CNS during the early stages of the disease and is hypothesized to traverse the blood-brain barrier during the initial acute primary infection stage. Although the initial CNS invasion by HIV is asymptomatic in most individuals, affective and cognitive

Text continues on page 965.

TABLE 31-6 ■ CARDIOVASCULAR RISK FACTORS AND HIV

RISK FACTOR	INTERVENTION	RESULT
Cigarette smoking	Interpersonal counseling	Increased quitting rates.
HTN	Dietary and physical activity counseling	Reduced blood pressure.
	Calcium channel blockers, other antihypertensive agents	Drug interactions between calcium channel blockers and protease inhibitors.
Dyslipidemia	Dietary and physical activity counseling	Modest improvements in lipids.
	Statins, fibrates, fish oil, niacin	Statins improve endothelial function. Multiple drug interactions with HAART.
Disordered glucose metabolism	Dietary and physical activity counseling	Improvement in glycemia.
	Metformin and thiazolidinediones	Metformin reduces insulin resistance and visceral adipose tissue. Thiazolidinediones may improve subcutaneous adipose tissue.
Use of HAART	Modification of initial HAART based on metabolic profile and CVD risk	Modest effects on lipids and insulin resistance. Statins and fibrates may be more effective.
	Switching HAART to reduce metabolic side effects	

CVD, Cardiovascular disease; *HAART,* highly active antiretroviral therapies; *HTN,* hypertension.

BOX 31-2 ■ NEUROPATHOLOGY OF HIV INFECTION

CENTRAL NERVOUS SYSTEM (CNS)

Mechanism of CNS infection is unclear, but HIV seems unable to cross blood-brain barrier alone. It probably crosses in macrophages and T cells and most directly affects subcortical structures (basal ganglia, thalamus, brain stem).

AIDS dementia complex, a subcortical dementia, is different from cortical dementia such as Alzheimer disease.

Estimated 70% of infected individuals have cognitive, motor, and behavioral constellation that makes up the AIDS dementia complex.

PERIPHERAL NERVOUS SYSTEM (PNS)

Sensory—In early and middle stages, distal lower extremities are largely involved, with paresthesia and decreased temperature sensitivity. In advanced stages, the patient has decreased ankle and knee reflexes; diminished temperature and vibration sensitivity and proprioception; and hyperesthesia.

Motor—Most closely resembles Guillain-Barré syndrome (progressive muscle weakness → paralysis, decreased deep tendon reflexes). Splints and ankle-foot orthoses may prevent deformities.

AUTONOMIC NERVOUS SYSTEM (ANS)

Arrhythmias, especially tachycardia.

Abnormal blood pressure, orthostasis (may be aggravated by isometric exercises).

ANS involvement has been associated with dementia, myelopathy, and peripheral sensory neuropathies.

TABLE 31-7 ■ HIV AND NEUROLOGICAL CONDITIONS

STAGE 1 HIV DISEASE (CD4 >500 CELLS/MCL)	STAGE 2 HIV DISEASE (CD4 200-499 CELLS/MCL)	STAGE 3 HIV DISEASE (CD4 <200 CELLS/MCL)
Aseptic meningitis	Cognitive impairment	HIV encephalopathy (dementia)
Acute encephalopathy with seizures and confusion	Distal sensory polyneuropathy	CNS toxoplasmosis
Inflammatory demyelinating polyneuropathy (Guillain-Barré syndrome)	Myelopathy	CMV infection
Cranial nerve palsies (e.g., Bell palsy)	Myopathy	Primary CNS lymphoma
Herpes zoster (shingles)		PML
Distal sensory polyneuropathy		

Continued

TABLE 31-7 ■ HIV AND NEUROLOGICAL CONDITIONS—cont'd

CONDITION	COMMENTS AND SYMPTOMS	PROGNOSIS AND TREATMENT
AIDS dementia complex (ADC; HIV-associated encephalopathy)	Occurs primarily in persons with more advanced HIV infection (CD4 <200 cells/mcL); mild cognitive impairment may occur in earlier stages. Symptoms: encephalitis (inflammation of the brain), behavioral changes, and a gradual decline in cognitive function (decreased concentration, memory, and attention). May develop severe global dementia with memory loss and language impairment. Progressive slowing of motor function (decreased balance, weakness, decreased coordination) and loss of dexterity and coordination.	When left untreated it can be fatal. If ADC develops during treatment with HAART, additional or alternative agents should be tried. Neuroprotective therapies or global memory-enhancing agents such as memantine (Namenda) or donepezil (Aricept) may be useful in some individuals. Patients must often take multiple medications, many of which can affect thinking and memory and make the symptoms of ADC worse.
CNS lymphomas	Cancerous tumors that either begin in the brain or result from a cancer that has spread from another site in the body. Almost always associated with the Epstein-Barr virus. Symptoms: headache, seizures, vision problems, dizziness, speech disturbance, paralysis, and mental deterioration. May develop one or more CNS lymphomas.	Prognosis is poor owing to advanced and increasing immunodeficiency.
Cryptococcal meningitis	Manifests as meningitis, a space-occupying lesion, or meningoencephalitis; the fungus first invades the lungs and spreads to the covering of the brain and spinal cord, causing the inflammation. Symptoms: fatigue, fever, headache, nausea, memory loss, confusion, photophobia, stiff neck, altered vision, drowsiness, and vomiting. Develops when CD4 cell counts fall below 100 cells/mcL.	If untreated, patients with cryptococcal meningitis may lapse into a coma and die. Treatment relies on amphotericin B (Fungizone), which may be combined with flucytosine (Ancobon). An alternative for less severe cases is fluconazole (Diflucan), which is also the drug of choice for long-term prophylaxis (preventive therapy). Amphotericin B is an alternative maintenance therapy for people who relapse on fluconazole or do not tolerate it. Hydrocephalus can occur at times and requires a ventriculoperitoneal shunt (surgical drain of spinal fluid). Visual loss can be addressed by optic nerve surgery.
Cytomegalovirus (CMV) infections	Herpesvirus that causes infection of the brain, spinal cord, meninges, or nerve roots can lead to neurological problems such as encephalitis (inflammation of the brain), myelitis (inflammation of the spinal cord), retinitis (inflammation of the retina of the eye), polyradiculitis (inflammation of the spinal nerve roots), peripheral neuropathy, or mononeuritis multiplex. Infection of the spinal cord and nerves can result in weakness in the lower limbs and some paralysis, severe lower back pain, and loss of bladder function. Findings include low-to-normal glucose, normal-to-high protein, and increased numbers of white blood cells.	Untreated CMV encephalitis is almost always fatal and causes death within days to weeks. Anti-CMV drugs must be started immediately, often based on a suspected rather than proven diagnosis. Treatment relies on two drugs, ganciclovir (Cytovene) and foscarnet (Foscavir), used alone or in combination when monotherapy fails. Lifelong maintenance treatment is often necessary.

TABLE 31-7 ■ HIV AND NEUROLOGICAL CONDITIONS—cont'd

CONDITION	COMMENTS AND SYMPTOMS	PROGNOSIS AND TREATMENT
Herpesvirus infections	The herpes zoster virus (causes chickenpox and shingles) can infect the brain and produce encephalitis or myelitis. Signs of shingles include painful blisters (like those seen in chickenpox), itching, tingling, and nerve pain.	Antiherpes drugs: standard treatment for shingles is the drug acyclovir; new medications include famciclovir and valacyclovir. Nerve blocks: anesthetic drugs and/or steroids can be injected either into peripheral nerves or into the spinal column (central nervous system). Drugs normally used to treat depression, epilepsy, or severe pain are sometimes used for the pain of shingles; nortriptyline (antidepressant) is most frequently used for shingles pain; pregabalin is an epilepsy medicine used for pain after shingles. Skin treatments: several creams, gels, and sprays may provide temporary relief from pain; capsaicin has shown good preliminary results; the patch form of the anesthetic lidocaine provides pain relief for some people with shingles.
Neurosyphilis	Sexually transmitted infection caused by the spiral-shaped *Treponema pallidum* bacterium; *T. pallidum* gains access to the body through tiny abrasions of the skin or mucous membranes; this organism may invade the CNS a few months after initial infection. May proceed rapidly from the primary stage (skin chancres, or lesions, appearing about 21 days after infection) to secondary syphilis (skin rash) and tertiary syphilis (infection of different organs, including the brain) as early as 2 months after exposure. Tertiary syphilis may cause hearing loss, dizziness or vertigo, headache, failing vision, cognitive impairment, personality changes, peripheral polyneuropathy, gait imbalance, seizures, or stroke.	Choice of antibiotic depends on the stage of syphilis and follows general guidelines. Most common are different forms of penicillin. Although HIV-infected patients with neurosyphilis respond to antibiotics, they are less likely to have serological improvement than HIV-negative individuals; HIV-associated neurosyphilis may be more difficult to treat and more aggressive.
Progressive multifocal leukoencephalopathy (PML)	Characterized by widespread demyelinating lesions (loss of the insulating myelin sheath around nerves in the brain and spinal cord) and caused by the JC papovavirus. Symptoms include various types of mental deterioration, vision loss, speech disturbances, ataxia (inability to coordinate movements), paralysis, brain lesions, and coma; some may have compromised memory and cognition, and seizures may occur when CD4 cell counts fall below 200 cells/mcL. Onset is usually weeks to months.	Relentlessly progressive; death usually occurs within 6 months of initial symptoms. Typically progresses to severe dementia and death over several months. Whether HAART improves survival remains controversial. Survival correlates with suppression of plasma HIV viral load and higher $CD4^+$ cell counts. Death may result not from PML, but from end-stage immunodeficiency. Some positive response has been reported with use of cidofovir (Vistide).
Psychological and neuropsychiatric disorders	Occur in different phases of the HIV infection and AIDS and may take various and complex forms. Some illnesses, such as ADC, are caused directly by HIV infection of the brain, whereas other conditions may be triggered by the drugs used to combat the infection. Patients may experience anxiety disorder, depressive disorders, increased thoughts of suicide, paranoia, dementia, delirium, cognitive impairment, confusion, hallucinations, behavioral abnormalities, malaise, and acute mania.	Treatment options include antidepressants and anticonvulsants. Psychostimulants may also improve depressive symptoms and combat lethargy. Antidementia drugs may relieve confusion and slow mental decline, and benzodiazepines may be prescribed to treat anxiety. Psychotherapy may also help some patients.

Continued

TABLE 31-7 ■ HIV AND NEUROLOGICAL CONDITIONS—cont'd

CONDITION	COMMENTS AND SYMPTOMS	PROGNOSIS AND TREATMENT
Stroke and hemorrhage	Causes include hypertension (high blood pressure), blood vessel abnormalities (aneurysms, vein or artery malformations), hypotension (low blood pressure), coagulopathies (defective blood clotting), thrombotic thrombocytopenic purpura (TTP; characterized by low platelet counts and blood clots), elevated lipids (contributing to coronary artery disease), viral infections of the heart muscle, herpes zoster (shingles), hepatitis C, and cocaine or heroin use. Characterized by the abrupt onset of weakness, language problems, or sensory loss; symptoms often occur on only one side of the body. Imaging studies help differentiate stroke, hemorrhage, infection, and tumors.	Treatment parallels that in the HIV-negative population. If a stroke is diagnosed within three hours after onset, the person may be a candidate for an infusion of tissue plasminogen activator (tPA), an agent that dissolves clots and opens blood vessels. tPA is contraindicated in cases of brain hemorrhage. Lipid-lowering drugs (statins), blood thinners such as warfarin (Coumadin), or antiplatelet agents such as aspirin or clopidogrel (Plavix) are indicated. Specific causes of stroke may require other forms of treatment. Brain hemorrhages occasionally may need to be treated with surgery to remove the mass of blood. Prognosis after a stroke or brain hemorrhage depends on the size and location of the damage; recovery is greatest during the initial few weeks, but improvement often continues for months; inpatient and outpatient rehabilitation is often helpful. Preventive treatment parallels that in the HIV-negative population and includes antiplatelet agents or blood-thinning drugs, removal of plaque from the walls of carotid arteries, and newer techniques of endovascular stenting.
Toxoplasmosis	Caused by the parasite *Toxoplasma gondii.* Signs and symptoms include encephalitis, fever, severe headache that does not respond to treatment, weakness on one side of the body, seizures, lethargy, increased confusion, vision problems, dizziness, problems with speaking and walking, vomiting, and personality changes. Onset is over days to weeks.	Condition is treatable, most improve by day 14 of therapy. Generally responsive to intravenous (IV) antibiotics, and response to therapy is often rapid; agents of choice are sulfadiazine combined with pyrimethamine and folinic acid; for people with sulfa intolerance, clindamycin is an alternative. Steroids may be used to reduce associated swelling in the brain. After the initial regimen is completed, oral maintenance treatment, usually TMP-SMX (Bactrim, Septra), is continued indefinitely to suppress reactivation of the parasite. Prognosis is linked to parallel treatment with HAART to raise the CD4 cell count.
Vacuolar myelopathy	Causes the protective myelin sheath to pull away from nerve cells of the spinal cord, forming small holes called *vacuoles* in nerve fibers. Symptoms include weak and stiff legs and unsteadiness when walking; walking becomes more difficult as the disease progresses, and many patients eventually require a wheelchair.	Prognosis is poor, options are limited, and care is primarily supportive. May improve after starting HAART to stabilize spinal cord damage; maximally potent HAART is required. L-Methionine (also known as *SAMe,* a common dietary supplement) is an experimental treatment.

TABLE 31-7 ■ HIV AND NEUROLOGICAL CONDITIONS—cont'd

CONDITION	COMMENTS AND SYMPTOMS	PROGNOSIS AND TREATMENT
Primary central nervous system (PCNS) lymphoma	Characterized by the growth of abnormal lymphocytes, or white blood cells (B cells and T cells). Occurs in the brain, rarely in the spinal cord, and causes brain lesions and changes in mental functioning. In almost all cases, Epstein-Barr virus (EBV) is found in the lymphoma-related lesions or the CSF. Often associated with CD4 cell counts below 100 cells/mcL. Signs and symptoms are impaired cognition, aphasia (loss of ability to use or understand language), hemiparesis, and seizures. Onset is often more subtle, and progression slower.	Prognosis for PCNS lymphoma is generally poor. Whole brain radiation therapy (radiotherapy) has been the mainstay of treatment; it provides for a median survival of 2-5 months. Steroids are required for at least 48 hours before radiotherapy to minimize swelling; steroids should be continued throughout the course of treatment. High-dose methotrexate has been used with some success, given as frequently as every week for five cycles; combining methotrexate and radiotherapy can achieve survival of 1-2 years. Experimental chemotherapy agents include thiotepa (Thioplex) and procarbazine (Matulane). HAART should be continued.
Meningitis	Inflammation of the meninges, the membranes surrounding the brain and spinal cord. Signs and symptoms are malaise (vague body discomfort), fever, stiff neck, photophobia, and headache; less common are cranial neuropathies (one-sided facial weakness or double vision), confusion, drowsiness, and personality changes. HIV invades the brain early and may cause meningitis within days to weeks after infection. Chronic meningitis, or episodes of acute (rapid onset) meningitis for which no cause is found, can occur anytime during the course of HIV disease.	Treatment and prognosis vary by the specific cause of meningitis, severity at presentation, delay from symptom onset to treatment, and status of immunosuppression.
Tuberculosis meningitis	Bacterial disease caused by *Mycobacterium tuberculosis,* which can be suspended in tiny droplets in the air and transmitted person to person by inhalation. May cause persistent headache, fever, confusion, hemiparesis, seizures, stiff neck, double vision, or hearing loss. Hydrocephalus associated with tuberculosis may lead to drowsiness or stupor and, later, coma. Spinal cord damage can occur if the vertebrae (bones that encase the spinal cord) are infiltrated by TB (Pott disease) or as a result of abscesses inside or outside the spinal cord.	Triple antibiotic therapy—isoniazid, rifampin (Rifadin), and pyrazinamide—for 12-24 months is required; it is important that all doses be taken as directed. In cases of drug-resistant TB, a fourth drug, ethionamide (Trecator), should be added to this regimen. HAART should be continued. Significant interactions can occur between rifampin and protease inhibitors (PIs), so an alternative anti-TB drug may be necessary.
Distal sensory polyneuropathy	Damage to sensory nerves in the extremities (feet and hands), is the most common type of HIV-associated neuropathy. Nerves may be injured directly by HIV or by HIV-induced macrophages that secrete neurotoxic substances. May also be caused by nutritional and vitamin imbalances or drug toxicity, especially use of d4T (stavudine, Zerit), ddI (didanosine, Videx), or ddC (zalcitabine, Hivid). Occurs at any stage of HIV disease.	Treatment of symptoms may include local ointments (capsaicin, Aspercreme), antidepressant medications (amitriptyline [Elavil]), or antiepileptic medications (gabapentin [Neurontin], lamotrigine [Lamictal], carbamazepine [Tegretol]). Duloxetine (Cymbalta; an SSRI antidepressant) is FDA approved for painful diabetic polyneuropathy and is currently being used for HIV-associated painful polyneuropathy. Pregabalin (Lyrica; an antiepileptic drug) is under FDA review. Drugs should be chosen that are unlikely to interact with or influence the effectiveness of anti-HIV drugs. Lidoderm patches may provide partial pain relief without any systemic side effects and can be combined with oral drugs.

Continued

TABLE 31-7 ■ HIV AND NEUROLOGICAL CONDITIONS—cont'd

CONDITION	COMMENTS AND SYMPTOMS	PROGNOSIS AND TREATMENT
Inflammatory demyelinating polyneuropathy (IDP)	Inflammation of the myelin sheath that surrounds the spinal and peripheral nerves. Acute form of IDP (AIDP), also known as *Guillain-Barré syndrome* (GBS). Characterized by rapid onset and progression over hours to weeks. Chronic form (CIDP) has slower onset and progression over weeks to months, sometimes with a relapsing course. Both forms are autoimmune conditions in which the immune system attacks nerves. Causes varying degrees of weakness and sensory loss, which can develop in the limbs. Nerves around the head may also be affected and cause symptoms such as facial weakness and double vision. Other symptoms may include pain and diminished reflex responses; may have difficulty with urination and bowel movements, and occasionally respiratory paralysis, irregular heartbeat, and dangerously high or low blood pressure.	Treatment and response rates are similar to those seen in the HIV-negative population. Intravenous immunoglobulin (IVIG), a highly concentrated antibody infusion from many pooled blood donations, is the mainstay of therapy. Plasma exchange, or plasmapheresis, may be helpful; in this procedure antibodies are removed from the blood. Chronic IDP may also necessitate use of corticosteroids such as prednisone.
Mononeuritis multiplex	Painful condition that involves isolated nerves over the arms, legs, or trunk; nerves are affected asymmetrically. The involvement of more than two nerves is generally seen in people with advanced HIV. Patients complain of burning or shooting pain down an arm or leg, then, even as it is resolving, another burning pain will emerge over another nerve pathway down a different arm or leg. Weakness in the distribution of specific nerves is common. Nerves can be affected in the head and the body.	Occurring early in HIV infection. May resolve with HAART. IVIG or plasma exchange should be considered in early or late HIV stages. Late-stage HIV disease may require anti-CMV medications (ganciclovir, foscarnet).
Polyradiculopathy	Damage to the nerve roots where the nerves exit the spinal cord to form peripheral nerves. Polyradiculopathy may be caused by CMV, or less likely by lymphoma; may also be idiopathic (of unknown origin). Rapidly progressive ascending numbness, pain, and weakness affecting the legs, and later occasionally the arms, is characteristic of the CMV form. Early bowel and bladder control problems may suggest the syndrome. More benign, slower clinical progression characterizes the idiopathic form.	CMV polyradiculopathy is rapidly fatal without therapy. Treatment with foscarnet or ganciclovir may improve or stabilize the condition. HAART also may be useful. The idiopathic form may improve spontaneously without treatment.

TABLE 31-7 ■ HIV AND NEUROLOGICAL CONDITIONS—cont'd

CONDITION	COMMENTS AND SYMPTOMS	PROGNOSIS AND TREATMENT
Myopathy	HIV-associated myopathies fall into several categories: some are caused by drug toxicity, for instance, from cholesterol-lowering drugs (statins), ddI, or AZT (zidovudine [Retrovir]); others are caused by a variety of bacterial, viral, and other infections; still others, such as polymyositis (inflammatory disease of muscles), are caused by an abnormal immune response; HIV wasting syndrome may result from HIV infection itself. Progressive muscle weakness is the typical presentation, with the speed of progression depending on the cause.	If medications are the likely cause, they may need to be stopped or replaced. Muscle infections are treated with drugs specific to the responsible bacterium, virus, or other infectious agent. When inflammation results from an overactive immune system, corticosteroids may be a treatment option.

CMV, Cytomegalovirus; *CNS,* central nervous system; *CSF,* cerebrospinal fluid; *FDA,* U.S. Food and Drug Administration; *HAART,* highly active antiretroviral therapies; *PML,* progressive multifocal leukoencephalopathy; *SSRI,* selective serotonin reuptake inhibitors; *TB,* tuberculosis; *TMP-SMX,* trimethoprim-sulfamethoxazole.

deficits may develop.[93] It is not possible in this context to discuss the neuropathological features of each of the many secondary infections and neoplasms of HIV illness. It is important to realize, however, that the clinical manifestations of these pathological processes overlap with one another and with the signs and symptoms of primary HIV infection of the CNS; lesions of the CNS can be the site of more than one opportunistic disease process simultaneously. In Table 31-8, a wide variety of organisms or conditions responsible for the neurological manifestations associated with HIV infection are listed. These include primary and secondary viral, protozoan, fungal, and *Mycobacterium* infections, as well as neoplasms and iatrogenic conditions. Infectious processes may cause large lesions in the brain, such as meningitis, encephalitis, or both. Such infections cause neurocognitive impairments that develop as dementia, amnesia, or delirium.[93] Thirty percent to 40% of healthy adults have contracted toxoplasmosis, caused by *Toxoplasma gondii.*[34,94] Unchecked by the immune system, toxoplasmosis results in CNS dysfunction—namely, altered cognition, headache, focal neurological deficits, encephalitis, and seizures. Cerebellar disorders associated with HIV infection are typically the result of discrete cerebellar lesions resulting from opportunistic infections such as toxoplasmosis and progressive multifocal leukoencephalopathy or primary CNS lymphoma.[95] CNS lymphoma results in cognitive dysfunction and presentation of fever, focal neurological impairments, headache, seizures, and motor deficits.[93]

Evidence supports that the neurotoxic effect of HIV is more likely to affect the basal ganglia, the frontal neocortex, the white matter tracts connecting the regions (such as the fronto-striato-thalamocortical loops), the temporal cortices (including the hippocampus), and the parietal cortices.[96] A relationship between stroke and AIDS has been reported.[97,98] The most common cause of cerebral infarction in both clinical and autopsy series was nonbacterial thrombotic endocarditis. Intracerebral hemorrhages were usually associated with thrombocytopenia, primary CNS lymphoma, and metastatic KS.

HIV-related conditions in the spinal cord include not only HIV myelitis, opportunistic infections, and lymphomas but also vacuolar myelopathy, which affects predominantly the dorsolateral white matter tracts. The cause of vacuolar myelopathy is not understood, and it has not been unequivocally linked with HIV infection.[99] Vacuolar myelopathy may affect up to 30% of untreated adults with advanced HIV/AIDS, and the incidence may be even higher in children infected with HIV.[100] Unless it is treated with effective antiretroviral therapy, vacuolar myelopathy of the spinal cord associated with moderate clinical disability develops in many patients with AIDS.[101]

Treatment for CNS impairments includes an eclectic blend of rehabilitation strategies. Neuromuscular disturbances may first appear as movement disorders. Subtleties of altered movement can be detected early and during subsequent treatment phases. A neurological examination can be performed to determine a diagnosis and prognosis. This may include the level of the lesion, neuromuscular deficits, need for assistive devices, ability to perform ADLs, and functional abilities. Various quality-of-life assessments used with the HIV population can be found in Table 31-9.

Peripheral Nervous System. Possible neurological complications associated with HIV disease that may affect the PNS include meningitis, ataxia, myelopathy, and encephalitis. PNS diseases have been reported in up to 50% of HIV-infected individuals, resulting in distal polyneuropathy, Guillain-Barré syndrome, and mononeuropathy.[102]

Distal symmetrical polyneuropathy (DSP) is the most common form of neuropathy in HIV infection. The most frequent complaints in DSP are numbness, burning, and paresthesias in the feet. These symptoms are typically symmetrical and often so severe that patients have contact hypersensitivity and gait disturbances. Involvement of the upper extremities and distal weakness may occur later in the course of DSP. Neurological examination shows sensory loss to pain and

Text continues on page 970.

TABLE 31-8 ■ COMMON OPPORTUNISTIC DISEASES IN HIV INFECTION

DISEASE AND PATHOGEN	SITES OF INFECTION	SYMPTOMS	MEDICATIONS AND SIDE EFFECTS	DISEASE-SPECIFIC PRECAUTIONS
PCP—*Pneumocystis jiroveci,* a protozoan found in air, water, and soil, carried by domestic animals, and possibly latent in most people.	Lungs; sometimes spreads to the spleen, lymph nodes, and blood in late disease	Fever, cough, shortness of breath, chills, chest pain, sputum production	Trimethoprim-sulfamethoxazole: rash, itching, Stevens-Johnson syndrome, extreme fatigue, dysphagia, fever, leukopenia, sore throat, thrombocytopenia, hepatitis, hematuria, diarrhea, dizziness, headache, anorexia, nausea, vomiting Intramuscular or intravenous pentamidine isethionate: azotemia, serum creatinine elevations, pain and induration at intramuscular sites, abscess or necrosis at injection sites, elevated liver function test results, leukopenia, nausea, vomiting, hypotension, syncope, blood sugar imbalances Aerosolized pentamidine isethionate: investigational Dapsone: nausea, vomiting, abdominal pain, vertigo, blurred vision, tinnitus, insomnia, fever, headache, phototoxicity, lupus, anemia Sulfadoxine-pyrimethamine: allergic skin reactions, nausea and vomiting, glossitis, stomatitis, headache, peripheral neuritis, mental depression, fatigue, weakness	None
Toxoplasmosis—*Toxoplasma gondii,* a protozoan found in air, water, soil, and some cats and other animals. Most often acquired by ingestion of uncooked infected lamb or pork, unpasteurized dairy products, raw eggs, or vegetables. Mothers can give it to unborn children. Other human-human transmission does not occur.	Produces lesions in the CNS; may also involve heart and lungs	Fever, chills, headache, visual disturbances, lethargy, confusion, hemiparesis, seizures	Sulfadiazine: same as for trimethoprim-sulfamethoxazole Pyrimethamine: anorexia, vomiting, megaloblastic anemia, leukopenia, thrombocytopenia, glossitis	None
Cryptosporidiosis—*Cryptosporidium,* a protozoan primarily acquired through oral contact with feces of an infected animal, or oral sexual contact with an infected person	GI tract	Copious diarrhea, abdominal pain, anorexia, nausea, vomiting, dehydration, weight loss, weakness, fever	Spiramycin: nausea, vomiting, diarrhea, abdominal pain Eflornithine: investigational	Gloves and gown or apron when handling feces Private room when patient has poor hygiene

TABLE 31-8 ■ COMMON OPPORTUNISTIC DISEASES IN HIV INFECTION—cont'd

DISEASE AND PATHOGEN	SITES OF INFECTION	SYMPTOMS	MEDICATIONS AND SIDE EFFECTS	DISEASE-SPECIFIC PRECAUTIONS
Isosporiasis—*Isospora belli,* a protozoan primarily acquired through eating uncooked beef or pork or through oral sexual contact with an infected person	GI tract	Diarrhea, abdominal pain, nausea, vomiting, anorexia, weight loss, weakness, fever	Trimethoprim-sulfamethoxazole: see under PCP—*P. jiroveci*	Gloves and gown or apron when handling feces Private room when patient has poor hygiene
Mycobacterium avium-intracellulare infection—*M. avium-intracellulare,* a bacterium found in soil, water, animals, eggs, and unpasteurized dairy products and other foods. Infection is atypical and noncommunicable.	Disseminated	Fever, malaise, night sweats, anorexia, diarrhea, weight loss	Isoniazid: paresthesia and peripheral neuropathy, elevated liver function test values, anorexia, nausea, vomiting, fatigue, malaise, weakness Rifabutin: hepatotoxicity, neutropenia, nausea, vomiting, diarrhea, rash, itching Clofazimine: reddish-brown discoloration of skin, conjunctiva, sweat, hair, urine, and feces; abdominal pain, diarrhea Ethambutol: reversible blurring of vision, anaphylaxis, skin irritation, nausea, vomiting, fever Cycloserine: convulsions, drowsiness, headache, tremor, other CNS disturbances Ethionamide: nausea, vomiting, peripheral and optic neuritis, mental depression, postural hypotension, rash Rifampin: urine discoloration, heartburn, nausea, vomiting, abdominal cramps, headache, drowsiness, fatigue Streptomycin: nausea, vomiting, vertigo, numbness of the face, rash, fever, itching, elevated white blood cell count	Gloves and gown or apron when handling wound drainage
Candidiasis—*Candida albicans,* a fungus that inhabits the oropharynx, vagina, large intestine, and skin, causing no harm as long as immunity remains undamaged; may occur as a secondary infection in conjunction with herpes simplex virus lesions.	Anywhere skin or mucous membrane is damaged, including through intravenous therapy and pressure monitoring sites	Thrush, esophageal, perianal irritation, vaginitis, proctitis; inflammation around fingernails can be disseminated	Clotrimazole: abdominal pain, diarrhea, nausea, vomiting Nystatin: diarrhea, nausea, vomiting, stomach pain Ketoconazole: hepatitis, gynecomastia, nausea, vomiting, decreased libido, diarrhea, dizziness, drowsiness, photophobia, rash, itching, sleepiness Amphotericin B: fever, shaking chills, hypotension, anorexia, nausea, vomiting, headache and tachypnea	None

Continued

TABLE 31-8 ■ COMMON OPPORTUNISTIC DISEASES IN HIV INFECTION—cont'd

DISEASE AND PATHOGEN	SITES OF INFECTION	SYMPTOMS	MEDICATIONS AND SIDE EFFECTS	DISEASE-SPECIFIC PRECAUTIONS
Cryptococcosis—*Cryptococcus neoformans,* a fungus found in air, water, soil, raw fruits and vegetables, and pigeon droppings found on window ledges and nesting places; acquired by inhalation.	CNS, lungs; can be disseminated	Altered cognition, low-grade fever, headache, nausea, vomiting, meningeal signs	Amphotericin B: fever, shaking chills, hypotension, anorexia, nausea, vomiting, headache and tachypnea Ketoconazole: see under Candidiasis	None
CMV infection—cytomegalovirus, an organism found in saliva, semen, cervical secretions, urine, feces, blood, breast milk. It causes problems only when immunity is compromised.	Disseminated	Fever, profound fatigue, muscle and joint aches, night sweats, impaired vision, cough, dyspnea, abdominal pain, diarrhea	Ganciclovir: leukopenia, bone marrow depression, elevated liver enzymes, edema, nausea, muscle aches, headaches, anorexia, disorientation, rash, phlebitis	Private room if the patient has enteritis and poor hygiene. Gloves and gown or apron for handling excretions and secretions if soiling is likely
Herpes simplex virus (HSV) infection—HSV-1 is spread by contact with infected oral secretions. HSV-2 is spread by contact with infected genital secretions. Patient can spread either variety by touching lesions then touching other body parts.	Mouth, perianal area; can be disseminated	Painful burning, itching vesicular lesions; sometimes colitis, pericarditis, esophageal infection	Acyclovir: rash, diarrhea, light-headedness, headache, nausea, vomiting, thirst, fatigue	Gloves and gown or apron for handling secretions from lesions Private room if infection is disseminated or severe
Progressive multifocal leukoencephalopathy (PML)—JC virus; transmission routes unclear	Brain	Impaired speech, vision, and thought; ataxia and limb weakness; advanced disease can cause profound dementia	No known effective treatment	None

CMV, Cytomegalovirus; *CNS,* central nervous system; *GI,* gastrointestinal.

TABLE 31-9 ■ QUALITY-OF-LIFE ASSESSMENTS IN HIV DISEASE

INSTRUMENT	AUTHOR	DIMENSIONS	LENGTH	ADMINISTRATION
AIDS Health Assessment Questionnaire (AIDS-HAQ)	Lubeck and Fries (1991-1992)	Physical function, mental health, cognitive function, social health, energy and fatigue	30 items	Self-administered (5 minutes)
AIDS Specific Functional Assessment (ASFA)	Rapkin et al (1991-1993)	Evaluates usefulness of functional assessment	Varies	Self-administered, care provider
Idiographic Functional Status Assessment (IFSA)	Rapkin et al (1991-1992)	Patient-generated activities associated with pursuit of following goal types: a. achievement b. problem-solving c. avoidance-prevention d. maintenance e. disengagement	75 items	Self-administered

TABLE 31-9 ■ QUALITY-OF-LIFE ASSESSMENTS IN HIV DISEASE—cont'd

INSTRUMENT	AUTHOR	DIMENSIONS	LENGTH	ADMINISTRATION
Medical Outcomes Study HIV Instrument (MOS-HIV or MOS-30)	Wu et al (1991)	Health, pain, physical functioning, role functioning, social functioning, mental health, fatigue, energy, health distress, cognitive functioning, health transition, general quality of life	30 items	Self-administered (5 minutes)
HIV Patient-Assessed Report of Status and Experience (HIV-PARSE)	Berry et al (1991)	Physical health, mental health, general health	38 items	Self-administered (5 minutes)
Functional Multidimensional Evaluation of People with HIV (VFM/HIV)	Marazzi et al (1992)	Self-sufficiency with ADL, economic resources, social resources, physical health, mental health	12 items	Self-administered
Neuropsychiatric AIDS Rating Scale (NARS)	Boccellari et al (1992)	Assesses patient's orientation, memory, motor ability, behavioral changes, problem-solving ability, and ADL	Varies	Health care provider
HIV Overview of Problems Evaluation System (HOPES)	Schag et al (1992)	Global, physical, psychosocial, medical interaction, significant others, sexual components	139 items	Self-administered (15 minutes)
HIV-Related Quality-of-Life Questions (HIV-QOL)	Cleary et al (1993)	Mental health, energy and fatigue, fever, limitations of basic ADL and intermediate ADL, disability days, all symptoms, sleep symptoms, neurological symptoms, memory symptoms, pain	30 items	Self-administered (5 minutes)
HIV Quality Audit Marker (HIV-QAM)	Holzemer et al (1993)	Captures nurse data collector's judgment of status of patient based on observations, interviews, and recorded interviews	Varies based on duration of interview	Nurse
HIV Visual Analog Scale	Nokes et al (1994)	Rates HIV-related symptom severity and general well-being	Varies	Nurse Self-administered
HIV Assessment Tool (HAT)	Nokes et al (1994)	Physical symptoms related to HIV disease, social and role functioning, psychological well-being, and personal attitudes related to well-being	34 items	Self-administered
Multidimensional Quality of Life Questionnaire for Persons with HIV (MQOL-HIV)	Avis and Smith (1994)	Mental health, physical health, physical functioning, social functioning, social support, cognitive functioning, financial status, partner intimacy, sexual functioning, medical care	40 items	Self-administered (10 minutes)
Medical Outcomes Study HIV Health Survey (MOS-HIV)	Wu, Rivicki, Jacobson, and Maltz (1997)	General health perceptions, role functioning, mental health, quality of life, pain, social functioning, health distress, physical functioning, energy and fatigue, cognitive function, and health transition	35 items	Self-administered or via interview (5-10 minutes)

Continued

TABLE 31-9 ■ QUALITY-OF-LIFE ASSESSMENTS IN HIV DISEASE—cont'd

INSTRUMENT	AUTHOR	DIMENSIONS	LENGTH	ADMINISTRATION
HIV/AIDS-Targeted Quality of Life (HAT-QoL) Instrument	Holmes and Shea (1998)	Overall function, sexual function, disclosure worries, health worries, financial worries, HIV mastery, life satisfaction, medication concerns, provider trust	42 items	Self-administered (15 minutes)
World Health Organization-Quality of Life HIV Instrument (WHOQOL-HIV)	Mental Health: Evidence and Research Department of Mental Health and Substance Dependence, World Health Organization, Geneva	Physical, psychological, level of independence, social, environmental, spiritual, general quality of life and health, symptoms of HIV, social inclusion, death and dying, forgiveness and fear of death	115 items	Self-administered
Functional Assessment of Chronic Illness Therapy—Spiritual Well-Being (FACIT-Sp-12)	Brady et al; Peterman (2002)	Faith, meaning, and peace	12 items	Self-administered
The Self-Efficacy for Managing Chronic Disease 6-Item Scale	Lorig and Sobel (2001)	Covers several domains that are common across many chronic diseases—symptom control, role function, emotional functioning, and communicating with physicians—with less subject burden than other surveys	6 items	Self-administered

temperature in a stocking-glove distribution, increased vibratory thresholds, and diminished ankle reflexes compared with knee reflexes.[85,103] Patients with AIDS frequently have concurrent CNS disorders and neuropathy, characterized by hyperactive knee reflexes and depressed ankle reflexes.

The incidence of DSP increases with advancing immunosuppression, in parallel with decreased CD4 counts.[104] Thirty-five percent of patients with AIDS may have electrophysiological or clinical abnormalities.[105] Furthermore, pathological evidence of DSP is present in almost all patients who die of AIDS.[106] Various theories regarding the mechanism of DSP have been proposed. It was formerly thought that direct HIV invasion of the nervous system caused DSP[94]; however, most investigators now believe that this is not the sole cause.[104] A "dying-back" neuropathy affecting all fiber types, with prominent macrophage infiltration of the peripheral nerve, has been described.[106] Additional theories include HAART drug toxicity, neurotoxic effects of cytokines, toxicity of HIV proteins, and mitochondrial damage.[107] Cytokines, tumor necrosis factor, and interleukin-1 have been identified in the peripheral nerves of patients with AIDS.[108]

Balance and Postural Mechanisms. Balance disturbances may be seen with HIV involvement of either the CNS or the PNS. Polyneuropathy caused by AZT (AZT polyneuropathy) and CMV, which is a common pathogen in AIDS (inflammatory polyneuropathy), may manifest in the form of a generalized asymmetrical demyelination and chronic denervation of muscles.[109] Demyelination and denervation of nerves that supply postural muscles may weaken such muscles and result in balance problems (e.g., distal pain, paresthesia, numbness, or core weakness). It is also possible that, apart from muscle demyelination and denervation, the pathological process, which also includes macrophage infiltration of neural structures, could spread to affect the vestibular neural complex of the inner ear, which is important in the maintenance of both static and dynamic balance. Our clinical experience shows that sensory changes are common in the lower limbs of neuropathic HIV/AIDS patients. The balance problems of these patients are likely to be connected to a lack of adequate proprioception from the legs during stance, and it is well known that diminished sensory information makes gait control more difficult. Refer to Chapter 22 for a discussion of balance dysfunction.

Peripheral neuropathy weakens the neuromuscular system and causes a limitation in functional activities. These effects on the neuromuscular system manifest in disturbances of postural control. An appropriate posture should be regarded as the starting position for a functional activity. However, compromise of the postural pattern is so characteristic of HIV peripheral neuropathy that it is diagnostic for HIV-1 infection.[110] The neurological abnormality resulting from peripheral neuropathy in HIV/AIDS produces postural disturbances[111] that may take various forms that worsen with the severity of the neuropathy[112] and compromise functional activity at various levels. This means that as the condition of HIV/AIDS patients deteriorates, balance deficits may increase.

According to Husstedt and colleagues,[113] peripheral neuropathy in HIV disease progresses much more rapidly than that associated with diabetes or hereditary polyneuropathies. Again, because of demyelination as the HIV infection progresses, distal symmetrical peripheral neuropathy increases, resulting in a depression of certain motor functions such as gait and manual dexterity, and a worsening of the condition is caused by demyelination.[113] There is therefore a need to treat HIV neuropathy as soon as it is diagnosed, to avoid complications that lead to impairments in functional mobility.

One group[61] has identified peripheral neuropathy and its complications as causes of functional limitations in individuals with HIV disease. A patient who, for instance, has balance impairment resulting from peripheral neuropathy may not function effectively with ADLs. Functional impairments may impede a patient's ability to return to gainful employment. For individuals with HIV disease, peripheral neuropathy and its resulting pain may be a limiting factor in the ability to return to work. Any intervention that can aid in the reduction of functional limitations should be incorporated into the rehabilitation plan of care.

Pain

A factor closely related to HIV neuropathy is pain. Pain is one of the most prominent and distressing symptoms in patients with HIV disease, and it has a significant effect on quality of life and psychological state. Pain may affect patients at any stage of the disease process; however, it is more frequent during the advanced stages. The occurrence of pain during HIV infection varies from 30% to 80%. Pain is the result of a complex process that involves psychological and neurophysiological mechanisms, and therefore it should be assessed with use of sensitive tools that examine its multidimensional nature. One model that evaluates the evaluative, affective, and sensory aspects of pain is the McGill Pain Questionnaire. This assessment tool is useful in evaluating HIV disease–related pain because different causes and nonsensorial factors related to the disease often make clinical assessment of pain difficult.[114]

Most HIV patients require various pain treatment interventions. Distal symmetrical peripheral neuropathy has been shown to be the most common peripheral neuropathy complaint in patients with HIV-1 infection.[115-117] Peripheral neuropathy is one of the most common types of pain in HIV-infected men,[118] and peripheral neuropathies occur in as many as 40% to 60% of patients with HIV disease. Peripheral neuropathy is the most prevalent neurological complication associated with HIV. CNS or PNS involvement has been found in 30% to 63% of patients across the arena of HIV and is often related to antiretroviral therapy.[119] When neuropathy results in distal painful paresthesia, imbalance in stance and gait may result from compensatory measures aimed at relieving pain in dynamic standing activities. Postural compensations may further exacerbate musculoskeletal, cervical, thoracic, or lumbosacral back pain.

Pain management is a critical part of the overall care of individuals with HIV disease. Pain is the second most common reason for hospitalization of patients with AIDS.[120] A study of 72 AIDS patients found that 97% had pain related to the disease process.[121] Newshan and Wainapel,[121] who surveyed 100 patients who had pain associated with AIDS, showed that the two reported pain types were abdominal and neuropathic pain. In a longitudinal study of HIV-positive men, painful peripheral neuropathy was one of the most common types of pain.[118]

DSP results in painful paresthesias that are challenging to treat with pharmacological interventions. Oral gabapentin and cutaneous lidocaine patches are often prescribed to manage pain associated with peripheral neuropathy. Clinical experience shows that conventional transcutaneous electrical nerve stimulation may exacerbate or relieve peripheral pain in patients with HIV infection. Another consideration for treatment is low-voltage electroacupuncture.[122] Manual therapy to improve ankle and foot range of motion along with other compensatory areas is recommended for pain management and return to function. (See Chapters 32 and 39 for additional information.)

Psychopathology

Medical and neuropsychiatric sequelae of HIV infection present a spectrum of diagnostic and treatment challenges to health care practitioners. Both HIV infection and the various opportunistic infections that manifest in patients as the result of an immunocompromised state can affect the CNS. Epidemiological studies indicate that greater than 60% of HIV-positive individuals will experience at least one major psychiatric disorder during the course of their infection. Depression is the most common disorder, closely followed by anxiety and substance abuse disorders.[123] Therefore therapists need to be familiar with the diagnosis and management of HIV infection–related medical and psychiatric disorders. These disorders have a great impact on the outcomes of rehabilitation.

Careful consideration of psychological function is warranted during clinical encounters with HIV-infected persons. AIDS-related psychopathologies mimic many previously described consequences of primary HIV infection, opportunistic infections, and drug side effects. These psychiatric complications can be affective or organic. Indicators include disturbances in sleep and appetite patterns, diminished memory and energy, psychomotor retardation, withdrawal, apathy, and emotional liability. Anxiety disorders (particularly posttraumatic stress disorder), adjustment reactions, reactive and endogenous depressions, and obsessive disorders frequently result.[124-126] Refer to Chapter 6 for additional recommendations regarding psychological adaptation and adjustments to nervous system dysfunction.

With use of the American Psychiatric Association's *Diagnostic and Statistical Manual of Mental Disorders,* Fourth Edition, Text Revision, one study found Axis I disorders (excluding substance abuse) in 61.9% of the subjects.[127] Indeed, the virus's affinity with subcortical structures of the CNS that regulate affect and mood supports research indicating a prevalence of manic episodes that is 10 times higher than in the general population.[128] Manic episodes have been identified at all stages of the disease process and may also occur in response to AZT therapy.[16,46,129] When associated with HIV infection, mania appears to be secondary to structural CNS changes.[130,131] Described manic episodes generally respond well to psychiatric medications and may not recur.[46,132-134]

Analyses of new-onset psychosis among HIV-positive individuals yielded the following information. Psychotic episodes are preceded by a period (days to months) of affective and behavioral changes.[135] Admitting diagnoses to psychiatric units included "undifferentiated schizophrenia, schizophreniform disorder, 'reactive psychosis,' atypical psychosis, depression with psychotic features and mania."[135] Some psychiatric diagnoses were revised during the course of hospitalization to "AIDS encephalitis, cryptococcal meningitis, or 'organic psychosis.'"[136] Eighty-seven percent of the subjects in one study displayed delusions that were usually persecutory, grandiose, or somatic. Affective disturbances were present in 81% of the subjects. Hallucinations and thought process disorders were each prominent in 61% of patients. Several subjects received the diagnosis of AIDS during their psychiatric hospitalization.[136]

Remarkable progress has been made in recent years in the therapeutics of HIV-associated dementia. Viral replication in and outside the CNS has been reduced by HAART. This has resulted in partial repair of cellular immune function with improvement in, and prevention of, neurological deficits associated with HIV disease.[137] Extensive use of PIs is associated with dramatic declines in overall mortality and morbidity, including HIV-associated dementia.[37,138]

Neuropathological abnormalities seen in the brain tissue of patients with HIV-associated dementia are usually diffuse and predominantly localized to the white and deep gray matter regions. Myelin pallor and inflammatory infiltrates composed of macrophages and multinucleated giant cells are the hallmarks of this disease process, although a spectrum of lesions has been identified from encephalitis to leukoencephalopathy.[139,140] The characteristic clinical feature of HIV-associated dementia is disabling cognitive impairment, often accompanied by behavioral changes, motor dysfunction, or both.[140] Degrees of impairment have been recorded, and a five-part staging system was subsequently developed.[141-143] Motoric manifestations of AIDS dementia complex include gait disturbances, intention tremor, and abnormal release of reflexes.

Differentiation between psychiatric and physiological manifestations is complicated. Psychiatric and organic disorders are initially indistinguishable on the basis of behavior and may exist concurrently. Furthermore, other primary disease processes and drug reactions imitate psychopathological conditions. Differentiation is nonetheless essential because many disorders respond well to established therapies, both psychological and pharmacological, once differential diagnoses have been established. Awareness of the intricate interplay of all factors is essential for competent rehabilitative efforts for those infected with HIV.

Pediatric HIV Infection

Pediatric HIV infection differs from that most commonly seen in adults. Symptoms develop much earlier in pediatric patients compared with adults. Children infected with HIV may be classified as "rapid progressors" or "slow progressors." Rapid progressors are children infected with HIV who manifest symptoms within the first 12 to 24 months of life. These children progress quickly to AIDS-defining conditions and have a rapid decline in CD4 count. Children who are slow progressors have a more gradual progression of symptoms and are likely to show evidence of immune system compromise by 7 to 8 years of age. A small percentage of children remain healthy and have only nominal or no symptoms of the disease and a normal to slightly decreased CD4 count through 9 to 10 years of age.[144]

The prediction of 6 million pregnant women and 5 to 10 million children infected with HIV-1 by the year 2000[145] may have been an underestimate. An accurate understanding of the timing of HIV transmission from mother to fetus is important for the design of intervention strategies. The AIDS Clinical Trial Group Study (ACTG) 076 trial, which included treatment from the fourteenth week of gestation in women with CD4 counts of more than 200/mm^3, prompts other considerations.[146] Onset of HIV-1 infection in children has a wide spectrum of clinical manifestations.[147] Thus prevention of transmission from mother to fetus via HAART is a critical component of managing this worldwide epidemic.

Pediatric HIV is neurotrophic in nature in that the virus most often initially affects the CNS rather than the PNS. As the virus spreads, pediatric HIV patients can have CNS disorders that include encephalopathy, pyramidal tract signs, receptive and expressive language difficulties, cognitive deficits, psychomotor impairments, and upper respiratory infections.[144] Neuroimaging shows HIV has an influence on neurological function in the basal ganglia, frontal cortex, and other connecting structures in the CNS. Studies also support that there is an environmental component which contributes to developmental and behavioral issues in HIV-positive children.[148]

In the first year of life, severe immunodeficiency develops in 15% to 20% of pediatric patients with serious recurrent infections or neurological dysfunction, whereas in school-age children the disease progresses more slowly and the risk for development of HIV-related encephalopathy becomes less.[149] Some infants have features of severe immunodeficiency, whereas others have nonspecific findings, such as hepatosplenomegaly, failure to thrive, unexplained fever, parotitis, and recurrent gastroenteritis. Adenopathy is common, and salivary gland enlargement occurs more frequently than in adults. Otitis media and measles, despite immunization, are also more frequent complications in children.[56,81] Cardiac involvement in children with HIV infection is a well-known entity and occurs clinically more often in patients with advanced disease.[150]

Studies have shown that children with HIV demonstrate behaviors often associated with attention-deficit/hyperactivity disorder (ADHD) including impulsivity, hyperactivity, difficulty attending, and decreased ability to focus on stimuli. In one study, the most common behavioral issues were psychosomatic disorders (28%), learning disorders (25%), hyperactivity (20%), impulsive-hyperactive disorder (19%), conduct problems (16%), and anxiety (8%); standardized intelligence scores were lower compared with established population norms. Hyperactivity was more common in children with a Wechsler IQ lower than 90, anxiety issues were more common in children older than 9 years, and conduct disorders were more often seen in children with CD4 counts less than 660 cells/mcL.[148]

Children are susceptible to disorders seen in adults—herpesvirus infection, pneumonia, toxoplasmosis, meningitis, and encephalitis. HIV encephalopathy is noted to have the most serious side effects because of its progressive deteriorating pattern and associated CNS abnormalities,[17] although static encephalopathy can be characterized by severely delayed cognitive functioning and neuromotor skills without deterioration.[151] Manifestations in children include cerebral atrophy, ataxia, rigidity, hyperreflexia, and the inability to achieve or sustain developmental milestones. Although the HIV neurodevelopmental involvement causes a prognostic worsening, most studies of pediatric cases of neuro-AIDS demonstrate that an early diagnosis followed by adequate antiretroviral therapeutic regimens can lead to significant, even if temporary, improvement.[149]

Rehabilitation of the pediatric patient requires a multidisciplinary approach to meet the medical, emotional, and psychosocial needs of these children and their families. Children are encouraged to give form to their psychological experiences through play, writing or telling stories, and creating works of art.[152]

REHABILITATION INTERVENTIONS

The examination procedures for HIV illness are broadly outlined in the following paragraphs. Of course, each case varies and the evaluation process is individualized according to the specific needs of the client (Box 31-3).

What is the relationship of the person with HIV infection to the environment, both at present and in the future? The rehabilitation therapist should keep this question in mind throughout the examination process. In this context the term *environment* is meant to include not only the physical aspects of surroundings but also the psychological and emotional climate in which the individual functions (see Table 31-1).

The examination process has a different focus for different stages of the disease. If the client is in the early stages of the disease, the therapist should determine whether she or he is still managing in accustomed life roles. Important issues may include new or adapted vocational and leisure skills. During the advanced stage, the focus may change to more basic daily functional concerns. The therapist must remember, however, that the client may place more importance on participation in avocational interests than on independent self-care. This choice not only is valid but must be respected and supported by health care professionals. If the patient is evaluated in an inpatient setting, another crucial determination to be made is whether the person is to be discharged to home or some other supervised setting. It is critical to determine what kind of community-based support networks are available to the individual. Case managers are often adept at identifying home and community resources available and will assist in setting up these resources before the patient's discharge.

Astute evaluative questions about the psychosocial status of the client include the following:

- Does the client's perception of his or her status and prognosis agree with that of the treatment team?
- What is the client's predominant coping style?
- Who are the client's caregivers?
- What is the social support system?
- What is the client's home environment?
- What is the client's prior level of function?

The support system can be a critical issue for many people with HIV infection, especially those who are part of the high-risk groups, such as homosexual and bisexual men and intravenous drug users.[153] Many of these people have traditional networks of family, spouse, and friends; a significant number have equally strong nontraditional support systems. Some

BOX 31-3 ■ EVALUATION PROCEDURES FOR HIV ILLNESS

A. Baseline data (premorbid functional level)
   1. Accustomed life roles
   2. Medical comorbidities
B. Stage in disease process
C. Psychosocial issues
   1. Coping mechanisms
   2. Social support system
   3. Financial resources
D. Cognitive/perceptual status
   1. Reality orientation
   2. Memory
   3. Organizational skills
   4. Visual perception
   5. Motor planning
   6. Safety awareness
   7. Judgment
E. Communication
   1. Oral language
   2. Written language
   3. Language comprehension
F. Sensorimotor status
   1. Balance
   2. Gait
   3. Coordination
   4. Proprioception
   5. Kinesthesia
   6. Sensation and pain
   7. Muscle tone
   8. Strength
   9. Reflexes
G. Activities of daily living (ADLs)
   1. Grooming and hygiene
   2. Feeding
   3. Bathing
   4. Dressing
   5. Housework
   6. Community management
   7. Other self-care regimens (e.g., medications)
   8. Avocational interests
   9. Activity tolerance

will be lacking in the kinds of support needed to cope with the devastating physical and emotional effects of the disease.

It is possible to use models developed for oncology and progressive neurological disorders for HIV involvement of the CNS and PNS. An orthopedic approach may be taken when pain is a presenting factor or biomechanical alterations are a result of other disease processes. Functional fluctuations that characterize HIV infection and secondary infections must be understood; therefore the therapist must appreciate the effects that HIV infection has on various systemic complications.

The examination of an individual who has HIV disease should include standard cognitive, perceptual, and motor function evaluative tools. The idiosyncratic nature of the disease may necessitate more detailed evaluation of these specific areas. Recommended cognitive and perceptual evaluations are both formal and observational. Safety, judgment, functional mobility, ADL management, community management skills, and independent financial management skills need to be assessed. Evaluation of the systemic complications of HIV infection is necessary for optimal rehabilitative planning and treatment team efficacy.

The ADL evaluation is best made within the context of the immediate and projected life roles of the individual. Maximal independent functioning is the goal of rehabilitation, whatever the stage of illness. If the person is at home or is being discharged to home, a crucial component of the ADL examination is the assessment of community management skills; consider an individual's access to transportation, socialization opportunities, shopping, and banking. The ability to negotiate health care and insurance systems and participate in community activities is critical to returning to independence. Many people with HIV infection and their caregivers have minimal experience with disability because of their age or social status. This, combined with the stressors of illness, can create unrealistic expectations and unnecessary frustrations.

Treatment Process

The neuromuscular rehabilitation treatment procedures for HIV infection and an overview of treatment techniques for opportunistic infections are presented in Boxes 31-4 and 31-5.

Cognitive deficits in attention, concentration, and memory necessitate consistency, structure, and environmental cues to minimize confusion. Safety and judgment deficits can be countered by environmental adaptations. Lethargic clients benefit from sensory enhancement. Maintenance of endurance, strength, and passive and active range of motion are important components of any motor function treatment plan. Neuromuscular facilitation and inhibition, positioning, and splinting are feasible modalities to normalize tone as needed. Gait training, the use of assistive devices, training in motor planning, balance activities, and endurance exercises may be appropriate.

In addition to techniques and modalities, active listening, empathy, and unconditional positive regard are important aspects of the therapeutic process. The clinician must set aside personal biases and beliefs to accurately hear the perspective of the individual client. The use of expressive modalities facilitates the development of coping skills while providing appropriate exploration and release of powerful emotions. Human touch can counter the powerful and isolating effect of fear of contagion. Rehabilitation therapists can demonstrate and educate caregivers about the safety and benefit of touch.

Motoric manifestations of AIDS dementia complex include gait disturbances, intention tremor, and abnormal release of reflexes. Rehabilitation and progression of independent functional mobility become more complex in these patients secondary to the cognitive involvement.

Pain management is best approached with a behavioral and a physical approach. Pain reduction is achieved through training in breathing techniques, visualization, progressive muscle relaxation, autogenics, music, meditation, and engagement in meaningful activities. Various forms of electrotherapy such as

BOX 31-4 ■ NEUROMUSCULAR REHABILITATION TREATMENT PROCEDURES FOR HIV INFECTION

A. Psychosocial intervention
   1. Facilitation of the expression of grief
   2. Validation and education of caregivers
B. Cognitive and perceptual intervention
   1. Rehabilitation
   2. Maintenance
   3. Compensation (including communication)
C. Sensory and motor intervention
   1. Sensory stimulation
   2. Maintenance of strength, range of motion, and endurance
   3. Tone normalization
   4. Functional mobility (including assistive devices and adaptive equipment)
   5. Balance and coordination activities
D. Pain control
   1. Psychological modalities
   2. Behavioral modalities
   3. Physical modalities
E. Training in activities of daily living (ADLs)
   1. Leisure or avocational skill development
   2. Community management skills
   3. Transfer training
   4. Recommendations for adaptive equipment
   5. Self-care retraining
   6. Energy conservation
   7. Work simplification
F. Continuity of care
   1. Discharge planning and follow-up care
   2. Community linkages
   3. Social support services

BOX 31-5 ■ MOST COMMON OPPORTUNISTIC INFECTIONS AND REHABILITATION INTERVENTIONS IN HIV-INFECTED PATIENTS

PCP—Most common opportunistic infection. Infectious agent unclear but probable latent infection; 65% to 85% of healthy adults possess PCP antibodies. Fever, dyspnea, and hypoxia ⟶ diaphragmatic breathing, energy conservation.*

Candida albicans—Present in healthy people, immunocompromised status ⟶ yeast infections of oral, esophageal, and vaginal mucosal tissues ⟶ teach good oral care with soft brush, bland diet, salt water rinses.

Cryptococcus neoformans—A yeast that manifests in CNS as abscesses and meningitis. Headache, altered mental states, nausea, vertigo, somnolence, seizures, and coma ⟶ pain management, safety and gait training, cognitive and sensory stimulation.

Cryptosporidiosis—Infects GI tract ⟶ chronic diarrhea and malabsorption, contributes to wasting syndrome ⟶ nutritional and hydration strategies.

Wasting syndrome—Involuntary loss of 10% of baseline body weight, weakness, chronic diarrhea, and unexplained fever ⟶ Nutrition, hydration, energy conservation.

Toxoplasmosis—Affects CNS in 30% to 40% of cases; headache, altered cognition, encephalitis, seizures, focal deficits ⟶ imposed structure, concrete tasks, pain management.

CMV—Present in 40% to 100% of healthy adults. Can affect GI and respiratory tracts but most often affects ocular structures ⟶ unilateral or bilateral decreased visual acuity, field cuts and blindness ⟶ compensatory skills, safety tasks and mobilities, home evaluation, supportive service referrals.

Mycobacterial infections—Two are most pertinent: *Mycobacterium avium* complex (MAC) and *Mycobacterium tuberculosis* (causes TB). MAC affects 18% to 56% of those with HIV, but autopsies reveal that this is a low estimate. MAC infection is not latent but is a primary infection. It appears late in HIV infection, begins in the GI or respiratory tract, and then disseminates. Pneumonia, fever, weight loss, malaise, sweats, anorexia, abdominal pain, and/or diarrhea may occur. TB appears early, with latent reactivation in 90% of HIV-infected patients. Pulmonary TB affects an estimated 75% to 100% of HIV-infected persons infected with the TB bacillus. It also infects lymph nodes and bone marrow in 60% of these patients, and it also infects CNS, cardiac, and mucosal tissues. Fever, weight loss, malaise, cough, lymph node tenderness, and night sweats ⟶ energy conservation, nutrition, hydration, and caregiver and patient education in safe management of infection. The infection is communicable; wear a mask, follow respiratory isolation protocol.

AIDS-KS—Frequent neoplasm and most frequent in homosexual men; it is rare in women and intravenous drug users. Purple skin or visceral lesions are present. Associated are deficient lymphatic transport, nodal tumors, and lymphedema ⟶ swollen, painful lower extremities. Nutrition, pain management, task simplification, mobility, and training in ADLs.

ADLs, Activities of daily living; *AIDS-KS,* AIDS–Kaposi sarcoma; *CMV,* cytomegalovirus; *CNS,* central nervous system; *GI,* gastrointestinal; *PCP, Pneumocystis jiroveci* pneumonia; *TB,* tuberculosis.

electroacupuncture, thermal agents, and manual therapy are useful therapeutic tools. (See Chapters 9, 32, and 39 for additional treatment ideas.)

The impact of HIV infection can be evident in cerebral, emotional, psychosocial, and other physical domains, affecting the patient infected with HIV and those around her or him. The prognosis and psychological and physical consequences of HIV infection are associated with significant emotional distress and clinical syndromes, such as adjustment disorders, depression, and anxiety in some patients.[154] Increasing focus is being placed on the potential impact of HIV infection–related stress on the course of infection because of the observed and postulated relationship between psychosocial stress, neuropsychological functioning, and immune status.[155] Minimizing stressful events throughout the management of chronic HIV infection can be approached in various ways, such as meditation, relaxation, and various forms of exercise.

Exercise

Exercise is an intervention commonly used by movement specialists to address a multitude of impairment and functional limitations. Thus, understanding of the implications of the HIV disease process on exercise prescription is important. A review of published studies[156] on the effects of exercise on individuals with HIV disease revealed the following: (1) although intense bouts of exercise may result in transient immunosuppression, there is no evidence that regular exercise by individuals with HIV disease results in a detrimental effect on the immune system over time, (2) some studies have shown actual improvement in immune system function in response to regular exercise, (3) improved cardiovascular function has been observed in response to aerobic exercise, and (4) resisted exercise may be effective in counteracting the effects of wasting syndrome and improving strength and lean body mass. A systematic review of progressive resistive exercise (PRE) showed that PRE or a combination of PRE and aerobic exercises lead to statistically significant increases in weight, arm girth, and thigh girth. Trends were also found supporting an improvement in submaximum heart rate and exercise time. In addition, PRE was found to contribute to improved strength and psychological status. PRE was found to be safe and beneficial for medically stable HIV-positive adults.[157]

From a psychoneuroimmunological perspective, psychological stress has been implicated among the cofactors that contribute to the immunological decline in HIV disease. Good evidence supports the stress management role of exercise training as a means to explain a buffering of these suppressive stressor effects, thereby facilitating a return of the CD4 cells. Early intervention with exercise, in compliance with guidelines, is most prudent to stave off opportunistic infections throughout the spectrum of HIV disease.

Precautions and Concerns during Exercise

It is important to address any orthopedic or neurological concerns before embarking on an exercise or movement therapy program. If musculoskeletal problems exist or other pain symptoms are present, a concerted effort to modulate pain is necessary for the successful completion of an exercise regimen.[158] If HIV-related peripheral neuropathy exists, it is important to implement proper foot care and supportive shoes when weight-bearing activities are performed.[61,159] In addition, appropriate safety measures, such as guarding during balance activities, should take place when working on exercise programs with patients who have decreased stability.

There is some concern about aerobic exercise increasing the body's metabolic rate and thus increasing additional muscle loss. However, with a balanced diet and incorporation of a sound nutritional program, this should not pose a problem for the asymptomatic person with HIV disease. If wasting is present, the cause needs to be addressed and treatment rendered.[47] One study determined the contribution of total energy expenditure to weight changes in individuals with HIV infection–related wasting. The researchers observed a significant positive relation between total energy expenditure and the rate of weight change. During rapid weight loss, total energy expenditure fell from an average 2750 kcal per day to 2189 kcal per day. The key determinant of weight loss in HIV infection–related wasting, they concluded, was reduced energy intake, not increased energy expenditure.[160]

If fatigue is present as a symptom, a differential diagnosis for anemia, low testosterone levels, or specific vitamin deficiencies must be made before any exercise regimen is begun. Proper caloric intake must be adequate to meet the energy expenditure required for the activity. Seeking the advice of a nutritionist is recommended for proper guidance.

Evidence of autonomic neuropathy (a peripheral neuropathy that affects involuntary body functions including heart rate, blood pressure, perspiration, and digestive functions) on provocative testing is common in HIV infection, with estimates of incidence ranging from 30% to 60%.[161,162] Underlying cardiac parasympathetic dysfunction may need to be assessed throughout the course of HIV disease. One method described by Mallet and co-workers[163] is the use of the 4-second exercise test, which consists of pedaling an uploaded ergometer at maximal individual speed from the fourth to the eighth second of a 12-second maximal inspiratory apnea. From an electrocardiogram, vagal activity is estimated through a ratio. In that study, subjects were subjected to respiratory sinus arrhythmia, which is a valid method to detect vagal dysfunction. The researchers found that there was a tendency for lower values of the vagal function test in HIV-positive subjects. Vital sign monitoring is prudent throughout any exercise regimen. Exercise can help control long-term side effects including altered body composition; elevated cholesterol, triglyceride, and blood glucose levels; and elevated blood pressure.[164] Certain comorbidities associated with HIV disease, such as inflammatory myopathy, acute infectious arthritis, or compromised cardiac status may result in restrictions on exercise prescription.[156]

A supervised training program should be consistent with recommendations of the American College of Sports Medicine. Guidelines have been established for the spectrum of the stages of HIV disease.[25] During the stage of asymptomatic HIV disease, there are no limitations on maximum graded exercise testing. Exercise should consist of resistance training, cardiovascular training, flexibility training, balance training, and mind-body training.[164] In this stage, all metabolic parameters are within normal limits for most individuals. Thus, unrestricted activity is generally encouraged. Most sports do not pose a significant risk of HIV transmission. However, sports such as boxing, in which there is a risk of open wounds and contamination with infected blood, should be viewed with great caution.[156]

Exercise is safe and beneficial for most individuals with HIV disease; however, caution is warranted with symptomatic HIV disease and advanced HIV disease. In symptomatic HIV disease, there may be reduced exercise capacity, $\dot{V}O_2max$, and oxygen (O_2) pulse max. There may also be other cardiovascular and pulmonary problems, anemia, and peripheral muscle abnormalities. Pain, side effects of medications, psychosocial issues, and unplanned events may also create obstacles to exercise for individuals in the symptomatic stage of HIV disease. For individuals with cardiac myopathy or hyperlipidemia, submaximal aerobic capacity testing should be followed with a staged cardiac rehabilitation program[92] because of the risk of cardiac failure in patients with compromised cardiac status.[165]

Patients with AIDS have dramatically reduced exercise capacity, vital capacity, $\dot{V}O_2max$, and O_2 pulse max. Elevated heart rate and breathing reserve persist in this stage. Neurological dysfunction, opportunistic infections, and progressive disability indicate a need for careful monitoring of the exercise program during this stage of the disease. In general, individuals with advanced HIV disease should remain physically active and exercise on a symptom-limited basis. Precautions related to comorbidities should be implemented. Individuals in this stage of the disease are at greater risk for exercise-induced injuries as a result of chronic tissue changes in both muscle and peripheral nerve. For individuals with severe morbidity and extensive disability, treatment should emphasize enhancement of basic functional tasks, ADLs, and energy conservation.[156]

Psychoneuroimmunology: Prevention and Wellness in HIV Infection

Psychoneuroimmunology is the field that investigates the interrelationships among psychological constructs (e.g., stressors and mood states) of the neuroendocrine and immune systems. Although all the precise mechanistic links among these varied components of psychoneuroimmunology are not yet fully elucidated, psychoneuroimmunology does offer a useful framework for our understanding of how stressors play a role in immunomodulation. The progression of HIV disease can be modulated by psychosocial factors and by factors such as the viral strain, genetic characteristics of the host immune system, co-infections with other pathogenic organisms, and health maintenance habits (diet, exercise, medical treatments).[166] These factors may have a profound influence on the occurrence and progression of ill health in chronic diseases such as HIV infection or AIDS.

Findings of studies related to psychoneuroimmunology suggest that it may be useful to evaluate the influence of behavioral factors on immune functioning and disease progression in HIV-infected individuals.[167-169] The stress response is physiologically mediated by certain immune parameters (catecholamines and glucocorticoid hormones). A study by Leserman and colleagues[170] in 2002 concluded that "stressful life events, dysphoric mood, and limited social support" are correlated to the increased rate of progression from HIV to AIDS.[170] Behavioral interventions with immunomodulatory capabilities may help restore competence and thereby slow the progression of HIV disease, especially at the earliest stages of the infectious continuum.

A growing body of literature indicates that many different stressors have deleterious effects on the immune system.[171] It has been well documented in healthy individuals that changes in immune function and disease susceptibility are correlated with times of "psychic distress."[166] These stressors in the case of people living with HIV infection may be attenuated by an exercise training program. Research indicates that continued aerobic exercise training may result in increased CD4 cell counts, heightened immune surveillance, and a potential for a slowing of disease progression.[169] Other researchers have demonstrated similar benefits of exercise for individuals infected with HIV who are at more advanced stages of disease. However, these are studies conducted on traditional modes of exercise and do not investigate alternative activities such as yoga or tai chi. Exercise within the context of psychoneuroimmunology appears to be a promising approach in the treatment of illness and promotion of health in chronic HIV disease.

Complementary Therapies in HIV Infection

There is substantial evidence to suggest that traditional exercise, particularly aerobic exercise, can provide notable physiological and psychological benefits for most individuals, especially those with chronic diseases. However, the mode, duration, and intensity of many traditional standardized exercise programs may not always be entirely appropriate during chronic illness. The stage of disease and the type of illness itself may preclude more strenuous exercise activities at various times. During such times, less traditional movement therapies may prove to be more appropriate and efficacious. In fact, movement therapy includes a number of similar constructs used in physical therapy and can be quite complementary to an individual's program of more traditional exercise.[172,173] Refer to Chapter 39 for additional information.

The HIV epidemic has resulted in an increasing use of alternative therapies, some more traditional than others.[165] Estimates show that 53% of HIV-positive individuals in the United States report the use of at least one complementary and alternative medicine (CAM) therapy.[174] The exploration outside the medical model has fostered investigations by the Office of Alternative Medicine at the National Institutes of Health.[175] Eisenberg and colleagues[176] reported that prayer and exercise combined accounted for more than 60% of all alternative therapies used. Other therapies include relaxation techniques (13%), massage (7%), imagery (4%), and spiritual healing (4%). Traditional exercise such as aerobic and weight training is incorporated in the medical model through exercise physiology and rehabilitation. However, various movement therapies (such as martial arts) are often viewed as less traditional and outside the established medical model. In a study by Bastyr University (1998), various movement therapies were used by people living with HIV disease. This study evaluated the use of alternative therapies within the previous 6 months. Yoga had been used by 15.5%, tai chi by 4.8%, and qi gong by 3.6% of the participants. Research[172] demonstrated beneficial physiological and psychological effects of the use of tai chi and aerobic exercise (see Chapter 39). In 1993 researchers at the University of Maryland School of Nursing in Baltimore concluded that there was a positive correlation between patient health and participation in prayer and meditation. Relevant factors included participants' "perception of their physical, emotional, and spiritual health; and their participation in exercise and the use of special diets."[177] A study done at Rutgers University in 1999 looked at guided imagery and progressive muscle relaxation on HIV. Health status was significantly different after treatment. Guided imagery produced the most positive effects in the middle stage of the disease. The combination of imagery and muscle relaxation is suggested to improve health status, and it should be initiated early in the disease process.[178] Recent studies indicate that pain level is a good predictor of the use of CAM therapies; individuals with pain decreased by CAM therapy are less likely to use illegal or untested drugs. Patients experiencing depression were more likely to use illegal or untested drugs and therapies.[174]

Social Interactions and the Association with Disease Management

The process of grieving is often mistakenly associated solely with the death of another. It is a natural reaction to loss, including the loss of one's own health and diminished independence. Loss of abstract human qualities, such as perceived attractiveness and productivity, results in grief. Such emotions are often difficult for a client to articulate. It is the therapist's responsibility to be sensitive to the client's individualized grief pattern (see Chapter 6).

Placement issues accompany discharge planning from acute health care facilities. The rehabilitation professional is often called on to make recommendations regarding the level of assistance the client will need. All of the previously discussed areas of cognitive-perceptual, sensorimotor, and ADL management combined with available psychosocial and practical support influence these recommendations. Options include a return to independent living and work, assisted independent living with help from a loved one, home with supportive services (often supplied by community-based AIDS organizations), home with hospital-based home care, hospice, Level I (inpatient acute) rehabilitation, Level II (subacute) rehabilitation, and an extended care facility.

Literature on long-term survivors with AIDS is replete with anecdotal evidence linking survival to one or more of the following: (1) holding a positive attitude toward the illness, (2) participating in health-promoting behaviors, (3) engaging in spiritual activities, and (4) taking part in advocacy activities related to the HIV community.[141,179-180] Positive relationships have been demonstrated between hardiness and perception of physical, emotional, and spiritual health and participation in exercise and the use of special diets.[181-183]

Research provides support for the hypothesis that interpersonal relationships influence patterns of physiological functions. Data from experimental studies have shown that social contact can serve to reduce physiological stress responses.[184,185] Community-based studies have also shown negative associations between reported levels of support and physiological parameters such as serum cholesterol, uric acid, and urinary epinephrine levels.[185] Studies of immune function have demonstrated that social relationships have both positive and negative impacts on immune function. Loss of a partner to cancer or HIV infection, family caregiving for patients with Alzheimer disease, and divorce or poor marital quality all show negative associations with immune function, whereas more supportive relationships are associated with better immune function.[171]

Exercise and movement therapy in a group context may provide the socialization necessary to foster these physiological changes and adherence to an exercise regimen. Another area of potential socialization is the workplace. The quality-of-life issues for people with HIV/AIDS are becoming more complicated as more people with the disease achieve higher CD4 counts and lower viral load levels. Improvement in health status is directly related to the improved effectiveness of newer treatment regimens, and many individuals are improving enough to either continue working or reenter the work force. Exercise and movement therapy may augment the stress and fatigue that may be associated with the adjustment to the workplace.

SUMMARY

Research and resultant treatments are extending lives so that more people require rehabilitative services that maximize function and quality of life. Medical management has focused on the treatment of reducing viral load, preventing secondary illnesses, and improving the immunological status of chronic HIV disease. Examination of the neuromusculoskeletal system and interventions for individuals with HIV disease are similar to those for other progressive neuromusculoskeletal disorders. HIV disease should be addressed like other life-altering diseases such as cancer, but with an emphasis on cognitive and perceptual function. Rehabilitation interventions focus on specific impairments, disabilities, and psychosocial ramifications of the disease. Adaptive compensations, mobility, ADL retraining, pain control, and community management skills constitute a well-developed treatment plan.

The epidemic is a major challenge on a personal as well as a professional level because of the continued natural fear of contagion. The illness originally appeared in subcultures that are often disenfranchised. Social, racial, and economic status and controversial behaviors contribute to prejudice, fear, and limited access to health care. Rehabilitation professionals have responded significantly to this challenge. Continued advocacy and compassion combined with professional enlightenment will, in a small way, alter the course of the disease.

Future Directions for Research

The issue of HIV disability warrants a careful investigation into our current health care system. Some long-term survivors of HIV disease who formerly received disability ranking are potentially ready to return to work. However, their grave concern about the long absence from work, reflected in the resume, and fears about potential opportunistic infections while on the job require specific strategies. Vocational rehabilitation and on-the-job counseling are necessary for optimal return to work. The systemic issues of acquisition of disability and the loss of all benefits when one relinquishes disability are quite complicated and overwhelming. The diagnosis of advanced HIV disease is the determining factor for disability, and many people living with HIV disease with CD4 counts less than 200/mcL have experienced considerable improvement in their immunological status with a concomitant drop in viral load. Prognosis for these individuals has great variability. Promoting quality of life may be greatly enhanced through the use of complementary therapies. An integral aspect of self-perception is often the role played in society. The workplace affords individuals a sense of identity and a self-sustaining purposefulness. Therefore our health and governmental systems need to conduct further research on return-to-work outcomes, with ease of transition and on-the-job accommodations when necessary. Future directions in the AIDS epidemic as we see people living longer will be the full return to function in all domains of ADLs and return to productive work.

CASE STUDIES

Three case studies are presented to help the reader understand and identify various stages of this clinical problem and how each stage may require a different therapeutic focus.

References

To enhance this text and add value for the reader, all references are included on the companion Evolve site that accompanies this textbook. This online service will, when available, provide a link for the reader to a Medline abstract for the article cited. There are 192 cited references and other general references for this chapter, with the majority of those articles being evidence-based citations.

CASE STUDY 31-1 ■ ASYMPTOMATIC HIV DISEASE VERSUS SYMPTOMATIC HIV DISEASE: MARIO

EXAMINATION

History

Mario is a 48-year-old male chemistry teacher who tested positive for HIV 6 years ago. Currently, his absolute $CD4^+$ cell count is 475/mcL, and his viral load (HIV RNA) is 40,000 copies/mL. Mario runs 5 miles three times per week for exercise. Recently he began to experience some pain and tingling in the soles of his feet that is most noticeable after running. His weight has been stable. He has noticed a mild deficit in short-term memory over the past year, which he attributes to middle age. He has a history of rotator cuff tendonitis but is otherwise healthy and denies other symptoms. His wife and 28-year-old son serve as his primary emotional support system. The rest of his family lives in Italy, his native country. He is a Roman Catholic and attends church regularly. Current medications include aspirin as needed after running.

CASE STUDY 31-1 ■ ASYMPTOMATIC HIV DISEASE VERSUS SYMPTOMATIC HIV DISEASE: MARIO—cont'd

Tests and Measurements

Left extremity sensation testing with Semmes-Weinstein monofilaments[186] reveals diminished light touch sensation over the distribution of the medial plantar nerves bilaterally. A lower-extremity neural tension test (straight leg raise with dorsiflexion) and a Tinel test over the tarsal tunnel have positive results bilaterally and reproduce tingling along the medial arches of the feet. Screening of the lumbar spine, hips, and knees is negative. Foot and ankle range of motion and strength are normal. Pain is not provoked with passive stretching of the plantar fascia. Lower-extremity reflexes are normal, and no abnormal reflexes are present. Excessive pronation is noted during the gait cycle; gait is otherwise normal. In standing, an excessive calcaneal valgus angle is noted; normal medial arches are observed in non–weight bearing. Foot pain on a visual analog scale is 0/10 at rest and 5/10 after running.

EVALUATION AND DIAGNOSIS

Bilateral distal sensory disturbances may be caused by DSP in individuals with HIV disease. However, this is typically associated with side effects of HAART, and the patient has not yet been placed on these drugs. Furthermore, sensory loss with DSP typically involves multiple peripheral nerves and occurs first in the most distal distribution. The patient's toes have no sensory impairment. Myelopathy should be considered in patients with chronic HIV disease who appear to have peripheral neurological symptoms; however, Mario does not demonstrate any signs that would suggest myelopathy as the cause of his foot symptoms. Examination is significant for signs and symptoms of flexible pes planus, which may be contributing to tarsal tunnel syndrome bilaterally. His gait pattern of excessive pronation is likely contributing to compression on the tibial nerve within the tarsal tunnel when he runs.

Prognosis, Goals, and Outcomes

Mario is expected to have full recovery with interventions directed at reducing biomechanical stress on the tarsal tunnel during running. Mario's goal is to run for 5 miles without any symptoms. Outcomes will be measured with patient's self-report of global improvement, the visual analog scale for pain associated with running, and changes in clinical signs (lower-extremity neural tension test, Tinel test, and monofilament sensory testing).

Intervention Plan and Recommendations

Mario will receive low Dye taping[187] to decrease his pronation and provide temporary relief of symptoms. Orthotics will be fabricated to reduce pronation and adverse stress on the tarsal tunnel. Mario will replace running with aerobic training on a stationary bike until his orthotics are adequately broken in, after which he can resume running. Before discharge he will receive instruction in general lower-extremity and plantar fascia flexibility exercises. If foot symptoms are recalcitrant to biomechanically based interventions, further consultation with Mario's HIV specialist will be warranted to rule out possible tibial nerve mononeuropathy related to his HIV disease.

The therapist will encourage Mario to see a mental health professional because of the complaints of memory loss. A mental health professional may use the HIV Dementia Scale,[188] or other instruments may be used to assess the patient's cognitive function and rule out the possibility of early signs of HIV dementia. If any of Mario's symptoms are determined to be related to his HIV disease, he will be re-staged to symptomatic HIV disease.

CASE STUDY 31-2 ■ ADVANCED HIV DISEASE (AIDS) AND A PLAN FOR THE FUTURE: RUBY

EXAMINATION

History

Ruby is a 23-year-old woman of African American and Hispanic descent. Ruby has an 8-year history of intravenous drug abuse and bipolar disorder. She was tested for HIV disease 5 years ago, at which time she was hospitalized with a diagnosis of *P. carinii* pneumonia and oral thrush. At that time, her absolute $CD4^+$ cell count was 15/mcL and her viral load was 750,000 copies/mL. Her opportunistic infections were successfully treated with antibiotics, and HAART was initiated. Within a few months, her viral load was undetectable and her absolute $CD4^+$ level had climbed to 400/mm^3. Since then she has had intermittent periods of homelessness and is currently residing with a friend. She stopped adhering to her HAART regimen several months ago, during a period of depression. Recently Ruby has worked as a prostitute to earn money for crack cocaine. Ruby was admitted to the hospital 12 days ago with complaints of abdominal bloating and severe left shoulder pain. Her behavior was clearly agitated. A large abscess was present over the left deltoid. Medical workup revealed that Ruby had a staphylococcal infection in the left anterior deltoid and infectious arthritis of the left glenohumeral joint. It was determined that she was 4 months pregnant. Her psychiatric status was significant for a manic episode. Her $CD4^+$ count was 175/mcL and viral load was 200,000 copies/mL. Ruby's shoulder infection was treated with intravenous methicillin, and recent magnetic resonance imaging of the shoulder region was negative for osteomyelitis. Medical clearance for examination and interventions for the shoulder was obtained from her infectious disease physician. She was placed on psychotropic medication for mood stabilization. Pending results of genotype testing, Ruby was placed on a new regimen of HAART. Genotype testing is needed because she likely has mutant strains of the virus as a result of poor adherence to the previous course of HAART. HAART will be implemented quickly, with the goal of achieving undetectable viral loads by the time of birth. Consultation with nutrition services was ordered to ensure adequate nutrition during the remainder of her pregnancy.

Continued

CASE STUDY 31-2 ■ ADVANCED HIV DISEASE (AIDS) AND A PLAN FOR THE FUTURE: RUBY—cont'd

Ruby has disclosed that her arm infection was probably caused by injecting drugs. She has been referred to see an addiction counselor and the social worker. Current medications: none.

Tests and Measurements

Ruby has a nonhealing wound over the left anterior deltoid region that was 1.5 cm × 1.1 cm with a depth of 0.5 cm. The wound appears to be clean with 100% granulation tissue, and the most recent laboratory report is negative for *Staphylococcus.* Ruby reports that the swelling and redness in her left shoulder have resolved, and no swelling or redness is observed during the examination. Left shoulder strength is 3/5 (fair) for abduction, internal rotation, and external rotation and 4/5 (good) for other motions. Passive range of motion (PROM) of the left side is limited as follows: external rotation 70 degrees, abduction 160 degrees, and internal rotation 45 degrees. Her score on the Disabilities of the Arm, Shoulder and Hand questionnaire (DASH)[189] is 85/100 for the left upper extremity. Screening examination of the cervical spine is clear; however, hypertonicity is noted in the elbow and wrist and the finger flexors on the left side. PROM of the elbow, wrist, and hand is within normal limits; however, slight resistance is noted with quick passive stretching of flexor muscles. Ruby has weakness in grasp and demonstrates a mild flexor synergy pattern with attempts to elevate the left arm.

EVALUATION AND DIAGNOSIS

As a result of the findings of the examination, neurology is immediately consulted and brain magnetic resonance imaging (MRI) is performed. The MRI reveals a mild right cerebrovascular accident involving the middle cerebral artery. Physical and occupational therapy will be initiated to address the following findings: impaired integumentary integrity associated with partial-thickness skin involvement over the left anterior deltoid region; impaired glenohumeral joint mobility, muscle performance, and range of motion associated with connective tissue dysfunction (adhesive capsulitis as sequela of infectious arthritis); and impaired motor function (spasticity and weakness in the left upper extremity) associated with nonprogressive disorder (right cerebrovascular accident) of the CNS.

Prognosis, Goals, and Outcomes

Ruby's outcomes will be strongly influenced by her complex psychosocial status. She states that she is highly motivated to have a healthy baby and learn how to become a stable provider, which may help her adherence to HAART and drug rehabilitation. Continuing communication among all team members (infectious disease, obstetrics-gynecology, social work, addictions counseling, physical therapy, and occupational therapy) will be critical to optimize her care. Because of multisystem involvement and multiple impairments, it is expected that Ruby will require 6 to 8 weeks of therapy. Goals specific to physical therapy include the following: facilitate wound healing and prevent reoccurrence of infection, restore full PROM to the left shoulder, improve strength and function throughout the left upper extremity, achieve independence in performance of ADLs with the left upper extremity, improve the DASH score,[189] and minimal functional limitation as per the Barthel Index score.[190] Outcomes will be measured with continuing assessment of wound characteristics, the DASH score,[189] the Barthel Index score,[190] shoulder PROM measurements, and strength assessment of upper-extremity musculature.

Intervention Plan

Wound healing will be facilitated with dressing changes and use of topical agents as prescribed by her physician. Glenohumeral impairments will be addressed with joint mobilization, therapeutic exercises, and functional retraining. Upper-extremity impairments involving tone and weakness will be addressed with motor learning techniques, functional activities, and strengthening exercises. Ruby will receive daily physical and occupational therapy until she is discharged from the hospital. Social work will facilitate discharge to a structured group home for women because Ruby's current roommate is using drugs and working as a prostitute. On discharge from the hospital, Ruby will return for outpatient therapy at a frequency of three times per week. She will continue to follow up with the social worker regarding vocational counseling.

CASE STUDY 31-3 ■ ADVANCED HIV DISEASE (AIDS) AT THE END STAGE OF LIFE: WALTER

EXAMINATION

History

Walter is a 68-year-old man who was diagnosed with AIDS in 1987. He lost his life partner to the same disease in 1990. He has no living relatives. At the time of his diagnosis, Walter had toxoplasmosis, KS, AIDS wasting syndrome, and anemia. He was one of the first patients to receive AZT, which, along with other medications used to treat the opportunistic infections, proved to be lifesaving. As new classes of drugs became available and were added to his regimen, Walter's viral loads and $CD4^+$ cell counts were usually stable. Over time, viral resistance developed to many of the drugs. Recently, he was placed on enfuvirtide (Fuzeon), an injectable receptor site inhibitor that is used when other drugs and salvage therapy have been exhausted. His current $CD4^+$ count is 25/mcL with a viral load of 200,000 copies/mL. Walter has multiple side effects and complications of long-term HIV survival, including peripheral neuropathy in the hands and feet, chronic fibromyalgia, myelopathy, liver toxicity, and severe lipodystrophy. He has marked wasting of fat in the face and extremities, severe truncal obesity, and a dorsocervical fat mass. Walter has also been undergoing treatment for hypertension and hyperlipidemia. Over the past decade, Walter's Medical Outcomes Study HIV Health Survey[191] scores have indicated progressive

CASE STUDY 31-3 ■ ADVANCED HIV DISEASE (AIDS) AT THE END STAGE OF LIFE: WALTER—cont'd

disability and worsening quality of life. Walter has been hopeless and depressed about his physical appearance and level of function. Before admission to the hospital, Walter lived alone in a modest studio apartment. He employed a daily home health aide to assist with food preparation and personal hygiene. Walter had been ambulating short distances in his apartment, often using a walker because of fatigue and unsteadiness. Walter's gait became increasingly ataxic over the past month. Last week, he had a seizure that resulted in admission to the hospital. Testing revealed progressive multifocal leukoencephalopathy (PML). Walter's physician expects that this brain infection, combined with his immunosuppression, will lead to death within a few months. Current medications: Fuzeon (enfuvirtide; HAART component), Kaletra (lopinavir and ritonavir; HAART component), Truvada (emtricitabine and tenofovir disoproxil fumarate; HAART component), Oxycontin (oxycodone; for chronic pain), Norpramin (desipramine; a tricyclic antidepressant), Pravachol (pravastatin; a cholesterol-lowering agent), and Prinivil (lisinopril; an angiotensin-converting enzyme inhibitor and diuretic).

Tests and Measurements

Inspection of the integumentary system reveals redness over the sacrum; otherwise the skin is intact. Diminished light touch sensation is noted in a stocking-glove distribution over the hands and feet. A Hoffman reflex, consistent with his myelopathy, is present in the upper extremities. Walter rates his pain at rest as ranging from 4/10 to 6/10. His pain drawing indicates low back, bilateral hand, and bilateral foot pain. Pulse oximetry reveals 96% oxygen saturation. Vital signs sitting: heart rate 70 beats/min, blood pressure 130/70 mm Hg, and respiratory rate 16 breaths/min with no apparent distress. Rate of perceived exertion at rest (RPE, Borg Scale) is 1/10. Pitting edema (+1) is noted in the ankles and feet.

Walter is independent with all bed mobility. Sitting balance is good. Standing balance is fair. Contact guard is required for sit-stand transfer and for ambulation a distance of 10 feet with a rolling walker. Vital signs after ambulating 10 feet: heart rate 110 bpm, blood pressure 150/70 mm Hg, respiratory rate 24 breaths/min, RPE 5/10, and oxygen saturation 96%. He demonstrates erratic foot placement and a wide base of support during gait. His Functional Independence Measure (FIM)[192] score is a 4. Because of fatigue and pain, strength and range-of-motion assessments are abbreviated. The following strength data are obtained (all measured bilaterally): shoulder abduction 3/5 (fair), elbow extension 4/5 (good), knee extension 3/5 (fair), and dorsiflexion and plantarflexion 4/5 (good). Passive range of motion data (bilateral): dorsiflexion 5 degrees; knee flexion 125 degrees (full knee extension not available, 10-degree flexion contracture noted); hip flexion 120 degrees; hip extension 10 degrees; shoulder flexion and abduction 140 degrees; and elbow, wrist, hand within normal limits.

EVALUATION AND DIAGNOSIS

Walter exhibits multiple impairments related to his advanced HIV disease (affecting multiple systems) and PML (a progressive disorder of the CNS). Summary: impaired integumentary integrity associated with superficial skin involvement, pain, impaired sensory integrity, impaired joint mobility and range of motion (knees, shoulders), impaired muscle performance, impaired gait, impaired balance, and impaired endurance.

Prognosis, Goals, and Outcomes

Walter's prognosis for survival is poor. It is likely that he will deteriorate slowly over the upcoming months. Goals and outcomes will thus focus on optimizing quality of life during Walter's remaining days. Specifically, goals are to reduce pain; prevent sequelae of immobility (such as pressure wounds, pneumonia, deep venous thrombosis, joint contracture, deconditioning, and atrophy); achieve independent sit-stand transfers and short-distance (15 feet) ambulation with a wheeled walker; improve endurance (RPE of 2 to 3 after ambulation); maintain independence with bed mobility; and promote safety.

Intervention Plan

Physical therapy will first be provided at bedside. If the patient wishes, treatment may be provided in the physical therapy department. Interventions will include relaxation techniques, passive range of motion and grade I joint mobilization (knees and shoulders), gait training with a wheeled walker, balance activities, and gentle strengthening and endurance exercises as tolerated. Occupational therapy will be consulted to address bed mobility and self-care tasks. Walter's vital signs will be closely monitored during therapy because it is possible that his ANS dysfunction may become evolved as a result of the CNS infection.

Walter's physician will be contacted regarding Walter's pain ratings. It is likely that increased dosage of pain medication is warranted as a result of reports of moderate pain at the current dosage. Walter will be seen by a dietician. The social worker will plan for transfer to a hospice setting.

In hospice care, physical therapy will focus on basic functional activities, such as transfers, gait, and endurance. Palliative interventions (moist heat, gentle massage) will be provided as needed for pain control. Caregiver education will be provided regarding prevention of the effects of immobility and safe functional mobility. In the hospice setting, Walter will have the opportunity to work with a spiritual counselor. Walter has expressed an interest in exploring Eastern medicine for pain control. Therefore a consultation with an acupuncturist will be arranged.

CHAPTER 32 Pain Management

ANNIE BURKE-DOE, PT, MPT, PhD

KEY TERMS

ANS pain: complex regional pain syndrome
acute pain
behavioral manipulations: exercise, operant conditioning, hypnosis, biofeedback
chronic pain
CNS pain: thalamic pain
cognitive strategies: relaxation exercises, body scanning, humor
nociceptor
pain intensity measurements: visual analog scale (VAS), simple descriptive pain scale (SDPS), pain estimate, faces pain scale
pain localization tools: pain drawing
pain modulation: gate control theory, neurotransmitters, neuromodulators
pain pathway
pain quality measurements: McGill Pain Questionnaire (MPQ), pediatric verbal descriptor scale, caregiver checklists
point stimulation

OBJECTIVES

After reading this chapter the student or therapist will be able to:

1. Describe the pain pathways.
2. Describe how pain is modulated within the nervous system.
3. Identify the causes of acute and chronic pain.
4. List the signs and symptoms of CNS, ANS, and peripheral pain and give an example of each.
5. Perform a comprehensive pain evaluation, including taking a pain history, measuring pain intensity, measuring pain character, and examining the client.
6. Design a comprehensive pain management program that addresses the objective and subjective aspects of the pain experience.

Chronic pain has a profound impact on all aspects of an individual's life. It influences relationships with family members, friends, co-workers, and health care providers. It affects the ability to fulfill responsibilities, to work, and to participate in social activities. Perhaps more than any other factor, the presence of chronic pain and the response to it determine the overall quality of an individual's life.

Chronic pain is prevalent. The National Institutes of Health (NIH) estimate that 100 million Americans suffer from chronic pain.[1] The prevalence of chronic noncancer pain in patients seen in the primary care setting shows an approximate range of 5% to 33%,[2] and a 2006 American Pain Foundation survey found that fewer than 40% of people with chronic noncancer pain reported that their pain was under control.[3] Studies of physicians, nurses, and therapists who treat individuals with chronic pain show that most do not have even a basic understanding of the concepts of pain management.[4-6] The result is inadequate or inappropriate care[6-8] of individuals who report having pain.

The use of the International Classification of Functioning, Disability and Health (ICF) model as a framework for understanding the relationship among impairments, activity limitations, and participation restrictions has been covered previously (refer to Chapter 1 as well as many chapters in the second section of this text). In terms of the application of the ICF model to pain, the clinician must understand that many impairments within various body systems cause pain and can limit activity and participation. The ability to identify appropriate rehabilitation approaches to improve activity and participation depends to a great extent on the clinician's ability to identify different impairments that cause pain, or the resulting impairments and activity and participation problems caused by pain.

This chapter deals with the complex issue of acute and chronic pain management. In the first section, an overview of the anatomy and physiology of pain is presented. In the second section, examination and evaluation of pain are explained. In the third section, a number of treatment interventions are suggested. Finally, case studies are presented to guide clinicians through the problem-solving process for designing pain management programs.

DEFINING PAIN

The primary purpose of pain is to protect the body. It occurs whenever there is tissue damage, and it causes the individual to react to remove the painful stimulus. Pain is also a sensation with more than one dimension. To the individual, pain is both an objective and a subjective experience. The objective dimension is the physiological tissue damage causing the pain. The subjective dimensions include the following[9]:

- A perceptual component: the client's awareness of the location, quality, intensity, and duration of the pain stimulus

- An affective component: the psychological factors surrounding the client's pain experience, including the client's personality and emotional state
- A cognitive component: what the client knows and believes about the pain resulting from his or her cultural background and past pain experiences (both personal pain experiences and those of others)
- A behavioral component: how the client expresses the pain to others through communication and behavior

All of these components taken together constitute the client's pain experience. Thus all must be addressed for a successful pain management program. When the subjective components of the pain experience are ignored, it is entirely possible that the client's underlying tissue damage may be corrected without her or his pain perception being cured.

In addition, recognizing that pain is more than simply a physical injury or disease process helps clinicians explain some of the inconsistencies observed in patients with chronic pain. Why is a client's pain report out of proportion to the magnitude and duration of the injury? Why is pain intolerable to one person and merely uncomfortable to another? And why is pain tolerable in one instance but overwhelming to the same individual when experienced at a different time?

The answers lie in the interconnectedness of the nervous system and the fact that pain transmission involves several higher centers. To select the most appropriate intervention, it is important for clinicians to have at least a general idea of the pain pathways. An overview of pain anatomy and physiology is discussed next.

PAIN ANATOMY

Pain arises from the stimulation of specialized peripheral free nerve endings called *nociceptors.* Injurious stimulation to the skin, muscle, joint, viscera, or tissue can trigger these peripheral terminals, whose cell bodies are located in the dorsal root ganglia and trigeminal ganglia. The density of nociceptors varies between as well as within these tissues. Nociceptors are extremely heterogeneous, differing in the neurotransmitters they contain, the receptors and ion channels they express, their speed of conduction, their response properties to noxious stimuli, and their capacity to be sensitized during inflammation, injury, and disease.[10]

Nociceptors found in interstitial tissues become excited with extreme mechanical, thermal, and chemical stimulation,[11] whereas nociceptors found in vessel walls become excited with these stimuli plus marked constriction and dilation of the vessels.[12] These receptors respond directly to some noxious stimuli and indirectly to others by means of one or more chemicals (histamine, potassium, bradykinin) released from cells in the traumatized tissues.[13]

Thermal nociceptors are triggered by intense hot or cold temperatures (>45° C or <5° C). They have fibers that are of small diameter and thinly myelinated with moderately fast conduction signals of 5 to 30 m/s. Mechanical nociceptors are triggered by intense pressures applied to the skin, such as a pinch. They also have thinly myelinated, moderately conducting fibers with speeds of 5 to 30 m/s.

Polymodal nociceptors are triggered by more than one sensory modality (mechanical, chemical, or thermal). These nociceptors have small-diameter, nonmyelinated fibers that conduct more slowly, generally at velocities less than 1.0 m/s. Stimulation of these receptors causes sensations of diffuse burning or aching pain. The difference in the fibers' size and lamination determines the speed at which impulses will travel to the brain.

These three types of nociceptors are broadly distributed in the skin and tissues and may work together. One example would be hitting one's shin against a table: a sharp "first pain" is felt immediately, followed later by a more prolonged aching, sometimes burning, "second pain."[13] The fast, sharp pain is transmitted by A delta fibers that carry information from thermal and mechanical nociceptors. The slow, dull pain is transmitted by C fibers that are activated by polymodal nociceptors.

Nociceptive input travels on A delta and C fibers into the dorsal horn of the spinal cord, where the gray matter is laminated and organized by cytological features. The first-order A delta and C fibers synapse with second-order neurons in lamina I (marginal layer), II (the substantia gelatinosa [SG]), and V. The second-order neurons do one of three things. A small number synapse with motor neurons, causing reflex movements (e.g., withdrawing the hand from a hot object). Others synapse with autonomic fibers, causing responses such as changes in heart rate and blood pressure and localized vasodilation, piloerection, and sweating. Most, however, travel a multisynaptic route to the higher centers by means of the ascending tracts.[11,14]

There are four major classes of neurons[15] responding to pain in the dorsal horn: low-threshold nociceptive-specific neurons designated class I; wide dynamic range (WDR) neurons designated class II; high-threshold nociceptive neurons designated class III; and a fourth, nonresponder group of neurons that develop spontaneous activity with exposure to endogenous inflammatory cytokines, designated class IV. Nociceptive-specific neurons are most abundant in superficial lamina; their receptor fields are discrete and vary from one to several square centimeters.[16] WDR neurons, in contrast, respond to a wide range of stimuli from A delta, A beta, and C fibers in a graded manner (i.e., the rate of firing escalates with increasing intensity of stimulation), can be found in all lamina, and are the most prevalent cells in the dorsal horn.[16] Because of their unique response to innocuous or nociceptive input, as well as their larger receptor field, WDR neurons play an important role in the central sensitization and the plasticity of the spinal cord.[16]

Nociceptive input crosses at the cord level to the anterolateral quadrant of the ascending contralateral spinothalamic tract (Figure 32-1). The axons of the anterolateral quadrant are arranged so that the sacral segments are most lateral, with the lumbar segments more medial and the cervical segments most central. This arrangement may be important clinically in that symptoms may be provoked according to dermatomal maps to some degree.[17] Pain dermatomes overlap to several adjacent dorsal roots so boundaries can be less distinct, requiring the clinician to distinguish the pain and dysfunction.

The anterolateral tract is divided into three ascending pathways: the spinothalamic, spinoreticular, and spinomesencephalic. The spinothalamic tract conveys information about painful and thermal stimulation (location and intensity) directly to the ventral posterior lateral nucleus of the thalamus, as well as sending collaterals off at the brain stem to join the spinoreticular tract. Axons within the spinoreticular tract synapse on neurons of the reticular formation of

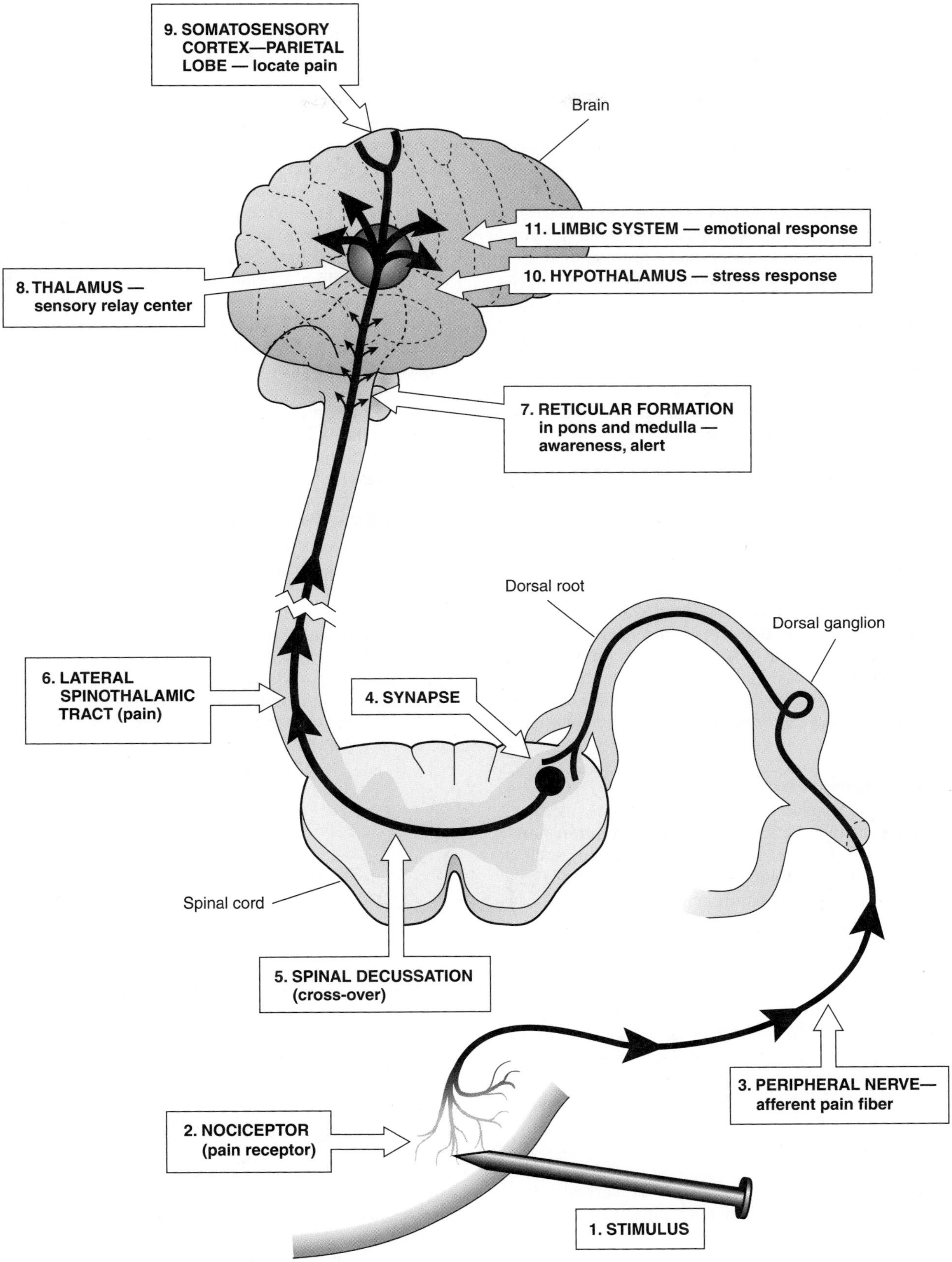

Figure 32-1 ■ Pain pathway. (From Gould BE: *Pathophysiology for the health professions,* ed 2, Philadelphia, 2002, WB Saunders.)

the medulla and pons, which relay information to the intralaminar and posterior nuclei of the thalamus and to other structures in the diencephalon, such as the hypothalamus (emotional response to pain).

Axons in the spinomesencephalic tract relay information to the mesencephalic reticular formation and periaqueductal gray matter by way of the spinoparabrachial tract. It then projects to the limbic system, which is involved with the affective component of pain (central modulation of pain).

The thalamus processes and relays information to several higher centers.[12] Each projection serves a specific purpose. Axons of the spinothalamic tract project information to both the lateral and medial nuclear groups of the thalamus. The lateral nuclear group of the thalamus is where information about the location of an injury is thought to be mediated.[13] Injury to the spinothalamic tract and the lateral nuclear group of the thalamus causes central neuropathic pain, which is discussed in further detail later.

Projections from the spinoreticular tract to the medial nuclear group of the thalamus are concerned with processing information about nociception, and they also activate nonspecific arousal systems. These pathways project from the thalamus to the basal ganglia and many cortical areas.

Projections to the postcentral gyrus (sensory cortex) are responsible for pain perception. It is from this projection that pain can be localized and characterized. Projections from the thalamus to the frontal lobes and limbic system are concerned with pain interpretation. It is from all these projections that an individual perceives pain as hurting. Projections from the thalamus, as well as from the limbic system and sensory cortical areas, to the temporal lobes are responsible for pain memory; and projections from the thalamus to the hypothalamus are responsible for the autonomic response to pain.

PAIN TRANSMISSION

Ascending transmission of pain impulses is mediated by the action of the chemical excitatory neurotransmitter glutamate (A delta and C fibers) and tachykinins such as substance P (C fibers). Glutamate and neuropeptides have distinct actions on postsynaptic neurons, but they act together to regulate the firing properties postsynaptically.[13] Tachykinins' activity is thought to prolong the action of glutamate, as levels are increased in persistent pain conditions.[16] The substrates of nociception that exist at the spinal level are complex in that more than 30 different neurotransmitters acting on more than 50 different receptors have been identified in the spinal cord and associated with some pain-related phenomenon.[18] Modulation of these substrates will assist in the effectiveness of therapeutic interventions and will be discussed next.

PAIN MODULATION

Nociceptive transmission is modulated at several points along the neural pathway by both ascending and descending systems.

The Gate Control Theory

The SG contains an ascending gating mechanism to block nociceptive impulses from leaving the dorsal horn of the spinal cord. The first-order neurons for both nociceptive and nonnociceptive information synapse with second-order neurons in the SG. The second-order neurons for both types of information project to specialized neurons named *T cells* (transmission cells) in lamina V. For pain transmission to occur, T cells must be stimulated while the SG is inhibited. The input from A delta and C fibers stimulates the T cells and inhibits the SG (Figure 32-2). Therefore A delta and C fiber input opens the gate, allowing pain transmission to the higher centers. On the other hand, when the SG and T cells are both stimulated, the T cells are inhibited and the gate is closed to pain transmission. The input from nonnociceptive A beta fibers carrying information from pressoreceptors and mechanoreceptors stimulates both the T cells and the SG. Therefore A beta fiber input closes the gate, blocking pain transmission.[17]

One example that illustrates the gate control theory is the use of transcutaneous electrical nerve stimulation (TENS) in an area that overlaps the injury. It works to reduce pain by activation of large-diameter A beta fibers that "closes the gate," thereby preventing pain transmission to the higher centers of the brain. This is also why shaking (vibrating) your hand after hitting your thumb with a hammer temporarily relieves pain.

Descending Pain Modulation System

There are at least two descending pain modulation systems. One involves the action of neurotransmitters, including serotonin, dopamine, norepinephrine, and substance P. High concentrations of brain serotonin108 and L-dopa (a precursor of dopamine)[19] have been found to inhibit nociception, whereas norepinephrine appears to enhance nociception.[20-23] The spinal mediators of descending nociceptive inhibitory influences include serotonin, norepinephrine, and acetylcholine (ACh). This may be relevant to the action of antidepressants in relieving pain in the absence of depression. Substance P is

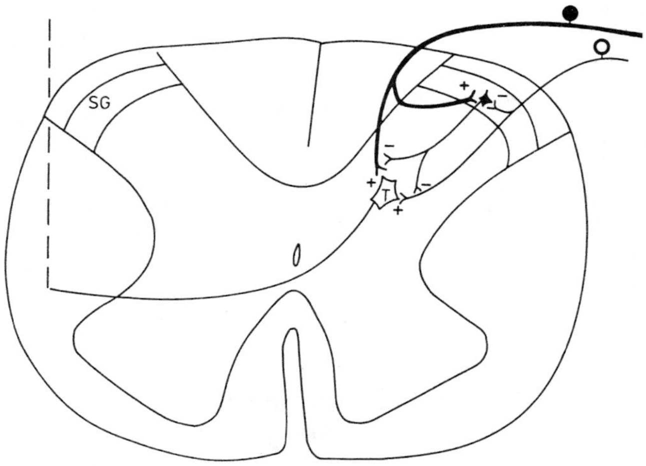

Figure 32-2 ■ Schematic representation of spinal structures involved in the gate control theory of pain transmission. Afferent input by means of both large- and small-diameter fibers is theorized to influence the transmission cell *(T)* directly and through small internuncial neurons located within the substantia gelatinosa *(SG)*. (From Nolan MF: Anatomic and physiologic organization of neural structures involved in pain transmission, modulation, and perception. In Echternach JL, editor: *Pain,* New York, 1987, Churchill Livingstone.)

thought to be the neurotransmitter for neurons transmitting chronic pain.[24]

The second descending modulating system is mediated by neuromodulators—chemicals capable of directly affecting pain transmission. The neuromodulators include enkephalin and β-endorphin, which are referred to as *endogenous opiates* because they have morphine-like actions and are found in areas of the central nervous system (CNS) that correspond to opiate-binding sites. Endogenous opiates are believed to modulate pain by inhibiting the release of substance P. They have been shown to have a profound effect on nociception and mood.[25-27] Their levels in the brain and spinal cord rise in response to emotional stress, causing an increase in the pain threshold and providing a possible reason that acute stress decreases acute pain.[28,29]

Although serotonin is not classified as an endogenous opiate, it exerts a profound effect on analgesia and enhances analgesic drug potency. High concentrations of serotonin lead to decreased pain by inhibiting transmission of nociceptive information within the dorsal horn,[30,31] whereas low concentrations result in depression, sleep disturbances, and increased pain.

The success of several therapeutic modalities, including noxious counterirritation (e.g., brief intense TENS or acupressure) and diversion (including hypnosis), is attributed to raising the level of endogenous opiates in the body.[29]

CATEGORIZING PAIN

Pain is grouped into several categories: acute, chronic, referred, central neuropathic, autonomic, and peripheral.

Acute pain is the normal predicted physiological response and serves as a warning. It alerts the individual that tissues are exposed to damaging or potentially damaging noxious stimuli. Acute pain is localized, occurs in proportion to the intensity of the stimuli, and lasts only as long as the stimuli or the tissue damage exists (1 to 6 months).[32] Although acute pain is associated with anxiety and increased autonomic activity (increased muscle tone, heart rate, and blood pressure),[33] it is usually relieved by interventions directed at correcting the injury. The pain experience is usually limited to the individual.[34]

Chronic pain is usually referred to as *intractable pain* if it persists for 6 or more months. It is defined as pain that continues after the stimulus has been removed or the tissue damage heals. Physiologically, chronic pain is believed to result from hypersensitization of the pain receptors and enlargement of the receptor field in response to the localized inflammation that follows tissue damage.[35] Chronic pain is poorly localized, has an ill-defined time of onset, and is strongly associated with the subjective components outlined previously. It does not respond well to interventions directed solely at correcting the injury. Chronic pain patients frequently report other symptoms, such as depression, difficulty sleeping, poor mental and physical function, and fatigue. The effects of the pain experience extend beyond the individual and affect the family, the workplace, and the social sphere of the individual.[34]

Referred pain is felt at a point other than its origin. Pain can be referred from an internal organ, a joint, a trigger point, or a peripheral nerve to a remote musculoskeletal structure. Referred pain usually follows a specific pattern. For example, cardiac pain is frequently referred to the left arm or jaw; the referral pattern for trigger points is exact enough to be used as a diagnostic tool and is often used by physicians to diagnose pathology. Referred pain is the result of a convergence of the primary afferent neurons from deep structures and muscles to secondary neurons that also have a cutaneous receptive field.[36,37]

Although it is now recognized that all neuropathic pain results in abnormal activity within the CNS,[38] pain initiated or caused by a primary lesion or dysfunction of the CNS[39] is referred to as *central neuropathic pain.* The involvement of the nervous system can be at many levels: nerves, nerve roots, and central pain pathways in the spinal cord and brain. In this circumstance, there is permanent damage to the nervous system (usually a peripheral nerve) and likely anatomical reorganization of spinal terminations of surviving axons or ectopic activity from a neuroma that contributes paroxysmal, persistent input to the spinal cord.[40] In addition to anatomical reorganization in the spinal cord, there could be some reorganization in the rostroventral medulla (RVM) as well, but more likely there is prolonged input to the RVM that sustains facilitatory influences that descend to the spinal cord. Less appreciated, descending facilitatory influences on spinal sensory processing could also be important to maintenance of chronic pain conditions, particularly those that persist in the absence of obvious tissue pathology.[40]

Central neuropathic pain is medically diagnosed by its defining neurological signs and symptoms; it is verified with neuroimaging tests that identify a CNS lesion and rule out other causes. It is important that the therapist be able to localize the level and differentiate between central and peripheral pain. Central neuropathic pain can be caused by vascular insult; traumatic, neoplastic, and demyelinating diseases; and surgery (including vascular compromise during surgery). Central neuropathic pain is distinct from nociceptive pain (nonneuronal tissue damage).

The onset of central neuropathic pain is usually delayed after the occurrence of the initial episode that results in damage to the CNS; onset of pain may occur during the phase of recovery from neurological deficits.[41] Pain originating from a cerebrovascular incident and spinal cord injury usually begins weeks or months after the insult, whereas pain originating from tumors may take years to begin.[38]

Individuals with central neuropathic pain may have difficulty describing their pain and report burning, aching, pricking, squeezing, or cutting pain after cutaneous stimulation, movement, heat, cold, or vibration. A normally nonnoxious stimulus, such as moving clothing across skin, becomes agonizing. In some cases the pain begins spontaneously.[42] Pain intensity varies, but it does seem to be associated to some degree with the location of the lesion.[38] Allodynia (pain from normally nonnoxious stimuli) and dysesthesia are common, and one of the characteristic features of central neuropathic pain is that the clinical symptoms persist long after the stimulus has been removed.

Central neuropathic pain is topographical. The site of the lesion determines the location of the symptoms. The pain may involve half the body, an entire extremity, or a small portion of one extremity.[38] It is frequently migratory. Thalamic pain is the classic example of central neuropathic pain.

Central neuropathic pain is difficult to treat. Surgery is not helpful for most individuals with central neuropathic pain, and medications have not been effective in permanently relieving the symptoms.[11] Therefore the treatment of clients with central neuropathic pain stresses coping strategies and prevention of loss of activity and participation. The ideal management of a chronic pain patient is by a multidisciplinary approach, including disciplines such as internal medicine, neurology, anesthesia, nursing, psychology, pharmacy, rehabilitation medicine, physical therapy, occupational therapy, and others. The limitation of this approach is that access to such a wide range of specialists is often available only at large medical centers and special pain clinics, which restricts access to a limited number of patients.

Under normal conditions there is a fine balance between the parasympathetic and sympathetic branches of the autonomic nervous system (ANS). Parasympathetic activity maintains homeostasis, whereas sympathetic activity functions to make "fight-or-flight" changes in response to stress. Stimulation of the autonomic efferent fibers is not normally painful. However, the balance between afferent input and the descending sympathetic nervous system (SNS) is disrupted when there is injury, resulting in exaggerated and prolonged sympathetic activity, allodynia, and hyperalgesia (increased response to normally painful stimuli)—hence, autonomic pain.

Allodynia is a product of the phenomenon of central sensitization.[43] After injury, new axons sprout from the sympathetic efferent neurons. These fire spontaneously and, because they synapse on the cell bodies of the primary afferent neurons, cause them to fire as well. In addition, the dorsal horn neurons themselves become more excitable. They show an enlargement in their receptive field and become more sensitive to mechanical, thermal, and chemical stimulation. The result is an increase in the neuronal barrage into the CNS and the perception of pain with usually nonpainful stimuli.[13]

Complex regional pain syndrome (CRPS) is an example of pain that arises from abnormal activity within the ANS.[44] CRPS has been classified into two distinct types[39]: CRPS type I (formerly *reflex sympathetic dystrophy*) follows mild trauma without nerve injury, and CRPS type II (formerly *causalgia*) follows trauma with nerve injury. CRPS type I generally begins within the month after the injury, whereas CRPS type II can occur any time after the injury.[45]

The main features of CRPS type I are constant burning pain that fluctuates in intensity and increases with movement, constant stimulation, or stress. There are also allodynia and hyperalgesia, edema, abnormal sweating, abnormal blood flow and trophic changes in the area of pain, and impaired motor function. CRPS type I is relieved by blocking the SNS, indicating that the pain is sympathetically maintained.[45]

CRPS type II occurs in the region of a limb innervated by an injured nerve. The nerves most commonly involved in CRPS type II are the median, sciatic, tibial, and ulnar; involvement of the radial nerve is rare. Pain is described as spontaneous, constant, and burning and is exacerbated by light touch, stress, temperature change, movement, visual and auditory stimuli, and emotional disturbances. Allodynia and hyperalgesia are common and may involve the distribution of more than one peripheral nerve. As with CRPS type I, edema, abnormal sweating, abnormal blood flow, trophic changes, and impaired motor function occur. The symptoms spread proximally and can involve other areas of the body. Evidence also points to sympathetic involvement in CRPS type II.[45]

The treatment of CRPS is complex and must be carefully coordinated among members of an interdisciplinary team including the neurologist (medications), psychologist (behavior), anesthesiologist (injections), and therapist (functional recovery). The therapist provides the core treatment to improve function. Therapists need to pay close attention to the following aspects of the disorder: (1) the degree of motor abnormalities, including restricted active range of motion (ROM), abnormal posturing, spasm, tremor, and dystonia; (2) true passive range restriction; (3) hyperesthesia and allodynia; (4) swelling and vasomotor changes; and (5) evidence of osteoporosis by radiograph.[46] Please refer to Case Study 32-1 for interventions for clients with CRPS.

Peripheral pain results from noxious irritation of the nociceptors. The character of peripheral pain depends on the location and intensity of the noxious stimulation, as well as which fibers carry the information into the dorsal gray matter. As noted previously, information carried on A delta fibers is sharp and well localized, begins rapidly, and lasts only as long as the stimulus is present, whereas information carried on C fibers is dull and diffuse, has a delayed onset, and lasts longer than the duration of the stimulus. The treatment of peripheral pain is covered in detail in Chapter 18.

The management of central versus peripheral pain is determined by the type of pain—acute or chronic—and the clinical features present, including clinical localization; time of onset; laboratory study localization; response to analgesics, including narcotics; response to antidepressants; and response to nerve block or neurectomy.[41] Differentiation among features will drive the treatment plan, but because some peripheral and central forms can coexist, diagnosis may be difficult.

The multidimensional aspects of chronic pain make it important to evaluate the causes as well as the emotional and cognitive sequelae.[47] Persistent pain is now considered to have a psychogenic component.[48] The longer an individual has pain, the more a psychological component may become dominant. Many emotional factors can strongly influence pain, such as pain thresholds, past experiences with pain, coping styles, and social roles. The emotional experience that we perceive with pain reflects the interaction of higher brain centers and subcortical regions, such as the amygdala and cingulate gyrus (limbic system).[49] Positron emission tomography of patients with chronic neuropathic pain demonstrates a shift of acute pain activity in the sensory cortex to regions such as the anterior cingulate gyrus.[50] Understanding the physical limitations imposed by chronic pain is an area that therapists commonly assess; it is the mind-body connection that is often less articulated by the client and more difficult for the practitioner.

Treatment of chronic pain should include a patient-centered approach, given the unique manifestations that occur in an individual's response to pain. Patient-centered models, such as the ICF model, provide a framework that embraces a multidisciplinary team approach practiced in pain clinics. In such models, chronic pain has been noted to include psychological factors such as feelings of fear, anxiety, and depression,[51] which are known to have the ability to modulate and exacerbate the physical pain experience.[52] For example, a client with chronic pain who has the fear that movement will increase pain may alter his activity, causing muscular shortening, spasms, and a spiraling course of more pain and disability. The focus in treating clients with chronic pain should be on improving functional physical activity, decreasing peripheral nociception and central facilitation, and providing cognitive and behavioral strategies to help in resuming normal activities.

EXAMINATION OF THE CLIENT WITH PAIN

The examination of a client with pain can be challenging because the therapist must frequently weed through the individual's emotions, behaviors, and secondary gains in an attempt to identify the source of the symptoms. Many clients are not referred to therapy until they have participated in weeks, months, or even years of failed interventions, and their expectations and patience are at low levels. They often approach therapy anticipating more instructions, more frustration, and more pain. Despite these obstacles, therapists must strive to complete pain evaluations that include measurable, reproducible information that identifies the source of pain and provides direction toward treatment that is both beneficial and cost-effective and that assists in establishing attainable goals. The time allotted for the examination may be dependent on the type of practice setting; many therapists send a comprehensive questionnaire to the client or ask the client to arrive early to complete important paperwork. It is essential to develop a trusting relationship, ensuring that the client feels that the therapist has listened to his or her concerns and has acknowledged his or her fears, and will participate in a plan for improving his or her physical, mental, and functional abilities.

Pain History

Every evaluation of a client with pain should begin with a comprehensive pain history. It is important to have a standardized format to decrease chances of missing important information and to minimize having the client "lead the interview." The following alphabetical mnemonic device may prove helpful (OPQRST):

- Observation: Observation of the client from the moment of entry until (and sometimes beyond) the moment of exit from the clinic. By observing the client outside of the evaluation, the therapist is able to assess the client's movement. The patient's nervous system will accurately express itself to the therapist, especially when the patient is asked to focus attention on a topic other than pain and the patient is not aware that movement is being observed.
- Origin and onset: Date and circumstances of the onset of pain. How did the pain start? Gradually or suddenly? Was there a precipitating injury? If so, what was the mechanism of injury? If not, can the client correlate the onset to a particular activity or posture?
- Position: Location of the pain. Have the client demonstrate where the pain is located rather than relying on description alone. In addition to being more accurate, demonstration allows another observation of the client's ability and willingness to move. Clients can also be asked to draw their symptoms on a schematic, such as the pain drawing, which is described later.
- Pattern: Pattern of the pain. Is the pain constant or periodic? Does it travel or radiate? Which activities and postures increase or decrease the pain? Does medication or time of day have any effect on the pain? Have there been any recent changes in the pattern? Does the client believe that the pain is improving, worsening, or remaining the same?
- Quality: Characteristics of the pain. Does the client use adjectives indicating mechanical (pressing, bursting, stabbing), chemical (burning), neural (numb, "pins and needles"), or vascular (throbbing) origin? Two tools for describing pain character are described later.
- Quantity: Intensity of the pain. How has the pain intensity changed since the onset? Several methods that allow for monitoring change in pain intensity are presented later.
- Radiation: Characteristics of pain radiation. Does the pain radiate? What causes the pain to radiate? Can the radiation be reversed? How?
- Signs and symptoms: Functional and psychological components of the pain. Has the pain resulted in any functional limitations? Has it caused any changes in the client's ability to participate in life, including employment and recreational activities? Does the client's personality contribute to the pain, or has the pain caused changes in the client's emotional stability? Does the client benefit from the pain? How? It may be necessary to interview the client's significant others or family members for an accurate picture.
- Treatment: Previous and current medical and therapeutic treatment and its effectiveness, including medications, home remedies, and recommendations for movement activities. It is also important to determine the client's attitude and expectations concerning therapy in addition to obtaining a treatment history.
- Visceral symptoms: Physical symptoms of visceral origin that can accompany and be responsible for the pain (Box 32-1). Visceral causes of pain require referral to the client's physician for further investigation before the initiation of treatment by a therapist.

Pain Measurement

Research has shown that pain memory does not provide an accurate measure of pain intensity.[53] Therefore pain measurement tools are designed to provide information about the intensity, location, and character of a client's symptoms at the time of the evaluation. This information can then be merged with the pain history, the disease or pathology history, and the physical findings to identify the cause of the pain. The disease or pathology management and its pain measurement will be the responsibility of the physician, whereas the movement limitations caused by the pain are the responsibility of the therapist. A number of pain measurement tools are available. These tools are used by professionals whose focus is pathology, as well as professionals whose responsibility is helping the patient to regain functional activities and life participation. The applications and limitations of several are discussed.

Measuring Pain Intensity

Pain intensity rating tools are scales that have the client rate the current level of pain by marking a continuum or assigning a numerical value to the pain intensity (Figure 32-3).

BOX 32-1 ■ VISCEROGENIC BACK PAIN

GENERAL SIGNS AND SYMPTOMS
- Pain does not increase with spinal stresses or strains.
- Pain is not relieved with rest.
- Visceral symptoms accompany back pain.

GASTROINTESTINAL TRACT SIGNS AND SYMPTOMS
- Pain is accompanied by altered bowel habits.
- Pain is related to eating.
- Peptic pain is relieved with vomiting.

KIDNEY SIGNS AND SYMPTOMS
- Increased pain with diuresis indicates hydronephrosis.

PELVIC SIGNS AND SYMPTOMS
- Low back pain associated with vaginal bleeding or discharge.

PROSTATE SIGNS AND SYMPTOMS
- Low back discomfort associated with micturition.

LUNG SIGNS AND SYMPTOMS
- Posterior thoracic pain associated with respiration in chronic obstructive pulmonary disease.

VASCULAR SIGNS AND SYMPTOMS
- Deep, boring, pulsating low back pain associated with a palpable abdominal aortic aneurysm.
- Back pain with or without calf pain after walking and relieved with standing still; possibly impaired lower extremity pulses and trophic skin changes associated with occlusive disease of the internal iliac artery or its branches.

Modified from Makofsky H, Willis GC: Non-mechanical and pathological causes of low back pain. *Phys Ther Forum* May 15, p 12, 1989.

Each of the first three tools described here has been found to be reliable over time when used to measure pain that is present at the time of the rating. In general, however, clients who are depressed or anxious tend to report higher levels of pain and clients who are not depressed or anxious tend to report lower levels of pain on all three of these scales.[54]

Visual Analog Scale. With the visual analog scale (VAS), the client rates the pain on a continuum that begins with "no pain" and ends with "maximum pain tolerable." This tool provides an infinite number of points between the extremes, making it sensitive to small changes in pain intensity. However, it has not been found reliable for individuals who have impaired abstract thinking skills[55] and may be unable to translate their pain intensity into a corresponding point on a line.

Simple Descriptive Pain Scale. With a simple descriptive pain scale (SDPS), the client rates the pain on a continuum that is subdivided using descriptors that gradually increase in intensity. Sample descriptors are "no pain," "mild pain," "moderate pain," "severe pain," and "maximum pain tolerable." This tool is more useful than the VAS for clients with impaired abstract thinking because it is easier for them to identify with the pain descriptors than with the line found in the VAS. However, clients have been found to favor the points corresponding to each descriptor rather than points between, resulting in a less sensitive tool than the VAS.[56]

Pain Estimate. With a pain estimate, the client assigns a numerical rating to the pain, staying within defined limits (most commonly between 0 and 100, where 0 represents no pain and 100 represents maximum pain tolerable). Because it provides a numerical range of scores, this tool is valuable for statistical analysis purposes. However, whereas some clients find assigning a numerical rating to their pain intensity easy,

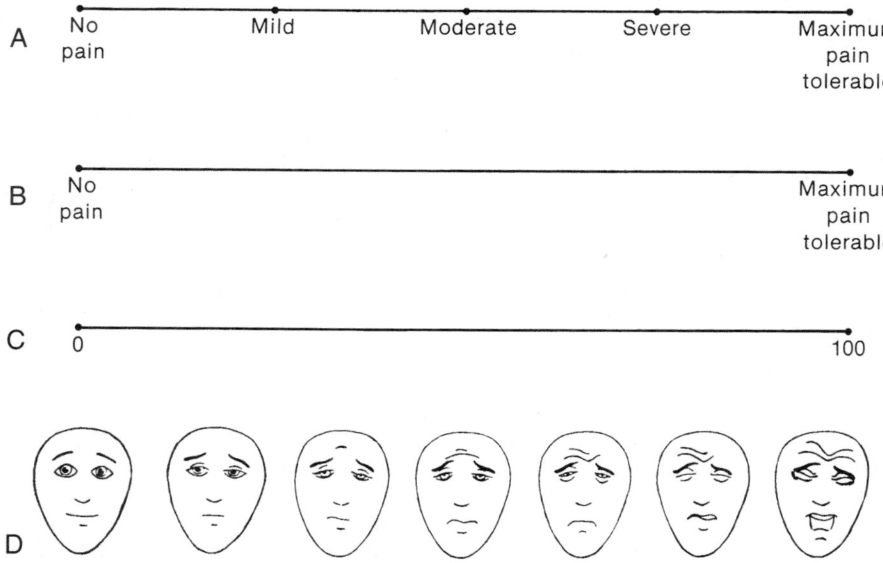

Figure 32-3 ■ Rating scales for measuring pain intensity. **A,** Simple descriptive pain scale (SDPS). **B,** Visual analog scale (VAS). **C,** Pain estimate. **D,** Faces pain scale. (**D** Reprinted from Bieri D, Reeve DA, Champion GD, et al: The faces pain scale for the self-assessment of the severity of pain experienced by children: development, initial validation, and preliminary investigation for the ratio scale properties. *Pain* 41:139–150, 1990, with permission from Elsevier Science.)

clients with impaired abstract thinking may have difficulty similar to that encountered with the VAS.

Faces Pain Scale. With the Faces Pain Scale, the client selects one of seven schematic faces representing gradually increasing pain intensities. The scale begins with a face representing no pain and ends with a face representing the most pain possible. This tool is designed for use with young children who do not have the ability to use any of the three previous tools. The Faces Pain Scale has been found to be valid across cultural lines[57] and to have a strong correlation with other pain measures.[56] It is simple to use, does not require verbal skills, and requires little instruction. It has been used successfully with children as young as age 3 and with individuals who are limited in verbal expression.

Localizing Pain Symptoms

Pain Drawings. The client is asked to draw his or her symptoms on a schematic of the human body using a provided list of symbols (Figure 32-4). The result is a diagram describing the nature and location of the client's pain, which can be compared with the client's verbal report. In addition to providing a database, the pain drawing has been found to be useful in identifying individuals who have a heavy psychological or emotional component to their pain, making it helpful also in identifying clients who would benefit from further psychological evaluation.[58]

Describing Pain Quality

McGill Pain Questionnaire (MPQ). One of the most popular scales to rate pain quality is the McGill Pain Questionnaire (MPQ), which includes 20 categories of descriptive words covering the sensory (numbers 1 to 10), affective (numbers 11 to 15), and evaluative (number 16) properties of pain (Figure 32-5). Sensory properties are measured using temporal, thermal, spatial, and pressure descriptors. Affective properties are measured using fear, tension, and autonomic descriptors. Evaluative properties are measured using pain experience descriptors.[59] Each word has a numerical value based on its position within its category.

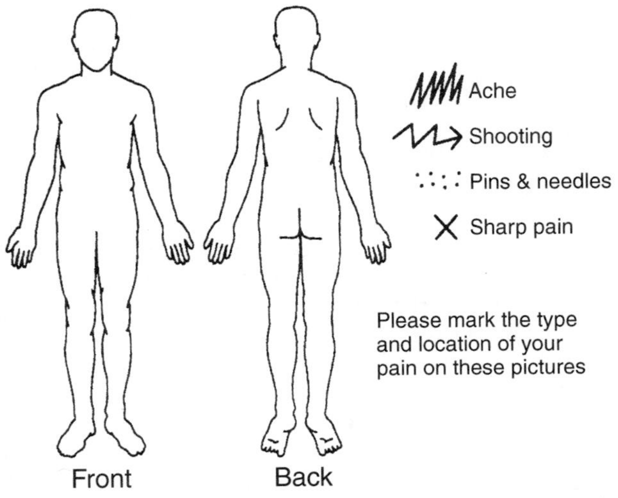

Figure 32-4 ■ Pain drawing for describing the nature and location of a client's pain symptoms. (From Cameron MH, editor: *Physical agents in rehabilitation,* Philadelphia, 1999, WB Saunders.)

The client is instructed to "select the word in each category that best describes the pain you have now. If there is no word in the category that describes the pain, skip the category. If there is more than one word that describes the pain, select the word that best describes the pain."[59]

The MPQ can provide the following types of information[59]:

- A pain-rating index based on the sum of the values of all the words selected
- A pain-rating index based on the sum of the values of all the words in a given category
- The total number of words chosen

The MPQ has been studied extensively and found valid for adults with acute and chronic pain as well as for those with a variety of specific pathological states.[60-62] It provides clues into the specific cause of pain because it describes the client's symptoms.

However, the MPQ does pose some disadvantages. It is time-consuming, requiring more time to complete than any of the previously described rating scales. Thus it is not appropriate for quick estimates of pain after treatment. Clients, especially children, are frequently unfamiliar with some of the descriptors and ask the evaluator to assist by defining words. However, reliability and validity of this test are based on examiner objectivity, and care must be taken to avoid the introduction of evaluator bias by helping the client to select appropriate descriptors.[59] This issue can be dealt with by telling the client, "If you do not recognize a word, it probably does not apply to you."

Pediatric Verbal Descriptor Scale. Because a child's description of pain is limited by a smaller vocabulary, Wilkie and associates[63] have developed a verbal descriptor scale specifically for use with children (Table 32-1). Their list includes 56 words commonly used by children aged 8 to 17 to describe their pain experience. The word list is divided into the four categories found in the MPQ. The evaluators' research has shown the list to be useful for children with a variety of diagnoses because it is relatively free of gender, ethnic, and developmental bias.

Caregiver Checklist. Clients who are unable to communicate verbally because of neurological disabilities may be unable to use any of the just-described pain measurement scales. However, because of pain associated with their medical conditions, extensive and repeated surgery, and behavioral oddities that might limit pain expression, these individuals are at high risk for having their pain go unrecognized. McGrath and colleagues[64] have attempted to develop and categorize a checklist of demonstrated pain behaviors identified by caregivers of severely handicapped individuals. Although their list did not pass validity criteria, the researchers propose that clinicians develop a client-specific checklist that could be used to gauge changes in the client's pain from the information gained during the caregiver interview portion of the evaluation of nonverbal handicapped clients.

In addition to qualifying and quantifying the client's pain, pain measurement tools have an additional value. They can be used to identify inconsistencies between a client's pain report and the clinician's objective findings. For example, a client with normal objective findings would not be expected to give a high pain report or draw symptoms over the entire pain drawing. Conversely, a client with a multitude of objective findings within the severe range would be expected to

What Does Your Pain Feel Like?

Some of the words below describe your present pain. Circle ONLY those words that best describe it. Leave out any category that is not suitable. Use only a single word in each appropriate category–the one that applies best.

1	2	3	4
Flickering	Jumping	Pricking	Sharp
Quivering	Flashing	Boring	Cutting
Pulsing	Shooting	Drilling	Lacerating
Throbbing		Stabbing	
Beating		Lancinating	
Pounding			
5	**6**	**7**	**8**
Pinching	Tugging	Hot	Tingling
Pressing	Pulling	Burning	Itchy
Gnawing	Wrenching	Scalding	Smarting
Cramping		Searing	Stinging
Crushing			
9	**10**	**11**	**12**
Dull	Tender	Tiring	Sickening
Sore	Taut	Exhausting	Suffocating
Hurting	Rasping		
Aching	Splitting		
Heavy			
13	**14**	**15**	**16**
Fearful	Punishing	Wretched	Annoying
Frightful	Grueling	Blinding	Troublesome
Terrifying	Cruel		Miserable
	Vicious		Intense
	Killing		Unbearable
17	**18**	**19**	**20**
Spreading	Tight	Cool	Nagging
Radiating	Numb	Cold	Nauseating
Penetrating	Drawing	Freezing	Agonizing
Piercing	Squeezing		Dreadful
	Tearing		Torturing

Figure 32-5 ■ The McGill Pain Questionnaire used to rate pain quality. (Reprinted from Melzack R: The McGill Pain Questionnaire: major properties and scoring methods. *Pain* 1:277, 1975, with permission from Elsevier Science.)

provide a high pain rating. In addition, as objective symptoms subside, it is expected that the client will report a similar decline on the rating scales. Inconsistencies between the client's pain descriptions and the therapist's findings should serve to alert the clinician that the client might require cognitive or affective intervention in addition to physical treatment.

PSYCHOSOCIAL ASSESSMENT

Psychosocial factors are key variables in the comprehensive assessment of chronic pain. Davidson and colleagues[65] determined seven factors using a "prototypical" pain assessment battery that included pain and disability, pain description, affective distress, support, positive coping strategies, negative coping strategies, and activity. Irving and Squire[66] described two key individual personality features that affect pain: catastrophizing and health-related anxiety. Persons who catastrophically misinterpret innocuous bodily sensations, including pain, are likely to become fearful of pain, which results in pain-related fear. Pain-related fear is associated with avoidance of movement and physical activity, which directly affects recovery of function. Pain-related fear is also associated with increased pain levels and an exacerbated painful experience. Two validated tools to screen for these features include the Pain Catastrophizing Scale (PCS) and the Tampa Scale of Kinesophobia (TKS).[67]

EXAMINATION OF THE CLIENT

The clinical examination should begin the moment the client enters the door. Clients frequently change posture and affect when they are being formally evaluated, and it is important to gain an accurate view of pain behavior during spontaneous activities to assess the validity of complaints. The following should be included in the examination:

- Observation of gait and movement patterns, including the use of assistive devices.
- Notation of body type and anomalies.
- Examination of sitting and standing posture, including both the normal posture and that assumed because of the pain. (Observe the client during activities, if possible, to differentiate movement patterns altered by intent versus automatic adjustments.)

TABLE 32-1 ■ PEDIATRIC VERBAL DESCRIPTOR SCALE

DIMENSION	WORD	DIMENSION	WORD	DIMENSION	WORD	DIMENSION	WORD
A	Annoying Bad Horrible Miserable Terrible Uncomfortable	S	Biting Cutting Like a pin Like a sharp knife Pinlike Sharp Stabbing	S	Itching Like a scratch Like a sting Scratching Stinging	A	Crying Frightening Screaming Terrifying
E	Aching Hurting Like an ache Like a hurt Sore	S	Blistering Burning Hot	S	Shocking Shooting Splitting	A	Dizzy Sickening Suffocating
S	Beating Hitting Pounding Punching Throbbing	S	Cramping Crushing Like a pinch Pinching Pressure	S	Numb Stiff Swollen Tight	E	Never goes away Uncontrollable
A	Awful Deadly Dying Killing						

Reprinted from Wilkie DJ, Holzemer WL, Tesler MD, et al: Measuring pain quality: validity and reliability of children's and adolescents' pain language. *Pain* 41:151–159, 1990, with permission from Elsevier Science.

S, Sensory; *A,* affective; *E,* evaluative.

- Inspection of the skin for pliability, trophic changes, scar tissue, and other abnormalities.
- Palpation of the soft tissue structures to identify changes in temperature, swelling, tenderness, and areas of discomfort.
- Palpation of the anatomical structures to determine end feel—the sensation felt at the end of the available movement.[68]
  - Bone to bone: hard normal, for example, at the end range of elbow extension.
  - Spasm: muscular resistance abnormal.
  - Capsular feel: rubbery normal at the extreme of full ROM; abnormal when encountered before the end of ROM.
  - Springy block: rebound abnormal.
  - Tissue approximation: soft tissue normal at the extremes of full passive flexion.
  - Empty feel: no physiological resistance, but client resists movement because of pain.
- Examination of ROM: active ROM testing is performed to assess the client's willingness to move and to identify any limitations or painful areas; passive ROM testing is used to further refine the observations.[68]
  - When active and passive movements are painful and restricted in the same direction and the pain appears at the limit of motion, the problem is most likely arthrogenic.
  - When active and passive movements are painful or restricted in opposite directions, the problem is most likely muscular.
  - When there is relative restriction of passive movement in the capsular pattern, the problem may be arthritic in nature.
  - When there is no restriction of passive movement but the client cannot perform the movement actively, the muscle may not be functioning, either from intrinsic problems within the muscle or interruption in the neural pathway (central or peripheral).
- Examination of muscle strength[68]:
  - When the movement is strong and painful, there is a minor lesion in the muscle or tendon.
  - When the movement is weak and increases the pain, there is a major lesion that needs to be identified with further testing.
  - When the movement is weak but does not increase the pain, there is the possibility of either complete rupture of the muscle or tendon or a neurological disorder.
  - When all resisted movements are painful, the pain may be organic or the patient may be emotionally hypersensitive.
  - When movement is strong and painless, the test results are normal.
- Assessment of bilateral neurological function:
  - Reflexes: peripheral lesions tend to diminish deep tendon reflexes (DTRs). CNS lesions tend to intensify DTRs, and testing frequently elicits a clonic reaction.[69] Note any asymmetries in response.
  - Sensation: test light touch, sharp (noxious) touch, and vibration. Pressure on a nerve usually affects

conduction on the large, myelinated fibers first. Therefore vibration is the first sensation to be diminished. Where there is decreased perception of touch and noxious stimuli, the lesion is more severe.[70] Note any asymmetries in response.
- Allodynia and hyperalgesia: delineate areas of allodynia and hyperalgesia to touch, hot, and cold. Exact descriptions of these areas, along with areas of decreased perception of vibration, will provide information concerning A beta versus C fiber involvement in the production of pain.[70]
- Stretch and pressure tests to nerve trunks.

It is not always possible to complete a pain evaluation in one session. Clients may not be able to tolerate all the required activities at one time, or there may be enough inconsistencies for the therapist to want a second appointment to refocus on specific tests. However, with the limitations on number of visits common with managed care, the therapist may feel pressured to identify a cause for the client's pain in the initial visit. This is not necessary. It is far better to take more than one visit and be accurate than to take only one visit and develop a treatment plan that is not appropriate for the client's needs.

REHABILITATION MANAGEMENT OF THE CLIENT WITH PAIN

There are three broad avenues of intervention for pain management: physical interventions, cognitive strategies, and behavioral manipulations.[71] Each avenue addresses a different aspect of the pain experience, and each requires a different level of participation from the client.

Physical interventions are directed at the client's body with the goal of healing the tissue injury. Examples include medication, surgery, and the therapy modalities. Physical interventions are of use most frequently with acute pain or recurrent pain resulting from reinjury. Physical interventions are often passive and, for the most part, soothing. When used long term, they promote dependence on the clinician. Therefore it is best to use them as a short-term adjunct in the overall treatment program.

Cognitive strategies are directed at the client's thoughts with the goal of changing the client's pain paradigms. Cognitive strategies include body scanning and reinterpretation of self-statements. Cognitive strategies are self-initiated and performed independently; therefore they encourage personal responsibility and independence.

Behavioral manipulations involve a behavioral change on the part of the client to bring about the desired response. They include exercise, biofeedback, hypnosis, relaxation exercises, and operant conditioning. There is usually a brief learning period until the client becomes proficient with these techniques; however, once learned, behavioral manipulations can be initiated and performed independently. Behavioral manipulations also encourage personal responsibility and independence.

A brief review of the benefits, indications, contraindications, and precautions for many of the interventions provided by therapists should provide an overview of the complexity of pain management. The purpose of this section is to provide guidance in the selection of one treatment option over another so that intervention will be based on sound physiological principles. Readers who wish to explore an intervention in greater depth are directed to the references listed at the end of this chapter.

Physical Interventions

Thermotherapy

The physiological effects of heat depend on the method of application, the depth of penetration, and the rate and magnitude of temperature change. In terms of the use of thermotherapy to control pain, several mechanisms have been established. Muscle spasm decreases as a result of decreased activity in gamma motor efferents, decreased excitability of muscle spindles, and increased activity of Golgi tendon organs.[72,73] This modality will often decrease peripheral pain. Ischemic pain is relieved by the influx of oxygen-rich blood into the dilated vessels, and muscle tension pain is decreased by interruption of the pain-spasm cycle. In addition, the pain threshold itself rises through gating at the spinal cord level.[74,75]

Several textbooks[76-80] on physical agents and rehabilitation discuss the physiological effects, precautions, contraindications, and method of application for these modalities. The reader is advised to refer to the textbooks for details.

Superficial heat can be applied by conduction, convection, or radiation. Conductive heating involves the exchange of heat down a temperature gradient by two objects that are in contact. The depth of penetration with conductive heating is usually 1 cm or less.[81] Moist heat packs and paraffin are examples of therapeutic conductive heating. Convective heating involves heat transfer through the flow of hot fluid. Therapeutic convective heating takes place during hydrotherapy and Fluidotherapy (Encore Medical Corporation, Austin, Texas). Molecules with a temperature greater than absolute zero are in an excited state and emit energy, thus creating radiant heat. Objects that are warmed by the energy are heated by radiation. Therapeutic radiant heat is applied with infrared or ultraviolet light. Because of the contraindications of ultraviolet light, this type of radiant heat is seldom used by therapists today in rehabilitation settings.

Clients can be taught how and when to apply superficial heat independently. Once they have demonstrated independence, responsibility for the application of superficial heat should be transferred to the client or her or his caregiver.

The deeper tissues can be heated using conversion, the alteration of one form of energy into another. Examples of heating by conversion include use of shortwave diathermy or ultrasound.

During shortwave diathermy, the client is placed into an oscillating magnetic field. The systemic ions create friction as they attempt to line up with the continuously reversing current, resulting in an increase in tissue temperature deep within the body. Shortwave diathermy is contraindicated for clients with metal implants because of the potential for the implant to become hot and burn the surrounding tissues. It is also contraindicated for clients with cardiac pacemakers because of the pacemaker's metal components and because the electromagnetic radiation may interfere with the pacemaker's operation. Shortwave diathermy should not be used for clients with cancer or multiple sclerosis or who are pregnant, and it should not be used over the eyes, the reproductive organs, or growing epiphyses. Female therapists should avoid prolonged exposure to shortwave diathermy because some research has demonstrated a possible negative effect on pregnancy outcome and fetal development.[82]

Ultrasound is another modality that heats deep tissues by conversion. As its name implies, ultrasound consists of sound waves delivered at a frequency too high to be perceived by human hearing. Sound waves are repeatedly refracted as they encounter tissues of differing acoustical resistance while traveling through the skin toward the bone (Figure 32-6). Tissues with high collagen content (tendon, ligament, fascia, and joint capsule) are heated more efficiently than tissues with low collagen content (fat, muscle). The extent of the temperature increase is related to the dose of ultrasound energy delivered. As the dose of ultrasound energy is increased by increasing the treatment duration or intensity, more energy is available to the tissues and the heating effect increases.[21] Moreover, the higher the frequency of ultrasound delivered, the more superficial the effect. Ultrasound delivered at 1 MHz heats tissues at depths to 5 cm, whereas ultrasound delivered at 3 MHz heats tissues in the upper 2 cm.[83]

The thermal effects of ultrasound can be used to increase tissue extensibility, cellular metabolic processes, and circulation; decrease pain and muscle spasm; and change nerve conduction velocity. The number of impulses traveling along the nerve decreases at low doses but begins to rise slowly beginning at 1.9 W/cm^2. Sounding of C fibers yields pain relief distal to the point of application, whereas sounding of large-diameter A fibers brings relief of spasm by changing gamma fiber activity, making the muscle fibers less sensitive to stretch.[84] Because it is impossible to treat C or A fibers selectively, ultrasound provides both pain relief and relief from muscle spasm, making it effective in the treatment of peripheral neuropathies, neuroma, and muscle spasm associated with musculoskeletal pathology, including sprains, strains, and contusions.[85]

In addition to thermal effects, ultrasound has nonthermal effects that come from the mechanical effects of the ultrasound wave on the tissues. Ultrasound causes cavitation, the development and growth of gas-filled bubbles, in the tissues. Ultrasound also causes tissue fluid to move or stream. The movement of fluid around the gas bubbles formed by cavitation is called microstreaming, and the movement of fluid within the ultrasound delivery area is called acoustic streaming. The nonthermal effects of ultrasound include accelerating metabolic processes, enzyme activity, and the rate of ion exchange, as well as increasing cell membrane permeability and the rate and volume of diffusion across cell membranes. These effects are thought to explain the role of ultrasound in enhancing the healing of soft tissue and bone.[86-88] The nonthermal effects of ultrasound can be achieved without raising tissue temperature by applying ultrasound in the pulsed mode.

Phonophoresis is the use of ultrasound to deliver pain-relieving chemicals to the tissues. Chemicals are delivered to the cells by the ultrasound wave, where they are broken down into ions and taken up into the cells (Figure 32-7). Common pain-relieving chemicals that can be administered with phonophoresis include 5% lidocaine ointment (Xylocaine) for acute conditions in which immediate pain relief is the primary goal, and 10% hydrocortisone cream or ointment for conditions in which pain is the result of inflammation.[89]

After phonophoresis, measurable quantities of these molecules have been found at tissue depths of up to 2 inches.[90] The contraindication to use of any chemical during phonophoresis is having an allergy to that chemical. Clients should be questioned about any adverse reactions to dental local anesthesia (lidocaine) or aspirin.

Cryotherapy

The physiological effects of cold make it superior to heat for acute pain from inflammatory conditions, for the period immediately after tissue trauma, and for treating muscle spasm and abnormal tone. Peripheral nerve conduction velocity in both large myelinated and small unmyelinated fibers decreases 2.4 m per degree centigrade of cooling. As a result, pain perception and muscle contractility diminish.[91] Peripheral receptors become less excitable.[91] Muscle spindle responsiveness to stretch decreases; as a result, muscle spasm diminishes.[84]

Local blood flow initially decreases, local edema decreases, the inflammatory response decreases, and hemorrhage is minimized. However, cold application for longer

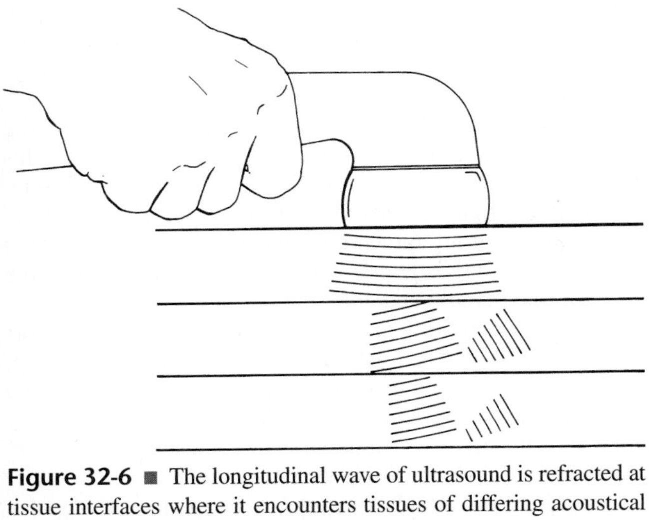

Figure 32-6 ■ The longitudinal wave of ultrasound is refracted at tissue interfaces where it encounters tissues of differing acoustical resistance. When the wave changes direction, energy is transferred to the tissues, resulting in the production of heat.

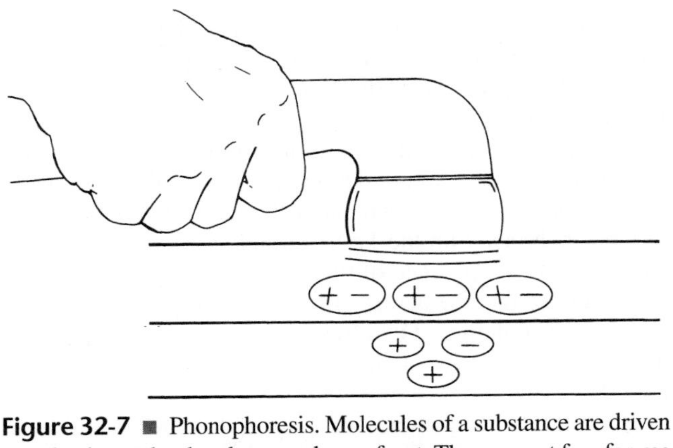

Figure 32-7 ■ Phonophoresis. Molecules of a substance are driven into the tissues by the ultrasound wavefront. They are not free for use by the body until they are broken down into chemical ions.

than 15 minutes results in increased local blood flow. Known as the "hunting response," this protective mechanism brings core temperature blood to the surface and prevents tissue injury resulting from prolonged cooling.[81] Cellular metabolic activities slow. The oxygen requirements of the cell decrease.[91]

As with heat, several precautions must be taken when using cold as a therapeutic modality. Cryotherapy is contraindicated in individuals with Raynaud phenomenon or cold allergy. Cryotherapy should not be used in individuals with rheumatic disease who, with the application of cold, have increased joint pain and stiffness. Cryotherapy should be used with caution in young, frail, or elderly individuals and those with peripheral vascular disease, circulatory pathological processes, or sensory loss.[92]

Cryotherapy is applied in three ways. Convective cooling involves movement of air over the skin (fanning) and is rarely used therapeutically. Evaporative cooling results when a substance applied to the skin uses thermal energy to evaporate, thereby lowering surface temperature. Most commonly, this substance is a vapocoolant spray. Conductive cooling uses local application of cold via ice packs, ice massage, or immersion. Cooling is accomplished as heat from the higher-temperature object is transferred to the colder object down a temperature gradient. Conductive cooling is the most commonly used form of therapeutic cold application.

Because muscles, tendons, and joints respond differently, the best method of cold application depends on which tissues are causing the pain.[93] Acute injuries are best treated with cryotherapy along with rest, compression, and elevation (RICE). Muscle spasm is decreased with cold packs and stretching. Trigger points, irritable foci within muscles, are best treated with vapocoolant spray, deep friction massage, and stretching. Tendinitis responds well to ice massage and exercise. Cold packs are often the only source of pain relief in acute disc pathology. The inflamed joints of rheumatoid arthritis frequently respond to cold packs or ice massage with decreased inflammation, increased function, and long-lasting pain relief.[92,94]

Clients and caregivers can be taught how and when to perform cryotherapy independently. Once they have demonstrated their proficiency, responsibility for the use of cryotherapy should be transferred to the client or the client's caregiver.

Transcutaneous Electrical Nerve Stimulation

TENS is the use of electricity to control the perception of pain. It appears that at a high rate TENS selectively stimulates the low-threshold, large-diameter A beta fibers, resulting in presynaptic inhibition within the dorsal horns,[95] either directly through the gating mechanism or indirectly through stimulation of the tonic descending pain-inhibiting pathways.[96] Research has shown that the neurons in the brain stem fire in synchrony with the TENS stimulation frequency,[97] and although the significance of this is not known at this time, it does indicate that the action of high-rate TENS is not limited to the dorsal columns. TENS delivered at a low rate is thought to facilitate elevation of the level of endogenous opiates in the CNS.[98]

Stimulation frequencies of 1 to 250 pulses per second (pps) decrease pain. Frequencies of 50 to 100 pps have proven most effective for sensory-level (high-rate) TENS, and frequencies of 2 to 3 pps are most effective for motor level (low-rate) TENS.[31] Stimulation at exactly 2 pps causes an increase in the pain threshold.[53] As the frequency is decreased, more time is needed before the onset of relief, but the effects are more long-lasting.[99] Pulse width duration determines which nerves are stimulated. Sensory nerves are stimulated at widths of 20 to 100 ms, and motor nerves at 100 to 600 ms.[100]

There is a variety of modes of TENS delivery. Each mode relieves pain through a specific physiological mechanism and is therefore most beneficial for a specific type of pain.

When TENS impulses are generated at a high rate (greater than or equal to 50 pps) with a relatively short duration, the stimulation is referred to as *sensory-level* or *conventional* or *high-rate TENS.* Sensory-level TENS produces mild to moderate paresthesia without muscle contraction throughout the treatment area. Sensory-level TENS is thought to control pain through the gating mechanism in the spinal cord. The onset of relief is fast (seconds to 15 minutes)[31] because the gate is closed at the onset of stimulation. The duration of relief after stimulation stops is short-lived (at best up to a few hours). Sensory-level TENS has been found to be beneficial for acute pain syndromes and for some deep, aching chronic pain syndromes. (Refer to Chapter 33.)

Stimulation using high-rate and long-duration impulses is called *brief-intense TENS.* Brief-intense TENS decreases the conduction velocity of A delta and C fibers, producing a peripheral blockade to transmission.[31] Brief-intense TENS is useful in the clinical setting for short-term anesthesia during wound debridement, suture removal, friction massage, joint mobilization, or other painful procedures.

When the impulses are generated at a low rate (less than or equal to 20 pps) and have a relatively long duration (100 to 300 microseconds), the stimulation is referred to as *motor-level* or *acupuncture-like* or *low-rate TENS.* Motor-level TENS produces strong muscle contractions in the treatment area with or without the perception of paresthesia. Motor-level TENS is associated with deployment of endogenous opiates within the CNS. The onset of relief is delayed 20 to 30 minutes, presumably the time it takes to deploy the opiates. Relief frequently lasts hours or days after treatment. Because motor nerves are not stimulated in isolation, sensory fibers are also excited, causing the gating mechanism to come into play.[100] Motor-level TENS has been found to be beneficial for chronic pain syndromes and when sensory-level TENS has not been successful.

Modulating TENS parameters is one way to avoid the negative aspects of each of the treatment modes. Rate modulation is most commonly used to avoid neural accommodation during TENS. By setting the initial pulse rate so that, even with the programmed decrement, it will remain within the treatment range, there will be continuous variation in the stimulus, and neural accommodation will be avoided.

Width modulation is most commonly used with motor-level TENS. By setting the initial pulse duration so that, even with the programmed decrement, the impulses are able to recruit the desired motor units, there will be a continuous variation in perceived strength of the muscle contraction, rendering motor-level TENS more tolerable.

Stimulation in which the impulses are generated in pulse trains is called *burst TENS.* Burst TENS is another form of TENS modulation. The stimulator generates low-rate carrier impulses, each of which contains a series of high-rate pulses. Because burst TENS is a combination of high-rate and low-rate TENS, it provides the benefits of each. The low-rate carrier impulse stimulates endorphin release, and the high-rate pulse trains provide an overlay of paresthesia. The advantage to burst TENS is that muscle contractions occur at a lower, more comfortable amplitude, and accommodation does not occur. Burst TENS is beneficial whenever motor-level TENS cannot be tolerated and sensory-level TENS is ineffective because of neural accommodation.[101]

TENS, like all electrical stimulation, is contraindicated for clients with pacemakers, in the low back and pelvic regions of pregnant women, and over areas with thrombus. TENS should be used with caution for clients who have decreased sensation in the area being stimulated and for clients who have difficulty with understanding or expression. TENS electrodes should not be placed over areas of skin irritation, the eyes, or the carotid sinuses. It also should not be used in the immediate area of an operating diathermy unit.

TENS appears to be of greatest benefit for acute conditions with focal pain, chronic pain syndromes, postoperative incision pain, and during delivery. It has been found least effective with psychogenic pain[102] and pain of central origin.[103] For additional information on TENS, see Chapter 33.

Clients and caregivers can be taught how and when to apply TENS independently. Once they have demonstrated independence, responsibility for the use of TENS can be transferred to the client or to the caregiver.

Iontophoresis

Iontophoresis is a process in which chemical ions are driven through the skin by a small electrical current. Ionizable compounds are placed on the skin under an electrode that, when polarized by a direct (galvanic) current, repels the ion of like charge into the tissues. Once subcutaneous, the ions are free to combine with the physiological ions, resulting in a physiological effect dependent on the characteristics of the ion (Figure 32-8). Ionizable substances that are known to be effective analgesics include the following[104]:

- Five-percent lidocaine ointment (Xylocaine) administered under the positive electrode for an immediate, although short-lived, decrease in pain. Iontophoresis with lidocaine is recommended before ROM exercises, stretching, and joint mobilization and when immediate relief of acute pain (as in bursitis) is the object of treatment.
- One-percent to 10% hydrocortisone and dexamethasone administered under the positive electrode for relief of inflammatory pain in conditions such as arthritis, bursitis, or entrapment syndromes. Iontophoresis with hydrocortisone has a delayed onset but a prolonged effect, and it frequently eliminates the underlying cause of pain.
- Two-percent magnesium (from Epsom salts) administered under the positive electrode for relief of pain from muscle spasm or localized ischemia. High levels of extracellular magnesium inhibit muscle contraction, including the smooth muscle found in the walls of the vessels, leading to localized vasodilation.
- Iodine (from Iodex ointment [Lee Pharmaceuticals, South El Monte, California]) administered under the negative pole for relief of pain caused by adhesions or scar tissue. Iodine "softens" fibrotic, sclerotic tissue, thereby increasing tissue pliability.
- Salicylate (from Iodex with Methyl Salicylate [Lee Pharmaceuticals] or Gordogesic Creme [Gordon Laboratories, Upper Darby, Pennsylvania]) administered under the negative pole for relief of pain from inflammation. Salicylate is effective for arthritic joint inflammation, myalgia, and entrapment syndromes.
- Two-percent acetic acid administered under the negative pole to dissolve calcium deposits.
- Two-percent lithium chloride or lithium carbonate administered under the positive pole to dissolve gouty tophi. In both acetic acid and lithium iontophoresis, the insoluble radicals in the deposits are replaced by soluble chemical radicals so the deposits can be broken down through natural processes.

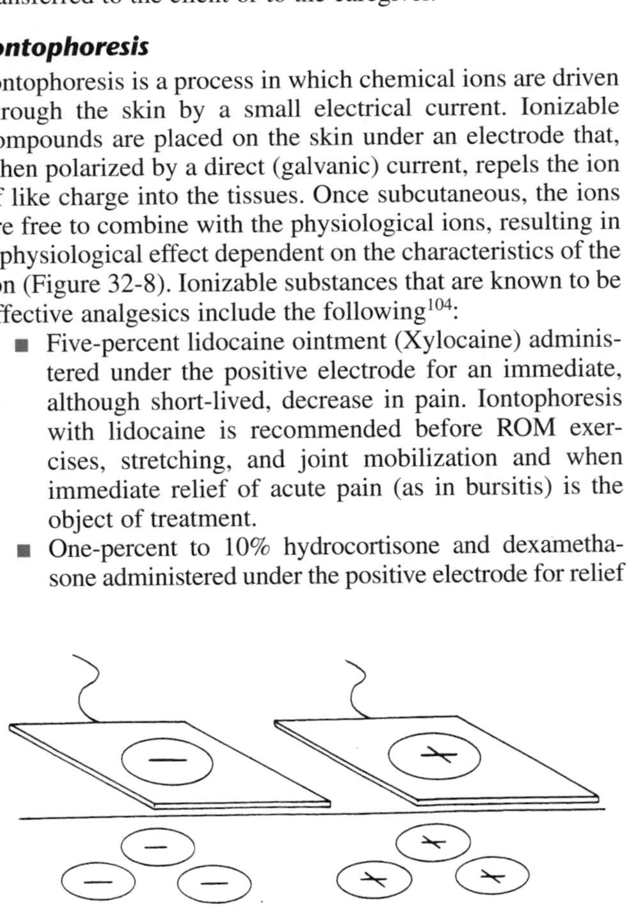

Figure 32-8 ■ Iontophoresis. Chemical ions are driven into the tissues by a small electrical current. Once subcutaneous, they are immediately free to take part in chemical reactions within the body.

The contraindication to the use of any ion is an allergy to that ion. Because most clients will not have had iontophoresis previously, it is important to inquire about experiences that might indicate an allergy. For example, intolerance to shellfish may be the result of an allergy to iodine, and a poor reaction to dental local anesthesia may indicate a problem with lidocaine. Moreover, because iontophoresis involves the application of direct current, the likelihood of polar reactions under each electrode is greater than with electrical stimulations using alternating current (for example, TENS), and therefore the risk for skin burns is greater.

Massage

Massage has been recognized as a remedy for pain for at least 3000 years. Evidence of its beneficial effects first appeared in ancient Chinese literature, and then in the writings of the Hindus, Persians, Egyptians, and Greeks. Hippocrates advocated massage for sprains and dislocations as well as for constipation.[105]

Massage decreases pain through both direct and indirect means. Massage movements increase circulation through mechanical compression of the tissues, resulting in reflex relaxation of muscle tissue and direct relief from ischemic pain. Massage also indirectly stimulates A delta and A beta fibers, causing activation of the gating mechanism and the descending pain-modulating system.[34]

Massage movements are classified by pressure and the part of the hand that is used.[106] The two massage movements that may cause a decrease in pain include stroking (effleurage) and compression (kneading or pétrissage). Stroking involves running the entire hand over large portions of the body. Stroking causes muscle relaxation and elimination of muscle spasm or improved circulation depending on the depth and force of the strokes. Compression is applied with intermittent pressure using lifting, rolling, or pressing movements meant to stretch shortened tissues, loosen adhesions, and assist with circulation.

Massage is useful in any condition in which pain relief will follow the reduction of swelling or the mobilization of the tissues. These include arthritis, bursitis, neuritis, fibrositis, low back pain, hemiplegia, paraplegia, quadriplegia, and joint sprains, strains, and contusions. Massage is contraindicated over infected areas, diseased skin, and thrombophlebitic regions.

Clients or caregivers can be taught how and when to perform massage. Once they have demonstrated independence in the appropriate technique, responsibility for the performance of massage should be given to the client or caregiver.

A specialized massage technique is lymphatic massage, which consists of light-pressure rhythmic strokes to encourage organizational flow of the lymphatic system. This type of massage can be beneficial with clients who have peripheral swelling with or without pain. A popular form of lymph massage called *manual lymphatic drainage* (MLD) is used after surgical procedures to reduce swelling (for example, mastectomy for breast cancer). Evidence-based studies show conflicting results regarding the efficacy of this technique, and more research needs to be done to validate it.[107-109]

Myofascial Release

Myofascial release (MFR) techniques are used to release the built-in imbalances and restrictions within the fascia and to reintegrate the fascial mechanism. The therapist palpates the various tissue layers, beginning with the most superficial and working systematically toward the deepest, looking for movement restrictions and asymmetry. Areas of altered structure and function are then "normalized" through the systematic application of pressure and stretching applied in specific directions to bring about decreased myofascial tension, myofascial lengthening, and myofascial softening,[110] thereby restoring pain-free motion in normal patterns of movement. MFR is useful in treating musculoskeletal injuries, chronic pain, headaches, and adhesions or adherent scars.[111] MFR has been shown to be effective in the treatment of chronic prostatitis (CP) and chronic pelvic pain syndrome (CPPS) in conjunction with paradoxical relaxation therapy (PRT).[112] More research is needed to provide evidence regarding the efficacy of MFR in pain control.

MFR is contraindicated over areas with infection, diseased skin, thromboembolus, cellulitis, osteomyelitis, and open wounds. In addition, it should not be used with clients who have osteoporosis, advanced degenerative changes, acute circulatory conditions, acute joint pathology, advanced diabetes, obstructive edema, or hypersensitive skin.[111] (See Chapter 39 for more in-depth information regarding MFR.)

Joint Mobilization

Joint mobilization consists of passive oscillations that restore normal accessory movements.[113] In addition, the rhythmical repetition of the motions provides pain relief through the spinal gating mechanism.[114]

The oscillations involved in joint mobilization are presented in Chapters 9 and 18. Grades I and II oscillations are performed to maintain joint mobility and for pain relief, making them the choice for subacute conditions in which pain and potential loss of motion are the primary considerations. Grades III and IV oscillations are performed to increase joint mobility and are indicated for chronic conditions in which regaining lost motion is the goal. Grade V thrusts are performed to regain full joint mobility.[113]

Joint mobilization is contraindicated with rheumatoid arthritis, bone disease, advanced osteoporosis, and pregnancy (pelvic mobilization), as well as in the presence of malignancy, vascular disease, or infection in the area to be mobilized.[53]

Light Therapy

Light therapy is described by Bot and Bouter[115] as a light source that generates extremely pure infrared light of a single wavelength. When applied to the skin, infrared laser light produces no sensation and it does not burn the skin. Because of the low absorption, it is hypothesized that the energy can penetrate deeply into the tissues, where it is assumed to have a biostimulative effect.[77,115,116] It has been suggested that laser therapy may act by stimulating ligament repair,[117,118] producing antiinflammatory effects,[119] increasing production of endogenous opioids,[120] reducing swelling,[121] and influencing nerve conduction velocity.[122] To promote wound healing and manage pain, rehabilitation centers use lasers with power outputs less than 500 mW at a power density of 50 mW/cm^2 and wavelengths ranging from 600 to 1500 nm.[77] Contraindications to light therapy include exposing photosensitive areas, hemorrhagic areas, any area that has undergone 4 to 6 months of radiation treatment,[116] neoplastic lesions, and unclosed fontanelles in children; the abdomen of pregnant women; areas over the heart, the vagus nerve, or sympathetic innervations routes to the heart of cardiac patients; or, locally, endocrine glands.[77,116,123,124] In addition, exposure to the cornea of the eye is contraindicated, so protective eye equipment should be worn by the patient and the therapist. Caution should be used for areas with compromised somatosensation, the epiphyseal plates in children, the gonads, and infected areas and with patients displaying fever, epilepsy, or mental confusion.[77,116,123]

Therapeutic Touch

A description of therapeutic touch can be found in Chapter 39. Therapeutic touch has been effective in treating painful conditions resulting from anxiety and tension. In a report by Keller and Bzdek, 90% of individuals treated with therapeutic touch experienced tension headache relief, and 70% had continued relief for more than 4 hours; only 37% of the placebo group expressed sustained relief.[125] A meta-analysis and systematic review on therapeutic touch revealed that the available studies have varying approaches and protocols on therapeutic touch, subject selection, and description. Although most of these studies confirm the efficacy of the technique, several studies also have demonstrated negative or mixed results.[126] Therapeutic touch, as well as other approaches, are being more widely accepted; however, the therapist must continue to be diligent in using outcome studies to substantiate the use of any complementary therapy. (See Chapter 39 for additional information.)

Point Stimulation

Refer to Chapter 39 for an in-depth discussion of point stimulation. It is interesting to note that acupuncture points frequently correspond in location to trigger points, which are tight, elevated bands of tissue that are extremely sensitive when palpated and have a characteristic pattern of radiation to remote regions of the body. Trigger points appear to be areas of "focal irritability" that are myofascial in origin and are usually the site of small aggregations of nerve fibers that produce continuous afferent input when stimulated.

Needling therapies include trigger point injections and trigger point dry needling and are used in myofascial pain conditions. Trigger point injections are usually restricted to medical doctors and their professional support staff.[127] Trigger point dry needling consists of superficial and deep dry needling, and the exact mechanism of pain relief is not known. It is thought that needling and injections may trigger changes in the end plate cholinesterase and ACh receptors,[127] may involve central pain mechanisms, and may activate enkephalinergic, serotonergic, and noradrenergic inhibitory systems in association with A delta fibers through segmental inhibition.[127] Acupressure (i.e., finger pressure applied to acupuncture or trigger points) is thought to decrease their sensitivity through the same mechanism. The therapist applies deep pressure in a circular motion to each point for 1 to 5 minutes, until the sensitivity subsides. Pressure must be applied directly to each point for the treatment to be effective. Acupressure can be accompanied by the use of a vapocoolant spray to provide additional sensory stimulation.

Sensitive points also can be stimulated using electricity. A point locator is used to identify points along the appropriate meridians that are sensitive to stimulation or more conductive to electricity. Each is then stimulated at the client's level of pain tolerance for 30 to 45 seconds. The points farthest from the site of pain are treated first.

Points that are most sensitive to stimulation are beneficial sites for TENS electrode placement. When point stimulation alone does not provide sufficient pain relief, TENS can be used between sessions for continuous stimulation for more prolonged relief. (See Chapter 39 for additional information on electrical acupuncture.)

Cognitive Strategies, Including Cognitive Behavioral Therapy

The extent to which an individual perceives and expresses pain is a result of his or her emotional state, expectations, personality, and cognitive view. Each individual feels and responds to pain differently. Melzack and Wall[114] identified the following three nonphysical components of pain that interact and determine how an individual will respond to pain:

- The individual's sensory and discriminative interpretation of the pain
- The individual's motivation and attitudes relating to the pain
- The individual's cognitive and evaluative thoughts and beliefs concerning the pain experience

Cognitive strategies are part of a holistic approach to health that looks at the total person and the interaction among the three components of body, mind, and spirit. Cognitive strategies recognize that the mind is not separate from the body, accept that there is a mental component to pain, and use the inner resources of the mind to influence the pain experience.

Cognitive strategies work in two ways. First, they activate the descending cortical modulating systems, and, second, they teach the individual to control, rather than be controlled by, the pain. Used in conjunction with other modalities necessary for physical relief, these approaches can play a significant role in long-term pain management and should not be overlooked in seeking a viable pain management alternative.

As mentioned previously, current research has given the medical community a much deeper understanding of chronic pain. Many new intervention approaches have been developed based on these new theories, and physical rehabilitation clinicians play a significant role in these new interventions. Of particular importance is the increasing role of clinicians in using cognitive behavioral therapy (CBT) in the management of individuals with chronic pain.[128] CBT for pain management involves the integration of cognitive, affective, and behavioral factors into the case conceptualization and treatment.[128] It is thought that a person's beliefs about pain are associated with various functional outcomes[129,130] and that changes in patients' beliefs about pain are related to changes in functioning.[131,132] Techniques potentially used may include coping skills, education and rationale about the course of an illness, relaxation, imagery, goal setting, pacing, distraction, and cognitive restructuring as well as homework assignments. A thorough discussion of this approach as it applies to physical rehabilitation is beyond the scope of this text. The work of Butler and Moseley provides clinicians a great resource on how to better explain pain to patients and clients, as well as to use the most current evidence on pain science and chronic pain management in treating individuals with chronic pain.[133,134]

Relaxation Exercises

People who are in pain experience stress. Chronic stress can trigger increased pain. Both pain and stress cause an increase in SNS activity, including increased muscle tension. Relaxation exercises can bring about muscle relaxation and a generalized parasympathetic response.[135] Benson[136] has named this effect the *relaxation response* and reports that it is accompanied by an increase in alpha brain waves.

Relaxation reduces ischemic pain by normalizing blood flow to the muscles by making way for more oxygen to be delivered to the tissues. In addition, relaxation reduces muscle tension, resulting in an interruption in the pain-spasm cycle.[137]

Relaxation exercises all have two elements in common: a single focus and a passive attitude toward intruding thoughts and distractions. The end product of relaxation is a lowered arousal of the SNS and a lessening of the symptoms caused by or worsened by stress.[138]

Deep relaxation can be achieved through progressive relaxation and attention-diversion exercises. Progressive relaxation involves alternately tensing and relaxing the muscles until, eventually, the entire body is relaxed. This activity teaches the individual how to recognize and relieve muscle tension within the body.

Attention diversion is an active process in which the individual directs her or his attention to nonnoxious events or stimuli in the immediate environment to achieve distraction from the pain. Attention diversion is categorized as passive or active. Passive attention diversion includes meditation and involves concentrating on a visual or auditory stimulus rather than the painful sensation, whereas active attention diversion involves active participation in a task (e.g., serial subtraction).

Meditation involves quieting the mind and focusing the attention on a thought, word, phrase, object, or movement. The individual becomes more alert to the constant stream of conversation taking place within the mind. Meditation calms the body through the relaxation response and keeps the attention focused in the present moment. Individuals in Eastern cultures have traditionally focused on a mantra, a word with spiritual meaning; however, there are no rules for where to focus the attention. The word or object should bring the individual a sense of peace and should allow the attention to be pleasantly directed toward the immediate moment.

Imagery is another form of attention diversion. During imagery the individual uses his or her imagination to produce images with pain-weakening potential. This can take two forms. In one, the individual imagines experiences that are inconsistent with the pain (e.g., imagining rolling in snow to alleviate burning pain). In the other, the individual imagines experiences that modify specific features of the pain experience (e.g., imagining that the pain is the result of a sports injury or that the sensation is "numbness" rather than pain).

Attention diversion works by activating the relaxation response and by diverting the individual's attention from the pain. However, attention diversion also has been found to activate the higher brain centers and may have an inhibitory effect on pain through the spinal gating mechanisms.[44,71] Lautenbacher and colleagues[139] found that individuals who used attention diversion for pain management reported decreased intensity and unpleasantness of their pain.

Clients can be taught to perform relaxation exercises independently and should be encouraged to perform them regularly because the benefits of these exercises are gained through regular practice.

Body Scanning

Clients with chronic pain frequently become one with their suffering; they do not view themselves as individuals with pain, but rather as painful individuals. Body scanning is a technique that endeavors to separate the individual from the pain.[140]

During body scanning, the client is taught to achieve a meditative state, then focus attention on each body area, one area at a time. The client is instructed to breathe into and out from each area, relaxing more deeply with each exhalation. When the area is completely relaxed, the client "lets go" of the region and dwells in the stillness for a few breaths before continuing. Painful areas are scanned in an identical manner as nonpainful areas. The client notes, but does not judge, changes in sensation, thoughts, and emotions during scanning of each area.

Individuals who practice this technique report new levels of insight and understanding concerning their pain experience. They separate the pain experience into the following three parts[140]:

- An awareness of the pain sensation and their thoughts and feelings about it
- An awareness of a separation between the pain sensation and their thoughts and feelings about it
- An awareness of a separation between themselves and their pain, because they are able to examine objectively the sensation and their thoughts and feelings about it

Once clients have accepted that they are not their pain or their reaction to the pain, they can determine how much influence and control pain will have in their lives.

Studies of chronic pain patients at the Stress Reduction Clinic at the University of Massachusetts Medical Center revealed that 72% of patients who used body scanning along with traditional medical interventions experienced at least a 33% reduction on their McGill-Melzack Pain Rating Index score.[140] In addition, at the end of an 8-week training period, the individuals perceived their bodies in a more positive light, experienced an increase in positive mood states, and reported major improvements in anxiety, depression, hostility, and the tendency to be overly occupied with their bodily sensations.

Humor

Ever since Cousins[141] reported in his book *Anatomy of an Illness* that he used humor to manage pain and enhance sleep during his illness, the role of humor in healing has been well studied. Humor has been found beneficial for both acute and chronic pain management.[96,142]

Laughter increases blood oxygen content by increasing ventilation. It helps to exercise the heart muscle by speeding up the heart rate and enhancing arterial and venous circulation, resulting in more oxygen and nutrients being delivered to the tissues.[143] Laughter decreases serum cortisol levels (cortisol levels increase with stress and are thought to have a negative effect on the immune response)[144,145] and increases the concentration of circulating antibodies.[143] As little as 10 minutes of belly laughter a day has been found to decrease the erythrocyte sedimentation rate and provide 2 hours of pain-free sleep.[144] Finally, laughter releases energy and emotional tension and is followed by generalized muscle relaxation.[143,146]

Therapeutic humor can be used to provide distraction from pain and as a coping mechanism to decrease the anxiety and tension associated with chronic pain. The muscle-relaxing effect can be used to interrupt the pain-spasm cycle.

Therapeutic humor should not be used with individuals who do poorly with humor. This includes individuals who despise or misunderstand humor, individuals who find joy threatening or guilt inducing, and narcoleptic individuals who become cataleptic with laughter.[147]

Very few clients will benefit from all these cognitive strategies, and it may take some trial and error to find the appropriate cognitive strategy for an individual client. Some clients will have no difficulty learning and practicing cognitive strategies, whereas others will not be able to perform any of these techniques independently. It may be beneficial to provide the client with an individualized relaxation tape or to have the client repeat coping affirmations over and over throughout the day. The success of cognitive strategies is dependent on applying the appropriate strategy to the appropriate client and fine-tuning the strategy so that it matches the client's needs.

In conclusion, it is important to reemphasize that all individuals with chronic pain have some degree of emotional or cognitive involvement, or both, in their pain experience. Many clients will live with pain regardless of the treatment they receive. Therefore it is imperative for health care practitioners to address the emotional and cognitive components of each client's pain to allow her or him to function at the highest level and as comfortably as possible and to find joy in each day.

General Conditioning through Exercise

Deconditioning is a major source of disability with chronic pain. Pain causes an intolerance for activity, which in turn leads to physiological and pathological changes in the organ systems. Exercise improves overall functional performance by improving ROM, muscle strength, neuromuscular control, coordination, and aerobic capacity, as well as offering higher self-esteem.

All three types of exercise are beneficial for pain management. ROM and stretching exercises restore normal joint mobility and correct muscle tightness. The joints are held in normal alignment and are subjected to normal stresses during movement. ROM and stretching exercises are indicated where there is decreased mobility.

Strengthening exercises increase muscle strength and cardiovascular endurance. When performed with high intensity for a short duration, strengthening exercises result in increased muscle mass, improved neuromuscular control, and improved coordination. When performed at low intensity for a long duration, they increase the aerobic capacity of the muscles.

Aerobic exercises improve cardiovascular fitness. More oxygen is supplied to the tissues because there is an increase in the number and size of capillaries and a decrease in the diffusion distance between the capillaries and the muscles. The tissues use oxygen more efficiently, and the individual has a higher energy level.

All exercise has an analgesic effect through the gating mechanism by stimulation of the A delta neurons and a pain-modulating effect through activation of the descending systems. Exercise of sufficient intensity has been known to increase circulating β-endorphin levels, but exercise-induced β-endorphin alterations are related to the type of exercise and special populations tested and may differ in individuals with health problems.[148,149]

It is important to include exercise in all pain management programs. Clients should be taught the appropriate exercises beginning with the first treatment session and encouraged to perform the exercises consistently when not at therapy. The ultimate end product of movement intervention is to empower the client to modulate and control all functional activities, enabling that individual to participate in life.

Operant Conditioning

Coping strategies are learned. Individuals with chronic pain express their pain with behaviors that provide them with consistent positive rewards. For example, wincing might result in attention from a family member, or limping might allow the individual to avoid performing a particular task. Over time, the individual with pain becomes conditioned to perform certain behaviors for the behavior's rewards rather than as a reaction to the pain. Similarly, individuals with chronic pain also can condition their nervous systems through learning. If an individual expects to experience pain as the result of a particular level of activity, the individual will always experience pain at that level of activity.

Operant conditioning addresses the learned (or conditioned) aspects of pain.[150] Operant conditioning involves unlearning or separating the behavior and the response from the pain experience. If the goal of treatment is to lessen social reinforcement of the client's pain behaviors (and thus extinguish those behaviors), the client and the family or other involved individuals are shown how their behaviors and responses provide social reinforcement for the client's reaction to pain. The involved individuals are provided with specific new responses to the client's behavior. Family members might be instructed to ignore wincing, groaning, or the verbal report of pain. They might be told not to perform activities that are the client's responsibility just because the client reports pain. In time, the client will become conditioned to the new response, and pain in those situations will diminish.

If the goal of treatment is to increase the client's pain-free activity level, operant conditioning can be used to condition the nervous system to a higher level of activity before responding with pain. If the client's usual pattern is to remain active until the onset of pain (negative reinforcement for activity) and then rest (positive reinforcement for pain), the client is instructed to remain active to just below the pain threshold and then rest (positive reinforcement for activity). In this way the nervous system unlearns the connection between activity and pain, and the client's activity level increases.

Hypnosis

Hypnosis is a state in which the body and conscious mind are deeply relaxed while the subconscious mind remains alert, focused, and open to suggestion.[138] This has been demonstrated physiologically by electroencephalography (EEG), which shows an increase in the number of theta waves, which are associated with enhanced attention.[151] When a hypnotized individual is given a suggestion that is in alignment with his or her existing belief system, it is accepted by the subconscious mind as reality. The suggestion is not filtered through the conscious mind, which is critical and judgmental. Hypnosis allows the individual to bypass her or his critical beliefs.[152] For example, if the individual believes that a certain activity will cause pain (critical belief), that activity is sure to cause pain. If, however, during hypnosis, the individual accepts the suggestion that the activity does not cause pain, the pain may decrease and even disappear.

When hypnosis is used for pain management, a client is first assisted to achieve complete relaxation, then given suggestions that reinterpret the pain experience. For example, a client might be guided to reframe the pain into a messenger and then be encouraged to listen to its message to gain understanding of the meaning behind the pain. Or a client might be guided to view the pain as an indication to stop a particular activity to avoid being injured. Or a client might be instructed to feel less pain. Finally, where harmless activities have become painful through learning, the client can be guided to disconnect the activity from his or her pain.

Biofeedback

Biofeedback is a training process in which the client becomes aware of and learns to selectively change physiological processes with the aid of an external monitor. A monitoring instrument is placed on the appropriate area of the body. The machine provides an initial readout. The client is instructed how to change the monitored process, and as change occurs, the machine "feeds back" that information. By mentally changing a biological function, the client learns to gain control over it. In time, the client learns to control the process without needing an assist from the instrument.

Muscle tension, pulse rate, blood pressure, skin temperature, and electromyography (EMG) and EEG readings are some of the physiological processes that can be consciously modified with biofeedback.[135]

Biofeedback is proving to be an effective pain management tool for headaches, muscle spasms, and other physical dysfunction that leads to or increases chronic pain (see Chapters 33 and 39).

GENERAL TREATMENT GUIDELINES

As noted earlier, chronic pain management using the medical model has not been found effective. Treatment limited to correcting pathology promotes dependence on the therapist, as well as making full resolution of symptoms the measure of success.

The ICF model addresses the functional losses associated with impairments. Therapeutic interventions are not focused on pathology, but they are directed at improving the individual's function and preventing or improving disability. This does not mean that the impairment is ignored, however. Most times, addressing the individual's functional losses involves treating the impairments that caused them.

For example, clients with chronic pain frequently become sedentary, leading to the impairments of limited ROM, muscle weakness, and deconditioning. These factors can then, of themselves, cause pain, creating a cycle that spirals upward until the individual becomes disabled. During therapy, interventions are directed at the impairments with the goal of restoring function. Therapeutic interventions are selected based on their ability to improve functional outcome. Impairments that do not affect function do not become the focus of therapy; therapeutic interventions that do not address functional deficits are not used.

The development of an appropriate treatment plan may seem overwhelming when the therapist is confronted with a client who has chronic pain that has not responded to previous interventions or who has a chronic condition that has pain as one of its characteristics. The key is to identify the client's functional deficits and then develop a treatment plan that addresses the causes of those deficits. In some cases this may mean not treating the pain itself but rather its causative factors.

For example, if the client has chronic pain because of joint hypomobility, the treatment plan includes interventions to increase joint mobility. Conversely, if the client's pain is caused by joint hypermobility, the treatment plan includes interventions to increase support around the hypermobile joints. Merely addressing the joint pain by applying modalities will do little to resolve the pain because it does nothing to correct the precipitating cause.

When a client has pain because of a chronic disease and the treatment plan will include instruction in pain-relieving interventions, it is important for the therapist to understand the specific causes of the pain to select the appropriate intervention. For example, pain from rheumatoid arthritis most commonly is the result of either joint inflammation or biomechanical stress on unstable joints. A client would be instructed in pain-relieving modalities for the former and instructed to wear splints to support the joints for the latter. One intervention would not be appropriate for both causes.

CASE STUDIES

Case Studies 32-1, 32-2, and 32-3 demonstrate a problem-solving approach to the treatment of clients with chronic pain.

CASE STUDY 32-1 ■ FIBROMYALGIA

K. E. is a 35-year-old computer programmer with a diagnosis of fibromyalgia. She reports a 6-month history of generalized muscular pain and fatigue that increase when she performs repetitive motions or holds a position for a prolonged period. K. E. is currently unable to work because she is no longer able to perform data entry without increased neck and shoulder pain. She states she awakens from pain and leg cramps several times during the night. She awakens each morning with a headache and low back pain; she does not get much relief from pain medication. K. E. states she has not been out with friends in several months. She states she is "nervous, unable to concentrate, and depressed." She has been evaluated by several physicians. All medical test results are negative.

K. E.'s objective examination reveals pain on digital palpation of distinct points in the muscles of her neck and shoulder girdles, over both lateral epicondyles and greater trochanters, in her gluteal muscles, and just above the medial joint lines of the knees. Pain is referred from the tender points distally. K. E. sits and stands with a forward head and elevated protracted shoulders, and her cervical ROM is restricted slightly at end range because of her posture and muscle guarding. Muscle strength is 4/5 throughout. All other musculoskeletal and neurological test findings are normal.

K. E. demonstrates the impairments of pain, poor posture, decreased cervical and shoulder ROM, and decreased endurance, resulting in the activity limitations of interrupted sleep and decreased tolerance for activity and participation restrictions of inability to work at her profession.

The long-term goals of treatment for K. E. are independence with self-management of pain, normalization of posture, restoration of normal sleep, independence with a home exercise program, and return to work and appropriate social activities. The short-term goals include decreasing K. E.'s pain, helping her to achieve proper sleep positioning, correcting her postural abnormalities, improving her limited endurance, and assessing and correcting the ergonomics of her workstation. K. E. also needs intervention to address the emotional and cognitive aspects of her condition.

The lowered pain threshold and magnified pain perception seen with fibromyalgia result from a complex combination of

CASE STUDY 32-1 ■ FIBROMYALGIA—cont'd

muscle tissue microtrauma, neuroendocrine abnormalities, and changes in the levels of CNS neurotransmitters. The muscles of individuals with fibromyalgia show abnormal energy metabolism, poor tissue oxygenation, and localized hypoxia. Their blood shows decreased levels of the inhibitory neurotransmitter serotonin and increased levels of the facilitatory neurotransmitter substance P. This combination, which is unique to fibromyalgia, is thought to cause changes in the dorsal horn neurons and eventually in the areas of the brain responsible for the sensory-discriminative and affective-motivational aspects of pain.[42]

Fibromyalgia pain has been shown to respond favorably to interventions that work through the gating mechanism. These include sensory-level TENS, light massage, muscle warming, and gentle stretching. K. E. can be taught to apply localized heat or to take a warm bath before gentle stretching of her tight muscles. She should be cautioned to stretch slowly to the point of resistance and to hold the stretch for 60 seconds to allow the Golgi tendon organs time to signal the muscle fibers to relax. Quick stretching to the point of pain will cause increased tightness and pain through the pain-spasm cycle. It is important for K. E. to understand that these measures address the pain of fibromyalgia but do not have any long-term effect on the course of her condition.

Individuals with fibromyalgia, and most individuals with chronic pain, experience a variety of emotions, including depression, anger, fear, withdrawal, and anxiety.[153] These individuals have been helped with hypnosis, biofeedback, and cognitive restructuring.[42,153] In addition to giving them a sense of control over their pain, these interventions are known to bring about an increase in the individual's level of endogenous opiates, thereby activating one of the descending pain modulation systems. K. E. can be taught to perform these techniques independently.

K. E. should be asked to demonstrate her sleeping posture. Because the muscles of individuals with fibromyalgia do not relax easily, K. E. should be shown how to use pillows to support her neck and back so that they are encouraged to relax while she sleeps. This will help to decrease the frequency of morning headaches and back pain and help her to sleep through the night. She might also benefit from a warm bath before going to bed.

K. E.'s therapist can use gentle MFR to help correct the biomechanical imbalances causing her poor posture. K. E. can then be taught to selectively stretch the shortened muscles of her neck and shoulder girdles using the technique already described and to selectively strengthen their weakened antagonists using light resistance. To counter deconditioning, K. E. should be placed on a nonimpact aerobic program (walking, pool exercises, or stationary bicycle) with a goal of 30 minutes three to four times a week at 70% maximum heart rate (220 minus her age). If she is unable to tolerate 30 minutes of exercise at one time, she can be started at 3 to 5 minutes twice or three times daily and gradually progressed to three sessions of 10 minutes, then two sessions of 15 minutes, and finally one session of 30 minutes. K. E. may require a significant amount of coaxing and education to motivate her to participate in exercise; many individuals with fibromyalgia do not wish to move because movement initially increases their pain.

Before she returns to work, K. E. should be assisted with the ergonomics of her workstation. Research[154] has shown that individuals who work at computers need to vary their positions throughout the day even if their sitting posture is appropriate. Further research[72,155,156] has shown that correct mouse placement is important to minimize stress to the arms and shoulders.

CASE STUDY 32-2 ■ PHANTOM LIMB PAIN

A. R. is a 60-year-old carpenter who underwent below-knee amputation of his right leg 4 weeks ago after a motor vehicle accident. He now reports a constant burning, piercing, throbbing sensation in the distal portion of his missing limb. He states that immediately after the amputation, he was aware of an itching or tickling in the missing portion of the leg, but the sensation gradually changed to pain. He notes that the leg feels as if it is shortening, as if the missing foot is moving closer and closer to his hip. A. R. has been fitted with a shrinker but does not wear it because of fear of increasing the pain. He does not believe he will be able to wear a prosthesis and is concerned because his employer will be unable to find work for him if he is wheelchair bound.

A. R.'s objective examination reveals a healing surgical incision and a poorly shaped stump. Right lower-extremity hip and knee strength are 3/5 and 2+/5, respectively. Sensation to light touch is diminished in the area of the incision. All other musculoskeletal and neurological test findings are normal. A. R. ambulates short distances using a walker but relies on a wheelchair for locomotion outside his home.

A. R. has the diagnosis of a below-knee amputation and demonstrates the impairments of phantom limb pain and decreased strength in the right lower extremity, resulting in the functional limitations of inability to prepare his leg for a prosthesis, inability to ambulate, and inability to work in his profession.

The long-term goals of treatment for A. R. are independent use of a prosthesis and return to work with modified job tasks. The short-term goals include resolution of his phantom limb pain, preparation of his stump for a prosthesis, at least 4/5 right hip and knee strength, and, when appropriate, gait and balance training with the prosthesis.

There are two theories of the cause for phantom limb pain. At one time it was thought that it occurred as the result of the formation of a terminal neuroma at the site of the amputation[11]; however, this theory did not explain phantom phenomena in individuals with congenital amputations or individuals with complete spinal cord injuries who also experience painful and nonpainful sensations in their missing or anesthetic limbs. This led researchers to look at the role of the CNS in phantom phenomena, and the latest theories suggest the previously

Continued

CASE STUDY 32-2 ■ PHANTOM LIMB PAIN—cont'd

described changes in the dorsal horn neurons and changes in the spinal cord caused by the sudden loss of afferent impulses after amputation.[157]

These theories are supported by the effectiveness of interventions that stimulate the large nerve fibers and provide inhibitory input through the gating mechanism. Phantom limb pain is relieved by stroking, vibration, TENS, ultrasound, heat applications, and the use of a prosthesis. A. R. can be taught a progressive desensitization program. He should be encouraged to wear the shrinker both to prepare his stump for a prosthesis and to decrease pain. Because phantom limb pain is adversely affected by emotional stress, exposure to cold, and local irritants, he should be taught to avoid these factors as much as possible.

A. R.'s adjustment to a changed body image, a changed lifestyle, and the use of a prosthesis can be aided with any of the cognitive strategies described previously. He might also benefit from referral to an amputee support group.

It is important for A. R. to be aware of his abilities and limitations so that he remains safe when he returns to work. If appropriate, the therapist should accompany A. R. to his job and perform a job task analysis, making suggestions for necessary modifications. If this is not possible, the therapist could discuss needed modifications with A. R. based on his descriptions of his job tasks.

CASE STUDY 32-3 ■ COMPLEX REGIONAL PAIN SYNDROME

P. S. is a 45-year-old right-handed secretary who sustained a Colles fracture of the right wrist 6 months ago. The wrist was placed in a cast for 6 weeks, during which time P. S. avoided using the extremity. Two weeks after the cast was removed, P. S. developed pain, swelling, and stiffness in the wrist and hand. She returned to her physician who diagnosed CRPS type I. She has received four sympathetic nerve blockades. The first provided 4 weeks of pain relief. The second and third provided 2 weeks of relief each. She has just received her fourth injection along with a referral for therapy.

P. S. is wearing a sling. She has 30-degree flexion contractures of her right fingers, along with swelling and stiffness of the wrist and hand. Her right wrist, elbow, and shoulder show limited motion as well. P. S. describes constant burning pain that becomes worse with any stimulation, even air blowing over the skin. She rates her pain as 4/10 since the block, but she states that the pain had slowly been escalating toward 10/10 before the injection. Her hand and wrist are cool, and the skin appears mottled and shiny. P. S. states that she is not using her arm and needs assistance at home for activities of daily living and household chores.

P. S. demonstrates the impairments of pain, swelling, stiffness, and decreased ROM of the right wrist and hand. These impairments cause activity limitations, decreasing her ability to use the right upper extremity for any functional activities, including activities of daily living, job tasks, and homemaking activities. In addition, because she is not using the extremity and carries the arm in a sling, P. S. is at risk for developing shoulder-hand syndrome.

The long-term goal of treatment for P. S. is restoration of pain-free use of her right upper extremity. The short-term goals include quieting the SNS, decreasing P. S.'s pain and edema, and restoring normal ROM of the shoulder, elbow, wrist, and hand.

Successful treatment of CRPS involves a coordinated effort by the physician and the therapist. The treatment of choice is interruption of sympathetic activity with nerve blocks and movement therapy.[158]

Interventions included in a pain management program for CRPS should be chosen for their ability to quiet the SNS as well as accomplish the desired outcome. For example, thermotherapy is more beneficial than cryotherapy because of its ability to decrease pain without stimulating a sympathetic response.[158]

A successful rehabilitation program for CRPS cannot be limited to therapy visits. Clients need to be instructed in interventions that they then perform three, four, or even five times daily. Therefore the therapist needs to become a guide, with the responsibility for performing the pain management program given over to the client or caregiver.

Pain reduction is the first priority. This can be accomplished through the gating mechanism or through the deployment of endogenous opiates. Thermotherapy and TENS have both been found effective for pain management with CRPS. If P.S. cannot tolerate electrode placement on the right arm, the electrodes can be placed on the opposite arm or along the spinal roots of the involved segments.[31,104] P.S. can be instructed in any of the superficial heating modalities. Stroking massage along the paravertebral muscles beginning in the cervical region and continuing to the coccyx has also been found effective in quieting the SNS.

Before P. S. can regain mobility of her wrist and fingers, the edema must be resolved. This can be accomplished with elevation, massage, lymphatic drainage, and compression. P. S. can wear a compression glove or, if she is able to tolerate it, receive intermittent compression to the arm. She should be instructed to keep the arm above heart level as much as possible.

P. S. should be advised to discontinue use of the sling and begin frequent weight bearing through her arm. Immobility increases the symptoms of CRPS. Movement of the extremity is important to increase proprioception and circulation, both of which have an inhibitory effect on the SNS.[158] Therefore P. S. should be encouraged to begin using her hand as much as possible throughout the day. If she is reluctant to use the arm, the therapist can design a functional activity program that allows her to use the arm during simple activities, which can be progressed as her symptoms improve.

There are two forms of exercise that are beneficial in CRPS. The first is active ROM exercises, which should be performed

CASE STUDY 32-3 ■ COMPLEX REGIONAL PAIN SYNDROME—cont'd

frequently throughout the day within the pain-free range to regain motion, increase circulation, and provide nonnociceptive input. Exercise of the specific ROM should be within functional activities. The activity itself will encourage ROM while the patient is concentrating on successfully completing the activity itself. The second form of exercise is stress loading,[159] which involves active compression and traction activities without joint motion. For example, P. S. can use a coarse-bristled brush to scrub a piece of plywood and apply as much pressure as possible without causing pain (compression activity). Or she can carry a briefcase or purse in her affected hand (traction activity). Compression and traction both provide increased proprioceptive input.

P. S. should also begin performing desensitization activities, which can be modified as she is able to tolerate more stimulation to her extremity. P. S. may benefit from biofeedback to gain control over the circulation in her arm and from relaxation activities to stimulate the relaxation response and enhance parasympathetic function.

Once P. S. becomes independent in the performance of her program, therapy can be decreased to once or twice weekly to monitor and modify her pain management regimen.

Acknowledgments

We would like to acknowledge the contribution of Linda Mirabelli-Susens to the writing of this chapter in the fourth edition of the textbook.

References

To enhance this text and add value for the reader, all references are included on the companion Evolve site that accompanies this textbook. This online service will, when available, provide a link for the reader to a Medline abstract for the article cited. There are 159 cited references and other general references for this chapter, with the majority of those articles being evidence-based citations.

CHAPTER 33 Electrophysiological Testing and Electrical Stimulation in Neurological Rehabilitation

ALAIN CLAUDEL, PT, DPT, ECS, ROLANDO T. LAZARO, PT, PhD, DPT, GCS, GEORGE WOLFE, PT, PhD, and JANET MARIE ADAMS, PT, MS, DPT

KEY TERMS

electromyographic feedback
electroneuromyography
functional electrical stimulation
kinesiological electromyography
nerve conduction velocity
neuromuscular electrical stimulation

OBJECTIVES

After reading this chapter the student or therapist will be able to:

1. Identify electrophysiological tests performed on clients with neurological disorders.
2. Describe the instrumentation and general procedures for electrophysiological testing.
3. Recognize normal and abnormal findings of various electrophysiological tests.
4. Recognize the differences in instrumentation, signal processing, and interpretation when performing electrophysiological testing versus kinesiological electromyographic testing.
5. Differentiate the basic mechanism underlying functional neuromuscular stimulation, electrical stimulation, and electromyographic biofeedback.
6. Describe the appropriate instrumentation, signal processing, and interpretation for kinesiological electromyographic testing.
7. Describe the indications and contraindication for the use of neuromuscular stimulation, electrical stimulation, and electromyographic biofeedback.

The goal of this chapter is to enhance the clinician's ability to recognize indications for the most commonly used electrophysiological tests and to integrate knowledge of these test indications and findings into the management of clients with neuropathological dysfunction. The first section presents a basic description of the electrophysiological tests, including nerve conduction studies (NCSs), electromyography (EMG), kinesiological electromyography (KEMG), and the underlying neuroanatomical structures being tested. Normal and abnormal findings are discussed, with emphasis on how knowledge of these tests can assist the therapist in client evaluation. The second section provides an introduction to the physiology, indications, contraindications, equipment, and applications of electrical muscle stimulation (EMS), neuromuscular electrical stimulation (NMES), and electromyographic biofeedback (EMGBF). The information integrates electrotherapeutic interventions into program planning for common neurological body system problems, their subsequent functional limitations, and perceived decrease in quality of life. Published evidence examining efficacy is included to assist the therapist in making choices about the use of these tools in the clinic. The third section provides a series of four case studies that illustrate the usefulness of electromyographic testing in patients with a variety of medical diagnoses.

ELECTROPHYSIOLOGICAL TESTING

Physical therapists (PTs) are uniquely positioned to understand and perform electrophysiological testing. This is because PTs examine patients with pain, numbness, and/or weakness and also because they have a superior knowledge of neural and muscular anatomy and physiology. Electrophysiological testing is a sensitive and specific tool designed to assist in the diagnosis and the development of treatment plans for patients with diseases of the peripheral nervous system (PNS) and of the muscle itself.

An informed perspective on the application of these tests will benefit the therapist's interaction and communication with other members of the medical and health management community. At the completion of the electrophysiological consultation, the clinician who performed the test generates a report. Understanding this report can guide decisions in planning and modification of intervention programs or will assist in referring to other health care practitioners. A review of components of such report follows.

Electrophysiological tests are usually performed by neurologists, physiatrists, and PTs who have education, training, and experience in these procedures. Most PTs practicing in the area of clinical electrophysiology are board certified by the American Board of Physical Therapy Specialties.[1] Some states (such as California) require additional licensing.

The general goal of electrophysiological testing is to answer the following questions:

- Is there a lesion in the PNS and/or muscles?
- Where precisely is that lesion?
- What is the extent of the lesion?

Most of the electrophysiological tests described involve the application of an external electrical stimulus to a nerve or muscle and observation and assessment of the muscle or nerve response. Other tests such as needle EMG and single-fiber electromyography (SFEMG) involve the monitoring and recording of the electrical activity produced by the muscle tissue at rest or during contraction.

The electrophysiological tests most commonly used are motor and sensory NCSs, including F-wave and H-reflex latency measurements; repetitive stimulation; somatosensory evoked potential (SSEP) tests; and needle EMG. Most often, a patient referred for electrophysiological testing will undergo at least two motor nerve conduction tests, at least two sensory conduction tests, and at least one limb needle EMG. The American Association of Neuromuscular and Electrodiagnostic Medicine (AANEM) has published evidence-based guidelines, which may be found on the AANEM website at www.aanem.org/Practice/Practice-Guidelines.aspx.[2] A review of the client's history, a relevant systems review, and a physical examination guide the examiner in the selection and sequencing of appropriate tests. In other words, muscle strength and tone, sensation, range of motion (ROM), neurological signs, and cognition are crucial in selecting and administering electrophysiological tests. Electrophysiological testing is considered by all authors on the subject as an extension of the clinical examination.[3,4] It does not replace a careful history and physical examination of the patient. It does, however, establish the precise state of the nerves and muscles and can thus determine the location of a lesion more precisely than the clinical examination alone, particularly in cases of mild weakness or ill-defined sensory changes. In very clearly defined pathologies, electrophysiological tests are not necessary (except perhaps for medicolegal reasons). For example, in the case of a unilateral ankle dorsiflexion weakness coupled with a clearly defined L5 nerve root compression on magnetic resonance imaging (MRI) of the lumbar spine, the electrophysiological test may be of little added value. However, for a similar clinical presentation (foot drop) and no clear-cut imaging, the electrophysiological tests will differentiate between a peroneal palsy, a sciatic nerve neuropathy, a lumbosacral plexopathy, or an L5 radiculopathy.

Finally, evidence-based practice recommends that the practitioner have a good understanding of the implication of the sensitivity and specificity of each test to rule it in or out for a specific condition.[5]

Anatomical Review

In order to best understand the systematic interpretation of data from the electrophysiological examination of nerves, the reader is invited to review the following foundational principles. These are explored in much greater detail elsewhere in this text.

At the Cellular Level

A nerve is composed of axons covered with a sheath of myelin. Depolarization inside the axon is an "all-or-nothing" phenomenon in which an action potential moves along the surface of the cell membrane. This action potential is an electrical wave caused by a flow of ions across the cell membrane. A local current opens a sodium channel, allowing Na^+ ions to rush inside the cell. The electrical resistance to this wave is inversely proportional to the diameter of the axon. Larger nerves conduct faster than smaller nerves. In order for efficiency as an organism to be achieved, nerve conduction must be fast. In complex organisms with billions of axons, increasing the nerve diameter is not a viable option; hence, the role of the myelin sheath. The myelin is produced by Schwann cells. These are special satellite cells that separate axons from the endoneural fluid. The myelin acts as a capacitor: the conduction "jumps" between gaps in the myelin called *nodes of Ranvier.* This saltatory conduction allows human nerves to be 50 times smaller but conduct four times faster than unmyelinated nerves.[6] Consequently, recording and analyzing the *conduction velocity* of nerves primarily reflects on the state of the myelin. The amplitude of the response (if a supramaximal stimulation is delivered) is a reflection of the number of axons available to the stimulation.

The physiology of the nerve is such that when there is an injury to the axon, the portion of the axon distal to the injury will degenerate (wallerian degeneration). This is important because all muscles innervated by branches of the nerve distal to the lesion will show signs of denervation approximately 11 days after the lesion. Consequently, assessing a patient too early after a lesion may lead to false-negative results.[6,7]

At the Anatomical Level

The accurate performance and interpretation of the electrophysiological test—particularly the needle EMG—is significantly contingent on knowledge of the precise innervation of each muscle. As an example, an ulnar neuropathy at the elbow (UNE) clinically may be indistinguishable from a C8 radiculopathy. However, the astute clinician will remember that the cell body of the sensory nerve lies in the dorsal root ganglion, which is typically not involved in a radiculopathy. The therapist will also know that the abductor pollicis brevis is a C8- and median nerve–innervated muscle. Consequently, an ulnar nerve neuropathy is distinguishable from a C8 radiculopathy in that the ulnar sensory test will have decreased amplitude in the UNE and the abductor pollicis brevis will be denervated in the C8 radiculopathy. As a matter of fact, the clinician will keep in mind the innervation of each muscle while conducting the test. Electrophysiological testing is hence a dynamic process during which the choice of the next nerve to test or muscle to sample is predicated on the result of the previous test.[6,7]

As a result, the electrophysiological examination is not a single, stereotyped investigation but an evolutionary one during which several tests (nerve conduction, both sensory and motor, and EMG of several muscles) can be applied to a clinical presentation.[3,8]

Nerve Conduction Tests

A general overview of NCSs is presented to provide an understanding of their application and indications. Many excellent texts are available for details of the techniques.[9-13]

Motor and sensory NCSs can provide data that are helpful in establishing the presence and location of pathological conditions in the PNS. The tests may indicate the anatomical level, such as a plexopathy, versus a localized peripheral mononeuropathy. Individual and multiple nerves may be assessed, and the findings compared with responses of the same nerves contralaterally. The site of pathology may be localized, such as median nerve compression at the wrist versus a lesion of the lateral cord of the brachial plexus.

Nerve conduction velocity is faster in myelinated fibers because of saltatory conduction. Disorders involving peripheral demyelination can thus be differentiated from impairments primarily involving axonal degeneration. A mild localized compressive disorder (neurapraxia) may be distinguished from a more severe lesion in which the axons and surrounding connective tissue have been completely disrupted (neurotmesis).[11,14] In the event that the findings of

NCS and EMG are normal, the clinician may be able to rule out most conditions involving the PNS and look for central nervous system (CNS) or other pathology. Knowledge of the rationale for NCSs and EMG should help the therapist decide when the tests may be indicated and understand the reasoning behind reports of tests that have already been performed on clients.

Motor Nerve Conduction

In motor NCSs the peripheral nerve is stimulated at various sites and the evoked electrical response is recorded from a distal muscle supplied by the nerve (a measure of orthodromic conduction). Surface electrodes are usually used for both stimulating and recording. An example of electrode configuration for a motor NCS is shown in Figure 33-1 (ulnar nerve study). The response represents the electrical activity of muscle fibers under the recording electrodes and is called the *compound muscle action potential* (CMAP). It is also called the *M wave* or *M response.* Measurements are taken of the latency (the time in milliseconds required for the impulse to travel from each stimulus site to the recording site) and the amplitude of the response in millivolts (mV). The shape and duration of the response are assessed, and motor nerve conduction velocity is calculated for each segment of interest by dividing the distance between stimulus sites (in millimeters) by the difference in latency measured at each respective site.

Velocities, latencies, and the shape and amplitude of the responses (Figure 33-2) are studied and compared with established normal values and often with values taken from tests of the uninvolved extremity (when possible). In infants and children, nerve conduction is slower than in adults and reaches adult values by age 4 years.[13] Nerve conduction velocities gradually slow after age 60 years but generally remain within the outer limits of normal.[11,13]

Sensory Nerve Conduction

Sensory nerve conduction can be measured from many superficial sensory nerves, such as the superficial radial and sural nerves. It can also be measured from mixed motor and sensory nerves. The stimulus is applied over the nerve in question, and the recordings taken from electrodes placed over a distal sensory branch of the nerve. The recordings are called *sensory nerve action potentials* (SNAPs). An example of recording and stimulation sites is shown in Figure 33-3. Both orthodromic and antidromic conduction can be assessed. Response latencies and amplitudes are measured, and sensory nerve conduction velocities are calculated for each segment by dividing the distance between two adjacent stimulus and recording sites, or two stimulus sites, by the latency (conduction time) between these same sites. Sensory nerve responses are considerably smaller than motor responses. Their amplitudes are generally measured in microvolts (μV). Sensory recordings are more sensitive than motor recordings in cases of mixed sensory-motor neuropathies.

F-Wave Latency

When a motor nerve is stimulated in the periphery, both orthodromic (peripherally to the muscle) and antidromic (centrally toward the spinal cord) impulses are generated. A proportion of the antidromic impulses will, as it were, "bounce off" the axon hillock and return as a recurrent discharge along the same neurons to activate the muscle from which the recording is taken. This activity is termed the *F wave* (Figure 33-4), and it is observed as a small wave occurring after the M wave.[11,13,14] No synapse is involved.

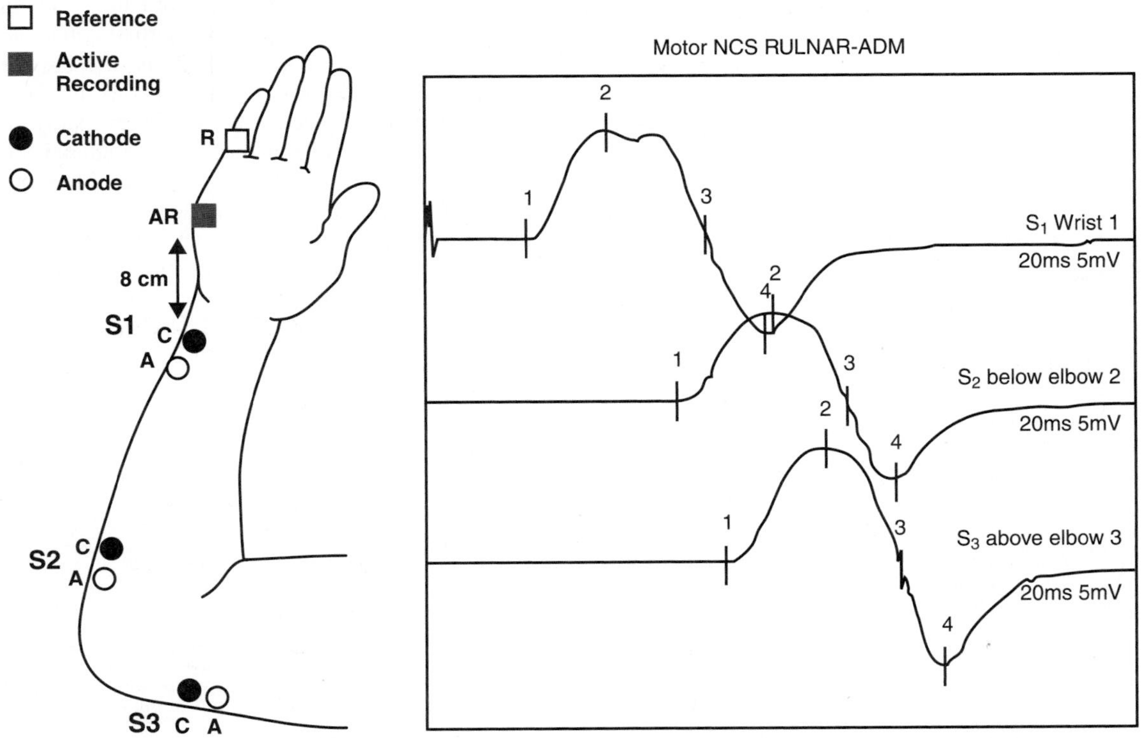

Figure 33-1 ■ Electrode location for ulnar motor nerve conduction.

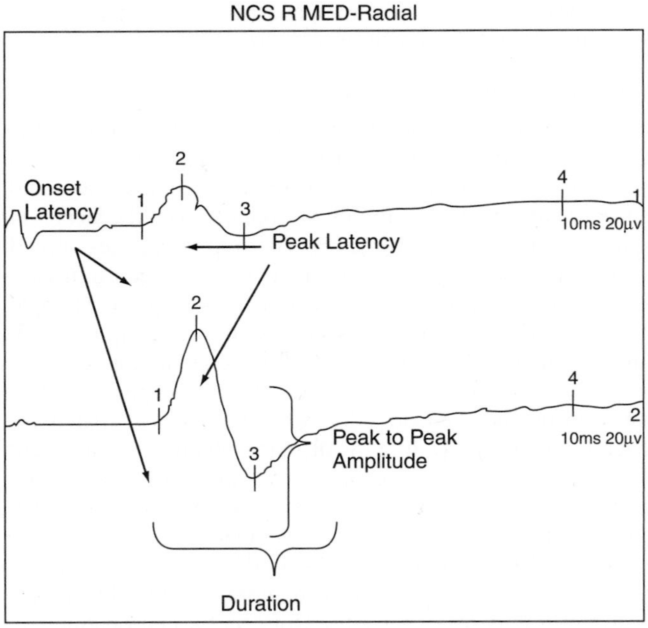

Figure 33-2 ■ Velocities, latencies, and the shape and amplitude of the responses.

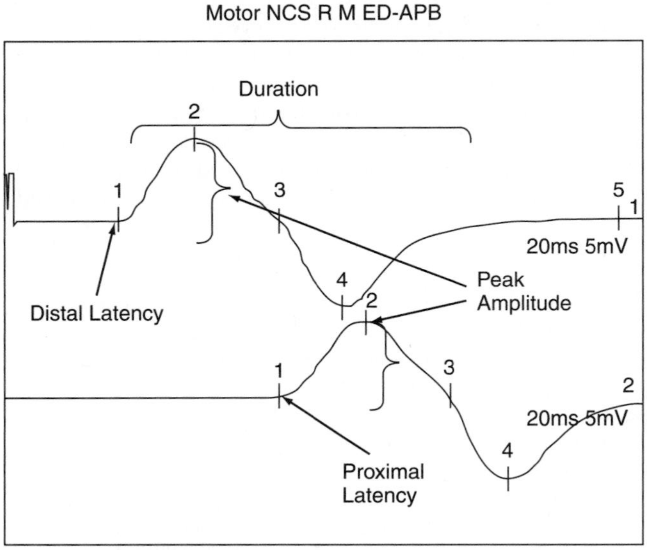

Figure 33-3 ■ Example of recording and stimulation sites.

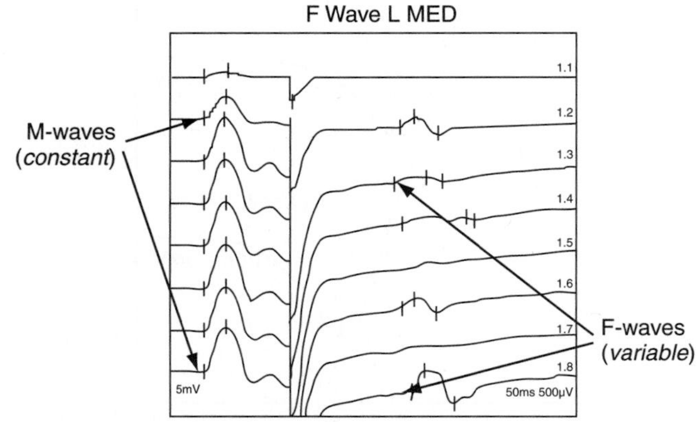

Figure 33-4 ■ Example of F-wave study.

Thus the F wave is not a reflex response, but rather only a measure of conduction along the motor neuron. Specific conditions of electropotential must exist at the soma-dendritic cell membrane to reactivate the efferent axon; therefore the occurrence of the F-wave response is inconsistent and variable in latency and waveform.[15]

The F-wave latency can be useful in evaluating conduction in conditions usually involving the proximal portions of the peripheral neurons (e.g., radiculopathy, Guillain-Barré syndrome [refer to Chapter 17], or thoracic outlet syndrome [refer to Chapter 18]). Its value, however, has been questioned by some authors because of its variability. Normal values of F-wave latency are 22 to 34 ms in the upper extremity (stimulating at the wrist) and 40 to 58 ms in the lower extremity (stimulating at the ankle), depending on the height of the subject, with a bilateral difference in latency of no greater than 1 ms.[16]

H-Reflex Response

The H-reflex response latency (Figure 33-5) is a measure of the time for action potentials elicited by stimulating a nerve in the periphery to be propagated centrally over the Ia afferent neurons to the spinal cord, to be transmitted across the synapse to alpha motor neurons, and then to travel distally over these neurons to activate the muscle. The response therefore measures conduction in both the afferent and efferent neurons.[11,13] It is also referred to as a "late" response (the other being the F wave).

The H reflex is constant in latency and waveform, and it occurs with a stimulus usually below the threshold level required to elicit the M-wave response (Ia afferent fibers are larger in diameter than alpha motor neurons and thus more sensitive to electrical stimulation). This monosynaptic reflex response is most easily found by stimulating the tibial nerve at the popliteal area and recording from the soleus muscle. Braddom and Johnson[17] reported a mean latency of 29.8 ms (±2.74 ms) for the tibial nerve in normal adults, and a bilateral difference of no more than 1.2 ms. The H-reflex latency is a valuable measure of conduction over the S1 nerve root in differentiating suspected proximal plexopathy and radiculopathy from a herniated disc or foraminal impingement. Sabbahi and Khalil[18] have reported a technique for recording the H reflex from the flexor carpi radialis muscle when stimulating the median nerve. In normal human beings older than 1 year, the H reflex is usually seen only in the tibial, femoral, and median nerves. It can be elicited from several nerves in infants and in conditions of CNS dysfunction in adults.

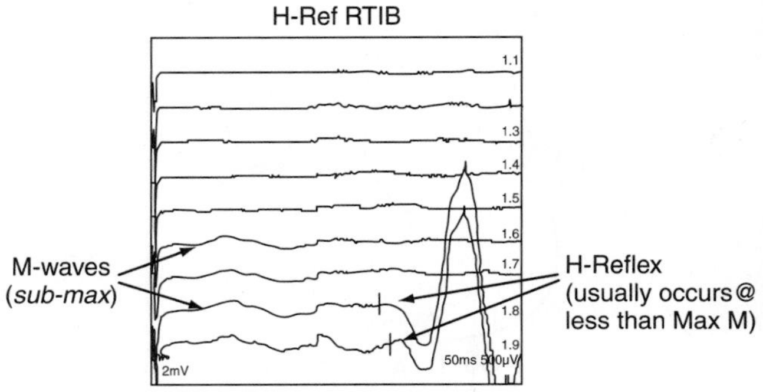

Figure 33-5 ■ Example of H-reflex study.

Repetitive Stimulation Tests

The repetitive nerve stimulation (RNS) test is used to evaluate transmission at the neuromuscular junction (motor synapse) in patients with diffuse weakness. RNS tests are helpful in the differential diagnosis of disorders such as myasthenia gravis and Lambert-Eaton myasthenic syndrome (LEMS). One protocol uses a series of supramaximal electrical stimuli applied to a peripheral nerve at a distal site (e.g., median or ulnar nerve at the wrist) at a rate of three to five per second for five to seven responses. Changes in amplitude of the muscle response are assessed. Precise technical requirements are specified to prevent movement artifacts and other testing errors. Detailed descriptions of the RNS test can be found in other texts.[11,19] Under normal conditions the amplitude does not change more than 10% from that of the initial response in a series of 10 stimuli recorded before and after resistive exercise. An amplitude decrease in the fifth or sixth response of more than 10% is considered abnormal and is compatible with a physiological defect at the postsynaptic receptor site of the neuromuscular junction, as in myasthenia gravis.

In another RNS protocol, stimuli are applied to a nerve, first at a slow rate, then at a faster rate, usually 10 to 20 per second for up to 10 seconds. Normally, the amplitude can decrease up to 40% from the initial amplitude. In some defects at the presynaptic site, the response may be lower than normal during a slow stimulation rate but show a significant amplitude increase at the higher rate. Increases in amplitude greater than 100% over the initial response are consistent with presynaptic neuromuscular junction defects such as seen in LEMS, which has a strong association with small-cell bronchogenic carcinoma, and in botulism. In 1957 Eaton and Lambert[20] reported this phenomenon as a myasthenic syndrome.

Gilchrist and Sanders[21] reported another protocol referred to as a *double-step RNS test.* This test measures amplitude before and after a temporarily induced ischemia of the extremity. They found the double-step RNS test to be slightly more sensitive than the routine RNS test, but only 60% as sensitive as the SFEMG technique. The RNS test is a good alternative test for neuromuscular transmission when the SFEMG is not available, but the examiner must meticulously adhere to technical details when conducting the test.

Blink Reflex

In some conditions (e.g., facial palsy) or to establish the presence of a widespread neuropathy, it may be necessary to assess the conduction in the cranial nerves. The stimulation of the supraorbital nerve (branch of the trigeminal nerve, cranial nerve V) elicits two separate responses of the orbicularis oculi muscles, one early and ipsilateral (R1) and one late and bilateral (R2), via the facial nerve (cranial nerve VII). The early R1 response involves a synapse in the pons, whereas the late bilateral R2 responses involve a more complex pathway involving the pons and lateral medulla. Analysis of the respective latencies of each response will help in determination of the following:

- Trigeminal neuralgia (cranial nerve V) or Guillain-Barré: all responses delayed
- Acoustic neuroma or Bell palsy (cranial nerve VII): ipsilateral responses delayed
- Pontine lesion: absence of R1
- Medullar lesion: absence of R2
- Others

Hence, the blink reflex is a nerve conduction test that assesses a portion of the CNS and has shown some utility in assisting in the diagnosis of multiple sclerosis (see Chapter 19) and Wallenberg syndrome.[7]

Clinical Evoked Potentials

Electrical potentials elicited by stimulation of nerves or sense organs in the periphery can be recorded from various sites as the impulses are transmitted centrally along the neuronal pathway and from the representative area of the brain.[11,22-24] SSEP procedures are particularly useful in assessing the integrity of afferent pathways in the CNS. They are helpful in differentiating among lesions in areas such as the plexus, spinal cord, brain stem, thalamus, and cerebral cortex. Evoked potential tests have the advantage of providing data about the integrity of both peripheral and central neuronal pathways, including transmission across axodendritic synapses.

The SSEP is valuable in assessing damage and continuity of spinal cord tracts in early spinal cord injury (SCI). For example, if an electrical stimulus is applied at the popliteal area over the tibial nerve, responses can be recorded with surface electrodes placed over the spine at the L3 and C7 spinal segments and from the lumbar representation of the contralateral sensory cortical area. Conduction time and other parameters of the response waveforms can be measured from the recordings.

This simplified example of an SSEP illustrates how conduction over sensory peripheral nerves and afferent pathways to the cerebrum can be studied. The median nerve is usually tested to evaluate the integrity of peripheral and central pathways and their synaptic connections as the impulses travel from the upper extremity to the contralateral cortical area.

In visual evoked potential (VEP) procedures, visual stimuli such as variable light flashes of changing patterns are applied to one or both eyes under highly controlled conditions. The response is recorded from the scalp over the representative area of the cerebral cortex.[11,23,24] The term *pattern reversal evoked potentials* (PREPs), a more descriptive term for these procedures, is recommended by the American Electroencephalographic Society.[22] These tests and other VEP procedures are useful in assessing pathology of retinal photoreceptors, the optic nerve, and postchiasmal pathways. Abnormal conduction findings have been reported when VEP studies are used in demyelinating disorders such as multiple sclerosis and optic neuritis. The examiner may conclude that the patient is cortically blind because no response is recorded on the visual cortex. Although many causes for a stimulus not reaching the visual cortex are possible, the end result is considered blindness. If the cause for cortical inactivity is swelling or a neurochemical imbalance within a nuclear relay structure, once corrected, the individual may experience normal vision. A change in the reaction of the patient to the visual environment may reflect increased awareness and a change in coma scale rating. Similarly, just because an individual turns toward a light or visual stimulus does not mean an evoked potential reaches the visual cortex. Instead, the eyes as receptors and the visual tract to the brain stem may be intact even though a problem in the synaptic connections between or within the thalamus and visual cortex may exist.

Auditory evoked potential tests are used to evaluate neurological function of the cochlear division of the auditory nerve (eighth cranial nerve), central auditory pathways and synapses in the brain stem, and the receptor areas on the cerebral cortex.[11,22-24] Brain stem auditory evoked potentials are frequently referred to as BAEPs. A series of high-intensity clicks is applied to auditory receptors in the ears through headphones, and several components of the response waveforms are recorded by using surface electrodes over the representative cortical areas. The BAEP is an effective test procedure for localizing and evaluating acoustic neuromas and other space-occupying lesions in the brain stem. This test is also used for assessment of brain damage in patients who are comatose as a result of traumatic brain injury (TBI). Robinson and Rudge[25] recommend caution in using BAEP tests for this purpose because other factors, such as defective receptor organs, can cause abnormalities in BAEPs.

The evoked potential tests described in this chapter all require application of appropriate external stimuli that are rapidly repeated many times. The response is electronically averaged to sort out the desired signal from interference signals. The conduction times (latencies), waveform shape and amplitude, and sometimes conduction velocities are measured and compared with normal values. Absence of a response, increased latencies, decreased amplitudes, and slowing of conduction velocities are all abnormal findings. Normal values and details of techniques for the evoked potential tests are described elsewhere.[11,22-24]

Therapists with special interest and training administer the SSEP tests for neurological applications more frequently than other types of evoked potential tests. Because of the highly specialized techniques necessary to administer VEP tests for ophthalmological applications and BAEP tests for hearing dysfunction, they are usually performed by persons who specialize in these procedures.

Needle Electromyography

Needle EMG complements the motor and sensory NCSs; it is most sensitive in the detection of denervation.

Unlike NCSs, which use the electrical stimulation of the motor nerves to elicit muscle contraction, the needle EMG is used to record and analyze muscle activity at rest and during voluntary activation. It is particularly useful in identifying pathology of the lower motor neurons and of the muscle itself. EMG can also be used to identify abnormalities of motor neuron recruitment that are associated with certain disorders of the CNS especially when NCS findings are normal—as would be the case in radiculopathies. The primary recording studied is the insertional activity, along with activity at rest and the motor unit action potential (MUAP), which is produced by the depolarization of single motor units during voluntary or reflex activity. Spontaneous electrical activity of single muscle fibers at rest is termed *fibrillation* and is diagnostic of denervation. For recording of muscle activity, small-diameter needles are inserted within the muscles to be studied. Three electrodes are required: active (negative), reference (positive), and ground. The needles may be *monopolar,* requiring a second needle or surface electrode for reference, or *bipolar,* containing both the active and reference electrodes (usually concentric in cross section). The ground electrode is typically placed on the surface of the skin. Most commonly the needles used are disposable. The activity detected in the muscle is displayed on the video display terminal of a computer (and can be stored and printed later). It is simultaneously played through an audio amplifier. The electromyographer can often identify pathological conditions by the characteristic "sounds" of the electrical activity of the muscle. Many excellent resources are available for readers interested in details of the equipment and procedures for EMG.[9-11,26,27] Details of contraindications and special precautions are described by Currier and colleagues.[27]

In an EMG examination, four conditions are evaluated at each location: (1) activity during needle insertion (normally a brief burst (250 ms) of high-frequency activity that abates when the needle ceases motion), (2) activity during rest (electrical silence is normal unless an electrode is placed directly over a motor endplate), (3) activity during minimal and gradually increasing voluntary contraction (biphasic or triphasic MUAPs of small amplitude composed of slow-twitch type I fibers that increase in frequency and are joined by higher-amplitude potentials as larger, predominantly fast-twitch type II motor units are recruited), and (4) activity during maximal activation (an *interference pattern* caused by the blending of potentials in which individual MUAPs cannot be identified), characterized as full (complete), reduced, or absent. Several locations in an individual muscle may be studied. The specific muscles to be studied are determined by clinical findings, and results must always be interpreted in the context of the total complex of signs and symptoms. In determining the specific location of a lesion, muscles located both proximally and distally to the suspected lesion site must be assessed. Studies may be repeated at intervals to determine if changes consistent with recovery (such as reinnervation) or exacerbation are present. EMG is typically used to help determine the presence (and extent) of the following:

- Denervation
- Reinnervation
- Myopathic or neuropathic signs
- Distribution or specific location of peripheral nerve pathology

Needle EMG is sensitive in determining the state of the axons. When axons are interrupted, there is denervation of the muscle cell. The findings in denervation and partial denervation include increased insertional activity, fibrillation potentials or positive sharp waves at rest, and a reduced or absent interference pattern. CNS dysfunction can result in no resting potentials, but if motor control was impaired a decreased or abnormal interference pattern might be apparent because of difficulty in recruitment (Figure 33-6). Needle EMG also informs the clinician about muscle cell disorders such as myopathies. The primary finding in the case of a myopathy is fibrillation potentials and small-amplitude polyphasic MUAPs.

Although client cooperation during EMG testing is important, some aspects of muscle electrical activity can be studied in the client who is very young (infant), who is unable to move, or who has only involuntary or reflex activity. Insertional and resting potentials can always be evaluated. MUAPs appear during the contraction of muscle fibers activated both voluntarily and involuntarily in both isotonic or isometric conditions. In normal conditions MUAPs are seen with

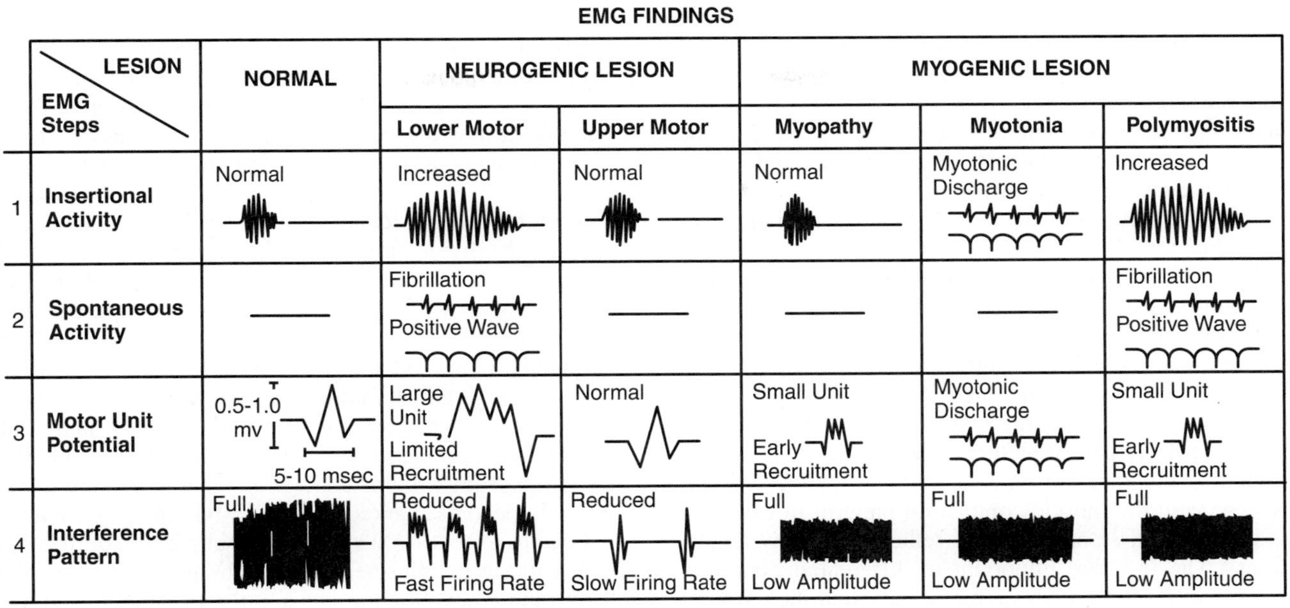

EMG FINDINGS
LESION
EMG Steps
NORMAL
NEUROGENIC LESION
Lower Motor
Upper Motor
MYOGENIC LESION
Myopathy
Myotonia
Polymyositis
1
Insertional Activity
Normal
Increased
Normal
Normal
Myotonic Discharge
Increased
2
Spontaneous Activity
Fibrillation
Positive Wave
Fibrillation
Positive Wave
3
Motor Unit Potential
0.5-1.0 mv
5-10 msec
Large Unit
Limited Recruitment
Normal
Small Unit
Early Recruitment
Myotonic Discharge
Small Unit
Early Recruitment
4
Interference Pattern
Full
Reduced
Fast Firing Rate
Reduced
Slow Firing Rate
Full
Low Amplitude
Full
Low Amplitude
Full
Low Amplitude

Figure 33-6 ■ Typical findings in lower and upper motor neuron disorders and myogenic lesions. Myotonia shares many features common to myopathy in general in addition to myotonic discharges triggered by insertion of the needle or with voluntary effort to contract the muscle. Polymyositis shows combined features of myopathy and neuropathy, including (1) prolonged insertional activity, (2) abundant spontaneous discharges, (3) low-amplitude, short-duration, polyphasic motor unit potentials, and (4) early recruitment leading to a low-amplitude, full-interference pattern. (From Kimura J: *Electrodiagnosis in diseases of nerve and muscle: principles and practice,* ed 3, New York, 2001, Oxford University Press.)

voluntary movement; however, reflex activation of muscle also produces MUAPs with certain normal characteristics. In CNS disorders hypertonic or spastic muscles will produce recognizable MUAPs when they are actively contracting. The electromyographer can elicit a contraction by tapping on the muscle or tendon. For example, consider a client who is recovering from a traumatic head injury with residual spastic hemiplegia. She is unable to cooperate with the EMG exam. The client has abnormal extensor responses in the lower extremity with the exception of the ankle and foot, which appear flaccid. An EMG of the leg and foot muscles detects abnormal resting potentials, including fibrillation and positive sharp waves in muscles innervated by the peroneal nerve. Tapping on the muscles fails to elicit MUAPs. Muscles in the tibial nerve distribution have no resting potentials and respond with bursts of identifiable MUAPs when the tendon is tapped. These findings would guide the physician and therapist in looking for a possible peripheral nerve lesion in addition to the CNS dysfunction. The treatment program in this situation would differ from that for a client without peripheral nerve pathology.

In summary, results of the needle EMG are best presented in the form of a table that indicates the following:

- Insertional activity: may be increased in acute denervation and myopathic processes
- Spontaneous activity at rest: present (positive sharp waves and fibrillation potentials) in denervation
- Fasciculations: may be present in motor neuron disorders
- Analysis of MUAPs:
  - Amplitude: Low amplitude is seen in myopathy or nascent potential; large amplitude is a sign of chronicity.
  - Phases: Normal MUAPs are biphasic or triphasic. Polyphasia is indicative of denervation-reinnervation.
  - Recruitment pattern: A less-than-full recruitment is indicative of fewer motor units discharging, as can be seen in axon loss.
  - Firing rate: If elevated, fewer motor units are contracting more often to provide the same tension in a denervated muscle.

Justification and analysis of the basic principles and results after EMG studies should assist therapists managing clients with neurological dysfunction in planning and modifying therapeutic management programs. As electrical tests are being conducted, the findings are continuously studied and used by the physician and examiner as a guide in continuing with or modifying the plan for future tests based on whether they fit the characteristics usually identified with specific pathological conditions. As previously stated, the results of the electrodiagnostic tests must be correlated with other clinical findings and data.

Summary of Clinical Electroneuromyographic and Nerve Conduction Studies

Instruments with computer-assisted analysis are now commonplace for studying electromyographic signals in great detail.[11,28-30] Parameters of the waveform, including amplitude, duration, frequency spectrum, number of turns, or phase polarity reversals and area (the integral or total voltage of the waveform) can be automatically analyzed. The data are then compared electronically with predetermined patterns of electrical changes, which correlate with categories of neuromuscular disorders such as myelopathies and neuropathies.

The following is a summary of the more characteristic EMG and nerve conduction changes associated with selected groupings of neurological disorders. The intent is to assist in the understanding of reports of these studies and recognize changes that may be seen in sequential tests during the course of the disorders. The following is a simplified grouping of electrical changes; actual electrodiagnostic studies show considerably more detail and frequent variations of these findings.[9-11,26,27]

Electrical testing in CNS disorders typically shows normal motor and sensory nerve conduction. In the EMG, spontaneous activity is typically not seen, and individual motor units seen on muscle contraction usually have normal parameters. The recruitment pattern may show a slower-than-normal MUAP discharge frequency with an incomplete and irregular interference pattern. In the presence of tremor and other involuntary movements, bursts of MUAPs occur, consistent with the muscle contraction pattern. In cases involving the brain stem, the blink reflex may show abnormalities.[7] The tests are important in differential diagnosis between a CNS and a PNS problem, but often they are not used when clinical examinations demonstrate the problem to be definitively in the CNS.

In myelopathies, which include upper and lower motor neuron disorders (e.g., amyotrophic lateral sclerosis [ALS], poliomyelitis, cervical spondylitis, and syringomyelia), motor and sensory nerve conduction is usually normal, although mild slowing may be present.[11] The characteristic EMG changes, which usually appear in the more chronic stages of the disorders, are increased amplitude and duration of MUAPs because of the variable impulse conduction time in sprouting axon terminals. An increased number of polyphasic potentials with increased duration is usually found. Spontaneous activity is often seen, and on strong contraction fewer rapidly firing large MUAPs are recruited, resulting in a single-unit or partial interference pattern. In ALS, fasciculations and denervation potentials are typically found. The distribution of the EMG abnormalities determines the extent of the condition.

Peripheral neuropathies show a variety of electrical changes depending on the type and location of the pathology. In a proximal pathology (e.g., radiculopathy), motor and sensory nerve conduction generally remain normal, except F waves and H-reflex responses in specific spinal segments. If motor nerve roots are compromised, spontaneous activity and increased polyphasic potentials appear, and reduced recruitment of MUAPs results in an incomplete interference pattern. In more chronic stages MUAP amplitude and duration can be increased. As the lesion improves, spontaneous activity decreases and the recruitment patterns become more normal. If only sensory roots are injured, no EMG changes occur. Again, the distribution of the EMG abnormalities (all in one myotome) is pathognomonic, especially in the presence of denervation potentials in the corresponding paraspinal muscles.[31]

Lesions of peripheral nerves, which range from a focal mononeuropathy to plexopathy, frequently show abnormalities in motor and sensory nerve conduction depending on which components of the nerve are involved. In the EMG, spontaneous activity, particularly fibrillation and positive sharp waves, is common. If the lesion is complete, no MUAPs are found. The presence of even a few MUAPs suggests a more optimistic prognosis. Often the location of the lesion can be identified by the distribution of the electrical changes. With regenerating axons, low-amplitude polyphasic MUAPs gradually appear. In the chronic stage, the amplitude and duration of MUAPs are often increased. Spontaneous activity decreases with reinnervation, but it may persist for several years.

Generalized, systemic peripheral polyradiculoneuropathies can be divided into primarily demyelinating, primarily axon loss, or mixed axonal-demyelinating polyneuropathies. Some involve mostly sensory nerves (e.g., hereditary sensory neuropathy types I to IV, Sjögren syndrome, Friedreich ataxia), and others mostly motor nerves (e.g., chronic inflammatory demyelinating polyneuropathy [CIDP], lead neuropathy), but most involve both sensory and motor nerves. In the primarily demyelinating type, such as Guillain-Barré syndrome, motor and sensory nerve conduction and F waves become markedly slow. EMG changes usually do not occur, except for a reduced recruitment pattern consistent with weak muscle contraction or conduction block (when the demyelination is such that the impulse does not propagate). With primarily axonal polyneuropathies, such as uremic neuropathy, isoniazid or cisplatin toxicity, and lead poisoning, motor and sensory nerve conduction is mildly slowed or may remain normal. The duration and amplitude of the response, however, decrease. During advanced stages, many polyneuropathies develop both demyelinating and axonal pathology (e.g., diabetic neuropathy, which is by far the most commonly encountered polyneuropathy). On EMG, spontaneous activity is commonly seen. These electrical changes generally become more severe with worsening of the pathology, but they also improve if the pathology is reversed. From a patient management standpoint, remyelination occurs at a much more expedient pace than reinnervation.[32-34]

Again, the scope of the NCS electromyographic test is to determine the presence and extent of a neurological dysfunction. Attributing a cause to the dysfunction (e.g., diabetes versus alcoholism) requires other tests.

With myopathic disorders, motor and sensory nerve conductions are generally normal unless neural tissue is also affected. In advanced stages, however, severely atrophied muscles can produce decreased amplitude and distorted nerve conduction responses. The characteristic findings on EMG are short-duration, low-amplitude potentials. Some spontaneous potentials, particularly fibrillations and positive sharp waves, may be found but are much more frequent in the inflammatory myopathies such as polymyositis. Specific myotonic potentials appear in certain myopathic disorders (e.g., myotonia congenita). The recruitment pattern shows many low-amplitude MUAPs, appearing in a full pattern, with little voluntary effort. This type of recruitment pattern is referred to as *early recruitment.*

Neuromuscular junction disorders involve the synapse between axons and myocytes. In LEMS the pathology is in the presynaptic membrane (decreased release of acetylcholine [ACh]), whereas in myasthenia gravis the pathology involves the postsynaptic membrane. The two are differentiated by the response to RNS or jitter with single-fiber EMG (see later). In LEMS the amplitude of the responses increases with repetitive stimulation (more quanta of ACh released), whereas in myasthenia gravis the responses decrease (all ACh receptors saturated). Sensory NCS findings are typically normal.

Table 33-1 provides a summary of typical findings.

Single-Fiber Electromyography

Electrical activity can be recorded from two or more muscle fibers innervated by the same motor unit by using a specially designed single-fiber needle electrode. SFEMG is, at this time, the most sensitive test for evaluation of neuromuscular transmission defects such as myasthenia gravis and myasthenic syndrome. It is also used to evaluate peripheral neuropathies, motor neuron diseases, and myopathies. It is typically provided only in tertiary centers and requires a high level of patient participation.

During a carefully controlled minimal voluntary contraction, a 25-μm–diameter needle is inserted into the muscle, and several potentials from muscle fibers within the recording area are stored. Equipment with a trigger and delay line is necessary to "time lock" the tracings of the potentials. The slightly different conduction time or interpulse interval (IPI) required for impulses to be transmitted from a single motor neuron to each of its terminal endplates, cross the neuromuscular junction, and activate the muscle fiber is called *jitter*. This time difference is collected from several tracings and is converted into a mean consecutive time difference (MCD), which normally ranges from 5 to 55 ms. Values shorter or longer than this range are considered abnormal. The impulses from some axons to their muscle fibers may fail to be transmitted. This is referred to as *blocking*. Another capability of SFEMG is the measure of fiber density, that is, the average number of muscle fibers within the needle recording area. Fiber density is increased in reinnervation and also with certain myopathies because of axonal collateralization or splitting.[28]

Macroelectromyography

A variation of SFEMG uses a macroelectrode to record the majority of muscle fibers of a single motor unit as they are triggered by an initial potential, which is then time locked with all the other muscle fiber potentials recorded from a different part of the same or a nearby needle.[11,29,30,35,36] Two recording channels are used. Maximal amplitude of the potentials from several muscles has been reported by Stalberg.[35] The findings are analyzed, along with findings of jitter, fiber density, and conventional EMG, to evaluate the status and prognosis of various neurological and neuromuscular disorders, such as motor neuron disease, peripheral nerve lesions, and myopathies.

In summary, the astute PT in the presence of a patient reporting weakness and/or numbness will refer that patient appropriately for electrophysiological testing based on the findings of a judicious clinical examination. In reading the report of an electrophysiological consultation, the PT will first correlate the results with the findings of the physical examination of the patient, determine whether the studies performed are complete (i.e., there are sufficient data to rule in the condition but also sufficient data to rule out other conditions), and correlate the findings with the conclusion. There is evidence that PTs performing NCSs and EMG tend to follow guidelines consistently.[37]

Kinesiological Electromyography

KEMG measures muscle activation during movement, whether it is purposeful, involuntary, dynamic, or relatively static. It is the method by which the therapist-examiner determines a muscle's (or muscle group's) onset, cessation, relative intensity, and activation sequencing during functional activities such as walking. Because normal movement depends on the CNS's ability to execute motor programs through muscle action, KEMG provides the therapist with insight, in real time, into motor function, motor control, and motor learning.

Persons with neuromuscular disorders typically exhibit control errors, including the inability to initiate, execute, or terminate movement. Selective control may be absent or abnormal with errors in muscle timing, intensity, and sequencing. Spasticity or synergistic muscle action may impede smooth execution of tasks and prevent purposeful movement. With

TABLE 33-1 ■ SUMMARY OF TYPICAL FINDINGS

DISORDER	MOTOR CONDUCTION	SENSORY CONDUCTION	ELECTROMYOGRAPHY
Motor neuron disease (e.g., amyotrophic lateral sclerosis [ALS])	Reduced amplitudes	Normal	Acute plus chronic neurogenic changes, fasciculations
Radiculopathies	Normal	Normal	Acute neurogenic changes in myotome
Plexopathies	Reduced amplitudes	Reduced amplitudes	Acute neurogenic changes in specific pattern
Axonal neuropathy	Reduced amplitude in affected nerve(s)	Reduced amplitude in affected nerve(s)	Acute neurogenic changes in affected nerve
Demyelinating neuropathy	Reduced conduction in affected nerve	Reduced conduction in affected nerve	Normal
Neuromuscular junction disorder	Decrement (myasthenia gravis [MG]) or increment (Lambert-Eaton myasthenic syndrome [LEMS]) with repetitive stimulation	Normal	Occasional myopathic motor unit action potentials (MUAPs)
Myopathies	Normal	Normal	Small-amplitude polyphasic MUAPs

increased emphasis on evidence-based practice, KEMG can provide objective documentation of abnormal control and intervention outcomes and provide insight into optimizing strategies for improved functional performance. Many orthopedic surgeons rely on KEMG testing to supplement clinical evaluation in planning surgical interventions (muscle transfers and releases) in children with cerebral palsy,[38] in patients with TBI,[39] and in those who have had a stroke.[40]

KEMG interpretation depends on the examiner's understanding of the instrumentation chosen for testing, including electrode selection, recording techniques, signal processing, and time and intensity normalization.[41] Coupled with three-dimensional motion (infrared camera and motion capture) and force plate analysis, external moments are calculated that define internal force demands on muscles during functional activities such as walking. KEMG delineates the muscles that participate in meeting the internal force demand.

Recording Instrumentation

KEMG can be performed by using surface or fine wire electrodes (intramuscular). Controversy exists about the choice of electrodes, with the selection dependent on the clinical or research question. If the examiner is interested in "muscle groups" (e.g., dorsiflexors, quadriceps) then surface electrodes are appropriate. Fine wire electrodes are optimal if activation of individual or deep muscles is desired (e.g., posterior tibialis, iliacus). Fine wire allows for specificity of muscle action required for surgical decisions related to muscle transfers, releases, or muscle lengthening.[38,39,42]

Needle or Fine Wire Electrodes (Indwelling or Intramuscular). A pair of 50-μg fine wire electrodes, also referred to as *indwelling* or *intramuscular electrodes,* are introduced through the skin and into the muscle with a 25-gauge hypodermic needle. The 50-μg, Teflon-coated wires are threaded through the needle's core; 2 to 3 mm of the wire's distal end are stripped of insulation and, once inserted, record adjacent motor unit activity. Before insertion the electrodes are sterilized. Inserted through the skin and into the muscle of interest, the barbed end "hooks" the muscle fibers when the needle is withdrawn. Accurate placement requires that the examiner have extensive knowledge of three-dimensional anatomy and excellent palpation skills. A maximal concentric voluntary contraction is elicited to anchor the wires into the muscle fibers, preventing displacement during subsequent contraction. This ensures sampling the same motor unit pool during subsequent tasks, trials, or conditions. Electrical stimulation is an essential testing element to verify electrode location. Wire electrodes allow a more precise definition of muscle timing (onset and cessation) by reducing the incidence of intramuscular crosstalk.[43] Disadvantages include decreased reliability and insertional pain caused by skin penetration.[44-46] In several states the examiner must possess specialized KEMG licensure to penetrate the skin with a needle.

Surface Electrodes. When the clinical question can be answered by using surface electrodes, electrical stimulation of motor points often defines optimal electrode placement over the muscle or group of muscles of interest. A maximal voluntary contraction (MVC) is elicited to confirm that optimal placement has been achieved. Standardizing electrode placement, size, interelectrode distance, and skin preparation enhances test-retest repeatability,[47] with submaximal contractions more reliable than maximal contractions.[48] Skin displacement under the recording site may introduce movement artifact, which can be minimized by securing the electrodes to the skin with tape. To improve interday reliability, electrode placement should be marked (with ink) and standardized electrodes used. When both recording electrodes are contained in the same housing, interelectrode distance is standardized and movement artifact attenuated. Advantages of using surface electrodes include improved reliability and the ease with which they can be applied without causing patient discomfort.[44-46] Specialized licensure is not required.

Instrumentation for Kinesiological Electromyography Acquisition

KEMG signal acquisition requires either a telemetry unit (FM modulation) or a hard-wired system that relies on a "cable" tethered to the subject to transmit signals from the electrode site to the receiver. The subject's performance and nature of movement strategies performed may be altered by the cabling. Telemetry allows the subject unrestricted movement; KEMG signals are transmitted through the air from a small unit worn around the subject's waist. The optimal characteristics of the receiver include a bandwidth frequency of 40 to 1000 Hz and an overall gain of 1000 Hz.[41]

Signal Processing. KEMG processing has become highly automated with the advent of high-speed computers and customized software. Once the signal has been acquired, it is stored digitally and processed by various computer programs. The "raw" signal is full wave rectified (all the negative values become positive), and a linear envelope is generated within a designated time interval. The area under the curve is mathematically integrated, and an average EMG profile is generated. Muscle-specific onset, cessation, and relative intensity are defined with a variety of software. According to a recent study, KEMG timing (onset and cessation) is optimally identified by using the intensity filtered average (IFA) and packet analysis (PAC) when compared with ensemble average (EAV).[49] Despite a smaller recording volume with wires, Bogey and colleagues[49] demonstrated no significant difference in signal amplitude when multiple insertion sites within the same muscle were compared.

Normalization. Any acquired "raw" EMG signal needs to be referenced to a standard value. This is accomplished by dividing the raw EMG during a functional task such as walking by a reference value. The MVC serves this purpose. Subjects exert a maximal voluntary effort for each muscle that determines the maximal EMG activity possible. All subsequent efforts are compared with this maximal effort and expressed as a percentage of maximum (%MVC). In patients with neurological dysfunction who lack selective motor control, a maximal effort can be elicited in either an extensor or flexor synergy by using the upright motor control (UMC) test developed at Rancho Los Amigos National Rehabilitation Center, grading the effort as "weak," "moderate," or "strong" in synergy.[50] Maximal efforts are elicited for 3 to 5 seconds, and the software determines the maximal activity for a 1-second interval. The muscles' activation during a functional activity is subsequently expressed as a percentage of MVC.

Interpretation of Kinesiological Electromyography

Kinesiological Electromyography and Strength. KEMG testing does not directly measure muscle strength, and the examiner should resist equating raw EMG signal amplitude directly with muscle force or torque output. Grading the strength (manual muscle testing [MMT] or UMC test) of each maximal effort must accompany the interpretation of the muscle participation during a functional task.[51] For example, patients with postpolio syndrome (refer to Chapter 35) produce large-amplitude KEMG signals that often reflect the maximal exertion of a "weak" muscle (e.g., "MMT—Poor" or 2/5). Large-amplitude EMG signals represent activation of large motor units typical of reinnervation, not force output. Despite large-amplitude signals, the muscle is functionally weak. In other words, a 100% MVC normalized KEMG record for a muscle may represent the maximal effort of a "poor" or 2/5 muscle.

Muscle Tone versus Spasticity. Therapists should resist making inferences about *tone* from KEMG testing. As previously stated, KEMG reflects the contractile activity of motor units. Muscle tone refers to the amount of *resting* tension in a muscle because of its viscoelastic properties. Because tone is not a function of motor unit activity, it cannot be measured with KEMG.[41] In contrast, spasticity, defined as a hyperactive quick stretch response, can be recorded by KEMG because it reflects prolonged muscle activation (>0.1 s). Clonus has a distinct frequency characterized by a prolonged 5- to 8-Hz signal. Using signal duration in response to quick stretch, Cahan and colleagues[52] identified significant decreases in spasticity in selected lower-extremity muscles in children with cerebral palsy after selective dorsal rhizotomy. In these children spasticity interfered with agonist activation during walking.

In conclusion, KEMG is useful for delineating patterns of muscle activation in motor performance, reflecting the integrity of the neuromuscular control mechanism. The examiner's interpretation should also consider additional factors such as the type of contraction; speed of movement; joint acceleration; and a host of physiological, biomechanical, anatomical, and neurological elements beyond the scope of this chapter.

ELECTRICAL STIMULATION AND ELECTROMYOGRAPHIC BIOFEEDBACK

NMES and EMGBF are often used as tools in the management of neurological dysfunction. EMGBF can be used both alone and in conjunction with stimulation. The primary goal of use is improvement of function by improving voluntary motor control. To that end, strengthening and alteration of abnormal tone are also common goals of treatment. EMGBF is discussed later in this chapter. More detailed explication of treatment protocols is included in a variety of published work.[53-64]

Electrical stimulators used in physical rehabilitation practice may be either small, portable, battery-operated units or larger line-powered clinical instruments. The clinical units often will offer a variety of stimulus forms and options for modulation of currents. Portable units provide the ability for patients and caregivers to carry out prescribed stimulation at home. Clinical units allow the therapist to customize programs to optimize treatment outcomes.

Neuromuscular Electrical Stimulation

In NMES, muscle contraction is elicited by depolarization of the motor neurons. Electrodes may be placed over the muscle to be stimulated or over the motor nerve that controls the muscle. Firing order of neurons is a result of neuronal size, proximity of the electrical stimulus, and the intensity of stimulation.[65] Muscle recruitment patterns triggered by electrical stimulation differ from those observed in normal muscle activation. In a voluntary muscle contraction, motor units fire asynchronously, with a larger proportion of type I, fatigue-resistant muscle fibers of the smaller motor units being recruited first. The order of muscle fiber firing occurs as a result of motor neuron size and the anatomy of synaptic connections.[66] Conversely, an electrically stimulated muscle contraction elicits initial responses from larger motor units, which contain a greater number of fatigable, type II muscle fibers. The type II fibers are innervated by larger-diameter neurons that have a lower threshold for electrical stimulation than smaller neurons.[67] A study of healthy subjects demonstrated recruitment of these higher-threshold motor units at relatively low NMES training levels. In voluntary exercise a much greater exercise intensity is required for activation of these larger motor units.[67]

Synchronous recruitment of muscle fibers is obtained with electrical stimulation. This does not occur with volitional activation. During a sustained volitional contraction motor units periodically "drop out" and then "drop in" to reduce fatigue. With NMES, once recruited the motor units will continue to fire until the stimulus is ended. This, coupled with the early recruitment of fatigable motor units, accounts for fatigue being a major problem in the use of NMES. It also is one reason functional activities performed under control by stimulation are much less smooth and balanced than when they are performed volitionally. At the same time, relatively low levels of NMES can recruit motor units that volitionally would be recruited only with maximal effort. This provides support for observed increases in strength with low NMES training intensities.[68] Numerous potential benefits have been identified for NMES. Among them are improvement in ROM, edema reduction, treatment of disuse atrophy, and improvement of muscle recruitment for muscle reeducation.[56]

Parameters of Stimulation

With any electrical stimulation used for patients with neuromuscular dysfunction, three parameters must be considered within the waveform: pulse (or phase) duration, pulse frequency, and pulse amplitude. Depending on the intent of the electrical stimulation, instruments are available that allow all of these to be independently adjusted.

Waveform

NMES units use alternating currents. The waveform of the stimulus produced by most NMES units is either a symmetrical or an asymmetrical biphasic pulse. The two phases of each pulse continually alternate in direction between positive and negative polarity. Although an ideal waveform has not been identified, most studies have shown the symmetrical biphasic waveform to be more comfortable than either the asymmetrical biphasic or the monophasic waveform.[53,69,70]

Duration

Phase or pulse duration (also called *pulse width*) refers to the amount of time of a single pulse or phase. Stimulators with a pulse duration of 1 to 300 μs (0.3 ms) can be used to activate muscles with intact innervation. Waveforms of shorter durations require a greater current amplitude to produce a muscle contraction (because the current is on for a shorter period of time). They may be more comfortable but may not possess enough charge for good contraction levels. Longer-phase durations may be used but are less comfortable. In NMES units, pulse durations may be started at 100 μs, then increased to 200 to 300 μs if tolerated well by the patient.[71,72] Denervated muscles require significantly longer phase durations (20 to 100 ms) because of the longer chronaxy of muscle cells compared with motor neurons.

Frequency

Pulse frequency (or *pulse rate*) refers to the number of electrical pulses applied per unit time. In applications seeking to provide muscle contraction, the stimulus rate should be 35 to 50 pps. This is a typical critical frequency at which a muscle will respond with a smooth contraction (also called a *tetanic frequency*). Higher frequencies than this can result in early onset of fatigue. NMES used for spasm reduction may use a higher frequency, with the intent of fatiguing the muscle and decreasing spasm, which will result in decreased pain levels.

Amplitude

The amplitude (intensity) of the stimulus should be sufficient to achieve the desired strength of contraction. Battery-operated units usually indicate the amplitude only in a relative way (nonquantitatively) because the output of the battery declines over time. Depending on the impedance of the electrodes, coupling agent, skin and soft tissue, the amount of current required at one location could be quite different than at another to produce the same degree of muscle contraction. This is why the amplitude of the stimulus is usually described according to the strength of the sensation felt by the patient. *Mild, moderate,* or *maximum sensory* refers to the intensity of the stimulation as felt by the patient, without eliciting a motor contraction. Similarly, *mild, moderate,* and *maximum motor* describe the amplitude of the stimulus needed to produce those visible muscular contractions using electrical stimulation. If the intent is to strengthen the muscle or increase endurance, the client is usually asked to participate by voluntarily contracting the muscle being stimulated when the stimulation is on. The amplitude of stimulation should be graded based on the response of the patient, aiming at production of the clinically desired force output.

Additional Parameters: Ramp Time and On-Off Time Ratio

On Time and Off Time. NMES for facilitation of muscle contraction should be used to supplement exercise, and goals for stimulation should be consistent with the goals of the exercise program. To simulate isotonic or isometric muscle contractions, as in voluntary movement for exercise, the stimulator must have the capability of setting cycles of on and off times. Each period of muscle contraction is followed by a period of relaxation (Figure 33-7).[2,56] In most cases a shorter on time than off time is desirable to avoid fatigue. For example, a 10-second on time may be followed by a 50-second off time in a cycle, resulting in an on-off ratio of 1:5. Packman-Braun[73] investigated ratios of stimulation to rest time with NMES for wrist extension in a group of hemiplegic patients. Results supported the on-off time of 1:5 as being the most beneficial in training programs of 20 to 30 minutes because of the deleterious effects of fatigue with lower ratios (1:1, 1:2, 1:3, 1:4). If the goal is to reduce edema by providing a muscle pumping action, a ratio of 1:1 or 1:2 may be preferred,[73] as the intent is to decrease the edema by continuous muscle pumping action. Lower ratios may be used when the goal is neuromuscular reeducation or endurance training.

Ramping. Ramping is another modulation that can be set by the therapist. Ramp-up is the time it takes each train of pulses to increase amplitude or intensity sequentially from zero to maximum. Ramp-off is the period set at the end of the train of maximal intensity pulses to decrease sequentially from maximum to zero amplitude (see Figure 33-7). Ramp time can be adjusted so that the stimulation more nearly resembles a pattern of gradually contracting and relaxing muscles. For clients with hypertonicity or spasticity and a goal of facilitation and strengthening the antagonist muscle, a longer ramp-up time may avoid or minimize activation of the stretch reflex in the hyperactive agonist muscle.

Duty Cycle. The term *duty cycle* is sometimes confused with the on-off time ratio. Duty cycle is the percentage of

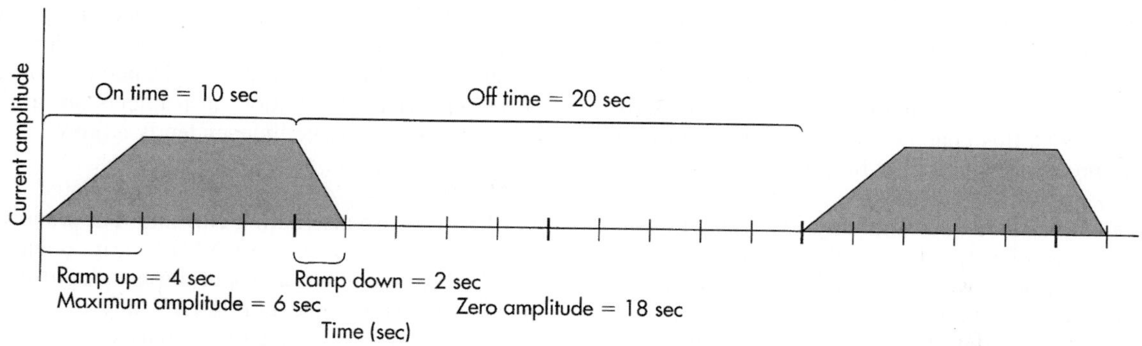

Figure 33-7 ■ Example of the relation between ramp times and on/off times. Each division on the horizontal axis equals 2 seconds. Note that the ramp-up time is considered part of the on time, whereas the ramp-down time is considered part of the off time. (Reprinted from DeVahl J: NMES in rehabilitation. In Gersh MR, editor: *Electrotherapy in rehabilitation,* Philadelphia, 1992, FA Davis.)

time a series or train of pulses is on out of the total on and off time in a cycle.[2,53] For example, if the train of pulses is on 10 seconds and off 30 seconds, the total cycle time is 40 seconds. The duty cycle would be 25% (10 seconds of the total 40-second cycle). The actual on time and off time of the pulses in a cycle is a more informative description than either the duty cycle or the on-off ratio.

Muscle Reeducation

After an insult or injury affecting the CNS, problems with motor control frequently manifest. One of the common goals of therapy is to facilitate movement in the areas where control is lacking. If active movement is not present, NMES allows movement to occur by stimulation, which may be followed by resumption of active movement, possibly triggered by the sensory (visual and proprioceptive, among others) experience that accompanies the stimulation. When active movement is present but is weak or not well controlled, the therapist may choose to use NMES to supplement and strengthen the muscular contraction already present. Some evidence exists that NMES can increase activity in the somatosensory cortex and that the cortical activity is correlated with improvement in functional tasks.[74] In the presence of hypertonicity, the muscles serving as antagonists to the spastic muscle may be targeted for NMES, not only to strengthen the antagonist but to inhibit the spastic muscle by reciprocal inhibition.

Functional Electrical Stimulation

The term *functional electrical stimulation* (FES) has been used casually to describe various applications of NMES. However, FES is defined by the Electrotherapy Standards Committee of the Section on Clinical Electrophysiology of the American Physical Therapy Association as the use of NMES (on innervated muscles) for orthotic substitution.[2] Baker and Parker[75] use the term to describe external control of innervated, paretic, or paralytic muscles "to achieve functional and purposeful movements." Although NMES is generally considered to have therapeutic applications, such as increasing ROM, facilitation of muscle activation, and muscle strengthening, the key to application of FES is to enhance or facilitate functional control. It is used with clients with SCI, TBI, cerebrovascular accident (CVA), and other CNS dysfunction who have intact peripheral innervation.

An example of FES application is the electrical stimulation of the peroneal nerve to enhance ankle dorsiflexion during gait in patients with hemiplegia.[76] Two of the more common applications of FES on the market include the WalkAide system (Innovative Neurotronics, Austin, Texas) and Bioness (Bioness, Valencia, California). In terms of neurological dysfunctions, research has been published that indicates efficacy of these devices and FES in general in improving functional performance in people with CVA,[77-80] multiple sclerosis, TBI, SCI,[81,82] and cerebral palsy.[83] Moreover, numerous other uses of FES have been described, ranging from isolated motor control activities, such as decreasing shoulder subluxation and reducing scoliosis, to highly technical computerized gait and bicycling capabilities, sometimes referred to as *computerized FES* (CFES).[84-92] The trigger that activates muscle contraction in synchrony with the functional activity can be manually initiated by the client, set within the stimulator to automatically trigger on and off cycles, or programmed into a complex computer system for bicycling or gait.

Stimulation is generally applied in short-duration pulses with a frequency sufficient to provide smooth, tetanizing muscle contractions and adjusted to cycle on and off, with adequate ramp functions, as indicated by the speed and time needed to synchronize the stimulation with the functional activity. The length of the intervention depends on the purpose and may vary from a few contractions during the functional activity, building to multiple 30-minute sessions working up to several hours, repeated daily or three to five times per week. With the more complex computerized systems used with clients with complete spinal cord lesions, electrically activated functional movements are the mechanism to achieve physiological and psychological benefits. In some situations, assisted function is also an important goal, although functional community ambulation is not yet a reality.[88,90,93-100] Hooker and co-workers[94] evaluated the physiological effects of use of FES-assisted leg cycling in SCI. Compared with resting levels, significant increases were found in cardiac output, heart rate, stroke volume, respiratory exchange rate, pulmonary ventilation, and other physiological phenomena. CFES for cycle ergometry and ambulation has also been shown to increase muscle mass, electrically induce muscle strength and endurance,[89,101,102] increase circulation and aerobic capacity, decrease edema, and have a beneficial impact on self-image.[90,102,103] Jacobs and colleagues[100] compared the metabolic stress of FES-assisted standing versus frame-supported standing. Cardiorespiratory stress was significantly higher with FES, and the authors concluded that FES-assisted standing alone may provide a stress sufficient to meet minimal requirements for exercise conditioning.

The demonstrated benefits of FES clearly indicate that it is a valuable tool for supplementing functional activities. The practicality and cost of applications of the more complex computerized systems need further study, especially in terms of function in community activities. (Refer to Chapter 38 for additional discussion.)

Electromyographic Biofeedback

Biofeedback is a general term used to describe the use of visual or auditory representation of physiological processes to allow an individual to modify those processes. EMGBF makes available to the client information regarding the electrical activity of muscle. EMGBF has several well documented applications, including alteration of physiological responses such as heart rate, temperature, and muscle tension.[54] These applications may prove beneficial for clients with neurological dysfunction. An example would be relaxation to modify pain perception. The focus of this review is the use of EMGBF for improvement of active movement, which may include reduction of hypertonicity in addition to muscle reeducation. EMGBF units range from basic single-channel portable models to clinical units with multiple channels and multiple options for provision of feedback.

EMGBF may be used to assist a client in attaining greater levels of muscle activation in paretic muscle, decrease levels of muscle activation in spastic muscle, or attain a balance between agonist and antagonist muscle pairs.[104] For most practicing clinicians, EMG levels are monitored through the use of surface electrodes. Monitoring of activation of deep muscles is often not feasible. Attention to size and specific electrode placement is critical to ensure feedback that will be useful. Smaller electrodes allow specific placement, although higher impedance will be encountered. Skin must be carefully prepared to take this into account.[105] Because the EMG information recorded represents the sum of action potentials from motor units between the electrodes, large interelectrode distance will increase the area of muscle recorded. This may be desirable for large muscle groups or when minimal activity is present.

Smaller interelectrode distances are preferable if interference from "crosstalk" or "volume conduction" from muscles or motor units not part of the target group is a risk. Basmajian and Blumenstein[105] provide an excellent review of electrode placements.

Reduction of Hypertonicity

DeBacher[106] described a progression of intervention with EMGBF designed to reduce spasticity. The program uses three stages of intervention: (1) relaxation of spastic muscles at rest even in the presence of distraction, mental effort, or use of muscles not targeted for EMGBF training; (2) inhibition of muscle activity during passive static and dynamic stretch of the spastic muscle, beginning with static stretch at the extremes of motion, then progressing to passive movement speed at a speed of 15 degrees per second; and (3) isometric contractions of the antagonist to the spastic muscle, with relaxation of the spastic muscle, progressing to prompt muscle contraction and relaxation of the spastic muscle, and grading of muscle contractions with movement for various force output requirements. Use of the technique in a small sample of young adults with cerebral palsy demonstrated improvement in resting levels of involuntary muscle activity.[107] Improvements in function, however, were not demonstrated.

Inhibition of a spastic muscle alone may not be enough to improve function. Often the spastic muscle itself, once hypertonicity has diminished, is weak or has low functional tone. Weak antagonists to the affected muscle may contribute to the functional limitation. EMGBF to reinforce activity in the weak muscle may be done concurrently with its use to modify the tone in the agonist.[108] EMGBF can be useful in helping a client decrease abnormal muscle activation, but persistence of control problems may be related to lack of force production, deficits in speed of muscle activation, and lack of reciprocal interaction of muscle groups.[109]

Muscle Reeducation

Therapists may opt to use biofeedback to provide information about the quality of the muscle contraction directly to the client. The client can then attempt to alter the contraction in accordance with guidelines provided by the therapist, whether the focus is to facilitate stronger contraction, decrease apparent hyperactivity, or modulate a balance of muscle activity during a functional task.

Concurrent assessment of muscle activity (CAMA) is an application of EMGBF in which the therapist uses biofeedback as an adjunct in evaluation of client response to therapeutic exercise.[110] In this procedure the therapist decides which muscle group(s) are desired for activation and adjusts the position of the client or the therapist intervention accordingly to get the correct responses. CAMA allows for the judgment of the effectiveness of a particular activity based on actual EMG responses rather than presumptions of what the intervention should cause. In a placebo-controlled study of hemiplegic patients, the addition of EMGBF to hand exercises based on the Brunnstrom approach resulted in significant improvement in active ROM in those using biofeedback compared with sham.[111]

Several authors suggest the use of biofeedback signals from homologous extremity muscles as a model for what the hemiplegic client needs to alter muscle activity in a particular function.[112,113] This has been described as a "motor copy" and was compared with a more targeted training procedure. Indications showed that the motor copy resulted in better carryover in function than the comparison therapy in follow-up evaluations. A similar training study showed indications of benefits of the procedure, but the results were not statistically significant because of the small group size.[112] At least two studies support patterning or copying EMG from other muscles as a potentially useful tool for individuals with C4-7 SCI.[114,115] A meta-analysis that compared EMGBF with conventional physical therapy for upper-extremity function in individuals after stroke reviewed only six studies and concluded that neither approach was superior to the other.[116]

Feedback Considerations

EMGBF has the benefit of being provided simultaneously with the client's movement, consisting of accurate and objective information about muscle activity (given careful electrode application), and not requiring the same level of therapist skill as verbal feedback provision. EMGBF therefore may be beneficial for clients with deficient sensory feedback systems. The frequency of feedback provision, however, may require close scrutiny by the therapist.

Experiments examining feedback frequency in the learning of motor tasks support the use of less than 100% relative frequency for the subject to learn the task. Feedback provided on every trial may improve performance but degrades learning in normal subjects.[117] In a study of stroke patients attempting a pursuit tracking task, biofeedback was used for the experimental group (electrodes over the spastic biceps), whereas the control group performed the task without feedback.[118] Posttests revealed that the use of continuous feedback had a negative transfer effect on learning of the movement task, suggesting that the experimental learners became dependent on the external feedback in performance of the task. The clinician must therefore carefully structure the use of external feedback so the client begins to develop a sense of muscle activation or relaxation that is present without the EMGBF apparatus. This may be accomplished by turning the screen away from the client and turning off the auditory signal as the patient progresses.

Integrating Neuromuscular Electrical Stimulation and Electromyographic Biofeedback

The use of EMG-triggered NMES, in which NMES is initiated once the client has achieved a predetermined level of EMG activity in the targeted muscles, is an application that has been shown to have merit,[119,120] although a more recent systematic review showed no statistically significant differences between EMG-NMES and usual care in improving upper-extremity function of the affected extremity in people who had had a stroke.[121] Threshold levels of EMG activity could gradually be increased as the client gains the ability to activate muscles independently, with eventual discontinuance of the NMES as strength and active control allow. The success of this application has been shown in patients with hemiplegia in terms of increasing EMG activity and subsequent improvement in ROM and function in the involved arm and leg.[119] In another study, patients who had had a stroke more than 1 year previously significantly improved wrist and finger extension strength and function after treatment with EMG-triggered stimulation compared with controls.[120]

A variation of this application is NMES triggered by positional feedback, such that NMES is initiated once the patient actively moves through a portion of the available ROM at a joint.[122] The therapist may set the threshold angle in accordance with the patient's goals and abilities. This method has been shown to be effective in improving wrist motion after stroke, although it was not as effective in altering control of the knee in a similar patient group.[123]

Although discussions of EMGBF, NMES, and FES are often presented separately, the use of these modalities can be intertwined to achieve desired muscle control. NMES or FES may be initiated in the absence of active control (although lower levels of muscle activation may be discovered and facilitated with EMGBF). Once return of active control begins, EMGBF may be used to refine the control. An increase in muscle EMG should not be assumed to translate automatically to an improvement in functional use of that muscle in daily activities. Consequently, NMES and EMGBF need to be integrated into daily functional activities so that appropriate muscle activity is elicited and used in its appropriate functional context.

Applications

The application of the common principles of EMGBF and NMES to different patient populations emphasizes the role of the therapist in tailoring intervention to meet specific client needs.

Many investigators have evaluated the use of NMES and EMGBF in clients who have had a stroke.[108,124-126] FES has been used extensively with clients with SCI. Other populations that demonstrate neuromuscular impairment or dysfunction have not been as thoroughly studied. This may be because the heterogeneity of these groups may create difficulty in research design.

Upper-Extremity Management

Electromyographic Biofeedback

EMGBF has been extensively studied, but success of the treatment is mixed, with difficulty in interpretation. A reduction in co-contraction has been observed,[127] as well as improvement in several neuromuscular variables[124,128,129]; however, a lack of significant improvement in functional skill was noted. Given the challenge of improving upper-extremity functional ability after stroke, Wolf and Binder-Macleod[129] suggested consideration of several key factors in predicting which clients may benefit from EMGBF: "Those patients who achieve the most substantial improvement in manipulative abilities initially possess voluntary finger extension; comparatively greater active ROM about the shoulder, elbow, and wrist; and comparatively less hyperactivity in muscles usually considered as major contributors to the typical flexor synergy." Attention to the chronicity of motor dysfunction also appears critical in anticipating success with EMGBF, as clients 2 to 3 months after stroke demonstrated stronger functional gains after intervention with biofeedback compared with clients 4 to 5 months after stroke. A placebo-controlled study of EMGBF showed statistically significant improvement in active ROM of the hand in clients who received EMGBF in addition to exercise.[111] A study by Doğan-Aslan[130] and colleagues found improvements in the Ashworth scale, Brunnstrom stage, upper-extremity function test, wrist extension ROM, and surface EMG potentials in their subjects who were treated with EMGBF in conjunction with neurodevelopmental treatment (NDT) and conventional treatment in a population of subjects with hemiplegia secondary to stroke.

Neuromuscular Electrical Stimulation

Common upper-extremity applications of NMES for the patient with a stroke include reduction of shoulder subluxation (FES) and facilitation of elbow, wrist, and finger extension and motor control.

FES for shoulder subluxation reduction appears beneficial for prevention of pain and subluxation, especially if used during the early stages of recovery. The functional benefits over the long term are not always clear, and cost-benefit ratios need to be considered. Baker and Parker,[75] Faghri and colleagues,[85] and Chantraine and colleagues[131] have reported success in management of shoulder subluxation after stroke by using gradually increasing stimulation times that ultimately reached 6 to 7 hours per day. On-off ratios were typically 1:3.

Use of NMES after stroke to facilitate motor control and function has been studied, but many studies lack controls. The extensors of the fingers and wrist are typically the targeted muscle groups. de Kroon and colleagues[61] reported a systematic review of literature that included six randomized controlled trials. A variety of stimulation parameters were used. Three studies tested subjects with acute conditions, and three tested subjects with chronic conditions. Outcome measures for motor control included the Fugl-Meyer Motor Assessment (four studies) and strength (two studies). Functional outcomes were reported by two studies, one using the Action Research Arm test and one using the Box and Block test. The authors concluded that there was a positive effect of stimulation on motor control. Only two studies reported functional outcomes, but both were positive. Of significance is the fact that only six studies met the criteria for review in terms of rigor.[119,120,122,132-134]

FES has also been investigated as an upper-extremity orthosis after hemiplegia, using movement of the uninvolved shoulder to trigger stimulation of elbow extension and hand opening.[135] After an extensive training period, patients were able to demonstrate functional use of the involved hand for basic reach and grasp.

Systems with more than two channels of stimulation have proved difficult for patients to use.[136] Popovic and colleagues[137] reported two studies in which they used NMES to treat patients after stroke. They termed the intervention *functional electrical therapy* (FET). The stimulation was used during an exercise program composed of voluntary arm movements and opening and closing, holding and releasing objects with the stimulation serving as an electric prosthesis. Treatment was 30 minutes daily for 3 weeks in one study[137] and 6 months in the other.[138] Outcomes were reported as better than controls. Initially higher-functioning subjects benefited more than those who were rated as low functioning. Unfortunately, outcome measures in these studies were not standardized.

A study of use of daily NMES in the form of neuroprosthetic FES (NESS Handmaster) stimulation of hand and finger extensors in patients with subacute strokes (6 to 12 months after onset) was reported by Ring and Rosenthal.[139] All subjects were receiving physical and occupational therapy three times a week. The stimulator was used at home. Those receiving stimulation had significantly greater improvements in spasticity, active ROM, and functional hand test scores compared with control subjects. The authors concluded that supplementation of outpatient rehabilitation with NMES improves upper-limb outcomes.[139]

Three-month interventions with EMG-triggered NMES, low-intensity NMES, proprioceptive neuromuscular facilitation (PNF) exercise, or no treatment were compared in a group of chronic stroke patients.[140] At 3 and 9 months after treatment, Fugl-Meyer scores improved 18% for the PNF group, 25% for the patients receiving low-intensity NMES, and 42% for the group receiving EMG-triggered NMES. The control group did not change.

These findings lend support to the use of NMES and EMGBF and NMES alone as adjuncts to physical therapy. Typically, higher-functioning patients have shown the greatest impact. Results have tended to show greater effect in patients with acute or subacute conditions, but longer-term patients sometimes benefited as well.

With the advent of the use of technology in neurological rehabilitation (see Chapter 38), an increasing number of investigations have been done to incorporate new technology with electrical stimulation to improve functional performance. Sayenko[141] described the use of a video game–based training system combined with NMES in a person with chronic SCI. Results indicated improvement in the strength and endurance of the paralyzed lower extremities of the individual after the intervention.

Lower-Extremity Management

Electromyographic Biofeedback

Several studies evaluating EMGBF for retraining lower-extremity control after stroke have focused on improvement of tibialis anterior control and reduction of gastrocnemius muscle activity. Results support increases in strength and ROM in ankle dorsiflexion with carryover into ambulation and maintenance of this improvement on follow-up evaluation.[142-144]

Wolf and Binder-Macleod[124] examined a number of variables at the hip, knee, and ankle in a controlled group study of the effects of EMGBF. Subjects were assigned to one of four groups: lower-extremity EMGBF, upper-extremity EMGBF, general relaxation training, and no treatment. No significant changes were observed between experimental and control groups for EMG levels and ROM at the hip, but improvements were noted in knee and ankle active motion for the experimental group. Although subjects in the experimental group increased their gait speed, these changes were not significantly different from findings in the comparison groups.

Use of EMGBF with the intent of improving ambulation may require use of feedback during the task of ambulation instead of during static activity, as demonstrated by this study. Positional biofeedback regarding ankle position and traditional EMGBF were compared in a group of hemiplegic subjects.[145] A computerized system provided audiovisual feedback during ambulation for both groups. Pretreatment and posttreatment measures of ankle motion, gait, and perceived exertion were conducted for the two treatment groups and a control group. The group receiving positional feedback increased walking speeds relative to the other groups, with improvements maintained at follow-up intervals of up to 3 months. The consideration of integrating feedback into functional ambulation bears further investigation.

Neuromuscular Electrical Stimulation

Peroneal nerve stimulation has been documented as an assistance for patients with hemiplegia to improve ambulation.[76,146-148] Long-term stimulation with implanted electrodes has proved effective in improving gait patterns, but difficulties in achieving balanced dorsiflexion, infection, and equipment maintenance were drawbacks.[148,149]

Shorter-term use of peroneal nerve stimulation as an adjunct to traditional physical therapy may be considered. In a controlled study examining the use of 20 minutes of peroneal nerve stimulation six times per week for 4 weeks, the stimulated group demonstrated dorsiflexion recovery three times greater than the control group, as measured by an average of 10 maximal dorsiflexion contractions. These improvements were regardless of site of lesion, age, or time since lesion.[146] Surface electrode stimulation is effective, and gait parameters can be improved with its use.[150,151] If, however, a foot drop is the only major impediment to ambulation, lightweight plastic orthoses are a functional and much less expensive choice of intervention.

Multichannel electrical stimulation has been used in the management of ambulation in patients who have had a stroke.[140,152-155] Although more effective than traditional gait training in some cases in terms of gait velocity and stride length, at follow-up evaluations 8 to 9 months after therapy the difference between groups had faded. However, the expense and availability of such systems make their use unlikely at this time.

NMES used for ankle dorsiflexion triggered by heel switch during gait and biofeedback to improve active recruitment of ankle dorsiflexors or relaxation of ankle plantar flexors has been studied in hemiplegic clients.[156] Patients who received a combination of these interventions demonstrated significantly improved knee and ankle range parameters more rapidly than those using a single modality. This improvement was maintained over a 1-month period. Although all groups improved in gait cycle times, results in the combined intervention group were better. This may be attributable to the synergy of biofeedback and stimulation.[51] Granat and colleagues[157] also studied peroneal muscle stimulation effects on gait parameters after stroke. After intervention the subjects showed significant control of eversion on all surfaces. The Barthel Index score also improved after intervention. However, no improvement occurred when the patients were not using the stimulator.

Evidence-Based Practice

Much of the literature evaluating the use of EMGBF and NMES involves patients with CVA. Although these studies have shown many significant results, interpretation of these findings in relation to what is recommended for clinical intervention is not as clear-cut. Improvements in generation of EMG activity and active movement are well documented, but the functional implications of these gains are not as well established. Clearly, in the current practice environment much of the focus is on function, so these techniques to improve muscle activation patterns must be put to functional use in the context of therapy. The therapist must consider the relevant factors that may predict success and critically evaluate outcomes during trial use of these modalities. Cost-benefit analyses must accompany any intervention using technology with the goal of regaining movement as quickly as possible and eliminating the use of equipment when practical.

Stroke (See Chapter 23)

Wolf and Binder-Macleod[124] examined client characteristics that are critical to success with biofeedback training for upper- and lower-extremity control after stroke. In a group of 52 clients with stroke, no significant relations between outcome and age, sex, number of EMGBF treatments, or side of hemiparesis were found. Lower-extremity treatment was associated with a greater probability of success, and this success did not seem related to chronicity of stroke sequelae. In contrast, success of upper-extremity treatment did appear to be related to length of time since onset of stroke, and poorer outcomes were noted if clients had received therapy to the involved arm for more than 1 year before EMGBF training. Improvements in elbow and shoulder function were obtained in this group of patients, but improvement in functional use of the hand was limited. Aphasia imposed a slight limitation to achieving improvement, but proprioceptive deficits were more significant in restricting functional gains. The role of client motivation in success with EMGBF training was emphasized. On follow-up over a 12-month period, the improvements made in the initial intervention were maintained in 33 of 34 clients evaluated.

A number of studies have been published discussing the muscle recruitment problems observed after CVA.[108,125,126] Knowledge of these problems is a prerequisite for determination of the appropriate application of EMGBF and NMES. Delayed recruitment of the agonist and antagonist is a relatively consistent finding. Other findings include delayed termination of muscle activity once initiated,[158] presence of co-contraction of agonist and antagonist muscles,[125,126] lack of co-contraction,[108] and maintenance of agonist muscle contractions.[125] These reports emphasize the potential value of EMGBF in determining the best mode of intervention.

Jonsdottir and colleagues[159] found that the application of EMGBF in a task-oriented manner, incorporating motor learning principles, resulted in improvements in gait velocity, stride length, and peak ankle power in a population of individuals with hemiparesis. Sander and colleagues[160] found that NMES application to the tibialis anterior muscle for 30 minutes three times a week for 4 weeks was effective in improving strength of the affected lower extremity.

Lourencao and colleagues[161] studied the effects of biofeedback with FES and occupational therapy on upper-extremity function of individuals with hemiplegia. Results indicated significant improvements in upper-extremity ROM and functional recovery with the addition of biofeedback in the treatment regimen.

Lastly, a systematic review was conducted by Woodford and Price[162] on the use of EMGBF for recovery of motor function in individuals with stroke. The authors found evidence from a number of small studies that indicate that EMGBF resulted in improvement in gait, function, and muscle power compared with the usual physiotherapy interventions. The authors emphasized limitations in the results because of the small amount of evidence and problems with methodological designs and differing outcome measures.

Traumatic Spinal Cord Injury (See Chapter 16)

NMES has a variety of applications for clients who have sustained SCI. Muscle strengthening may occur for muscles innervated by segments just above a complete SCI, or a variety of strengthening applications may be appropriate in the case of incomplete SCI. EMGBF may be used to identify muscle activity in weak musculature, as a tool to judge improvement in muscle activation, and as a method of facilitating increased strength.[163] Applications of EMGBF for individuals with SCI also include facilitation of unassisted ventilation in high-level quadriplegia[164] and use of biofeedback for muscle reeducation with incomplete SCI in the acute stages when immobilization may be required.[165]

The use of NMES, EMGBF, and other physical therapy was examined in a group of clients with incomplete cervical SCIs over a total treatment period of 16 weeks. Clients were randomly assigned to one of four groups receiving physical exercise, NMES, or EMGBF. Group 1 received EMGBF followed by physical exercise, group 2 received EMGBF followed by NMES, group 3 received NMES followed by physical exercise, and group 4 received 16 weeks of exercise only. Measurements of muscle strength, self-care ratings, mobility scores, and voluntary EMG were conducted at baseline, treatment midpoint, and conclusion of all interventions. All groups demonstrated improvement across the treatment period on all measures except voluntary EMG; however, no significant differences were seen among the four groups.[166] At least one other study compared conventional intervention, EMGBF, electrical stimulation, and combined stimulation with biofeedback over a 6-week period in individuals with quadriplegia. An examiner who was blinded to the intervention protocol evaluated 45 subjects in the four treatment groups. All groups improved in the parameters evaluated, and no significant difference among groups was noted.[167] These results again emphasize the need to consider carefully cost as well as time and effort for setup and equipment operation in intervention planning.

A study by Carvalho and colleagues[168] studied the use of treadmill gait training with NMES to improve bone mass in people with SCI. Their research study included 21 males with chronic quadriplegia between C4 to C8, randomly assigned to a control and treatment groups. Those in the treatment group received treadmill training with NMES, unweighting the body of 30% to 50% of body weight. The training was done for 20 minutes, twice a week for 6 months. Results showed that gait training with NMES, even with 30% to 50% unweighting, resulted in the improvement of bone mass in the subjects with chronic quadriplegia. In another study also by Carvalho,[169] NMES with partial body weight support resulted in hypertrophy of the quadriceps femoris muscle also in a population of subjects with quadriplegia. In both studies, NMES was helpful in producing stimulation that allowed for the subjects to advance their lower extremities while walking with body weight supported on the treadmill.

In a few studies, the application of NMES appears to be beneficial in improving impairments associated with SCI. Bittar and Cliquet[170] found that the use of NMES on the quadriceps and anterior tibialis of individuals with SCI was beneficial in that it allowed the feet and ankles to be placed in a better biomechanical position for ambulation. In addition, a study by de Abreu and colleagues[171] found improvements in the cross-sectional area of the quadriceps after NMES to these muscles.

In a study by De Biase[172] EMGBF training was noted to have resulted in increased EMG response of the rectus femoris muscle in 20 subjects with chronic SCI.

Upper-Extremity Management

The use of electrically stimulated hand orthotic systems for patients with C6 or higher level SCI have been refined to allow greater functional independence for a select group of patients.[87,96,97,115,173-175] Because hand function does not occur in a cyclical pattern, the onset and termination of stimulation must be controlled by the patient in some manner, with a myoelectric or contact closing switch.[96] Multichannel stimulation is then applied with intramuscular electrodes for the flexors and extensors of the fingers and thumb, with computer-configured interplay between the different muscles to achieve a functional grasp. A chest-mounted position transducer (operated by shoulder elevation or depression and protraction or retraction) allows the user to initiate stimulation and lock the stimulation to maintain a grasp as well as unlock it for release. A toggle switch mounted on the chest allows a choice between electronically stimulated lateral or palmar grasp patterns.[87,97] Some investigators have used contralateral shoulder slings as well as elbow accelerometers to trigger the needed stimulation.[176,177] Multiple authors have described successful implantation and use, with a few drawbacks, of upper-extremity FES prostheses.[178-181] Use of this type of system may allow patients with SCI at the C5 level to operate at the same level of independence (or even a higher level) as those with C6 quadriplegia with tenodesis, gaining the ability to perform more activities of daily living (ADLs) without an attendant. Patients with SCI at the C6 level may be able to manipulate a greater variety of objects without special adaptations.

Lower-Extremity Management

Standing. In an excellent review of the use of FES for the purpose of standing patients with SCI, Gardner and Baker[182] described the easiest approach to stimulating the quadriceps femoris to allow paraplegic clients to stand. More complex systems may incorporate stimulation of the gluteus maximus, gluteus medius, hamstring, adductor magnus, gastrocnemius, and soleus muscles for longer-duration and better-quality standing performance. Multichannel surface and implantable systems have been and continue to be developed for assistance in sit-stand and transfer activities.[183-185] Surgical procedures, client selection, and technology are also factors cited in successful interventions. Despite these efforts, the duration of standing with electrically stimulated systems ranges from a few minutes to several hours. The client with SCI may be able to use this technology to perform functional activities that require standing. The use of these systems depends on the functions unavailable to a client without use of the technology, and the ease with which a system can be used and maintained. Peripheral to, but no less important, are the reactions of joints to these interventions. Two studies[186,187] have reported positive benefits to the structure and functions of lower-extremity joints of adolescents with SCI after participating in FES programs. A recent study has also identified that the physiological responses to standing in SCI may provide a cardiorespiratory stress sufficient to meet minimal requirements for exercise conditioning.[100]

Cycling. The use of systems to stimulate reciprocal lower limb motions electrically has increased for stationary cycling. The benefits of these interventions for the client with SCI may relate to prevention of cardiovascular disease in the wheelchair-dependent client. Physiological changes noted with electrically stimulated cycling include improvement of peripheral muscular and cardiovascular fitness, as demonstrated by increased power output after training with leg cycle ergometry.[85,94,95,101,102] Combining FES and lower-extremity cycling with upper-extremity ergometry induced a higher level of cardiovascular fitness than lower-extremity ergometry alone.[188] Exercise session frequency as little as two times a week induced positive changes in cardiovascular fitness.[189] When testing of clients with paraplegia or quadriplegia is conducted with arm crank ergometry after a training program with electrically stimulated leg cycle ergometry, clients do not demonstrate differences in pretest and posttest measures of hemodynamic and pulmonary responses. These findings may relate to the specificity of the leg exercise training or the presence of a peripheral rather than a central circulatory response to the training procedure.[95] As previously noted, many cardiovascular factors can be improved and the improvements retained for at least 8 weeks after a program of FES ergometry.

Ambulation. As technology continues to progress, the use of electrically stimulated systems for ambulation may become more practical and useful for the patient with SCI.[98,190,191] Acceptance and use of the systems by clients outside the clinic have been mixed, but the systems have been shown to have positive effects on characteristics of ambulation.[149,192] Improvements in functional applications and use will also take place as the ability to select appropriate candidates improves.[193,194] Benefits of these systems may include increased muscle bulk, a reduced risk of pressure sores and osteoporosis, and psychological benefit. Generally, improvements in functional ability are expected to produce positive psychological factors. Addressing these factors directly, Bradley,[195] in a study measuring the effects of participation in an FES program on the affect of 37 individuals with SCI, demonstrated that positive affect was not significantly altered. Significant changes in negative affect occurred, however, with particular items of hostility and depression evident in those individuals in the treatment group who had unrealistic expectations. The author noted that these individuals need to be identified and monitored through the course of rehabilitation. Other drawbacks relate to the expense of the equipment and personnel and the lack of long-term efficacy studies. The speed with which a client with a complete SCI is able to walk with electrically stimulated systems remains relatively low (2 to 54 m/min) compared with normal rates of 78 to 90 m/min.[196,197] Many of the published reports do not provide information on the maximal distance patients are able to walk with these systems, but reported distances range from 100 to 400 m.

Some clients may perceive the technology of electrically stimulated standing and walking as moving them toward a cure for their paralysis. With a complete injury, however, the stimulation occurs passively, without expectation that voluntary control will return.[195] In cases of incomplete injury, electrically stimulated ambulation may assist the client in using and bolstering active control so that movement without the stimulation is more feasible. In considering use of electrically stimulated cycling and ambulation, discussion of the goals of treatment and the costs of the procedure must be conducted openly with the client to allow an educated choice to be made about the use of this expensive technology.

Traumatic Brain Injury (See Chapter 24)

NMES may be a useful tool with clients having sustained brain injury, with potential benefits of managing contractures by increasing ROM, facilitating active control, and reducing spasticity by strengthening the antagonist of a spastic muscle.[198] In cases in which an understanding of the purpose and principles of NMES is not feasible for a client, the comfort of the stimulation may be critical in ensuring its continued use. Comfort may be enhanced by increasing the ramp-on time and selecting waveforms that allow stimulation at lower amplitudes yet still obtain the desired contraction.[36] Use of NMES with a client at Rancho Level IV and below is not appropriate because the client may not be able to understand the purpose and meaning of the stimulus and thereby may perceive the stimulus as noxious.

EMGBF applications for clients with brain injury can be similar to those used with stroke, given similar motor presentations.[199] Therapists must consider residual cognitive deficits after brain injury in determining the appropriateness of EMGBF.

Guillain-Barré Syndrome (See Chapter 17)

EMGBF in clients with Guillain-Barré syndrome demonstrated improvements in muscle strength in upper and lower extremities, although inconsistent improvement in functional use of the upper extremities was noted.[200,201] Treatment regimens consisted of EMGBF for 10 trials per muscle conducted in 45-minute treatment sessions twice a week, in one case for 78 weeks and in the other case for 46 weeks.[201]

Multiple Sclerosis (See Chapter 19)

In a case series, Wahls and colleagues[202] found improvements in ambulation of patients with primary or secondary progressive multiple sclerosis. The authors cited the possible positive effects of NMES application on muscle spasm, muscle pain, and disuse atrophy as possible reasons behind the improvements in ambulatory function in their subjects.

Pediatric Applications

Special considerations for pediatric clients need to be understood when addressing the use of electricity. Although contraindications and precautions are the same as for adults, acceptance and tolerance of these devices are not. Fear and apprehension of electricity, for both child and parent, must be addressed. The clinician must take extra care in explanation and demonstration, perhaps on themselves and possibly the parent, before placing the device on the child. Allowing the child as much control as possible in device operation may assist with acceptance. Of course, the attention span of the child must also be addressed.

Cerebral Palsy (See Chapter 12)

The use of NMES with children with cerebral palsy has been addressed to some degree, with several case study reports.[203-205] Carmick[203,204] described a variety of applications with children at 1.6, 6.7, and 10 years of age, integrating NMES into a treatment regimen that focused on a "task-oriented model of motor learning." Improvements were noted in upper- and lower-extremity movement and functional use across a variety of tasks appropriate to the age and the movement dysfunction each child demonstrated. In a study by Nunes and colleagues,[206] the once-a-week application of NMES on the tibialis anterior muscle of 10 children with spastic hemiplegia resulted in improvements in gross motor function, passive ROM of ankle dorsiflexion, and muscle strength.

Ozer and collegues[207] studied the effect of using NMES combined with dynamic bracing and found the intervention to be more effective than either alone in reducing upper-extremity spasticity in their sample of children with spastic hemiplegic cerebral palsy. A similar study by Postans and colleagues[208] found that NMES combined with dynamic splinting reduced upper-limb contractures in children with cerebral palsy. In another study,[209] the application of NMES to the gluteus medius improved gait parameters in children with spastic diplegia.

Advancements in technology have allowed the use of EMGBF in increasing contexts, such as the computer-assisted feedback (CAF) system, which can be used to provide feedback about muscle activity during ambulation.[210] Data examining use of this system to provide feedback about the level of triceps surae activity during gait of children with cerebral palsy suggest potential improvements in gait symmetry, velocity, and appropriate muscle activation patterns as a result of this intervention. Use of this modality as an adjunct to physical therapy may prove beneficial.

Spina Bifida (See Chapter 15)

Five subjects with spina bifida (aged 5 to 21 years) were treated with daily NMES over an 8-week period to strengthen the quadriceps femoris muscles. Increases in maximal quadriceps torque production were observed in two of the five subjects in the treated limb. Improvements in functional activity speeds were noted for all of the subjects. Lack of improvement in torque production by three subjects was speculated to be related to lack of adherence to the exercise regimen and the heterogeneity of the subject sample.[211]

Spinal Muscular Atrophy (See Chapter 13)

One study has reported the use of low-intensity electrical stimulation in children with types II and III spinal muscular atrophy in an attempt to determine any effect on arm strength and function. After 6 to 12 months of stimulation no statistically significant differences were noted between experimental and placebo-control arms in strength, muscle mass, or function.[212]

Scoliosis

Axelgaard and Brown[84] demonstrated in the 1970s that surface NMES could reduce idiopathic scoliosis. Criteria for this treatment required curves measuring 20 to 45 degrees by the Cobb method, at least 1 year of growth remaining, idiopathic and progressive nature of the curve, cooperative and psychologically stable and compliant patient, and tolerance of the stimulation. Electrodes were placed laterally over the midaxillary line on the convex side. A paraspinous location on the convex side was sometimes used. Settings included a pulse duration of 220 μs, frequency of 25 pps, and an on-off ratio of 6 seconds on and 6 seconds off. The treatment time was gradually increased to 8 hours of stimulation per day (the stimulation was typically done at night if tolerated). High success and low dropout rates were reported.[213] Others, however, reported much lower success rates.[214] Intolerance of the treatment resulting in low compliance may be the cause of these differences. This disorder is much more common in adolescent girls. When NMES first was introduced for scoliosis, the uncomfortable and cosmetically undesirable Milwaukee brace was still the norm for treatment. With more advanced materials and orthotic management that is much more acceptable cosmetically, the use of NMES in scoliosis management has significantly declined.

Contraindications and Precautions

Any electrical stimulation application is contraindicated for clients who have epilepsy or demand-type pacemakers. In addition, contraindications exist to applications over the transthoracic area or the uterus in pregnancy as well as in a cancerous area and the carotid sinus. Other factors require precaution but are not strict contraindications, such as sensory deficits, skin problems (sensitivity to stimulation, electrodes, or gel; edema; open wounds), tolerance of stimulation intensity sufficient to elicit muscle contraction, client's capability to participate in the training process, and financial considerations.[56-58,215]

Matthews and colleagues[216] reported changes in blood pressure and heart rate suggestive of autonomic hyperreflexia when electrical stimulation was applied in seven subjects with SCI above the T6 level. FES to the quadriceps produced the noted changes as stimulation intensity was increased. The mechanism for this reaction is unclear. Clinicians should monitor vital signs in clients with SCI (and possibly all clients), at least during the initial application of electrical stimulation.

Use of stimulation modalities by clients outside clinical therapy sessions requires a degree of cooperation and motivation to take care of the stimulation unit, use it as instructed, and observe precautions. Long-term use of NMES (e.g., FES) may not be feasible for clients who do not have the financial resources (insurance or otherwise) to rent or purchase a unit or do not have reasonable access to support for equipment maintenance.

EMGBF does not require as many precautions because the procedure only monitors muscle activity. This form of feedback by the client requires a basic level of attention and cognitive skill to understand the meaning of, as well as act on, the feedback to change muscle performance. Client motivation and interest in use of this modality are also required because the client must be able to develop sensitivity to the degree of muscle activation independently so that feedback is no longer required. EMGBF may be used in some instances that do not require the cognitive skills of the client to use this information, such as an evaluative tool for the therapist to gather information about muscle activation to plan intervention strategies.

SUMMARY

The concepts, descriptions, and applications of electrodiagnosis presented in this chapter are intended to enrich the therapist's comprehension of these studies as applied to clients with neurological conditions. Integration of the results of these tests in differential diagnosis and in subsequent planning of intervention is invaluable.

Clearly the use of NMES and EMGBF has numerous possibilities with clients of all ages who have sustained neurological insult or injury. Improvement of motor control has been supported in some applications, although well controlled group research in populations other than stroke and adult SCI is lacking. This underscores the need for further investigation to support the evidence for these modalities. As the therapy environment continues to change in response to time and funding constraints, therapists must carefully evaluate the benefits of a variety of available tools to assist their clients in regaining motor control and functional ability. A benefit of FES or EMGBF is the ability of the client to work autonomously (i.e., at home) after becoming familiar with the treatment regimen, with the therapist periodically updating a home program. This protocol allows physical and occupational therapy time to be used for direct intervention. NMES and EMGBF may efficiently assist in attaining improvement in control, and may also be used in the context of functional activities, but these tools alone will not create functional changes. The case studies that follow further integrate these concepts in actual cases.

CASE STUDIES

Part 1: Electrodiagnosis

The following are cases studies from patients seen in the electrophysiology lab. The reader will receive the full benefit of studying the cases by first reading the evaluation and establishing a set of differential possible diagnoses and dysfunctions of the nervous system. The reader can then progress through the report, test by test and challenge the differential diagnoses. The conclusion of the study is provided. NOTE: Please refer to Appendix 33-A for a key to all the abbreviations found in the figures and tables used in the Case Studies.

CASE STUDY 33-1

The patient is a right-handed 55-year-old general contractor. He reports that 3 months prior, he purchased an exercise cycle which he started using quite vehemently. Following this bout of exercise, he started noticing muscle soreness in his hamstrings and right calf. He now reports fatigue and twitching of the muscles in both shoulders and right leg. He also has an achy back in the middle of his thoracic spine. There is no numbness. He does not have any particular stressors except for the decrease in business brought about by the change in the economy. He never lost control of his sphincters. His thinking is clear.

Prior medical history is significant only for skin cancers which were excised from his back last year and a meniscal tear. He has no known allergies and is lactose intolerant. On questioning, the patient does report hunting and eating the game he kills but has no other exposure to heavy metals.

Physical examination shows that walks unassisted but has a slight foot drop on the right side. From an orthopedic standpoint there is some crepitus with mobilization of the left shoulder; otherwise, ROM is full, including in the cervical spine. There is no Lhermitte sign. Inspection shows significant fasciculations in the right quadriceps and both upper arms; a mild facial asymmetry from a previously fractured upper maxilla on the left side; easily palpated dorsalis pedis pulse on both sides; and mild atrophy of the right calf, which is 1.5 cm smaller than that of the left side. Grip strength is 80 lb on the right side and 60 lb on the left side. MMT reveals a decrease in the strength of the extensor and flexor hallucis longus on the right side, 3+/5 (4/5 on the left side); right tibialis anterior, 3/5 (4/5 on the left side); right to gastrocnemius, 3−/5; right quadriceps, 4−/5; and intrinsic muscles, 4/5 on both sides. The patient fully detects the 3.61 Semmes-Weinstein monofilament in the lower extremities and the 2.83 monofilament in the upper extremities, which is normal. Muscle stretch reflexes are 2+ in the upper extremities and 1+ in the lower extremities; there is no Hoffmann sign in either hand; plantar cutaneous reflex is equivocal; cranial nerve scan is normal including extraocular movements. Speech is normal.

SUMMARY OF NERVE CONDUCTION FINDINGS

Motor distal latencies are normal in all nerves tested. Conduction velocities in all segments are normal. Amplitudes of the responses are slightly decreased or at the lower limit of normal. Sensory distal latencies, amplitudes, and conduction velocities are all within normal limits.

F-wave latencies are slightly delayed in the right peroneal and tibial nerves and normal in the left peroneal and right median nerves.

H-reflex latencies are delayed on both sides.

SUMMARY OF ELECTROMYOGRAPHIC FINDINGS

Insertional activity was increased in the right vastus medialis, tibialis anterior, gastrocnemius, extensor feature brevis, and left tibialis anterior. Fasciculations were found in the right deltoid, triceps, first dorsal interosseous, vastus medialis, and extensor digitorum brevis, as well as in the left gastrocnemius and thoracic paraspinals. Denervation potentials were found in every muscle sampled (including the tongue) except the right biceps. Analysis of the MUAPs showed them to be polyphasic in the first dorsal interosseous of the right hand, right tibialis anterior, right gastrocnemius, left extensor digitorum brevis, and left tibialis anterior. Recruitment pattern was reduced in the right biceps and in the tibialis anterior, gastrocnemius, and extensor digitorum brevis on both sides. Firing rate of the MUAPs was fast in the extensor digitorum brevis on both sides as well as in the right gastrocnemius and tibialis anterior. Refer to Tables 33-2 to 33-6, and Figures 33-7 and 33-8 for a summary of various nerve conduction studies performed on this patient.

CONCLUSIONS

The results of this study are abnormal. Findings include normal sensory distal latencies, nerve conduction, and amplitudes; normal motor distal latencies and nerve conduction, slightly reduced amplitudes; widespread denervation potentials in three limbs, paraspinals, and the tongue; fasciculations. This is consistent with an acquired motor neuron disorder.

Based on this study, laboratory tests, and the physical examination, the referring neurologist diagnosed patient 1 with ALS.

PROGNOSIS

Poor.

INTERVENTIONS

The patient was issued ankle-foot orthoses, first on the right side, then the left. He later required a walker, then a powered wheelchair and CPAP. He died 12 months after this study.

TABLE 33-2 ■ MOTOR NERVE CONDUCTION STUDY

NERVE/SITES	REC SITE	LAT MSEC	AMP 1-2 MV	DISTANCE CM	VEL M/S	TEMP °C	AMPL %
R MEDIAN—APB							
Wrist	APB	3.80	4.7	8		30.9	100
Elbow		7.80	4.1	23	57.5	30.8	87.1
Axilla		9.30	3.4	10	66.7	30.9	71.9
L COMM PERONEAL—EDB							
Ankle	EDB	4.55	2.6	8		31.1	100
Fib Head		11.35	1.7	31	45.6	30.9	64.4
Knee		13.30	1.6	9	46.2	30.8	60.8

Continued

TABLE 33-2 ■ MOTOR NERVE CONDUCTION STUDY—cont'd

NERVE/SITES	REC SITE	LAT MSEC	AMP 1-2 MV	DISTANCE CM	VEL M/S	TEMP °C	AMPL %
R COMM PERONEAL—EDB							
Ankle	EDB	5.40	2.8	8		31.3	100
Fib Head		12.35	2.4	29	41.7	31	85.3
Knee		14.65	2.7	10	43.5	30.9	95.4
R TIBIAL (KNEE)—FHB							
Bel. Ankle	FHB	5.85	1.8	8		30.5	100
Ab. Ankle		8.25	1.9	10	41.7	30.5	106
Knee		17.55	1.3	38	40.9	30.4	73.9

TABLE 33-3 ■ SENSORY NERVE CONDUCTION STUDY

NERVE/SITES	REC SITE	LAT 2 MSEC	AMP PK-PK μV	VEL PK M/S	DISTANCE CM	TEMP °C
R RADIAL—VS MEDIAN—THUMB						
Forearm (Radial)	Thumb	2.70	6.8	44.4	12	32.3
Wrist (Median)	Thumb	3.40	14.7	35.3	12	32.4
L SURAL—LAT MALLEOLUS						
Calf	Lat Malleolus	3.20	2.9	37.5	12	30.5
Calf	Lat Malleolus	3.35	0.42	35.8	12	30.5
R SURAL—LAT MALLEOLUS						
Calf	Lat Malleolus	3.60	0.29	33.3	12	31.1
Calf	Lat Malleolus	3.70	0.17	32.4	12	31.1

TABLE 33-4 ■ F-WAVE STUDY

NERVE	MIN F LAT MS	MAX F LAT MSEC	MIN F AMP MV	MAX F AMP MV	MIN F-M MSEC	MAX F-M MSEC
L COMM PERONEAL—EDB	52.05	56.85	0.10	0.17	46.30	51.15
R COMM PERONEAL—EDB	54.50	56.55	0.16	0.27	48.60	50.70
R TIBIAL (KNEE)—FHB	58.10	64.90	0.00	0.04	50.10	56.85
R MEDIAN—APB	27.65	61.65	0.05	0.15	23.75	57.70

TABLE 33-5 ■ H-REFLEX STUDY

NERVE	RESP. NO MAX M	RESP. NO MAX H	H LAT MSEC	H AMP MV	H/M AMPL %
L TIBIAL—Gastrocnemius	11	9	34.20	0.3	3.54%
R TIBIAL—Gastrocnemius	21	22	35.30	0.4	9.94%

TABLE 33-6 ■ EMG SUMMARY TABLE

	SPONTANEOUS				MUAP			RECRUITMENT	
	IA	FIB	PSW	FASC	AMP	DUR	POLYPH	PATTERN	FIRE RATE
R. TONGUE	N	2+	None	None	N	N	N	N	N
R. DELTOID	N	1+	None	1+	N	N	N	N	N
R. BICEPS	N	None	None	None	N	N	N	Reduced	N
R. TRICEPS	N	1+	1+	1+	N	N	N	N	N
R. EXT DIG COMM	N	2+	1+	None	N	N	N	N	N
R. FIRST D INTEROSS	N	1+	2+	1+	1+	N	1+	N	N
R. VAST MEDIALIS	1+	1+	2+	1+	N	N	N	N	N
R. TIB ANTERIOR	2+	2+	2+	None	N	N	1+	Discrete	Fast
R. GASTROCN (MED)	2+	1+	3+	None	N	N	2+	Reduced	Fast
R. EXT DIG BREVIS	1+	2+	2+	1+	N	N	N	Reduced	Fast
L. EXT DIG BREVIS	N	2+	None	None	2+	N	2+	Reduced	Fast
L. GASTROCN (MED)	N	1+	2+	1+	N	N	N	Reduced	N
L. TIB ANTERIOR	2+	2+	2+	None	N	N	3+	Reduced	N
L. VAST MEDIALIS	N	1+	1+	None	N	N	N	N	N
R. THOR PSP (M)	N	1+	1+	1+	N	N	N	N	N
R. LUMB PSP (M)	N	1+	None	None	N	N	N	N	N

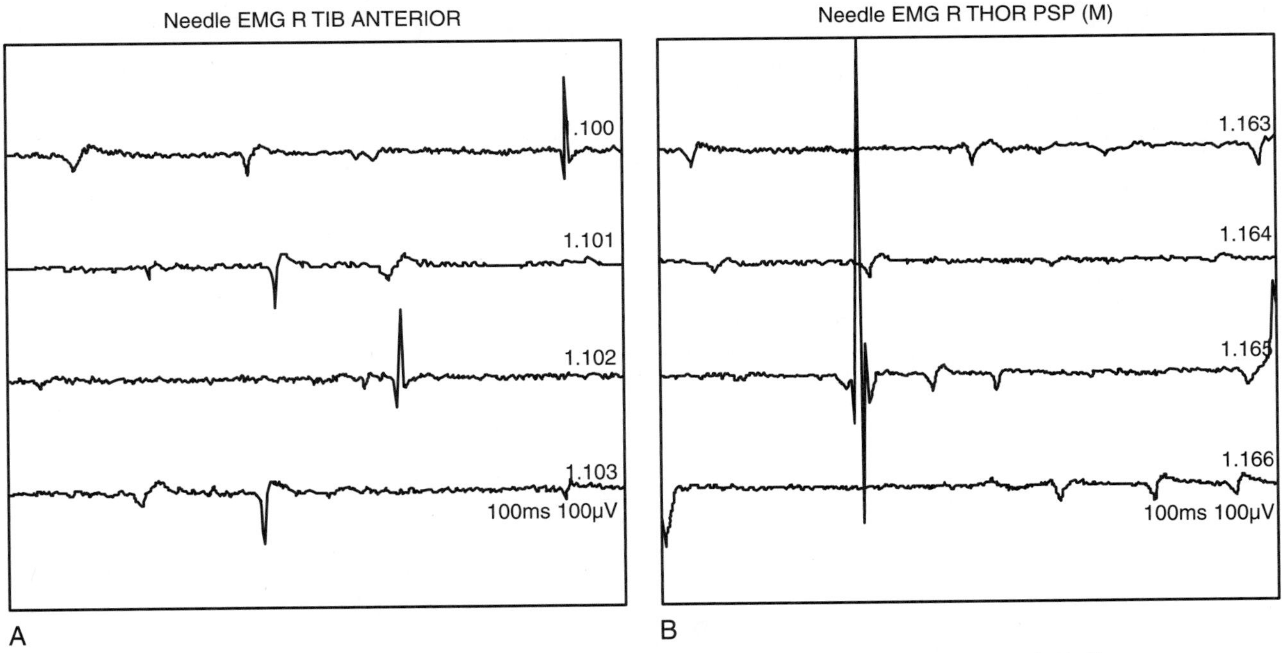

Figure 33-8 ■ Needle electromyography. **A,** Positive sharp waves and fibrillation potentials. **B,** One fasciculation and positive sharp waves.

CASE STUDY 33-2

The patient is a right-handed, 49-year-old administrative assistant. She reports a 1-year history of numbness in the right hand. Initially, this numbness was present only intermittently. The numbness involves mostly the thumb and index and long fingers. Recently the numbness has been present every morning. This impairs her ability to sleep. The patient also reports difficulty with writing. She has a positive flick sign. Finally, she reports that ibuprofen has been of some help in the sense that she no longer wakes up in the middle of the night. She has no numbness in her toes. There are no complaints regarding her cervical spine.

Prior medical history is essentially unremarkable and includes only uterine fibroids. The patient has had a hysterectomy. There are no known allergies.

Physical examination shows that the patient walks unassisted with a normal gait pattern. Inspection shows slight

Continued

CASE STUDY 33-2—cont'd

arthritic changes at the base of the right thumb but no noticeable muscle atrophy in the intrinsic muscles or thenar eminence. Grip strength is 45 lb on the left side and 55 lb on the right side. Sensation is slightly decreased: the patient detects the 3.61 Semmes-Weinstein monofilament at the tip of the fingers of the right hand. Result of the Phalen test is positive, and the reverse Phalen test causes wrist pain; the Finkelstein test also causes wrist pain. "Okay" sign is normal. Cervical ROM is full in all directions; result of the Spurling test is negative. Muscle stretch reflexes are 2+ and symmetrical. Cranial nerve scan is normal.

Based on this physical examination, what is your clinical impression?

SUMMARY OF NERVE CONDUCTION FINDINGS

The median motor distal latency is prolonged compared with the ipsilateral ulnar motor distal latency (2.05 ms difference). Amplitudes of the median motor responses are decreased. The ulnar motor distal latency, amplitudes, and conduction velocities are within normal limits.

The median sensory distal latencies are significantly delayed. Radial and ulnar sensory distal latencies are normal. The combined sensory index (CSI) is 7.1 (cutoff value for normal conduction for the CSI is 1.3).

Median F-wave latencies are at the upper limit of normal for a patient this height. Ulnar F-wave latencies are normal.

SUMMARY OF ELECTROMYOGRAPHIC FINDINGS

Insertional activity was normal in all muscles sampled. A few denervation potentials were found at rest in the abductor pollicis brevis (fibrillation potentials). Analysis of the MUAPs showed them to be of normal configuration, phases, and recruitment in all muscles tested except in the abductor pollicis brevis. In this muscle, motor units were slightly polyphasic. Refer to Figure 33-9, and to Tables 33-7 to 33-10 for a summary of various nerve conduction studies performed on this patient.

CONCLUSIONS

This study is abnormal. Findings are consistent with a moderate to severe mononeuropathic process involving the right median nerve at or distal to the wrist. This is evidenced by delayed median motor and sensory distal latencies, decreased amplitudes of the median motor responses, and abnormal electromyographic findings in the abductor pollicis brevis only.

Because the ipsilateral ulnar motor and ulnar and radial sensory NCS findings are normal and because the needle EMG findings are limited to the abductor pollicis brevis, a polyneuropathic, plexopathic, or a radiculopathic process is unlikely in the right upper extremity.

PROGNOSIS

Excellent. The patient and her surgeon elected to go ahead with a carpal tunnel release.

INTERVENTIONS

The patient started rehabilitation after surgery and went on to a full recovery in 2 months.

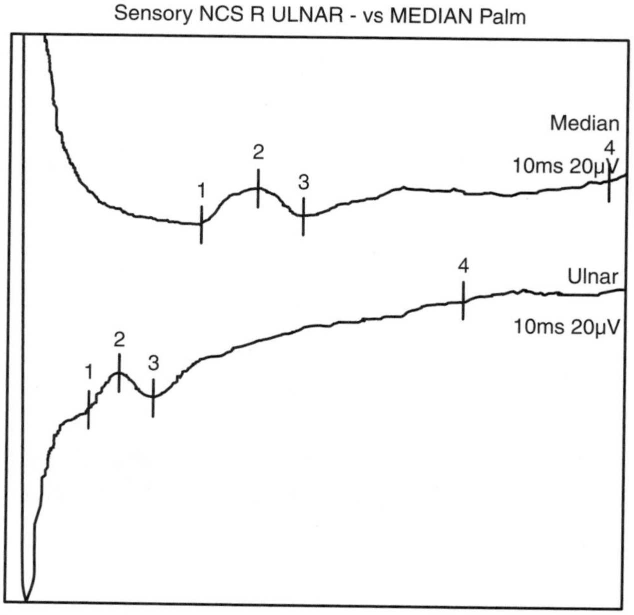

Figure 33-9 ■ Sensory nerve action potential (SNAP) difference: median *(above)* and ulnar *(below)*.

TABLE 33-7 ■ MOTOR NERVE CONDUCTION STUDY

NERVE/SITES	REC SITE	LAT MSEC	AMP 1-2 MV	DISTANCE CM	VEL M/S	TEMP °C	AMPL %
R MEDIAN—APB							
Wrist	APB	5.55	3.9	8		32.8	100
Elbow		9.60	3.8	21	51.9	32.7	97.4
Axilla		11.00	4.6	9	64.3	32.7	117
R ULNAR—ADM							
Wrist	ADM	2.50	9.1	8		32.3	100
B. Elbow		6.15	8.0	21	57.5	32.3	88
A. Elbow		7.80	7.7	9	54.5	32.3	84.9

TABLE 33-8 ■ SENSORY NERVE CONDUCTION STUDY

NERVE/SITES	REC SITE	LAT 2 MSEC	AMP PK-PK MV	VEL PK M/S	DISTANCE CM	TEMP °C
R RADIAL—VS MEDIAN—THUMB						
Forearm (Radial)	Thumb	2.85	8.3	42.1	12	33.6
Wrist (Median)	Thumb	4.75	15.3	25.3	12	33.8
R ULNAR—VS MEDIAN DIG IV						
Median	IV	6.10	8.5	23.0	14	33.6
Ulnar	IV	3.05	13.6	45.9	14	33.6
R ULNAR—VS MEDIAN PALM						
Med Palm	Wrist	4.10	10.4	19.5	8	33.2
Uln Palm	Wrist	1.90	8.7	42.1	8	33.2

TABLE 33-9 ■ F-WAVE STUDY

NERVE	MIN F LAT MSEC	MAX F LAT MSEC	MIN F AMP MV	MAX F AMP MV	MIN F-M MSEC	MAX F-M MSEC
R MEDIAN—APB	28.95	32.25	0.00	0.15	23.55	26.75
R ULNAR—ADM	25.10	27.65	0.07	0.29	22.50	25.05

TABLE 33-10 ■ EMG SUMMARY TABLE

	SPONTANEOUS				MUAP			RECRUITMENT	
	IA	FIB	PSW	FASC	AMP	DUR	POLYPH	PATTERN	FIRE RATE
R. DELTOID	N	None	None	None	N	N	N	N	N
R. TRICEPS	N	None	None	None	N	N	N	N	N
R. EXT DIG COMM	N	None	None	None	N	N	N	N	N
R. FLEX CARPI RAD	N	None	None	None	N	N	N	N	N
R. 1st D INTEROSS	N	None	None	None	N	N	N	N	N
R. ABD POLL BREVIS	N	1+	None	None	N	N	1+	N	N
R. CERV PSP (L)	N	None	None	None	N	N	N	N	N

CASE STUDY 33-3

The patient is a right-handed, 86-year-old retired internist. He consults today for assessment of the strength in his lower extremities and numbness in his right hand. He reports having difficulty going up the 13 steps he has at home and states that his right thumb and index and middle fingers feel like "Band-Aids are on too tight at the tip of the fingers."

Prior medical history includes Waldenström macroglobulinemia, gastrectomy for recurrent bleeding, 7+ years of taking amiodarone, hypothyroid.

Physical examination shows that the patient walks with a bilateral foot drop and increased base of support. MMT shows decrease in the strength of ankle dorsiflexors on both sides, noted 3+/5; right quadriceps, 4/5; foot intrinsic muscles, 3/5; hand intrinsic muscles, 3+/5; right triceps muscle, 3+/5. All other muscles groups have normal strength. Grip strength is 30 lb on the right side and 35 lb on the left side. Sensation is decreased to the 3.61 Semmes-Weinstein monofilament at the sole of the right foot; the patient detects the 4.31 filament. It is also decreased to the 2.83 monofilament at the palm of the right hand; the patient detects the 3.61 filament. ROM of the left shoulder is impaired in abduction. Cervical ROM is within normal limits. Spurling's test is negative. Toes are down-going with the plantar cutaneous reflex; there is no Hoffmann sign in the hands. Muscle stretch reflexes are 2+ in the quadriceps and upper extremities, 1+ at the ankle. Cranial nerve scan is normal. Romberg sign is positive. Refer to Figure 33-10, and Tables 33-11 to 33-15 for a summary of various nerve conduction studies performed on this patient.

CONCLUSIONS

The study findings are abnormal. Findings are consistent with an axonal loss, mixed sensorimotor polyneuropathic process. This is evidenced by normal motor and sensory distal latencies, absent or significantly reduced amplitudes in both motor and sensory responses, delayed F-wave and H-reflex latencies, denervation in the distal more than the proximal muscles, and no findings in the lumbar paraspinals.

PROGNOSIS

Fair to good. Improvement expected over the next 4 to 6 months with medical management of the polyneuropathy.

INTERVENTIONS

The patient started balance rehabilitation and muscle strengthening and ultimately met his goal of safely climbing up and down his stairs.

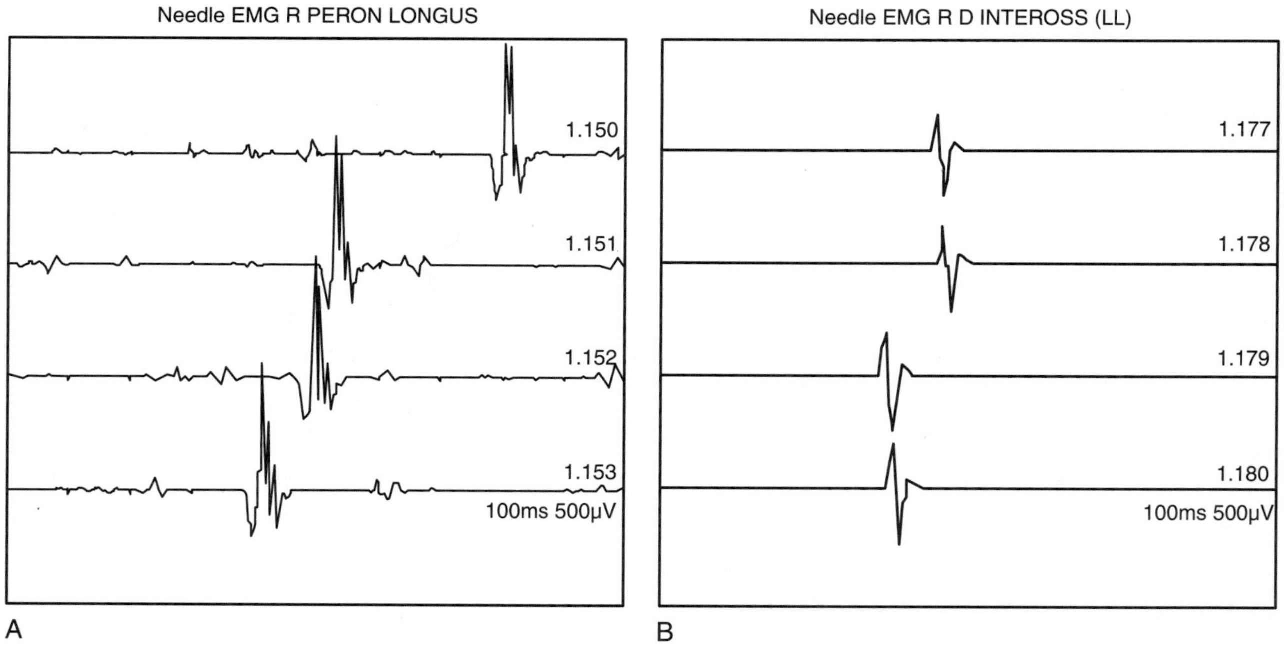

Figure 33-10 ■ Needle electromyography. **A,** Polyphasic motor unit action potentials (MUAPs) in the right peroneus longus. **B,** Essentially one MUAP in the foot dorsal interossei.

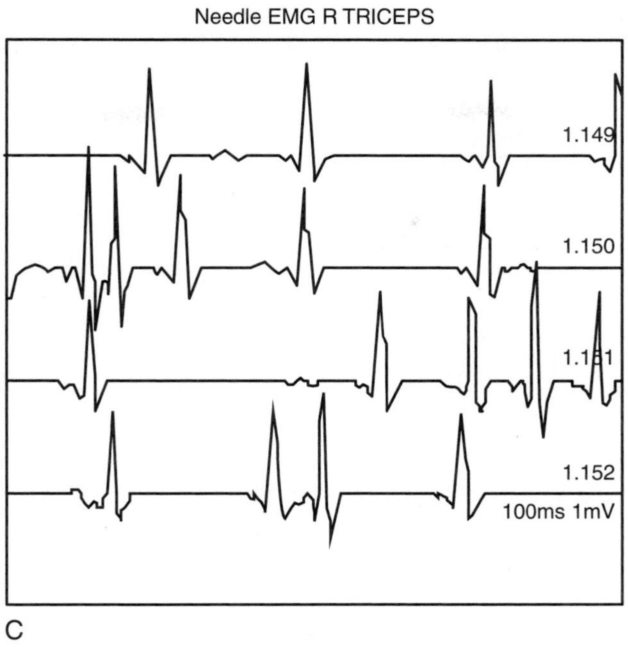

Figure 33-10, cont'd ■ **C,** Fast firing MUAPs.

TABLE 33-11 ■ MOTOR NERVE CONDUCTION STUDY

NERVE/SITES	RESP	REC SITE	LAT MSEC	AMP 1-2 MV	DISTANCE CM	VEL M/S	TEMP °C	AMPL %
R MEDIAN—APB								
Wrist		APB	3.75	3.1	8		33.8	100
Elbow			8.75	1.8	25.5	51.0	34	57.7
Axilla			10.65	1.3	10	52.6	34.3	43.2
R ULNAR—ADM								
Wrist		ADM	3.00	6.2	8		33.9	100
B. Elbow			7.05	6.6	20	49.4	33.5	106
A. Elbow			9.25	5.5	10	45.5	32.4	87.9
R COMM PERONEAL —EDB								
Ankle	No	EDB	NR	NR			31.9	
R TIBIAL (KNEE)—FHB								
Bel. Ankle		FHB	5.35	0.7	8		31.1	100
Ab. Ankle			7.80	0.5	10	40.8	31.1	78.4
Knee			18.20	0.5	32	30.8	31.1	66.4
R COMM PERONEAL —TIB ANT								
Fib Head		Tib Ant	2.95	**0.7**	8		31.3	100
Knee			5.20	**0.7**	10	44.4	30.9	102

TABLE 33-12 ■ SENSORY NERVE CONDUCTION STUDY

NERVE/SITES	REC SITE	LAT 2 MSEC	AMP PK-PK MV	VEL PK M/S	DISTANCE CM	TEMP °C
R RADIAL—VS MEDIAN—THUMB						
Forearm (Radial)	Thumb	3.50	1.3	34.3	12	32.1
Wrist (Median)	Thumb	3.75	8.5	32.0	12	32
R ULNAR—VS MEDIAN—DIG IV						
Median	IV	4.25	2.0	32.9	14	32.8
Ulnar	IV	5.80	2.3	24.1	14	32.5
R SURAL—LAT MALLEOLUS						
Calf	Lat Malleolus	3.70	0.46	32.4	12	31.6
Calf	Lat Malleolus	4.05	0.79	29.6	12	31.6

TABLE 33-13 ■ F-WAVE STUDY

NERVE	MIN F LAT MSEC	MAX F LAT MSEC	MIN F AMP MV	MAX F AMP MV	MIN F-M MSEC	MAX F-M MSEC
R TIBIAL (KNEE)—FHB	60.35	65.30	0.01	0.03	4.35	55.40
R MEDIAN—APB	31.25	82.10	0.04	0.26	27.30	78.10
R ULNAR—ADM	35.25	74.45	0.03	0.29	32.00	71.10

TABLE 33-14 ■ H-REFLEX STUDY

NERVE	RESP. NO MAX M	RESP. NO MAX H	H LAT MSEC	H AMP MV	H/M AMPL %
R TIBIAL—Gastrocnemius	13	11	33.50	1.1	102%
L TIBIAL—Gastrocnemius	14	14	35.20	0.6	37.2%

TABLE 33-15 ■ EMG SUMMARY TABLE

	SPONTANEOUS				MUAP			RECRUITMENT	
	IA	FIB	PSW	FASC	AMP	DUR	POLYPH	PATTERN	FIRE RATE
R. VAST MEDIALIS	N	None	None	None	N	N	N	N	N
R. DELTOID	N	None	None	None	N	N	N	N	N
R. TIB ANTERIOR	N	None	None	None	N	N	2+	Reduced	Fast
R. PERON LONGUS	N	None	None	None	N	N	3+	Reduced	Fast
R. GASTROCN (MED)	N	None	1+	None	N	N	1+	Reduced	Fast
R. EXT DIG BREVIS	-	None	None	None	-	-	-	No activity	-
R. D INTEROSS (LL)	N	1+	None	None	N	N	N	Discrete	N
R. TRICEPS	N	3+	3+	None	N	N	N	Reduced	Fast
R. EXT DIG COMM	N	1+	1+	None	N	N	N	Reduced	N
R. FIRST D INTEROSS	N	1+	2+	None	N	N	N	Reduced	N
R. LUMB PSP (L)	N	None	None	None	N	N	N	N	N

Part 2: Neuromuscular Electrical Stimulation and Electromyographic Biofeedback

CASE STUDY 33-4

A 68-year-old woman is referred 3 weeks after left middle cerebral artery CVA with residual right hemiparesis affecting the upper extremity to a greater degree than the lower extremity. The client's left extremities appear well controlled with at least functional strength. She exhibits a two-fingerbreadth right shoulder subluxation, with pain at the extremes of shoulder flexion (150 degrees), abduction (135 degrees), and external rotation (30 degrees), and hypertonicity in a stereotypical flexor synergy pattern affecting the shoulder horizontal adductors and internal rotators and elbow, wrist, and finger flexors. She is beginning to develop upper-extremity movement with the ability to shrug her shoulder, abduct, and flex through partial range (with elbow flexed), full-range elbow flexion, partial-range elbow extension against gravity, and no wrist or finger extension. Right lower-extremity ROM is within normal limits, although control is limited at the ankle (dorsiflexion only with hip and knee flexion, no eversion actively) and knee control is decreased (reduced eccentric quadriceps control, difficulty isolating knee flexion with hip extension). Ambulation is accomplished with the use of a quad cane and an articulating AFO on the right for limited distances with standby assistance. This client lives at home with her husband, who is very supportive of her rehabilitation. Both of them are retired, but they have an active calendar of participation in volunteer and leisure activities. Insurance coverage is good.

PROGNOSIS

Independent or isolated motor function is promising for continued improvement in the condition of the client. Lower-extremity impairments are expected to be minimized as the return of motor control progresses. Quad cane use should continue until isolated hip and knee action improves. A need for AFO is expected for an indefinite time period.

INTERVENTION

Interventions including EMG or NMES would assist in accelerating improvement in functional control. Table 33-16 provides the various intervention options using NMES-EMGBF for this patient.

TABLE 33-16 ■ NMES/EMGBF OPTIONS

CLIENT PROBLEM	GOALS	MODALITY PARAMETERS	MEASURES TO DETERMINE EFFICACY	CONSIDERATIONS
Shoulder subluxation	Decrease subluxation to 1 fingerwidth, with pain manageable within patient's daily routine.	Portable FES for home use, begin with 10:30 second on-off ratio for 15-minute periods tid, amplitude to generate muscle contraction without shoulder elevation. Increase on time and treatment time as tolerated so that reduction is maintained majority of day.	Trial use for 1 month. Measure amount of palpable subluxation, pain-free ROM; if improvement is not observed, discontinue FES, with instruction to maintain shoulder flexibility, consider lapboard or arm tray when sitting, support when standing.	1. Requires rental of portable FES unit; patient/family compliance is needed for success in home program. 2. Cost of rental of FES and supplies. 3. Frequent use for reduction of subluxation requires close monitoring of skin for possible reactions to stimulation, gel, or electrodes. 4. Integrate scapular movement and stabilization exercises into program
Lack of active ankle dorsiflexion	Increase active control of ankle dorsiflexion with knee extended, allowing heel-strike without AFO for short-distance ambulation.	FES twice daily for 15-minute duration; 10:20 second on-off ratio with slow ramping on-off; as active movement improves, consider EMGBF to further focus attention on balanced dorsiflexion (with eversion). Use of heelswitch requires decreased ramp time to minimum patient can tolerate. Switch should activate at heel-off to control dorsiflexion through the swing phase.	Monitor each session for increased active dorsiflexion in sitting, standing, and ambulation. Integrate use of heelswitch during ambulation without AFO. Trial use over 2 to 3 weeks. Discontinue if not seeing increase in voluntary control; compensate with AFO.	1. If client rents unit for shoulder subluxation, may also use stimulator at home instead of requiring time during therapy session. 2. Similar cost, convenience issues as above. 3. Additional education necessary if stimulator settings are to be switched for dorsiflexion and shoulder subluxation interventions.

Continued

TABLE 33-16 ■ NMES/EMGBF OPTIONS—cont'd

CLIENT PROBLEM	GOALS	MODALITY PARAMETERS	MEASURES TO DETERMINE EFFICACY	CONSIDERATIONS
Lack of full active wrist and finger extension	Control of active wrist and finger extension to allow release in gross grasp.	NMES and/or EMGBF twice a day for 10-minute sessions initially, with gradual increase in duration up to 20 minutes if fatigue does not alter the quality of the contractions. Other parameters as described for ankle dorsiflexion.	Trial period of 2 to 3 weeks; discontinue if voluntary motion is not changing significantly. Active movement in finger extensors with wrist in neutral position. Functional ability to release grasp of objects of varying shapes and sizes.	May use portable stimulator as described for ankle or shoulder interventions, with similar considerations.
Muscle imbalance, lack of right upper-extremity functional movement	Decrease hypertonicity in flexor muscle groups; increase extensor control for gross arm movements (e.g., positioning).	EMGBF to decrease flexor muscle activity (resting and with passive movement) and increase extensor activity.	Speed and control with reciprocal elbow motions, especially with extension. Use of this motion for functional activity (e.g., positioning the arm, reaching activity).	Focus on increased extensor control may prove more effective than simply decreasing flexor hyperactivity.

References

To enhance this text and add value for the reader, all references are included on the companion Evolve site that accompanies this textbook. This online service will, when available, provide a link for the reader to a Medline abstract for the article cited. There are 216 cited references and other general references for this chapter, with the majority of those articles being evidence-based citations.

APPENDIX 33-A ■ Key to Abbreviations

The following is a key to the abbreviations used in the Case Studies in this chapter.

μV = microvolts
ABD POLL BREVIS = abductor pollicis brevis
ADM = abductor digiti minimi
Amp PK-PK = peak to peak amplitude
AMP = amplitude
APB = abductor pollicis brevis
AR = active recording
bel. = below
ab. = above
CM = centimeters
COMM PERONEAL = common peroneal nerve
D INTEROSS = dorsal interroseus
EDB = extensor digitorum brevis
EMG = electromyography
EXT DIG BREV = extensor digitorum brevis
EXT DIG COMM = extensor digitorum communis
FASC = fasciculation potentials
FLEX CARPI RAD = flexor carpi radialis
FHB = flexor hallucis brevis
FIB = fibrillation potentials
Fib head = head of the fibula
FIRST D INTEROSS = first dorsal interosseus
GASTROCN = gastrocnemius
H AMP = H reflex amplitude
H LAT = H reflex latency
H/M APML = Ratio between the amplitudes of the H-reflex and the M wave or motor response
IA = insertional activity
L = left
LAT MALLEOLUS = lateral malleolus
LAT = latency
LL = lower leg
LUMB PSP = lumbar paraspinals
M/S = meters per second
MAX F AMP = maximum F wave amplitude
MAX F LAT = maximum F wave latency
MAX F-M = Maximum difference in F wave and M latencies
Med = median
MIN F LAT = minimum F wave latency
MIN F-M = Minimum difference in F wave and M latencies
msec = milliseconds
MUAP = motor unit action potentials
MV = millivolts
PERON LONGUS = peroneus longus
POLYPH = polyphasic
CERV PSP = cervical
PSW = positive sharp waves
R = right REC SITE = recording site
SNAP = sensory nerve action potential
TEMP = temperature
THOR PSP = thoracic paraspinals
TIB ANTERIOR = tibialis anterior
VAST MED = vastus medialis
VEL PK = peak velocity
VEL = velocity
vs = versus
Uln = ulnar

CHAPTER 34 Orthotics: Evaluation, Intervention, and Prescription

HEIDI TRUMAN, CPO, and WALTER RACETTE, CPO

KEY TERMS

ankle-foot orthosis (AFO)
knee-ankle-foot orthosis (KAFO)
thoracolumbosacral orthosis (TLSO)
anterior or toe lever arm
double-adjustable ankle joint

OBJECTIVES

After reading this chapter the student or therapist will be able to:

1. Identify and analyze the force systems produced by the use of an orthosis.
2. Comprehend the prescription rationale gained from an orthotic evaluation for individuals with neuromuscular dysfunctions.
3. Identify and differentiate the variables considered by the orthotist to optimize outcomes during orthotic intervention.

OVERVIEW

An orthosis is an external device that produces a force that biomechanically affects the body to correct, support, or stabilize the trunk, the head, and/or an extremity. The goals in patient care with orthotic use vary from temporary application to permanent usage to maintain improvement. Orthoses are named by the sections of the body to which they are applied. For example, an orthosis that controls and covers the ankle and foot is called an *ankle-foot orthosis* (AFO). The abbreviations for the device are used by professionals in clinical documentation. Many factors enter into the decision regarding use and type of orthosis, and these will be discussed later. It is essential that the least complicated and most cost-effective orthosis be applied to the patient. The rehabilitation team must build a priority list of desired outcomes and accept that sometimes all of the items on the list may not be achieved by either the orthosis or the patient-team combination. At the very least, care must be attempted in stages because the patient's condition changes or other medical concerns may arise. For example, an excessive number of custom-made and custom-fit plastic AFOs have been issued because they are "more cosmetic and lighter" than AFOs made of metal and leather material. There are times when all higher-priority goals can be achieved so that down the list the goals of cosmesis and light weight can be considered (Table 34-1). However, in the case of neuropathy of the foot, significant risk would be incurred by providing a total contact AFO made of plastic to keep it lightweight. A double-upright metal AFO with a well-fitting extra-depth shoe with a custom accommodative insert would fit the patient's needs and take into consideration the sensory and motor changes within the lower extremity. Effective coordination and communication between health professionals in development of patient goals is essential during the evaluation process. For example, a design criteria omission as simple as placing a loop closure on the side that the patient cannot reach will prohibit the use of the orthotic device. A sound understanding of biomechanical and orthotic principles as well as skilled patient management techniques must be used to be successful with patients who require orthoses.

There are similarities in orthotic management of orthopedic and neurologically impaired patients; however, the neurological population presents additional factors that challenge prescription criteria and outcomes for the rehabilitation team. Lack of proprioception, impairments in sensation, and spasticity are some of these special considerations. Concurrent medical issues, problems with communication, and caregivers may complicate patient management.

The advancements in and access to medical technology have had a profound effect in the field of orthotics. The evolution of plastic, composite, and metals fabrication technology has dramatically improved the ability to control, support, and protect all areas of the human body. Today, patients are fit for custom and prefabricated orthotic devices that provide a variety of functions in both a timely and cost-effective manner. These factors have led physicians to routinely prescribe orthoses for a wide range of medical conditions, whereas in prior decades lack of availability and shortage of experienced orthotists restricted patient access and narrowed the use of orthoses.[1] Orthoses are important options for postoperative management, acute fracture management, and adjunct treatment, in addition to more traditional uses. For many, the proliferation of the prefabricated orthosis signaled a dilution of quality orthotic care, but in reality it has had the opposite effect. These readily available, cost-effective orthoses have not taken orthoses out of the hands of the orthotist but rather have moved them into the minds of treating professionals. There has been continued growth of new and improved orthoses and expansion into other areas of treatment previously lacking in orthotic management. For example, positional and corrective orthoses can be used for premature and newborn infants, and a wide range of sizes of orthoses that previously were made only in adult sizes have become available for pediatric patients. As with any new technological advancement, there has been incorrect application and use. It is not that many of these prefabricated orthoses are difficult to

TABLE 34-1 ■ COMPARISON OF METAL AND PLASTIC ORTHOSES

FACTOR	METAL AND LEATHER	POLYPROPYLENE	LAMINATION OR GRAPHITE	POLYETHYLENE
Adjustability	Yes	Yes, with heat	No	Yes, with heat
Patient changes shoes	No	Yes	Yes	Yes
Weight-bearing strength	Yes	Yes	Yes	No
Skin at risk	Yes	Yes, close observation	No	Yes
Best spinal use	No	Yes	No	Yes
Long-term wear	Yes	Less	Yes	Least
Weight (lightest at 1)	4	2	3	1
Adjustability to changing clinical picture	Yes	Limited unless initial articulation fabricated	No	No
Short-term need	Yes	Yes	Yes	Yes
Requires corrective force with good patient sensation	Fair	Good	Fair	Good
Patient compliance, ability, or direction	Best	Questionable	No	Fair
Ability of clinician to change angulation, ankle or knee	Best	Limited*	No	Not indicated for weight bearing
Upper-extremity fabrication-direct mold highest frequency	Limited	Yes	Limited	Yes

*Use in combination with metal joints produces best results.

apply; rather, there has been lack of a clear understanding of the indications, contraindications, and limitations these devices present to the orthotist and other health professionals such as occupational and physical therapists.

Advancements in technology have allowed the use of lighter, stronger materials in the fabrication of lower-extremity orthotics. Specifically, the substance called *preimpregnated carbon* is a graphite fabric with an exact amount of resin and catalyst already incorporated into the material. With the fibers properly directed over a model, it can be formed with heat. Graphite in other forms has been used in both prosthetics and orthotics for years. However, it had limited acceptance in orthotics because it did not significantly reduce the weight of the orthosis compared with other materials. It also lacked the properties to enable modification of the orthosis after the lamination process. The preimpregnated graphite has a dramatically reduced weight, still maintains its strength, and gives the orthotist the opportunity to use the dynamics of loading and response during the gait cycle. This allows for assistance in both the swing and stance phases of gait (Figure 34-1). A clinical example at the end of this chapter demonstrates this need in patient management.

Another significant advancement in component technology has been the introduction of weight-activated orthotic knee joints. Although available in prosthetics for decades, the development of a lightweight, compact knee joint that would allow a patient to have knee stability during stance[2] and clearance during swing phase has been elusive until recently. Before this, the available knee joints for knee-ankle-foot orthoses (KAFOs) involved some type of locking mechanism that remained locked throughout the gait cycle. The joint provided stabilization of the weak quadriceps

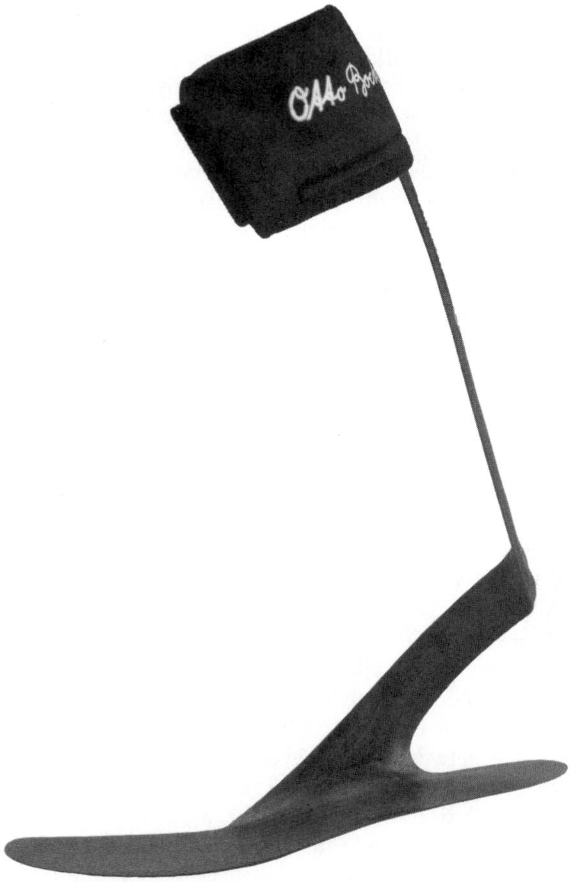

Figure 34-1 ■ New lightweight materials. (Courtesy Otto Bock Healthcare.)

musculature during stance but kept the knee in a fully extended position, making advancement of the limb in swing more difficult for the patient. There are specific indications and contraindications for stance control KAFOs, but early results are promising. This feature can significantly reduce energy output,[3] as it is not necessary to raise the center of gravity to clear the locked knee during swing phase. This improves patient safety when walking on uneven surfaces. New technology for externally powered knee orthoses has just entered the market. These "bionic legs" are robotic aids worn during therapy sessions for gait training. They assist and augment the strength of the patient's muscle and are most typically used in post–cerebrovascular accident (CVA) rehabilitation. Once the patient has achieved functional improvements, the use of the orthosis is discontinued.

Other advancements in orthotic technology include the development of neuroprosthetic devices. These devices act through circuitry and programming to substitute for a deficit in the neural system. Functional electrical stimulation (FES) is a method of applying low-level electrical currents to motor nerves to restore function. In the 1960s the application of FES for foot drop was demonstrated by using a simple single channel to stimulate the common peroneal nerve to activate the ankle dorsiflexors. FES has widespread applications in many other neuroprosthetic devices such as cardiac pacemakers, cochlear stimulators, bladder stimulators, and phrenic nerve stimulators. Until recently, FES devices to provide ambulation assistance were large, unreliable, complex, and restricted to use in a therapy setting. The FES used in neurological rehabilitation attempts to unmask existing voluntary control (if any) and/or initiate dormant activity of the nerves and muscles. For FES to be used, the patient must have an upper motor neuron lesion. This means the nerve-to-muscle pathway is intact and the reflex arc is undamaged. Goals of FES address many rehabilitative outcomes. FES can reduce spasticity, synergy patterns, swelling, and blood clot formation as well as maintaining range of motion (ROM). FES used in gait can improve overall walking abilities by dorsiflexing the foot during swing to provide foot clearance, control initial contact, increase safety, decrease energy expenditure, and retrain muscles. FES has some application in the upper extremity as well, although at this time it is purely in a therapeutic setting. Currently, there are several FES units for foot drop on the market. These devices are used by patients in their daily lives and are not limited to the rehabilitation setting. The WalkAide from Innovative Neurotronics (Figure 34-2) and NESS L300 from Bioness (Figure 34-3) both function to provide dorsiflexion during the swing phase by stimulating the peroneal nerve. An ideal candidate for these devices must have an upper motor neuron lesion, good control of the knee joint, and drop foot. Common neurological conditions in which these devices are used are CVA and multiple sclerosis (MS). Both devices involve some sort of sensor to determine when the patient is initializing the swing phase of the gait cycle and send an electrical stimulus to the nerve to dorsiflex the foot. Advantages of functional FES over traditional orthotic management for foot drop are that it shifts an orthotic device from being a passive support to providing active assistance. FES stimulates the patient's muscles to lift the foot, rather than acting as a passive splint to hold the foot.

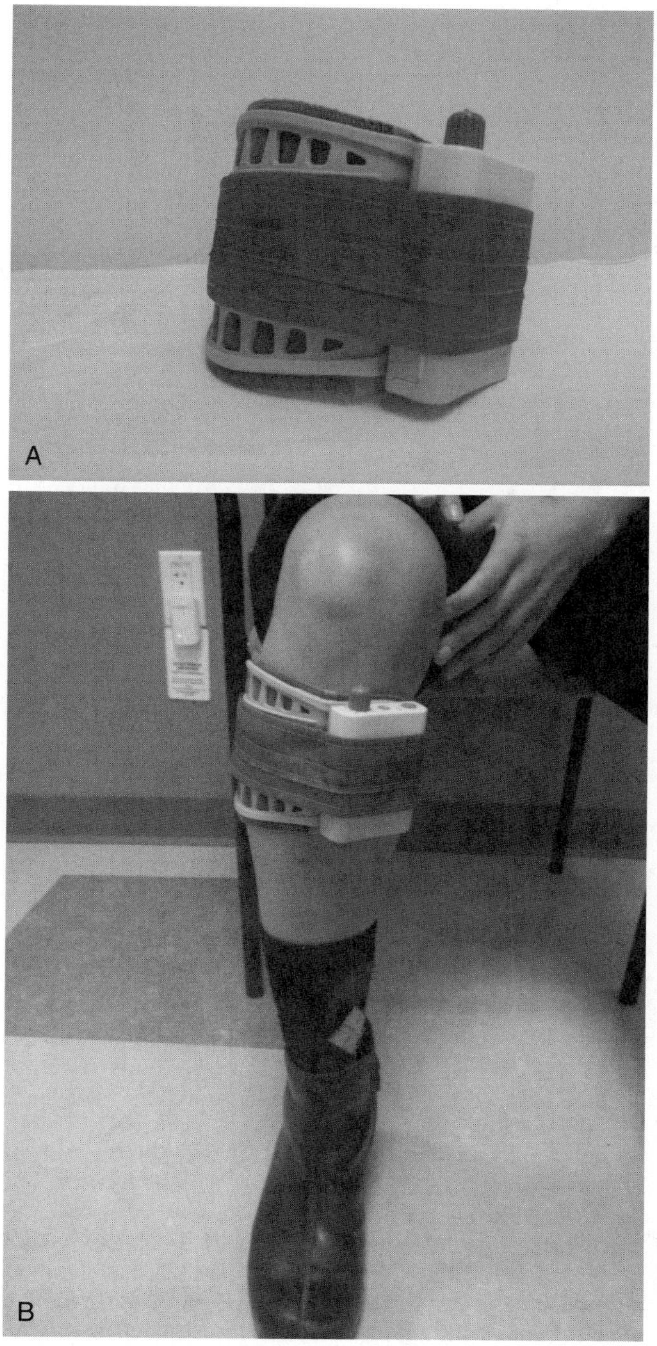

Figure 34-2 ■ **A,** The WalkAide functional electrical stimulation unit (Innovative Neurotronics, Austin, Texas). **B,** WalkAide unit on a patient.

Future developments in the field of orthotics will provide external power and support for patients lacking muscular control. There are already prototypes of systems that can be applied to a patient with paraplegia to allow him or her to stand and walk. "Bionic" orthotics will incorporate microchips and computer programming to provide a degree of artificial intelligence to devices. This will allow the orthosis to change its setting according to the patient's input or position during the specific task or part of the gait cycle. In more traditional types of orthotics, the materials used will continue to become lighter, stronger, and more versatile.

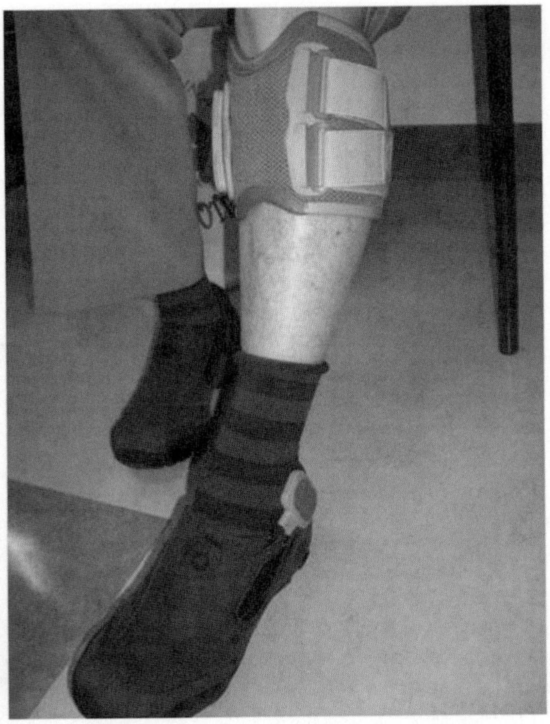

Figure 34-3 ■ The NESS L300 Foot Drop System.

No discussion of the delivery of health care services within the United States would be complete or accurate without acknowledging the effects of governmental and private regulations. The earlier discussion regarding a dramatic increase in usage has raised the medical justification debate about the use of orthotic intervention.

Governmental regulations have dramatically changed the course of the orthotic profession, beginning with the Medicare program, to diagnosis-related groups (DRGs), managed care, and, soon, qualified providers. Medicare was the first national program to cover the cost of both orthotic and prosthetic devices. Before that time only a special few had access to "braces and limbs." DRGs put the responsibility of paying for prescribed orthoses into the hands of the local hospital. Once a specific diagnosis was made, the government would pay a specified amount as reimbursement, leaving the decision of how to manage the patient's care with the physician and hospital. This policy change created many new innovations. Hospitals, interested in reducing the length of hospital stays, challenged physicians to change the way they treated their patients. Patients are no longer immobilized for long periods in hospital beds and are sent home sooner, or sent to a less acute setting or a skilled nursing facility. The use of orthotic devices to expedite care and for precautionary care during hospitalization has increased dramatically. The use of halo fixation systems, thoracolumbosacral orthoses (TLSOs), fracture orthoses, and contracture-preventing orthoses are a few examples of orthotic care that is helping to reduce length of stay. Another significant effect of the DRG decade on orthotics was the need to reduce delivery times and be as cost-effective as possible. Orthoses needed to be delivered in hours, not days. Careful evaluation developed to determine whether a prefabricated, custom-fit, or custom-made orthosis was most appropriate. A prefabricated orthosis is one that is available in "off-the-shelf" sizing and is intended for temporary use. Commonly used prefabricated items are commonly kept in stock by the orthotic provider. Custom-fit orthoses are customizable devices that can be modified to optimize the fit to each individual patient. These devices are intended for use on a more definitive basis, and are often appropriate when the patient has adequate sensation and normal anatomy. Custom-made orthoses require very specific measurements or models of the patient to be obtained for the most specific fit and to accommodate any deformity. These devices are time and labor intensive and are worn definitively when the patient's condition is permanent or when his or her condition or anatomy does not facilitate fitting of a more basic device. Challenges to improve traditional methods of fabrication, better materials, and higher usage spawned the rapid growth of a wide range of orthoses for patient care. There is no reason to believe that this trend will slow as the population ages.

Professional relationships between physical and occupational therapy and orthotics are critical as the evolution of managed care continues. Identifying patient functional goals and a variety of evidence-based care is critical for patient care and clinical outcomes. Orthotic use must be based on proven evidence-based care specific to the profession. In that spirit, a broad overview of the evaluation, prognosis, and intervention of orthotics in neurological rehabilitation is presented.

BASIC ORTHOTIC FUNCTIONS

Alignment

Alignment of the extremities and spine is a common function in orthotic prescription. The orthosis can provide either temporary or permanent function. A TLSO may be prescribed for stabilizing alignment after spinal fusion in the case of an unstable spinal cord injury (refer to Chapter 16). A supramalleolar orthosis (SMO) is commonly prescribed to hold the foot in proper alignment. When the goal of orthotic intervention is to correct alignment to a position well tolerated by the overlying soft tissue and/or the malalignment is a result of a muscle weakness, the new position should stabilize the joint. Clinicians need to remember that aligning one joint may result in the proximal or distal joint being placed in malalignment. An example of this is a genu valgum knee, which may seem easily corrected. However, changes in alignment result in adjustments by the other joints up and down the kinetic chain. Questions such as "Does the subtalar joint have the mobility to pronate?" must be asked and answered.

Stability

Stability is often required for the patient with neurological deficits. These patients frequently lack the muscle control and strength necessary to maintain trunk balance or to ambulate. Patients with muscular dystrophy benefit from TLSOs to help maintain trunk stability, achieve sitting balance, and perform safer transfers. However, the decision regarding an orthosis must take into consideration maximum stability and flexibility while not restraining breathing capacity. An AFO that limits both dorsiflexion and plantarflexion can stabilize the ankle and the knee for the patient who has had a CVA. Although this patient may initially require medial and lateral ankle stability, controlling the anterior posterior lever arms at the ankle can also provide knee stability and prevent future knee impairments. The orthosis functions in the sagittal plane by producing a posterior force that extends the knee during the stance phase of gait, as most patients requiring this type of stabilization have a foot-flat gait instead of a normal initial heel-strike pattern.

Contracture Reduction

Contracture reduction is the goal for many orthotic applications in patients with neurological involvement. The increase in the use of these types of orthoses has been dramatic, as even slight increases in contractures can make the difference between nonambulatory function and ambulatory community participation. Increased awareness and proactive use of prefabricated orthoses have become routine during periods of inactivity, associated surgical procedures, and "sound side" prevention. These types of orthoses can be either dynamic or static and are used in conjunction with various therapeutic modalities to reduce the contracture. Dynamic contracture-reducing orthoses use a spring-type mechanism that applies a low force to a joint over an extended period of time to gain ROM. Static-type orthoses range from serial casts, in which a manual stretch is placed over the joint, to custom-made cylindrical devices designed to spread force over larger areas, to custom-fit devices with some type of quick adjustability. Dynamic-type orthoses are usually contraindicated for the patient with a neurological disorder. Low-tension stretch can trigger spasticity and create skin breakdown because of the high pressure on localized skin areas. The exception for this would be individuals with lower motor neuron impairments and residual hypotonicity. Any tension orthosis needs to be monitored when there is sensory loss, regardless of the cause. To achieve results in contracture reduction, one must be cautiously aggressive, as the amount of force required to improve ROM often threatens the soft tissue's ability to tolerate the pressure of the orthosis. Experience, frequent sessions, and close communication with other members of the rehabilitation team and the family and patient are critical factors in the success of the use of orthotic devices.

EVALUATION

The examination and evaluation of the neurologically impaired patient must be comprehensive. One must not read a diagnosis and assume a total clinical picture. The diagnosis should alert the evaluator to movement patterns associated with the impairment, and these should be used to confirm potential findings. Complete patient evaluations do not end with determination of ROM, muscle testing findings, assessment of proprioception, skin sensitivity evaluation, or assessment of the integrity of the affected limb or spine. The individual ordering an orthotic device must assess the total picture to determine what limitations orthotic care may impose on other important functions, activities, and patient participation in life. The evaluation must include a patient management assessment. What is the patient's or family's motivation? How much equipment can the patient tolerate, and with how much can he or she function? What chance of success does the patient or family have once they have left the clinical setting? How significant are the risks associated with orthotic intervention? As stated, the total evaluation of the patient and the patient's environment is important in developing the treatment plan, as is the communication among the physical therapist, occupational therapist, and orthotist. Whether done together or (more realistically) at separate sites, the details of the treatment plan must be discussed. The patient with neurological impairment often presents a series of complex issues: biomechanical, communication, visualization, and so on. Incomplete information or a lack of effort at communication among these professionals will not lead to a comprehensive treatment plan and ultimate outcome optimization.

During evaluation, review of the diagnosis and gathering of patient history are extremely valuable. A complete medical diagnosis will indicate important information to the team. For example, if a patient with poliomyelitis is to be seen, the orthotist is aware that it is a lower motor neuron lesion and that proprioception is intact (see Chapters 17 and 35). These patients have the benefit of skeletal balance in standing and ambulation and therefore require durable orthotic construction. Compare this with a similar result in muscle testing and ROM assessment for an individual with T12 level paraplegia. Assuming this is a complete lesion, patients with this upper motor neuron lesion lack proprioception. They require other means to get feedback about standing balance and require a lightweight orthosis, as they rarely use orthoses as a major means of locomotion. Although gathering patient history is a vital part of the evaluation, it is, more importantly, an opportunity to establish a productive patient management environment. Patients and family members have important information regarding the initial injury, previous medical care, reasons they sought additional care, and desired outcomes of new treatment. Most of this information can be gathered efficiently as either the therapist or the orthotist begins other professional evaluations. These are important patient and family management skills. One must hear from the patient or family why they came to see the health care professional and their expectations of care. The therapist should not assume the family's goals without asking, as often patient and family goals are higher than the clinicians' expectations. Communicating at a level that is understandable both is vital and demonstrates to the patient and family that the therapist is a concerned professional, thereby engendering trust and confidence. Complete and timely documentation of these findings is becoming increasingly vital to the evaluation and treatment plan. Whether communicating with others on the rehabilitation team, insurance carriers, or legal professionals, documentation and building medical justification are essential in treating all patients.

Evaluation of the Spine

Each area of the spinal column presents various combinations of motion and function. Beginning at the lumbar level as the base for upright position, the spinal column (1) protects vital organs, (2) serves as a supporting structure for the lungs to expand, (3) provides a base for the upper extremities to reach from, (4) acts as a scaffold for objects to be carried, (5) protects the nervous system pathway for the body, (6) and controls the upright position and motions of the head. The individual segments of the spine have relatively few complicated orthotic challenges. However, it is rare that only one segment is involved in the patient with neuropathic impairments. It is more common for two or more segments of the spine to be involved in orthotic fitting. For example, supporting the head in a functional position is a major goal of orthotic intervention, but to accomplish this the orthosis must encompass the thoracic as well as the cervical spine in order to distribute the forces to minimize skin pressures.

When evaluating the cervical spine and head, one must (in addition to muscle testing) determine at what angulations an upright position of the head cannot be recovered. Limiting the head from assuming nonfunctional positions such as extreme extension is an easier orthotic function than holding the head upright. Many patients with neurological problems may have the strength to move in a 15- to 20-degree range of flexion and extension, lateral bend, and rotation but do not have the strength to recover the head from greater angles. Even the most pressure-tolerant soft tissue about the head does not tolerate long-term pressure from an orthosis; intermittent control and relief are a critical part of the design. Pressure directly on the ear is not tolerated at any time.

The thoracic and lumbar spine is almost always treated concurrently with an orthosis in the patient with a neurological deficit. The major reasons for orthotic intervention in this area are to stabilize the trunk for balance, to protect surgical correction or stabilization, and to maintain respiration. The pelvis is generally used as a base to prevent distal migration of the orthosis whether the patient is sitting or standing. For this reason, one must closely evaluate the degree of deformity, prominence of bony structure, skin sensation, and condition of soft tissue coverage. Many neurologically impaired patients also have other medical issues that need to be considered in orthotic design, such as a colostomy, gastrointestinal (GI) tubes, pressure sores, and other factors. Scoliosis and kyphosis are common biomechanical impairments within this patient group. Balance between correcting the spinal deformity to maintain respiratory function by use of a tightly fitting TLSO and the skin pressure it creates must be reached by the rehabilitation team. The evaluation of the spine and potential need for orthotic intervention would not be complete without recognizing the effect the desired orthosis may have on the extremities, whether the patient is ambulatory or non–weight bearing. What movements of the spine are present during ambulation, and would immobilizing the spine significantly affect the patient? Will the orthosis restrict needed shoulder elevation and arm movements? Variation in materials used for fabrication of a spinal orthosis can often significantly improve the desired outcome, increase the wear time, ease the donning process, and improve skin care. From a patient and family management standpoint, one must consider many variables in potential design of the orthosis. Can the patient or family apply the orthosis and remove it when appropriate? Do they understand potential areas of pressure? What is the home situation like?

Evaluation of the Upper Extremities

Evaluation of the upper extremities requires multiple inputs from health care professionals, patients, family, and teachers because of the wide range of specific functions an individual performs daily. Unique to the upper extremity, multiple functions generally require multiple orthotic devices for activities of daily living (ADLs). Typical functions of orthoses of the upper extremity include maintenance of functional wrist and hand position, reduction of contracture or tone, transfer of force available in one area to another, and support of subluxations resulting from denervation. It is common for the neurologically impaired patient to require several orthoses with different functions for use throughout the day. Strength, ROM, condition of soft tissues, and sensation are all important evaluation factors. In addition, ambulatory status, bilateral or unilateral condition, status of vision, and condition of the spine and head must be factored into the indications and contraindications in assessment of the orthotic needs of the patient. Much more critical muscle tests must be performed in the upper extremity as opposed to the lower extremity, as minor increases or decreases in strength will dramatically alter orthotic need. For example, the C5 quadriplegic has the ability to function with a wrist-hand orthosis by providing enough wrist extension to use the tenodesis effect, which can produce a three-jaw-chuck type of grip. The difference between a functioning and nonfunctioning orthosis is minor, not only because there is limited muscle strength, but also because minor inefficiencies in the tenodesis splint (from friction or malalignment) could reduce function to below acceptable levels. Patients with unilateral involvement have far different needs than the bilaterally involved. The patient with a CVA with unilateral involvement may have an intervention of a positional wrist-hand orthosis to prevent contracture and injury and a supportive shoulder orthosis to prevent shoulder subluxation (Figures 34-4 and 34-5). In these cases the other extremity becomes dominant, and there is little need to fabricate complex orthoses for the use of the affected extremity. The patient with bilateral involvement presents a much different picture. Consideration for grooming, feeding, mobility, and so on must be factored into the desired expectation during evaluation. The case of the patient with neurological impairments who requires orthotic intervention is complex, as this patient typically has involvement in the trunk, head, and

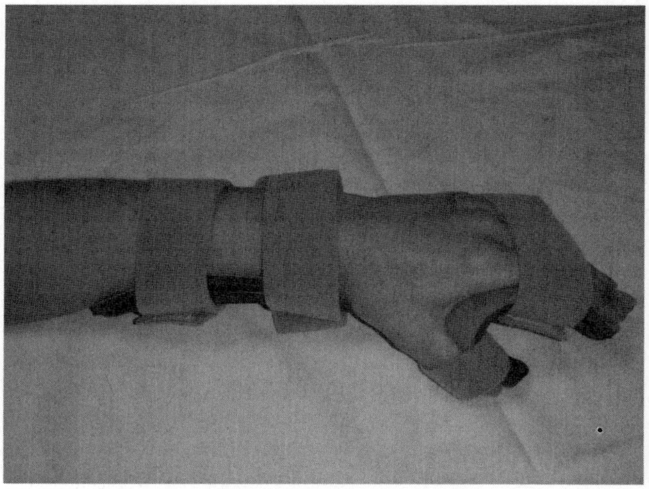

Figure 34-4 ■ Resting hand splint.

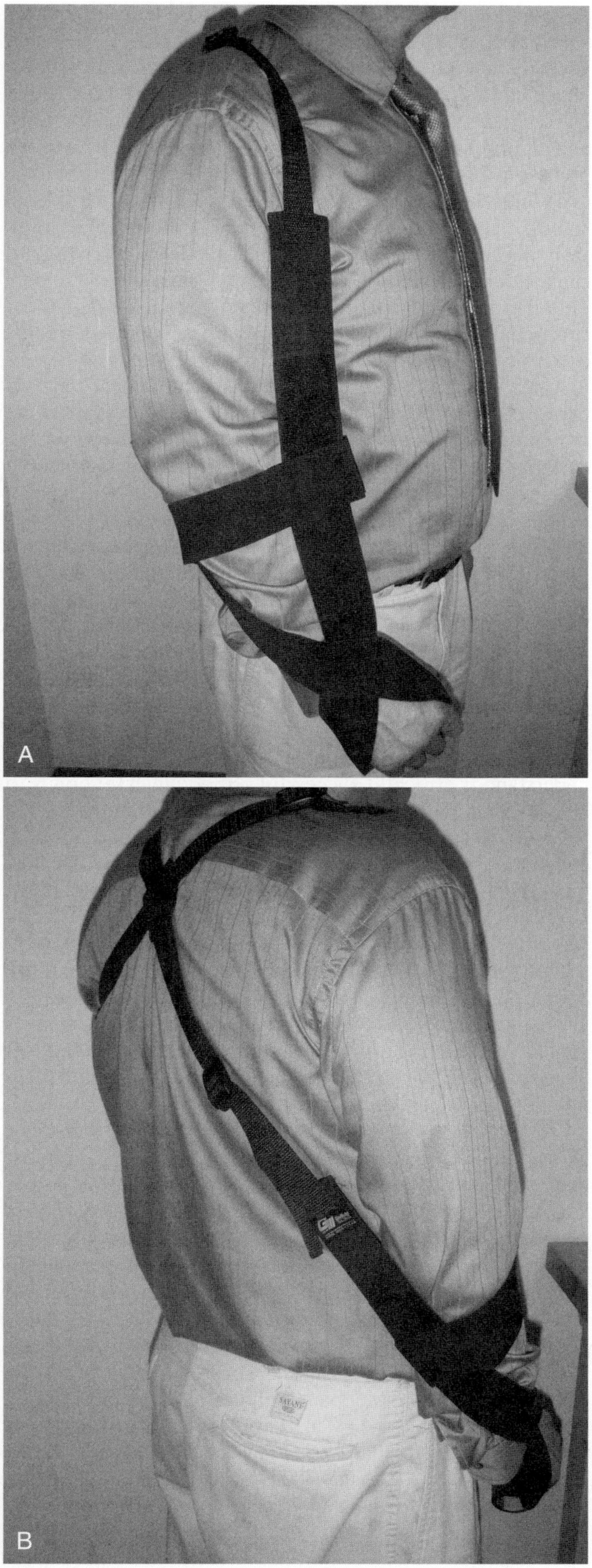

Figure 34-5 ■ Shoulder splint to support the shoulder against subluxation and pain. **A,** Sagittal view. **B,** Posterior view.

lower extremity. These patients require specialized wheelchairs and seating systems. Evaluation is most effective with all rehabilitation team members present to establish a treatment plan. Orthotic treatments maximize what limited muscle strength and ROM the patient may have. Orthoses that are used during the day to maximize function are often replaced with positional orthoses at night to preserve gains and prevent decline in ROM. The occupational therapist provides most of the functional and positional orthoses for the upper extremity. In today's rehabilitation environment, many occupational therapists work directly with orthopedic hand specialists and trauma physicians. They use low-temperature materials to mold custom devices specifically designed for protecting surgical reconstruction or promoting or maintaining ROM or for use as assistive devices.

Evaluation of the Lower Extremities

Evaluation of the lower extremity offers additional challenges owing to the role of ambulation and its value to independence for the patient and family members. ROM, strength, existing deformity, proprioception, muscle tone, and soft tissue condition and sensation must be evaluated. Where appropriate, weight-bearing evaluation and gait analysis are completed. Patient and family assessment as it relates to the ability to comprehend and follow instructions is extremely important, as the potential for injury may outweigh the benefit of orthotic intervention to transform a patient from being non–weight bearing to having limited ambulation. Lack of ROM at the hip and knee will significantly decrease the duration of potential ambulation or may totally inhibit ambulation. Lack of ROM at the hip and knee is more critical than lack of strength. In the foot and ankle, the need for normal ROM is even more critical for efficient standing balance and ambulation. Orthoses of the lower extremity provide a combination of force lever arms acting about a joint axis at the knee, hip, or ankle. These joints are significantly compromised by the lack of ROM. These force lever arms within the lower extremities substitute for the lack of strength. For example, by blocking dorsiflexion of the ankle, the toe or anterior lever arm provides a posteriorly directed force in the sagittal plane during stance that stabilizes the knee. If the patient lacks the ability to get the ankle even to neutral, this tightness provides its own lever arm, which will result in a variety of undesirable forces and actions. Genu recurvatum, foot or ankle varus, a shortened stride length on the nonaffected side, and the heel rising out of the shoe are common signs of this problem. These issues are further complicated when lack of proprioception, spasticity, and lack of sensation are present. Lack of ROM at the ankle creates many symptoms in the lower extremity but is often overlooked during evaluation as the cause of these problems. Genu varus and genu recurvatum are common deformities of the patient with neurological impairments. A number of factors create these problems. In addition to the ankle ROM, leg length differences, lack of quadriceps strength, and lack of proprioception can create deformities about the knee. The patient with poliomyelitis may have both a short extremity and weak knee extensors, which lead to genu recurvatum and genu valgus. However, reducing the genu recurvatum without protecting against undesirable knee flexion would be a mistake. Patients with lower motor neuron disease have excellent proprioception, which is the reason they protect the unstable knee by hyperextending it. They may even use force from their upper extremity by pushing posteriorly on the femur with the hand. A similar patient with upper neuron impairments, for example a patient who has had a CVA, has a similar knee presentation. However, the usual cause of this patient's deformity is different. Reduced or lack of strength and ROM limitations about the hip limit effective ambulation and leave the patient much more reliant on trunk stability and upper-extremity ambulatory aids. Hip flexors are more critical than hip extensors, as they serve to advance the limb in reciprocal gait, whereas lack of hip extensors is compensated for by the strong hip ligaments, which tighten for stability in extension. A lack of ROM to at least neutral extension about the hip creates major challenges for the patient, even if the patient has excellent upper-extremity strength. This lack of ROM will not allow stability in standing once force is removed from the upper-extremity ambulatory aids. Creating hands-free standing balance is a highly desirable outcome of orthotic intervention. The patient is then able to use both upper extremities for ADL tasks.

ORTHOTIC INTERVENTION

Several factors play key roles in the success of orthotic intervention. To improve function without complication or patient risk, the clinician must be sure to address the patient's major complaint; the reason the patient and family came to see the therapist or orthotist must be clearly established to ensure compliance with orthotic intervention. It is important to establish a baseline of function so that results of intervention are measurable. In some situations the patient benefit is clear and immediate, whereas in others, concentrated instruction, orthotic modification, and time are required before improved function can be observed or measured. The process of donning and doffing the orthosis as independently as possible enhances the overall goal for the patient and family and must be well thought out by the experienced clinician. The clinician must be conservative in setting these expectations. It is important to remember that what happens in the clinical setting may not be easily reproducible in the home situation. The orthotic interventions must be kept as simple as possible: what is the least amount of orthotic intervention that will provide the expected goal? Although an obvious statement, the balance between too much and not enough can challenge the clinician's skill and experience. The use of trial orthoses can provide valuable information during the evaluation, and these are generally available commercially for short periods. Various types of heat-moldable plastics have been beneficial for many individuals. At times, however, their use adds risk and complication without improvement compared with traditional AFOs fabricated with metal and leather attached to the patient's shoe. For example, if the patient requires ankle and knee stability yet lacks sensation in the foot and ankle, the double-upright metal orthosis attached to the patient's shoe creates much less risk for possible skin breakdown than a rigid total contact plastic orthosis (see Table 34-1). With a plastic orthosis, the family must find a shoe big enough to easily fit the orthosis. Technological advancements have led to a number of additions to the arsenal of orthotists. Prefabricated orthoses with better sizing and materials have given the clinician additional tools for evaluation and for devising permanent orthoses. Preimpregnated graphite AFOs are now available in multiple sizes and provide toe pickup during swing phase and some knee-stabilizing characteristics during stance phase. Although very lightweight, these orthoses provide dynamic stance phase control. Introduction of biomechanical forces to the extremities may cause unwanted movements or restrictions, and careful selection of components is essential to keep the focus on the orthotic plan. For example, a patient with a CVA may need more anterior lever force to provide knee stability, so one would plantar flex the orthotic ankle joint. However, this knee-stabilizing effect in stance phase would cause a toe drag during swing phase. A simple fix is to provide the opposite side with a ¼-inch heel and sole lift for additional clearance during swing phase of the affected extremity (Table 34-2).

Clinicians need to set realistic, manageable patient-centered treatment goals. All too often, treatment plans are only in the minds of the clinicians and are either never or too poorly communicated with the patient and family. Clinicians should assume that the patient and family members will expect benefits of the intervention that will far exceed what the therapist knows are possible. The time to address those gaps is certainly before treatment, not when the patient and family realize that expectations regarding functional gains may not be realistic. If failure is the reason a patient recognizes that the intervention was wrong, the therapists have lost the patient's trust and the potential for future intervention guidance. Discussing realistic achievable goals of treatment, after assessing all factors, the home situation, and individual motivation, with the patient and family in language they understand is critical if successful orthotic intervention is to be achieved. The goal of orthotic care for a patient with CVA is to provide safe standing balance for transfer and minimal ambulation in the home. Patients and their families will realize the major benefit this will have on the home situation. However, without this identified as the goal before orthotic care, they may leave the therapeutic environment wondering why the patient cannot walk normally and participate in life activities that require longer distance ambulation skills.[4] This clinical error is an all too frequent patient management mistake. Integrating orthoses with physical and occupational therapy motor relearning and neuroplasticity should help optimize functional recovery.

To provide a cost-effective orthosis in a timely manner with today's vast number of orthotic devices, the orthotist must stay abreast of the wide array of choices at his or her disposal to meet the needs of the patient. The reality of cost containment is not a recent event in the orthotic profession, as funding for these devices has always been challenged. This has necessitated the development of more cost-effective alternatives, such as the prefabricated orthosis. The introduction of heat-moldable plastics into orthotics in the late 1960s and early 1970s on a custom basis replaced, to a large extent, the need to mold leather and/or metal to fabricate an orthosis (see Table 34-1). This improved the total contact fit and dramatically reduced the time and skill level required for manufacturing. Today's orthotist has a multitude of devices from which to choose to meet the needs of the patient. Options range from custom-made devices using a patient mold to prefabricated custom-fit devices. A thorough understanding of the indications and contraindications for each of these devices is essential in order to meet patient needs. A lack of understanding of biomechanical principles, of the

TABLE 34-2 ■ INDICATIONS FOR COMMON ORTHOTIC MODIFICATIONS AND ADDITIONS

MODIFICATION OR ADDITION	DESCRIPTION
SACH modification	This modification is done by cutting out a triangular wedge in the heel of the shoe and inserting a softer material. The solid ankle cushion heel (SACH) modification is used to dampen the effect of the heel or posterior lever arm at heel strike. This force produces an anterior force to destabilize the knee, which may be undesirable.
Heel and sole buildup	Adding a ¼-inch heel and sole buildup to the unaffected side can create additional swing clearance needed on the affected side. This modification is indicated if additional dorsiflexion of the orthotic joint creates knee instability or if the patient lacks dorsiflexion range of motion.
Rocker-bottom heel and sole modifications	There are several different styles of rocker-bottom buildup. Although the roll built into this modification may differ, the basic results are the same—to add motion and translate the center of gravity forward when the ankle and/or knee joint is locked.
Long tongue stirrup, extended steel shanks	A stirrup is the metal attachment to the shoe. The use of a long tongue (a steel extension that goes distally between the bottom of the shoe and the heel and sole) is necessary to transfer the force created by restriction of ankle motion. Without this type of fabrication, the force produced at midstance will not be controlled. A steel shank produces the same control but is not part of the stirrup and may be used in combination with a rocker bottom.
Medial or valgus control T-strap; lateral or varus control T-strap	These straps, leather on traditional double-upright orthoses or plastic or padding control T-strap modifications on plastic AFOs, produce a force to reduce valgus (a medial T-strap) or varus (a lateral T-strap). A medial T-strap attaches to the shoe medially, and the beltlike strap goes around the lateral upright and is tightened. The lateral T-strap attaches to the lateral side of the shoe and applies a medially directed force by being tightened around the medial upright of the AFO.
Heel buildup	A heel buildup is used to accommodate heel cord tightness. The tibia must be at least 90 degrees to the floor for safe balance and ambulation. Common signs of the need to build up the heel are genu recurvatum and the heel slipping out of the shoe. The amount of heel buildup must be matched with the same heel and sole buildup on the opposite side for balance.
Instep or figure-of-8 straps	This orthotic modification is used to keep the heel seated in the shoe or plastic ankle-foot orthosis when a tight heel cord is present. These straps fit across the dorsum of the foot with a posterior attachment point.
Swedish knee orthosis	This prefabricated knee orthosis is an effective method to prevent genu recurvatum. It is typically indicated after a CVA for the patient who lacks proprioception and whose knee hyperextends, creating pain and slackening the knee ligaments. It can be used temporarily as a training orthosis or on a more definitive basis when persistent pain and instability are present.

limitations of prefabricated orthoses, and of custom fitting can lead to failure and increase the impairment problems existing within the patient environment. All orthoses produce a force field, some desirable and some undesirable. It requires an experienced clinician to make the most appropriate choices, as too often the failure of treatment is blamed on an orthosis. Usually such failure is the result of an inappropriate initial selection of orthotic components, lack of discernment between custom-made and custom-fit devices, or misidentification of the patient as an orthotic candidate. Prefabricated custom-fit orthoses are cost-effective only if they produce the desired goal over time. As a general rule, one should consider prefabricated custom-fit orthosis for patients who have an anatomically "normal" biomechanical structural environment and who will use the orthosis for only a short time. Custom-made orthoses for extremities or the spine are usually prescribed for patients who have deformity or unusual size or who must use the device indefinitely.

CLINICAL EXAMPLES

Paraplegia

Orthotic intervention for a patient with paraplegia is generally considered for the lower extremities at the T12 level in the complete lesion.[5] Complete lesions higher in the cord leave the patient without enough trunk stability to use bilateral orthoses effectively. Although a thoracic extension can be added to bilateral KAFOs, this addition greatly increases the difficulty of donning the orthosis independently, and most patients will have great difficulty getting from sitting to standing.

The most appropriate orthoses for a T12 complete paraplegic are bilateral KAFOs. The patient generally uses a swing-to or swing-through gait, and successful use of orthoses requires excellent standing balance. There are three significant design requirements for these KAFOs: shallow thigh and calf bands, bail or French knee locks, and double-adjustable ankle joints.

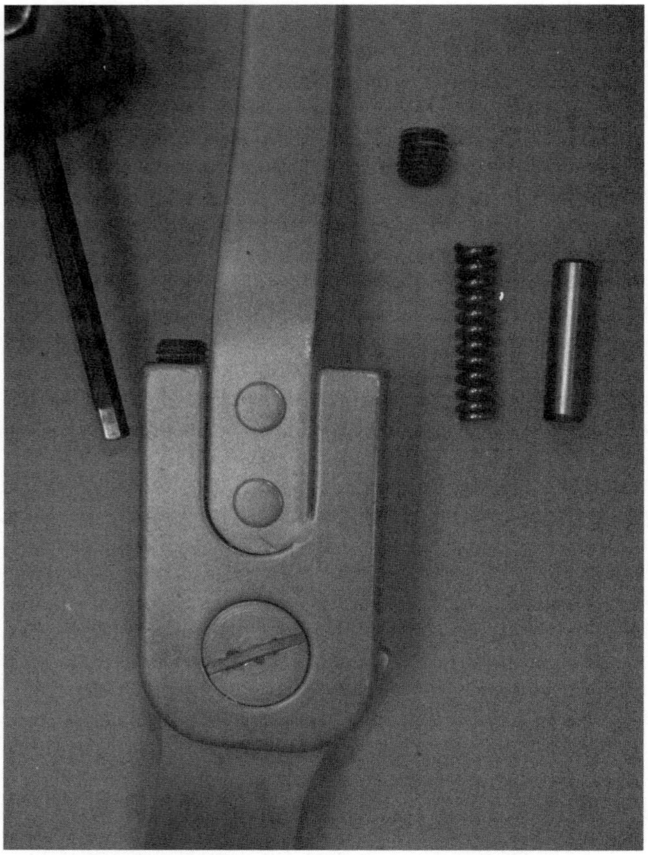

Figure 34-6 ■ Double-adjustable ankle joint. The channels on the anterior and posterior sides allow for easy adjustment of dorsiflexion and plantarflexion range of motion. Springs can also be added to provide dynamic assistance to the movements.

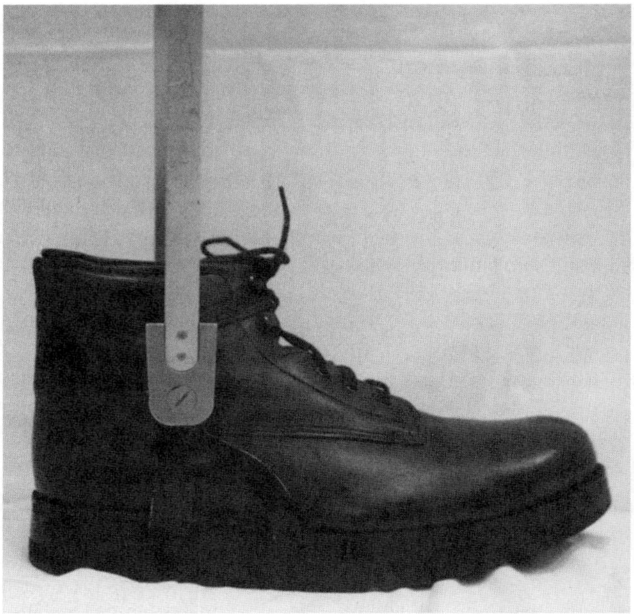

Figure 34-7 ■ Modifications necessary to control the ankle setting in a client with spinal cord injury (Scott-Craig shoe or stirrup modifications).

A double-adjustable ankle joint has channels on the anterior and posterior sides of the joint. This allows the orthotist to easily adjust dorsiflexion and plantarflexion position and ROM, or even provide dynamic assistance via a spring added to the channel of the joint (Figure 34-6). The shallow bands force the center of gravity forward, inducing lordosis so the patient can rest on the iliofemoral or Y ligaments of the hip. The knee joint locks are automatic because the patient requires the upper extremities for standing. The bail or French joint will lock as the patient stands and bends over the rigid ankle joint, forcing the knee joints into extension. The lock then can catch on the back of a wheelchair seat or other chair to release the lock and bend at the joint when the patient sits. The foot-ankle complex forms the basis for balance. A few degrees of adjustment at the double-adjustable ankle joint can make the difference between safe standing balance and limited standing balance. The long tongue stirrup extends at least to the heads of the metatarsals and farther if the patient is taller and heavier than normal (see Table 34-2). The use of a strutter bar from the upright of the stirrup extending to a transverse bar at the heads of the metatarsals with a long tongue stirrup (Scott-Craig design, Figure 34-7) ensures that the necessary rigidity is provided. A point between effective standing balance and ambulation is reached after training and ankle adjustment. Patients must have full ROM at the hips, knees, and ankles for use of these devices to be successful.

CASE STUDY 34-1 ■ A. M.

A. M. is a 21-year-old man with incomplete T12-level paraplegia secondary to a gunshot wound. A. M. has normal upper-extremity strength and ROM. He has had surgery for spinal fusion. Trunk strength is 4/5, left hip is 3/5, knee is 2/5, right hip is 1/5, and right knee is 0/5. ROM is full at hips, knees, and ankles. A. M. can transfer independently and has the goal of household ambulation, although he is aware that it "takes a lot of work." A. M. was fitted with a right KAFO with shallow bands, drop lock knee joints, and double-adjustable ankle joints locked in 5 degrees of dorsiflexion (Figure 34-8). Drop locks were used instead of bail locks because of the use of a unilateral KAFO. A. M. had balance, strength, and a foot orthosis on the left side. The left lower extremity was fitted with an AFO and double-upright and double-adjustable ankle joints adjusted to match the right orthosis. The distal attachment to the shoes was with long tongue stirrups and strutter bars. The patient was able to ambulate with forearm crutches.

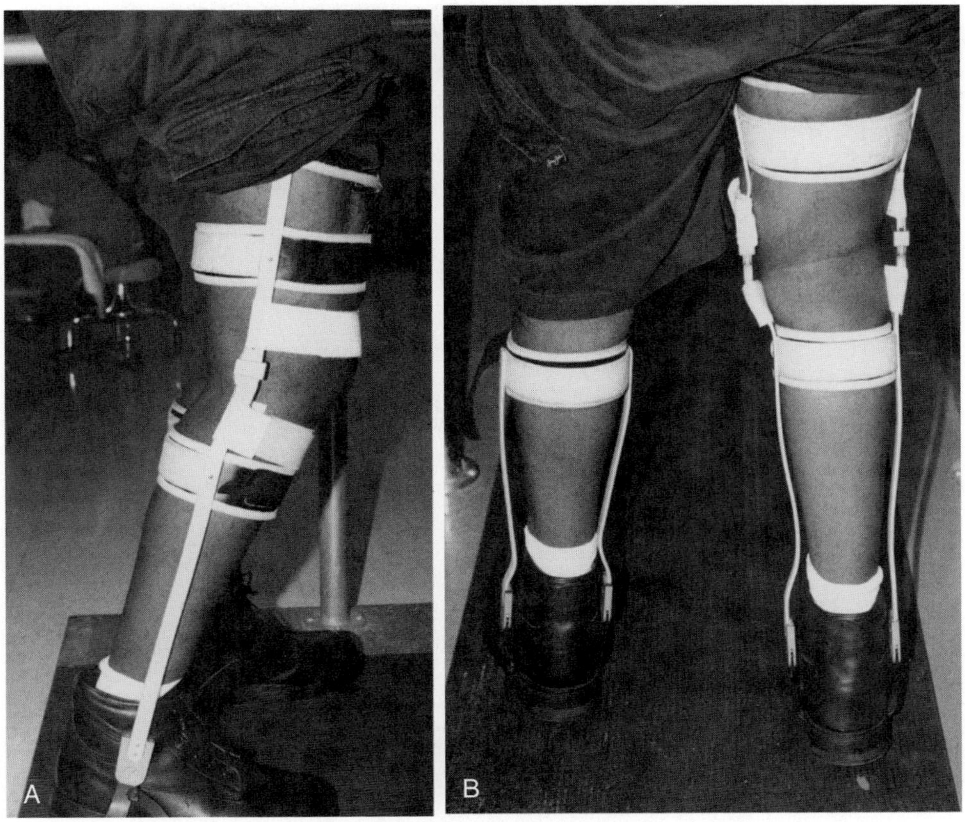

Figure 34-8 ■ Patient standing wearing a right knee-ankle-foot orthosis. **A**, Lateral view; **B**, posterior view.

Hemiplegia

Patients who have had a CVA can vary widely in their need for orthotic intervention, from a simple AFO to assist toe clearance, to an AFO to stabilize both ankle and knee, to an orthosis used temporarily for training purposes.[6,7] The use of a KAFO in the patient with hemiplegia is rarely indicated. Even though the more affected patient does not have knee stability, he or she rarely ambulates with a heel strike that would destabilize the knee and therefore can use an AFO with an anterior limited-range ankle joint. In addition, patients cannot don the KAFO with the use of only one upper extremity. With hip flexor weakness and knee instability on the affected side, the orthotic intervention may be to assist in transfers rather than to facilitate gait. As a general rule, orthotic intervention for the client with a CVA ranges from a static toe pickup orthosis to a double-adjustable ankle joint with the ankle locked. The use of dynamic components is not effective, because they will initiate spasticity. The lack of ROM into dorsiflexion or even to neutral causes the most significant problems for these patients. An ankle that lacks dorsiflexion ROM prevents advancement of the center of gravity and produces a lever arm that induces genu recurvatum and pain, and either the heel comes out of the shoe or the ankle rolls into varus. Because these patients lack proprioception, this constant force directed posteriorly will, over time, be significant. The patient will develop pain in the knee and not ambulate, the heel cord will shorten more, and the cycle will continue. Heel cords rarely gain length after the patient has been discharged from the rehabilitation setting, and one must consider the family and home situation. Heel buildups on the affected side are used to bring the tibia into 90 degrees. Buildups of 1 to 1½ inches are not uncommon. Remember to balance the opposite shoe. When selecting between different orthotic components, it is best to choose the more stable orthosis. The use of trial orthoses during evaluation is invaluable and helpful initially. As the patient improves, he or she may require less orthotic management or no orthosis at all. A three-point pressure orthosis for the knee, such as a Swedish knee cage (Figure 34-9), is also a valuable training orthosis and, in the case of some post-CVA patients, is used daily when the degree of recurvatum exceeds the patient's ability to control the posteriorly directed force. The stirrup (the metal attachment to the patient's shoe) of the AFO must be firm and extend under the sole and heel to the heads of the metatarsals. Although this adds weight to the orthosis, it is necessary to transmit knee-stabilizing forces. Stirrups attached under the heel will only allow undesirable motion and will not provide the required stability.

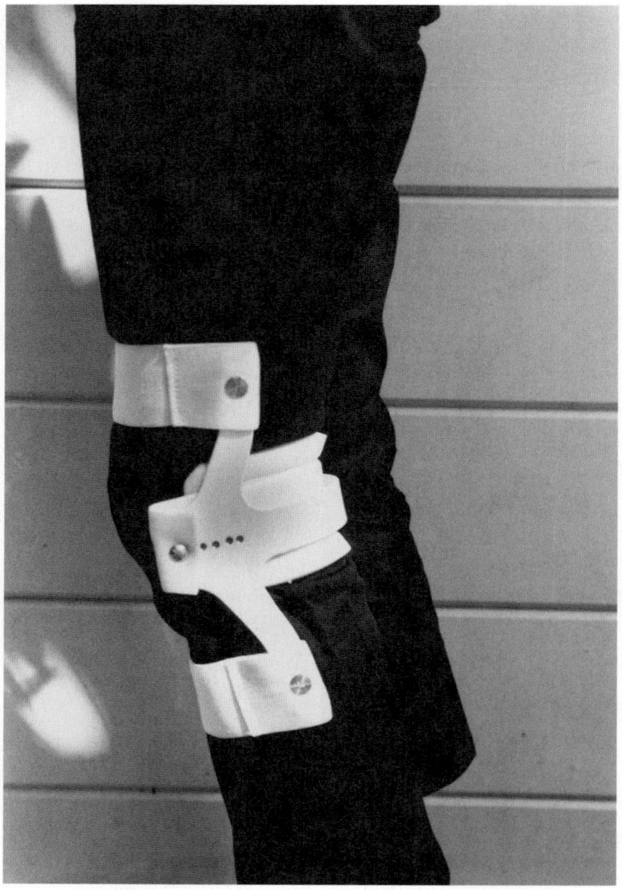

Figure 34-9 ■ Prefabricated three-point pressure knee orthosis (Swedish knee cage) to control genu recurvatum.

CASE STUDY 34-2 ■ D. M.

D. M. is a 58-year-old woman who had a left CVA, resulting in a right hemiplegia, almost 2 years ago. She was evaluated at the request of her physician because of increased knee pain and poor standing balance. D. M. was fitted with a plastic AFO fixed at 90 degrees 14 months ago. She was wearing the orthosis, but the heel would not stay in her shoe. Evaluation showed that the patient lacked 15 degrees from getting the foot to neutral (the ankle was therefore in 15 degrees of plantarflexion), had 0/5 dorsiflexion or plantarflexion, and had 3-/5 knee extension and flexion. She also walked with the aid of a quad cane and had 10 degrees of genu recurvatum and slight genu varum at midstance. Her goal was to walk with less pain and to be more stable. D. M. was fitted with bilateral upright, double-adjustable locked ankle joints with long tongue stirrups and a 1½-inch heel buildup (Figure 34-10). The left shoe was built up 1½ inches in the heel and sole to balance the right shoe (Figure 34-11). A Swedish knee orthosis also was used initially to help train the patient and to provide hyperextension control. Although the double-adjustable ankle joint does give total flexibility to change the angle, a 90-degree posterior stop also can be used. Patients who lack this much ROM provide an "anatomical" anterior stop.

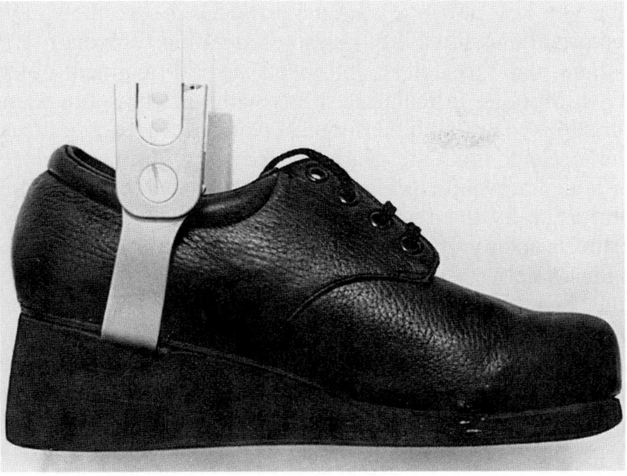

Figure 34-10 ■ Shoe modification with double-adjustable ankle.

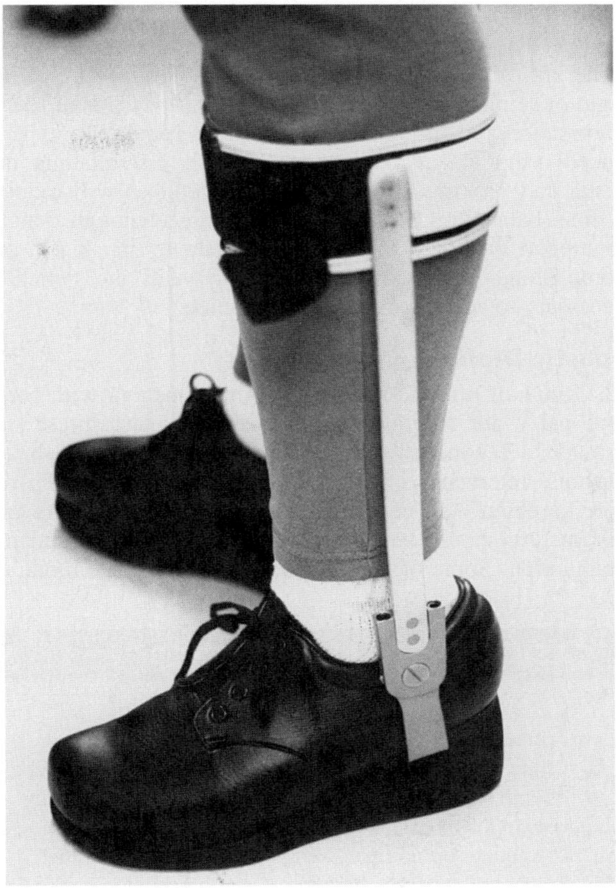

Figure 34-11 ■ Left double-upright, double-adjustable ankle-foot orthosis with balancing right buildup.

CASE STUDY 34-3 ■ M. H.

M. H. is a 59-year-old woman with a history of a CVA 1 year ago. She has left hemiplegia. She works as a facilities manager and walks through her office building several times per day. She underwent extensive therapy after the CVA and has good strength; ROM is within normal limits at her hip and knee. At her left ankle, M. H. has 3+/5 plantarflexion strength but 0/5 dorsiflexion or eversion strength, and she has extensor tone into plantarflexion and inversion. She ambulates very cautiously owing to her inability to dorsiflex and evert the foot during the swing phase of gait. She has a high risk of falling because of her ankle instability and has sustained multiple inversion sprains at the ankle.

M. H. was tested using an FES device and had an appropriate response to the stimulus. She was fitted with an FES device for foot drop. This unit consists of a cuff and control unit around her proximal calf, attached to electrodes on her skin near the fibular head. It allows her to ambulate barefoot and/or with various types of footwear, as it is programmed using the angle of her leg to determine the transition from stance to swing phase in gait. The unit is inconspicuous and lightweight. Her walking velocity, safety, and stability are significantly improved with the FES unit. She uses it throughout the day on a daily basis.

Paralytic Spine

Many neuropathic diagnoses affect the spinal column. Spinal muscle atrophy, tetraplegia, myelomeningocele, and Duchenne muscular dystrophy can all require orthotic intervention. Although materials, padding versus no padding, trim lines, length of time used, and optional area openings can vary with different conditions, most spinal stabilizing orthoses are TLSOs. Orthoses used for postsurgical stabilization tend to be of more rigid material to support the healing spine. The paralytic spine that is not surgically stabilized can have either a flexible or a rigid curvature. An orthosis for a patient with a rigid curvature is used to avoid further deformity and differs from that used by the patient with a flexible curvature. If the curve is flexible, the orthosis will be used to hold some of the correction that can be obtained. Patients with paralytic spine deformity usually undergo casting for custom orthoses, and although non–weight-bearing supine casts can greatly reduce the curve, many patients will not tolerate the pressure once in the upright sitting position. Orthotic intervention usually has one or more of the following goals: (1) improved sitting balance, (2) support of surgical stabilization, (3) prevention of further spinal deformity, (4) use as an assistive positional device for better use of head and upper extremities, and (5) improved respiratory function.

Most TLSOs for these patients are total circumferential designs that use rigid materials (polypropylene) to less rigid materials (polyethylene) or a combination of padding with a rigid or semirigid frame internal to the heat-formable foam. Fabrication and fitting of these orthoses require an experienced orthotist and adherence to detail. Establishing the distal and proximal trim lines of the orthosis will require a fine balancing act between providing enough length to support the spine without breaking down the skin in accomplishing that goal. Several clinic visits are typically necessary to achieve the desired outcome.

Spastic Diplegic Cerebral Palsy

The goals of orthotic intervention in the patient with cerebral palsy are to control tone, prevent contractures, and provide a secondary support after a surgical procedure.[8] Orthotic intervention for these individuals varies from region to region. As a general rule, the orthosis used to prevent contracture should be different from the orthosis used for ambulation. Some of the new designs incorporate modules that can key into one another or be used separately. This feature allows flexibility, assists in donning (especially in a patient with spasticity), and meets several treatment objectives. Modular articulating joints with various settings and functions to use with thermoplastic orthoses greatly increase the options that are available today. With the goals of orthotic intervention stated earlier, total contact–type orthoses are generally the desired option. As with any total contact orthosis and hypersensitive or hyposensitive skin, a cautious balance between correction or holding and skin tolerance must be reached. The fitting of and follow-up for these types of orthoses require experience, knowledge, and patience. Combinations of padding, wedging, straps, and heat relief methods are often necessary to enable the patient to wear the orthosis for a significant amount of time on a daily basis. A patient with spastic diplegic cerebral palsy relies heavily on her or his orthosis and wears it out faster than most other orthotic patients. In the case of a child, she or he may grow out of the orthosis before it wears out. This should be considered in the design and fabrication.

CASE STUDY 34-4 ■ S. G.

S. G. is a 13-year-old girl with spastic cerebral palsy with involvement of all four extremities. She is nonambulatory with significant scoliosis. Her hip ROM is from −25 degrees to 135 degrees of flexion. S. G. is fully dependent and lacks upper-extremity use.

The goal of orthotic intervention was to prevent further deformity, maintain the thoracic and lumbar column height for internal organ function, and provide trunk stability for seating balance in her wheelchair. She was fitted with a custom TLSO fabricated from a cast impression (Figure 34-12). It has ¼ inch of padding with a polypropylene outer layer, which has been modified over bony prominences for skin tolerance.

S. G. wears her TLSO not only while seated in her chair, but also in bed. Frequent checks of the skin were made during the first few weeks of use to establish trim lines and window type modifications. She continues to be checked periodically for comfort and control as she grows to ensure that the TLSO's fit and function are appropriate.

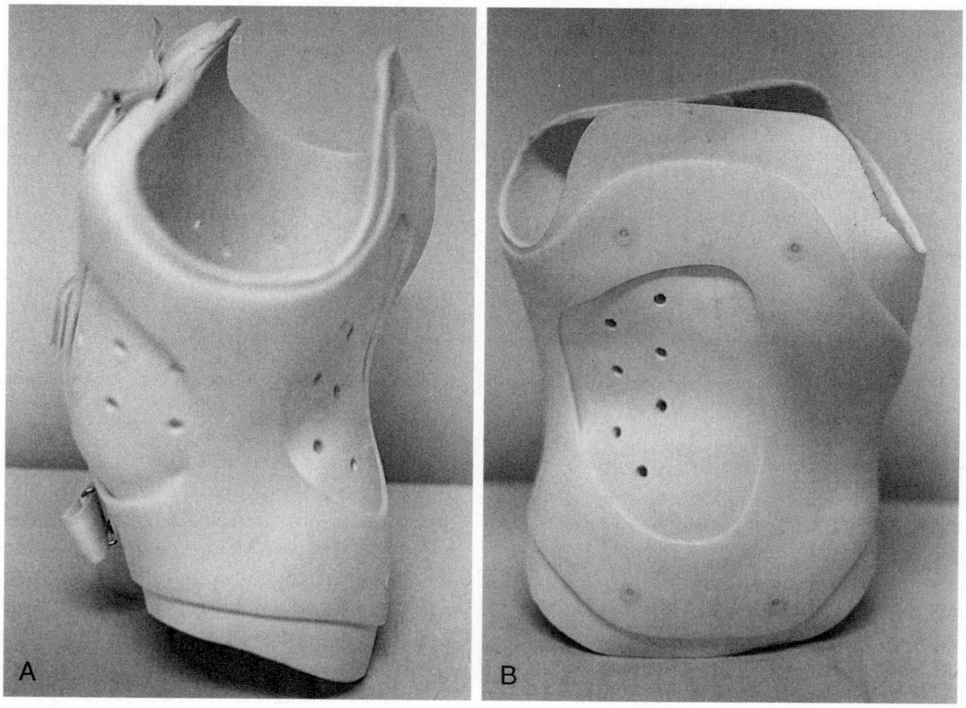

Figure 34-12 ■ Thoracolumbosacral orthosis with anterior opening. A, Lateral view. B, Posterior view. Cutouts in rigid plastic to inner soft foam are for expansion and comfort.

CASE STUDY 34-5 ■ R. B.

R. B. is a 41-year-old woman with spastic diplegic cerebral palsy. She has tight heel cords bilaterally, with −5 degrees from neutral ROM at the ankle. Plantarflexion strength is 3+/5, and dorsiflexion strength is 3/5 bilaterally. The patient has 5 to 7 degrees of varus in the calcaneus. The left lower extremity is asymptomatic. The right side has pain in the midfemur and at the knee. She has a bilateral genu valgum deformity of 5 to 7 degrees (Figure 34-13, *A*). ROM at the knees is full, and strength of the quadriceps and hamstrings is good. Her hips are normal except for some internal rotation; leg lengths are equal and sensation is good.

Because the right lower extremity was painful at the knee and ankle (Figure 34-13, *B*), the patient was fitted with an AFO that extended medially and proximally to the medial tibial condyle; ankle joints that had a posterior adjustment to limit plantarflexion; and a medial heel wedge and heel buildup of $\frac{5}{8}$ inch. The ankle was fitted with a submalleolar orthosis that fit inside the AFO (Figure 34-13, *C* and *D*). The submalleolar orthosis controlled enough pronation of the ankle along with the medial heel wedging and exerted a varus force at the knee (Figure 34-13, *E*). The heel buildup reduced the posteriorly directed force from midstance to toe off. The patient's symptoms were reduced, allowing her to be more active (see Table 34-1).

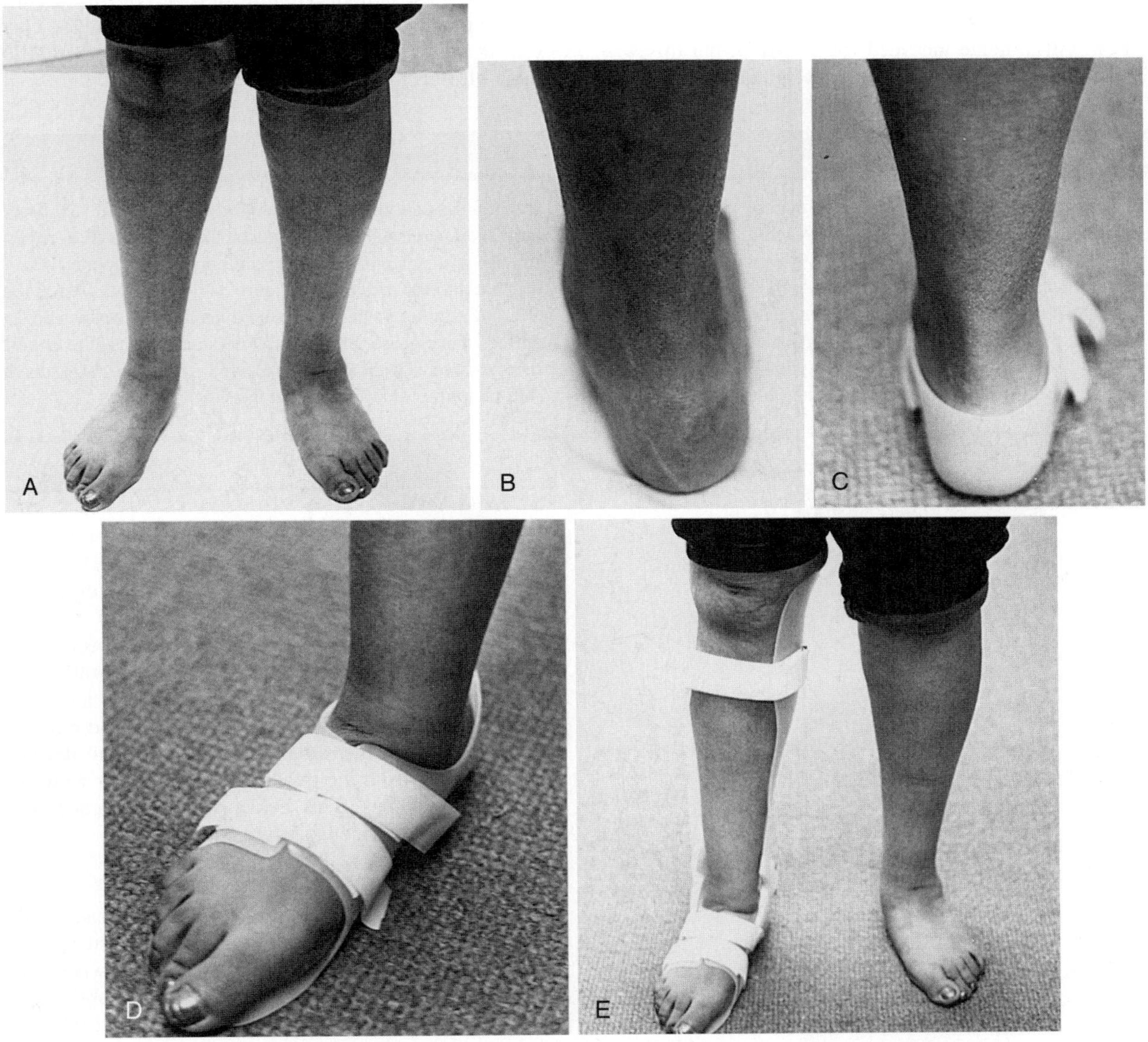

Figure 34-13 ■ **A**, Painful right genu valgus and pronation. **B**, Posterior view of right ankle. **C** and **D**, Client wearing submalleolar orthosis with pronation corrected. **E**, Patient in submalleolar ankle-foot orthosis extended to knee to control genu valgus.

Multiple Sclerosis

As MS progresses and further demyelination occurs, increased interruption of normal nerve impulses creates deficiencies in muscle control, vision, balance, sensation, and mental functions. Orthotic considerations for a patient with MS can vary as the patient's symptoms fade, recur, and change over the years with the disease. Clinical presentation may vary from month to month. Fatigue plays a major role in the symptoms, and the patient's expectations and willingness to use orthotic devices ebb accordingly. Typical patient reaction is reluctance to use any form of ambulatory aid or orthosis until safety is a major issue. Patients and family usually seek help when falls become more frequent. Lack of toe clearance during swing phase and poor knee stability and push off in stance phase are the most common problems that can benefit from orthotic intervention. Because of the nature of symptom fade and recurrence and the increase with fatigue, the weight and simplicity of orthotic intervention must be major considerations. In many instances the evaluation will indicate the need for a KAFO, but this will be rejected by the patient because of its weight and complexity. The benefit of the KAFO for knee stability and foot and ankle control is counteracted by the patient's inability to advance the limb during swing phase and control the extremity, as well as a perception that he or she does not need that type of control. Most patients also will reject the use of a double-upright, double-adjustable metal orthosis for the same reason, and although their strength varies from day to day, they will judge need when they are at their strongest rather than their weakest. Traditionally, plastic AFOs are used to control foot drop and provide some medial and lateral ankle control. These orthoses also can provide some knee stability if the plastic is robust enough and if the medial and lateral trim lines are advanced anteriorly past the malleoli. This anterior force stops the center of gravity's forward progression at midstance, and, again, many patients reject this type of orthosis. The recent development of prefabricated AFOs made of graphite has met the needs of many of these patients (Figure 34-14). This ultralight orthosis fits inside the patient's shoe. It will provide toe clearance during swing phase and some dynamic knee stability and push off during stance phase.

CASE STUDY 34-6 ■ D. K.

D. K. is a 38-year-old mother of three young boys and works outside the home. She was diagnosed with MS at the age of 30. Until 4 years ago she was managing the symptoms with medication and having minimal ambulatory problems. With the birth of her son, she had to cease use of medication, and the symptoms recurred and weakness increased. At age 36 she was limiting her activity outside the home because of safety issues—she was falling and unstable in standing and walking. She was evaluated at that point and was fitted with a right AFO, as she had foot drop and knee instability and lacked the ability to recover her balance if she caught her toe. A prefabricated graphite AFO was fitted to the patient (see Figure 34-14). D. K. now has toe clearance during swing phase and dynamic knee extension during stance phase. Shortly after beginning to use the orthosis, she was able to walk safely on uneven ground and walk down stairs step over step for the first time in 3 years.

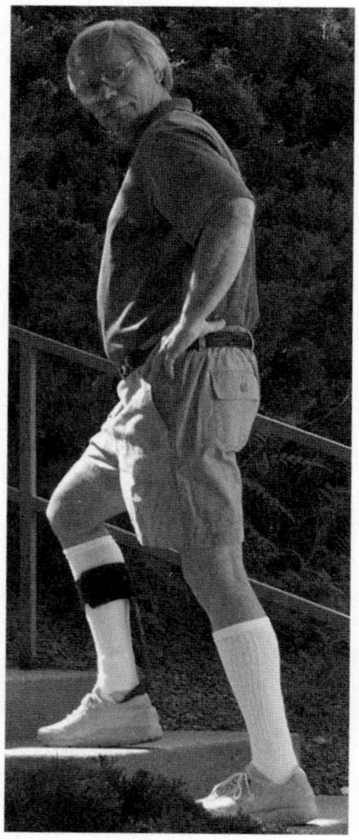

Figure 34-14 ■ Example of an ankle-foot orthosis, which provides stance-phase advantages in addition to swing-phase assistance. (Courtesy of Otto Bock HealthCare.)

SUMMARY

All orthoses create a force system. It is important to understand and integrate the appropriate force to achieve the desired outcome of intervention. A thorough initial evaluation and knowledge of the multiple orthotic options available are vital to reaching treatment goals. There has been a dramatic improvement in material technology, along with far greater access to orthotics and a much wider range of indications for orthotic intervention. This should challenge the rehabilitation team to establish measurable goals and then to develop new goals leading from the treatment interventions with the most effective outcomes. This evidence-based practice will help provide better service for future patients.

References

To enhance this text and add value for the reader, all references are included on the companion Evolve site that accompanies this textbook. This online service will, when available, provide a link for the reader to a Medline abstract for the article cited. There are 8 cited references and other general references for this chapter, with the majority of those articles being evidence-based citations.

CHAPTER 35 Management of Chronic Impairments in Individuals with Nervous System Conditions

MYLA U. QUIBEN, PT, PhD, DPT, GCS, NCS, CEEAA

KEY TERMS

adaptation
aging
fatigue
health promotion
orthotics
postpolio syndrome

OBJECTIVES

After reading this chapter the student or therapist will be able to:

1. Analyze how the aging process may affect people with lifelong functional limitations and challenges in life participation.
2. Analyze the unique challenges faced by people with chronic motor impairments such as those associated with cerebral palsy, genetic malformations, developmental disabilities, postpolio syndrome, spinal cord injury, and traumatic or acquired head injury during the aging process.
3. Evaluate this population of patients/clients with sensitivity and skill, incorporating precautions and effectiveness of interventions.
4. Provide a framework for the examination process for individuals with chronic conditions.
5. Present holistic intervention considerations for individuals with chronic motor impairments.
6. Identify gaps in knowledge and research in the management of aging individuals with chronic neuromuscular conditions.
7. Appreciate the complexity of examination, evaluation, and management of the aging patient with chronic motor impairments.

Improvements in health care delivery, research, medicine, nutrition, and knowledge of health and physical activity have resulted in a new challenge for health care professionals—a growing population of individuals who have sustained and survived an initial injury to the central nervous system (CNS) with resulting secondary impairments and functional limitations and who are now experiencing the added effects of aging.

The aging process typically leads to gradual physiological changes in muscle strength, flexibility, and joint mobility and changes in balance and endurance. Physical activity and a healthy lifestyle have been shown to address age-related changes by delaying the decline and deterioration; however, age-related changes such as osteoarthritis and vascular changes are still likely to occur to varying degrees despite a healthy lifestyle. Healthy but sedentary older individuals report more problems in activities of daily living (ADLs) than do those who continue to be physically active and who previously had an active lifestyle.[1-3]

In an individual with preexisting impairments and functional limitations, the aging process may present new or additional loss of components of functional activities and participation—a new challenge to the individual who may have had the opportunity to successfully participate in life activities in earlier adulthood. Individuals with existing disabilities undergo a similar aging process; however, the typical changes associated with aging are superimposed on the body system problems and functional limitations caused by the initial CNS injury.

In the realm of chronic problems in life participation, individuals who experienced the effects of polio in their younger years give clinicians an enlightening example of the chronic interaction among neurological and functional impairments, recovery, effects of aging, and health care. As a chronic condition, individuals who dealt with polio can teach therapists to reconsider and reevaluate their approach to individuals who are now experiencing activity limitations, impairments, and ineffective postures and movement. The challenges of aging with chronic body system problems or impairments are encountered by individuals who have postpolio syndrome (PPS); those who acquired CNS insult at birth (developmental disabilities including cerebral palsy [CP; see Chapter 12] and Down syndrome [see Chapter 13]); and those who acquired injury through disease or trauma sometime in the life span development process (traumatic brain injury [TBI; see Chapter 24], multiple sclerosis [MS; see Chapter 19], and spinal cord injury [SCI; see Chapter 16]).

The discussion of chronic impairments brings several questions to the forefront:

- What is the course of age-related medical conditions common in individuals with chronic impairments?
- Do age-related conditions vary among the developmental or genetic diseases or among conditions occurring at one point during the life span?
- What are the prevalence and/or incidence of secondary conditions in individuals with chronic impairments?

- Have specific treatment protocols for health provision for this population been identified?
- What is the state of dissemination of information related to aging and health to people affected by these conditions?
- How has the effect of aging with chronic body system problems changed the ability of these individuals to participate in life as well as their perceived quality of life?

As an emerging population, individuals with chronic impairments have not been on the receiving end of research. Much of what is known about nervous system disorders is in the pediatric realm and in the initial stages of care immediately after the initial injury or diagnosis. It is only recently that studies have begun to look at the health care implications of aging with chronic conditions. Therefore, definitive answers to the questions posed previously are still nonexistent or in the early stages of conception. Based on a review of existing literature, the consensus appears to be that there is a dearth of definitive information on the health status and effect of age-related processes among individuals with chronic conditions from developmental or genetic disorders or from injury sustained at one point in the life span such as TBI and MS. Moreover, there is agreement that further evidence-based research is needed in this emerging population.

This chapter aims to provide a holistic view of the management of the chronic problems of individuals with nervous system impairments, with consideration given to the effects of aging and compensation over time. Movement emerges from the interaction among the individual, task, and environment,[4] with several variables and degrees of freedom. Therefore physical therapists (PTs) and occupational therapists (OTs) need to examine and address multisystem impairments and contributions to movement while appreciating the changing dynamics of a highly complex movement system.

DIAGNOSES WITH UNDERLYING CHRONIC CONSEQUENCES

Developmental Conditions

With increasing life expectancy, mainly as a result of innovations in health care, a unique group of individuals with chronic conditions are subject to age-related changes. Individuals with developmental disabilities constitute a growing segment of the aging society. This is a broad topic, in part because of the many conditions that are categorized as developmental disability. According to the Administration on Developmental Disabilities and the Administration for Children and Families,[5] developmental disabilities are severe, chronic functional limitations attributable to mental or physical impairments or a combination of both, that manifest before age 22 years and that are likely to continue indefinitely. These result in substantial limitations in three or more of the following areas: self-care, receptive and expressive language, learning, mobility, self-direction, capacity for independent living, and economic self-sufficiency. These individuals also have a continuous need for individually planned and coordinated services.[6] The definition envelops a wide range of conditions leading to significant and lifelong disabilities. This group includes those with genetic and neurological conditions, two of the more common of which are CP (see Chapter 12) and Down syndrome (DS; see Chapter 13).

The question of whether unexpected changes among people with neurodevelopmental disabilities occur as they age and how these changes compromise functioning with progressive aging is of massive importance with the emergence of a population of individuals with developmental disabilities with increased life expectancy and concurrent increase in older-age–related diseases. According to Heller[7] the number of adults with intellectual and developmental disabilities aged 60 years and older is projected to nearly double from 641,860 in 2000 to 1.2 million by 2030 owing to increasing life expectancy and the aging of the Baby Boomer generation. With the aging of adults with developmental and genetic disorders a new societal issue looms, as individuals with developmental disabilities have a lifelong need for external support. Much is unknown about the long-term effects of aging and maturation in adults with these conditions.

Adults with several types of developmental disabilities have life expectancies similar to those of the general population, excluding adults with particular neurological conditions and with more severe cognitive deficits. Recent studies show the mean age at death ranges from the mid-50s for adults with severe disabilities or DS, to the early 70s for those with mild to moderate intellectual disabilities.[8-10]

Concurrent with an increased life span, some evidence exists that certain individuals with developmental disabilities have experienced an increase in age-related diseases. Of the limited information available, research has shown that aging affects certain genetic and neurologically based intellectual and developmental disabilities that may increase the risk of age-related pathologies and lead to an increased occurrence of coincident conditions.[11] Of several developmental conditions, DS has been the subject of a substantial body of research. DS is known for resulting in advanced aging that includes a higher risk for Alzheimer disease and select organ dysfunctions.[11-13]

Evidence exists that adults with CP, considered a life span disability, lose functional abilities earlier than individuals who are able-bodied.[14] For CP, evidence is also increasingly pointing to specific age-related outcomes such as the effects of deconditioning, limitations with performance reserve, and possibly a shorter life span.[11] In adults with CP, secondary conditions commonly described in research primarily are related to the long-term effects on the musculoskeletal system, such as pain, degenerative joint disease, and osteoporosis.[11,15,16] Secondary impairments in CP can progress subtly and may not appear until late adolescence or adulthood.[15] Age-related health conditions are also seen in other genetic and neurological disorders as the affected individuals age. However, the nature of these risks lacks extensive substantiation in the literature.

Overall, knowledge of adult health issues for older people with developmental disabilities is limited.[7] Several reasons contribute to the lack of knowledge. Limited health care programs exist for this population, likely because this is an emerging population. Most of the existing literature is in the pediatric domain rather than dealing with age-related issues. Although these individuals were likely seen by therapists for various functional limitations throughout their lives, the professional training that health care providers have received regarding the care of these individuals has focused on early childhood and school-aged children. As a result, many adolescents and adults with developmental disabilities have difficulty accessing appropriate health care information regarding secondary conditions resulting from their specific disabilities. Moreover, in general, older individuals with developmental disabilities have more difficulty in finding, accessing, and paying for high-quality health care.[7] Communication difficulties also limit the understanding of the experiences of aging adults with developmental disabilities. Evidence exists, however, showing that obesity and inactivity are more common in individuals with developmental disabilities than in the general population.[17] Bazzano and colleagues[17] identified several reasons for this health discrepancy, including individual and community factors, physical challenges, segregation from the community, lack of accessible fitness facilities and developmentally appropriate community programs, and cognitive deficits.

Given trends of increasing survival and longevity observed among individuals with developmental disabilities, it is sensible to consider a more in-depth look at the aging process among a variety of neurodevelopmental conditions and the need for a holistic approach. Although some literature exists regarding life span changes with these disorders, particularly DS and CP, there is lack of confirming evidence for most of these conditions. Horsman and colleagues[14] advocate for research on the expectations regarding aging for adults with CP, including preventive measures to lessen the effects of secondary impairments. This recommendation applies to developmental life span conditions and other chronic conditions that are subject to age-related changes that may be magnified or made worse by existing impairments and limitations. Evidence-based research is necessary to better understand the long-term effects of aging on adults with developmental and chronic conditions. The challenge then is to provide a holistic examination that involves a multisystem approach and to provide appropriate referrals as necessary to address the multiple needs of individuals with developmental disabilities.

Neurological Conditions Acquired in the Life Span: Spinal Cord Injury, Traumatic Brain Injury, Postpolio Syndrome

In the realm of management of chronic movement dysfunction, PPS—the late effects of polio—becomes a model case for other chronic neuromuscular conditions. There is much to learn from the complex nature of the late effects of polio and the effects of aging on an already stressed system. The cause must be briefly discussed to further understand the possible effects of aging. PPS can affect polio survivors years after recovery from the initial polio infection and is characterized by multifaceted symptoms that lead to decline in physical functioning.[18] PPS manifests with progressive or new muscle weakness or decreased muscle endurance in muscles that were initially affected by the polio infection and in muscles that were seemingly unaffected; generalized fatigue; and pain.[18] The exact cause of PPS remains unknown on the basis of review of the literature. Although it is not clear what exactly causes the new symptoms, there appears to be a consensus that insufficient evidence implicates the reactivation of the previous poliovirus.[19] Underlying causes have been proposed in a variety of hypotheses from several authors, with aging playing a key role.[20-24]

The suggestion that aging contributes to PPS is supported in the literature.[21,25,26] By the fifth decade of life, loss of anterior horn cells begins, and by age 60 years the loss of neurons may be as high as 50%.[27] Age-related changes superimposed on the already limited motor neuron pool after polio appear to be important factors in the development of PPS. With the effects of the normal aging process, the remaining anterior horn cells are further reduced to a point at which the deficits caused by the initial insult cannot be overcome. The loss of even a few neurons from a greatly exhausted neuronal pool potentially results in a disproportionate loss of muscle function.[20,28] The loss of motor neurons from aging alone may not be a considerable factor in PPS because studies[20] have failed to link chronological age and the onset of new symptoms. Rather, it is the length of the interval between the onset of polio and the appearance of new symptoms that seems to be more critical.

Another plausible hypothesis alludes to overuse and fatigue of the already weakened muscles as a factor in the development of new muscle weakness.[19,29,30] A study by Trojan and colleagues[30] provides support to this hypothesis. Their results suggest that length of time since acute polio, joint and muscle pain, physical activity, and weight gain are factors associated with PPS. Years of overuse after recovery from polio causes a metabolic failure leading to an inability to regenerate new axon sprouts. The exact cause of degeneration of axon sprouts is not known. Evidence to support this hypothesis can be inferred from muscle biopsies, electrodiagnostic tests, and clinical response to exercise.[20] McComas and colleagues[31] suggested that neurons that demonstrated histological recovery from the initial virus were possibly not physiologically normal and were potentially vulnerable to premature aging and failure.

Other proposed hypotheses include persistence of dormant poliovirus that was reactivated by unknown mechanisms, an immune-mediated response, hormone deficiencies, and environmental contaminants.[20] Another hypothesis points to the loss of anterior horn cells during the initial polio as a factor.[19,21] Findings from Trojan and colleagues[30] support the hypothesis that the severity of the initial motor unit involvement, seen as weakness in acute polio, is critical in predicting PPS. Individuals at greatest risk for PPS had severe attacks of paralytic polio, although individuals with milder cases also had symptoms.[20] These hypotheses have not been completely examined, and currently the evidence is not strong enough to support any one possible cause. Clinically it is difficult to assume that only one factor causes symptoms. The chronicity of the disease lends weight to the possibility that more than one factor contributes to the individual's symptoms.

Medical practitioners must take into account the effects of existing comorbidities and aging in the examination and management of PPS. The complexity and nonspecificity of symptoms warrant consideration of all possible contributors to the symptoms of PPS. Based on the recent literature, there appears to be some confusion regarding terminology pertaining to PPS. Compounding the general symptoms are the common problems in aging: decreasing muscle strength and endurance, joint problems, and myriad health deficits leading to functional losses. Physiological aging, overuse, and comorbidities play contributory roles in disrupting the state of stability after the initial infection.

McNaughton and McPherson[32] state that the simple descriptive labels "late problems after polio" and "of late deterioration after polio" are less limiting and do not imply a direct link with the previous polio diagnosis. Post-Polio Health International[33] uses the terminology "late effects of polio and polio sequelae" as the most inclusive category. *Late effects of polio* and *polio sequelae* pertain to health problems that are a result of chronic impairments from polio and may include degenerative arthritis from overuse, bursitis, or tendinitis. A subcategory under this heading is PPS leading to decreased endurance and decreased function.

Currently no definitive test exists in the literature to diagnose the late effects of polio or PPS. It remains a diagnosis of exclusion, and as such the diagnostic process for PPS is challenging and may be long. Halstead and Gawne[34] identified cardinal symptoms of PPS as new or increased muscle weakness, fatigue, and muscle and joint pain with neuropathic electromyographic changes in an individual with a definite diagnosis of polio. Diagnostic electromyography (EMG) may be required or used when the muscle pattern or history is atypical.

The criteria most commonly used for establishing a medical diagnosis of PPS were developed by Halstead[35] and are as follows:

1. A confirmed history of paralytic polio in childhood or adolescence
2. Partial to complete muscle strength and functional recovery
3. A period of at least 15 years of neurological and functional stability
4. Onset of two or more new health problems listed in Table 35-1
5. No other medical conditions to explain these new health problems

TABLE 35-1 ■ MOST COMMON NEW HEALTH PROBLEMS IN 132 CONFIRMED POSTPOLIO INDIVIDUALS WITH A DIAGNOSIS OF POSTPOLIO SYNDROME

	NO.	%
HEALTH PROBLEMS		
Fatigue	117	89
Muscle pain	93	71
Joint pain	93	71
Weakness		
Previously affected muscles	91	69
Previously unaffected muscles	66	50
Cold intolerance	38	29
Atrophy	37	28
ADL PROBLEMS		
Walking	84	64
Climbing stairs	80	61
Dressing	23	17

Modified from Halstead L, Wiechers D, editors: *Research and clinical aspects of the late effects of poliomyelitis,* White Plains, NY, 1987, March of Dimes, p 17.
ADL, Activity of daily living.

Dalakas[36] identified additional inclusion criteria in the diagnosis: residual asymmetrical muscle atrophy, with weakness, areflexia, and normal sensation in at least one limb and normal sphincteric function and deterioration of function after a period of functional stability unexplained by primary or secondary condition.

Several individuals who recovered from polio during the early epidemics were encouraged to exercise for years and to use heroic compensatory methods for function. An exhaustive regimen of daily stretching and strengthening, demanding compliance from individuals and their support systems, was strongly encouraged. Orthotics and assistive devices were promoted as a means toward independent mobility. The outcomes of rigorous training were individuals who adapted and compensated with their remaining capabilities. Compensations include use of muscles at high levels of their capacity, substitution of stronger muscles with increased energy expenditure for the task, use of ligaments for stability with resulting hypermobility, and malalignment of the trunk and limbs. With the late effects of polio or a diagnosis of PPS, many of these individuals may have extreme difficulty dealing with these new problems because of the attitude of "working hard" to reeducate weakened muscles and compensate for loss of function after the initial diagnosis.[37-40] The new symptoms of PPS, which limits their motor function and likely impairs established personal and societal roles, require that they not work hard or overexert themselves. These two approaches are contradictory and can leave an individual frustrated and confused over therapeutic recommendations.

Spinal Cord Injury and Traumatic Brain Injury

For persons with SCI and TBI, a trend is seen toward increasing awareness on the effects of aging on the functional status of this group. Owing to medical advances, patients are now living 20 to 50 years past their time of injury. Numerous studies have been done describing quality-of-life issues for people with TBI; however, those studies seldom look specifically at changes in functional levels or what can be done to ameliorate the declines.[41-43]

McColl and colleagues,[44] studying the impact of aging on people after SCI, have identified major categories of problems related to aging, such as musculoskeletal problems and joint, sensory, and connective tissue changes; chronic urinary tract infections; heart, respiratory, and other chronic diseases; secondary complications of the initial lesions, such as syringomyelia; and problems related to social and cultural acceptance and access or barriers. Evidence on specific age-related changes is presented in the section on examination.

Decreases in perceived health status and in functional abilities with increases in additional assistance for ADLs have been documented for aging individuals with SCI.[45-49] In a study of 150 people aging with an SCI, nearly 25% reported decreases in the ability to perform functional activities that they had been able to handle after the acute rehabilitation phase. The subjects who reported decreases in functional ability were generally older (45 years compared with 36 years) and had longer postinjury periods (18 versus 11 years). The most common symptoms reported by the individuals with decreases in functional status were related to fatigue, pain, and muscle weakness. The ADLs reported to be more difficult were transfers, bathing, and dressing. To maintain their functional levels, those with declines in functional ability reported needing additional equipment.[45]

The need for further assistance with ADLs was echoed in a study by Gerhart and colleagues of individuals with SCI 20 years after the initial injury.[46] The study showed that 22% of the subjects reported an increased need for support with ADLs. Compared with a general group of nondisabled men and women aged 75 to 84 years in which 78% of the men and 64% of women did not need help with ADLs, the population of persons with SCI needed increasing support to remain independent, and the need for help occurred at a younger age. On average, those with quadriplegia required more help with ADLs around the age of 49 years, whereas those with paraplegia were able to maintain their functional level until age 54 years. The groups showing functional decreases reported greater fatigue, increased muscle weakness, pain, stiffness, and weight gain.[46] Other studies support the findings that 5, 10, and 15 years after the initial SCI, an association with the need for additional help with increasing age existed.[47]

Liem and colleagues,[48] referencing an international data set of people with SCI, investigated a subset of 352 people at least 20 years after their injury. Thirty-two percent of the subjects reported needing increased help with transfers and housework compared with their functional abilities at acute hospital discharge. With increasing age, women had a higher incidence of reported musculoskeletal impairments, which may have been related to biomechanical differences between men and women (e.g., 40% lower upper body strength).

In addition to the need for ADL support, neurogenic bowel and bladder symptoms also worsen with age in some people with SCIs. With changes in general health status, polypharmacy, decreased activity, and poor nutritional patterns, bowel problems (particularly constipation) become more of an issue. Although constipation seems like a minor issue relative to paralysis, those with SCIs report significant abdominal distention and pain, an increased incidence of perineal and sacral skin breakdown, and in some cases autonomic dysreflexia. In addition to the discomfort of chronic bowel dysfunctions, the required bowel care programs may take more time, which can lead to increased psychosocial issues associated with anxiety about bowel accidents in social and work situations and may take time away from social activities for both the person with an SCI and the caregiver. For those with continuing bowel problems that interfere with life and work activities, a colostomy may be an option that increases independence from caregiver support during the bowel program.[50] Another complicating factor related to bowel dysfunction is the typical treatment for pain complaints. Because the origin of pain is often illusive, the most common treatment involves oral medications rather than referrals for therapeutic interventions. Pain medications, especially opioids, increase gastrointestinal difficulties in nondisabled populations,[51] and the problem for patients with SCI is compounded.

Charlifue and colleagues,[52] drawing on the National Spinal Cord Injury Database of 7981 individuals with SCIs that occurred from 1973 to 1998, found a slight decrease in perceived health status the longer one lived after SCI. Evidence was also found that those injured later in life had a higher number of rehospitalizations after injury than those injured at a younger age. Despite palpable problems with the statistical issues within the sample, the study clearly indicated that the best predictor of a complication is a previous history of that complication. On the basis of their results, Charlifue and colleagues[52] suggest that prevention of complications is the best approach to improve quality of health and quality of life for people aging with SCI.

Individuals with TBI are often neglected by professional health care and insurance providers after the acute rehabilitation period. According to Levin,[53] before 1980, individuals with brain injuries were considered "dead on arrival." Persons who would have died from the TBI several decades ago are now living into old age and are coping with the changes caused by the aging process superimposed on their physical limitations and cognitive problems. Of great concern is the possible relationship between a history of brain injury and increased cognitive changes along the dementia continuum.[54] Cognitive decline in the nondisabled population is a problem, but the additive effect for a person with a previous TBI may seriously impair the person's coping mechanisms when dealing with his or her own health and self-care needs.[55]

Extensive work has been done on rehabilitation programs and quality-of-life issues related to head injury and, to a lesser extent, cerebral vascular accidents.[56] (See Chapters 23 and 24 for interventions for head injury and hemiplegia.) Unfortunately, the focus of rehabilitation after a TBI has been on the acute and rehabilitation stages of treatment and not the chronic problems that follow this group of patients into their older years. As with other chronic conditions, few patients see a therapist after they are discharged from rehabilitation unless they have new acute events such as musculoskeletal problems or a medical condition that causes a change in functional status.

Although TBI is a lifetime disability, little attention has been paid to the needs of aging persons with a TBI who may have recurring needs for physical and cognitive rehabilitation and retraining over the life span. Individuals who sustain a TBI in the older years will likely have different needs from those injured at a younger age. In a study on the effect of age on functional outcome in mild TBI, Mosenthal and colleagues[57] found that those injured later in life (after age 60) had longer inpatient rehabilitation periods and lagged behind younger patients in functional status at the point of discharge; however, similar to the younger individuals who sustained a head injury, the over-60 individuals showed measurable improvement during the 6-month study period. Therefore, aggressive management of older patients with TBI is recommended, and older patients may require continuing management owing to the overlying issues of the aging process.[57] This is echoed in the National Institutes of Health (NIH) consensus document on the treatment of people with TBI, which suggests that specialized interdisciplinary treatment programs need to be put in place to deal with the medical, rehabilitation, family, and social needs of people with TBIs who are over the age of 65 years. The document also concludes that access to and funding for long-term rehabilitation is necessary to meet long-term needs; however, it recognizes that changes in payment methods by private insurance and public programs may jeopardize the recommendations.[58]

Although the authors of the NIH document recognize the need to deal with the aging processes associated with TBI, there continues to be a lack of services and trained professionals available, especially at the community level.[59] As with the SCI population, work is now being done to investigate the relationships among TBI, aging, and health. Breed and colleagues[60] found that older individuals with TBI were more likely than their age-matched nondisabled peers to report metabolic, endocrine, sleep, pain, muscular, or neurological and psychiatric problems. Their findings support those of Hibbard and colleagues[61] and Beetar and colleagues,[62] which suggest that medical personnel need to be prepared to treat a broad range of health issues in the aging TBI population. Fewer of the studies on long-term outcomes and issues in TBI extend to the 10- and 15-year postinjury periods that have been examined for patients with SCIs. In studies 5 years after the initial TBI, improvements in physical and social functions were noted in most areas for at least the first 2 years after injury, with the exception that those with a history of alcohol or drug abuse did less well. One could assume that continued abuse of alcohol or drugs would bode ill for individuals aging with a TBI.[63] In one study of 946 children and adolescents who sustained a TBI, Strauss and colleagues[64] found that patients with severe and permanent mobility and feeding deficits had higher mortality rates, with a 66% chance of surviving to age 50 years. In contrast, survivors with fair or good mobility had a life expectancy only 3 years shorter than that of the general population. However, because both severely and mildly injured individuals with a TBI can live well into and beyond their 50s, the impact of aging on the physical and cognitive deficits must be dealt with assertively to prevent superimposed disability.

Because aging individuals with an SCI or a TBI may have health problems similar to those of any aging population, primary impairments in muscle strength and endurance may be magnified. Therefore individuals with these chronic conditions who make repeat visits regarding medical problems such as musculoskeletal, cardiac, respiratory, and renal diseases should be referred for a comprehensive therapy examination and program that focuses on education, lifestyle changes, and health and wellness promotion interventions.

EXAMINATION OF INDIVIDUALS WITH CHRONIC IMPAIRMENTS

Estimates of the U.S. Department of Health and Human Services indicate that 40 to 54 million Americans have some type of chronic condition or disability.[65,66] Conditions are diverse and may be related to trauma or chronic conditions such as MS.[66] Trends of increasing survival and longevity are now being observed among individuals with chronic conditions as they experience aging processes. It is timely to consider how to manage individuals with chronic impairments.

Examination of individuals with chronic impairments and disabilities is challenging to say the least. Not only are the impairments and functional limitations diverse, but the combinations of these impairments and limitations are many and unique to each individual owing to societal, personal health, environmental, and psychological considerations. Moreover, the effects of aging will likely affect individuals differently depending on existing impairments, functional limitations, current health status, and each individual's attitude toward health and maintaining their functional status and lifestyle. This entails a more thorough, methodical, multisystem examination with a meticulous health interview and wellness model (see Chapter 2).

EXAMINATION: SYSTEMS MODEL

Aging with existing neuromuscular disorders, be it from a late-onset pathology or from a developmental condition, is a challenge for both the individual and the health care professional. There is a small body of literature on the later-life complications of early-onset acquired disabilities. Several problems may result from complex interactions among physical, medical, environmental, behavioral, and psychosocial factors.

Aging may confound late-onset symptoms or magnify the deficits from the initial CNS insult. With the trend of increasing longevity and survival rates from improvements in health care, it is necessary to look at how the health care provider approaches the examination of individuals with chronic impairments and activity limitations. As individuals with chronic neuromusculoskeletal impairments age, there will be an increasing number of comorbidities, and sorting out the cause of each new symptom will be increasingly complicated.

Bottomley[67] identifies essential components of a comprehensive geriatric assessment as psychosocial, functional, mental, and social health elements. These components are applicable to individuals with chronic neuromuscular impairments, who with aging are experiencing new symptoms or a magnification of preexisting impairments. Box 35-1 shows a sample examination template for this population.

BOX 35-1 ■ EXAMINATION PROFILE FOR CHRONIC NEUROMUSCULAR IMPAIRMENTS

Examination: Systems Model

- Examination guidelines
- Health history
- Systems review
- Tests and measures
  - Musculoskeletal: strength, range of motion, and muscle length
  - Balance and coordination
  - Pain
  - Tone
  - Cardiovascular functioning
  - Integumentary
  - Mobility
  - Posture
  - Sensory deficits
  - Sleep
  - Temperature intolerance
  - Psychosocial considerations
  - Functional assessment

Challenges of Examination of Individuals with Chronic Conditions

Assessment of individuals with chronic nervous system conditions is challenging because of the diversity of impairments, the nonspecific nature of symptoms, and the complex interaction of several factors, including the heterogeneous effects of aging. Depending on their underlying health conditions, individuals with chronic conditions may have higher risks than others of developing preventable health problems.[66] In comparing nondisabled individuals with persons with disabilities, Iezzoni[68] found that the latter group is much more likely to have higher obesity and overweight rates and higher rates of depression, anxiety, and stress. Twenty-seven percent of adults with major physical and sensory impairments are obese, compared with 19% of those without major impairments.[68] Thirty-four percent of individuals with major difficulties in walking reported frequent depression or anxiety compared with 3% among those without disabilities.[68] Information on predisposition to conditions such as these is important for the health care provider during the health interview and examination process.

The examination of individuals with chronic impairments presents a different challenge than examining patients or clients with acute diagnoses. For both cohorts, the task of the health care provider is to determine the effect of the active pathology on the varied systems and function. However, for the individual with chronic impairments, an added challenge exists such that the impact of the active pathology is viewed with the underlying preexisting deficits in function and/or impairments that may leave the individual with a narrow margin for health.

Individuals with developmental and genetic disabilities and with conditions acquired through diseases or trauma sometime in the life span development have activity limitations and participation restrictions that are diverse and unique to each individual. Therefore some individuals may have higher risks than others of developing certain preventable health problems or may be more susceptible to developing secondary conditions owing to the long-term effects of the primary impairments from the original health condition.

The absence of specific medical diagnostic tests adds to the dilemma, as does the continuing uncertainty of the underlying cause and the lack of curative intervention. Health care professionals' limitations in knowledge of age-related medical disorders that are common in people with these conditions, including the prevalence and incidence of medical conditions with neurodevelopment disabilities also add to the complexity. Box 35-2 provides several important pointers for examining this population of patients and clients.

The individual with chronic impairments who is currently facing an active pathology likely has adapted to his or her existing system impairments and activity limitations. Depending on their underlying health conditions, some individuals with chronic conditions may have higher risks than others of developing preventable health problems.[66] Thus, from an examination viewpoint, the critical task of the health care provider is determining what new changes to the individual's current abilities and disabilities have been brought on by the active pathology. These changes will likely affect the current functional abilities (e.g., mobility, ADLs), as will preexisting system impairments such as deficits in strength and endurance, pain, and so on. Regardless of the level of deficit, these individuals have some prior knowledge of deficits that affect function, which may help or may hinder their willingness to participate.

BOX 35-2 ■ EXAMINATION POINTERS

- Comprehensive: A systems approach to address the number, complexity, and diversity of the deficits is a must. Essential components are physical, functional, mental, and social health.
- Interdisciplinary: Consideration for the functional, medical, vocational, and psychosocial issues warrants a coordinated evaluation of a team versed in addressing the unique needs of individuals with chronic neuromusculoskeletal conditions and disabilities.
- Patient/client centered: Factors that influence performance, such as fatigue, must be considered during the examination. Recognition of the individual's and family's values and goals is essential.
- Thorough: Assessment may take several hours and extend for two to four visits[232,233] to better integrate the evaluation process and allow the patient to fully participate, contend with the recommendations, and engage in long-term management.

On the other hand, for the patient/client who has been otherwise healthy and functional and now has an acute diagnosis, active pathology may bring on impairments and limitations that are "new" experiences to the individual. The level of education should thus be adapted to the individual, and education performed on a case-by-case basis.

Moreover, the psychosocial aspect of a new pathology and its effect on function may be very different in an individual who has dealt with chronic impairments and limitations versus one who has been active up until the disease process. As with the level of education, the health care provider's approach to a patient/client should always be professional and respectful, with open lines of communication and active listening.

PTs may develop diagnostic focuses regarding functional limitations different from those of OTs. These variances depend on the functional activity limitations identified by the patient and the professional.[69,70] An example of the physical therapy diagnostic process can be found in Appendix 35-A.

It is critical for the clinician to examine all possible contributors to symptoms reported by the individual with chronic impairments. A thorough review of systems may identify symptoms that are related to the primary medical diagnoses, but equally important, it may identify symptoms that are associated with one or more existing comorbidities that have developed over time since the initial nervous system insult.

Health History

Therapists typically collect health history information as part of a comprehensive examination. The history information along with the symptom investigation and review of systems and physical examination will provide guidance in the differential diagnosis process (see Chapters 7 and 8) and in the choice of examination and intervention techniques.

The information from the history will be useful in determining the possible cause of current difficulties or symptoms for which the patient/client is now seeking intervention (Box 35-3). Fatigue or pain may be present from unnecessary and inefficient movement strategies or from high levels of activity. Information on the habitual sleeping, sitting, standing, and walking postures along with ineffective use of devices may alert the clinician to possible factors contributing to the patient's current symptoms or difficulties.

Systems Review

A systems approach to the examination is essential because individuals with chronic conditions have a multitude of possible impairments with superimposed age-related conditions. This situation is best illustrated when examining individuals with PPS. The patient presentation in this condition is a complex interaction of all systems along with the effects of aging, previous interventions, and environmental, psychosocial, and medical aspects of care. The initial diagnosis of polio, which is critical in the diagnostic criteria, will need to be established. This may be difficult because approximately 10% to 15% of individuals who were believed to have or were diagnosed with polio did not have it, and some individuals with mild weakness were diagnosed as having nonparalytic polio.[35,71]

Boissonnault[72] discusses the review of systems as a vital component in the PT's role in medical screening and differential diagnosis (see Chapter 7). OTs are responsible for this same vital component. Possible multisystem involvement warrants review of all systems to determine if current problems are associated with existing comorbid conditions or occult disease or are indeed late manifestations of the initial disease process, as in the case of polio.

BOX 35-3 ■ COMPONENTS OF PATIENT/CLIENT HISTORY

- Demographics, include body mass index
- Growth and developmental history (particularly in those diagnosed with developmental disabilities and those with acquired diagnoses such as polio in childhood or spinal cord injury as an adolescent)
- Past medical-surgical history: include information on interventions and outcomes from initial diagnosis
- Family medical history: critical in ruling out possible contributors to symptoms such as pain from rheumatoid arthritis; critical for possible genetic contributor to original diagnoses
- Social and vocational history: include work status, modifications to work or home environment, and support system
- Living environment: include adaptive equipment, modifications done or necessary to home
- General current health status
- Current functional status, activity level, and perceived quality of life

Providing further substantiation for the need for a methodical and multisystem approach are findings of high rates of secondary conditions related to obesity and inactivity common in individuals with developmental disabilities. These secondary conditions include type 2 diabetes, cardiovascular disease, and metabolic syndrome, diagnoses that affect multiple systems.[17] Individuals with developmental disabilities also have four to six times the preventable mortality of the general population.[9,73] As therapists are entering into the decade of becoming primary care providers, anyone with a preexisting functional problem may walk into a PT or OT clinic searching for help. The importance of medical screening cannot be overemphasized.

The nonspecificity of symptoms seen in individuals with chronic movement dysfunction lends credibility to the need for review of all body systems. Fatigue, for example—a symptom frequently seen in individuals with chronic conditions of MS and PPS among others—is associated with several systems, such as endocrine, nervous, psychological, and cardiopulmonary involvement.

Tests and Measures

Through system assessment by the PT and/or OT, each individual with chronic movement problems should have an opportunity to participate in development of a unique clinical profile. This profile should reflect the strengths and limitations of that individual. Simultaneously these data should aid both the patient and the therapist in identifying realistic treatment goals and selecting the most appropriate intervention strategies. The choice of outcome measures will depend on the individual's current functional skills, the medical status, and the desires and expectations of the individual. Because the severity of symptoms is variable and nonspecific, the clinician is strongly urged to perform a thorough examination and take into consideration factors that may influence performance specific to that individual's functional impairment problems, such as fatigue and pain.

Critical to the examination process is the determination of secondary conditions. Secondary conditions have been defined as injuries, body system impairments, functional limitations, or disabilities that occur as a result of a primary condition or pathology[15,74-78] as well as physical problems that were caused by small insults to one of the body systems not related to the primary condition. Musculoskeletal problems account for many of these secondary conditions; thus the musculoskeletal examination is of critical importance in individuals with developmental disabilities. Gajdosik and Cicerello[77] outlined numerous conditions that may affect the adult with CP; some can lead to significant loss in function and pain from complications such as fractures and osteoporosis. Other musculoskeletal conditions, including scoliosis, subluxations, dislocations, patella alta, foot deformities, pelvic obliquities, and contractures, further complicate the life progression of an adult with developmental disabilities.[77] Frequently these chronic conditions may have their origins in childhood, but because of the lack of sensory awareness may go undetected until later adolescence, adulthood, or well into advancing age when the body no longer has the ability to compensate for these abnormal biomechanical forces. Furthermore, as the aging process progresses, less regeneration of damaged tissue occurs, leading to greater cumulative trauma in joints and other load-sensitive structures.[78] Again, these conditions need to be closely monitored over time to ensure appropriate intervention, optimizing an individual's function and minimizing damage to various tissues.

Fatigue

Fatigue is one of the most common symptoms reported by individuals with chronic conditions such as PPS[79] and MS.[80] Movement and performance of daily activities are more energy consuming for individuals with disabilities and may cause greater fatigue.[81] Evidence also points to individuals with disabilities aging faster than those without disabilities; cardiovascular data from individuals with SCI indicate that persons with SCI may age faster than those without SCI.[82,83] Cook and colleagues[81] identified the lack of age-specific general population norms as an obstacle in the understanding and estimation of the influence of aging on the fatigue of individuals with neuromuscular conditions.

It is likely that that an earlier increase in fatigue with age might be observed in other chronic neuromuscular conditions; however, the effects of chronological age on fatigue in individuals with disabilities are not entirely clear.[81] In a recent study, Cook and colleagues[81] assessed fatigue and age in four clinical populations of individuals with PPS, SCI, MS, and muscular dystrophy (MD), comparing self-reported fatigue experience in different age cohorts with age-matched, U.S. population norms. A total of 1836 surveys were used in data analysis.

The authors concluded that individuals with disabilities reported higher levels of fatigue than the general U.S. population, regardless of age or disability type.[81] Interestingly, the authors noted that the causes of fatigue likely vary by disability type—that is, MS, PPS, and MD are more likely to cause fatigue through a combination of central neurological processes, the effect of sleep disorders such as periodic limb movements (PLMs),[84] or increased physical effort, whereas in SCI fatigue may be a side effect of medications or result from sleep disorders.[81]

Results revealed not only that individuals with disabilities have a higher risk of experiencing fatigue than those without disabilities, but also that the risk for increased fatigue, compared with normative values, increases with age.[81] The reported mean fatigue levels were the highest observed in older PPS age cohorts among the disability samples. In the MS group, fatigue was higher than in any other clinical group except PPS. The highest fatigue reported in the MS sample was in the 35- to 44-year-old age cohort, with lower fatigue in older cohorts except for those 75 years of age and older, but the older group had a small sample size. In the SCI group, peak reported fatigue was in the 55- to 64-year-old age cohort. The results for the SCI group younger than 55 years old were very similar to those for the general population.[81]

In the general population, very little change in fatigue levels for most adults was found moving from young (65 years) to middle (75 years) old age, whereas in the disability samples the authors saw a slight but consistent increase toward greater fatigue at this point in the life span.[81] This increase in fatigue could be associated with current physical decline associated with disease progression.[81] The authors concluded that more research is needed to determine the specific effects of fatigue on the functioning of persons aging with disabilities and to further explore interventions that may shield against or reduce any negative effects that occur.[81]

Bruno and colleagues[79] state that fatigue has been identified as the most commonly reported, most debilitating, and least studied symptom in the postpolio sequelae. Generalized fatigue is typically described as overwhelming exhaustion or flulike aching accompanied by marked changes in level of energy, endurance, and mental alertness.[20] The lack of energy with minimal activity is often described as "hitting a wall," thus the term "polio wall." Polio survivors differentiated between the fatigue associated with weakness and a "central fatigue" that leads to attention and cognitive problems.[79] Severe fatigue affects not only physical function but mental function as well—hence the controversial suggestion that the fatigue associated with postpolio is caused by impaired brain function rather than the diffuse degeneration of motor units and motor junctions.[79]

Descriptors for fatigue associated with PPS are significantly different.[85] The fatigue of PPS may not appear at the time of the activity, and recovery does not occur with typical rest periods. It has also been described as a sudden and total wipeout. In a few instances headaches and sweating appear, suggestive of autonomic nervous system overload.[86] Fatigue commonly occurs in the late afternoon or early evening. Fatigue that tends to last all day is atypical in PPS[35] and should alert the therapist to consider other possible diagnoses.

Similar to the fatigue of PPS, MS fatigue profoundly disrupts multiple aspects of general well-being.[80] Krupp[87] reported that 67% of individuals with MS reported fatigue as a major limiting factor in their social and occupational responsibilities compared with no reports in healthy adults. The fatigue of MS is unique in that it is exacerbated by heat, as are many MS symptoms. Fatigue may be acute, chronic, or intermittent or persistent, whether related to a specific diagnosis such as MS, CP, or polio or having no relation to the initial medical diagnosis. It is necessary to consider the role of other symptoms related to the specific medical diagnosis during the examination of fatigue.

The evaluation of fatigue includes the various factors that can induce or worsen fatigue. The history and examination also are used to assess for new medical diagnoses or the possibility of infection, an impending relapse, heat exposure (in the case of MS), and side effects from medications.

Differential diagnoses for fatigue are extensive and may include disorders of several systems, including psychological, cardiopulmonary, neurological, and endocrine disorders, and medication use. Specific conditions that may cause fatigue include depression, myasthenia gravis, hyperparathyroidism, congestive heart failure, sleep apnea, cancer, and infections. Numerous medications commonly used in symptom management can cause fatigue, including antispasticity agents, tricyclic antidepressants, and β-blockers. The challenge is to differentiate the fatigue caused by typical activities from the fatigue of chronic conditions.

Pain

Individuals with chronic diseases often have pain as a common symptom, most likely from long-term atypical biomechanical forces on joints and muscles or from long-standing disease processes. Many developmental disabilities have a component of disordered movement, from hypomobility in the case of DS to hypermobility in the case of spastic CP. These abnormal joint stresses and strains cause long-term damage to the musculoskeletal system.[77,88,89] The natural degradation of joint structures with aging coupled with weakness and atypical ground reaction forces leads to higher incidence of musculoskeletal pain.[90-92] Please refer to Chapter 32 for additional discussion of pain.

Pain that occurs with chronic conditions may be muscular or it may be joint related, or both. The source of pain needs to be considered because pain may limit the individual's functional abilities and lead to further decline. Muscle pain is often described as a deep, aching pain similar to the pain experienced during the initial infection. The pain is frequently aggravated by physical activity, stress, and cold temperature. Pain is unusual in that it does not occur at the time of activity but rather 1 to 2 days after a precipitating event.

Joint pain in itself usually results primarily from long-term microtrauma from abnormal biomechanical forces. An example might be the overuse of the shoulder girdle muscles and joint from a lifetime of use of Loftstrand crutches to compensate for lower-extremity impairments after polio. Joint pain is frequently associated with physical activity but is rarely associated with inflammation. Interventions are complicated by the presence of osteoporosis, lack of compensatory substitutions to rest the injured part, and, often, poor response to exercise. Failing joint fusions, uneven limb size, progressive scoliosis, poor posture, and abnormal mechanics may also contribute to pain.[93]

Although pain is not a hallmark of many chronic conditions such as DS and MS, it may occur in some individuals with long-term impairments and thus should be part of a comprehensive examination. Pain frequently associated with MS is related to postural problems and inefficient use of muscles and joints to compensate for loss of function or spasticity.

More than 65% of individuals with PPS have reported neck, shoulder, and back pain radiating to the hip and leg.[94] This pain is expected because the incidence of major postural abnormalities and gait deviations is also high, as shown in Table 35-1.

Differential diagnosis for acute muscle and joint pain includes consideration of chronic musculoskeletal conditions leading to wear and tear and disorders with significant muscle or joint manifestations. The list is extensive and may include osteoarthritis, tendinitis, bursitis, fibromyalgia, rheumatoid arthritis, and polymyalgia rheumatica. The challenge is determining whether muscle or joint pain occurs from long-term wear and tear or from an acute or exacerbating occurrence.

Strength

Examination of strength is another critical component of the examination of individuals with chronic impairments. Long-standing weakness is an expected occurrence from decreased physical activity common in individuals with disabilities and chronic diseases. Strength deficits may result from several causes other than disuse such as upper motor neuron weakness, fatigue, compensatory movements, pain, or spasticity. It is likely, however, that aging individuals with chronic conditions have adapted to the initial weakness associated with their diagnoses, as in the case of people with SCI or PPS who have led productive and functional lives since the initial diagnosis or acute onset.

Typical aging involves the losses of muscle strength, loss of power, and sarcopenia—processes that may intensify or build on the initial losses of strength. Delineation of weakness from age-related processes versus weakness as part of the disease process or that from lack of physical activity common in people with chronic impairments is difficult if not impractical from both research and clinical perspectives. Too many variables need to be controlled and accounted for unless specific muscle groups were examined initially and the findings well documented, which may have been the case for people with PPS. Many individuals with PPS have extreme difficulty dealing with these new problems because they were taught that hard work was the only way to correct physical problems that followed acute polio. These new problems, which also limit motor function, require that these individuals not work hard. These two concepts are contradictory and can leave an individual frustrated and confused over therapeutic recommendations.

Manual muscle testing of the entire body, although time-consuming, may be necessary to determine the muscular involvement. Muscle testing, however, may not always reveal the full extent of muscle involvement, and functional assessment may provide a better picture of individuals' potential and true difficulties. Performance and participation in daily activities will provide a better picture of a person's strengths and impairments. Therefore, current functional activities are critical in determining whether current mobility difficulties are related to the aging process, represent an exacerbation of initial disease processes such as in PPS, or are signs and symptoms of new medical concerns.

Weakness and Postpolio Syndrome. Weakness may occur in both previously affected and clinically unaffected muscles; however, it is primarily prominent in muscles most severely affected in the initial infection.[35] It is typically asymmetrical and may be proximal, distal, or patchy.[93] Weakness is primarily observed in repetitive and stabilizing contractions rather than with single maximum efforts. The decreased ability of the muscles to recover rapidly after contracting may be a factor. Recovery of quadriceps muscle strength after fatiguing exercise was significantly less in symptomatic PPS subjects compared with asymptomatic and control subjects.[95] Overuse of muscles in relation to their limited capacity has long been associated with these new problems.[96-98] New weakness and atrophy have been attributed to metabolic overload of the giant motor units, with more pruning of muscle fibers than axon sprouting.[99,100]

New muscle involvement may also cause signs and symptoms such as muscle fasciculations, cramps, atrophy, and elevation of muscle enzymes in the blood. Yet many of these physical signs and symptoms are also present in other neuromuscular problems such as amyotrophic lateral sclerosis (ALS; see Chapter 17). Fasciculations occur at rest and during contraction and tend to persist even when muscle pain and fatigue have been resolved. Muscle cramps are common in fatigued muscles and are alleviated by decreased activity. The new weakness may or may not be accompanied by atrophy. New postpolio muscular atrophy of muscles is sometimes reported. It is very noticeable when it occurs in the gastrocnemius or the anterior tibialis owing to the effect on everyday ambulation. Elevation of muscle enzymes, indicative of muscle damage, has been found in individuals with PPS and has been related to the intensity of work.[97,101,102]

Gross muscle testing may mask the true involvement because several muscles that were initially believed to be uninvolved were truly subclinically affected by polio. The pattern of definitive manual test findings (spotty, flaccid, and asymmetrical paresis or paralysis) is also used to confirm the initial polio diagnosis.

Several polio survivors are able to function at high levels of activity with few strong muscle groups as a result of the random, diffuse nature of the motor deficits and the body's ability to compensate with uncommon muscle and joint function. This delicate balance may be maintained for years, and a disruption from late-onset weakness of a significant muscle group can lead to disproportionate functional losses.

Superimposed pathological problems have been proposed as a possible cause of the later exhibition of new signs and symptoms in postpolio survivors. Several conditions may contribute to weakness, including arthritis, fibromyalgia, deconditioning from disuse, and coronary heart disease.[103]

Range of Motion and Muscle Length

Limitations in joint motion from muscle contractures and from shortening of ligamentous joint structures are common in individuals with chronic disabilities. Likewise, hypermobile joints may also result from compensatory techniques forcing more mobility. An evaluation of the individual's activity levels and goals is vital before intervening with muscle and joint deficits. In some instances during the convalescent stage of the initial diagnoses, as in polio or SCI, selective tightness was allowed to give some stability to joints with paralyzed muscles. In addition, the body may develop useful contractures to maintain or regain function. The presence of spasticity, particularly in severe cases, may have also contributed to the development of contractures in older adults with CP, SCI, MS, or TBI. Before making attempts to stretch contractures, therapists should carefully evaluate the functions that may be lost if gains in range of motion (ROM) are achieved. Equally important is to evaluate what functions would be gained and what the cost would be. Consider that after 20 to 40 years these contractures resist any significant elongation, and aggressive intervention may cause more harm and loss of function.

Box 35-4 lists the secondary conditions that may develop in an individual with CP. These impairments not only cause pain but also limit mobility and interfere with performance of ADLs and leisure activities. Thus a thorough evaluation of musculoskeletal status and periodic monitoring are imperative to maintaining quality of life and social participation for these individuals.

BOX 35-4 ■ SECONDARY CONDITIONS DEVELOPED BY INDIVIDUALS WITH CEREBRAL PALSY

PATHOLOGICAL CONDITIONS
- Fractures
- Osteoporosis
- Cardiovascular disorders
- Degenerative joint disease
- Spinal cord compression
- Dental problems
- Seizures
- Pulmonary dysfunction

IMPAIRMENTS
- Constipation
- Contractures
- Depression
- Emaciation
- Obesity
- Incontinence (bowel and bladder)
- Pain
- Ulcers
- Dysphagia
- Gastrointestinal problems
- Low self-esteem
- Nerve entrapments
- Overuse syndrome
- Balance problems

FUNCTIONAL LIMITATIONS OR ACTIVITY RESTRICTIONS
- Inability to indicate toileting needs
- Dependence on others for activities of daily living
- Limitations in mobility
- Difficulties using public transportation

DISABILITIES OR LIMITATIONS IN LIFE PARTICIPATION
- Difficulties living independently
- Limited recreational opportunities
- Problems with social relationships and intimacy
- Social isolation
- Difficulty with role as patient when medical professionals fail to make accommodations for treatment
- Underemployment

Modified from Gajdosik CG, Cicerello N: Secondary conditions of the musculoskeletal system in adolescents and adults with cerebral palsy, *Phys Occup Ther Pediatr* 21:49-68, 2001.

Tone

Examination of tone is a focal component of the examination of individuals with chronic neuromuscular conditions. This group of individuals may demonstrate a wide range of tone deficits from hypotonia seen with DS, to hypertonicity seen in persons with TBI, SCI, MS, or CP, to a mixed type with episodes of high and low tone.

Spasticity can interfere with mobility and may coexist with weakness. It may cause pain and atypical postures, predispose the individual to contractures (particularly those with severe spasticity), and interfere with hygiene and self-care. On the opposite end of the tone spectrum, persons with DS have hypotonia that may or may not limit mobility. Tone deficits in DS are not a primary limiting factor to mobility and physical activity, as the characteristic finding of marked hypotonia tends to gradually diminish with age.

Cognitive Function

Cognitive deficits may be a major disabling feature in genetic and developmental conditions such as DS and CP. Similarly, cognitive dysfunction may be a key symptom in chronic conditions such as MS, TBI, and SCI. The degree of cognitive deficits affects not only health management but also the long-term planning for aging processes in persons with chronic disabilities and conditions. The need for lifelong external support is a considerable issue for those who are unable to independently care for themselves as they age. The degree of cognitive deficits in this population may range from memory deficits to mental retardation; the degree of cognitive and perceptual deficits determines participation in functional activities and self-care, mobility, compliance, and even health status.

Standardized outcome measures exist to measure cognitive impairments; the examiner is cautioned to consider the validity and reliability of outcome measures for specific populations before use. The reader is referred to chapters discussing specific diagnoses for detailed outcome measures. Because cognition is multidimensional, examination for deficits will need to be directed at different components of cognition. Screening may be as simple as a three-item recall or short questions determining the ability to follow commands, attention, level of consciousness, orientation, judgment, construction, and higher memory function.

Mobility and Posture

In individuals with chronic impairments, addressing inefficient alignments and postures is of critical importance, particularly if this area was not addressed early in their care. The dire effects of such malalignments and compensations described in the following paragraphs eventually affect functional abilities.

Asymmetrical or abnormal gait patterns, crutch walking, and propelling manual wheelchairs for several decades are frequently the major sources of the pain, weakness, and fatigue in people with chronic movement dysfunctions after a medical problem such as TBI, SCI, CP, PPS, or cerebrovascular accident (CVA). The incidence of pain in a group of 114 patients with confirmed PPS increased from 84% in those who were ambulatory without orthotics to 100% in those who used crutches or wheelchairs for locomotion.[94] A high prevalence of osteoarthritis in patients with PPS was documented in the hand and wrist by radiography.[104] More than twice the number of subjects with PPS had osteoarthritis of the wrist or hand than would be expected in a healthy population of the same age. The risk factor was significantly increased with lower-extremity muscle paralysis and use of assistive devices.

In an electromyographic study of walking in clients with PPS, Perry[105] demonstrated overuse and substitution activity of the vastus lateralis, biceps femoris, and gluteus maximus muscles when the soleus is nonfunctional. Such substitution and overcompensation in the long term, however, lead to microtrauma of ligaments and joint structures and exhaustion of neuromuscular units.

In addition to sitting in poorly supporting chairs, sofas, auto seats, and wheelchairs, the individual with chronic impairments may have trunk muscle paresis or asymmetries of the pelvic base and may spend up to 16 hours per day in the seated position. The typical posture is slumped, hanging on posterior vertebral ligaments with loss of lumbar and cervical curves. Neck, shoulder, and back pain are therefore commonly reported.

Levels and types of mobility will be diverse in individuals with chronic neuromuscular impairments. Mobility may range from independent ambulation to gait with an assistive device all the way to wheelchair dependency, depending on existing impairments and cognitive function. Thorough examination should determine the current mobility levels and possible modification needs depending on new impairments or functional limitations. It may be necessary to include a seating examination in persons who are wheelchair dependent or sit for the majority of the awake hours.

Balance and Coordination

Deficits in balance and coordination in individuals with chronic conditions predispose these people to falls and limit safe mobility. As individuals with these conditions age, typical age-related changes in balance may add to the existing deficits and magnify functional limitations and impairments. Coordination and balance deficits need to be examined under functional conditions and in the context of the individual's daily activities. Standardized outcome measures are also available to objectively measure impairments; however, the reliability and validity of such measures in specific populations may be deficient. Use of outcome measures may provide a multidimensional look into deficits and provide objective baseline measures to track progress with intervention as well as progression of the movement dysfunction.

Environmental Temperature Intolerance

Consideration for the effects of heat and/or cold may be necessary when working with individuals with chronic diseases, and the examination must include a component of temperature intolerance. Two specific diagnoses embody this phenomenon: PPS for cold intolerance and MS for the negative effects of environmental heat.

Regulation of body temperature is often a problem for individuals with MS (see Chapter 19). Earlier, it was noted that a feature of fatigue unique to MS is that the fatigue is exacerbated by heat. Other MS symptoms may also be aggravated by heat. The Uthoff phenomenon[106] is an adverse response to external heat, causing fatigue or deterioration of symptoms; it often occurs with exercise. Specific recommendations for cooling during exercise intervention may be necessary to counteract the deleterious effects of heat. It is important that the examiner meticulously determine during the health interview the symptomatic effects, if any, of increased temperature in the aging individual with MS.

Sensory deficits per se are not hallmark features of polio; however, cold intolerance is a commonly reported late-onset symptom. Involved extremities in individuals with PPS are frequently abnormally cold as a result of sympathetic nerve cell involvement leading to decreased vasoconstriction and venoconstriction with heat loss to the environment.[107] The impairment may become worse with PPS. Environmental adaptation can create an easy solution to this problem as long as the individual with PPS is aware first of the problem and second of the adaptations necessary to avoid thermoinstability within the extremities.

Preventing versus responding to the inadequate vasoresponse to cold empowers the individual to develop environmental control.

Sleep Disturbances

It is common knowledge that elderly individuals report and manifest sleep disorders.[108,109] Thus, this body system problem certainly can be associated with aging individuals with chronic movement dysfunction. Disturbances in sleep are a common symptom in persons with chronic neuromuscular diseases. Sleep deprivation is a contributing factor to fatigue in individuals with MS. Similarly, more than 50% of individuals with PPS have been found to have sleep disturbances.[110] These disturbances may be caused by pain, stress, hypoventilation, or obstructive apnea.[111-113] Bruno[114] proposed a high incidence of abnormal movements in sleep in nearly two thirds of polio survivors, with 52% reporting sleep disturbance caused by these movements. All seven of subjects with PPS in the study demonstrated abnormal movements in sleep. The author points to the importance of eliminating sleep disorders as a cause of fatigue before the diagnosis of postpolio sequelae is made, particularly because it remains a diagnosis of exclusion.[114]

In addition to the typical symptoms of muscular weakness, pain, and fatigue associated with PPS, some individuals also develop sleep disorders such as periodic limb movements (PLMs).[84] PLMs in sleep are repetitive episodes of muscular contractions with durations of 0.5 to 5 seconds; frequencies of five or more per sleep hour are deemed pathological. The association of PLMs with insomnia or daily sleepiness suggests the diagnosis of PLM disorder.[84] Whereas PLM has been related to the pathophysiology of PPS,[114] the occurrence of PLM in PPS is not well known.[84] In a recent retrospective study of 99 patients with PPS, researchers assessed the frequency of PLMs during sleep, including other sleep-quality variables such as total sleep time, efficiency of sleep, apnea-hypopnea index, and awaking index.[84] Sixteen patients showed a PLM index that was considered pathological. The authors concluded that a close relationship between PLM and PPS exists; however, the prevalence of PPS with or without PLM and its combination with apnea-hypopnea is not clearly established, a finding in agreement with the conclusions of Jubelt and colleagues.[84,115]

A thorough history and review of systems including a sleep history may reveal the potential causes and guide the therapist in the clinical decision-making process for referral and consultation. Sleep apnea, which occurs frequently in polio survivors, and other sleep disorders including abnormal movements in sleep, may be revealed with specific questioning, triggering the referral process. The therapist plays a role when the sleep disorder is associated with the area of pain management.

Life-Threatening Conditions

Limited knowledge exists of adult health issues for older individuals with developmental disabilities. Secondary medical conditions warrant further examination, particularly in aging adults with chronic conditions. Acute onset of new symptoms may suggest exacerbation of disease or decreased functional reserves or may arise from long-standing effects of impairments from the initial disease process.

In the case of PPS, bulbar muscle dysfunction[93] may also result from the new weakness. Life-threatening conditions such as hypoventilation, dysphagia, sleep apnea,[116] and cardiopulmonary insufficiency require management by medical specialists.[111,117,118] These problems occur in people with previous bulbar poliomyelitis who may or may not be using ventilatory assistance and in those with severe kyphosis or scoliosis. Respiratory failure may occur primarily in individuals with residual respiratory insufficiency and minimal reserves.[115]

Functional Assessment

Performance in functional activities often provides a better picture of the losses stemming from chronic impairments. Decreases in strength are not usually revealed in a single-effort maximum contraction such as required in the manual muscle test. Resistive force during testing is a necessary element for two grades, 5 (normal, "N") and 4 (good, "G"), whereas the other four grades are nonresistive and mostly nonfunctional, and few examiners are now tested for reliability.[119] In a 1-year follow-up using quantitative muscle force testing, no differences were found in muscle strength, work capacity, endurance capacity, or recovery from fatigue of the quadriceps in either asymptomatic or symptomatic groups with PPS.[120] Nevertheless, there is at best a slow decline in functional ability, which clients may describe as loss of muscle strength. Clinically, individuals seeking therapy report functional loss or limitation more easily than a specific loss of muscle strength.

Functional assessment of individuals with chronic movement limitations provides a more practical and clearer picture of the abilities and limitations related to the initial condition or stemming from new impairments. Functional activities are visible and reportable performances of relevant tasks in the context of the individual's culture.[121] Functional tasks imply a specific goal and can range from simple to complex activities. In functional motor performance, the specific task and environmental context is as important as the individual functional movement (refer to Chapter 8). Consideration for these factors is necessary during examination. Detailed functional assessment is outlined by Howle[122] and Zabel.[123]

Functional limitations are difficulties in performing specific tasks. Difficulty in performing daily tasks including mobility and transfers may stem from overuse of muscles and joints that are already performing beyond their typical use, pain, fatigue, muscle weakness, weight gain, cognitive impairments, and decreases in functional endurance, among others. It can be logically inferred that individuals living with chronic movement impairments will reach a tipping point at which the performance of current activities will be hindered or the way activities are performed will require modification.

Decreases in functional activities over time for varied chronic conditions[35,45-49,124] have been documented in the literature. As early as 5 years and up to 20 years after the initial SCI, individuals have reported decreases in functional activities and increased need for assistance with ADLs.[45-48] An association with the need for increasing support with advancing age in individuals with SCI is seen in the literature.[45-47]

TABLE 35-2 ■ MAJOR POSTURAL ABNORMALITIES IN SITTING, STANDING, AND WALKING IN 111 CONFIRMED POSTPOLIO CLINIC CLIENTS

POSTURE	ABNORMAL DEVIATION	NO.	%
Sitting (n = 111)	Absent lumbar curve	64	54
	Forward head (loss of cervical curves)	50	45
	Uneven pelvic base*	29	26
	Structural scoliosis	38	34
Standing (n = 76)	Absent lumbar curve	52	68
	Uneven pelvic base*	40	53
	Weight bearing on stronger leg	29	38
Walking (n = 76)	Abnormal gait deviations	76	100
	Major lateral trunk oscillations	33	43
	Obvious forward lean	40	53

Modified from Smith L, McDermott K: Pain in post-poliomyelitis: addressing causes versus effects. In Halstead L, Wiechers D, editors: *Research and clinical aspects of the late effects of poliomyelitis,* White Plains, NY, 1987, March of Dimes.

*Pelvic asymmetry was ½ inch or more.

According to Agre and Rodriquez,[125] postpolio survivors with significant weakness perform daily activities at a different level of effort than other individuals; muscles of polio survivors may have to work near maximal effort during activities that individuals without polio can execute at relatively lower levels of effort. Individuals with PPS commonly report difficulty in walking, stair climbing,[35] and dressing (Table 35-2). Westbrook[124] described a 5-year follow-up study examining physical and functional abilities and health status of 176 individuals with PPS. During the course of the study, most subjects reported increases in muscle weakness, muscle and joint pain, and changes in walking. Notably, the participants reported more difficulty in four of the eight daily living activities (stair climbing, walking on level surfaces, transfers in and out of bed, and meeting the demands of home or work). Most of the participants (87%) also reported problems in meeting the demands of their job and completing household tasks. Clearly, the ability to perform motor tasks essential to completing one's goals and desires is multifactorial. Therefore, functional limitations are usually related to a combination of systems impairments.

In persons with PPS, to determine whether the cause of the new weakness is overuse or possibly disuse, a detailed assessment is required of home, work, recreational, and community activities.[126] This paradigm of multidimensional assessment is applicable to all individuals with chronic movement problems. If the client is merely asked what his or her activity level is, the response may lead to assumptions that weakness is from disuse. With specific questioning, one usually finds that the client is doing an extraordinary amount of physical activity. It is vital to establish a total picture of the client's activities in sitting, standing, walking, lifting, carrying, climbing stairs, using a telephone or a computer, and performing daily activities such as self-care and home management.

PSYCHOSOCIAL CONSIDERATIONS

The challenges of chronic diseases are ongoing as the individual ages. Despite new pharmacological interventions, several genetic, developmental, and neuromuscular conditions remain incurable with uncertain courses as the person ages. Although individuals and their families cope effectively with the initial disease process, the incidence of depression is common in the presence of chronic disease and impairments. The impact of chronic conditions on family, marital life, and socioeconomic and financial functions is persistent. The clinician's attitudes, beliefs, support, and understanding will play a major role in the management of individuals with chronic impairments.

Most individuals living with chronic impairments and functional limitations have learned to adapt not only with their movement strategies, but also with the psychological and socioeconomic impact of the initial diagnoses. Not only have these individuals learned to live with the challenges of their initial diagnosis and its movement-related, functional, financial, and psychosocial impact, but their families and caregivers have likewise done so. It may not be surprising, then, that changes to once-established routines, either from acute medical conditions or from gradual but significant changes from the aging process, are resisted and negatively viewed. These individuals will possibly need more assistance, move slower, and need to cut back from activities once engaged in; the consequent changes in philosophy and lifestyle will not likely be welcomed by most individuals and their support systems.

Over the past years, several authors have addressed the prevalence of PPS, its causes, and the effects of aging on the development of PPS.* Some literature addresses the effects of aging on developmental and genetic disabilities, yet information on how aging affects individuals with existing impairments is still not conclusive. Because persons who are aging with chronic disabilities is an emerging population owing to improvement in health care delivery and nutrition, evidence on the consequences of the aging process remains uncertain. Similarly, the psychological effects are not as widely addressed in the literature. Not much is known about the quality of life of older adults with congenital or childhood-acquired

*References 19, 21, 25, 26, 31, 32, 35, 36, 71, 79, 93, 104, and 127-131.

disabilities. Psychological adjustment is difficult with any disease with an unpredictable course, and differentiating organic psychological problems from adjustment issues may complicate the management of individuals with chronic diseases.

As a chronic disease, PPS provides an informative example of the interaction among neurological and functional impairments, recovery, effects of aging, and health care. Much has been written about the psychological and psychosocial issues with PPS that is applicable to other chronic disabilities as well. A brief synopsis of the psychosocial considerations of PPS follows.

Postpolio Syndrome

Although the physical manifestations of and interventions for PPS are recognized, psychological symptoms become evident in polio survivors. Bruno and Frick[37] described psychological symptoms such as chronic stress, depression, anxiety, compulsiveness, and type A behavior in polio survivors; these symptoms not only cause distress but limit these individuals in making lifestyle changes to manage late-onset symptoms. Currie and colleagues[103] made generalizations about adults with childhood-onset or congenital disabilities spanning a range of disability types. Understanding the background of individuals with PPS and a few of the myths that helped to shape their lives is beneficial in their care. Fear of the disease was rampant during the early epidemics. Despite safety measures, children and adolescents contracted polio. Part of the coping strategy was encouraging the child to high levels of physical achievement; approval and rewards were gained by walking farther or faster and keeping up with or exceeding the performance of other children. The best treatment available for all polio victims at that time was from the March of Dimes, which entailed hospitalization for months at a time away from the individuals' families and communities. The situation led to feelings of abandonment, anxiety, and total dependence on strangers. The "polio patient" was expected to be a "good patient" and to "work hard." Indeed, these patients did work hard to reeducate weakened muscles and compensate for lost function.[37-40] Courage, determination, and cheerfulness were attributes to be prized, self-pity was viewed unfavorably, and talking about the functional loss was not encouraged. Later in the recovery process, parents made decisions to have their children undergo multiple surgical procedures to allow removal of heavy braces so that they would "look normal" and "fit in." One can understand why clients react so negatively to the suggestion of orthotics.

Coping Strategies

The psychosocial issues confronting persons with PPS often are more disruptive than the physical problems.[22,23,71,132-134] An increasing population of polio survivors is experiencing, with aging, an unanticipated late onset of new symptoms. Associated with loss of physical function and independence are social and psychological problems stemming from the inability to perform personal and societal roles. Previous research suggests that well-established, often compulsive behavior patterns may impair the ability to deal effectively with the new threats to functional independence. Bruno and Frick[24] confirmed the presence of psychological stress in survivors, noting that type A behavior and stress could precipitate or exacerbate postpolio sequelae. In a later study in 1991[37] the same researchers suggested that the acute experience conditioned survivors into lifelong patterns of compulsive type A behavior, a behavior pattern that impairs the ability to cope with new late postpolio symptoms. Kuehn and Winters[135] also noted that symptom distress and intensity were less in individuals with greater coping resources. In this study[135] in Sweden of 113 patients with postpolio sequelae, results revealed that the prevalence of distress was highest in the physical dimensions of physical mobility, pain, and energy and lowest in social isolation. The high scores for the triad of dimensions were similar to the findings of previous studies.[116]

Individuals with PPS developed several styles to cope with their disability. Maynard and Roller[136] described coping styles according to severity of muscular involvement. Survivors with little or no obvious physical involvement were able to hide atrophy with clothing and avoided activities that revealed the weakness. Many individuals invested much energy in projecting normality and were so adept at denial that they disconnected themselves from the polio experience; often spouses do not know of the history of polio. This group can develop the most severe cases of PPS. The denial renders them detached from other individuals with PPS and thus difficult to assist.

Polio survivors with obvious physical involvement such as a limp or an atrophied extremity or who use an assistive device have usually pushed themselves to function at normal or supernormal levels. These individuals will tolerate high levels of pain before acknowledging the late effects of polio. The third group, the most severely impaired of the individuals with PPS, may have respiratory involvement or more mobility deficits. Several use or have used wheelchairs for mobility and required great effort and persistence to gain independence in self-care activities. The members of this group integrated their functional problems into their self-image and have led active, productive lives.

In a 5-year study of 176 individuals with PPS, it was unexpectedly found that participants' stress levels decreased over time.[124] The author hypothesized that eventually, lifestyle modifications and treatment contributed to the coping process. Kuehn and Winters[135] in their study found that more than half of their subjects of working age had gainful employment. Moreover, no difference in employment rate as a result of distribution of polio involvement was found, implying that this was not a deciding factor. The authors hypothesize that persons with severe polio involvement were either forced to choose or encouraged to take up an appropriate profession early in life, whereas those with less involvement had not needed such planning. Nevertheless, vocational issues encompassing satisfactory accessibility and equipment are an important part of management.

Response to New Diagnosis. The response to the diagnosis of PPS can range from relief to despair. Relief comes to polio survivors who have been told their symptoms were psychosomatic. Despair occurs when survivors are given a program of lifestyle changes and management suggestions that are opposed to the adage they followed during the initial infection. The proposed philosophy shift from "no pain, no gain" to energy conservation and rest may be viewed unfavorably or with disdain. Polio survivors who have led active lives may have significant difficulty adjusting their lifestyle to new symptoms and decreasing abilities, and psychological support may be indicated.[137]

The stresses of the diagnostic process also add to the challenges. Most health care professionals have limited understanding of the initial polio experience and the late effects of polio, and therefore the diagnostic process of PPS may take time and involve a series of physician consultations.[37,38,138-140] Publicity from support groups has helped refer clients to PPS clinics or to specialists with knowledge of PPS.[140]

Fear of the threat to independence, inadequate knowledge about the physiological changes, and the expectation of functional loss may contribute to the anxiety of polio survivors. Individuals with PPS will feel anxious about the prospects of changing roles with their families, friends, and co-workers.[38,136,139] Defenses and coping strategies that have been successfully used for years have broken down, and the individual experiences overwhelming anxieties and conflicts.[139]

Compliance. The patient-clinician relationship is an important determinant of compliance. Several authors[24,37,141] have identified compliance as a significant problem in type A polio survivors. Although a few individuals with PPS readily accept suggestions for lifestyle changes, a few immediately make changes, and a few refuse to consider any changes at all, most will eventually make changes but will require support, patience, and time to process. Compliance is an issue encountered not only in individuals with PPS but in many individuals with chronic conditions. Clinicians' sensitivity, support, and respect will play a major role in the response of the patient/client to management suggestions. Acknowledging the individual's current activities, values, and goals is an important step in establishing a relationship with the patient/client. Allowing clients to express feelings about the new challenges, their prior high levels of physical achievement, and previous treatment is equally important.

A health care provider perceived to be knowledgeable, interested, and concerned significantly increases compliance with recommendations.[142] Compliance of the client with PPS may be improved by the therapist's ability to suggest management strategies that are accepted as conventional and the ability to alleviate pain in the initial examination. Conservative management should be attempted first before more aggressive or life-changing interventions such as orthoses, mobility changes, or motorized carts, which they may have used in the past and eventually discarded. Therapists can also be a source of information about support groups.[140] Support groups offer information about every facet of living with chronic impairments, and these members may be positive role models to help not only the newly diagnosed individual in the transition process but also the aging individual with chronic disease and impairments deal with issues with maturation and advancing age.

HEALTH-RELATED DISPARITIES IN AGING ADULTS WITH CHRONIC DISABILITIES

Individuals aging with chronic impairments and conditions are exposed to the effects of aging and maturation differently than the general population. Persons with disabilities often start at the lower end of the health continuum owing to secondary conditions that overlap with the primary disability.[143] Few will argue that despite medical advances and public health initiatives, the reality is that health disparities, including decreased access to high-quality health care, health promotion, disease prevention, and health literacy, are still present and reflect areas that need to be addressed. Outlined here are some health disparities facing adults with chronic disabilities and conditions.

- Compared with the general population, higher rates of disability and obesity are seen among adults with developmental delay.[66,144,145] Of adults with major physical and sensory impairments, 27% are obese, compared with 19% of those without major disability.[68]
- Cardiovascular disease is one of the most common causes of death among aging adults with developmental delay.[17,146,147]
- Evidence supports the earlier appearance of age-related health conditions in individuals with developmental delay. Conditions include cognitive decline, incontinence, and sensory losses.[148] Examples of health conditions that may be influenced by aging in persons with developmental delay were discussed earlier regarding individuals with CP[149] (who may have increased issues with musculoskeletal deformities, progressive cervical spine degeneration, dental problems, bladder or bowel dysfunction, or osteoporosis) and individuals with DS (who have a higher prevalence of early-onset Alzheimer disease compared with the general public).[13,150]
- Generally, individuals with intellectual and developmental disabilities have poorer health and more difficulty in finding, accessing, and paying for higher-quality health care.[7]
- Adults with developmental disabilities also have limited access to medical care, which may result in lack of obesity screening, counseling, and management.[151]
- Higher rates of depression, anxiety, and strong fears and stress are seen in persons with chronic disabilities. Iezzoni[68] found that 34% of adults with major impairments in walking reported frequent depression or anxiety, compared with 3% in those without disabilities.

MANAGEMENT OF CHRONIC IMPAIRMENTS

Aging with Chronic Impairments

The management of individuals with chronic impairments is challenging, not only because of the possibility of multisystem involvement warranting a holistic approach, but also because much is unknown about effects of the aging process on chronic neuromuscular impairments.

Aging adults with chronic conditions may be more vulnerable to conditions that will make their old age potentially more difficult with an increased possibility for infirmity and dependence.[7] Individuals with chronic and disabling impairments are often at an increased risk for the development of secondary conditions and further disability that can lead to further decline in independence and functional status and to mobility deficits. It has been suggested that people with chronic conditions such as living with developmental delay, may age differently based on the nature and severity of their disability, other coexisting health problems, and secondary chronic conditions. With increased life expectancy, health care professions will likely see an increase in the care of those aging with chronic impairments. There is then a unique challenge for health care professionals to develop and implement programs for the management of aging adults with chronic impairments to effect optimal health status.

The heterogeneity of aging adults with chronic neuromuscular impairments lends to the need for individualized management programs. The aging process is unique for each individual, as is the recovery process in people with chronic conditions and the overall manifestation of late-onset or secondary symptoms. Therefore intervention will be dependent on the individual's current symptoms, functional needs, level of activity limitations, and values or goals.

Although evidence exists regarding interventions for individuals with chronic disease, overall, there is a dearth of information on specific treatment strategies if one considers the magnitude of associated diseases and the increasing population of individuals aging with chronic functional limitations and impairments. The reason for this is multifactorial; it may stem from the mismatch between the increase in number of individuals with chronic diseases that is resulting from longer life expectancies because of advancements in medicine and the gaps in our knowledge about the effects of aging in this population. The limitation on specific knowledge about interventions is echoed by Marks and colleagues, who state that there is a lack of framework for assessing health-related interventions for individuals aging with developmental delay.[152]

A finite number of research and treatment centers have been established to deal with comprehensive care issues for individuals with disabilities.[153] The statement by Kailes[154] regarding the lack of helpful information related to exercising for those aging with a disability is troubling yet accurate. Considering the extensive evidence showing that many of the physical limitations that occur as part of aging in nondisabled people can be prevented or delayed by changing health habits, Kailes[154] suggests that individuals with disabilities need (1) appropriate fitness assessment measures that can be used with various types of disabilities, (2) exercise guidelines that are appropriate for age and types of limitations, (3) exercise facilities that are accessible, integrated, and not separate from those of nondisabled populations, and (4) exercise equipment that incorporates universal design features.

Unfortunately, in today's health care environment, many individuals with PPS, SCI, TBI, or developmental disabilities do not have access to specialists, including PTs, who understand their complex movement limitation–related needs and how these limitations affect participation in life. Care is fragmented, and physicians and therapists, if involved in the care at all, seldom have a comprehensive picture of the person's needs. Although one might assume that the managed-care system would provide coordination of care within the provider system, the reality is that there may be more restrictions in care, particularly for disability-related care that may require a period of continuing rehabilitation treatment and retraining. Even providers within the group seldom communicate because the group is composed of practitioners who accept the insurance contract rather than practitioners working together to improve health. In my experience, hardly any individuals aging with neurological conditions such as TBI, CVA, or SCI seek therapy past their initial episode of care in the acute phase of the condition. This reality is confirmed in the literature; today persons with SCI or TBI are followed in comprehensive specialty centers or clinics as they age.[155,156]

Multisystem Approach

Individuals with chronic neuromuscular conditions have multidimensional impairments across multiple systems. Chronicity of impairments in one system likely and eventually affects other systems. For example, an individual with limited physical mobility because of impairments in the neuromuscular system likely has decreased levels of physical activity, which in turn are correlated with lower muscle strength, which is associated with a greater degree of disability. Although the initial impairments may be in the neuromuscular system, over time the condition will affect the cardiovascular system from inactivity and potentially the integumentary system. An increased likelihood of multisystem effects in an individual with chronic impairments is a reality. Therefore a multisystem, holistic approach to management is warranted.

The rehabilitation clinician is in a unique position to provide holistic care to the client with chronic impairments. In the realm of management of chronic movement dysfunction, PPS becomes a model case for other chronic neuromuscular conditions—there is much to learn from the complex nature of the late effects of polio, and designing an intervention program may be as challenging as the evaluation because of the interactions of the systems and the influences of the environment, medical treatment, and aging. Before beginning physical or occupational therapy, it is necessary for the team to first identify and treat other medical and neurological conditions that may produce the reported symptoms.[157]

The individual's values and goals are the most significant variables to take into consideration in designing the interventions. Improvement will largely depend on the patient's commitment and thus compliance. Relatively simple interventions may result in distinctive positive changes. Conservative management should be attempted first before major life-changing interventions. Psychological considerations play a major role in designing an acceptable and appropriate management plan that will encourage compliance. Lifestyle modifications may not be favorably viewed by some individuals who have "conquered" the disease and pushed themselves to be independent, as in the case of those with PPS or SCI in their younger years. Prescription of interventions that are perceived to be "radical" should be done with sensitivity and caution. The rationale for interventions should be carefully considered in light of the client's current functional status and goals. Introduction of orthoses, assistive devices, and mobility modifications is often difficult for the individual with chronic impairments to accept, given the long, arduous effort expended over years to avoid such devices and the movement adaptation achieved without such devices.

The long-term goals for individuals with chronic conditions center primarily on self-management of home exercise programs and appropriate lifestyle changes to reduce physical demands. No definitive, curative intervention currently exists for chronic neuromuscular conditions ranging from developmental delay (DS, CP) to those acquired through trauma or disease sometime in the life span

(SCI, TBI, PPS); therefore symptom management is a key element in both the short and long terms. Short-term goals focus on the symptoms present and may address the following areas:

- Modified strengthening and conditioning
- Postural correction
- Energy conservation
- Lifestyle modifications
- Mobility and locomotion
- Balance during functional activities
- Walking aids, mobility devices, orthoses
- Pain reduction
- Improved functional endurance
- Ability to transfer
- Respiratory care
- Weight control

The information is presented with an evidence-based approach and will specifically address the management of adults with PPS, SCI, and TBI. When possible, the intervention approaches first offered should focus on several problems at one time (Table 35-3). The importance of individualized programs that address the variability of symptoms cannot be overemphasized. The reader is referred to specific references for further details on management prescriptions.

Before discussion of specific intervention strategies, a shift in the philosophy of management of chronic disease and disability is presented. Within the past decade, in an effort to affect the trajectory of further decline from chronic conditions, there appears to have been a shift toward the promotion of health rather than the control of the disease itself.

HEALTH PROMOTION

Health Promotion with Chronic Conditions

Emerging in the public health arena is a call for attention to the growing population of aging adults with chronic disabilities and for reducing health disparities involving this aging population. There is consensus on a need to address issues related to the health and care of aging individuals with developmental and intellectual disabilities related to primary care, health promotion, health literacy, and health care providers.[66,152]

Decreasing health disparities affecting aging adults with chronic impairments is an increasing area of focus, as evidenced by its inclusion in the national health goals for individuals with disabilities outlined in several documents such as the Healthy People 2020 initiative,[158] the New Freedom Initiative,[65] the U.S. Department of Health and Human Services document *Closing the Gap: A National Blueprint to Improve the Health of Persons with Mental Retardation,*[159] and the U.S. Surgeon General's Call to Action to Improve the Health and Wellness of Persons with Disabilities.[160] Healthy People 2010 cautioned that people with disabilities would be expected to experience disadvantages in health compared with the general population. Five years after the release of the U.S. Surgeon General's Call to Action, it was reported that some individuals with disabilities still lacked equal access to health care, and health promotion has been outlined as a goal to be achieved by people with disabilities.[160]

TABLE 35-3 ■ EVIDENCE-BASED APPROACH TO THE MANAGEMENT OF POSTPOLIO SYNDROME

Generalized weakness	Lifestyle changes
	Therapeutic nonfatiguing strengthening exercises
	Aerobic exercise
	Orthoses
	Assistive devices
	Avoidance of overuse
	Weight loss
Pain	Therapeutic heating modalities*
	Cryotherapy*
	Activity reduction and lifestyle changes
	Pacing of activities
	Stretching
	Weight loss
	Assistive devices
	Orthoses
	Motorized mobility devices
	Nonsteroidal antiinflammatory drugs†
Dysphagia	Dietary changes or restrictions
	Breathing techniques
	Swallowing techniques
	Monitoring fatigue and timing eating when not fatigued
Fatigue	Lifestyle changes
	Energy conservation techniques
	Nonfatiguing exercise programs
	Lightweight orthoses and assistive devices
	Pacing of activities
	Frequent rest breaks
	Naps during the day
	Motorized mobility devices
Cardiopulmonary conditioning	Aquatic exercise training
	Endurance training
	Cycle or arm exercises
Psychosocial concerns	Postpolio support groups
	Interdisciplinary approach
	Counseling from psychologists, psychiatrists
	Vocational counseling
	Behavior modification
Pulmonary dysfunction	Preventive measures
	Noninvasive ventilatory assistance
	Pulmonary therapy
	Breathing exercises: glossopharyngeal breathing

Modified from Trojan D, Finch L: Management of post-polio syndrome. *NeuroRehabilitation* 8:93–105, 1997; Jubelt B, Agre J: Management of post-polio syndrome. *JAMA* 284:412–414, 2000.

*Effectiveness of heat and cold modalities are patient specific and must be used with caution.

†Antiinflammatory drugs have been shown to be effective in pain management in medical treatment of postpolio syndrome. The specific drug and dosage must be prescribed by the physician.

Health promotion is defined by Pender[161] as activities motivated by the desire to increase well-being and actualize human potential. It includes self-initiated behaviors and stresses the need to enhance the responsibility and commitment of each person to achieve a healthy lifestyle. Health promotion was reflected in Healthy People 2010. Healthy People 2020 includes individuals with disabilities in all health promotion efforts as an emerging area in disability and health, reflecting a continuation of the initiative's prior goals for the well-being of persons with disabilities.[158]

Shift to Health Promotion

In 1997, Patrick[162] found that research on health promotion for individuals with health disabilities was almost nonexistent. Fast-forward to 2011: a shift from disability prevention to health promotion has emerged, and literature on health promotion efforts for persons with a variety of chronic diseases is emerging.

In contrast to health protection or disease-management behaviors, which are motivated by the desire to avoid illness or its effects, health promotion is not disease or injury specific.[161] Whereas both wellness and disease-management interventions may focus on improving similar health behaviors, a critical difference between these approaches has been proposed by Stuifbergen and colleagues.[163] They assert that the significant difference is in how the individual is viewed with regard to the interaction between his or her chronic disability and the purpose or intention of the change in behavior—that is, control and management of disease versus maximizing quality of life and health. Furthermore, whereas wellness interventions have wellness or health in the forefront and the disease in the background,[164] wellness and health promotion interventions allow the individual to choose behaviors that improve and/or sustain the quality of life within the perspective of living with chronic conditions.[165]

Part of the national initiative to improve the health of aging adults with developmental disabilities, the U.S. Surgeon General's Call to Action to Improve the Health and Wellness of Persons with Disabilities[160] stated that persons with disabilities can promote their own health through developing or maintaining healthy lifestyles. Embedded in this statement is the responsibility of the individual for his or her own health trajectory. This responsibility is shared with health care providers and support persons. A need to develop skills to improve health literacy related to health care issues is paramount to this responsibility[152] and to encouragement of active participation. Health literacy is defined by Selden[166] as the degree to which individuals have the capacity to obtain, process, and understand basic health information and services necessary to make apt health decisions.

Early education combined with opportunities for lifelong learning can help individuals develop the skills and confidence needed to improve or manage healthy lifestyles with aging.[152] Similarly, health care professionals need to improve, maintain, and use clear communication.

Health promotion and disease prevention activities should consist of specific health education programs and preventive or screening programs.[152] In the paradigm shift to health promotion, some interventions have focused on a single behavior such as exercise or nutrition or a combination of interventions for a more inclusive lifestyle approach.[163,165,167]

Community-Based Programs

With approximately 54 million persons with disabilities[65] targeted by public health initiatives, assistive technology advancements, and cultural changes, many barriers still exist to access to community-based programs.[65] Community-based interventions for health promotion are ideal for those with developmental disabilities because they address social inclusion, self-efficacy, and sustainability.[168] However, few community-based lifestyle interventions targeting those with developmental disabilities exist.[17] Developing and implementing accessible programs in the community setting for adults with long-term disabilities remain challenging.[152]

Today, adults with chronic movement dysfunction have more of an opportunity to participate in sporting events and recreational activities. Therapists need to be involved in the process to ensure optimum benefit of these activities for clients to be not only successful but also safe. As research supports fitness training for persons with chronic disabilities and impairments, more effort will be needed to maximize the availability of community-based facilities to meet the demand. Again, therapists can be instrumental not only in the design of equipment but also in advocacy efforts by educating governmental officials and third-party payers regarding the needs of those aging with chronic conditions. Therapists not only possess the knowledge of the physiological effects of exercise but also understand biomechanical principles critical to ensuring safety in fitness and recreational activities. Therapists can work with these individuals on maximizing strength, flexibility, body mass indices, and cardiorespiratory reserves. This focus will not only increase functional capacity and social participation of the adult with functional limitations but will lower the risk of medical comorbidities associated with the effects of physical inactivity.

Health Promotion Interventions: Evidence and Challenges

Iezzoni[66] identified several barriers faced by persons with disability to accessing health care and public health interventions. Physical access, communication, financial barriers, and discriminatory and stigmatizing attitudes were identified as externally imposed barriers.

Although there has been a shift in philosophy and growing interest in health promotion in individuals with chronic impairments, the supporting evidence on the effectiveness of these interventions has not been examined in depth. Although there are published studies on health promotion in people with chronic diseases, several challenges arise. Studies often involve varied chronic diseases such as cancer, heart failure, arthritis, or human immunodeficiency virus (HIV) infection, with few studies examining individuals with chronic neuromuscular conditions. The studies often involve small experimental interventional strategies, use small population samples, and have varied intervention delivery from individual, group, or community-based programs. Moreover, Stuifbergen and colleagues[163] found that despite the benefits of health promotion for improving or maintaining function and independence in older adults, very few studies had samples of older subjects. Iezzoni[66] asserts that improving access to health promotion and disease prevention should be a national public health priority.

A mounting body of evidence regarding the positive impact of health promotion and wellness interventions on individuals with chronic conditions is seen in the literature.[163] Although these studies report significant effects and used multiple outcome measures, they had small population samples that encompassed varied chronic conditions not specific to those with neuromuscular impairments alone. Moreover, types, lengths, and delivery of interventions varied greatly from community-based to independent settings. Therefore, generalization and comparison across studies are difficult to say the least. It is noteworthy that a review of the literature supports the benefits and positive effects of health promotion and wellness interventions; however, in agreement with the findings of Stuifbergen and colleagues,[163] minimal information exists about the long-term effects or efficacy of interventions.

INTERVENTION STRATEGIES

A paucity of evidence specifically addresses precise exercise or intervention plans in individuals with chronic impairments. This lack of data is evident in specific neurological populations: SCI and TBI, to name two. Although no published studies were found on exercise plans and aging in SCI, the interest in promoting exercise and lifestyle changes to prevent secondary medical problems has been identified. Similarly, most studies are conducted in the early years after TBI, and although TBI is a lifetime disability, little attention has been paid to the needs of aging people after a TBI who may have recurring needs for physical and cognitive rehabilitation and retraining over the life span. The information presented is directed more toward PPS, for which a body of evidence supports specific intervention strategies. In a recent review on the treatment of PPS through the Cochrane Collaboration, Koopman and colleagues[18] found inadequate evidence from randomized controlled studies pointing to definitive conclusions on the effectiveness of different treatment options for individuals with PPS. Their results indicate that pharmacological intervention, specifically drugs such as lamotrigine and intravenous immunoglobulin (IVIG), and nonpharmacological interventions, specifically muscle strengthening and static magnetic fields, may be beneficial but need further research.[18]

As with other chronic neuromuscular conditions, there currently exists no curative treatment for PPS,[18] and therefore rehabilitation management is regarded as the key intervention. The succeeding discussion presents strategies for the rehabilitation of chronic neuromuscular dysfunction with the goals of improving and/or maintaining functional capacities and decreasing secondary impairments magnified by aging or the chronicity of the condition.

Although primarily directed at PPS, most of, if not all, the intervention strategies are applicable to people with other chronic impairments; there are commonalities to all chronic neuromuscular conditions that need to be identified and analyzed from a long-term quality-of-life perspective. Individuals who are aging with these chronic functional limitations should be allowed to age with the dignity given to any other individual. The challenge to therapists will be to step out of the model of regaining functional skill through repetitive practice and into the model of maintaining function, energy conservation, and empowerment of that function to the individual needing service. The client is and should be the individual who determines what aspect of functional activities are critical to quality of life and what compensations are acceptable and unacceptable as part of an adult life expectation. From that information and the analytical understanding of what is happening to the CNS of these individuals, clients and therapists together can establish realistic goals and intervention strategies that will optimize and maintain the potential motor function of those individuals.

Therapeutic Exercise

Strengthening and Conditioning

Evidence suggests that both physical activity and strength are significant factors in severity of disability.[169] It has been shown that muscle strength has a significant role in a spiraling model of decline. Specifically, lower muscle strength is correlated with a greater degree of disability. In terms of function, difficulties in motor activities are reported by those with poor strength. It is logical, then, that the management of chronic disabilities involves a strengthening program.

A mounting body of evidence supports strengthening exercises for individuals with PPS,[93,170-174] contrary to the initial approach of no exercise because of fear of overuse or symptom exacerbation. Generally, survivors with PPS who exercised and avoided overuse demonstrated positive results without detrimental effects. Several types of nonfatiguing strengthening exercises, aerobic exercise, and the evidence supporting them have been examined. Willen[175] suggests that water exercise may be beneficial because it decreases the biomechanical stresses on the muscles and joints. Specific exercise prescription is dependent on several factors such as the current level of function, other presenting symptoms, and the client's interests.

Jubelt and Agre[93] note that the most important advance in the treatment of weakness in PPS involves the findings of several studies that mild to moderate weakness can be improved with nonfatiguing exercises. The benefits of nonfatiguing exercises using both submaximal and maximal contraction with limited number of repetitions are documented in the literature.[93,170]

Isokinetic and isometric dynamometers have been used to record maximum muscle forces (or torques) in PPS subjects before and after resistive exercise programs designed to increase muscle strength. Two of the studies were of single cases,[176,177] and two had 12 and 17 subjects.[171,172] Both of the multisubject studies tested the quadriceps femoris. Einarsson[171] investigated the effects of a standardized, 6-week, maximal effort and isometric strength training program on the quadriceps muscles of 12 individuals with postpolio muscles, nine of whom met the criteria for PPS. Einarsson[171] reports an average gain of 29% in isometric strength and 24% in isokinetic strength over a period of 6 weeks; muscle biopsy specimens revealed no muscle damage. In addition to the feeling of well-being in most of the subjects during and after the training program, 10 of 12 subjects stated a feeling of increased strength in the trained muscle. In subsequent follow-ups 6 to 12 months after intervention, gains in strength did not decrease, and several subjects reported better performance in daily activities such as climbing stairs, walking, and standing from a chair.[171]

Fillyaw and colleagues[172] reported a strength gain of 8% over a 2-year period. An isometric contraction was used for testing, and concentric-eccentric contractions were used for the exercise. These results do not compare with the strength gains of 100% and higher made by healthy subjects undergoing training but rather compare with serial testing when no exercise was done.[173,174] For example, Munin and colleagues[173] measured the affected and unaffected quadriceps muscle every 6 months over 3 years to document muscle weakness in persons with PPS. They reported increases in muscle strength up to 25%. In older persons without polio, test performance gains of the quadriceps increased an average of 174% in 90-year-old subjects[178] and 107% in 60- to 72-year-old men.[179] In these two studies, thigh muscle area (as documented by computed tomography) increased by 9% and 11%, respectively, indicating an increase in muscle bulk.

The effects of nonfatiguing resistance exercises are well documented in the literature. Fillyaw and colleagues[172] in a study of 17 subjects with PPS concluded that muscle strength may be increased in individuals with PPS and suggested supervision of exercise programs by PTs and quantitative muscle testing every 3 months to guard against overuse weakness. Agre and Rodriguez[180] suggested that a supervised exercise program could safely increase strength in subjects with PPS with at least a grade 3+ strength. Their program of a supervised 12-week nonfatiguing quadriceps strengthening program with rest intervals revealed no detrimental effects. Most of the participants reported improvements in quadriceps strength, endurance, and work capacity, and half noted increased strength recovery with rest periods after activity, walking, and stair climbing. A nonfatiguing weight lifting program for at least 24 weeks was examined in six subjects with PPS by Feldman and Soskolne.[181] The results showed increased strength in 14 of the 32 muscle groups with maintained strength in 17 muscles.

Alternate-day, low-intensity, muscle-strengthening quadriceps exercises showed no adverse effects, with reported findings of increased endurance, strength, and work capacity. As a result of the low-intensity program, no increased muscle strength was found, although half of the participants sensed increased strength recovery after exercise.[182] The same protocol but with a more vigorous program of 4 days per week revealed improvements in muscular work performance and endurance without unfavorable effects noted.[182]

Because there are neural adaptations specific to the type of muscle contraction used for measurement and training, it is difficult to determine the differences in true increases in strength from the ability to improve performance on a specific test. Another term for this phenomenon or improvement in performance is *motor learning* (see Chapter 4). The theory states that the subject learns to perform the measurement or the exercise better without true gains in strength. This happens even with an apparently simple weekly maximum isometric contraction.[183] Evidence of this phenomenon can be seen when improvements are made in the opposite untrained muscle group (transfer of training), when the apparent strength gains are maintained for months after cessation of the training, and when there are no increases in the size of the muscle. The greatest improvements in test performance occur when the muscle contraction is the same for both the test and the training. Smaller increases are seen when the measurement and training muscle contractions are different and when measures to decrease the effect of motor learning have been used.

The neural adaptation specific to the type of measurement or training is illustrated in the following study on older men.[179] Multiple tests to assess strength were performed. The training program required lifting and lowering 80% of the weight of one repetition maximum (1 RM), which was assessed weekly. After 12 weeks, there were average increases in quadriceps muscle strength of 104% for the 1 RM, 7% for maximum isometric, 8% for maximum isokinetic at 60 degrees per second, and 10% for isokinetic at 240 degrees per second. In addition, there was an increase in cross-sectional area of the quadriceps of 10%, and muscle biopsy showed approximately a 30% increase in muscle fiber size.[184] This study illustrates some of the complexities of designing or evaluating studies that attempt to measure changes in muscle strength.

In chronic movement dysfunction, high tone is a symptom that may be considered a deterrent to exercise. As therapeutic procedures became based on motor control, motor learning, and neuroplasticity theories, strengthening of spastic muscles may still be underused.[185,186] In the past, placing resistance on a spastic muscle was thought to increase the spasticity. This tenet was interpreted to preclude anyone from advocating strength training in these individuals.[185,187] Interestingly, the literature identified that one of the major problems of CP is weakness. Clinicians during the 1960s and 1970s believed that the answer to this weakness underlying spasticity was to increase proprioceptive and tactile stimulation.[185,187] Current research would say that true strengthening would not occur through feedback alone and that resistance on muscle tissue is a necessary variable for strength training.[90,188,189] Damiano and colleagues[91,190-192] have shown that resistance training does not affect spasticity negatively and in fact improves many functional measures of gait. On the basis of these findings, clinicians should evaluate individual patients to determine whether the level of weakness is affecting functional performance or the attainment of personal goals. If indeed the individual's weakness is found to be clinically significant, then strength training is indicated. Strength training within functional patterns should lead to the greatest carryover.

Physical Activity

The literature clearly documents the benefits of physical activity, and in polio survivors with PPS, activity that falls within a safe range is beneficial to overall functional performance (Box 35-5). In a study involving women with disabilities in the Women's Health and Aging Study,[169] the authors found an inverse relationship between disability and physical activity, with the most disabled women being more inactive. In addition to diseases and musculoskeletal pain being directly associated with motor disability, lower levels of physical activity associated with poorer muscle strength contributed to a greater degree of motor disability.

Physical inactivity and obesity have been shown to be more common in individuals with developmental disabilities than in the general population.[17,145] Specifically, Rimmer and Wang[193] in a study of 306 individuals with physical and mental disabilities found that the rate of obesity in those with intellectual disabilities was twice as high as in the

BOX 35-5 ■ FUNCTIONAL EXERCISE: KEY POINTS

1. Consult with a health care team before starting an exercise program. A physical and occupational therapist can provide valuable insight and recommendations on activity type and intensity.
2. Avoid overuse of muscle groups.
3. Judicious exercise programs of low to high intensity can result in positive results. Include warmup and cool-down periods.
4. Short periods of activity are encouraged.
5. Allow for adequate rest between bouts of activity.
6. Alternate days may be necessary for full recovery (depending on activity type).
7. Individualized therapy program to address unique needs is critical.
8. Use energy conservation and joint protection techniques in regular routines.
9. Incorporate breathing, relaxation, mental imagery, and meditation exercises into daily activities.
10. Be cognizant of the body's alignment during exercise and functional activities.
11. Incorporate postural exercises and correction to address malalignments and unnecessary use of muscles and joints.
12. Compliance with clinical recommendations can significantly reduce symptoms and prevent further decline.
13. Listen to your body—pain is typically your body's way of alerting you to slow down or to stop.

general population. More alarming was the finding that the rate of extreme obesity (body mass index [BMI] equal to or greater than 40 kg/m^2) was approximately four times higher among individuals with disabilities than in the general population. Moreover, individuals experience high rates of secondary conditions associated with obesity and inactivity, such as type 2 diabetes, cardiovascular disease, and metabolic syndrome.[146]

Although few studies have been done on the impact of exercise or the best type of exercise for people aging with a TBI, Gordon and colleagues[194] studied 240 people living in the community with a TBI. They compared exercisers and nonexercisers with a TBI and exercisers and nonexercisers without a TBI. Typical exercise activities were swimming, jogging, biking, or sports that increased heart rate for more than 30 minutes at least three times per week for a 6-month period. Their findings suggest that although exercise did not decrease functional impairments related to the TBI, people who exercised reported fewer physical, emotional (less depression), or cognitive complaints (sleep problems, irritability, memory problems, and disorganization). Of interest was that the exercisers in the group with a TBI had more severe brain injuries than those who did not exercise. In their online TBI consumer report, Gordon and colleagues[195] recommend aerobic and nonaerobic exercises as beneficial. They also suggest that individuals with TBIs check out local exercise centers, independent living centers, or adult education classes and seek out videotapes that might provide encouragement or support for engaging in exercise. There is no mention of referrals to PTs or OTs for guidance in setting up exercise or lifestyle change programs or locating resources within the community.

Cardiopulmonary Conditioning

Because cardiovascular disease is one of the most common causes of death among aging adults with developmental delay,[17,146,147] and physical inactivity and obesity occur at higher rates in this population, cardiovascular conditioning is a critical part of the management of individuals with chronic impairments. The following information pertains to interventions for individuals with PPS, as the evidence is strong for this population. Although limited information exists for those with SCI or TBI, one can logically infer that some benefits are likely to occur with aerobic activities in these groups.

Aerobic testing using modified protocols to reduce fatigue has been used on the treadmill,[196] bicycle ergometer,[197] and arm ergometer[198] in individuals with PPS. There were no cardiorespiratory training effects in the first study, probably owing to the low intensity of the exercise, but the duration and distance of walking increased.[173] The two ergometry studies showed an increase in maximum oxygen consumption of 15% and 19%, which is a training effect comparable to normal values for age. There were, however, no changes in blood pressure or heart rate, particularly the expected decrease in resting heart rate that occurs with aerobic training. Although the intensity of the exercise protocols had to be reduced for some of the subjects, none had to terminate the exercise because of overuse symptoms, nor did these symptoms occur at the end of the studies. A problem in evaluating these studies is that it is not always clear whether the study subjects with PPS were asymptomatic, symptomatic (PPS), or mixed.

An endurance training program in subjects with PPS demonstrated beneficial cardiovascular and strength effects without adverse consequences.[199] Aerobic exercise such as using a bicycle ergometer, walking, or swimming may be useful, but the client must be interested in the activity to increase compliance.[157] Willen and colleagues[175] in a recent study of 28 individuals with late effects of polio found that a program of nonswimming dynamic exercise in warm water twice weekly resulted in decreased heart rate at submaximal work level, less pain, and positive functional impact. As with the previous studies on exercises, no adverse effects were noted. Their general fitness training, however, did not result in changes in muscle strength or endurance. Previous studies documenting improvements in muscle function and aerobic capacity were designed for three or more times per week; the authors hypothesize that a twice-a-week program was not enough to show improvements in the subjects' aerobic capacities or muscle strength.

The literature indicates that exercise within constraints can lead to several beneficial physiological and psychological adaptations in individuals with PPS.[157,170] It appears that therapeutic exercise is beneficial when performed without causing undue pain and fatigue. As with any intervention, a comprehensive examination will assist in developing a well-rounded and individualized program tailored to the specific needs of the individual with PPS.

Pulmonary Status

Older individuals with neuromuscular diseases may have increased vulnerability to respiratory complications.[103] Respiratory insufficiency and sleep apnea may mandate intermittent or constant use of ventilatory devices. Nighttime noninvasive positive pressure ventilation may be beneficial.[200] Pulmonary therapy and breathing exercises may help some individuals avoid tracheostomy.[103] In individuals with PPS who have respiratory impairments, respiratory muscle training may be beneficial in improving respiratory muscle endurance and general well-being.[201]

The role of the therapist is to modify activities and teach glossopharyngeal breathing, manually assisted coughing, or bronchial drainage as indicated.[202,203] If trunk supports are considered, vital capacity should be checked with and without an abdominal binder to determine the effect on breathing. The therapist's attention should also be directed toward prevention of problems that may occur from bed rest and maintaining as much function as can be permitted.

Fatigue Management

Use of muscles at high levels for extended periods will result in muscle overload. To perform the same activity with weak muscles, the muscles need to contract at a higher percentage of their capacity than is normally required. For example, in walking, clients with PPS contract their muscles at both higher intensities and for prolonged or even continuous periods in the gait cycle.[98] Energy expenditure for the task is increased, and the prolonged contractions keep the capillaries compressed to limit needed muscle nutrition. Clients with PPS are often observed using nearly maximum voluntary contractions to perform a daily activity. The muscles of individuals with PPS cannot maintain these high levels of activity indefinitely.

A general program addressing fatigue may include nonfatiguing daily activities and energy conservation techniques. Relaxation, breathing, and meditation exercises may also be useful. Lifestyle changes that incorporate methods that decrease physical demands and prevent further decline in function are the most efficacious way to target fatigue impairments. In a study by Agre and Rodriquez[120] symptomatic subjects with PPS demonstrated the ability to perceive muscular exertion. This is indicative of a mechanism to monitor local muscle fatigue that may be used to avoid exhaustion. Their study of pacing, defined as interspersed activity with rest, revealed less local fatigue and significantly greater strength recovery in subjects who paced their activities than when they worked at a constant rate to exhaustion. The Borg Rating of Perceived Exertion (RPE) is an outcome measure that may be used to judge effort (see Chapter 30). Finch and colleagues[204] in a study of individuals with PPS found that after one training session subjects reliably used the RPE in an exercise test to monitor their effort and complete the test. Finch and colleagues[205] have gone on to establish reliability and construct validity on an effort-limited treadmill test for individuals with PPS.

Peach and Olejnik[206] on reevaluation found that compliance with recommendations affected fatigue; it was resolved or improved in a group of individuals who complied with recommendations and was unchanged or increased in the group of individuals who did not.

Sleep Disturbance

Sleep disturbance is a significant age-related change, with an estimated 50% of older adults reporting difficulty initiating or maintaining sleep.[108,109] Several factors may contribute to reports of sleep disturbance, ranging from relatively apparent reasons to more medically complex reasons such as sleep apnea. Habitual sleeping patterns may provide important information. Sleep disturbances from medical or psychiatric conditions (e.g., chronic pain, dementia) or a primary sleep disorder that may be age related or a combination of these may further produce changes in sleep that may be reflective of typical normal developmental processes.[108] Loss of sleep with aging is often a result of the decreased ability to sleep in older adults.[109] According to Neikrug and Ancoli-Israel,[109] this diminished ability is less a function of age and more a function of other age-related factors such as medical and psychiatric diagnoses, increased medication use, and a higher frequency of specific sleep disorders.

A history of pain or numbness that is worse at night or on rising points to sleeping surfaces that are too firm or sleeping with joints in close-packed positions (usually the neck and shoulders). These problems are correctable with foam mattress covers or air pressure mattresses, cervical pillows, and modification of sleeping postures.

Given the frequency and significant number of older adults with sleep problems, health care professionals need to be more aware of sleep disturbances.[109] Changes in sleep quality and quantity in later life influence quality of life and level of function[108]; thus it is critical to distinguish typical age-related changes in sleep from pathology-related sleep disturbances. More complex reasons for sleep disturbance such as sleep apnea may necessitate referral to specialists.

Decreasing the Workload of Muscles

Energy Conservation Techniques

Energy conservation techniques provide the easiest way to decrease the work of muscles without loss of function. Analysis of all activities by type, time, distance, and intensity is valuable in designing interventions. Such an inventory forms the basis for setting priorities and determining where and how individuals wish to use their limited neuromuscular capacity.[126]

Questions addressed include the following:

1. Can one trip do for two or three?
2. Can the activity be performed in a less strenuous way, such as by sitting or using a rolling basket?
3. Can the activity be broken up into parts with change of activity or rest?
4. Are there easier ways to perform the activity with modern comforts and technology, including motorization and electronics?
5. Can someone else perform some of the physical aspects of the activity?

Particular attention should focus on activities that produce fatigue and pain. Specific suggestions may address breaking tasks into subtasks, making environmental adaptations such as to work height and locations, taking frequent rest breaks during activities, and using adaptive or ergonomic equipment.

Orthotics and Assistive Devices

Reduction of muscular overuse and fatigue may be accomplished with lightweight splints and braces, adaptive equipment, walkers, or crutches.[93,103] The use of orthotics and/or assistive devices is individualized and specific to the patient, whose goals, along with the therapist's expertise, will ultimately determine the use of devices. For example, unlike most individuals with chronic mobility impairments, individuals with PPS may have strong and usually negative feelings about orthotics. The use of orthotics or assistive devices may be challenging for the individual newly diagnosed with PPS and facing a relatively "new disability." Polio survivors may have previously relied on devices or may have refused such devices earlier in life and consenting to using them again may symbolize defeat and acceptance of losses.

As with every intervention, a thorough explanation of the specific rationale and goals for the intervention not only will be helpful in gaining the client's trust but will also improve compliance. Rationale for orthotic use includes preventing falls and potential fractures, limiting joint motion and preventing pain, restoring weight bearing on the weaker extremity to decrease the work of the less affected leg in locomotion, improving posture and decreasing back pain, and decreasing energy expenditure.

Thoughtful consideration for the appropriateness of orthoses or assistive devices is critical; such devices should not be haphazardly prescribed or given as the only intervention of choice. They should be prescribed cautiously. Ineffective and inappropriate use of such devices will lead to malalignments, ineffective movement strategies, and postures that will cause more harm. Therapists should carefully evaluate the functions that may be lost or gained and the emotional and physical cost of the use of these devices.

Most individuals have long discarded braces and assistive devices and have relied on compensatory techniques for walking (Figure 35-1). If an orthosis has been used and is essential for walking, it often becomes a part of the individual's body image; thus the client may be resistant to changes in braces or devices. For other individuals, prior attempts to use plastic orthoses may have been painful or resulted in no functional use, and thus these patients may

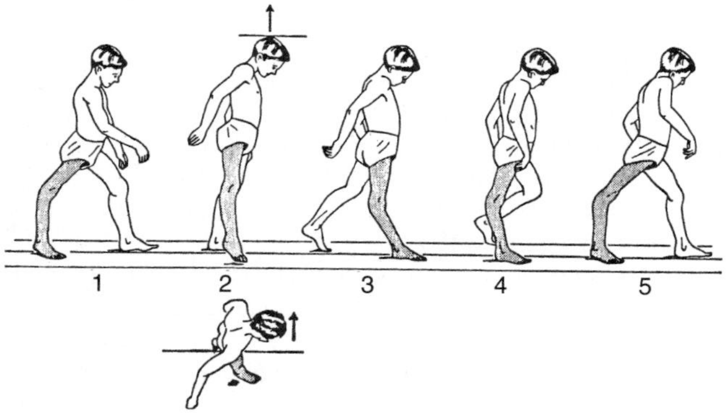

Figure 35-1 ■ The functional compensations of a boy with paralysis of the right lower extremity show increased energy expenditure and progressive ligamentous laxity. (Adapted from Ducroquet R, Darroquet J, Darroquet P: *Walking and limping—a study of normal and pathological walking,* Philadelphia, 1968, JB Lippincott.)

previously have rejected the potential of such devices. Thus it may be difficult to persuade the long-term user to consider orthoses or an orthotic change. When given the appropriate orthosis or prescription, however, polio survivors may benefit significantly enough to improve their current symptoms. A retrospective study of lower-extremity orthotic management for ambulation in 104 postpolio clinic patients by Waring and colleagues[207] revealed that 78% of patients noted that the appropriate orthotic prescription improved the ability to ambulate, increased apparent walking safety, and decreased pain.

In instances in which both the talocrural and subtalar ankle joints were fused surgically, the increased stresses on the posterior structures of the knee or the transverse tarsal joint for ambulation eventually lead to hypermobility and pain in these areas. Rocker bottom shoes may assist with restoring motion for walking. An ankle-foot orthosis (AFO) may address pain in the transverse tarsal joint, whereas a knee-ankle-foot orthosis (KAFO) may help with knee pain.

AFOs are recommended for dorsiflexor weakness resulting in dropfoot or slapfoot, for plantar flexor weakness with absent heel rise, and for mediolateral instability. Individuals with PPS have difficulty with solid AFOs because of the structural design; they are typically made with 5 to 10 degrees of dorsiflexion and are then placed in a shoe with a slight positive heel, thus increasing the angle of the posterior shell to the floor. In standing and walking, this causes a knee flexion torque, with potential buckling of the knee if the quadriceps muscle is weak. Clients may attempt to straighten the knee by pushing back against the posterior shell of the AFO, potentially causing pain. In such instances, AFOs should be made in slight plantarflexion so that the tibia is perpendicular to the floor in the usual shoes worn. This is the normal position of the ankle for toe and heel clearance.[208] In cases of plantarflexion contracture, more plantarflexion is required in the AFO. Most jointed AFOs are of limited value because of the bulk and weight. Moreover, they require a larger shoe and do not provide much control for the ankle. Jointed AFOs allow adjustment to find the best angle in function.

A floor reaction AFO prohibits all ankle motion and can place forces to control the knee.[209-211] The orthosis prevents dropfoot, promotes heel rise, provides an extension torque on the proximal tibia to supplement weak quadriceps muscles, and can limit hyperextension of the knee. It requires precision in fabrication for the knee extension torque to occur only when the tibia is perpendicular to the floor during gait. When used with rocker-bottom shoes, the client with a flail foot can walk with a more typical gait pattern. Subjects with ligamentous laxity of the knee, excessive tibial torsion, or paralysis of the quadriceps muscles are poor candidates for this type of AFO.

Shoe inserts, heel lifts, and molded foot orthoses can provide a number of inconspicuous corrections. Positive heel shoes with a broad base, such as cowboy boots, stacked or Cuban heels, or the Swedish clog,[212] decrease the amount of dorsiflexion and plantarflexion motion and the work needed for ambulation. Rocker-bottom soles, which provide mechanical heel rise to assist the calf muscles, can be added to shoes and are commercially available. Work boots, dress boots, or basketball shoes may provide needed ankle stability.

Asymmetrical standing is typical in individuals with unilateral lower-extremity paralysis or pain. Standing is accomplished with more weight on the stronger limb, which must perform continuous, high-level isometric contractions (Figure 35-2). Unloading the stronger leg requires restoration of weight bearing on the more involved leg using a KAFO or in some instances an AFO that prevents advancement of the tibia in the stance phase (Figure 35-3).[94,209-211]

An obvious forward-leaning posture is seen in some ambulatory individuals with PPS. This posture requires continuous contraction of the erector spinae muscles and leads to back pain, often radiating to the hip and leg. The forward-leaning posture is found in people with quadriceps muscle paresis and in those with ankle weakness. Those with quadriceps weakness must move the center of gravity of the body anterior to the knee axis to lock the knee and prevent knee flexion in stance. This posterior force also produces ligamentous instability and genu recurvatum (see Figure 35-1). In some instances, lightweight athletic knee braces allowing 10 to 15 degrees of hyperextension provide adequate control. More often, a KAFO with an offset knee joint allowing necessary hyperextension is required.[213-215] People with dorsiflexor muscle paralysis or ankle instabilities walk in the forward-leaning posture to watch the floor and foot placement to avoid tripping and falling. Athletic ankle supports or boots may be sufficient to control some ankle instabilities. Molded and posted plastic AFOs with or without ankle joints are needed for more control. Flexible plastic AFOs and the dynamic spring dorsiflexion assists can correct simple dropfoot.[94] Once the forward-leaning posture is addressed, the individual can walk upright and back pain will lessen and may disappear within days.

Walking with lateral trunk shift in the stance phase (gluteus medius gait) produces abnormal forces and joint dysfunction from the spine to the foot. In addition to a strengthening program, these forces may be reduced with use of a forearm crutch or a cane (see Figure 35-2).

Long-term crutch walkers with or without orthoses and those with slow, precarious, or labored gait should be evaluated for appropriateness for use of motorized vehicles as their primary form of locomotion, whereas orthotic corrections or applications may be indicated to assist with transfers and short-distance walking.

Changes in Locomotion

In individuals with chronic neuromuscular impairments, the extent of impairment is influenced by the degree of neurological deficit in motor control, tone, and strength. In neurological disorders such as CP, deficits in tone may cause the individual to walk with a flexed-knee stance, which has higher biomechanical requirements and greater forces in the lower extremities.[216] Perry and Burnfield[216] stated that the most substantial increases occurred with knee flexion beyond 15 degrees. It is noteworthy that as the degree of knee flexion contracture increases, the amount of oxygen rate and oxygen cost progressively increase while comfortable walking speed decreases. Oxygen rate is the amount of oxygen consumed per minute and is related to the length of time that exercise can be performed.[216] Oxygen rate indicates the intensity of physical effort during exercise.[216] Oxygen cost pertains to the amount of energy used for walking; since it is typically greater than normal for a patient depending on the degree of disability, gait efficiency is less than 100%.[216] In children with spastic diplegia with

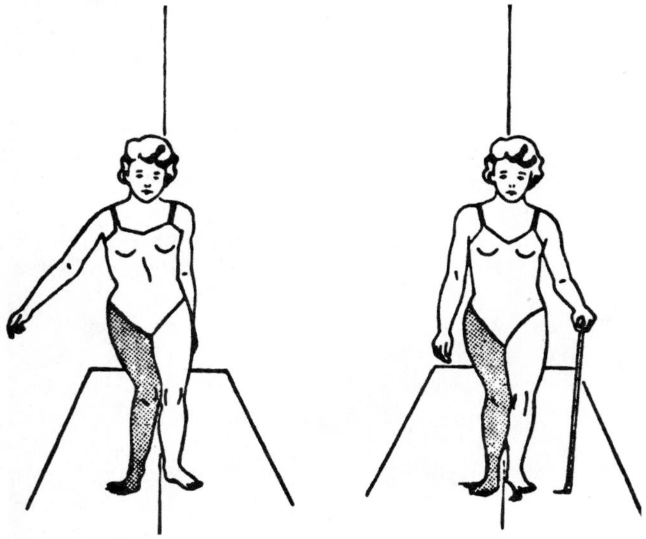

Figure 35-2 ■ Lateral trunk shift in a postpolio individual to illustrate abnormal forces occurring in the back, knee, and ankle with resulting joint dysfunction and pain. Prevention of these abnormal forces and some correction can be provided by use of a cane or forearm crutch. (Adapted from Ducroquet R, Darroquet J, Darroquet P: *Walking and limping—a study of normal and pathological walking,* Philadelphia, 1968, JB Lippincott.)

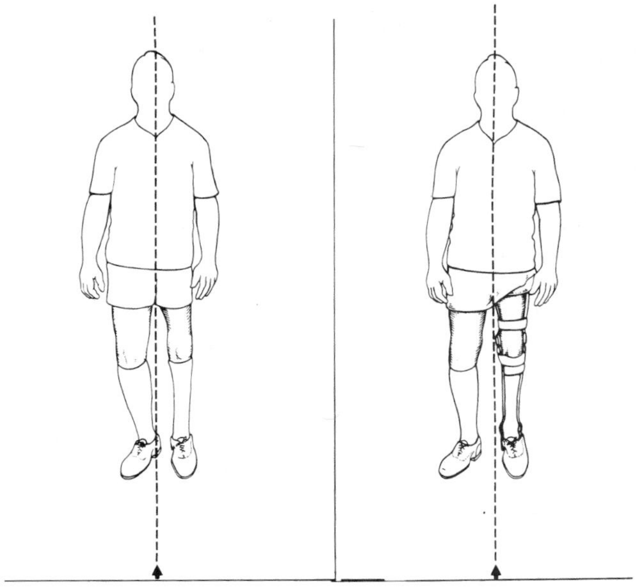

Figure 35-3 ■ This man has paralysis of the left lower extremity with severe fatigue, low back pain, pain and weakness in the right lower extremity, and decreased function. He can be seen to bear weight and stand on the right leg. Application of a left knee-ankle-foot orthosis (KAFO) with a free knee joint (with a drop lock for use in prolonged standing and walking on rough terrain) and a limited-motion ankle joint unloaded his right leg and permitted him to walk in an erect posture. His pain disappeared and he has regained function at work and in social activities.

moderate to severe disability with both lower extremities affected leading to a flexed hip and knee posture, the mean heart and oxygen rates were notably higher than normal and were consistently elevated even when upper-extremity assistive devices were not required.[217] The bilateral stance of flexed hip and knees requires considerable muscular effort from antigravity muscles even at slow speeds to prevent collapse in the child with spastic diplegia. Moreover, Perry and Burnfield[216] state that the elevated oxygen rate may be attributed to the limited motor control to perform the compensatory gait substitutions due to bilateral lower-extremities involvement. In contrast to typical children, the oxygen rate increases with age in children with spasticity. This is consistent with the increased size and body weight in older children and the difficulty with impaired motor control and spasticity. As the child ages, walking becomes more burdensome, and as Perry and Burnfield[216] state, the child may prefer to walk less and rely more on a wheelchair. This scenario illustrates the challenges associated with aging with chronic impairments and may very well be reflected in other neuromuscular diagnoses.

Despite severe difficulties with locomotion from overuse, asymmetrical gait patterns and movement, or ineffective use of assistive devices, changes or modifications are hard for many people with chronic mobility problems, such as many polio survivors, to consider. As locomotion becomes more arduous or painful, many begin to limit outside activities rather than modify individual methods of locomotion. Resistance to lifestyle changes is common in the PPS population and leads to needless suffering and functional decline.[206]

Prevention of this spiraling disability and restoration of lost function require a marked decrease in the amount of walking or propelling a chair and a change to methods of locomotion that do not cause pain, weakness, and fatigue. Independent ambulators or those with inadequate assistance may need to use a cane, forearm crutches, trunk support, shoe corrections, or new orthoses. Clients who have been walking for years with crutches with or without orthoses develop shoulder, elbow, and wrist injuries, as well as new muscle weakness, muscle pain, and fatigue. Use of personal mobility vehicles (motorized carts) for distance locomotion or as the primary form of locomotion may need to be explored, with walking reserved for transfers and short distances only. Lightweight manual wheelchairs only perpetuate the problems and eventually create new ones; use may lead to development of repetitive stress injuries of the shoulder, elbow, wrist, and hand. These people need to obtain electric wheelchairs or motorized carts if suitable. Manual wheelchairs at best only postpone problems. Use of motorized mobility devices will need to be explored to prevent fatigue, muscle overuse, and further damage to joints.

Use of motorized vehicles for locomotion should be considered and explored with sensitivity and caution. Specific rationales should be thoroughly understood by a seemingly resistant client, and perceptions regarding the use of such vehicles should be addressed. Changes in methods of locomotion may be justified to increase safety and prevent costly falls, to reduce energy expenditure and decrease fatigue, to prevent further repetitive injury and pain, and, most important, to increase function and quality of life. Those who do make these difficult changes in their methods of locomotion seem to undergo a metamorphosis from pain and dysfunction to renewed activity and increased function.

Management of Postural Deviations

Altered biomechanics from atypical postures or faulty physiological neuromuscular processes over time may lead to deviations that may cause pain and further functional limitations. In polio survivors, common biomechanical deficits abound, including genu recurvatum, genu valgum, inadequate dorsiflexion in swing, mediolateral ankle instability, and dorsiflexion collapse during stance, as described by Clark and colleagues.[213] These deviations are very likely to be seen in persons with other neuromuscular diagnoses. Strengthening exercises may be used to correct these impairments initially, with orthoses as an alternative management.

Postural exercises incorporated with breathing and stretching exercises are a way to address ineffective postures identified in all positions. Mental imagery, which may avoid impairments from fatigue, may be used early in addressing postural correction. Mechanical restoration of the lumbar curve in all seating and all settings and activities can address the problem if contractures do not limit motion. Properly fitted clerical chairs, ergonometric chairs, anterior tilt seats, gluteal pads, and several types of lumbar rolls, back supports, and seating systems may be beneficial (Figure 35-4).

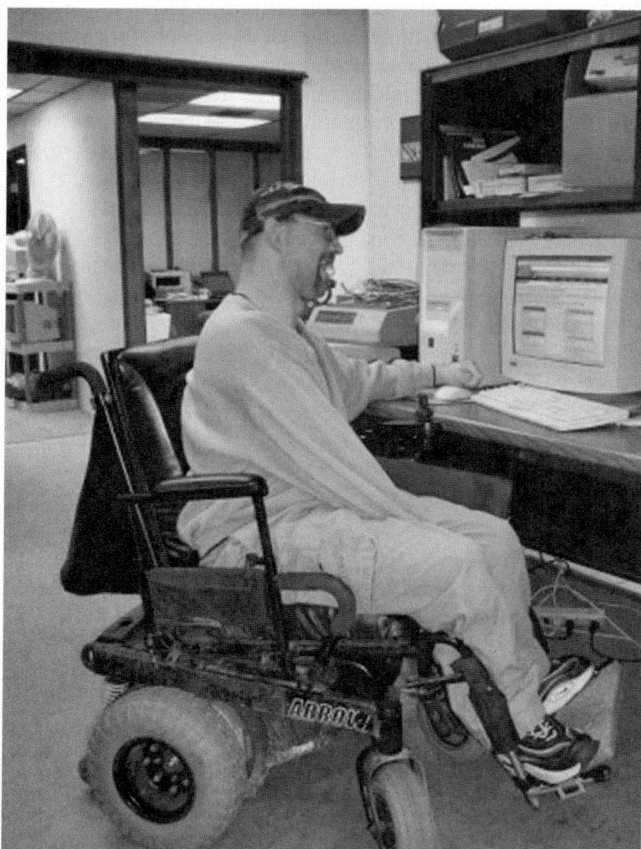

Figure 35-4 ■ Man with athetoid cerebral palsy working at his computer. His power chair has been modified with a back support and a seat cushion for proper positioning.

Individuals with abdominal muscle paralysis may benefit from custom-made thoracolumbar corsets, with the posterior rigid stays bent to produce a normal standing lumbar curve. Paretic or paralyzed neck muscles can be rested and supported by soft foam collars or supportive microcellular neck collars. People with severe trunk muscle paralysis or scoliosis with or without spinal fusion often support the trunk or relieve pain by pushing down with their hands or elbows on chairs, on tables, and on their hips. In time, such self-traction results in pain and weakness in their arms. Chair inserts and fixed supports as well as custom-made corsets, back braces, and molded body jackets should be considered. The rigid trunk supports, however, take away mobility used for function. Usually such supports can be worn for part of the day in activities in which trunk mobility is not essential.

For persons with abnormal biomechanical alignment resulting from spasticity, orthopedic deformation, or severe muscle imbalance, care must be taken to maintain proper alignment throughout the exercise. Additional positioning equipment may be required to assist the person in exercising independently. For example, persons with lower-extremity spasticity frequently exhibit medial rotation of their femurs and bilateral pronation. Combined with asymmetrical patterns of weakness and tightness, a squatting motion produces an excessive valgus angle at the knee. Ensuring satisfactory alignment throughout the arc of motion improves the efficacy of the exercise. Conversely, without this attention to biomechanical alignment, these imbalances and deformities can be exacerbated.

Limitations in Range of Motion

A thorough evaluation of muscle length and range of motion (ROM) is critical in the overall management of life activities in individuals with chronic mobility impairments. The clinician should consider that not all tightness or limitation in motion is detrimental. Selective tightness may have provided some stability to otherwise unstable joints with paralyzed muscles, and useful contractures may have been developed by the body to achieve function. An excellent example can be seen in individuals who contracted polio as children. Muscle involvement was primarily in one lower extremity with a decrease in growth of that extremity as a result of diminished weight-bearing forces. If the individual has at least a G− (4−) manual muscle test grade in the plantarflexors, the person will walk on the toes (in some plantarflexion) to decrease large drops in the center of gravity, resulting in increased energy expenditure for walking. Over the years, a plantarflexion contracture develops that can provide up to 3 to 4 inches for weight bearing on the shortened extremity. With a custom-made shoe, gait is similar to walking in a high-heeled shoe. This can be far more energy efficient than if motion were permitted to have dorsiflexion ROM.

Gentle myofascial release can also be beneficial for recent secondary impairments of muscles to decrease pain and muscle spasms, increase nutrition to the area, and slightly lengthen muscles.

Weight Management

Adults with chronic impairments, particularly those with developmental disabilities, are at high risk for obesity and its sequelae. Weight reduction, when appropriate, addresses this health disparity and is an effective way to decrease the muscle workload, but it is one of the most difficult. Clinicians recommend a modest weight loss of 5% of body weight as an achievable and maintainable goal that may result in decreased hyperlipidemia, hypertension, and glucose intolerance.[218] Weight loss is slow without exercise, but it can be accomplished. Weight control needs to be incorporated as a permanent modification of nutritional habits rather than achieved in a short-term diet. Dietetic counseling and support groups are important components of this challenging lifestyle modification.

In a study of 431 community-dwelling individuals with developmental delay who participated in a community-based health promotion intervention, two thirds of participants maintained or lost weight (mean of 2.6 pounds, median 7 pounds, range 2 to 24 pounds) over a 7-month, twice-weekly program.[17] The authors stated that even without the weight loss, the decreased abdominal girth achieved by participants may be predictive of a decrease in cardiovascular risk factors.[218]

Pain Management

Pain management in the patient with chronic movement dysfunction is dependent on the cause of the muscle or joint pain. As an example of how pain management contributes to secondary health problems, patients with SCI who reported pain from musculoskeletal problems and overuse were seldom referred for therapeutic interventions but were treated primarily with prescription medications to treat painful conditions. This medical management often resulted in increased problems, such as constipation, fatigue, irritability, and frustration.[219] The cause of pain must be carefully determined to establish appropriate intervention and management strategies. Typical interventions for pain include activity reduction, therapeutic heating modalities, cryotherapy, stretching, or energy and joint conservation techniques.

If chronic overuse is the only or major underlying cause of the symptoms present, conservative measures can often slow or prevent further deterioration and may even lead to improved function. Conservative measures include reducing mechanical stress, pacing activities, supporting weak muscles, stabilizing abnormal joint movements, and improving biomechanics of the body. Interventions that address fatigue and weakness such as nonfatiguing functional activities, energy conservation,[126] more frequent rest periods, or change of activity[220] are also useful in pain management. Antiinflammatory agents have been used to supplement conservative measures.

Joint conservation techniques may include use of ergonomic devices, elevated chairs, bathtub bench or shower stool, and weight control. Recommendations for the neck and upper extremities include seating and workstation corrections, telephone headsets, rolling carts for carrying items, newspaper support for reading, ergonomic computer screens, wrist rests, and keyboards.

Successful intervention for joint pain, however, requires identification and elimination of the cause of the pain. This is frequently difficult because the person with chronic movement dysfunction may not have the strength in other parts of the body to compensate and carry out an essential function, or the person may be unable or unwilling to make necessary lifestyle changes. Intervention techniques may include inhibiting muscle spasm, stretching fascia and muscles, decreasing edema and increasing nutrition in joint structures, and mobilizing or stabilizing joints.[221] At some point, relaxation, meditation, modified tai chi (see Chapter 39), aquatic therapeutic exercise, or body awareness techniques such as Feldenkrais[183] may be beneficial.

Local pain and dysfunction can be treated as athletic injuries from overuse, but they require major modifications and careful monitoring of performance, pain, and fatigue. Many joint pain problems can be relieved and controlled by home program interventions such as rest for the injured part, mechanical postural corrections, cold packs, nonsteroidal anti-inflammatory drugs, orthotics, and pain-free ROM exercises.

With regard to McConnell taping, although no radiological evidence shows changes in actual alignment of bone, individuals without neurological diagnoses have experienced a 50% to 78% reduction in patellofemoral pain during activities.[221,222] In the Postpolio Clinic of the Institute for Rehabilitation and Research in Houston, Texas, these taping techniques relieved anterior knee pain for several months at a time in all individuals with PPS who were selected to receive the taping. Relief occurred, although the ability to strengthen surrounding muscles was limited or impossible. The therapy program should also include assisting the client in carrying out the home program and lifestyle changes, along with the development of a continuing program of appropriate exercises.

As with the management of fatigue, compliance of the individual with chronic impairments with suggested recommendations plays a significant role in pain management. In those with PPS, Peach and Olejnik[206] found that muscle pain was resolved in 28% and improved in 72% of people who complied with recommendations. In those who were noncompliant, muscle pain was improved in 14%, unchanged in 57%, and increased in 29%.

Alternative Pain Management

Pain sensitivity must be acknowledged by clinicians when providing therapy that may be perceived as painful, such as stretching, and in the treatment of acute pain.[223] Persons with chronic movement dysfunction have undergone extensive orthopedic surgery in attempts to overcome their initial deficits, as in the case of some polio survivors, and some have pain or hypersensitivities at the surgical sites. Desensitization exercises may decrease the hypersensitivities if the client is willing to devote the necessary time. The most frequent old surgical sites of pain are in the trunk from surgery for scoliosis, the ankle near a subtalar arthrodesis, and the foot with hypermobility of the transverse tarsal joint. In most instances of foot pain, stabilization of the ankle and foot in a custom-made AFO and use of a rocker-bottom shoe has relieved the pain and permitted weight bearing and walking.[212] Custom-made corsets and trunk supports in chairs may help with the pain at previous surgical sites in the trunk. Transcutaneous electrical nerve stimulation may be helpful for pain control (see Chapter 32). Most individuals, however, stop using these devices because masking the pain permits them to physically overdo, leading to further injury to their bodies.

Static magnetic fields have become a familiar alternative approach in the treatment of athletic injuries as well as in persons with PPS who have localized pain. In a double-blind randomized clinical trial, Vallbona and colleagues[224] applied active (300 to 500 Gauss) and placebo magnets in a group of 50 subjects with PPS and chronic pain. The magnets were applied to the palpable pain pressure point for 45 minutes. There was a significant ($P > .0001$) and prompt decrease in pain in the group receiving the active magnets compared with those who received the placebo.[224]

Cold and Heat Intolerance

Strumse and colleagues[225] investigated the effect of climate on the outcomes of individuals with PPS. In a randomized controlled trial of 88 individuals diagnosed with PPS, subjects received one of three interventions: (1) warm climate rehabilitation (dry and sunny, temperature around 25 degrees Celsius or 77 degrees Fahrenheit) consisting of individual and group therapy with daily treatment in a swimming pool, physical therapy, and an individually adapted training program for 4 weeks, (2) cold climate rehabilitation consisting of indoor treatment as described for the first intervention in a rehabilitation center in Norway with rainy or snowy weather with temperatures around 0 degrees Celsius or 32 degrees Fahrenheit, or (3) the usual health care program (control). This study was included in the review by the Cochrane Collaboration, and the authors concluded that there is low-quality evidence of no beneficial effect of rehabilitation in warm and cold climates 3 months after intervention.[18] The reviewers suggest that a more thorough description of the components of the program and outcome assessment for the usual control group would have clarified the short-term effects on both rehabilitation groups and the results of the study. The study could not demonstrate a positive effect of rehabilitation in warm or cold climate for PPS, and further studies are warranted.[18]

Most individuals with chronic conditions who have cold intolerance have learned to control heat loss as best as they can with clothing, massage, and local heat. For interventions, however, cold intolerance can pose a potential problem with the use of cold modalities in the treatment of injuries and pain. Most persons with PPS are hesitant to use local cold on any part of the body. They may typically use heating pads and hot water, which feel good at the time but may perpetuate or increase the edema, inflammation, and pain. Local cold is often more effective and is well tolerated by most people with PPS. Successful application of cold requires more client education about the use of cold and demonstration of the effects.

In persons with MS who are sensitive to environmental heat or an increase in body temperature, specific recommendations for cooling during exercises may be necessary to counteract the deleterious effects of heat. Aquatic exercises and swimming in a cool pool with temperatures at or below 82 degrees may be beneficial for cooling. Use of cooling vests, ice packs, air conditioning, and hydration during activities is also recommended.[226-228] An example of a specific exercise recommendation is the use of a Schwinn Airdyne bicycle to help with cooling while cycling.[226]

Other Interventions

The reader is referred to specific pharmacological texts and specific chapters within this text for detailed pharmacological interventions for specific neuromuscular diagnoses. As emphasized earlier, the management of chronic conditions is individualized and dependent on the unique needs of the individual based on the interaction of multisystem involvement. Thus the pharmacological management of persons with chronic conditions is also individualized and wide-ranging. Although there are classes of medications that are commonly used across varied neurological conditions (e.g. spasticity medications), the use of medication is still symptom and patient dependent. A literature review of pharmacological approaches for PPS revealed that controlled trials of pyridostigmine and prednisone have not been beneficial.[25,229,230] Currently there is no specific pharmacological agent widely recommended to address the multiple symptoms of PPS.

As part of the evaluation, oral motor function is an important component in terms of sensation, speech, and swallowing. Because of their prevalence in persons with developmental delay, dysphagia and aspiration potential need to be carefully explored in the history. Owing to disturbances in muscle tone, these individuals often have difficulty with feeding, which may lead to serious medical complications and potential death. In general, intervention may consist of performing breathing exercises, using swallowing techniques, monitoring fatigue levels, avoiding eating when fatigued, and initiating dietary restrictions or changes. For those with dysphagia, specific management will warrant a thorough evaluation by a speech therapist. Recent advances in treatment including deep pharyngeal neuromuscular stimulation and neuromuscular electrical stimulation offer persons with poor motor control and weakness in pharyngeal musculature opportunities to improve safe oral feeding[231] (Figure 35-5).

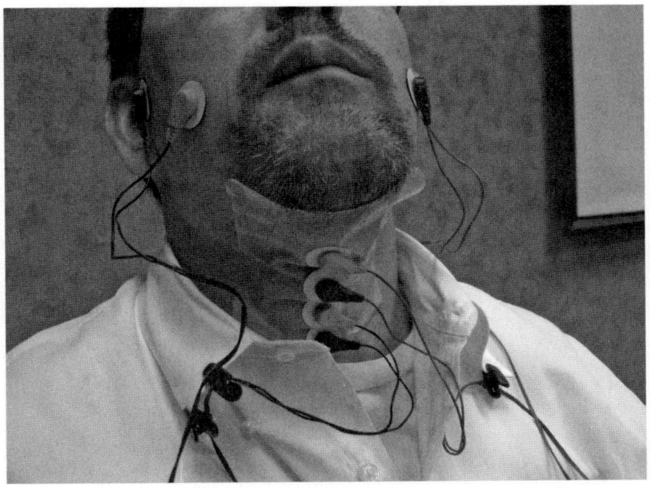

Figure 35-5 ■ Man with spastic cerebral palsy receiving neuromuscular electrical stimulation for facial and pharyngeal activation to improve swallowing and motor control in face.

Acknowledgements

I would like to thank Laura K. Smith, PhD, PT; Carolyn Kelly, MS, PT; Robert Eskew, PT, MS, PCS; and Ann Hallum, PT, PhD, who contributed to this chapter in the previous editions of this text.

References

To enhance this text and add value for the reader, all references are included on the companion Evolve site that accompanies this textbook. This online service will, when available, provide a link for the reader to a Medline abstract for the article cited. There are 233 cited references and other general references for this chapter, with the majority of those articles being evidence-based citations.

CASE STUDY 35-1 ■ AGING WITH TRAUMATIC BRAIN INJURY

Mark was 19 years old when he was involved in a motor vehicle accident in which a drunk driver hit Mark's car while he was stopped at an intersection. He had severe injuries that included fractures of the left femur, both forearms and wrists, and right ankle; multiple internal injuries; "swelling" of the spinal cord; and increased intracranial pressure necessitating removal of part of his skull. He had sustained frontotemporal brain injury with no injuries to the spinal cord despite severe injuries from the accident. He had complicated postsurgical sequelae and was in a coma for 3 weeks. He stayed in the acute hospital for another 3 weeks and was sent to inpatient rehabilitation, where he stayed for 4 months. At discharge he was able to stand and walk short distances at home with minimal assistance, although primarily he used a power wheelchair as his main mode of mobility. Although his upper extremities were functional, he had to learn how to write and use his dominant extremity all over again. He had dysphagia and dysarthria, yet was able to communicate functionally. Mark reports he had difficulty with memory and other cognitive deficits, and those were as hard to deal with as the physical impairments from his injury. He continued outpatient physical, speech, and occupational therapy services for another 3 months and worked on the physical, cognitive, and psychological effects of his injury. He stayed with his parents who at that time became his primary caregivers as he transitioned to a new lifestyle.

In the 20 years after his injury, Mark learned to live with the chronicity of his injury and its secondary effects. He learned to walk with a walker then a cane and eventually walked without an assistive device with a slow, ataxic gait. He learned to use public transportation and navigate his way in the community by using landmarks for spatial orientation. He was involved with support and volunteer groups for several years that provided him the socialization and support he needed, particularly in the early stages of his injury. He married in his mid-20s, and his wife assists him with daily activities as needed, although Mark says he is independent with "everything" except with instrumental ADLs, specifically balancing the checkbook, grocery shopping, and cooking. They live in a one-level home with steps at the front and side entries and have done "some modifications" with bars and a shower chair installation in the bathrooms and wider doors in the bedrooms. Mark says he has seen a PT "maybe once or twice" in the subsequent years for back pain or walking but has not received continued care since his long episodes of therapy after the initial injury. He candidly states that he gets by with all physical abilities although it is "hard at times" and does not currently engage in a specific health or

Continued

CASE STUDY 35-1 ■ AGING WITH TRAUMATIC BRAIN INJURY—cont'd

exercise program. He says he has "learned to live with it" and shares some sadness at being unable to finish his education and care for his parents, who are now in their early 80s.

Now at 48 years old, Mark reports he is starting to feel more fatigued with walking and has noticed the need for more frequent rests. He continues to walk without an assistive device for indoors and short distances but uses a single-tip cane for long distances in the community and outdoors. He and his wife are saving to renovate the front and side entries of the home, which currently have five steps and handrails. Although Mark is able to navigate the steps on his own, he has noticed more difficulty over the years. In the previous year, he fell once on the steps and once in the community as he stepped off a curb. He now uses a "memory" notebook more frequently. He volunteers at the local library three times a week and continues to use public transportation as his primary mode of transportation. "I'm slower, but I get there," he states. He "feels" the secondary impairments from his initial injuries—for example, contractures of the hamstrings, decreased ROM of the ankles and shoulders, postural impairments, gait deficits, and memory deficits—"more now that I'm getting old." He has more frequent bouts of back and hip pain from a combination of biomechanical changes from chronic impairments and possible contributions from aging. He has not sought physical therapy services despite the symptoms, difficulties, and changes in the past couple of years. Although he is interested in seeking physical therapy services, he has not done so, thinking that he will not quality for services because of the chronicity of his condition. He volunteers at a local physical program where he is provided pro bono services at least twice a year.

Points for discussion (suggested answers can be found online) include the following:

- What further secondary impairments and functional limitations do you anticipate?
- What recommendations regarding lifestyle changes would you give Mark?
- If he decides to seek physical therapy services, what recommendations would you give for a holistic program?
- What specific systems need to be examined and addressed in the intervention?
- What services are available for individuals with chronic conditions? Community and hospital or outpatient-based services?
- What health care and community services *should* be available to individuals with chronic conditions?

CASE STUDY 35-2 ■ PERSONAL REPORT: POSTPOLIO SYNDROME*

Today my life is filled with optimism and hope. This was not the case long ago. I am 58 years old and have been diagnosed with PPS. I contracted polio at the age of 2 years, but for the first time in my life I feel disabled.

It is difficult for me to determine when the symptoms began. My life has been filled with caregiving, of first my mother-in-law, who was ill for the last year of her life, and then my parents, who had special needs. I had a vague awareness that I was slowing down, not able to do some of the things that I had always done. But at that point in my life, the focus was not on me. It seems like when I was able to take a deep breath again, I was in a lot of pain.

I was able to see a doctor who specializes in PPS. She recommended a new leg brace and she also recommended physical therapy. The new brace, while better for my body, is asking it to do different things. I basically am trying to learn how to walk all over again. My pain stems from weakness and tight muscles in my unaffected limb. My unaffected leg has been stressed by many years of overuse. The pain I experience is mainly in my hip and occasionally in my knee. Because of the stress of this pain, my stamina is less than it once was; my balance is not good, and just the task of moving from point A to B is a challenge. I found that I needed to use crutches to help take weight off of my leg. The pain that I felt a little over a year ago became the focus of my life. It affected everything I did. My day was reduced to struggle to even shower and dress, let alone do anything else. I had to depend on my husband to do more and more.

During this period I would allow myself, if I was having a really bad day, to just do nothing. Some days I wouldn't even get out of bed until 11:00 AM. This didn't happen too often, but if it did, I allowed myself to not feel guilty. I think that this helped with my mental state. Yes, some days I would get frustrated and impatient and other days depressed, but it never lasted for too long. I have seen, on a personal level, what positive thinking can do. My parents were told that I would never walk again. I walked.

Having had polio, I learned at an early age how to "figure things out." If I couldn't do things one way, I perhaps could another. I think that this mindset has helped with my newest challenge. After meeting with my PT, she helped to map out a plan to achieve my goals. My goals are simple; I want to walk without pain and without crutches. I want to cross my left leg over my right knee to tie my shoe. I want to build up my stamina so that I can go shopping. I want to be in the best health that I can be in. I want to remain independent.

I am learning that achieving my goals may be a long process. It has been a little over a year and I still have a long way to go. I have gained some strength, my stamina has increased, and I am a bit more flexible, but more important, the pain level some days is just an afterthought. I am starting to regain my life.

I have learned in the past year how important it is to listen to your body. I have learned how to manage my work, rest, and exercise time. I understand that to achieve my goals it has and will take a lot of hard, sometimes painful, work. I also understand the importance of working toward my goal and achieving it. I consider myself to still be a relatively young woman who has a lot left to do in my life. Life is a gift, and that is what I want to do—live mine fully.

*Orva Klopfer, as relayed to Holly Klopfer Holton, PT, DPT.

CASE STUDY 35-2 ■ PERSONAL REPORT: POSTPOLIO SYNDROME—cont'd

Points for discussion (suggested answers can be found online):

- If this individual were to seek physical therapy consultation, what history information should the therapist ask?
- What screening questions should the therapist ask?
- What specific systems should the therapist screen?
- What specific tests and measures are appropriate for this case?
- What possible interventions are possible for this individual?
- What considerations should be taken into account when planning for intervention?

APPENDIX 35-A ■ Movement Diagnosis Process Used by Physical Therapists

The *Guide to Physical Therapy Practice*[69] outlines specific examination guidelines based on a diagnostic classification using preferred practice patterns. In the process of determining the appropriate physical therapy diagnosis, the pathophysiological features of poliomyelitis, current functional status, and impairments are invaluable. As an acquired viral disease that primarily affected the central nervous system (CNS), polio infected a broad age range, with the initial infection lasting a finite time. Individuals with postpolio syndrome (PPS) are then classified according to the Neuromuscular Pattern and fall into two categories:

Pattern C: Impaired Motor Function and Sensory Integrity Associated with Nonprogressive Disorders of the Central Nervous System—Congenital Origin or Acquired in Infancy or Childhood, Adolescence

Pattern D: Impaired Motor Function and Sensory Integrity Associated with Acquired Nonprogressive Disorders of the Central Nervous System Acquired in Adolescence or Adulthood

Individuals for whom the specific patterns are used may not have all of the symptoms listed as commonly reported. As Weiss[233] notes, although impaired sensory integrity is not a common deficit after polio, these patterns should still be more appropriate than any of the identified patterns that clearly apply to individuals without polio or patterns that specifically include polio in their exclusion criteria.

The examination element of the patient/client management model distinctly identifies three components: history, systems review, and test and measures (see Chapters 7 and 8). The application of these components in the management of individuals who have had polio can be found in this chapter beginning with the section on health history.

CHAPTER 36 Impact of Drug Therapy on Patients Receiving Neurological Rehabilitation

ANNIE BURKE-DOE, PT, MPT, PhD, and TIMOTHY J. SMITH, RPh, PhD

KEY TERMS

adverse drug reactions
disease
drug interactions
drug therapy
impairment
pharmacist

OBJECTIVES

After reading this chapter the student or therapist will be able to:

1. Identify how drugs may positively or negatively affect the behavior of individuals within a neurological rehabilitation setting.
2. For a given disease state, comprehend how drugs may affect that disease state and the implications on an individual's potential for neurological rehabilitation.
3. When considering one or more impairments, recognize the influence of drug therapy on these impairments and on an individual's potential for neurological rehabilitation.
4. Recognize the importance of a collaborative approach in resolving drug-related issues and how those issues affect an individual's potential for neurological rehabilitation.

Drug therapy is one of the most rapidly expanding therapeutic interventions in the health care system. Whereas monotherapy (the use of one drug for treatment of a single disease state) is preferred, complex pathologies and comorbid conditions usually render this goal impossible. In addition, most of the problems associated with multidrug therapy at one time were generally isolated to geriatric patients, but such problems have expanded because of more aggressive drug treatment in all age groups. Only rarely will an occupational or physical therapist manage a client who is not receiving drug therapy for conditions either related or unrelated to the therapist's scope of practice. Drugs used for the management of a wide variety of disease states may have unintended or undesirable effects on a therapeutic plan for a client undergoing neurological rehabilitation. Although the occupational or physical therapist may not be responsible for monitoring all aspects of a client's therapeutic plan, the scope of drug-related complications must be recognized. A client's pharmacist, who is acutely aware of the prescribing practices of the client's physician(s), may be instrumental in resolving the drug-related impact of any medication on a therapeutic plan. The client will benefit greatly from an effective collaboration that includes the therapist and a pharmacist. Focusing on drug effects, diseases, and impairments, this chapter addresses these interactions from three perspectives. First, the chapter discusses what the body does to a drug (pharmacokinetics) followed by what a drug does to the body (pharmacodynamics). Second, the chapter covers a disease- or pathology-driven model that focuses on the pharmacological approaches used in drug therapy of major diseases that are often concurrent with rehabilitation. Finally, the chapter presents an impairment, activity, or functional limitation–driven model that focuses on the effects of drugs on the impairment and resulting functional deficit and the impact on the therapeutic plan. Although defining every problem associated with a class of drugs or among patients with a particular impairment is not possible within the scope of this chapter, highlighting common difficulties is important.

CLINICAL PHARMACOLOGY

Medications do not affect all clients in the same way, and rehabilitation specialists should be concerned whether a drug achieves or falls short of achieving its therapeutic response. Many situations may alter a drug's response, including drug dose, drug interactions, and a client's comorbidities, and the effect on functional recovery can be positive or negative. In order to understand the impact of prescriptions, the pharmacology of medications used by clients will be discussed. Pharmacology—or the science of drug origin, nature, chemistry, effects, and uses—is commonly divided into two important areas: pharmacokinetics and pharmacodynamics.[1] *Pharmacokinetics* refers to how drugs are absorbed, distributed, biotransformed (metabolized), and eliminated in the body, whereas *pharmacodynamics* can be defined as the study of the biochemical and physiological effects of drugs and their mechanism of action.[1] Many clients in the rehabilitation population will be undergoing pharmacotherapy, and clinicians need to understand how drugs work in the body and how drugs work differently in different populations to optimally manage clients.

In looking at pharmacokinetics, how the drug is absorbed into the body from its site of administration must be considered. Drugs may cross many membranes before reaching their target and can be affected by factors such as drug size, physical state, and dispensing temperature.[2] The absence or presence of food in the digestive tract, characteristics of the membrane, and the drug's ability to bind to plasma proteins can also play a role in the rate of absorption and distribution. Some medications such as Sinemet for Parkinson disease can be absorbed more slowly with a high-protein meal, thus decreasing their availability and potentially affecting function.

When a drug binds to a plasma protein such as albumin, the drug is held in the bloodstream and thus is unable to reach its target cells.[1] The term *bioavailability* is often used to describe how much of a drug will be available to produce a biological effect after administration.

Metabolism is the next step in pharmacokinetics, involving the biochemical pathways and reactions that affect drugs, nutrients, vitamins, and minerals. The first-pass effect is an important phenomenon because many drugs absorbed across the gastrointestinal (GI) membrane are routed directly to the liver.[1] The liver is then the primary site of metabolism before distribution to target organs. Variations in drug response and metabolism may be caused by genetic factors, the presence of disease, drug interactions, age, diet, and gender.[2] Drug doses in the elderly and young are often reduced to compensate for their physiological differences. Any drug or disease that affects metabolism has the potential to affect drug activity. Excretion is the last step in pharmacokinetics and removes drugs from the body. Most substances that enter the body are removed by urination, exhalation, defecation, and/or sweating.[1] The main organ involved with excretion is the kidney. *Elimination* is another term for excretion and is often measured so that dosages of drugs can be determined more accurately. The rate of elimination is helpful in determining how long a particular drug will remain in the bloodstream and thus indicates for how long the drug will produce its effect.

Pharmacodynamics focuses on how the body responds to drugs; it deals with the mechanism of a drug's action or how drugs exert their effects. Successful pharmacotherapy is based on the principle that in order to treat a disorder, a drug must interaction with specific receptors in its target tissue. Drugs activate specific receptors and produce a therapeutic response. Optimal treatment with medications will result only when the physician is aware of the sources of variation in responses to drugs and when the dosage regimen is designed on the basis of the best available data about the diagnosis, severity, and stage of the disease; presence of concurrent diseases or drug treatment; and predefined goals of acceptable efficacy and limits of acceptable toxicity.[1] Rehabilitation professionals are poised to assist the other members of the medical team with the data needed to assist in determining the effectiveness of a pharmacotherapeutic plan.

DISEASE PERSPECTIVE

A number of diseases and their treatment regimens may be concurrently managed while a client is in a neurological rehabilitation environment. The pharmacological interventions for these conditions and their implications from both a physiological and a disease or pathology model are addressed. Although not a comprehensive list, these include Parkinson disease, cancer, seizure disorders (epilepsy), cardiovascular disorders, disorders of mood, autoimmune disorders, diabetes, infectious diseases, pulmonary diseases, and GI disorders.

Parkinson Disease

Parkinson disease is a degenerative disorder involving a progressive loss of dopaminergic neurons in the substantia nigra. This deficit in dopaminergic function results in resting tremor and difficulty in the control of voluntary movement. Cardiovascular function, bowel motility, and cognitive function are often compromised. Although not directly associated with the motor system pathology, the functional deficits are emotionally devastating to the patient, resulting in depression and other mood disorders. The predominant pharmacological approach in the management of Parkinson disease is the enhancement of dopaminergic function in the affected brain regions. Among the earliest successful approaches was the use of levodopa (L-dopa), a precursor of dopamine in the central nervous system (CNS). The use of this agent (and all agents to date) only enhances the dopaminergic function in remaining neurons. This approach has no effect on the progressive loss of neurons. In addition to central conversion of L-dopa to dopamine in the substantia nigra, a similar conversion occurs in the limbic system, a brain center associated with the regulation of behavior. Excessive dopaminergic influence in the limbic system has been associated with aberrant behaviors, including paranoia, delusions, hallucinations, and related psychiatric disturbances that may influence sleep and mood. These behavioral changes are obviously antagonistic to any therapeutic plan. In addition to L-dopa, a dopamine precursor, agents that inhibit the breakdown of dopamine, enhance the release of dopamine, or have dopaminergic agonist activity will have similar behavioral effects (Box 36-1). Dopaminergic agents may produce postural hypotension and syncope by virtue of their ability to produce vasodilation on the basis of CNS and peripheral actions.[3,4] If clients are unable to take their medication, an increasing danger exists (with extended therapy) that movement may be impossible and the normal chest wall expansion and contraction may be compromised (see Chapter 30).

BOX 36-1 ■ AGENTS FACILITATING DOPAMINERGIC ACTIVITY IN THE MANAGEMENT OF PARKINSON DISEASE*

AGENTS CONVERTED TO DOPAMINE
L-dopa (in Sinemet)

AGENTS THAT STIMULATE RELEASE OF DOPAMINE
amantadine (Symmetrel)

AGENTS THAT REDUCE BREAKDOWN OF DOPAMINE
carbidopa (in Sinemet)
entacapone (Comtan)
rasagiline (Azilect)
selegiline (Eldepryl)
tolcapone (Tasmar)

AGENTS THAT ARE DOPAMINERGIC AGONISTS
apomorphine (Apokyn)
bromocriptine (Parlodel)
pergolide (Permax)
pramipexole (Mirapex)
ropinirole (Requip)

ANTICHOLINERGIC AGENTS
benztropine (Cogentin)
diphenhydramine (Benadryl)
trihexyphenidyl (Artane)

*The effects of these agents on muscle tone are complex and dose dependent.

Because Parkinson disease is progressive in nature, clients may have different presentations depending on the stage of the disease and the presence of pharmacological interventions. In the early months of the disease, the motor signs may be particularly subtle, and patients may report only slowness, stiffness, and trouble with handwriting. Particular attention to the history of tremor, slowness of fine motor control, a hunched and slightly flexed posture, and micrographia may lead the physician to diagnose Parkinson disease in its early phases.[5] As Parkinson disease advances, patients have increasing difficulty in activities of daily living and gait as well as bradykinesia and distal tremor.

Once a definitive diagnosis has been made, controlling symptoms of the disease and the side effects of medications is balanced with the level of functional involvement. The physician and client may discuss the option of a number of medications (see Box 36-1) but must determine the best approach on the basis of the clinical presentation. One limitation is the side effect of involuntary movements (dyskinesias). These dyskinesias can be difficult to control and are different from the involuntary movements caused by the disease itself. As mentioned earlier, dopamine agonist regimens that do not cause dyskinesias can also be prescribed, but their effect on symptoms is not as potent.[6] Often physicians may begin treatment with a dopamine agonist and continue with the agonist as long as symptoms are satisfactorily controlled. Later the physician can initiate treatment with L-dopa when the disease is in the advanced stages. With the elderly client who has cognitive deficits, combination therapy may be the initial choice. Once a medication regimen has been initiated, the client and therapist may notice improvement in Parkinson disease symptoms and therefore functional abilities. After taking a medication over time, clients may find that the effect of the medication begins to wear off before the next dose is scheduled. At this point consultation with the rehabilitation team is recommended to potentially change the medication timing or release ability or combine the treatment with other antiparkinsonian medications.

Great emphasis is placed on treating the motor features of Parkinson disease, but clients may have nonmotor manifestations, including depression, anxiety, cognitive impairment, and dementia. Often the client does not mention these difficulties because he or she does not link them to Parkinson disease. Clients may demonstrate some of these difficulties, and the therapist should recognize the symptoms and refer the client for further follow-up.

The major problems that patients have after 5 years of treatment for Parkinson disease are fluctuations (both motor and nonmotor), dyskinesias, and behavioral or cognitive changes.[7] The mechanisms behind these complications relate both to the underlying Parkinson disease and to the effects of medications. Motor fluctuations take several forms. Most commonly, a predictable decline in motor performance occurs near the end of each medication dose ("wearing off"). Patients change gradually from "on" with a good medication response into an "off" period 30 minutes to 1 hour before the next medication dose is due. Often patients have involuntary movements (dyskinesias) as a peak-dose complication, and sometimes similar movements occur at the end of the dose. Sudden and severe cataclysms of motor fluctuation occur rarely, with ambulatory patients becoming immobilized over a period of seconds ("sudden on-off").[8] Because these fluctuations occur throughout the day, accurate detection requires the cooperation of the patient, who must be trained to complete diaries of function.[9] These journals generally divide the 24-hour day into 30-minute segments to detect good medication response ("on"), poor medication response ("off"), disabling dyskinesias, and sleep.

In general, therapists working with clients taking antiparkinsonian medication must be aware of both the positive and the negative side effects of medications to meet functional goals and outcomes effectively. Learning the difference between tremor and dyskinesia is crucial. The therapist must coordinate therapy sessions during good medication response times to assist optimal outcomes. In addition, clients should be monitored for postural hypotension, dizziness, and cognitive changes. Therapists have the unique opportunity to determine the best timing, frequency, and duration of the treatment, and understanding the impact of a client's drug regimen will only enhance the outcome. Therapists must also be aware that exercise increases metabolism. Increased metabolism may use up the medication faster; thus an individual who generally remains symptom free (no off times between doses) will again exhibit signs of the disease (distal tremors and axial or proximal rigidity). These increases in symptoms may be a drug dosage problem, not signs of further degeneration of the basal ganglia. All changes in symptoms should be discussed with both the pharmacist and the physician.

Cancer

Cancer is a general term for classifying disorders associated with abnormal and uncontrolled cell growth. Virtually any organ system in the body can be affected, either as the primary site of the disorder or as a secondary site associated with metastasis. Cancer may interfere with neurological rehabilitation in various ways. Tumors within the brain may interfere with cognitive and motor function as well as autonomic and metabolic control (see Chapter 25). Peripherally, tumors may interfere with peripheral nerve function and associated motor control or may produce pain. In addition, drugs that reduce cancer pain may interfere with cognitive and motor function.[10] Among these, morphine and related opiate derivatives are notable (Box 36-2). A significant degree of tolerance to the CNS depressant effects of these agents will develop with long-term administration. In cancer chemotherapeutic regimens, many antiemetic agents are used. These include dopaminergic antagonists (which may produce motor deficits similar to Parkinson disease), dronabinol (a chemical component of marijuana, which can affect cognitive function), as well as high-dose corticosteroids (which affect mood). Some antitumor agents may be neurotoxic; a reduction in deep tendon reflex, paresthesias, and demyelination is associated with vincristine (Oncovin).[11] Naturally, any change in drugs that involves a cancer treatment regimen (directly or indirectly) requires the approval of the client's oncologist.

The main role of rehabilitation specialists is to help patients with cancer recover from the physical changes that accompany their illness, promote function in activities of daily living, and help provide adaptations to activities within the limits of each patient's function and the illness. Clinicians

BOX 36-2 ■ EXAMPLES OF NARCOTIC ANALGESICS, MORPHINE, AND RELATED AGENTS*

alfentanil (Alfenta)
buprenorphine (Buprenex)
butorphanol (Stadol)
codeine
fentanyl (Duragesic)
hydrocodone (Vicodin)
hydromorphone (Dilaudid)
levorphanol (Levo-Dromoran)
meperidine (Demerol)
methadone (Dolophine)
morphine (MS-Contin)
nalbuphine (Nubain)
oxycodone (Roxicodone)
oxymorphone (Numorphan)
pentazocine (Talwin)
propoxyphene (Darvon)
remifentanil (Ultiva)
sufentanil (Sufenta)
tapentadol (Nucynta)
tramadol (Ultram)

*Effects on motor systems are systemic or indirect.

should be aware of chemotherapy side effects and the side effects of medications given to treat the toxic effects of chemotherapy.

A number of chemotherapeutic and nonchemotherapeutic medications are used to fight cancer. Most therapies against cancer operate on the simple principle that because cells in tumors are actively dividing, agents that kill dividing cells will kill tumor cells.[12] Tissues that rapidly divide in the body are therefore at risk, including hair, mucosal lining, bone marrow, immune cells, and skin epithelial cells. Nonchemotherapy medications called *biological response modifiers* (BRMs) are naturally made by the body but delivered in large quantities and at higher doses than what the body is capable of producing.[13] Interferon and interleukin are two of the most commonly used medications. Monoclonal antibodies are also used as chemotherapy to suppress the immune system.

Chemotherapy often has side effects that affect the integumentary, GI, hematological, and neurological systems. Each type of therapy has potential side effects as well as more general side effects of the treatment regimen. As a result of chemotherapeutic treatment of cancer, patients often have muscular weakness, fatigue, pain, immobility, and reduced flexibility. Often the therapist will have to be supportive and flexible with treatment plans to accommodate for changing physiological, psychological, and social factors during treatment.

GI symptoms such as nausea and vomiting may occur, and medications such as Compazine and Reglan may be given to help control these episodes. Symptoms of diarrhea may be addressed through prescriptions or the use of over-the-counter (OTC) medications including milk of magnesia and magnesium citrate. The development of mucositis or esophagitis is also possible. A prescription solution of three medications (Benadryl, nystatin, viscous lidocaine) can help relieve the pain, inflammation, and potential associated fungal infections. Bone marrow suppression from chemotherapeutic regimens may lead to increased risk of infections, increased risk of bleeding, and increased fatigue and lack of exercise capacity resulting in musculoskeletal weakness. Patients undergoing chemotherapy may receive one or more medications to signal the bone marrow to increase output of white blood cells (Neupogen), stimulate the production of red blood cells (Epogen), and stimulate increased production of platelets (Neumega). These therapies may be instituted to help the patient more quickly reverse suppression of bone marrow and allow the chemotherapy to continue without interruption.[14] Generalized symptoms include fever, body aches and pains, and feelings of ill health and fatigue. No specific medications are used to improve these symptoms. In general, taking medications such as acetaminophen, ibuprofen, or narcotics for fever and pain may help. The use of exercise as an adjunct therapy for cancer treatment–related symptoms has gained favor in oncology rehabilitation as a promising intervention.[15,16] Exercise is thought to help improve endurance and functional abilities.[15] The major side effects associated with BRMs and monoclonal antibodies are generalized as well and include fever and flulike symptoms with associated arthralgia and myalgia. Other side effects include lymphedema characterized by fluid retention caused by disruption of lymphatic drainage or removal of lymph nodes. As mentioned earlier, neurological changes may occur, with the development of neurological signs as well as forgetfulness, suicidal ideation, and depression. The rehabilitation professional is an important team member in oncology because he or she potentially affects quality of life.

Seizure Disorders (Epilepsy)

Epilepsy is associated with a diverse group of neurological disorders resulting in motor, psychic, and autonomic manifestations. Many antiseizure medications may produce drowsiness, ataxia, and vertigo (Box 36-3). Some may produce cognitive disorders in children and adults.[17,18] Although these adverse effects may be exhibited throughout therapy, they are most troublesome during initiation of drug therapy, addition of a drug, and dosage escalation. Sudden discontinuation of antiseizure medications may result in status epilepticus, which may be fatal. Many antiseizure medications are finding successful applications outside epilepsy, especially in the area of pain management.

The practicing clinician working with clients who have a history of seizure disorders must be prepared for the onset of a seizure and be aware of any adverse side effects of medications. Adverse side effects are typically determined on a clinical basis, signifying the importance of recognition by the health care provider. Many of the common side effects can also have negative implications for motor learning, especially while the client is getting used to the medication or the dosage is being elevated or tapered.

The treatment of seizure disorders with pharmacotherapy is typically intended to control the seizure activity completely without producing unwanted side effects. Pharmacological intervention usually begins with one medication (monotherapy); if this drug is unsuccessful a second is added while dosage of the first is tapered. Or a combination may be

BOX 36-3 ■ ANTICONVULSANTS*

acetazolamide (various brand names)
carbamazepine (Tegretol)
clonazepam (Klonopin)
diazepam (Valium)
ethosuximide (Zarontin)
felbamate (Felbatol)
fosphenytoin (Cerebyx)
gabapentin (Neurontin)
lacosamide (Vimpat)
lamotrigine (Lamictal)
levetiracetam (Keppra)
lorazepam (Ativan)
oxcarbazepine (Trileptal)
phenobarbital (various brand names)
phenytoin (Dilantin)
pregabalin (Lyrica)
primidone (Mysoline)
rufinamide (Banzel)
tiagabine (Gabitril)
topiramate (Topamax)
valproic acid (Depakene)
vigabatrin (Sabril)
zonisamide (Zonagran

*Effects on motor systems are direct and may decrease tone at higher doses. Direct effects on muscle are minimal. This list includes benzodiazepines that have antiseizure applications.

needed. The effects of the medications vary and may include enhancing the inhibitory effects of γ-aminobutyric acid (GABA) (benzodiazepines); reducing posttetanic potentiation, thereby reducing seizure spread (iminostilbenes); or modulating neuronal voltage-dependent sodium and calcium channels (hydantoin).[19] The overall result is a reduction in abnormal electrical impulses in the brain. The choice of antiseizure drugs primarily depends on the seizure type and, if possible, the diagnosis of a specific syndrome. If seizures are recurrent and occur during critical periods of childhood, adolescence, and early adulthood, they may result in significant impairments in function and increased disability.

Some side effects may be slow to develop and difficult to diagnose because seizures can often be mistaken for sedation or cognitive dysfunction, especially in children, who may not report drug side effects. Practitioners can also mistakenly accept reversible drug toxicity as a necessary consequence of a seizure disorder. The number of seizures occurring during physical or occupational therapy should be tracked to assist in determining appropriate pharmacotherapy.

One common antiseizure medication, valproic acid (Depakene), may cause nausea, vomiting, hair loss, tremor, tiredness, dizziness, and headache. Valproic acid has also been reported to aggravate absence seizure in clients with absence epilepsy.[20] Metabolic side effects may include an increase in glucose-stimulated pancreatic insulin secretion, which may be followed by an increase in body weight.[21] Long-term valproic acid use is known to increase bone resorption in adult epileptic patients and lead to a decreased bone mineral density.[22]

Another seizure medication, carbamazepine (Tegretol), is considered a safe drug but has a long list of adverse events, most commonly ataxia and nystagmus.[23] Other systems frequently involved are the skin, the hematopoietic system, and the cardiovascular system. Gabapentin (Neurontin) is another well-tolerated antiseizure medication with proven clinical efficacy and a low incidence of adverse events in clinical trials. Common side effects include dizziness, fatigue, and headache. Phenytoin (Dilantin) has adverse reactions including ataxia, nystagmus, slurred speech, confusion, dizziness, and, at high doses, peripheral neuropathy.

Benzodiazepines (e.g., diazepam) are useful in managing status epilepticus, but their effects are not long lasting so they are often used along with a primary anticonvulsant. The most frequent side effects are dose-related sedation, difficulty with concentration, dizziness, and difficulty walking.

Pharmacological adverse events that occur under the influence of seizure medications must be recognized by the rehabilitation specialist to participate in a team approach to patient care. Therapists can assist in determination of effectiveness of a specific treatment regimen, appropriate timing of rehabilitation interventions, and the overall progress of the client during rehabilitation.

Stroke, Hypertension, and Related Disorders

Stroke, by virtue of the interference with blood flow and oxygenation, produces both reversible and irreversible neurological deficits (see Chapter 23). The loss of function associated with stroke has at least two major causes. The first involves loss of oxygenation to a critical brain region, followed by glutaminergic rebound and excessive calcium influx with apoptosis (programmed cell death). Current drugs and those under development are aimed at restoring blood flow and inhibiting glutaminergic hyperexcitability and intracellular apoptotic mechanisms.[24] The second pathogenic issue is related to reperfusion injury associated with oxygen radicals and associated cellular damage. In this case, free radical scavengers have shown some promise in animal models of stroke.[25] To reduce the damage associated with thromboembolism in such cases, tissue plasminogen activator has been recommended. However, this agent is most effective when given within an hour after the vascular insult. Drugs with other mechanisms used to improve the prognosis of stroke are under development. However, drugs used for concurrent conditions (atherosclerosis and hypertension) before and after a stroke are complicating factors for optimal outcomes from rehabilitation. These drugs include β-adrenergic antagonists, which reduce heart rate and correspondingly reduce exercise tolerance. Occasionally, calcium channel blockers, α-adrenergic blockers, and related agents may cause similar effects, including weakness, dizziness, syncope, and cognitive disorders. Changes in serum electrolytes induced by diuretics and the angiotensin-converting enzyme inhibitors may affect the heart, the vasculature, and skeletal muscle and ultimately cause impairments in areas such as strength of contraction.[26] Box 36-4 lists many of these drugs. Many of the cholesterol synthesis inhibitors (agents used to reduce serum cholesterol) may induce muscle weakness (Box 36-5).[27,28] Abrupt discontinuation of antihypertensive medications may result in a hypertensive crisis, dramatically increasing the risk of stroke and related disorders.

BOX 36-4 ■ COMMONLY USED ANTIHYPERTENSIVE AND CARDIOVASCULAR DRUGS*

β-ADRENERGIC BLOCKING DRUGS
acebutolol (Sectral)
atenolol (Tenormin)
betaxolol (Kerlone)
bisoprolol (Zebeta)
carteolol (Cartrol)
esmolol (Brevibloc)
metoprolol (Lopressor)
nadolol (Corgard)
nebivolol (Bystolic)
penbutolol (Levatol)
pindolol (Visken)
propranolol (Inderal)
sotalol (Betapace)
timolol (Blocadren)

AGENTS THAT AFFECT α- AND/OR β-ADRENERGIC SYSTEMS
carvedilol (Coreg)
clonidine (Catapres)
doxazosin (Cardura)
guanabenz (Wytensin)
guanadrel (Hylorel)
guanfacine (Tenex)
labetalol (Trandate)
methyldopa (Aldomet)
prazosin (Minipress)
silodosin (Rapaflo)
tamsulosin (Flomax)
terazosin (Hytrin)

CALCIUM CHANNEL BLOCKING DRUGS
amlodipine (Norvasc)
bepridil (Vascor)
clevidipine (Cleviprex)
diltiazem (Cardizem)
felodipine (Plendil)
isradipine (DynaCirc)
nicardipine (Cardene)
nifedipine (Procardia)
nimodipine (Nimotop)
nisoldipine (Sular)
verapamil (Calan)

AGENTS THAT AFFECT THE RENIN-ANGIOTENSIN SYSTEM

Angiotensin-Converting Enzyme Inhibitors
benazepril (Lotensin)
captopril (Capoten)
enalapril (Vasotec)
fosinopril (Monopril)
lisinopril (Zestril)
moexipril (Univasc)
perindopril (Aceon)
quinapril (Accupril)
ramipril (Altace)
trandolapril (Mavik)

Angiotensin Antagonists
candesartan (Atacand)
eprosartan (Teveten)
irbesartan (Avapro)
losartan (Cozaar)
olmesartan (Benicar)
telmisartan (Micardis)
valsartan (Diovan)

*Effects on motor systems are predominantly systemic or indirect.

Clinicians caring for patients with stroke, hypertension, and cardiac disorders will benefit from understanding the impact of any medication on the therapeutic plan. These clients may be taking any number of medications to manage the acute and subacute complications of cardiovascular impairments and their resulting sequelae. Other complications after stroke that may require pharmacological intervention include urinary tract infections, musculoskeletal pain, deep vein thrombosis, pressure sores, shoulder subluxation, and depression. All these medications have their own issues, and health care providers must be aware of adverse events and any alteration in function of the heart that may occur in relation to exercise.

BOX 36-5 ■ HYPOLIPIDEMIC DRUGS (HMG-CoA REDUCTASE INHIBITORS)*

atorvastatin (Lipitor)
fluvastatin (Lescol)
lovastatin (Mevacor)
pitavastatin (Livalo)
pravastatin (Pravachol)
rosuvastatin (Crestor)
simvastatin (Zocor)

*May rarely produce muscle damage through a direct effect on the muscle.

Anticoagulants such as heparin, warfarin, and aspirin (so-called *blood thinners*) are used to prevent another stroke after the first one has occurred. Side effects may include bleeding, allergic reactions, thrombocytopenia, and, in the case of aspirin, stomach irritation.[29] Blood thinners make the client more susceptible to bruising; therefore care must be taken in client handling and choice of activity. Antiarrhythmics are used to restore normal conduction patterns of the heart. Antiarrhythmic drugs may make some clients experience lightheadedness, dizziness, or faintness when they get up after sitting or lying down (orthostatic hypotension).[30] Antiarrhythmic drugs may also cause low blood sugar or changes in thermoregulation.[31] The most common side effects are dry mouth and throat, diarrhea, and loss of appetite.[32] These problems usually go away as the body adjusts to the drug and do not require medical treatment. Therapists must be prepared for hypotensive events and the need to educate clients on positions that will reduce the effects of orthostatic hypotension.

Hypertension is a common disorder that is frequently encountered when treating patients in the rehabilitation environment. Antihypertensive medications are used to lower blood pressure (see Box 36-4) by limiting plasma volume expansion, decreasing peripheral resistance, and decreasing plasma volume. Often clients under medical management will undergo changes in dose and additions or deletions of medication, which may lead to problems during rehabilitation. Side effects of these medications may include increased frequency of urination, increased urinary excretion of potassium, orthostatic hypotension, hypotension, dehydration, tiredness, fatigue, cold hands and feet, and dizziness.[33] When working with a client taking antihypertensive medications, health care providers should monitor for side effects, clinical signs, and the client's perceived exertion. Generally, people on antihypertensive medications require careful cardiovascular monitoring during any physical activity.

Many clients may become depressed after a neurological disorder such as stroke or a cardiac event.[34] It may be attributable to a natural loss of physical function or a neurochemical response to changes in brain chemistry. Clients with signs and symptoms of depression (sadness, anxiousness, hopelessness, suicidal ideation) should be referred for further follow-up by the physician. Many antidepressant medications take at least 2 weeks to achieve a therapeutic level. Antidepressants may cause temporary side effects (sometimes referred to as *adverse effects*) in some people. These side effects are generally mild. Any unusual reactions, side effects, or behaviors that interfere with functioning should be reported to the doctor immediately. The most common side effects of tricyclic antidepressants (TCAs) are dry mouth, constipation, bladder problems, sexual problems, blurred vision, dizziness, and drowsiness.[35] The newer antidepressants have different types of side effects, including headache, nausea, nervousness, insomnia, agitation, and sexual problems.[36] Therapists working with clients who are depressed may need to delay rehabilitation until the depression is well managed.

Hyperlipidemia is considered a modifiable risk factor for heart disease and stroke. Many clients may be receiving pharmacological treatment to reduce their cardiovascular risk. Several types of drugs are available for cholesterol lowering, including statins, bile acid sequestrants, nicotinic acid, and fibric acids.[37] The statins are considered first-line drugs and are generally well tolerated but can produce myopathy under some circumstances.[37] An elevation of creatine kinase level is the best indicator of statin-induced myopathy and should be checked for when clients report leg pain. Bile acid sequestrants also produce moderate reductions in cholesterol. Sequestrant therapy can produce a variety of GI symptoms, including constipation, abdominal pain, bloating, fullness, nausea, and flatulence. Nicotinic acid (niacin) therapy can be accompanied by a number of side effects. Flushing of the skin is common with the crystalline form and is intolerable for some persons. However, most persons have tolerance to the flushing after more prolonged use of the drug. The fibrates have the ability to lower serum triglycerides and are generally well tolerated in most persons. GI symptoms are the most common reports, and fibrates appear to increase the likelihood of cholesterol gallstones.[37]

Overall, clients taking cardiovascular medications need careful monitoring for any drug impact on cardiorespiratory or metabolic responses in relation to rehabilitation activities. Thus the effects of drugs must be considered in developing the rehabilitation plan (see Chapter 30).

Anxiety and Depression

Agents used in the management of anxiety, whether from acute or chronic disease, must be carefully titrated. Among these agents are the benzodiazepines, whose anxiolytic (anxiety-reducing) dosage range immediately precedes a dose that may affect motor skills and cognitive function (Box 36-6). In subjects of all ages, but especially the geriatric population, administration of benzodiazepines may produce paradoxical excitement, confusion, and behavioral changes.[38] Geriatric subjects also have an increased incidence of injury from falls concurrent with use of benzodiazepines and other sedative-hypnotic drugs. Although benzodiazepines may have variable effects on learning and declarative memory, these effects may differ among the benzodiazepines, displaying considerable variation among individuals. If producing sleep alone is desired, zolpidem (Ambien) and zaleplon (Sonata) are attractive alternatives because these agents do not have anxiolytic effects. Although the anxiolytic agent buspirone (Buspar) is relatively free of benzodiazepine-like effects, the onset time for the desired anxiolytic effect is characteristically delayed.[39] Lack of compliance with anxiolytic agents may increase panic attacks and reduce effective interactions with a therapist.

The emergence of the selective serotonin reuptake inhibitors (SSRIs) has revolutionized the treatment of depression. The older agents, such as the TCAs, are just as effective in the management of several forms of depression; however, their adverse effect profile is somewhat different. TCAs often produce drowsiness and orthostatic hypotension, effects that complicate any rehabilitation regimen.[40] Although these effects may be produced by SSRIs, their incidence is much reduced. Certain TCAs, by virtue of their ability to inhibit the reuptake of norepinephrine in adrenergic nerve terminals, may be used at lower doses for neuralgia. Although these low-dose regimens are usually not associated with the side effects previously mentioned, some patients may be more sensitive to these effects than others. This requires increased vigilance for the care team in determining iatrogenic versus pathological sources of somnolence and syncope. A partial list of antidepressants is presented in Box 36-7. Noncompliance with antidepressant therapy may result in lack of interest in any therapeutic regimen.

BOX 36-6 ■ ANXIOLYTIC BENZODIAZEPINES*

- alprazolam (Xanax)
- chlordiazepoxide (Librium)
- clorazepate (Tranxene)
- diazepam (Valium)
- halazepam (Paxipam)
- lorazepam (Ativan)
- oxazepam (Serax)

*Note that benzodiazepines indicated for sleep induction are not included in this list. The above agents reduce muscle tone through a direct effect on motor systems at higher doses.

BOX 36-7 ■ ANTIDEPRESSANTS: EXAMPLES OF TRICYCLIC ANTIDEPRESSANTS (TCAs) AND SELECTIVE SEROTONIN REUPTAKE INHIBITORS (SSRIs)*

TCAs
amitriptyline (Elavil)
amoxapine (various trade names)
clomipramine (Anafranil)
desipramine (Norpramin)
doxepin (Adapin)
imipramine (Tofranil)
nortriptyline (Pamelor)
protriptyline (Vivactil)

SSRIs
citalopram (Celexa)
escitalopram (Lexapro)
fluoxetine (Prozac)
fluvoxamine (Luvox)
paroxetine (Paxil)
sertraline (Zoloft)

*These agents may produce complex direct and indirect effects on motor systems with minimal effects directly on muscle.

Patients with stroke and other neurological diagnoses often have depression, which reduces motivation and decreases compliance with a therapeutic regimen. Although obviously linked, the degree of functional restoration after a stroke does not always correlate with resolution of depression.

Many patients with neurological disorders are diagnosed with or experience anxiety and depression. The cause of affective symptomatology can be the result of cognitive and emotional deficits or impairment of brain function from the existing pathology.[34] In the rehabilitation environment many patients may show signs and symptoms of anxiety or depression that can make the process of recovery more difficult. The rehabilitation professional must recognize the manifestations of both anxiety and depression such as fear of dying or "going crazy," heart palpitations, shortness of breath, difficulty concentrating, depressed mood, diminished interest or pleasure in activities, sleep disturbance, changes in appetite, psychomotor retardation and agitation, and suicidal ideation.[41] Anxiety and depression may limit the client's full participation in recovery of function and are associated with poorer outcomes.[36,42]

Anxiety and depression can be managed well when treated with the medications discussed previously, but some drugs—including centrally acting hypotensives (methyldopa), lipid-soluble β-blockers (propranolol), benzodiazepines, and other CNS depressants—may cause a depressed mood.[1] Therefore review of the medication regimen in someone with depression is useful in case one of the medications may be implicated.

Pharmacological treatments for anxiety and depression should be administered at a dosage and time that ensure the best patient response during rehabilitation treatments. Antianxiety medications (see Box 36-6) act within a short time after ingestion, producing their effects of sedation and relaxation and thereby reducing anxiety. Higher levels may cause drowsiness, sleep, and anesthesia and are associated with falls, which may not be ideal when trying to promote recovery of function. Antidepressant medications (see Box 36-7) typically take weeks for therapeutic levels to be achieved in the brain and an improvement in mood to be demonstrated. Rehabilitation may be appropriate for a client taking these medications when they have improved the client's mood and outlook. Side effects of antidepressants can also cause some difficulties, including lightheadedness, drowsiness, short-term memory loss, disturbed sleep, clumsiness, sedation, and low blood pressure.

Some evidence has shown that recovery from brain injury may be positively influenced by antidepressants[43,44] and that antidepressants can play a role in brain plasticity.[45] These studies suggest that recovery of function after brain injury can be influenced by experience and pharmacological intervention. Rehabilitation specialists need to be prepared to assess responses to pharmacotherapy, recognize adverse effects, manage minor side effects, and seek appropriate assistance for adverse events.

Arthritis and Autoimmune Disorders

In rheumatoid arthritis (RA), autoimmune mechanisms play an important role in the inflammatory process and progressive joint destruction. Because of the constant pain associated with movement, clients will seek nonprescription drugs (including dietary supplements) that often escape prescription drug monitoring programs in pharmacies. It is important for all health professionals to recognize this issue, particularly with RA. In the management of RA, the therapeutic approach may influence the progress of rehabilitation. Aggressive treatment with glucocorticoids may reduce joint pain and facilitate movement, but it may produce changes in mood and muscle wasting.[46] Although this is reversible and limited to systemic administration of high-dose corticosteroids, its impact cannot be overlooked and certainly affects physical or occupational therapy prognosis. Prednisone and related glucocorticoids may often produce a false sense of well-being that may exceed the ability of the patients to engage safely in certain exercise regimens. From the patient's perspective, this pharmacological effect is perceived as a "cure" and does not provide the motivation to continue with exercise therapy. The same problems may exist with the use of corticosteroids in other autoimmune disorders.[47]

Nonsteroidal antiinflammatory agents (NSAIDs) (Box 36-8) have long been used for the relief of pain with arthritis; however, depletion of prostaglandins in the gastric mucosa produces bleeding, which has limited their usefulness.[48] The development of newer agents that are more selective for isoforms of cyclooxygenase (COX-2 inhibitors) that are involved in joint inflammation is a major advance. An example is celecoxib. Although bleeding disorders are dramatically reduced, the incidence of ataxia with these agents may be increased.[49] Unfortunately, cardiovascular toxicity risk has led to the withdrawal of most of the COX-2 inhibitors from the market. Clients with neurological diseases or pathological processes with problems requiring antiinflammatory medications may develop side effects that interact with and complicate existing motor deficits. Failure to comply with the arthritis medication regimen will likewise reduce effective movement.

Clinically, clients with the onset of RA may have a number of systemic manifestations, including fatigue, anorexia,

BOX 36-8 ■ COMMONLY USED NONSTEROIDAL ANTIINFLAMMATORY AGENTS (NSAIDs) AND SALICYLATES*

aspirin or acetylsalicylic acid
celecoxib (Celebrex)
diclofenac (Voltaren)
diflunisal (Dolobid)
etodolac (Lodine)
fenoprofen (Nalfon)
flurbiprofen (Ansaid)
ibuprofen (Advil, Motrin, Nuprin)
indomethacin (Indocin)
ketoprofen (Orudis KT, Oruvail)
ketorolac (Toradol)
meclofenamate (various trade names)
mefenamic acid (Ponstel)
meloxicam (Mobic)
nabumetone (Relafen)
naproxen (Aleve, Naprosyn)
oxaprozin (Daypro)
piroxicam (Feldene)
sulindac (Clinoril)
tolmetin (Tolectin)

*Only at higher doses will these agents affect motor systems directly. Most problems are through systemic or indirect effects.

generalized weakness, and musculoskeletal symptoms followed by synovitis. These forewarning symptoms may continue over weeks or months before more specific symptoms occur. The initial evaluation of the patient with RA should document symptoms of active disease (e.g., presence of joint pain, duration of morning stiffness, degree of fatigue), functional status, objective evidence of disease activity (e.g., synovitis, as assessed by tender and swollen joint counts, and the erythrocyte sedimentation rate), mechanical joint problems (e.g., loss of motion, crepitus, instability, malalignment, or deformity), the presence of extraarticular disease, and damage detected radiographically.[50] Neurological complications of RA may occur in the CNS (cerebral vasculitis), the peripheral nervous system (nerve compression), the neuromuscular junction (myasthenic syndrome), and muscle (myopathy).[51] Depending on the stage of involvement, the client may be undergoing nonpharmacological modalities (education, weight loss, range-of-motion exercises) and pharmacological therapy including analgesics, NSAIDs, steroids, disease-modifying antirheumatic drugs (DMARDs), and BRMs.

The goals of pharmacological treatment of RA are to prevent or control joint damage, prevent loss of function, decrease pain, and improve joint function.[50] NSAIDs assist in analgesia and decrease inflammation, thus allowing the therapist to work on range of motion and strengthening, but they do not alter the disease process. Because NSAIDs regulate the production of chemicals (prostaglandins) in the body that help trigger inflammation by inhibition of an enzyme (COX), they sometimes lead to unwanted side effects previously discussed. Data suggest that although selective COX-2 inhibitors have a significantly lower risk of serious adverse GI effects than do nonselective NSAIDs, they are no more effective than nonselective NSAIDs, are related to cardiovascular events, and may cost as much as 15 to 20 times more per month of treatment than generic NSAIDs.[52,53]

Steroids are synthetic forms of naturally occurring hormones produced by the adrenal glands and are typically administered orally or by injection. They provide rapid and powerful reduction of pain and inflammation, thus resulting in improved function. Recent evidence suggests that low-dose glucocorticoids slow the rate of joint damage and therefore appear to have disease-modifying potential.[54] Side effects include blood sugar elevations, cataracts, hypertension, increased susceptibility to infection and bruising, osteoporosis, and weight gain, depending on the dosage and length of treatment. They are often used at disease onset or with disease flares as a temporary aid in obtaining control. Disabling synovitis frequently recurs when glucocorticoids are discontinued, even in patients who are receiving combination therapy with one or more DMARDs. Therefore many patients with RA are functionally dependent while taking glucocorticoids and continue them long term.[50]

An important foundation in the treatment of RA is the use of DMARDs, which are medications that reduce signs and symptoms, reduce or prevent joint damage, and preserve the structure and function of the joints. Their use alone or in combination has been reported to allow patients to remain active and productive.[55] The most common DMARDs in current use include methotrexate, sulfasalazine, hydroxychloroquine, leflunomide, and cyclosporine. Others include gold salts, azathioprine, and D-penicillamine. Side effects may include diarrhea, eye damage, liver damage, nausea, and vomiting and depend on the DMARD taken.

Finally, BRMs are a newly developed class of medicines that restore or stimulate the immune system to fight disease. BRMs target specific parts of the immune system that destroy joints. Some do so by blocking the effects of tumor necrosis factor (TNF), a protein involved in RA through the inflammatory cascade, and are credited with improving signs, symptoms, and function in patients with RA.[56]

Rehabilitation therapy is important in maintaining physical function in clients with RA. With combinations of medications, health care providers can reach goals of increasing or maintaining joint mobility; decreasing pain; improving functional abilities; improving cardiovascular fitness; and educating clients on the use of assistive devices, joint protection, and energy conservation.

Infectious Diseases

Both bacterial and viral diseases may produce neurological disorders (see Chapter 26). The neurological impact of treatments and prophylactic measures must be understood. Although this may be readily apparent for drugs, vaccines have also been implicated in causing similar problems. The association of a hypotonic-hyporesponsive episode with the pertussis vaccine is such an example.[57]

In the course of treating bacterial diseases, many antibiotics and antiinfective agents may compromise sensory, motor, and cognitive function. These functions may be compromised temporarily or permanently and may be patient specific. First, in the critically ill patient, aminoglycosides (gentamicin, tobramycin, and amikacin) and vancomycin may produce ototoxicity, such as hearing loss (reversible and irreversible) and vestibular damage (dizziness, vertigo, and ataxia). Minocycline is also associated with vestibular toxicity.[58] Extra precautions may be necessary to prevent falls during and after therapeutic exercise sessions. Fall-prevention programs must be developed in these cases as well as with the use of sedative-hypnotics, as previously noted.

A wide variety of viral diseases interfere with neurological function. Polio is historically the most widely recognized (see Chapter 35). Acquired immunodeficiency syndrome (AIDS) may manifest as a wide variety of neurological disorders (see Chapter 31). A recent finding is that protease inhibitors, which reduce the assembly of viral particles, may dramatically reduce and possibly reverse the neurological manifestations of AIDS.[59] Although adverse effects associated with antiviral and antibiotic agents may be intolerable, noncompliance may result in increased resistance of the virus or microorganism to retreatment.

The guiding principle of chemotherapy for infection is selective toxicity, in which the agent must cause more harm to the pathogen than to the host. Problems associated with antimicrobial therapy include resistance to drugs, side effects, allergies, and suppression of normal flora. Clinicians ask clients to exercise under conditions in which they may potentially have a compromised immune response because of trauma, a pathological condition, or surgery. These conditions may make clients more susceptible to infection, slow healing, and slow recovery.[60]

An increasing number of strains of antibiotic-resistant bacteria are now emerging, in large part because of the overuse and misuse of antimicrobial drugs by health care providers.[61] Overuse of antimicrobial drugs exerts a selective pressure among bacteria, encouraging the emergence of antibiotic-resistant strains by eliminating antibiotic-sensitive strains, promoting the establishment of bacteria with rare mutations of resistance, and permitting the spread of resistant strains from infected individuals.[62] One example is the use of antibiotics for upper respiratory tract infections caused by viruses. This has been shown to have no beneficial impact on the course of the disease.[63] Infection control in the rehabilitation environment is essential to stop the spread of disease. Therapists must be diligent with infection control procedures such as handwashing, updating vaccinations, and cleaning all equipment. Educating clients to use antibiotics only when needed and complete the entire course of medication can potentially slow the proliferation.

Common adverse effects from the use of antimicrobials and antiviral drugs include nephrotoxicity and ototoxicity (aminoglycosides), GI complications (cephalosporins, clindamycin), thrombophlebitis and vertigo (tetracyclines), jaundice (erythromycin), photophobia (vidarabine), neurotoxicity (metronidazole), and allergic reactions (β-lactam antibiotics). The therapist must be aware of adverse side effects to assist with early recognition and referral to the physician.

Antibiotics kill various normal commensal bacteria in the gut, altering the balance and allowing overgrowth of pathogens.[64] This change of bacterial flora is believed to result in increased toxins from pathogens and can cause infection with resistant microbes.[64] When clients are taking drugs to fight infection or undergoing procedures or surgeries that place them at risk for infection (indwelling catheters), they can be more susceptible to infectious agents. Abscesses or contamination as a result of the normal flora into a normally sterile body site is often the reason for perioperative antimicrobial prophylaxis.[65] Rehabilitation specialists will most likely see many clients who are undergoing chemotherapy with antiinfective medications and play a crucial role in preventing and controlling infectious disease in the health care setting. Therapists need to update their knowledge foundation with evidence-based protocols for specific diagnoses and treatments as well as understand when infections may or may not need antimicrobial medications. In addition, education of patients about why antimicrobial agents are not indicated in specific situations, how to alleviate symptoms, and what signs indicate further follow-up may help them understand the growing problem of antibiotic resistance.

Diabetes

Diabetes, as a disorder of insulin production and sensitivity, has two major forms. Type 1 has an autoimmune component based on destruction of pancreatic islets, but success in modulating this pathogenic feature has been limited. As a result, clients with type 1 diabetes are necessarily insulin dependent. The pathogenic features of insulin insensitivity characteristic of type 2 are not well understood, but a wide array of therapeutic agents have been developed for management of this condition. Although the metabolic states of type 1 and 2 pathologies may differ somewhat, the chronic pathologies associated with poorly controlled hyperglycemia are remarkably similar. The development of peripheral neuropathy (see Chapter 18) is a progressive problem in patients with diabetes. This neuropathy compromises sensory and motor control. In addition to long-term management of diabetes from a glucohomeostatic perspective, other agents show promise. Treatment of diabetic neuropathy with trazodone or mexiletine is an example.[66,67]

A more acute problem is swings in blood glucose level from inappropriate diet, exercise, insulin, and oral hypoglycemic drug administration. The balance of these factors is important, and monitoring of blood glucose level is essential. Swings in blood glucose level are often associated with changes in behavior and sensorium. This may pose a safety concern because cognitive and motor function may be impaired as a result. An increase in exercise will decrease the blood glucose concentration, thereby reducing insulin requirements. These factors should be carefully considered in any exercise regimen for the client with diabetes.[68] A list of oral hypoglycemic agents is presented in Box 36-9. Lack of glucose control because of noncompliance with medications that are useful in controlling diabetes will only return the client to an accelerated course to peripheral neuropathies and related sequelae.

In the clinical setting the health care practitioner must remember that the main goal of diabetes management is to prevent both the small-vessel complications (e.g., retinopathy and neuropathy) and large-vessel complications (e.g., heart disease and amputation) of the disease linked with elevated blood glucose levels. Diabetes is therefore often controlled through intensive, tailored treatment regimens of diet and physical activity, oral agents, and insulin.[69] Each of these regimens is designed to potentially reduce hyperglycemia and can result in hypoglycemia if not monitored.

Initially, the physician and client with diabetes can work together on a treatment plan to manage the disease. An important first step includes diet, physical activity, and a

BOX 36-9 ■ ORAL HYPOGLYCEMIC AGENTS*

SULFONYLUREAS
acetohexamide (Dymelor)
chlorpropamide (Diabinese)
tolazamide (Tolinase)
tolbutamide (Orinase)
glimepiride (Amaryl)
glipizide (Glucotrol)
glyburide (Micronase)

RELATED AGENTS
repaglinide (Prandin)
nateglinide (Starlix)

*May produce direct and indirect effects on motor systems through hypoglycemia.

program to reduce body weight by 5% to 10%.[70] The effects of exercise as a cause of hypoglycemia deserve particular consideration because physical activity represents the most variable factor in the routine of many clients, especially those in rehabilitation.[71] With vigorous exercise, glucose use can increase severalfold, and this increase can persist long after the completion of the exercise, resulting in a fall in blood glucose long afterward. Although diet and activity are important cornerstones for diabetes care, oral agents and/or insulin may eventually be required to achieve glycemic control.

Five classes of oral agents are available to help or make the body use its own insulin, including sulfonylureas (chlorpropamide), meglitinides (repaglinide), biguanides (metformin), glitazones (rosiglitazone), and α-glucosidase inhibitors (acarbose). These classes of medications have specific regimens and may be prescribed as monotherapy or taken in combinations that may include insulin. Side effects vary from weight gain to GI symptoms to hypoglycemia. Hypoglycemia as a side effect of pharmacotherapy is of concern in the rehabilitation setting because abnormally low glucose levels can cause alterations in cognition, cardiovascular hemodynamic changes, and an increased risk of physical injury.[72] The signs and symptoms of hypoglycemia can vary from person to person and may depend on how fast the blood sugar drops. Early signs include shaking, sweating, fatigue, and weakness. Later signs may include confusion, combativeness, and exhaustion that inhibits eating, which may lead to loss of consciousness.

Insulin is a primary therapy in type 1 diabetes, in which the body has no ability to produce its own insulin. When oral antidiabetic agents no longer assist in maintaining glycemic targets, insulin is usually instituted in the diabetic with low production or resistance to insulin (type 2 diabetes).[73] Many forms of insulin are available, and administration is typically through subcutaneous injection or insulin pumps. Insulin can be long acting or short acting and is often used in combinations to maintain the optimal level of glycemic control. Hypoglycemia is the primary problem associated with insulin use because of its ability to lower blood sugar.[73]

Health professionals working with clients who have diabetes should consider a number of strategies for prevention of hypoglycemia and be able to analyze the risk and benefits of exercise. Because glycemic control is individualized, each client must be addressed uniquely, and as a member of the health care team the rehabilitation specialist can potentially assist in education of all those involved in the care of the client. The following are guidelines published by the American Diabetes Association (ADA) and should be implemented in clients with known type 2 diabetes.[74] Medical evaluation of the client before exercise begins is important to determine the extent of involvement and complications present. Prepare the client for exercise by monitoring glycemic control before, during, and after exercise. Exercise is contraindicated if fasting glucose levels are more than 250 mg/dL and ketosis is present; use caution if glucose levels are greater than 300 mg/dL and no ketosis is present. The patient should ingest added carbohydrate if glucose levels are less than 100 mg/dL. Document when changes in insulin or food intake are necessary, and learn the glycemic response to different exercise conditions (e.g., light, moderate, heavy). Food intake should include consumption of carbohydrates as needed to avoid hypoglycemia. Carbohydrate-based foods should be readily available during and after exercise.

Clinicians need to have an understanding of what causes diabetes, the effects of medications and exercise on the regulation of blood sugar levels, signs and symptoms of hypoglycemia, and what should be done in a diabetic emergency.

Pulmonary Diseases

Many clients with neurological problems have pulmonary disease as well (see Chapter 30). The treatment of pulmonary diseases presents an unusual challenge. Many drugs used for treatment of asthma, emphysema, and chronic obstructive pulmonary disease (COPD) are intended to have direct effects on the lung, yet systemic effects are often unavoidable. Adrenergic bronchodilators, such as albuterol, epinephrine, and metaproterenol, may increase heart rate and tremor.[75] If tremor first manifests because of a neurological insult, then these drugs may exaggerate the motor impairment. Although ipratropium is an anticholinergic with bronchodilating properties, the associated systemic anticholinergic effects (such as urinary retention with prostatic hypertrophy) are not well tolerated in geriatric men.[76] Prednisone and related corticosteroids may dramatically reduce the degree of pulmonary hyperresponsiveness but often produce systemic effects as previously noted. These are often reduced (but not necessarily eliminated) with the use of inhaled corticosteroids such as beclomethasone, budesonide, flunisolide, and triamcinolone. Although the use of xanthines in asthma is declining, theophylline in asthma and obstructive pulmonary diseases can produce changes in cognitive function, including delusions and hallucinations with higher doses. General CNS stimulation, including nervousness, insomnia, and seizures, is well recognized.[77] Tremor and nausea are often produced with theophylline, even with clinical dosage regimens commonly accepted. Finally, the increase in diuresis caused by theophylline in patients with prostatic hypertrophy is certainly troublesome. The metabolism of this drug is often changed by other medications, which complicates therapy. These changes in drug metabolism may increase toxicity or decrease efficacy.[78] Newer classes of disease-modifying agents known as *leukotriene modifiers* (montelukast and zafirlukast) are being favored in many regimens for the management of asthma. Although cardiovascular and neurological side effects of these drugs appear to be dramatically reduced when compared with other agents, they have been implicated in several important drug interactions.[78] Lack of compliance with these medications decreases pulmonary gas exchange, ultimately decreasing motor performance.

Clients may have signs and symptoms of lung dysfunction during exercise, including nonproductive cough, dyspnea, alterations in breathing rate and chest expansion, changes in skin color, as well as changes in auscultation and percussion findings. Symptomatic pharmacotherapy may be required to reduce disease-related symptoms such as shortness of breath and improve exercise tolerance.[79] The client should begin exercise after medications to improve exercise tolerance. Often with chronic lung disease, exacerbations may be caused by an infection; therefore antibiotics may be prescribed.[80] In addition, thinning and mobilization of secretions in airways with mucolytics and chest therapy may be necessary.[81] Oxygen therapy is a secondary therapy that may be necessary for hypoxemic patients.[80] This therapy reduces the hematocrit level to more normal levels, moderately improves neuropsychological factors, and ameliorates pulmonary hemodynamic abnormalities.[82] Oxygen therapy may be indicated during exercise for patients whose levels become desaturated during low-level activity.[83] Understanding the use of pharmacological treatments for pulmonary dysfunction can assist the rehabilitation professional in promoting improved strength, exercise tolerance, and functional abilities in clients with pulmonary dysfunction.

Gastrointestinal Disorders

Among the wide variety of agents used in the treatment of GI disorders, problems with agents affecting GI motility are among the most frequently encountered. Antiemetics that are dopaminergic antagonists, such as prochlorperazine (Compazine), chlorpromazine (Thorazine), and promethazine (Phenergan), may produce extrapyramidal side effects resembling Parkinson disease through the drug's actions on the basal ganglia.[84] Dronabinol (Marinol), a cannabinoid derivative from marijuana, is an effective antiemetic but may produce cognitive and sensory disturbances, including drowsiness, dizziness, ataxia, disorientation, orthostatic hypotension, and euphoria.[85] The selective serotonin antagonists dolasetron (Anzemet), granisetron (Kytril), and ondansetron (Zofran) are effective and valuable antiemetics, especially in cancer chemotherapy. The most common adverse effect is severe headache.[86] The benzodiazepine lorazepam is an effective adjunct for control of emesis. Problems associated with benzodiazepines have been previously discussed. Corticosteroids such as dexamethasone should be included among the antiemetic agents; their adverse effects have also been previously discussed.

In producing normal motility, metoclopramide (Reglan), domperidone (Motilium), and cisapride (Propulsid) are often used. The adverse effects of metoclopramide are primarily through dopaminergic antagonism. Domperidone was developed to reduce these CNS effects and has been used to treat diabetic gastroparesis with some success.[87] Cisapride, a restricted-use prokinetic agent, may have a wide variety of CNS effects, including dizziness, mood disorders, vision changes, hallucinations, and amnesia, although with low incidence compared with concerns of arrhythmias induced by this drug.[88] Compliance with medications that reduce problems with the GI system may have little direct effect on motor performance but may prove troublesome to the client's quality of life.

In the rehabilitation setting, GI signs and symptoms are common problems for many clients. The side effects of drugs reported in formularies show that almost all oral preparations are the potential cause of some form of GI disturbance.[89] Signs and symptoms include upper GI effects such as nausea, vomiting, indigestion, gastric reflux, and stomach pain or lower GI effects such as diarrhea, constipation, colonic pain, and blood in stools. These symptoms may be caused by an underlying GI condition (gallstones and acid reflux) or side effects from medications (nausea and vomiting). Because GI problems can be prevalent and challenging, cause poor compliance, and be a signal for a more serious condition, the causes and potential approaches used to ameliorate the symptoms must be understood.

Medications can modify GI absorption, cause dysmotility, damage the mucosal lining, or change the bioavailability and resulting effectiveness of drugs. Some drugs modify the absorption or activity of nutrients, ions, and drugs. Drugs such as metformin (used in the treatment of diabetes) may reduce the absorption of vitamin B_{12}, with the potential development of megaloblastic anemia, necessitating exercise precautions.[90] Other drugs that damage the mucosal lining (methotrexate, allopurinol, neomycin, colchicine, methyldopa) may reduce nutrient absorption, leading to deficiencies.[64] One class of agents, NSAIDs, is estimated to be regularly used by 5% to 10% of the U.S. population, with more than 70 million prescriptions filled annually and more than 30 billion OTC tablets sold.[91] These drugs are implicated in patients reporting gastric dyspepsia (pain or discomfort in the upper abdomen), and concomitant administration of proton pump inhibitors (which block production of stomach acid) and prostaglandin analogs (which protect the stomach lining) may often reduce mucosal erosion.[64]

Drugs that cause dysmotility of the small intestine such as TCAs (for depression), anticholinergics (for asthma), calcium channel blockers (for heart failure), and opiates (for pain) may be commonly administered to patients within the rehabilitation population.[64] The large intestine is more likely to have reduced motility, with abdominal pain, constipation, nausea, vomiting, and abdominal distention present. Many patients require increased activity, change of dietary habits, or laxatives to improve motility.[92] Precautions must be taken because of the potential for chronic use of laxatives, fluid and electrolyte imbalance, steatorrhea, protein-losing gastroenteropathy, osteomalacia, and vitamin and mineral deficiencies.[64]

It is important to note that some supplements and fluids (e.g., grapefruit juice) taken with medications can potentially cause changes in the bioavailability of drugs. Concurrent ingestion of iron causes a marked decrease in the bioavailability of a number of drugs such as tetracycline (an antibiotic), methyldopa (an antihypertensive agent), levodopa (for Parkinson disease), and ciprofloxacin (an antimicrobial).[93] Grapefruit juice is also known to change the bioavailability of some medications, leading to an elevation of their serum concentrations; these drugs include cyclosporine (an immunosuppressive agent), calcium antagonists (for hypertension), and coenzyme A reductase inhibitors (statins).[94]

Most medications have the potential to cause some form of GI difficulties, whether taken systemically, topically applied, or given by the parenteral route.[64] Most adverse effects can be reduced with identification of the causal relation, proper administration of the drug, and administration according to all the guidelines on the label. Therapists may suggest specific timing of medication administration to relieve symptoms and increase participation in therapy. The role of physical and occupational therapists should be recognized in observing adverse drug events to warn patients of early signs of potential problems, provide education, and refer for further follow-up by the pharmacist or physician.

AN IMPAIRMENT PERSPECTIVE

In this section of the chapter, different forms of neurological impairments are discussed and appropriate drugs are identified that either reduce or increase the degree of impairment. Although not a comprehensive list, these impairments include sensory impairments, motor problems, cognitive deficits, problems with balance and coordination, cardiovascular impairments, and problems with muscle tone; a brief overview of neuroplasticity is included. Remember that pharmacists have been educated and work closely with physicians who have been educated in a disease or pathology model. A large portion of physicians' practice is related to drug therapy as it is related to disease and pathology. Looking at drugs from an impairment, functional activity, life participation model is not the role of either the physician or the pharmacist. Thus movement specialists, whose model for care is based on function and quality of life, need to bridge the gap between these concepts because the outcome of the interactions dramatically affects the potential of the individual after any CNS dysfunction.

Sensory Impairment

Drugs that affect hearing, vision, and touch may influence any type of sensory, cognitive, and motor impairment. In any impairment, the processing of accurate sensory information is crucial to modify and adjust procedural programming during movement. A subject must be able, through visual, manual, or auditory cues (even through olfactory means), to relate to or recognize the relevance of the external environment, engage the specific motor programming centers that reach consensus regarding the specific motor response, and produce the series of signals that may progress uninterrupted through spinal mechanisms and the motor endplate to a regional muscle group for an appropriate response. Any impairment or drug that affects any component within these systems, whether early or late in this sequence, will affect the motor performance. Clients with sensory integrative problems are often given medications such as those for attention-deficit disorder, anxiety, seizure, and depression.[95] As previously discussed, certain drugs may influence hearing (as previously indicated regarding infectious diseases) or produce tinnitus (e.g., aspirin), which may be distracting and thus ultimately affect motor performance.[58] Changes in the visual field (e.g., with ethambutol and anticonvulsants) are likewise important. Analgesics and topical anesthetics may dangerously affect surface heat or cold discomfort and undermine avoidance cues. However, elimination of excessive pain (peripheral and central) may enhance cognitive focus and learning as well as allow an individual to move as part of daily living, which will help maintain power, range, balance, and thus quality of life. The CNS functions with the consensus of multiple interactions. Because the branched as well as sequential nature of systems links sensory and motor functions, the peripheral effects of drugs commonly modify the function of central systems. This is a relatively unappreciated reason why drug therapy can modify rehabilitation techniques both positively and negatively (see Chapter 9). Therapists must be aware of medications when working with clients who have sensory impairments. Medications can increase or alleviate signs and symptoms, as well as produce unwanted side effects. Clients may benefit from alterations in the environment to limit sensory sensitivities, timing of treatment to coincide with the most effective dose of medications, and monitoring for unwanted side effects.

Cognitive and Central Motor Control Impairment

Disorders of mood (anxiety and depression) reduce initiative in the rehabilitation process. In this context, anxiolytics and antidepressants may have a positive impact. However, if the dose is not carefully titrated, drowsiness and anterograde amnesia will cloud effective response and learning. Both antidepressants and many of the benzodiazepines may cause these effects, as previously discussed. Behavioral disorders, especially those associated with untreated psychoses or dementia, impede cognitive function. Although antipsychotics may correct these disorders, the dopaminergic antagonism associated with these may interfere with the function of the basal ganglia and facilitation of movement. Many newer antipsychotic agents (also known as the *atypical antipsychotics*) have, in addition to dopaminergic antagonism, serotonin antagonist activity, which may reduce the extrapyramidal side effects of the earlier agents when analyzed as movement dysfunction (Box 36-10) (see Chapter 20). The therapist should be monitoring for signs of depression, which is common in clients who have had loss of function. Effective management of depression is dependent on finding an appropriate formulation and therapeutic dose, which may take weeks, and clients will need education and support. Extrapyramidal motor signs should be monitored and reported to the health care team.

Vertigo, Dizziness, Balance, and Coordination

Many agents with histamine antagonist and anticholinergic activity have been used for treatment of vertigo and dizziness. Meclizine and related antihistamines are primary examples. Occasionally, sinus congestion can result in impaired vestibular function and dizziness. In the absence of hypertension or related autonomic dysfunction, an indirect-acting adrenergic agonist such as ephedrine or pseudoephedrine can reduce this congestion and improve this condition (see Chapter 22).[96] Dizziness is a common clinical problem, affecting at least a third of the population in one form or another at some point during their lives.[97] Medications should be reviewed in all patients with dizziness, as numerous medications can be associated with this effect, including alcohol and other CNS depressants, aminoglycoside antibiotics, anticonvulsants, antidepressants, antihypertensives, chemotherapeutics, loop diuretics, and

BOX 36-10 ■ EXAMPLES OF ANTIPSYCHOTIC AGENTS

STANDARD ANTIPSYCHOTICS*

chlorpromazine (Thorazine)
fluphenazine (Prolixin)
haloperidol (Haldol)
loxapine (Loxitane)
molindone (Moban)
perphenazine (Trilafon)
pimozide (Orap)
thioridazine (Mellaril)
thiothixene (Navane)

ATYPICAL ANTIPSYCHOTICS

aripiprazole (Abilify)
asenapine (Saphris)
clozapine (Clozaril)
olanzapine (Zyprexa)
quetiapine (Seroquel)
iloperidone (Fanapt)
paliperidone (Invega)
risperidone (Risperdal)
ziprasidone (Geodon)

*May produce a parkinsonian-like effect through dopaminergic antagonism.

salicylates.[98] Clients should be monitored for orthostatic hypotension and hyperventilation. Depending on the cause of dizziness, clients with dizziness may benefit from canalith repositioning procedures,[99] vestibular exercises,[100] instrumental rehabilitation training on a moving platform,[101] positional education (sitting at bedside before standing), use of compression garments, dietary changes (salt and fluid intake), and use of simple physical counter-maneuvers such as squatting to temporarily but rapidly raise blood pressure.[102] Symptoms of dizziness and balance dysfunction should be reported to the health care team for determination of the underlying cause and best management strategies.

Cardiovascular Impairment

In the management of hypercholesterolemia, the 3-hydroxy-3-methylglutaryl coenzyme A (HMG-CoA) reductase inhibitors (see Box 36-5) may produce myopathies to various degrees. Changes in hemodynamics caused by antihypertensive regimens must be monitored because these agents can produce syncope and lower exercise tolerance. Weakness from intermittent claudication is a challenge that can be managed in part with cilostazol.[103] Any drug that is used to decrease spasticity as a consequence of stroke and related cerebrovascular disorders may impair motor control and thus affect motor learning. A discussion of these drugs is outlined in the next section (see also Chapters 23 and 30). Cardiovascular impairments are common in the rehabilitation setting. Knowing the pharmacological management for and side effects of medications related to the cardiovascular system will assist the therapist in providing high-quality care. Clients will benefit from education on modifiable and nonmodifiable risk factors, monitoring blood pressure and heart rate, signs of heart failure, vascular effects of modalities, and responses to exercise and positional changes.

Spasticity and Muscle Tone

Muscle spasms may be controlled with centrally acting and peripherally acting agents, all of which produce drowsiness, dizziness, and muscle weakness to various degrees.[104] Commonly used agents are listed in Box 36-11. Pharmacological management of muscle tone, spasticity, and coordination of movement is of primary importance in neurological rehabilitation.

With regard to spasticity, several additional options are available. Tizanidine (Zanaflex) is the newest of the α-adrenergic agonists available to reduce spasticity, primarily through activation of descending noradrenergic inhibitory pathways.[105] Clonidine (Catapres) has similar actions. Intrathecal administration of baclofen (Lioresal) produces an antispasmodic effect through enhancement of GABAergic function, both central and spinal.[106] Likewise, enhancement of GABAergic function and reduced spasticity can be realized through the antiseizure drug gabapentin.[107] Selective motor neurons can be inactivated through local injection of botulinum toxins.[108] These agents inhibit the release of acetylcholine at the neuromuscular junction. The investigational agent 4-aminopyridine has been shown to reduce spasticity in patients with spinal cord injury.[109]

The involvement of serotonin in maintenance of muscle tone and spasticity is complex and controversial. Cyproheptadine, a relatively nonselective serotonergic antagonist, can reduce spasticity and maintain muscle tone.[110] However, SSRIs used as antidepressants may occasionally increase spasticity,[111] and clozapine (Clozaril), a selective serotonin antagonist, may produce muscle weakness.[112]

In addition to spinal cord injuries, multiple sclerosis (MS) may cause spasticity as a complication. Although several interferons have been used in the management of MS, interferon beta-1b has been shown to increase spasticity (see Chapters 19 and 24).[113] Therapists often work closely with clients who are undergoing treatment with antispasticity medications. Knowing the underlying cause of the spasticity in the client with neurological impairments (disruptions of inhibitory control) and using concomitant rehabilitation therapy may assist with decreasing pain and improving range of motion and functional ability. Therapists should have an understanding of the desired effects of agents and the adverse effects, including sedation and addictive properties.

BOX 36-11 ■ MUSCLE RELAXANTS AND ANTISPASMODICS*

baclofen (Lioresal)
carisoprodol (Soma)
chlorzoxazone (Paraflex)
cyclobenzaprine (Flexeril)
dantrolene (Dantrium)†
metaxalone (Skelaxin)
methocarbamol (Robaxin)
orphenadrine (Norflex)
tizanidine (Zanaflex)

*Direct effects on motor systems to reduce tone.
†Direct effects on muscle to reduce tone.

Neuroplasticity

The effects of drugs on plasticity are highly controversial. In Alzheimer disease a loss of plasticity may occur through deficits in hippocampal and cortical function, leading to memory loss (see Chapters 4, 5, and 27). Many anticholinesterase agents improve memory, which may provide evidence that they enhance neuroplasticity.[114] At the time of this publication, the primary agents used in the management of Alzheimer disease are anticholinesterase agents. Within the past few years, agents affecting the glutaminergic system have shown promise.[115] Based on the putative molecular mechanisms of the pathology, inhibitors of β-amyloid formation and related modulators may hold additional promise.[116] This rapidly evolving area of research may provide interesting avenues for treatment of Alzheimer disease. Neuroprotective agents that aim to prevent neuronal death by inhibiting one or more pathophysiological steps in the process that follows brain injury or ischemia are currently under development for neurological disorders including stroke, spinal cord injury, traumatic brain injury, and Parkinson disease. In addition, studies on enriched environments are providing knowledge related to neuronal capacity for regeneration and repair in the adult and ageing brain and spinal cord.[117] The future of neuroplasticity in rehabilitation may be enriched when medications that protect or promote neurological recovery can be paired with techniques to improve function.

RESEARCH AND DEVELOPMENT PROSPECTS

The prediction of which areas of pharmacological research will have the most valuable impact on the management of neurological disorders and the resulting residual impairments is difficult. Drug development is a continuous process, although this text must have a definitive end point. Many drugs with outstanding promise for treating neurological diseases will have adverse effects that may be less acceptable than the neurological problem (or in fact may be lethal in rare cases) and may require removal from the market. In spite of these disappointments, many reasons for optimism exist.

Among the burgeoning areas of biotechnology that will have an influence on neurology will be the discovery, characterization, and application of neuronal growth factors, related growth modifiers, and cellular implants, which may have the long-term promise of either partially or completely restoring nerve function. Among these are stem cell implants, whose function and development have been tested in a limited number of patients.[118] It is also likely that drugs will continue to play an important role as adjuncts in disorders partially treated with stem cell therapies. Although these developments are unlikely to have extensive application within the next few years, over a period of decades these and related developments will take root and revolutionize our understanding and treatment of a wide variety of neurological disorders.

The pharmacist stands as a valuable resource for physical and occupational therapists today and will continue to do so in the future. Pharmacists must participate in the management of drug therapies that may be related to each area discussed in this chapter. Therapists should consult the pharmacist about new drug developments and discuss potential problems that these new drugs may have on neurological rehabilitation. This is especially true when new drugs not mentioned in this text are being administered to clients. These discussions can illuminate intended and adverse effects that may affect interventions and change patient outcomes. These drugs may cause improvements as well as exacerbations in movement function. Some of those changes are disease or pathology related. Other changes are attributable to spontaneous return, new learning, and neuroplasticity within the CNS. Changes can also occur because of drug therapy. Those changes, as stated, can be both positive and negative. The scope of practice for occupational and physical therapists does not involve differentiating which change is caused by which process, but these professionals certainly can recognize functional changes. When changes are positive, the team needs to be made aware, and most likely everyone will take credit for the changes. When the changes take away function, families and therapists are often the first to identify those changes. The pharmacist and physician will need to determine why the system is deteriorating. The therapist is responsible for sharing those negative behavior changes with the team and monitoring for future changes when drug regimens have been altered.

SUMMARY

The vast array of drugs, along with their intended and unintended consequences, can pose significant challenges to all clinicians. An awareness of the client's perspective in dealing with diseases and impairments can yield valuable information to prevent and/or manage the adverse impact of drugs on rehabilitation. One component of this perspective is the client's desire to self-medicate in addition to undergoing clinician-prescribed therapy. The pharmacist can often provide guidance that can be effectively relayed to a client's therapist(s). This degree of vigilance can yield greater rewards for the client in terms of effective management of multiple diseases and reduced interference with rehabilitation. Resolving problems with therapies requires a team approach. When drugs are involved with management of these problems, the client's physician, pharmacist, therapist, nurse, and caregiver must be aware that drugs pose a certain degree of risk with every positive step. The team must work closely to address adequately inquiries into possible drug problems and opportunities for therapeutic success.

CASE STUDIES

In a previous edition of this text, two patients in case studies were pharmacologically managed for cognitive decline with donepezil (Aricept) 10 mg (1 tablet) daily. This information was shared with their physical therapists, and their therapy was successfully maintained until the patients' deaths. Important lessons have been learned since the last edition from the management of these two cases and have also changed the way one author (H. R.) now writes referrals for physical or occupational therapy for any patient identified with a cognitive problem. This recommendation should be applied to any patient who is treated for memory loss or is suspected of having a cognitive loss. The plan for physical or occupational therapy intervention must also consider the mental-cognitive abilities of those who will care for the patient at home—the spouse, other family members, or an outside care provider. Sometimes home programs are not always completed because the patient does not understand or the family member in charge forgets the instructions or does not remember to have the patient do activities that help regain functional movement and thus activities of daily living. The primary care provider may also be in the early stages of dementia. The plan should include illustrations and clear and easy-to-follow pictorial instructions of the exercises or functional activities. These must be given and discussed with the care provider for more effective reference and follow-up. If during the course of a scheduled medical and occupational or physical therapy visit the care provider does not come with the patient, request that the care provider accompany the patient on subsequent visits.

Other drugs related to donepezil are available for dementia. These need closer attention to titration to acceptable dosage levels (e.g., rivastigmine [Exelon] 1.5 mg, 3 mg, 4.5 mg, and 6 mg, administered twice daily; galantamine [Razadyne] 4 mg, 8 mg, and 12 mg, administered twice daily; and memantine [Namenda] 5 mg and 10 mg, administered twice daily). The combination of Aricept and Namenda is well accepted for extending cognitive function. Regardless of the drug used, the impact of progressive dementia will exceed drug efficacy and adversely affect occupational and physical therapy. This reinforces the necessity for family and care provider involvement in all phases of therapy.

The two case studies presented in this section illustrate the importance of obtaining a complete medical history before initiating therapy. Unfortunately, and all too often, physical and occupational therapists are asked by the referring physician to look only at a specific problem, for example, "improve upper limb mobility," and are not given background medical history other than perhaps a one-word descriptor such as "stroke" or a short note such as "weakness in upper and lower extremities." Unless the therapist has access to a full medical history, including prescription and OTC drugs, the therapy requested may be less than fully successful because many drugs have adverse side effects that may alter cognitive function or the patient's ability to learn and redevelop impaired motor functions.

Therapists must know and understand the underlying pathophysiology of the referred patient's diagnosis to evaluate the impairment that is causing motor dysfunction. In addition, therapists need to understand how drugs affect the specific physical impairment that is altering the quality of life through day-to-day activity—in some cases hour by hour—functioning. For example, drugs given to patients can either alter or promote their depression and can interfere with intellectual, cognitive, and pain levels, all of which can alter their ability to fully participate in physical and occupational therapy. Often patients' cognitive abilities are modified by either their organic problem or the medical drug therapy. If a cognitive impairment is present, the therapist needs to assess how severe it is to adjust instructions and plan of therapy to a level at which the patient can succeed. The cognitive level, along with the primary medical diagnosis, shapes the physical and occupational therapy prognosis.

Knowledge of the drugs currently being used by the patient provides guidance in structuring therapy and may determine whether the plan of care will be effective. For example, will a patient taking pain medicine have a cognitive level that permits a full understanding of what is being asked during therapy? Will drug therapy provide adequate pain management to enable physical manipulation by either the therapist or the patient in response to the commands? When is the pain medication administered, and is the time in relation to the appointment appropriate? How long does the drug work, and does it have negative effects on cognition?

These are only a few examples of the kind of questions that therapists need to ask to design and implement therapy programs that enhance patients' abilities to recover motor functions, prevent physical regression, and perhaps even retard or stop some aspects of mental regression caused by either drug therapy or endogenous depression. Clinicians must keep in mind the potential for both positive and negative drug-induced changes and ways that these can alter or improve the overall physical and mental status of the patient. The following case studies further illustrate the interactions among the disease, pharmacological management, and physical or occupational therapy interventions.

References

To enhance this text and add value for the reader, all references are included on the companion Evolve site that accompanies this textbook. This online service will, when available, provide a link for the reader to a Medline abstract for the article cited. There are 118 cited references and other general references for this chapter, with the majority of those articles being evidence-based citations.

CASE STUDY 36-1 ■ MULTIPLE SCLEROSIS

C. G. is a 42-year-old white man with relapsing remitting MS who had an Extended Disability Status Score (EDSS) of 1 when first seen. He now has an EDSS score of 3.1. C. G. is no longer able to work. He had been a building contractor, and for a short period after his MS diagnosis he continued working until he lost the use of his legs. He is currently confined to a wheelchair, is incontinent for both bowel and bladder, has lost the ability to stand, and is unable to dress or transfer from any seated position, such as to toilet himself or shower independently. In addition, he is no longer able to prepare his own meals during the 8 to 10 hours per day he spends alone from his family.

HISTORY

C. G. had been treated unsuccessfully with two of the interferon drugs (interferon beta-1a and beta-1b [Avonex and Betaseron]) used to retard MS progression. He is now taking glatiramer (Copaxone), a third MS-suppressive drug, and his condition is currently stabilized. Unfortunately, he has sustained considerable damage to both his brain and spinal cord.

Although MS is a crippling disease of motor and cognitive functions, C. G. remains cognitively intact but has slowed thinking. He also has lapses in immediate recall and occasional indiscretions of judgment that result in inappropriate conversation with outside family members. He expressed suicidal ideation and was treated effectively with paroxetine (Paxil) for his depression. Paxil, an SSRI, was specifically chosen because of its minimal cognitive blunting effects.

All of C. G.'s identified disabilities occurred gradually, but with a sudden progression of his disease his motor impairments progressed from poor lower extremity ambulation and postural control to involvement of his upper extremities and dependence on a wheelchair. He needed therapy initially for ambulation

CASE STUDY 36-1 ■ MULTIPLE SCLEROSIS—cont'd

and more recently for wheelchair use and transfer techniques. As his MS status deteriorated, control of his upper extremities began to decline. Again therapy was ordered to teach him alternate ways to accommodate to these new losses in upper motor control and strength. He was retaught how to get dressed, use the toilet, shower, and feed himself.

Drugs used in the management of MS patients must be considered in any therapy plan, but most clinicians do not share this information or list it only as a part of the patient's chart. At the initial referral of C. G. for gait training, he was taking baclofen (Lioresal) for management of muscular spasms and associated pain. This drug, however, has the potential to increase weakness and fatigue as well as introduce some CNS depression. This is important information because C. G.'s MS was already responsible for motor weakness, but the need to reduce painful muscle spasticity outweighed the loss of muscle strength. If the therapist had not known that C. G. was taking baclofen, the physical therapy plans would have been significantly jeopardized because the therapist would have assessed C. G. as being weak simply because he had MS. The therapy plan needs to include exercises and maneuvers that compensate for the drug-induced motor weakness. C. G. was also taking oxybutynin (Ditropan) for bladder control, a drug that has a potential side effect of drowsiness; in C. G.'s case the Ditropan dose was minimal and was not a cognitive concern. As noted, he had been placed on paroxetine, which also can contribute to muscle weakness, but in his case this did not increase his upper extremity weakness.

C. G. was referred to therapy for functional training, such as transferring from his wheelchair to a bed, shower stool, or toilet; dressing; and eating. Understanding the patient's environmental status, which includes his family situation, is also important in creating a therapy plan. C. G.'s therapy was through home health and incorporated a plan appropriate to C. G.'s environment. C. G. is married and has two children. His wife must work to support the family. The children are not yet in high school and are gone much of the day. Thus C. G. must manage self-care while the family is away during the day. Understanding how drug therapy enhances or interferes with physical or occupational therapy interventions is the only way to optimize the interaction of both and enhance the quality of life for C. G.

POSTSCRIPT

Unfortunately, with MS the demyelinating of neurons is relentless and progressive. At this writing, C. G. has begun to lose additional upper extremity mobility after an MS exacerbation 6 months after his last occupational therapy treatments. He has recently been taught to use assistive tools to grasp and pull items to him, such as books, utensils, and doorknobs. The assistive tools were introduced by the therapist treating C. G., thus extending C. G.'s self-reliance and security during time alone.

CASE STUDY 36-2 ■ PARKINSON PLUS SYNDROME

Mrs. N. is a 72-year-old married woman with Parkinson plus syndrome whose disease status has progressed over the past 5 years, resulting in impaired gait, periods of severe rigidity, dystonia, occasional oculomotor dysfunction, significant behavioral and cognitive changes, and some speech impairment. She is a highly educated woman who had been a speech and special education therapist and administrator. In addition to the aforementioned problems, she now has attention span difficulty, is emotionally labile, and tends to ramble on tangentially to questions posed or simply on her own. Mrs. N. is still oriented to time and place, but to a large extent she is now housebound.

Mrs. N. is currently wheelchair dependent and has had extensive therapy over the past 5 years to keep her mobile and reduce muscle atrophy. She has been given hydrotherapy to facilitate both limb motion and flexibility. Her right hand and both arms are frequently immobilized for short periods of time by rigidity as a result of levodopa blood level peaks. These have been recently modulated by the addition of ropinirole (Requip, a dopamine agonist), and this drug, along with therapy to decrease upper extremity impairments, has improved her ability to carry out voluntary hand and arm movements. Mrs. N's limb movements are characteristically slow and deliberate as a result of the pathological features of Parkinson disorders. She does not have any cogwheeling of the biceps, hands, or head frequently seen in Parkinson patients. Her muscle mass is reduced as a result of disuse atrophy and noncompliance with home-instructed daily exercise. She continues, with poverty of motion, to feed herself but depends on her husband for assistance in dressing and transferring from her wheelchair to the toilet, bed, and shower despite the fact she could do these maneuvers on her own if she chose to do so.

She remains in a long-term stable relationship with a highly supportive husband, who is slowly being driven to exhaustion by her constant demands for attention. She scores well on mental status examinations and does not yet demonstrate marked signs of dementia but frequently has appeared slightly groggy. Mrs. N.'s chief complaint has been one of poor motor control and strength in both her upper and lower extremities. She is still able to stand but now requires assistance during walking. She is unable to sleep normally, finds rolling over or changing position in bed to be difficult, and wakes her husband to rotate her frequently throughout the night.

Her Parkinson disease is being less than successfully treated with standard antiparkinsonian therapy, that is, levodopa and carbidopa. With the addition of Requip, she has improved somewhat. One of the telltale characteristics of a Parkinson plus syndrome is that patients do not respond as well to levodopa therapy as do persons with pure Parkinson disease. Thus the importance of adjunctive physical and occupational therapy to assist Mrs. N. in maintaining mobility cannot be overstated.

Mrs. N. has several other problems that affect her quality of life and her therapy. She, like many other patients with a parkinsonian syndrome, has significant joint pain for which she uses OTC drugs (NSAIDs) in addition to gabapentin

Continued

CASE STUDY 36-2 ■ PARKINSON PLUS SYNDROME—cont'd

(Neurontin, an anticonvulsant drug with neuropathic pain-relieving properties). Mrs. N. has painful muscle spasms that have been moderately well managed with baclofen. She has a nocturnal sleep problem that is lessened by using zolpidem tartrate (Ambien), which helps her get 3 to 4 hours of quality sleep. However, her daytime inactivity has resulted in significant nighttime sleep disturbance that even zolpidem does not always cover.

Unfortunately, Mrs. N., like so many patients with chronic problems, has sought secondary sources for relief of pain and fractured sleep without informing her medical and physical-occupational therapy team until she began to experience a new set of problems caused by polypharmacy or prescriptive or OTC agents. She has been reluctant in the past to disclose her use of these additional agents, several of which have clouded assessment of her therapy. This is not an uncommon occurrence with patients who have progressively degenerative conditions.

Clinicians must routinely ask about patients' drug use and specifically about the use of OTC drugs at each visit. For example, Mrs. N. reported at one recent visit that she was having a hard time following her therapist's instructions and participating in the sessions. She was sure the therapist was "not paying proper attention to my needs." This not being the case, the therapist asked, "So, Mrs. N., refresh my mind and save me some time from looking it up. What medicines are you now taking?" She responded, "Sinemet, as you told me to; Requip; Ambien at bedtime; Synthroid; Klonopin; and a new pill I got at the health food store for sleep." She was taking two drugs—Klonopin and the OTC drug melatonin—both of which would account for the therapist's response that Mrs. N. appeared groggy and was not able to follow directions. The Klonopin she got from a psychiatrist friend of the family. She had put herself on these three sleep drugs, one long acting and the other two short acting, but in combination additive. In addition to this, the drug gabapentin, which was managing her neuropathic pain at a dose of 1200 mg/day, contributed to her level of drowsiness—a known side effect of gabapentin. Mrs. N. was already taking the short-acting non–sensorium-clouding zolpidem, which had been given to her for her sleep disorder. Zolpidem does not cause daytime hangover drowsiness. The key to her new daytime lethargy was found in the Klonopin and melatonin.

The offending drugs were discontinued with an explanation of why she should not add drugs. Mrs. N. subsequently returned to therapy, and her therapist found her once more able to participate in the therapy plans that had been worked out for her. Asking patients to review the drugs they are taking is vital to the entire health care team and to their ultimate success.

With the recently confirmed diagnosis of Mrs. N.'s Parkinson plus syndrome, all that can now be offered to her is supportive therapy, both medical and physical. She is in a class of Parkinson patients who do not respond well to the antiparkinsonian drugs. Her medical management now depends on her participation in physical and occupational therapy and her resisting the temptation to add other drugs that will only cloud her senses and not improve the underlying pathology. Mrs. N. and her husband have now accepted this, and she is doing better.

CHAPTER 37

Use of Medical Imaging in Neurorehabilitation

ROLANDO T. LAZARO, PT, PhD, DPT, GCS, and DARCY A. UMPHRED, PT, PhD, FAPTA

KEY TERMS

Computed tomography (CT)
Imaging
Magnetic resonance image (MRI)
Radiograph

OBJECTIVES

After reading this chapter the student or therapist will be able to:

1. Recognize the various ways the brain can be labeled according to the slice and what differences in the types of cuts help identify the slice or image.
2. Transition from viewing a subject in various spatial positions to seeing the skeletal frame in that position to visually recognizing the entire nervous system when the subject is placed in the same position.
3. Recognize various slices of the central nervous system; what nuclear masses are visible in that slice; how the ventricles change from one slice to another; and how sagittal, horizontal, and coronal slices present those nuclear masses and/or ventricles differently.
4. Recognize the difference in diagnostic capabilities of radiography, computed tomography (CT), magnetic resonance imaging (MRI), and nuclear medicine scans.
5. Identify neuroradiological descriptive terminology.
6. Recognize normal and abnormal neuroanatomy on radiographs, CT scans, and MRI images.
7. Analyze information obtained from imaging of the central nervous system and integrate this information into the neurological clinical presentation and the patient's intervention.
8. Recognize and analyze how a medical diagnosis using imaging may and may not be reflected in the movement diagnosis made by a physical or occupational therapist.

The increasingly complex role of physical and occupational therapy practitioners in health care delivery has increased the need for these clinicians to acquire knowledge and skills that will further enhance their ability to make appropriate decisions involving patient/client management. The recognition of direct access practice in many states and the increasing role of physical and occupational professionals as primary care providers have heightened the need for these clinicians to recognize and analyze how different medical tests and procedures affect movement and function. This differential analysis is critical in order for these professionals to know when to refer a client to another health care practitioner, when to refer and treat, when to merely treat, and when to neither refer nor treat (see Chapter 7).

Indeed, with the advent of doctoral education in physical and occupational therapy, entry-level knowledge of content such as pharmacology, radiology, and medical screening has become an accreditation requirement. Therapists are recognizing the value of information obtained from medical imaging studies in the appropriate delivery of physical and occupational therapy services. Orthopedic radiology is now a common part of curricula; however, content on neuroradiology, more specifically the application of neuroradiology in practice, is lacking. In a study by Little and Lazaro,[1] it was found that many of the physical therapy practitioners in California use medical imaging in their practice. When looking at the types of imaging, the majority of respondents felt comfortable using results (and radiology reports) from radiographs obtained because of a musculoskeletal problem. This study showed the lack of access to and confidence in using medical images of the central nervous system (CNS).

In certain instances it may be easier for therapists to recognize musculoskeletal problems when viewing medical images because the abnormality in the structure directly correlates with what is manifesting as a movement problem. When images of the CNS are viewed, these correlations may be much more complex owing to the relationship of nuclei, tract systems, ventricular balance, and basic neurochemistry. For example, when looking at a bone fracture (Figure 37-1, *A*) versus a vascular insult (Figure 37-1, *B*), it is clear that the fracture and its effects on the bone, muscle, or skin can easily be visualized and interpreted. The second image of the CNS has many surrounding structures that must be identified in relation to the vascular insult.

In 2007 the journal *Physical Therapy* produced a special issue on neuroradiology in physical therapy practice. It is encouraging to note that this issue offered physical therapy clinicians an opportunity to understand the modalities used in the imaging of the brain and the spinal cord (for details, see the article by Kimberley and Lewis[2]). However, the rest of the articles presented the application of neuroradiology in physical therapy research,[3,4] and although these articles provided valuable information for the practicing clinician, the articles did not specifically give insights as to how clinicians

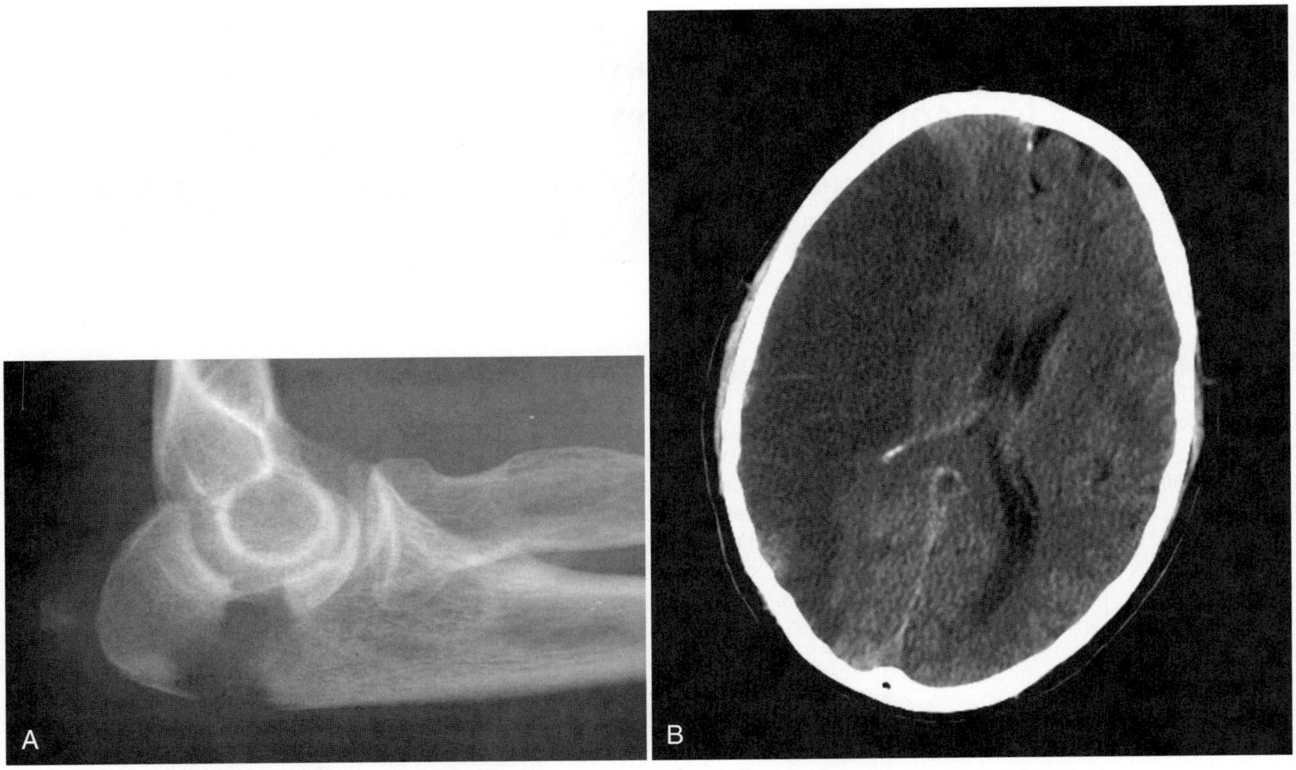

Figure 37-1 ■ **A,** Radiograph showing a fractured olecranon. **B,** Computed tomography scan showing an infarct of the middle cerebral artery. (**B** from Wikipedia. http://en.wikipedia.org/wiki/File:INFARCT.jpg.)

can use knowledge of neuroradiology in their actual patient/client management.

VISUALIZING THE CENTRAL NERVOUS SYSTEM

Before jumping into viewing images of the nervous system, the reader needs to be very familiar with the position and type of slices presented in those images. Figure 37-2 illustrates the three types of slices common to the nervous system. The horizontal slices shown in Figure 37-3 are cuts made horizontally through the brain beginning with a superior slice at the level of the beginning of the lateral ventricles. This individual would be lying supine if the brain were cut as shown. If a person were standing, the horizontal slice would be horizontal to the ground with the frontal lobes facing forward (toward the nose) and the occipital lobe in the back. The slices cut horizontally are always perpendicular to the brain stem and spinal cord or perpendicular to the upright position of the brain regardless of the position of the head in space. All right and left slices will look exactly the same as long as the nervous system has not sustained any insult. Figure 37-4 shows the position of an upright human and what the skeleton would look like in the same position. Can you visualize what the horizontal slices would look like? The horizontal section would be perpendicular to this upright position. When viewing radiological slices in horizontal, the slices will often be on a slight angle with the lower portion slightly forward. Most of these films are taken when individuals are supine, which places the brain off vertical so a correction is made. The film usually slices horizontally through the brain as if the head were slightly tucked, similar to the image of the adult in Figure 37-4, *A*. Also, some radiologists want a slightly different angle to the slice because they are looking for specific orientations. When viewing these films, try to look at the radiological slice pattern (scanogram), if shown. Figure 37-3 shows a progression of horizontal slices as if the individual were supine and the slices began anteriorly with emphasis on ventricular changes as part of the progression. Many of the medical images of the brain are viewed as horizontal (or axial) slices or views. The person is lying supine when undergoing computed tomography (CT), magnetic resonance imaging (MRI), or positron emission tomography (PET). Therefore the imaging process cuts 90 degrees off the horizontal plane of earth in order to achieve horizontal slices of the brain. Remember to look at the scanogram, if available, to identify the position of the head in relation to the cuts.

Coronal slices in the right hemisphere look similar to those in the left hemisphere except that the top of the slice will not look like the bottom on either side (see Figure 37-2). The two sides will reflect each other, with the tops being alike as well as the bottoms. Depending on where the cut is made, the result will be cortex on the outside, tracts (white matter) projecting downward, and gray matter again inferior and medial within the slices as the thalamus, basal ganglia, caudate, hippocampus, and so on are viewed. These slices begin at the top and cut down through both sides of the brain, with the slice ending on the inferior section. The progression of the slides can go from front (frontal lobe) to back (occipital lobe) or back to front. If visualized in a standing subject, the slice would begin in the superior frontal area and slice

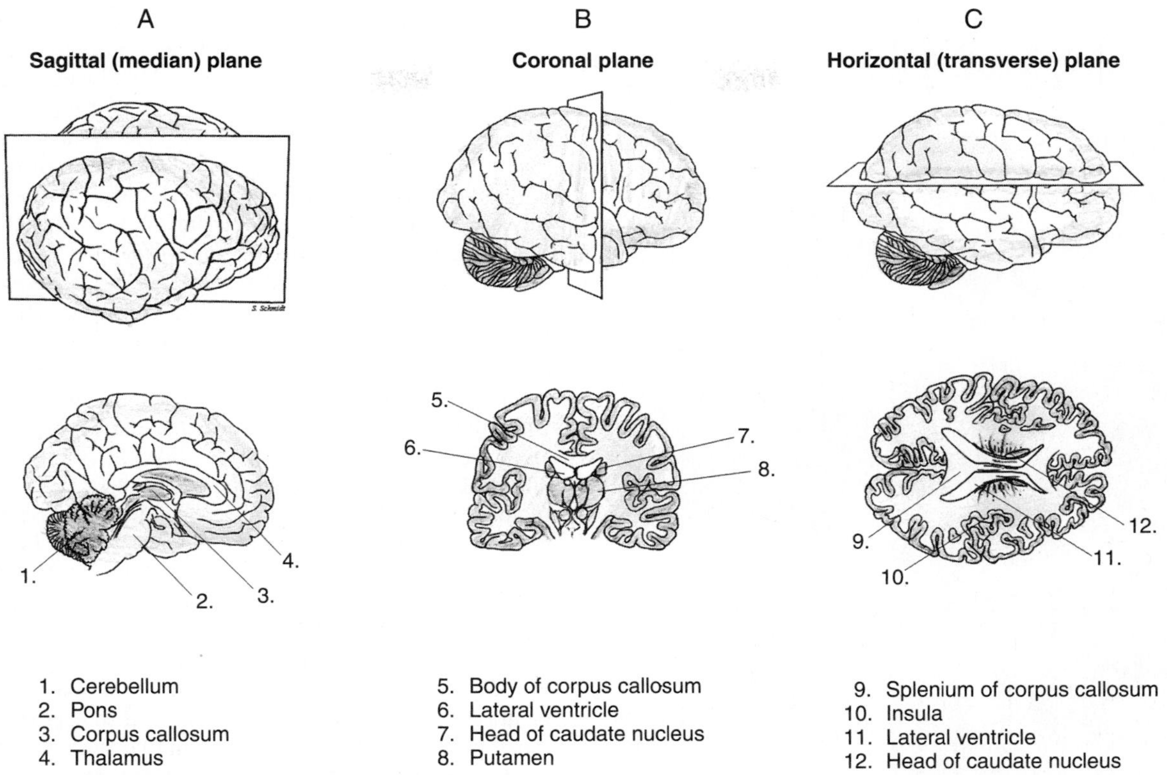

Figure 37-2 ■ Orientation of brain slices. **A,** Sagittal. **B,** Coronal. **C,** Horizontal. (Courtesy Stephen Schmidt, PT, OCS, FAAOMPT.)

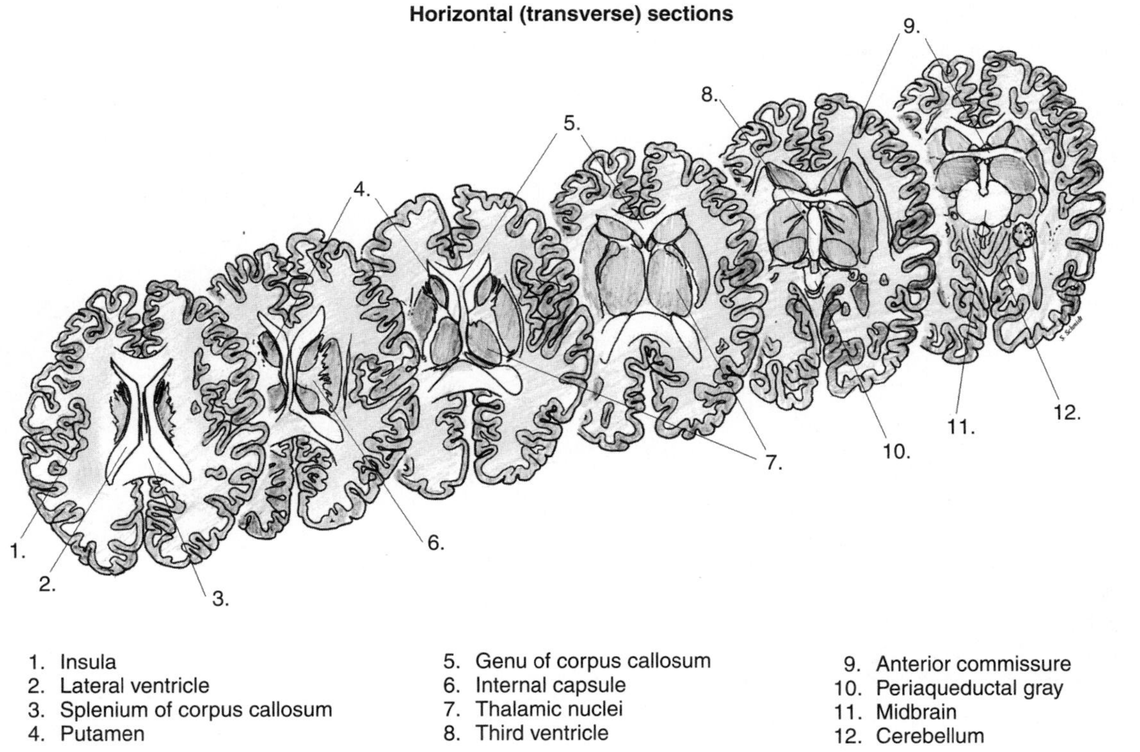

Figure 37-3 ■ Illustration of horizontal slices. (Courtesy Stephen Schmidt, PT, OCS, FAAOMPT.)

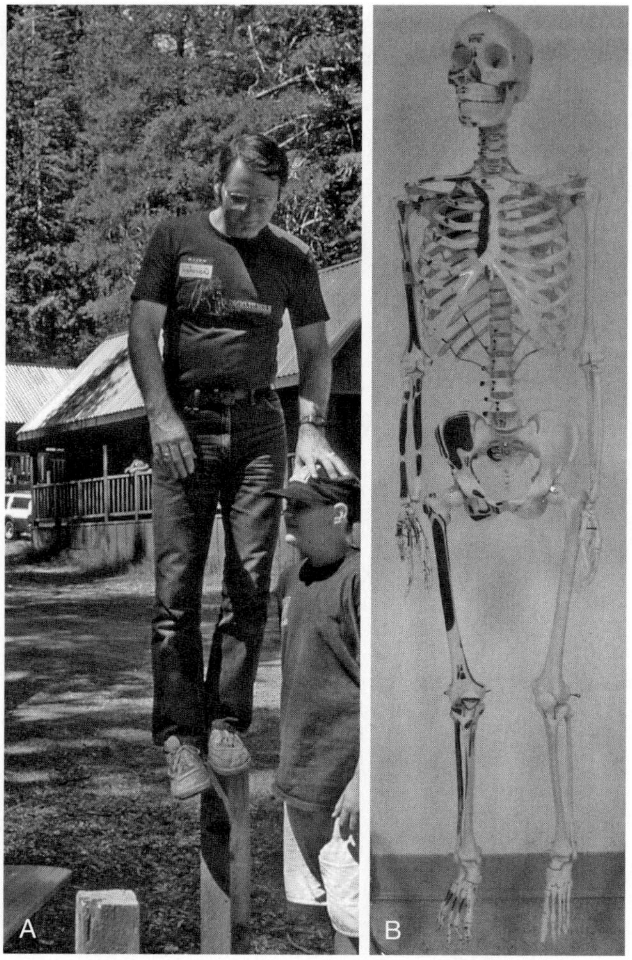

Figure 37-4 ■ **A,** Photograph of a human standing. **B,** A skeleton standing.

downward through the brain toward the feet, thus cutting equally on both sides. These slices can proceed in the posterior (backward) direction of the brain but always cutting from the top toward the bottom with equal distribution on each side. Figure 37-5 progresses from the front of the brain toward the back using the ventricles as a point of reference.

For sagittal cuts (see Figure 37-2), most cuts start by slicing down through the central fissure separating both sides of the brain. This cut is called a *midsagittal section.* Each sagittal slice proceeds outward toward the lateral aspect of the brain on each side respectively, depending on which side is being sliced. Anatomically, you begin as if you were slicing down through the middle of the face and the back of the head when a person is standing. Each sagittal slice moves from the inside outward toward the ear or laterally away from the midsagittal slice. Each slice cuts though the front and back of the brain from top to bottom and proceeds from medial to lateral. Sagittal images usually begin on either the right or the left side and continue slicing toward the middle to the midsagittal section separating the two sides of the brain, and then proceed toward the outside on the opposite side of the brain from the beginning slice.

Another way to conceptualize the nervous system is by visually sequencing from a view of a human in a specific position to the skeleton of a human in that position to an intact plastinated nervous system in that same position. The reader is encouraged to try to visualize what the horizontal, coronal, and sagittal slices might look like given the spatial position of the individual. Once you can easily recognize the various types of slices and where the slice was made when viewing the nervous system, you are ready to begin viewing radiological images.

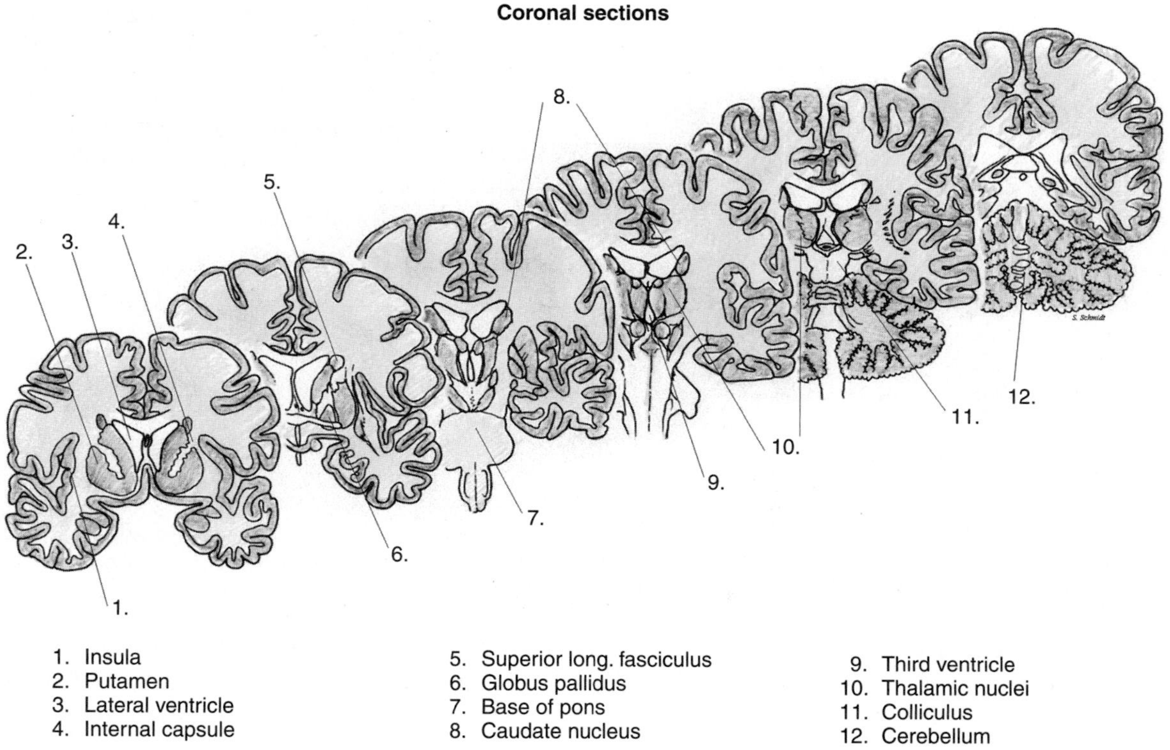

Figure 37-5 ■ Illustration of coronal slices. (Courtesy Stephen Schmidt, PT, OCS, FAAOMPT.)

IMAGING OF THE CENTRAL NERVOUS SYSTEM

It is beyond the scope of this chapter to discuss the physics behind the more common imaging modalities (see article by Kimberley and Lewis[2] for background). The purpose of this chapter is to provide the clinician a method of systematically evaluating medical images of the CNS, and, more important, to provide examples of how clinicians can use these images to guide practice.

CT and MRI remain the two most common modalities for imaging the CNS. CT scans of the brain are widely used in acute neurological injuries in which the speed of the examination is of primary importance. A common application of this is in acute traumatic brain injuries, when rapid assessment of information about hematoma formation and brain swelling is imperative to make appropriate decisions regarding medical management. Although there is less anatomic detail in CT than in MRI, the level of detail being generated by a CT is generally sufficient for the appropriate management of the patient with an acute injury. Because CT also administers the highest dose of radiation (as it is a series of x-ray exposures), it causes a higher risk of development of conditions associated with increased levels of radiation exposure.

Owing to its increasing availability, MRI can also be an ideal choice for imaging the brain and the spinal cord. MRI provides excellent resolution and can also be performed with contrast to enhance the detail even more. MRI, however, generally takes longer than CT to perform, and it requires the subject to avoid excessive movement while the machine is actively scanning. Also, because MRI uses powerful magnets, the use of this modality in patients with metal implants is contraindicated. With regard to cost, MRI is still more costly than CT, but this expense is rapidly coming down as more hospitals and clinics are investing in this technology.

As mentioned earlier, contrast media can also be used in both CT and MRI to enhance the image, although that will increase the scanning time. There are also additional risks associated with contrast, such as possible allergic reactions to the medium being used to enhance the image.

Clinical Decisions Regarding the Need for Imaging Studies

Obviously, patients with acute neurological symptoms should be seen by a medical practitioner, but individuals with chronic neurological problems should have imaging films that reflect those anatomical lesions as well as the movement dysfunction associated with those medical diagnoses. When the movement dysfunction changes in the direction of increased impairments, then new images may need to be obtained. A therapist may be in a situation in which recommending that new images be taken is appropriate. After the radiologist has read and interpreted the new films, decisions can be made as to whether the patient needs to be referred to another practitioner such as a neurologist. From the standpoint of the therapist, it is critical that a therapist analyze how his or her evaluation matches or does not match the movement diagnoses seen in the clinic and reported by the patient, the family, or the advocate for the individual. If there is a mismatch, it is the therapist's responsibility to bring the information and the question to the attention of the physician of record who is treating the patient and then to the team. For example, if the radiological report clearly states a cerebellar problem but the movement dysfunction more closely represents basal ganglia involvement, there is a mismatch. Thus, further exploration by those health care providers needs to be pursued in order to more accurately develop treatments from all individuals involved in the care of that person. However, it is *never* the responsibility of a therapist to correct a physician's medical diagnosis or any other diagnosis outside the scope of a therapist's practice. It is the responsibility of the physical or occupational therapist to report the inconsistencies between the imaging report or medical diagnosis and the specific movement dysfunction seen and reported in the therapy situation.

GENERAL GUIDELINES FOR REVIEWING MEDICAL IMAGES

Radiodensity

Because CT scans, like conventional radiographs, are images formed by the absorption of x-rays by the body at different densities, evaluation of CT images is the same as evaluation of conventional radiographs. Structures in the body that absorb a lot of x-ray energy are *radiopaque* and will be white on the image. Structures that absorb less x-ray energy will be different shades of gray. Air does not absorb any x-rays and will be black on the film, and is said to be *radiolucent.* Bone is an example of a radiopaque structure and will be white on the image. Because the skull is composed of bones of varying thickness, portions of this structure that have more bone will be whiter than those with less bone. Contrast media can be positive (white; heavy metals such as gadolinium) or negative (black; air, however, is not used as a contrast medium in the CNS). Brain matter and spinal cord will be varying shades of gray. The sinuses are normally filled with air and will therefore show as black, whereas the ventricles are filled with cerebrospinal fluid and will be a shade of gray on a CT image.

There are a few steps to follow when evaluating neuroradiological images. These steps are presented in the following sections.

Step 1

Gather All Pertinent Information Regarding the Patient's Neuroimaging Studies

As mentioned earlier, because of the complexity of the structure and function of the CNS, it would be appropriate to have a radiologist and a neurologist or neurosurgeon to read the images first and make a report before the physical or occupational therapist reviews the images. Previous neuroimaging scans and reports will also provide additional information regarding the progression or improvement of the conditions, or the involvement of other structures that may have implications for the patient's care. Review the report thoroughly, making note of the structures that were reported to be normal as well as the ones that were reported to be pathological. This will provide insight as to the patient's potential movement disorders, as well as functions that may be normal for the patient. This review can also reveal a mismatch between the report and the presented movement diagnosis.

Step 2

Be Familiar with Background Information, and Orient Yourself Correctly to the Image

After reviewing the imaging report, the clinician then examines the actual images. The clinician must be familiar with the basic background information presented on the image. Normally the film will contain information such as the patient's name, age, and medical record number; the date of the scan; and the name of the hospital or facility that performed the procedure (Figure 37-6). The date of the scan is particularly important when attempting to establish relationships between what can be seen on the image and the patient's presentation. There might be a mismatch between what is shown on the image and what the patient is doing because of either resolution of the condition or worsening of the pathology. Comparing scans taken at different intervals will also assist the clinician in arriving at some general impressions on the rate or recovery (or lack thereof) or prognoses following physical rehabilitation.

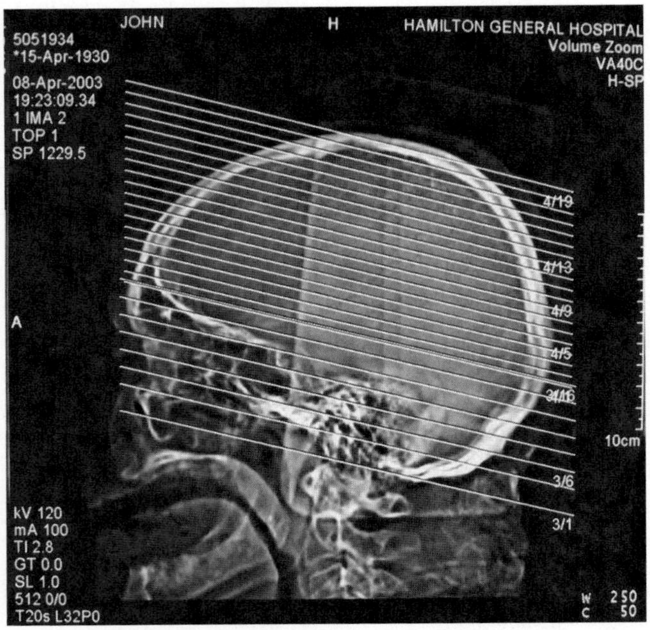

Figure 37-6 ■ Computed tomography scan of the brain with identifying information. (Courtesy Dr. John Wells. How to Read a CT Scan of the Brain. www.neurosurvival.ca/ComputerAssistedLearning/readingCTs/scanogram.htm.)

Markers may also be available. The use of markers significantly simplifies analysis by allowing the examiner to easily orient the film correctly. Common markers include *R* and *L* for right and left, respectively, and *A* and *P* for anterior and posterior.

Often a scale is provided for the clinician to relate the size of the structures on the image to actual size.

Next, the clinician should be familiar with some of the basic technical detail. CT and MRI can provide multiple "slices" of the brain, much like slices in a loaf of bread. Often a single large film containing all the images arranged in order can be found. Usually, the first image on the left top most corner is the "scout view" or scanogram and serves to illustrate the orientation and thickness of each slide. Depending on the suspected pathology, the slice orientation could be frontal, coronal, or sagittal, based on the specific structure in question.

Certain views of the CT image can also be produced by the radiology team by manipulating certain image parameters. These "windows" are presented in Figure 37-7. A bone window shows bone the best and is helpful when a skull fracture is suspected. A brain window shows brain matter the best and is used when the suspected pathology is caused by or affects the brain matter (tumors, atrophy of the nuclear masses, or general atrophy of the brain itself). A subdural window is beneficial when suspecting the presence of subdural hematoma or swelling of the brain. With MRI, the images can also be "weighted" (for example, T1 versus T2). T1-weighted images show better gray matter–white matter contrast, whereas T2-weighted images might show edema better. As mentioned earlier, contrast may be used with either CT or MRI to improve visualization of the structures in question.

Step 3

Do a Quick Scan-through, Then Examine Thoroughly

After getting familiar with the basic information, the clinician should then make a "quick scan" of the image, noting the pathology that quickly stands out. After doing so, a more thorough analysis of each film in the series must be done. Multiple windows and/or successive slices are often helpful in visualizing the extent of the pathology. The

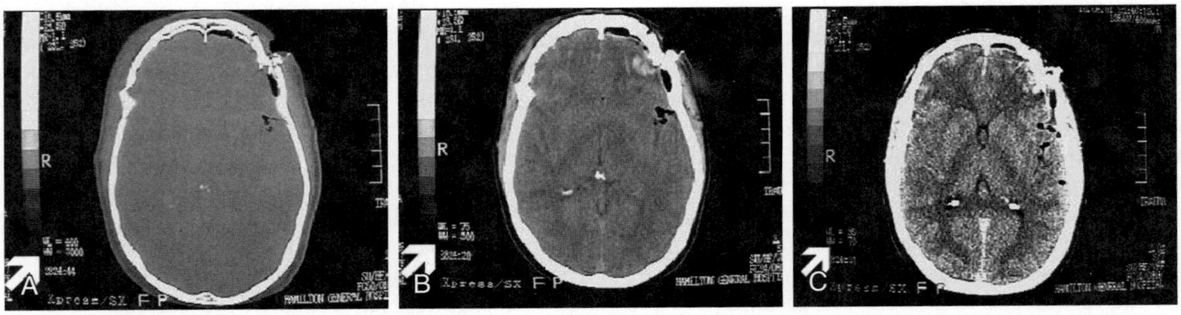

Figure 37-7 ■ Computed tomography scan of the brain showing three different windows. **A,** Bone window. **B,** Subdural window. **C,** Brain window. (Images courtesy Dr. John Wells. How to Read a CT Scan of the Brain. www.neurosurvival.ca/ComputerAssistedLearning/readingCTs/windows.htm.)

clinician mentally constructs a three-dimensional image of the brain from the two-dimensional scan. In a CT scan, knowledge of radiodensity is helpful in making this accurate representation, as is knowledge of normal structure and function of the CNS.

Several resources recommend slightly different methods of analyzing an image. The following are suggestions to make the process more organized and efficient.

1. Examine the symmetry.[5] Compare both sides of the brain as represented on the image. In orienting the images, the right side of the brain is usually shown on the left. Look for a midline shift by drawing an imaginary line from the anterior falx cerebri to the posterior falx cerebri. Identify the side of the greatest shift and measure it (in centimeters or millimeters). It would also be helpful to look for signs of mass effect (when structures on one side are "pushed" to the other side, or a possible atrophy on the structures on one side that pushes the structures on the other side across the midline). Additional structures to inspect for symmetry include the basal ganglia, thalamus, and corpus callosum.
2. Examine the size and shape of the structures.[5] This is particularly helpful when looking at the integrity of the ventricles and cisterns. When filled with excessive fluid as in hydrocephalus, the ventricles enlarge disproportionately. This enlargement is seen in babies as a result of a variety of pathologies (see Chapter 15) and in children and adults after brain trauma (see Chapters 23 and 24). Likewise, in atrophy of the brain tissue the ventricles may also become enlarged; this is often seen in elderly adults as the brain loses gray matter and the ventricles enlarge to fill in the extra space (see Chapter 27). Examining the size and shape of the sulci may also be beneficial when looking at atrophy of the specific structure, thereby accounting for the abnormalities of movement being observed.
3. Look for lesions in the brain. Space-occupying lesions such as brain tumors or hematoma can be visualized (Figure 37-8). Because the brain has such a finite size to fit snugly within the cranial vault, any lesion in the brain has the potential to push brain structures to the midline or to displace the structure and create more serious pathology. Plaque formations secondary to multiple sclerosis can also be visualized as bright white spots in the gray matter (Figure 37-9).
4. Examine densities.[5] As mentioned previously, different tissues will have different densities, and these differences are what forms the generated images. Hyperdensities may include blood, tumors, or enhancing lesions, whereas common hypodensities include air, non-enhancing tumors, and chronic hematoma.

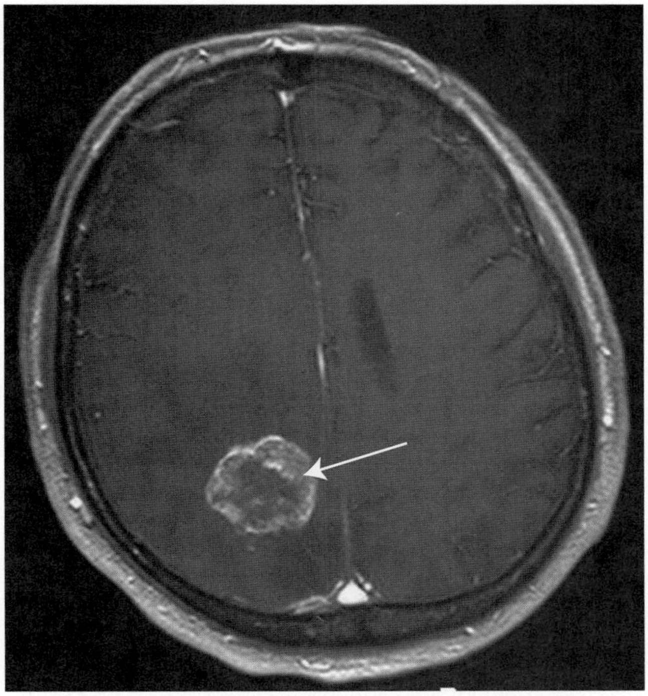

Figure 37-8 ■ T1-weighted magnetic resonance image with intravenous contrast showing a brain tumor. (From Wikipedia. http://en.wikipedia.org/wiki/File:Hirnmetastase_MRT-T1_KM.jpg.)

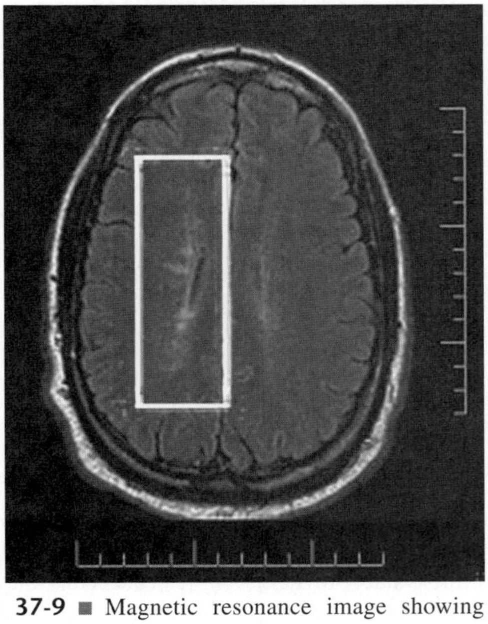

Figure 37-9 ■ Magnetic resonance image showing plaque formation caused by multiple sclerosis. (From Wikipedia. http://en.wikipedia.org/wiki/File:Dawsonsfingers.jpg.)

Step 4

Establish Relationships between the Structures Involved and the Presenting Impairments, Movement Dysfunctions, and Activity Limitations

There are two possible clinical scenarios in which the medical imaging information is reviewed. First, the therapist may be reviewing the medical imaging information before seeing the patient for the initial examination or evaluation. If this is the case, the therapist is expected to use this information in relation to other medical information in the chart (from physician's history and physical examination, nursing notes, and so on) to get an initial sense of what the patient may be able or unable to do. This will allow the therapist to plan for the appropriate tests and measures to perform during the examination (Case Study 37-1).

CASE STUDY 37-1 ■ A PATIENT WITH A BRAIN TUMOR*

The patient was a 71-year-old woman with history of glioblastoma multiforme, the most aggressive form of brain tumor (refer to Chapter 25). It has been reported that a second recurrence of this condition is associated with a less favorable prognosis.[6] The patient had previously undergone tumor resection, chemotherapy, and radiation. She had then been found to have another recurrence of the left frontal glioblastoma multiforme of 4 cm (Figure 37-10), for which she had undergone a stereotactic resection (Figure 37-11) of the tumor. After this surgery she underwent intensive inpatient rehabilitation.

Her past medical history included history of radiation therapy, seizure disorder, diabetes mellitus, hypertension, anemia, and leukopenia. Medications include Dilantin, Lipitor, dexamethasone, fosinopril, and metformin.

The patient's primary caregiver was her husband. They were both retired, living in a single-story home with two steps to enter. She had two supportive daughters who lived nearby and were available for support as needed. Before the most recent hospitalization, the patient had been at a supervised level of assistance with ambulation outdoors and independence for household ambulation, with no assistive device required.

The medical images revealed a resected parietal lobe tumor in the left side of her brain. In the imaging report it was noted that there was significant edema in the surrounding area and that mainly white matter tracts were affected. However, no midline shift or mass effect was noted. In addition, the tumor was reported to be located near the Broca and Wernicke areas but superficial to the ventricles.

Based on the information provided by the imaging reports and the associated medical images, the clinician developed several initial impressions about the patient's presentation and care. First, the note about significant edema indicated more diffuse, global effects on movement and function; associated structural impairments rather than only dysfunctions specific to parietal lobe damage would be expected. The lack of midline shift or mass effect indicated a more favorable prognosis for survival for the patient. The information about the tumor being located near the speech areas indicated the possibility of deficits in expressive and receptive communication. Finally, damage to the parietal lobe indicated the potential for agraphia, aphasia, and agnosia. Because the parietal lobe is also largely important for perception and interpretation of somatosensory information, the formation of the idea of a complex purposeful motor act may also have been impaired.

The initial examination confirmed and supported all the expected movement deficits and clinical presentation of the patient. She underwent intensive occupational, physical, and speech therapy to improve her functional mobility and ambulation, self-care and activities of daily living, and also speech, swallowing, and communication. There was a concerted effort among the rehabilitation team and the patient's family to optimize communication strategies while minimizing patient frustration. For example, more complex tasks such as transfers were broken down into smaller components and then practiced extensively as components and as whole functions. The transfer task was broken down into three steps: (1) locking the brakes, (2) removing the legrests, and (3) standing and turning to sit on the destination surface. These step-by-step instructions were written on the patient's whiteboard; practiced during speech, physical, and occupational therapy; and communicated to the family and rehab team. Hand-over-hand guidance and facilitation were also included during instruction, as was use of mental rehearsal to remediate executive and visuomotor deficits to improve motor sequencing and problem solving while decreasing perseveration and frustration.[7] The rehabilitation team worked closely together to standardize treatment techniques, increase opportunity for task carryover, and decrease the patient's frustration with learning. Speech therapy started to integrate pictures and words representing tasks learned in physical and occupational therapies. In addition, therapy became more focused on repeated task training of three or four essential skills versus multiple activities, games, and skills.

This case example demonstrated how medical imaging information not only confirmed the expected presenting deficits in movement, function, communication, and learning of the patient but also included information that guided the rehabilitation team in selecting interventions that optimized function for this patient.

*Case adapted from Parikh M: *The use of medical imaging in neuromuscular physical therapy practice: a case report.* Samuel Merritt College Physical Therapy Case Report Presentations, May 2007.

The second clinical scenario involves the use of medical imaging information to guide clinical decisions during the actual occupational or physical therapy session. One of the major goals of this step is to make sure that the movement dysfunctions presented by the patient match the information obtained from the medical images. The therapist is expected to act accordingly and to demonstrate sound judgment, especially when the mismatch indicates a possible life-threatening situation. For example, if the imaging results indicate a small focal area involvement but the patient demonstrates significant impairment in movement and function, the mismatch may be indicative of a worsening and potentially life-threatening condition that must be communicated to the physician and other members of the medical team.

As mentioned earlier, the complexity of the structure and function of the nervous system makes interpretation of imaging information very challenging. There may be situations in which images may not fully explain what the patient or client is able to do in terms of function and movement (as illustrated in Case Study 37-2).

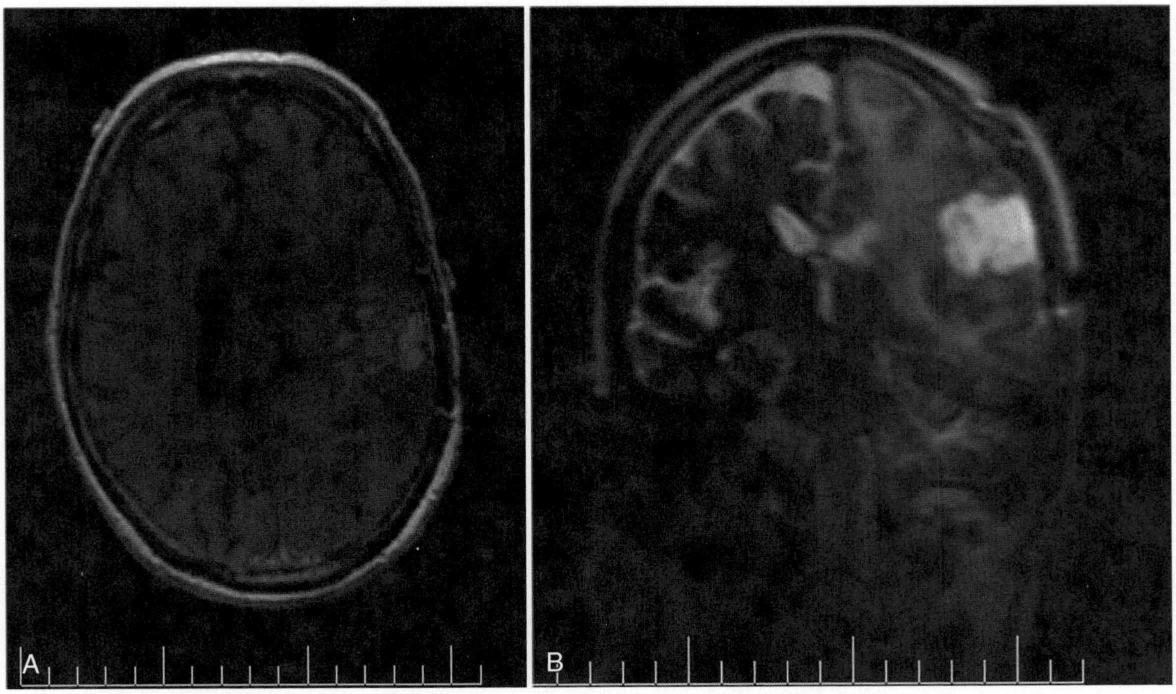

Figure 37-10 ■ **A,** Axial view showing tumor. **B,** Coronal view showing tumor.

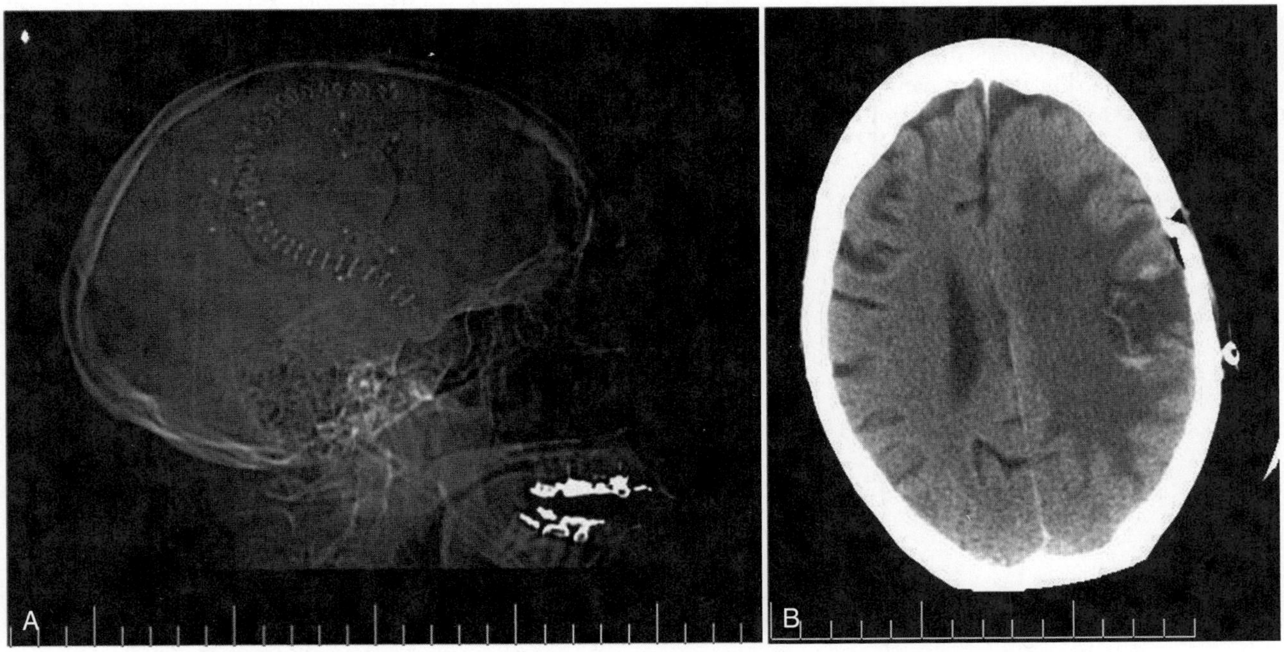

Figure 37-11 ■ Images after surgery for tumor resection. **A,** Lateral view. **B,** Axial view.

CASE STUDY 37-2 ■ A PEDIATRIC PATIENT WITH DEVELOPMENTAL PROBLEMS AT 18 MONTHS

The patient was a full-term baby. The doctors identified through ultrasound that the child had an unusually large head and were expecting problems. At birth, they had placed the child in the neonatal intensive care unit (NICU) and obtained CT scans of his head. It had been identified that he did not have closure of his lateral and third ventricles. Their prognosis had been that the child would die within days after birth. They had encouraged the family to take him home and spend as much time with him as they had before his death.

One author of this chapter was called in to help colleagues establish realistic expectations and treatment protocols for this child. The child was 18 months of age at the time of this therapist's first visit. The child's motor development was very delayed owing to the large size of his head (hydrocephaly). He was also nonverbal, and the doctors had concluded that he had an extremely low level of intelligence. He had loving parents who played with him, fed him, bathed him, and interacted with him all day. They felt he had more ability than the pediatrician had stated.

This video case study illustrates a situation in which there is a mismatch between the medical diagnosis/medical imaging results and what the client presents in terms of function and movement. This case will engage and guide the therapist in a clinical decision-making process of analyzing the client's movement and functional capabilities and relating those to the integrity of the specific areas of the nervous system that are responsible for the movement or behavior. It is recommended that the reader first look at and analyze the motor function of this child at 18 months and then 6 months later, looking specifically for increased motor function and potential. During the interim, the child did receive weekly therapy, but most of the practice was done at home with the parents interacting with the child. Analyze the movement from a motor learning and neuroplasticity perspective as you determine the potential for motor control. Then look at the MRI images that lead the doctors to diagnosis the medical problem and the prognosis of death. Then ask yourself what could be happening to cause such a mismatch between a movement and a medical diagnosis?

Note: The continuation of the case, including the video clips and imaging results, can be found on the companion website.

References

To enhance this text and add value for the reader, all references are included on the companion Evolve site that accompanies this textbook. This online service will, when available, provide a link for the reader to a Medline abstract for the article cited. There are 7 cited references and other general references for this chapter, with the majority of those articles being evidence-based citations.

CHAPTER 38 Integrating Technology into Clinical Practice in Neurological Rehabilitation*

KATIE BYL, PhD, NANCY N. BYL, PT, MPH, PhD, FAPTA, MARTEN BYL, PhD, BRADLEY W. STOCKERT, PT, PhD, SEBASTIAN SOVERO, MS, CLAYTON D. GABLE, PT, PhD, and DARCY A. UMPHRED, PT, PhD, FAPTA

KEY TERMS

actuators
assistive robotics
biomechatronics
brain-machine interfaces
cognitive human robotic interaction
computerized learning-based gaming
controllers
emotional entertainment robotics
empowering robotic exoskeletons
empowerment
engineering terminology
exoskeleton
game consoles
human robotic interfaces
kinematics
mechatronics
microprocessors
motion controllers
orthotic robotics
personal simulators
physical human-robotic interaction (sensory and motor)
prosthetic robotics
rehabilitation robotics
robotics
robot-mediated therapy
sensors
service robotics
software programs
telecare
telemedicine
virtual reality training
vocational robots
wearable robots (WRs)
wireless

OBJECTIVES

After reading this chapter the student or therapist will be able to:

1. Summarize the need, demand and principles for integrating advanced robotic technology in neurological rehabilitation.
2. Define common terminology used in the field of rehabilitation robotics and technology.
3. Classify the different types of advanced technology used in neurorehabilitation.
   a. Rehabilitation robots and assistive technology including:
      i. Service robots for movement
      ii. Service robots for physical assistance and indoor and outdoor navigation
      iii. Nonwearable robotic assistive device for mobility, unweighting, and object manipulation
      iv. Wearable robotic assistive device for upper-limb object manipulation
      v. Wearable robotic assistive device for lower-limb mobility and gait training
      vi. Communication robotics to enable interpersonal interaction
      vii. Interactive entertainment robotics for companionship and emotional support
   b. Advanced clinical technology including:
      i. Virtual reality training systems for improved neural recovery of upper- and lower-limb function
      ii. Computerized learning-based gaming systems for home training of individuals with physical disabilities and memory impairments
      iii. Computerized patient simulators for teaching clinical diagnoses and intervention strategies to medical professionals
      iv. Computer technology for teaching home exercise programs to patients
4. Use the guidelines for integrating robotics and assistive technology into a patient's rehabilitation program.
5. Summarize the challenges and basic engineering principles involved in creating rehabilitation robotics and interfacing with advanced technology to help individuals to design:
   a. Robots that operate independently
   b. Controllers, actuators, and sensors required for service and assistive rehabilitation robots
   c. Human interfaces (physical, sensory physical, cognitive, and brain machine)
   d. User-friendly interfaces and controllers to maximize kinematics (e.g., force, velocity, timing)
   e. Rehabilitation robotics based on the materials and control technology currently available
   f. Safe robotics for rehabilitation
6. Discuss the benefits of performing a cost-effectiveness analysis when considering the application of robotic technology in rehabilitation.
7. Describe the challenges of commercializing robotic devices.
8. Discuss the future of advanced technology and rehabilitation.

*The authors would like to thank Susan L. Whitney, PT, PhD, DPT, NCS, ATC, FAPTA, for her contribution of the case study on virtual reality training for a patient with unilateral vestibular hypofunction. Dr. Whitney is a professor at the University of Pittsburgh, Departments of Physical Therapy and Otolaryngology.

This chapter presents and discusses the integration of computer-assisted technology as one approach to maximize independence and quality of life in older adults and people with moderate to severe physical impairments. Rehabilitation robotics and computer-assisted technology use brain interfaces, sensorimotor interfaces, virtual reality (VR) environments, and learning-based gaming programs to remediate sensory, motor, and cognitive impairments and improve memory skills and physical abilities required for independent mobility and self-care at home, in the community, at work, and during the performance of recreational activities.

INTRODUCTION TO THE APPLICATION OF ROBOTICS AND TECHNOLOGY IN REHABILITATION

General Overview

The purpose of this chapter is to excite rehabilitation professionals about the integration of technology in rehabilitation and the potential to expand possibilities for healing, adaptation, compensation, and recovery for individuals with neurological impairments. Robotics and technology are considered supplemental to "one-on-one rehabilitative therapy," not a replacement for individual therapy. This chapter will provide an overview of technology and rehabilitation robotics appropriate for consideration within neurological rehabilitation. The chapter will not provide a detailed analysis of all of the technology that is available or an exhaustive bibliography referencing all of the studies that have been carried out in the area of rehabilitation robotics.

The objective of rehabilitation technology is to empower clinicians and individuals to take responsibility and control of the environment, facilitate physical and cognitive recovery, and comply with learning-based practice to drive neural adaptation and neural reorganization. The principles underlying technology and rehabilitation are summarized in Box 38-1. Since the early 1990s, medical science has been able to minimize damage to the nervous system postinjury. It is known that the central nervous system (CNS) possesses the potential for spontaneous healing and recovery. Learning-based sensory and motor training can be used to drive recovery of function. Rehabilitation robotics are a logical addition to supervised, one-on-one therapeutic interventions.[1-9]

Robotic technology can provide service, unweighting, passive assistance, active assistance, variable and on-demand assistance, or a combination of service and assistance.[10] Computerized and robotic technology provides the foundation for patients to practice and attend to purposeful, goal-oriented, progressive tasks spaced over time. This technology can also minimize the risk of injury during retraining. Robotic interfaces, actuators, and controllers can convert sensory, physical, and cognitive signals to control robots, permit perception of spatial relationships, mobilize individuals in space, assist in object manipulation, provide emotional support, and allow individuals to call for help and communicate with others. In addition, through creative virtual training environments and gaming technology, patients can improve memory, motor skills, and movement quality. In addition, patient simulators can help medical professionals learn diagnostic processes, treatment interventions, and manual techniques. Computer-assisted technology can also improve our ability to teach home exercise programs to patients. Over the next 10 years, robotic technology will expand the opportunities for clinicians to assist patients to achieve maximum independence and quality of life with less dependence on others.

History Supporting the Use of Technology in Neurological Rehabilitation

The idea of interfacing technology with rehabilitation was introduced into practice by George J. Kelin in the 1940s. Kelin was a productive inventor from Canada who invented the power wheelchair for patients with quadriplegia, the microsurgical staple gun, and a wide range of industrial gearing systems. He also contributed to internationally important innovations in aviation and space technology. During the early 1970s, a new field emerged known as *mechatronics,* which combines mechanical, electrical, and control engineering design principles to produce a diverse range of useful practical devices.[11,12] The science of biomechatronics then developed as a unique engineering discipline responsible for integrating neuromusculoskeletal appliances with biological systems to control and facilitate human-machine interactions as well as developing interfaces, sensors, actuators, and energy supplies to create functional devices for human use.[13]

The first conference on rehabilitation robotics was held in 1990. There are now multiple conferences each year on rehabilitation robotics. In 1999 the Robotics and Automation Society created the Rehabilitation Robotics Technical Committee to improve definitions and understanding about rehabilitation and assistive robotics.[14] The scope of this technical committee has been recently specified as rehabilitation and assistive robotics. This modification is the direct outcome of the scientific progress and maturity reached in this broad research area. The goal of rehabilitation robotics is to investigate the application of robotics to therapeutic procedures for achieving the best possible motor, cognitive, and functional recovery for persons with impairments associated with aging, disease, or trauma (e.g., stroke, neuromotor disorders, brain trauma, orthopedic trauma, cognitive disease).

In particular, service robotics include aids for supporting independent living of persons who have chronic or degenerative limitations in motor and/or cognitive abilities, such as the severely disabled and the elderly. Such robotic devices are typically key components of more general assistive and supportive systems. These service robots usually integrate telematic, mechatronic, and other technological devices such as smart house designs and advanced human-machine interfaces. On the other hand, innovative, passive assistive, and active and dynamic assistive robotic devices are being integrated into rehabilitation programs to maximize recovery and functional independence skills.

Some clinicians have been skeptical of robotics in rehabilitation. Some health care providers worry that robots will replace therapists; others worry that robots are unsafe.[8] However, researchers have persisted in developing innovative hardware, new control strategies, improved compliance, and feed-forward and adaptive control systems, as well as computerized modeling. In addition, new assistive, wearable robotic arm devices have been developed (e.g., MIT-Manus, the MIME, the ARM, and the iARM) to more carefully outline

BOX 38-1 ■ PRINCIPLES SUPPORTING ADVANCED TECHNOLOGY AND REHABILITATION ROBOTICS IN NEUROREHABILITATION

PRINCIPLE I

Goals for advanced technology and rehabilitation robotics include the following:

A. *Indirectly augmenting* functional independence of individuals with impairments by:
   1. performing mobility tasks for individuals at the home (e.g., using automatic motorized wheelchairs to move individuals from room to room; transitioning individuals from bed to chair and from chair to standing; moving patients who are standing; smart houses; calling for help)
   2. minimizing the need for assistance from another individual
   3. performing functional activities of daily living (ADLs; e.g., getting objects, cooking food, doing dishes, bathing, transferring)
   4. helping perform difficult or repetitive tasks at work (e.g., assembly line tasks; lifting and moving heavy objects)

B. *Directly improving* human motor skill capabilities of individuals with impairments to enable them to:
   1. perform functional tasks independently
   2. improve voluntary control
   3. perfect quality of movement
   4. learn new skills

PRINCIPLE II

Advanced technology and rehabilitation robotics should maximize neural adaptation and reorganization through the creation of practice opportunities that:

A. are attended, repetitive, purposeful, goal oriented, progressive, and spaced over time
B. are fun, interesting, and practical
C. are task oriented
D. provide feedback on accuracy of task completion
E. can be matched to patient abilities

PRINCIPLE III

The objectives of assistive rehabilitation robotic devices need to be clearly defined in terms of:

A. unweighting a limb to reduce patient effort required for movement
B. actively canceling mechanical limitations on movement of the patient and robot arm dynamics (e.g., friction, inertia, and weight under gravity)
C. gently and progressively moving a limb to assist patient effort to perform a task
D. stabilizing a joint to enable a patient to produce a controlled movement
E. assisting the patient to improve the accuracy and quality of a movement
F. assisting the sequencing of movements
G. providing resistance to strengthen movements

PRINCIPLE IV

Robotic technology must be:

A. safe for training
B. reliable in performance
C. able to reduce risks of injury (e.g., falls)
D. able to minimize injury during use

PRINCIPLE V

Robotic technology should be:

A. adaptable (across patient needs, side, type of actuation)
B. able to integrate interfaces, actuators, and controllers sensitive to the ability of the individual

PRINCIPLE VI

Robotic devices need to be:

A. reasonably priced and cost-effective
B. versatile
C. durable
D. repairable
E. easy to use

PRINCIPLE VII

Wearable robotic devices must be:

A. lightweight
B. easy to get on and off
C. portable
D. cosmetically acceptable
E. interfaced to patient ability (sensory, motor, cognitive, brain)
F. minimally harmful to the skin
G. dynamically adaptable to performance capabilities

PRINCIPLE VIII

Robotic technology for rehabilitation needs to be defined by:

A. location of the control system relative to the patient (controlled at a distance from the user [e.g., Web, Skype]), controlled in proximity to the user [e.g., by a therapist or engineer], or controlled by the user [e.g., wearable device or interface])
B. environmental connection of the device and the patient (fixed to a nonmobile surface [e.g., wall], attached to a mobile platform [e.g., wheelchair], freely mobile with the patient [wearable])
C. type of control system (e.g., joystick, sensor, breath)
D. type of interface (physical, sensory, cognitive, brain)
E. type of anatomical connection (e.g., by end effector only, end effector and multiple points of attachments with serial links or temporal links)

PRINCIPLE IX

Brain controlled interface rehabilitation robotics must be:

A. considered after all other alternatives have been unsuccessful
B. minimally intrusive despite surgery
C. physically accessible via remote control outside the brain
D. controlled with minimal patient risk and with safety
E. potentially controlled by cognition or the patient's mental effort
F. able to extend patient's independent task performance

and address the engineering challenges related to what the robot can do, the logical physical targets for active assistance, and the joints and the types of movements that can safely be assisted.

There is no question that the demand for rehabilitation robotics is currently increasing, particularly with soldiers with traumatic injuries returning from war zones and with aging baby boomers. With the proliferation of innovative hardware, new control strategies, improved compliance systems, error amplification strategies, adaptive controls, and optimization of neurocomputational modeling, robotics and technology can provide assistance within virtual environments to speed up learning and recovery.

To endure, rehabilitation technology and robotic devices need to be reasonably priced, versatile, safe, reliable, durable, reparable, and easy to use. If devices are wearable, they also need to be lightweight, easy to don and doff, portable, and cosmetically acceptable. Robotic devices must also be adaptable across a variety of users and environments. Depending on their purpose, rehabilitation devices can operate at a distance from the user, be in proximity to the user, or be attached to the user. The device may be controlled through a motor, sensory, or brain interface. The device can perform tasks for individuals, passively move an individual, stabilize movement, assist and direct a movement, resist a movement, and even be "intelligent." The primary technological challenge that remains is the complexity of controlling the accuracy, direction, balance, and force of robotic devices across the multiple body segments to successfully accomplish a task. This is a particular challenge when creating wearable robotics for human use.

The field of rehabilitation robotics is still considered to be in its infancy. However, with the increasing demand for effective rehabilitative strategies, many new and exciting innovations are being developed. There are many robotic systems in various stages of research and development, but only a few are commercially available. Improvements in engineering, materials, human physical interfaces, software, and robotic designs will require constant analysis and adjustment in the future. It is projected that the market for personal robotic devices will be worth $15 billion by the year 2015.[15,16] The challenges of robotic engineering are broad. Clinicians will need to participate in research to help document cost-effective outcomes as well as to develop efficient screening criteria to match patient needs with available robotic devices. One of these challenges will be to bridge the gap between the mechanical attributes of robotic sensors, actuators, controls, microprocessors, force, velocity, friction, unweighting, pressure tolerance, software design, and flexibility with the human limb, brain, and nervous system. Important issues related to safety, materials, technology, and the quality of matching machine and human movements must constantly be considered. These engineering issues are discussed later in this chapter.

CLASSIFICATION OF REHABILITATION ROBOTS

General Principles

There is a variety of ways to classify computerized technology for rehabilitation. For this chapter, we will group robotic technology first in terms of how robotics are used with or by the client relative to rehabilitation. This classification system is summarized in Figure 38-1 and Box 38-2. Rehabilitation technology can be further classified by a variety of variables summarized in Box 38-3. Rehabilitation robotics can also be classified by type of interface used. Some classification systems classify technology by multiple parameters.

Service robots usually focus on task performance, movement assistance, and stability. These devices can be fixed, can be movable, or can be attached to a wheelchair (Box 38-4). Assistive robotic devices help patients perform a task with direct or indirect assistance. Some of the assistive robotics are nonwearable but assist through unweighting or movement assistance (Box 38-5). Wearable robotics are specifically designed to be worn by patients to assist movements. These are designed for the upper or lower limb (Box 38-6). There are some new assistive training devices for the spine such as the Valedo Shape, Valedo Motion, and Hocoma devices (Figure 38-2). Prosthetic devices help patients maintain function despite the loss of a limb. Vocational robotics can enhance performance at work either in terms of repetitive motions or high-force task production that would otherwise be dangerous to humans. Communication robotic devices are designed to improve communication potential for subjects who cannot adequately speak or hear. Emotional support robotics are designed to provide emotional support for isolated individuals at home.

VR training technology (with and without robotics) provides the opportunity to simulate simple and complex environmental and clinical situations to facilitate learning (Box 38-7). Game-oriented computerized learning systems are currently popular for fun and recreation, but they can also facilitate memory as well as sensory and motor skill development. Finally, computerized technology can also enhance teaching home exercises to patients.

In this chapter, we will not address prosthetics for amputees, vocational robotics, communication robotics, emotional support robotics, or socially assistive devices,[17,18] as these areas are considered specialty oriented and may or may not be included in traditional neurorehabilitation programs coordinated by physical or occupational therapists. However, information about the impact of the sound of the robot voice on patient motivation and compliance may be relevant to effectiveness. It is also important to acknowledge there are a number of motorized chairs, lifts, and walkers available that can be used to transition a patient from sitting to standing, or provide unweighting while walking or working on balance. Examples can be found in Box 38-8. Many of these systems are electromechanical systems controlled by the patient or the therapist. These devices are not usually programmable and are not classified as "rehabilitation robotics" or "advanced technology." However, these types of devices are very beneficial for helping patients maintain walking and training to improve safety and quality of gait at home and with supervision. It is important for therapists to be sure these types of assistive devices have been integrated into a patient's rehabilitation program and at home before recommending more sophisticated technology.

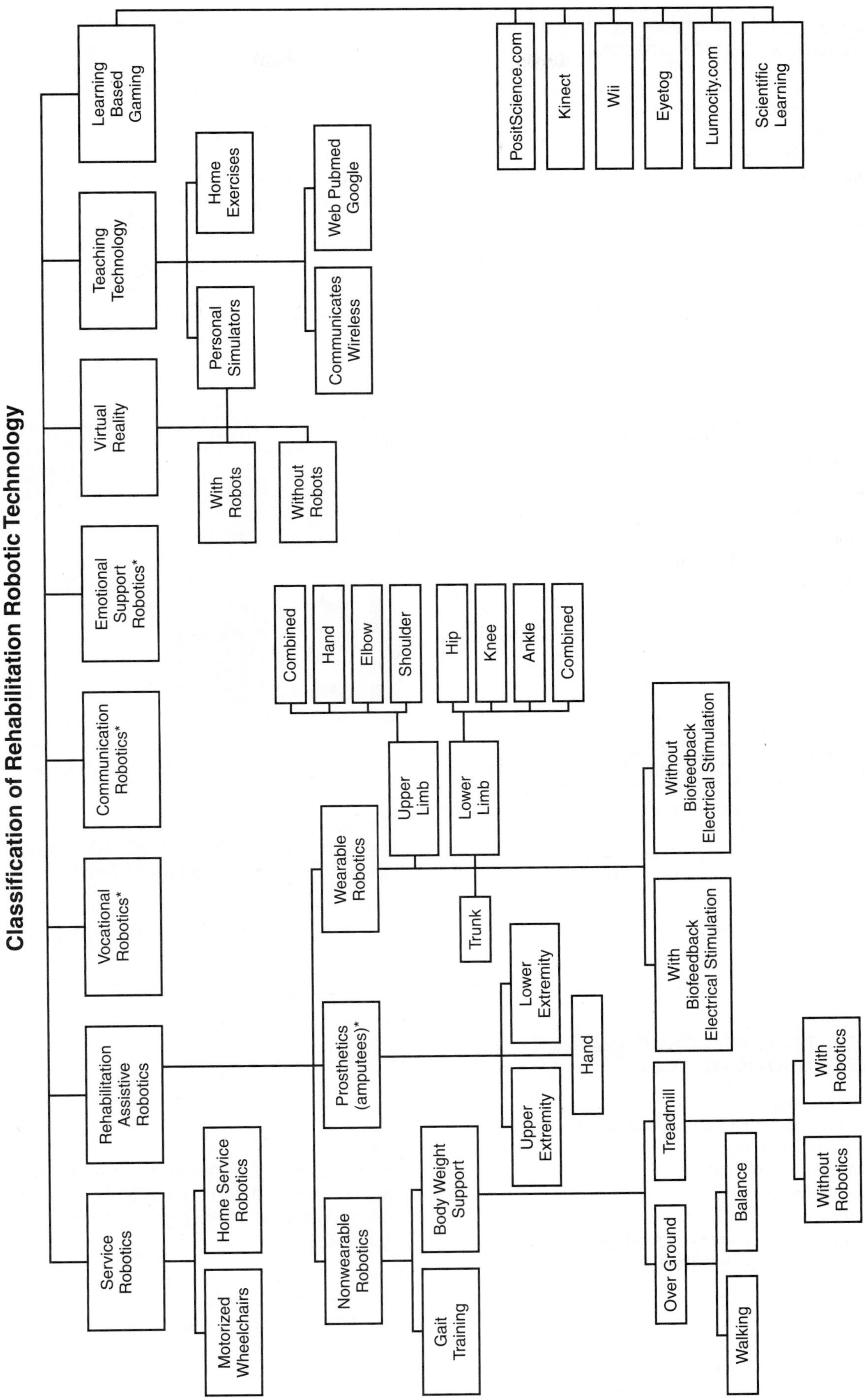

Figure 38-1 ■ Classification of Rehabilitation Technology. * Topic not discussed in this chapter.

BOX 38-2 ■ CLASSIFICATION ACCORDING TO HOW THE ROBOTICS ARE USED

- Service robotics
- Assistive robotics
- Vocational robotics
- Prosthetic robotics
- Emotional robotics
- Communication robotics
- Virtual reality technology and robotics (including personal simulators)
- Learning-based gaming technology
- Technology for teaching

BOX 38-3 ■ REHABILITATION TECHNOLOGY CLASSIFICATION

- Purpose
- Anatomical part serviced (upper or lower limb)
- Wearability
- Attachment: fixed and stationary, attached to wheelchair, or freely movable
- Interface used to operate

BOX 38-4 ■ TYPES OF SERVICE ROBOTIC DEVICES

- Fixed—preprogrammed task performance
- Mobile service—mechanical slaves
- Wheelchair-mounted—upper-limb manipulators
- Automatically guided wheelchairs (AGWs)
- "Smart houses"—designed for independence

BOX 38-5 ■ TYPES OF NONWEARABLE ASSISTIVE ROBOTIC DEVICES

- Body-weight–supported mobile walking aids
- Robotic devices for physical support (indoors, outdoors)
- Robotic devices for physical support, unweighting, and mechanical stepping in place
- Robotic devices for unweighting and controlled destabilization
- Robotic devices for unweighting and gait training
- Robotic devices for unweighting and robotic stepping on a treadmill

BOX 38-6 ■ CHARACTERISTICS OF WEARABLE ASSISTIVE ROBOTIC DEVICES

- Fixed or wheelchair mounted (upper limb)
- Freely movable
- Assist in virtual task or actual task practice (single or multiple tasks)
- Interface sensory, physical, cognitive, or brain
- Unilateral or bilateral
- Assist single joint or multiple joints
- Can integrate neuromuscular stimulation for muscle activation (skin or implanted electrodes)
- May use biofeedback to encourage muscle recruitment

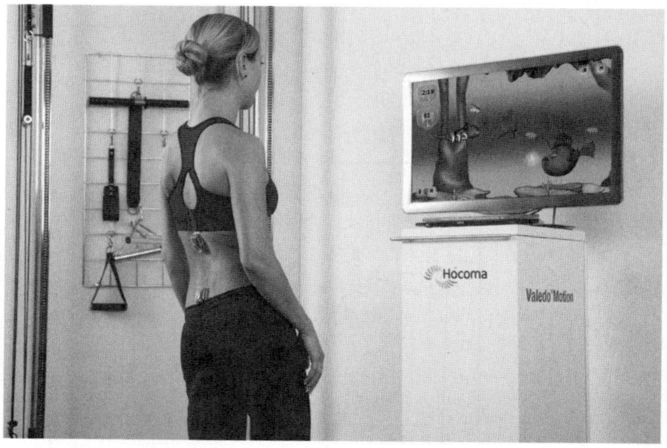

Figure 38-2 ■ ValedoShape and ValedoMotion—new spine robotic training devices for movement and stability with neuromuscular stimulation. (Courtesy Hocoma, Volketswil, Switzerland.)

BOX 38-7 ■ EXAMPLES OF HOW VIRTUAL REALITY CAN ASSIST LEARNING

- Creating simulated environments for teaching patients how to perform different tasks, such as driving
- Using patient simulators to teach health professionals how to diagnose and treat patients
- Using gaming computerized technology to facilitate neural reorganization
- Using computer technology to teach how to do home exercises

BOX 38-8 ■ EXAMPLES OF ASSISTIVE DEVICES NOT CONSIDERED ADVANCED TECHNOLOGY OR REHABILITATION ROBOTICS TO ENHANCE MOBILITY

- Up n' Go walker
- New Up n' Go walker
- Mobility Research walker
- Guldmann harness system

Description of Robotic Systems by Type

Service Robotic Systems that Provide Movement Assistance

Service robotics assist individuals with severe disabilities. Most commonly, the robot performs everyday activities (e.g., assisting with eating, drinking, object replacing, ambulating). There are three main types of schemes: desktop-mounted robots, wheelchair-mounted robots, and mobile autonomous robots. In general, these robots are used in the home, are interconnected to a variety of control systems, and are programmed to the environment and consequently are not very portable.[19-21]

These types of robotic devices are generally used by patients with severe physical impairments and are generally preprogrammed to perform certain tasks. There are also some autonomous robots in which the cognitive interface between the user and the robot is used to tell the robot to perform a new task or to help the patient perform the task. These robotic systems are successful if the robot, the user, and the manipulated objects remain in the same initial set position every time a concrete task is performed. With the wheelchair-mounted manipulator, the relative position of the user with respect to the manipulator needs to remain the same. Although there are a variety of simple service-based robotic devices, most are complex, and setting them up at home generally requires a computer or engineering specialist.

Several examples of service robotics are described in Box 38-9.[22-30] A major issue is patient control options for service robotic devices. For example, through the use of

BOX 38-9 ■ SUMMARY OF SERVICE ROBOTICS

I. FIXED UPPER-EXTREMITY SERVICE ROBOTIC DEVICES

A. The earliest robots were fixed-site robots.

B. Fixed robotics were located in a *nonmovable* workstation.

1. The arm was preprogrammed to carry out selected routines which the user selected by pressing appropriate buttons (e.g., Seamone and Schmeisser at Johns Hopkins University, 1974).
2. These workstations led to early Desktop Vocational Assistive Robots
3. These units were good for selective, predictable tasks.

C. Stanford University researchers, Boeing, and researchers responsible for several advances in France made significant improvements, particularly in integrating existing robotic systems.

D. Later, special manipulators were constructed to better fit the environment and the task.

E. The most well known systems for feeding were the Handy 1, My Spoon, and Neater Eater.[22]

F. Today, these devices have been advanced with powered programmable devices (devices can provide maximum control for those with minimal voluntary ability and assistance for individuals who are trying to retrain the arm to work in a functional task).

II. MOBILE SERVICE UPPER-LIMB ROBOTS

A. Mobile service upper-limb robots are actually mechanical slaves. They are instructed to perform tasks.

B. The technology must be adequate to operate autonomously.

C. These units are expensive both in development and maintenance and usually require an engineer to set them up in the house and maintain their function over time.

1. The best known was developed in California at Stanford (the MoVAR system).[23]
2. This has a mobile base and a console to give feedback to the user to improve control.
3. The HelpMate robot is another mobile service robot that a disabled person can use to carry things from one place to another. If there is a cluttered environment within the home, that external environment negates the practical use of this robot.
4. The KARES II robot system[24] uses a visual server to help provide assistance with movement (e.g., an eye mouse and a haptic suit with the arm mounted on a remote-controlled mobile base).
5. The Wessex robot allows different tasks to be performed in different rooms.

III. WHEELCHAIR-MOUNTED UPPER-EXTREMITY MANIPULATORS

A. Wheelchair-mounted manipulators were first designed at the VA Prosthetics Center in New York (1984).

1. This sophisticated wheelchair-mounted manipulator is able to reach from the floor to the ceiling.
2. It has 7 degrees of freedom and a gripper hand.
3. This device may be sold to a rehabilitation facility to enable training of multiple users at that site. It is also sold to individual users. It is relatively expensive.

B. The Raptor[25] was produced at a lower cost (only 4 degrees of freedom).

C. Exact Dynamics has also created a robotic manipulator (iARM) that is designed to help provide independence to people with severe disabilities.

D. Exact Dynamics also produces the Dynamic Arm Support (DAS), which compensates for the forces of gravity, making the arm practically weightless. These devices are currently being used in rehabilitation settings for training and for research.

IV. AUTOMATICALLY GUIDED WHEELCHAIRS (AGWs)

A. Powered wheelchairs can have autonomous intelligence systems attached.

B. AGWs are service rehabilitation robots intended to move the individual with severe disability.

Continued

BOX 38-9 ■ SUMMARY OF SERVICE ROBOTICS—cont'd

C. Computer sensing devices can be set up to handle emergencies and assist with task performance.
D. The robot must receive instruction about the destination point.
   1. These work best in a fixed, predictable environment and operate on an information decoding system whereby sensors identify the position and compare that position to the destination.
   2. The algorithm must create a collision-free path from the starting point to a target.
   3. Some robotic devices detect location and perform object avoidance behaviors through the use of ceiling-mounted or doorframe-mounted cameras.
   4. In some cases the user may be able to modify the environmental situation by programming in new obstacles.

V. REHABILITATION SERVICE ROBOTS: SMART HOUSE DESIGN

A. For individuals with physical disabilities and older individuals, these smart devices allow residents to live independently with minimal or no human assistance.
B. There are a number of smart devices that can be installed in the house that are linked to one another to process information from the inhabitant to make decisions and take actions in case of emergency.
C. Smart house designs continue to be an area of development, particularly with the increasing number of aged individuals who are no longer able to manage independently.
   1. One example is the Robotic Room developed at the Sato Laboratory of the Research Center for Advanced Science and Technology in the University of Tokyo.[26]
   2. The Robotic Room consists of a ceiling-mounted robot arm (long-reach manipulator) and an intelligent bed with pressure sensors for monitoring the person's posture.
      a. Modules monitor respiration without attachments.
      b. Cameras detect positions of the ends of the quilt on the bed.
      c. There is a second robot that is mobile to perform transportation tasks. The cameras on the ceiling detect robot positions.
      d. The interface of the robot consists of three ceiling-mounted video cameras to detect orientation of the user's hand. When the user points at the robot, the television, curtains, and so on will be controlled.

VI. FUNCTIONAL INTEGRATION OF MULTIPLE ROBOTS IN THE INTELLIGENT HOME ENVIRONMENT

A. In the intelligent home environment, there are additional rehabilitation robotics designed to work with home-installed devices.
B. Placed in the correct arrangement, these robotic devices are controlled in a coordinated manner.
   1. The M3S (multiple master–multiple slave) is a communication robot installed in the home.
   2. This robotic system started with the TIDE Project[27-29] and has set the standard for this type of robots.
   3. Users can assemble a specific complete modular system.
   4. In case of emergency, the user can halt the operation of the whole system ("dead man switch").
   5. The ICAN Project (Integrated Control for All Needs) developed the functional integration aspects of the system.[23]
   6. The main objective is to propose an optimal control over all home-installed devices by a single interface device (e.g., joystick or switch input).
   7. ICAN is a collaborative project in Europe and continues to receive government support.[30]

headpieces on robotic devices, information can be detected from flexion and extension, rotation, and side bending of the head to operate wheelchairs, TV sets, telephones, doors, and security systems. There are also some new interfaces that are sensitive to facial movements and optoelectronic detection of light-reflective head movements.[31] Other interfaces are sensitive to eye movements or use voice recognition, brain control,[32,33] and gesture recognition.[34] These interfaces not only may allow control of the robot but also may be applied to move a limb or perform a task.

Service robotics are recommended when patients have achieved their maximum potential and still need assistance to live independently. A therapist may continue to work with a patient at home in order to maintain range of motion, minimize skin problems, and review whether the robotic technology is still providing the necessary assistance. However, an engineer will usually assume the primary responsibility for maintaining and adjusting the robotic equipment.

Assistive Robotics

Nonwearable Assistive Robotic Devices. Nonwearable assistive robotic technology can be programmed for unweighting, facilitating compliance, providing assistance to perform a task (at home or at work), manipulating the environment, communicating (general interaction or calling for help), or improving memory and learning. Nonwearable assistive robotic technology includes devices that can sense the user's force and velocity of reactions and facilitate assistance. These robotic devices may also be programmed to implement different movement exercises to fit the needs of the user.

A variety of parameters such as range of motion, sequential motions, force, and speed can be adjusted. A few of these devices have become commercially available, but many continue to be used for testing in the laboratory. At present and in the foreseeable future, the emphasis is on enabling devices that encourage dynamic patient movements for training or for enabling independence. These types of devices do not include electromechanical devices such as motorized bicycles in which different speeds can be set (see the discussion of screening patients for service robotics).

Types of Nonwearable Assistive Robotic Devices. There is a variety of nonwearable assistive robotic devices. Some of these nonwearable assistive robotic devices are summarized in Box 38-10.[35-43] This group of robotic devices primarily includes powered wheelchairs with autonomous intelligence, body-weight–supported mobile walking aids, robots for body support with indoor and outdoor navigation, hands-off service robotic devices, and body-weight–supported treadmill systems (BWSTSs) with and without robotics.[37,41-45]

BOX 38-10 ■ NONWEARABLE ASSISTIVE ROBOTIC DEVICES FOR GAIT TRAINING

I. BODY-WEIGHT–SUPPORTED MOBILE WALKING AIDS

A. Newly designed rehabilitation robotic systems can function as walking aids to help those who cannot walk independently.
B. Some mobile walking aids can walk the client, but others can also be used for training the patient to walk.
  1. There are several electric motor-based gait rehabilitation systems.
  2. Generally, gait rehabilitation systems include a robotic manipulator, a mobile platform, and a sensor system.
  3. The robotic manipulator controls the amount of body-weight support.
  4. The robot is mounted on a mobile platform that not only can support the user's weight but can be adjusted to the height of the subject and provide stability when walking.
  5. The robot has sensors to detect the status of the user (direction and velocity).
  6. The mobile platform moves the whole system according to the subject's motion with objects in the way of the moving platform detected by ultrasonic sensors on the front of the system.[43]
    a. The mobile platform can vary from having a carlike design to having a mobile base with driving and steering wheels and differential driving mobile bases.
    b. The front-wheel-drive carlike model has a complex mechanical design and can be very expensive.
    c. The synchronous driving and steering mechanisms are complex but can approximate human walking, especially when the path is not linear.
    d. Differential driving mechanisms require two independent driving wheels.
    e. The mechanical architecture is simple and practical to implement but may require more maintenance.
    f. There are training and following modes.
    g. The challenge is to have sensors that can control stop and go of the user.
    h. The supervisor can push an emergency stop button, but if the user is generally weak and does not have adequate balance reaction, the patient could fall when the mobile unit stops suddenly.
    i. Example: the gait rehabilitation system:
      (a) Used to study the impact of unweighting on gait parameters and patient exertion and heart rate.[37]
      (b) Researchers have demonstrated that with increasing amounts of unweighting, there is an increase in single leg support and a decrease in double leg support, in terms of the percentage of time a given leg contacts the ground during steady-state walking.
        (1) At 0% unweighting, single leg stance was 34.5%.
        (2) At 20% unweighting, single leg stance was 38%, with 23% on both limbs.
        (3) At 40% body unweighting, single leg stance was 42.5%, and 17.5% of time included bilateral support.
      (c) With increased unweighting and comfortable walking speed, there is a decrease in heart rate.
        (1) Heart rate was 97 at 0% unweighting.
        (2) Heart rate was 90 at 20% unweighting.
        (3) Heart rate was 85 at 40% unweighting.
        (4) Heart rate would vary to some extent by speed of walking and treadmill slope.[37]
C. If the device is primarily used to facilitate standing to prevent contractures and skin ulcers, it may be classified as a stander rather than a walking aide.

II. ROBOTS FOR PHYSICAL SUPPORT

A. Indoor navigation
  1. These devices assist users with limb and trunk weakness and visual impairments; usually the patients are older.
  2. These machines usually have a motorized base to give physical support to the user.
  3. The robot control system identifies its specific location and puts out voice synthesized navigation instructions or warnings about obstacles on the intended routes.
  4. The robot automatically detects the user intention regarding walking speed and direction of movement.
  5. Examples include the HITOMI,[38] the PAM-AID,[39] and the WHERE (walking and moving helper robot system).[37]
B. Indoor and outdoor navigation
  1. These devices provide physical support for unweighting, harness or robotically controlled protection from falling, and the ability to step.
  2. The robot protects against falling when the end-range body sway has been exceeded.
  3. These devices are best for improving postural righting reactions without falling.

Continued

BOX 38-10 ■ NONWEARABLE ASSISTIVE ROBOTIC DEVICES FOR GAIT TRAINING—cont'd

C. Unweighting with robotic-controlled stepping
   1. These devices can include harness support and unweighting while the user stands on an electromechanical platform system.
   2. The feet are attached to assistive computerized devices that force stepping of the feet.
   3. Training is done on the device (e.g., electromechanical gait trainer developed by Hesse).
   4. With practice in stepping, the goal is to improve efficiency and effectiveness of walking.
   5. Studies with this device confirm it is safe and there are improved outcomes as measured by increased walking speed and endurance.

D. Unweighting with robotic-controlled destabilization
   1. One device that has been tested at the University of Chicago is the KineAssist (IMAGE).[40] (See Figure 38-6.)
   2. The KineAssist is a robotic gait training device that emphasizes balance recovery training during gait training.
   3. The goal is to provide partial body-weight support and postural control on the torso while the patient walks over ground.
      a. This device is on a mobile, multidirectional base that allows the patient to walk over ground, indoors or outdoors.
      b. The trunk and pelvis are free to move, the legs are accessible, and the arms are free.
      c. A servomotor follows the patient in forward, rotation, and sideways walking.
      d. It has a robotic arm that is linked to the patient's trunk.
      e. The robotic arm can be set to allow the patient to move easily and even exceed the limit of stability.
      f. The robot can also be programmed to specifically interfere with stability.
      g. The patient can lose balance and "fall," but the robotic arm will stop the fall after a defined range.
      h. The patient can experience what is needed to keep from falling when the limit of stability has been reached.
      i. With practice the patient can improve postural righting and balance.

III. HANDS-OFF SERVICE ROBOTS

A. These are devices that can be placed on the less affected side to restrict motion of a limb.

B. The objective is to force the patient to use the affected limb (similar to constraint-induced therapy in which the least-affected limb is constrained with a mitt or a cast; see Chapter 9).

C. Usually the robot is programmed to perform specific tasks with the patient assisting.

D. The robot could give feedback by nodding, talking in a synthesized voice, or using a prerecorded friendly human voice with humor and engagement that could be matched to some extent to the patient's personality.

E. Patients appear to perform better when they receive a robot voice for feedback and the robot personality is matched to the patient.

IV. BODY-WEIGHT–SUPPORTED GAIT TRAINING SYSTEMS

A. Without computerized assistance for stepping
   1. Body-weight–supported gait training systems are designed to unweight the body to enable the patient to walk more easily.
   2. The purpose of unweighting is to decrease ground reaction forces, protect against falling, improve balance, and improve walking speed over ground (see Table 38-4).
   3. Most of these devices integrate self-regulated stepping by stimulating the automatic stretch stimulus to activate the pattern generator for stepping at the spinal cord level.
   4. With unweighting, it is possible to maintain physical activity while undergoing healing and recovery.
   5. Progressive unweighting and reweighting may also be important for maintaining bone mineralization during healing.
   6. Unweighting may also make it possible for patients to perform more complex tasks such as one-footed balance, end range reaching without falling, and coordinated movement patterns such as skipping, dancing, ice skating, and roller skating without the risk of falling.
   7. With unweighting:
      a. Patients can slowly build up endurance and strength as well as perform tasks that are difficult when fully weighted (e.g., rising on toes, squatting, jumping, skipping).
      b. When unweighting is used over the treadmill, it is possible to increase the treadmill speed so the individual who is training can achieve higher speeds of walking or running.
   8. A variety of unweighting systems are available for gait training. Most use a harness system; however, in 2011 new unweighting systems that use a harness and a leg system, air, or a bike seat were introduced.
      a. Some emphasize walking over a treadmill and some over ground.
      b. Some emphasize balance training and some emphasize gait training.
      c. Most unweighting systems are comfortable at up to 20% to 30% of unweighting.
      d. Some body-weight–support systems can comfortably unweight the body up to 80% (AlterG), and some 100% (e.g., GlideTrak, Gait Trainer).
         i. In 2008, the AlterG air-distributed unweighting treadmill systems were approved by the U.S. Food and Drug Administration (FDA) for physical rehabilitation and gait training.
            (a) The patient stands on the treadmill in an enclosed waist-high pressurized bag air-chamber.
            (b) During use, pressure inside the chamber is increased until the pressure difference across the waist seal generates

BOX 38-10 ■ NONWEARABLE ASSISTIVE ROBOTIC DEVICES FOR GAIT TRAINING—cont'd

an upward "lifting" force, evenly distributed to the lower body to counter gravitational body weight.
(c) As pressure within the chamber is increased, a greater proportion of the patient's body weight is supported (a range of 0% to 80% for patients weighing 140 to 300 pounds).[14]
(d) The unit can be ordered with portholes to allow the therapist to reach into the bag to assist the patient.
ii. In 2010 the concept of a bicycle was used for unweighting.
(a) The GlideCycle unweights the patient by supporting the patient through the pelvis on a posted seat similar to a bicycle with anterior bar support against the ilium.
(b) The patient is essentially standing in a cone of support to stride with the legs.
(c) This system can be used on a treadmill or over ground. The legs are free to move in a stride-type fashion.
(d) When the patient swings the arms, an increased demand is placed on balance.
(e) Stepping the legs can be easily facilitated by a therapist.
(f) When the unweighting is performed over ground on a two-wheel or four-wheel bicycle, the individual can be outside and enjoy the terrain, still unweighted.

B. Body-unweighting treadmill systems with computer assistance for stepping and walking
1. Some body unweighting systems include a robot to assist with stepping.
a. The Lokomat (Hocoma) is a body-unweighting treadmill system that uses a harness for unweighting, suspending the patient over a treadmill.
i. An exoskeleton, robotic manipulator is attached to the patient's legs with many sensors to detect the status of the user and step the legs.
ii. With linear potentiometers attached, the user's walking direction and velocity are analyzed, and then parameters are computer generated to assist the patient in walking.
(a) Walking is facilitated by setting the speed of the treadmill and setting the parameters of leg movement.
(b) Use of the device is referred to as "robot-assisted walking therapy" and involves passive movement.
(c) At the early stage of spinal cord injury, the goal is to stimulate neural adaptation and recovery.
(d) In the late stage of healing after spinal cord injury, the objective is to facilitate good metabolism, prevent contractures, decrease bone demineralization, and facilitate well-being.
2. Other laboratory model robotic gait trainers use a system of cuffs and straps to help walk the legs.[41,42]
a. One system is a simple strap system (ARTHuR).
b. Another system includes a combination of straps and computerized control systems (PAM and POGO).
c. The KNEXO is a bilateral lower-limb robot-assisted exoskeleton developed by Pieter Beyl in Brussels.
i. This includes an evaluation platform and a gait training device.
ii. It has a high-force pleated pneumatic artificial muscle (PPAM) system to enable full knee support during treadmill walking.
iii. It has a zero torque mode for unassisted walking and reference knee pattern recording.
iv. It has a tunable assistive mode with safe interaction with human movement. Stepping is facilitated over a treadmill.
d. STRING-MAN[42]
i. Novel system for gait rehabilitation
ii. Developed in Berlin
iii. Purpose is to restore posture and gait functions
iv. Provides partial body-weight support
v. Supports patient to autonomously perform gait training
vi. Assesses and supports patient initiative
vii. Quantifies measurement of motor function
e. Passive gravity balancing leg orthosis (University of Delaware)[35,36]
i. Boom to support hip motor.
ii. Has a hip linear actuator.
iii. Spring-loaded winch to support device weight.
iv. Walker used to support the device.
v. Used over the treadmill but will be used over ground.
vi. Load cell on hip linear-actuator.
vii. Knee linear actuator.
viii. The orthosis is connected to a walker, and its trunk has four degrees of freedom with respect to the walker (vertical and lateral translation, rotation about vertical axis and horizontal axis perpendicular to sagittal plane).
ix. Hip joint has two degrees of freedom with respect to the trunk, one in the sagittal plane and the other for abduction-adduction motion.
x. Knee has one degree of freedom with respect to the thigh segment.

Purpose of Nonwearable Assistive Robotic Devices. Nonwearable assistive robotic devices were designed primarily to facilitate mobility and gait training. More specifically, body-weight–supported gait training systems were initially designed to unweight the body, decrease ground reaction forces (GRFs), and protect against falling (Figure 38-3). Under these assisted conditions, it is easier for patients to achieve intense levels of exercise such as walking, skipping, and running with less pain and less trauma to the joints.[46] These systems also allow runners to exceed the speed of overground running while being protected from falling.[47] Unweighting also allows patients to increase their heart rate more slowly while running or jogging at a higher speed.[47] For patients with spinal cord injuries, body unweighting over a treadmill was a translation of basic science findings to clinical practice. In animal studies, walking ability could be restored after induced spinal cord injury by facilitating the spinal generator for stepping through movement of the treadmill belt.[48-50] Through unweighting, it is also possible to maintain metabolic activity while allowing healing and recovery after joint inflammation, muscle injuries, degenerative joint conditions, bone fractures, surgical repairs, joint replacements, osteoporosis, stroke, or head trauma. Most of the research on bone density is based on studies involving patients with spinal cord injuries. In these studies, walking on a BWSTS does not significantly increase bone density. However, those who walk on the BWSTS lose less bone density than those who do not exercise on the treadmill.[51,52] On the other hand, although body-weight–supported treadmill training (BWSTT) may not necessarily increase bone density, particularly in patients with spinal cord injuries, exercise (with or without BWSTT) can increase muscle mass and/or prevent atrophy. On the other hand, in one study the use of shorter, frequent mechanical loading sessions was correlated with enhanced bone mass.[53] More research is needed to determine the time and frequency of standing and walking exercises and their beneficial effects on bone density.[54]

Key Features of Unweighting. A key feature of BWSTT is the degree, comfort, and convenience of adjustable support.[55] Whereas harness systems are the most commonly used for unweighting, when high levels of body support are needed or patients are jogging, these harnesses can be uncomfortable and cause pressure chaffing. This has led to the development of new body-weight–support systems such as the AlterG trainer (Figure 38-4), which uses a lower-body air distribution system, or the GlideTrak and Glide Cycle, which use a suspended bicycle seat–type unweighting system (Figure 38-5). The movement of the treadmill support surface provides an automatic stretch stimulus for the individual to step. In addition, the speed can be modified to stimulate faster or slower lower-extremity movements, which is very beneficial for individuals who need to vary the rate and responsiveness of their motor movements, such as clients with Parkinson disease, aging adults, or individuals with balance impairments. See Table 38-1 for a summary of the characteristics of some of the current unweighting systems.

Effectiveness of Body-Unweighting Treadmill Training. Various biomechanical studies have been done to confirm the parameters of unweighting. After use of early lower-body positive pressure support (LBPPS) prototypes, Grabowski[46,47] reported that GRFs were reduced while metabolic power demands were maintained during running. Individuals could achieve faster running speeds when under conditions of unweighting. With slow-speed running on the LBPPS (1.0 to 1.5 mph), it is possible to reduce GRFs by 50% when the body is unweighted to 27% to 48% of normal body weight. At faster speeds (3 to 5 m/s; 6.6 to 11 mph), individuals must be unweighted to 25% of their body weight to maintain a GRF similar to that during walking over ground.

During progressive levels of unweighting, Ruckstuhl[55] compared cardiorespiratory performance, gait parameters, and comfort between a laboratory prototype device similar to the LBPPS AlterG trainer and a traditional harness BWSTS. Subjects reported significantly greater comfort using the AlterG trainer and greater tolerance for high unloading. Subjects had significantly lower heart rates when training on the LBPPS versus the harness-based body

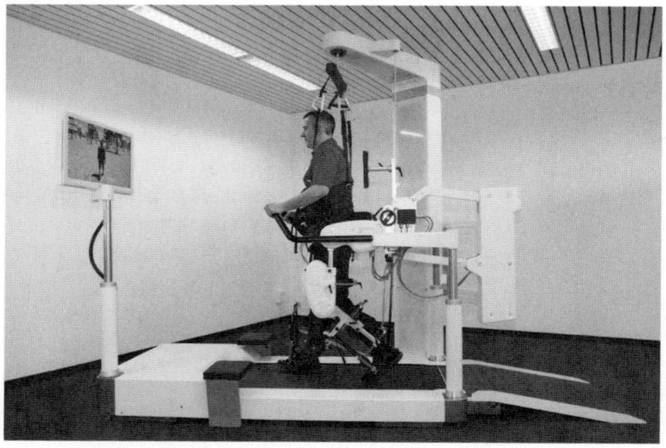

Figure 38-3 ■ Body-weight–support trainer or body-weight–supported treadmill trainer: Lokomat robotic system. (Courtesy Hocoma, Volketswil, Switzerland.)

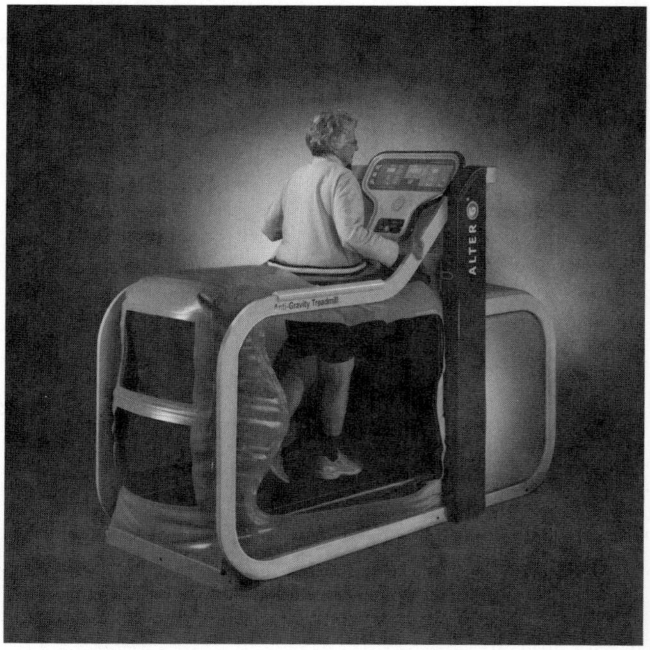

Figure 38-4 ■ Body-weight–supported treadmill trainer: AlterG. (Courtesy AlterG, Freemont, Calif.)

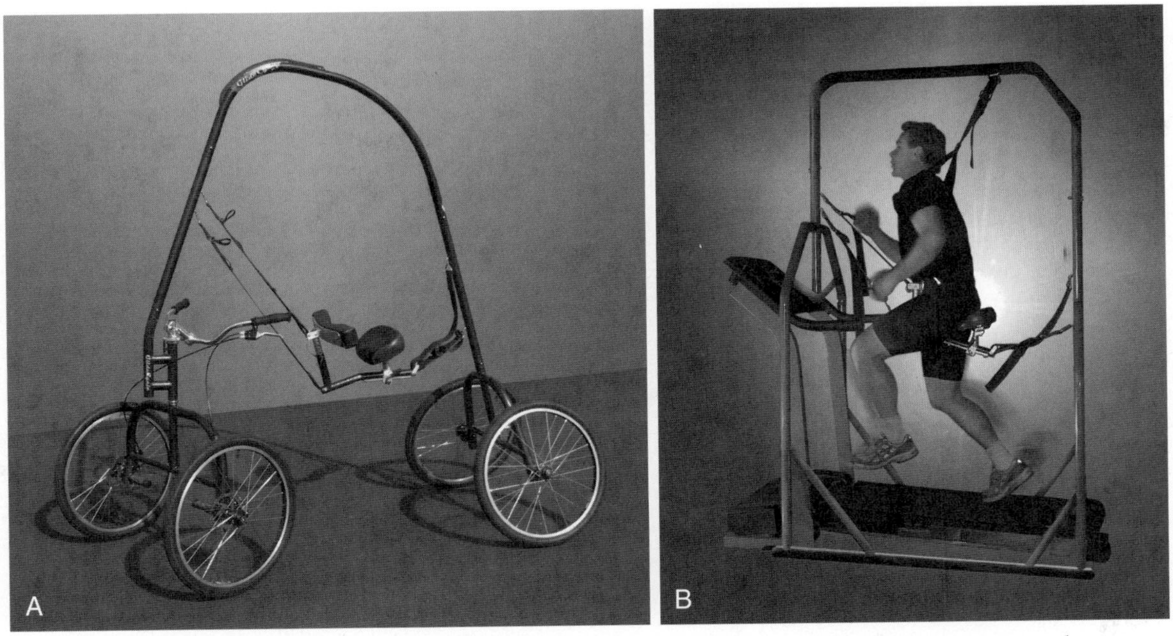

Figure 38-5 ■ Body-weight–supported treadmill trainers. *A,* ClideCycle GC-4 over ground unweighting system. *B,* GlideTrak treadmill bicycle unweighting. (Courtesy GlideCycle, Ashland, Ore.)

support system. Other clinical studies have been carried out to confirm the benefits of body unweighting for patients with neurological problems (Box 38-11).

The outcomes studies on BWSTT (in patients after stroke, after spinal cord injury, and with Parkinson disease) have generally positive findings. BWSTT enhances gait speed, endurance, and potentially quality.[56-58] It is important to force patients to walk at community-level velocities of at least 0.8 m/s (faster than 2.0 mph).[59-63] With forced intensity, patients are more likely to achieve physiological and possibly neuroprotective benefits.[64,65] For those who make the greatest gains, the improvement has been noted as increased single-limb support, particularly on the most affected limb of individuals after stroke.[66] Although there are positive mobility benefits of BWSTT for patients with spinal cord injuries,[58,59,67-73] guidelines still have not been generated regarding the best parameters for training (e.g., speed, amount of unweighting, time of intervention). Furthermore, one randomized clinical trial found that intense task-specific gait training over ground was equally as effective as intense body-weight–supported gait training for patients after stroke and after spinal cord injury.[74] In another study, BWSTT produced similar gains in mobility compared with locomotor training at home.[56] However, there were more falls in those patients who were started on locomotor training early rather than late. In addition, although the outcomes of improved gait performance are similar for BWSTT and aggressive bracing-assisted walking over ground for patients poststroke, the patients with the most severe impairments made the greatest gains with BWSTT.[75] Other researchers have reported statistically significant gains in balance, balance confidence, and quality of life after chronic poststroke patients were trained on a BWSTS. However, over the long term the gains were not necessarily considered to meet the criteria for minimal detectable change.[76] It appears that the gains in speed after BWSTT should be 0.16 m/s to achieve a *minimal clinically important difference*.[77] Furthermore, there may be additional training activities that can be done to increase the effectiveness of BWSTT, such as VR training,[78] electrical stimulation,[79] constraint-induced therapy and/or robotics,[70] or dual-task learning-based training.[80]

One BWSTS device allows the individual to walk overground while having one arm attached to the apparatus. The KineAssist gait trainer–destabilizer is an example of this type of body-supported gait trainer (Figure 38-6). Its primary function is to retrain balance to prevent falling. It is considered a BWSTS because the attached arm perturbs the individual while walking and can also provide some support. It perturbs the individual to fall and then catches the individual before he or she falls to the ground.[40]

Wearable Assistive Robotics

General Issues of Wearable Robots. Wearable assistive robots are person oriented. The distinctive aspect of the wearable robot is that the exoskeleton is mapped onto the body or limb(s) with touch, pressure, visual, auditory, or movement sensors. The exoskeleton is worn by the individual, but the internal or external interface must be mapped to the anatomy, a cognitive control mechanism, or the brain. Wearable assistive robotic technology extends, complements, empowers, replaces, or enhances the function or capability of the individual. Ideally, the wearable orthotic moves with the individual in open space. However, some of these devices are in the developmental phase and are temporarily tethered to electronic systems or workstations.

Key Elements of Wearable Assistive Robotic Devices. Two major issues in wearable robotic devices are safety and dependability. A third major issue is the quality of the interface with the patient and the control of the assistive robotic device. In designing a wearable robotic device, biological principles must be followed. It is important for the robot to be adaptable with minimal weight, muscle fatigue, and energy consumption. In addition, there should be minimal

TABLE 38-1 ■ NONWEARABLE ASSISTIVE UNWEIGHTING GAIT TRAINING SYSTEMS

NAME	TYPE OF UNWEIGHTING			ROBOT ASSISTED	SURFACE FOR TRAINING			ENVIRONMENT		FREEDOM OF TRUNK	CHALLENGE TO BALANCE
	BIKE SEAT	HARNESS	AIR		GROUND	TREADMILL	PLATFORM	INDOORS	OUTDOORS		
AlterG			x			x		x		Good	Stable
Biodex		x			x	x		x		Partial	Stable
Gait Stepper		x		x			x	x		Partial	Stable
Gait Trainer		x		x	x			x		Partial	Stable
GlideTrak	x				x	x		x	x (bike)	Good	Unstable
KineAssist		x		x (arm)	x			x	x	Partial	Unstable
Lokomat		x		x		x		x		Limited	Stable
Mobility Research		x			x	x		x	x	Partial	Stable
Bioness ZeroG		x			x	x		x		Good	Unstable
Guldmann harness system		x			x	x		x		Good	Unstable

BOX 38-11 ■ BRIEF SUMMARY OF TRENDS FROM RESEARCH ON EFFECTIVENESS OF NONWEARABLE BODY-WEIGHT–ASSISTED GAIT SYSTEMS

CHRONIC POSTSTROKE PATIENTS

Body-weight–supported treadmill training (BWSTT) (10% to 30% unweighted, two to five times per week for 3 to 12 weeks, with or without one-on-one gait training with a physical therapist or gait-assisted treatment including neuromuscular stimulation or ankle-foot orthosis) is associated with increased gait speed, increased time on the affected limb, and increased endurance during training when the speed of the treadmill is increased to speeds faster than the patient would normally walk.

Patients who make the greater gains in gait speed after BWSTT (e.g., 0.08 m/s) also have greater increases in terminal stance hip extension angle and hip flexion power (product of net joint moment and angular velocity) and higher intensity of muscle firing of the soleus.[77]

PATIENTS WITH PARKINSON DISEASE

Walking with BWSTT guarding on a circular treadmill with and without unweighting has been shown to decrease freezing. However, the exact parameters for training (frequency and intensity) to produce long-term effects for unweighting are yet unknown. This area of research is in its infancy.

Patients with mild to moderate Parkinson disease exercising at moderate to high intensity using BWSTT (two to three times per week for 8 to 12 weeks) have increased endurance, enhanced quality of gait, improved balance, and reduction in falls.[80]

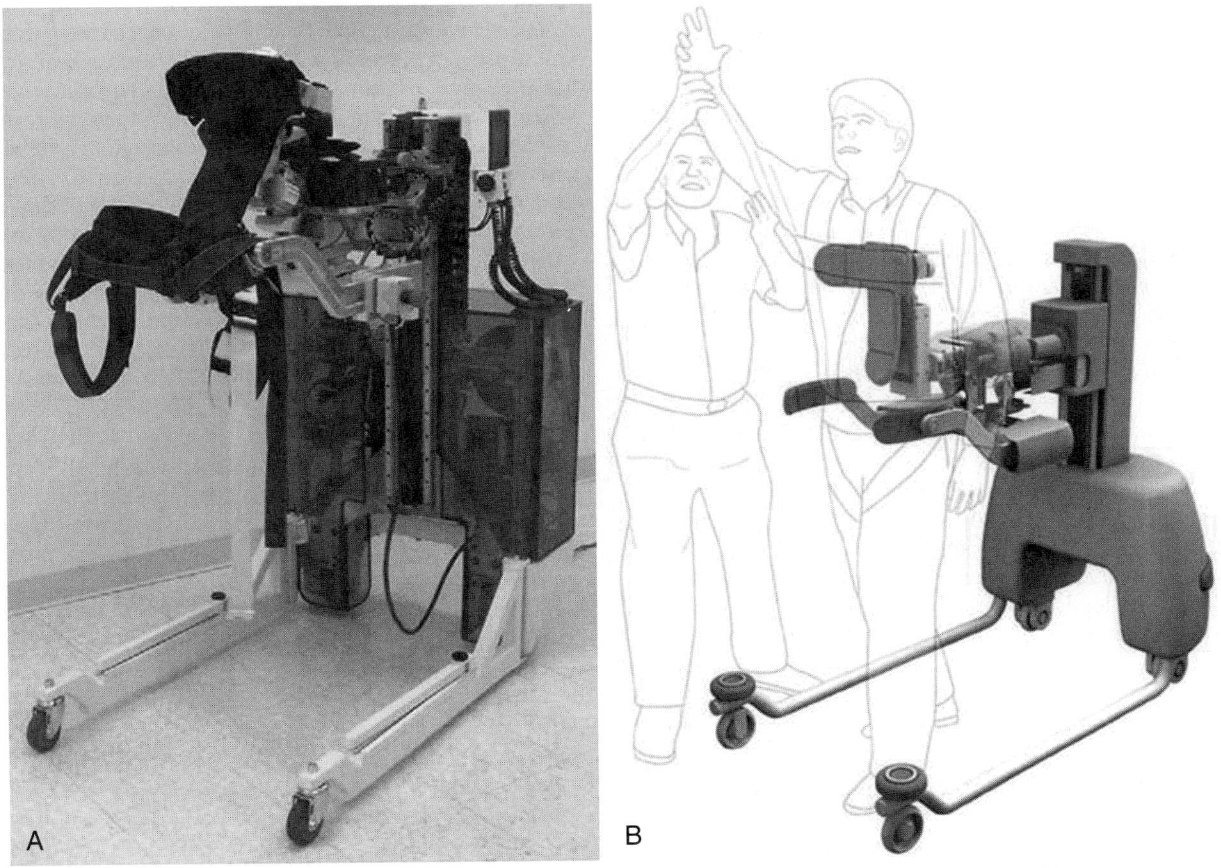

Figure 38-6 ■ KineAssist gait trainer–destabilizer. (Courtesy Kinea Design, Evanston, Ill.)

damage imposed on the tissues while the biological systems have high functionality. The extremities can be used to perform multiple tasks, and the redundancy of the joints and degrees of freedom (shoulder, elbow, and wrist) allow human subjects to perform tasks in a variety of ways, creating high functionality. The robot must be adaptable, have minimal weight, be slim, create minimal muscle fatigue, conserve energy, and be easy to control. In addition, there should be minimal damage imposed on the tissues while the biological systems have high functionality. Consistent with biomechanical function of the upper limb, the upper limb must be able to perform multiple tasks with redundancy of the joints and degrees of freedom from the shoulder to the elbow to the wrist. This redundancy, integrated within different environments, provides the opportunity for variation in movement, high functionality, and minimum energy costs.[81]

With the nervous system as a model responsible for processing sensory (afferent) information (e.g., tactile and kinesthetic [muscle length, joint compression]) to generate a movement (efferent), the system is based on an internal model of processing, with action potentials generated after excitation. This action potential triggers muscle contractions at the motor end plate. Three types of muscle fibers can be facilitated: skeletal, smooth, and heart muscles. The heart muscle is controlled by the autonomic nervous system. When excited, the muscles change shape (especially length) owing to the sarcomeres' contractile elements producing a force that is dependent on the volume of the muscle and its innervation. A little force recruits the slow fibers first. With increased force, faster fibers are excited. The excitability of the muscle fiber is not linear; however, passive length-tension relationships are linear.

The sensorimotor mechanisms are essential to this model. The muscles are actuators with built-in sensors that measure length, rate of change of length, and force. These muscle receptors are part of the proprioceptive sensory system. With muscle movement leading to joint movement, the Golgi tendon organs (GTOs) are activated. When the GTO is compressed, it is excited and limits firing to avoid muscle tearing and joint damage. The intrafusal muscle spindles sense the length of the muscle fibers, and the extrafusal fibers sense the length of the muscles. These fibers control the stretch reflex and the inhibitory reflex caused by the GTOs.

The biomechanics of the human limbs must also be considered part of the model. The limbs move in a three-dimensional space. The concavity and convexity of the joint surface control limb movement. This movement can be altered by using the limb in an open or closed chain condition.

In addition to the neural, muscle, and sensory components, there are other issues that modify patient responses. First is the strength of the stimulus. Second is the consequence of the action. Third is the tendency to minimize complexity of movement. Fourth is the imitation of movements and actions of others (e.g., following someone). Then there is the replication of the movements and the ability to accomplish the task in the same way more than once. However, it is not easy to model the biological system owing to the many redundancies and complexities. Engineering models tend to try to simplify the systems.

Assistive robotic devices for rehabilitation need to be slim, lightweight, and easy to control mechanically. If the device is mounted on a wheelchair, it needs to be mechanically integrated with the control of the wheelchair and consume minimal power.

Walking efficiency is one area that has been studied for many years. Walking, for example, is a translation of the center of mass over the base of support, with progressing, controlled falls, prevented by having the swing leg come through and quickly plant the heel or foot to catch the fall. Usually a certain speed (cadence and step length) is selected to minimize metabolic energy.

Classification of Wearable Assistive Robotic Devices. Wearable assistive robots can be classified in a number of ways. Most simply, they can be classified by body part, such as the upper limb, lower limb, or trunk. They can also be classified by how they are powered (e.g., static orthotics for stability, prosthetic robots, or empowered exoskeletons for task performance or mobility for gait training). Empowered exoskeletons, called *extenders,* are controlled by the individual and are usually designed to enhance the performance of the subject beyond natural ability. This is a type of master slave. These robotic devices usually require an external force. Most often, these master slave robotics are used in space and certain types of research rather than rehabilitation and will not be elaborated on in this chapter.

In designing a wearable robotic device, biological principles must be followed. The wearable robot must be adaptable with minimal weight, muscle fatigue, and energy consumption. It should be compact, miniaturized, portable, and energy efficient. In addition, there should be minimal damage imposed on the tissues. Redundancy of the joints and degrees of freedom allow a variety of ways patients can perform a task. However, these redundancies may be hard to control. Wearable robotic devices will vary by type of human interface system incorporated (e.g., brain neurons, cognitive, sensory [tactile, pressure], physical [movement], or breath). At a minimum, the physical interface of a wearable robot requires an actuator and a rigid structure to transmit forces to the neuromusculoskeletal system.

Some common types of wearable assistive devices are summarized in Box 38-12[10,11,82-114] for the upper extremities

BOX 38-12 ■ WEARABLE ASSISTIVE ROBOTICS FOR THE UPPER LIMB

I. WEARABLE ASSISTIVE ROBOTIC DEVICES: FIXED, ATTACHED TO WHEELCHAIR, OR MOBILE[83]

A. Workstation assistive robots (fixed site)
  1. Manipulator fixed to a wall or a surface.
  2. Manipulator may be able to move in different paths.
  3. Control system has information about the objects in the immediate environment.
  4. Usually unilateral.
  5. Some are preprogrammed to perform functions for the user.
     a. DeVAR (Desktop Vocational Assistive Robot).
     b. RTX, Tim Jones, United Kingdom, 1985; paved the way for rehabilitation robotics
     c. RAID, Stanford University Telematics for the Integration of Disabled and Elderly people (TIDE)
     d. Handy 1 (Rehab Robotics) feeding aid–based robot
     e. My Spoon (Secom, Tokyo, Japan)
     f. Neater Eater (Buxton, United Kingdom)

BOX 38-12 ■ WEARABLE ASSISTIVE ROBOTICS FOR THE UPPER LIMB—cont'd

B. Wheelchair-mounted robots for training
   1. Usually unilateral.
   2. First arm robot developed by Neville Hogan and his research group at Massachusetts Institute of Technology (MIT).[86,87]
   3. The primary commercially available model for this is the Manus.
      a. Currently manufactured by Exact Dynamics as iARM, ARM, and MIT-Manus.
      b. Supports the shoulder and arm and assists movement of the arm.
      c. Has a handpiece that can be used to help manipulate objects.
      d. Upper-limb robot goes anywhere end-user takes the chair.
      e. Can be switched for right and left.
      f. See task practice for more information.
   4. Raptor Rehabilitation Technologies, Division of the Applied Resources Corporation
      a. Lower cost than Manus
      b. Four degrees of freedom
   5. Spitting Image (Jim Hennequin in United Kingdom)
   6. Armeo (Hocoma) attached to chair and workstation (see virtual task practice)
   7. WREX—Wilmington Robotic Exoskeleton (new model WREX II)
      a. Can be attached to most common wheelchairs and seating systems (three different mounts and forearm support).
      b. Exoskeleton approximates normal human anatomy.
      c. Linear elastic bands are used for balance, provide antigravity lift, and assist movements.
      d. Can be switched for right and left.
      e. WREX II has a motor to assist the rubber bands to lift heavier things.

C. Temporarily mounted but freely moving upper-limb robot: Jacob Rosen, University of California, Santa Cruz
   1. Mounted to wall during development stage.
   2. Can be used for unilateral or bilateral training.
   3. See description under virtual task practice.

D. Freely moving wearable assistive upper-limb exoskeleton
   1. MoVAR, Stanford University (the DeVAR on wheels)
   2. KARES II robot system, developed at KAIST in Korea, with arm mounted on mobile base
   3. Wessex robot (Bath Institute of Medical Engineering)
   4. Myomo mPower 1000 for the elbow (see under biofeedback-assisted devices)
   5. Armeo (see virtual practice)
   6. Bioness L200 for the wrist (see under neuromuscular stimulation–assisted upper-limb robotics)

II. WEARABLE ASSISTIVE ROBOTIC DEVICES FOR TASK PRACTICE

A. Virtual reality task practice
   1. Armeo—Hocoma
      a. Robot fixed to chair.
      b. Used to perform virtual tasks at a workstation.
      c. Supports affected arm and hand.
      d. Facilitates self-initiated and intensive, repetitive movements within a three-dimensional environment.
      e. Games are fun and provide feedback to facilitate motivation.
   2. University of California, Santa Cruz upper-limb exoskeleton
      a. Robot includes two arms; patients can train with one or both arms.
      b. Exoskeleton has six degrees of freedom at the shoulder and four at the elbow and wrist.
      c. Does not include a robotic hand.
      d. Exoskeleton hooked to wall frame.
      e. Patient performs virtual tasks.
      f. Robot unweights the arm, decreases joint friction of the device, and on some games assists the patient in performance.
      g. Robot measures kinematic data associated with the task performance.
      h. Subject works in open space, but the exoskeleton is fixed to a support stand on the wall.
      i. Has potential to be connected to a brain interface.
   3. L-Exos system (University of Pisa, Italy)
      a. Five degrees of freedom and force feedback.
      b. Used to study the benefits of robotic-assisted virtual reality–based rehabilitation for chronic poststroke patients.
      c. Patient sits with the right forearm (not left) in the exoskeleton.
      d. Video projector displays a virtual scenario: a reaching task.
      e. A motion task constrained to a circular trajectory and an object manipulation task are practiced.
      f. Designed to be used in a fixed workspace.
      g. On some tasks, the robot provides assistance; on other tasks, no guided assistance is provided, but the therapist can elect to unweight the arm.
      h. Device is controlled by two concurrent impedance controls.
      i. Reaching and following accuracy are calculated.
      j. Patient cannot use the device to move around and perform a variety of daily activities.

B. Real task practice
   1. Single task robots—The single-task robots carry out predefined tasks (e.g., eating) activated by simple input devices. The most successful example is the Handy 1.[83]
   2. Multitask robots
      a. Manus Assistive Robotic Manipulator (iARM, ARM, MIT-Manus, Exact Dynamics)[84]
         i. Wearable orthotic is activated and monitored based on myoelectric and visual signals.
         ii. Robot is attached to the wheelchair; is available where the wheelchair is located.

Continued

BOX 38-12 ■ WEARABLE ASSISTIVE ROBOTICS FOR THE UPPER LIMB—cont'd

iii. Patient puts on the exoskeleton and is able to use a gripper end-effector to perform tasks.
iv. Manus-HAND includes fingers with three joints.
v. Crossed tendon mechanism is used to control the amount of flexion and extension movements.
vi. Movement of the wrist is separate from movement of the hand.
vii. Dexterous nature of the hand is limited by the current actuation technology.
viii. Force sensors are present on the thumb and two fingers.
ix. There is real-time identification of electromyographic commands and computation of control loops and force biofeedback.[99]
x. Has a two-fingered gripper end-effector.
xi. Has six plus two degrees of freedom.
xii. User can control the Manus ARM by accessing menus on standard devices (e.g., keypad, joystick, or switch).
xiii. Patient can move each joint individually.
xiv. Vision system has two cameras mounted with the camera at the shoulder providing the perspective of the occupant and a camera within the gripper to provide a closer view of computer control.
xv. Task includes a gross reaching movement to the target and then fine motor control of the end effector to manipulate the object.

b. Mirror Image Mobilization Enabler (MIME) System (Department of Veterans Affairs Research and Development, Palo Alto, Calif).
   i. Bimanual robotic device
   ii. Uses an industrial available robot (PUMA) to apply forces to the paretic limb during three-dimensional movements to perform actual tasks
c. In Japan, two exoskeleton-based systems were developed at Saga University.
   i. One-degree-of-freedom interface was designed for the elbow using a robot to interpret human subject intention.
   ii. A newer two-degrees-of-freedom interface is used to assist human shoulder joint movement.
d. In Switzerland, the ARM was also developed with three degrees of freedom for shoulder and one degree of freedom for elbow actuation.
   i. Patient performs task-oriented repetitive movements.
   ii. Receives visual, auditory, and haptic feedback.
e. The Salford Exoskeleton is based on a pneumatic muscle actuator system (pMA) and provides power over weight ratios.
f. Gentle/S robotic assistance (Europe)—integrates haptic technologies with high-quality virtual environments to drive practice in patients with upper-limb impairments.[85]

III. BIOFEEDBACK AND UPPER-LIMB ROBOTIC DEVICES: ACTUAL TASK PRACTICE

A. Myomo mPower 1000 exoskeleton for the elbow
   1. It is a wearable assistive robotic device for facilitating control of the elbow.
   2. It is programmed to sense patient effort (muscle firing) with elbow flexion and extension before providing assistance to the patient.
   3. mPower 1000 is approved by the U.S. Food and Drug Administration (FDA) for use in the home or in the clinical setting.
   4. Designed to pick up patient effort and then assist with elbow movement for patients after stroke, spinal cord injury, multiple sclerosis, cerebral palsy, muscular dystrophy, or traumatic brain injury.
   5. Based on MIT-developed technology.
   6. Fits like a sleeve on the arm.
   7. Has sensors that are in contact with the skin and the muscles to detect even faint muscle signals.
   8. When the person tries to move and the muscle fires, the robot will engage to assist in completing the desired movement.
   9. Unit can be programmed to assist with elbow flexion, elbow extension, or both elbow flexion and extension.
   10. Sensor electrodes are placed over the biceps and triceps.
   11. Therapist selects the desired mode, and the patient practices object manipulation and task activities with assistance of one or both muscles.
   12. Device is battery powered and allows the patient to move around when practicing.
   13. The patient and the therapist create the tasks.
   14. Robotic device does not include an end effector such as a hand or a claw.
B. Hand Mentor (Kinetic Muscles)—another upper-extremity assistive robotic device that assists patients with repetitive practice of hand and wrist movements
   1. Electrodes are applied to the forearm within a wearable exoskeleton to sense muscle contraction.
   2. The patient is asked to participate in recruiting the muscles with some biofeedback regarding success.
   3. With or without voluntary muscle contractions, the assistive device helps the patient move the wrist.
   4. Device is used while the patient sits in a fixed place or position.
   5. Functional task activities are not performed.
   6. There is no end effector for the hand.
   7. Patient focuses on extension or flexion of the wrist.
   8. Unit must be plugged into the wall.
   9. Designed primarily to train patients poststroke, but could be used for patients with other neurological diagnoses.
C. AMES—assisted movement with enhanced sensation (upper limb)
   1. Developed by Paul Cordo (Oregon).
   2. Uses biofeedback regarding voluntary joint torque.

BOX 38-12 ■ WEARABLE ASSISTIVE ROBOTICS FOR THE UPPER LIMB—cont'd

3. Sensation of motion enhanced by tendon vibration.
4. Initial trials with acute poststroke patients with severe impairments.
5. Effective at restoring functional movement in upper extremity in profoundly disabled acute poststroke patients.
6. Does not restore functional movement at fingers or wrist joints.
7. Product moving into the commercial market.
8. Some further development underway to try to convert electromyographic signals from voluntary muscle contractions into useful biofeedback on a graphic display.
9. Unit has a lower-limb robotic device attached.

IV. NEUROMUSCULAR STIMULATION AND WEARABLE UPPER-LIMB ROBOTICS TO ASSIST TASK PRACTICE

A. Neuromuscular stimulation to facilitate upper-limb movements with assistive robotic devices
   1. Surface electrodes
      a. Bioness L200
         i. Surface electrodes on wrist muscles
         ii. Assistive robotic device for stimulation of wrist flexors and extensors of the wrist
         iii. Programmable
            (a) Patient must have an intact peripheral nervous system.
            (b) Operates on a battery, and the hand can be used as part of training.
            (c) Muscles are stimulated, and the patient is instructed to move in the direction of the stimulation.
            (d) One challenge is contractures of the finger flexors. When wrist extension is stimulated, the fingers go into flexion.
            (e) Another challenge is excessive spasticity in the finger flexors making it difficult to open the hand even with stimulation of the extensors of the wrist and fingers.
      b. Handmaster system (NESS, Ra'anana, Israel)[82]
   2. Muscle-implanted electrodes for neuromuscular stimulation with assistive robotic devices (no commercial products in 2011).
   3. Subdural implanted electrodes in brain to provide electrical stimulation to control limbs for patients after spinal cord injury. Current area of research in 2012 with promise for functional use in the clinic.

V. BRAIN-CONNECTED WEARABLE UPPER-LIMB ROBOTICS

A. Brain interfaces are being developed.
   1. Control is by direct brain connections (surface electrodes).
   2. When there are no other options to help patients control a limb or an exoskeleton using usual interfaces, the brain may become the primary connection.
B. Brain-machine interfaces.
   1. Involve the control of a robot through a direct implantation of an electrode in the brain.
   2. The patient only has to "think" about performing a task and the exoskeleton can move the limb with an end effector to perform the task.
   3. Is the newest form of advanced technology and is currently directed toward the upper limb.
   4. Research in this area is being completed at a variety of neuroscience and neurorehabilitation research laboratories.
   5. Collaborations developing to use existing robotic devices and develop a brain interface.
   6. Challenges regarding how long the electrode can remain in the brain (implanted in cortex or basal ganglia or embedded in subdural space).

(Figure 38-7) and Box 38-13[10,11,35,42,115-121] for the lower extremities (Figure 38-8). In general, they are divided into three categories of wearable robots: single-task robots, workstation robots, and wheelchair-mounted manipulators (see Figure 38-7). They can also be classified by whether they use neuromuscular stimulation or biofeedback to assist the movement (Figure 38-9). Some patients use these wearable assistive robotics for training and recovery. Those who have reached a plateau in recovery may continue to use these assistive robotic devices for ongoing functional assistance and safety.

In 2012, there were a variety of wearable upper-limb robotic devices on the market, and most were unilateral (see Box 38-12). At the same time, there were fewer lower-limb wearable robotic devices on the market; however, a variety of lower-limb exoskeletons are under development[10,11,35,94] (see Box 38-13).

Wearable Assistive Robotic Devices with Neuromuscular Stimulators. Wearable assistive robotics with neuromusculoskeletal stimulation are available for both the upper and lower limbs. Ideally, both muscle stimulation and active voluntary muscle contractions are used to increase functional use. These robotic devices may facilitate muscle contractions in one or more directions around one joint such as the elbow, wrist, or ankle.

The primary impairment that can be addressed with neuromuscular stimulation is muscle weakness, but the patient may also have neuromotor control problems or abnormal synergies of movement. These devices work only when peripheral nervous system function is preserved. However, in the case of patients with spinal cord injuries, multiple electrodes may need to be used to sequentially activate a series of muscle contractions to enable walking. Similar robotic devices are available for patients poststroke. The electrodes are placed on the skin within the wearable robotic device and programmed for stimulation during specific movements.

Effectiveness of Wearable Assistive Robotic Devices. The effectiveness of wearable assistive robotic devices is promising. Assistive robotic devices for the lower limb have

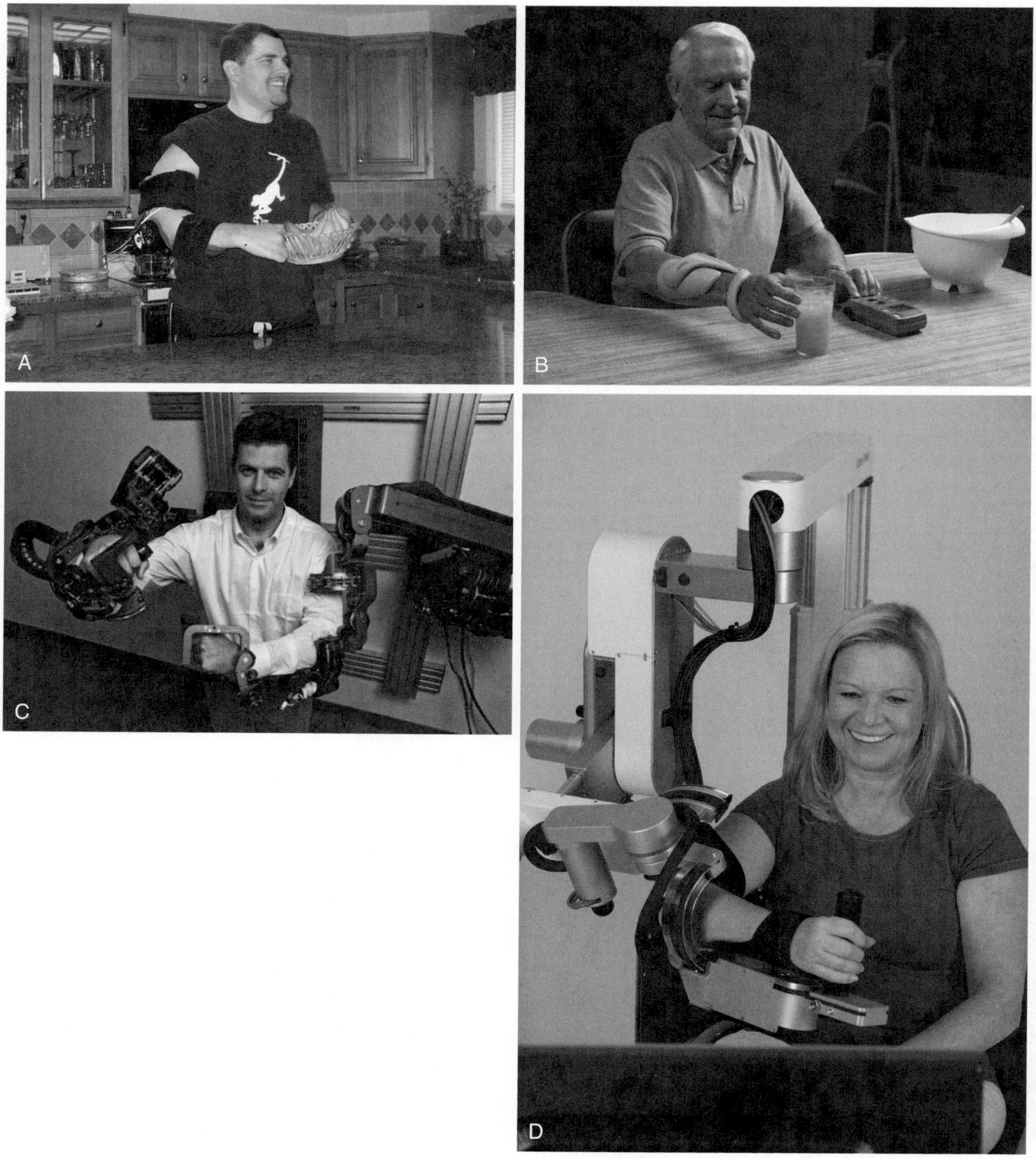

Figure 38-7 ■ Wearable upper-limb assistive robotic exoskeleton devices. **A,** Myomo upper-limb robotic assistive device. **B,** Bioness L200 arm and wrist trainer. **C,** Shoulder, elbow, and wrist upper-limb assistive robotic bilateral device. **D,** Armeo robotic arm. (**A,** courtesy Myomo, Cambridge, Mass; **B,** courtesy Bioness, Valencia, Calif; **C,** courtesy Jacob Rosen/Jim Mackenzie, UCSC; **D,** courtesy Hocoma, Volketswil, Switzerland.)

BOX 38-13 ■ GAIT TRAINING WEARABLE ASSISTIVE ROBOTIC DEVICES FOR THE LOWER LIMB

I. LOWER-EXTREMITY GAIT TRAINING WEARABLE ASSISTIVE ROBOT

A. Unilateral exoskeleton
1. Tibion Bionic Leg
   a. A wearable, unilateral, assistive robotic device, commercially available in 2009.
   b. Exoskeleton is noninvasive: rigid and soft material.
   c. Exoskeleton can fit right or left leg.
   d. Uses sensors, a microprocessor, an actuator, and customized software to automatically detect a user's action (e.g., walking or climbing stairs).
      i. Actuator provides power assistance and resistance at knee.
      ii. Sensory interface: responds to pressure (weight) in shoe insert to signal microprocessor to provide appropriate assistance:
         (a) Extends knee when sensor is loaded.
            (1) Heel strike: loads sensor and extends knee
            (2) Load on sensor: extends knee when rising to standing
         (b) Releases knee extension when sensor is unloaded during heel off in swing phase of gait.
         (c) Provides resistance (eccentric flexion) when sensor loaded and patient moving from standing to sitting or descending a stair.
      iii. Combines a drive force system with an external support system.
   e. Programmable to the individual patient in terms of:
      i. Patient weight
      ii. Amount of loading (threshold to activate) robotic device
      iii. Amount of assistance in knee extension
      iv. Amount of resistance (eccentric control of knee flexion)
   f. Battery operated.
   g. Weighs approximately 5 pounds.
   h. Effective[115]
      i. Helps with teaching patients to put weight on affected limb (especially those with neglect).
      ii. Provides assistance with transitional movements.
      iii. Enhances walking speed, endurance, and quality of gait.
      iv. Seems to have carryover to assist ankle dorsiflexion.
      v. Can also be used with an ankle-foot orthosis (AFO).
      vi. Patients can practice walking indoors and outdoors independently.

B. Bilateral robotic-assisted lower-extremity exoskeletons
1. REX (robotic exoskeleton)
   a. Bilateral robotic exoskeleton for walking.
   b. "Step-in" exoskeleton.
   c. Device supports an upright posture and robotic-assisted walking.
   d. Does not require a backpack or crutches.
   e. Two large legs support and lift the user.
   f. User controls the system with joysticks at his or her side on the exoskeletons.
   g. Can be used by individuals who can self-transfer and operate hand controls.
   h. Used mostly with patients with spinal cord injuries.
   i. Suitable for patients with other orthopedic and neurological conditions.
   j. Uses a rechargeable battery (runs for 2 hours; takes 3 to 4 hours to recharge).
   k. Costs approximately $150,000 and is available only in New Zealand and England.
   l. Programmable; provides assistance for both legs through sensors, microprocessors, and actuators controlled by a joystick.[116]
2. Ekso—Berkeley, California
   a. Initially referred to as eLEGS in Home Rehabilitation System; designed by Homayoon Kazerooni, University of California, Berkeley; manufactured by Berkeley Bionics)
   b. Original step-in bilateral exoskeleton was used in war to assist a soldier to carry people and objects
   c. Ekso Bionics (formerly Berkeley Bionics)
      i. Integrates sensors in the crutches and the feet with computer-generated stepping of the legs, including flexion of the knee.
      ii. Enables paraplegic patients to walk with a four-point gait.
      iii. Model for gait training is being designed for patients poststroke.
      iv. Patient has to have enough strength to rise from the chair or a wheelchair.
      v. Easy to step into exoskeleton.
      vi. Computer and battery carried in backpack.
      vii. Primary advantages are that this exoskeleton:
         (a) Can be used indoors and outdoors
         (b) Allows individuals to take their first steps after five to ten sessions of training
         (c) Can be worn over regular clothes
         (d) Has a battery that lasts about 6 hours
         (e) Allows users to attain a speed of 3 km/hr, which is close to the speed of a community ambulator
      viii. Currently available to institutions for clinical use and for research.
      ix. Scheduled to become commercially available for personal use and training in 2012.
         (a) Price range: $90,000 to $100,000.
         (b) Clinical tests are underway for patients with spinal cord injuries and stroke.[117]
3. ReWalk
   a. Bilateral robotic exoskeleton.
   b. Motorized gears move the legs.
   c. Computer-equipped backpack with battery to power the device for 3 to 4 hours.
   d. Motion sensors and onboard processing monitor the upper-body movements and center of gravity.

Continued

BOX 38-13 ■ GAIT TRAINING WEARABLE ASSISTIVE ROBOTIC DEVICES FOR THE LOWER LIMB—cont'd

e. When user shifts the body, the device steps in the proper direction.
f. Patient uses stabilizing crutches.
g. Developed by Argo Medical Technologies.
h. Available for institutional training.
i. ReWalk for personal use will be available by the end of 2012.[118]

4. Cadence Biomedical
   a. Cadence Biomedical walking system developed by Brian Glaister (Seattle, Washington) to assist with gait training in patients with weakness or loss of control of the lower limbs
   b. Bilateral exoskeleton using springs to activate assistance at the hip and the ankle
   c. Can be used unilaterally
   d. Approved by the U.S. Food and Drug Administration for gait training.
   e. Requires casting to fit the spring system into an exoskeleton.
5. STRING-MAN—wire robotic gait system
   a. Integrates robotic technology with control algorithm.
   b. Developed at Fraunhofer IPK, Berlin.[42]
   c. Combines body-weight support with controlled weight suspension and postural control.
   d. Provides automatic, comfortable, efficient, and adjustable preparation of the patient.
   e. Has programmable system for controlling biomechanical patterns of gait.
   f. Facilitates patient's own initiatives and effort (assistive).
   g. Initial studies have been small but positive trends.

C. Lower-limb assistive robotic devices with neuromuscular stimulation
   1. Surface electrodes
      a. WalkAide
         i. Facilitates dorsiflexion and eversion through electrical stimulation.
         ii. Activates firing via the peroneal nerve when tibia moves anteriorly just after roll off and through swing phase.
         iii. Commercially available for rent or purchase.
         iv. Programmable: amplitude, frequency, timing.
         v. Unit includes electrodes in a cuff; can be worn on left or right.
            (a) Has a walking mode and an exercise mode
            (b) Adjust amplitude to encourage joint effort of patient activation and electrical stimulation
            (c) With time and improved dorsiflexion and eversion, may no longer be needed.
      b. Bioness L300
         i. Facilitates dorsiflexion and eversion through electrical stimulation.
         ii. Activates firing via the peroneal nerve when heel lifted off ground at push off.
         iii. Commercially available for rent or purchase.
         iv. Programmable: amplitude, frequency, timing.
         v. Unit includes electrodes in a cuff with controller around neck or in pocket.
         vi. Can be worn on left or right, but best if patient has a left cuff and a right cuff.
         vii. Has a walking mode and an exercise mode.
         viii. Adjust amplitude to encourage joint effort of patient activation and electrical stimulation.
         ix. With training, there has been improvement in dorsiflexion and eversion; sometimes device is no longer needed.
      c. Bioness L300 Plus for foot drop and thigh weakness
         i. Stimulates the quadriceps for knee extension
         ii. Can be worn with the Bioness L300 for the ankle (usually they are sold together)
         iii. Triggered with heel strike
   2. Implanted neuromuscular stimulation
      a. Implant electrodes for single or multiple muscle groups.
      b. For the ankle, implant electrodes for peroneal stimulation.
      c. For sequential gait in patients with spinal cord injuries, implant a series of multiple electrodes for walking.
      d. Facilitates sequential gait in patients with spinal cord injuries.
      e. Eight- to 12-channel units have been implanted in several research studies for patients with partial cervical spinal cord injuries.
      f. System has been well tolerated and reliable.
      g. Has been associated with increased endurance and walking speed after 12 weeks of training.
      h. Improves efficiency with practice.
      i. Advantages: decreases skin irritation, can decrease amplitude necessary for activation.
      j. Disadvantages: needles may be uncomfortable; can get infected.
      k. Expensive and not necessarily user friendly for patient to use alone.

D. Biofeedback-facilitated assistive robotic devices
   1. Foot Mentor (Kinetic Muscles)
      a. Uses the same Mentor Pro device as the Hand Mentor.
      b. Has different programs to facilitate foot dorsiflexion and extension exercises.
      c. Picks up biofeedback cues from patient when asked to engage the muscles.
      d. Assists the patient into the desired movements.
      e. Practice at a fixed workstation.
      f. Unit must be plugged in.
   2. AMES—assisted ankle movement with enhanced sensation
      a. Uses biofeedback of voluntary joint torque.
      b. Sensation of motion enhanced by tendon vibration.
      c. Effective at restoring functional movement in lower extremity in profoundly disabled chronic stroke patients.
      d. Did not restore functional movement at the ankle joint.
      e. Continued development to try to convert electromyographic signals into useful biofeedback on a graphic display.

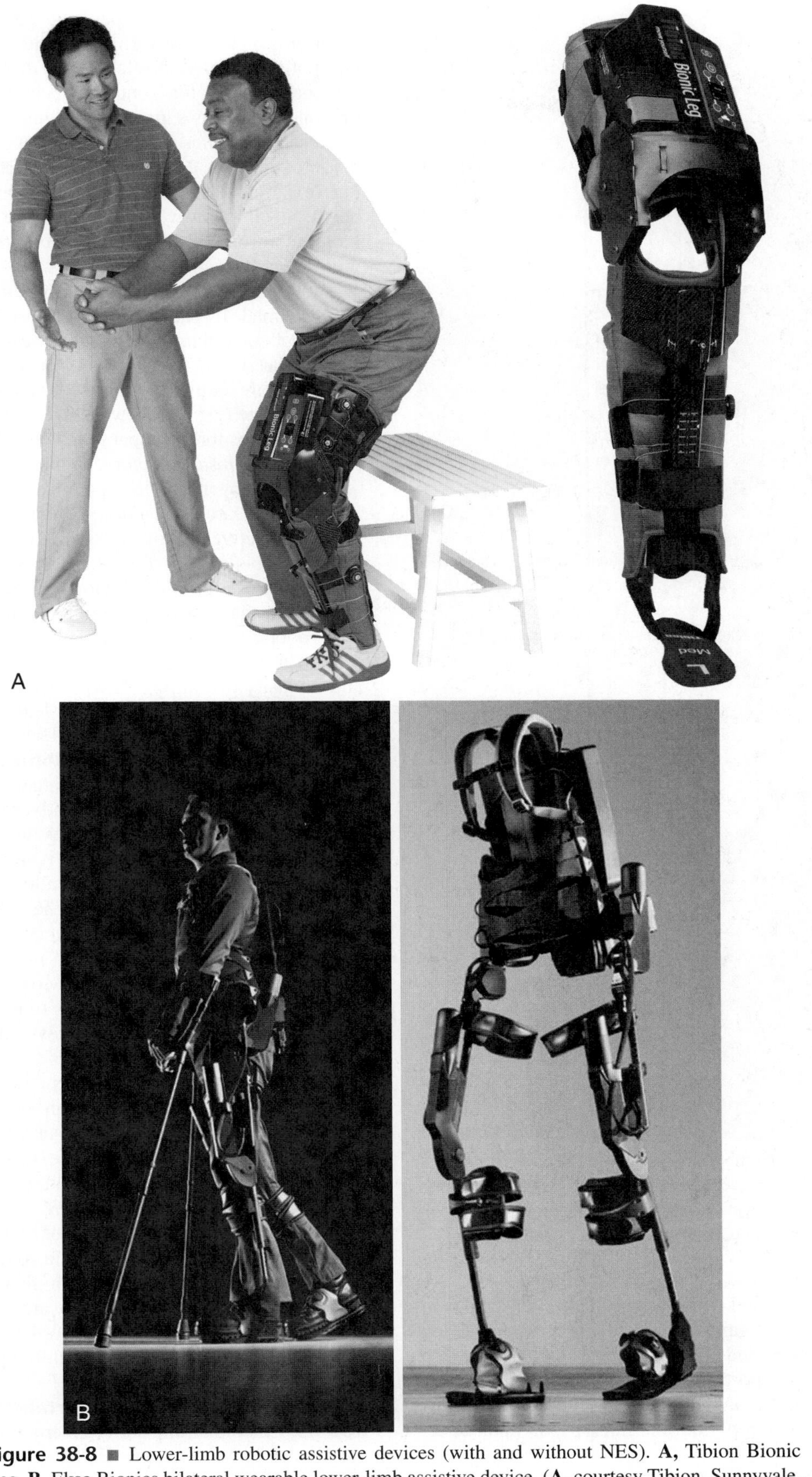

Figure 38-8 ■ Lower-limb robotic assistive devices (with and without NES). **A,** Tibion Bionic Leg. **B,** Ekso Bionics bilateral wearable lower-limb assistive device. (**A,** courtesy Tibion, Sunnyvale, Calif; **B,** courtesy Ekso Bionics, Richmond, Calif.)

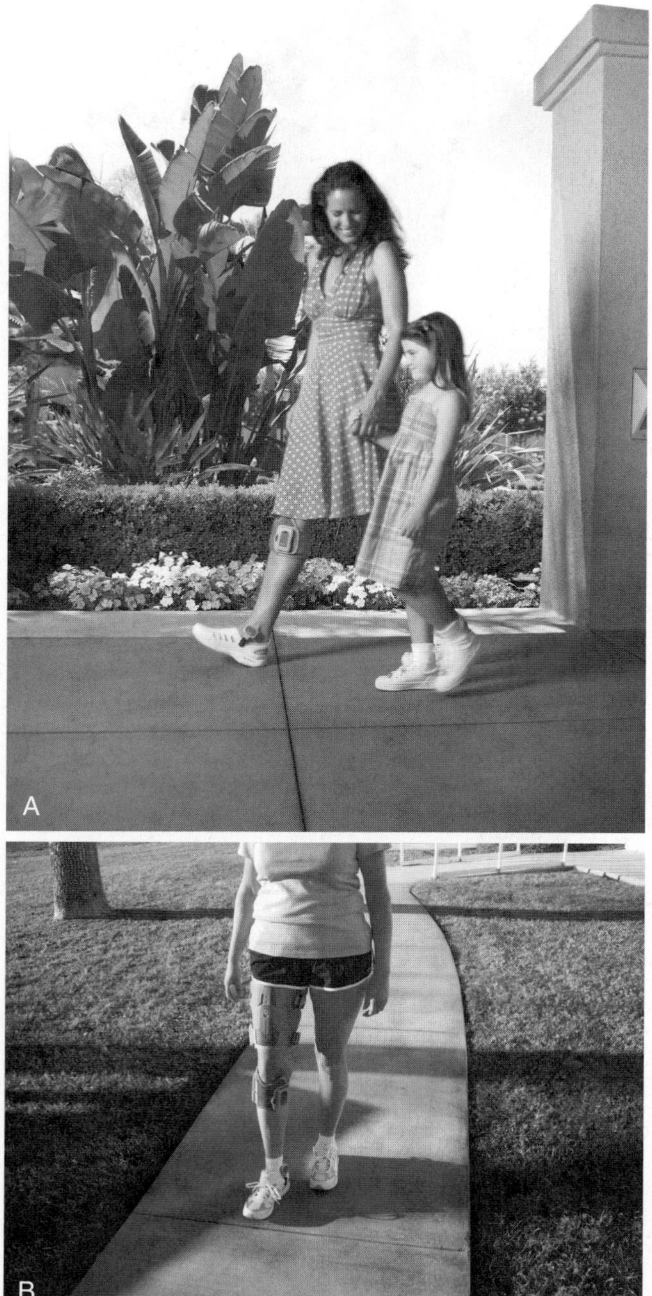

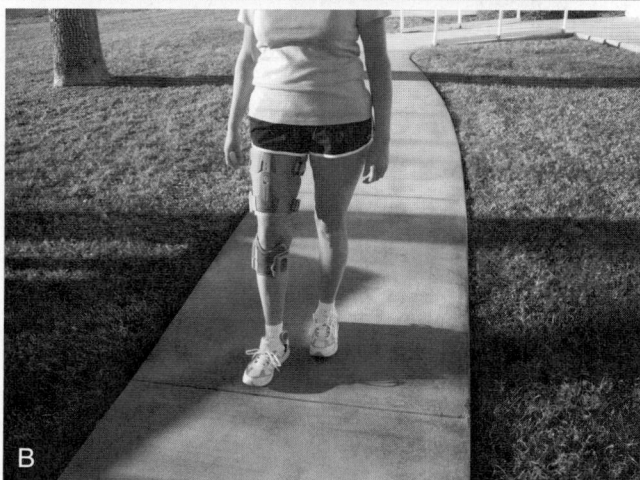

Figure 38-9 ■ Lower-limb assistive robotics with neuromuscular stimulation. Bioness wearable lower-limb assistive robotic device with neuromuscular stimulation. **A,** Foot drop system. **B,** Knee extension system. (Courtesy Bioness, Valencia, Calif.)

been positively associated with short- and long-term gains in gait speed, quality of gait, endurance, time in single leg stance, toe clearance, and balance.[35,115,119,120] There is also positive evidence supporting the effectiveness of training with a neuroprosthetic ankle-foot gait trainer, with short- and long-term gains reported in gait speed, endurance, safety, and quality.[122-126]

For upper-limb assistive robotic training, there are positive trends for improving motor control, particularly in patients poststroke.[84,96,105,106,127-143] Unfortunately, based on a systematic review of upper-limb robotics,[132,133] improved function in task performance and object manipulation was not necessarily correlated with improved motor control. The gains in motor control appear to be greatest when one-on-one care is supplemented with robotic training.

Research studies also report improved motor control with the integration of a neuroprostheses in functional arm training (e.g., includes neuromuscular stimulation or biofeedback).[82,144-146] However, although there are greater gains in motor control, these gains are not necessarily associated with improved function.[146]

For both upper- and lower-limb neuroprostheses, greater gains are made by patients with the most spontaneous recovery before robotic training. In addition, earlier training appears to be associated with greater gains in motor control. Training needs to be repetitive and intense (several hours a week) for a period of time (e.g., 2 to 8 weeks). Unfortunately, some of the robotic devices for the upper limb do not have an end effector, limiting the gains in object manipulation.

For both upper- and lower-limb assistive wearable robotics, more research is needed in a variety of areas: comparing the effectiveness of unilateral versus bilateral training; functional benefits of wearable exoskeletons for the upper limb that have an end effector to allow better object manipulation; the benefits of one-on-one therapy supplemented with robotic training compared with one-on-one therapy or robotic training alone; timing of the robotic intervention; and intensity of training. It will also be necessary to determine whether a device should be leased for temporary use or purchased for long-term use.

Vocational Rehabilitation Robotics. Vocational rehabilitation robots are primarily designed to perform everyday activities. The user is significantly impaired and unable to independently perform everyday work activities without assistance. These robots help individuals perform occupational activities including the operation of equipment. These devices should be considered by the broader physical rehabilitation clinical team including social workers, employers, and psychologists.

Communication Devices. Most communication devices include communication aids (e.g., hearing aids, voice amplification systems, computer keyboards). However, there are some assistive robotic devices that are currently being used that are appropriate for patients who are deaf or blind. For example, the Dexter hand can act as a finger-spelling hand for patients who are deaf or blind. Because finger spelling is not understood by the general population, the Dexter also enables a person to input normal text and the Dexter converts it to finger spelling.

Another important element for communication is the ability to read a book. Designing a robot to turn pages has been very challenging. Although there are page-turning robotic devices on the market, they are expensive, bulky, and not reliable. New computerized book reading devices serve as an alternative for those with limited physical capacity to turn pages.

Emotional Interactive Entertainment and Friendly Robots. Emotional interactive entertainment robots (EIARs) are similar to VR systems. EIAR systems are designed for communication and emotional support.[147] EIAR devices can increase emotional comfort and give emotional relief to people who live alone.

Entertainment robots are mechatronic devices that exhibit animal-like behaviors.

For example, within the project Home Information Infrastructure House (HII) house, National Panasonic introduced a user-friendly home interface for older people as a memory jogger (e.g., cuddly toys). The speech synthesis can reproduce phrases and can be programmed to remind users to take their medications at a particular time. Failure to respond can activate a direct call to a caregiving staff member who can then check on the user. BECKY,[148] a friendly robot from Korea, demonstrates different behaviors according to the emotional status of the user. The seal robot and the cat robots from Japan[149,150] provide interactions between hospitalized human patients and the pet robots. The Autonomous Robotic Remedial Activity (AuRoRA) Project[151,152] applied robots to education and therapy for children with autism.

SCREENING PATIENTS FOR THE INTEGRATION OF ROBOTIC TECHNOLOGY

General Screening

The criteria used to determine which patients might benefit from rehabilitative technology will change over time. Screening is partly an art that includes sensitivity to the individual and the family, as well as a science. Before screening a patient for robotic technology, clinicians need to be certain that all standard assistive devices have already been integrated into the individual's rehabilitation program. Ultimately, guidelines should be developed to match the potential of the individual with the prognosis for independence, with and without dependable, user-friendly technology.

An objective evaluation is needed to match a patient with a commercially available robotic device. This evaluation must include a thorough assessment of anatomical, physiological, cognitive, and sensory impairments. Whenever possible, standardized tests should be used to document strength, flexibility, endurance, balance, coordination, synergistic responses, hypertonicity, gait, balance, posture, and postural righting skills. These impairments need to be integrated into functional and task-specific assessments of motor learning, motor control, activities of daily living (ADLs), work requirements, and recreational needs. Then each patient should be screened by defined objectives relative to outcomes in terms of quality of life and independence. Subjective and emotional issues such as attention, motivation, history of positive health behaviors, durability, depression, desire for independence, and commitment to learning must also be considered. Many of these assessment tools are described in Chapter 8. The challenge is to determine if achieving rehabilitation goals requires integration of advanced technology and whether the patient has the potential to be trained to benefit from the prescribed technology.

Specific Screening by Type of Robotic Device

Table 38-2 summarizes some screening criteria that could be used by the therapist to determine if a patient can include rehabilitation technology into the plan of care in order to maximize function. This table also summarizes the level of function required by the patient to be able to effectively use robotic technology to improve independence and quality of life. The criteria to assess patient needs and abilities are classified by type of robotic technology. The criteria are neither all-inclusive nor exclusive but serve as a starting point for a therapist to make a recommendation for this type of technology to be considered.

Screening Patients for a Service Robotic Device (e.g., Motorized Wheelchair)

Motorized wheelchairs are the most common type of "service" technology used in rehabilitation. Motorized wheelchairs are designed for patients who have extreme weakness of the legs, upper limbs, and trunk and who cannot use a manual wheelchair to achieve an element of independence. One of the most important issues to consider is how the individual patient will control the wheelchair. Frequently this is a team decision including the patient, the family, the therapist, and the supplier.

When a patient is going to use a motorized wheelchair outdoors, consideration must also be given to car accessibility and public transportation. Many individuals will use a motorized wheelchair at home and around the neighborhood and use a manual wheelchair when traveling out in the community. For community integration with the motorized wheelchair, some special adaptations will be needed for the car. A drive-in ramp or a lift plus a seat belt for the person and the chair are minimum requirements. It may be possible to install driving controls for the hands instead of the feet and create a wheelchair-accessible van if the person has sufficient cognitive ability but has minimum control of the legs but good control of the hands and arms. This control system requires the ability to grasp and release the steering wheel, turn a key in both directions or push a start button, and turn the steering wheel to the right and left with sufficient control of the head to look to the side and back to control the van in order to back up.

For those with limited ability to control a motorized wheelchair, automatically guided wheelchairs (AGWs) can facilitate transportation in the indoor environment. The AGW relies on verbal commands from the user and/or programmed responses. The programs are usually goal oriented. With these "go to goal" wheelchairs, the patient gives the command through a sound, a word, or pressure, and the navigational system automatically manipulates the chair to the goal. The AGW will work best in a structured or semistructured environment in which the locations of objects in the environment are fixed. These devices usually have passive sensitivity, with sensors programmed for object location. Often the actuating and force sensors as well as the relays are mounted on the ceiling of the room. The sophistication of the sensors creates a variance in the cost of these chairs. The chair also needs to be integrated with other home service robots. Therefore a team including patient, family, therapist, and representative from the company providing the service robots should be involved in determining what is needed.

There are also new power assist wheelchairs (PAWs) for patients with acceptable upper-limb function. Shoulder strain is often an issue in patients who are very active in a manual chair. Thus the new PAWs are designed to minimize shoulder strain. They have been adapted specifically for patients with paraplegia after spinal cord injury.

If a patient also requires a home service robotic system to perform all ADLs and instrumental activities of daily living (IADLs) for the patient, a team would also be necessary to screen the patient to determine all the patient's needs as well

TABLE 38-2 ■ SCREENING PATIENTS FOR INTEGRATING ADVANCED TECHNOLOGY OR REHABILITATION ROBOTICS INTO NEUROREHABILITATION

SCREENING CRITERIA	SERVICE ROBOTIC DEVICES	ASSISTIVE ROBOTIC DEVICES	
		NONWEARABLE— MOBILITY AND UNWEIGHTING	WEARABLE—MOBILITY AND OBJECT MANIPULATION
Criteria for determining potential **benefit** for patient to integrate advanced or robotic technology	*Patient with severe physical impairments challenged to be independent without personal assistance:* 1. Has significant weakness of trunk and limbs (0, trace, poor) 2. Has minimal voluntary control of trunk and limbs 3. Cannot use a manual chair independently 4. Requires personal assistance to transfer to and from chair 5. Cannot step without maximum assistance 6. Unable to walk or stand independently 7. Unable to meet ADL needs without personal assistant 8. Is cognitively alert and aware	*Patient with mobility impairments compromising safety, full independence, and quality of life:* 1. Has impaired ability to walk 2. Has poor or slow balance responses 3. Demonstrates unstable single-limb support (unilateral or bilateral) 4. Is at risk of falling 5. Could benefit from fall protection when standing 6. Is weak (has poor strength) 7. Has difficulty initiating stepping 8. Lacks high-quality voluntary control for walking 9. Has involuntary synergistic movements 10. Has reduced flexibility 11. Uses an assistive mobility device 12. Needs to reduce ground reaction forces when walking or during intense exercise owing to pain, inflammation, osteoporosis, joint replacement, incoordination, and so on 13. Walks very slowly (household ambulatory but limited community ambulation) 14. Must maintain cardiopulmonary and metabolic health 15. Could benefit from stimulation of neurotransmitters and endorphins	*Patient with impairments compromising mobility and/or independent task performance at home, at work, or during recreation:* 1. Is unable to perform common daily tasks for independence without an assistive device or personal assistance 2. Needs assistance at one or more joints 3. Needs assistance to complete a task 4. Takes excessive time to complete task 5. Needs assistive device to ensure stability to walk 6. Has experienced a fall or an injury when performing a daily task (e.g., toileting) 7. Cannot live safely alone without personal assistance 8. Cannot cross the street in time 9. Needs more controlled forced task practice 10. Needs assistance to improve quality 11. Is not afraid of computerized or electromechanical devices 12. Is learning "abnormal" movements 13. Lives alone, but safety is in question 14. Drives but needs some assistance with transfers and/or arm or leg movements

Screening criteria to determine if patient has the **ability** to use advanced or robotic technology	*Patient has potential to achieve independent wheelchair mobility and ADLs at home with reduced human assistance:* 1. Has cognitive ability to control motorized and robotic devices 2. Has the sensory, physical, and cognitive abilities to control a motorized chair (e.g., via joystick, head movement, button press, breath, piezoelectricity, voice) without human assistance 3. Can activate an automated harness system to transfer into a wheelchair 4. Can sit in a chair with or without positional assistance 5. Has sufficient understanding and ability to activate robotic service and emergency devices to be independent without human assistance (smart house designs)	*Patient has the potential to improve walking quality and speed, endurance, and independence with progressive practice or training:* 1. Has cognitive ability to participate in training 2. Has sufficient attention and understanding to cooperate in gait training 3. Has adequate head and trunk control to maintain postural uprightness when legs moving 4. Has sufficient strength in legs to stand up when unloaded or protected from falling 5. Has some sensation in lower limbs or can see legs 6. Has partial movement in major muscle groups in lower limb (hip, knee, ankle) 7. Has sufficient range of motion to get into standing or walking position 8. Can transfer onto the treadmill or transfer from chair to standing 9. Tone does not prevent the feet from staying on the ground or stepping when unloaded 10. Has ability to step when standing over ground or over treadmill 11. Steps after perturbation of the treadmill 12. Can swing leg through clearing floor or treadmill (with or without AFO). 13. Stepping speed can be changed with treadmill speed 14. Can tolerate training several hours a week	*Patient has the sensory, physical, and cognitive ability to control a wearable device to achieve independence in mobility and/or object manipulation*: 1. Has intellectual ability to understand how to use the wearable assistive orthotic device 2. Has the ability to don the wearable assistive device (or has someone at home to help) 3. Is motivated to use a wearable assistive robotic device to improve independence 4. Has basic stability of the head and trunk to move the limb(s) (even if positioning device is required) 5. Involuntary movements do not interfere with robotic assistance 6. Has adequate standing balance (with or without cane or walker) to work with a wearable assistive orthotic gait training exoskeleton 7. Has the range of motion to allow full or partial task function 8. Has adequate sensation to sense rubbing and chaffing of orthotic device 9. If inadequate sensation, has sufficient vision, audition, touch, or cognition to monitor wear and control of interface 10. Has adequate strength to lift the weight of the exoskeleton 11. Has sufficient voluntary control to assist the exoskeleton 12. Able to use the robotic assistive device several hours per day 13. Has the physical, sensory, sensorimotor, and/or cognitive skills to control the interface of the assistive robotic device 14. If unable to meet 13, may be eligible for advanced technology using a brain interface

Continued

TABLE 38-2 ■ SCREENING PATIENTS FOR INTEGRATING ADVANCED TECHNOLOGY OR REHABILITATION ROBOTICS INTO NEUROREHABILITATION—cont'd

SCREENING CRITERIA	SERVICE ROBOTIC DEVICES	ASSISTIVE ROBOTIC DEVICES: NONWEARABLE— MOBILITY AND UNWEIGHTING	ASSISTIVE ROBOTIC DEVICES: WEARABLE—MOBILITY AND OBJECT MANIPULATION
Screening criteria to determine **temporary versus permanent need** for technology	*Patient has:* 1. Goals and objectives to be functionally independent without personal assistance 2. Predictable disease- or impairment-specific issues that are not going to change or may get worse 3. A support system (family or community) to check on status at home 4. Home that can be modified to accommodate robotic equipment	*Patient has:* 1. Goals and objectives to be functionally independent without personal assistance 2. Predictable disease- or impairment-specific issues that necessitate regular exercise to maintain independence 3. A progressive neurodegenerative condition that could be slowed with regular exercise 4. A support system (family or community) to check on status at home 5. Access to public transportation to access resources 6. The ability to drive (e.g., take driver's training or simulation; car modification) to maintain independent access to needed resources	*Patient has:* 1. Goals and objectives to be functionally independent without personal assistance 2. Predictable disease- or impairment-specific issues that require regular exercise to maintain and maximize independence despite injury or disease 3. Ability to maintain if not maximize independence despite injury 4. Ability to use robotic technology to improve functional recovery 5. Ability to put on and remove the assistive devices 6. Ability to slow down progression or maintain or improve function despite neurodegenerative condition that could be slowed with protected, guarded, stress-reduced intense exercise 7. A support system (family or community) to check on status at home 8. Access to public transportation to achieve community independence 9. Ability to maintain independent community driving with regular training, simulation, car modification
Screening criteria to determine **safety**	*Patient has:* 1. Ability to call for emergency help if devices do not work 2. Secondary harness systems to prevent falling with robot-assisted transfers 3. Ability to manipulate control devices to stop or encourage function of the robot 4. Ability to turn off the robot when inappropriate movements develop	*Patient can:* 1. Safely step on and off the treadmill 2. Tolerate the tension of the harness or unweighting system 3. Spontaneously step as triggered by the moving treadmill 4. Express concern if exercising beyond his or her limits 5. Manipulate the parameters of the treadmill 6. Tolerate the end range parameters for performance (e.g., high speed)	*Patient has:* 1. Adequate sensation to notice increased pressure or chaffing or skin sensitivity to electrodes 2. Ability to decrease the hypertonicity that interferes with function or causes pain 3. Sufficient cognitive awareness to recognize abnormal robotic behaviors (e.g., forced movement in abnormal directions) 4. Ability to stop excessive, abnormal movements 5. Ability to initiate self-directed movements with robotic assistance

Screening criteria to determine **accessibility** of advanced or robotic technology	*Patient has:* 1. Access to financial resources to afford advanced technology 2. Access to technology that is currently commercially available 3. Access to technology that is currently accessible in his or her geographical area 4. Opportunity to arrange for technical help to maintain equipment 5. Evidence available in terms of cost-effectiveness 6. Insurance that will help cover costs	*Patent has:* 1. Resources to purchase needed equipment for home use 2. Resources to pay to use equipment in the community 3. Equipment that is commercially available in his or her community 4. Equipment available in the community 5. Evidence on cost-effectiveness of the technology 6. Insurance that will help pay for lease or purchase	*Patient has:* 1. Resources to obtain assistive robotic devices 2. Access to commercially assistive robotic devices in his or her area 3. Ability to have equipment brought to his or her residence 4. Access to someone to fit, maintain, and repair the device 5. Evidence on cost-effectiveness 6. Insurance to assist with payment
Screening criteria to determine **cost-effectiveness** of advanced technology or rehabilitation robotics	*There are clinical research trials reporting:* 1. Objective outcomes as measured by decreased personal assistance, which can be documented in terms of hourly costs saved 2. That resource investment costs can be amortized across 5 years 3. That patients could gain 5-10 years of independent function at home 4. That the patient would be able to sustain independence at home (versus in skilled living environment) in the last few months of life	1. Objective outcomes focused on maintaining independence at home in lieu of an extended care facility 2. Patient can minimize falls and decrease risks for inpatient stay resulting from fall injuries 3. Patient able to sustain safe, independent indoor navigation without personal assistance 4. Patient able to get out of house and move in community independently or with public transportation	1. Objective outcomes focused on maintaining independence at home 2. Patient can perform ADLs and community activities safely 3. Patient uses assistive devices to minimize risk of falls 4. Patient remains committed to brain and physical fitness 5. Patient maintains safe, independent indoor and outdoor navigation without personal assistance 6. Patient able to get out of house and move in community independently or with public transportation

ADL, Activities of daily living; *AFO,* ankle-foot orthosis.

as to assess the availability and accessibility of resources. The team needs to include a representative from the company that would be creating the "smart house" to enable the patient to be independent with minimal personal assistance. Refer to Appendix 38-A for potential Web addresses for various companies offering this type of service.

Specific Screening of Patients for Assistive Nonwearable Robotic Technology: Example of Body-Weight–Supported Gait Training Technology Systems

The patient needs to go through general and specific screenings to determine the appropriateness of integrating a nonwearable assistive robotic device into the rehabilitation program (see Table 38-2). The patient who is most likely to benefit from body-weight–supported gait training is the patient who has the prognosis for functional independence but needs to train to improve quality, endurance, speed, and stability of gait. Thus many patients with problems described within this text might benefit from this type of training. Those who do not have the potential for independent ambulation could still benefit from training on a BWSTS. In these cases, the training would be directed toward enhancing metabolic health, providing a sense of well-being, increasing circulation, and minimizing secondary impairments associated with excessive sitting such as decubitus ulcers and bone demineralization. These patients may need robotic, human, or harness assistance to achieve standing or stepping as well as bracing of the neck and trunk when upright. Patients with joint pain in the back or knee may also benefit from wearing supports when standing or exercising.

If a patient does not demonstrate the ability to bear weight on a single limb, then robotic control of the lower limbs may be the preferred mechanism to facilitate secondary benefits. When all the movements are passive, however, there will be minimal gains in terms of neural adaptation and reorganization. On the other hand, it may counter the secondary problems of bone demineralization and decubitus ulcers and be of value as a maintenance strategy.

In spite of advancements in rehabilitation robotic technology, some patients may still have difficulty taking advantage of this type of therapeutic assistance (Box 38-14). In patients with challenging impairments, for safety the use of an overhead harness to access the treadmill may be required, in addition to close supervision by one or more therapists.

Specific Screening of Patients for Wearable Assistive Devices

Most patients with temporary or permanent sensory, motor, or structural impairments can benefit from training with a dynamic wearable assistive device. However, there are currently no guidelines that can be applied to assist a clinician with objective screening. Some screening criteria have been developed to try and match patients to devices, with a focus on safety.[10,11,86,94,153-157]

Screening must be sensitive to the characteristics of the individual and consistent with factors in Table 38-2. After identifying the parameters of performance and the potential benefits of assistive wearable technology, the patient, the family, the therapist, and sometimes the orthotist should determine what assistive robotic devices or advanced technological equipment are available to meet the patient's needs. The team also has to assess where the devices are located, whether they are accessible, whether the device should be rented or purchased, and whether the insurance company will help pay for the rental or purchase of the device.

BOX 38-14 ■ MATCHING PATIENTS TO EFFECTIVE WEARABLE ROBOTIC DEVICES

In attempting to match a patient to an effective wearable assistive robotic device, several questions must also be asked about the dynamics of the robot providing assistance:

1. How much force can the robot safely exert to overcome resistance from hypertonicity?
2. How strong does the patient need to be to overcome the weight of the wearable assistive robotic device?
3. Does the robot need to be programmed across multiple joints to move with high-quality movements?
4. Does the robot need to stop if the individual does not initiate movement in the exact pattern of the programmed assistance?
5. Is there negative learning when there is a mismatch between the patient's movements and the robotic assistance?
6. Can the amount of assistance provided be dynamically controlled by the robot while being based on the patient's need for task performance?
7. Can the therapist or the patient easily modify the assistance given by the wearable robotic device?

Ideally patients will use a wearable robotic assistive device to try to drive neural adaptation to recover function. Thus some patients may "train out" of the robotic device as they recover more function. Obviously, it would be better for these patients to rent rather than purchase the orthotic. Other patients would benefit from purchasing the assistive device because the robotic device improves function and independence despite ongoing impairments. Long-term use is also common when a patient has a degenerative condition, when the impairments are likely to get worse rather than better, and when with assistance independence can be prolonged.

In addition to the general and specific screening criteria, it is important to note that some assistive robotic devices may target control of one specific joint. However, given the biomechanical links, flexibility and sensory and motor characteristics must be assessed at each major joint above and below the primary assisted joint. For example, the Tibion Bionic Leg (see Figure 38-8, *A*) focuses on assisting the knee, but the patient's hip and ankle also should be assessed. The less affected side also needs to be evaluated. To maximize the benefit of a wearable assistive device, patients should ideally have some ability to voluntarily initiate movement and a grade of poor or greater strength to be able to assist in the movement.

Wearable robotics must be programmed to assist patient function but also to stop to avoid harm. This requires a balance between the dynamic nature of the wearable assistive device and a patient's weakness, lack of voluntary motor control, and the presence of involuntary muscle activity including hypertonicity (e.g., spasticity, dystonia, rigidity, tremor) (Box 38-14). For example, how much force would the assistive device need to provide to overcome involuntary tone? Other relevant questions must then be asked: If a robotic device is programmed to assist with flexion and the patient initiates movement into extension or abduction, will the robot have to stop assisting the limb to prevent harm? If the robot stops assisting, is there a negative effect caused by the mismatch of force between the patient and the robot? Does the patient need consistent assistance or variable assistance? How will the therapist, the robot, or the patient determine how much assistance is needed? In one case a patient may need unweighting of only a limb, and in another case both unweighting and assistance may be needed. In theory, the amount of assistance needed should decrease with recovery of function. Thus it is helpful if the wearable assistive device can easily be adjusted by the therapist or the patient.

Despite the advancements in rehabilitation robotics, some patients will still have difficulty wearing an assistive orthotic. For example, wearable assistive orthotic devices may not work well for patients with severe sensory impairments, severe balance problems, a fear of falling, or inadequate assets to control the device or for elderly patients who are afraid of computerized technology (see Box 38-15). Sophisticated rehabilitation robotic devices may also not be recommended for patients who are disoriented, who have severe pain or neural hypersensitivity, or who cannot don the apparatus independently (Box 38-16).

It may be appropriate and helpful for patients with severe sensory and motor impairments to train using VR technology with or without assistive technology. Patients may begin with mental imagery and practice before engaging in physical practice, without and then with the integration of wearable robotic devices. It is also possible to begin the training with the assistive technology while in a harness system to protect from falling. In addition, depending on the severity of balance and voluntary abilities, it may be necessary for patients to train with technology under careful direct supervision. In cases in which balance and motor control are good but can be improved, it may be possible for patients to train at home with wireless telemetry-type supervision.

BOX 38-15 ■ IMPAIRMENTS THAT INTERFERE WITH UNWEIGHTED GAIT TRAINING

Individuals with the following impairments may not be good candidates for use of body-unweighted gait training:

1. Severe cardiopulmonary disease
2. Severely high blood pressure
3. Unstable blood pressure when standing or walking
4. Uncontrollable seizures
5. Uncontrolled diabetes
6. Complete loss of sensation
7. Unhealed incisions
8. Pressure sores
9. Severe and fragile osteoporosis
10. Unexplained swelling or lymphedema of the lower limbs
11. Severe contractures of the legs
12. Vegetative state
13. Inability to communicate
14. Uncooperativeness
15. Lack of head control

BOX 38-16 ■ INTERFERENCE WITH COMPLIANCE WITH WEARABLE ASSISTIVE ROBOTIC DEVICES

Specific cognitive or emotional impairments might interfere with compliance with and benefits of retraining with a wearable assistive robotic device. Patients with such impairments include the following:

1. Patients who are afraid of computerized or advanced technology
2. Patients who are confused, hallucinating, or unable to understand how to don the device or how the robotic device works
3. Patients with excessive hypersensitivity of the skin, severe pain, or complete loss of sensation to touch

If the patient does not meet the cognitive screening criteria for using either physical or cognitive sensors to control a wearable robotic, then a more sophisticated psychocognitive screening may be necessary. In these cases, biomagnetic imaging may be appropriate to determine if the individual could benefit from a wearable exoskeleton that has been mapped directly to the brain. Brain-mapped wearable robotic exoskeletons are available for patients with severe motor impairments. This brain-mapped wearable robotic allows the individual to use specific brain signals to help the individual achieve control of the limbs and the trunk to complete tasks. These brain-mapped wearable exoskeletons are still in the developmental stage. Most are not yet available on the commercial market.

OTHER ADVANCED TECHNOLOGY: CONTRIBUTION TO NEUROREHABILITATION

Virtual Reality Technology

Definitions and Benefits of Virtual Reality Technology

One of the most important issues in neurorehabilitation is creating the most effective training environment. To achieve maximum neural adaptation, training must be specific, task oriented, repetitious, spaced in time, progressed in difficulty, and salient to the outcomes targeted. VR technology allows the creation of the most applicable practice environment in which novelty, complexity, obstacles, task appropriateness, and progressive changes can be manipulated. With some virtual training, a therapist can conveniently immerse a patient into computer-generated multisensory, task-appropriate environments. This environmental variety can be stimulating, engaging, and fun, while enhancing compliance in practice. VR training can be not only adapted to the impairment or the acuity or chronicity of recovery but also directly related to the type of functional outcome desired. In addition, VR can be programmed for intensity and duration of training. Furthermore, VR training can be supplemented with traditional or robotic therapy. One additional attribute, and equally important, is that changes can be made efficiently in the virtual world while the patient and the therapist are in the same location.

VR is becoming increasingly popular as a way to enrich the environment for retraining the brain. It can be used as an assessment measure, a training tool, an outcome tool, or a combination of all three. One of the greatest aspects of virtual environmental manipulation is that it can be done safely and rapidly without changing the venue of the patient or the therapist. Real-world situations surrounding task performance can be re-created while precisely and systematically manipulating environmental obstacles and constraints. Without danger to the individual, task difficulty can be increased. Sensory parameters can be changed, adapted, and scaled to the user's changing abilities. Object properties can also be changed easily, along with reliable changes in object location and orientation. In these VR environments, it is possible to study how individuals interact with objects and situations, particularly when changes are made in conditions within the virtual world. For example, for walking, it is possible to re-create real-work obstacles to develop adaptive responses—for instance, a perceived rock that needs to be stepped over. A variety of patient populations can be integrated in VR retraining paradigms; however, it cannot be assumed that VR training will be equally effective with patients with different types of movement impairments or medical diagnoses. VR can be designed to target regional neural reorganization or improve task functions.[94,157-166]

A variety of VR paradigms were available at the time this chapter was prepared. These paradigms can be defined for an individual for supervised training, for multiple users, or for practice at home.[167] The types of VR training will continue to expand. In order to be able to compare outcomes with different approaches to VR training, there needs to be a way to categorize the paradigms. One way may be to organize the training according to the type of learning paradigm facilitated. Refer to Box 38-17 for examples of some of these learning paradigms. Ultimately guidelines need to be developed to match the training paradigm with the patient impairments. A therapist will need to assess not only motor impairments but also emotional, cognitive, and perceptual impairments, especially when working with individuals who have sustained some CNS insult. This will not be a simple process. In addition to variability in patient impairments, the match needs to consider patient personality and age; user friendliness, costs, availability, accessibility, and location of equipment; ease of use; and supervision needed.

Does Virtual Reality Simulate Reality in the Physical Environment?

One important question is whether movement kinematics produced in virtual environments are associated with the same kinematics in the real physical environment for healthy subjects and those with impairments (e.g., poststroke).[157,159,160,168] In a VR study of reaching, grasping, transporting and releasing a ball, with one exception both healthy subjects and subjects with a hemiparesis used similar movement strategies in the VR environment as they did in the real environment. Both healthy controls and patients with hemiparesis used less wrist extension in the VR tasks, but healthy subjects reduced wrist extension more than subjects with a hemiparesis. In a three-dimensional VR environment, subjects had to place targets in different places with different combinations of arm joint movement. The task was to point quickly and accurately to each of six targets in a random sequence. Very few movement kinematic differences were reported in the different environments for healthy subjects and for poststroke subjects. Healthy subjects made faster movements, pointing more accurately with straighter endpoint paths than poststroke patients. The poststroke patients demonstrated less accurate movements and a curved path to the target with less trunk displacement. In another research study, there was an increase in movement time, and the movement endpoint trajectories were more curved in the virtual environment than in the physical environment for both healthy subjects and poststroke patients.

One criticism has been that VR environments lack real-life haptics, defined as the sensory interface of the patient and the object being manipulated. Some of the new virtual training systems now integrate haptic assistance, adaptive antigravity support, or even robotic technology to enhance motor outcomes. In one laboratory, traditional dynamic posturography was adapted to VR.[169] The objective of this study was to test and train postural righting behaviors in different virtual environments to simulate real-work conditions. It was hypothesized that shifts in spatial perception, visual inputs, and force perturbations would elicit normal positive postural reactions to right the body. Keshner and Kenyon[169] reported measurable gains in postural orientation with this type of training in the virtual environment.

Mental imagery is another way to manipulate the environment. This manipulation can be considered a variant of VR training. In this case, the patient mentally imagines performing tasks such as object manipulation or walking. This mental imagery can be guided or spontaneous. It can also include progressive and repetitive practice. It can also be combined with VR training and actual task practice.[146,157,170-175]

Effectiveness of Virtual Reality Training

The major question regarding the interface of VR and the real world is whether task practice in a progressive, strategically manipulated environment is associated with a greater return of function compared to task practice alone. Is it possible that a virtual training environment would help patients specifically recover more recalcitrant skills—for example, could it drive greater neural adaptation to achieve higher levels of arm function in patients poststroke? Large research studies on the effectiveness of the different VR paradigms are still in their infancy. There has been some quantification of the physiological mechanisms of VR and the effectiveness of VR rehabilitation technologies based on laboratory testing, case studies, and small controlled trials, and large randomized clinical trials are needed to examine the benefits of different types of VR training in different types of VR paradigms.[160] If the evidence suggests that VR training

BOX 38-17 ■ EXAMPLES OF LEARNING PARADIGMS THAT COULD BE FACILITATED WITH VIRTUAL REALITY

- Movement initiation
- Action execution
- Feedback reinforcement
- Haptic feedback
- Augmented repetitive practice videocapture virtual reality
- Exoskeleton robotics integrated with simultaneous virtual reality
- Mental practice and virtual reality

significantly enhances the recovery of function beyond task practice alone, then studies on cost-effectiveness are needed. VR systems can be expensive. The incremental gains in performance must make a clinically significant difference in patient function in the community. If this can be documented, then guidelines for neurorehabilitation may need to integrate VR technology as a standard aspect of rehabilitation, particularly in the early stages of retraining.

Small randomized clinical trials have been carried out using VR training with and without robotics. The findings are positive in support of improved motor control. The results are less clear with regard to improved function.[158,161-163,176-178]

One study of effectiveness has been reported by researchers using the commercially available Rehabilitation Gaming System (RGS) VR system.[179] This system specifically targets functional training to maximize plasticity after a neural insult. It is a noninvasive multimodal system of stimulation. It has been tested primarily for rehabilitation of the upper extremity of patients after stroke. RGS provides VR tasks in which the movements of two virtual arms are controlled by the subject's own arm movements. The RGS system incorporates a variety of tasks, graded in complexity and difficulty. The games can be adapted to the capability of the individual. RGS VR tries to model gaming in order to heighten arousal and performance as well as potentially being entertaining. The user is asked to reconstruct different elements of a variety of IADLs. The hypothesis is that action execution combined with observation of correlated movements in a virtual environment may activate undamaged primary or secondary motor areas, which will facilitate improved function.

The behavior in the virtual environment appears to be consistent with the behavior in the real world.[158,160] Furthermore, effectiveness of the RGS VR was enhanced when the observation of hand movements was consistent with the orientation of the observer. For example, first-person perspective appeared to be more effective than third-person perspective in terms of driving cortical activation during performance of virtual tasks. Also, the first-person perspective appeared to recruit the motor system to a greater extent, allowing for integration of kinematic information. The integration of kinematic information in motor learning appeared to result in a higher degree of representation and more effective functional reorganization. The researchers also observed that the behavior in the virtual environment was consistent with the behavior in the real world.[158,160] The differences between paretic and nonparetic limbs were preserved. Each training task included 300 repetitions. Three hundred repetitions produced robust and accurate data. Given these data, it was possible to calculate the error distribution for the paretic and nonparetic arm. For both limbs, there was measurable arousal before a missed event. This finding suggests that this type of training or therapeutic environment could be another way to provide feedback. For example, just before the patient is likely to fail, the patient would be made aware of that potential rather than being given feedback about failure on the task itself. The physiological effects on heart rate were not consistently related to the stress of completing a task. On objective and functional tasks, the RGS VR group showed similar absolute improvement from baseline to week 5 compared with individuals in the control groups, who did not interface with a VR environment. However, in the second 6 weeks, the patients in the RGS VR group showed a higher mean increase in all of their outcome scores on functional measures, whereas the control subjects tended to plateau after 5 weeks.

Small randomized clinical trials have also been conducted on the effectiveness of mental imagery and improved motor control and task function.[170,171,173,175,180] Usual therapy enriched with mental locomotor, kinesthetic, visual, or auditory practice was associated with greater gains in mobility for healthy patients and those with impairments. Specifically, elderly patients and poststroke patients made greater gains with a combination of auditory step rhythm imagery in addition to locomotor imagery. Other researchers have reported that poststroke patients had greater reductions in measured impairments and improvement in task-specific function in the upper limb after regular physical therapy and mental practice than after regular physical therapy alone.[175] However, although motor control improved with robotic-assisted virtual training using the WREX upper-limb robot, there was no correlation between these reported motor benefits and performance improvements.[159]

CASE STUDY 38-1 ■ BEFORE AND AFTER VESTIBULAR REHABILITATION TRAINING USING A VIRTUAL REALITY ENVIRONMENT

Mrs. S. was a 52-year-old woman who came to the clinic with a diagnosis of unilateral vestibular hypofunction and a chief complaint of being unable to go into large crowds or stores or to shop without feelings of dizziness and disorientation. Clinical and laboratory findings revealed bilaterally reduced vestibular evoked myogenic potentials and a unilateral caloric weakness on the right. The patient reported onset of her symptoms one month ago with tinnitus and difficulty walking in crowds and in grocery stores. She was referred to physical therapy by a neuro-otologist. Mrs. S. signed informed consent to participate in a virtual reality (VR) treatment trial. The VR treatment trial consisted of testing of her function and symptoms pretreatment, during six intervention sessions, immediately posttreatment, and at a 6-month follow-up.

PROCEDURES

The Virtual Reality Protocol

Each VR session consisted of six 4-minute exposures walking and "shopping" on the treadmill. The Balance Near Automatic Virtual Environment (BNAVE) was used as the Virtual Intervention.[181] (See Figure 38-10.)

The BNAVE consists of three walls that surround the person with a treadmill in the center. The patient was instructed to push the instrumented grocery cart (which had a force sensor on the push bar of the grocery cart) at the speed at which she wanted to ambulate through the store. The upper speed limit of the treadmill was fixed at 1.2 m/s. The specially designed treadmill was built to be wider than a normal treadmill to accommodate the turning required at the end of the grocery store aisle.

Continued

CASE STUDY 38-1 ■ BEFORE AND AFTER VESTIBULAR REHABILITATION TRAINING USING A VIRTUAL REALITY ENVIRONMENT—cont'd

The three rear-projected scenes were merged to form one image on the BNAVE screens with the hope that persons would be immersed and "feel" as though they were shopping in a grocery store.[181] During the 4-minute exposures to the scene, Mrs. S. was introduced first to the easiest aisle (the white paper products). There were 16 different aisles, and they were designed to be increasingly more complex either via a greater number of products on the shelves, more vibrant colors, or a greater population density of products per square inch.

Mrs. S. was asked throughout the VR experience to "find" certain products in each aisle. She reported verbally when she found the product on the shelves and then continued walking. Some patients are able to continue to "walk" and "shop" at the same time. Mrs. S. was able to fairly smoothly ambulate through the store without stopping. She would occasionally slow down significantly if she was having difficulty finding a particular product and then would continue walking in the "store."

Safety

The patient was secured to an overhead harness to prevent a fall. In addition, the therapist held a switch and could stop the treadmill if there was any indication that Mrs. S. was having a problem. The patient could also stop pushing on the grocery cart in order to stop the treadmill, plus the technician who ran the computer also had the ability to immediately stop the treadmill with a stroke of a key.

One last safety measure was incorporated into the design of the study. If the patient's leg went too far back toward the edge of the treadmill, the motor turned off the treadmill immediately in order to prevent a fall. A physical therapist stood behind and toward the side of the patient and monitored the patient's condition.

OUTCOMES

Mrs. S. tolerated the treatment well and the sessions never were terminated because of patient intolerance of the visual surround. Mrs. S. provided subjective ratings on a visual analog scale at the beginning and end of each VR treatment session (Table 38-3).[182] The following symptoms were rated: nausea, headache, dizziness, and visual blurring. No nausea was experienced, but she did rate symptoms of headache, dizziness, and visual blurring over the six sessions. Headache was experienced during only the first VR exposure. Dizziness decreased from 1.8 (10 is the maximum score) to 0.1 at the end of the last session. Visual blurring had the highest rating at the start, at 1.9; at the end of the last session her visual blurring was self-reported to be 0.1. She appeared to be better able to tolerate the virtual experience over the six treatment sessions. Over the six treatment sessions, she was able to progress from the first aisle to aisle 16, the most difficult aisle, where the products were much smaller and more closely packed on the shelves.

At the beginning of physical therapy, Mrs. S. was asked to complete the Dizziness Handicap Inventory (DHI),[182] the Situational Characteristics Questionnaire parts A and B (SCQ-A and SCQ-B),[183] the Dynamic Gait Index (DGI),[184] the Functional Gait Assessment (FGA),[185] the Timed Up-and-Go Test (TUG),[186] a gait speed assessment, and the Sensory Organization Test (SOT) of computerized dynamic posturography.[187,188] Data for all of the these tests before therapy, after therapy, and at 6-month follow-up for Mrs. S. are included in Table 38-4. Scores on all measures were better after the 6-week VR intervention program except for the TUG, and the scores remained relatively stable at 6 months. Lower scores on the DHI, SCQ-A, SCQ-B, and TUG indicate improvement, and higher scores on the DGI, the FGA, gait speed, and the SOT are "better" scores.

Mrs. S. was very satisfied, as she was able to shop again without symptoms. A clinically meaningful change on the DHI has been reported to be 18,[182] and Mrs. S. improved 34 points. The Activities-specific Balance Scale (ABC) change from 29% to 69% over the course of the VR intervention was probably meaningful, as Lajoie and colleagues[189] have reported that scores of less than 67% are related to increased risk of falling. Her DGI score improved by 4, which has also been reported to be clinically meaningful.[182] Gait speed over the course of the intervention improved only by 0.07 m/s, and 0.1 m/s has been reported as a clinically meaningful change.[185] Overall, Mrs. S. made positive changes after the VR physical therapy intervention.

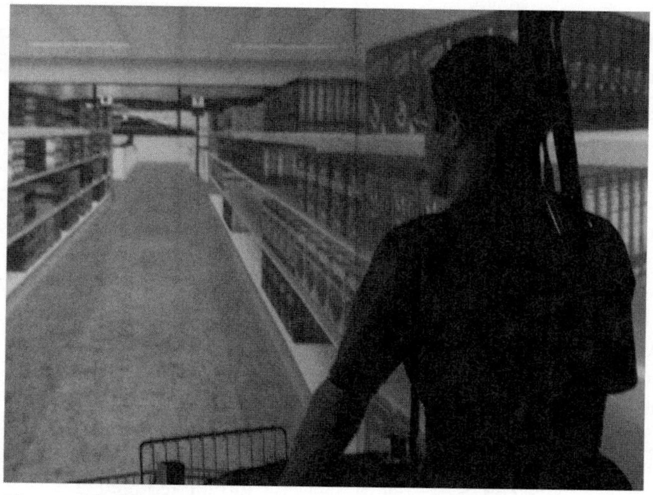

Figure 38-10 ■ The Balance Near Automatic Virtual Environment (BNAVE). A patient walking on the treadmill through the virtual grocery store while pushing a cart. The vest was worn to ensure safety.

TABLE 38-3 ■ WITHIN SESSION MEASURES: VISUAL ANALOG SCALE (VAS) AND SIMULATOR SICKNESS QUESTIONNAIRE (SSQ) ACROSS SIX TREATMENT SESSIONS (BEFORE AND AFTER SCORES)

		VISIT 1		VISIT 2		VISIT 3		VISIT 4		VISIT 5		VISIT 6	
		BEFORE	AFTER	BEFORE	AFTER	BEFORE	AFTER	BEFORE	AFTER	BEFORE	AFTER	BEFORE	AFTER
VAS	Nausea	0	0	0	0	0	0	0	0	0	0	0	0
	Headache	0.5	0.3	0	0	0	0	0	0	0	0	0	0
	Dizziness	1.8	1.5	0.1	0.9	0	0.5	0	1.5	0	0.1	0	0.1
	Visual blurring	1.9	2.2	0.5	1.3	0.5	1	0	1.2	0.4	0.2	0.3	0.1
SSQ	Disorientation	6	6	3	6	3	5	1	3	3	2	3	4
	Nausea	1	1	2	2	1	3	1	1	1	3	2	1
	Oculomotor stress	6	4	4	5	4	5	4	4	4	4	4	3

TABLE 38-4 ■ SELF-REPORT AND PERFORMANCE MEASURES FOR MRS. S. BEFORE AND AFTER THERAPY AND AT 6-MONTH FOLLOW-UP

	ABC	DHI	SCQ-A	SCQ-B	DGI	FGA	TUG	GAIT SPEED	SOT
Before treatment	29	52	72	37	17	19	8.9	0.90	68
After treatment	69	18	18	9	21	26	9.6	0.97	81
Six-month follow-up	91	14	20	8	20	24	10.2	1.08	74

ABC, Activities-specific Balance Confidence Scale; *DHI*, Dizziness Handicap Inventory; *SCQ-A* and *SCQ-B*, Situational Characteristics Questionnaire parts A and B; *DGI*, Dynamic Gait Index; *FGA*, Functional Gait Assessment; *TUG*, Timed Up-and-Go Test; *SOT*, Sensory Organization Test.

Patient Simulator Robotics

Purpose

One area of robotics contributing both to improved rehabilitative care and education of rehabilitation professionals is the development of human programmable patient simulators. This section of the chapter describes programmable patient simulators that are currently available. Human programmable patient simulators can be used to replicate common physiological symptoms, as well as acute, critical care events that require quick, safe, and appropriate intervention so that when rehabilitation professionals encounter a similar situation with a patient they can respond more effectively.

Introduction

Simulation using task trainers, actors, and standardized patients is not new to the education of rehabilitation professionals. What is new is robotics.

Currently available robotic patient simulators can be programmed to demonstrate clinical signs and symptoms consistent with a diverse group of clinical conditions. The patient simulator can be programmed to present signs and symptoms that require a participant to analyze and differentiate the urgency of the situation, make a diagnosis, determine an appropriate intervention, and see the consequences of the action or inaction without compromising patient safety. A wide variety of clinical conditions and situations can be presented in an effort to ensure that during each simulation the participant has an opportunity to practice and receive feedback regarding performance. Simulation experience is critical for practicing how to respond to common as well as rare but critical events—for example, acute myocardial infarction (MI). The learner's ability to respond appropriately during a simulated event can increase the likelihood that rehabilitation professionals are adequately prepared to respond efficiently and effectively when encountering an actual emergency situation.

Technology

At the beginning of 2011 there were two primary manufacturers of human programmable patient simulators: METI Learning (www.meti.com/products_ps_hps.htm) in Sarasota, Florida, and Laerdal Corporation (www.laerdal.com/doc/86/SimMan) based in Wappingers Falls, New York. In this chapter on rehabilitation robotics, the properties and capacities of programmable patient simulators are discussed based on currently available models. This analysis will hopefully help rehabilitation professionals evaluate the benefits of new robotic simulators for professional education.

Features

The number of features available on programmable human patient simulators continues to increase the degree of realism (fidelity) and reflect both basic and advanced clinical features that are extremely useful for training rehabilitation professionals. In addition, there are several noteworthy observable features that can be used to elevate the degree of realism during simulation.

Size. The size of the adult human programmable patient simulator mannequins is similar to an average-sized full grown adult, but the weight is significantly less than average (approximately 85 pounds). In addition to adult models, there are baby simulators, child simulators, and birthing simulators. Some models are wireless. This discussion focuses on the features and properties of the adult high-fidelity simulators available in 2011.

Limb and Chest Mobility. The upper and lower extremities of most programmable patient simulator models have very limited passive mobility with the exception of the shoulders, hips, knees, and ankles which approach "normal" for an adult. The limited mobility of the limbs allows for some range of motion and bed exercises to be simulated, but clinicians will note the completely passive nature of the movement and that the limb weight is significantly less than normal. The chest wall moves and the excursion of the chest can be programmed to be symmetrical or asymmetrical. In addition, the rate and depth of ventilation can be manipulated during the course of a simulation.

Physiological Features. Many programmable patient simulators have the capacity to produce realistic physiological features. A library of normal and abnormal breath sounds, heart tones, bowel sounds, and other symptoms is available for simulating a variety of clinical conditions. The sounds and tones produced can change during the course of a simulation to reflect a change in "patient" status.

The simulator mannequins are typically connected to a series of lines and tubes to simulate a critical care environment (e.g., arterial line, intravenous line, electrocardiograph wires, nasal cannula). This allows the simulation participant an opportunity to identify the lines and tubes, verify their status, and practice "clearing" them. The simulator is connected to a patient monitor similar to those found in critical care settings. The monitor can be changed to display a number of different physiological variables including arterial blood pressure, pulmonary blood pressure, respiratory rate, cardiac rhythm, hemoglobin saturation, oxygen consumption, pH, temperature, and others. The value and number of variables shown on the monitor can be programmed to change during the course of the simulation to mimic clinical conditions and/or a change in patient status.

Pulses are palpable in a variety of locations including carotid, brachial, radial, femoral, popliteal, and dorsalis pedis pulses. The pulse is synchronized with the electrocardiogram (ECG), and the pulse strength can be varied and changed during a simulation. When a simulation participant palpates the pulse, a notation is made in the computer log that specifies which pulse was palpated and at what point in time during the simulation the pulse was taken. In addition, when blood pressure is low, some pulses (e.g., the dorsalis pedis) are no longer palpable, simulating the clinical condition of hypotension.

High-fidelity patient simulators are capable of vocalizations. The simulation operator is able to speak through a microphone and/or use audio files to produce sounds that appear to come from the mouth of the mannequin. Cyanosis is simulated through the use of a light contained within the mouth that makes the lips and gums appear blue. The eyes can form tears, the eyelids blink, and the pupils are reactive to light. The skin in the forehead is capable of diaphoresis. In some areas the skin has "wound modules" that can be inserted and connected to ports that contain "blood" used to simulate bleeding from the wound site.

Cerebrovascular System Features. High-fidelity patient simulators can be programmed to replicate and display signs and symptoms (physiological features) consistent with an acute cerebrovascular accident (CVA). The simulator has the potential to display a slurred speech pattern, a drooping eyelid, asymmetrical pupils, and emotional lability. The simulator can state that its arm or leg feels heavy and that it cannot feel the limb. The patient monitor can be programmed to show a variety of changes consistent with an evolving CVA such as blood pressure, heart rate, and respiratory rate.

Cardiovascular and Cardiopulmonary System Features. The onset of an acute MI is a scenario commonly used in simulation. The patient simulator can be programmed to complain of chest pain while simultaneously developing diaphoresis. The patient monitor can show the changes in the blood pressure, heart rate, respiratory rate, and cardiac arrhythmias consistent with an acute MI. This scenario can be used to practice recognizing the signs and symptoms related to acute conditions as well as to practice health care team responses to acute crises. The advanced features of the cardiovascular system include the capacity to bleed from a variety of portals; the system permits health care personnel to practice advanced cardiac life support (ACLS) protocols and to practice team responses to medical emergencies. The ACLS features built into the patient simulators measure and record the rate and depth of chest compressions. In addition, the physiological response to a variety of drugs and clinical conditions is programmed into some models, allowing participants to witness the response to the administration of medications as well as adverse drug reactions and/or the acute onset of a clinical condition (e.g., acute MI). The advanced clinical features for the pulmonary system include the ability to intubate (esophageal and endotracheal) and insert chest tubes into the mannequin, allowing students and clinicians an opportunity to practice their clinical skills with "patients" who are intubated and/or have a chest tube.

A variety of cardiac arrhythmias are programmed into the patient simulators, allowing the operator to alter the ECG tracing on the patient monitor during the course of a simulation. All of this physiological information is stored in the computer log and can be used during the debriefing session after the simulation to enhance the learning experience for participants.

Programmability of Patient Simulators

In addition to the features discussed previously, high-fidelity simulators have the capacity to be defibrillated and undergo cardioversion. The physiological response to many drugs and clinical conditions is programmed into some models so that participants can witness the acute response to the administration of medications as well as adverse drug reactions and/or the acute onset of a clinical condition (e.g., acute MI).

Costs of Establishing a Simulation Laboratory

The costs associated with establishing a simulation laboratory will vary with the type of programmable patient simulator selected, additional equipment required and/or desired, and the amount of training needed. The price for a mid-fidelity programmable patient simulator is $10,000 or higher depending on the features; high-fidelity programmable simulators can cost $100,000 to $200,000 for top-of-the-line models with state-of-the-art features. However, the price of the simulator(s) is only a portion of the setup costs. Establishing a simulation laboratory will also require (1) space designed for the simulation laboratory; (2) audiovisual equipment; (3) networking infrastructure; and (4) training in how to operate the system. The cost for each of these individual components can vary markedly depending on the type of equipment and infrastructure present as well as the level of sophistication desired in terms of audiovisual and networking capacity.

Summary

Each new generation of programmable human patient simulators has improved our ability to teach excellence in analysis and problem solving in acute, critical care situations. Programmable patient simulators have advanced in (1) the degree of realism provided by the technology and (2) the ability of the operator to manipulate and alter the "patient" status at any point in time. These simulators are now placed in multidisciplinary clinical teaching centers in academic health care institutions. They are also incorporated into community-based training courses for practicing health care professionals. A high degree of realism can be provided during simulation using currently available robotics when high-fidelity simulators are placed in a realistic mock intensive care unit. The combination of a high-fidelity patient simulator and a realistic environmental setting provides an opportunity to train rehabilitation professionals to recognize and respond to changes in patient status and to practice working as members of a health care team without compromising patient safety.

Technology and Computer-Assisted Gaming for Learning at Home

Most of the programs developed for improving memory, learning, and physical skills are based on the principles of scientific research on how the brain learns. Scientific expertise is combined with new technologies, innovation, and creative game playing. At a minimum, the effectiveness of this modality of learning must meet the criteria listed in Box 38-18.

A number of game formats are available to improve memory and physical abilities (Tables 38-5 and 38-6). Some of the programs involve the purchase of training CDs, some are free applications for smart phones, and others can be accessed from the World Wide Web by paying a monthly fee. Some gaming programs include packages of hardware and software, and others require purchase of individual components. Some components are mobile and others are nonportable. Some are for one user and others for multiple users.

Fitness of the Brain

Over the last few years, keeping physically fit has been emphasized for general positive health and aging. The evidence is accumulating that people can sharpen their brains. The computerized gaming industry has made a significant contribution to creating fun, interactive gaming activities for children and adults. Although some of the games can be played just for fun, others can improve physical fitness, memory, balance, and fine motor skills.

Current research suggests that regular brain exercises[190] and regular physical exercise can increase attention, improve efficiency and reliability of information processing, and maintain the length of our telomeres (a method of measuring aging).[191] Intense, forced exercise may also be neuroprotective in terms of maintaining memory skills and motor function and decreasing depression, particularly in patients with neurodegenerative disease such as Parkinson disease.[64,65] However, to be successful, the learner must invest some time to keep the brain fit and active. Not only should individuals participate in fun, rewarded, progressive learning activities, but older individuals need to be willing to learn something new each day, avoid habit and routine, take some risks, get out of the house, and have fun. Some companies offering brain fitness programs are summarized in Table 38-5.

BOX 38-18 ■ LEARNING-BASED CRITERIA FOR COMPUTER-ASSISTED GAMING FOR LEARNING AT HOME

1. There is an opportunity to practice with appropriate frequency and intensity.
2. The practice is matched to the ability of the learner.
3. The task is advanced in difficulty to challenge but not exceed learner ability.
4. Task practice and skill development are cross-trained, including redundancy to help facilitate lasting improvement.
5. Motivation is maximized with timely and positive feedback and reward.
6. The learning environment is safe enough that individuals will take some learning risks.
7. The content of training is age appropriate, engaging, and fun.
8. The learner is committed to complete the learning series.

Motivation for proactive brain training may be further enhanced by changes in social practices. For example, Geico (one U.S. insurance agency) noted that there were fewer automobile accidents in older individuals when they maintained their memory skills. As a result of this information, the company offers a discount on automobile insurance if individuals over the age of 55 years perform standardized brain fitness and driving simulated exercises.

Physical Motor Skills

A variety of gaming systems can be used to enhance physical motor skills of children and adults. In 2011, the most well known commercialized programs included Nintendo (e.g., Wii), Sony (EyeToy, PlayStation 2 and 3), and Microsoft Xbox 360 (Kinect). Each company produces new games on a regular basis. The games vary among the companies, but there are some similarities. Each company has sports games, balance games, competitive cognitive games, and physical skill performance games. All systems include games that can be played by one person or by two or more individuals. For the most part, scores are kept for the games, and the player tries to improve performance every time he or she plays. Feedback regarding success is provided both during the game and at the end.

These computerized game-oriented training systems can supplement "one-on-one" training in a rehabilitation environment. For each individual, the games should be selected to achieve a particular performance goal matched to the ability of the individual and integrated into the broader neurological rehabilitation program. Selecting the best system depends on costs, capability of the individual, space limitations, cognitive ability of the individual, and setup requirements. Some of the games can be played with the person standing or sitting. The similarities and differences among the systems by Nintendo, Sony, and Microsoft are summarized in Table 38-6.

In addition to commercially available game training for improving physical abilities, some researchers are developing special game training programs for patients with neurodegenerative diseases such as Parkinson disease. In one case, therapeutic interactive games are being designed to improve gait and balance in patients with Parkinson disease. Red Hill Studios has partnered with Dr. Glenna Dowling at the University of California, San Francisco and Dr. Marsha Melnick to develop a wearable suit with more sensitive sensor controllers in multiple sites. After donning the suit, the individual engages in virtual games that challenge body and limb movements. These types of programs are not yet commercially available but are likely to continue to be developed in the near future. It is important for individuals to remain both physically and cognitively fit as they age, and integrating these types of games is important not only for aging individuals but also for individuals aging with chronic impairments, progressive disease processes, and newly acquired medical conditions. Aging will become a part of most individuals' future as long as their health or life activities do not limit their life expectancy. As the world's population ages, the potential to use these types of preventative strategies not only enlarges in everyday life but should become common practice in neurorehabilitation.

TABLE 38-5 ■ EXAMPLES OF GAMING-TYPE PROGRAMS FOR IMPROVING BRAIN FITNESS

COMPANY	PURPOSE OF PROGRAM	DESCRIPTION OF PROGRAM	MODALITIES ADDRESSED	SPECIFIC PROGRAMS	EQUIPMENT NEEDED AND PROGRAM REQUIREMENTS
Posit Science (www.positscience.com)	Programs built on the principle that the brain is adaptable across the life span based on continued challenges and engaging, attended activities. Purpose of programming is to improve alertness, attention, accuracy of short- and long-term memory skills as well as speed of remembering and thinking.	Computerized, fun, rewarded game-type programs created as a translation of the research on neuroplasticity carried out by Michael Merzenich. Exercises provide feedback on progressive accomplishments. Total of 40 hours of learning exercises and programs. Can track multiple users. Posit Science is also working on the development of other sensorimotor training modalities to improve balance, fine motor control, and sensory processing.	Brain Fitness emphasizes accurate, reliable, and quick auditory and spatial memory. InSight uses useful field-of-view "visual training technology" to help individuals increase processing speed and peripheral vision, improve driving skills, and be safe.	Brain Fitness (auditory and spatial memory. InSight (visual and visual perceptual memory).	Computer (PC or Mac), keyboard, Internet access, headphones, mouse. Must register program online after opening. Can purchase multiuser systems. When there are questions, it is possible to visit the Cognitive Club at www.cognitiveclub.com to find an answer, ask questions of other users, or send a message to Posit Science; or users can call a customer service agent.
Lumosity www.lumosity.com	The programs are built on the theoretical construct that the brain is adaptable and new neurons can be trained across the life span. The exercises are appropriate for the young and the old, with an emphasis on improving cognitive thinking through spatial working memory and visual attention. The games progress in difficulty as the individual plays.	The three neuroscience and cognitive psychological specialists who created this software program were Kunal Sarkar, Michael Scanlon, and David Drescher.	Game-oriented learning. New games are developed and posted on a regular basis. The games are interesting and motivating. The games can be easy or hard. Games can progress in difficulty. The goal is to force the brain to learn.	Programs change with new ideas. Programs can be personalized to client defined issues.	Computer, Internet access, keyboard, mouse. Membership based; anyone can join. Can purchase monthly or lifetime membership. Member can go online at any time to engage in training. It is possible to download the games to a smart cell phone to create opportunities to train any at any time.
Scientific Learning	Program based on the translation of science on neuroplasticity to training kids with dyslexia and other reading and learning problems. The product enhances brain fitness (memory, attention, processing, and sequencing) as well as cognition (accelerated acquisition of knowledge, improved ability to use and organize information, and readiness to improve strategies for lifelong learning).	The company was also founded by Michael Merzenich, William Jenkins, and Paula Tallal. The program is called Fast ForWord.	The Fast ForWord program is sold to school districts for working with children with reading problems. Some of the programs can be initiated and practiced at home. The programs are particularly beneficial for learners who have difficulty paying attention and difficulty remembering what they are taught.	The evidence suggests that learners can progress 1-2 years in reading in as little as 8-12 weeks. The success of this program appears to be integrating brain fitness exercises with standard-based curriculum-based instructions.	Computer, Internet access, keyboard, mouse, headset. Primarily available at the school. Families can purchase home reinforcement programs. Parents can help their children by using online instructions.

TABLE 38-6 ■ COMPARISON OF LEARNING-BASED GAMING SYSTEMS TO IMPROVE PHYSICAL ABILITIES (2012)

NAME	CONTROLLER	CAMERA	MICROPHONE	SENSOR METHOD	LIGHTING	NUMBER OF PLAYERS	OTHER USES	ADVANTAGES	DISADVANTAGES	OPTIONS
Wii (Nintendo)	Hand-held	No	No	Accelerometer. Must hold controller and move; need to encourage large movements. Each person must have controller.	Normal room lighting	One to six; tracked by controller numbers.	Can get Weather Channel	Portable if on a movable platform; price includes full program. Games are fun. Allows competition between players. Can use indoors or outdoors.	Each player has to hold own controller; tracks simple movements, not complex movements. A cartoon figure is shown, not the user.	In 2012 the reasonable price included controller, balance platform, and two games.
EyeToy (Sony)	Movement	Yes, but needs webcam	Yes	Movement of body and limbs of individuals.	Has a lighted ball	At least two and can be more. Players are camera monitored.	Can use screen for TV	Portable if monitor and cameras on a mobile platform. Cannot be used in sunlight. Games are fun. User sees self, not a cartoon. Monitors more complex movements than Wii.	Limited camera recognition of multiple players. No other uses (e.g., cannot use with TV or CDs).	In 2012, must buy as separate parts; more expensive than Wii.
Kinect	Movement	Yes; complex camera; can track multiple players	Yes	Movement of body and limbs of individuals.	Needs some extra lighting for the camera	Up to six individuals, tracked with camera.	Can use for TV, CDs, and going online	Monitors more than one person. Monitors complex motions. Fun to play games. Large movements followed. Players see themselves. Allows high exertional movements. Can also be used as TV and to play CDs. Company released applications for research purposes (www.pointscloud.org).	Not portable. Must use indoors. Cannot be used in sunlight. Hard to interface with exoskeleton, as must see whole person.	In 2012, the Xbox 360 is more expensive than Wii and EyeToy. Must buy separate parts.

Effectiveness of Learning-Based Gaming to Improve Cognitive Ability and Physical Motor Skills

General exercise in addition to learning-based training can improve mental alertness and sense of well-being. As our society ages, the combination of engaging in forced exercise and forced learning can be effective in maintaining physiological function despite aging or chronic disease. The use of gaming strategies to enable progressive learning-based training is fun and positively correlated with improved skills.[175,179,190,192-204] If an individual were to force himself or herself to engage in new learning activities every day along with general, forced moderate- to high-intensity exercise, then gaming-type learning would not be necessary. On the other hand, when a learning activity is fun, individuals are more likely to be compliant.

Using Technology to Create Home Exercise Programs

A less complex but nonetheless important aspect of merging technology is the link between teaching a home exercise program to patients by using verbal or written instruction or demonstration, and the availability of the World Wide Web network, through which complex exercises can be explained, simple and complex movements can be demonstrated, and compliance can be recorded. Clinicians are able to identify, select, and change home exercises based on patient need, then direct the patient to view the program for visual feedback and reinforcement. Patients can then easily practice and review how to do those exercises each time they choose to perform the home program.

The current reimbursement system in health care (see Chapter 10) limits the billable time a physical therapist can spend with the patient. When a practitioner has to make a choice between providing professional expertise for hands-on care (e.g., manual therapy, neuromuscular facilitation, advanced balance, and mobility training) versus instructing patients on therapeutic exercises the patient needs to do at home, the therapist frequently chooses the former rather than the latter. All too often, the patient's exercise instructions include a quick demonstration of the exercise and a sheet of exercise instructions, with or without illustrations. This limited instruction usually occurs because the therapist does not have an efficient way to teach the desired exercises or reinforce the quality of exercise performance when the patient goes home. Fortunately, the advances available on cell phones, the Internet, videophones, and other personal devices offer a possible solution that links technology to potential home exercise programs. Similarly, we have learned that individuals activate the brain not only when physically practicing a new movement but also when watching movements, imagining movements, and mentally rehearsing movements. Thus, clinicians should consider the integration of visually enhanced Web-based teaching programs to more effectively and efficiently teach home exercises to patients.

Background

Early theories of motor learning viewed feedback as a simple stimulus-response event that was used to reinforce learning and conditioned responses.[205] Later, the importance of the information contained in the feedback was found to be more important than the reinforcement characteristics. As a result of this research, motor learning was divided into three artificial phases of learning: declarative-cognitive (i.e., a verbalizable representation of the movement), associative (i.e., comparing and contrasting the current task and performance with prior memories), and autonomous (i.e., relatively automatic performance of the well learned task with minor modifications).[206,207] Refer to Chapter 4 for additional concepts and applications regarding principles of motor control, motor learning, and neuroplasticity.

There is one major exception and conflicting method of learning that appears to "skip" the declarative or cognitive stage of learning: learning by observation and imitation. Although learning by imitation appears to skip the verbal instruction stage, a human would be able to verbally describe the movement. In some pathological instances, such as severe autism, there are exceptions to this ability to imitate, but for the most part observational learning is pervasive in the natural world.[208,209]

Research into observational learning has spanned the last 150 years. Initially it was concluded that observational learning was of no importance and not helpful.[210,211] Other authors have described it as useful but not cognitive in nature.[212,213] Badets and colleagues[214] argued in favor of a role for observational learning aiding in the cognitive phase of learning and that it is useful in error detection. Observational learning has also been described as highly beneficial for the associative phase of learning, most beneficial when combined with physical practice. It has been found to be very similar to actual practice in terms of learning benefits, performance, retention (memory), and cortical activation patterns.[215,216] With the increased availability of neuroimaging techniques, more research has been done looking at areas of brain activation during *performance* of a motor skill, *mental imagery of* the performance of a motor skill, and *observation* of a motor skill.[217-219]

In research studies using relatively simple hand and finger tasks, the activated areas of the brain were generally expected regions, including all the major motor cortices and the cerebellum.[217] Similar tasks were then used to test the cortical activation levels of the brain when the subject was instructed to imagine performing the movement. The resulting cortical activation levels were also similar, with the expected exception of the primary motor strip that would activate the response. Other researchers have reported that the same major areas of the brain are activated when imagining or observing movement (or parts of movement) as when performing the movement.[215] About 30% of the neurons are activated during imagined compared with actual task performance.

Most of the previously cited work has been performed based on hand and finger movements. The ability to generalize the findings to more complex movements of the body may be questioned. However, Brown and colleagues[220] performed work using a dance movement of the foot and lower extremity. This task used a relatively simple component of an Argentine tango dance step. The activation patterns were very similar to those found in hand tasks.[221]

Research studies[222-224] have repeatedly reported that observing movement with the intent to learn the movement engages the brain in a similar pattern as performing the task. In general, this research supports a contention that when teaching a patient an exercise, rehabilitation practitioners

TABLE 38-7 ■ VARIOUS HOME EXERCISE PROGRAMS, WEB LINKS, AND USER VARIABLES

NAME	LINK	DESIGN HEP	MODIFY HEP	ADD A PATIENT	ASSIGN HEP TO PATIENT	MANAGE PASSWORDS	SEND NEWSLETTERS
HomeExPro	www.homeexpro.com	Y	Y	Y	Y	Y	Y
Fizio	www.fizio.com	Y	Y	Y	Y	?	?
Perfect Fit Health	www.perfectfithealth.com	Y	Y	Y	Y	Y	Y
HomeStretch	www.homestretchhealth.com	Y	Y	Y	Y	Y	?
Physiotec	www.physiotec.ca	Y	Y	Y	Y	Y	?
Exercise Prescriber	www.exerciseprescriber.com	Y	Y	Y	Y	?	N

A, Animation; *HEP*, home exercise program; *N*, no; V, video; *Y*, yes; *?*, unknown at this time or in process of integrating.

should first demonstrate the exercise to the patient. A second study[225] suggests that using written instructions for teaching a motor task may help with the sequencing of the task; however, written instructions do not provide the observational practice that is provided by a moving image. This is particularly important to remember when patients may have experienced some type of brain insult. In an applied study, Weeks and colleagues[226] reported superior performance, motivation, and perceived confidence of subjects when performing simple and complex exercises after viewing videotaped instruction compared with reading written instruction.

Technologies Can Assist Patient Exercise Performance

In this day of moving pictures and digital video, it may be time to leave behind text-based movement instruction, with the exception of the listing of complex sequences of movements. Clinicians can videotape the exercises they want patients to perform or demonstrate the exercises for their patients during a video conference using smart phones, iPads, and Skype. The exercises can even be animated. Therapists' options are now almost limitless.

Current technology allows the clinician to instruct the patient through the use of the Web by doing the following:

- Designing home exercise programs for later use with multiple patients
- Modifying existing home exercise programs
- Entering minimal patient identifying information to keep track of the individual patient while avoiding any Health Insurance Portability and Accountability Act (HIPAA) infringement problems
- Assigning a home exercise program to a patient and providing a brief handout containing a username, password, and some minimal printed information about the exercise program
- Controlling the period of time for which the current home exercise program is considered valid or acceptable by changing, updating, or extending the time period for which the patient has access to the exercises
- In some situations, recording the number of times the patient accesses the program in order to determine compliance

Several companies provide home exercise instruction using a Web link. Each company has its strengths and weaknesses (Table 38-7). Some have newsletters that can be scheduled to be emailed to patients as reminders. Some providers allow the clinician to make a DVD of their patient's exercise program. One provider even allows users to upload their own video for the patient to watch at home, similar to YouTube services. Some of the websites are multilingual, and all will create specific exercises on request of the therapist or clinic using their services. The potential of all current as well as future companies is limited only by the vision of the individuals developing the services as well as the technology available at the time. Technology is constantly evolving and can only improve the potential methods therapists use to teach home exercise programs to patients.

How to Use Web-Based Home Exercise Programs with Patients

One option for demonstrating exercises for the patient has been developed by HomeExPro (www.homeexpro.com). In this system, the therapist has the option of selecting from a catalog of therapeutic exercises. The clinician can then combine a group of exercises into a customized home exercise program for the patient. The clinician can actually provide the patient a link to a personalized exercise program that only he or she can see by entering a username and password. As the patient improves, the clinician can change the exercise program, the frequency, and/or the intensity in order for the patient to optimally benefit from the individualized home program.

HomeExPro and similar companies offer the user an excellent method of giving the patient additional instruction regarding his or her home exercise program as well as being a reminder to continue those exercises without a therapist being present. Using corresponding links, clinicians should be able to determine whether a patient is accessing the exercise program. In the future, placing a camera recording the patient during the exercise itself may be able to give the clinician feedback regarding whether the patient is not only completing the exercises but doing them accurately.

Examples of a Specific Exercise Routine Using Online Access. Access to the two exercises can be found on the Elsevier Evolve site. These two exercises were chosen because

PRINTED MATERIALS	MULTILINGUAL	MULTIPLE CAMERA ANGLES	DVD	BLOG	VIDEO OR ANIMATION	SEND MESSAGES	UPLOAD VIDEOS
Y	Y	Y	Y	N	A	N	N
?	Y	N	N	?	V	Y	Y
Y	N	N	N	Y	A	Y	N
Y	Y	N	N	Y	V	?	Y
Y	Y	N	N	?	A	?	N
Y	N	N	N	Y	V	Y	N

they both might be used by a therapist for instructing a patient in a home program after a neurological insult. These two exercises were developed by Dr. Clayton Gable, who collaborated with others to develop Home Exercise Pro. These exercises are not necessarily typical of exercises developed by programs identified in Table 38-7. Most exercises have been illustrated to augment home exercises given to patients with orthopedic-type impairments. The two exercises presented illustrate the possibility of developing more thorough home exercise programs for patients with neurological movement impairments.

Conclusion

This section has briefly presented evidence that observation of an exercise in motion is better for motor learning, quality of movements, and recall of therapeutic exercise than printed instructions. There are many possible methods available to rehabilitation professionals to overcome the limitations of printed material.

Clinicians might consider making their own library of video exercise programs. However, this endeavor is complex. There are many steps to consider, such as the lighting, the camera angle, the model to be used within the video program, and what generic exercises should be included within the video library. Production of such a library can be expensive to develop and maintain. Another approach would be to use commercially available videos of exercises. However, by using available videos, the clinician has no control over the content of the video and even less control over the camera angle and other factors that can affect the patient's ability to learn the exercise from the video.

There are numerous resources on the Internet for exercise instruction. However, most of them are designed for individuals without pathology or patients with common conditions such as low back pain. In addition, the expertise reflected in publicly available exercise videos varies tremendously. The exercises may be presented by someone who had personal experience with acute back pain and found some exercises that helped. Or the exercises may be presented by extraordinarily well qualified professionals offering excellent information. Very few patients can differentiate the expertise of those individuals presenting the exercise programs.

Another problem with the common approaches to video or a media-based approach to therapeutic exercise is the lack of customization. The very best low back pain exercise program in a therapist's library or on the Internet may not be appropriate for a specific patient, especially if that patient has additional impairments owing to CNS involvement. The Web-based companies included in Table 38-7 can help mitigate this risk with customized exercise programs. The ability to control the patient's access to his or her home exercise program via password management also gives the therapist control over the length of time that particular exercise program is considered valid. Additional home exercise programs developed by professional clinicians and available online will become an important tool for physical and occupational therapists as familiarity and ease of access grow.

The costs of the service for the Internet-based presentation of therapeutic exercise vary broadly. Some providers offer a limited version of their service for free. Others offer access to a full-service website for free to students. None of the providers actually charge patients. The cost is absorbed by the clinic or practice that purchases the service each month. These prices range from $15 to $150 USD per month for basic to the highest level of service. Although the higher-end price might seem high, there is no limit on the number of home exercise programs that can be generated per month by a practice. The potential to purchase the service for three to five clinics within a practice with three or four providers at each clinic makes the cost per patient drop to very little. This cost could easily be incorporated into the cost of service, and the outcomes from the home program bring recognition to the practice.

The needs of the therapeutic setting should determine which of the various options best matches what is needed for the specific patients seen by the clinicians within that practice. Although it seems obvious that private practices could benefit from this type of technological access, hospital-based rehabilitation centers or outpatient rehabilitation practices could also take advantage of programs that would help patients regain functional movement. Even if the patient is practicing independently in a rehabilitation gym, this type of reinforced learning can be an alternative to having a clinician constantly attend to that patient. Options are going to change as technology enhances access to online exercise programs that optimize motor learning and enhance desired outcomes.

LEARNING MORE ABOUT THE ENGINEERING PRINCIPLES IN REHABILITATION ROBOTICS

The usefulness of a rehabilitative and assistive robotic device will always be limited by its design. A robot's passive mechanical structure, sensing capabilities, types of actuation, and control are all key issues for both performance and safety. The way a robot is interfaced to a human, both physically and cognitively, can determine its effectiveness. This section discusses each of these issues briefly. The intention is to give a general overview of rehabilitation robotic engineering, to enable a medical professional to converse with the engineers who develop such devices, and to educate physical and occupational therapists who are challenged with the task of selecting robotic technology regarding relevant issues.

Robot Dynamics, Kinematics, and Control

The position, force, and control of a robot end effector are key concerns during human movement tasks and thus key categories within the field of robotics. The term *end effector* will be defined more precisely; however, for now assume that it is simply a tool of interest (e.g., a fingertip) that exists at the end of a potentially complicated limb and interacts with something in the outside world (e.g., a key on a keyboard). The success of the end effector depends on the relationship between force and motion. This relationship is known as *mechanical impedance.* It quantifies the resistance a mechanical system provides against motions when a force is applied.

Intuitively, one might assume the most useful goal for most motor tasks is to control *both* force and position. In daily lives, individuals want to accurately contact objects, but they also want to apply the appropriate contact forces. For example, if the end effector of interest is a human fingertip and the goal is to hit a note on a piano keyboard, then one must have accurate positioning to hit the correct notes, but one must apply the correct level of force so that each note is played just as loudly *(forte)* or softly *(piano)* as desired.

In a way, the physics of the real world necessitates a tradeoff to achieve both positional accuracy and desired force as simultaneous goals. It is generally impossible to achieve both exact position control and exact force control along the same direction (axis) of motion, except perhaps in specially contrived situations in which the environment is perfectly known and the goals are artificially chosen. For example, imagine an individual wishes to push down on the surface of a pillow, as shown in Figure 38-11, until he feels 1 pound of force, and that he also wishes to push down until his hand is 1 inch below the resting surface of the couch. A reasonable model for the pillow is that it is a spring with the following relationship between force *(F),* displacement (Δx), and the spring constant of the pillow (k_p):

Equation 38-1

$$F = k_p \Delta x$$

As seen in Equation 38-1, it may turn out that the spring constant of the pillow is such that pressing down with a 1-pound weight depresses the pillow more than 1 inch (if the pillow is soft, with a small value for k_p) or less than 1 inch (if the pillow is very firm). Alternatively, one might create a fantastically strong robot that can compress the pillow downward by precisely 1 inch "come hell or high water," but the force that is required to do so depends entirely on the properties of the pillow, not on the clever robot. It will always require more force to compress a firm pillow 1 inch than to compress a softer pillow the same amount, by definition.

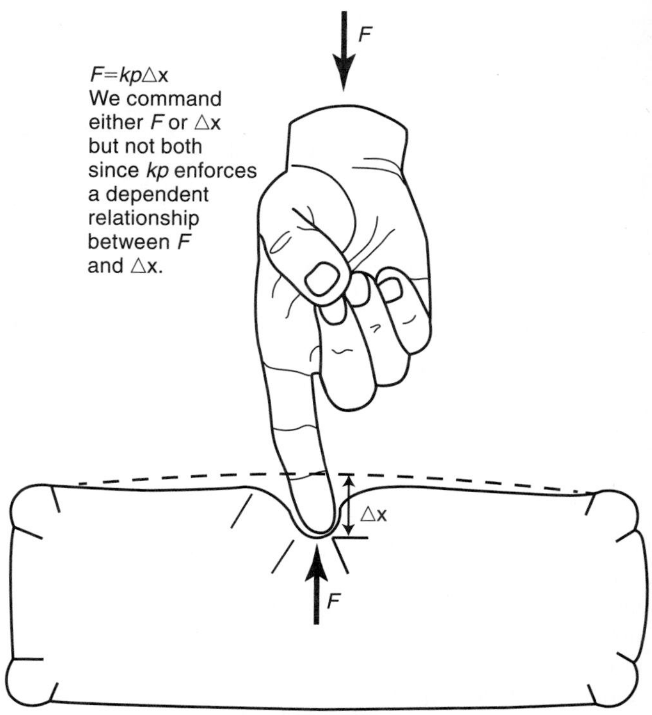
F
F=kpΔx
We command
either F or Δx
but not both
since kp enforces
a dependent
relationship
between F
and Δx.
Δx
F

Figure 38-11 ■ Pressing a finger into a pillow is an example of how it is not possible to directly control both the position of an end effector and the force applied by the end effector. Because the stiffness of the pillow is unknown, either the force applied or the desired displacement Δx can be controlled.

Hybrid Position and Force Control

In many real-world situations, a human is required to control both force and position during a task. Take, for example, the task of pushing a button, shown in Figure 38-12. In this task a human is required both to control the position of the finger in the x dimension precisely and to simultaneously control the force applied to the button in the y direction. As in the previous example, it is not possible to specify both position and force independently along the x-axis. Nor can one accomplish both for motion along the y-axis. However, it *is* possible to choose *either* position or force to control in x and to choose *either* position or force to control in y. In Figure 38-12, for example, we control position in x and force in y. There is a wide range of tasks in which an individual wishes to control force in one direction while controlling position in a plane perpendicular to this direction. Classic examples include washing a window, sanding a floor, writing text, or painting a canvas. In each case, an individual needs to press *into* a surface with controlled force while tracing a desired trajectory of positions *across* the surface.

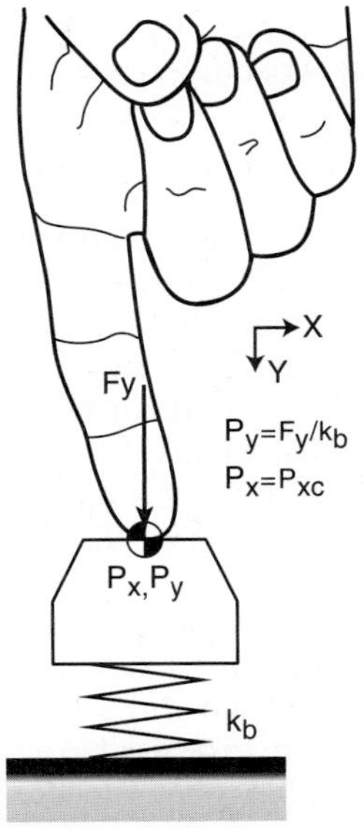

Figure 38-12 ■ Pressing a button is an example of a task in which a human must simultaneously control both position and force. In this case, the position of the finger in the *X* dimension must be precisely controlled while the amount of force applied to the *Y* dimension is also controlled. Creating control strategies for robots that replicate this behavior, particularly when environmental parameters such as k_b are unknown, is a significant challenge and is the focus of ongoing research and development.

Humans accomplish such tasks fairly easily because during early motor development children have learned to seamlessly prescribe motor control strategies for force control and position control with seemingly little active thought. Hybrid position and force control is a well-known technique used to accomplish this interaction in a robot arm. Such control techniques are still a significant engineering challenge when real-world environmental parameters, such as the spring force coefficient, k_p, are unknown before contact. Individuals often know from the context of the situation that scraping paint, for example, will require much greater forces than frosting a cake. Anticipating the resistance of the environment is still an important problem in mobile robot manipulation.

Now, imagine that instead of pillows and buttons, the capable robot is interacting with a human. As in the case of interacting with pillows, different humans will tend to resist a robot's motions with different amounts of force. A well-designed robot will anticipate the response of a human before a robot-human interaction occurs. Humans anticipate this natural variability in human response intuitively, and this guides decisions about how to interact with other people in daily life. For example, one might decide to use a very different style of motion to shake hands with a professional athlete than with a 2-year-old child or a 102-year-old senior. An individual knows intuitively that he or she is controlling important aspects about both position and force in moving a hand during a handshake. From the point of view of an engineer, human limbs have rather sophisticated kinematics, dynamics, sensing, and control, which allow individuals to perform a wide range of tasks—typically without requiring much high-level thought.

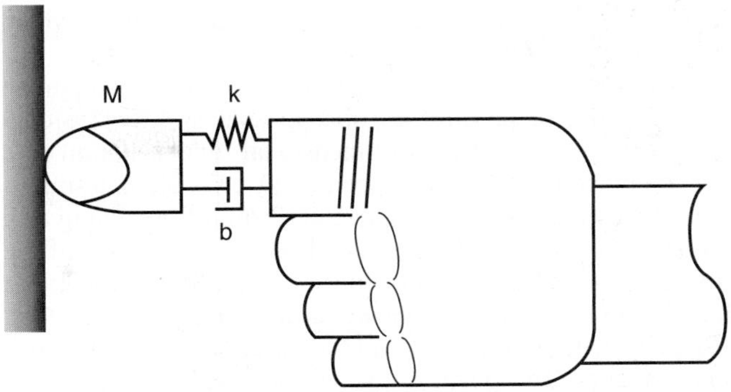

Figure 38-13 ■ One way humans safely explore their environment is to treat their end effector, in this case a finger, as a spring. Either engineers can replicate this effect using a complex suite of actuators, sensors, and computation, or they can add series compliant elements to the limb.

Series Compliance in Robot Limbs

Engineers have come up with several approaches that attempt to replicate the human ability to interact "gently" with an unknown environment. Take the example shown in Figure 38-13, in which a person is pushing a finger against a wall of unknown properties. One model of how a human does this is that the human end effector, in this case a finger, is treated as a spring with a stiffness *k*. As one explores the properties of the wall, the finger is allowed to interact *gently* with the wall, preventing both damage to the wall and injury to the end effector. In robots, the same effect can be achieved through a suite of sensors, actuators, and computation, which must work perfectly together to "simulate" a passive spring, or one can simply include a real passive spring in line with, or in engineering language *in series* with, the rest of the limb. This is an increasingly popular strategy, and the included spring is technically known as a *series compliant element.* Intuitively, a series compliant element in a limb plays the role of bumper on a car. If the car hits something unexpected, the bumper can absorb the shock to reduce damage to the car. In humans, the softness of the skin, connective tissue, and muscle provides a natural series elastic element between the stiff bones and the outside world. In the past 20 years, engineers have increasingly realized that including compliance in robot limbs can improve both performance and safety as a robot interacts with its environment. An excellent and approachable paper that discusses the advantages of including series elastic elements in real-world robotics was presented by Pratt and colleagues at the 4th International Symposium on Experimental Robotics.[227]

Underdetermined Kinematics

One of the other major challenges faced by engineers building multilink robots is that the robot limbs are typically underdetermined as they interact with the environment. In underdetermined systems, the number of degrees of freedom exceeds the number of constraints on the system. For example, engineering constraints may define how a grasper at the end of an arm is to be positioned and oriented, but the engineer may be allowed to use all the limb joints (and perhaps motions of the robot body, as well), which means that many possible solutions exist. In such cases, engineers must give the robot a practical strategy for determining which solution(s) work best for a particular situation.

An example of an underdetermined problem is a person reaching out to pick up an object, such as a coffee cup. Figure 38-14 shows a two-dimensional representation of a person reaching for a cup at position (X_c, Y_c). Here, a simplified, four-link model of a human performing a reaching task is used. One link is the distance between the center of the torso to the center of the shoulder L_1, a second represents the upper arm L_2, a third is the lower arm L_3, and the fourth link, L_4, goes between the wrist and the virtual center of the gripping fingers. The position of the hand with respect to the body can then be calculated based on the orientation of the torso θ_1, the shoulder angle θ_2, the angle of the elbow θ_3, and the angle of the wrist θ_4 as shown in Equation 38-2.

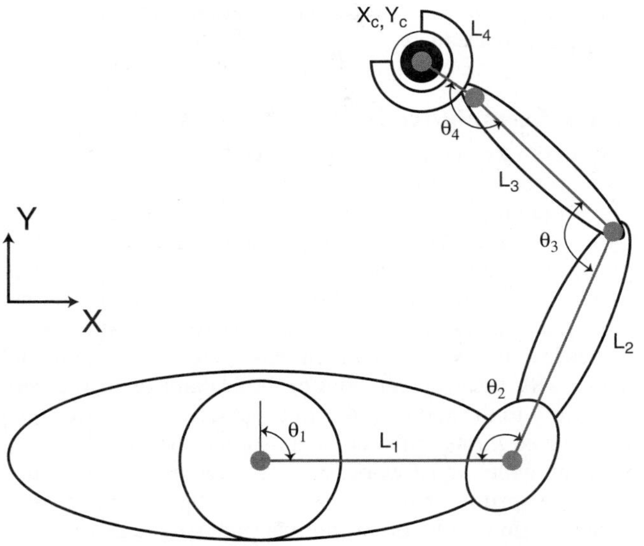

Figure 38-14 ■ A person reaching for a cup of coffee is an example of an "underdetermined" system.

Equation 38-2

$$(X_c,Y_c) = f(L_1,L_2,L_3,L_4,\theta_1,\theta_2,\theta_3,\theta_4)$$

Here, the linkage lengths are all set constants, whereas the angles are all controlled variables. Thus this system has four degrees of freedom (the angles) but only two constraints (the *X* and *Y* positions of the cup). Even with the body position fixed, there are an infinite number of joint angle combinations that would allow the person to successfully pick up the cup of coffee. Allowing for repositioning of the body provides even more flexibility in how to grasp the cup.

Challenges an engineer faces when trying to control a humanoid robot reaching for a cup of coffee include deciding what trajectory the hand will follow in such a situation and what joint angles are to be used to achieve the trajectory. If the robot is a wearable robot intended to assist a human, the choice of poses and trajectories is also critical to the safe operation of the robot. Figure 38-15 shows three sets of joint angles that would position the end effector to pick up the cup. Figure 38-15, *A,* shows the person in an achievable and comfortable pose. Figure 38-15, *B,* shows the person in an achievable but potentially uncomfortable pose. Lastly, Figure 38-15, *C,* shows a pose that might be possible for a robot but is not achievable for a normal human. Although all three solutions may be mathematically feasible for a robot device, solution A is likely the preferred solution for compatibility with human biomechanics. Correctly identifying optimal solutions for robot manipulation is a nontrivial engineering challenge that involves problems in both kinematics and dynamics.

In the next few sections, some common terminology in robotics will be defined and engineering solutions for controlling a multilink limb will be investigated. As a side note, the reader should consider that solutions for upper- and lower-limb control are distinct in some important ways. In particular,

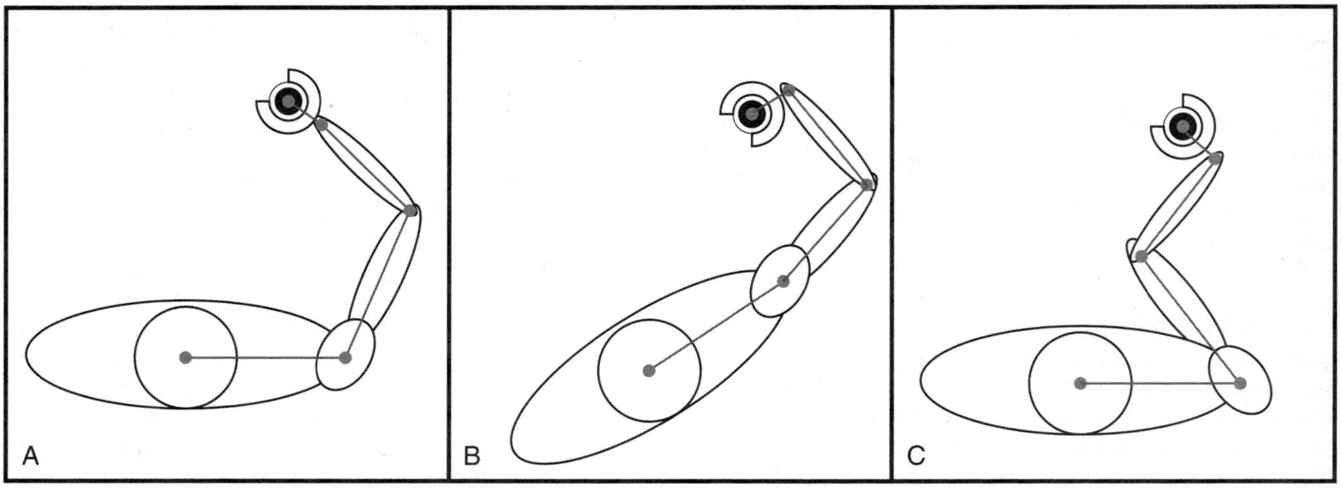

Figure 38-15 ■ Because a person reaching for a cup of coffee is an "underdetermined" system, the same end effector position can be achieved with an infinite combination of joint angles. **A,** A set of joint angles that might be selected that results in a "comfortable" and achievable pose. **B,** A set of joint angles that is achievable but results in an "uncomfortable" pose. **C,** An unachievable set of joint angles.

walking involves a more repetitive, cyclical motion that is punctuated with intermittent contact with the ground, whereas upper-limb tasks generally involve smoother, more variable motions—usually without such dramatic collision with the environment, as compared with heel strike, stance phase, and push off during the gait cycle.

Robot Kinematics

Both human and robot kinematics determine how angles of the joints map to positions of the limbs; they are a *geometric* description of a system. Kinematics gives the mathematical relationships from angles of joints to positions of particular points on the limbs or body. In problems of robot manipulation, one is often primarily interested in how a particular tool, gripper, or anthropomorphic hand at the end of a limb interacts with the environment. This end-part of a robot limb is typically referred to as the *end effector.* For an engineer, it is most useful to consider the end effector more formally to be a particular point located on a link near the end of a robot limb, along with the rotational orientation of this link. For example, it might be the tip of a pencil, used for drawing. A traditional goal in factory robotics is to get an end effector to track a desired reference trajectory over time, such as following a set of desired positional motions. Engineers have gotten good at commanding positions of robot limbs. In common language, however, when one sees a task being performed in an overly repetitive way, one may derogatorily refer to such motions as seeming *robotic.* Many real-world tasks require control of both position and force, as well as some intelligence about the context of the situation. Controlling position alone is not always adequate in robotics.

In rehabilitation robotics, it is often important to determine not only where an end effector of a robot is, but also what forces it applies and where intermittent points are located between the robot body and the end effector. For example, contact with a human must be gentle, and it may also be important to attach a human to a robot limb at multiple points of contact, to ensure that a patient is comfortable, is recruiting the correct muscle groups, and is achieving the correct range of motion for various joints.

In robotics, engineers care about both *forward kinematics*, which map the angles of the joints to the position of the end effector, and *inverse kinematics* (IK), which is the problem of determining what set of angles to use to get the end effector into a desired position and orientation. (For example, Figure 38-15 gives three IK solutions for grasping a cup.) As previously discussed, there are generally multiple solutions to the IK problem of placing an end effector at a desired position. This is true for both a robot limb and a human one.

Velocity Kinematics: The Jacobian

Just as robotics engineers are concerned with the geometric (i.e., kinematic) mapping from joint angle positions to Cartesian *(x, y, z)* coordinates in a robot, they also care about the mapping from joint angle *velocity* to the velocity of an end effector in Cartesian coordinates. In general, robots have many actuated joints, and six coordinates are needed to fully define the position and orientation of an end effector: three positions (*x*, *y*, and *z* coordinates in space) and three rotations (pitch, roll, and yaw). To help with all the bookkeeping for these mathematical relationships, engineers typically represent these equations in matrix form. The *Jacobian* is an important matrix in robotics that describes the velocity mapping, or "velocity kinematics," between joint angle velocities and the translational and rotational velocities of a robot end effector.

The Jacobian is simply a tool to understand how the current configuration of a robot influences the relationship between actuator velocities and the end effector velocities. Physics dictates that the Jacobian also describes how the current configuration determines the relationship between static torques applied by motors and static forces exerted at the end effector.

Because the Jacobian is such a fundamental concept in robotics engineering, it may be worth having some intuition about the information it conveys. A toy example will be used to describe the basic physics that the Jacobian captures. In Figure 38-16, a seesaw-style pivot point is used to represent the geometric relationship between a motor actuator, at the pivot point, and the *y* position of the end effector, y_{ee}. For the configuration at the left, the velocity relationship between the rotational speed of the motor, $d\theta/dt$, and vertical velocity of the end effector, dy_{ee}/dt, is $dy_{ee}/dt = R \bullet d\theta/dt$. Here, *R* is the Jacobian. (Usually the Jacobian is a much larger matrix, but this is a special case in which it is a 1 × 1 matrix.) If the arm length, *R,* were two times the shown value, the end effector would move twice as fast for a given motor speed. However, for a given motor torque, the longer arm would be capable of supporting only half (½) the weight at the end effector. To generalize, changing the velocity relationship by a factor of *N* always changes the force relationship by a factor of $1/N$; the same rate of mechanical work (force times velocity) is performed as the robot starts to move.

In Figure 38-16, the orientation of the arm matters, as well as its length. Given a particular motor speed, the vertical velocity of the end effector, dy_{ee}/dt, is greater for the orientation shown at the left, with the arm in horizontal abduction, than for the configuration at the right. To visualize this, imagine if the angle, θ, were nearly vertical. Then all motion of the end effector would be left-to-right instead of up-and-down. The vertical velocity, dy_{ee}/dt, would be exactly zero when the arm is aligned to be perfectly vertical.

The concluding message for this section is that the range of speeds and forces a robot arm is capable of producing depends not only on the actuators used, but also on the current configuration of the robot. This is intuitive from our

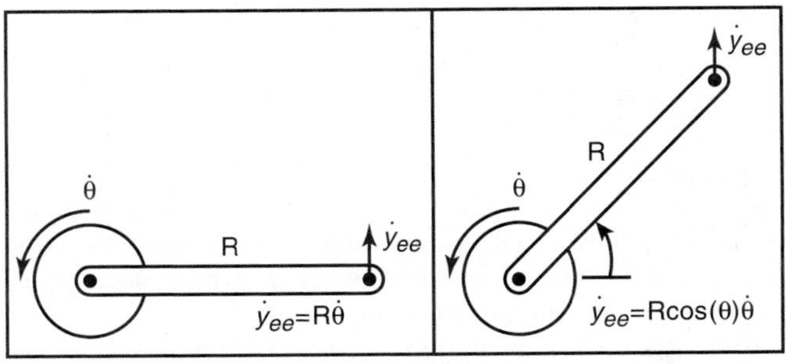

Figure 38-16 ■ A robot arm essentially acts like a lever. The Jacobian matrix is used to describe the leverage relationship between actuator angular velocities (or torques) and limb velocities (or forces).

daily life, as well. It is more difficult to support a heavy object with arms fully extended than by using a more comfortable configuration with arms closer to the trunk. As another example, the speed when hitting a tennis ball depends not only on the strength of the muscles but also on how the individual commands joint trajectories of the arms, exploiting velocity kinematics to achieve a high-speed swing.

Robot Dynamics

Dynamics is the study of how forces affect motion in a system. By contrast, kinematics is not concerned with forces. Rather, kinematics describes only geometric relationships.

The most fundamental concept in dynamics is that force equals mass times acceleration, or, in equation form, $F = ma$. This relationship is known as *Newton's second law of motion.* It means that a body at rest will stay at rest unless a force is applied. Furthermore, a body in motion keeps moving with the same velocity unless a force is applied to change that motion. In practice, there are many forces (e.g., friction, viscous damping, or air resistance) that tend to apply natural forces to slow down objects that are in motion. These are some of the many ways in which forces act to change velocity over time.

Equations of motion (EOMs) are used to describe the forces in a dynamic system and the way these forces affect the acceleration(s) of various degrees of freedom (e.g., joint angles of a robot). In robotics, EOMs are typically described using matrix equations. Without delving into the details of such equations, it is still useful to examine the general structure of the EOMs for a typical robot manipulator. Although exact variable notation will vary, the usual form for such matrix equations is as shown in Equation 38-3.

Equation 38-3

$$\tau = M(\theta)\ddot{\theta} + V(\theta,\dot{\theta}) + G(\theta)$$

The parentheses in Equation 38-3 merely show whether each matrix is a function of position (θ) only or of both position and angular velocity ($\dot{\theta}$). Thus engineers can simply rewrite the equation as follows:

$$\tau = M\ddot{\theta} + V + G$$

On the left-hand side are the controlled input torques (i.e., rotational efforts), τ, which are generally supplied by electric motors in most modern robot manipulators for rehabilitation robotics. On the right-hand side are the natural dynamics of the mechanical system. M represents the mass distribution, known formally as the *inertia matrix,* of the links of the robot, which depends on the robot configuration. V gives all the velocity-dependent torques. These include losses caused by friction and viscous damping, as well as centrifugal forces and Coriolis forces caused by rotations of joints. Finally, G is the torque resulting from gravity. Note that G also depends on the geometry of the robot: holding an arm fully extended outward requires greater torque, to counteract gravity, than does holding an arm near one's side. G captures this relationship more exactly.

The term $M\ddot{\theta}$ is analogous to ma in Newton's $F = ma$ equation. All other terms τ together represent the net torque (analogous to F). That is, the torques that affect angular accelerations of the robot links include both the controlled input torque, (i.e., τ, V, G) and the natural dynamics of the system prescribed by V and G. One popular approach in robot manipulator control is to attempt to "cancel out" the natural dynamics of the robot, to the extent possible. For example, if engineers can set the motor torques such that $\tau = G$, then apparent effects of gravity can be cancelled out, to make a robot arm seem weightless. Similarly, engineers can attempt to cancel out the forces caused by friction and other velocity-dependent terms that are captured in V.

Although canceling out the natural robot manipulator dynamics may sometimes be an elegant solution in theory and in simulation, it requires a very good model of the natural dynamics of the robot. In practice, this may be difficult to achieve, and the true dynamics may vary over time, as a robot ages or is deliberately modified or updated. Joints may begin to stick more, and a user may wish to modify a robot by attaching additional components (cameras, straps, or other tools) that may change the mass and inertia of the limbs.

The overall dynamics of a robot depend on both its natural dynamics, given by $M\ddot{\theta} + V + G$, and on the control laws that determine motor torques, τ. In general, it is safer, when practical, to obtain as much of the possible dynamics of a system as possible through the use of natural dynamics, as will be discussed later. Control is always extremely important, however, and the next section describes some general control techniques used in rehabilitation robotics.

Robot Control Techniques

For a given degree of freedom, engineers can control either position or force of a robot end effector. (Recall our earlier example of pushing a pillow, illustrated in Figure 38-11.) Force and position at the end effector are related through the *mechanical impedance* of the environment. Classical factory robotics, developed in the 1970s and 1980s, emphasized position control of end effectors. The goals of such control were to have higher repeatability and, often, to apply high forces at the end effector. For example, a robotic device might be used to machine a part for an assembly. Here the grinding or cutting forces during the machining process would be quite high, and the tool would need to move in a very exact pattern.

For applications in which a robot interacts with humans and in human environments, forces must be more gentle, and the control over force is typically more important than control over exact position trajectories. Forces may be dictated either directly, through force control, or indirectly, through impedance control. In traditional force control, one designs a controller to specify, directly, the force that an end effector exerts. This might be useful in regulating the pressure exerted by a roller, for example. In manipulating a human or object, however, it is often desirable to keep the robot limb motions close to some nominal positional path, as well. Here, it may be more desirable to control the force "indirectly," by employing control to actively set the mechanical impedance of the robot limb. Recall that a mechanical impedance enforces a relationship between forces exerted and the motions (position, velocity, and acceleration) that occur. Intuitively, an impedance controller can create a "force field" to push a patient arm gently, if it deviates only mildly from a planned trajectory, and to provide firmer resistance if a patient tends to move in an erratic manner or to drift too far from a desired range of motions. The impedance of a robot assistant interacting with a human can also be adjusted over time, to provide more or less guidance and correction as a person regains strength and/or relearns motor skills.

Hogan introduced the concept of impedance control for manipulation over 25 years ago in his seminal work.[228] Despite theoretical advances (largely during the 1980s and early 1990s) in force and impedance control, most industrial robotics for manufacturing purposes have continued to favor position control over either force or impedance control. As robotics has moved out of highly controlled factory settings and into real-world environments, two particular factors have encouraged the use of force feedback techniques. First, unlike many factory assembly machines, robots in clinics or in the home must now interact directly with humans. Therefore they must be gentle. Second, real-world environments involve a lot more uncertainty than a factory setting. Because the mechanical impedance of the objects a robot will touch will vary drastically (e.g., a very stiff wall or doorway versus a soft curtain or pillow), it could be quite dangerous to command only position references to a robot limb. A position-controlled robot could simply put a hole in the wall if it were too strong, and it might not produce enough force to open a simple door if it were simply designed to be "less strong." Controlling the impedance of the robot limb allows for a much greater range of physical interactions in the real world.

There are many ways to define the exact goals for a rehabilitation robot controller, corresponding to the task of the device. It may be used to provide physical therapy, to retrain motor skills in a human, or more directly as a means of surrogate motor compensation for performing daily activities. In both cases, one must assume that the robot will interact directly with a human and, potentially, with objects (e.g., walls, doors, chairs, coffee cups, remote controls) in human environments. Because of the wide range of possible situations that may arise, safety and dependability are significant challenges in developing control techniques for such robotic devices, and thus discussion of safety issues is very important with human-robotic interactions.

A wide body of literature exists on control methods for both human and robot motor tasks.[229-244] Two good introductory texts on general engineering principles for robot kinematics, dynamics, and control are *Introduction to Robotics: Mechanics and Control* by J. J. Craig[245] and *Robot Modeling and Control* by M. W. Spong and colleagues.[246]

Human-Robot Interactions and Interfaces

There are two important classes of interplay between humans and rehabilitation robots: *physical* and *cognitive.* The first type discussed is physical human-robot interaction (pHRI); later, cognitive human-robot interaction (cHRI) is described. In both cases the interactions that are possible between a human and a robot depend on the *interface* that links them, which consists of both hardware and software. In most cases the cHRI and the pHRI are not independent. For example, typing at a keyboard allows the user to have a cognitive interaction of communicating information to a computer through a physical interaction of depressing buttons on a keyboard. Table 38-8 lists some common terms associated with cognitive and physical interactions.

Physical Interactions

From an engineer's point of view, physical interaction is the *exchange of mechanical work*[229]: how systems push (or pull) one another and subsequently move. In rehabilitation robotics, we care both about how a robot is physically related to a human, for example, while providing assistance, and how

TABLE 38-8 ■ COMMON TERMS FOR HUMAN-ROBOT INTERACTIONS, INTERFACES, AND DEVICES[11]

TERM	DESCRIPTION
Human-machine interface (HMI)	The HMI is the means by which a human and a machine interact. This interaction can include touch, sight, sound, heat transference, exchange of electrical signals, or any other physical or cognitive function. The HMI is also commonly known as a man-machine interface (MMI) or human-computer interface (HCI).
Brain-computer interface (BCI)	The BCI is a direct communication pathway between the brain and an external device. This interface may be either unidirectional or bidirectional.
Physical human-robot interaction (pHRI)	A pHRI is the physical interaction between a human and a robot that explicitly involves the flow of power. This interaction may be either unidirectional or bidirectional.
Cognitive human-robot interaction (cHRI)	A cHRI involves the transmission of information between the human and the robot with the goal of allowing the human to control a robot. This interaction may be either unidirectional or bidirectional.
Physical human-robot interface (pHRi)	A pHRi is the interface by which the robot and the human exchange power. Typically a pHRi is based around a rigid structure with actuators that transmit forces to and from the human.
Cognitive human-robot interface (cHRi)	A cHRi is used to exchange information between the human and robot. In the human-to-robot direction, data are acquired through sensors that may measure bioelectrical and biomechanical variables such as neural activity and limb position. The robot-to-human direction can involve direct neural stimulus, physical stimulus, visual stimulus, and auditory stimulus.
Neural interface (NI)	This is an all-encompassing term for artificially stimulating or sensing neural activity.
Brain-machine interface (BMI)	In this interface, the brain directly communicates with some sort of machine. BMI is often used interchangeably with brain-computer interface (BCI), in which the brain is communicating directly with a computer.
Neural prosthetics (NP)	A prosthetic device under the direct control of the brain.
Neural motor prosthetic (NMP)	Here, the motor cortex is used to drive a prosthetic device directly.

a robot physically contacts the environment, for example, to help manipulate objects during daily activities.

In describing dynamics and control, there are two distinct meanings for the word *passive.* Often, *passive* is meant simply to indicate that no actuation is used: *passive* in this context means *not actively controlled.* However, passivity is also used within the controls literature to indicate a dynamic system, either actuated or unactuated, in which one *can imagine* creating an equivalent dynamic system entirely out of stable, passive mechanical elements: traditional springs, masses, and dampers.

By using actuated control instead of using unactuated parts, one can actively modify the stiffness, damping, and apparent inertia of an actively controlled system as desired. For example, in impedance control, one can use active control to create a dynamic system that responds in essentially the same way as a passive one that is built only from springs, dashpots, and inertias. There are significant advantages of using active control instead of a truly nonactuated mechanical device. For example, one can tune the mechanical impedance over time, to provide more or less of the total effort required for a person to perform a given motion. Also, one can change the set point for an actively-simulated mechanical impedance (e.g., spring) element, to track a desired continuous motion.

An alternate strategy is to attempt to compensate for the anticipated dynamics of the environment. One may know from experience that it will take a lot of force to push against a particular door—for example, if it is heavy (great inertia), if it sticks (great friction), or if it has a strong spring-loaded closing mechanism (great stiffness). By anticipating the properties of the door, one can plan ahead and attempt to "cancel out" the natural dynamics of the situation. This type of compensation amounts to *feed-forward* control. Attempting to cancel out the natural dynamics of the environment can be destabilizing, however, if the environment is not perfectly known. Therefore in any realistic situation, one must also use appropriate *feedback* control to ensure stability. The combination of feed-forward (anticipatory) control and feedback (error-driven) control is the basis of most human and robotic motor control.

As an example, imagine you wish to pick up a flower vase, assuming it is full of water and heavy. If it is actually nearly empty and weighs much less than expected, a person might attempt to grasp it and lose control by throwing it into the air. As another example, imagine grasping a rope to pull a heavy object or to play "tug of war" with someone. If there is suddenly no resistance to motion, a person can easily lose control and might even fall down backward.

Similarly, a robot that expects to encounter a particular human response during an interaction may react in an unexpected way if the human dynamics are not as anticipated. In a worst-case scenario, as both robot and human react to try to recover from an unexpected situation, they may interact in such a way as to cause unwanted or dangerous oscillations or to push and pull in such a way that the robot arm acts like the person who has overcompensated when lifting the lightweight vase. Although our controller might have performed just fine had the vase been full, we must always plan for a worst-case scenario (robust control) when the environment is unknown, to ensure stability of the system. This scenario could also occur when a human attempts to move in the opposite direction to what is anticipated by the robot controller. If the task requires shoulder flexion for example, and the human moves the shoulder into extension or abduction rather than flexion, to err on the side of safety the robot may have to stop assisting the patient when the arm moves incorrectly. This can lead to a nontherapeutic "push-pull" situation.

Control engineers have, of course, studied the requirements for stability for robot manipulators in depth. One basic—and intuitive—rule of thumb is that a device is generally both dynamically safer and more forgiving if the dynamics of the device can be implemented through mechanical elements, rather than through clever control to achieve similar dynamics through powered actuators. This has two big advantages. First, the easiest way to implement dynamics with the "passivity" property desired for our dynamics is to use passive (i.e., unactuated) mechanical elements. Second, active control solutions would require additional sensing and powered actuators. However, sometimes actuated control is the only practical way to allow for flexibility in unweighting part of a patient and providing a range of resistance or support during motion. Even if a device is actively controlled with sophisticated actuators, it is possible to do so with a control strategy that mimics a passive system. Such a system would correspondingly be classified as demonstrating the desirable passivity property mentioned earlier.

Force and Pressure Loads from Physical Interfaces

During pHRI, forces are of course exerted between the human and the robot, for example to achieve desired task-specific motions and/or to facilitate motor training. There are several factors to consider in how these forces are applied to a person. The interface should be both comfortable and safe, and it should not unnecessarily inhibit the range of human motion.

Pressure is the measure of force distributed per unit area. As an example, a snowshoe is used to distribute the weight of a person across a larger area, thus lowering the pressure applied to the snow. By contrast, a high-heeled shoe concentrates force onto a small area, increasing pressure, which is why pointed heels can leave prominent marks on carpeting. Distribution of force is also important in dictating the pressure characteristics of human-robot interactions. Applying too much pressure to human skin can cause discomfort or pain, and it can also cut off the flow of blood. Force loads should therefore be distributed across a region of skin to avoid high contact pressure. One should also avoid applying concentrated loads where there is little natural, fleshy tissue to buffer contact and to help in distributing loads. Contact with bony regions can concentrate forces, increasing pressure, and can cause pain and injury. As a simple experiment, find a bony region of your forearm or, alternatively, along your shin. If you slowly press this region against the edge of a desk or table nearby, you should notice that the pressure from the tabletop can quickly become uncomfortable. The same experiment on a fleshier part of the body is significantly more tolerable. Contact should also be avoided or minimized in sensitive tissue regions rich with surface nerves. Contact between a human and robot should also be planned such that forces push downward directly on the skin, to avoid pain or discomfort from undesirable twisting (shear forces) and chafing.

More detailed coverage of this important topic can be found in the text by Pons[11] in Chapter 5 in the discussion of wearable robots and biomechatronic exoskeletons.

Manipulation and Locomotion: Dual Problems

Limbs can be used for either manipulation or locomotion. From an engineering perspective, these are essentially twin problems. In manipulation, one uses limbs (usually arms) to move other objects in the environment. In locomotion, limbs (usually legs) are used to move oneself around with respect to the environment. In both cases, accomplishing a desired task requires generating joint trajectories and forces to achieve desired motions.

However, there are also obvious differences between the two tasks. Most manipulation tasks require coordination between gross and fine motor skills. Manipulation also generally involves smooth, continuous motions. Humans are capable of learning a vast range of motor skills with the arms and hands. These include putting on clothing, using utensils for eating, and performing a tremendous number of other daily activities. In manipulation, one uses limbs to move other objects in the environment.

By contrast, locomotion is punctuated by periodic discontinuities. One leg is used for support and stability while the other leg swings in free space to position itself for the next heel strike. At each step, the two legs swap roles, following a near-repeating pattern over time. Contact with the ground may trigger signals to reset the timing of this periodic cycle. There is usually very little variability in step length during normal human walking, and the swing foot end effector typically swings only a couple of centimeters clear of the ground below.[247] Stated briefly, although we have the capacity to vary our gait if desired, the basic task of locomotion is distinct from and more periodic than that of manipulation, and it is likely that robot technologies for upper and lower limbs should correspondingly differ, to match these differences.

Humans use both feedback and feed-forward in controlling both locomotion and manipulation. As mentioned, in *feed-forward* control, one commands movements based on past experience. Essentially, one anticipates the motor commands that are required to achieve a desired limb motion. By contrast, *feedback* control uses error signals, such as the difference between the desired and actual position of a limb, and motor commands are generated to reduce these sensed errors. Generally speaking, the advantage of feed-forward control is speed: it takes significant time for information (e.g., vision, touch, proprioception) to be transmitted and processed by the brain or a feedback mechanism.

Feedback is important because of the variability that exists from trial to trial in performing a task. Manipulation tasks generally involve direct interaction with the environment. There are many parameters defining this interaction that may be slightly different each time a given task is performed. For example, the pose of one's body may be oriented a bit differently, and the object one wishes to manipulate may have a different trajectory over time and/or a different mechanical impedance than anticipated. Also, one may not be able to perform a given motion in exactly the same way owing to muscle fatigue or other variability in human capabilities.

Both therapists' and engineers' understanding of the roles of feed-forward and feedback in various motor tasks is still incomplete. For example, although both feed-forward and feedback control are traditionally considered to be important in both upper- and lower-limb tasks, recent literature suggests that feedback control without feed-forward control is theoretically sufficient for maintaining a stable, upright posture.[248] This is a particularly interesting result, given the significant time delays (roughly on the order of ⅒ of a second) involved for regulation of balance by the CNS. Understanding what is theoretically necessary for stable balance control in turn has direct application in the design of reliable devices and control algorithms for neuroprostheses,[249] rehabilitation robotics, and other equipment relying on human-robot interaction to accomplish motor tasks.

This section has provided only a brief overview of some of the issues in common between and differentiating locomotion and manipulation. Additional references on human and other animal locomotion and manipulation are available to those interested in additional reading.[250-259]

Cognitive Interfaces

Cognitive interfaces are another means by which information is passed between the human and the robot. A cognitive human-robot interface (cHRi) is an interface that allows information to be passed between a human and a robot. As noted earlier, the cHRi is rarely independent of the physical human-robot interface (pHRi), with many types of cHRi accomplished through a pHRi. For example, the human-to-robot direction of the cHRi can be accomplished through the use of keyboards and mice, the measurement of limb positions, voice activation, eye tracking, or measurement of neural activity. Similarly, the robot-to-human directions of the cHRi can be accomplished through mechanical stimulation (vibration or force feedback), auditory stimulation (voice or tonal feedback), visual feedback (flashing lights, or graphics on a screen), or direct neural feedback. Cognitive interface design is a developing field with technical contributions coming from many different fields including but certainly not limited to clinical medicine, neuroscience, biology, engineering, and computer science. As one might expect with such a diverse range of contributors, the terminology defining the cognitive interface has many overlapping and conflicting terms used to define the characteristics of the cognitive interface, with each contributing specialty having a preferred terminology. In this section the reader will not be given a comprehensive description of all possible cognitive interfaces. Instead the reader is provided an introduction to the engineering challenges and some of the associated terminology.

From an engineering perspective, there are two classes of cognitive interface(s): direct and indirect. In a direct interface, the cognitive interface attempts to replicate the original relationships between the input measurement and the output robot motion. An example of a direct measurement is using electroencephalography to monitor motor cortex activity that corresponds to arm motion and then using that measurement to control a prosthetic arm. In an indirect interface, measurements are taken of signals or motions that are *not* normally used to control a particular activity directly. An example of this would be using voice commands to control a lower-limb prosthetic. Clearly these are "fuzzy" distinctions because humans rarely use a single modality to achieve a task. For example, an individual can choose to move a box by picking it up himself, direct control; or he can ask a colleague across the room who is closer to the box to bring it to him, via indirect control.

Neural Interfaces

A relatively new type of direct interface is the emerging field of neural interfaces. Although neural interfaces may seem far-fetched, the U.S. Food and Drug Administration (FDA) estimates that as of December 2010, approximately 219,000 individuals worldwide had received cochlear implants.[260] The cochlear implant relays sounds from a microphone to directly stimulate the auditory nerve to restore hearing. Neural interfaces currently have a huge potential to expand in capabilities owing to recent innovations of computer technology. Computers supporting brain-machine interfaces (BMIs) can now record and process large amounts of neural data.

When creating a neural interface, there is a tradeoff between the invasiveness of a device and the fidelity of the signal. Although measuring with electrodes directly placed in or on the brain yields high-fidelity signals, the hazards of surgery have motivated researchers to use indirect measurements. One of the least invasive methods is to use the electroencephalogram (EEG). Electroencephalography measures scalp voltages, which correlate to neural firing on the surface of the brain. The drawback of electroencephalography is that there is little time and spatial sensitivity to individual neurons. The readings for individual sensors can be considered gross time and spatial averages of the neural activity occurring next to the sensor. A notable example of how electroencephalography can be used cheaply and easily is the Mindflex by Mattel, which uses a modified EEG to control a fan. Whereas this may seem promising, the practicality of electroencephalography is limited owing to the intense concentration and training that each subject must undergo to control this device. One limiting example is that subjects are unable to talk or multitask when using this interface, further limiting its utility.[261] Figure 38-17 shows an EEG recording net being used on a study participant.

As mentioned earlier, placing the electrical sensors on the exterior of the skull significantly reduces sensor sensitivity owing to both signal attenuation as a result of distance (electric and magnetic field strength are inversely proportional to distance squared) and "smear" in the nonuniform tissues between the source and sensor. Thus the performance of an electrical sensor is substantially increased with the more invasive option of implantation.[262] Implanted electrodes on the surface of the brain (Figure 38-18) are capable of measuring the neuron action potential (the electrical signal across the neuron's membranes). The close proximity to the neuron gives good signal sensitivity, enhances spatial localization, and allows higher data rates than external sensors. One must be aware that although embedded electrodes have good neuron specificity, they do not measure many neurons. The number of neurons being sampled is important for neural-controlled prosthetics because even the most routine task, such as moving one's hands, uses millions of neurons.

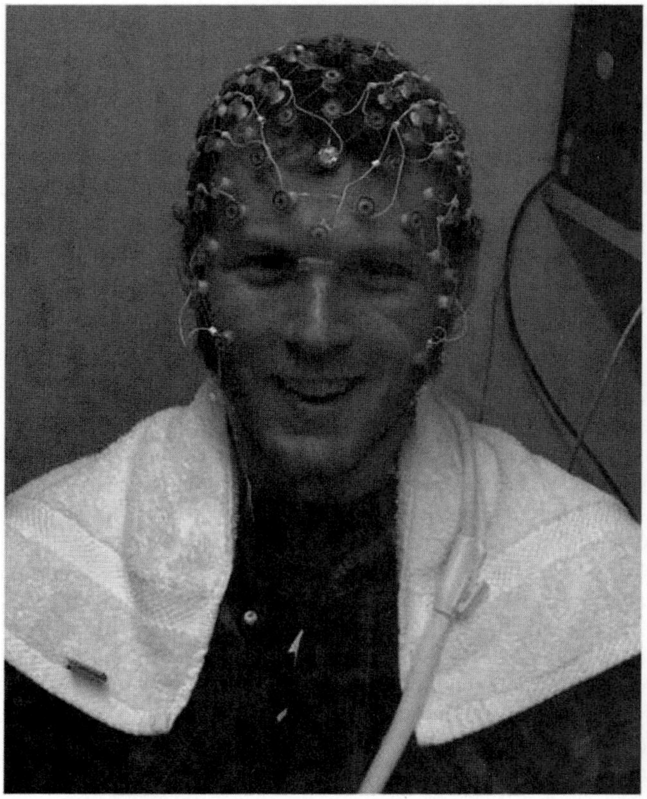

Figure 38-17 ■ A subject with an electroencephalogram net placed on his scalp for a research experiment. There is some variability in the placement of the net, which may affect the calibration required each time the net is placed.

Although researchers have been able to decode hand movement commands with only six neurons, this comes at the sacrifice of reliability in the measurement. Generally, the more neurons measured, the more reliable the motor signals that may be decoded.[263] Figure 38-18 shows an example of an intracranial sensor. Sarpeshkar and colleagues[264] have identified some of the challenges

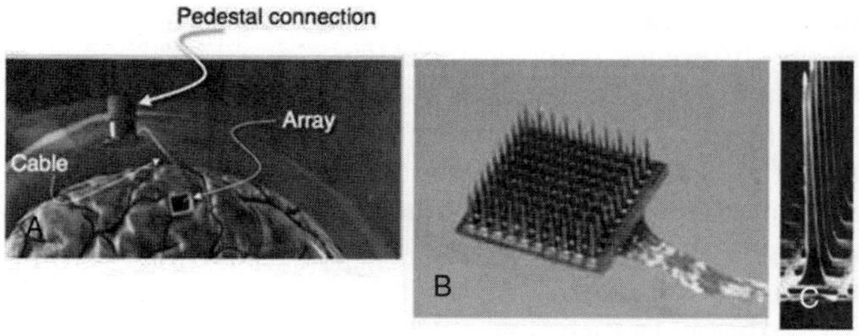

Figure 38-18 ■ An electrode array design by Richard Normann and colleagues in 1998. **A,** The mounting pedestal that runs through the skull. **B,** The array of 100 tapered 1.5-mm–long microelectrodes arranged in a 10 × 10 grid. **C,** Electron microscope view of the electrode. (From Donoghue JP, Nurmikko A, Black M, Hochberg LR: Assistive technology and robotic control using motor cortex ensemble-based neural interface systems in humans with tetraplegia, *J Physiol* 579(Pt 3): 603–611, 2007.)

associated with intercranial devices. These include the following:

- Size restrictions—The device must be safely contained within the skull.
- Material biocompatibility—There is a growing list of materials that have been tested, but long-term use and subject-specific sensitivities remain issues.
- Heat dissipation—These devices must not generate excessive heat that could damage surrounding tissues.
- Power consumption—Frequent battery replacement is not practical owing to complications and risks from operating on the skull. In addition, high power consumption may lead to excessive heat dissipation.
- Risk of infection—Implementation of the device requires a surgical procedure, and infection is always a risk with surgery.

Another commonly used method of creating a neural interface is functional magnetic resonance imaging (fMRI). An fMRI is a specialized magnetic resonance imaging (MRI) scan in which measured change in blood flow in the brain or spinal cord is correlated with neural activity. In contrast to electroencephalography, this method has good spatial resolution over a large area of the brain. Drawbacks to fMRI are that it does not directly measure a neuron firing and that the slow response of blood flow to neuron firing does not make this practical as a real-time neural interface. For example, in 2004, researchers used fMRI to allow subjects to neurally control a mouse in four directions. Although selecting "north" versus "west" may seem like a simple enough command, it took on average 2 minutes and 15 seconds for the users to enter a single command.[265] Also note that MRI machines are not practical outside of a research or clinical setting because of the high cost and large size of the instruments and limitations on the types of materials (i.e., nonmagnetic) that can be used near an MRI machine owing to the strong magnetic fields generated.

Biomechanical Interfaces

As with the definition of cognitive interfaces, there is no universal definition of what a *biomechanical interface* is. For the purposes of this chapter, a biomechanical interface will be defined as a subtype of cognitive interface in which various measurements are used to estimate the mechanical state and intentions of a biological system (in this case a human) and then use traditional engineering assumptions to translate those state measurements into signals that control a robot or machine. In the context of this discussion of direct versus indirect measurement, a biomechanical interface is usually an indirect measurement. Thus, although it could be argued that electromyography should be categorized as a neural interface (a direct measurement), it is more typically employed in practice as a biomechanical interface, because the amplitude of muscle activation that is output must then be interpreted to estimate the desired robot actuator force or actuator motion.

There are many means of achieving a biomechanical interface, including the following:

- The aforementioned electromyography, which measures muscle activation levels
- Wearable sensors and exoskeletons that directly measure joint angles and body postures and indirectly measure joint torques and limb forces
- Motion capture systems such as the Kinect system from Microsoft that uses cameras to measure the pose and motion of the subject
- Semiactive prosthetics that sense the wearer's intent based on the magnitude and frequency of a single input angle

All of these interfaces share the characteristics that they take a series of mechanical (or electrical) measurements and then fit those measurements to an engineering model, which is then used to estimate the desired state of a robot or prosthesis and the most likely intentions of the user. These engineering models are often called *finite-state machines* (FSMs), in which the current state of the system is used to determine the forces and actions required to move the system from its current state into a desired next state. As an example, walking gaits are often described using a series of phases that are performed in a consistent order in normal walking. An FSM can be used to describe this repeating series of phases, allowing a robot controller to anticipate the next motions required to continue walking normally.

Just as in the case of neural interfaces, there are many challenges associated with successfully achieving a functional and safe biomechanical interface. Sometimes it is not possible to directly measure, nor to indirectly estimate, all of the states (e.g., joint angles and angular velocities) in a dynamic system. Such systems are not fully observable. Also, it is often not possible to actuate each degree of freedom (e.g., joint angle) independently. Such systems are not fully actuated—that is, they are underactuated. One of the keys to successful interface design is to select a combination of measurements, modeling assumptions, and control outputs that allows for the stable operation of a robot when neither full observability nor full actuation is possible.

For example, if a robot arm is assisting a human in a reaching task, such as grasping a cup (see Figure 38-15), the exact orientation of all the joints in the arm will probably not be known and forces will not be applied directly to all joints to help to control the motion. Proper use of a biomechanical interface in such situations depends on proper interpretation of the context in which a device is being used.

Context

One of the things a cognitive interface must successfully communicate is context. Let us return to the planar arm example. So far we have discussed this problem in the context of picking up a cup of coffee. In this context, we would like to have good position control of the hand while we minimize the velocity of the hand as we pick up the coffee to avoid spilling it. What if, instead, we were attempting to hit a nail with a hammer? In this context, we would still want to have good positional accuracy but we would like to maximize the velocity of the hammer so that we have good energy transfer from the hammer to the nail. In both cases, the system would have the same state variables and state measurements, but the cognitive interface needs to understand the context in order to achieve the desired outcome.

The common feature of nearly all cognitive interfaces is that both the human and machine components must be trained. An important takeaway point is that the human needs to learn how the machine responds, and typically the machine also needs to be trained such that the parameters of the state model match those of the controlling human.

Safety Issues for Robotic Technology

There is a tremendous range of issues relating to safety when interfacing robotic technology with a human. For example, a robot may unintentionally encourage poor kinematic positioning and orientation of a patient limb, part of the robot may collide with a person, or the forces applied at an attachment point may be dangerously high or may unintentionally excite or accentuate tremor-style oscillatory motions. In addition, intentions of a user may be misinterpreted, faults may occur in power or other wiring, a device may be improperly calibrated, or bugs may exist in software. Although all are important concerns, this section will focus on inherent engineering design aspects for the device when used as intended, as opposed to the wide variety of possible failure modes that might occur in any electromechanical device.

In the following section, safety issues caused by mechanical design, type of actuation, and/or control techniques employed are highlighted. This summary will parallel the earlier discussions of kinematics and dynamics for robots by briefly summarizing engineering design issues related to each. More detailed information on pHRI safety may be found in the article "An Atlas of Physical Human-Robot Interaction"[266] or in the text *Wearable Robots: Biomechatronic Exoskeletons.*[11]

Kinematics and Geometry of the Device

Kinematically, it is important to avoid positioning a patient in such a way that joints may be encouraged or forced into abnormal, painful, and/or damaging configurations. Recall from the earlier discussions that there are typically multiple solutions to get a desired end effector to a particular position. It is correspondingly important how and where a robot limb interfaces with a human arm or leg. If they are joined at only their respective end effectors, for example, one runs the risk of hyperextension of human joints because the robot simply does not track exactly what is happening to all joints along the way to the human end effector. There various other, common sense issues involving the shape or geometry of the device. For example, sharp corners or edges should be avoided to minimize any damage that might occur owing to unplanned collisions between the robot and the human. A much more thorough discussion of this topic can be found in Chapter 5 of *Wearable Robots: Biomechatronic Exoskeletons.*[11]

Dynamics and Stability of Man-Machine Systems

Once a robot interacts with another dynamic system or the environment, stability depends on the coupled dynamics of the two systems together.* Time delay may also cause instability,[238,243,268] as may backlash in the transmission mechanism.[131] There may be time delays in the system owing to the slow response time of the human in the loop (i.e., slow compared with the sensing and computation of a robot). *Backlash* refers to the play that exists in mechanical gears or other transmission elements: when a motor first reverses direction, it may first need to "take up the slack" that exists in real-world gears before a reversal in the motion of a robot joint actually occurs.

Several principles can be employed to make the mechanical impedance (mass, damping, and stiffness) of the device safer. Robotic limbs should have low mass and inertia. Imagine a robot limb, in a worst case scenario, as being roughly similar to a baseball bat: a lightweight design will cause less damage during unintended impacts. In addition, both the joints and the "skin" of the robot (if any) can employ mechanical compliance and damping. Essentially, this provides shock absorption for the human-robot interface. One way to achieve both a lightweight and a compliant arm is to hide motors or other actuators within the body or base of the robot and to control the joints through the use of cables. Practically speaking, cables (e.g., like the ones used to control bike brakes by squeezing levers on the handlebars) stretch when they are pulled. Thus the cables naturally act as both a means of transmission and a compliant spring element in a design. This mechanical compliance may limit the speed with which robot limb motions can be commanded. However, for rehabilitation robotics, this compliance versus speed tradeoff is likely a reasonable one to make, because desired motions are generally smooth and slow.

In summary, when considering engineering issues in rehabilitation robotics, both passive and dynamic mechanical structure as well as active control of forces and positions are important for both performance and safety. Where and how a robotic device interfaces with a human is also important, both physically and cognitively. These are all areas of active research. Furthermore, a variety of solutions are currently employed or are under development for research and commercial purposes. This field will continue to grow and be refined. As this field expands, therapists will more likely interact with engineers in order to provide the best practice for individuals who might potentially benefit from robotics.

ANALYZING COST-EFFECTIVENESS AND EFFICIENCY OF REHABILITATION ROBOTICS

Costs of Rehabilitation Robotics

At this time, the cost of rehabilitation robotics is very high. There are not a lot of robotic devices available; thus there has been little price reduction based on quantity. The costs vary from $3000 to more than $300,000 depending on whether the device is individualized to one person or whether the device can be used in locations to serve many individuals. Technology between $75,000 and $90,000 is considered to be in the low range. The appearance of the robot is important from esthetic and psychological points of view. Safety is a major consideration. Because rehabilitation robotics are complicated devices and are produced in small numbers, at this time the costs are high. It is also not clear whether insurance companies will ultimately contribute to the purchase of these assistive devices or whether the cost will be the problem of the end user. However, as demand, acceptance, use, and production increase, it is expected that the manufacturing prices could go down. This is an especially volatile market when there is economic stress.

If research confirms increased function and increased independence with rehabilitation robotics and there is a decrease in the need for long-term care support in a nursing home, and less demand for one-on-one therapeutic treatment, it is possible that initial investment in the device may be considered cost-effective. This has been the case with

*References 231, 232, 235, 239, 243, 267.

cochlear implants. For example, for children and elders, the investment in the implant is associated with maintained functional hearing, improved communication, safety, and greater independence. Thus third-party payers have determined the investment in the implant is cost-effective.

Effectiveness of Robotic Technology

The commercialization of rehabilitation robotics and assistive devices will depend both on the costs of the device as well as the effectiveness. When deciding to pursue the integration of rehabilitation technology and robotics, a number of questions should be answered by the user, the health care provider, and the health care system in order to determine cost-effectiveness (Box 38-19).

The Manus upper-limb assistive robotic device (Manus ARM) can be used as an example of practicality and cost-effectiveness.[269] The Manus ARM is an assistive robot that is mounted to a wheelchair. It has six degrees of freedom and a gripper to capture objects (up to 1.5 kg). It is controlled by a keypad, a joystick, a headband or spectable-mounted laser pointer, or a mouse. Initial evaluation programs have been developed to analyze cost-effectiveness. Two studies were conducted in the Netherlands relative to the cost-effectiveness and safety of the Manus ARM. The Manus ARM allows a

BOX 38-19 ■ QUESTIONS TO ASK TO DETERMINE COST-EFFECTIVENESS OF REHABILITATION ROBOTICS AND ADVANCED TECHNOLOGY

I. UTILITY OF THE ROBOTIC DEVICE

A. With what types of activities will the robot assist?
B. Are the activities and tasks enabled important for everyday life and movement freedom?
C. Is there still a gap between academic laboratory research activities and practical, efficient robotic applications at home (e.g., eating, bathing, manipulating objects)?
D. Can the robot help the patient maintain privacy to perform personal activities (e.g., changing clothes, bathing, and toileting)?
E. Can the robot assist with movement across a broad spectrum of movement impairments?
F. How much does the robot contribute to completing the full task (e.g., can the robot help prepare the food, serve the food, and assist the patient in eating) ?
G. How many hours in the day will the robot be able to replace a human helper (e.g., many hours—just a few hours, or possibly enough hours to afford complete independence except for house cleaning and yard work)?
H. Compared with the time required for common tasks, what are the time constraints of robotic assistance (e.g., does it take an hour to eat a sandwich, or 10 minutes; is the intensity of effort the same)?
I. Does the human interface require additional sensory attachments initially or continually to enable individuals to use it?
J. What is the reliability of the robot? Does it break down a lot? Is it easy to have it repaired? What is the feedback of previous users?
K. Does the robot effectively assist in task performance, or does it get in the way?
L. Does the robot perform needed tasks accurately, or are there risks for destroying other objects in the area or work surfaces?
M. Do patients effectively learn to improve their performance of a task, or is the task practice irrelevant?
N. How much noise is there when the robot is operating (e.g., does it interfere with conversation or bother others)?
O. What kind of energy is needed for robot operation, and how long does the energy source last?
P. What space does the robot access (e.g., can it easily fit into the house without special modifications)?
Q. What is the limit of the space the robot can access to help perform functional tasks?
R. How much does the robot weigh, and what are the parameters of its size?
S. If the robot attaches to a wheelchair, how hard is it to mount and what space does it occupy (e.g., does it limit the ability of the wheelchair to go through fixed spaces)?
T. How much time during the day will the robot be used?
U. Is the robot gripper precise enough to be functional?

II. QUESTIONS TO ASK ABOUT EASE OF CONTROL

A. Can the robot be used only at home in the house, or can it be transported to other sites?
B. How easy is it to get the robot into the car?
C. Does it take special training to use the robotic device?
D. How long does it take the user to get comfortable and efficient in using the device (e.g., does it get easier to use the more it is used)?
E. Are instructions for use in languages other than English?
F. What type of controls are demanded (e.g., does it mostly require attention at execution, or does it require attention throughout task completion)?
G. Is there any automatic part of the task performance?
H. Is the robot flexible in responding to commands, or does the command have to be precise and delivered in only one mode?
I. Can the robot be used in a variety of environments (e.g., home, school, work)?
J. Are there speeds of execution differences for certain tasks?
K. What type of sensor attachments are needed?

III. QUESTIONS TO ASK ABOUT APPEARANCE AND PRACTICAL USE

A. Does the robotic device attract negative attention when out in the community or when people come to visit at home?
B. Will the robot fit into the household without disrupting others (e.g., if used in the kitchen or the

Continued

BOX 38-19 ■ QUESTIONS TO ASK TO DETERMINE COST-EFFECTIVENESS OF REHABILITATION ROBOTICS AND ADVANCED TECHNOLOGY—cont'd

bathroom, does it interfere with others functioning in the same space)?

C. If the robotic device must be applied to equipment, does it keep others from using the equipment (e.g., if hand devices are integrated in the car, can others still use the car using the foot pedals)?

D. What is the extent of construction or changes needed in the house to accommodate the assistive device (e.g., sensors and actuators mounted on the ceilings)?

E. Can the robot be integrated with other robotic subsystems in terms of control features?

F. Will it be required to have multiple robots, or is the robot a complete system?

G. Can the robot pick up information from the user about errors, problems, possible injuries, or unmet needs?

H. Are there multisensory control systems embedded (e.g., vision, movement, auditory, verbal)?

I. If the device is to help with functional activities at home, can it also be used for a health monitoring or alert system?

J. Does the control system interfere with other household activities (e.g., does the electrical or magnetic monitoring system interfere with TV signals or mobile phone signals)?

K. Is the system potentially flexible to integrate with other service systems that are expected to develop in the future?

IV. QUESTIONS TO ASK ABOUT INITIAL AND MAINTENANCE COSTS

A. How much does the robotic device cost at initial purchase?

B. What type of maintenance is required on the robotic device, and how much does it cost (labor and parts)?

C. Is the user able to meet some of the costs both initially and on an ongoing basis?

D. Will insurance help cover the costs for initial purchase as well as maintenance?

E. Is the price of the robotic device increasing or decreasing?

F. What is the demand for the robotic device; can it help a variety of people, particularly the aging population?

G. Will the assistive robotic technology allow the patient to maintain independence at home (e.g., instead of having to go to a nursing home)?

H. Is there evidence the price will go down with increased demand and supply (e.g., or is the technology itself so complex that the price will continue to stay high regardless of supply)?

variety of ADLs to be carried out at home including drinking from a glass, removing an item from a desk, scratching one's head, discarding an item into the trash, handling a floppy disk, shopping, and posting a letter.

In order for insurance companies to pay for the Manus ARM, the user must meet certain qualifications:

- Possess very limited or nonexistent arm and/or hand function
- Be dependent on the assistance of another person for help
- Use a power wheelchair
- Have sufficient cognitive skills to operate and control the ARM device
- Possess a strong determination to gain independence
- Possess adequate social and environmental support to achieve independence, such as caregivers, friends, and relatives

If the criteria are met, then the user is given an opportunity to use the ARM using different control devices. The appropriate control device is selected. Most individuals use the joystick and their original wheelchair. The ARM is purchased with a 5-year service warranty.

The process of approval and purchase can take several months. The installation takes several days. Each client is trained in his or her own home, where safety issues are discussed. Additional training sessions may be arranged at 2-week intervals with a 3-month evaluation.

In the Netherlands, the support for assistive robotics is funded by a governmental exploratory grant, not by Social Security or a social health insurance system. Follow-up studies indicate that at least 0.7 to 1.8 hours per day of caregiver help can be saved.[270] However, this estimate of cost savings may be an underestimate. For example, the cost for the standard ARM (plus 3-year warranty) is about $30,000. With the savings on caretaker help, the return on the investment was 1 to 1.5 years. The cost savings were even higher if the user returned to work.[271]

COMMERCIALIZATION OF REHABILITATION ROBOTICS

The greatest impediments to rehabilitation robots are the high cost, low efficiency, and welfare regulations. Despite these limitations, some rehabilitation robots have become commercially available for patients to use on a daily basis.

Increasing demand for the rehabilitation robotics will depend not only on costs, but on clarifying the benefits of the robotic device. This must be done with adequate protection of privacy. It should be possible to list the activities that need to be assisted, the user's movement freedom, what kind of movement impairments the robot can address, the importance of each activity for everyday use, and whether the robot can contribute to the completion of the task.

There are many other questions that need to be asked to determine cost-effectiveness and how to promote the use of these devices. Further details are also needed regarding the time required for the user to learn how to operate the robot, whether the robot control demands some user instructions each moment of the task execution, what level of automatic task performance is needed, and whether the robot responds to exact user commands or can respond correctly even if there is some inexactness (see Box 38-19).

FUTURE REHABILITATION ROBOTICS

Neural Plasticity

Activity-dependent plasticity will continue to underlie neurorecovery. More and more technology and robotic devices will become available over the next 10 years. It is conceivable that neurorehabilitation clinics of the future may need to become "gyms" for rehabilitation. Therapists will need to tailor the exercise routine to the patient's needs to optimize recovery but at the same time will increase clinic productivity by seeing more than one patient at a time; they will incorporate current rehabilitation robotics to enable more effective, controlled, and progressive practice. Efforts must also be made to optimize efficient and effective operation of the robots to make them more accessible.

Advances in Technology

Rehabilitation robotics will continue to grow over the next 10 years as our population ages, medical care advances in saving lives, science continues to document plasticity and recovery, there are changes in technology, and wireless opportunities expand.[272]

Advances in technology in the future will be driven by an increasing demand for robotic technology to assist in the rehabilitation of an increasing number of elderly and an increasing number of individuals with impairments. Advances in computer technology, software programming, and materials will also drive an increase in the development and types of robotics. Visionary developers and the marketplace will drive leading-edge solutions for challenging problems.

There must be a drive in the current health care market to encourage investors to provide financial support for the development of visionary robots. Research on the cost-effectiveness of rehabilitation robotics will also drive development. If rehabilitation and service robots can decrease the number of caregivers needed and decrease the costs of transportation of patients with impairments, the demand and need for robotic devices will increase. Furthermore, with the emphasis on telecommunication systems, wireless technology, and Internet-based possibilities, patients with impairments may be able to train at home as well as work at home, particularly if they can be safe and independent in that environment using smart robotic devices.

Robotic technology for rehabilitation will also increase as materials, computer chips, design engineering advances, wireless communication electronics, computers, and robustness of sensory, transducers, and actuators improve. The computer devices must continue to be smaller, lighter, more convenient, easy to control, and more mobile. This advancement in computerized technology is definitely taking place right now with advances in cell phones and Global Positioning System (GPS) technology, high-speed storage systems, flexible display technologies, and alarm systems. This area of advancement is well underway.

Most people think of robots as stiff and inflexible, connected and run by motors. As wearable robotic devices are improved to better interact and adapt to humans, then the character of the material may have to soften and become more flexible—like a shirt rather than a metallic or wire-based exoskeleton. One can imagine the possibility of putting on a shirt with unobtrusive motors to help a patient lift an object; wearing robotic boots with actuators to prevent accidents for patients who tend to fall; or wearing a special helmet with sensors that can sense danger and actuators that can correct the situation.

Brain-Machine Interfaces

There are already high-frequency electrical stimulation devices that can be placed on the surface of the spinal cord to facilitate locomotion (see Chapter 16). Deep brain stimulators now exist to help decrease abnormal involuntary movements, improve motor control, or control seizures (see Chapter 20). As advances are made in understanding brain specialization, neuronal networks, and communication pathways through the brain and the spinal cord, more rehabilitation robotic devices that facilitate CNS-machine interfaces will also grow in popularity and availability. Intel, Google, and Microsoft have already created brain-machine divisions to work on developing noninvasive methods to sample high-resolution brain activities to make BMIs a practical robotic reality.

For example, the Walk Again Project is a project that links living brain tissue to a variety of artificial tools to develop and implement the first BMI that is capable of restoring full body mobility to patients with severe body paralysis. A full neuroprosthetic device is a wearable robotic device wired to the premotor cortex and the primary motor cortex. It was designed by Gordon Cheng.[273] The objective is to give the patient control over his or her upper and lower limbs to sustain and carry his or her body weight. This device requires the safe implantation of high-density microelectrode cubes in the human brain. This robot can provide reliable, long-term simultaneous recordings of the electrical activity of thousands of neurons distributed across multiple brain locations.

Ideally, to make the BMIs clinically relevant and affordable, the large-scale brain activity recordings will have to be stable for at least a decade without need for surgical repair. The BMIs will have to incorporate low-power multichannel wireless technology transmitting the collective information generated by thousands of individual brain cells to a wearable processing unit about the size of a modern cell phone. A BMI will have to run independent computational program models to optimize function through actuators distributed across the joints of a robotic exoskeleton to mimic reflexes and trigger postural and gait adjustments in response to unexpected changes in the terrain. Electromechanical circuits will enable motor adjustments. The major blocks to the advancement of robotics are the high financial investments that will be required, variability in human factors, and safety issues.

Wireless Opportunities

Information and communication technologies will be integrated to extend opportunities for patients to rehabilitate at home under wireless conditions of supervision and advisement. Telemedicine has grown over the last few years to extend care into rural communities and allow sharing of databases and information across multiple sites for integrative management of individual patients. Real-time interactions (verbal and visual) will be possible between participants and providers through videoconferencing. However, other methods will need to be incorporated to maintain the dynamic interaction between clinicians and clients. User-friendly telemedicine designs are just in their infancy. In addition, shifting the paradigm from one-on-one management to self-care management will also need to be integrated into telemedicine methods. Telemedicine may help shift our resources to efficiently and effectively manage the rehabilitation needs of elders and other patients with impairments.

CONCLUSION

Although the field of rehabilitation robotics is still in its infancy, it has already made important contributions to many individual patients' quality of life. Regaining functional control over impaired movements will remain a primary objective for patients with movement dysfunctions after CNS insult, whether through traditional physical or occupational therapy services, retraining using a nonwearable robotic, movement assistance from a wearable exoskeleton, or some combination of those three areas. Finding the most efficacious and cost-effective way for physical and occupational therapists to provide services for individuals with movement dysfunction will incorporate the potential use of robotics as intervention options. To what extent robotics will be integrated into inpatient and outpatient rehabilitation as the intervention of choice will depend on many factors discussed in this chapter. This chapter was developed to provide to the reader the opportunity to widen clinical understanding and envision clinical options for patients who will be receiving occupational and physical therapy services in the future. The options are numerous, and whether to use or not use robotics as part of clinical services is not easily answered with a yes or no. But no matter the final decision regarding choice of intervention strategies, having options always helps provide a therapist with alternative treatment approaches when traditional approaches do not seem to be effective.

References

To enhance this text and add value for the reader, all references are included on the companion Evolve site that accompanies this textbook. This online service will, when available, provide a link for the reader to a Medline abstract for the article cited. There are 273 cited references and other general references for this chapter, with the majority of those articles being evidence-based citations.

CASE STUDY 38-2

Lena is a 30-year-old occupational therapist employed by a transitional care and rehabilitation center, a 55-bed inpatient care center that is part of a large nursing and rehabilitation care network. She had a major stroke 13 years ago, resulting in profound right-sided hemiparesis, which physicians at the time predicted she was unlikely to reverse.

After about 2 weeks in local hospitals, she began a month of inpatient and 3 years of outpatient physical, occupational and speech therapy. Her arm and hand function came back faster than her gait. During this time, she had multiple surgeries on her right leg and ankle owing to repetitive ankle sprains, decreased balance, decreased strength, and decreased motor control.

Her experience as a patient inspired her to pursue a degree in occupational therapy. After completing her studies, she took a position as an occupational therapist at a skilled nursing facility. After a few years, she realized that she was limping and tripping more often. Simultaneously, a speech therapist brought in some information about a new lower-limb exoskeleton, the Bionic Leg by Tibion. She called the company to find out how she could take advantage of training with this technology. The following is a transcript of an interview with Lena and her physical therapist (Dr. A.).

Question: What was your reaction to putting the Tibion Bionic Leg on for the first time?

Lena: It seemed too good to be true. Almost immediately I could walk without my ankle-foot orthosis [AFO] without tripping. I could see improvement from the very first session.

Question: How long was that first session? Did you see any carryover?

Lena: My first session was an hour and a half. There was a lot of repetition, and I was exhausted. But afterward, I did see a little carryover for 15 to 20 minutes. And the more I've used the Bionic Leg since that time, the longer the carryover lasts. At this point I have used the Bionic Leg for about 16 sessions, twice a week for 8 weeks.

Question to Dr. A.: Can you describe your impressions of Lena's gait when you first evaluated her?

Dr. A.: My impression was that Lena could walk with a better gait pattern. Lena had a lot of muscle wasting in her right leg, much more noticeable in her leg than her right arm. This recovery pattern is somewhat unusual for a patient poststroke. Part of this could possibly be explained by her work as an OT and her insight about how to rehabilitate her arm. On the other hand, the location of the ischemia was also important. Her arm appeared to be spared a little more than her leg.

If Lena was sitting in a chair and using her arms to talk to you, you would never know she had a stroke. But as soon as she would rise from the chair to walk, she had a very typical gait for a patient poststroke. She had circumduction of the hip, decreased weight-bearing time on the right affected lower limb, hyperextension of the knee, and a tendency to drag her toes when she would swing the right leg. Her gait was very asymmetric. When she would complete the swing phase of gait, given the circumduction, her leg was out to the side and it was difficult to shift her weight over her center of support to roll off the forefoot and prepare for the next step. She was off balance and had to make a quick step with the left leg.

In addition, Lena could not lift or dorsiflex her ankle or extend her toes. This weakness and ankle instability was addressed surgically with a tendon transplant to aid dorsiflexion and modification of the ligaments to increase stability. She had a dynamic (spring-loaded, hinged) AFO to keep her ankle in neutral dorsiflexion to

Continued

CASE STUDY 38-2—cont'd

minimize tripping. She had minimal strength in knee flexion (with hypertonicity in extension) and weak hip flexors. This imbalance in strength and motor control made it very hard to go up and down stairs reciprocally. She reported great frustration at having to go one step at a time. She works as a busy professional under a tight schedule and needs to be able to move quickly.

Question to Lena: As both a therapist and a patient, how do you evaluate the results of the first 16 Bionic Leg sessions?

Lena: I have more endurance and a more efficient and effective gait pattern. I can walk faster and straighter. I don't turn my foot out as much as I did, and I can roll or push off my right forefoot, which helps facilitate knee flexion, hip flexion, and dorsiflexion for the next step. I am able to clear my toes when walking and also when going up and down stairs, reciprocally.

Dr. A.: She has gained more flexibility in her gait. Interestingly, this included increased arm swing and increased trunk and pelvic rotation. She's improved her awareness of balance. She has learned to walk sideways and walk forward kicking a ball as if she were playing soccer. She has decreased circumduction of the right leg and improved the symmetry of the single-leg stance as she walks. She also has learned to decrease foot slapping after heel strike.

Question to Lena: It sounds as though someday, if you keep up this kind of progress, you might get rid of the AFO.

Lena: That's what I'm hoping—something I never thought would be possible. I had come to the conclusion that I would need the AFO for life. On the other hand, I remain guarded because of my ankle surgery.

Question to Dr. A.: What impact has the Bionic Leg had on Lena's gait speed? Just seeing her walking in your clinic is very impressive. Is she likely to ever be able to run?

Dr. A.: We initially kept her speed relatively slow when wearing the Tibion Bionic Leg, both walking over ground as well as walking on a regular treadmill and then walking on a BWSTS. Our goal has been to improve quality of gait including the integration of sagittal plane movements rather than circumduction at the hip joint. After improvement in quality and stability, we began to push Lena to the limit of her abilities (forced intense exercise). When you push people to the limit of their ability, it is important to avoid facilitating the abnormal patterns. One way to push the limits and try to promote quality of gait is with unweighting. Unweighting on a treadmill provides the opportunity to decrease GRFs, decrease the risk of falling, improve balance, and maximize gait symmetry and quality.

Once Lena was walking with a better pattern of gait over ground, we had her walk on a treadmill with the Bionic Leg. Then we slowly increased the speed of the treadmill. She progressed to 4.0 mph with good quality, good sagittal plane movement, and a stable ankle.

Patients with motor control problems and hypertonicity must initially learn to concentrate 100% on walking. If they are walking and talking they can trip, risking a fall. With hypertonicity and weakness, often there is a decrease in the speed of postural righting reflexes to protect against falling. This was the case with Lena. If she was not thinking about her walking, she returned to her bad habits and tended to trip. She needed to practice enough to make these patterns automatic without conscious awareness.

Lena is clearly a community ambulator (>1.0 mph). Our functional objective is to help her become a better, safer, more integrated community ambulator. She works very hard, but she has to think about it. With every step, she's got to say, okay, where's my balance? Where's my weight? She needs to integrate quality of gait without attention.

Lena: Thinking and concentrating is especially true when I'm going down stairs, stepping off curbs, and looking out for uneven sidewalks. I'm always looking down. Only recently, I've started to be able to walk more spontaneously without thinking about every step. I am hoping that one day my walking will be more spontaneous.

Dr. A.: The gait pattern she demonstrated when she walked into our clinic the first day was partly compensatory and partly learned. When she used the Bionic Leg, it helped her to replace the abnormal learned gait pattern with a better pattern. She could also use the mirror to reinforce a better pattern of gait.

Question to Lena: You've commented that your gait is better since you started training with the Bionic Leg. Have you seen your toe clearance improve with training with the Bionic Leg?

Lena: I can see improved toe clearance since I started therapy with the Bionic Leg. In fact, if I'm not wearing shoes, when I'm at home, I'm now able to clear my toes on my own without wearing the AFO.

Dr. A.: Right before Christmas, I noted the carryover and integration of her gains in mobility. With less cognitive attention to her walking, her gait pattern was more symmetrical with less circumduction, a longer stride, and better toe clearance. Her mom and dad both commented about the improvement in the speed and quality of her gait.

Lena remains critical of her own achievements and she would like to be even better. However, the fact that she is walking faster, walking better, and tripping less and can walk at home without her AFO indicates her progress. She's a very dedicated patient, and I'm optimistic she will achieve the highest goals she has set for herself. I wish all patients had Lena's commitment and motivation.

NOTE from Dr A.: Lena progressed in training to be able to jog aerobically for 30 minutes at 3.5 to 4.0 mph while unweighted to 50% of her weight. Unfortunately, she developed a repetitive strain injury in the unaffected foot (left), interpreted as a stress fracture (without MRI to confirm). She was treated with steroid injections and non–weight bearing and was fitted with new orthotics. Over 3 months without training, she put on weight and developed some pain in her unaffected knee. She thinks this is a result of the additional weight and a tendency to return to

Continued

CASE STUDY 38-2—cont'd

her abnormal, asymmetric pattern of gait with increased circumduction. However, she has maintained the speed of her walking and she performed her balance tasks within normative time. She wants to resume forced intense exercise in a body-weight–supported environment to restore the quality of her gait as well as improve endurance and lose weight. She also notes that she has less pain and is happier when she is exercising more aggressively.

Although this is a case of a specific patient and a specific exoskeleton, the reader needs to be aware that the principles presented within Chapter 4 in the discussion of motor learning and motor control, and discussed throughout the entire text, have been used to facilitate neuroplasticity in this patient. Repetition of practice of the correct motor programs has been shown both in the literature and with this specific individual to create change even after 13 years poststroke. However, just as aerobic exercises are recommended for positive health for all individuals, especially as we age, aerobic and specific exercises have to be an ongoing investment for Lena as well. Exercise also has to be specific, and general exercises have to be an investment for the rest of her life. The case study was presented to help the reader identify and analyze how rehabilitation robotics can help individuals improve motor control for gait. Each therapist needs to analyze which of the many available therapeutic robotic tools can best assist an individual to maximize quality of life and independence after CNS insult. The reader is referred to the online video where the effectiveness of this exoskeleton can be observed.

APPENDIX 38-A ■ Websites for Learning More about Smart House Designs

www.smartthinking.ukideas.com/Publications.html
Publications for creating smart homes with smart home technology

http://hiddenwires.co.uk/resourcesarticles2010/articles20100104-10.html
Manuals and information for creating smart house designs in the United Kingdom

www.cen.eu/cen/Services/Business/Value/Documents/Project11SmartHouseServices.pdf
Smart house guidelines for the elderly and the disabled

www.servicemagic.com/sem/category.Specialty-Services-Disability-Chairlifts-Elevators.10431.html?entry_point_id=11832226&kw_id=house+disability&c_id=5433166634&m=cammgooglemain&entry_point_id=11832226
Search for architects for smart house designs in your area

CHAPTER 39

Complementary and Alternative Therapies: Beyond Traditional Approaches to Intervention in Neurological Diseases and Movement Disorders

DARCY A. UMPHRED, PT, PhD, FAPTA, CAROL M. DAVIS, DPT, EdD, MS, FAPTA, and MARY LOU GALANTINO, PT, PhD, MSCE

KEY TERMS

alternative therapies
belief based theories
complementary models
complementary therapy interventions
energy-based theories
evidence-based practice
movement diagnosis
movement therapies
transdisciplinary models

OBJECTIVES

After reading this chapter the student or therapist will be able to:

1. Differentiate the four historical to modern worldviews of health care delivery.
2. Analyze how complementary and alternative-based health care practices overlap with allopathic traditional medical models and movement diagnoses.
3. Analyze how mind, body, and spiritual interactions have the potential to lead to health, healing, and quality of life.
4. Compare and contrast the various therapeutic models discussed and identify similarities and differences between these and the traditions of Western medicine, OT and PT practice, and the International Classification of Functioning, Disability and Health (ICF) World Health Organization (WHO) model.
5. Appreciate the role of complementary and alternative approaches in the examination and intervention of individuals with movement-based problems as a result of neurological disorders.
6. Use evidence-based practice to measure outcomes in body system functions, functional activities, and life participation.

The use of complementary and alternative methods (CAMs) in the treatment of patients with neurological disorders and resultant movement problems is evolving into common practice. Clinicians and patients/clients are seeking nontraditional approaches to relieve signs and symptoms of neurological diseases, syndromes, and movement disorders as well as to attempt to alter the progression of diseases of the central nervous system (CNS) through unconventional movement therapies and manual therapeutic approaches. It is important that professionals working within a traditional rehabilitation environment understand the principles and practices of complementary, alternative, and even transdisciplinary approaches to the treatment of movement problems because many of these therapeutic approaches are being proposed as options in the management of body system problems and restrictions in daily life activities and independence resulting from neurological problems. The clinician needs to be cautious in the application of these treatment modalities. We do not want to accept alternative therapies as intervention solutions without significant evidenced-based research substantiating the use of these approaches. The reader must also be reminded that evidence comes from effectiveness, and many complementary approaches have established effectiveness.[1]

This chapter presents a sampling of alternative therapeutic models and philosophies that are available and could potentially assist patients/clients who have movement dysfunction because of CNS pathology. Most of the techniques discussed in this chapter have been firmly established by sound research; some less–evidenced-based models are also included to widen the scope of therapeutic models. Clinicians are continually being exposed to the therapeutic potentials of less scientifically established theories and therefore need to be aware of their existence and potential. Creating evidence-based practice is not an all-or-none principle, nor do we suggest that models that do not have a strong research base are ineffective. We do suggest that to adopt a model because of belief or the charisma of the founder will be and should be challenged by colleagues today and in the future. Models whose theoretical constructs are based on sound rationale or that link effective-based practice across multiple areas need to be scrutinized and approached cautiously but should not be nullified as potential alternatives. In time, if those models maintain their sound base, more research will be developed and their efficacy established. New models will also be created in the future that link and integrate theories with practice, and our professions will continue to evolve and offer better-quality care to the consumer.

HISTORICAL PERSPECTIVE

Jennifer M. Bottomley
Darcy A. Umphred

A historical perspective of how complementary and alternative therapeutic approaches have evolved to become increasingly part of the medical and rehabilitation landscape can be helpful to obtaining a broader scope of how they link to allopathic medicine of today. The language and rationale encountered in alternative methods can seem confusing and foreign to clinicians unfamiliar with modalities outside of the realm in which they were taught. With many of our patients/clients seeking alternative methods of intervention beyond what the traditional Western medical model can offer, the time has arrived for us to explore and understand the scientific basis for the apparent effectiveness of these interventions. The positive results experienced by many patients/clients who have received alternative interventions cannot be ignored. This is the impetus for the growing acceptance of alternative forms of therapy by the general public and many health care practitioners. Can we scientifically explain the effects of complementary and alternative interventions? And if so, how can we best integrate complementary and alternative approaches into our accepted, current, and changing approaches to neurological rehabilitation?

Looking at the evolution of health care throughout the world over hundreds and even thousands of years, general categories or worldviews have developed that best categorize philosophy of management of individuals with health care issues and their respective rationales for practice. In the following paragraphs a further discussion of these four worldviews will help the reader identify how the practice of health care today still fits within the second worldview but has begun to fractionate into the third worldview as linear research based on two variables does not explain the multiple variables involved both in disease or pathology and in recovery of function. In their book *The Second Medical Revolution,* Laurence Foss and Kenneth Rothenberg described levels of academic learning as being three tiered.[2,3] Starting at the top, the third tier comprises the applied studies and subjects for therapists, such as therapeutic exercise and electrotherapy. The second tier is the pure sciences on which these subjects are founded, such as anatomy, chemistry, physiology, and biology. The first tier is the "assumption of reality" (day-to-day observations) on which the pure sciences are based. This first tier consists of the basic assumptions found in "worldviews" today. Different worldviews yield different scientific bases, whether pure or applied. Alternative approaches used in medicine and rehabilitation are well established in "premodern" and "postmodern" worldviews. This is in contrast to the "modern worldview" customarily taught in current Western medical training. To present these methods in overview, it would be helpful to discuss these worldviews and how physical therapy (PT) and occupational therapy (OT) may fit into the scheme.

Essentially, there are four worldviews[4]: the premodern, modern, "fracturing or splintering," and postmodern views. The first worldview developed during prehistoric times and lasted until the sixteenth century. This is called the *premodern view.* In this perspective, time is cyclical rather than linear. In other words, it was believed that the sun, the moon, and the stars circle around the earth, the tides ebb and rise cyclically, and the seasons circle back again and again, using the same patterns each time, connecting with "deep time." Deep time is compared with profane time. Profane time is tangible, as in the time it takes rice to boil; or visible, as in the sundial; or sensible, as in the heartbeat. In deep time such perceptions are suspended, profane time stands still, and one becomes a part of time. It is in deep time that premodern man finds reality. Infused in this thinking is that life and death, the earth and the sky, are mysterious or mystical. In other words, they contain truth beyond human comprehension.

This is a hard perspective for many to grasp, yet the role of the scientist is to be a passive observer. Numbers were used to describe observed events, such as the days between the circling of the sun and the moon, and the number of hours between the ebb and high tide, but "there was no widespread assumption in the western world that natural processes in general had any intrinsic relation to numbers, to mathematics."[5] In other words, in Western science, these perspectives were not tangible, visible, or sensible…and so, historically, science moved on.

The second worldview, which began with Copernicus, is known as the *modern worldview.* It is the one with which the majority of the Western population would be most familiar and feel at home. In this view time is linear, progressing from start to finish. "The world is a rational, predictable, clockwork universe. Every bit of it can be predicted if you know one part of it. Purpose in life is to describe, generalize, predict, and control. Human beings are fairly mechanistic, separate, discrete entities from the rest of the universe."[4]

René Descartes (1596-1650), French philosopher and mathematician, and Isaac Newton (1642-1727) were two of the most important figures ushering in the "modern era." To Descartes, the world was logical, predictable, and intrinsically expressible through mathematics. The whole was obviously equal to the sum of the parts—categorical and hierarchical. The role of the scientist became that of an active, experimental, objective observer. If the numbers did not fit, it could not be real.

The modern era of the second worldview spanned the 1500s through the twentieth century. However, the near perfection of the view began to falter in the early 1900s with important discoveries in the field of physics. Although the hold of the second worldview on Western culture is still immense, it is splintering, as can be seen within our own professions.

Worldview 3 is about this fracturing, about the realization that the categorical, orderly clockwork is not a complete or necessarily accurate picture. It is a prelude to worldview 4. A small but growing number of people see the world in worldview 3, and fewer yet in worldview 4, but the effects are starting to be felt.

Worldview 4, postmodern, is complex, integrated, and nonlinear. It is about self-organizing and self-regulating systems, looking for patterns, and knowing that a small variation in the pattern can produce large changes. Time is a dimension, interwoven with the dimensions of space. Time and space can change, expand or shrink, speed up and slow down. Rituals are an important means for creating order. The whole is greater than the sum of the parts, and "we know and yet don't know." Worldview 4 has a lot of similarities with worldview 1. The pure sciences that arise from this worldview include systems theory, quantum physics, cybernetics, string theory, and fractal mathematics, which in turn affect many other fields of study, such as meteorology, ecology, business and economics, medicine, theology, movement science, and computer science, to name but a few. Research parameters, technology, and interpretation differ significantly from the assumptions of worldview 2 because scientific description is no longer considered purely objective, but rather *epistemology* (the view from which knowledge is gathered) is becoming "an integral part of every scientific theory."[6] Western medicine has begun to shift from the second worldview into the third worldview because a total linear approach to explain efficacy has not proven inclusive and cannot always explain why individuals do and do not recover from disease or pathology or the functional loss they produced. The professions of PT and OT have run into the same dilemma as Western medicine and are also making similar shifts. The incorporation of alternative or complementary approaches that take into consideration the mind, body, and spirit is becoming more acceptable as colleagues embrace the shift in thought process. Change will come. The rate and the depth of that change will depend on the openness of all of us to accepting different research methodology and outcomes while still embracing those linear research models of today that we believe lead to efficacy or evidence-based practice.

Today we practice within the paradigms of our professions, which have in the past aligned with Western medicine. Thus, for our ease, we can first start where we are, look at the medical profession, and discuss models or strategies that parallel the worldviews.

The roots of Western medicine extend back to Hippocrates, 400 BC, who provided a holistic picture of the state of health, writing that "Health depends upon a state of equilibrium among the various internal factors which govern the operations of the body and the mind, the equilibrium in turn is reached only when man lives in harmony with his external environment" (p. 23).[2] The basic assumption in this perspective is that health depended on a balance with mind-body and nature or the environment, and disease was a disturbance of this balance. Preserving the balance was the priority for the practitioner. Three means were used to ascertain the characteristics of an illness: a dialogue with the patient, observational assessment of the patient's appearance, and palpation of the soft tissues and pulses. The most important component of this approach was considered the dialogue with the patient/client. It was believed that the "meaning" of the illness to the patient/client, and his or her attitude and expectations were valuable diagnostic and prognostic factors. This coincides closely with the World Health Organization (WHO) International Classification of Functioning, Disability and Health (ICF) model accepted by rehabilitation professionals around the world.[7]

Descartes largely initiated the shift from a preservative approach for mind-body-environment integrity to the conventional curative thinking found in medicine today. He conceptualized reality as having two separate domains, one the body or matter, the other the mind. "The body is a machine," said Descartes, "so built up and composed of nerves, muscles, veins, blood and skin, that though there were no mind in it at all, it would not cease to have the same [functions]" (p. 32).[2] His ideas were closely tied to newtonian physics, which conceives the universe as a harmonious and well ordered machine. These concepts gave rise to the view that matter and nature were separate from humans, and thus one could observe without affecting what was being observed. The physician, then, could have complete objectivity when assessing the patient. The patient could be viewed as a biological organism whose function was reducible to interrelating physical parts.

The resulting medical model, known as *biomedicine,* was fully in place by the middle of the nineteenth century. Its characteristics may be considered as follows:

1. Disease or dysfunction is a "deviation from the norm of measurable biological parameters" (p. 23).[2] A patient/client is a biological organism whose dysfunction is reduced to the identified deviations. Treatments or procedures are then used to cure or at least improve the deviations, which in turn improves the biological condition.
2. Objectivity provides the basis for diagnosis or assessment and the subsequent rationale for treatment. Patients'/clients' descriptions of what they are experiencing and the clinician's observation are considered "subjective" and not given as great a value as the "objective" findings, such as laboratory or other measured tests.
3. Eventually biomedicine can address virtually all medical problems at least adequately, if not fully, through more knowledge and research.

It goes without saying that the biomedical model has produced stunning and tremendous accomplishments. Yet its restriction to physical causes of disease, in light of diseases and dysfunctions that are more widely recognized as having multiple causes, is creating a search for other answers. More of the public and some physicians and other health professionals are turning to alternative forms of intervention and healing. As stated in *Life* magazine in September 1996, "Why have alternative therapies in this country started to migrate from the margins to the center? One reason is that as allopathic medicine, a term commonly used to describe western techniques, becomes better at what it *can* do well, its limitations become more conspicuous. Allopathy is clearly superb at dealing with trauma and bacterial infections. It is far less successful with asthma, chronic pain and autoimmune diseases."[8]

Many of the alternative practices used in a medical setting today clearly come from premodern worldview sources, such as acupuncture, yoga, meditation, herbal remedies, and prayer. Just how some of these therapies work to restore health is difficult to perceive from a linear worldview 2 perspective. Frequently what happens is that alternative approaches are used to address areas of limitations in the biomedical model, in a complementary fashion. Alternative practices used this way do not supplant traditional medicine; rather, they support and enhance the options available in health care. A new worldview and medical model would not necessarily arise from this relationship, yet the conceptual framework is no longer cohesive. Ideas from ancient sources, as well as postmodern sources, are changing the previously complete and adequate image of the second worldview and consequent medical model. Grappling with these issues places one in worldview 3.

Evidence of these dynamics is apparent in the professions of PT and OT. In neurorehabilitation, for example, proprioceptive neuromuscular facilitation and neurodevelopmental techniques were developed in the middle of the twentieth century at a time when "rehabilitation" was being established as an integral part of unquestioned biomedical order. Both approaches, in their early form, worked primarily with the nervous system, and both used hierarchy and order. Patients/clients were to progress through a sequence of skills, such as the *developmental sequence,* that was invariable. The hierarchy was also found regarding the role of the therapist as the professional who could identify the pathokinesiology and "fix" it with the appropriate technique. The patient was the recipient of the treatment. With the advent of *motor control, motor learning, and neuroplasticity theories* over the last couple of decades, these fixed approaches have changed because the new concepts have influenced them. The developmental sequence, now termed *learning sequence,* no longer uses a strict hierarchy based on movement development of a child. Its treatment approach is moving away from emphasizing the therapist's role in identification and resolution of pathological movement and moving toward a science of functional movement that is based to a large extent on the role of the patient in his or her own capacity to problem solve, self-monitor the motor control system, and help establish outcome expectations on the basis of function, not pathological conditions. Last, an entirely new entity of neurorehabilitation has been formed recently as a result of concepts from motor control, motor learning, dynamical systems theory, and the understanding of neuroplasticity, which is known as the *task-oriented* or *functional approach.* Masters of the past used the available science to justify their respective approaches, but the one thing that all masters seemed to hold in common was a close relationship with their clients. They all let that relationship and the needs of the client determine how treatment progressed irrespective of the verbal explanation given for any sequential progression of treatment. They wanted the client to become functionally independent and have the highest quality of life that was possible for that individual. Those masters in the past did not have the science of today to explain why a treatment was effective. The fact that they created an environment that brought about the functional change in the patients would suggest that they intuitively used motor learning, motor control, and neuroplasticity because their patients improved in function over time.

One of the tenets of dynamical systems theory, as noted in the journal of the American Physical Therapy Association (APTA) in 1990, is that "biological organisms are complex, multidimensional, cooperative systems. No one subsystem has logical priority for organizing the behavior of the system" (p. 770).[9] The nervous system, then, is no longer a dominant subsystem with neurological patients. Rather, it is part of a self-organizing system that has multiple subsystems such as arousal, gravity, learning style, body weight, center of gravity, cardiovascular function, and so on. "No one subsystem contains the instructions for [an action]. . . . The behavior of the system is instead an emergent property of the interaction of multiple subsystems" (p. 771) (see Chapters 4 and 5).[9]

Added to these developments was the emergence in the 1980s of a new field of therapy intervention: vestibular habilitation for posture and balance, which is multisystem and multifunctional and inherently demands the use of motor control and learning principles and understanding of the mechanism of neuroplasticity and interactive systems theories. Systems concepts are used for both balance and the task-oriented approach, the concept being that "movement emerges from an interaction between the individual, the task, and the environment"[10] (see Chapters 11 through 17 and 19 through 31).

Orthopedic, or manual, PT appears to be firmly committed to the biomedical model, yet there is interest found in "being holistic," and treatment and exercise approaches are continually being developed that endeavor, to various degrees, to work with movement and function in a broader and more integrated manner (see Chapter 18).

Thus we find that today therapists are incorporating systems concepts, motor control, and motor learning theories into practice and experimenting with ancient sources of healing, such as yoga, tai chi, acupressure, and meditation, as well as refining skills in the traditional biomedical aspects of therapy. For our professions, holistic approaches have created and will continue to create change, and change can be confusing, threatening, and exciting all at the same time.

Worldview 2 still remains the dominant model within the Western allopathic health care delivery system. Two distinct observations may be made that show the prevalence of a worldview 2 approach. The first is that many colleagues continue to consider themselves to be objective observers separate from our patients. The second is that we endeavor to understand ancient, modern, and postmodern therapeutic concepts and research, frequently from a linear, mechanistic, categorical worldview 2 epistemology. Yet such a view at times does not suffice to explain what is happening. That is the dilemma of worldview 3.

Further changes will be experienced when a critical mass of the population turns fully, in all aspects of personhood, to "worldview 4," which, again, has great similarities to worldview 1. A big difference, though, is that at this time in history, we have scientific methods for understanding our nonlinear, complex, evolving, multidimensional, multilevel, continually interacting, irreducible world. Through systems theory we can handle, with sophistication, this multitude of complex detail, by working with its "sweeping simplicity and order in overall design."[3] Throughout the twenty-first century, as the growth of worldview 4 continues to evolve on many levels and in many fields of endeavor, it is entirely possible that it and its sciences will indeed replace, and not simply complement, worldview 2. And from there, the future has yet to be conceptualized and belongs to future students willing to venture beyond what is comfortable to best meet the health care needs of a world society.

ALTERNATIVE MODELS AND PHILOSOPHICAL APPROACHES

Darcy A. Umphred

Approaches to patient management that do not fall within a traditional allopathic medical model are often considered alternative or complementary. Although many of these therapeutic approaches have not been able to show effectiveness or efficacy in totality as an approach to medical management, neither has Western medicine. Although the *evidence-based method of medicine* is the accepted term for identifying outcome measures by reliable and valid instrumentations and interventions, there is controversy within the literature as to the validity of evidence-based medicine.[8-16] Personally, I have been a patient for the last two decades with interactive health issues that medical practitioners cannot explain. I have been told by at least seven excellent medical specialists that, when looking at their specific area of specialization, they have never seen the specific system problem that my body system presented. Thus, not knowing what it is, each doctor does not know specifically how to treat the problem. Medical doctors know there is some genetic basis and understand the specific system problem from a descriptive perspective, but cannot explain how and why the system problems interact. Thus a syndrome exists without a medical diagnosis. My medical case was submitted to the National Institutes of Health (NIH) as a potential syndrome for which they might find a diagnosis. NIH returned the case saying they do not have the ability to determine the diagnosis because it is much too complex. Doctors have had to stretch beyond their comfort zone to help me and work with me in order for me to remain on this plane we call life.

Medical practice is evolving, as are the practices of PT and OT. Future research will help validate many aspects of Western medicine, and some areas will be discarded. The same will happen to OT and PT practice. Similarly, research will demonstrate the effectiveness of many components of complementary approaches, although some components will need to be eliminated and new creative ideas and therapeutic techniques developed. One research problem encountered with complementary approaches is that these approaches consistently focus on the patient as a total human being with all the interactions of all bodily systems. This philosophy of the whole does not coincide with the linear, reductionistic physical research accepted by Western medicine, in which one variable is studied while another is controlled. PT and OT involve the same approach to research, in which one approach may be compared with another, such as overground walking versus body-weight–supported treadmill training. One may or may not be more efficacious, but the investigations as to why it is or is not, and what other variables are affecting the results of the study may be needed. These answers are still beyond our understanding. Until research models are developed and instrumentation becomes available that measures multiple systems at multiple levels of consciousness simultaneously, it will be difficult to prove the strengths of many aspects of alternative approaches to patient management. That does not mean the evidence is not there. It means our research skill may not have developed to the level of measuring all the influences that are interacting simultaneously during a complementary approach intervention. Finding those research models with supporting instrumentation is and will continue to be a challenge to therapists who choose to incorporate these interventions as part of their professional management of patients with neurological disabilities. If doctors had made the decision to stay within their respective branches of evidence-based medicine, I (D. Umphred) would no longer be editing this textbook. There are many holes in our understanding of movement science, just as there are holes in medical science. Answers to questions often do not come from research scientists but from clinicians finding solutions to specific patient problems. Once those potential solutions have been identified, research may be able to refine and identify the specific components that are affecting change as long as the tools are available to accurately identify the initial problem(s) and the intervention(s) creating change.

All of the models for patient management presented in this chapter have a common thread. All approaches focus on helping the patient/client maintain or regain a quality of life that is within that person's potential. The specific philosophy or conceptual framework embraced by any one approach varies. As various approaches are introduced in the following sections, subheadings will help the reader categorize similarities of philosophies. Even with the discussion of any or all of these approaches, whether accepted by our professions as the best available today or considered complementary, it still seems that we are looking through holes at what is total. The whole or total is made of all possible interventions that have, are having, and will have efficacy. When we no longer need to view problems with a specific model influencing our approach but are able to base our decisions on truth, we will finally be able to access what is truly available to us as practitioners and give the best possible guidance and suggestions to our patients to help them regain or maintain motor function as they experience life on a daily basis.

Movement Therapy Approaches

Equine-Assisted Therapy

Kerri Sowers, USEF National Paraequestrian Classifier

Introduction to Hippotherapy and Therapeutic Riding. At the 1952 Helsinki Olympic Games, a Danish dressage rider named Liz Hartel won the silver medal and inspired a renewed interest in the field of hippotherapy and therapeutic horseback riding (THR). Liz used horseback riding as a form of rehabilitation to aid her recovery from poliomyelitis, which left her lower extremities paralyzed.[17,18] The use of horses in therapy to improve physical and mental health has its founding roots in Greek culture. The term *hippotherapy* originated from the Greek word *hippos,* meaning "horse."[19] The renewed interest in hippotherapy and THR grew first in Europe and was especially popular throughout England. In 1969, the North American Riding for the Handicapped Association (NARHA) was founded; this organization established standards for the developing THR centers in the United States.[17-20] Recent studies conducted in North America show that approximately 90% of children with disabilities participate in THR programs, and the remaining 10% participate in hippotherapy sessions.[21]

It is crucial to understand the differences between hippotherapy and THR, as both programs are commonly offered at the same facility and are often mistakenly thought to accomplish the same goals. The American Hippotherapy Association (AHA) defines hippotherapy as "a term that refers to the movement of the horse as a tool by physical therapists, occupational therapists and speech-language pathologists to address impairments, functional limitations and disabilities in patients with neuromuscular dysfunction. Hippotherapy is used as part of an integrated treatment program to achieve functional outcomes."[20] During hippotherapy, the horse is used as a modality or treatment tool; the therapist and his or her assistants control the horse in order to effect a change in the patient/client. In contrast, THR teaches the client specific riding skills that allow the rider control of the horse's movement; the focus is on teaching horseback riding skills to riders with disabilities. AHA attempts to clarify the difference by stating that hippotherapy "treatment takes place in a controlled environment where graded sensory input can elicit appropriate adaptive responses from the client. Specific riding skills are not taught as in therapeutic riding but rather, a foundation is established to improve neurological function and sensory processing."[20]

Benefits, Indications, and Precautions. Hippotherapy and THR are felt to be beneficial because the equine walk provides a multidirectional input resulting in movement responses that closely mimic the movement of the pelvis during the normal human gait. The movement is both rhythmic and repetitive and allows for variations in speed and cadence. In hippotherapy the horse is used as a dynamic base of support (BOS) to assist in improving trunk control, postural stability, core strength, and righting reactions to improve balance.[22] Vestibular, proprioceptive, tactile, and visual sensory inputs are incorporated during a hippotherapy session. As stated by the AHA, "the effects of equine movement on postural control, sensory systems and motor planning can be used to facilitate coordination and timing, grading of responses, respiratory control, sensory integration skills and attentional skills."[22]

Hippotherapy is indicated for neuromuscular conditions characterized by reduced gross motor skills, decreased mobility, abnormal muscle tone, impaired balance responses, poor motor planning, decreased body awareness, impaired coordination, postural instability or asymmetry, sensory integration deficits, impaired communication, and limbic system dysfunction (impaired arousal or attention skills).[18,22,23]

Common conditions that may benefit from hippotherapy and THR include autism spectrum disorder, cerebral palsy, developmental delay, genetic syndromes, learning disabilities, sensory integrational disorders, speech-language disorders, traumatic brain injury (TBI), and cerebral vascular accidents.[22]

There have been a multitude of suggested therapeutic benefits from hippotherapy and THR, which affect many body systems. Suggested physical benefits include improvements in endurance, symmetry, and body awareness; development of trunk and postural control; improvements in head righting and equilibrium responses; normalization of muscle tone; mobilization of the pelvis, lumbar spine, and hip joints; and improved sensory awareness. Suggested cognitive, social, and emotional benefits include improvement in self-esteem, confidence, interaction with others, concentration, attention span, and communication skills.[18,19,24]

Contraindications for the use of hippotherapy or THR include excessive hip adductor or internal rotator tone accompanied by potential hip subluxation or dislocation, lack of head control (in large children or adults), pressure sores, spinal instability, or anxiety around animals.[18,24]

Regulations. AHA offers a Clinical Specialty Certification for therapists demonstrating advanced knowledge and experience in the practice of hippotherapy. Physical therapists, occupational therapists, and speech-language pathologists must have been practicing in their profession for 3 years (6000 hours) and have had 100 hours of hippotherapy practice within the 3 years prior to application. Certification is valid for 5 years; once applicants pass a multiple choice test they are entitled to used the designation HPCS.[22,25]

APTA recognizes hippotherapy as a treatment tool to address impairments and functional limitations in patients with neuromusculoskeletal dysfunction. APTA recommends that PT sessions that incorporate hippotherapy be billed as neuromuscular education, therapeutic exercise, or therapeutic activities based on the treatments completed. The American Occupational Therapy Association (AOTA) also recognizes hippotherapy as an interventional tool, which can be billed as neuromuscular education, therapeutic exercise, therapeutic activities, or sensory integrative activities.

Evidence and Clinical Implications. Research and studies concerning the use of hippotherapy and THR are limited but expanding. At the time of publication of this text, there have been no large, well designed, randomized controlled trials investigating the use of hippotherapy or THR. There have been several fair-quality randomized controlled trials and many nonrandomized trials that do support the use of hippotherapy in children with cerebral palsy. One systematic review investigating the use of hippotherapy and THR found improved gross motor function; normalization of pelvic motion; improvements in weight shifting, postural and equilibrium responses, muscle control, and joint stability; improved recovery from perturbations; and improved dynamic postural stabilization.[21] Studies have supported that hippotherapy can improve postural stability in individuals with multiple sclerosis (MS) and can assist in treatment of balance disorders.[26,27] Hippotherapy has also been shown to reduce lower-extremity spasticity in patients with spinal cord injury.[28] Support for hippotherapy has been shown by improvements in the areas of muscle symmetry, gross motor function (as measured by valid and reliable tools), energy expenditure, and postural control. Researchers suggest that hippotherapy will lead to improved head righting and equilibrium reactions and dynamic postural control, normalization of abnormal muscle tone or symmetry, improved muscle control, and better endurance. In addition, hippotherapy has the potential to contribute to psychosocial well-being and improved motivation by allowing interaction and acceptance with another living being and the opportunity to be mobile while astride the horse; being positioned high up on a horse gives the child the chance to be at eye level with his or her peers, and the fun of riding encourages participation and enjoyment of the therapy sessions. Continued research into hippotherapy and THR using larger, randomized controlled studies that investigate specific outcomes and account for the variations within a variety of neuromusculoskeletal conditions will be necessary to conclusively determine all potential benefits that exist.

Feldenkrais Method of Somatic Education

James Stephens

The Feldenkrais method is about learning the following:

> I do not treat patients. I give lessons to help people learn about themselves. Learning comes from the experience. I tell them stories [and give them experiences of movement] because I believe learning is the most important thing for a human being" (p. 117).[29] [parentheses added by the author].

Development of the Feldenkrais Method. As a boy in Palestine, Moshe Feldenkrais developed a method of hand-to-hand combat that was used by settlers for self-defense. Later, as a student in Paris where he trained in physics at the Sorbonne, he studied judo and became the first person in Europe to receive a black belt. When he injured his knee playing soccer, he relearned pain-free walking on his own. Later he studied with F. M. Alexander, Elsa Gindler, and Gurdieff. He also studied psychology, progressive relaxation, bioenergetics, and the hypnosis methods of Milton Erickson. And he was familiar with the physiology of his day: Sherrington, Magnus, Fulton, and Schilder. With this background, Feldenkrais developed two approaches to facilitating learning that are now known as Awareness Through Movement (ATM) and Functional Integration (FI).[30]

Feldenkrais was ultimately interested in the development of human potential. He saw that, although all people encounter trauma and difficulty in their lives, those who are most successful develop new, adaptive behaviors to overcome those difficulties. He proposed that a type of learning that reconnected the brain to the control of the musculoskeletal system would be the most effective way to approach this problem of adaptation. His initial thinking in this area is set out in his first book, *Body and Mature Behavior: A Study of Anxiety, Sex, Gravitation, and Learning*.[31]

Background Theory—Dynamical Systems Theory. For Feldenkrais, learning was an organic process in which cognitive and somatic aspects were completely integrated and interactive. Presented first in 1949, this idea prefigured our current sense of dynamic systems functioning of the brain and body.[32] The learning should proceed at its own pace in an individualized way following the learner's intention and guided by the learner's perception that the performance of the task, movements of the body, and interaction with the environment become easier.[31] This interactive cycle of action and perception has been described well by the motor learning model proposed by Newell.[33]

Learning is a complex process with overlays from the intention of the learner, interference from environmental distraction, misperception of the task and the body, desire related to self-image, fear of injury, or incorrect performance. Thus it is possible to learn poorly, incorrectly, or in such a way as to interfere with performance and not improve it. This kind of process has been suggested by Byl and coworkers[34] as the underlying cause of focal dystonia. One of the definitions Feldenkrais gave for learning took this process into account: "Learning is the acquisition of the skill to inhibit parasitic action (components of the action unrelated to the intention behind an action but resulting from a secondary intention) and the ability to direct clear motivations as a result of self-knowledge."[31] An adult engaged in learning to walk again after a stroke with a fear-related reluctance to bear weight on the involved limb would be an example of such a secondary intention.

The process of learning proposed by Feldenkrais is one of discovery. The outcome desired is one of increased awareness. Vereijken and Whiting[35] have proposed that discovery learning, in which learners are free to explore any range of solutions in learning to perform a task in any way that they want, is as effective as or more effective than any formal approach to motor learning involving controlled schedules of practice or feedback. This process of discovery has the added dimension of allowing learners to focus on the perceptual understanding of the body/task/environment as a component of the learning process. In the Feldenkrais method this discovery and perceptual learning process is explicit.

Our understanding of how experience and learning restructure almost all areas of the CNS is expanding rapidly.[36] A large focus of current thinking in rehabilitation is how to translate neuroplasticity concepts into more effective techniques for rehabilitation.[37-39] The method developed by Feldenkrais and practiced by people around the world who are trained in this method is clearly explained by these new principles, creating new approaches to rehabilitation.

Approaches to Feldenkrais Method. The two approaches to facilitating learning created by Feldenkrais, ATM and FI, are similar in principle and process although they differ in practice. They are essentially two methods for communicating a sensory experience that the client can consider and act on. The first requirement of the process is to create an environment that is comfortable, safe, and conducive to learning, whether the learner is being moved passively or creating the movement experience voluntarily. The second requirement is that the amount of effort associated with making the movements be reduced greatly so that it is possible to make fine discriminations about the effects of force acting on the system from outside, from inside, or both. The goal is to develop a rich understanding of changes throughout the system produced by small perturbations. This understanding becomes the basis for creating new solutions to movement problems as the client progressively approaches functional movements that she or he desires to perform.[40]

In FI the practitioner will manually introduce small perturbations into the learner's system after placing the learner into a safe position closely approximating some desired activity to be learned. Here the practitioner is providing the force inputs and the client is asked to attend to the changes created in response to the perturbation. For example, the practitioner might press gently into the bottom of the client's foot and ask the client to notice where in the body movement and pressure are felt as a result. This will be repeated a number of times and then some other forces or movements will be introduced. The guiding idea for the practitioner might be to build sensory experiences in the body that are associated with a particular movement, such as rolling. This goal is rarely explicitly expressed to the client and is left to emerge in the client's understanding of the experience: "Oh, now I am rolling," or "This feels like rolling to me." Also there is no strict expectation by the practitioner about what specific movement might emerge. Thus it is possible to create novel and unexpected outcomes of how a particular task might be best performed by this particular person at this time. This allows for a process of assessment that is continually evolving as the intervention is unfolding.[40]

In ATM the practitioner verbally provides suggestions for movements for a client to explore and asks the client to focus on the sensory outcomes throughout the body. Thus the client introduces the experimental forces into his or her own system with the intention of understanding how the body as a whole responds. The underlying idea, however, is the same. In my practice, I use FI as a form of communication when clients do not understand how a force might act on the body or when they are unable to produce a range of movements that we might desire to explore. An example might be in a case where spasticity prevents fine discrimination in both sensory and motor realms.

In practice with an individual client, it is common to move back and forth between ATM and FI during the same session. The session is usually focused on the development of understanding and performing a specific function: turning, rolling, standing, stepping, and so on. ATM is a verbal process in which clients perform their own movements; thus a practitioner can work with many individuals simultaneously. At the same time individuals within the learning group are free to respond differently from one another in ways that may be appropriate only for them as individuals.[41] Because ATM is under the active control of the client, this method is often a more effective tool in reestablishing voluntary control (Case Study 39-1).

CASE STUDY 39-1 ■ SUE: HEREDITARY SPASTIC PARAPARESIS

Sue was a toe walker as a young child. She remembered her father sitting in a chair all the time, his legs too stiff and weak to walk. In her mid 20s, she too began to develop weakness and stiffness in her legs. At the age of 36 years she was diagnosed as having "uncomplicated" hereditary spastic paraparesis (HSP).

Uncomplicated HSP involves extreme spastic weakness, some loss of sensation in the lower extremities, and hypertonic bladder reflexes. It progresses slowly over many years without exacerbations or remissions. Individuals experience progressive difficulty walking and often require canes, walkers, or wheelchairs. They typically retain normal strength and dexterity of the upper extremities, have no involvement of speech, chewing, or swallowing, and have a normal life expectancy.

Sue was first seen in our outpatient clinic when she was 38 years old. She worked as an office manager at a local college. Her office was up a set of stairs that was becoming more difficult to negotiate. She also owned a horse that she had not been able to ride because she was no longer able to mount because of her increased spasticity. Sue was a large, muscular woman at 5 feet 10 inches and 175 pounds.

On initial examination she reported pain in her right knee with weight bearing (8/10) and pain in her low back (5/10). Her proprioception appeared to be intact. She had decreased passive range of motion (ROM) in dorsiflexion bilaterally and hyperextension of her knees bilaterally, greater on the right. There was tightness in the iliotibial band and hip adductors, flexors, and rotators bilaterally and the extensors of the back from the lumbar through the cervical spine. Her muscle strength was 3+ to 4−/5 at all joints of both lower extremities, with the right being generally weaker than the left. She also had mild weakness in her trunk flexors (3+/5). There was sustained clonus in plantar flexors bilaterally and one beat clonus in her quads on the right. She had normal active ROM throughout her upper extremities with normal (5/5) strength throughout. Sue stood statically with her hips externally rotated, knees hyperextended, hips forward with her back extended in a stiff swayback posture. Her shoulders were retracted and tight. She was unstable to a moderate challenge and reported falling frequently. Her gait was stiff with knees hyperextended and toe drag bilaterally. She achieved swing by doing a lateral trunk tilt with contralateral circumduction with each leg, no arm swing and a foot flat landing. She used a straight cane for balance. Her self-paced gait speed was greater than 75 ft/min (1 mph = 88 ft/min). She reported "it feels like I have a stick up my back and if I try to go faster, my knees lock and I'm really in trouble." Sue was assessed to be a good candidate for a Feldenkrais intervention, and a series of FI and ATM lessons was planned.

The first FI lesson was an exploration of the organization of turning and rolling from supine. I began this exploration with Sue supine and observed her postural organization in that position. She lay with her arms flat at her sides, palms up. Her legs were adducted and externally rotated and her back arched away from the mat table. I put a small towel roll under her neck and back and a 4-inch roller under her knees to allow her extensors to relax somewhat. I began the exploration by rolling her head gently and found a lot of resistance to that movement. Attempts to do small amounts of turning of a leg or bending of the knee also met with similar resistance. I then began working through a process of manually shortening muscles that were tight and overworking. I began with neck extensors by gently holding the cervical spine in a slightly more extended position progressing to the extensors of the trunk by compressing the ribs from the side to cause a slight lateral flexion first on the right then on the left. The relaxation focused last on the legs by holding the knee and hip in a slightly more externally rotated and flexed position first on the right, then on the left. Going back to the neck, pressure was exerted down through the first rib on the right to cause a slight lateral flexion to the left through the spine. This movement was now easier than before, with force being translated further down the spine into the lumbar area. Next the pressure was combined with rolling of the head to the right, first passively, then with small active movements. The instruction was to turn the head only as much as could be done with almost no effort. The same process of compression of the spine and turning of the head was repeated from the left side of the neck. The interaction then progressed to the right leg by pushing through the right foot so that the force translating up the leg caused lateral flexion of the spine to the left, then again from the left leg. The right foot was then turned to initiate external rotation and flexion of the right leg first passively and then actively. Sue began to be able to control that small movement on the right leg with minimal effort and then repeated on the left. We then began to link the movement of the legs, trunk, and head together in a sequence in which she began to be able to roll her head to the right, flex her right leg and left leg together toward the right, and allow her trunk to flex and turn toward the right. During this process, Sue's attention was directed to sensing the movement and timing of different body segments; to feel the forces created in her body by the movement of one segment and how they impeded or facilitated movement of other segments. This lesson ended with Sue being able to roll more easily onto her side from supine than she had been able to do in a long time. This session took about 45 minutes, during which I was doing some work with another patient at the same time. When Sue came up to standing after this lesson, she reported feeling like she was stuck into the ground solidly. She felt shorter, softer, and better balanced. Her feet were flatter on the floor, and when she walked she did not drag her toes on the floor.

At the beginning of the second session on the following day, Sue was tested again on the treadmill and was now able to walk about 120 ft/min. The second lesson began again in supine and reinforced and developed the movements of the first lesson. Sue learned to slowly roll to her right side, moving her arms at the same time so that she could take weight on them, flex her legs until they came over the side of the mat table and then push

CASE STUDY 39-1 ■ SUE: HEREDITARY SPASTIC PARAPARESIS—cont'd

herself up to sitting all in one motion and then reverse this process slowly until she was lying supine again. She learned to roll herself into a fetal position back and forth from the left to the right without her legs stiffening in between, and when she sat up she was able to actively flex her legs up to put her shoes on, which she had not been able to do for at least a year. After this lesson she reported that she had been able to move her foot easily from the gas to the brake in the car without slipping and that she was able to get onto and ride her horse for the first time in several years.

In the third lesson, we worked more purely with ATM because Sue was now able to control more movement more easily herself. During this lesson Sue learned to roll with minimal effort to the left and right while holding her knees and then to reach to her ankles and roll while holding her ankles without stiffening her neck in the process. Flexing her hips had become easy.

The fourth lesson involved standing, weight shifting, and turning. The instructions related to keeping movements small and slow and maintaining a feeling of softness that she now had developed. She explored movements of allowing her knees to flex while she shifted weight to one foot and moving her body over the weight-bearing foot to get a sense of how she could distribute weight differently across her foot on the basis of changing the configuration of her upper body and movements of her hips. These movements included exploring the effects of intentionally stiffening and softening her back and neck to feel any changes that happened in control of her weight bearing, knee flexion, and ankle. Weight on one side was increased while the other was unweighted, and the unweighted leg was lifted in a controlled manner, easily and effortlessly, feeling the support of the skeleton for the process of lifting. At the end of this lesson, Sue was able to lift her foot easily up onto the 19-inch-high surface of the mat table and bring it back to the floor without disturbing her balance. At home she was now able to step up onto her horse from a low step without other assistance.

In the fifth and final session, more time was spent doing an ATM lesson related to standing balance, turns in walking, and bending to the floor. In this session and at the end of the previous one, we also spent time in transfer training with toilet, tub, car, and floor transfers and gait training on smooth and uneven surfaces and for speed on the treadmill. She still used a cane for balance (or a single hand support on the treadmill) but now was able to walk on the treadmill at 175 ft/min, well more than double her initial speed, without dragging her toes or hyperextending her knees. She did complain of some back pain and calf pain, but this was determined to be from exercising muscles that had not been used in years and resolved after several days. I recorded the ATM lessons with a lapel microphone and recorder as we did them and gave her the tapes to use at home as part of her home exercise program.

Three months after discharge, as a passenger in her sister's car, Sue was in an auto accident and sustained a herniated disk at C5-6. After this she had decreased mobility for several months. During this time she lost her understanding of how to control her movement and returned to us 6 months after her initial visit to review what she had done earlier. After several series of lessons over a period of several months, she achieved a level of function higher than previously so that she was able to walk and go up and down stairs without any support.

Evidence of Effectiveness. The theory underlying the Feldenkrais method predicts that there should be changes in perception of the body or body image. Although there have not been a lot of studies in this area, there are several that support this prediction. Elgelid[42] reported positive changes in body perception, as evaluated by the semantic differentiation scale in a group of four subjects after a series of ATM lessons. Dunn and colleagues[43] reported that subjects who had had a unilateral sensory imagery ATM lesson perceived their experimental sides to be longer and lighter and demonstrated increased forward flexion on that side, linking the changes in perception to changes in motor control. Batson and coworkers[44] have shown that ability to image movement is improved in people poststroke after a series of ATM lessons, and furthermore that there is a high positive correlation between the Movement Imagery Questionnaire (MIQ) score and improvements in balance assessed by the Berg Balance Scale.

There is not a lot of literature evaluating the efficacy of the Feldenkrais method in general and even less specifically for people with neurological diagnoses, as a result of the complexity of the problems and the multiple system involvement of the individuals. Evidence-based studies on effectiveness are more easily identified. In a review, Stephens and Miller[40] divided the literature into four different areas: pain management, postural and motor control, functional mobility, and psychological and quality-of-life impact. Much of the literature is in case report format. A small amount of the literature is controlled study format, with some of that using randomized control groups. The work on pain management suggests that the Feldenkrais method may be especially effective in treating pain that is biomechanical in origin. This concept may be applied to work with pain in patients with neurological diagnoses, especially pain caused by biomechanical malalignment. No research has been done in this area with neurological patients. Hall and colleagues[45] found improvements in balance (Berg Balance Scale [BBS]), mobility (Timed Up-and-Go Test [TUG]), functional activity (Frenchay, Short Form 36 [SF-36]), and vitality (SF-36) in a large group of elderly women compared with control subjects as a result of a 16-week ATM intervention. These results have been confirmed by Vrantsidis and colleagues[46] and Connors,[47] also using ATM with a group of elderly women. In the areas of psychological and quality-of-life impact, Kerr and colleagues[48] have shown decrease in state anxiety in subjects who participated in ATM lessons, and Laumer and colleagues,[49] working with young women with eating disorders, have demonstrated positive changes in self-concept, self-confidence, and behavior resulting from participation in ATM lessons. Many of these findings are beginning to be reproduced in clinical populations with neurological diagnoses. Most of the studies to date have been done with people with MS. Colleagues are beginning to look at ATM effectiveness in patients after a stroke (cerebrovascular accident [CVA]).

Research

Multiple Sclerosis. The initial study, done in Germany in 1994, looked qualitatively at the effects of a 30-day ATM experience on a group of people with MS. The investigators concluded that ATM improved overall well-being, resulted in greater self-reliance of the participants, and led to better self-acceptance and a more positive self-image.[50] After that, Johnson and colleagues[51] studied the effects of FI in people with MS. Although they did not find any significant mobility changes, they did report a decrease in perceived stress in the FI compared with the massage controls. Stephens and colleagues[41] reported the cases of four individuals who participated in the same ATM classes over a period of 10 weeks. Three of four reported large improvements in their Index of Well-Being score. All subjectively reported improvements in gait. However, there were no measures of gait that consistently improved across the group. Instead, it was found that changes were appropriate to the participant's individual needs and resulted in a greater sense of control. In a follow-up to this study, using a randomized controlled group design, Stephens and colleagues[52] found improvements in postural control and balance confidence measures, along with a strong tendency toward an increase in self-efficacy and decreased falling. It was also found[53] that the ATM group had significant improvements in memory of recent events and perception of positive social support. It is interesting to note that they also had a decrease in pain effects.

Cerebrovascular Accident. The original publication in this area is the classic work, *The Case of Nora,* in which Feldenkrais explained his work in great detail and described improvements in sensation, perception, and mobility of a woman several years after a right-sided CVA.[54] More recently, results from pilot studies are just beginning to be reported in patients with diagnoses of CVA. Connors and Grenough[55] reported a decrease in spatial neglect as measured by line and star cancellation tests in a patient after a series of ATM lessons. Nair and colleagues[56] reported the recovery of upper-extremity function and the return to playing golf in a 68-year-old man after an 8-week program of ATM and FI. This Feldenkrais program was begun only after a 9-month program of traditional rehabilitation had left him with a nonfunctional hand. The Feldenkrais program included mental imagery and bimanual activities. This subject was also studied before, during, and after the Feldenkrais program with functional magnetic resonance imaging. The magnetic resonance imaging analysis showed that there was a return to higher activity in the involved contralateral primary motor cortex with activity of the right hand compared with higher activity in the ipsilateral M1 and SMA that has been shown in other reports of CVA recovery[57] before the Feldenkrais sessions began. This finding suggests a return to more normal brain function even after a period of 1 year after the stroke. A small pilot study (three subjects)[58] found an average 33% decrease in movement times on the Wolf Motor Function Test. In another pilot with four subjects, Batson[59] found significant improvements in Dynamic Gait Index ($P = .033$, 55% average) and the BBS score ($P = .034$, 11% average) and a 35% improvement on the Stroke Impact Scale (SIS). A larger study is in progress to further assess these findings.

Other Medical Diagnoses. There are some preliminary findings with other neurological diagnoses. Shelhav-Silberbush[60] reported improvements in motor, sensory, kinesthetic, perceptual, and learning functions in two case studies of children with cerebral palsy. Shenkman and colleagues[61] reported improvements in balance, gait, and functional movement in two people with Parkinson disease as a result of interventions that were based partly on a Feldenkrais approach. Gilman and Yaruss[62] have reported significant improvements in several young children who had problems with stuttering. Ofir[63] reported improvements in flexibility, mobility, and level of dependence in two young women who had sustained traumatic brain injuries.

Conclusion. The Feldenkrais method, in its two forms, embodies a process of somatic learning that aims to develop the perceptual capabilities of clients as it underlies the control of movement. Recent literature suggests that predicted results of improved body perception and motor control are supported in work with people with neurological diagnoses. These findings are encouraging and suggest that the Feldenkrais method will make positive contributions to our understanding and methods of rehabilitation. However, we must approach these findings with caution because many are from case studies or pilot studies done with a small number of people. Research continues to substantiate these claims at a higher evidence-based level. Refer to Box 39-1.

The Pilates Method

*Brent Anderson**

German-born Joseph H. Pilates developed his unique form of movement therapy in the early 1900s. As a young man, Pilates was affected by a multitude of illnesses that left him physically weak. In an effort to strengthen his frail body, Pilates studied yoga, martial arts, Zen meditation, and ancient Greek and Roman exercise. His experiences led him to develop his own unique method of physical and mental conditioning. In 1926 Pilates brought his movement exercise program with him to New York City. Joseph Pilates's studio was soon embraced by many artists and choreographers from the dance companies of Martha Graham, George Balanchine, and Jerome Robbins. At the time, traditional allopathic medicine lacked the knowledge of how to restore injured dancers to their prior level of activity. Pilates encouraged nondestructive movement early in the rehabilitation process and worked to correct underlying biomechanical problems. This early movement intervention without pain was believed to hasten the healing process and allowed dancers to quickly return to the stage.

Almost a century later, the Pilates method has gained popularity within the rehabilitation setting because of its assistive nature in restoring functional movement. Rehabilitation practitioners are currently using the method in a variety of fields including orthopedics,[64-67] pain management, women's health,[68] neurological rehabilitation, geriatrics, pediatrics,[69,70] and even acute care. Most Pilates exercises in the rehabilitation setting are performed on specifically designed apparatus: the Reformer (Figure 39-1), the Cadillac table (Figure 39-2), the Wunda Chair (Figure 39-3), and the Ladder Barrel (Figure 39-4). The apparatus regimen evolved from Joseph Pilates's original mat

*The author wants to thank Matt Butler for his contribution to the Pilates section in the fifth edition of this textbook.

BOX 39-1 ■ RESOURCES AND TRAINING

1. Only people who have graduated from accredited training programs may practice the Feldenkrais method. Training in the Feldenkrais method in North America is overseen and accredited by the Feldenkrais Guild of North America (FGNA).
2. For information about training programs and the Feldenkrais method, contact the FGNA at (800) 775-2118 or e-mail to info@feldenkraisguild.com. There are more than 1000 certified practitioners in the United States and Canada. To find a certified practitioner in your local area, go to the FGNA website: www.feldenkraisguild.com.
3. In 2004, the International Feldenkrais Federation (IFF) founded the *IFF Academy Feldenkrais Research Journal* as an online resource for research on the Feldenkrais method. You can find this journal on the Web at http://iffresearchjournal.org.

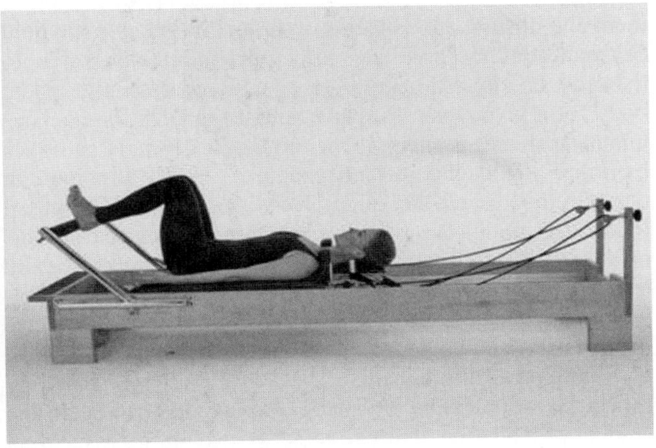

Figure 39-1 ■ The Reformer apparatus used in Pilates.

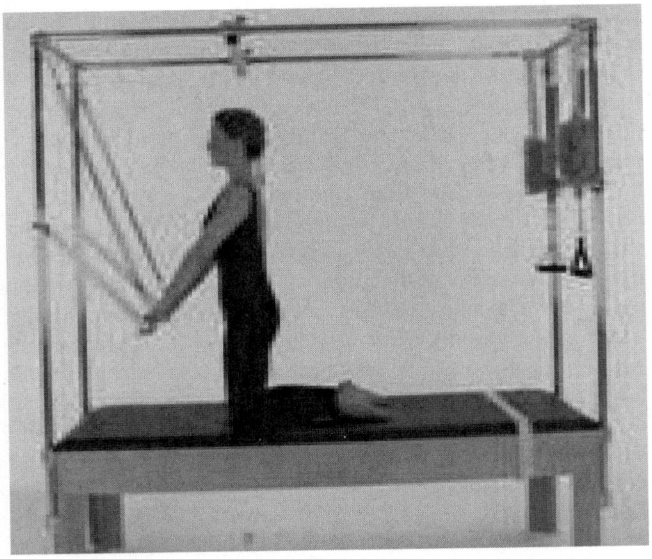

Figure 39-2 ■ The Cadillac table apparatus used in Pilates.

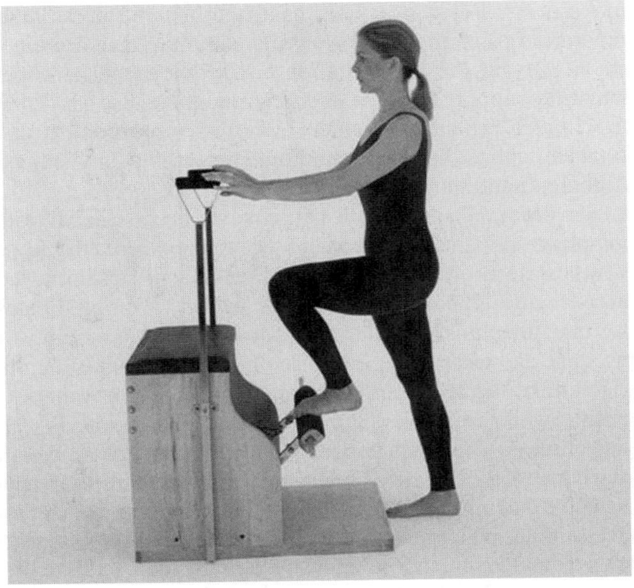

Figure 39-3 ■ The Wunda Chair apparatus used in Pilates.

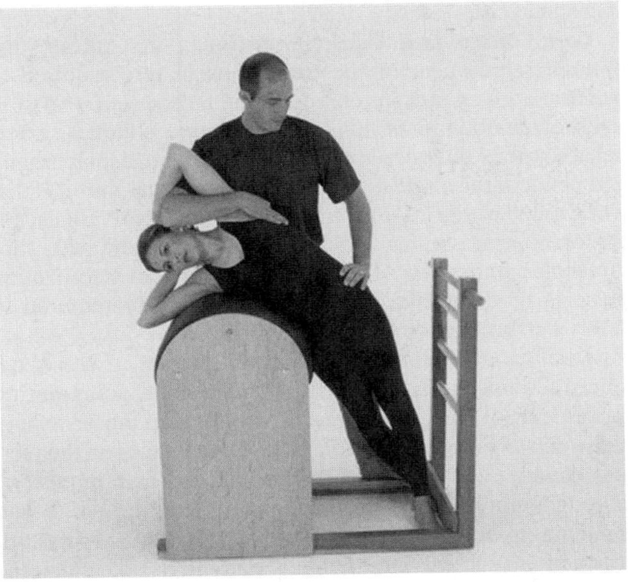

Figure 39-4 ■ The Ladder Barrel apparatus used in Pilates.

work, which was shown to be too difficult for many injured individuals. On the apparatus, springs and orientation to gravity are modified to assist an injured individual to successfully complete movements that would otherwise be difficult or limited. Ultimately, by altering the spring tension or increasing the challenge of gravity, an individual may progress toward functional movement safely, efficiently, and without pain.

Pilates Principles. Joseph Pilates espoused only three guiding principles according to the Pilates Method Alliance: (1) Whole Body Healthy, (2) Whole Body Commitment, and (3) Breath. A number of the first-generation Pilates practitioners known as *the Elders* expanded Pilates principles to include concentration, control, precision/coordination, isolation/integration, centering, flowing movement, breathing, and routine. Polestar Pilates has modified the eight first-generation principles into six principles that have a greater practicality in the rehabilitation environment and stronger scientific support than the classic principles. The six Polestar Pilates principles include breathing, core control and axial elongation, spine articulation, efficiency of movement, alignment, and movement integration.*

Breathing. Faulty breath patterns can be associated with complaints of pain and movement dysfunction.[71] Pilates movements create an environment where breath facilitates improved air exchange, breath capacity, and posture. During Pilates exercise, breathing is used to facilitate stability and mobility of the spine and extremities. Because of the movement of the rib cage on the thoracic spine, inhalation can promote spinal extension while exhalation can promote spinal flexion. Breath may or may not facilitate movement based on where the breath is occurring. If accessory breath were to occur while attempting spine extension, it would not have a positive movement on the spine articulating into extension. It is then important to realize that the direction of movement in the ribs facilitated by breath determines whether or not breath facilitates movement or not. Likewise, breath may assist with stability of the spine through the coordinated contraction of the diaphragm and the lower abdominal muscles, which both attach to the lumbar spine and pelvis.[72,73]

Core Control and Axial Elongation. Core control is the optimal recruitment of the trunk musculature required to perform a given task in relation to the anticipated load. The transversus abdominis, internal abdominal obliques, external abdominal obliques, multifidi, erector spinae, diaphragm, and pelvic floor muscles are key organizational muscles that work together during movement in healthy individuals.[74-76] Motor control studies indicate that the coordinated, subthreshold contraction of these local and global stabilization muscles modulate the level of spinal stability required to safely perform activities of daily living.[77]

Axial elongation is the proper alignment of the head, spine, and pelvis that provides optimal joint spacing during movement. Correct joint spacing avoids working or resting at the end of range, which can place undue stress on the inert and contractile structures of the trunk and extremities.[78,79] Through emphasis on axial elongation of the spine and maintaining appropriate joint spacing, soft tissue surrounding the joint can move more freely and the risk of injury can be minimized. Recent discussion has challenged the Pilates approach to core control, attempting to minimize its benefit. As yet, there have been no studies that show that the use of the local stabilizing muscles interferes with or minimizes core stability compared with increasing the intraabdominal pressure by pushing out into the abdominal wall and the hypertrophy of the musculature inside the thoracolumbar fascia. This is more likely to represent rigidity and stability and might serve a population lifting severely heavy weights.

Spine Articulation. Spine articulation is the equal distribution of movement throughout the cervical, thoracic, and lumbar spine. As a motor control principle, spine articulation is where distribution of movement equals distribution of force. It has been suggested that repetitive movement at a hypermobile spinal segment may result in microtrauma or macrotrauma.[80-82] Hypermobility is often a result of a lack of movement in a neighboring segment or joint.[83] Pilates exercise attempts to facilitate a change in movement strategy during functional tasks. Patients are trained to distribute movement in the spine over a greater number of spinal segments, thereby decreasing potentially harmful forces at the hypermobile segment. The ability to segmentally move the spine decreases unwanted stress and shear of the spinal segments and increases the efficiency and fluidity of movement. The clinical findings of decreased low back pain as a result of Pilates exercise may be due to changed strategy that reduces the stress afforded to the pathological segment.

Efficiency of Movement. Efficiency of movement is the minimization of unnecessary muscle contractions that tend to interfere with healthy movement. The excessive recruitment of antagonist muscles is obstructive and significantly increases the amount of energy required to perform a task.[84,85] This principle can be applied to functional movement skills as well as performance skills. Inefficient motor recruitment can often be recognized by the amount of tension or faulty posture in the head, face, neck, and shoulder girdle, in relation to the thoracic spine and trunk.

Alignment and Weight Bearing of Extremities. Alignment and posture are concepts often incorporated in the field of rehabilitation. The Pilates principle of *alignment* refers to the most energy-efficient posture (static or dynamic) of the body for a given task. Proper postural organization can significantly decrease energy expenditure during daily activities by improving mechanical advantage.[86,87] Faulty alignment in the extremities and the spine can be a source of decreased ROM, loss of joint congruency, early fatigue of muscle groups, or abnormal stresses on inert structures and may potentially cause degeneration and injury.[88,89]

Pilates provides a closed chain environment that facilitates compression and decompression forces on the axial skeleton and extremities through a full ROM. Adjusting the spring resistance or patient's orientation to gravity can alter the amount of load. The ability to regulate load on the basis of an individual's physiological limits, set by age or pathological condition, allows practitioners to more safely and effectively stress the skeletal and soft tissue systems. Theoretically, these forces can help stimulate osteoblastic activity and provide nutrition to a larger surface area of the joint and its surrounding connective tissue.[90-92]

Movement Integration. Many forms of rehabilitation focus on treating limitations of anatomical structures and neglect the neuromuscular reeducation required to learn to regain the motor control necessary to perform a complex task. Pilates provides a more holistic approach by emphasizing the synthesis of mind (motor control) and body (physical strength and flexibility) to achieve fluid movement. Mobility, control, and coordination of the extremities with the trunk and the trunk with the extremities are examined and trained through motor learning and repetition of practice. In addition to the physical and mental capacity to complete a task, the environment in which a task is performed can greatly affect the success of movement organization.[93,94] Pilates provides an environment that can be modified on the basis of a patient's impairments and limitations, providing a safe, successful, and pain-free movement experience.

Clinical Application. Within the Pilates environment, faulty movement strategies are broken down into components

*The six modified Pilates principles were developed by the Polestar Pilates method.

and addressed through task-oriented interventions. By adaptation of the environmental constraints, such as gravity, assistance, and BOS, the degrees of freedom that must be controlled by the nervous system are reduced.[95] The successful manipulation of the environment can hasten the functional reeducation process and allow exercises to be safely progressed until the desired outcome is achieved. Pilates practitioners are also trained to be able to modify any exercise so it is pain free for the patient. It has been suggested that successful, pain-free movement, in addition to enhancing physical attributes, helps to alleviate anxiety.[96,97] By decreasing anxiety levels and improving self-efficacy, the development of chronic pain and dysfunction related to the injury may be prevented.[98-100]

The potential causes of faulty movement patterns include congenital defects and abnormalities, habitual adaptations, and compensation because of injury. Motor control problems associated with the pathological condition need to be addressed before the application of therapeutic interventions that are temporary coverups for problems that have deeper roots. For example, a pathological condition at the L4/L5 segment could be a result of faulty movement patterns in the hips and other lumbar vertebrae. The lack of movement in surrounding joints might be the mechanism of the lesion; however, treatments are often focused on the site of the lesion rather than the mechanism of the lesion.

One problem often encountered in the rehabilitation setting is flawed movement progression. On a spectrum of movement progression, practitioners often jump from passive movement to resistive movement too quickly. Through facilitation of assistive movement, a pattern can be practiced without irritating the lesion. Assisted movement with the use of springs can allow for a decrease in unwanted muscle activity or guarding that is often associated with pain, weakness, or abnormal tone. As the pattern progresses and symptoms decrease, assistance decreases and dynamic stabilization can be emphasized to challenge the newly acquired mobility or stability in a more functional and gravity-dependent position. Resistive movements are introduced only after adequate dynamic stability of the trunk is demonstrated through controlled movements that prevent excessive loading of the injured tissue. The five environmental conditions in Pilates that are altered to allow a therapist to facilitate motor changes are the following[93,101]:

1. Narrow or widen the BOS.
2. Raise or lower the center of gravity.
3. Lengthen or shorten the length of the levers.
4. Decrease or increase the degree of assistance (spring tension).
5. Progress from a foreign environment to a familiar environment.

Traditional modes of muscle conditioning focus on isolating specific muscles and producing a maximal voluntary contraction. Although this has been found to positively alter the targeted muscle, the gains achieved have not always been shown to correlate with functional return. Pilates progresses patients through stages of motor learning via neuromuscular reeducation of functional movement patterns and emphasizes efficient recruitment of motor units. The patient is first trained to become aware of or gain a perception of current movement strategies. Then the patient must cognitively learn a new strategy. Finally, the patient must practice or take action until efficient with the new strategy of movement. Task-specific interventions are progressed from a foreign to familiar environment by altering the level of assistance and the patient's orientation to gravity.

Summary. Pilates is an effective exercise system that works well in conjunction with traditional PT and OT practice. The Pilates-evolved apparatuses allow patients to safely perform exercises that improve strength, flexibility, balance, coordination, and motor control in an environment that can be easily progressed as they advance in their rehabilitation process. In addition, Pilates is thought to address the psychosocial components of an injury that lead to chronic pain or disability by decreasing anxiety and improving self-efficacy.[98,99] Early return of functional movement after an injury helps to physically and mentally empower individuals with regard to the demands of life and is crucial in the long-term success of patient outcomes. The Pilates environment is a clinical tool that can be used by practitioners to provide patients with a safe, successful, and pain-free way of restoring function and quality of life.

Tae Kwon Do

Clinton Robinson, Jr., 9th Degree, Grand Master
Darcy A. Umphred, 4th Degree

Philosophy. The overall philosophy of Tae Kwon Do (TKD) can be summed up in the student oath recited by all practitioners at the beginning of each class: *"I shall observe the tenets of Tae Kwon Do: courtesy, integrity, perseverance, self-control, and indomitable spirit."* The tenets are to be practiced outside as well as inside the training hall in all aspects of life. All aspects of these tenets reflect CNS control and neuroplasticity and incorporate cognitive, emotional, and motor aspects into an integrated whole. The oath continues with, *"I shall respect the instructors and seniors,"* which refers to having respect for all people—our teachers, our parents, our peers, our students, our patients—all individuals with whom the student may interact throughout a lifetime. *"I shall never misuse Tae Kwon Do."* No matter what motor skill a student develops, it is not to be used to build one's ego or to injure another unnecessarily. *"I will be a champion of freedom and justice."* Individuals are expected to develop a sense of responsibility for those less fortunate than themselves and to be active participants in the development of humanity as a whole. These tenets are basic philosophies of both OT and PT. Empowering our patients to overcome their movement limitations and once again actively participate in life should be the goal of all therapeutic treatment outcomes. *"I will build a more peaceful world."* Understanding that change begins with self, and developing and integrating the mind, body, and spirit while helping others do the same, will set an example not only in the classroom but in our society both nationally and worldwide, so that others may improve themselves. The profession of OT has identified similar educational outcome criteria for students who graduate from an accredited educational program. PT has begun to integrate the mind, body, and spirit into outcomes, but as of today PT has not embraced the interactions of those three human characteristics as part of the accreditation criteria set forth by the Commission on Accreditation in Physical Therapy Education (CAPTE). Yet there are commonalities between the practice of TKD and some of the expectations of students in educational programs in both PT and OT.

The overall goal of TKD training is the development of self-sufficiency through rigorous physical and mental practice. With this training, an inner balance or peace can be attained, thus balancing all aspects of a person's life. Students are expected to strive for their own personal excellence versus comparing that skill with another's. Thus, individuals with physical challenges are always encouraged to participate. Their challenges and expectations are different, but achieving personal excellence gives them the same respect and confidence that any other student would receive. Thus, TKD as a movement science empowers participants to gain or regain a feeling of empowerment over the mind, the spirit, and the physical body. It engages all students to participation in a community of people who all begin as novices and advance only as each respective mind, body, and spirit grows as a whole unit. At times an individual may have physical restrictions that limit the ability to do specific techniques, but that never limits one's ability to grow and advance as a human being and continue to learn as a student of TKD.

Philosophy of Training. Training in TKD consists of three primary components: forms, breaking of solid objects, and sparring. Other martial arts focus on some of the same components. The practice of tai chi focuses on the first component, forms. But with practice a TKD student not only will have the skill to perform a sequential pattern or combinations of simple and complex movements (forms), but also will overcome a perceived obstacle (board), and interact with another person using quick movement techniques with control (sparring).

Poomsee. Poomsee is a prearranged dance of defensive and offensive techniques against an imaginary opponent. The practice of poomsee increases the practitioner's memory, coordination, balance, and body awareness. All poomsee components have predetermined patterns of movements with a proper beginning and ending point that include various stances, along with hand and kicking techniques. The complexity and difficulty of these forms increase as the student progresses. Simple movements and combinations of patterns challenge beginners, and appropriate levels of complex patterns challenge the highest-ranking black belts. Thus all individuals studying TKD are challenged to be in a state of growth and learning.[155]

Kyukpa. Kyukpa is breaking of solid objects such as boards, concrete, and bricks using a body part as a weapon. Kyukpa represents overcoming limitations and obstacles and facing fear. It requires tremendous concentration and belief in one's abilities. In addition, it allows participants to demonstrate the power they have attained, thereby increasing self-confidence. Self-confidence is the primary attribute in conflict resolution skills and leads to the understanding that there are few situations in life in which physical confrontation is necessary. Board breaking helps teach the student that an object, such as a board, is only an obstacle if you, the student, empower that object to have that role. Once the board is broken and the limb has passed through the obstacle, it no longer is an obstacle. This philosophy reflects life and plays a role in the establishment of values and motivation by teaching practitioners to go beyond the known and through the obstacles that life poses.

Kyorugi. Kyorugi is actual sparring between two people using both defensive and offensive techniques learned through fundamental TKD practice. Kyorugi can be further broken down into two types. (1) In *one-step sparring,* practitioners take turns initiating a prearranged attack—one person attacks while the other defends. This allows the practitioners to engage each other without risk of injury to either party. It also allows them to practice proper distancing and execution of the techniques. This develops confidence in the ability to use the techniques properly if the need arises. (2) In *free sparring,* neither opponent knows what the other is going to do. Although free sparring may appear dangerous to one untrained in TKD, it is a relatively safe activity. Free sparring requires respect for your partner and absolutely controlled motions at all times. It is an exercise in which the aim is for all involved to increase their skill level.[156] It develops the practitioner's quick motor responses, confidence in his or her abilities, and overall awareness as well as a cooperative learning environment.

Although both offensive and defensive techniques are viewed as equally important, all training is begun with blocking techniques to indicate that TKD never allows any initial offensive attack in its technique. Blocking techniques are practiced diligently so that they may function equally as offensive techniques. This way one can defeat an opponent, whether in the classroom or in real life, without either suffering or inflicting serious injuries. This builds self-confidence and replaces a perception of the "role of a victim."[157] Defensive techniques are not only power against power but truly reflect power of the attacker and deflection by the opposition. This deflection can stop the attacker, redirect the power back onto the attacker, or incapacitate the attacker in order for the opposition to get away. The skill in redirecting the force and intent of an attacker is not too different from redirecting a patient's motor pattern into a direction that would be functional as a motor program. The TKD practitioner and the therapist are working with the pattern of movement presented to them. The intent of the TKD student would be to disempower the attacker, and the intent of the therapist would be to empower the patient.[158-160]

In TKD training, all students begin in the same place. There is no concern for one's status in life. The white belt is used to denote the beginning student. With all students beginning at that level, it allows another aspect of training that is critical to all students and individualized. Training encompasses setting and achieving goals or empowering oneself toward excellence and to one's own quality of life. In TKD, there is a belt ranking system, and the object is to progress through the various levels of proficiency, culminating in attainment of the black belt. Everyone, regardless of social status or physical skill, has the same opportunity to advance in TKD. Students who persevere and obtain a first-degree black belt learn that they have only begun their circle of growth and learning. With additional years of training, students may advance in black belt ranks that should reflect a greater understanding and acceptance of those initial tenets. The circle of growth will always lead to further integration of mind, body, and spirit and an inner peace and balance.[161] The balance of mind, body, and spirit is the core of other complementary therapy paradigms and ultimately seems to be an element linked to health and healing.[162]

Tae Kwon Do and Complementary Therapy.[154,161,163-167] Although TKD is a martial arts style whose original intent was not to heal a body system condition or to allow one to regain a functional movement activity lost after some acute health care crisis, the concepts and procedures learned, repetitively practiced, and transformed into life behavior have established the foundation for health and healing in individuals. Most students in TKD fall within a health and wellness model of life. *Their choice to participate is not based on a bodily system problem as often seen in a PT or OT clinic. These individuals are looking to participate from a wellness perspective and expect that Tae Kwon Do will enhance their balance and their cardiopulmonary and musculoskeletal systems through exercise.* Yet many individuals have experienced some aspect of musculoskeletal system problems during their lives. These individuals, as a result of life activities, have forced the CNS to adapt and accommodate to prior bodily system problems such as ligament tears or *physical or emotional* trauma from bullying in school. These experiences create change whether the deficits are motor, cognitive, or affective.[168,169] Similarly, with identified chronic motor limitations that have caused functional *activity* restriction after a birth trauma, an external head trauma, or an internal insult, TKD can help maintain existing motor function, cognitive integrity, emotional balance, and a feeling of self-worth in the face of a long-term and possibly progressive neurological problem. All these components encourage an individual to participate in life and base advancement not only on the standards of TKD but also the individual goals set by each student.

As in all martial arts, TKD requires active participation by the student. When any TKD movement pattern is examined, certain motor control components are seen to be interacting. There are a variety of activities that generally occur during a class. First there are warmup exercises, after which the student will work on (1) her or his respective form or poomsee or hyung (dancelike patterns that may have 18 to 100 different movement sequences), depending on the level of advancement; (2) sparring, which is done either with one partner moving with an identified pattern while the other stays in one position or with both moving and learning to respond to the movements or feints of the other; or (3) learning to focus and perform specific strikes or blows that will lead to skills in board or brick breaking or defending oneself against a life-threatening attack.

During warmup, a student stretches and builds up power, using specific movement, balance, timing, concentration, and cardiopulmonary functions that set the stage for the remainder of the class. When doing the forms, the student will need to work on balance, postural tone, the state of the motor generator, synergistic patterns of movement, trajectory, speed, force, directionality, sequencing, reciprocal patterns, and the context within which the movement is being done. Similarly, memory of the specific pattern, movement sequences, and direction of the movements requires concentration. As the student progresses in rank, the specific patterns become more and more complex, increase in number of specific movements, and frequently change from quick movements to slow, controlled patterns. This repetition of practice and increase in difficulty leads to higher skill and cortical representation.[170,171] If other students are also practicing in class, then each individual needs to be aware of the total environment to respect the space of all other students. This unique individual experience during a group activity allows for variance during each class and thus should lead to greater motor learning and cortical representation.[171,172]

When students are learning and practicing either one-step sparring or free sparring, they are not only working on learning combinations of movement patterns and how they interact or conflict with those of their partners, but they are also learning how to control their emotional responses to threatening situations. Little in life is worth hurting another—a basic principle of TKD. During sparring, the potential for injury is directly correlated with the control over the force and direction of movement of each individual. That control can be dramatically affected by emotion (see Chapter 5). Once students learn to control the emotional aspect, their skill and techniques become procedural, which allows their cognitive analytical ability to drive responses (see Chapter 6). The student is then ready to begin study of the mind, body, emotional, and spiritual connections that need to intertwine and become harmonious if the student is to learn the true meaning of TKD. Sparring *should be* a controlled situation in which injury or damage to another person is never acceptable. Research over the last 10 years has pointed out the danger a student faces during TKD competition. Mistakes both in techniques themselves and in emotional force placed behind the techniques do create a potential danger to students.[173-178] Therefore safety gear is required at all TKD competitive events for color belt students. Mouth guards are always required no matter the level of the student. As in other contact sports, injuries do happen, but fortunately most are minor, and a quick recovery the result. During class the instructor is never to spar above the skill level of the student, nor is the student to enter into a sparring match with the intent to show the teacher or another student just how good he or she is. In reality, when a student does take that emotional stance, the motor skills reflect only just how much more that student needs to learn. Feedback from others is a powerful learning tool for students at all levels. It is the teacher's responsibility to help redirect students' emotional stances and help to teach that TKD represents control, not lack thereof. Board and brick breaking is the activity in which a student can demonstrate force production as it interlocks with trajectory, speed, and position in space. If any of these perceptual or motor variables are incorrect, the student will not succeed at going through the obstacle. These skills are taught and practiced not to damage or destroy the wood or brick, but rather to learn to go beyond or through the obstacle. Once the specific body part used as a trajectory goes beyond the obstacle, it no longer remains an obstacle and the student feels great satisfaction. In reality, to be successful at these tasks, the hand, elbow, or foot that is used to go through the brick or wood is only an extension of the body. Success is based on the learner's ability to tie the entire body's motor response, its rotation, its balance, its trajectory, its force, and its speed into a motor program that will project through one or more obstacles as a knife cuts butter. If the student, emotionally, believes that the obstacle will not break, it will not! The student will stop the movement before completing the task and often empower the wood or brick as a successful obstacle versus empowering herself or himself to overcome that obstacle as if it were not there. This concept is a critical element of TKD. It is also a critical component of any client's learning of any motor program, turning the program into a functional activity, and improving one's quality of life and ability to participate in that life's adventure. If a patient's CNS is convinced that the movement is not possible, then that individual will fail. Without internal motivation by an individual to accept the possibility of success, acceptance of failure is embraced. This internal environment plays a key role in any individual's overcoming what he or she perceives as an obstacle in life.[179] It is the role of the TKD teacher and the therapist teacher to empower the student to the possibility of success while creating an external environment that will enhance the probability of that success.[155,170] To ask TKD students to perform motor skills above their level of competence can lead to injury and the embracing of failure. Failure often stops the motivation to continue to learn. Patients in a therapeutic environment are no different. They need an environment that creates safety, promotes success, and empowers the individual to overcome life obstacles.

Those who respond best to TKD training to maintain motor function are individuals who are motivated to move, enjoy interactions with others, have cognitive integrity, and have some control over their motor system. When instructing a TKD club of individuals who had all had traumatic head injuries, the teacher, a TKD instructor and therapist who had worked for more than 25 years in the area of neurological rehabilitation, found that using therapeutic skills through TKD movement patterns augmented the students' learning and helped them to regain motor function through guided activities without the students ever realizing there had been any kind of therapeutic intervention. To those students, they were learning and advancing in a martial arts style, were tested and judged according to their development of skills, and felt accomplished as adults participating in an adult activity. Carryover and improvement in balance, postural integrity, reciprocal patterns of movement, and control of trajectory, force, and speed, as well as development of emotional stability and confidence, could be easily identified and evaluated by the use of standard objective measurement tools if so desired. Expected outcomes would be improvement in those areas of motor control just mentioned. As long as the student continued training, improvement would be expected and carryover into other life activities anticipated. These are the principles of neuroplasticity and have meaning both within the predisease or wellness model as seen in TKD[37,180] and after acute injury, disease, or insult to the CNS.[181-185] Whether sequential movements are taught as new movements as in TKD or require relearning of functional movements taught by physical and occupational therapists, the end result leads to an individual participating in a life activity.

As therapists, we want individuals who have been discharged to continue with movement activities that encourage their participating in life as a whole individual. TKD provides an excellent movement-based activity that leads to physical fitness[186-192] and has been studied in relation to changes in vitamin and hormonal levels in elite athletes.[193-196] One systematic review studied martial arts training, looking at a variety of martial arts styles including TKD and tai chi. Both styles lead to an increase in health status of participating individuals.[197]

When considering the elderly population, a group frequently referred to both PT and OT for movement and balance disorders, TKD training has been shown to improve balance, walking abilities, and somatosensory organization in standing.[198,199] Owing to immobility, muscle weakness, and decrease in balance in standing, the elderly population certainly presents a fall risk within the community. Falls obviously can lead to hip fractures and months of medical and therapeutic interventions. Looking at a martial art that encourages participants to stretch to their respective limits of stability both with fast and slow movement patterns, a valid question must be asked: "Would TKD be harmful to this population, especially if the participants had osteoporosis?" Two research studies investigated that question and determined that training in martial arts such as TKD can teach fall training, prevent hip fractures, and be safe for individuals with osteoporosis.[200,201] Literature has shown that accelerated patterns of the head and pelvis during upright walking can lead to falling in community-dwelling elderly people.[202] Individuals with Parkinson disease show evidence of body system problems causing impaired head and trunk control, thus increasing their risk of falling.[203] During TKD practice as a beginner or advanced student, individuals learn to use the head and hips in rotational patterns while maintaining an upright posture and moving their upper extremities.[204,205] It has also been shown that as students increase their skill with practice and time, they also increase their "neural efficiency," which increases their reaction time and the ability of their brains to make spatial judgments.[206] All these components should help maintain the physical capabilities of an elderly individual while providing a social environment in which to practice.

TKD not only affects the physical and mental capabilities of the learner, but it also has the benefit of changing one's mood to a more positive feeling.[207] This emotional response helps to motivate all students to return to practice and once again regain that positive reaction. This drive becomes deeper and deeper as an individual advances from a white belt to degrees within the black belt ranks.

Over the last decade many research articles have been written that look at one aspect of TKD training, whether it be strength, balance, coordination, motivation, cardiac fitness, emotional self-control, or the effect on the many other bodily systems that interact during a TKD workout. The reader must understand that it is all those elements that make up a TKD student, teacher, or master. In the future, more research will identify this martial art as a potential form of physical exercise for all populations of individuals who have comorbidities after CNS injury (Case Study 39-2). Physicians and therapists should consider recommending this martial art as an exercise activity for individuals who wish to maintain or regain their abilities to participate in life activities.[198] Until then, students of all ages will be welcomed into TKD studios and encouraged to reach beyond their perceived potential. The age ranges of TKD students now include the elderly population, with classes focusing on strength, balance, and core work without the need for strenuous sparring or board breaking.[208] A TKD instructor will modify each senior's class experience to allow each individual to reach his or her potential without injury or trauma.

CASE STUDY 39-2 ■ A TAE KWON DO CLASS OF SIX INDIVIDUALS AFTER TRAUMATIC HEAD INJURY

This case study is not of an individual patient but rather a group of individuals who had previously had TBI. (Refer to Chapter 24.) All participants were at least 2 years postinjury. They received services at an Easter Seals facility, where they participated in adult swimming twice a week as well as having unlimited use of the gym and strength training equipment. They all had inquired about receiving martial arts training from that specific facility. Holding a fourth-degree black belt in TKD and as a physical therapist whose focus had always been directed toward individuals with brain injury, I was asked if I was willing to instruct these individuals in TKD twice a week. I agreed to volunteer as long as the students agreed to continue for 3 months. The students ranged in age from 23 to 35 years, and all were male. Four of the students had had one TBI; one student had experienced two TBIs, and one had sustained three. Four students had been injured initially in auto accidents, and two in motorcycle accidents. One student had received his second injury in a fight. The individual who had experienced three head injuries had sustained all three on his motorcycle. All students communicated using English, and all were independent in basic activities of daily living. Two members shared an apartment, three lived in a group home, and one lived with his parents. They all were on public assistance for their primary income, although three worked part time in a job-training program. Four students had a high school education, and two had Associate of Arts (AA) degrees.

Each individual student had slightly different movement problems; however, they all had balance and postural issues as well as impairments in force and directional control of their upper and lower extremities during gross mobility skills and during activities that required fine motor functional control in the upper extremities. As they were all friends and worked out together on exercise equipment at the facility at least three times a week, they all looked physically fit with large muscle mass in the arms, shoulder girdles, hips, and quadriceps. All were independently ambulatory, although one did have mild gait ataxia during the swing phase of either leg. Similarly, that individual exhibited mild ataxia in the upper extremities but had learned to compensate using pure muscle power to slow the movements. All participants stated that falling was an issue but that they did not know exactly what caused them to fall. Three of the participants had mild to moderate hypertonicity primarily in the lower extremities and axial muscles and thus moved slowly and with cognitive attention. No individual could do rapidly alternating movements when performing alternating punches or blocks with the upper extremities. Initially no student's balance allowed him to independently stand on one foot while kicking with the other. All students would either fall or take a step with the kicking foot in order not to fall. No formal evaluation was done to assess baseline motor control because it was not a therapeutic environment but rather a training environment for a martial art that was considered a sports activity for fun.

As stated earlier, the TKD instructor had a fourth-degree black belt as well as having been a physical therapist for over 20 years. She wondered, if she used her handling skills while teaching TKD, would the students recognize her PT skills? Or would they accept only that she was the instructor and thus was teaching them the skill of TKD? The answer to that question came quickly. The students acknowledged her martial arts skill and were amazed at their own ability to learn. They never thought that they were doing anything other than learning TKD while in the class.

Three basic kicks were taught. A *front kick* required the student to balance on one leg while picking up the opposite leg in hip, knee, and dorsiflexion and then extending the entire leg forward with the foot in plantarflexion while the toes remained in dorsiflexion. The leg remains in neutral rotation throughout the entire kick. Obviously, the higher the instructor asked a student to kick, the more difficult it became for the student. The second kick is called a *sidekick.* This kick requires the student to first abduct with slight external rotation and flex the hip with the knee flexed and foot in dorsiflexion and slight inversion, then to extend the hip and knee into full extension, abduction, and neutral to slight internal rotation while the foot remains in strong dorsiflexion and slight inversion so that the strike from the kick is at the heel. The higher the kick, the more abduction the student must control and maintain throughout the kick. Refer to Chapter 5, Figure 5-10, in which the instructor is performing a sidekick while in the air, but has chosen to hold back full extension. If he did not have control and chose to finish the kick, the individual standing would probably have her neck broken. The last kick is called a *roundhouse kick* and it requires that the leg be picked up into hip abduction, external rotation and extension with the knee flexed and the foot in flexion and eversion. The kick then progresses from hip extension into hip flexion as the hip rotates out of external rotation to slight internal rotation with knee extension. The foot can strike either with the top of the foot in total plantarflexion-inversion or with the ball of the foot with the ankle in plantarflexion-inversion while the toes remain strongly flexed. The height of the kick will depend on the ability of the student to control and contract the flexors and abductors while performing the kick from the beginning to the end. Figure 5-11, in Chapter 5, is an example of the roundhouse kick at the end of the excursion. All kicks were practiced first with the instructor guiding the students' movements. Then the students were asked to visualize the kick and to perform the movement independently as they progressed. The instructor could easily correct errors in movement using handling. With time and practice each student was able to perform all three kicks. Initially, they were asked to do the movements slowly with control. This required each student to gain the postural power to control his trunk and weight-bearing leg while holding and controlling the kicking leg as it moved in space from the initial position to the end. In time each student was asked to control this pattern while kicking at a target in space. Finally, the mitt or bag target was moved after each kick, requiring the student to adjust to the changing requirement for the second kick.

The upper-extremity patterns taught were reciprocal punches, overhead blocks, low or groin blocks, and knife hand strikes. The reciprocal punches began with the arm first, beginning at the side with the shoulder in external rotation and adduction, elbow flexed, the wrist in supination-neutral extension-flexion and the fingers strongly flexed. The arm then

Continued

CASE STUDY 39-2 ■ A TAE KWON DO CLASS OF SIX INDIVIDUALS AFTER TRAUMATIC HEAD INJURY—cont'd

moves into shoulder internal rotation and flexion with elbow extension, forearm pronation, and neutral position of the wrist, with the fingers remaining flexed. The final position of the arm should be directly in front of the person. The arm should be straight with the line of force coming from initial scapular retraction to scapular protraction as the force goes down through a straight arm with the wrist stabilized and the fist clenched. The other arm begins at the end of the first arm's trajectory and then is moved back toward the initial position of the first arm. All upper-body movements, whether a punch, a downward block across the body to block a punch or kick to the groin, a strike to the side, or an overhead block to protect the head from a round kick or a punch, required learning these new motor patterns with the final goal of controlled movement by each student. All patterns required a combination of movements that began in one type of rotation at the shoulder and wrist and ended in the reverse pattern. The diagonal patterns required a combination of flexion, extension, and rotation and were taught either as a blow to an opponent attack or as a block from an opponent punch or kick. Initially none of the students could perform any of the kicks or blocks taught, and they enjoyed kidding each other about coordination and balance problems. As the activities were considered fun, no one expected anything other than enjoyment and success from the practice.

In reality, no student had the coordination to perform any of the kicks or upper-body movements, *but* they were told truthfully that no TKD student can perform these movement with coordination when they start at the beginner level as white belts.

Obviously, increasing the ROM in the axial joints was an important aspect of their martial arts training, as was gaining stability in the distal joints in order to prevent injury. All students had previously learned to gain control over their axial joint activities by reducing ROM and building muscle mass. Although their axial muscles could produce power for short periods of time, learning to develop control throughout an entire movement pattern was difficult, especially if the student was asked to hold the kicking leg or the punching arm in a position for 30 seconds, 1 minute, or longer. The instructor was able to help the students learn to slow down movements while retaining control over each movement itself from the beginning to the end of the range. Through handling techniques that guided the student through these specific movement patterns, or the use of resistance by the instructor to slow down the movement, the student learned not only the specific patterns required for TKD, but also to control various degrees of speed of each movement. With practice and motor learning, each student began to gain motor control. The focus was on accuracy of the kick itself and not on the force produced. In fact, the students were asked not to produce a high level of force until they had the control over the movement itself.

As the students practiced kicking against a heavy suspended punching bag or against a padded mitt held by the instructor or another student, they all improved in their ability to perform these movements. They were then taught to perform these movements in patterns similar to a dance, which in TKD is considered a form. This combination of movements encouraged forward motion as well as turning in both left or right directions. As they practiced shifting their weight from foot to foot or balancing over one foot while kicking with the other, their posture and balance automatically improved. At the end of each week the instructor would ask each student how many times he had lost his balance or fallen during the week? The numbers went from multiple times per day, to daily, to a few times per week, to very seldom over a 3-month period of practicing TKD with formal instruction two times per week.

The therapist-instructor could see that the ambulatory skills of each student had also improved, as did their balance, even though the students were not in class to improve motor control over either of those activities. As the students learned to perform the upper-body patterns first slowly and then with more speed and power, they all talked about how activities such as eating were so much easier and more social. They would also comment that they didn't have to think about controlling the fork or keeping the food on the spoon. Other activities of daily living were also improving. They thought the instructor asked those questions just because she was social and interactive, not because she was using her PT skill to help them regain motor control, and wondered if there was carryover. It was truly a wonderful learning experience for the therapist because she watched motor learning and neuroplasticity change the way these people moved and interacted. They practiced on their own and together. They encouraged one another while enjoying the learning. They would laugh at their lack of coordination but also acknowledged the improvement they saw in each other. They were taught to work together, with one performing a kick or punch while another blocked or redirected the movement. These activities caused a huge variety of perturbations with inconsistent force and direction, requiring the student to spontaneously respond while remaining in vertical control of his body in space and ready for the next movement. They knew they not only gained control over their bodies but also had the ability to avoid injuring their partners and friends.

Each student's skill improved to the extent that all of them were ready to advance from a white belt to a yellow belt rank. They were able to enter a regular class with other TKD students and had earned the respect from all the students in the new class and the belt they wore with pride. This experience certainly proved to one therapist that integrating normal TKD activities while using the professional skill of a clinician helped six individuals dramatically improve motor control in their daily lives and positively affected the way they felt about themselves.

Yoga

Mary Lou Galantino

Yoga is an ancient Indian mind-body practice that has been around for more than 2000 years.[209] It focuses on a combination of meditation, mindfulness, self-exploration, breathing control, and body movement to improve flexibility, focus, balance, and strength. The two types of yoga popular in the United State are Hatha and Iyengar. Hatha involves holding the body in particular postures known as *asanas* for periods of time while controlling breathing rate and focus.[210] Iyengar yoga uses the aid of supports, props, and belts to allow better control to perform the *asanas*.[211,212] Although yoga has been accepted in other countries for centuries, the evolution in the United States has been a recent phenomenon. Research on the effect of yoga in the musculoskeletal areas is promising,[212-214] yet research in the neurological population is still in its infancy and in need of larger randomized clinical trials. This section will present a general analysis of the benefits and efficacy of yoga for individuals with a variety of common neurological issues.

Carpal Tunnel Syndrome. Physical and occupational therapists treat carpal tunnel syndrome (CTS), an upper-limb neuropathy caused by compression of the median nerve. Symptoms involve numbness, tingling, and pain from repetitive movements that respond to a variety of treatments.[215,216] Two studies specifically explored the use of yoga to treat subjects with CTS. A yoga trial with 42 individuals (median age 52, range 24 to 77 years) tested the effectiveness of a yoga regimen on CTS symptoms. Those in the experimental yoga group were given 11 postures designed to stretch and strengthen the upper limbs, along with relaxation techniques, twice a week for 8 weeks at a local geriatric center. A control group was given wrist splints or no treatment at all.[217] Significant improvements in grip strength, pain reduction, and Phalen sign were noted. However, no statistically significant change was recorded in sleep improvement, Tinel sign, or median nerve conduction. Participants showed improvements in pain and function 4 weeks later.[217] A second study investigated the impact of yoga in patients with osteoarthritis. Twenty-six patients (52 to 79 years) performed 1-hour yoga sessions each week for 8 weeks. Subjects reported significant improvement in joint and hand pain during activity.[218] Larger randomized clinical trials could provide definitive evidence for patients with CTS.

Stroke and Hemiparesis. Strokes are the number one cause of adult disability in the United States and Europe, with 4.7 million individuals in the United States living with the sequelae of stroke. Extreme difficulties encountered while performing simple movements result in a sedentary lifestyle in this population. Resultant muscle atrophy further potentiates fall risk.[219]

A pilot study with four subjects observed the impact of yoga as a treatment for impairments poststroke. Baseline measurements included the BBS, Timed Movement Battery (TMB), and SIS version 2.0. Three of the four participants in this study had statistically improved BBS scores indicating improved balance, improved self-selected speed on the TMB indicating improved ability to perform everyday tasks, and positive changes in quality of life based on the SIS.[219]

Other factors may have affected the outcome of this pilot study, including differing adherence to the home exercise program with varying participation levels, degree of impairment, and fear of pain, which reduce participation with certain asanas. This preliminary study showed that those who adhered to the program improved more than those who did not follow it as closely. Yoga appears to have some level of positive impact on function in poststroke patients; however, future research is needed to confirm these findings.[219]

Multiple Sclerosis. Individuals with MS can suffer from virtually any neuropathy, fatigue, ataxia, and chronic or acute pain. Cognitive, digestive, visual, and speech problems may also occur. Although there is no cure for MS, patients have life expectancies similar to those unaffected by the disease, and yoga may be an option to manage the various impairments encountered through the years.[220] It is interesting to note that 65% of those diagnosed with MS use some CAM, with yoga being the most popular.[221] Perhaps the best study to date was a 6-month study that compared Iyengar yoga and exercise interventions. Participants underwent multiple cognitive assessment tests such as the Stroop Color and Word Test and the Cambridge Neuropsychological Test Automated Battery to test reaction times in performance of certain tasks that are difficult for individuals with MS. These tests measure attention and visual and auditory abilities to determine the impact of cognitive abilities. Alertness, mood, fatigue, and quality of life were also measured using tests such as the Profile of Mood States (POMS), the SF-36, electroencephalography, and physical activities such as a timed walk.[220] Of those who completed the study, both the exercise and yoga intervention groups had greater quality of life based on data from self-assessment forms (SF-36), a reported increase in vitality and energy, and a decrease in fatigue.[220] This is the first study on the use of yoga for patients with MS, and the findings need to be confirmed using larger randomized controlled trials.[220]

Epilepsy. Yoga, as well as other mind-body practices, has shown promise in helping control seizures. One yoga meditation trial reported a 62% decrease in seizure occurrence at 3 months, 86% at 6 months, and 40% of the subjects becoming seizure free.[221,222] The patients in this study had hyperventilation-related epilepsy caused by anxiety, so the meditation and controlled breathing exercises along with the asanas may have led to a better understanding of how the subjects could control their diaphragm, resulting in the high success rates. In this study, electroencephalographic data recorded a large shift in frequency from 0 to 8 Hz to 8 to 20 Hz, with an increase in A-band power and a decrease in D-band power. These results showed improvement in control and power of breathing. It is hypothesized that the yogic meditation regulates the limbic system, providing better control over endocrine secretions and lowering the chance of over-firing neurons.[222] Another investigation tested the use of yogic meditation for 1 year versus a control of no meditation in patients with drug-resistant epilepsy.[223] Data showed significant differences between the experimental and control groups, with the experimental group having significantly lower seizure activity over the observation period.[222]

A study done in an epilepsy care center in 2006 assessed the efficacy of yoga meditation protocol (YMP) as an adjunctive treatment in patients with drug-resistant chronic epilepsy.[224] It was a supervised trial based on the frequency of complex partial seizures, which was assessed after 3, 6, and

12 months. There were 20 patients, who sat in a relaxed position with legs crossed (sukhasana) and focused on deep, slow, controlled breathing (pranayama) for 5 to 7 minutes, followed by silent meditation.[224] Patients were instructed to perform YMP daily for 20 minutes in the morning and evening at home and at supervised sessions.[224] Individuals with greater than or equal to a 50% reduction in the rate of monthly seizures were classified as responders, whereas patients with less than this percentage in seizure reduction were classified as nonresponders.[224] After the first 3 months there was a reduction in the frequency of seizures in all but one patient. Fourteen patients continued the YMP for 6 months or more and were tested again. Of these, six had been seizure free for a 3-month period, and three had been seizure free for 6 months.[224] The authors of this study concluded that yoga was a less expensive and an adverse effect–free way to treat patients with drug-resistant forms of epilepsy.

Human Immunodeficiency Virus. A pilot study examined the use of a yoga intervention for individuals with human immunodeficiency virus (HIV) infection who experienced pain and anxiety.[225] Results indicated a decrease in pain and anxiety symptoms and a reduction in amount of pain medication after an 8-week yoga program.

Another study examined the effect of yoga practice that included breathing, movement, and meditation techniques for 47 participants with HIV disease. Positive changes were noted in mental health on the Mental Health Index (MHI), and general physical health on the Medical Outcomes Study HIV Health Survey (MOS-HIV).[226] The Daily Stress Inventory showed a decrease in stress after the yoga program. Improvements in activities of daily living were reported by all yoga participants.

Fear of Falling and Insufficient Balance. A recent study investigated the use of a 12-week yoga practice for adults over the age of 65 years old with fear of falling and balance problems. Sessions of yoga postures and breathing exercises were completed in sitting and standing.[227] Fear of falling was measured using the Illinois Fear of Falling Measure and balance was captured with the BBS before and after the yoga intervention. Results showed a 6% decrease in fear of falling, 4% increase in static balance, and 34% increase in lower-body flexibility.[227]

An observational cohort study explored the effect of yoga on balance, fear of falling, and quality of life in 26 postmenopausal and osteoporotic women over age 55 years. Results of the Quality of Life Questionnaire of the European Foundation for Osteoporosis (QUALEFFO) and a neuromuscular test battery revealed improvements in all aspects of the QUALEFFO for the yoga participants, as well as improved ability to stand on one leg and improved perception of general health.[228] Yoga may prove to be a promising intervention to improve balance and reduce fear of falling.

Conclusion. Available data on the use of yoga as a therapeutic intervention for people with various neurological disorders are sparse. However, preliminary data show promise for the use of yoga as a treatment for CTS, stroke, MS, and epilepsy and for fall prevention. Most studies have small sample sizes but do show trends toward improved function and reduced impairments. In general, yoga can assist in the establishment of the mind-body connection and awareness of self. Greater self-awareness may explain why patients report improvements in quality of life, improved ability to better manage their disease, and a deeper understanding of their own bodies. Relaxation that results from yogic meditation fosters stress management and may improve the outlook on long-term management of neurological conditions. Yoga may serve as an alternative to traditional exercise and can be adapted for elderly patients who are unable to perform strenuous exercise. Yoga can be modified to accommodate patients with almost any physical or cognitive disability, and potentially provide mental enhancement, which can create a significant relaxation effect. Further research is needed specific to the effects of yoga practice in neurological populations.

Energy Therapy Approaches

Therapeutic Touch

Ellen Zambo Anderson

Therapeutic Touch (TT) is a complementary therapy categorized by the National Center for Complementary and Alternative Medicine as a therapy based on the concept of energy fields (biofields).[229] It is practiced by nurses, rehabilitation specialists, and others for the purposes of reducing pain and anxiety, accelerating the healing process, and promoting a sense of well-being.[230]

Assumptions. There are four assumptions that form the foundation for TT as an intervention that can facilitate healing and health. The first assumption, described by Delores Krieger, RN, PhD, the developer of TT, is that the body is an open energy system. The open system allows energy, often referred to as *subtle energy,* to flow within and through the body. This flow allows for a dynamic interface with the environment.[231] The second assumption suggests that individuals are bilaterally symmetrical so that the right and left, front and back mirror each other. This symmetry allows for a balanced energy flow. The third assumption is that an imbalance or an irregular flow of subtle energy is associated with physiological impairments, illness, and disease. The fourth assumption is that the body can initiate and achieve a process of self-healing through manipulation of biofields and restoration of subtle energy balance and flow.[231]

The concept of internal and external subtle energies and their relationship to health and illness can be found in many whole medical systems such as Ayurveda,[232] traditional Chinese medicine,[233] and Navajo medicine.[234] More specifically, the assumptions of TT described by Krieger have their roots in the ancient concepts of prana and chakras.[235,236] Prana, which is coined *chi* or *qi* in other systems of medicine, is the universal life force or energy that circulates through the universe and all living things. Chakras are the centrally aligned energy centers that are able to receive, transform, and send prana throughout the body. A blockage, interruption, void, or imbalance of prana is thought to exist when there is pathology or disease. Restoration of an individual's energy flow and balance is important for self-healing and health.[237]

Krieger, along with her colleague Dora Kunz, investigated the phenomenon and characteristics of people known as "healers" and concluded that healers possess a heightened sensitivity to their clients' state of health and being and are able to effect change through intention and energy. Through her description of sensing and effecting change in an individual's energy or biofield, Krieger has elucidated a four-step process that defines TT as a distinct therapeutic intervention different from other energy-based therapies such as reiki and Healing Touch.

Procedure. TT is often performed with the patient or client fully dressed and sitting. Despite the name, TT can be administered without actually touching the patient because TT practitioners are able to sense and manipulate the patient's subtle energies from a distance of 2 or more inches away from the patient's body. The first step in the TT process is called *centering*. During centering, practitioners center their consciousness so that a state of integration and quiet can be achieved. From the state of centeredness, practitioners initiate the assessment step by placing their hands 2 to 3 inches from the client's head and slowly moving their hands down the patient's body, noting the patients biofield. Practitioners may perceive the patient's energy as hot or cold or sense that a patient's energy is blocked in a particular area. Perceived disturbances in a biofield suggest that the practitioner should return to that area later in the process.

Krieger has described the next step in the TT process as "unruffling the field."[231] To unruffle the field, TT practitioners sweep away bound up or congested energy, which allows the patient's energy field to become open and unrestricted. Opening the energy field sets the stage for the final step of the TT process. During the final step, TT practitioners direct and modulate the transfer and flow of energy so that the patient's energy fields can achieve balance and symmetry and healing can occur. Krieger points out that TT does not "cure" people of their diseases. Rather, she suggests that TT can have positive effects on energy fields and the flow of energy, and that these effects create an environment in which the patient's own self-healing processes can be optimized.[230,231] Sessions usually take 20 to 30 minutes, but TT practitioners have reported that frail patients and children can benefit from as little as 5 to 8 minutes of TT; other patients may require 60 minutes of TT to achieve a state of relative energy balance.

Scientific Literature. The application of TT for persons with neurological diseases and disorders has not been widely investigated in the scientific literature. Researchers have, however, investigated the efficacy of TT for the reduction of anxiety and pain in a variety of patient populations and for the reduction of disruptive behaviors in persons with AD.

Anxiety. *Anxiety* is a general term associated with nervousness, fear, apprehension, and worrying. An anxiety disorder differs from feelings of anxiety associated with a specific event and is characterized by an irrational dread of everyday situations or excessive and long-standing anxiousness regarding nonspecific events and objects.

Robinson, Biley, and Dolk[238] performed a systematic review of the effect of TT on symptoms related to anxiety disorders but were unable to identify any studies in which subjects met the definition of anxiety disorder as defined by the *Diagnostic and Statistical Manual of Mental Disorders* (DSM-IV) or the International Classification of Diseases (ICD-10). In all of the studies of TT and anxiety included in the review, Robinson and colleagues[238] noted that pretest anxiety was measured in all subjects, but these subjects did not have "anxiety disorder" as their primary diagnosis. This systematic review helps to show that individuals with neurological disorders and other medical diagnoses may not be diagnosed with an anxiety disorder but may experience some anxiety as they face the challenges of their condition.

Several researchers have investigated the effect of TT in different patient populations such as those with severe burns,[239] cardiovascular diagnoses,[240,241] and breast cancer.[242,243] Turner and colleagues[239] found that for hospitalized patients with severe burns, TT was associated with a reduction in anxiety with no adverse effects. Quinn[240] and Heidt[241] investigated the application of TT in persons with cardiovascular conditions and determined that compared with sham TT, subjects who received TT reported significant reductions in anxiety on the State-Trait Anxiety Inventory (STAI). Women with breast cancer were studied by Samarel and colleagues[242] and Frank and colleagues.[243] Samarel and co-workers[242] found that women who received 10 minutes of TT and 20 minutes of dialogue before surgery reported significantly lower preoperative anxiety than women who received quiet sitting and dialogue, but no differences in anxiety were observed postoperatively. Frank and colleagues[243] found that TT was helpful for reducing restlessness, fear, and nervousness in women who were scheduled to undergo a stereotactic core biopsy (SCB) but that the results were similar between the TT group and the sham TT group.

The application of TT with older adults has been reported by Simington and Laing[244] and Lin and Taylor.[245] Both research studies found that older subjects who received TT had significant postintervention reductions of anxiety as measured by the STAI. In the study by Simington and Laing, TT was paired with a backrub in the experimental group. The control group received just a backrub.[244] In the study by Lin, TT was compared with sham TT.[245] For inpatients with psychiatric diagnoses, TT was compared with sham TT and relaxation therapy.[246] The researchers found that TT was more effective than sham TT but no more effective than relaxation therapy for reducing anxiety in this population.

A review of the TT literature and anxiety suggests that TT's efficacy for reducing anxiety is inconclusive. Several researchers have reported benefits of TT, yet others have found no effects when comparing use of TT with a control group or with use in patients with another condition. Reasons for the inconclusive results may be differences in the criteria for anxiety and variability in the measurement instruments. Other reasons may include research design issues such as assignment methods, blinding, and the frequency and duration of the TT intervention and comparison conditions.

Pain. Patients' pain can severely interfere with their ability to function efficiently and effectively. Nonpharmacological methods for managing pain have the potential for assisting patients in their rehabilitation and achievement of functional independence without adverse effects. Investigations of TT for pain associated with neurological conditions are extremely limited. In a case report of a subject with long-standing phantom limb pain, Leskowitz[247] found that TT was effective in reducing the subject's pain from an 8 to 10 out of 10 on a visual analog scale (VAS) to a 0 in one session. Self-administered TT was then able to maintain pain at a 0 to 1 on a VAS in which 10 is the maximum intensity. Before TT, medication, stress management, hypnosis, transcutaneous electrical nerve stimulation (TENS), and ultrasound had been successful in temporarily reducing the subject's pain to 6 to 8, but long-term pain management with these approaches was inadequate.

TT was investigated in subjects with chronic pain associated with fibromyalgia syndrome[248] and CTS.[249]

Denison[248] found no significant improvement on the Short-Form McGill Pain Questionnaire (SF-MPQ), VAS, or Fibromyalgia Health Assessment Questionnaire (FHAQ) after subjects received 6 weekly sessions of TT. TT and sham TT groups both demonstrated immediate significant improvement in median motor nerve distal latencies, pain scores, and relaxation scores; however, there were no significant differences between the two groups on any of the outcome measures.

Other researchers have investigated the use of TT with older adults,[245,250] cancer pain,[242,243,251] osteoarthritis,[252,253] headache,[254] postoperative pain,[255,256] burns,[239] and various chronic pain complaints.[245] The results of studies that have included TT and measures of pain suggest that TT may be helpful in managing phantom limb pain, headaches, and pain associated with burns. There are, however, inconsistencies across the studies that raise questions about both significant and insignificant findings. Inclusion of a control group, use of sham TT, sample size, measurement instruments, and the duration and frequency of TT are factors related to the studies' validity that limit the ability to draw firm conclusions about the efficacy of TT for reducing pain.

Disruptive Behaviors. TT has been investigated for its effect on disruptive behaviors in persons with AD. Although most patients with neurological conditions do not typically manifest AD, alterations in cognitive functioning and behavior are often observed. In a within-subjects study by Woods and Dimond,[257] long-term care residents with AD received 5 to 7 minutes of TT twice a day. Disruptive behaviors were measured using the Brief Agitation Rating Scale (BARS). The researchers found a significant reduction in overall agitation and in two specific behaviors, vocalization and pacing during the treatment and posttreatment period. In a randomized controlled trial, TT was also applied 5 to 7 minutes twice a day with persons with AD.[258] Similar to the observations of Woods and Dimond,[257] TT was found to be helpful for significantly decreasing overall behavioral symptoms of dementia including restlessness and vocalizations when compared with the usual care and placebo group. Hawranik, Johnston, and Deatrich[259] studied TT's effect on three forms of disruptive behavior—physical aggression, physical nonaggression, and verbal agitation—in persons with AD. They found a significant reduction in physical nonaggressive behaviors but no differences in physically aggressive and verbally agitated behaviors in subjects who received TT compared with subjects who received sham TT or routine care. These studies have provided some preliminary evidence for TT's potential use for modifying at least some forms of agitated behaviors. Application of TT to patient populations other than AD for the reduction of disruptive behaviors needs to be investigated.

Conclusion. As a noninvasive, nonpharmacological intervention, TT may be helpful to patients with AD who demonstrate disruptive behaviors and patients with pain or anxiety. Research that investigates the mechanism by which TT may alleviate pain and the physiological changes that may occur with TT will advance the acceptance of TT as a useful modality and suggest patient diagnoses that might benefit from the incorporation of TT into a rehabilitation plan of care.

Physical Body Systems Approaches

Craniosacral Therapy

John Upledger
Mary Lou Galantino

Craniosacral therapy (CST) is a gentle, noninvasive, yet powerful and effective treatment approach that relies primarily on hands-on evaluation and treatment. It focuses in the normalization of bodily functions that are either part of or related to a semiclosed hydraulic physiological system, which has been named the *craniosacral system.*

Structure of the Craniosacral System. The anatomy of the craniosacral system includes a water-tight compartment formed by the dura mater, the cerebrospinal fluid (CSF) within this compartment, the inflow and outflow systems that regulate the quantity and pressure of the bones to which the dura mater attaches, the joints or sutures that interconnect these bones, and other bones not anatomically connected to the dura mater. The bones of the cranium and the second and third cervical vertebrae, the sacrum, and the coccyx are also included in the structures of the craniosacral system.[260,261] In combination with the message sent to the patient through the intentional touch of the therapist is the corrective work that is done on a basic physiological level by gentle hands-on manipulations applied both directly and indirectly to the craniosacral system. The semiclosed hydraulic system includes the dural sleeves, which invest the spinal nerve roots outside the vertebral canal as far as the intervertebral foramina, and the caudal end of the dural tube, which ultimately becomes the cauda equina and blends with the coccygeal periosteum. The fluid within the semiclosed hydraulic system is CSF. The inflow and outflow of CSF are regulated by the choroid plexuses within the brain's ventricular system and arachnoid granulation bodies, respectively. CSF outflow is not rhythmically interrupted, but its rate may be adjusted by intracranial membrane tension patterns, which are broadcast primarily by the falx cerebri and tentorium cerebelli to the anterior end of the straight venous sinus, where an aggregation of arachnoid granulation bodies is located. This concentration of arachnoid granulation bodies is known to affect venous backpressure, which has an effect on the rate of reabsorption of CSF into the blood-vascular system.[262-264]

Technique. The therapist, after mobilization of bony restrictions, focuses on the correction of abnormal dural membrane restrictions, perceived CSF activities, and energy patterns and fluctuations as they relate to the craniosacral system. It is during this time that the patient often moves from a phase of being corrected and having obstacles removed to a phase of self-healing, with the therapist serving as a facilitator of the process. The tenets of CST include the concept that the dura mater within the vertebral canal (dural tube) has the freedom to glide up and down within that canal for a range of 0.5 to 2.0 cm. This movement is allowed by the slackness and directionality of the dural sleeves as they depart the dural tube and attach to the intertransverse foramina of the spinal column.[260]

A basic assumption in CST, as it has evolved, is that the patient's body contains the necessary information for the discovery of the cause of any health problem. The treatment relies primarily on hands-on evaluation and treatment. The hands-on contact is tender and supportive. It is accompanied by a sincere intention to assist the patient in any way that is possible. In short, the therapist serves primarily as a facilitator of the patient's own healing processes. The rapport that develops during the patient-therapist interaction lends itself powerfully to the positive therapeutic effect that many patients experience.

Western medicine imparts a therapeutic modality for curative measures, whereas CST fosters facilitation, wherein the client directs the treatment session. The inherent participation of the patient through CST promotes a holistic approach to healing. Conventional medical diagnosis will usually be more closely related to what the therapist views as the result rather than the cause. For example, the therapist would search for a cause of strabismus within the intracranial membrane system and the motor control system of the eyes, rather than considering the strabismus as a diagnosed condition to be corrected by surgery. The cause of strabismus can be found as an abnormal tension pattern in the tentorium cerebelli. The therapist then searches for the cause of the abnormal tentorial tension pattern. Quite often, these tension patterns are referred from the occiput or from the low back or the pelvis. If this is the case, the CST "diagnosis" would be intracranial membranous strain of the tentorium cerebelli as a result of occipital or low back or pelvic dysfunction, individually or severally, resulting in secondary motor dysfunction of the eyes (strabismus). The therapist would focus on the sacrum, the pelvis, the occiput, and then the tentorium cerebelli. Correct evaluation and treatment would be signified by a "spontaneous correction" of the strabismus.

Somatoemotional release is a technique that involves the bodily, and usually conscious, reexperiencing of episodes, the energies for which have been stored in the totality of body tissues. A powerful emotional content is typically connected with this technique, and it has proved to be extremely effective in cases of severe posttraumatic stress disorder. It was tested through qualitative research with a group of six Vietnam veterans in 1993. It proved to be successful in all six of these patients.[260,261,265,266]

Outcomes. Objective responses to CST are based on the removal of obstructions to smooth and easy physiological motions of the patient's body, the absence of energy cysts, the free movement of the dural tube in the spinal or vertebral canal and the rate and quality of the craniosacral rhythm, the absence of pressing responses during the somatoemotional release process, and statements from the deeper levels of consciousness through dialogue with various images encountered in the session that "all is well."[260,261,265]

Subjectively, clients report an increased sense of well-being, improved sleep patterns, reduced manifestation of stress, reduction in or disappearance of pain, increased energy levels, and fewer episodes of transitory illness. How long it takes to achieve these results is extremely variable and dependent on the complexity of the layers of adaptation, the defense mechanism, and the level of spiritual evolution of the patient.

Use in Treatment Intervention. CST is useful as a primary treatment modality and as an adjunct to a wide variety of visceral dysfunctions. It works well to balance autonomic function, specifically reducing sympathetic nervous tonus. It has proved beneficial in chronic headache problems, temporomandibular joint problems,[267] whiplash sequelae, and chronic pain syndromes. We have used it as an intensive treatment for persons rehabilitating from head injuries, craniotomies, spinal cord injuries, poststroke syndromes, transient ischemic attacks, seizure disorders, and a wide variety of rare brain and spinal cord dysfunctions.[268-271] Little positive effect has been reported in people with amyotrophic lateral sclerosis. However, some remarkable success has been seen in patients with MS.[270]

CST has been used extensively and effectively in a great number of children with spastic cerebral palsy, seizure disorders, Down syndrome, and a wide variety of motor system disorders, including problems with the oculomotor system, learning disabilities, attention deficit disorder, speech problems, childhood allergies, and autonomic dysfunction.[272-274]

We have used CST for people living with HIV disease who have HIV-related peripheral neuropathy and other chronic musculoskeletal and neurological problems. Pain management techniques can be used by the therapist and also taught to the family members to implement for a home program.[275] Future studies addressing the interaction of the immune system with the craniosacral system would be helpful in elucidating the neuroendocrine response to this technique. CST has been found to be an effective means for treating lower urinary tract symptoms and improving quality of life in patients with MS.[276]

Clinical experiences also suggest that CST is a powerful evaluative and treatment modality for patients with vertigo who have not responded well to or have not found relief from traditional medical treatments. Osseous, dural membrane, and fascial restrictions leading to asymmetric temporal bone movement and hence vertigo are some of the dysfunctions of the craniosacral system. More clinical trials are necessary to verify that CST is an effective treatment as well as to determine the full range of symptoms for which CST is beneficial.

Recent studies have found a connection between patients with fibromyalgia and CST. CST improved quality of life in this population, reducing the perception of pain and fatigue and improving night rest and mood with an increase in physical function.[277]

The latest research includes using CST along with other osteopathic techniques to treat chronic lateral epicondylitis as opposed to treating it with traditional orthopedic techniques. The results have revealed increased strength and decreased pain for both osteopathic and orthopedic groups. The assumption is that osteopathic techniques such as CST can be successful in treating chronic lateral epicondylitis[278]; however, future studies will need to isolate CST to ultimately reveal its efficacy in treatment for this problem.

To date, there have been several studies refuting the value of CST. One example is in *The Scientific Review of Alternative Medicine.* According to this group of researchers, interexaminer reliability among CST practitioners is zero.[279] Other studies suggest that the sutures that CST practitioners are attempting to mobilize are fused in the adult population, and therefore the techniques are ineffective.[280-284] Future studies are necessary for CST to achieve recognition as a valid and reliable treatment option.

Training. The prerequisites for training in CST by the Upledger Institute are quite simple. It is believed that any kind of therapist who has a license to see and treat patients/clients might find CST, in its more basic form, a useful adjunct to practice. Therefore a license as a health care practitioner is all that is required to enroll in the Upledger Institute's CST seminar series.

There are six levels of training within the series that are required before one can enroll in the advanced-level workshops. The workshops are all 4 or 5 days in length and are about evenly divided between academic work and hands-on supervised practice. The training program is designed to develop the sense of touch, motion, and energy perception slightly before the academic material is presented.

A certification process started in 1995 is now in place. There is a newly formed International Association of Healthcare Practitioners of which the American CranioSacral Therapy Association is a subdivision. The American CranioSacral Therapy Association, a nonprofit organization, was founded by a group of therapists and concerned laypersons in 1994. Its stated objectives are to bring CST into public awareness, to enhance networking among practitioners who use CST, to develop a certification program that will result in the recognition of CST as a specialty for persons who are licensed as health care practitioners in other fields, and to ultimately develop CST as an independently licensed and freestanding profession.

Reimbursement by third-party carriers is done largely on a case-by-case basis. A few insurance companies have recognized CST, but there is much work to be done on this front. The Upledger Institute published a book listing all the practitioners who have completed training. It is available to all health care professionals.

Myofascial Release (Barnes Method)

Carol M. Davis

Before beginning the discussion on myofascial release, a discussion of the research on fascia is appropriate. This discussion applies to the topic of CST and myofascial release as well as any other therapeutic technique within which fascia is affected. As fascia is part of the human body, both occupational and physical therapists need to accept that it influences their treatment and analyze its importance as a body system that can cause functional problems, prevent an individual from participating in daily living activities, and limit quality of life.

Research on Fascia: A Summary of Recent and Rediscovered Research on the Nature and Function of the Fasciae. Since the last edition of *Neurological Rehabilitation* was published, much has been learned, rediscovered, and published about the nature and function of the various connective tissue fasciae in humans. Fascial tissue turns out to be quite complex, is intimately involved in the moment-to-moment function of all of our cells, and is intricately involved with central, peripheral, and autonomic nervous system tissue. It is no longer useful to view the body or the fascial system as a mechanical system alone. Nonlinear system dynamics are at work as we now understand the involvement of fascia with the neuroendrocrine system, the brain, and the neurological plexus in the lining of organs such as the stomach and gut. Fascia must be viewed by practitioners and patients not as static, but as innervated, alive, functional, fluid, and self-regulatory. Involving the patient or client in the process of manipulation of fascia and its embedded tissue enhances the response of the tissue and the patient.[285]

Central to the complete understanding of the effectiveness of energy-based myofascial release for the relief of pain and the facilitation of healing are the following points:

- There are 12 different fasciae or connective tissues in the body, each with varying concentrations of collagen, elastin, and ground substance.[286]
- "Our richest and largest sensory organ is not the eyes, ears, skin, or vestibular system, but is in fact our muscles with their related fascia. Our central nervous system receives its greatest amount of sensory nerves from our myofascial tissue."[285]
- "The presence of smooth muscle cells within fascia, along with the widespread presence of myelinated and unmyelinated sensory and motor nerve fibers and capillaries has led to an hypothesis that fascia is an actively adapting organ with functional importance, rather than a passive structural organ alone. This may be the root of myofascial pain syndromes."[285]
- There are nine or 10 sensory nerve endings in the fascia for every one sensory nerve ending in the muscle. Thus fascia plays a major role in helping us to sense where we are in space and sense our inner tissue in ways not fully appreciated previously.[287]
- Fascia contains myofibroblasts that can tense or release in fascial sheets.[288]
- Fascia has been hypothesized to play a role as the seat of consciousness in the body-mind system.[289] As one example, there are 10 times as many connective tissue cells as nerve cells in the brain. Previously thought only to provide support and nutritional pathways to nerve, the latest brain scan research indicates glial cells "light up" during certain brain states, particularly emotional states. They have been shown also to play a role in regulating neuropeptides and neurotransmitters, thus thought to play a role in helping to regulate mood.[290]
- Fascia plays a role in the maturation of stem cells. The fascia that surrounds all cells as the cell wall, and the fascia of the extracellular matrix, which is the environment of all cells in the body, determine the pressures sustained on developing stem cells into their mature forms.[291]
- Three specialized stretch receptor nerve endings in fascial structures play a role in helping us to be able to sense what is happening in our tissue moment to moment as well as when receiving manual therapy. Golgi tendon organs in both tendons and in aponeuroses give feedback about the straightening of the fibers in the tendon. Paciniform endings in the myotendinous junction, joint capsules, and ligaments report vibration and rapidly changing pressures in the fascial net. Ruffini endings respond to deep and sustained pressure.[285]
- Fascia is piezoelectric tissue. Myofascial release that emphasizes sustained pressure and tension over fascial restrictions generates a flow of electrical activity, or information, throughout the fascial system. Electrical impulses are generated in the collagen by compressive and distraction forces within the musculoskeletal system. These impulses trigger a cascade of cellular, biomechanical, neural, and extracellular events as the body adapts to external stress. In response to internal stress,

components of the extracellular fluid change in polarity and charge, affecting fascial motion.[292]

- With myofascial release, the extracellular matrix softens from "gel" to "sol," allowing the fascial restriction to melt and release pressure on pain-sensitive tissue, and to rehydrate to allow for conduction of flow of photons and vibration.[293] It is hypothesized that this action facilitates the cell-to-cell communication required in homeostasis and self-regulation and thus facilitates the body-mind's ability to heal itself.[294]

Myofascial Release. Myofascial release is a manual ("hands-on") energetic therapy designed to treat the fascia that surrounds every cell and tissue in the body as a living crystal matrix within which all of our cells are embedded.[289] John Barnes, the physical therapist credited for developing this holistic, physical and energy-based treatment technique, has pointed out that it is a mistake to think of muscle as being a tissue in and of itself. Just as we now recognize that the mind and body cannot be separated, we also realize that there is no such entity as muscle; rather, the fascial-muscle unit is the more accurate anatomical and physiological entity. As Janet Travell[295] first described it, the fascia that surrounds each muscle fiber and fibril is inextricably interconnected with the muscle, and it is impossible to treat the muscle alone. Until the fascial barriers are released, the muscle, no matter how often stretched or contracted, will tend to resume its original shape. If that shape is distorted by a central or peripheral nervous system pathological condition, as is so often the case with our clients, or distorted from hypertonicity, if the muscle group has taken a postural position of ease from prolonged positioning or emotional protection, or if the fascia surrounding the cells of skin nearby is contorted from a surgical scar, then the muscle is not free to contract in the way it was created to function.

It is also important to emphasize that fascia has been referred to as the structural base of the "living matrix" of all cells in the body.[289] Fascia surrounds not only skin and muscle cells, but each and every cell in our bodies and even penetrates each cell as a cytoskeleton. In sum, the cellular matrix is connected with the extracellular matrix by way of fascia. Thus, as therapists when we touch the skin, "we contact a continuous interconnected webwork that extends throughout the body" (p. 47).[296]

The Physiology of the Fascial System. To understand how myofascial release is administered and why it seems to result in such positive outcomes to patients, it is necessary to understand the physiology of the fascial system. This section should enhance understanding of the fascial system as discussed earlier. Because fascia exists as a three-dimensional web surrounding all our cells, from the top of our head to the bottom of our feet, functional biomechanical movements depend on intact, properly distributed fasciae.[296] There are three topographical groupings of twelve different types of fascia,[286] and each kind of fascia is composed of connective tissue of similar structure. The fascia just below the dermis is known as *superficial fascia.* The fascia that surrounds and fuses with bone, muscle, nerves, blood vessels, and organs is termed *deep fascia.* The third grouping of fascia is the *dura,* which surrounds the brain and spinal cord. All 12 forms of fascia are composed of collagen, elastin, and a ground substance of polysaccharide composition. This connective tissue plays a vital role in holding the body together. Without fascia, the body could not remain intact and erect, supported by bones, joints, tendons, and ligaments alone. The fascia functions much like the stays of a tent, supporting the structure of the body but also facilitating metabolism and blood and lymph flow and separating organs and other structures from one another, down to the cellular level.[296]

Intervention. In contrast to traditional stretching of tissue, during myofascial release practitioners and their clients experience a sensation of softening, or melting similar to melting butter, or stretching, like pulling taffy under the palms of the therapist. Once tight tissue is located by palpation or observation, the slack is taken out of the tissue under the hands, and the therapist gently leans into his or her hands and waits for the tissue to respond. Within 90 to 120 seconds, the therapist's hands will sink deeper, and a feeling of flow results. The therapist then simply follows that twisting and deepening flow of tissue until it stops (indicating a fascial barrier), when she or he again waits, maintaining slight tension until the tissue begins to flow again, and the therapist can follow the fascia, as it flows or releases, to the next collagenous barrier. The collagen fibers seem to be rearranging themselves back to a position of alignment, or self-correction. Often an area of heat and redness under the release occurs, but curiously, at times an area of erythema occurs distant from the release itself.[297] It is hypothesized that the feeling of flow occurs when the polysaccharide ground substance of the fascia becomes more in solution, less gel-like, by way of a piezoelectric effect. Mechanical pressure from the therapist's hands is converted to chemical energy. Recent research has shown that "actin filaments and microtubules…could function as conduits for the spread of biochemical agents" once they are mechanically stimulated. In other words, human cells have been filmed instantly messaging one another by way of mechanical energy being transmitted to biochemical messages.[298]

The effect of myofascial release can be enhanced by prolonged, corrective positioning with use of postural wedges or therapeutic balls, or both, to sustain the appropriate pressure to release the fascia over time. For example, for a rotated pelvis, wedges will sustain a correcting derotation while the patient is lying supine or prone.[298] In addition, once fascia has been released, it is important to maintain fascial length and to exercise muscles to strengthen resistance to the fascia tightening up once again in gravity. Yoga, Pilates, TKD, and tai chi are excellent exercises to use to maintain length of released fascia. Inversion tables also assist in maintaining fascial length but should not be used for patients restricted from inverting, such as patients or clients with uncontrolled blood pressure or glaucoma.

The purpose of myofascial release is to lengthen the fascia that has been abnormally constricted, thus allowing a more efficient and effective contraction of muscles, release of trapped energy, a more barrier-free blood and lymph supply to nerves and organs, an upright posture that responds in a neutral way to the forces of gravity, and a body-mind that is more in balance from a less restricted flow of body energy, or chi. Myofascial release, along with soft tissue mobilization, therapeutic exercise, and movement reeducation, is an excellent holistic therapeutic approach for musculoskeletal, neuromuscular, and integumentary disorders in function.

Myofascial Release Intervention. Myofascial release treatment consists of a thorough examination of the client, including an in-depth history of symptoms and a thorough musculoskeletal and neuromuscular examination, noting pain; impairments in strength, ROM, or endurance; and any disorders in function. The client's posture and specifically the position of the pelvis are noted. In many people, the hips will appear uneven, palpation of the anterior superior iliac spines will reveal an iliac rotation, and many times there will be a leg-length discrepancy associated with pelvic rotation. In the case of stroke, TBI, or cerebral palsy, abnormal tone will have resulted in fasciae frozen along with their spastic muscles as a result of disorganized nerve conduction. No matter what the cause of the fascial tightening, the treatment remains to release the connective tissue, the fascia. This is done with manual releases, soft tissue mobilization techniques, traction, positioning on wedges, facilitation of whole-body release (unwinding or somatoemotional release), craniosacral techniques, and a technique called "rebounding." The technique of rebounding, which is especially useful with CNS pathological conditions, involves a passive rocking of tissue, exploiting the hydrophilic aspect of tissue to the maximum. As the therapist rhythmically rocks chest, legs, thorax, or arms, the tissue reverberates with the rhythm of the motion, often resulting in a spontaneous release of tense and hypertonic tissue. Patients respond positively to this technique.

The actual techniques of myofascial release, a holistic complementary therapy, may at first appear to be exactly like mechanical manual therapies, but soon the novice recognizes the need to quiet the mind and body and learns to wait and feel gently with an enhanced proprioceptive sense for the tissue to "move up into the hands" and then gently to follow it as the collagen releases or melts and the fascia lengthens with twists and turns. It is an art that is greatly enhanced by a calm and centered proprioceptive listening that is not linear or mechanical in nature but energetic and holistic.[299] Palpating for the cranial rhythm takes the same centered, quiet "listening with one's hands." Eventually, we learn to feel with the whole self.[300]

As science increasingly focuses on researching the effects of subatomic particles on tissue, and on the nature of "consciousness" and "mind," the hypothesis that consciousness resides not in the cranium, but in the fascial matrix will be further clarified. Energy-based myofascial release facilitates the release of holding patterns, and the emergence of body memories and buried emotions and awarenesses that were difficult to access, allowing patients to become increasingly aware, thus helping to restore balance and homeostasis. In this way, energy-based myofascial release is far more than a structural therapeutic process, but facilitates a reorganization of the entire awareness of one's self within the body-mind.[296]

Models of Health Care Belief Systems

American Indian Healing Traditions of North and South America

Richard W. Voss

Bob Prue, Member of the Rosebud Sioux Tribe

American Indians are understandably wary of the written word. Some may criticize the inclusion of this section in this chapter. This criticism is understandable because the written word objectifies understandings out of the cultural context and can be manipulated outside the relationship in which the understanding was shared. However, not to include a discussion of American Indian views about medicine and health care is also a concern because it perpetuates the invisibility of American Indian peoples. The purpose here is to honor the continuing journey of understanding between medical science practitioners and traditional American Indian medicine practitioners to see how these two medicine paths can help restore health to the people and to bring about increased understanding—wo 'wableza—among peoples.

Contemporary American Indian Health Care and Traditional Healing: North and South American Indian or Indigenous Perspectives. In a report to NIH, *Alternative Medicine: Expanding Medical Horizons,*[301] the Lakota (a Sioux people) were cited for the use of healing ceremonies by specialists who are essentially shamanic in their approach to treatment. To understand American Indian medicine ways, one cannot rely solely on written accounts. Although written ethnographical studies may provide a wealth of descriptive data, it is best to talk to authoritative sources personally. Professionals interested in learning more about traditional approaches to help and healing should contact any one of the federally recognized tribal headquarters and the tribally sponsored American Indian colleges and universities for more specific information. Many colleges conduct summer courses on Lakota culture and philosophy that are open to non–American Indians, as well as American Indians, interested in learning the culture. This information may be found on the Internet under tribal colleges and federally recognized tribes.

Today, many of the old American Indian healing traditions are experiencing a renaissance and are beginning to be viewed with a renewed sense of respect and credibility as an alternative and complement to more invasive or secular Western medical models of treatment.[301-307] For example, on the Cheyenne River Sioux Reservation at Eagle Butte, South Dakota, the tribe has incorporated traditional methods and approaches to a variety of social service programs, including services for at-risk youth and care for people with alcoholism, which is viewed as a problem with social, emotional, physical, and spiritual dimensions.[303,304,306,307] These traditional methods include the inipi, or purification ceremony (popularly called the "sweat lodge"), the hanblecaya, or pipe fast (often called the "vision quest"), and the wiwang wacipi, or the Sundance. The inclusion of these ceremonies within the treatment process has collectively been called the "Red Road approach."[303,304,307]

A number of medical facilities on various reservations include medicine men as consultants on a formal and informal basis,[307-310] and the use of traditional ceremonies in health care settings is encouraged and respected.[311] Where the ceremonial burning of sage (a common medicinal herb burned for purification) had been discouraged in the past, hospital staff report increased acceptance of this practice and now arrange appropriate space for traditional ceremonial practices both within the health care facility and outside on hospital grounds.[310,312] One Lakota friend commented on his recent hospitalization at an allopathic hospital. He was visited by a medicine man that placed a bundle of sage under his pillow. This made him feel better and showed how simple cooperation among allopathic medicine, health care practices, and alternative, complementary health care practices can be.

A Lakotacentric Perspective on Health. A traditional American Indian perspective on health care and medicine begins with the spiritual reality of the human being who is part of all creation and dependent on creation. Traditional understanding views human beings as intimately related to plants and all other creations in the natural world that sustain life. Reality is not linear, it is circular. Everything is connected to everything else. Good and bad, sickness and health, physician and patient are not separate processes, they are all related aspects and part of the whole. For the Lakotas and other traditional American Indian peoples there is no split or dualism in reality or creation. This traditional view challenges the intervention model and offers a prevention model as the starting place for social health and assistance. The emphasis from a Lakotacentric view is on building up the immune system and seeing the important role of the community in promoting good health care and well-being, a cultural emphasis often overlooked in conventional health care practices.

Traditional Lakota values of health and well-being emphasize the participation of the family in the healing process, including the extended family and the larger kinship community, to bring about good health to the individual. The health of the individual is connected to the health of the community, so there is an important tribal dimension to this understanding. For traditional Lakota people the health and healing process is not impersonal but highly personalized and individualized around specific needs. The roles of medicine practitioners are multidimensional and include those of healer, counselor, politician, and priest.

Another important contribution of the Native American perspective on health is that it provides a rich topology of spirit. The human creation, like all creations, is a spirit being composed of multilayered aspects of spirit. "Spirit" here is not some supernatural reality outside the human being but an intrinsic dimension of everything that is, including the human creation (person). To speak of human beings is to speak of spiritual reality. For traditional American Indians, medical treatment or any kind of social, human, or mental health service is first and foremost a spiritual endeavor.

Ayahuasca: A Spiritual Pathway to Consciousness and Healing. Traditional Indian peoples of South America have similar and yet distinctive traditions of help and healing where the rain forest provides the pharmacopoeia of medicinal plants, bark, herbs, and vines. Of course, the forest itself is viewed as a powerful source of spiritual healing. During a recent field study to the Tambopata River area of the southeastern Peruvian Amazon (through the Amazon Center for Environmental Education and Research), I had an opportunity to meet with various shamans, their patients, and public health care representatives at a local community center where the regional public school and health care station are located. It is interesting to note that all members of the health care staff rotate, making visits to the area community members, including both indigenous traditional people, who mainly live dispersed through the forest (Amazon), and mestizo or mixed-blood settlers, many of whose families have lived in the river settlements since the mid 1970s.[313] Both indigenous natives and mestizo settlers seek assistance from the shaman, the curanderos, and the health station outpost, staffed by nurses and a visiting physician. The South American indigenous community I visited in the Tambopata River region of the southeast Peruvian Amazon used both herbal remedies and spirit-calling ceremonies, often incorporating the use of forest tobacco and other vegetation gathered from the forest as a means of purification. The use of ayahuasca, a concoction or tea made from various plants, tree bark, and vines gathered from the forest, is administered to both patient and shaman and is a common shamanic practice throughout Amazonia, according to the shamans I interviewed.[313] A detailed description of an ayahuasca ceremony is reported by Salak,[314] providing a fascinating participant observer's experience of an ayahuasca ceremony. A brief audio-video capture of the beginning of an ayahuasca ceremony may be viewed at www.nationalgeographic.com/adventure. Clinical applications of ayahuasca are being studied by Jacques Mabit, Director del Centro de Rehabilitacion de Toxicomanos (Rehabilitation and Detoxification Center) at the Takiwasi Center, Peru. Mabit combines the traditional use of ayahuasca and psychotherapy techniques, and holistic methods (consciousness expansion methods such as fasting, hyperventilation, and nonaddictive plants), largely in treatment of coca paste addictions. The center is funded by the French government. Conventional allopathic medicines are not used, except in unusual circumstances.

Riba and colleagues[315] have published their neuropsychobiology study on the effects of ayahuasca, so traditional medicine has captured both the imagination and the attention of medical science.

Physical detoxification is accomplished through the use of medicinal plants. Conventional Peruvian approaches to addiction treatment are based on prison or military models, which have raised human rights concerns among health care workers. All studies on the clinical use of ayahuasca have European or South American sponsorship, and most have been published in Spanish.[316]

Health Risks Associated with Ayahuasca. Religious groups in the United States have obtained a First Amendment exemption to use ayahuasca in their ceremonies. Despite the U.S. government's opposition to the use of dimethyltryptamine (DMT), which is the main chemical substance found in ayahuasca, the government could not meet the burden of showing that ayahuasca posed a serious health risk to church members who use it in their ceremonies.[317] Gable reports that there have been no deaths caused by hoasca or any other traditional DMT/β-carboline ayahuasca brews. Furthermore, he writes, "The probability of a toxic overdose of ayahuasca is seemingly minimized by serotonin's stimulation of the vagus nerve, which, in turn, induces emesis near the level of an effective ayahuasca dose. The risk of overdose appears to be related primarily to the concurrent or prior use of an additional serotonergic substance. People who have an abnormal metabolism or a compromised health status are obviously at greater risk than the normal population, and might prudently avoid the use of ayahuasca preparations" (p. 29).[317]

Although there is generally no known harm to ingesting ayahuasca in a ceremonial context, common sense about nonceremonial use is called for. Using watchers to sit with the person while using ayahuasca and of course not allowing driving or use of heavy machinery is common sense. Therefore a harm reduction approach is called for. That said, the pharmacology of ayahuasca is such that "selective serotonin reuptake inhibitors can have potentially harmful interactions with MAO inhibitors, so people taking these kinds of medications are advised to avoid ayahuasca" (p. 301).[318] This is consistent with Gable's findings. There are no significant associations between the typical dosage of ayahuasca in ceremonial usage and long-term psychosis. Gable reports that "Many or most of UDV [União do Vegetal] psychiatric episodes were transient in nature and resolved spontaneously" (p. 30).[317]

Gable notes, "The ritual context in which ayahuasca is ingested provides some control of dosage and subsequent psychological effects. Because the natural sources used in preparation of the tea do not allow UDV members to standardize their hoasca brew with respect to DMT or β-carbolines, the person conducting the ceremony drinks the brew before administering it to UDV members as a means of testing for potency. Different amounts of the brew are initially offered to individual participants, and, depending on reactions, a participant may be offered a second cup at his or her request" (p. 26).[317]

Another area of concern is risk of dependency on ayahuasca. There is no convincing evidence that ayahuasca leads to physiological dependence. Of course, this is an area worth careful attention in continuing research, although Gable notes that the general psychopharmacological profile of huasca "suggests that it lacks the abuse potential of amphetamines, cocaine, opiates or other widely abused substances." Elsewhere, Gable notes that "tryptamine derivatives such as DMT (found in ayahuasca) result in erratic patterns of self-administration indicating that 'these compounds have weak reinforcing effects, or alternatively, mixed reinforcing and aversive effects.'" (p. 31).[317] Gable notes, "The unpredictable occurrence of frightening images and thoughts, plus predictable nausea and diarrhea, makes it a very unlikely candidate for a 'club drug'" (p. 32).[317] On the other hand, Grob reported that "all of the 15 UDV subjects claimed that their experience with ritual use of hoasca as a psychoactive ritual sacrament had had a profound [positive] impact on the course of their lives." Most of the UDV members had a history of moderate to severe alcohol use prior to joining the UDV" (p. 30).[317]

Traditional Acupuncture

Jeffrey Kauffman

It has been gratifying to see Western medicine, as it is practiced by allopathic physicians, come around to include many of the holistic practices that were once considered quackery. This is happening with chiropractic, massage, and other forms of body work; nutrition and diet; and exercise practices such as hatha yoga and tai chi, and so on. A research study designed by David Eisenberg of Harvard Medical School, published in the *New England Journal of Medicine* in 1993 and again in 1998,[319,320] showed just how extensive alternative or holistic practices are and how a large percentage of patients are using these practices, with or without knowledge of their personal physicians. Alternative health therapeutic modes are on the rise, are being used by more and more of the general population of the United States, and are being more and more accepted by Western medical practitioners. Many medical schools now have courses teaching alternative healing practices to medical students.

The question arises as to why people are drawn to therapeutic approaches outside the medical sphere. The answer is relatively straightforward. They are not getting everything they need in health care from traditional allopathic, Western-trained medical doctors. People are looking for something that works better. More and more people are disenchanted by the lack of compassion of a large percentage of the medical profession. This involves the patient being approached by the physician as a disease rather than a person, as a gallbladder case or a case of appendicitis or chronic fatigue instead of Sherri Jackson or Marvin Jones. This involves the hurried 5- to 10-minute visits created and encouraged by health maintenance organizations. It involves the use of pharmaceuticals over the use of any other therapeutic modality. The side effects of such medications add to the problem. Along with the decrease in or lack of compassion comes the inability of many physicians to develop rapport with their patients.

There is one other important principle that separates allopathic medicine as it is practiced in the United States from holistic healing, and that is the attention paid to the symptoms. Allopathic medicine traditionally treats the symptoms. In fact, the diagnosis is usually the symptom with the name changed to something that has "-itis" on it at the end as a suffix. For example, *arthritis* means inflammation of the joints, *appendicitis* means inflammation of the appendix, and *iritis* means inflammation of the iris. Tension headache or migraine headache is simply a headache. It means an ache or pain in the head. Western medicine is essentially treating the symptoms, most commonly with drugs. Even the medications are named after the symptoms, for example, antiinflammatories, antihypertensives, antimetabolites, antacids, antiarrhythmic agents, and diuretics (to increase output of fluid through the urine).

On the other hand, holistic healing is aimed at determining the cause of the disease (even the Western medical term *disease* means dis-ease or lack of ease). In determining the cause of dis-ease, one looks for the underlying imbalances that all human beings have. None of us is born with a perfect body-mind that never breaks down. We all have an underlying imbalance or constitutional imbalance that is the weak or vulnerable area of our body-mind that will always be the first to show symptoms and illness when we are under pressure or stress.

The pressure or stress coming from the outside world, outside of our body, can be in the form of physical agents such as physical trauma (accidents), which cause bruised tissues, strained or torn ligaments, or broken bones; toxic agents from the environment, such as poison or chemicals in the water or foods or air; carcinogens from contaminants; or poor nutrition and poor diet, not taking in enough nutrients or taking in too much of a particular kind. There are also external causes that are related to weather, such as excessive exposure to heat or cold, humidity or dryness, or wind or dampness; being struck by lightning; or near drowning. These causes were much more prevalent 200 years ago and even more so further back in the past. In modern civilization the much more common causes of illness come from the inside. These would be in the mental or emotional spheres. Generally, it is an emotion that is in excess or deficient in the person's life, such as too much fear or not enough, too much grief or not enough expression of grief, too much anger or not enough, too much joy (that's right, too much joy or inappropriate joy) or not enough, too much sympathy or not enough. Feelings and emotions that are in excess or in deficient states affect particular organs, which in turn can cause imbalance, symptoms, and disease in a particular organ, which then manifests as a heart attack or arthritis or constipation or cancer, and so on. For example, too much anger or not enough anger imbalances the gallbladder and/or the liver, making those organs susceptible to gallstones or hepatitis, respectively; too much grief or not enough affects the lungs and the colon, and could cause bronchitis or asthma or constipation. This occurs with our thoughts as well; we can focus to excess on particular negative thoughts, which creates imbalance, illness, and disease.

There is also the most important sphere for all human beings, which is the spirit. There can be, and often are, imbalances in this realm that have everything to do with not recognizing one's true value, which means not acknowledging the spirit that lives inside each and every human being. When one is aware of the spiritual energy inside and focuses on it daily, then that person knows and experiences the infinite energy of spirit whose nature is bliss. Unfortunately, most human beings have lost sight of this and consequently are suffering deep inside because of a lack of recognition of self-worth or self-esteem. The latter comes from knowing the Divinity inside. This, in turn, causes physical or mental disease.

There are also genetic causes of disease that are not adequately addressed. Generally, this is rather a cross that the person must bear; balancing and integrating the body, mind, and spirit still help that person lead an enjoyable and valuable life. Imbalances can also come from excess or deficiencies of other things such as too much work or not enough, too much exercise or not enough, too much sex (or not enough?), too much food or not enough. These are usually related to underlying emotional imbalances as well. Holistic modes of therapy address either these external causes or the internal causes, or preferably both.

Once alternative health practices are well entrenched in medical training in medical colleges, their efficacy can be proved easily over a 5-year period by simply measuring monies spent on pharmaceuticals and the quantities of pharmaceuticals used before, during, and after holistic programs are introduced. This would also include measuring and comparing outpatient visits to physicians, visits to emergency departments, hospital admissions, need for surgery, and some kind of standard for measuring quality of life. Improvements in some of these categories have already been proved in research studies done by Herbert Benson,[321] who noted the effect on patients using his relaxation response (a form of meditation) on a daily basis for 3 years.

History. Acupuncture as it is practiced in the United States is a huge conglomerate of different styles of acupuncture coming from China, Japan, Korea, Thailand, Vietnam, and Western Europe. The styles differ radically depending on who is doing the acupuncture, where he or she learned it, and how much individuality has been instilled into the practice. Within this discussion, the similarities among practices are described, followed by an in-depth analysis of the style that I use.

Acupuncture is one of the five categories that make up Chinese medicine. The other four are herbal medicine, diet and nutrition, exercise, and massage. Acupuncture is a healing method that tunes a human being. Just as a piano tuner tunes a piano or one tunes a guitar or an auto mechanic does a tune-up on a car, it is possible to tune a human being. After this process, or intervention, is done, the body-mind functions more efficiently in a balanced, harmonious fashion. As a result, the aches and pains often are eliminated and illnesses and diseases reversed. Acupuncture can be used by itself and, even better, in combination with other holistic and traditional Western medical methods.

Methods. Acupuncture involves the use of tiny needles made of stainless steel, their diameter two or three times the width of a human hair, sharpened by a diamond. These needles are put into particular points on the surface of the body. There are at least a thousand of these points all over the human body. They have a lower electrical potential compared with the surrounding skin, as is evidenced by a galvanometer. These points are also known as *acupuncture points, acupressure points, trigger points,* and perhaps by other names as well. These points are about 1 mm in diameter and are located pretty much in the same place for everyone, according to bony landmarks, skin landmarks, anatomical structures such as nipples, umbilicus, fingernails and toenails, eyes, ears, nose and mouth, and so on. The points can be found with practice by the trained finger of the practitioner. There are electrical instruments that can help locate these points, but their reliability has not been established. Needles are put into these acupuncture points, and after being inserted, the needles are turned either clockwise or counterclockwise one revolution. They are either taken out immediately or left in for a period of time, depending on the individual patient's imbalance and illness.

Examination and Evaluation. Deciding where to insert the needles is really the key and the most difficult and important part of acupuncture diagnosis. This is where styles of acupuncture come into play. There is a spectrum of acupuncture styles or methods that ranges from completely symptomatic to perfectly holistic, just as there is in traditional Western medicine. The symptomatic methods involve simply putting needles into acupuncture points at anatomical sites that are specifically related to symptoms. For example, for shoulder pain, or arthritis or bursitis, an acupuncturist using a symptomatic method would select acupuncture points that are in or around the shoulder area. Headache would be treated with needles in the head area. Constipation would be treated with needles in the belly area. Hemorrhoids would be treated with needles around the anus and coccygeal area. This method pays little attention to where the constitutional imbalance exists within each person. An opposite philosophy, which is called *holistic acupuncture,* treats the underlying constitutional imbalance within the person. Described earlier, such imbalances are considered the vulnerable, or weak, links in the chain in each human being, that part that always gives out first because it is not as strong or disease resistant as the rest of the body-mind. The type of acupuncture I use is a holistic form. Specifically, it is called *five-element acupuncture.* It is based on the Law of Five Elements, which is a law of nature that comes from Chinese philosophy and is one of the basic foundations of Chinese medicine. It is sometimes known as the *Five Phases* and is considered the most holistic form of acupuncture available.

The Law of Five Elements. The Law of Five Elements states that there are five elements in nature (fire, earth, metal, water, and wood) and that these elements all relate to one another in a particular fashion (Figure 39-5). The diagram in Figure 39-5 shows an outer creative cycle (known as *Shen*)

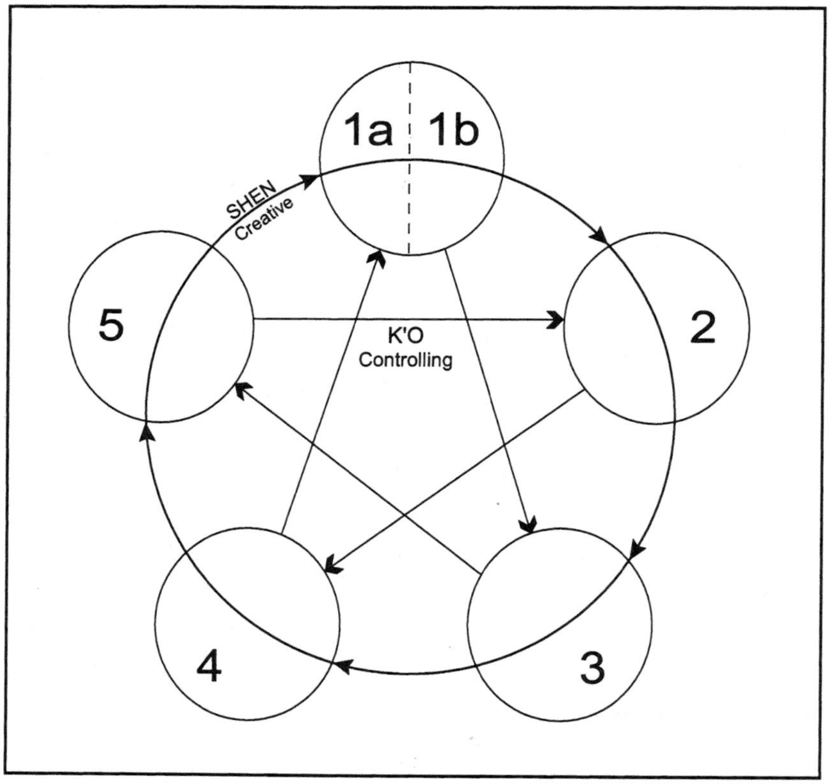

Figure 39-5 ■ Law of five elements: demonstrating the Shen (creative) and K'o (controlling) cycles.

that goes in a clockwise fashion and demonstrates that fire creates earth, earth creates metal, metal creates water, water creates wood, and wood creates fire again. Also, a star-shaped control, or destructive, cycle (known as *K'o*) shows that fire destroys or controls metal, metal does the same to wood, wood to earth, earth to water, and water to fire. These two cycles, the creative and destructive cycles, are necessary to keep balance in nature. These five elements are also found in human beings because the body is composed of elements that come from nature and return to nature when the body dies. The emotions and feelings in our personality align themselves with these same elements (Figure 39-6).

People in Western society have not been taught to think of their bodies in elemental forms, but nevertheless these elements are there. The concept of fire is present in each and every cell. The cells burn glucose to survive and this is referred to as "burning calories." It is this burning that causes our body temperature to remain at 98.6° F throughout most of our lives. It is not difficult to picture each cell of the body having a little bonfire in the center with mitochondria sitting around roasting pieces of glucose on a stick. Obviously, water is present in our bodies. Students in grammar school are taught that our bodies are 98% water with all the tears and urine and lymph and blood. Similarly, metal can be found in the body in the form of calcium in the bones and iron in the blood, in our teeth, and so on. The concept of wood is most easily seen in the fingernails and toenails, which are similar to the bark of a tree. Also, the ligaments and tendons are much like a strong fiber. The concept of earth is best seen in the gastrointestinal tract. Picture taking a microscopic journey down the gastrointestinal tract starting from the mouth, going down the esophagus into the stomach and the intestines; the further down you get, the more the material seems earthlike, until it is excreted into the outside world.

Each of the elements has a particular color that emanates from the face, a particular emotion that comes from the personality, a particular odor that comes from the body, and a particular sound that comes from the voice, as well as a particular taste, season, climate, secretion, and body part or system that it fortifies.

Every human being has a constitutional imbalance in one of these elements. The explanation for how this happens lies in spiritual law. Suffice it to say that this imbalance is well engrained some time during the first 5 years of life. Diagnosing this constitutional imbalance is both an art and a science and is done primarily by determining the color, emotion, odor, and sound belonging to each human being. The reader probably has noticed these colors, emotions, odors, and sounds previously with friends or even with strangers. Yet the realization that these are diagnostic clues that reveal a person's constitutional imbalance may not be as self-evident. The person who is always angry, no matter what, is displaying the emotion that goes with the wood element. The person who is always happy, joyful, bubbling over (or the opposite, more commonly seen—very sad, depressed) goes with the element of fire. The person who is always sympathetic and loves to take care of you or is always caring for children is displaying the emotion of sympathy, and that goes with earth. The person who is always grieving, who has tremendous loss and cannot seem to get over it, goes with the element of metal. The

	1a	1b	2	3	4	5
Element	Fire		Earth	Metal	Water	Wood
Meridian	Small Intestine	Three Heater	Stomach	Colon	Bladder	Gall Bladder
Organ	Heart	Heart Protector	Spleen	Lung	Kidney	Liver
Color	Red		Yellow	White	Blue	Green
Emotion	Joy		Sympathy	Grief	Fear	Anger
Odor	Scorched		Fragrant	Rotten	Putrid	Rancid
Sound	Laughing		Singing	Weeping	Groaning	Shouting

Figure 39-6 ■ Law of five elements linking fire, earth, metal, water, and wood with interlocking variables.

person who is always fearful, paranoid, and afraid of life fits into the water element. People have different sounds to their voice. People who laugh excessively and are always humorous go with the fire element. People who shout a lot, their voices very powerful and strong, knocking you over, go with the wood element. People who have a singsong quality to their voice go with the earth element; groaning goes with the water element; and a weeping sound of the voice, although the person is not crying, goes with the metal element. You have probably smelled people who have a strong body odor and wondered why they did not bathe or use deodorant. There are five different odors and each one belongs to one of these elements. And perhaps you have seen a person who is green with envy or ash white, white as a sheet, or has pallor in the face. Each one of these colors goes with an element as described in the diagram (see Figure 39-6).

Each element also has organs relevant to it, with energetic pathways, called *meridians,* which are housed by that element. These pathways, or meridians, are just under the surface of the skin, throughout the body, and serve as channels for an electrical form of energy that flows in all human beings. This energy is the life force. In Chinese it is called *chi.* In the East Indian culture it is known as *prana.* This life force is always circulating round and round the body-mind along these pathways. And the acupuncturist can get in touch with this energy at certain points on these meridians, which are the acupuncture points.

Intervention. Once the examination is complete and the diagnosis is made, paying close attention to the color, emotion, odor, and sound and the elemental constitutional imbalance determined, it is simply a matter of treating the points along the meridians that are housed by that element on a week-to-week basis. Generally, this tunes the human being and everything starts to function more efficiently and more harmoniously, enhancing the person's quality of life.

There are 12 major meridians, two in each element, except for fire, which has four. Each of these meridians is named after the organ to which it is connected, which is also described in the diagram. Each meridian has 9 to 67 points on it. Each point has a name described by the Chinese that has been translated into English. It is the names and the functions of the different points that allow the acupuncturist to decide which points are to be used on which day and time and treatment. For example, the point Kidney-24 is actually named *spirit burial ground* and can be used to help a person suffering from grief, having lost a loved one. Taking the history at each visit, and determining blockage of the chi energy flowing in the meridians, is used as well to select the points used in treatment.

As patients get better, not only do their symptoms decrease in intensity and dissolve and often totally disappear with time, their emotional and feeling states also change for the better. People tend to become happier and peaceful and calm, more able to handle stress. They often will say, "I feel better in myself." The reason for this is that the patient is not just having her or his symptoms treated. This form of acupuncture, the five-element style, treats the body, the mind, and the spirit and integrates these three spheres of the human being. The point names are particularly revealing. There are names connected to nature and physical objects such as *small sea, greater mountain stream, blazing valley, sea of chi,* and *skull breathing.* There are also point names that have to do with emotions and feelings, such as *palace of weariness, gate of hope, rushing the frontier gate, intermediary, little merchant,* and *abdominal sorrow.* And then there are the points that relate to the spiritual qualities of life, such as *spirit burial ground, heavenly ancestor, heavenly pond, heavenly window, gate of destiny, inner frontier gate, soul door,* and *spirit deficiency.* When these spirit points are used, the person's spirit is buoyed up—it turns back on.

Each treatment lasts 15 to 60 minutes, depending on the individual practitioner. The practitioner can also include any of the following in the treatment sessions: conversation, history taking, massage, joint adjustments, instructions on diet and nutrition, psychosocial counseling, exercise recommendations, and so on. The initial visit takes longer because a history and physical examination are done and sometimes the initial treatment as well. This depends on the technique and abilities of the practitioner. Generally, the treatments are done twice a week for the first two to four visits and then once a week as the patient starts to get better. The interval continues to lengthen to every 2 to 4 weeks, and as the patient improves, the optimal interval is once every 3 months—once every season, the patient comes in for a tune-up for maintenance and prevention. Generally, a series of 10 treatments is a good way to start this type of therapy. Improvement in the patient's condition may be noticed as soon as the first treatment is done. It may take five or 10 treatments before it is noticed by the patient. Depending on the ability of the practitioner, improvement in the patient's condition generally occurs in 80% to 90% of patients. This, of course, also depends on the severity of the patient's imbalance and illness.

When acupuncture treatment is combined with psychosocial counseling, nutritional advice, exercise instruction, massage, or other forms of body work, in which the person is touched with warmth, peace, and love by another human being, great healing can take place.

Benefits of Intervention. Five-element acupuncture can be used for all sorts of clinical problems: physical, mental, emotional, and spiritual. Any and every type of person can and does respond. There are always exceptions to this, but the general rule is one of success. This includes acute problems and chronic problems, outpatients and hospitalized patients. In China, all patients with stroke are automatically treated with acupuncture as well as the more traditional Western methods. It works on babies, toddlers, adolescents, and the elderly. It can be used as a primary form of therapy to which other therapies are added, or it can be an adjunct to surgery, radiation, and medication or to other holistic therapies.

Future Treatments. The amount of time it takes for a person to heal depends on how long the person has been ill. A rule of thumb is that for every year a person has had a particular physical or mental problem, it is going to take about a month's worth of treatment, with each session done weekly. So, if a person has had arthritis for 20 years, 20 months of treatment should be expected.

On the other hand, if symptoms have been present for only a month or two, it is possible that they could go away with one or two treatments unless they are the result of some kind of serious illness, such as the sudden onset of cancer or heart disease or something that has been present for 1 or 2 years but has been subclinical. The general average is 10 treatments over a 4- to 8-week period, with a good possibility of illness being relieved partially or almost completely during that period, depending on the severity.

Summary. In summary, acupuncture is a healing therapy that is both an art and a science that comes from the Orient, specifically starting in China approximately 4500 years ago. There are many styles of acupuncture, and the most holistic style is known as *five-element acupuncture.* It truly helps to integrate the body, mind, and spirit. When acupuncture is combined with teaching the patient how to live a more healthy lifestyle, including eating a healthy diet, reducing stress, making healthy choices, thinking healthy thoughts, and including fun and relaxation, true healing can occur. Because of the chronic and degenerative nature of many illnesses in the United States, it is possible that total healing would not occur. Nevertheless, this type of therapy, along with the adjuncts mentioned earlier, should definitely help to create a healthier human being.

Allopathic Links to Models of Health Care Belief Systems

Electroacupuncture

Mary Lou Galantino

Acupuncture, a part of traditional Chinese medicine, has been used for more than 4500 years. Mapping of 12 meridian points, which are named primarily after the visceral organs they transverse, incorporates 361 regular points. There are also "Ashi points," which are typically tender points that are used for treatment of pain syndromes.[322] The acupuncturist must make a decision as to which acupuncture points to stimulate on the basis of a specific diagnosis. The goal is to balance chi, which is considered vital energy. If there is an imbalance caused by disease, the altered flow of chi can be detected and subsequently treated through needles or electrical stimulation over specific acupuncture points.

Therapeutic Effects of Electroacupuncture. The use of acupuncture is growing in popularity in most Western countries,[323] and the effectiveness of electroacupuncture as a modality for the treatment of pain has been shown by significant decreases in VAS scores.[324] The therapeutic effects of acupuncture have generally been applied for the treatment of pain; with the increasing acceptance of acupuncture as an effective modality for pain relief, the scope of research on this modality has widened considerably to include other health care conditions. The intensive research efforts on other therapeutic effects of acupuncture have produced encouraging results.[325-327] These results point to a reduction in pain, improvement in motor function, better balance, and improved gait; the results therefore have a neurophysiological interpretation. The effect of spasticity has been explored by researchers for multiple diagnoses such as spinal cord injury and stroke. Electroacupuncture has been found to have more of an effect on spasticity the earlier treatment is implemented, ideally within 3 weeks of injury. Findings reveal positive short- and long-term effects[328-330]; however, future research needs to include frequency of treatment and specific points of stimulation for a more comprehensive understanding. Some of the possible mechanisms by which acupuncture may affect motor function include the following:

1. Stimulation of the release of endogenous opioids.[331]
2. Changing of the amplitude of end plate potential, thus facilitating the events at the neuromuscular junctions. It has been suggested that peripheral factors contributing to the potentiation of a reflex (e.g., the H reflex) may affect the afferents and the neuromuscular junction.[332]
3. Stimulation of the sensory system, which will result in integrative actions at the spinal cord level, where acupuncture may facilitate the stretch reflex arc through both the gamma and alpha motor neurons. Facilitation may depend on the intensity and timing of the stimuli used to activate muscle afferents.[333]
4. Revealed on neuroimaging of acupuncture in patients with chronic pain, changes in cerebral blood flow associated with pain and acupuncture analgesia that correspond to areas of the brain involved in such phenomena.[333]

Training for acupuncture varies throughout the United States (refer to section on traditional acupuncture). Because needling is considered an invasive technique, physical therapists are prohibited from using it. Therefore an alternative to needle acupuncture is noninvasive electroacupuncture or electrical neurostimulation. Concerning the effects of electrical neurostimulation, there are various interpretations of the methods and underlying physiological mechanisms. One mechanism is neural.[334] Another study has indicated that electrical stimulation applied to acupuncture points may activate both neurological and endocrine functions that control pain.[334] Anderson and Lundeberg's study supported the release of β-endorphin and oxytocin, which are important for the control of pain and the regulation of blood pressure and body temperature.[334]

Research. Research on the effects of electroacupuncture on HIV-related neuropathy found significant reduction in pain, which suggests an excitatory effect on the neuromuscular system. Such an effect may be on membrane potential (possibly through influencing ionic transport) and improvement in body fluid circulation.[335] The effect on the sympathetic system is often reported and more or less explained. The same explanation is proposed for the action of electrical stimulation on pain,[336,337] with some effects on pain-mediating neurotransmitters at the level of the spinal cord and an endogenous modulation from the brain stem.[338]

Even in patients after cardiac surgery, relief of pain through electroacupuncture was shown to reduce the use of opioids such as fentanyl.[339] One case report showed excellent results in chronic pain reduction over a 2-year period in a patient with a pacemaker. In answer to the initial question regarding safety, electroacupuncture was shown to be an excellent alternative for individuals with pacemakers.[340]

Studies have shown that electroacupuncture may enhance the effect of strength training on motor function. One study compared upper-limb motor functional improvement in chronic stroke survivors who received a combination of electroacupuncture and strength training with that of subjects who received strength training alone. After the combined treatment, the quantitative spastic level, active wrist extension ROM, and Fugl-Meyer upper-limb motor score changed significantly. No significant changes were noted in isometric wrist strength. The strength training alone resulted in no significant changes to any measured variable. These results indicate that the combined acupuncture and strength training treatment reduced muscle spasticity and may have improved motor function for chronic stroke survivors with moderate or severe muscle spasticity.[341]

Although two mechanisms underlying the physiological mechanisms of electroacupuncture were presented previously, it would be prudent for physical therapists to consider maximizing the benefits of electrical modalities in various musculoskeletal and neurological disorders.[342] One prospective study[343] investigated the physiological effects of stimulation of acupuncture points ST36 and ST39 of the stomach meridian with Dynatron 200 microcurrent. Hemodynamic functions and skin temperature were monitored, with no significant differences found. However, further research is necessary to elucidate the nature of physiological effects of specific surface electrodes and various types of stimulation to determine the efficacy of electroacupuncture treatment.

Music Therapy

Therese Marie West

Music therapy is the clinical and evidence-based use of music interventions to accomplish individualized goals within a therapeutic relationship by a credentialed professional who has completed an approved music therapy program.[433]

Although music is not a "universal language" in the sense that a particular piece of music would have the same meaning and effect for any person anywhere, music *is* a universal human phenomenon. Most people today could describe ways in which music might be used to enhance health or well-being, and we find evidence of the use of music as part of healing practices throughout history.[434,435] Within a first worldview perspective, magical or mystical powers were attributed to music, and healing occurred within a context of social structures and shared beliefs. Music was often a part of rituals conducted by a shaman or healer who served as a spiritual intercessor or guide in a process designed to reestablish balance and harmony for the individual. Music, sometimes with dance, served as a gateway to altered states of consciousness and entry to deep altered states of consciousness, where creative experiences manifested multiple sources of information not available through observation alone. This process supported insights about the causes of and remedies for physical, emotional, social, and spiritual imbalance. Where patient, healer, family, and community members participated together in healing rituals involving the use of music, treatment occurred within the natural environment and social fabric of everyday life. Examples of music healing within a first worldview perspective can still be found within indigenous cultural groups to this day.

The rise of the second worldview brought new values that emphasized logical and rational approaches to the use of music to address health issues. During this phase in history, we see the first examples of published work asserting the theory that music could influence emotions and mood states and thereby improve physical or mental health.[434] Anecdotal evidence and case reports were used to support emerging theories and practices into the early twentieth century. In the latter part of the twentieth century, we began to see the scientific method applied systematically to the study of music in relation to single variable changes in (1) disease and pathological states or (2) functional activities and willingness to participate in rehabilitation treatment settings. Researchers continue to explore possible mechanisms through which music may contribute to improved physical or mental health via its influence on various factors such as emotional responses, mood states, relaxation, activation, or motivation.

History of Music Therapy. In the United States, music therapy began to develop as a profession after World War II, when it was found that music could facilitate both physical rehabilitation and recovery from emotional trauma in veterans returned from the war. Although early music therapists were often musician volunteers, music educators, or musician-physicians, it had become clear that specific education and training were needed, and music therapy curricula and academic programs were developed beginning in the mid 1940s. The first professional music therapy organization (the National Association for Music Therapy [NAMT]) was formed in 1950. A second professional organization, the American Association for Music Therapy (AAMT), formed in 1971. The NAMT and AAMT merged in 1998 to form the American Music Therapy Association (AMTA). The AMTA sets standards for education and clinical training in music therapy programs accredited at more than 70 colleges and universities in the United States and Canada. The Certification Board for Music Therapists (CBMT) was accredited in 1986 by the National Commission for Certifying Agencies and certifies music therapists to practice throughout the

United States. Certification is via a competency-based certification process that includes specialized coursework, 1200 hours of supervised clinical training, and a certification board examination. There are currently more than 5000 music therapists maintaining the MT-BC (Music Therapist, Board Certified) credential and participating in at least 100 hours of continuing education for recertification every 5 years to maintain and increase competencies for practice in this rapidly evolving field.[436] The development of music therapy in the United States parallels the stages of health care development as discussed earlier (see the discussion of historical perspective in this chapter). Stage 2 worldviews were dominant during the formative years of music therapy as a profession in the United States. The concurrent emergence of behavioral psychology, along with a need to provide validation of specific music therapy treatments, led to an emphasis on outcomes understood via behavioral measurements. Meanwhile, the complex and multifaceted interactions between humans and their music remained mysterious as clear evidence for mechanisms eluded early researchers. Although basic science study is now part of the continuing research, applied or clinical research has continued to dominate the literature in music therapy, and there is a great deal of work ahead to better understand many of the powerful effects of music observed in clinical settings. Therapists observe that patients who are unable to speak as a result of stroke or AD are often able to sing coherently when presented with familiar music. How is it that the gait of a patient with Parkinson disease improves markedly in the presence of a rhythmic auditory stimulus[437]? How does music-evoked imagery (such as experienced with the Bonny Method of Guided Imagery and Music) alter physiological and psychological indicators of stress[438,439]? Modern research developments in brain neuroscience, gait assessment technology, and psychoneuroimmunology are improving researchers' ability to study mechanisms as well as treatment outcomes. Meanwhile, an important focus in the field of music therapy is the development of clinically validated treatments for specific problems and populations. In the United States, music therapy is recognized as "an established health profession in which music is used within a therapeutic relationship to address physical, emotional, cognitive, and social needs of individuals. After assessing the strengths and needs of each client, the qualified music therapist provides the indicated treatment including creating, singing, moving to, and/or listening to music. Through musical involvement in the therapeutic context, clients' abilities are strengthened and transferred to other areas of their lives."[440]

Specialization. Music therapists develop specialized areas of practice, treating across the life span from perinatal to palliative care, in schools, hospitals, skilled nursing, rehabilitation, outpatient, or community settings. The goals they address support progress in developmental tasks, rehabilitation of physical and cognitive functioning, adaptation and coping, pain management, recovery from trauma, and quality of life. Music therapists work in private practice, as members of interdisciplinary teams, and as consultants and collaborators. Therese West is one of many music therapists who has worked in rehabilitation settings in co-treatment, consultation, or collaboration with speech-language pathologists, physical therapists, and occupational therapists, as well as with a wide range of practitioners from other professions in medicine and mental health arenas. During early clinical collaborations in rehabilitation settings from the mid 1980s to the early 1990s, West found little research to support an understanding of observed phenomena in the rehabilitation clinic setting and had to depend largely on basic skills of music therapy assessment, careful documentation, and evaluation of treatment outcomes and effectiveness. In recent years, the music therapy profession has focused on increasing the quality and scope of research to support empirically validated best practice with reliable outcomes for a number of specific populations of interest to professionals in rehabilitation settings. Rehabilitation music therapists now have the benefit of empirically supported treatment protocols and continuing research regarding effectiveness and safety of music therapy methods.

Music Therapy in the Neonatal Intensive Care Unit. Low–birth-weight and premature infants are at high risk for developmental disabilities, and given the vulnerabilities of their neurological systems, early sensory experiences in the neonatal intensive care unit (NICU) environment are of particular interest to music therapy researchers. A number of studies have explored the uses of music in the NICU, and results suggest that various clinically significant outcomes may result from carefully controlled application of music treatments for the premature infant. Physiological (autonomic nervous system) responses related to infant stress states (blood pressure, heart rate, respiration rate) have been shown to respond to various music stimuli, with favorable responses to sedative music.[441,442] Improvements in behavior state, weight gain, and decrease in length of hospital stay have been reported after treatment with recorded vocal music[443] and parent training in music and multimodal stimulation (MMS).[444] A collection of writings on basic theories, research, and clinical practice of music therapy in the NICU from 16 different countries offers an overview of the development of this practice area around the world.[445] Jayne Standley, a senior researcher and collaborator in the development of empirically supported treatments for premature and low–birth-weight infants in the United States, presents specific music therapy protocols for pacification, stimulation, and parent-infant interaction.[446] Music therapy treatment protocols have been reviewed and refined with particular attention to audiological issues and safety concerns[447] and with attention to nursing care models designed to meet individual developmental needs of newborn infants.[448] The MMS procedure is a comprehensive program engaging the premature infant, parents, and caregivers using auditory, tactile, visual, and vestibular stimulation to support optimal premature infant development.[449] Research is continuing, and as longitudinal studies are conducted we will know more about longer-term developmental outcomes that may correlate with the immediate benefits associated with music therapy in the NICU.

Music Therapy in Neurological Rehabilitation. Music therapists have been working in neurological rehabilitation settings in the United States for more than 25 years. Tomaino[450] describes her long professional collaboration with the neurologist Dr. Oliver Sacks and shares insights developed through extensive clinical application of music in the individualized assessment and treatment of various neurological diseases and injuries. Music can access intact neurological functions and is used to facilitate relaxation, to increase attention and motivation, to improve the readiness for (priming) and timing of motor activities, and to enhance communication and emotional expression while providing supports for coping and adaptation. Tomaino[450] describes the music therapy process from assessment and treatment planning through treatment and evaluation of outcomes, focusing not only on physical and behavioral changes but also on the engagement of the whole person through a trust-based therapeutic relationship. Familiar music can provide the patient a sense of safety, with predictable elements of rhythm, melody (prosody), words and lyrics, and structure across time within socially and culturally relevant contexts. Musical elements are systematically applied to support functioning in cognition and memory, speech and communication, gait, and upper-extremity activities.

Music therapy has been used in many rehabilitation settings to support cognitive functioning in areas such as attention, sensory filtering and focusing, memory, sequencing, and executive functioning. Ongoing development of theoretical foundations for clinical uses of music in the cognitive treatment of those with brain insult or injury is supported by brain imaging and in vivo functional studies providing evidence of shared mechanisms among musical and nonmusical perceptual and cognitive brain functions[451] and effects of music on electroencelphalographic activities in cortical networks.[452]

West has observed the phenomenon commonly reported in rehabilitation music therapy, where persons with various aphasias are able to sing, but not able to speak fluently. The patient is often able to sing clearly in time with the singing of the music therapist, who adapts the tempo and other elements as needed. There appears to be an entrainment process, not only rhythmically, but also in elements of prosody and articulation. The mechanisms are not yet fully understood, but at least one study suggests that singing in synchrony with an auditory model (choral singing) may be more effective than choral speech in improving word intelligibility because choral singing may entrain more than one auditory-vocal interface.[453] Kim and Tomaino[454] have developed and pilot tested a music therapy treatment protocol for persons with nonfluent aphasia, integrating extensive clinical experience with recent findings from experimental studies using cognitive-behavioral, electrophysiological, and brain imaging techniques. Whereas specific brain structures have been well established for speech and language, and were thought to be distinct from music processing areas, it now appears that music and language may share some aspects of neurological processing in bilateral hemispheric activities.[454] The evolving brain research may help us better understand our clinical observations and will most certainly support increasingly effective treatment protocols for expressive aphasia.

One particularly valuable discovery in music therapy for neurological rehabilitation is the fact that rhythmic elements of music can influence the timing and execution of motor sequences in both gross motor and fine motor activities. A neuroscience approach to understanding potential effects of rhythmic auditory stimulation (RAS) and motor-rhythm synchronization phenomena in neurological rehabilitation is supported by a well developed body of basic research and clinical studies with a number of rehabilitation populations.[455-458]

Research. One study demonstrated the ability of RAS to enhance treatment when it is added to a conventional PT gait program for acute hemiparetic stroke patients.[459] These patients showed significant increases in velocity and stride length and reductions in EMG amplitude variability of gastrocnemius muscle in the RAS-enhanced treatment group compared with the standard PT (control) group.[459] Studies have also demonstrated benefits of RAS treatments in gait rehabilitation for patients with TBI[460] and Parkinson disease.[437] Research continues to investigate possible applications for RAS in other areas of rehabilitation, such as speech motor control in patients with Parkinson disease, where the largest improvements have been found in patients with the most severe impairments and only minimal benefits in mildly affected patients.[461] The specificity of such findings highlights the importance of careful diagnostic assessment and an understanding of both problem and treatment specifics as we develop evidence-based best practices for music therapy or any other complementary or alternative treatment. Controlled clinical research continues to support the development of music therapy treatment protocols that demonstrate reliable physical outcomes for specific problems encountered in neurological rehabilitation settings.

Other kinds of music therapy investigations commonly conducted at earlier points along the pathway to empirical validation include qualitative research, case studies, and pilot studies. Although empirical research investigates specific outcomes, music therapists often look to qualitative research to help them identify and analyze processes and refine treatments on the basis of their effectiveness in the clinical or community setting. A group of Australian music therapists investigated themes in songs written by patients with TBI.[462] Such investigations give clinicians insight into the inner experience of the patient and may enable the practitioner to be more effective and supportive of patients' coping and recovery processes.

Case studies illustrate the potential of music therapy to enhance coping and adaptation to enormous losses experienced by patients poststroke. Erdonmez[463] describes the piano performance–based treatment of a 54-year-old man whose quality of life as a successful general medical practitioner, linguist, and talented keyboard player was abruptly changed by a stroke with massive damage in left temporal and parietal lobes. New motor skills were developed, as he learned to master with his functional left hand the complex musical tasks originally composed for the right hand. He learned new music and new adaptive skills, and treatment resulted in improvements in speed and manual dexterity. The results of this case study reinforce today's concepts of neuroplasticity and encourage further research into the possibility that music therapy may facilitate development of new neurological pathways and motor strategies. Simultaneously, music therapy gently supports the patient in coping with losses, adapting to limitations, and reconstructing a life with meaning and enjoyment. McMaster[464] describes a course of individual music therapy treatment for a woman in her early 40s who, after the rupture of a tumor in her heart resulting in a CVA, was blind, without speech, and severely disabled in many areas of functioning. Through a music therapy program, this woman was able to protest and grieve her many losses, discovered and received validation of her inner resources and creativity, and experienced new accomplishments. These experiences supported her sense of self and enabled her to mobilize her physical, emotional, and spiritual strengths to face life in a body that would never return to what she had always known.

Although loss of short-term memory and other cognitive limitations resulting from neurological insult may be considered contraindications for traditional psychotherapy approaches, Goldberg and colleagues[465] explored the use of music-evoked imagery with a brain-damaged woman whose behavioral problems had resulted in psychiatric hospitalization. This adaptation of the Bonny Method of Guided Imagery and Music supported a creative interaction between the patient and therapist. These interactions allowed the patient to explore in novel ways losses, role changes, and challenges in accepting help from others. Although these researchers were not able to gather follow-up data, immediate positive behavioral changes observed in the milieu suggested that the imagery may have facilitated psychological processing and change not accessible by verbal therapy alone. Short[466] suggests that the Bonny Method, through the spontaneous imagery process, can allow patients to convey information about how they are feeling physically and emotionally with regard to the rehabilitation process. She also proposes that the content of the images evoked by the music can be analyzed by the Bonny Method therapist, to discover emergent themes relevant to the clinical treatment. More research is needed to help music therapy researchers, educators, and clinicians understand how music imagery treatments affect neurological functioning.

Music Therapy as a Complementary Modality. Meanwhile, music therapy continues to play an important role in holistic care, even while some phenomena yet elude our scientific methods. West was asked to assess two different teenage boys, hospitalized and in comatose states after head injuries. The treating neurologist was preparing to recommend longer-term follow-up disposition for these young patients, and while considering all the medical evidence at his disposal, this physician also wanted to see what music therapy might discover in terms of responsiveness to stimuli. Although one patient showed no response of any kind to any auditory or tactile stimuli, the second patient proved to be a most interesting example of the mysterious recovery. His neurological tests indicated that his prognosis would be very poor; "persistent vegetative state" was the expectation. In the absence of any evidence that he could benefit from more intensive rehabilitation services, he would be sent to a facility where he would receive long-term custodial care but no therapies. During the music therapy assessment, this young man began to show signs of responsiveness to musical stimuli. A professional skeptic, West was reluctant to consider his eye gaze changes, head movement, and smiling to be meaningful responses to the music without additional testing. These could be random events coincident with the stimuli. West presented music in a popular style familiar to the patient (according to family sources) and gently applied tactile rhythmic stimulation to his hands, arms, legs, and feet in time with the music. The patient began to move his own extremities in rhythmic time to the music and continued to do so when the therapist removed her hands. The therapist carefully documented the procedures and patient responses and returned a report to the referring physician. Over the next few days, the patient's responsiveness increased dramatically. The neurologist had this young man placed in a rehabilitation treatment setting. A month later, he had begun to walk and showed promise of significant recovery of functions in a number of areas, including speech. This patient was initially medically evaluated as having little potential for recovery, yet after music therapy he was interactive and a participant in life. This case is a good example of how music can access and bring forward what is yet intact (whole) within a person whose body has been damaged by illness or injury.

Although basic and clinical research activities are increasing an understanding of "how" and "for what, when, and for whom" music therapy can be of specific benefit in neurological rehabilitation and medicine, music therapists are also facing the new challenges and opportunities of new worldviews. Music therapy is among the complementary modalities provided as part of a response to increasing demand for holistic and patient- and family-centered health care. Because music interacts with every domain of human experience (physical, cognitive, emotional, social, and spiritual), it has the potential to influence multiple needs simultaneously, in a unified way that respects both the uniqueness of the individual and the deep common ground of the person within the whole.

CASE EXAMPLE OF INTEGRATION OF VARIOUS APPROACHES

Carol M. Davis
Darcy A. Umphred
Therese Marie West

The intervention with the following patient reflected awareness by the therapist of using myofascial release, CST, and the Feldenkrais method, as well as more traditional therapeutic interventions. The reader must remember that any one of the other approaches presented within this chapter might also have been implemented as part of this client's treatment given another therapist's experience, education, and therapeutic sensitivity, as well as the cultural biases of the client and family. No judgment is being placed on the method or methods selected for this client or any other. What are critically important are the objective outcome measures after the intervention (Case Study 39-3).

CASE STUDY 39-3 ■ MRS. P. K.

Mrs. P. K., a 66-year-old woman, presented herself 2 years ago, once she let her diagnosis of Parkinson disease penetrate her consciousness. It was inconceivable to her that she might have the same illness that affected her grandmother and the same illness that the attorney general could not seem to mask in front of the public. As a seasoned lobbyist, she worked with politicians and traveled in powerful circles. Using her intellect and her considerable skill in negotiation, she successfully persuaded powerful people to see things her way for the benefit of her clients. A woman of small stature (5 feet tall and 105 pounds), Mrs. P. K. feared that her illness would be seen as a weakness and was adamant that under no circumstances was anyone to know that she had Parkinson disease. Fortunately for her, her only symptom was a slight right upper-extremity tremor on waking each morning and some "stiffness," especially in flexion and extension of her right shoulder and extension of her right knee. This aspect of the case is critical. Her endless motivation to exercise was based on this fear of exposure, which she regarded, in spite of her therapist's attempts to work through this with her, as a death knell for her professional life.

Mrs. P. K. had exercised much of her life and walked a mile on her treadmill each morning at 3.8 miles/hr. Her husband was familiar with massage and Rolfing, and, at her request, he stretched her hips and lower extremities each day as prophylaxis against the return of a low back pain problem from years earlier. Initial examination revealed the following deficits:

- Active right shoulder flexion 130/170
- Active right wrist flexion 45/85
- Cervical rotation, right 60/80
- Cervical rotation, left 45/80

Gait. Mrs. P. K. tended to walk with a narrow stance, heels close together, but with good heel strike. She was unable to ascend or descend stairs, looking straight ahead without severe slowing. She had little head movement or thoracic rotation; her gait looked rather robotic.

Skin. There was slight edema on the right side of the face, with slight swelling of the upper right lip.

Posture. Mrs. P. K.'s pelvis was rotated down to the right, she had a slightly forward head, and although she did not have rounded shoulders per se, the fascia was drawn tight over her pectorals toward her sternum. The fascia of her legs was taut and revealed a lack of tissue hydration.

Mrs. P. K. had no limitations in function. Her primary clinical goal was to prevent physical manifestations of the onset of the rigidity caused by Parkinson disease. If and when the disease itself progressed, we reasoned that the more fluid her tissue was, and the more physically fit she was, the less the impact of a dopamine deficiency, and the more efficient her medication (selegiline) would be in reducing the impact of a dopamine deficiency and controlling the progression of her symptoms. An intervention plan was developed that included a combination of traditional exercises for Parkinson disease, complemented by myofascial release and CST, and Feldenkrais exercises to increase her awareness of her movement.

After we received the referral from her neurologist, her treatments were scheduled for twice monthly, with home exercises. We explained how myofascial release "works" to keep the fascia loose but that how it seems to facilitate a sense of calm and peacefulness when done in conjunction with craniosacral rhythm was not known. Given the lack of basic science evidence, she still willingly signed her informed consent. The plan of intervention integrated myofascial release techniques (along with Feldenkrais exercises) with her traditional therapeutic interventions focusing on the body system problems (impairments) caused by Parkinson disease and their effect on functional movement. These exercises stressed active rotation, spinal segmental exercises, and controlled, active relaxation of the antagonists. Her prognosis was good, for she was beginning intervention in the early stages of the disease, which would preclude secondary complications; she was fully functional and she was physically fit, if not well hydrated, and was motivated. She was encouraged to drink more water.

Treatment began with several minutes of bouncing on the Swiss ball, working on spinal segment articulation and spinal proprioception, and on lateral and backward balancing to relearn where her center of gravity was in her cone of stability. Next, with the assistance of the therapist, she moved to the bolster, where she lay supine with knees flexed and worked on lower-extremity extension and balance. On the mat she worked with Feldenkrais exercises and rotation of her shoulders and hips in opposite directions, with head rotation, and reviewed the pelvic exercises in her home program to help her differentiate her pelvis from her hips and to keep her lumbosacral junction and sacroiliac joints mobile.

From there she moved to the plinth, where wedges were positioned to derotate her pelvis in the supine position. Myofascial treatment then began with gentle palpation of her cranial rhythm; she was asked to relax, take three large breaths, and in her mind's eye, "go on vacation." (Music therapy could be easily introduced at this time to assist her nervous system with relaxation.) This was difficult for her, for her mind is active, constantly thinking about work. As she relaxed, her breathing slowed, and her cranial rhythm became more pronounced. At this point, the thoughts of the clinician became centered and progressed through various activities. First, there was focused intention and reflective thought that asked that energy from the clinician be used to bring about the highest good for the client. Conscious centering included taking deep breaths, visualizing a grounding of the clinician, and seeing that energy flow deep into the earth. Next, the clinician focused attention within the heart (heart chakra according to medical intuitives) and felt deep appreciation for the client, and for the opportunity to help her by use of holistic techniques.

This exchange of healing energy was an important moment for both client and clinician. It might be conjectured that the therapist consciously tapped into the universal healing energy that surrounds all of us at all times and became a kind of transformer for that energy to be used to facilitate the flow of the client's own chi or healing energy that had been disrupted. No matter the verbal explanation used for this interaction, it created a strong bond of trust and respect that would continue to influence the outcome of the interventions.

The clinician continued treatment by moving into an occipital lobe release, followed by cranial releases and a sphenoid release, reasoning that this would assist the myofascia in the cranium to help ensure proper alignment of the cranial bones and to facilitate blood supply to and from the CNS. At this

Continued

CASE STUDY 39-3 ■ MRS. P. K.—cont'd

point in the treatment, the clinician would usually allow clinical perception or clinical intuition to guide decision making regarding the next movement. In reality, the therapist might just follow the guidance of the client's innate healing or centering aptitude. Occasionally, more time was spent on the neck and upper thorax, with supine or side-lying scapular releases and cervical spine work. Sometimes, after the wedges were removed and the symphysis pubis was in place, a leg pull or diaphragm release was done. If the clinician noticed tightness or imbalance, or if the client indicated that the "fascial voice" was speaking to her, for example, along her right rib cage as the leg pull was carried out, the clinician would follow the lead of what was happening in the body of the client, disregarding any obvious symptoms that needed attention.

This concept is an important facet of myofascial release and many other complementary medical practices. Myofascial release would prescribe that, clinically, it is often shortsighted to go directly to the area of symptoms for treatment, for the problem is often caused by fascial restrictions distant from that area. Specifically, myofascial release as a type of complementary therapy seems to involve subtle or low-intensity nonmaterial stimuli known as "energy medicine." Although various explanations are offered for energy medicine in terms of a vital force or life energy, there is no agreed-on scientific understanding or precise meaning of these ideas in Western scientific concepts. Two proposed mechanisms for healer interventions are (1) that consciousness is causal, that is, the conscious intention of the healer through prayer or other means may physically improve the health and well-being of the patient and (2) that subtle energies may be exchanged or otherwise be involved, for instance, a condition of physical resonance between the energy fields of healer and patient, which may mediate the beneficial effects.

During the 2 years of Mrs. P. K.'s, treatment, she had a partial left rotator cuff tear and pain in the right fibular head area of her knee, both of which responded positively to myofascial release: cross-hands release work and soft tissue mobilization. Routinely, her right wrist was mobilized after an arm pull, and both scapulae were released in side lying after cross-hands release to the pectoral area.

On days when the pelvic area stiffness could not be relieved, 5 to 10 minutes of the myofascial release technique of rebounding was used, in which her body and extremities were passively rocked back and forth. This helped the stiffness to release, after which Mrs. P. K. always remarked how much more "alive" her body felt. The treatment usually ended on the plinth with a side-lying dural tube release, helping her balance her energy gently.

Once the myofascial release and craniosacral work was completed, Mrs. P. K. might be asked to lie prone for further scapular extension exercise or go onto all fours for "cat and camel" spinal mobility work, with wrist extension, along with partial push-ups to work on active elbow extension. From there she would go to the stairs, where she practiced step-over-step maneuvers, forward and back and with "grapevine twists," working on fluidity of motion and on masking her tendency to keep her right fingers extended in a parkinsonian posture. A critical component of her intervention was working on her ability to trust herself without needing to watch her feet.

Her home program consisted of pelvic mobility exercises and opposite rotation of arms and legs with cervical rotation. Extra shoulder exercises were added for her rotator cuff injury, and passive lower-extremity stretch over the side of the bed for iliotibial band release for her knee problem, along with fibular head mobilizations. She also lay supine on a 6-inch rubber ball, which she would roll segmentally up her spine to music to help with segmental mobilization. She then walked the treadmill for 1 mile.

The 3-month follow-up on impairment outcomes revealed the following:

- Active right shoulder flexion 45/180
- Active right wrist flexion 5/85
- Cervical rotation, right 70/80
- Cervical rotation, left 60/80

Gait: There was improved step width distance between the heels. Stair agility was much improved, with ability to ascend and descend on most days looking straight ahead. Her braiding motion was smooth and continuous without needing to look at her feet. In Mrs. P. K.'s own words: "I feel stronger and more limber inside and outside. I feel I look better and function better."

Skin: The edema in the face was reduced and on most days was not noticeable at all.

The degenerative progression of Parkinson disease varies with the individual, but Mrs. P. K. has been fortunate. With careful regulation of her medication, her home program, and her twice-monthly therapy sessions, there has been extraordinary success in preventing any obvious signs of rigidity from manifesting, which was her goal and thus a primary target outcome for the clinician. No one knows how much of the relief of symptoms was a result of her medication, although she was taking the medication for 3 months before she began therapy without showing the results achieved with therapeutic intervention. With this therapeutic intervention demonstrating effective outcomes, it could be argued by both clinician and client that myofascial release and CST helped keep the fascial system elongated and functioning in a self-corrective way. Similarly, integrating traditional personalized exercises with complementary interventions has enhanced the accomplishment of the client's goals for therapy and helped her to regain and maintain a higher quality of life.

The case of Mrs. P. K. offers an opportunity to consider how other complementary and alternative therapies might also be added to her overall plan of care. For instance, music therapy could potentially support three areas of her treatment: (1) music-assisted relaxation during the myofascial treatment, (2) music added as a reinforcing and motivating element for her home exercise program, and (3) individual music therapy to support emotional coping and adaptation during the course of the Parkinson disease.

The music therapist would first assess Mrs. P. K.'s responses to music and her music preferences, as well as her comfort in using musical experiences for relaxation or for emotional expression. For treatment areas 1 or 2, the music therapist would work in consultation and collaboration with the treating physical/myofascial therapist. A co-treatment approach is ideal, but the music therapist can also serve as a consultant, providing musical materials to be used by the physical or occupational therapist. It is important to consider musical elements such as rhythm, harmony, and tone qualities, as well as highly individualized responses such as nonmusical memories and associations that are elicited by the

CASE STUDY 39-3 ■ MRS. P. K.—cont'd

music. Once the music is developed and refined with input from the patient, this music may be recorded for the patient to use during clinic treatments or at home. The music therapist carefully selects appropriate musical styles and instrumentation and matches the music to the breathing rate, tension level, and other individual parameters to enhance relaxation responses. For goal 2, the flow, tense-release, and tempos in the music are carefully selected to support movements during exercising and to provide a pleasant, energizing, and motivating stimulus. Finally, as mentioned in goal area 3, music therapy may augment rehabilitation team treatments by supporting the patient in tasks related to the psychological and emotional aspects of coping with disease and may assist the individual to continue experiencing well-being and improved quality of life. Music may enhance the sensory richness of mental imagery and can support sensory-kinesthetic imagery and body awareness. An advanced technique such as the Bonny Method of Guided Imagery and Music can be used to develop an increased awareness of bodily states through the language of imagery. This work can help the patient develop more sensitive awareness of the body's unique and individual form of nonverbal communication.

The integration of all these methods brings mental, emotional, and spiritual components of self into a more integrated approach for adaptation to change, whether it be caused by a progressive disease, aging, or any other event. One can move beyond merely coping, to thriving and living to full potential. Finally, all these types of therapeutic interventions can continue to provide familiar, comforting, and soothing support when the patient eventually enters the palliative care phase. Certainly, traditional and complementary approaches discussed within this chapter could also be integrated into the previous case. It is not within the scope of this chapter to integrate and synthesize all complementary approaches as if a large holistic approach was available to everyone. However, it is within the hopes of the authors that colleagues will recognize that integration has the potential to exist in future health care environments, but it will evolve only when therapists and patients are willing to accept that there is always more to learn. There are always more options for the patient than any one therapist has available, and new approaches will continue to evolve and become options in the future.

The final case study of Mrs. P. K. was presented not to negate but rather to integrate traditional therapeutic interventions with complementary approaches. With limitations in health care benefits, consumers experience frustration regarding access to providers such as physical, occupational, speech therapists. Many chronic problems remain unanswered by allopathic medicine. Many clients are looking elsewhere for answers and for hope. When individuals no longer can look toward the Western medical system to regain or maintain health or healing, the only available options exist outside traditional Western medicine. As individual practitioners we can be part of that transition or be left behind with traditional Western medicine. It is interesting that branches of Western medicine are turning toward complementary philosophies and some medical schools are incorporating this training into student physicians' education. If PT and OT remain tethered to the portion of Western medicine that is linear, is reductionistic, and focuses on research that is univariable, not system interaction based, then these two professions have the same potential future as traditional medicine. That future is not clear, but certainly traditional medicine is going to play a significantly reduced role in health care delivery. Our future in neurorehabilitation is up to the breadth and limitations of our leaders and to the willingness of our younger colleagues to follow or become leaders themselves. The future possibilities for both professions are enormous, not only in integrating complementary and alternative medicine into intervention for clients with chronic and degenerative illnesses, but also in acute care and in health and wellness maintenance. The answers to what is the best evidence-based practice lie in functional outcome measurements. Innovative research will play a role in the future direction of competency-based interventions. Until measurement tools are available to analyze the interactions of multiple variables simultaneously, clinicians must continue to use existing objective outcome measures to determine whether an intervention should be stopped, continued, or altered. Selecting intervention strategies on the basis of belief only, without simultaneously measuring objective outcomes, will always lead to questions regarding whether the intervention was worth the financial investment. The challenge will be to remain open and willing to discover new alternatives while staying grounded in the ethical responsibility to establish an evidence base for the practice of PT and OT.

CONCLUSION

Darcy A. Umphred

Before the clinician embraces any complementary approach, the individual needs to identify which philosophy or paradigm matches her or his own belief system and aligns with her or his own emotional safety issues. Tethering an understanding of any complementary approach to an established scientific base will allow clinicians to stretch beyond their comfortable paradigms. When treating patients, clinicians are not recommended to jump from one theory to another or from one intervention strategy to another without clinically reasoning why those choices have been made. Therapists, during their professional education, are taught to use the Western medical model to have an understanding and a scientific basis for disease and pathology. Similarly, the student and clinician are taught to develop the ability to evaluate and analyze both normal and abnormal movement and synthesize what components within and outside the body will influence those movements. Emphasis is placed on movements that lead to the functional ability to interact in daily living and work environments and those movements that the client considers critical for quality of life. The last category encompasses any activity the client values, such as golf, gold panning, fly fishing, birdwatching, hiking in the mountains, scuba diving, hunting game for food or sport, or any other activity important to the client. The therapeutic variables that might influence the quality of movement of that client may or may not be a result of the disease or pathology commonly considered the reason for medical management (Figure 39-7). No one who studies and works

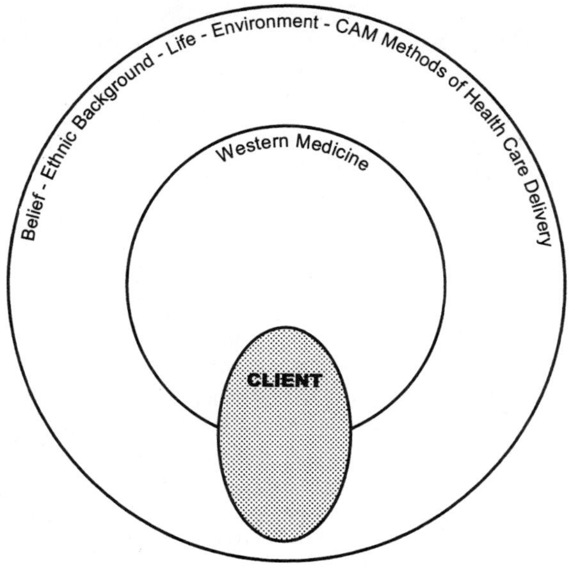

Figure 39-7 ■ Client enters Western medicine owing to disease or pathological condition or with functional limitations that prevent participation in life.

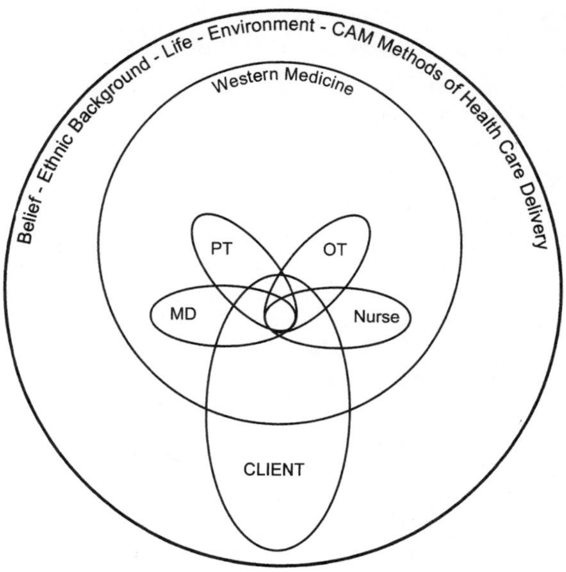

Figure 39-8 ■ Transdisciplinary interactions within Western medical model.

with individuals who have had a CNS injury would imply that the medical management of that injury or disease is not critical to the outcome of the patient's motor recovery and/or quality of life. Simultaneously, clinicians in the past and today's students and clinicians with an in-depth scientific knowledge of motor control, motor learning, and neuroplasticity observe, analyze, and influence motor, emotional, and cognitive recovery in patients that physicians might not expect. When treating patients with neurological insults of any kind, students are taught to accept that there is a transdisciplinary interaction among professional disciplines and that each profession not only uniquely affects the client but also has an interactive effect that is dependent on other professions and their respective impact on the patient's health, wellness, and potential to attain a maximal quality of life (Figure 39-8). When complementary and alternative approaches to health care are introduced into this model, then our colleagues need to determine which approaches interact with Western medicine and which do not (Figure 39-9). Why one approach interacts with the patient and another does not is based on the client's beliefs, needs, and responses to intervention as well as the clinician's beliefs and knowledge. Because the professions of OT and PT have always been tethered to Western medicine, therapists need to critically analyze the interactions of those approaches that clearly overlap with our existing paradigm before we let go of the tether and venture totally into the unknown (Figure 39-10). Those components of alternative approaches that obviously overlap with acceptable practice need to be identified and their effectiveness established (Figure 39-11). Evidence-based practice is considered the norm today and not just a gold standard. Yet, clinicians must also accept that evidence is based on comparison of one variable against another and that our research tools cannot look at all variables simultaneously as seen when observing and interacting with a patient. Thus, clinicians need to be constantly vigilant in observing, feeling, and analyzing what variables

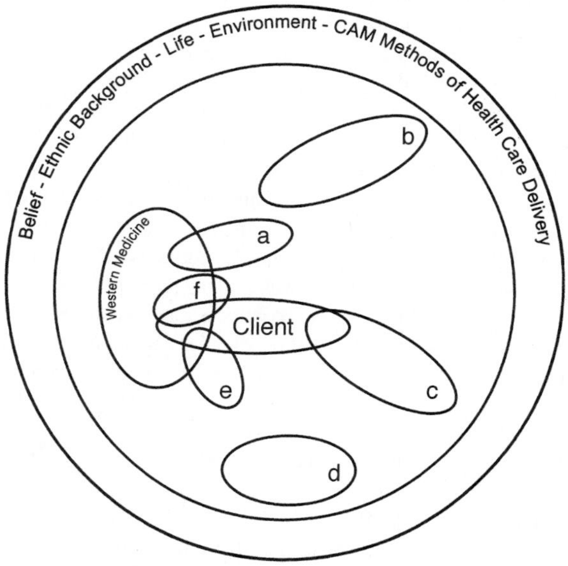

Figure 39-9 ■ Complementary and alternative methods (CAMs) of health care delivery. Some CAMs interact with Western medicine: *a, f, e*. Some alternative models do not interact with Western medicine: *b, c, d*. Some alternative models meet needs of the client: *c, e, f*. Some alternative models do not meet the needs of the client: *a, b, d*.

seem to be affecting the patient's recovery of functional movement. Just accepting that a treatment will create change because the evidence suggests so does not guarantee that the specific patient will benefit optimally from the intervention. Thus, when considering using an "alternative treatment approach," therapists need to remain critical in their analytical skill in order to determine whether the patient is actually improving. With the establishment of those clear clinical correlations (those that match Western science models and those that show improvement in the patient), the remaining

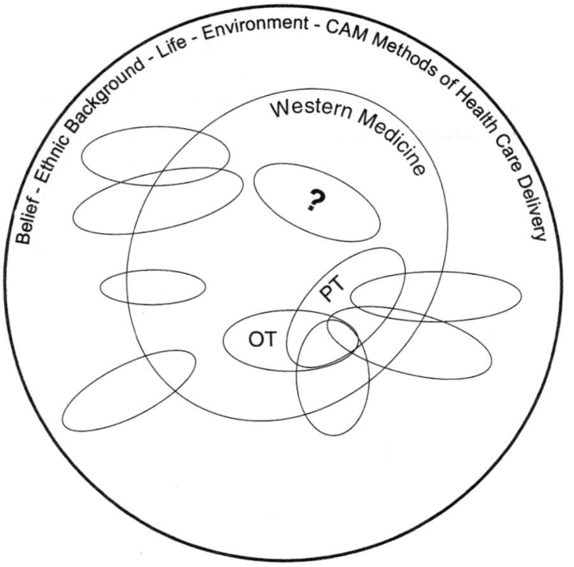

Figure 39-10 ■ Complementary and alternative methods (CAMs) interacting with Western medicine. Some models interact to a large extent with Western medicine and some to a small extent. Some models interact with both Western medicine and other complementary models. The extent of complementary interactions with either physical or occupational therapy or both reflect which models fall within respective scopes of practice and thus become part of the professional's treatment tools.

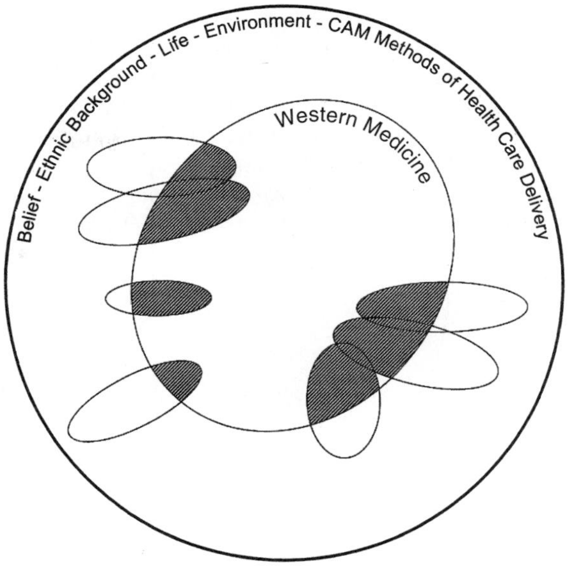

Figure 39-11 ■ The portion of each alternative or complementary model that overlaps with allopathic medicine and traditional occupational and physical therapy has been the focus of this chapter. As efficacy is established for those components that interlock, therapists will more readily accept these approaches as part of their practice.

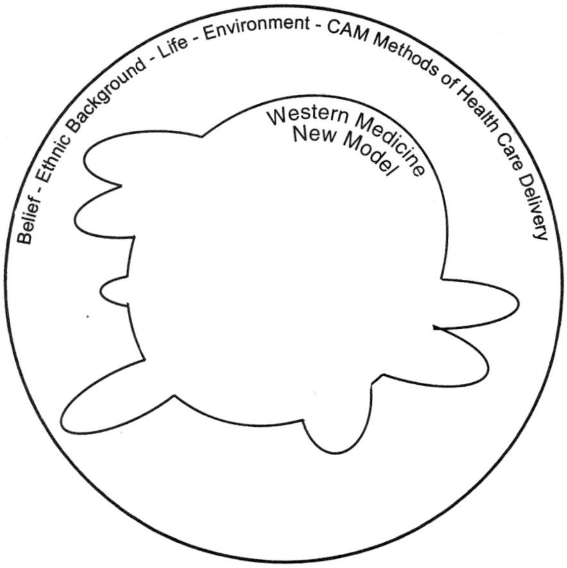

Figure 39-12 ■ New model of Western health care delivery beyond complementary therapies. As the overlapping components of each alternative model are accepted as part of existing Western health care delivery practice, the barriers to the remaining aspects of these models become transparent. With barriers disappearing a new model with a different shape and different alternative becomes what will be known as traditional medicine in the future.

components of identified alternative paradigms seem naturally to become part of the established delivery system. As a result, a new model for Western health care practice as identified by PT and OT is formed, which continues to allow the therapist to be tethered while enlarging or stretching a professional comfort zone to encapsulate alternative models without feeling as if the grounded neuroscience background is jeopardized (Figure 39-12). A clinician must always be cognizant of the fact that no matter what methods, philosophies, or interventions he or she selects to help a client reach a desired functional outcome, there is no way to eliminate the fact that other aspects of human system processing may also be active and affecting the outcome. For a century, master clinicians have been observed treating clients. Often colleagues comment that, although those masters seem to use the same methods, they get different outcomes. The question is, are those masters using other alternative interventions without those techniques ever being brought to consciousness? That is, if as a therapist I use myofascial techniques along with traditional intervention, am I also affecting craniosacral rhythm, or affecting chakras and energy fields and setting the stage for the nervous system to learn by optimal augmentation, which allows that nervous system to select better options for motor responses? If so, what truly is leading to somatosensory retraining, motor learning, neuroplasticity, and eventual improved motor control? It may be that master clinicians use *all* approaches but only verbalize the paradigm with which they are most comfortable and that they are most capable of verbally explaining. The adventure is a process of learning, enlarging one's skill to provide the best service to clients and differentiating what is effective within the clinical setting from what is believed to be effective. Differentiating true behavior on a client-by-client basis from what one is taught should happen is the reason for effectiveness of master clinicians. *Best practice is constantly evolving and changing.* As movement specialists we have the responsibility to evolve as well. That change needs to come flexibly tethered to knowledge, motor skill, emotional openness, and freedom to venture beyond a comfort zone while objectively measuring positive change in the functional abilities of our clients and thus improving their quality of life. For in-depth discussion on the topics of tai chi and biofeedback, please refer to: Davis CM: *Complementary therapies in rehabilitation: evidence for efficiency in therapy, prevention, and wellness,* 3rd ed, chapters 10 and 11, Thorofare NJ, 2009, Slack Inc.

References

To enhance this text and add value for the reader, all references are included on the companion Evolve site that accompanies this textbook. This online service will, when available, provide a link for the reader to a Medline abstract for the article cited. There are 352 cited references and other general references for this chapter, with the majority of those articles being evidence-based citations.

Index

A

B

F

H

I

J

K

L

O

P

U

W